Diagnostic Immunohistochemistry

Diagnostic Immunohistochemistry

THERANOSTIC AND GENOMIC APPLICATIONS

THIRD EDITION

David J. Dabbs, MD
Professor and Chief of Pathology
Department of Pathology
Magee-Women's Hospital
University of Pittsburgh School of Medicine
Pittsburgh, Pennsylvania

SAUNDERS
ELSEVIER

SAUNDERS
ELSEVIER

1600 John F. Kennedy Blvd
Ste 1800
Philadelphia, PA 19103-2899

DIAGNOSTIC IMMUNOHISTOCHEMISTRY

ISBN: 978-1-4160-5766-6

Notice

Knowledge and best practice in this field are constantly changing. As new research and experience broaden our knowledge, changes in practice, treatment and drug therapy may become necessary or appropriate. Readers are advised to check the most current information provided (i) on procedures featured or (ii) by the manufacturer of each product to be administered, to verify the recommended dose or formula, the method and duration of administration, and contraindications. It is the responsibility of the practitioner, relying on their own experience and knowledge of the patient, to make diagnoses, to determine dosages and the best treatment for each individual patient, and to take all appropriate safety precautions. To the fullest extent of the law, neither the Publisher nor the Editor assumes any liability for any injury and/or damage to persons or property arising out of or related to any use of the material contained in this book.

The Publisher

Library of Congress Cataloging-in-Publication Data
Diagnostic immunohistochemistry: theranostic and genomic applications / [edited by] David J. Dabbs.—3rd ed.
p. ; cm.
Includes bibliographical references and index.
ISBN 978-1-4160-5766-6
1. Diagnostic immunohistochemistry. I. Dabbs, David J.
[DNLM: 1. Immunohistochemistry—methods. 2. Diagnostic Techniques and Procedures. 3. Neoplasms—diagnosis. QW 504.5 D536 2009]
RB46.6.D33 2009
616.07'583—dc22 2009018160

Acquisitions Editor: William R. Schmitt
Developmental Editor: Kathryn DeFrancesco
Publishing Services Manager: Linda Van Pelt
Design Direction: Ellen Zanolle

Printed in China

Last digit is the print number: 9 8 7 6 5 4 3 2 1

This book is dedicated to the patients we serve
and to my colleagues in pathology and oncology,
especially those who inspire me in very special ways.

CONTRIBUTORS

N. Volkan Adsay, MD
Professor and Vice Chair
Pathology and Laboratory Medicine
Director of Anatomic Pathology
Emory University Hospital
Atlanta, Georgia

Nancy J Barr, MD
Assistant Professor of Clinical Pathology
Department of Pathology
Keck School of Medicine
University of Southern California Medical Center
Los Angeles, California

Olca Basturk, MD
Pathology Resident
Department of Pathology
New York University School of Medicine
New York, New York

Parul Bhargava, MD
Instructor in Pathology
Harvard Medical School
Medical Director, Hematology Laboratory
Beth Israel Deaconess Medical Center
Boston, Massachusetts

Rohit Bhargava, MD
Assistant Professor of Pathology
Co-Director, Surgical Pathology
Magee-Womens Hospital
University of Pittsburgh School of Medicine
Pittsburgh, Pennsylvania

Mamatha Chivukula, MD
Assistant Professor of Pathology
Associate Director of Immunohistochemistry Laboratory
Magee-Womens Hospital
University of Pittsburgh School of Medicine
Pittsburgh, Pennsylvania

Cheryl M. Coffin, MD
Goodpasture Professor of Investigative Pathology
Vice Chair for Anatomic Pathology
Department of Pathology
Vanderbilt University
Executive Medical Director of Anatomic Pathology
Vanderbilt Medical Center
Nashville, Tennessee

Jessica M. Comstock, MD
Visiting Instructor
University of Utah School of Medicine
Attending Physician
Primary Children's Medical Center
Salt Lake City, Utah

David J. Dabbs, MD
Professor and Chief of Pathology
Department of Pathology
Magee-Womens Hospital
University of Pittsburgh School of Medicine
Pittsburgh, Pennsylvania

Sanja Dacic, MD
Associate Professor
Department of Pathology
UPMC Presbyterian Hospital
University of Pittsburgh School of Medicine
Pittsburgh, Pennsylvania

Ronald A. DeLellis, MD
Professor and Associate Chair
Department of Pathology and Laboratory Medicine
Alpert Medical School of Brown University
Pathologist in Chief
Rhode Island Hospital and The Miriam Hospital
Providence, Rhode Island

Jonathan I. Epstein, MD
Professor of Pathology, Urology, and Oncology
The Reinhard Professor of Urologic Pathology
Johns Hopkins University School of Medicine
Director
Division of Surgical Pathology
Johns Hopkins Medical Institutions
Baltimore, Maryland

Nicole N. Esposito, MD
Assistant Professor
Department of Pathology and Cell Biology
College of Medicine
University of South Florida
Assistant Member
Anatomic Pathology Division, Breast Program
H. Lee Moffitt Cancer Center
Tampa, Florida

Eduardo J. Ezyaguirre, MD
Assistant Professor
Department of Pathology
University of Texas Medical Branch
Galveston, Texas

Alton B. Farris III, MD
Assistant Professor
Department of Pathology
Emory University School of Medicine
Atlanta, Georgia

Jeffrey D. Goldsmith, MD
Assistant Professor of Pathology
Harvard Medical School
Staff Pathologist
Beth Israel Deaconess Medical Center and Children's Hospital
Boston, Massachusetts

Samuel P. Hammar, MD
Clinical Professor of Pathology
University of Washington
Seattle, Washington
Staff Pathologist
Harrison Medical Center
Director
Diagnostic Specialties Laboratories
Bremerton, Washington

Jason L. Hornick, MD, PhD
Associate Professor of Pathology
Harvard Medical School
Associate Director of Surgical Pathology
Department of Pathology
Brigham and Women's Hospital
Boston, Massachusetts

Jennifer L. Hunt, MD
Associate Professor
Harvard Medical School
Associate Chief of Pathology
Director of Quality and Safety
Massachusetts General Hospital
Boston, Massachusetts

Marshall E. Kadin, MD
Professor of Dermatology
Boston University School of Medicine
Boston, Massachusetts
Director of Immunopathology and Imaging Core
Center for Biomedical Research Excellence
Roger Williams Medical Center
Providence, Rhode Island

Alyssa M. Krasinskas, MD
Assistant Professor of Pathology
UPMC Presbyterian Hospital
University of Pittsburgh School of Medicine
Pittsburgh, Pennsylvania

Alvin W. Martin, MD
Clinical Professor of Pathology
University of Louisville School of Medicine
Medical Director
CPA Laboratory
Norton Healthcare
Louisville, Kentucky

Paul E. McKeever, MD, PhD
Professor of Pathology
Chief
Section of Neuropathology
Department of Pathology
University of Michigan Medical Center
Ann Arbor, Michigan

George J. Netto, MD
Associate Professor of Pathology, Urology, and Oncology
Johns Hopkins University School of Medicine
Baltimore, Maryland

Yuri E. Nikiforov, MD, PhD
Professor and Director
Division of Molecular Anatomic Pathology
UPMC Presbyterian Hospital
University of Pittsburgh School of Medicine
Pittsburgh, Pennsylvania

Marina N. Nikiforova, MD
Assistant Professor
Department of Pathology
Associate Director
Molecular Anatomic Pathology Laboratory
University of Pittsburgh Medical Center
Pittsburgh, Pennsylvania

James W. Patterson, MD
Professor and Director of Dermatopathology
University of Virginia Medical Center
Charlottesville, Virginia

Joseph T. Rabban, MD, MPH
Associate Professor
Department of Pathology
University of California, San Francisco
San Francisco, California

Shan-Rong Shi, MD
Professor of Clinical Pathology
Department of Pathology
Keck School of Medicine
University of Southern California Medical Center
Los Angeles, California

Sandra J. Shin, MD
Assistant Professor of Pathology and Laboratory Medicine
Weill Medical College of Cornell University
New York, New York

Robert A. Soslow, MD
Professor of Pathology and Laboratory Medicine
Weill Medical College of Cornell University
Attending Pathologist
Memorial Sloane-Kettering Cancer Center
New York, New York

Paul E. Swanson, MD
Professor and Director of Anatomic Pathology
University of Washington Medical Center
Seattle, Washington

Clive R. Taylor, MD, PhD
Professor of Pathology
Senior Associate Dean for Educational Affairs
Keck School of Medicine
University of Southern California
Los Angeles, California

Diana O. Treaba, MD
Assistant Professor of Pathology
Alpert Medical School of Brown University
Director of the Hematopathology Laboratory
Rhode Island Hospital and The Miriam Hospital
Providence, Rhode Island

David H. Walker, MD
Professor and Chairman
Department of Pathology
University of Texas Medical Branch at Galveston
The Carmage and Martha Walls Distinguished University Chair in Tropical Diseases
Executive Director, UTMB Center for Biodefense and Emerging Infectious Diseases
Director, WHO Collaborating Center for Tropical Diseases
Galveston, Texas

Jeremy C. Wallentine, MD
Hematopathology Fellow
University of Utah School of Medicine
University of Utah Health Sciences Center and ARUP Laboratories
Salt Lake City, Utah

Mark R. Wick, MD
Professor and Associate Director of Surgical Pathology
Director of Diagnostic Immunohistochemistry
Division of Surgical Pathology
University of Virginia Medical Center
Charlottesville, Virginia

Sherif R. Zaki, MD
Branch Chief
Infectious Disease Pathology Branch
Centers for Disease Control and Prevention
Atlanta, Georgia

Charles Z. Zaloudek, MD
Professor of Pathology
Department of Pathology
University of California, San Francisco Medical Center
San Francisco, California

FOREWORD

Many are the "special" techniques that pathologists have used over the years to confirm, complement, and refine the information obtained with their "old faithful" armamentarium; that is, formalin fixation, paraffin embedding, and hematoxylin-eosin staining. These special techniques have come and gone, their usual life cycle beginning with an initial period of unrestrained enthusiasm, turning to a phase of disappointment, and finally leading to a more sober and realistic assessment. Many of these methods have left a permanent mark on the practice of the profession, even if often this was not as deep or wide-ranging as initially touted. These techniques include special stains, tissue culture, electron microscopy, immunohistochemistry, and molecular biology methods. Much was expected of the first three, and infinitely more is anticipated of the last, but it is fair to say that as of today no special technique has influenced the way that pathology is practiced as profoundly as immunohistochemistry, or has come even close to it. I don't think it would be an exaggeration to speak of a revolution, particularly in the field of tumor pathology. Those of us whose working experience antedated diagnostic immunohistochemistry certainly feel that way. The newer generations of pathologists who order so glibly an HMB-45 or a CD31 stain to identify melanocytes and endothelial cells, respectively, have very little feeling for the efforts made to achieve those identifications in the past. The virtues of the technique are so apparent and numerous as to make it as close to ideal as any biologic method carried out in human tissue obtained under routine (which usually means under less than ideal) conditions can be. To wit: It is compatible with standard fixation and embedding procedures; it can be performed retrospectively in material that has been archived for years; it is remarkably sensitive and specific; it can be applied to virtually any immunogenic molecule; and it can be evaluated against the morphologic backgrounds with which pathologists have long been familiar.

As with many other breakthroughs in medicine, immunohistochemistry started with a brilliant yet disarmingly simple idea: to have antibodies bind the specific antigens being sought and to make those antibodies visible by hooking to them a fluorescent compound. All subsequent modifications, such as the use of nonfluorescent chromogens, the amplification of the reaction, and the unmasking of antigens, merely represented technical improvements, although certainly not ones to be minimized. It is because of these technical advances that the procedure spread beyond the confines of the research laboratories and is now applied so pervasively in pathology laboratories throughout the world. Alas, it has its drawbacks. Antigens once believed to be specific for a given cell type were later found to be expressed by other tissues; cross-reactions may occur between unrelated antigens; nonspecific absorption of the antibody may supervene; entrapped non-neoplastic cells reacting for a particular marker may be misinterpreted as part of the tumor; and—most treacherously—antigen may diffuse out of a normal cell and find its way inside an adjacent tumor cell. Any of these pitfalls may lead to a misinterpretation of the reaction and a misdiagnosis. Ironically, this may lead to a final mistaken diagnosis after an initially correct interpretation of the hematoxylin-stained slides. A good protection against this danger is a thorough knowledge of these pitfalls and how to avoid them. An even more important safeguard is a solid background in basic anatomic pathology that will allow the observer to question the validity of any unexpected immunohistochemical result, whether positive or negative. There is nothing more dangerous (or expensive) than a neophyte in pathology making diagnoses on the basis of immunohistochemical profiles in disregard of the cytoarchitectural features of the lesions. Alas, this is true of any other special technique applied for diagnostic purposes to human tissue, molecular biology being the latest and most blatant example. However, when applied selectively and judiciously, immunohistochemistry is a notably powerful tool, in addition to being refreshingly cost effective. As a matter of fact, pathologists can no longer afford to do without it, one of the reasons being that failure to make a diagnosis because of the omission of a key immunohistochemical reaction may be regarded as grounds for a malpractice action.

Any listing of the virtues of immunohistochemistry would be incomplete if it did not include the visual pleasure derived from the examination of this material. I am only half kidding when making this remark. There is undoubtedly an aesthetic component to the practice of histology, as masters of the technique such as Pio del Rio Hortega and Pierre Masson liked to point out. It is sad that these superb artists of morphology left the scene without having had the opportunity to marvel at the beauty of a well-done immunohistochemical preparation. As their more fortunate heirs, let us enjoy this excellent book, edited by one of the foremost experts in the application of the immunohistochemical technique and written by a superb group of contributors—a book that summarizes in a lucid and thorough fashion the current knowledge in the field, in terms of both the technical aspects and the practical applications.

The first edition of this book, published in 2002, rapidly became one of the standard works in the field. The second edition featured a more standardized format, a wider coverage of organ systems, and an extensive update of markers. It incorporated a large number of useful tables listing the various antibody groups, an algorithmic approach to differential diagnosis, and key diagnostic points for all the major subjects. Special attention was paid to the detailed description of the so-called predictive-type markers (such as HER2/neu in breast carcinoma and CD117 in GIST), which are playing an increasingly important role in the evaluation of tumors by the pathologist.

In this third edition, a new chapter has been added that describes, in a simplified and condensed fashion, the rationale, technology, and applications of molecular anatomic pathology techniques to aid the surgical pathologist in acquiring a basic understanding of these molecular tests.

A new, very timely chapter on immunocytology has been included by Dr. Chivukula, which discusses proper cytologic technique for fixation and processing specimens obtained for hormone receptors and HER2/neu testing.

Overall, each organ-based chapter addresses the state-of-the-art body of knowledge and is summarized in bulleted format for ease of understanding.

There are several new completely rewritten chapters with new authors, all of them experts in their respective fields, including N. Volkan Adsay, Jonathan Epstein, Alyssa M. Krasinskas, Alvin W. Martin, George Netto, and Yuri E. Nikiforov. The latest recommendations for proper fixation and processing of hormone receptor testing are authoritatively discussed by Dr. Clive R. Taylor.

The title of this new third edition has been changed to *Diagnostic Immunohistochemistry: Theranostic and Genomic Applications* to emphasize the fact that immunohistochemistry is no longer used solely for diagnosis. Rather, the growing body of knowledge of cancer genomics, transcriptomics, and the new therapeutic armamentarium of biologics forces pathologists to be cognizant of the emerging field of therapeutic and genomic applications of immunohistochemistry. Accordingly, each chapter of the book includes a synoptic coverage of theranostic and genomic applications. As a result, each organ-based chapter provides detailed information on how gene-based disease can be diagnosed through the microscope with immunohistochemistry. In a similar vein, the presence or absence of markers predictive of the beneficial effects of targeted therapies is determined, launching the age of theranostic immunohistochemistry.

Last but not least, each chapter provides a bridge to new molecular anatomic pathology menus for pathologists, in order to empower them with additional diagnostic modalities whenever immunohistochemistry falls short.

In summary, the authors have again brilliantly succeeded in producing an authoritative, comprehensive, and updated book that pathologists will find next to indispensable as a theoretical backbone for the various methods discussed and of invaluable assistance in their daily work.

Juan Rosai, MD
Milan, Italy

PREFACE

The title of this third edition of *Diagnostic Immunohistochemistry* has been lengthened to include the terms "Theranostic and Genomic Applications." Fundamentally, the continuing challenge of this book is to assemble the vast body of knowledge of immunohistochemistry into a work that has meaning for the diagnostic surgical pathologist. The discipline of immunohistochemistry for the surgical pathologist has been evolving rapidly since the first edition of this book, and it can further be broken down into subsets of theranostic and genomic applications. The diagnostic aspect of immunohistochemistry in surgical pathology is straightforward. Pathologists use this tool to assign lineage to neoplasms that include carcinomas, melanomas, lymphomas, sarcomas, and germ cell tumors. The term "theranostics" is used to describe the proposed process of diagnostic therapy for individual patients—to test them for possible reactions to a new medication and/or to tailor a treatment for them based on a test result. Theranostics is a rapidly emerging field in oncology, and pathologists need to be prepared to serve oncologic patients with a vast and emerging array of individualized patient therapies. The prototype for understanding the concept of theranostics is hormone receptor testing for breast cancer and HER2/neu analysis. These were among the first and most widely known immunohistochemical tests with theranostic applications. With the proper application of these immunohistochemical tests, individualized therapy in the form of selective estrogen receptor modulation therapy for the patient with an estrogen-receptor positive breast carcinoma can be designed. Trastuzumab is administered for the patient with a HER2-positive breast carcinoma.

In addition, the genomic application of immunohistochemistry (i.e., genomic immunohistochemistry) is a tool for the surgical pathologist to facilitate recognition of specific genomic aberrations in the patients' tissues by identifying (or not identifying) the presence or absence of specific proteins or immunohistochemical profiles that directly imply, or connote, a specific genomic abnormality, aberration, or gene signature. A prototype for genomic application could be immunohistochemical testing for microsatellite instability in colorectal carcinomas, where the surgical pathologist applies antibodies to detect proteins for MLH1, MSH2, MSH6, or PMS2. The presence or absence of this protein is in essence a genetic test, a direct genomic application for immunohistochemistry. A genetic signature application might include the identification of basal-like breast carcinoma, in which the signature profile typically is a high-grade ER, PR and HER2 negative, CK5 positive, CK14 positive, CK17 positive, variably EGFR positive tumor. Furthermore, immunohistochemical surrogate markers for gene expression profiles for breast carcinomas can further identify the gene expression profile subsets of carcinomas as luminal A, luminal B, and HER2 categories.

It becomes clear that immunohistochemistry is a powerful tool with overlapping features among diagnostic, theranostic, and genomic applications. Theranostic applications may also be genomic, and genomic immunohistochemistry may also be theranostic. These categories admittedly are artificial and simplistic but give the surgical pathologist and the student of surgical pathology a conceptual framework for recognition of the enormous power of the immunohistochemical test.

Molecular testing in surgical pathology has many important diagnostic, theranostic, and genomic applications as well, but it is the immunohistochemistry platform that lays the groundwork for our understanding of what is normal and what is diseased in tissue by virtue of the direct visualization of molecular morphology.

In this edition, most chapters have been completely revised, and there are several new authors. There is a new chapter on molecular anatomic pathology, with new authorships in non-Hodgkin lymphoma; immunohistology of the gastrointestinal tract; immunohistology of the pancreas, bile ducts, gallbladder, and liver; and immunohistology of the genitourinary system. An additional new chapter on immunocytology is patterned after the chapter that appeared in the first edition.

Each chapter format may include subsections that discuss relevant theranostic and genomic applications of immunohistochemistry. These are included to highlight to the pathologist that these important applications go beyond traditional diagnostic immunohistochemistry for individual organ systems.

Immunohistochemistry has undergone a tremendous change, with new stresses and demands throughout the last decade. A critical factor affecting the surgical pathologist/immunohistochemist is the proper standardization of procedures in the laboratory to assure the highest quality immunohistology for diagnostic, theranostic, and genomic applications. Recent recommendations by the CAP-ASCO and additional new recommendations for hormone receptor testing have highlighted the importance of proper standardization of procedures and internal and external quality assurance programs.

Once again, the challenge of putting this work together has been to assure that the base of knowledge in each chapter is relevant and robust long after the ink has dried. The contributions of expert authors in each discipline are unique to this work. The continuing goal of this book is to provide a reference for pathologists who practice contemporary surgical pathology and cytopathology.

With few exceptions, each chapter is designed to be a stand-alone work. Inherent in this design is a body of information that is reproduced and redundant throughout each chapter. Each chapter is comprehensive in a diagnostic sense, which should limit the need to do extensive cross-checking to other chapters. Each section is punctuated by key diagnostic points that summarize the section and that serve as a rapid summary reference for the most important points in that section.

The positive feedback on this work continues to grow exponentially. I welcome personally any feedback regarding this book, no matter how small, even to point out typographical errors or informational errors. Please contact me at ddabbs@upmc.edu or dabbsihc@gmail.com.

My special thanks go to the dedicated investigators and pathologists across the globe who have given me feedback on this work.

David J. Dabbs, MD

HOW TO USE THIS BOOK

The first chapter of this book details the techniques and development of immunohistochemistry. This includes critically important updates of standardization as applied to theranostic testing, especially hormone receptor testing. The new second chapter on diagnostic molecular anatomic pathology is to be used as a reference guide to understanding molecular anatomic tests mentioned throughout this textbook. Molecular anatomic pathology has grown exponentially over the past decade, and the discipline supplies critically important testing that supplements diagnostic, theranostic, or genomic applications beyond immunohistochemistry. Each chapter, where relevant, will have subsections titled "Beyond Immunohistochemistry: Anatomic Molecular Diagnostic Applications."

The third chapter, "Immunohistology of Infectious Diseases," has been completely restructured. The remaining chapters continue as an organ system approach to diagnostic, theranostic, and genomic applications of immunohistochemistry. Each chapter has a liberal number of "immunohistograms" depicting immunostaining patterns of tumors, along with numerous tables, well structured for easy reference. Diagnostic algorithms are used where relevant. Many areas of the text are punctuated by summary "Key Diagnostic Points." Diagnostic pitfalls are also cited where particularly relevant.

To maintain constant terminology throughout the chapters, the following abbreviations in the text and tables are used unless otherwise specified:

+, the result is almost always strong, diffusely positive;
S, sometimes positive;
R, rarely positive, and if so, rare cells are positive;
N or a (-), negative result.

These are exciting times indeed for the discipline of immunohistochemistry as well as for the rapidly evolving molecular tests that will significantly affect patients' lives. This work should be viewed as a focal point, a punctuation mark in the continuous quality improvement of the knowledge base for immunohistochemistry for surgical pathologists.

David J. Dabbs, MD

CONTENTS

1 **Techniques of Immunohistochemistry: Principles, Pitfalls, and Standardization 1**
Clive R. Taylor • Shan-Rong Shi • Nancy J. Barr

2 **Molecular Anatomic Pathology: Principles, Technique, and Application to Immunohistologic Diagnosis 42**
Marina N. Nikiforova • Yuri E. Nikiforov

3 **Immunohistology of Infectious Diseases 58**
Eduardo J. Ezyaguirre • David H. Walker • Sherif R. Zaki

4 **Immunohistology of Soft Tissue and Osseous Neoplasms 83**
Mark R. Wick • Jason L. Hornick

5 **Immunohistology of Hodgkin Lymphoma 137**
Parul Bhargava • Marshall E. Kadin

6 **Immunohistology of Non-Hodgkin Lymphoma 156**
Alvin W. Martin

7 **Immunohistology of Melanocytic Neoplasms 189**
Mark R. Wick

8 **Immunohistology of Metastatic Carcinomas of Unknown Primary 206**
Rohit Bhargava • David J. Dabbs

9 **Immunohistology of Head and Neck Neoplasms 256**
Jennifer L. Hunt

10 **Immunohistology of Endocrine Tumors 291**
Ronald A. DeLellis • Sandra J. Shin • Diana O. Treaba

11 **Immunohistology of the Mediastinum 340**
Mark R. Wick

12 **Immunohistology of Lung and Pleural Neoplasms 369**
Samuel P. Hammar • Sanja Dacic

13 **Immunohistology of Skin Tumors 464**
Mark R. Wick • Paul E. Swanson • James W. Patterson

14 **Immunohistology of the Gastrointestinal Tract 500**
Alyssa M. Krasinskas • Jeffrey D. Goldsmith

15 **Immunohistology of the Pancreas, Biliary Tract, and Liver 541**
Olca Basturk • Alton B. Farris III • N. Volkan Adsay

16 **Immunohistology of the Prostate, Bladder, Kidney, and Testis 593**
George J. Netto • Jonathan I. Epstein

17 **Immunohistology of Pediatric Neoplasms 662**
Cheryl M. Coffin • Jessica M. Comstock • Jeremy C. Wallentine

18 **Immunohistology of the Female Genital Tract 690**
Joseph T. Rabban • Robert A. Soslow • Charles Z. Zaloudek

19 **Immunohistology of the Breast 763**
Rohit Bhargava • Nicole N. Esposito • David J. Dabbs

20 **Immunohistology of the Nervous System 820**
Paul E. McKeever

21 **Immunocytology 890**
Mamatha Chivukula • David J. Dabbs

Index 919

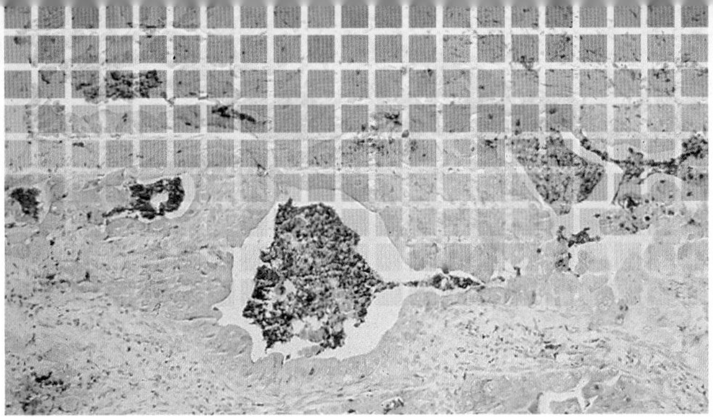

1

Techniques of Immunohistochemistry: Principles, Pitfalls, and Standardization

Clive R. Taylor • Shan-Rong Shi • Nancy J. Barr

- Introduction 1
- Basic Principles of Immunohistochemistry 2
- Antibodies as Specific Staining Reagents 2
- Blocking Non-specific Background Staining 4
- Detection Systems 5
- Quality Control and Standardization 13
- Tissue Fixation, Processing, and Antigen-Retrieval Techniques 18
- Techniques, Protocols, and "Troubleshooting" 22

INTRODUCTION

Immunohistochemistry (IHC), or immunocytochemistry, is a method for localizing specific antigens in tissues or cells based on antigen-antibody recognition; it seeks to exploit the specificity provided by the binding of an antibody with its antigen at a light microscopic level. IHC has a long history, extending more than half a century from 1940, when Coons developed an immunofluorescence technique to detect corresponding antigens in frozen tissue sections.[1] However, only since the early 1990s has the method found general application in surgical pathology.[2-5] A series of technical developments led eventually to the wide range of IHC applications in use today. The enzymatic label (horseradish peroxidase), developed by Avrameas[6] and by Nakane and colleagues,[7] allowed visualization of the labeled antibody by light microscopy in the presence of a suitable colorogenic substrate system. In Oxford, Taylor and Burns developed the first successful demonstration of antigens in routinely processed formalin-fixed paraffin-embedded (FFPE) tissues.[5] A critical issue in the early development of immunoperoxidase techniques was related to the need to achieve greater sensitivity. Greater sensitivity would facilitate staining of FFPE tissues—from a simple one-step direct conjugate method to multiple-step detection techniques such as the peroxidase antiperoxidase (PAP), avidin-biotin conjugate (ABC), and biotin-streptavidin (B-SA) methods—and would eventually lead to amplification methods (such as tyramide) and highly sensitive "polymer-based" labeling systems.[4,8-20] We will describe these methods in detail later in this chapter.

As the IHC method has evolved, its use in diagnostic pathology has expanded such that the use of one or more IHC "stains" is routine in surgical pathology, especially with respect to tumor diagnosis and classification. Furthermore, IHC has been adapted to the identification and demonstration of both prognostic and predictive markers, with corresponding requirements for semi-quantitative reporting of results. The widespread use of IHC and the demands for comparison of qualitative and semi-quantitative findings among an increasing number of laboratories have resulted in a growing focus on method reproducibility and have led to a new emphasis upon standardization. This standardization serves as an underlying theme of this chapter, and we will discuss it in detail in the Quality Control and Standardization section.

The development of the hybridoma technique[21] facilitated the development of IHC and the manufacture of abundant, highly specific monoclonal antibodies, many of which found early application in staining of tissues. Initial success in cryostat sections was eventually extended to routinely processed paraffin, celloidin, or other plastic-embedded tissue sections. Only when the IHC technique became applicable to routine FFPE tissue sections did it usher in the "brown revolution."[22] The critical significance of rendering the IHC technique suitable for routine paraffin sections was illustrated in 1974 by Taylor and

Burns, who showed that it was possible to demonstrate at least some antigens in routinely processed tissue.[5] These initial studies led to serious attempts by pathologists to improve the ability to perform IHC staining on FFPE sections.[5,23-28] Although great effort has been expended in the search for alternative fixatives (formalin substitutes) to preserve antigenicity without compromising preservation of morphologic features, no ideal fixatives have been found to date. Larsson states, "An ideal immunocytochemical fixative applicable to all antigens may never be found."[29] In addition, preservation of morphologic features is not comparable with formalin fixation, causing problems in interpretation and diagnosis.

Enzyme digestion was introduced by Huang as a pretreatment to IHC staining to "unmask" some antigens that had been altered by formalin fixation.[30] However, the enzyme digestion method, while widely applied, did not improve IHC staining of many antigens, a subject well reviewed by Leong and colleagues.[31] Another drawback of enzyme digestion was that it proved difficult to control the optimal "digestion" conditions for individual tissue sections when stained with different antibodies. These difficulties in standardization provided a powerful incentive for the development of a new technique, with the requirements that it should be more powerful, more widely applicable, and easier to use than enzyme digestion. In addition, it should enhance immunohistochemical staining of routine FFPE tissue sections in a reproducible and reliable manner. The antigen-retrieval (AR) technique, based on a series of biochemical studies by Fraenkel-Conrat and coworkers,[32-34] was developed by Shi and associates in 1991.[35-40] In contrast to enzyme digestion, the AR technique is a simple method that involves heating routinely processed paraffin sections at high temperature (e.g., in a microwave oven) before IHC staining procedures. An alternative method that does not use heating was developed for celloidin-embedded tissues.[36-38] The intensity of IHC staining was increased dramatically after AR pretreatment,[39-43] as evidenced by more than 100 articles published subsequently. Various modifications of the AR technique have been described; the majority of these use different buffer solutions as the AR solution in place of metal salt solutions, which may have a potentially toxic effect.[39,40,43-54] Worldwide application of AR-IHC in pathology has validated the feasibility of AR-IHC and expanded its use in molecular morphology, while raising some basic questions and practical issues that are subject to ongoing evolution of the method.[2,3,33,40,55-61]

It is the authors' view that there is no immediate prospect of replacing formalin in "routine" surgical pathology. Even if there was agreement as to a superior fixative, the logistics of converting all laboratories nationwide, yet alone worldwide, are formidable. Formalin is thus what we have to work with for the foreseeable future. For this reason, in this chapter we will focus on IHC as applied to archival FFPE tissue sections for diagnostic pathologic study. In addition to basic principles and practical technical issues, the limitations and pitfalls of IHC are discussed, with the intention of providing "food for thought" in the further development of IHC, particularly with respect to standardization and ultimately quantitative IHC applications.

BASIC PRINCIPLES OF IMMUNOHISTOCHEMISTRY

Surgical pathologists have long recognized their fallibility, although they have not always publicized it.[2,3,26] They have, however, sought more certain means of validating morphologic judgments. A variety of "special stains" were developed to facilitate cell recognition and diagnosis; most of these early stains were based on chemical reactions of cell and tissue components in frozen sections (histochemistry). In certain circumstances, these histochemical stains proved to be of critical value in specific cell identification. More often, they served merely to highlight or emphasize cellular or histologic features that supported a particular interpretation without providing truly specific confirmation. When the new field of immunohistochemistry was created by combining immunology with histochemistry, a wide variety of truly specific special stains were generated. This subject, which has been discussed in thousands of papers, will be discussed in this book.

The aims of IHC are akin to those of histochemistry. Indeed, IHC builds on the foundations of histochemistry; it does not replace histochemistry but rather serves as a valuable adjunct that greatly extends the variety of tissue components that can be demonstrated specifically within tissue sections or other cell preparations. As emphasized by pioneers in this field of functional morphology, "the object of all staining is to recognize microchemically the existence and distribution of substances which we have been made aware of macrochemically."[62] The basic critical principle of IHC, as with any other special staining method, is a sharp visual localization of target components in the cell and tissue, based on a satisfactory signal-to-noise ratio. Amplifying the signal while reducing non-specific background staining (noise) has been a major strategy to achieve a satisfactory result that is useful in daily practice.

After more than two decades, advances in IHC have provided a feasible approach to performing immunostaining on routinely processed tissues, such that this method is now "routine" for the performance of IHC "special stains" in surgical pathology laboratories using FFPE tissues (see Appendix 1A). However, demands for improved reproducibility and for quantification have led to a growing recognition that IHC has the potential to be more than just a special stain. If properly controlled in all aspects of its performance, IHC can provide a tissue-based immunoassay with the reproducibility and quantitative characteristics of an ELISA (enzyme-linked immunosorbent assay) test, which not only detects the presence of an "analyte" (protein or antigen) but also provides an accurate and reliable measure of its relative or real amount (see Quality Control and Standardization section).

ANTIBODIES AS SPECIFIC STAINING REAGENTS

An antibody is a molecule that has the property of combining specifically with a second molecule, termed the *antigen*. Further, the production of antibody by an

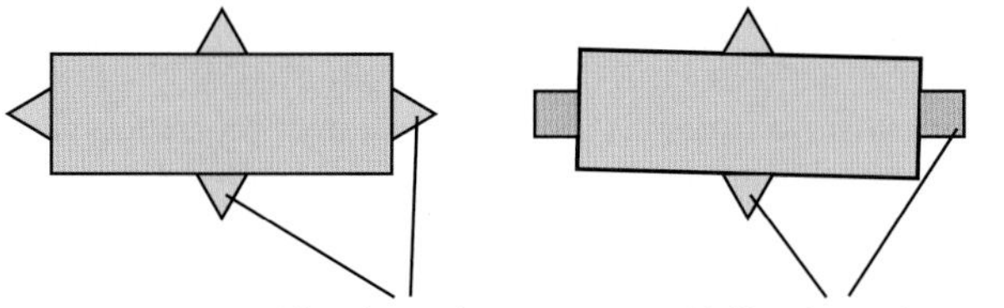

FIGURE 1.1 Antigens and antigenic determinants. An antigenic molecule may be considered to consist of an immunologically "inert" carrier component and one or more antigenic determinants of like type *(left)* or diverse types *(right)*. *From Taylor CR, Cote RJ, eds. Immunomicroscopy: A Diagnostic Tool for the Surgical Pathologist. 3rd ed. Philadelphia: Elsevier; 2005:6.*

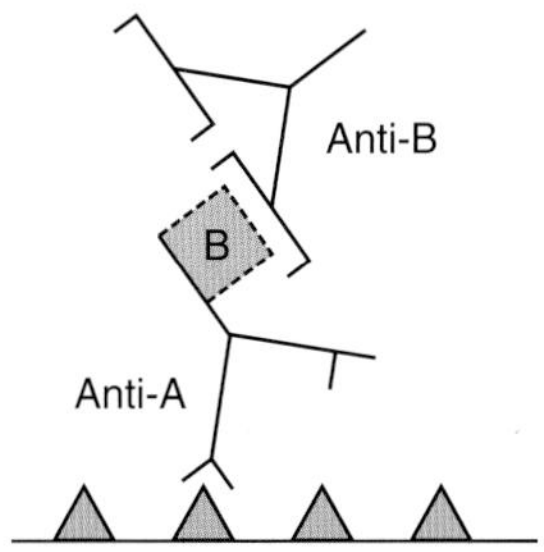

FIGURE 1.2 Antibodies as antigens. Anti-A antibody binds specifically to antigen A in the tissue section. Antigen B (B) is depicted as a second antigenic determinant that is part of the anti-A molecule; anti-B antibody, made in a second species, will bind to this determinant. Thus anti-B (the so-called secondary antibody) can be used to locate the site of binding of anti-A (the primary antibody) in a tissue section. *From Taylor CR, Cote RJ, eds. Immunomicroscopy: A Diagnostic Tool for the Surgical Pathologist. 3rd ed. Philadelphia: Elsevier; 2005:9.*

animal is induced specifically by the presence of antigen; this forms part of the basic immune response. Antigen-antibody recognition is based on the three-dimensional structure of protein (or other antigen), which may be compromised by formalin-induced modification of protein conformation ("masking") and restored in part by AR. We will discuss this process later in this chapter.

Antibodies are immunoglobulin molecules consisting of two basic units: a pair of light chains (either a kappa or a lambda pair) and a pair of heavy chains (gamma, alpha, mu, delta, or epsilon). An antigen is any molecule that is sufficiently complex that it maintains a relatively rigid three-dimensional profile and is foreign to the animal into which it is introduced. Good antigens are proteins and carbohydrates that are sufficiently complex to possess a unique three-dimensional "charge-shape" profile. In fact, such molecules may bear more than one unique three-dimensional structure capable of inducing antibody formation (Fig. 1.1). Each of these individual sites on a molecule may be termed an *antigenic determinant* (or *epitope*), being the exact site on the molecule with which the antibody combines. For a protein, the term *epitope* corresponds to a cluster of amino acid residues that binds specifically to the paratope of an antibody.[63] Although it is part of the protein, an epitope cannot be recognized independently of its paratope partner.[63] Antigenic determinants (epitopes) may be classified as continuous and discontinuous. The former are composed of a continuum of residues in a polypeptide chain, whereas the latter consist of residues from different parts of a polypeptide chain, brought together by the folding of the protein conformation.[64] This is an interesting issue that may reflect the variable influence of formalin fixation on antigenicity, and variations in the effectiveness of AR.

Antibody molecules are proteins; thus any rigid part of an antibody molecule may itself serve as the antigenic determinant to induce an antibody. IHC techniques exploit the fact that immunoglobulin molecules can serve both as antibodies (binding specifically to tissue antigens) and as antigens (providing antigenic determinants to which secondary antibodies may be attached) (Fig. 1.2).

Evaluation of an antibody for use in IHC is based on two main points: the sensitivity and the specificity of the antibody-antigen reaction for IHC. The development of the hybridoma technique[21] provided an almost limitless source of highly specific antibodies. Monoclonal antibodies do not guarantee antigen specificity; however, since different antigens may share similar or cross-reactive epitopes, the "practical" specificity reflected by IHC is excellent for most monoclonal antibodies. In contrast, a "polyclonal antibody" is an antiserum that contains many different molecular species of antibody having varying specificities against the different antigens (or antigenic determinants) used to immunize the animal. It is important to remember that polyclonal antibodies may also include varying amounts of antibodies to a whole range of antigens (including bacteria and viruses) that the immunized animal encountered before its use as a source of antibody. As a result, polyclonal antibodies often give more non-specific background staining in slides than encountered using monoclonal antibodies. By the same token, however, the presence of a mixture of different antibodies may on occasion confer an advantage to the use of polyclonal antibodies in the staining of certain "hard-to-detect" antigens in fixed tissues. For these reasons, the use of highly purified antigen preparations to produce high-affinity conventional polyclonal antibodies (antisera), which are then subjected to multiple absorption procedures to maximize specificity, is of value for certain applications. However, note that immunodiffusion assays used by manufacturers in the assessment of such antisera specificity may fail to detect "trace" antibody specificities; this becomes apparent only when the antiserum is applied to tissue sections containing many different antigens.

Comparison of sensitivity and specificity between polyclonal and monoclonal antibodies indicates that polyclonal antibody may be more sensitive but less specific than monoclonal antibody. The reason may be that polyclonal antibody (actually a composite of many antibodies) may recognize several different binding sites (epitopes) on a single protein (antigen), whereas a monoclonal antibody recognizes only a single type of epitope. Sophisticated amplification techniques, coupled with the use of the AR technique, have reduced the practical importance of this distinction. Although the specificity of monoclonal antibody is, as noted, not absolute because of cross-reactivity with non-target molecules,[65] most commercially available monoclonal antibodies are highly reliable for IHC. Most monoclonal antibodies in current use are derived from murine clones. Recently a number of rabbit-derived monoclonal antibodies have appeared on the market. Some of these appear to offer advantages over murine clones for detection of certain antigens by IHC. Selection of the "best antibody" is described briefly in the following paragraphs, and we will discuss it in more detail in the "Detection Systems" and "Quality Control and Standardization" sections. It must be emphasized that the ultimate specificity control for both monoclonal and polyclonal antibodies should be the observation of the expected pattern of staining in control tissue sections, with the corresponding lack of unexpected or inexplicable staining reactions (see Quality Control and Standardization section). Johnson[65] also recommended correlation of the staining result of a "new antibody" with the literature for antigen distribution, and comparison of the staining of the test antibody with that of a second antibody known to bind to the same antigen but to a different epitope. In recent years, recombinant DNA techniques have been used to develop antibodies that may demonstrate improved practical specificity following stringent affinity purification using recombinant protein epitope signature tags (PrESTs).[66]

BLOCKING NON-SPECIFIC BACKGROUND STAINING

There are two aspects to the blocking of background staining of tissues that may be attributable either to non-specific antibody binding or to the presence of endogenous enzymes. Non-specific antibody binding is generally more of a problem with polyclonal antibody, because multiple "unwanted" antibodies may exist in the antiserum. The greater the optimal working dilution, the lesser the problem. Another form of non-specific binding may result from the fact that antibodies are highly charged molecules and may bind non-specifically to tissue components bearing reciprocal charges (e.g., collagen). Such non-specific binding may lead to localization of either the primary antibody or the labeled moiety (conjugate, PAP, and so on), producing "false-positive" staining of collagen and other tissue components of sufficient degree to obscure specific staining (Fig. 1.3A). Preincubation with normal serum usually reduces these kinds of non-specific binding. In theory, proteins in the normal serum occupy the charged sites within the tissue section, excluding (or at least reducing) non-specific attachment of antibodies added subsequently. In practice, it is customary to use normal serum of the same species as the secondary antibody (in conjugate and ABC methods) because this normal serum neither interferes with nor participates in the immunologic reactions that occur as part of the IHC procedure.

Blocking endogenous enzyme activity is also important. The degree of susceptibility of an enzyme to denaturation and inactivation during fixation varies. Some enzymes, such as peroxidase, are preserved in both paraffin and frozen sections; others, such as alkaline phosphatase, are completely inactivated by routine fixation and paraffin-embedding procedures. Any residual activity of these endogenous enzymes must be abolished during immunostaining in order to avoid false-positive reactions when using the same or similar enzymes as labels. Peroxidase activity is present in a number of normal and neoplastic cells, including erythrocytes, neutrophils, eosinophils, and hepatocytes. When performing an immunohistochemical study in tissues rich in blood cells, such as bone marrow, it is recommended that a "peroxidase-blocking" step be used, coupled with a "substrate control" (i.e., a section treated only with the hydrogen peroxide–chromogen mixture to visualize the

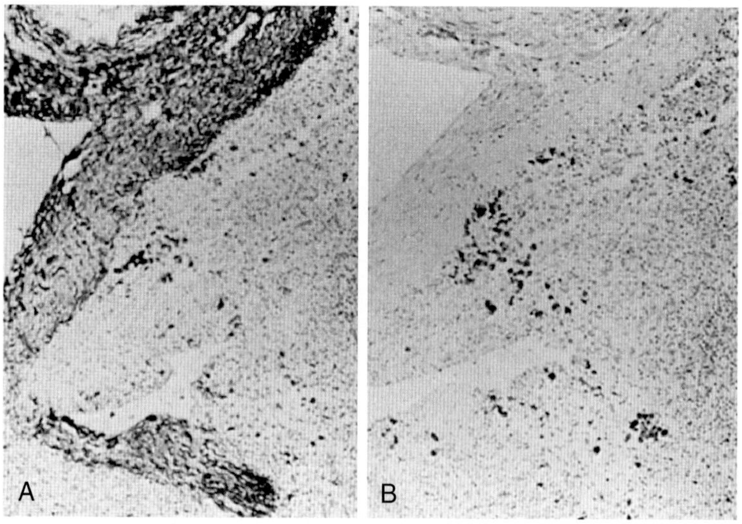

FIGURE 1.3 Example of the effectiveness of "blocking" non-specific binding of primary and secondary antibodies. **(A)** A section of spleen stained for IgG by the PAP method; scattered positive plasma cells *(black dots)* are seen, but there is heavy staining of collagen bands. **(B)** The adjacent parallel section treated in an identical fashion except that normal serum from the same species as the linking antibody (in this case normal swine serum to match the swine antirabbit Ig-linking antibody) was added before the primary antibody. In this instance, the plasma cells are seen even more clearly because the heavy non-specific staining of collagen is markedly diminished. Paraffin sections, DAB with hematoxylin counterstain. (×60.) *From Taylor CR, Cote RJ. Immunomicroscopy: A Diagnostic Tool for the Surgical Pathologist. 2nd ed. Philadelphia: WB Saunders; 1994:68.*

extent of endogenous peroxidase activity). Otherwise, alternative methods, such as alkaline phosphatase, glucose oxidase, or immunogold labeling, may be used to avoid the possibility of confusion with any endogenous enzyme activity. To risk stating the obvious, the blocking of endogenous enzymatic activity must be carried out before the addition of enzyme-labeled secondary reagent; otherwise, the enzyme label is also inactivated by the blocking procedure, resulting in a false-negative result. Various approaches have been devised to inhibit peroxidase activity, primarily using solutions of hydrogen peroxide (H_2O_2).[67-69] For general purposes, we have obtained satisfactory results with a 15-minute incubation in a methanol-H_2O_2 combination. Many manufacturers also include proprietary reagents and protocols that effectively neutralize endogenous peroxidase in both manual and automated methods; in these instances, one should validate the recommendations of the manufacturer for satisfactory performance and follow them strictly.

For those who encounter difficulty or wish to explore other approaches, a more detailed discussion follows. Some investigators[70-72] believe that the methanol-H_2O_2 approach is too drastic and may cause some denaturation of antigen. Straus[71,72] advocated the use of phenylhydrazine by using a combination of phenylhydrazine, nascent H_2O_2 (freshly produced by a glucose oxidase-glucose mixture), and sodium azide to effectively inhibit endogenous peroxidase activity with little damage to surface antigens of lymphocytes.[73] A mixture of H_2O_2 (0.3%) in 0.1% sodium azide was also found to be a simple and effective technique.[74] More recently, cyclopropanone hydrate was shown to inhibit endogenous peroxidase without adverse effects on antigenicity.[75] Robinson and Dawson[76] adopted a different approach, first developing the endogenous peroxidase with 4-chloro-1-naphthol (giving it a blue-gray color), then performing the IHC staining procedure, with a peroxidase label and diaminobenzidine (giving a contrasting brown reaction product). Taylor used a similar strategy 30 years ago in the initial reports describing the feasibility of demonstrating immunoglobulin antigens in paraffin sections; alpha-naphthol pyronine was used for endogenous peroxidase (pink), followed by diaminobenzidine (brown) for the horseradish peroxidase label.[5,23]

DETECTION SYSTEMS

Antibody molecules cannot be seen with the light microscope or even with the electron microscope unless they are labeled or flagged by some method that permits their visualization. Essentially, detection systems attach certain labels or flags to primary or secondary antibodies in order to visualize the target antibody-antigen localization in the tissue sections. A variety of labels or flags have been used, including fluorescent compounds and active enzymes that can be visualized by virtue of their property of inducing the formation of a colored reaction product from a suitable substrate system. Such methods have worked well in light microscopy and can be adapted to electron microscopy if the products are rendered electron-dense by suitable treatment. Alternatively, labels that are visible directly by electron microscopy may be used, such as gold, ferritin, or virus particles. Fluorescent labels also are making a comeback based upon improved microscope systems, digital imaging, and the availability of a variety of new fluorescent labels that do not fade. These approaches are discussed briefly with reference to double staining methods.

Another important goal of various detection systems is the enhancement of sensitivity through amplification of signal, as we will discuss later in this chapter.

Direct Conjugate-labeled Antibody Method

The method of attaching a label by chemical means to an antibody and then directly applying this labeled conjugate to tissue sections (Fig. 1.4) has been used widely in immunohistology. In preparing a labeled antibody conjugate, the aim is to attach the maximal number of molecules of label to each individual antibody molecule. It is desirable to label 100% of antibody molecules and to render none of them immunologically inactive by the labeling process. Similarly, the labeling process must not inactivate the antibody or the label (e.g., destroy the active site of the horseradish peroxidase enzyme). The final labeled reagent should not contain free molecules of unlabeled antibody or molecules of antibody linked to inactivated label.

These are exacting requirements that are difficult for individual scientists to meet "in house." However, conjugation methods have improved immensely since the early 1980s, and high-quality labeled reagents, including peroxidase, glucose oxidase, and alkaline phosphatase labels, are available from a number of commercial sources.

The direct conjugate procedure has the advantages of rapidity and ease of performance. With this procedure, the purity (i.e., mono-specificity) of the primary antibody or antiserum (polyclonal antibody) is of critical importance. As noted previously, an antiserum contains a range of antibody molecules of differing specificity in addition to the antibody having the desired specificity; all these antibodies are labeled during the conjugation procedure, and any or all may produce staining in tissue sections, leading to erroneous interpretation.

One practical disadvantage of the direct conjugate procedure is that to detect different antigens it is necessary to conjugate each of the appropriate primary

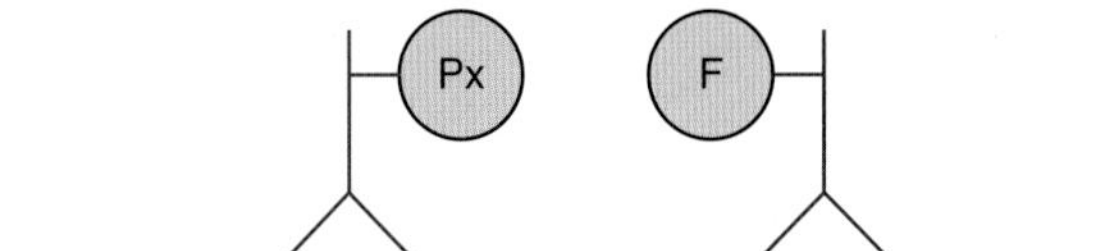

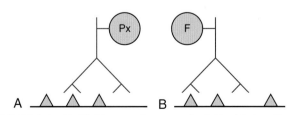

FIGURE 1.4 (A, B) Direct conjugate method. The label, or flag, is attached directly to the antibody having specificity for the antigen under study. Px, peroxidase; F, fluorescein. *From Taylor CR, Cote RJ, eds. Immunomicroscopy: A Diagnostic Tool for the Surgical Pathologist. 3rd ed. Philadelphia: Elsevier; 2005:19.*

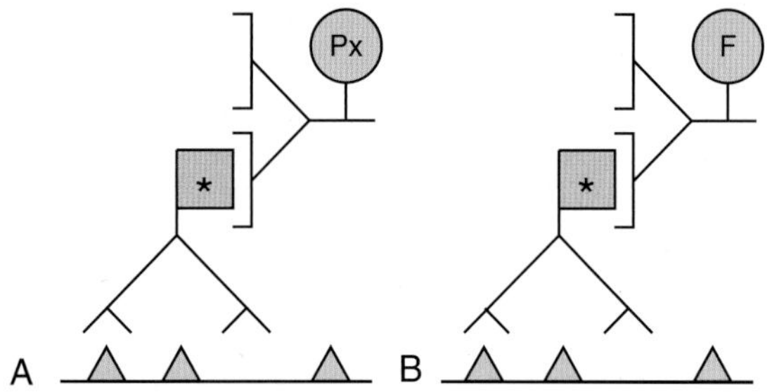

FIGURE 1.5 (A, B) Indirect conjugate (sandwich) method. The primary antibody is unlabeled. The method uses a labeled secondary antibody, having specificity against the primary antibody. (Boxed antigen determinant on primary antibody.) Px, peroxidase label; F, fluorescein label. *From Taylor CR, Cote RJ, eds. Immunomicroscopy: A Diagnostic Tool for the Surgical Pathologist. 3rd ed. Philadelphia: Elsevier; 2005:20.*

antibodies separately. Also, with regard to precious (scarce) antibodies, the direct conjugate procedure usually demands that the primary antibody be used at a relatively high concentration in comparison with indirect and unlabeled antibody methods.

Indirect, or Sandwich, Procedure

The indirect, or sandwich, conjugate procedure (Fig. 1.5) is a relatively simple modification of the direct conjugate method. It has the following advantages:

1. Versatility is increased in that a single conjugated antibody can be used with several different primary antibodies.
2. The labeling process is applied only to the secondary antibody.
3. The primary antibody can usually be used at a higher working dilution (than in the direct method) to achieve successful staining.
4. The secondary antibody, which is produced against immunoglobulin of the species from which the primary antibody is derived, is readily prepared with a high order of specificity and affinity. Many commercial sources are available for labeled secondary reagents, including polymer-based reagents.
5. The method lends itself to additional specificity controls in that the primary specific antibody may be omitted, or another antibody of irrelevant specificity may be substituted, providing a valuable assessment of the validity of any staining pattern observed.

All labeled antibody methods performed by the indirect procedure are analogous in principle; peroxidase and fluorescent indirect conjugate methods are illustrated in Figures 1.5A and B, respectively. The primary antibody that has specificity against the antigen in question (e.g., rabbit anti-A) is added to the section, and the excess is washed off. The labeled secondary antibody, which has specificity against an antigenic determinant present on the primary rabbit antibody (e.g., swine antibody versus rabbit immunoglobulin) is then added; it serves to label the sites of tissue localization of the primary antibody, which, in turn, is bound to the antigen.

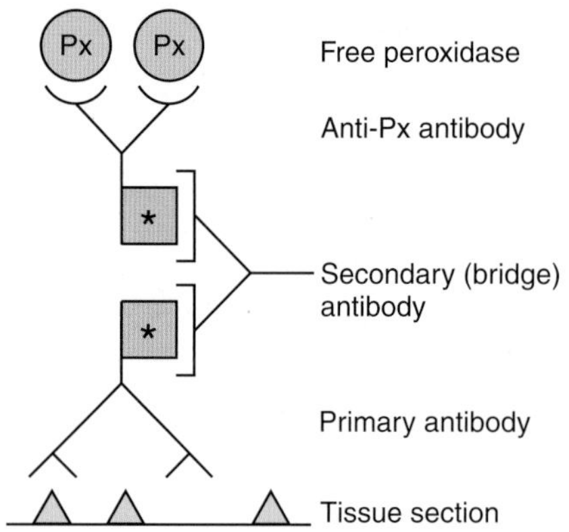

FIGURE 1.6 Enzyme bridge method. A second antibody is used to link (bridge) the primary antibody to an antiperoxidase antibody, which, in turn binds to free peroxidase. Boxed asterisk represents antigen determinant on primary and secondary antibodies. Px, peroxidase label. *From Taylor CR, Cote RJ. Immunomicroscopy: A Diagnostic Tool for the Surgical Pathologist. 2nd ed. Philadelphia: WB Saunders; 1994:12.*

Unlabeled Antibody Methods

ENZYME BRIDGE TECHNIQUE

The disadvantages of the chemical conjugation procedure may be entirely avoided by devising techniques whereby the labeled moiety is linked to the antigen solely by immunologic binding. To achieve this end, Mason and colleagues[77] developed a technique that has become known as the *enzyme bridge method* (Fig. 1.6). This method is rarely used today but is included for its value in research applications where chemical conjugation is undesirable.

PEROXIDASE ANTIPEROXIDASE METHOD

The PAP method (Fig. 1.7) also avoids the problems inherent in chemical conjugation. First employed by Sternberger and colleagues for the detection of antitreponemal antibodies,[78] the PAP system was reported to enjoy a sensitivity 100- to 1000-fold greater than that of comparable conjugate procedures. The principle of the PAP method is similar to that of the enzyme bridge method (see Fig. 1.6). The acronym PAP denotes the peroxidase antiperoxidase reagent that consists of antibody against horseradish peroxidase and horseradish peroxidase antigen in the form of a small, stable immune complex. Available evidence suggests that this immune complex typically consists of two antibody molecules and three horseradish peroxidase molecules in the configuration shown in Figure 1.7. The PAP reagent and the primary antibody must be from the same species (or from closely related species with common antigenic determinants), whereas the bridge or linking antibody is derived from a second species and has specificity against the primary antibody (e.g., rabbit anti-N) and the immunoglobulin incorporated into the PAP complex (e.g., rabbit antiperoxidase). In the example depicted in Figure 1.7A, the primary anti-N antibody is made in rabbit; the bridge antibody is made in swine (i.e., it is a swine antibody against rabbit IgG), whereas the PAP reagent is made

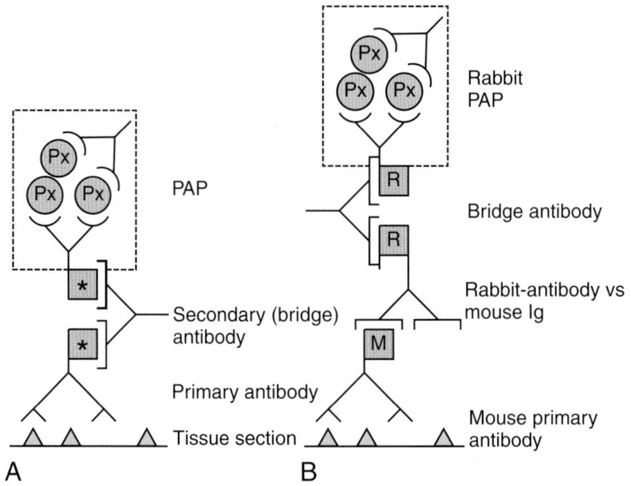

FIGURE 1.7 **(A)** Peroxidase-antiperoxidase (PAP) method (three-stage). PAP reagent *(dashed lines)* is a preformed stable immune complex; it is linked to the primary antibody by a "bridging" antibody. **(B)** PAP method (four-stage). PAP reagent *(dashed line)* is a preformed stable immune complex. Primary antibody in this example is murine (mouse Ig as in a monoclonal antibody [M]); this antibody is followed by a rabbit antimouse Ig (R), a bridge antibody (e.g., swine antirabbit Ig), and rabbit PAP. Px, peroxidase label. *From Taylor CR, Cote RJ. Immunomicroscopy: A Diagnostic Tool for the Surgical Pathologist. 2nd ed. Philadelphia: WB Saunders; 1994:12.*

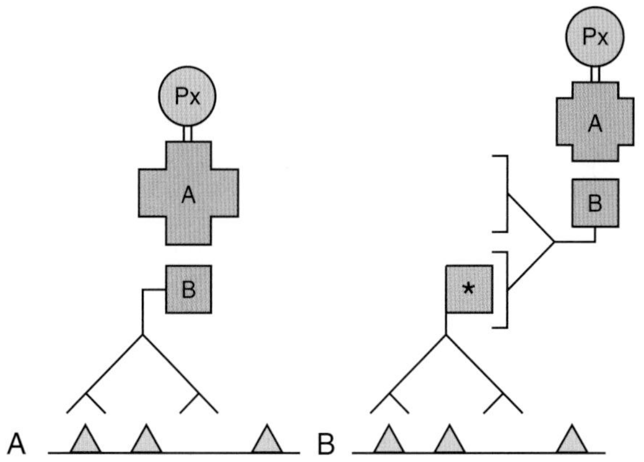

FIGURE 1.8 **(A)** Direct biotin-avidin method. The primary antibody is linked to biotin (B); an avidin-peroxidase-conjugate (A-Px) is then added. **(B)** Indirect biotin-avidin method. Used for monoclonal antibodies, the primary antibody is not conjugated; its localization is detected by a biotinylated secondary antibody. Boxed asterisk represents antigen determinant on primary antibody. Px, peroxidase label; A, avidin; B, biotin. *From Taylor CR, Cote RJ, eds. Immunomicroscopy: A Diagnostic Tool for the Surgical Pathologist. 3rd ed. Philadelphia: Elsevier; 2005:21.*

from rabbit antibody against horseradish peroxidase. This method enjoyed extensive use in routinely processed paraffin sections because of its high degree of sensitivity but has been replaced by streptavidin- and polymer-based systems (see the paragraphs that follow).

Biotin-Avidin Procedure

The biotin-avidin procedure (Fig. 1.8) exploits the high-affinity binding between biotin and avidin. Biotin can be linked chemically to the primary antibody (see Fig. 1.8A), producing a biotinylated conjugate that localizes to the sites of antigen within the section. Subsequently, avidin, which is chemically conjugated to horseradish peroxidase, is added; the avidin binds tightly to the biotinylated antibody, thus localizing the peroxidase moiety at the site of antigen in the tissue section. This method is rapid and has been used particularly in an indirect procedure (see Fig. 1.8B).

Two significant disadvantages exist. First, different batches of biotin and different batches of avidin have differing affinities for one other, and this drastically affects the sensitivity and reproducibility of the procedure. Second, some tissues contain significant amounts of endogenous biotin that may bind the avidin-peroxidase complex directly, thus producing non-specific (false-positive) staining. This can be combated by suitable blocking techniques, as described in the following paragraphs.

Avidin-Biotin Conjugate Procedure

Hsu and colleagues[14,15] developed a further modification of the biotin-avidin system that greatly enhanced its sensitivity. This method can be used as a direct or indirect technique. In the indirect technique (Fig. 1.9), the

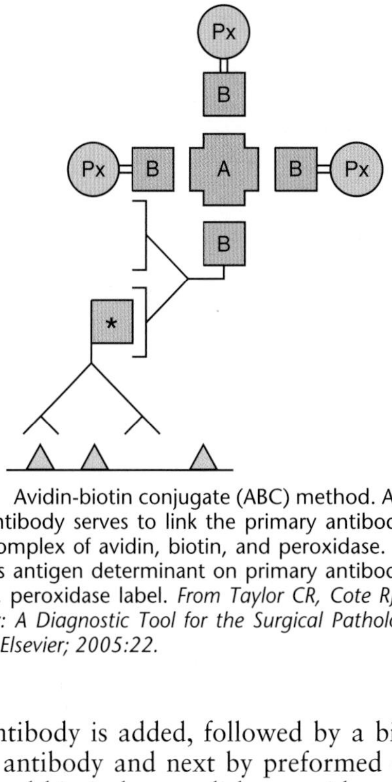

FIGURE 1.9 Avidin-biotin conjugate (ABC) method. A biotinylated secondary antibody serves to link the primary antibody to a large preformed complex of avidin, biotin, and peroxidase. Boxed asterisk represents antigen determinant on primary antibody. A, avidin; B, biotin; Px, peroxidase label. *From Taylor CR, Cote RJ, eds. Immunomicroscopy: A Diagnostic Tool for the Surgical Pathologist. 3rd ed. Philadelphia: Elsevier; 2005:22.*

primary antibody is added, followed by a biotinylated secondary antibody and next by preformed complexes of avidin and biotin horseradish peroxidase conjugate. This complex serves to localize several molecules of horseradish peroxidase at the site of the antigen. The time it takes to perform the ABC conjugate procedure compares favorably with that of the PAP method. Binding to endogenous biotin remains a problem.

Biotin-Streptavidin Systems

The B-SA method overcomes several of the problems associated with the ABC systems by substituting streptavidin for avidin and directly conjugating the streptavidin to the enzyme molecule. Streptavidin, a tetrameric

60-kD avidin analogue isolated from the bacterium *Streptomyces avidinii,* is capable of binding biotin with a very high affinity. Theoretically, this affinity is approximately 10 times higher than that of most antibodies for their antigens and provides very specific detection and amplification of the antigen-antibody binding event. The use of streptavidin is preferred to avidin for several reasons:

1. Streptavidin contains no carbohydrates, which can bind non-specifically to lectin-like substances found in normal tissue from kidney, liver, brain, and mast cells.
2. The isoelectric point of streptavidin is close to neutrality, whereas avidin has an isoelectric point of 10; thus, streptavidin conjugates exhibit less non-specific electrostatic binding than avidin conjugates.
3. Because the enzyme is directly conjugated to streptavidin in the B-SA system, it is a highly stable reagent that can be diluted and stored for long periods in an RTU form.

With these types of systems (Biocare, Shandon-Lipshaw, Immunon, Dako), the secondary and labeling reagents can be modified to maximize the amounts of biotin and enzyme label present, providing substantial increases in sensitivity. The improved sensitivity allows increased dilution of expensive primary antibodies. Either peroxidase or alkaline phosphatase may be used as the enzyme label.

Alkaline Phosphatase Labels, Double Stains, and Polyvalent Detection Systems

Increasingly pathologists are seeking to demonstrate more than one antigen in a single tissue section (slide), in part to reduce the number of slides stained, but particularly to facilitate interpretation of complex staining patterns in mixed cell populations. Double stains must produce contrasting colors to be effective in routine pathology. The simplest way to accomplish this has been to use a second enzymatic label (alkaline phosphatase), which has its own distinct range of chromogens. Many commercial suppliers now offer polyvalent detection systems (Biocare, Shandon-Lipshaw, Immunon, Dako, Ventana) that facilitate the detection of primary antibodies from two or more different species. Initially, double stains (or greater multiples) were performed sequentially, but recently the use of these newer approaches has allowed for concurrent performance. These systems provide primary and secondary reagents in "cocktails" of antibodies typically raised in different species (or hybridomas) to avoid troublesome cross reactions. Multiple stains are discussed more extensively later in this chapter.

There are several ways of introducing alkaline phosphatase labeled reagents, essentially paralleling those methods used with horseradish peroxidase. Ongoing improvements in polymer-based methods (discussed in the following section) are so dramatic that it appears likely that these methods will supersede PAP and streptavidin biotin methods as the primary method as well as for double stains. However, a brief description of special alkaline phosphatase applications follows.

ALKALINE PHOSPHATASE–ANTIALKALINE PHOSPHATASE METHOD

The principles of the alkaline phosphatase–antialkaline phosphatase (APAAP) technique are the same as those described for the PAP method (Fig. 1.10), except that the PAP complex is replaced with an APAAP complex.[79] The method has had three major applications: (1) staining of tissues with high levels of endogenous peroxidase, (2) double immunostaining in conjunction with peroxidase, and (3) staining of specific cell types that benefit from the bright red color of alkaline phosphatase substrates.[4] In general, the technical considerations for the PAP method we have discussed also apply to the APAAP method; the optimal concentration is determined by titration, as described for the PAP complex. Unlike the PAP complex, the APAAP complex consists of two molecules of antigen (alkaline phosphatase) bound to a single molecule of antibody, resembling the normal binding interaction of a bivalent antibody. APAAP complexes are stable for prolonged periods. As noted, polymer-based labels are now widely used.

Alkaline phosphatase labeling not only is useful as a second "double" stain but also may be preferred for tissues rich in endogenous peroxidase, such as bone marrow or lymphoid tissue containing infiltrating myeloid cells, particularly when using frozen sections. Because complete blocking of endogenous peroxidase in blood

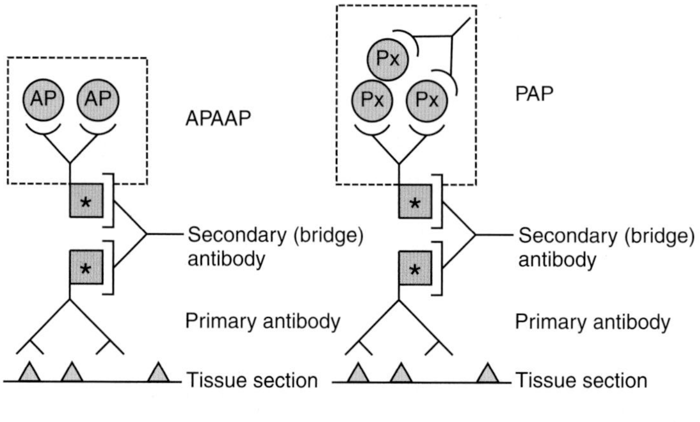

FIGURE 1.10 Alkaline phosphatase–antialkaline phosphatase (APAAP) and PAP methods showing the feasibility of double staining by the use of different primary and secondary antibodies, for example, mouse antivimentin, horse anti-mouse IgG, mouse APAAP *(left)*; rabbit antikeratin (polyclonal goat antirabbit IgG), rabbit PAP *(right)*. AP, alkaline phosphatase; Px, peroxidase. *From Taylor CR, Cote RJ, eds. Immunomicroscopy: A Diagnostic Tool for the Surgical Pathologist. 3rd ed. Philadelphia: Elsevier; 2005:20.*

and bone marrow smears may be difficult, and because blocking procedures may denature some of the antigenic determinants, the APAAP method has proved useful in staining bone marrow. The study by Erber and McLachlan[80] provides an excellent resource for those wishing to adopt this method.

For double immunostaining, it is convenient to use an alkaline phosphatase method in conjunction with an immunoperoxidase stain (see Appendix 1B). The use of alkaline phosphatase as the second label has the advantage of avoiding the cross-reactivity that may occur when two immunoperoxidase procedures are used together. In addition, one may carry out a simultaneous double immunostaining procedure using heterospecific antibodies such as polyclonal and monoclonal antibodies as the two primary antibodies under investigation (see Fig. 1.10). We will discuss this procedure in the context of cocktail methods. Sequential double immunostaining with the alkaline phosphatase method may produce excellent contrasting colors using fast red and fast blue stains.[81] In sequential double stains, care must be taken to avoid mixed-color staining (i.e., having the initial red color change to purple); to this end, the "weaker" staining antigen is usually stained first, and the second label applied may be developed for a shorter time (10 to 15 minutes, monitored by microscopy).

In some cases, the bright red color produced by alkaline phosphatase substrates (fast red or new fuchsin) may provide more distinct staining than the conventional peroxidase chromogens. The alkaline phosphatase method may be used successfully, for example, to demonstrate nuclear antigens or to stain cell smears in which only a few cells stain positively. This is exemplified by Wong and colleagues[82] in a study of estrogen receptors (ERs) in human breast carcinomas. In another example, Vardiman and coworkers[83] reported the detection of a small number of hairy cells using monoclonal antibody Leu-M5 (CD11c) and an alkaline phosphatase method to stain peripheral blood and bone marrow preparations from patients with hairy cell leukemia.

POLYMER-BASED LABELING, BASIC TWO-STEP METHOD

The demand for more sensitive, more reliable, and simpler methods for IHC continues to escalate. Traditional multi-step detection systems have several drawbacks including complex time-consuming protocols, difficulties in standardization, and difficulties with sensitivity and the ability to demonstrate hard-to-detect antigens. Simplification of these conventional multi-step detection systems, producing shorter protocols without compromising detection sensitivity, is theoretically possible and has long been desirable. Nevertheless, it is technically challenging. In practice, the reduction of the number of steps has always been unfortunately accompanied by a reduction in the sensitivity of the results. New approaches such as catalyzed reporter deposition or tyramine signal amplification (TSA)[8,9] immuno-polymerase chain reaction (immuno-PCT)[84] and end-product amplification[85] have improved sensitivity. However, these techniques are accompanied by more complicated protocols, by high or unacceptable non-specific staining, and by poor reproducibility, even within a single laboratory.

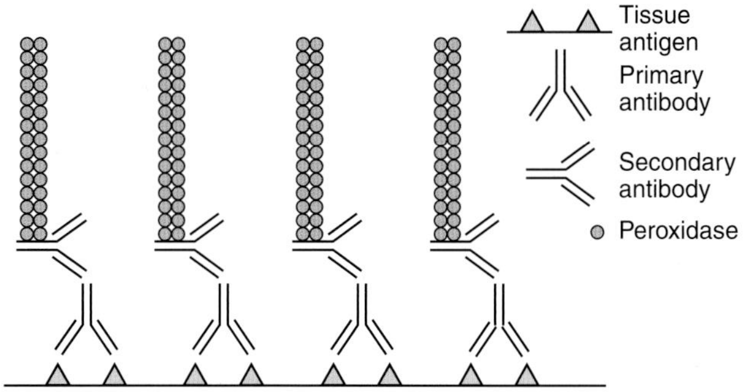

FIGURE 1.11 Schematic of polymer-based detection system. The enzyme-linker antibody has a more compact molecular shape than other polymer carrier-based conjugates and thus allows the attachment of multiple conjugates in close proximity to each other. The abundant conjugated enzymatic molecules are deposited in each antigenic location, which resembles a big-city skyline. *From Shi S-R, Guo J, Cote RJ, et al. Sensitivity and detection efficiency of a novel two-step detection system (PowerVision) for immunohistochemistry. Appl Immunohistochem Mol Morphol. 1999;7:201-208.*

The development of other amplification methods has circumvented some of these issues. These methods use linking antibodies and marker enzymes that are attached to a polymer backbone. The natural or synthetic polymers increase the number of enzymes or ligands that are coupled to the linking antibodies.[86-91] Examples of such carriers include dextran, polypeptides, dendrimers, and DNA branches. The advantage of these polymer-based detection systems is that they eliminate the problem of endogenous biotin by avoiding the biotinylated secondary antibody. Blocking of endogenous biotin is therefore not required, and the false-positive staining due to endogenous biotin is avoided.

The constant and encouraging trend toward simplicity with IHC methods persists, and it is the hope that such new methods will facilitate the goal of standardization of IHC. This goal is consistent with the overall philosophy that all other things being equal, simple techniques are better than complicated ones (Fig 1.11).

The enhanced polymer one-step staining (EPOS) system (Dako) was introduced in 1993 by Bisgaard.[91] It is a one-step direct polymer immunohistochemical staining method. In this system, a number of molecules of both monoclonal primary antibody and horseradish peroxidase (HRP) are covalently bound to an inert, high molecular weight dextran polymer (Dextran 1). This technique offers the advantage of combining the link antibody step and the detection complex incubation step into a single step. This results in a simpler and more rapid immunohistochemical staining process. However, utility of this system was limited because commercial availability of EPOS antibodies had been limited to approximately 20 different tissue and tumor markers. Nevertheless, testing with these antibodies could be performed on paraffin-embedded tissue sections, archival frozen material, and intra-operative frozen sections yielding sensitive and reproducible results.[92] Compared to prior standard multi-step procedures using direct HRP, PAP, ABC, or APAAP, which typically require 2 to 4 hours to perform, turnaround time with the EPOS system was significantly reduced to approximately 1 hour for routinely processed, paraffin- embedded material, and to less than seven minutes for intra-operative frozen section material.[93] Such a quick, simple, and reproducible technique offers obvious diagnostic and therapeutic advantages for routine work, particularly in an intra-operative clinical setting.

Two-step indirect polymer strategies have also been developed. These include the EnVision and EnVision+ systems, which were first developed by Dako in 1995 (Carpinteria, Calif), as well as PowerVision, marketed by ImmunoVision Technologies in 1999 (Daly City, Calif). In 2001, a second-generation, PowerVision+ system was introduced by ImmunoVision Technologies and several other manufacturers (e.g., Biocare).

Dako's EnVision system is a two-step staining technique. The tissue is first incubated with the primary antibody and is then incubated with a polymeric conjugate in sequential steps. The polymeric conjugate (EnVision complex) is large and consists of up to 100 peroxidase enzyme molecules and up to 20 secondary antibody molecules (goat antimouse or goat antirabbit). These molecules are bound directly to an activated dextran polymer backbone. Because it is a two-step process, this method offers the laboratory the flexibility of choosing a primary antibody whose concentration and incubation times may be individually optimized while benefiting from the simplicity and rapidity of a two-step assay. In one study, specific, reliable, and reproducible results for important intra-operative frozen section diagnoses could be obtained (in as little as 13 minutes in some instances).[90]

Other studies with this system have shown a sensitivity comparable to ABC techniques.[94] Subsequently, EnVision+ (EV+) was introduced. This was a modified EV system that showed increased sensitivity by using a mixture of dextran polymers. The EnVision system has been shown to offer many advantages over prior methods such as ABC and B-SA. It offered high sensitivity and allowed increased dilutions of the primary antibody. It has also been used for signal amplification in combination with *in situ* hybridization (ISH), where it has also been shown to increase sensitivity and shorten assay times.[95]

Other benefits of polymer-based methods are also worth noting. Since this is a biotin-free system, the problems of false-positive staining due to endogenous biotin are overcome.[96] Therefore, the efficiency of AR may be increased without the risk of evoking endogenous biotin activity. Furthermore, compared with three-step procedures, the technique is simpler, and assay time is decreased. Because of this, the risk of errors is reduced and reproducibility is increased.

Although sensitivity may be increased in many instances using polymer-based labels, others have reported that with some antibodies, particularly those that require proteolytic digestion or target unmasking, the EnVision method revealed slightly weaker staining and less sensitivity.[94] This outcome was believed to be due to problems of tissue penetration of the labeled polymer, most likely the result of spatial hindrance posed by the high molecular weight of the large polymeric conjugate. To circumvent this problem, Shi and colleagues[86] utilized a molecularly more compact enzyme-antibody conjugate (the PowerVision System) that consists of a high number of enzyme molecules attached to each linker antibody. With this system, molecular size is minimized by the use of small linear or minimally branched multi-functional reagents that polymerize under controlled conditions with linker antibodies and enzymes in a tight small space. Because of its more compact size, this enzyme linker antibody is able to attach to multiple conjugates in close proximity to one another, thereby avoiding the spatial hindrance problems and chromogen penetrance issues of some other systems.

A comparative study by Shi and colleagues[86] compared the PowerVision system with three multi-step detection systems available at that time: the ChemMate, LSAB2, and SuperSensitive kits. Three sets of experiments were performed to compare the different methods for immunohistochemical staining of routine FFPE tissue sections. In all three experiment sets, staining was performed under identical conditions, including the use of an optimized microwave AR technique. In these experiments, the polymer-based method outperformed other techniques in all aspects. The sections that were stained using PowerVision and an optimized AR protocol could be satisfactorily restored; this was not possible with the other three detection systems.

Improved "second-generation" polymer-based labels offer still higher levels of performance and seem destined to become the standard.[97,98] From a clinical practice standpoint, such methods are extremely useful, particularly when fast results are desirable. Some pathologists routinely use the polymer-based method to evaluate intra-operatively the surgical margins of melanoma specimens using Mohs micrographic surgery and MART-1 staining. Such a quick, sensitive method benefits the patient, pathologist, and surgeon, who can decide, based on IHC results, whether wider surgical margins need to be obtained.[99]

In summary, these polymer-based systems are usually two-step procedures, although they may be increased to a three-step procedure if more sensitivity is necessary. Generally speaking, the first step of these polymer systems consists of an unlabeled primary antibody, and the second step consists of a polymer containing numerous secondary antibodies as well as numerous molecules of enzymes. The structure of the secondary antibodies (opposite from that bound to the primary antibody) enables the omission of the linking step. The numerous HRP enzymes on the polymer conjugate oxidize and activate the chromogen—in most cases, a bronze-colored diaminobenzidine (DAB) chromogen. Because of the great number of HRP enzymes on the polymer, more DAB chromogen is activated. This results in brighter, more sensitive staining.

In addition to their relative simplicity, these polymer techniques offer other advantages as well over the more traditional three-step methods. Because these are biotin-free systems, they do not produce the non-specific background generated by endogenous biotin. Therefore, blocking of biotin is not required. According to various studies, the sensitivity of these polymeric methods is at least comparable and sometimes superior due to signal amplification, improved signal/background ratios, and increased detection efficiency. Because the methods are simpler and faster to perform, one is less likely to encounter procedural variability. Hence reproducibility and standardization are facilitated. Although the reagents are expensive, the cost may be offset by the ability to further dilute the primary antibodies and perform batch staining if applicable. The faster turnaround times free up labor costs and technician time, resulting in a streamlined, cost-efficient, sensitive, reproducible, and reliable test.

Note that successful application of any "ultrasensitive" detection system raises the possibility that it may be necessary to retitrate primary reagents to a higher working dilution in order to avoid non-specific staining.[100,101]

TYRAMINE SIGNAL AMPLIFICATION

Based on the principle of enzyme amplification for enzyme immunoassays adopted in the 1980s, Bobrow and associates developed a catalyzed reporter deposition technique (CARD) to achieve amplified signal for solid-phase immunoassay system and membrane immunoassays.[9,100] Subsequently, this CARD technique was introduced to IHC in 1992.[8]

Signal amplification in the CARD method is based on biotinylated tyramine deposition through free radical formation, which is catalyzed by oxidizing horseradish peroxidase. It is postulated that radicalized biotinylated tyramine will be covalently attached to electron-rich moieties (tyrosine, phenylalanine, tryptophan, and so on), resulting in additional biotinylated molecules being deposited at the site of antigen-antibody reaction (i.e., amplification of the signal) (Fig. 1.12).[102-105]

Application of tyramine signal amplification (TSA) for IHC has achieved positive immunostaining for some hard-to-detect antigens in archival paraffin-embedded tissue sections.[102] Several commercial TSA reagents are available (NEN Life Science Products, Boston, Mass; CSA system, Dako, Carpinteria, Calif). With use of these TSA kits, additional staining steps are performed after a regular horseradish peroxidase–conjugated detection system: incubating the slides with a biotinylated tyramine reagent, washing thoroughly, and then incubating the slides with horseradish peroxidase–conjugated streptavidin. Finally, chromogen (DAB, amino-ethyl carbazole [AEC], and so on) is used to visualize the amplified signal in the tissue sections. The so-called ImmunoMax technique recommended a combination of optimized AR and the TSA system for certain hard-to-detect antigens or for expensive primary reagents in using much higher dilution of the primary antibody.[102-108]

Although this TSA method has achieved satisfactory results in terms of significantly increasing intensity of IHC and ISH, it has not been widely applied in diagnostic pathology for several reasons,[103] including the following:

- Additional steps make the method more time consuming.
- Non-specific background staining may increase as the signal increases.
- Optimal AR treatment with existing methods may achieve equivalent results.
- Second-generation polymer-based methods are simpler and equally sensitive.

OTHER METHODS, CURRENTLY WITH LIMITED OR RESEARCH APPLICATION

Protein A, derived from *Staphylococcus*, has the remarkable ability to bind with the constant (Fc) portion of immunoglobulin molecules from several different species. The only absolute requirement is that the primary antibody binds with protein A; most IgG molecules bind protein A, although affinity varies among different IgG subclasses and in different species (Figs 1.13, 1.14). The protein A–peroxidase and related protein A-PAP methods do not match the sensitivity of the PAP, ABC, or streptavidin-based techniques, but they do have advantages that may warrant their use in specific circumstances.

The enzyme-labeled antigen method (Fig. 1.15) was devised as perhaps the ultimate in specificity among immunoperoxidase techniques. The principles of application of this method are illustrated in Figure 1.15. Only one antibody is used; the method exploits the fact that an antibody molecule possesses two valences, one of which may be bound to the antigen under study, with the second valency left free to bind with additional molecules of antigen added subsequently. The additional antigen is presented in a form that is directly conjugated with horseradish peroxidase; thus, this is a "labeled antigen" procedure.

The primary antibody is generally used at a relatively high concentration. This method therefore is not economical in use of the primary antibody and is best applied for the detection of antigens in which both antigen and antibody are in good supply. One major advantage is that the primary antibody need not be particularly pure because antibodies of irrelevant specificity will not be detected by this technique, even if they bind to the tissue section; lacking specificity for A antigen, they will not bind the A antigen–peroxidase conjugate and thus will not be visualized.

This method has proved particularly suitable for double-staining techniques whereby one seeks to stain two antigens simultaneously within the same section (Fig. 1.16) using two labeled antigens (e.g., kappa-peroxidase and lambda–alkaline phosphatase) together.

Titration of Primary Antibody and Detection System

The optimal dilution for use of an antibody in immunohistology is defined as the dilution at which the greatest contrast is achieved between the desired (specific) positive staining and any unwanted (non-specific) background staining. Selection is subjective and is based not simply

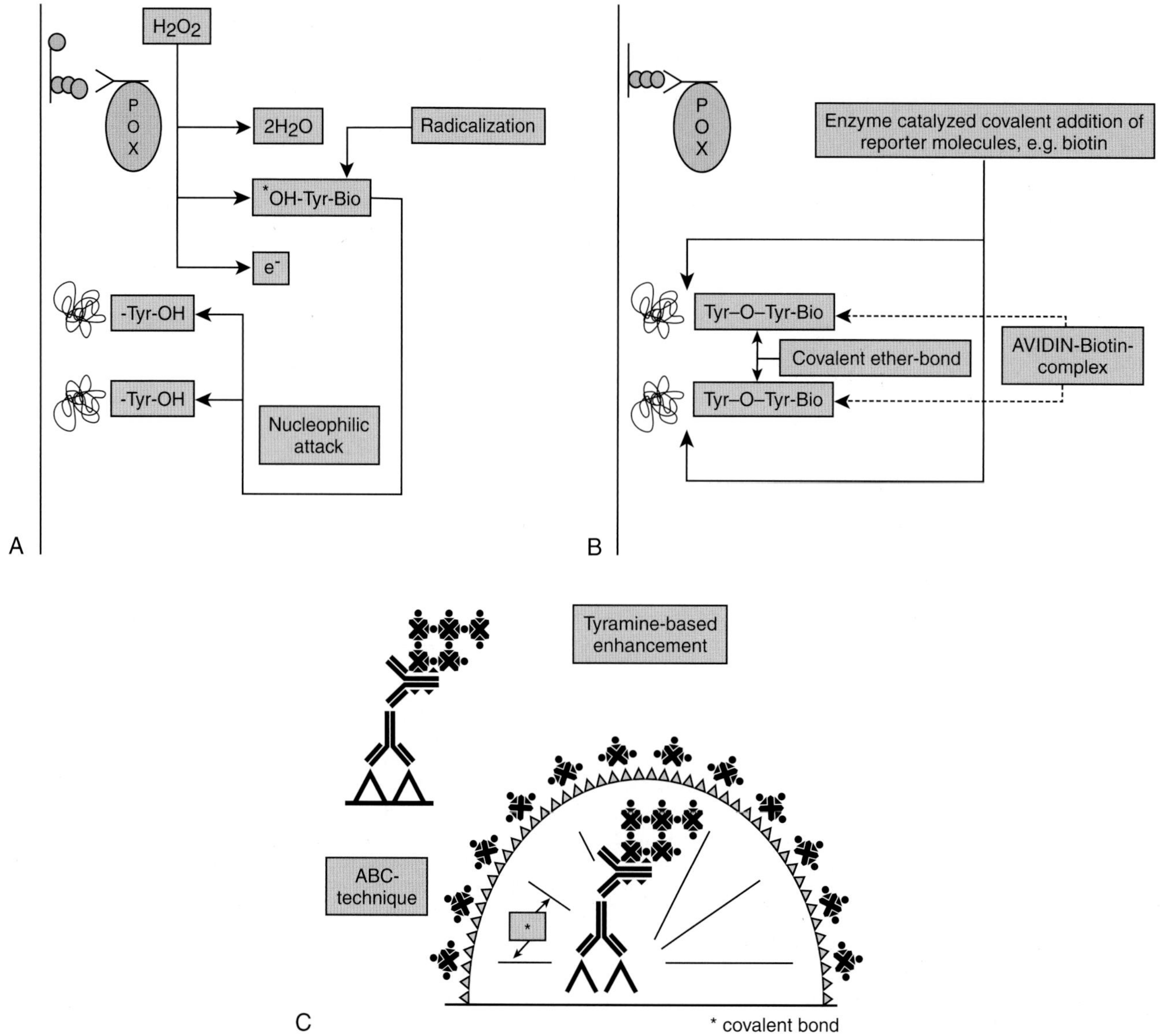

FIGURE 1.12 **(A)** Radicalization of tyramine amplification. **(B)** Tyramine-reporter deposition. **(C)** Comparison with the ABC method. *From Merz H, Ottesen K, Meyer W, et al. Combination of antigen retrieval techniques and signal amplification of immunohistochemistry in situ hybridization and FISH techniques. In: Shi S-R, Giu J, Taylor CR, eds. Antigen Retrieval Techniques: Immunohistochemistry and Molecular Morphology. Natick, MA: Eaton; 2000:228-229.*

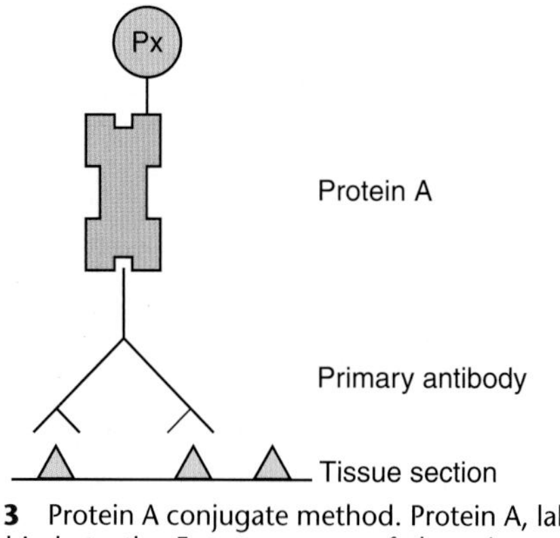

FIGURE 1.13 Protein A conjugate method. Protein A, labeled with peroxidase, binds to the Fc component of the primary antibody. Px, peroxidase label. *From Taylor CR, Cote RJ. Immunomicroscopy: A Diagnostic Tool for the Surgical Pathologist. 2nd ed. Philadelphia: WB Saunders; 1994:14.*

on the greatest intensity but rather on the greatest useful contrast. Titration is relatively straightforward in the direct method, with only a single antibody (Table 1.1). In two-layer methods, exemplified by the indirect and polymer-based labels, each of the separate immune reagents must be applied at optimal dilution. In addition, the dilutions of the primary and secondary antibodies (or labels) are interdependent in terms of contrast developed by the procedure as a whole. This fact necessitates comparison of the results obtained using several dilutions of the labeling reagent (secondary antibody) with several different dilutions of the primary antibody; comparison is achieved by checkerboard titration (Table 1.2). PAP methods and other multi-step procedures require more complex checkerboard titrations of each of these separate steps; sensitive polymer-based methods have superseded the use of these methods, and we will not discuss them further. Refer to previous editions of

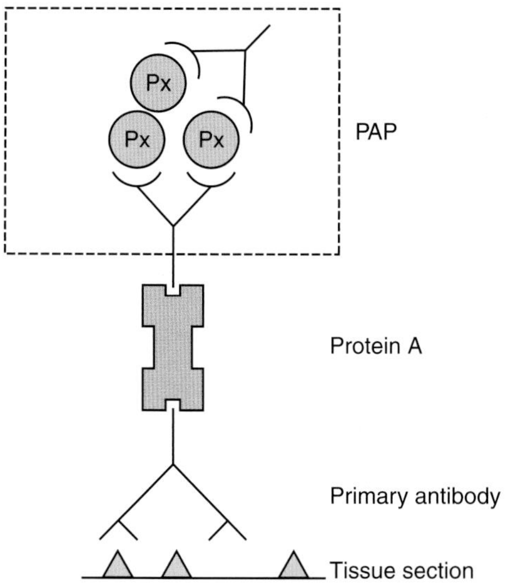

FIGURE 1.14 Protein A-PAP method. The protein A is used to link the primary antibody (Fc) to the antibody (Fc) within the PAP complex. Px, peroxidase label. *From Taylor CR, Cote RJ. Immunomicroscopy: A Diagnostic Tool for the Surgical Pathologist. 2nd ed. Philadelphia: WB Saunders; 1994:14.*

this book or Taylor and Cote (1994) if you require further details for research use.[4]

Once optimal dilutions have been determined, the stock of undiluted reagent should be divided into convenient aliquots for the preparation of working dilutions immediately before use. Generally speaking, it is not wise to store reagents in a highly diluted form unless additional protein or stabilizers are added to conserve activity, since reactivity may decline unpredictably. That stability of highly diluted reagents can be achieved is evidenced by the availability of commercial immunostaining kits that do contain prediluted reagents and have a defined but often limited shelf life.

A principal reason for the use of reagents freshly prepared from aliquots is the need to avoid repeated sampling of a single reagent tube (or bottle), as with a Pasteur pipette, since this practice almost invariably results in bacterial contamination and loss of reactivity that is both unpredictable and aggravating. Here the "pure" scientists might learn a lesson from their often maligned cousins in the commercial sector, who have to a large extent overcome the contamination problem by providing diluted reagents in sealed dropper bottles so that the reagent can be dropped directly from the reagent bottle. We have unashamedly borrowed this technique in our laboratory, and whenever we make up new dilutions of reagents for use over a period of several days, we use these small plastic dropper bottles.

QUALITY CONTROL AND STANDARDIZATION

Quality control as defined by the College of American Pathologists is "the aggregate of processes and techniques so derived to detect, reduce and correct deficiencies in an analytic process."[106] It is an integral component of a laboratory's quality assurance program,

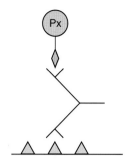

FIGURE 1.15 Labeled antigen method. The antibody is added in excess so that one valency is bound to the antigen in the section, leaving the second valency free to bind the labeled antigen that is added subsequently. Px, peroxidase label. *From Taylor CR, Cote RJ. Immunomicroscopy: A Diagnostic Tool for the Surgical Pathologist. 2nd ed. Philadelphia: WB Saunders; 1994:14.*

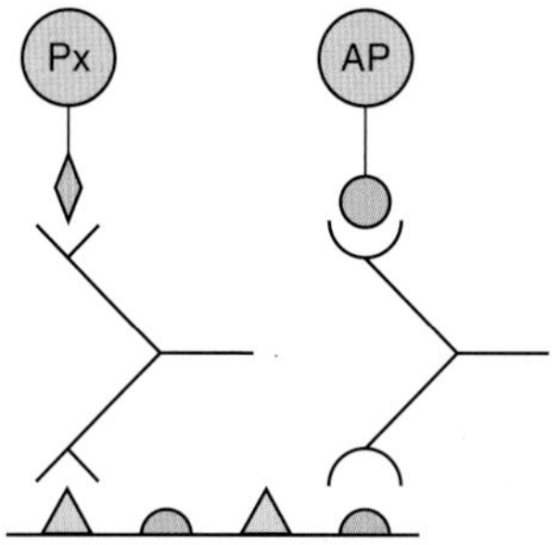

FIGURE 1.16 Labeled antigen double stain. Two different antibodies recognize their respective antigens in the tissue section and subsequently bind only the corresponding labeled antigen (labeled with peroxidase [Px] or alkaline phosphatase [AP]). *From Taylor CR, Cote RJ. Immunomicroscopy: A Diagnostic Tool for the Surgical Pathologist. 2nd ed. Philadelphia: WB Saunders; 1994:15.*

focusing mainly on procedural and technical aspects of the test under question. As it pertains to IHC, quality control standards should address and define each step of the "total IHC test" (Table 1.3), including tissue procurement, fixation, processing, sectioning, staining, and, finally, the interpretation and reporting of the staining results.

As part of a laboratory's quality control program, all steps of the test should be described separately, and parameters of each step established and monitored in order to ensure consistency of performance and reproducibility of results. Daily records of control results are maintained, and corrective actions are undertaken and documented when results are unacceptable. In practice the surgical pathology histology laboratory typically falls short of the ideal standards in key areas, especially with regard to tissue preparation. In this section, we will discuss quality control issues as they pertain to the validation of antibodies and the use of controls. We will also address measures that may be adopted to minimize variability deriving from inconsistent tissue preparation, including fixation.

Sample Preparation

Sample preparation has emerged as a key issue in recent years, in large part due to use of IHC assays for HER2 to qualify patients for Herceptin therapy in clinical trials,

TABLE 1.1 Representative Dilution Titration to Determine Optimal Titer of Antibody for use in Direct Conjugate Method

	Serial Dilutions of Primary Antibody					
Intensity of Staining* of:	**1/5**	**1/20**	**1/80**	**1/320**	**1/1280**	**1/2560**
Unwanted background[a]	++	+	±	±	±	±
Specific antigens[b]	+++	++++	++++	+++	++	+

*Intensity of staining scored on a semiquantitative scale 0 to ++++; ± indicates faint positivity of uncertain significance.
[a]Unwanted background staining may result from several different mechanisms (see text).
[b]Intensity of staining of specific antigen (e.g., with titration of anti-kappa antibody, specific staining would be present in plasma cells).
Adapted from Taylor CR, Cote RJ. Immunomicroscopy: A Diagnostic Tool for the Surgical Pathologist. 2nd ed. Philadelphia: WB Saunders; 1994:23.

TABLE 1.2 Determination of Optimal Titers for Indirect Immunoperoxidase Method—Checkerboard Titration

		Dilutions of Primary Antibody					
		1/5	**1/20**	**1/80**	**1/320**	**1/1280**	**Negative Control***
Dilutions of secondary antibody (conjugate)	1/10	slide 1	slide 2	slide 3	slide 4	slide 5	slide 16
		+++[a]	++++	+++	++	+	±
		(++)	(++)	(++)	(++)	(++)	(++)
	1/40	slide 6	slide 7	slide 8	slide 9	slide 10	slide 17
		+++	+++	++++	++++	++	–
		(+)	(+)	(+)	(±)	(±)	(±)
	1/160	slide 11	slide 12	slide 13	slide 14	slide 15	slide 18
		++	++	+	±	±	–
		(+)	(±)	(±)	(–)	(–)	(–)

Example of an 18-slide titration.
*Negative control (omit primary antibody, replace with pre-immune serum, or serum with irrelevant specificity; see negative controls).
[a]Intensity of specific staining is indicated on a scale of 0 to ++++; non-specific background is given on the same scale but is shown in parentheses e.g., +++ (+) indicates strong specific staining (+++) with moderate background (+).
Note: In this example, the optimal result is achieved with slide 9.
Adapted from Taylor CR, Cote RJ. Immunomicroscopy: A Diagnostic Tool for the Surgical Pathologist. 2nd ed. Philadelphia: WB Saunders; 1994:29.

TABLE 1.3 Components of the "Total Test" in IHC

Elements of Testing Process	Quality Assurance Issues	Responsibility
Clinical question, test selection	Indications for IHC; selection of stains	Surgical pathologist; sometimes clinician
Specimen acquisition and management	Specimen collection, fixation, processing, sectioning	Pathologist/technologist
Analytic issues	Qualifications of staff; intra- and inter-laboratory proficiency testing of procedures	Pathologist/technologist
Results validation and reporting	Criteria for positivity/negativity in relation to controls; content and organization of report; turnaround time	Pathologist/technologist
Interpretation, significance	Experience/qualifications of pathologist; proficiency testing of interpretational aspects; diagnostic, prognostic significance; appropriateness/correlation	Surgical pathologist or clinician, or both

Adapted from Taylor CR. Report of the Immunohistochemistry Steering Committee of the Biological Stain Commission. "Proposed format: Package insert for immunohistochemistry products." Biotech Histochem. 1992;67:110-117.

TABLE 1.4	Recommendations for Improved Standardization of Immunohistochemistry by the Ad-Hoc Committee[110] Recommendation
1	Fix all specimens promptly in 10% neutral buffered formalin.
2	Fix and process resections and core biopsies in an identical manner.
3	Only use 10% neutral phosphate buffered formalin.
4	Note that fixation is 8 to 72 hours for both core biopsies and resections.
5	Use formalin, not alcohol, to fix cytology specimens for ER assay.
6	Use conventional tissue processors to process breast tissue.
7	Ensure that the first formalin containers on the tissue processor are always newly replenished.
8	Ensure that tissue processor fluids do not exceed 37°C.
9	Be sure that paraffin in the tissue processor does not exceed 60°C.
10	Record and document fixation times in your report.
11	Use *in vitro* diagnostic kits that employ clone, 6F11, 1D5, or SP1.
12	Include positive and negative controls with each batch run.
13	Employ a threshold for positive result of 1% positive cells.
14/15	Report semi-quantitation, tabulating the intensity (0, 1+, 2+, 3+) and percent of positive cells.

during which unacceptably large variations were noted in tests performed by different laboratories. Since the 1990s, several conferences have convened on the topic of standardization, with a broad range of attendees. These included "experts" in IHC and representatives of the NCI (National Cancer Institute), CAP (College of American Pathologists), NIST (National Institute of Standards and Technology), and CMS (Centers for Medicare and Medicaid Services, which pays the bills in the United States). These meetings of minds served to focus attention on the need for improved reproducibility of IHC and particularly the enormous and unknown variability in specimen handling and preparation (fixation), but they have offered no practical or tangible results thus far. The NCI even issued requests for proposals (RFPs) in the area of sample preparation, again without tangible practical results.

While applauding these efforts and, in addition, noting that there have been serious searches for new, improved, and "molecularly friendly" fixatives, the authors conclude that no such fixative is likely to replace formalin in the next decade, at least to a significant degree. **Thus, FFPE tissues are what we have, and we must learn to work with them as best we can, to extract the maximum information available, in as consistent and reliable a manner as possible.**

One pragmatic approach has been the development of recommendations for all phases of the "total test," including definition of fixation as far as possible, and more rigid and uniform adherence to common protocols. The American Society of Clinical Oncologists (ASCO) in conjunction with College of American Pathologists (CAP) issued such guidelines with respect to HER2 testing.[107,108] These guidelines recognized the key importance of fixation time, assigning both minimum and maximum limits (namely, 6 to 48 hours for excised specimens), although the authors of the guidelines succumbed to clinical pressures for speed in allowing a one-hour fixation time for core biopsies. This concession appears to be unwise, and there is no scientific basis for it. Although penetration may have occurred in one hour, fixation (which is a "clock reaction") is unlikely to be complete. Yaziji and Taylor[109] nonetheless supported the basic idea of "everyone adopting guidelines," emphasizing that in performance of an IHC test, "begin at the beginning, with the tissue." The members of the Ad-Hoc Committee on Immunohistochemistry Standardization published a separate, very detailed set of guidelines with the goal of improving the reproducibility of testing for ER,[110] following principles previously set forth by the same group for standardization of IHC in general.[111] These recommendations began with the "total test" premise and then followed with a series of 14 recommendations relating to the pre-analytic, analytic, and post-analytic phases of performing and reporting an IHC test. These recommendations are summarized in Table 1.4.

Beyond following detailed guidelines, marked improvement in standardization may also be achieved by the use of reference standards, against which the impact (adverse or otherwise) of sample preparation (fixation) can be measured. This will be discussed in greater detail following the section on validation of reagents, protocols, and staining results.

Validation of Reagents, Protocols, and "Staining" Results

In a simplistic sense it would be best, in terms of reproducibility, if one manufacturer established an absolute monopoly in IHC, forcing uniformity of reagents and protocols upon us all. However, such dominance is unlikely to happen, so commonly used control systems (reference standards) can go a long way in bringing effective standardization.

TABLE 1.5 Types and Purposes of Daily Quality Control Materials for IHC

Type of Control	Antigen (Analyte)	Antibody (Reagent)	Purpose
Positive	Non-patient tissue or cells containing antigen to be detected and quantified Known expected result Fixed-processed in same way as a patient sample Fixed-processed in manner shown to preserve antigen under analysis	Antibody reagent (of the kit) constituted in same way as intended for patient sample	Control of all steps of the analysis Training user for appearance of positive reaction; comparison for semi-quantitation of reaction Validates all steps of analysis, including fixation and processing Validates all steps of analysis, except fixation or processing used by individual laboratory
Negative (specific)	Tissues or cells expected to be negative by antibody (of kit) Processed in same way as patient sample May be portion of patient sample	Antibody reagent (of kit) constituted in same way as intended for patient sample	Detection of unintended antibody cross-reactivity to cells or cellular components
Negative (non-specific)	Patient tissue with components that are the same as tissue to be studied Processed in same way as patient sample	Diluent (as used with antibody) without antibody Antibody not specific for antigen of interest in same diluents as used with kit antibody	Detection of unintended background staining

Adapted from Taylor CR, Cote RJ. Immunomicroscopy: A Diagnostic Tool for the Surgical Pathologist. 2nd ed. Philadelphia: WB Saunders; 1994:27.

For example, as part of the United Kingdom UKNEQAS program,[112,113] Rhodes and colleagues demonstrated improved reproducibility of IHC for ER and HER2-IHC detection through stringent quality control, an ongoing quality assurance program, and the use of standard reference materials based on a comparative study among laboratories in many different countries. In the United States, the ASCO/CAP guidelines[107,108] have made it a requirement that the HER2 detection test be done in a qualified accredited laboratory, with proficiency standards. Vani and colleagues[114] performed an elegant study that compared the proficiency of different laboratories, including peptide slides as standards (see the paragraphs that follow). They found that the almost 100% of the "failures" were due to errors in AR, errors in antibody titration/protocol, or both. This clearly identified where the focus must be for performing laboratories, and it showed the value of reference standards that can be compared across laboratories.

The use of reference standards for the quality control of reagents in the clinical laboratory is well established. For example, serum assay results can be validated by large standardized serum pools, such as those established by the College of American Pathologists "Check Sample" program. More recently, the development of reference standard controls for IHC has been under consideration. However, this undertaking is not that simple. Unlike serum samples, pathologic tissues cannot be pooled, and the supply of tissue samples is not infinite. Moreover, morphologically similar tumors are not necessarily antigenically identical. The use of multi-tissue blocks alleviates some of these problems, but these too contain only a limited amount of tissue, which will eventually become depleted. To overcome this, the development of infinite standard reference controls composed of artificial tumors or human tumor cell lines, or the use of defined peptide deposits, has been proposed.[114-117]

There is the potential to establish internal reference standards that will be of use in assessing the effectiveness of sample preparation and fixation, giving an indication of the suitability of the tissue for IHC studies; we will address this new area following the discussion of reagent and protocol validation and at the end of this chapter.

Reagent and protocol controls are essential in the validation of reagents, the evaluation of performance of the IHC protocol, and the staining result.[115] We will discuss these basic types of controls first (Table 1.5).

Validation studies are required for each test and antibody (including each new lot of antibody) that is used by a laboratory. Such testing is also required for RTU pretested reagents, including those that are part of a kit; however, this is less extensive because optimal dilutions and protocols have been established by the manufacturer. In this instance, the performing laboratory has only to show satisfactory performance on in-house tissues. With reagents purchased as concentrates, where manufacturer data may be very limited, detailed validation studies are imperative because the reagents may be of uncertain origin, composition, or concentration or specificity (or all of these).[115,118] Performance parameters to be addressed by these studies include the sensitivity, specificity, precision, accuracy, and reproducibility of the results. It is recommended that these initial studies be carried out on multi-tissue control blocks containing both known positive and known negative normal and tumor tissues, because this approach allows comparison of findings in many cells and tissues subjected to identical staining protocol on a single slide; it is also convenient and economical in time and use of tissue. The results obtained are reviewed and attest to the specificity and precision of the antibody under study. The specificity of antibody staining is shown by the "expected" absence of staining in certain cells, tissues, and tumors within the multi-tissue control blocks known not to contain the antigen (protein) in question. Precision, in contrast, attests to the validity of the entire procedure and is shown by the presence of both positive and negative elements as expected on the same control slide. A sensitive test is one that detects a small amount of antigen. This is shown by positive results using tissue with known low expression. Accuracy is determined by the evaluation of non-specific background staining. A negative reagent control can be used in place of the primary antibody to determine this. Finally, if there is no run-to-run variation in the results obtained, the test is reproducible.

The Biological Stain Commission (BSC), in conjunction with the Food and Drug Administration (FDA), published a set of guidelines for reagent package inserts. These guidelines include recommendations to manufacturers for the testing and marketing of reagents as well as for the use and purpose of positive and negative controls (see Table 1.5).[119] Because of the variability in tissue fixation, processing, and embedding (which are inherent aspects of the IHC test), the Biological Stain Commission concluded that it was unable to establish a single universal staining protocol. This, therefore, necessitates the concurrent performance and interpretation of controls in conjunction with the tests. These controls ensure proper technique and specificity of the staining method used and are essential for correct interpretation of immunohistochemical results.

Both positive and negative controls should be used. A positive control is one that is known to contain the antigen under question, ideally at a level of expression comparable to that being assayed in the test section. These controls should be fixed and processed in a manner that is analogous (ideally identical) to the tissue being tested. A false-negative test result can occur if the test tissue is over-fixed (resulting in diminished or absent antigenicity) and the control tissue is optimally fixed (and the test was optimized to the control tissue). For this reason, the manufacturers' positive control slides cannot be used as a substitute for positive control slides made in-house, because they are not processed in the same manner as the tissue being tested. They merely validate reagent performance but cannot verify proper tissue fixation and processing. Identical processing would be optimal in routine surgical pathology, but usually it is only achievable in laboratory experiments, if then. Later in this chapter, we will discuss the possibility of using internal reference standards to correct for variation in fixation.

From a general standpoint, the best positive controls are those that are processed in-house. It is most cost-effective to use surgical tissue controls that have been fixed and processed along with the regular workday's surgical specimens. Tissue (containing cells) with a level of expression comparable to the test tissue (cells) is preferred. As noted earlier, optimizing the test using normal tissue with a high level of expression may result in false-negative results on tumor tissue where expression may be variable or low. Moreover, the ideal positive control should not show uniformly intense positive staining. Rather, the intensity of staining should be variable, with weak staining in many areas. These weakly staining areas detect subtle changes in primary antibody sensitivity. This, too, helps to decrease the incidence of false-negative results. Many types of tissue can be used as positive controls. From a general standpoint, surgical material is preferable to autopsy tissue, as the latter may contain areas of autolysis that can affect staining results. For immunocytologic testing of body fluids and fine-needle-aspiration material, cytospins can be prepared and stored unfixed, or cell blocks can be fixed and embedded to be used as cytologic control material. The most important considerations in the selection of the appropriate control tissue are that it contains the antigen under question and that it is fixed and processed using the same protocol as the test specimen.

Negative controls are used to confirm the specificity of the method used and to assess the presence of non-specific background staining, defined by staining the test tissue in the absence of the primary antibody, for which there are multiple causes (described later). Absorption controls are "negative reagent controls" produced by absorbing the primary antibody (polyclonal or monoclonal) with the highly purified antigen that was used to generate the antibody. The objective is to eliminate staining; however the findings can be misleading owing to impurities in the antigen or the presence of unsuspected cross-reactive "epitopes."[120-122] The usual negative controls include substitution of the primary antibody with antibody diluent (buffer plus bovine serum albumin carrier protein) or with non-immune immunoglobulin, derived from the same species and used at the same dilution. The substitution of an irrelevant antibody can also be used as a negative control. In practice, when a panel of different antibodies is being tested on the same tissue, the results obtained from the different primary antibodies can be used as negative controls for each other. Finally, with regard to negative controls, if more than one protocol is used on a particular day (i.e., microwave AR pretreatment, protease-trypsin digestion), separate negative control slides should be run for each, in accordance with each protocol used.

As noted earlier, multi-tissue control slides (increasingly referred to as MTAs or multi-tissue arrays) have particular utility in first assessing a new antibody. Each multi-tissue control slide contains samples of tissues that are arranged in either a checkerboard or a sausage pattern. Multi-tissue array slides typically include maps designating the types of tissues present and their specific locations. While particularly useful for validation studies of new reagents, these may also be used for routine quality control purposes. Their disadvantage is a relatively high cost and the inability to control how different specimens that constitute the "array" were fixed and processed.[123-126] Some of these disadvantages have been addressed by improvements in the preparation of microtissue arrays, in particular the commercial availability of instruments that allow for the production of microarray blocks consisting of multiple fine tissue cores (e.g., Beecham Instruments, Hackensack, NJ). The MTA method provides a means of incorporating 200 to 300 cores of internally processed tissues into an MTA template. Because each core is small (generally 0.6 to 1.5 mm), a single initial biopsy tissue block can serve as a source for multiple core samples, while still preserving much of the original block for the archival files. The pros and cons of this technology are further discussed in *Applied Immunohistochemistry and Molecular Morphology* by Skacel and colleagues.[125]

Internal controls are present when the tissue being tested contains the antigen under question in adjacent normal cells or tissue. The presence of positive "internal control staining" in the expected cells indicates appropriate immunoreactivity. For ubiquitous antigens, such as vimentin, positive internal control staining may be used as this antibody's positive control. Moreover, because of its ubiquity, staining for vimentin is also helpful as a reporter molecule, that is, to assess fixation and processing of the tissue.[127] As discussed previously, variation in staining results can occur from over-fixation, under-fixation, or both. The intensity of staining of vimentin with monoclonal antibody V9 provides a crude indication of over-fixation and can also be used to monitor the recovery from formalin over-fixation by AR.

Internal Reference Standards for Quantification and the Evaluation of Sample Preparation

The human eye and the human mind have proven remarkably proficient in creating the art of surgical pathology and sustaining it for more than 100 years as the gold standard for cancer diagnosis. Remarkable though this may be, there are some areas of significant limitation. One is the lack of reproducibility of a morphologic interpretation not only among different observers, but also for the same observer over time.[3] The second is consistency in counting events (such as numbers of positively stained cells) and especially in the judgment of degree of intensity of a stain reaction; is it strongly, moderately, or weakly positive, or negative, or even weakly negative (whatever that might be). In both aspects, computer-assisted image analysis may hold significant advantages. Previously hampered by cumbersome software and limitations of "digitizing, storing and transmitting data," image analysis has a reputation for being time-consuming and expensive, an embellishment at best, and no substitute for the tutored eye. However, these limitations are quickly receding as integrated hardware/software systems have accelerated digitization and fostered the development of sophisticated programs (such as spectral imaging) that can simultaneously analyze and compare multiple colored signals (both IHC and immunofluorescent).[128,129]

It therefore becomes possible, in fact quite straightforward when coupled with polymer-based double stains, to consider performing every IHC stain for a target protein (antigen) in conjunction with staining for an internal control protein (reference analyte) to compare the intensity of one with the other by image analysis for relative (comparative) quantification, or even for absolute measurement by weight, once the staining protocol has been calibrated.[129] Furthermore, following experimental demonstration of the performance (relative loss) of antigenicity of the reference analyte (patented as Quantifiable Internal Reference Standards—QIRS[129]), under different conditions of fixation and AR, the intensity of reaction of the reference analyte as demonstrated by the calibrated system can be used to make corrections for observed loss of antigenicity due to sample preparation. This approach provides a potential method for correcting for variable fixation or processing, and it also provides a method of standardization that does not require the standardization of fixation per se—a task already described as difficult or impossible! Following the advice of Sherlock Holmes, further study of QIRS are being pursued: "—whenever one has excluded the impossible, whatever remains, however improbable, must be the truth."[130]

It is noteworthy, but unnoticed nonetheless, that the high standards of quality control testing that have long been employed in the clinical pathology laboratory have traditionally not been applied to tests that we perform across the hallway in surgical pathology. When the objective measure of surgical pathology was morphologic quality, this degree of rigor was not necessary. However, the growing list of "tests" of critical prognostic/predictive markers that are being introduced into anatomic pathology adds to the pressures for improved results. The IHC test is a slightly modified version of the ELISA test, but performed on a tissue section as opposed to in a test tube.[128,129] If similar rigor is applied to the performance of an IHC test, then similar accuracy and reproducibility may be achieved. For the results of any prognostic/predictive test to be clinically meaningful, rigorous quality control measures must be applied and followed. If for practical reasons we cannot "begin at the beginning," with proper specimen acquisition and handling protocols, then we can "begin at the end," by instituting a system of defined internal reference standards.[129]

From this discussion, one can see that the understanding and application of appropriate positive and negative controls is one of the most important yet often misunderstood aspects of IHC.[115] The proper use of these controls is essential for correct interpretation of immunohistochemical results.

TISSUE FIXATION, PROCESSING, AND ANTIGEN-RETRIEVAL TECHNIQUES

The following section reflects current practice, with formalin as the common fixative. Recommendations for increased documentation have already been emphasized (see Table 1.4).

Tissue preparation consists of fixation, subsequent dehydration, and embedding in paraffin wax to provide a rigid matrix for sectioning. Tissues that are to be embedded in paraffin wax are first fixed to optimize preservation, a process that profoundly affects the morphologic and immunohistologic results. The ideal fixative for IHC studies should not only be readily available but also be in widespread use to maximize the range and number of samples available for

IHC studies. The fixative should preserve antigenic integrity and should limit extraction, diffusion, or displacement of antigen during subsequent processing. Also, it should show good preservation of morphologic details after embedding in a support medium (e.g., paraffin).

Common fixatives used in histopathology are divided into two groups: coagulant fixatives, such as ethanol, and cross-linking fixatives, such as formaldehyde. Both types of fixative can cause changes in the steric configuration of proteins, which may mask antigenic sites (epitopes) and adversely affect binding with antibody. It is well recognized that cross-linking fixatives alter the IHC results for a significant number of antigens, whereas coagulant fixatives, especially ethanol, have been reported to produce fewer changes, although there remains some controversy.[35,131-133] In most surgical pathology laboratories, the fixative used is 10% neutral buffer formalin (NBF) (a cross-linking fixative). Subsequent processing usually includes a period in 100% ethanol; thus, tissues are effectively "double fixed" in both formalin and ethanol: if formalin fixation is inadequate, tissues will be in part alcohol fixed, with resultant "in section" variation in IHC staining. For tissues fixed in formalin, the intensity of staining is known to be fixation time–dependent for many antigens.[131,133,134] A long history of using formalin as a standard tissue fixative has revealed the following advantages; it will not be replaced easily, or soon:

1. There is good preservation of morphology, even after prolonged fixation; in this case, *good* is a somewhat subjective term encompassing the various artifactual changes that result in the morphologic features that "please" the pathologist, based on his or her previous experience and the manner of fixation-processing to which the pathologist has become accustomed.
2. Formalin is an economical chemical, much cheaper than most alternatives.
3. Formalin fixation sterilizes tissue specimens in a more reliable way than precipitating fixatives, particularly for viruses.
4. Carbohydrate antigens are well preserved.[135]
5. Cross-linking of protein *in situ* avoids leaching out of proteins that may diffuse in water or alcohol. Many low–molecular-weight antigens (peptides) are extracted by non–cross-linking fixatives such as alcohol, or methanol-based solutions, but they are well preserved in tissue by formalin.[29]

Today experience shows that formalin may be regarded as a satisfactory fixative for both morphology and IHC provided that an effective AR technique is available to recover those antigens that are diminished or modified.

Antigen Retrieval

A simple heat-induced AR technique is now widely applied in pathology.[39,40,57,59] Successful application of the AR technique for routine IHC staining of formalin-fixed tissues in diagnostic pathology has rendered the search for alternative fixatives to replace formalin less urgent. In 1997, Prento and Lyon[136] compared the performance of six commercial fixatives offered as formalin substitutes and concluded that the best IHC staining was obtained by combining formalin fixation with AR technique: none of the six proposed substitutes for formalin was judged adequate for histopathologic use (i.e., they did not give the good morphologic features to which pathologists had become accustomed). Williams and coworkers[137] investigated the effect of tissue preparation on IHC staining by using tonsil tissues that were subjected to variations in fixation, processing, section preparation, and storage. They demonstrated that the microwave AR technique ameliorated the problems resulting from variations in fixation, processing, and section preparation. They reported that 10% neutral buffered formalin, 10% zinc formalin, and 10% formal saline gave the most consistent results overall and showed excellent antigen preservation. In contrast, 10% formal acetic acid, B5, and Bouin's fixative all showed poor antigen preservation, even after AR treatment. Reduced effectiveness of AR when used with other fixatives has been documented by others.[138-140] Although storage of cut tissue sections was not an issue in the study of Williams and associates,[137] others have reported that decreased intensity of staining may occur for some antigens in slides stored for protracted periods.[141-147] It is our experience that storage-induced decreases in IHC staining are relatively uncommon, and most of these adverse effects also can be recovered by AR treatment. For example, combination of the AR treatment and use of a sensitive polymeric-labeling two-step detection system achieves satisfactory results for antibodies to p53 (Pab-1801), p21WAF1 (Ab-1, Oncogene Science, Cambridge, Mass), and p27Kip1 (DCS-72.F6, NeoMarkers Inc., Fremont, Calif),[18,86] even after prolonged storage.

The AR technique not only has utility for enhancement of IHC staining on archival tissue sections but also may contribute to standardization of routine IHC, conditional upon the AR method itself being optimized and standardized.[18,39,40,92,148] Recently, AR has also been adopted in formalin-fixed frozen cell/tissue sections successfully.[149,150] A key element in the appropriate use and standardization of the AR technique for IHC is understanding major factors that influence the effectiveness of AR, as described in the following paragraphs.

HEATING CONDITIONS

An optimal result for AR-IHC is correlated with the mathematical product of the heating temperature multiplied by the time of AR heating treatment: T (temperature of heating AR procedure) × t (period of heating time).

As noted previously, the heating AR-IHC method is based on biochemical studies of Fraenkel-Conrat and coworkers, who documented that the chemical reactions that occur between protein and formalin may be reversed, at least in part by high-temperature heating or strong alkaline hydrolysis.[32-34] We demonstrated that the use of conventional heating at 100°C may achieve results similar to those obtained by microwave heating and also that distilled water could be used as the AR solution, albeit with slightly less effect.[35] Subsequently, several publications reported similar results.[39,40,146,151-153] The chemical reactions occurring during the formalin fixation process remain obscure. Mason and O'Leary[151] demonstrated that the process of cross-linking does not result in discernible alteration of protein secondary structure, at least as determined by calorimetric and infrared spectroscopic investigation. They also noted that significant denaturation of unfixed purified proteins occurred at temperature ranges of 70° to 90°C, whereas similar temperatures had virtually no adverse effect on formalin-fixed proteins (i.e., formalin-fixed proteins are more heat stable). Subsequently, this same group studied the mechanism of AR using a purified protein RNase A and demonstrated that heating treatment may reverse formalin-induced cross-links for restoration of immunoreactivity.[154,155] Support for this conclusion soon followed from Sompuram and coworkers.[156,157] Thus, the AR heating technique appears to take advantage of the fact that the cross-linkage of protein produced by formalin fixation may protect the primary and secondary structure of formalin-modified protein from denaturation during the heating phase, while allowing reduction of cross-linkages at the surface of the molecule, thereby restoring antigenicity. Other theories, including protein denaturation,[44] do exist, and at the present time the mechanism must be considered unresolved.

In general, the heating conditions appear to be the most important factor in the effectiveness of AR.[38-42,55-58,152,153,157a,158-161] The evidence may be summarized as follows: Significant enhancement of immunohistochemical staining can be achieved by using high-temperature heating in pure distilled water,[35,152,162-164] and higher temperatures in general yield superior results.[39,40,56-59,152,159] Equivalent performance of AR-IHC can be obtained using different buffers as AR solutions if the pH value of AR solutions are monitored in a comparable manner, thereby demonstrating that individual specific chemical constituents are not necessary factors in yielding a satisfactory result.[48-50] Our early experience that even prolonged exposure of paraffin sections in citrate buffer solution (or indeed any buffer) without heating gave no noticeable AR effect has subsequently been confirmed by numerous studies.[53,55,165]

pH AND CHEMICAL COMPOSITION OF THE ANTIGEN-RETRIEVAL SOLUTION

The pH value of the AR solution is important for some antigens. From a comparative study in 1995,[50,51] we concluded that antigens fell into three broad categories with respect to the importance of pH on AR:

1. Most antigens showed no significant variation using AR solutions with pH values ranging from 1.0 to 10.0.
2. Certain other antigens, especially nuclear antigens (e.g., MIB1, ER), showed a dramatic decrease in the intensity of the AR-IHC at middle-range pH values but optimal results at low pH.
3. A small group of antigens (MT1, HMB-45) showed negative or very weak focally positive immunostaining with a low pH (1.0 to 2.0) but excellent results in the high-pH range (Figs. 1.17, 1.18).

Evers and Uylings[158] also found that the AR-IHC is both pH- and temperature-dependent. They concluded that it is not important what kind of solution is used as long as the pH is at an appropriate level. The chemical composition and molarity of the AR solution are cofactors that may influence the effectiveness of AR-IHC in certain instances and should be explored when satisfactory results cannot be obtained with the solutions usually used.[40,41,56-59,166,167] Namimatsu and colleagues[167] reported a novel AR solution of 0.05% citraconic anhydride solution at pH 7.4, heating at 98°C for 45 minutes, which they advocated as a universal AR method. Using their approach, we found that more than 90% of antibodies showed a stronger or equivalent signal, but occasional antibodies still gave a weaker staining intensity when compared to conventional AR solution, requiring use of the test battery in such instances.

In conclusion, major factors that influence the results of AR-IHC staining include heating temperature and heating time (heating condition $T \times t$) and the pH value of the AR solution.

TEST BATTERY APPROACH FOR ANTIGEN-RETRIEVAL TECHNIQUE

A test battery may be defined as a preliminary test of AR technique that examines the two major factors—heating condition ($T \times t$) and pH value—and is performed to establish an optimal protocol for the antigen being tested.[168]

Typically, three levels of heating conditions and pH values—low, moderate, and high—may be applied to screen for a potential optimal protocol of AR-IHC for a particular antigen of interest, as indicated in Table 1.6. The test battery method can also be performed in two sequential steps: (1) testing three AR solutions at different pH values, as listed earlier, with one standard temperature (100°C for 10 minutes) in order to find the optimal pH value of AR solution; and (2) testing optimal heating conditions based on the established pH value. We have demonstrated that different heating methods, including microwave, microwave and pressure cooker, steam, and autoclave heating methods,[39,40] can be evaluated in a similar fashion and adjusted to yield a similar satisfactory intensity of staining by AR-IHC.

The test battery serves as a rapid screening approach to identify an optimal protocol for each antibody-antigen to be tested. The goal is to establish the maximal retrieval level for formalin-masked antigens after undefined fixation times in order to standardize immunostaining results.[48-51] In addition, the use of a test battery may identify false-negative or false-positive AR-IHC staining results.

Newly available antibodies with improved staining characteristics also may obviate the need for special AR methods, and laboratories should pay particular attention to the claims of manufacturers in this regard, always validating such claims in-house.

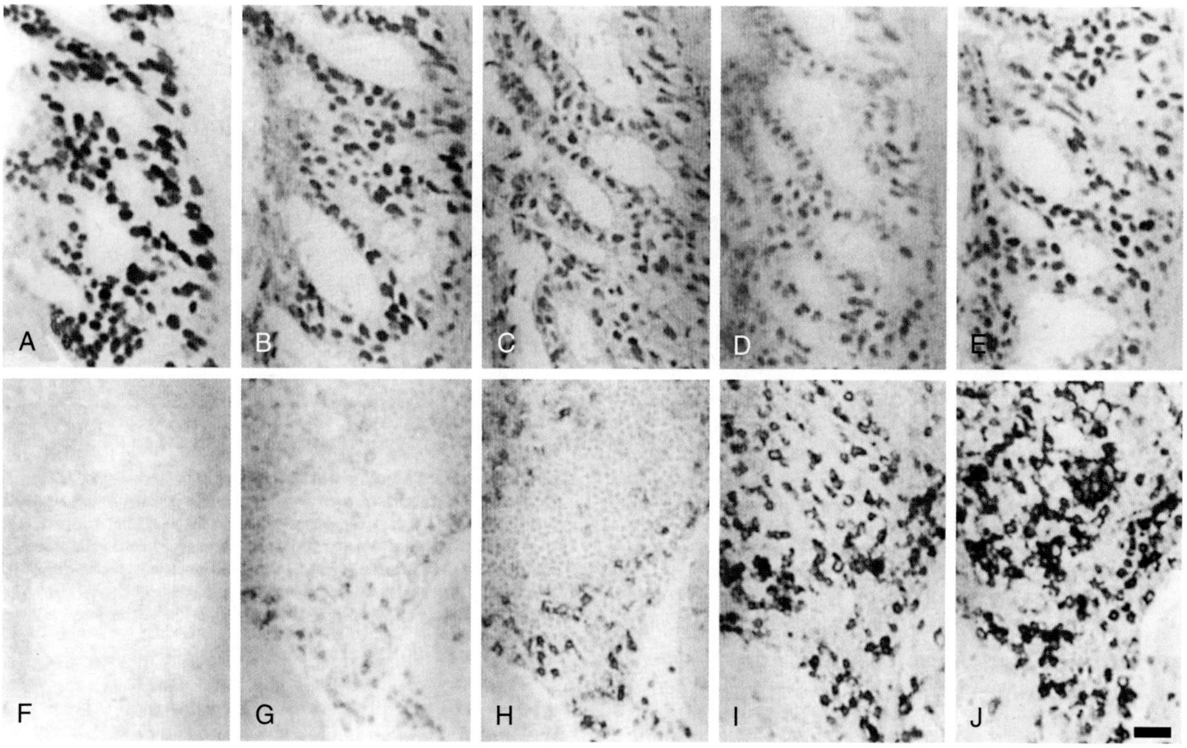

FIGURE 1.17 Comparisons of the intensity of AR immunostaining in routinely formalin-fixed, paraffin-embedded tissue sections with a monoclonal antibody (MAb) to ER in breast tissue **(A-E)** and Mab MT1 in lymph node **(F-J)**. Sodium diethylbarbiturate-HCl (SDH) buffer was used as the AR solution for both antibodies. The pH values of AR solution were pH 2, 3, 4, 6, and 8, which correspond to staining intensity of ++++, +++, +, ++, and +++, respectively, for ER with a type B pattern **(A-E)**. **F-J** show a type C pattern with SDH as the AR solution with a pH of 2, 3, 4, 6, 8, and intensity of staining –, +, ++, +++, and ++++, respectively, for MT1. Some nuclei showed very weak false nuclear staining **(F)**. DAB was the chromogen, and hematoxylin was the counterstain (original magnification ×100; bar = 20 mm). *Reproduced, with permission, from Shi S-R, Imam SA, Young L, et al. Antigen retrieval immunohistochemistry under the influence of pH using monoclonal antibodies. J Histochem Cytochem. 1995;43:193-201.*

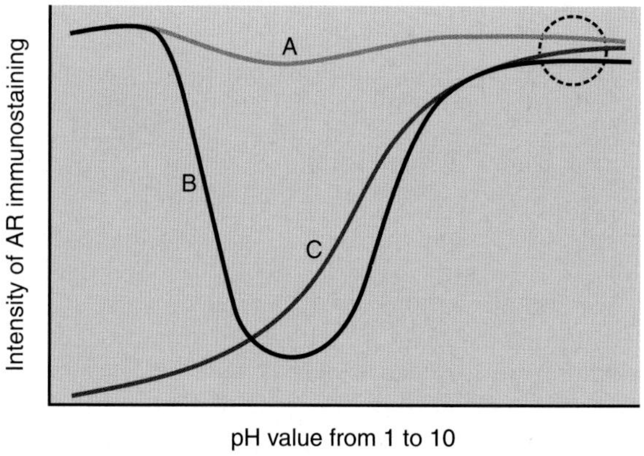

FIGURE 1.18 Schematic diagram of the three patterns of pH-influenced AR immunostaining. Line A (pattern of type A) shows a stable pattern of staining with only a slight decrease in staining intensity between pH 3 and pH 6. Line B (pattern of type B) shows a dramatic decrease in staining intensity between pH 3 and pH 6. Line C (pattern of type C) exhibits an ascending intensity of AR immunostaining that correlated with increasing pH values of the AR solution. Circle *(right)* indicates the advantage of using an AR solution of higher pH value. *Reproduced, with permission, from Shi S-R, Imam SA, Young L, et al. Antigen retrieval immunohistochemistry under the influence of pH using monoclonal antibodies. J Histochem Cytochem. 1995;43:193-201.*

TABLE 1.6 Test Battery Suggested for Screening an Optimal Antigen Retrieval Protocol

TRIS-HCl Buffer	pH 1 to 2	pH 7 to 8	pH 10 to 11
Super high, 120°C*	Slide 1	Slide 4	Slide 7
High, 100°C for 10 minutes	Slide 2	Slide 5	Slide 8
Mid-high, 90°C for 10 minutes[a]	Slide 3	Slide 6	Slide 9

*The temperature of super high at 120°C may be obtained by either autoclaving or microwave heating with longer time.

[a]The temperature of mid-high at 90°C may be obtained by either a water bath or a microwave oven monitored with a thermometer.

Note: One more slide may be used for control without AR treatment. The citrate buffer pH 6.0 may be used to replace TRIS-HCl buffer pH 7 to 8, as the results are the same.

Adapted from Shi S-R, Cote RJ, Taylor CR. Antigen retrieval immunohistochemistry: Past, present, and future. *J Histochem Cytochem.* 1997;45:327-343.

TECHNIQUES, PROTOCOLS, AND "TROUBLESHOOTING"

The following descriptions and protocols are focused on IHC techniques for archival paraffin-embedded tissue sections. The basic principles and protocols for fresh frozen tissue sections are the same as those for paraffin section, except that the AR and dewaxing procedures are not required for frozen tissue sections. Titrations (dilutions) may also differ and must be separately optimized.

Because the success of the IHC staining method depends on the correct application of both histologic and immunologic techniques, it is recommended that the user be familiar with the literature concerning the antigen under investigation before performing IHC staining. In particular, it is important to know the following information:

- Cellular localization of the antigen base
- Specificity of the primary antibody
- Results of previous IHC staining tests (from the literature, and especially from the experience of the performing laboratory) with respect to any adverse influence on the antigen from tissue fixation processing, and the value of any pretreatment procedure such as heat-induced AR.

In addition, detailed information regarding the reagents, particularly the primary antibody and detection system—such as the manufacturer, clone number of monoclonal antibody, and recommended concentration—is helpful in achieving a successful result. It is advisable to read the package insert provided by the manufacturer as well as key related literature.

Antigen Retrieval by the Microwave Heating Method[35,101]

1. Deparaffinized slides are placed in plastic Coplin jars containing AR solution; it is recommended that the same number of slides be used every time, using "blanks" if necessary to ensure consistent heating.
2. Jars are covered with loose-fitting screw caps and heated in the microwave oven for 10 minutes. The 10-minute heating time is divided into two 5-minute cycles with an interval of 1 minute between cycles to check the fluid level in the jars. If necessary, more AR solution is added after the first 5 minutes to avoid drying out the tissue sections. It is recommended that the heating time be standardized by beginning to count the time only after the solution has reached boiling in order to avoid discrepancies among laboratories when using various microwave ovens.
3. After completion of the heating phase, the Coplin jars are removed from the oven and allowed to cool for 15 minutes.
4. Slides are rinsed twice in distilled water and in phosphate-buffered saline (PBS) for 5 minutes and are then ready for IHC staining.

Various heating methods, including conventional heating in water bath, pressure cooker, steamer, and autoclave, may be used and may achieve results similar to those with IHC. Our studies have demonstrated that different heating methods can yield similar intensities of immunostaining if the heating conditions are adjusted appropriately.[39,40]

BLOCKING NON-SPECIFIC BINDING

Quenching endogenous peroxidase by an H_2O_2-methanol solution is performed immediately after the dewaxing procedure. Blocking of endogenous biotin may be performed before the biotin-conjugated link by using the avidin-biotin blocking reagent, or using skim milk as an alternative blocking reagent (incubate for 10 minutes).[139]

Normal serum taken from the same species as the secondary (link) antibody should be used to block non-specific binding sites, as discussed previously.

WASHING STEPS

Thorough washing is critical for each step, except for the blocking step of normal serum. PBS, 0.01 M at pH 7.4, is widely used, with the washing procedure carried out in a jar containing PBS and immersing slides for two 5-minute periods (total of 10 minutes). Alternatively, PBS may be flooded onto the slides in a humidity chamber for 10 minutes with one change. With automation of IHC staining technique, the washing procedure is also automated, and multiple washes are used. Some manufacturers provide proprietary diluents and washing solutions; if these are not purchased, the method must be carefully revalidated for performance.

INCUBATION OF PRIMARY ANTIBODY

The time of incubation depends on the sensitivity and concentration of the primary antibody used as well as the quality of the tissue section. Concentration of the primary antibody is based on a titration test as described previously, with reference to the manufacturer's instructions. In general, frozen tissue sections require less incubation time than do archival paraffin tissue sections. A commonly used incubation period is 30 minutes at room temperature. With multi-stage methods, successive incubation periods and washings result in a lengthy overall procedure. Some attempt has been made to shorten the procedure by performing incubations at 37°C in a hotplate humidity chamber; the incubation for each step may then be 10 minutes or less. Humidity chambers may be placed in an oven at 37°C, which is a less effective method than the hotplate because of the longer time needed for reagents to reach a temperature of 37°C. Some automated stainers also accelerate the process by operating at 37°C or 42°C. Microwave acceleration of the IHC staining technique has also been described for rapid IHC staining,[169-172] but generally it is not convenient.

Incubation of slides in a humidity chamber is advisable whatever the temperature. In practice, if a slide treated with antibody is permitted to dry, excessive non-specific background staining invariably occurs. Even when total drying does not occur, evaporation of the antibody solution on the slide may result in an effective increase in antibody concentration, producing unwanted background staining. Humidity chambers containing level slide racks may be purchased or can be made rather easily from glass rods and Plexiglas glued together with water-resistant bonds. Staining racks on which slides rest during incubation should be level to avoid drainage of antibody off the section to other areas of the slide.

Overnight (or extended) incubation may also be used in certain circumstances; here again, a humidity chamber partially filled with water is essential. We have used overnight staining to permit the use of a primary antibody at very high dilutions and have often achieved good results with reduced non-specific background staining (i.e., take an antibody that gives satisfactory results when incubated for 30 minutes, dilute it 10- or even 100-fold, and then incubate for 12 to 24 hours). This approach conserves precious antibody and reduces background staining owing to decreased non-specific attachment of antibody. (The antibody is present at a much lower concentration, favoring binding by high-affinity immunologic reactions.) With this method, only the primary antibody is given prolonged incubation; other reagents are used normally. Overnight incubation of primary antibody is a practical consideration for many service laboratories and can fit well into the working schedule, initiating staining requests in the late afternoon, incubating the primary antibody overnight, and completing the labeling steps early the next morning for examination by the pathologist.

TABLE 1.7 Immunohistochemistry: Commonly Used "Chromogens" or Reaction Products*

Procedure	Color	Solubility in Alcohol
Peroxidase		
Diaminobenzidine (DAB)	Brown	Insoluble
DAB with enhancement	Black	Insoluble
3-Amino-9-ethyl carbazole (AEC)	Red[a]	Soluble
4-Chloro-1-naphthol (4-CN)	Blue-black	Soluble
Hanker-Yates reagent	Blue	Insoluble
Alpha-naphthol pyronin	Red	Soluble
3,3′5,5′-tetramethylbenzidine (TMB)	Blue	Insoluble
Alkaline Phosphatase		
Fast blue BB	Blue	Soluble
Fast red TR	Red	Soluble
New fuchsin	Red	Insoluble
BCIP-NBT	Blue	Insoluble
Glucose Oxidase		
Tetrazolium	Blue	Insoluble
Tetranitroblue tetrazolium (TNBT)	Black	Insoluble
Immunogold		
With silver enhancement	Black	Insoluble

*Other proprietary "chromogens" are available, including purples and green, but those listed are those that are well documented. Various commercial products can be found in catalogs from several companies (e.g., BioCare, Dako, Ventana) and often have been formulated to be most effective when used with the same company's reagents and automated stainers. Use outside of these proprietary systems requires careful validation of effectiveness.

[a]AEC has two reaction sites: In the presence of enzyme excess both react, the color passing from red to green-brown.

Adapted from Taylor CR, Cote RJ. Immunomicroscopy: A Diagnostic Tool for the Surgical Pathologist. 2nd ed. Philadelphia: WB Saunders; 1994:67.

INCUBATION OF DETECTION REAGENTS

As noted previously, titration is necessary for optimum concentrations. A good place to begin is by following the manufacturer's instructions for concentration of each reagent and the exact protocol for the detection system. Incubation is carried out carefully, usually at room temperature for 30 minutes for each step (link and label). Dropping reagents on each slide to cover the tissue section completely is a simple but critical procedure. Caution must be taken to confirm that the whole tissue section is immersed in the reagent, including the margins, and that no air bubbles exist, particularly when using automation (e.g., the capillary action-based procedure).

SUBSTRATE AND CHROMOGEN

Several different chromogens (color-producing substrate systems) are available (Table 1.7). With horseradish peroxidase, DAB may be preferred because the brown reaction product is alcohol fast and thus is suitable for use with a wide range of counterstains and mounting media. AEC, which gives a red color, is alcohol soluble but is generally considered a lower-risk carcinogen than DAB and thus has been favored by commercial suppliers of immunohistologic reagents. For general purposes, we routinely use DAB or AEC for peroxidase. AEC produces a crisp red color that contrasts well with a hematoxylin counterstain; note that a "progressive" non-alcoholic hematoxylin should be used (e.g., Mayer's, not Harris') to avoid removal of the colored product, which is alcohol soluble. At high concentrations of antigen-antibody-enzyme, AEC may produce a brown-yellow color. (AEC has two reactive sites: When one is converted, it turns red; if both react with peroxidase, a green-brown product results.) It may be helpful to maintain the acetic acid buffer at pH 4.8 to minimize this effect. For AEC, the sections must be mounted in an aqueous medium (e.g., 80% glycerol). Aquamount contains small amounts of organic solvent and may cause slow diffusion or loss of stain. Dehydration through alcohol must be avoided. Glycerol-mounted preparations may be made permanent by sealing the edges of the coverslip with nail varnish. Alpha-naphthol pyronine (pink), 4-chloro-l-naphthol (blue), and Hanker-Yates reagent are other alternatives, together with a variety of "broad" chromogens (see Table 1.7).

DAB is also valuable for the electron microscopist because it is electron dense. For light microscopy, some investigators advocate osmication of the DAB reaction product, giving a more intense color. We have not found this necessary for light microscopy; indeed, we feel it may be a disadvantage because background staining is also enhanced, and the end result may be diminished contrast despite the more intense staining. A similar effect may be achieved by post-treatment with nickel sulfate or cobalt chloride, which produces excellent contrast.[173,174] If DAB is used, solutions should be prepared under a hood by a masked, gloved technician. Unused solution should be disposed of with an excess of water. At the working dilution used, the danger is considered minimal; it is the powdered form that evokes concern. Pre-weighed aliquots in sealed tubes are available from some manufacturers but are expensive. Ready-to-use liquid DAB is now provided commercially. It has the advantages of convenience, safety, and less potential for environmental pollution.

A range of substrates is also available for alkaline phosphatase; fast red, fast blue, and several commercial variants give excellent contrast and good morphology. Some substrates contribute to the sensitivity of the alkaline phosphatase systems by continuing to convert at the enzyme site, resulting in a granular accumulation of the colored product. If carried to excess, this granularity may obscure morphologic definition.

COUNTERSTAINING AND MOUNTING SLIDES

The final step in the process is counterstaining and mounting slides. Hematoxylin is used as the nuclear counterstain for most routine IHC staining. In the case of nuclear antigen immunolocalization, one must take caution to avoid overdevelopment of the hematoxylin stain. (A light hematoxylin stain is critical to allow any nuclear localization of chromogen to be discerned.) In our experience, the time of exposure to hematoxylin depends in part on how fresh the dye solution is. (A freshly prepared solution of hematoxylin requires a much shorter time than does exposure in an old solution.) It may be necessary to monitor the development of the stain by microscopy in order to determine the optimal time of counterstaining. For alcohol-soluble stains (e.g., AEC or fast red variants), an aqueous mounting medium is used. The mounting medium is warmed on a heating block until it liquefies. One of two methods is used: Either one drop is placed on the tissue section and a coverslip is lowered slowly onto the slide, or the coverslip is placed on a paper towel, one drop is placed in the center of the coverslip, and the inverted slide is lowered slowly onto the coverslip. In either case, care should be taken to avoid trapping an air bubble between the coverslip and the tissue section. For alcohol-insoluble stains (e.g., DAB or new fuchsin), a permanent mounting medium, such as Permount, may be used. The tissue section is first dehydrated by immersing the slide in graded alcohols: 90% and 100%, twice for each, followed by clearing in xylene (twice for 3 minutes each). Mount the coverslip on the slide as described earlier for aqueous mounting medium. Note that xylene and Permount should be used in a fume hood.

Double Immunoenzymatic Techniques

The identification of two antigens in fixed paraffin-embedded tissues is usually accomplished by immunoperoxidase staining of adjacent serial sections (Fig. 1.19). Although this approach suffices for general use, on occasion it may be difficult to identify with certainty the pattern of staining of a particular cell population in adjacent sections, especially if the cells under study are small or are scattered among other cells.

Double immunoenzymatic techniques (Fig. 1.20) permit the demonstration of two antigens concurrently within a single section. As described earlier with reference to alkaline phosphatase methods, double stains were usually performed sequentially; however, new polymer-based methods and polyvalent detection systems have made concurrent staining possible.

In the sequential method, the first sequence of staining for one antigen is completed with the development of the peroxidase reaction using DAB as the substrate. Staining for the second antigen is then carried out with a primary antibody of different specificity and a second, different substrate system for the peroxidase enzyme (for example, 4-chloro-1-naphthol); this produces a contrasting blue reaction product. The relative merits of elution of the first sequence of antibodies (after reaction with DAB) before titrating the second sequence of antibodies have been much debated. If desired, one can accomplish elution by incubating the sections with acid solutions (usually glycine–hydrochloric acid buffer at pH 2.2 or 1 N hydrochloric acid for 1 hour) or with an oxidizing solution (0.15 mol $KMnO_4$ and 0.01 N H_2SO_4 in 140 V of distilled water at pH 1.8), followed by reduction with 1% $NaSO_4$, for 1 minute. However, Sternberger and Joseph[19] were able to demonstrate two antigens without elution of the first set of reagents, despite the fact that both primary antibodies were of the same species and the same labeling reagents were used for both. The success of this system may be due to the fact that the polymerized product of DAB oxidation (used for the first antigen) blocks the catalytic site of peroxidase while also obscuring the antigenic reactivity of the first sequence of antibodies; this prevents interactions with the second sequence of antibodies and the second substrate system. Lan and colleagues[175] developed a simple, reliable, and sensitive method for multiple IHC staining by adding a microwave heating procedure (10 minutes) between each sequence of IHC staining (for elution of the previous sequence of IHC staining reagents), an approach that appears to ensure complete blocking of antibody cross-reactivity.

The possibility of cross-reaction of the second sequence of antibodies with the first sequence may be eliminated by the use of a double immunoenzymatic method in which two specific primary antibodies, produced in two different species, are used in combination with separate species-specific secondary antibodies coupled with

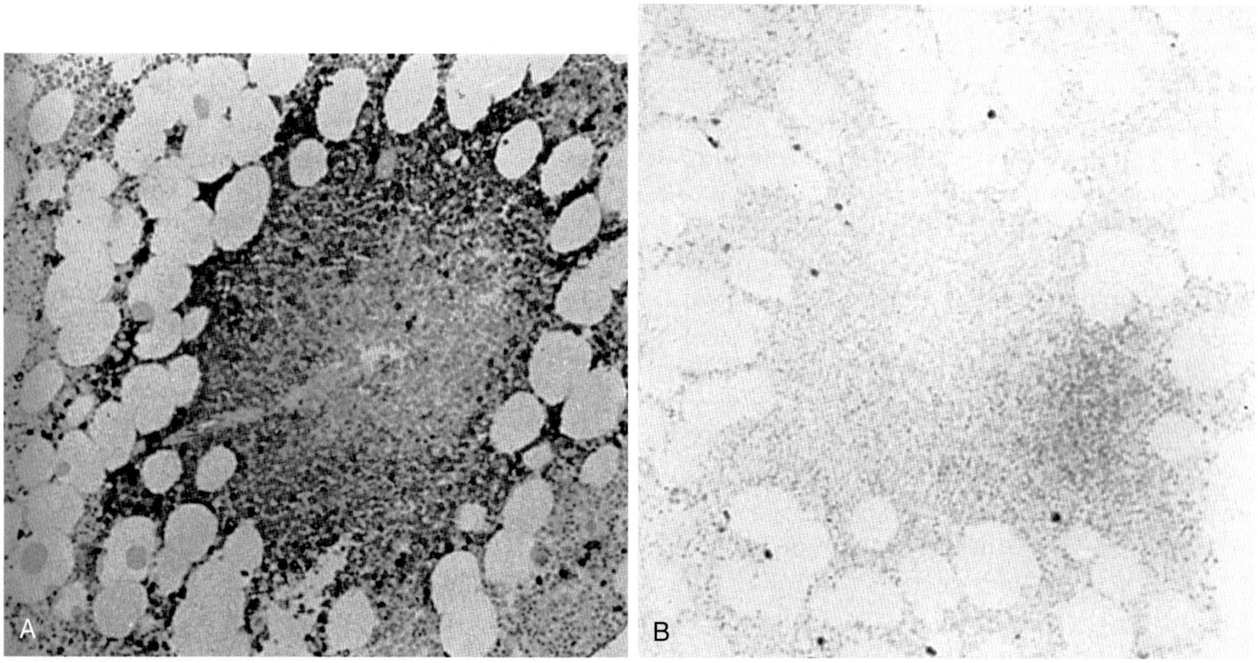

FIGURE 1.19 (A, B) B5-fixed section of bone marrow aspirate depicting a small solitary nodule consisting of lymphocytes and occasional plasmacytoid lymphocytes, with scattered plasma cells around it. Many of the lymphoid and plasmacytoid cells reacted strongly with anti-lambda antibody **(A)**. Anti-kappa reacted only with scattered plasma cells outside the nodule (**B**, small black dots). This patient eventually was shown to have a solitary plasmacytoid lymphocytic lymphoma in the small intestine (also lambda type). Paraffin sections, DAB with hematoxylin counterstain (×125). There was no serum paraprotein detectable at this time; presumably the number of tumor cells was insufficient for production of a detectable paraprotein; however, a "monoclonal" IgM appeared later in the course. *From Taylor CR, Cote RJ. Immunomicroscopy: A Diagnostic Tool for the Surgical Pathologist. 2nd ed. Philadelphia: WB Saunders; 1994:59.*

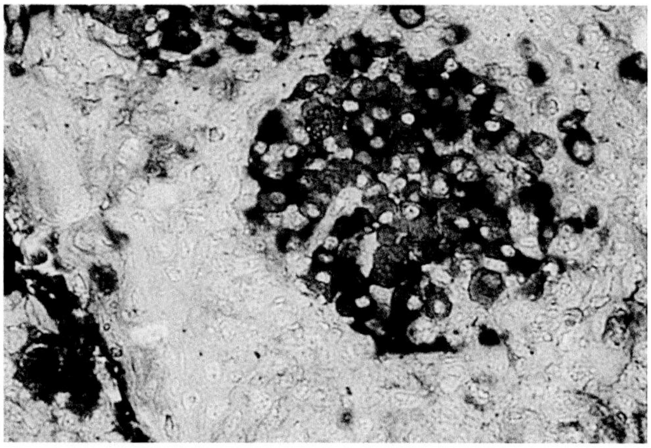

FIGURE 1.20 Double staining for kappa *(brown)* and lambda *(blue)* in paraffin section of a reactive lymph node using sequential horseradish peroxidase and alkaline phosphatase methods.

different enzymes (e.g., peroxidase and glucose oxidase, or peroxidase and alkaline phosphatase). This approach also has the advantage of expediency in that some of the reagents (e.g., the primary antibodies) can be added simultaneously.[176] This advantage is particularly exploited in new polymer-based methods, in which primary antibodies and secondary labeled reagents may be added as cocktails.

Considerable ingenuity has been manifested in adopting and adapting these techniques. For example, it is possible to demonstrate six different antigens on the same section.[177] Combinations of immunogold-silver staining (black) with immunoperoxidase-AEC (red-brown) or immunoalkaline phosphatase–fast red or fast blue produce excellent double or triple stains.[178] A combination of immunoperoxidase-AEC (red) with immunoalkaline phosphatase–fast blue (blue) provides excellent contrasting colors. In general, it is important to check carefully and control the development of the second (and third) colors by microscopy and to use detection systems of comparable sensitivity to obtain the best contrast of multiple colors in the same section. In practice, some double stains and most triple stains require computer-assisted image analysis methods for accurate interpretation of the intensity and localization of the double stain. In this respect, "spectral image analysis" is a particularly powerful and useful method that of itself renders double stains both practical and useful.[128,179]

The growing availability of image analysis systems has encouraged manufacturers to now offer a range of double or triple stains, often as RTU reagents for specific applications. In our experience, many of these reagents performed superbly; however, it is important to note that each part of the double or triple stain must itself be separately validated, and proper controls must be included.

One practical approach to double staining with monoclonal antibodies is given in Appendix 1A, but polymer-based systems are widely available today and generally simpler to perform.

Automation

Because of the great variability in specimen fixation and processing among laboratories, it has not been possible to establish a universal standard protocol for IHC. Instead, the goal has become the standardization of protocols within a single laboratory and across laboratories. As discussed earlier (the "total test"[115]), one can accomplish this by rigorously applying proper controls and strictly adhering to all aspects of the test, including preparing slides; preparing and applying reagents; monitoring incubation times; and so on. Such in-house standardization serves to ensure run-to-run reproducibility of accurate results. The newly recommended guidelines we have discussed are designed for this purpose. Another approach that is not mutually exclusive calls for automation.

Automated immunostaining devices started to appear in the early 1980s in order to meet increased diagnostic demands. Through pilot studies, improvement in software design, and innovations of hardware, this technology, although still evolving, is already in use in many IHC laboratories worldwide, with more than half a dozen recognized manufacturers of effective systems. Increasingly these systems are being integrated with other automated processes such as sample preparation, AR, staining, mounting, and automated cellular imaging systems, as we will briefly discuss.

With regard to the staining procedure itself, most steps in manual staining methods are technician dependent, and focused care by a skilled technician is required during each step to ensure the quality of the results obtained. There are more than 20 separate steps; these include preparing slides and reagents, blocking steps, AR, applying reagents and antibodies, monitoring incubation times, washing and wiping slides, and so on. Moreover, many of these steps are tedious and repetitive. Because of the large number of operator-dependent steps, the likelihood of technical error is increased. For example, a step may be accidentally omitted or performed in the incorrect sequence. The specimens may retain water after rinsing or, conversely, become dry during staining. Incubation times may be too short or too long, the antibody too dilute or too concentrated, or the substrate underdeveloped or overdeveloped. In addition to these technical variables, reagent variables must be considered, including the proper selection and use of antibodies with variable avidities as well as the selection of different chromogens, buffers, and enzymes. All these variables must be considered when using a manual staining method. With the advent of automation, manufacturers have addressed most of these issues and have standardized procedures.

Automated instruments are designed to imitate manual staining methods. Steps that lend themselves to automation include application of reagents, incubation of tissues, and rinsing of slides. These manipulations can be accomplished in several ways.[180] The slides can be arranged vertically and the reagents applied from above using gravity and top-to-bottom capillary action. Conversely, the reagents can climb up from a reagent-containing basin by bottom-to-top capillary action between two adjacent and clamped vertical slides. Using this second technique, the liquids are then eliminated by blotting the bottom of the slides. In a third method, the slides are arranged horizontally on a platform. Reagents and buffers are administered from above by a probe, disposable tip, or reagent test pack, and a horizontally administered air jet eliminates them as appropriate. These approaches have their advantages and disadvantages, and they have been exploited by different manufacturers. No general recommendation is possible other than to give a system (and the reagents that are designed for it) careful in-house trial before purchase. Price of the instrument is not necessarily a guide; over time, reagent use is often the major expense. Some systems are "closed" in a relative sense, easily admitting only pre-loaded protocols and proprietary reagents, whereas others are "open" to a greater or lesser degree. Generally, the more open the system, the more the individual laboratory has to do in-house to qualify the instrument, reagents, and protocols. Knowledge and availability of service technicians are vital for overall satisfaction.

Depending on the need of the individual laboratory, there are a variety of choices with different methods, analytic flexibility, and productivity.[181] However, certain performance criteria should be met by all. Before putting an automated immunostainer to use, parallel studies should be performed to confirm that the results obtained by automated technique are comparable to or better than those obtained previously by the manual method. Furthermore, staining results obtained from the automated instrument, using the same tissue and the same antibody (for example, the positive controls) should show intra-laboratory run-to-run reproducibility. Some machines permit the use of multiple antibodies and detection systems and provide random access to accommodate the diversity of antigens and recipes, with software that allows flexible programming and is user friendly. As noted, such machines are best employed in larger sophisticated laboratories. The ideal instrument should be easy to use and require minimal technician attention during a run. Should a problem occur, the machine should have an error tracking program and be able to report the problem. Regarding the dispensing of reagents, precise and reproducible microliter quantities of each reagent should be dispensed, resulting in complete tissue coverage. The evaporative loss and carryover of reagents should also be kept to a minimum. Many manufacturers supply proprietary reagents, enzymes, chromogens, and counterstains that must be used in conjunction with their instrument. Protocols requiring the strict use of proprietary reagents are not as flexible and cannot be customized. These RTU reagents tend to be more costly. However, the use of RTU bar codes permits computer-driven tracking and monitoring of reagent volume, lot number, and expiration date. These reagents, therefore, assist with matters pertaining to quality control, and they may save costs by means of reduced technician time and lack of errors. As described, open automated systems, in contrast, are more flexible and allow for the use of other reagents and protocols. These protocols can be customized and stored for use at any time. Each laboratory should make this decision carefully when choosing an option for an instrument. It is like purchasing a car—the technician is "selling" it to you and will present the instrument to its advantage.

The application of automation for immunostaining offers several advantages. The true value of automation is that it offers a uniform and standardized microenvironment, resulting in intra-laboratory run-to-run assay consistency. The costs and inconvenience of repeated procedures are, therefore, avoided. Moreover, small microliter amounts of expensive reagents can be dispensed accurately. This not only saves the cost of expensive immunologic reagents but also adds to accuracy. Moreover, automation allows for walk-away function and thereby frees not only the time but also the cost of skilled technicians. The use of automated instrumentation may also decrease the amount of technical training that is required through a user-friendly software interface. From a safety standpoint, the use of a consolidated and enclosed automated workstation increases biosafety by reducing exposure to, and facilitating the disposal of, hazardous chemicals. Other benefits of automation include increased throughput and decreased turnaround time by increasing the speed of reactions with heat and mixing. Finally, most systems also offer computer-driven accountability and reporting capabilities for each step of the staining procedure.[182,183]

Automated AR systems have very recently been introduced, sometimes integrated into or with the automated staining instrument. Antigen retrieval has been in use since the early 1990s. Nevertheless, because of the multiple variables inherent in this technique, standardization has been a challenge. These variables include the size and power of the microwave, the temperature of the retrieval solution, the duration of the retrieval, and the rate of cooling. Other variables include the number of slides and containers in the microwave as well as the size, color, and material of these containers. With this new automation, all these variables are controlled, and this results in more reproducible results.

As mentioned earlier, with automation quantitative IHC becomes possible. Many IHC tests are useful for diagnosis, prognosis, and therapy. Some require quantification for accuracy, and this is often achieved by crude semi-quantitative scoring methods that are unreliable. Automated IHC coupled with automated cellular imaging systems can be used for the detection of molecular markers, hormone receptors, or occult micrometastases in a more reliable reproducible manner.[184,185] Automated microscopy may be employed to evaluate target cells using greater than 100 different morphometric parameters, as well as spectral imaging for multiple stains,[128] with digital records of images and data. The results are quantitative and based on standardized scoring and reporting. Images of the cells, as well as the results, are stored permanently for later review or confirmation, or both, if necessary.

Despite the advent of these exciting new automated technologies, not all problems are corrected by automation, and in some respects the proliferation of automated stainers has aggravated problems of reproducibility, because now almost any laboratory can perform IHC staining, often without sufficient grounding or understanding of the principles. Thus, automation cannot overcome the improper selection of antibody ("stain") or tissue to be examined, faulty tissue fixation, or problems with processing or sectioning, all of which can compromise antigen detection and interpretation. It cannot replace a pathologist's expertise when selecting the appropriate tests to be performed or when interpreting tissue sections. It is, therefore, by no means a panacea for laboratories with poor quality control standards. Only a laboratory with high standards and proper controls can operate an automated machine effectively. However, automation can and does provide reproducible, standardized, and uniform results and serves as a prelude to quantitative IHC and computerized image analysis. It is time for the morphology and immunochemistry of tissue diagnosis to unite, not only for diagnosis but also for prognosis and therapy.

Technical Issues: "Troubleshooting"

Immunohistochemistry is a multistep diagnostic procedure involving the proper selection, fixation, processing, and staining of tissue.[186,187] The final interpretation of the results is the responsibility of an experienced pathologist. It is based on the presence, pattern, and intensity of colored chromogen products, which are deposited on the tissue as the result of specific antibody-antigen reactions in the cells. The resultant pattern of staining can be focal or diffuse, nuclear, cytoplasmic, or membranous. When the expected results are not obtained, one must troubleshoot the problem in a systematic way, and each single variable of this multistep diagnostic procedure should be addressed separately, one at a time (Tables 1.8 and 1.9).

Technical problems can be classified into two main categories: those that occur before staining and those that are related to staining. "Pre-analytic" effects of delayed fixation, over-fixation, under-fixation, or uneven fixation are well studied and have already been discussed. Conversely, the effects of tissue processing are less studied and less well understood. Currently, processing after fixation is accomplished in most laboratories by automated devices. Other than errors introduced by personnel or machine malfunction, the influence of processing on immunostaining results has not been studied thoroughly. One of the few problems in this area that has been described is due to inadequate tissue dehydration before paraffin embedding. This problem can be reduced by preparing fresh alcohol solutions on a more frequent and regular basis. Other processing problems include the use of incorrect slides, which can result in loss of tissue adherence. Imprecise sectioning can cause crinkling or folding of the tissue, which may result in reagent trapping and uneven staining patterns. Subsequent to processing, other non–staining-related problems pertain to pretreatment protocols (i.e., enzyme digestion, AR, or both). During pretreatment, technical problems are also unavoidable because of the variables involved.

The recognition of inappropriate staining can be divided into five main categories based on the pattern of staining results on the test tissue as well as the pattern of staining results on the positive control.[182,187] We will discuss troubleshooting considerations for each of the following five staining patterns:

- absence of staining of both the test tissue and positive control
- absence of staining of the test tissue with appropriate positive staining of the positive control
- weak staining of the test tissue with appropriate staining of the positive control
- the presence of background staining on the test tissue, the positive control, or both
- the presence of artifactual staining on the test tissue, the positive control, or both

TABLE 1.8 Troubleshooting Variables

Tissue	Pretreatment	Detection System
Patient tissue	Xylene	Link and label
Fixation	Alcohol	Compatibility
Processing	Water	Expiration date
Control tissue	Antigen retrieval	Chromogen
Fixation		Preparation
Processing		Incubation time
		Expiration date
Fixation	**Blocking**	**Results of Test**
Optimal fixation	Peroxidase block	Positive staining
Over-fixation	Biotin block	Negative staining
Under-fixation	Background block	Focal or weak staining
Delayed fixation		Background staining
		Artifactual staining
Processing	**Antibodies**	**Results of Control**
Dehydration	Prediluted-concentrated	Positive staining
Embedding	Expiration date	Negative staining
Sectioning	Storage	Background staining
Mounting	Contamination	Artifactual staining
Slides	Incubation	

ABSENCE OF STAINING OF BOTH SPECIMEN AND CONTROL

When neither the specimen nor the control stains, one must check to see if the procedure was followed correctly (i.e., that all the steps of the staining process were performed in the correct order), that the incubation times were sufficient, and that no reagents were accidentally omitted. Antibody titrations and dilutions should also be reviewed. This is particularly important for the primary antibody. One should also check the expiration dates and storage of the reagents. Using reagents beyond their expiration date can result in false-negative results. Moreover, antibodies stored in self-defrosting freezers are exposed to repeated freezing and thawing, and this can result in antibody breakdown. The rinse buffer should also be checked, because it may be incompatible with the reaction reagents. The buffer pH must be appropriate, and sodium azide should not be present in buffers that are used with peroxidase enzyme. The drying out of specimens can also result in absence of staining, and one needs to confirm that this did not occur. Was sufficient reagent applied to the sample to prevent dehydration? Was a humidity chamber used? Other possible causes of absence of staining include problems with the chromogen. One must confirm that the chromogen solution was properly prepared and that it is working. This can be accomplished by adding the labeling reagent to the small amount of the prepared chromogen and confirming that a color change occurs. Keep in mind that chromogen

TABLE 1.9 Technical Problems and Solutions: Absence of Staining or Weak Staining

Problem	Solution
Inadequate fixation	Avoid delay of fixation (>30 min) or over-fixation (>48 h)
Incomplete dehydration during processing	Check protocol for processing; perform regular reagent changes (i.e., alcohol)
Paraffin too hot	Monitor temperature of paraffin (<60°C)
Prolonged or excessive heating	Optimize antigen retrieval time
Staining steps not followed	Review procedure manual
Reagents not working	Check expiration dates; check storage parameters; check compatibility with other reagents; check pH
Antibody too dilute	Check antibody titration; increase concentration; lengthen incubation time; increase temperature of reaction; check amount of rinsing buffer left on slide
Drying out of tissue during processing	Keep specimen moist as indicated by procedure manual; prevent evaporation with humidity chamber
Insufficient incubation time	Lengthen incubation time to achieve desired intensity of staining; add heat; increase concentration of antibody
Chromogen not working	Add chromogen to labeling solution; monitor for change in color

solutions tend to deteriorate quickly. Finally, lack of staining can also occur because of improper pretreatment before IHC staining, counterstaining, or cover-slipping. For example, AEC should not be used with counterstains or mounting media containing alcohol, xylene, or toluene, because these chemicals can dissolve the soluble colored precipitates formed by the reaction of AEC chromogen and substrate. Following this type of review, the IHC procedure should be repeated with a positive control known to have performed well previously; if this fails, it is best to begin with entirely new reagents throughout.

ABSENCE OF STAINING OF SPECIMEN WITH APPROPRIATE POSITIVE STAINING OF POSITIVE CONTROL

If the positive control slide shows appropriate positive staining of the expected cells, one can assume that the procedure was performed correctly and that the reagents were working properly. In such instances, the problem is likely to be pre-analytic, rather than an aspect of the staining procedure itself. It may, therefore, be the result of improper tissue fixation, processing, pretreatment, or a combination of these. Keep in mind, however, that a single improper step may have occurred in protocol, limited to the test section.

Problems with formalin fixation include delay of fixation, over-fixation, under-fixation, and variable fixation.[186] For some antibodies, depending on the resistance of their target antigens to autolysis, a delay in fixation may cause loss of immunoreactivity and absence of staining. For this reason, fixation should begin as soon as possible, preferably within 30 minutes of removing the specimen. Over-fixation can result in absence of staining as well. Causes of this include the cross-linking of antigens as well as the presence of contaminant in the fixative. For these reasons, one should avoid formalin fixation in excess of 48 hours. In instances of under-fixation, only the periphery of the tissue has time to absorb the fixative. Toward the center of the specimen, the tissue will remain unfixed and raw. In these center areas, the specimen may undergo coagulative fixation by alcohol during tissue dehydration. This will result in variable staining, with more intense staining at either the center or the periphery of the specimen (depending on which has occurred, what antibody was used, and whether AR was used).

Absence of staining can also result from processing problems, although such problems are less studied and seemingly less important than those due to fixation. Potential processing factors include inadequate dehydration due to the use of old alcohol reagents. Moreover, heat-sensitive epitopes can be lost by embedding in paraffin that is too hot, or subjecting the tissue to prolonged heating. Therefore, the temperature of the paraffin should be monitored so as not to exceed 56°C (see Tables 1.8 and 1.9).

WEAK STAINING OF SPECIMEN WITH APPROPRIATE STAINING OF POSITIVE CONTROL

Improper fixation or processing, or both, of the test tissue may also cause weak staining of the specimen, whereas the control stains positively. All the causes explained previously for "absence of staining" apply to a lesser degree to the situation of weak staining. This serves to emphasize further the need for the control slides and the test tissues to be fixed and processed in an identical manner whenever possible. Other factors that may cause weak staining with appropriate positive control staining include a low concentration of antigen in the test tissue. If antibody concentration is found to be too low for the test tissue that had been fixed improperly, one can increase its concentration, lengthen the incubation time, or increase the temperature of the reaction. Any of these measures may intensify the weak staining and provide adequate results. Inappropriately diluted antibody can also be the result of leaving too much buffer rinse on the slide before the antibody is applied (see Tables 1.8 and 1.9).

BACKGROUND STAINING

Any positive staining that is not the result of antibody-antigen reaction is termed *non-specific background staining*. Such staining is demonstrated as inappropriate positive staining on the test tissue or the positive control. However, it is best confirmed by positivity on the negative control. There are a number of conditions that can cause this, the most common of which is the non-specific ionic binding of antibodies to charged connective tissue elements in the specimen, such as collagen. In these instances, such non-specific staining can be alleviated by the use of non-immune serum from the same animal species as the secondary antibody. The addition of salt to the buffer may also help.

Another common cause of background staining is the presence of peroxidase in the tissue being studied. If this peroxidase is not removed, positive staining will be found in red blood cells (pseudo-peroxidase) and white blood cells (endogenous peroxidase). Endogenous biotin is also found in certain tissues (i.e., liver and kidney) and may cause false-positive signals. This can be avoided in such situations by changing to another detection system that is free of avidin-biotin or by pre-incubation of the tissue with avidin. Poorly fixed tissues and areas of necrosis will also show background staining in these areas, as will tissue sections that are cut too thick. Some other causes of background positivity pertain to the antibody solution itself. Examples include solutions that contain particulates or inappropriately high concentrations of antibodies. In the former instance, the accumulation of particulates can be due to repeated freezing and thawing of the antibodies. Other less common causes of background staining involve problems related to tissue processing such as the incomplete removal of paraffin. This is recognized by diffuse background positivity that extends beyond the borders of the specimen. Background staining can also result from the incomplete rinsing of slides between steps or by the use of contaminated buffers. Finally, one other consideration that can cause non-specific positivity is overdevelopment of the chromogen-substrate reaction. This can result from incomplete solution or excess concentration of chromogen. Appropriate troubleshooting measures for these problems include filtering of the

TABLE 1.10 Technical Problems and Solutions: Background Staining

Problem	Solution
Non-specific protein binding	Use non-immune serum from same animal species as secondary antibody; add salt to buffer
Incomplete removal of paraffin	Use only completely deparaffinized slides
Poorly fixed or necrotic tissue	Make sure tissue is properly fixed; avoid sampling of necrotic areas
Thick preparation	Cut sections at 3 to 5 mm; prepare cytospins that are monolayer in thickness
Inappropriately concentrated antibody	Check titration; decrease concentration; decrease incubation time; decrease temperature of reaction
Endogenous biotin	Block with avidin
Incomplete rinsing of slides	Follow protocol for proper slide rinsing
Chromogen staining too intense	Monitor timing of chromogen-substrate reaction; filter chromogen; decrease chromogen concentration

TABLE 1.11 Technical Problems and Solutions: Artifactual Staining

Problem	Solution
Presence of chromogen or counterstain deposits	Filter the chromogen or counterstain
Black deposits in B5-fixed tissue	Remove the mercury before staining
Endogenous pigments confused with specific positive staining	Check the negative control for the presence of these pigments; use a chromogen of contrasting color
Microbiologic contamination	Change reagents often; use fresh reagents; check expiration dates

chromogen solution or decreasing its concentration (Tables 1.9 and 1.10).

ARTIFACTUAL STAINING

The presence of certain artifacts can result in unexpected and non-specific results. Artifacts include undissolved precipitates of chromogen or counterstain. The presence of these artifacts can be corrected by filtering. Sometimes, in B5-fixed tissues, black precipitates that are spread across the specimen are encountered. This results from incomplete de-Zenkerization of the tissue and can be corrected by removing the mercury from the tissue before staining. Not uncommonly, endogenous pigments, such as hemosiderin or melanin, are confused with true histochemical positivity. However, the presence of these pigments will also be seen on the negative control. If a negative control is not available for comparison, the use of a chromogen of contrasting color (such as AEC, which stains red) can be helpful in providing this distinction. Finally, other artifacts worth considering are the presence of microbial contaminants, such as yeast or bacteria (Table 1.11).

Because of the multistep nature of the immunohistochemical procedure, there are numerous technical problems that can arise. Fortunately, many of these can be managed fairly logically and easily with adherence to quality control guidelines and the strict application of positive and negative controls.[4,115,187] This is necessary for the correct interpretation of the results and for the avoidance of diagnostic pitfalls. For some examples of the staining problems discussed, see Figures 1.21 to 1.36.

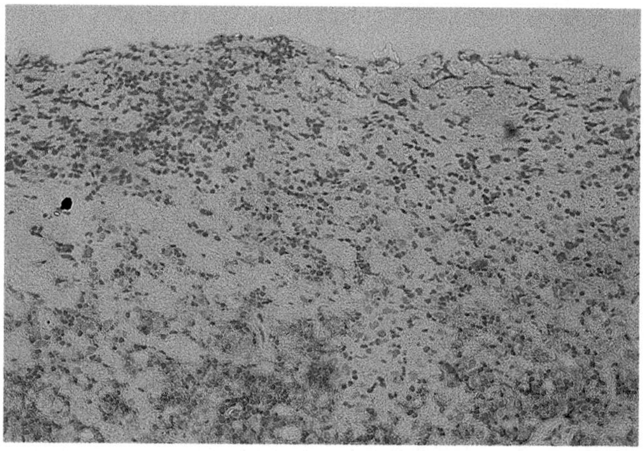

FIGURE 1.21 Section stained with autostainer using capillary action principle illustrating insufficient ascent of reagent.

Amplification Methods

The high level of detection sensitivity achieved by current labeling methods has generally made amplification unnecessary. A brief review of available approaches follows (Table 1.12, pg 35).

PRE-DETECTION AMPLIFICATION

In effect, the AR technique is an effective and simple technique of pre-detection–phase amplification.[4,39,40,55-58,86] It is generally accepted, although not well understood, that AR-induced amplification of signal is the result of

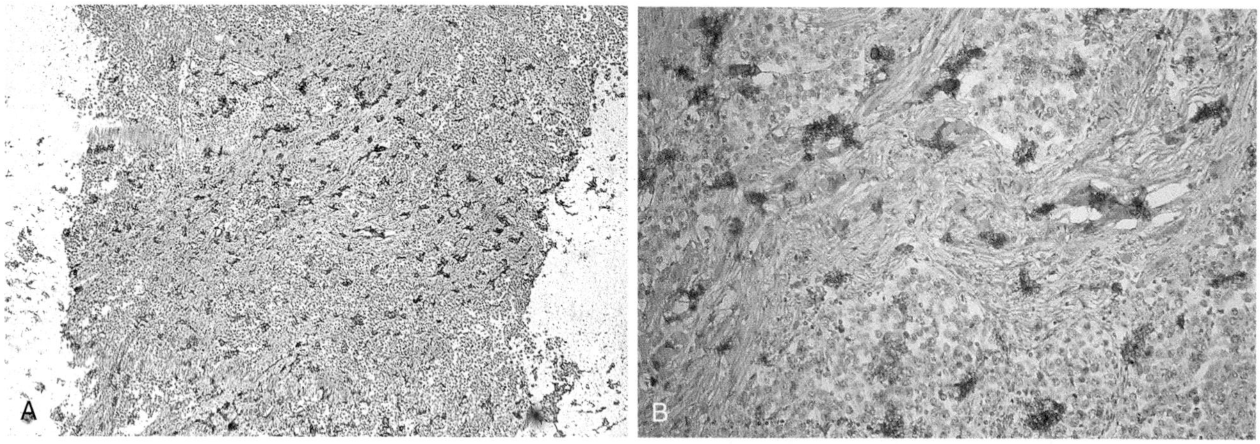

FIGURE 1.22 (A, B) "Chromogen freckles," which is an artifact that resulted from undissolved precipitates of chromogen.

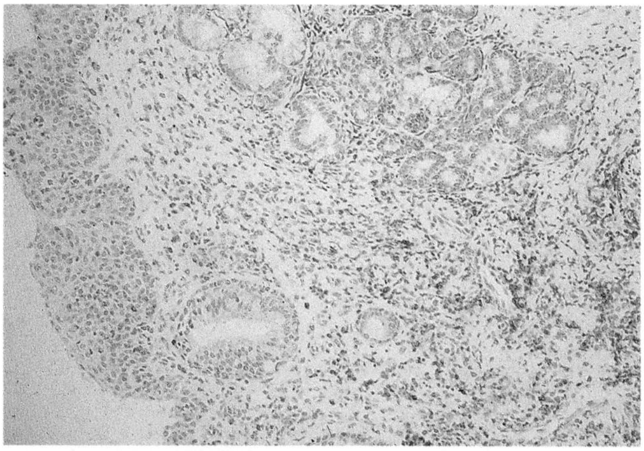

FIGURE 1.23 Section of parotid gland stained with CD3 showing scattered T-lymphocyte and non-specific cytoplasmic granular staining in the glandular epithelium.

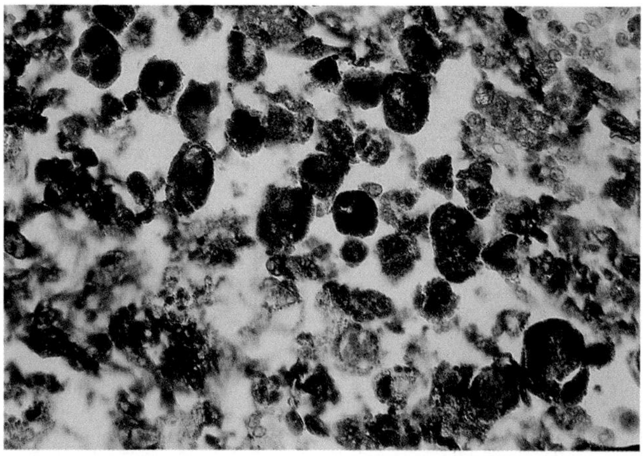

FIGURE 1.25 Pigmented melanophages, not to be confused with chromogen.

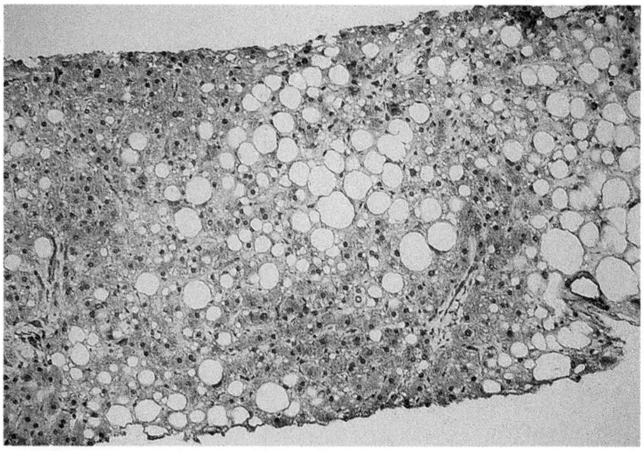

FIGURE 1.24 Section of liver illustrating endogenous biotin resulting in non-specific background staining.

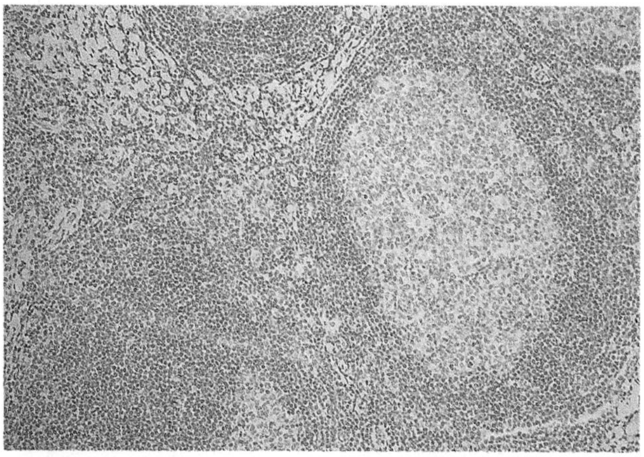

FIGURE 1.26 Section of lymph node with no primary antibody.

"restored" antigenicity contingent on recovery of certain epitopes in the formalin-modified protein structure.[60,61] To the extent that the AR technique serves to restore the natural antigen-antibody reaction, it favors specific binding and does not aggravate non-specific background staining, thereby providing the potential for an enhanced signal-to-noise ratio.

DETECTION PHASE AMPLIFICATION

As described earlier, development of staining methods has continued apace, reflective of drawbacks intrinsic to the three-step detection systems, including complex time-consuming protocols, difficulties in standardization, inefficient demonstration of certain hard-to-detect

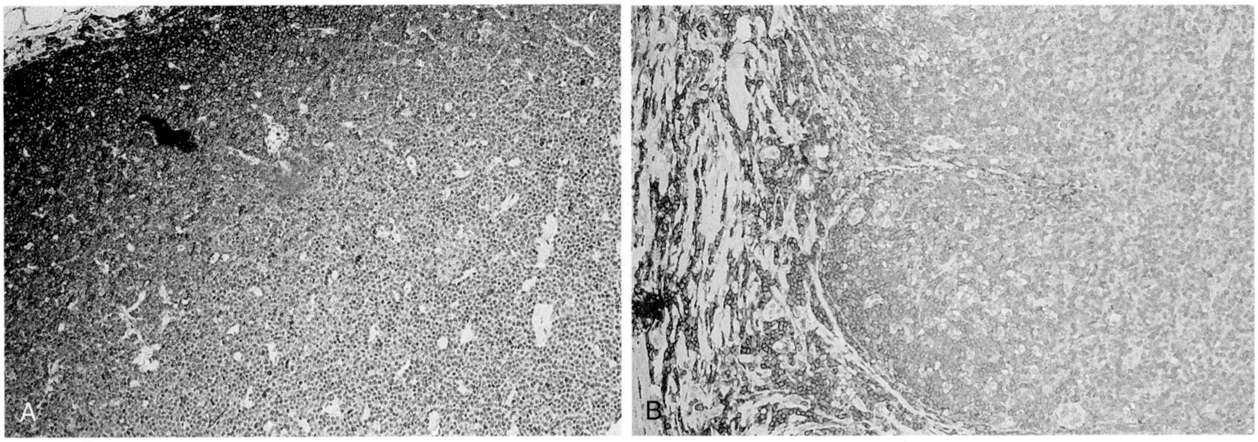

FIGURE 1.27 Section of lymph node stained with CD45 showing variable fixation artifact. Well-defined cytoplasmic membrane staining is seen in the subcapsular region **(A)** and toward the periphery of the section **(B)**, where the tissue is adequately fixed.

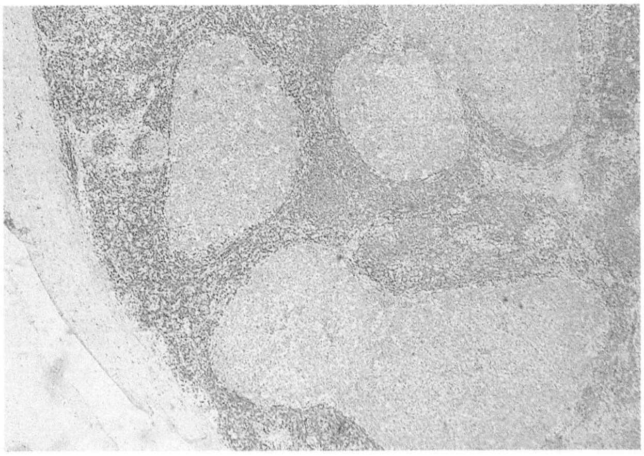

FIGURE 1.28 Another lymph node section stained with Bcl-2 showing similar variable fixation artifact with gradual loss of staining appreciated toward the center of the node.

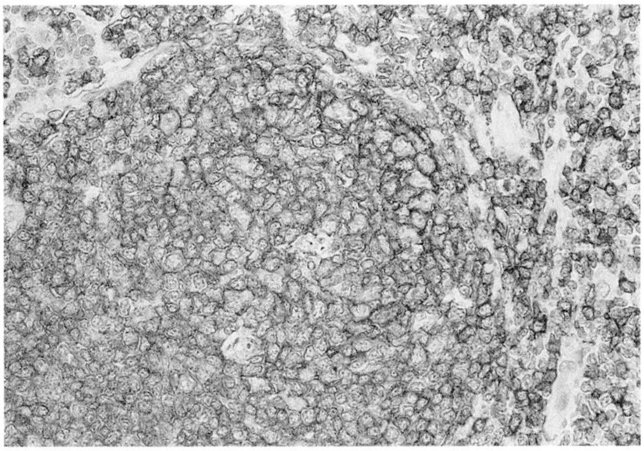

FIGURE 1.29 Sections of lymph node stained with CD20 showing bright cytoplasmic membrane staining of the B cells in the germinal center.

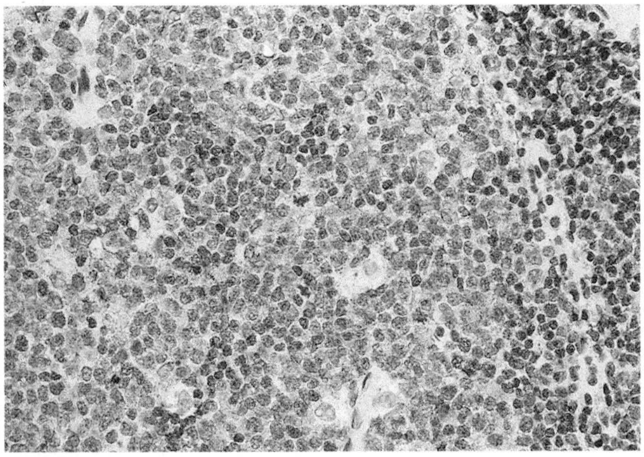

FIGURE 1.30 Similar lymph node section stained with CD20 showing suboptimal weak staining of the B cells in the germinal center, which is recognized by the presence of scattered tingible body macrophages.

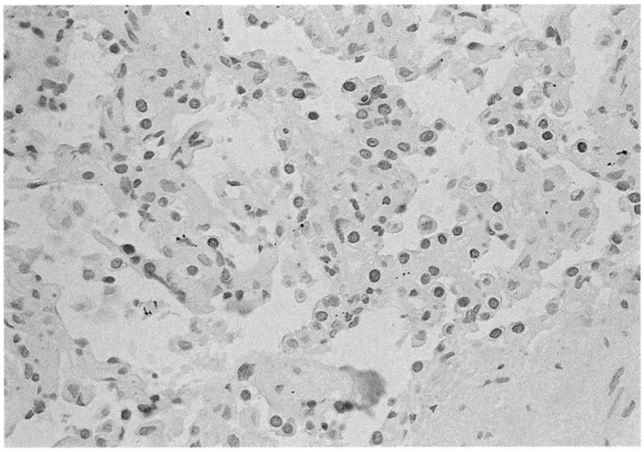

FIGURE 1.31 Section of normal lung tissue stained with TTF-1 (thyroid transcription factor), exhibiting specific nuclear positivity of the alveolar lining cells (pneumocytes).

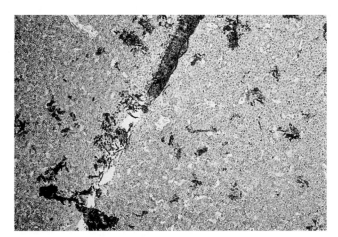

FIGURE 1.32 Section of lymph node stained with CD43 demonstrating processing problem with cleavage and folding of the tissue, which subsequently resulted in variable staining intensity and precipitation of the chromogen. All these artifacts can adversely affect interpretation.

antigens, and endogenous biotin or endogenous enzyme activity. As noted, several computer-assisted automated stainers have been manufactured to address the issues of consistency, high labor intensity, and cost. These developments have led to remarkable improvements in reproducibility and have facilitated the widespread use of highly sensitive detection methods that mostly use polymer-based secondary reagents, as described previously. The quality of reagents and kits available from the major and reputable manufacturers continues to improve, which has allowed rapid adoption of these sensitive labeling methods. Also, the package inserts and manufacturers' instruction or protocols are more comprehensive and of increased value in setting up the stain and interpreting the result. A major failing now is that technologists and pathologists often neglect to read the package insert, or if they read it they ignore the contents. For example, it is the authors' experience that the HER2 kit (Dako) is one of the most commonly abused

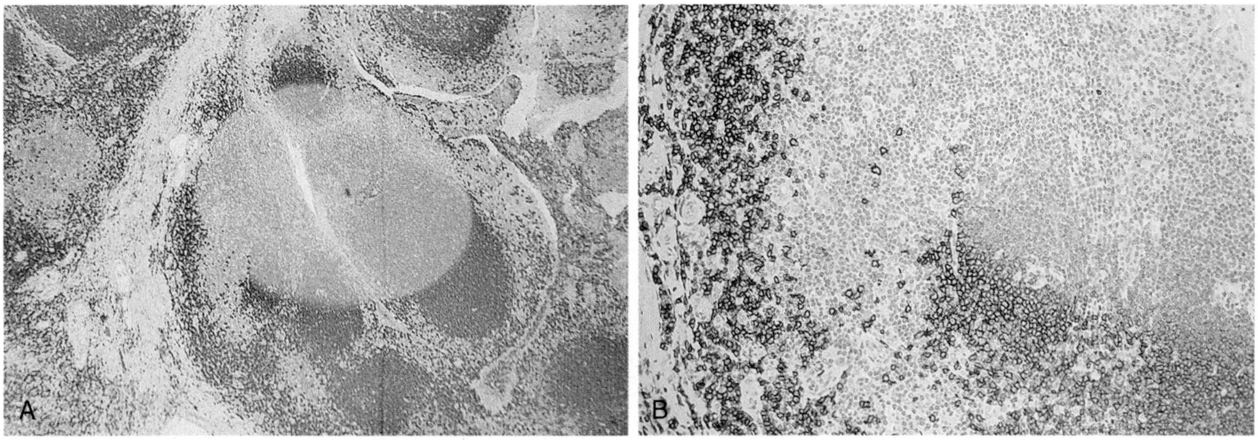

FIGURE 1.33 (A, B) Section of lymph node stained with CD20 showing low- and high-power views with "bubble artifact." This is the result of microscopic hydrophobic bubbles formed during staining process.

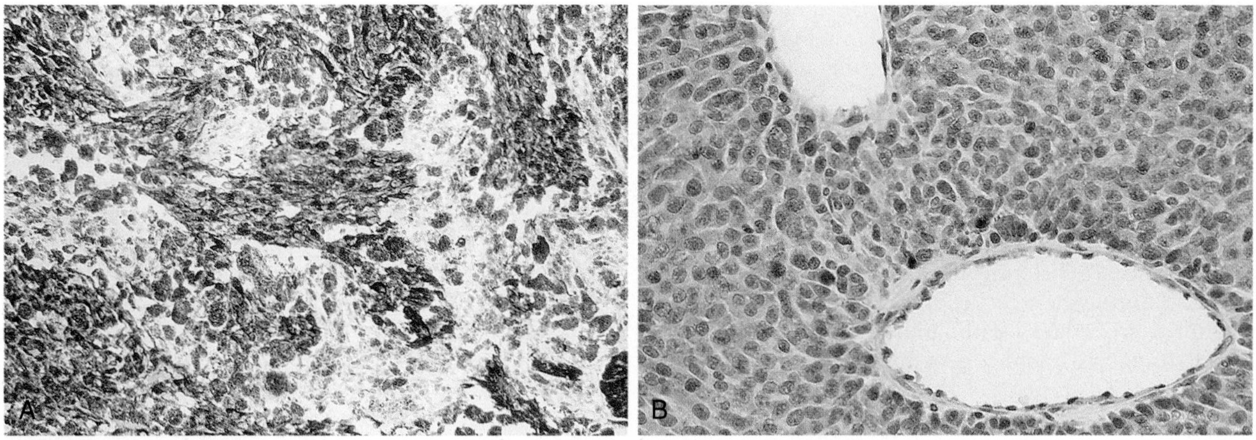

FIGURE 1.34 (A, B) Sections of malignant melanoma stained with S-100. The spindle-shaped neoplastic cells on the left are overstained to the extent that it is difficult to appreciate true nuclear staining. Similarly, spindle-shaped malignant cells around the blood vessels (on the right) show a gradation with different intensity of staining, resulting in more readily appreciated nuclear positivity.

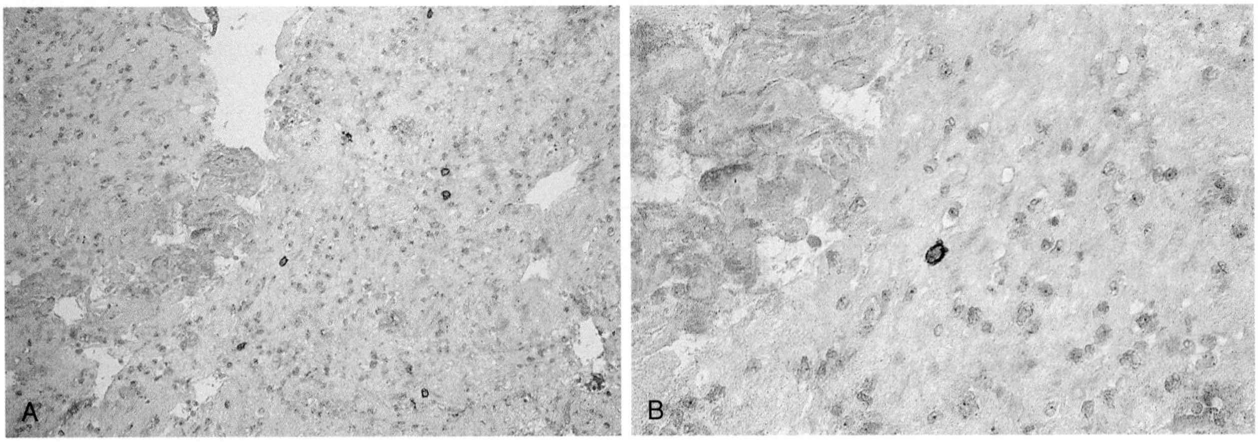

FIGURE 1.35 (A, B) Cell block section stained with CD20. There is high background staining of the amorphous proteinaceous material. The high-power view in **B** highlights positive B-lymphoid cells and aberrant nucleolar positivity of scattered T-lymphoid cells, which are negative for CD20.

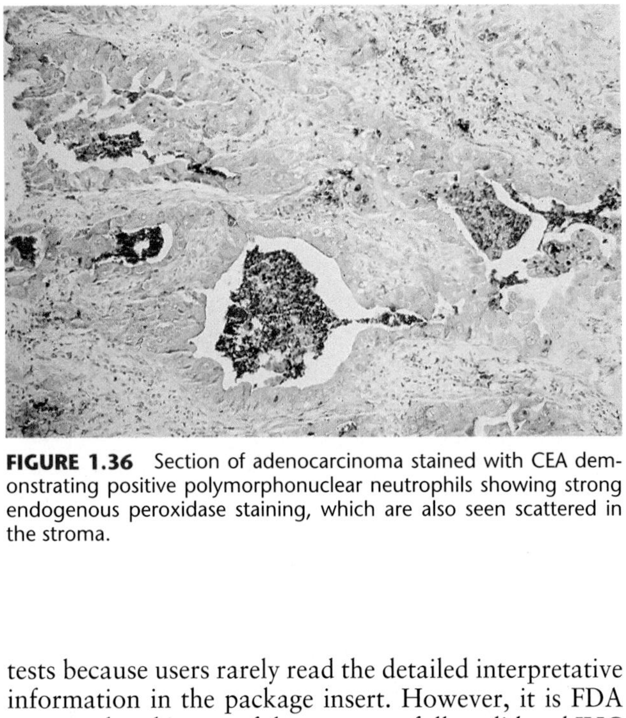

FIGURE 1.36 Section of adenocarcinoma stained with CEA demonstrating positive polymorphonuclear neutrophils showing strong endogenous peroxidase staining, which are also seen scattered in the stroma.

tests because users rarely read the detailed interpretative information in the package insert. However, it is FDA approved and is one of the most carefully validated IHC tests currently available.

POST-DETECTION AMPLIFICATION

Methods of post-detection phase amplification seek to intensify the chromogen reaction, as we have described with reference to chromogens. The two principal drawbacks are an increase in the complexity of the immunostaining procedure (with additional steps that are difficult to control) and a general increase in non-specific background staining. This latter effect often means that although the intensity of the stain is increased, the signal-to-noise ratio is not improved, and interpretation may even be more difficult. In general, we do not recommend this approach for routine use.

DEVELOPMENT OF REFERENCE STANDARDS AND STANDARD CURVES FOR CALCULATION OF ANTIGEN CONTENT IN TISSUE SECTION

We have discussed the current use of in-house controls and approaches to the development of QIRS[128,129] with respect to quantification, but also with an emphasis on correcting for variations in sample preparation. A number of investigators have reported improved control systems, including some with the potential for calibrating the IHC reaction. We will briefly discuss these systems next.

If properly used, controls enhance quality within any laboratory, but because they are "local" in production and availability, they do not ensure reproducibility among different laboratories. Universal reference standards, or controls, are therefore actively under investigation. Theoretically, it is possible to develop preparations of purified protein (antigen), which can be diluted to produce a series of known reference standards for both Western blotting and, when suitably prepared, for IHC. The peptide or protein deposits described by Sompuram, Bogen, and colleagues represent one promising approach in the production of known reference standards.[116,117,157] The technique of matrix models[188] has been used to create what is in effect an artificial control tissue for the protein (antigen) in question (see the paragraph that follows). In this approach, a conversion formula may be developed from a "standard curve" to determine the exact amount of antigen present in FFPE tissue sections under various conditions of immunostaining, including AR pretreatment, analogous to the method proposed for QIRS.[128,129] These types of peptide or matrix preparations may also be used as a pretest to establish a standardized protocol of IHC and may also serve as practical reference standards for quality control of IHC staining. The matrix model has advantages over an alternative Quicgel,[189] which is essentially an artificial tissue control block incorporating a breast cancer cell line, which is then added to the tissue cassette containing the clinical biopsy specimen. Histoids (Fig 1.37) are three-dimensional "faux tissue" pellets grown in centrifugal culture conditions. They provide another approach

TABLE 1.12 Classification of Three Basic Signal Amplification Approaches for IHC

Classification	Basic Principles and Mode of Action	Advantages and Problems
Predetection amplification		
Antigen retrieval (AR)	Restoration of formalin-induced modification of protein structure, resulting in dramatic amplification of signal while reducing the background simultaneously	Simplest and cheapest procedure (heating) among all methods of amplification, not effective for some antibodies/antigens
Detection amplification		
Multi-step detection systems; PAP, ABC, APAAP, B-SA	Increase the accumulation of labeling signal (enzyme or others) PAP, 2- to 50-fold; ABC, 2- to 100-fold increase	The polylabeling technique and polymer-based amplification systems are simpler, cheaper, and faster than other multi-step detection systems; as a biotin-free detection system, avoids the problem of the endogenous biotin reaction
Stepwise amplification	Repeating cycles of detection	
Polymeric and polylabeling amplification	Currently available kits of EnVision, PowerVision, and EPOS; average further dilution of primary antibody: 2- to 5-fold, our test: 1:160 further dilution of PCNA	
Postdetection amplification		
		Procedures are complicated, involving repeating cycles of reactions; labor and costs may be a drawback to widespread application; background staining increasing with amplification of signal
Enhanced DAB by metal, imidazole, and so on CARD	Enhance the color reaction HRP catalyzes deposition of biotinylated tyramine at the site of HRP	
Anti-end product (EP)	Anti-EP + biotinylated link + HRP label, 16-fold increase of signal	
Gold/silver enhancement method	Silver enhancement	

PAP, peroxidase-antiperoxidase; ABC, avidin-biotin conjugate; APAAP, alkaline phosphatase antialkaline phosphatase; B-SA, biotin-streptavidin; PCNA, proliferating cell nuclear antigen; EPOS, enhanced polymer one-step staining (Dako); CARD, catalyzed reporter deposition; HRP, horseradish peroxidase.

Adapted from Shi S-R, Guo J, Cote RJ, et al. Sensitivity and detection efficiency of a novel two-step detection system (PowerVision) for immunohistochemistry. *Appl Immunohistochem Mol Morphology.* 1999;7:201-208.

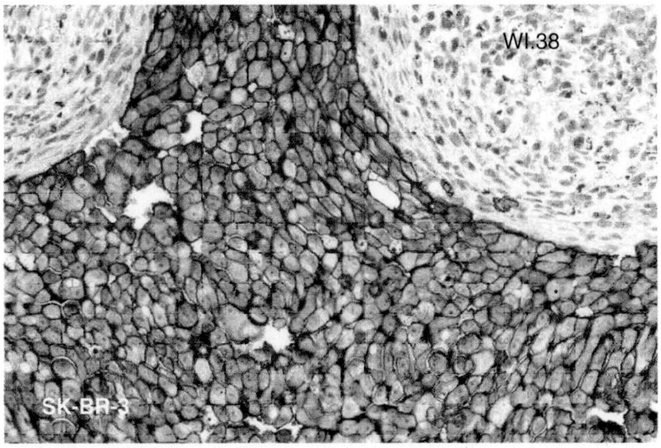

FIGURE 1.37 Faux tissue breast histoid, stained for HER2, showing good positivity of the breast epithelial elements (MCF-7 cell line), but lack of staining in fibroblasts. *Collaborative project, Dr. M. Ingram, Dr. A. Imam, Dr. C. Taylor, 2002, IMAT program grant, National Cancer Institute.*

to total process control. Histoids may be constructed to consist of two, three, or more cell lines co-cultured under standardized conditions to yield a faux tissue pellet (e.g., of fibroblasts, breast cancer cells, and endothelial cells), which may then serve as a reference standard (available in unlimited quantities) for the control of many commonly employed antibodies, including control of tissue fixation and processing steps. However, while potentially widely available to control the staining method, these controls cannot serve as controls for sample preparation (including fixation) unless they are included in every step of the preparation process. In this regard, the use of Internal Reference Standards, relying upon the demonstration of proteins that are intrinsic to each tissue under study, provide the only practical method proposed to date for evaluating sample preparation,[129] possibly also serving as a prelude to establishing quantification by IHC and ISH.

Certain manufacturers have begun to include control materials in test kits (e.g., Dako's HER2 kit), especially when graded interpretation (quantification) is required. These are valuable for determining levels of intensity. As described, computer image analysis methods are expected to continue to improve[128] and are far superior to the human eye for quantification, with the prerequisite that internal reference controls must be employed.

CONCLUSION

The widespread application of IHC has entirely transformed diagnostic surgical pathology "from something resembling an art into something more closely resembling a science."[3] However, as described, all is not entirely well. Reproducibility is a problem that is ameliorated by automation, when properly employed, and aggravated by the proliferation of automated devices that are not always used in controlled environments. Standardization has thus become the major focus and has been emphasized throughout this chapter, with reference to published practice guidelines. An ongoing major drawback of IHC is the lack of objective quantitative measurement for target antigens under investigation, especially for proper use of the prognostic markers that are described elsewhere in this book. In this respect, the use of QIRS has been described for calibration of the IHC method, analogous to ELISA tests in the clinical laboratory. Finally, while the focus has been on IHC, much of what has been written regarding standardization of IHC is equally applicable to the use of ISH methods in surgical pathology.

Pathologists have been practicing "molecular morphology" (the microscopic localization of protein, DNA, and RNA) since the late 1970s. To take the next leap forward, we need to "do it right." Reliable and true quantification is a goal that requires a demonstrable level of standardization and reproducibility, and the widespread use of reference standards and computer-assisted analysis of the reaction product.

Appendix 1A

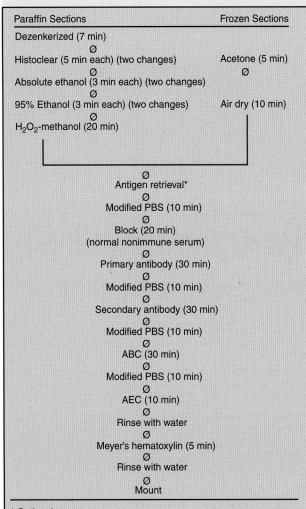

Paraffin Sections	Frozen Sections
Dezenkerized (7 min)	
Ø	
Histoclear (5 min each) (two changes)	Acetone (5 min)
Ø	Ø
Absolute ethanol (3 min each) (two changes)	
Ø	
95% Ethanol (3 min each) (two changes)	Air dry (10 min)
Ø	
H_2O_2-methanol (20 min)	

Ø
Antigen retrieval*
Ø
Modified PBS (10 min)
Ø
Block (20 min)
(normal nonimmune serum)
Ø
Primary antibody (30 min)
Ø
Modified PBS (10 min)
Ø
Secondary antibody (30 min)
Ø
Modified PBS (10 min)
Ø
ABC (30 min)
Ø
Modified PBS (10 min)
Ø
AEC (10 min)
Ø
Rinse with water
Ø
Meyer's hematoxylin (5 min)
Ø
Rinse with water
Ø
Mount

* Optional
PBS, phosphate-buffered saline; ABC, avidin-biotin conjugate; AEC, aminorthyl carbazole.
Adapted from Taylor CR, Cote RJ. Immunomicroscopy; A Diagnostic Tool for the Surgical Pathologist. 2nd ed. Philadelphia: WB Saunders; 1994:422.

Appendix 1B

Double Staining*

A satisfactory "sequential" double-staining method using mouse monoclonal antibodies has been in routine use in our laboratory for some time. The method is applicable both to frozen sections and to cytocentrifuge preparations.

Briefly, the procedure involves the sequential application of two different staining systems, both using a mouse monoclonal primary antibody. The first is an indirect ABC† peroxidase procedure, using biotinylated horse antimouse IgG linked to ABC peroxidase, with AEC as the substrate. The second is an indirect conjugate method using goat antimouse IgG linked with alkaline phosphatase, and fast blue as substrate. Controls reveal that there is no detectable binding of the second labeling system (goat antimouse Ig-alkaline phosphatase) to the first monoclonal antibody; this circumstance presumably is due to steric interference. Mounting is in buffered glycerol jelly in deference to the use of AEC, which is alcohol soluble.

This method for general use is being supplanted by polymer-based multiple staining methods, for convenience and quality of result. The reagents for these methods are available from several manufacturers and render the process quite straightforward, with the caveat that "proper controls" are essential for all elements of the multiple stain, and image analysis, such as spectral imaging (110a often is necessary to interpret results where the naked eye cannot).

*Adapted from Taylor CR, Cote RJ. Immunomicroscopy: A Diagnostic Tool for Surgical Pathologist. 2nd ed. Philadelphia: WB Saunders; 1994:424.
†ABC, avidin-biotin conjugate; AEC, amino-ethyl carbazole.

REFERENCES

1. Coons AH, Creech HJ, Jones RN. Immunological properties of an antibody containing a fluorescent group. *Proc Soc Exp Biol Med.* 1941;47:200.
2. Taylor CR. The current role of immunohistochemistry in diagnostic pathology. *Adv Pathol Lab Med.* 1994;7:59.
3. Taylor CR. An exaltation of experts: Concerted efforts in the standardization of immunohistochemistry. *Hum Pathol.* 1994;25:2.
4. Taylor CR, Cote RJ, eds. *Immunomicroscopy: A Diagnostic Tool for the Surgical Pathologist.* 2nd ed. Philadelphia: WB Saunders; 1994.

5. Taylor CR, Burns J. The demonstration of plasma cells and other immunoglobulin containing cells in formalin-fixed, paraffin-embedded tissues using peroxidase labeled antibody. *J Clin Pathol.* 1974;27:14.
6. Avrameas S. Enzyme markers: Their linkage with proteins and use in immunohistochemistry. *Histochem J.* 1972;4:321.
7. Nakane PK, Pierce GBJ. Enzyme-labeled antibodies for the light and electron microscopic localization of tissue antigens. *J Cell Biol.* 1967;33:307.
8. Adams JC. Biotin amplification of biotin and horseradish peroxidase signals in histochemical stains. *J Histochem Cytochem.* 1992;40:1457.
9. Bobrow MN, Harris TD, Shaughnessy KJ, et al. Catalyzed reporter deposition: A novel method of signal amplification: Application to immunoassays. *J Immunol Methods.* 1989;125:279.
10. Colvin RB, Bhan AK, McCluskey RT, eds. *Diagnostic Immunopathology.* 2nd ed. New York: Raven Press; 1995.
11. DeLellis RA, Sternberger LA, Mann RB, et al. Immunoperoxidase techniques in diagnostic pathology: Report of a workshop sponsored by the National Cancer Institute. *Am J Clin Pathol.* 1979;71:483.
12. Elias JM, ed. *Immunohistopathology: A Practical Approach to Diagnosis.* Chicago: American Society of Clinical Pathologists Press; 1990.
13. Heras A, Roach CM, Key ME. Enhanced polymer detection system for immunohistochemistry. *Mod Pathol.* 1995;8:165A.
14. Hsu SM, Raine L, Fanger H. A comparative study of the peroxidase-antiperoxidase method and an avidin-biotin complex method for studying polypeptide hormones with radioimmunoassay antibodies. *Am J Clin Pathol.* 1981;75:734.
15. Hsu SM, Raine L, Fanger H. Use of avidin-biotin-peroxidase complex (ABC) in immunoperoxidase techniques: A comparison between ABC and unlabeled antibody (PAP) procedures. *J Histochem Cytochem.* 1981;29:577.
16. Polak JM, van Noorden S, eds. *Immunocytochemistry: Modern Methods and Applications.* 2nd ed. Bristol, UK: Wright Publishing; 1986.
17. Sabattini E, Bisgaard K, Ascani S, et al. The EnVision system: A new immunohistochemical method for diagnostics and research: Critical comparison with the APAAP, ChemMate, CSA, LABC, and SABC techniques. *J Clin Pathol.* 1998;51:506.
18. Shi S-R, Cote RJ, Taylor CR. Standardization and further development of antigen retrieval immunohistochemistry: Strategies and future goals. *J Histotechnol.* 1999;22:177.
19. Sternberger LA, Joseph SA. The unlabeled antibody method: Contrasting color staining of paired pituitary hormones without antibody removal. *J Histochem Cytochem.* 1979;27:1424.
20. Vyberg M, Nielsen S. Dextran polymer conjugate two-step visualization system for immunohistochemistry. *Appl Immunohistochem.* 1998;6:3.
21. Kohler G, Milstein C. Continuous cultures of fused cells secreting antibody of predefined specificity. *Nature.* 1975;256:495.
22. Leong ASY. Commentary: Diagnostic immunohistochemistry—problems and solutions. *Pathology.* 1992;24:1.
23. Burns J, Hambridge M, Taylor CR. Intracellular immunoglobulins. A comparative study of three standard tissue processing methods using horseradish peroxidase and fluorochrome conjugates. *J Clin Pathol.* 1974;27:548-557.
24. Taylor CR. The nature of Reed-Sternberg cells and other malignant "reticulum" cells. *Lancet.* 1974;2:802.
25. Taylor CR. A history of the Reed-Sternberg cell. *Biomedicine.* 1978;28:196.
26. Taylor CR, Kledzik G. Immunohistologic techniques in surgical pathology: A spectrum of "new" special stains. *Hum Pathol.* 1981;12:590.
27. Pinkus GS. Diagnostic immunocytochemistry of paraffin-embedded tissues. *Hum Pathol.* 1982;13:411.
28. Swanson PE. Editorial: Methodologic standardization in immunohistochemistry: A doorway opens. *Appl Immunohistochem.* 1993;1:229.
29. Larsson LI, ed. *Immunocytochemistry: Theory and Practice.* Boca Raton, FL: CRC Press; 1988.
30. Huang SN. Immunohistochemical demonstration of hepatitis B core and surface antigens in paraffin sections. *Lab Invest.* 1975;33:88.
31. Leong AS-Y, Milios J, Duncis CG. Antigen preservation in microwave-irradiated tissues: A comparison with formaldehyde fixation. *J Pathol.* 1988;156:275.
32. Fraenkel-Conrat H, Brandon BA, Olcott HS. The reaction of formaldehyde with proteins. IV: Participation of indole groups. *J Biol Chem.* 1947;168:99.
33. Fraenkel-Conrat H, Olcott HS. The reaction of formaldehyde with proteins. V: Cross-linking between amino and primary amide or guanidyl groups. *J Am Chem Soc.* 1948;70:2673.
34. Fraenkel-Conrat H, Olcott HS. Reaction of formaldehyde with proteins. VI: Cross-linking of amino groups with phenol, imidazole, or indole groups. *J Biol Chem.* 1948;174:827.
35. Shi S-R, Key ME, Kalra KL. Antigen retrieval in formalin-fixed, paraffin-embedded tissues: An enhancement method for immunohistochemical staining based on microwave oven heating of tissue sections. *J Histochem Cytochem.* 1991;39:741.
36. Shi S-R, Tandon AK, Cote C, et al. S-100 protein in human inner ear: Use of a novel immunohistochemical technique on routinely processed, celloidin-embedded human temporal bone sections. *Laryngoscope.* 1992;102:734.
37. Shi S-R, Tandon AK, Haussmann RR, et al. Immunohistochemical study of intermediate filament proteins on routinely processed, celloidin-embedded human temporal bone sections by using a new technique for antigen retrieval. *Acta Otolaryngol (Stockh).* 1993;113:48.
38. Shi S-R, Cote C, Kalra KL, et al. A technique for retrieving antigens in formalin-fixed, routinely acid-decalcified, celloidin-embedded human temporal bone sections for immunohistochemistry. *J Histochem Cytochem.* 1992;40:787.
39. Taylor CR, Shi S-R, Chen C, et al. Comparative study of antigen retrieval heating methods: Microwave, microwave and pressure cooker, autoclave, and steamer. *Biotech Histochem.* 1996;71:263.
40. Taylor CR, Shi S-R, Cote RJ. Antigen retrieval for immunohistochemistry: Status and need for greater standardization. *Appl Immunohistochem.* 1996;4:144.
41. Boon ME, Kok LP. Breakthrough in pathology due to antigen retrieval. *Mal J Med Lab Sci.* 1995;12:1.
42. Evers P, Uylings HB, Suurmeijer AJ. Antigen retrieval in formaldehyde-fixed human brain tissue. *Methods.* 1998;15:133.
43. Gown AM, de Wever N, Battifora H. Microwave-based antigenic unmasking: A revolutionary new technique for routine immunohistochemistry. *Appl Immunohistochem.* 1993;1:256.
44. Cattoretti G, Pileri S, Parravicini C, et al. Antigen unmasking on formalin-fixed, paraffin-embedded tissue sections. *J Pathol.* 1993;171:83.
45. Leong ASY, Milios J. An assessment of the efficacy of the microwave antigen-retrieval procedure on a range of tissue antigens. *Appl Immunohistochem.* 1993;1:267.
46. Merz H, Rickers O, Schrimel S, et al. Constant detection of surface and cytoplasmic immunoglobulin heavy and light chain expression in formalin-fixed and paraffin-embedded material. *J Pathol.* 1993;170:257.
47. Shi S-R, Chaiwun B, Young L, et al. Antigen retrieval using pH 3.5 glycine-HCl buffer or urea solution for immunohistochemical localization of Ki-67. *Biotech Histochem.* 1994;69:213.
48. Shi S-R, Cote RJ, Yang C, et al. Development of an optimal protocol for antigen retrieval: A "test battery" approach exemplified with reference to the staining of retinoblastoma protein (pRB) in formalin-fixed paraffin sections. *J Pathol.* 1996;179:347.
49. Shi S-R, Cote RJ, Young L, et al. Use of pH 9.5 TRIS-HCl buffer containing 5% urea for antigen retrieval immunohistochemistry. *Biotech Histochem.* 1996;71:190.
50. Shi S-R, Imam SA, Young L, et al. Antigen retrieval immunohistochemistry under the influence of pH using monoclonal antibodies. *J Histochem Cytochem.* 1995;43:193.
51. Shi S-R, Gu J, Kalra KL, et al. Antigen retrieval technique: A novel approach to immunohistochemistry on routinely processed tissue sections. *Cell Vision.* 1995;2:6.

52. Suurmeijer AJ, Boon ME. Notes on the application of microwaves for antigen retrieval in paraffin and plastic tissue sections. *Eur J Morphol.* 1993;31:144.
53. Taylor CR, Shi S-R, Chaiwun B, et al. Strategies for improving the immunohistochemical staining of various intranuclear prognostic markers in formalin-paraffin sections: Androgen receptor, estrogen receptor, progesterone receptor, p53 protein, proliferating cell nuclear antigen, and Ki-67 antigen revealed by antigen retrieval techniques [see comments]. *Hum Pathol.* 1994;25:263.
54. von Wasielewski R, Werner M, Nolte M, et al. Effects of antigen retrieval by microwave heating in formalin-fixed tissue sections on a broad panel of antibodies. *Histochemistry.* 1994;102:165.
55. Shi S-R, Cote RJ, Taylor CR. Antigen retrieval immunohistochemistry: Past, present, and future. *J Histochem Cytochem.* 1997;45:327.
56. Shi S-R, Cote RJ, Young LL, et al. Antigen retrieval immunohistochemistry and molecular morphology in the year 2001. *Appl Immunohistochem Mol Morphol.* 2001;9:107.
57. Shi S-R, Cote RJ, Taylor CR. Antigen retrieval techniques: current perspectives. *J Histochem Cytochem.* 2001;49:931.
58. Shi S-R, Gu J, Kalra KL, et al. Antigen retrieval technique: A novel approach to immunohistochemistry on routinely processed tissue sections. In: Gu J, ed. *Analytical Morphology: Theory, Applications & Protocols.* Natick, MA: Eaton; 1997:1.
59. Shi Y, Li G-D, Liu W-P. Recent advances of the antigen retrieval technique. *Linchuang yu Shiyan Binglixue Zazhi (J Clin Exp Pathol).* 1997;13:265.
60. Shi S-R, Gu J, Taylor CR, eds. *Antigen Retrieval Techniques: Immunohistochemistry and Molecular Morphology.* Natick, MA: Eaton; 2000.
61. Shi S-R, Gu J, Turrens F, et al. Development of the antigen retrieval technique: Philosophy and theoretical base. In: Shi S-R, Gu J, Taylor CR, eds. *Antigen Retrieval Techniques: Immunohistochemistry and Molecular Morphology.* Natick, MA: Eaton; 2000:17-39.
62. Mann G, ed. *Physiologic histology.* Oxford: Oxford University Press; 1902.
63. van Regenmortel MHV. The recognition of proteins and peptides by antibodies. In: van Oss CJ, van Regenmortel MHV, eds. *Immunochemistry.* New York: Marcel Dekker; 1994:277-300.
64. Barlow DJ, Edwards MS, Thornton JM. Continuous and discontinuous protein antigenic determinants. *Nature.* 1986;322:747.
65. Johnson CW. Issues in immunohistochemistry. *Toxicol Pathol.* 1999;27:246.
66. Nilsson P, Paavilainen L, Larsson K, et al. Towards a human proteome atlas: High-throughput generation of mono-specific antibodies for tissue profiling. *Proteomics.* 2005;5:4327.
67. Streefkerk JG. Inhibition of erythrocyte pseudoperoxidase activity by treatment with hydrogen peroxide following methanol. *J Histochem Cytochem.* 1972;29:829.
68. Burns J. Background staining and sensitivity of the unlabeled antibody-enzyme (PAP) method: Comparison with the peroxidase-labeled antibody sandwich method using formalin-fixed paraffin embedded material. *Histochemistry.* 1975;43:291.
69. Weir EE, Pretlow TG, Pitts A. Destruction of endogenous peroxidase activity in order to locate cellular antigens by peroxidase-labeled antibodies. *J Histochem Cytochem.* 1974;22:51.
70. McMillan EM, Martin D, Wasik R, et al. Demonstration in situ of "T" cells and "T" cell subsets in lichen planus using monoclonal antibodies. *J Cutan Pathol.* 1981;8:228.
71. Straus W. Phenylhydrazine as inhibitor of horseradish peroxidase for use in immunoperoxidase procedures. *J Histochem Cytochem.* 1972;20:949.
72. Straus W. Use of peroxidase inhibitors for immunoperoxidase procedures. In: Feldman R, ed. *Proceedings of the first international symposium on immunoenzymatic techniques.* Amsterdam: Elsevier; 1976:117.
73. Andrew SM, Jasani B. An improved method for the inhibition of endogenous peroxidase non-deleterious to lymphocyte surface markers: Application to immunoperoxidase studies on eosinophil-rich tissue preparations. *Histochem J.* 1987;35:426.
74. Li C-Y, Zeismer SC, Lacano-Villareal O. Use of azide and hydrogen peroxide as an inhibitor for endogenous peroxidase method. *J Histochem Cytochem.* 1987;35:1457.
75. Schmid KW, Hittmair A, Schmidhammer H, et al. Non-deleterious inhibition of endogenous peroxidase activity (EPA) by cyclopropanone hydrate: A definitive approach. *J Histochem Cytochem.* 1989;37:473.
76. Robinson G, Dawson I. Immunochemical studies of the endocrine cells of the gastrointestinal tract. I: The use and value of peroxidase-conjugated antibody techniques for the localization of gastrin-containing cells in human pyloric antrum. *Histochem J.* 1975;7:321.
77. Mason TE, Phifer RF, Spicer SS, et al. An immunoglobulin enzyme bridge method for localizing tissue antigens. *J Histochem Cytochem.* 1969;17:573.
78. Sternberger LA, ed. *Immunocytochemistry.* Englewood Cliffs, NJ: Prentice-Hall; 1974.
79. Cordell JL, Falini B, Erber WN, et al. Immunoenzymatic label of monoclonal antibodies using immune complexes of alkaline phosphatase and monoclonal anti-alkaline phosphatase (APAAP) complexes. *J Histochem Cytochem.* 1984;32:219.
80. Erber WN, McLachlan J. Use of APAAP technique on paraffin wax embedded bone marrow trephines. *J Clin Pathol.* 1989;42:1201.
81. Wagner L, Worman CP. Color-contrast staining of two different lymphocyte subpopulations: A two-color modification of alkaline phosphatase monoclonal anti-alkaline phosphatase complex technique. *Stain Technol.* 1988;63:129.
82. Wong SY, Carrol EDS, Ah-See SY, et al. Detection of estrogen receptor proteins in breast tumors using an improved APAAP immunohistochemical technique. *Cancer.* 1988;62:2171.
83. Vardiman JW, Gilewski TA, Ratain MJ, et al. Evaluation of Leu-M5 (CDIIc) in hairy cell leukemia by the alkaline phosphatase anti-phosphatase technique. *Am J Clin Pathol.* 988;90:250.
84. Sano T, Smith CL, Cantor CR. Immuno-PCR: Very sensitive antigen detection by means of specific antibody-DNA conjugates. *Science.* 1992;258:120.
85. Chen B-X, Szabolcs MJ, Matsushima AY, et al. A strategy for immunohistochemical signal enhancement by end-product amplification. *J Histochem Cytochem.* 1996;44:819.
86. Shi S-R, Guo J, Cote RJ, et al. Sensitivity and detection efficiency of a novel two-step detection system (PowerVision) for immunohistochemistry. *Appl Immunohistochem Mol Morphol.* 1999;7:201.
87. Singh P, Moll F, Lin SH, et al. Starburst dendrimers: Enhanced performance and flexibility for immunoassays. *Clin Chem.* 1994;40:1845.
88. Van der Loos CM, Naruko T, Becker AE. The use of enhanced polymer one-step staining reagents for immunoenzyme double-labeling. *Histochemical J.* 1996;28:709.
89. Sabattini E, Bisgaard K, Ascani S, et al. The EnVisio++ system: A new immunohistochemical method for diagnostics and research. Critical comparison with APAAP, ChemMate, CSA, LABC and SABC techniques. *J Clin Pathol.* 1998;51:506.
90. Kammerer U, Kapp M, Gassel AM, et al. A new rapid immunohistochemical staining technique using the EnVision Antibody Complex. *J Histochem Cytochem.* 2001;49:623.
91. Bisgaard K, Pluzek K. Use of polymer conjugated in immunohistochemistry; a comparative study of a traditional staining method to a staining method utilizing polymer conjugates [abstract]. *Path Int.* 1996;46:577.
92. Rott T, Velkavrh D. Our experience with the enhanced polymer one-step staining in frozen sections. *Acta Otolaryngol.* 1997;(Suppl 527):114.
93. Tsutsumi Y, Serizawa A, Kawai K. Enhanced polymer one-step staining (EPOS) for proliferation cell nuclear antigen (PCNA) and Ki-67 antigen: Application to intra-operative frozen diagnosis. *Path Int.* 1995;45:108.
94. Heras A, Roach CM, Key ME. Enhanced polymer detection system for immunohistochemistry [abstract]. *Mod Path.* 1996;8:165A.
95. Wiedorn KH, Goldmann T, Henne C, et al. EnVision+, a new dextran polymer-based signal enhancement technique for in situ hybridization (ISH). *J Histochem Cytochem.* 2001;49:1067.

96. Vyberg M, Nielsen S. Dextran polymer conjugate two step visualization system for immunochemistry. A comparison of EnVision+ with two three step avidin biotin techniques. *Applied Immunochem Mol Morphol.* 1998;6:3.
97. Petrosyan K, Tamayo R, Joseph D. Sensitivity of a novel biotin-free detection reagent (Power vision+) for immunohistochemistry. *J Histotechnology.* 2002;25:247.
98. Hansen TP, Nielsen O, Fenger C. Optimization of antibodies for detection of the mismatch repair proteins MLH1, MSH2, MSH6 and PMS2 using a biotin-free visualization system. *Appl Immunohistochem Mol Morphol.* 2006;14:115.
99. Bricca GM, Brodland DG, Zitelli JA. Immunostaining melanoma frozen sections: the 1-hour protocol. *Dermatol Surg.* 2004;30:403.
100. Bobrow MN, Shaughnessy KJ, Litt GJ. Catalyzed reporter deposition, a novel method of signal amplification. II: Application to membrane immunoassays. *J Immunol Methods.* 1991;137:103.
101. Shi S-R, Gu J, Cote RJ, et al. Standardization of routine immunohistochemistry: Where to begin? In Shi S-R, Gu J, Taylor CR, eds. *Antigen retrieval technique: immunohistochemistry and molecular morphology.* Natick, MA: Eaton; 2000:255-272.
102. Toda Y, Kono K, Abiru H, et al. Application of tyramide signal amplification system to immunohistochemistry: A potent method to localize antigens that are not detectable by ordinary method. *Pathol Int.* 1999;49:479.
103. Mengel M, Werner M, von Wasielewski R. Concentration dependent and adverse effects in immunohistochemistry using the tyramine amplification technique. *Histochem J.* 1999;31:195.
104. Kawai K, Osamura RY. Antigen retrieval versus amplification techniques in diagnostic immunohistochemistry. In: Shi S-R, Gu J, Taylor CR, eds. *Antigen retrieval techniques: Immunohistochemistry and molecular morphology.* Natick, MA: Eaton; 2000:249-253.
105. Merz H, Ottesen K, Meyer W, et al. Combination of antigen retrieval techniques and signal amplification of immunohistochemistry in situ hybridization and FISH techniques. In: Shi S-R, Gu J, Taylor CR, eds. *Antigen retrieval techniques: Immunohistochemistry and molecular morphology.* Natick, MA: Eaton; 2000:219-248.
106. College of American Pathologists. *Standard for laboratory accreditation.* Skokie, IL: College of American Pathologists; 1987.
107. Wolff AC, Hammond EH, Schwartz JN, et al. ASCO/CAP Guideline Recommendations for Human Epidermal Growth Factor Receptor 2 testing in Breast Cancer. *J Clin Oncol.* 2007;25:118.
108. Wolff AC, Hammond EH, Schwartz JN, et al. ASCO/CAP Guideline Recommendations for Human Epidermal Growth Factor Receptor 2 testing in Breast Cancer. *Arch Pathol Lab Med.* 2007;131:18.
109. Yaziji H, Taylor CR. Begin at the beginning, with the tissue! The key message underlying the ASCO/CAP Task-Force Guideline Recommendations for HER2 Testing. *Appl Immunohistochem Mol Morphol.* 2007;15:239.
110. Yaziji H, Taylor CR, Goldstein NS, et al, and Members of the Standardization Ad-Hoc Consensus Committee. Consensus Recommendations on Estrogen Receptor Testing in Breast Cancer by Immunohistochemistry. *Appl Immunohistochem Mol Morphol.* 2008;16:513.
111. Goldstein NS, Hewitt SM, Taylor CR, et al, and Members of Ad-Hoc Committee on Immunohistochemistry Standardization. Recommendations for Improved Standardization of Immunohistochemistry. *Appl Immunohistochem Mol Morphol.* 2007;15:124.
112. Rhodes A, Jasani B, Balaton AJ, et al. Frequency of oestrogen and progesterone receptor positivity by immunohistochemical analysis in 7016 breast carcinomas: Correlation with patient age, assay sensitivity, threshold value, and mammographic screening. *J Clin Pathol.* 2000;53:688.
113. Rhodes A, Jasani B, Balaton AJ, et al. Study of interlaboratory reliability and reproducibility of estrogen and progesterone receptor assays in Europe. Documentation of poor reliability and identification of insufficient microwave antigen retrieval time as a major contributory element of unreliable assays. *Am J Clin Pathol.* 2001;115:44.
114. Vani K, Sompuram SR, Fitzgibbons P, et al. National HER2 proficiency test results using standardized quantitative controls: characterization of laboratory failures. *Arch Pathol Lab Med.* 2008;132:211.
115. Taylor CR. The total test approach to standardization of immunohistochemistry. *Arch Pathol Lab Med.* 2000;124:945.
116. Bogen SA, Sompuram SR. Recent trends and advances in immunodiagnostics of solid tumors [review]. *Biodrugs.* 2004;18:387.
117. Sompuram SR, Vani K, Hafer LJ, et al. Antibodies immunoreactive with formalin-fixed tissue antigens recognize linear protein epitopes. *Am J Clin Pathol.* 2006;125:82.
118. Cote RJ, Taylor CR. Immunohistochemistry and Related Marking Techniques. In: Damjanov I, Linder J, eds. *Anderson's Pathology.* 10th ed. St. Louis: CV Mosby; 1996:136-175.
119. Taylor CR. Report of the Immunohistochemistry Steering Committee of the Biological Stain Commission. Proposed format: Package insert for immunohistochemistry products. *Biotech Histochem.* 1992;67:323.
120. Burry RW. Specificity controls for immunocytochemical methods. *J Histochem Cytochem.* 2000;48:163.
121. Swaab DF, Pool CW, VanLeenwen FW. Can specificity ever be proven in immunocytochemical staining? *J Histochem Cytochem.* 1977;25:388.
122. Willingham MC. Conditional epitopes: Is your antibody always specific? *J Histochem Cytochem.* 1999;47:1233.
123. Battifora H. The multitumor (sausage tissue block): Novel method for immunohistochemical antibody testing. *Lab Invest.* 1986;55:244.
124. Battifora H, Mehta P. The checkerboard tissue block: An improved multitissue control block. *Lab Invest.* 1990;63:722.
125. Skacel M, Skilton B, Peltay JD, et al. Tissue microarrays: A powerful tool for high-throughput analysis of clinical specimens: A review of the method with validation data. *Appl Immunohistochem Mol Morphol.* 2002;10:1.
126. Mengel M, Kreipel M, von Wasielewski R. Rapid and large-scale transition of new tumor biomarker to clinical biopsy material by innovative tissue microarray systems. *Appl Immunohistochem Mol Morphol.* 2003;11:261.
127. Battifora H. Assessment of antigen damage in immunohistochemistry: The vimentin internal control. *Am J Clin Pathol.* 1991;96:669.
128. Taylor CR, Levenson RM. Quantification of Immunohistochemistry—issues concerning methods, utility and semiquantitative assessment. *Histopathology.* 2006;49:411.
129. Taylor CR. Quantifiable Internal Reference Standards for Immunohistochemistry; the measurement of quantity by weight. *Applied Immunohistochem Mol Morphol.* 2006;14:253.
130. Conan Doyle A. The Adventures of Sherlock Holmes, The Adventure of the Beryl Coronet. *Strand Magazine.* May 1892.
131. Battifora H, Kopinski M. The influence of protease digestion and duration of fixation on the immunostaining of keratins: A comparison of formalin and ethanol fixation. *J Histochem Cytochem.* 1986;34:1095.
132. Cuevas EC, Bateman AC, Wilkins BS, et al. Microwave antigen retrieval in immunocytochemistry: A study of 80 antibodies. *J Clin Pathol.* 1994;47:448.
133. Leong AS-Y, Gilham PN. The effects of progressive formaldehyde fixation on the preservation of tissue antigens. *Pathology.* 1989;21:266.
134. Shi S-R, Cote RJ, Chaiwun B, et al. Standardization of immunohistochemistry based on antigen retrieval technique for routine formalin-fixed tissue sections. *Appl Immunohistochem.* 1998;6:89.
135. Yokoo H, Nakazato Y. A monoclonal antibody that recognizes a carbohydrate epitope of human protoplasmic astrocytes. *Acta Neuropathol.* 1996;91:30.
136. Prento P, Lyon H. Commercial formalin substitutes for histopathology. *Biotech Histochem.* 1997;72:273.
137. Williams JH, Mepham BL, Wright DH. Tissue preparation for immunocytochemistry. *J Clin Pathol.* 1997;50:801.
138. Allison RT, Best T. p53, PCNA and Ki-67 expression in oral squamous cell carcinomas: The vagaries of fixation and microwave enhancement of immunocytochemistry. *J Oral Pathol Med.* 1998;27:434.

139. Miller RT, Kubier P, Reynolds B, et al. Blocking of endogenous avidin-binding activity in immunohistochemistry. *Appl Immunohistochem Mol Morphol.* 1999;7:63.
140. Zhang PJ, Wang H, Wrona EL, et al. Effects of tissue fixatives on antigen preservation for immunohistochemistry: A comparative study of microwave antigen retrieval on Lillie fixative and neutral buffered formalin. *J Histotechnol.* 1998;21:101.
141. Cote RJ, Shi Y, Groshen S, et al. Association of p27kip1 levels with recurrence and survival in patients with stage C prostate carcinoma. *J Natl Cancer Inst.* 1998;90:916.
142. Grabau KA, Nielsen O, Hansen S. Influence of storage temperature and high-temperature antigen retrieval buffers on results of immunohistochemical staining in sections stored for long periods. *Appl Immunohistochem.* 1998;6:209.
143. Jacobs TW, Prioleau JE, Stillman IE, et al. Loss of tumor marker-immunostaining intensity on stored paraffin slides of breast cancer. *J Natl Cancer Inst.* 1996;88:1054.
144. Kato J, Sakamaki S, Niitsu Y. More on p53 antigen loss in stored paraffin slides. *N Engl J Med.* 1995;333:1507.
145. Prioleau J, Schnitt SI. p53 antigen loss in stored paraffin slides. *N Engl J Med.* 1995;332:1521.
146. Malmstrom PU, Wester K, Vasko J, et al. Expression of proliferative cell nuclear antigen (PCNA) in urinary bladder carcinoma: Evaluation of antigen retrieval methods. *APMIS.* 1992;100:988.
147. Wester K, Wahlund E, Sundstrom C, et al. Paraffin section storage and immunohistochemistry. *Appl Immunohistochem Mol Morphol.* 2000;8:61.
148. Shi S-R, Liu C, Taylor CR. Standardization of immunohistochemistry for formalin-fixed, paraffin-embedded tissue sections based on the antigen-retrieval technique: from experiments to hypothesis. *J Histochem Cytochem.* 2007;55:105.
149. Shi S-R, Liu C, Pootrakul L, et al. Evaluation of the value of frozen tissue section used as "gold standard" for immunohistochemistry. *Am J Clin Pathol.* 2008;129:358.
150. Yamashita S, Okada Y. Application of heat-induced antigen retrieval to aldehyde-fixed fresh frozen sections. *J Histochem Cytochem.* 2005;53:1421.
151. Mason JT, O'Leary TJ. Effects of formaldehyde fixation on protein secondary structure: A calorimetric and infrared spectroscopic investigation. *J Histochem Cytochem.* 1991;39:225.
152. Igarashi H, Sugimura H, Maruyama K. Alteration of immunoreactivity by hydrated autoclaving, microwave treatment, and simple heating of paraffin-embedded tissue sections. *APMIS.* 1994;102:295.
153. Kawai K, Serizawa A, Hamana T, et al. Heat-induced antigen retrieval of proliferating cell nuclear antigen and p53 protein in formalin-fixed, paraffin-embedded sections. *Pathol Int.* 1994;44:759.
154. Rait VK, O'Leary TJ, Mason JT. Modeling formalin fixation and antigen retrieval with bovine pancreatic ribonuclease A: I—Structural and functional alterations. *Lab Invest.* 2004;84:292.
155. Rait VK, Xu L, O'Leary TJ, Mason JT. Modeling formalin fixation and antigen retrieval with bovine pancreatic RBase A II. Interrelationship of cross-linking, immunoreactivity, and heat treatment. *Lab Invest.* 2004;84:300.
156. Sompuram AR, Vani K, Messana E, et al. A molecular mechanism of formalin fixation and antigen retrieval. *Am J Clin Pathol.* 2004;121:190.
157. Sompuram SR, Vani K, Bogen SA. A molecular model of antigen retrieval using a peptide array. *Am J Clin Pathol* 2006;125:91.
157a. Yamashita S, Okada Y: Mechanisms of heat-induced antigen retrieval: analyses in vitro employing SDS-PAGE and immunohistochemistry. *J Histochem Cytochem* 2005;53:13.
158. Evers P, Uylings HB. Microwave-stimulated antigen retrieval is pH and temperature dependent. *J Histochem Cytochem.* 1994;42:1555.
159. Lucassen PJ, Ravid R, Gonatas NK, et al. Activation of the human supraoptic and paraventricular nucleus neurons with aging and in Alzheimer's disease as judged from increasing size of the Golgi apparatus. *Brain Res.* 1993;632:105.
160. Shi S-R, Cote RJ, Taylor CR. Antigen retrieval immunohistochemistry used for routinely processed celloidin-embedded human temporal bone sections: Standardization and development. *Auris Nasus Larynx.* 1998;25:425.
161. Werner M, Von Wasielewski R, Komminoth P. Antigen retrieval, signal amplification and intensification in immunohistochemistry. *Histochem Cell Biol.* 1996;105:253.
162. Katoh A, Breier S. Nonspecific antigen retrieval solutions. *J Histotechnol.* 1994;17:378.
163. O'Reilly PE, Raab SS, Niemann TH, et al. p53, proliferating cell nuclear antigen, and Ki-67 expression in extrauterine leiomyosarcomas. *Mod Pathol.* 1997;10:91.
164. Shin RW, Iwaki T, Kitamoto T, et al. Hydrated autoclave pretreatment enhances tau immunoreactivity in formalin-fixed normal and Alzheimer's disease brain tissues. *Lab Invest.* 1991;64:693.
165. Biddolph SC, Jones M. Low-temperature, heat-mediated antigen retrieval (LTHMAR) on archival lymphoid sections. *Appl Immunohistochem Mol Morphol.* 1999;7:289.
166. Miller RT, Swanson PE, Wick MR. Fixation and epitope retrieval in diagnostic immunohistochemistry: A concise review with practical considerations. *Appl Immunohistochem Mol Morphol.* 2000;8:228.
167. Namimatsu S, Ghazizadeh M, Sugisaki Y. Reversing the effects of formalin fixation with citraconic anhydride and heat: A universal antigen retrieval method. *J Histochem Cytochem.* 2005;53:3.
168. Shi SR, Liu C, Young L, Taylor CR. Development of an optimal antigen retrieval protocol for immunohistochemistry of retinoblastoma protein (pRB) in formalin fixed, paraffin sections based on comparison of different methods. *Biotech Histochem.* 2007;82:301.
169. Boon ME, Kok LP, Moorlag HE, et al. Accelerated immunogold-silver and immunoperoxidase staining of paraffin sections with the use of microwave irradiation: Factors influencing results. *Am J Clin Pathol.* 1989;91:137.
170. Chiu KY. Use of microwaves for rapid immunoperoxidase staining of paraffin sections. *Med Lab Sci.* 1987;44:3.
171. Choi TS, Whittlesey MM, Slap SE, et al. Advances in temperature control of microwave immunohistochemistry. *Cell Vision.* 1995;2:151.
172. Leong AS-Y, Milios J. Rapid immunoperoxidase staining of lymphocyte antigens using microwave irradiation. *J Pathol.* 1986;148:183.
173. Adams JC. Heavy metal intensification of DAB-based HRP reaction product. *J Histochem Cytochem.* 1981;29:775.
174. Hsu SM, Soban E. Color modification of diaminobenzidine (DAB) precipitation by metallic ions and its application for double immunohistochemistry. *J Histochem Cytochem.* 1982;30:1079.
175. Lan HY, Mu W, Nikolic-Paterson DJ, et al. A novel, simple, reliable, and sensitive method for multiple immunoenzyme staining: Use of microwave oven heating to block antibody crossreactivity and retrieve antigens. *J Histochem Cytochem.* 1995;43:97.
176. Mason DY, Sammons R. Alkaline phosphatase and peroxidase for double immunoenzymatic labeling of cellular constituents. *J Clin Pathol.* 1978;31:454.
177. Van Rooijen N. Six methods for separate detection of two different antigens in the same tissue section. *J Histochem Cytochem.* 1980;28:716.
178. Krenacs T, Laszik Z, Dobo E. Application of immunogold-silver staining and immunoenzymatic methods in multiple labeling of human pancreatic Langerhans islet cells. *Acta Histochem.* 1989;85:79.
179. Lehr HA, van der Loos CM, Teeling P, et al. Complete chromogen separation and analysis in double immunohistochemical stains using Photoshop-based image analysis. *J Histochem Cytochem.* 1999;47:119.
180. Herman GE, Elfont EA, Floyd AD. Overview of automated immunostainers. *Methods Mol Biol.* 1994;34:383.
181. Le Neel T, Moreau A, Laboisse C, et al. Comparative evaluation of automated systems in immunohistochemistry. *Clin Chim Acta.* 1998;278:185.
182. Fetsch PA, Abati A. Overview of the clinical immunohistochemistry laboratory: Regulations and troubleshooting guidelines. *Methods Mol Biol.* 1999;115:405.
183. Moreau A, Le Neel T, Joubert M, et al. Approach to automation in immunohistochemistry. *Clin Chim Acta.* 1998;278:177.

184. Bauer KD, Hawes D, de la Torre-Bueno J, et al. Analysis of occult bone marrow metastases using automated cellular imaging. *Mod Pathol.* 2000;13:220A.
185. Makarewicz K, McDuffe L, Shi S-R, et al. Immunohistochemical detection of occult metastases using an automated intelligent microscopy system. Presented at the 88th annual meeting of the American Association of Cancer Research, San Diego, CA, 1997:269.
186. Martin W, Chon A, Fabiono A, et al. Effect of formalin tissue fixation and processing on immunohistochemistry. *Am J Surg Pathol.* 2000;24:1016.
187. Rickers RR, Malinisk RM. Intralaboratory quality assurance of immunohistochemical procedures: Recommended practices for daily application. *Arch Pathol Lab Med.* 1989;113:673.
188. van der Ploeg M, Duijndam WAL. Matrix models: Essential tools for microscopic cytochemical research. *Histochemistry.* 1986;84:283.
189. Riera J, Simpson JF, Tamayo R, et al. Use of cultured cells as a control for quantitative immunocytochemical analysis of estrogen receptor in breast cancer: The Quicgel method. *Am J Clin Pathol.* 1999;111:329.

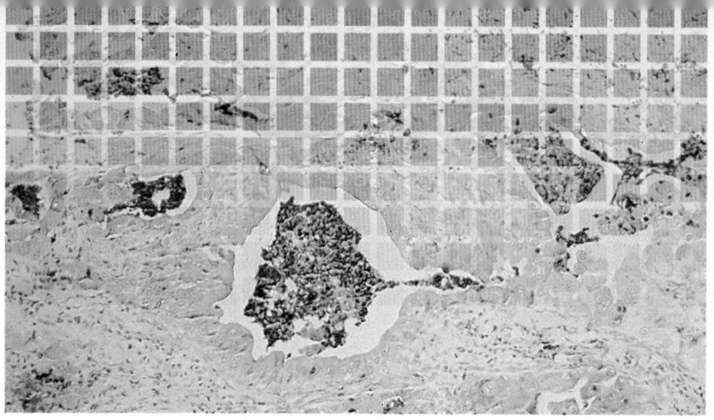

2

Molecular Anatomic Pathology: Principles, Techniques, and Application to Immunohistologic Diagnosis

Marina N. Nikiforova • Yuri E. Nikiforov

- General Principles of Molecular Biology 42
- Genetic Polymorphism and Mutations 44
- Specimen Requirements for Molecular Testing 44
- Common Techniques for Molecular Analysis 45
- Detection of Small-Scale Mutations 50
- Detection of Chromosomal Rearrangements 51
- Detection of Chromosomal Deletions/ Loss of Heterozygosity Analysis 52
- Detection of Microsatellite Instability 53
- DNA-Based Tissue Identity Testing 54

GENERAL PRINCIPLES OF MOLECULAR BIOLOGY

Immunohistochemistry is a common technique used to detect protein expression in various tissue samples. In the modern pathology practice, this methodology is expanded and complemented by molecular techniques that test for changes in nucleic acids (i.e., DNA and RNA) to assist the immunohistologic diagnosis.

In many of the chapters in this book, we will refer to theranostic and genomic principles that can be investigated with immunohistology and used directly for patient care. The underpinnings of these immunohistologic tests require an understanding of the molecular abnormalities of these disease states and how molecular methods apply to their study. In addition, the molecular methods discussed here may be valuable in diagnosis when immunohistologic results are nonspecific.

DNA

Genetic information in human cells is encoded in deoxyribonucleic acid (DNA), which is primarily located in the nucleus of each cell. DNA is a double-stranded molecule that consists of two complementary strands of linearly arranged nucleotides, each composed of a phosphorylated sugar and one of four nitrogen-containing bases: adenine (A), guanine (G), thymine (T), or cytosine (C). The order of these four bases encodes genetic information. Two strands of DNA run in opposite directions and are held together through pairing between specific bases. For example, adenine and thymine (A:T pairing) and guanine and cytosine (G:C pairing) form a double-stranded helix. As a result, the nucleotide sequence of one DNA strand is complementary to the nucleotide sequence of the other DNA strand.[1]

The human genome contains approximately 3 billion base pairs (bp) of DNA. The DNA is folded to fit within the nucleus. It is divided among chromosomes and compactly packed into chromatin by histones and other accessory proteins. Each normal somatic cell contains two copies of 22 different somatic chromosomes and two sex chromosomes (XX or XY). Less than 5% of DNA actually encodes protein and other functional products, such as tRNA, rRNA, miRNA, and other small nuclear RNAs.[2] The majority (>95%) of human DNA consists of non-coding sequences, typically repetitive sequences such as minisatellites, microsatellites, SINEs, and LINEs. Microsatellites are short tandem repeats with each repeat unit of 1 to 13 bp long. Minisatellites are tandemly repeated DNA sequences with the size of repeat unit of 14 to 500 bp. Microsatellite and minisatellite repeats are also known as short tandem repeats (STRs). Highly repetitive sequences containing thousands of repeated units are also found at the

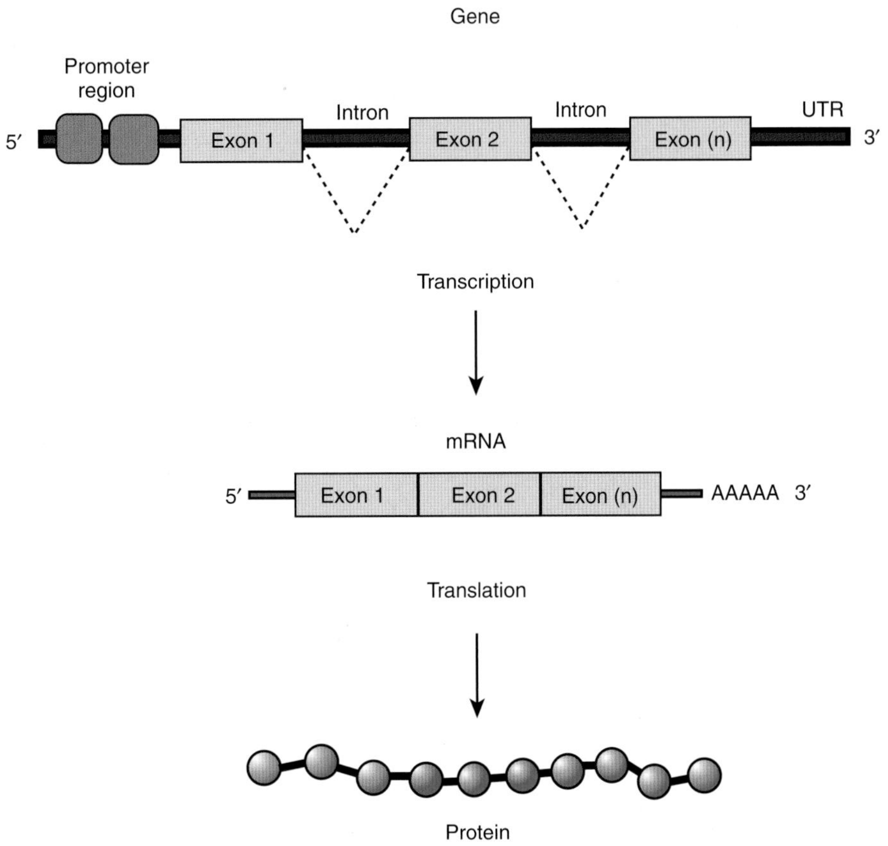

FIGURE 2.1 Gene structure on the DNA level and the process of transcription and translation. Genes are segments of DNA that contain protein-coding regions (exons), non-coding regions (introns), and regulatory regions including promoter and enhancer sequences. In the mature mRNA, only protein-coding parts, i.e., exons, are preserved, and they contain genetic information needed for the protein synthesis.

telomeric ends of the chromosomes and in the areas of centromere; they play a role in establishing and maintaining chromosome structure and stability.

In order to decode genetic information, the DNA is copied (transcribed) into mRNA, which then is translocated into the cytoplasm where it governs translation into protein (Fig. 2.1). Genes are segments of genomic DNA that encode proteins and other functional products. Each gene is typically present in a cell in two copies: One is on a maternal chromosome, and the other is on a paternal chromosome. Current estimations suggest that about 25,000 distinct genes are present in the human genome. Each gene typically consists of exons, which are protein-coding sequences, and introns, which are non-coding sequences located between the coding regions (see Fig. 2.1).[3] Transcription initiation codon and transcription termination codon flank the portion of a gene that codes for a protein. Gene transcription and silencing is facilitated by promoters and enhancers (DNA regions typically located close and upstream of the gene they regulate, but sometimes located a distance from the gene).

RNA

Ribonucleic acid (RNA) is a single-stranded molecule that consists of a chain of nucleotides on a sugar-phosphate backbone. However, in RNA the sugar is ribose rather than deoxyribose, and thymine is replaced by uracil. RNA is more susceptible to chemical and enzymatic hydrolysis and is less stable than DNA.[4]

There are several types of RNA that are different in their structure, function, and location. The most abundant types of RNA are ribosomal RNA (rRNA) and transfer RNA (tRNA), which compose up to 90% of the total cellular RNA. They are predominantly located in the cytoplasm and have important functions in protein synthesis. In a complex with specific proteins, rRNA forms ribosomes on which proteins are synthesized. During protein synthesis, tRNA is responsible for carrying and adding the amino acid to the growing polypeptide chain. Messenger RNA (mRNA) composes 1% to 5% of total RNA. Each mRNA molecule is a copy of a specific gene and functions to transfer genetic information from the nucleus to the cytoplasm, where it serves as a blueprint for protein synthesis. The gene sequence is first transcribed into the primary RNA transcript by RNA polymerase. This transcript is an exact complementary copy of the gene, including all exons and introns. Intron portions are spliced out from the primary RNA transcript while it is processed into mature mRNA (see Fig. 2.1).[5] Other types of RNA include heterogeneous nuclear RNA (hnRNA) and small nuclear RNA (snRNA). Recently, several classes of short RNAs have been discovered, such as the microRNA class (19- to 22-nt single-stranded molecules that function as negative regulators of the coding gene expression).[6,7]

Protein

The abundance of a particular protein within each cell depends on the expression levels of the gene (i.e., how many mRNA copies are transcribed from DNA) and stability of the protein. Proteins are synthesized on ribosomes in the cell cytoplasm. mRNA carries genetic information to the ribosomes. Ribosomes then direct the assembly of polypeptide chains by reading a three-letter genetic code on the mRNA and pairing it with a complementary tRNA that is linked to an amino acid. The three-bases code, called a *codon,* defines which specific amino acid is added by the tRNA to the growing polypeptide chain. After synthesis, the protein undergoes post-translational modification, such as chain cleavage, chain joining, addition of non-protein groups, and folding into a complex, tridimensional structure.

GENETIC POLYMORPHISM AND MUTATIONS

Variations in DNA sequence are common among individuals. Genetic polymorphism is an alteration in DNA sequences found in the general population at a frequency greater than 1%. Polymorphism may be associated with a single nucleotide change; this is known as a *single nucleotide polymorphism (SNP).* It may also be associated with a variation in a number of repetitive DNA sequences (e.g., minisatellites or microsatellites); this is called *length polymorphism.* Usually genetic polymorphism does not directly cause the disease but rather serves a predisposing factor.

Mutation is a permanent alteration of the DNA sequence of a gene that is found in less than 1% of population and most likely causes a disease. Mutations can be either *germline* (i.e., present in all cells of the body) or *somatic* (i.e., found in tumor cells only). Somatic mutations may provide a selective advantage for cell growth and initiate cancer development, but they are not transmitted to offspring. In contrast, germline mutations are passed on to the next generation.

Mutations can be classified based on size and structure into small-scale mutations (sequence mutations) and large-scale mutations (chromosomal alterations).

Small-scale mutations include point mutations, which are single nucleotide substitutions, and small deletion and insertion mutations. *Point mutations* can be further classified into (1) *missense mutations,* which lead to amino acid change and result in production of abnormal protein, (2) *silent mutations,* which do not lead to a change in amino acid, and (3) *nonsense mutations,* in which substitution of a single nucleotide results in formation of a stop codon and a truncated protein. *Deletion and insertion mutations* result in deletion or insertion of a number of nucleotides that is divisible by 3. This leads to a change in the number of amino acids and a shorter or longer protein, or to an insertion or deletion of a number of nucleotides that is not divisible by 3. This will cause a shift in the open reading frame of the gene, thus affecting multiple amino acids and typically producing a stop codon and protein truncation.

Large-scale mutations can be due to one of the following four causes:

1. *Numerical chromosomal change,* which is the loss or duplication of the entire chromosome
2. *Chromosomal rearrangement,* which is a translocation or inversion that initiates an exchange of chromosomal segments (between two nonhomologous chromosomes or within the same chromosome) and typically leads to activation of specific genes located at the fusion point
3. *Amplification,* the process in which a particular chromosomal region is repeated multiple times on the same chromosome (or different chromosomes) and results in an increased copy number of the gene located in that region
4. *Chromosomal deletion* or *loss of heterozygosity* (LOH), which occurs when deletion of a discrete chromosomal region leads to loss of a tumor suppressor gene residing in this area

Functional consequences of each mutation type vary. Generally, mutations result in either activation of the gene, typically forming an oncogene (e.g., *KRAS, RET*), or loss of function of a tumor suppressor gene (*TP53, PTEN, CDKN1A*).

SPECIMEN REQUIREMENTS FOR MOLECULAR TESTING

Molecular testing in surgical pathology can be performed on a variety of clinical samples, including fresh or snap-frozen tissue, formalin-fixed paraffin-embedded (FFPE) tissue, cytology specimens (fresh and fixed fine-needle aspiration [FNA] samples), blood, bone marrow, and buccal swabs. Specimen requirement depends on the type of the disease and on molecular techniques used for the analysis. Peripheral blood lymphocytes or cells from buccal swabs are typically used for detection of germline mutations responsible for a given inherited disease, such as *RET* mutations in familiar medullary thyroid carcinoma. Blood and bone marrow biopsy material is frequently used for detection of chromosomal rearrangements in hematologic malignancies (e.g., *BCR/ABL* in acute lymphocytic leukemia). Tumor tissue samples are required to detect somatic mutations such as *KRAS* point mutation in colorectal cancer, *SYT/SSX* rearrangement in synovial sarcomas, or *EGFR* mutation in lung adenocarcinomas.

Fresh or snap-frozen tissue is the best sample for testing because freezing minimizes degradation and provides excellent quality of DNA, RNA, and protein. Such specimens can be successfully used for any type of molecular analysis, including detection of somatic mutations, chromosomal rearrangements, gene expression arrays, miRNA profiling, and so on. FFPE tissue samples or fixed cytology specimens do not provide well-preserved nucleic acids; however, one can use these specimens for molecular testing in many test situations, particularly those that require DNA.

RNA molecules are less stable than DNA molecules. They are easily degraded by a variety of ribonuclease enzymes that present in abundance in the cell and in its environment. Therefore, only freshly collected or frozen samples are considered to be universally acceptable for RNA-based testing. RNA isolated from FFPE tissue is of poor quality and can be used for some but not all applications, particularly in a setting of clinical diagnostic testing.

The amount of tissue required for molecular testing depends on the sensitivity of the particular technique used and on the purity of the tumor sample (i.e., the proportion of tumor cells in a given specimen). Manual or laser capture microdissection can be used to enrich the tumor cell population.

For molecular testing of hematologic specimens, blood and bone marrow should be collected in the presence of anticoagulants EDTA or ACD, but not heparin. This is because even a small residual concentration of heparin will inhibit PCR amplification.

Conventional cytogenetic analysis requires fresh tissue. Fluorescence *in situ* hybridization (FISH) can be performed on a variety of specimens including frozen tissue sections, touch preps, paraffin-embedded tissue sections, and cytology slides.

COMMON TECHNIQUES FOR MOLECULAR ANALYSIS

Polymerase Chain Reaction

Polymerase chain reaction (PCR) is an amplification technique that is most frequently used in molecular laboratories. The introduction of PCR has increased dramatically the speed and accuracy of DNA and RNA analysis. The PCR is based on exponential and bidirectional amplification of DNA sequences using a set of oligonucleotide primers.[8]

Every PCR run must include the DNA template, two primers complementary to the target sequence, four deoxynucleotide triphosphates (dATP, dCTP, dGTP, dTTP), DNA polymerase, and $MgCl_2$ mixed in the reaction buffer. There are three steps in the PCR cycle (Fig. 2.2). First, the reaction mixture is heated to a high temperature (95°C), which leads to DNA denaturing (i.e., separation of the double-stranded DNA into two

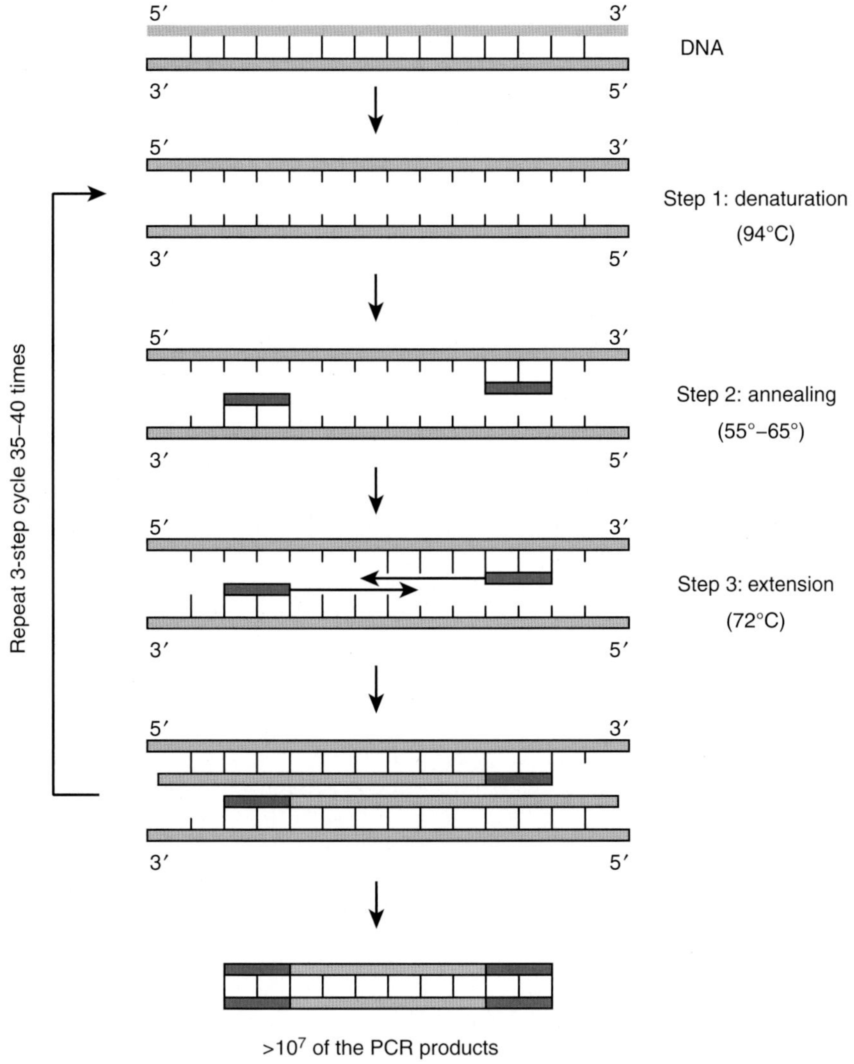

FIGURE 2.2 Schematic representation of a polymerase chain reaction (PCR). The three-step cycle of denaturation, annealing, and extension is repeated 35 to 40 times to generate more than 10^7 copies of the targeted DNA fragment.

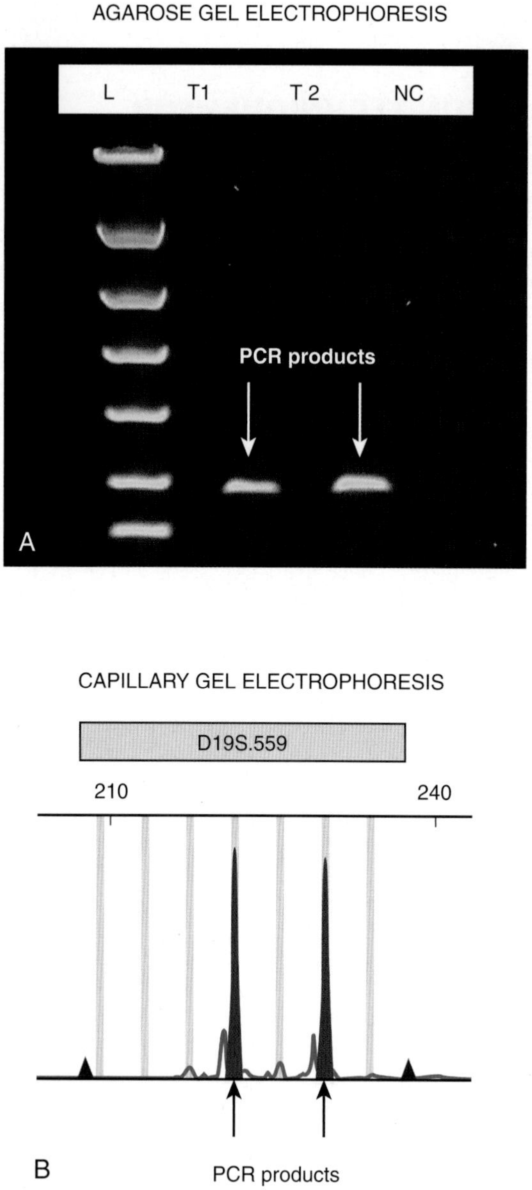

FIGURE 2.3 Post-PCR detection of amplification products. **(A)** Agarose gel electrophoresis showing two PCR products obtained using DNA from two tumor samples, T1 and T2, which are of similar size. L, DNA ladder (size marker); NC, negative control. **(B)** Capillary gel electrophoresis showing two PCR products of different sizes.

single strands). The second step involves annealing primers; the reaction is cooled to 55° to 65°C to allow primers to attach to their complementary sequences. In the third step, DNA extension, the reaction is heated to 72°C to allow DNA polymerase to build a new DNA strand by adding specific nucleotides to the attached primers. These three steps are repeated 35 to 40 times. During each cycle, the newly synthesized DNA strands serve as a template for further DNA synthesis. This results in an exponential increase in the amount of a targeted DNA sequence and production of 10^7 to 10^{11} copies from a single DNA molecule.

The efficiency of PCR amplification depends on many factors, including the quality of isolated DNA template, size of PCR product, optimal primer design, and optimal conditions of the reaction. High-quality DNA allows amplification of long products (up to 5 kb). However, when dealing with suboptimal-quality DNA (i.e., when DNA is isolated from fixed tissue or cytology preparation), one can only achieve a reliable amplification of relatively short DNA sequences (400 to 500 bp or shorter).

Once the PCR procedure is complete, the products of amplification should be visualized for analysis and interpretation. Agarose gel electrophoresis and ethidium bromide staining can achieve this; however, they cannot separate amplification products that differ in size by only a few nucleotides. Polyacrylamide gel electrophoresis or capillary gel electrophoresis can achieve a finer separation (Fig 2.3A,B). PCR amplification followed by gel electrophoresis is frequently used for detection of small deletions or insertions, microsatellite instability, and LOH. For detection of point mutations, the PCR products should be interrogated by other molecular techniques.

Reverse Transcription PCR

Reverse transcription PCR (RT-PCR) is a modification of the standard PCR technique that can be used to amplify mRNA. The first step is to convert isolated mRNA to a complementary DNA (cDNA) molecule using an RNA-dependent DNA polymerase (also known as reverse transcriptase) during a process called *reverse transcription (RT)*. The complementary DNA can be used as any other DNA molecule for PCR amplification. The primers used for cDNA synthesis can be either non–sequence-specific primers (a mixture of random hexamers or oligo-dT primers) or sequence-specific primers (Fig. 2.4). Random hexamers are a mixture of all possible combinations of six nucleotide sequences that can attach randomly to mRNA and initiate reverse transcription of the entire RNA pool. Oligo-dT primers are complementary to the poly-A tail of mRNA molecules and allow synthesis of cDNA only from mRNA molecules. Sequence-specific primers are the most restricted because they are designed to bind selectively to mRNA molecules of interest, which makes reverse transcription a target-specific process.

Reverse transcription and PCR amplification can be performed as a two-step process in a single tube or with two separate reactions.[9] RT-PCR performed on fresh-frozen tissue provides high-quality amplification and reliable results. However, when FFPE tissue is used for RT-PCR analysis, the results vary and depend on the level of RNA degradation and length of PCR amplification. To attain a more stable RT-PCR amplification from FFPE tissues, it is typical to choose a target that is less than 150 to 200 nt long.

RT-PCR analysis is employed in molecular laboratories to detect gene rearrangements and gene expression. RT-PCR may also be used to amplify several exonic sequences in one reaction. This is because it can benefit from the fact that all introns are spliced out in mRNA, which leaves the coding sequences intact and significantly shortens the potential product of

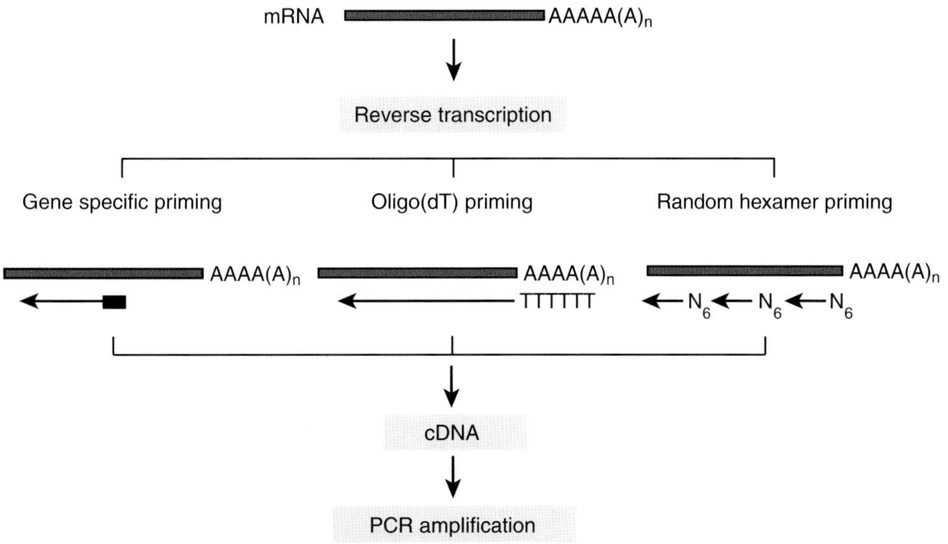

FIGURE 2.4 Principles of RT-PCR. During reverse transcription, mRNA is used to build a cDNA molecule by using either gene-specific, oligo (dT), or random hexamer (N_6) priming. cDNA then can be used as a template for PCR amplification.

amplification. However, it is important to recognize that RNA must be handled with great care during the entire process of reverse transcription in order to avoid degradation.[10] Amplification of a housekeeping gene must accompany each RT-PCR reaction as an internal control to monitor the quality and quantity of RNA in a given sample.

Real-Time PCR

Real-time PCR utilizes the main principles of conventional PCR but detects and quantifies the PCR product in *real time* as the reaction progresses. In addition to all components of conventional PCR, real-time PCR employs fluorescently labeled molecules for the visualization of PCR amplicons. It can be performed in two main formats. The first method incorporates DNA dyes (e.g., SYBR Green 1, SYTO 9, EvaGreen, or LC Green) into the PCR product. The second method takes advantage of fluorescently labeled probes such as FRET hybridization or TaqMan probes, which anneal to the PCR product.[11,12] During the PCR reaction, a PCR instrument detects an increasing amount of fluorescence, which results from an exponential increase in the amount of amplified DNA sequence. The instrument software allows one to construct an amplification plot of fluorescence intensity versus cycle number. During the early cycles, the amount of PCR product is low and fluorescence is not sufficient to exceed the baseline. As the PCR product accumulates, the fluorescence signal crosses the baseline and increases exponentially (Fig. 2.5). At the end of the PCR reaction, the fluorescence reaches a plateau as most of the reagents are consumed.

Real-time detection of amplification allows the real-time detection of PCR product and eliminates the need for subsequent gel electrophoresis. Another advantage is that it can use post-PCR melting curve analysis to detect sequence variations at the specific locus. For example, in the LightCycler probe format, hybridization probes bind to the PCR product in a head-to-tail fashion and initiate a fluorescence resonance energy transfer (FRET) from one probe to the other, and the detected fluorescence is proportional to the amount of amplified product.[13] During post-PCR melting curve analysis, the PCR product is gradually heated and fluorescence is measured at each temperature point. During this process, even a single mismatch between the labeled probe and the amplified sequence will significantly reduce the melting temperature (T_m), which is defined as the temperature at which 50% of the double-stranded DNA becomes single-stranded DNA. Therefore, the presence of a point mutation or single nucleotide polymorphism in the region covered by a fluorescent probe will be detected as an additional T_m peak on melting curve analysis (see Fig. 2.5).

Quantitative PCR (qPCR) is a variation of real-time PCR that can be used to evaluate gene expression levels or gene copy numbers. Quantitative assessment of the initial template used for PCR amplification can be attained by comparing the amount of PCR product of the target sequence with the PCR products generated by amplification of the known quantities of DNA or cDNA.

Real-time PCR is frequently used in molecular laboratories because it is a rapid, less laborious technique as compared to other techniques and does not require processing of samples after PCR amplification. This minimizes procedure time and risk of contamination by previous PCR products.

Restriction Fragment Length Polymorphism Analysis

Restriction enzymes (restriction endonucleases) are enzymes that cut DNA at specific nucleotide sequences known as *restriction sites*. The restriction sites are

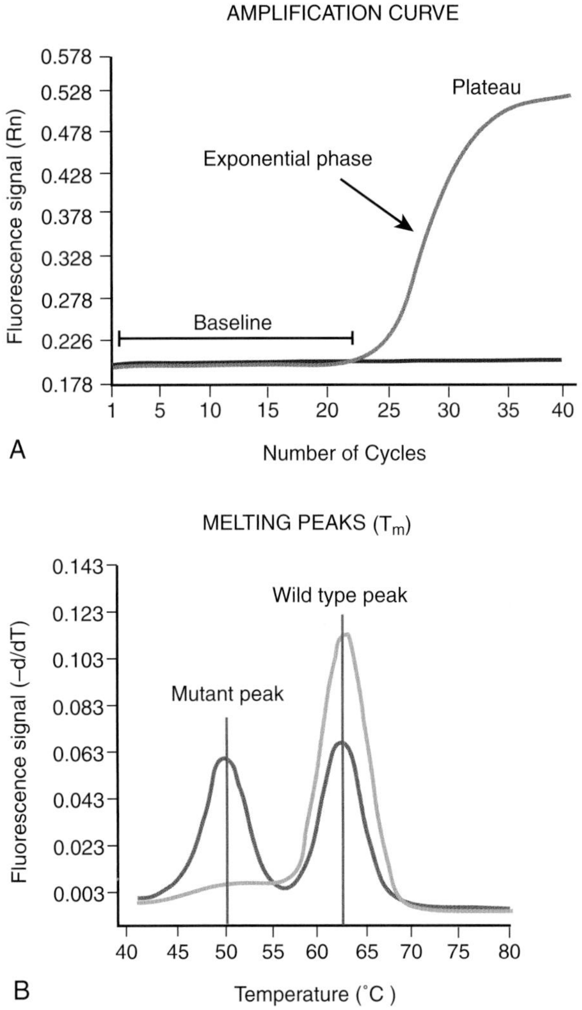

FIGURE 2.5 Real-time PCR. **(A)** Amplification plot showing low amount of fluorescence during the initial cycles of amplification (baseline), followed by exponential increase in fluorescence during the exponential phase, and final plateau at the end of PCR reaction. **(B)** Post-PCR melting curve analysis demonstrating a single melting peak in the normal DNA sample (wild-type peak) and two melting peaks in the tumor sample, one at the same melting temperature (T_m) as the wild-type peak and another lower T_m peak due to a one-nucleotide mismatch with the probe (mutant peak).

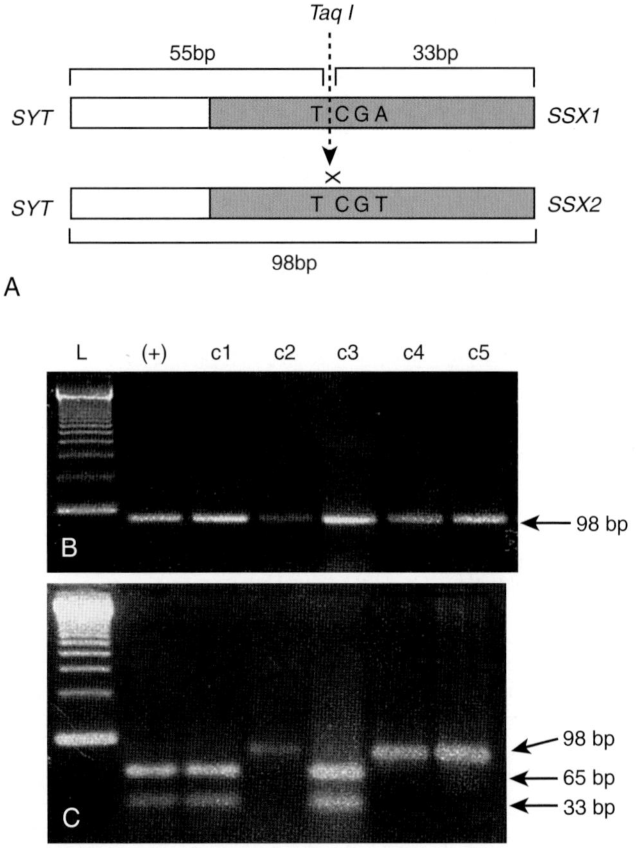

FIGURE 2.6 PCR-RFLP detection of *SYT/SSX1* and *SYT/SSX2* rearrangements in synovial sarcoma. **(A)** *Taq I* restriction enzyme cuts the *SYT/SSX1* fusion DNA into two fragments, 55 bp and 33 bp long. The *SYT/SSX2* fragment remains uncut, 98 bp in size. **(B)** Five synovial sarcoma DNA samples (c1 to c5) are PCR amplified with primers complementary to both *SYT/SSX1* and *SYT/SSX2* rearrangement types and reveal a 98-bp amplification band in the agarose gel. **(C)** After digestion with *Taq I*, the PCR products from tumors c1 and c3, as well as from the *SYT/SSX1* positive control (+), are cut into two fragments, indicating the presence of *SYT/SSX1* rearrangement, whereas the rest of the tumor samples remain uncut, consistent with *SYT/SSX2*.

usually 4 to 8 nt long and are palindromic (i.e., the DNA sequences are the same in both directions). Restriction fragment length polymorphism (RFLP) analysis exploits the ability of restriction enzymes to cut DNA at these specific sites. If a DNA sequence variation such as a point mutation alters (creates or destroys) the restriction site for a specific enzyme, it will change the size of the PCR product. This can be detected by gel electrophoresis.

RFLP is frequently used to detect known point mutations or single nucleotide polymorphisms (SNP).[14] It can also be used to separate two amplified sequences that are highly similar in nucleotide composition. Figure 2.6 illustrates the usage of PCR-RFLP to differentiate between *SYT/SSX1* and *SYT/SSX2* rearrangements, which are common in synovial sarcomas.

Single-Strand Conformation Polymorphism Analysis

Single-strand conformation polymorphism (SSCP) analysis is a post-PCR technique that can be used to screen for mutations that are not limited to a single hot spot but are randomly distributed throughout the exons. After the PCR amplification of the region of interest, the PCR products are denatured with heat and exposure to denaturing buffer and then subjected to polyacrylamide gel electrophoresis. If mutation is present within the amplified sequence, it will change the folding conformation of the sequence and its electrophoretic mobility. As a result, the wild-type and mutant sequences will migrate differently in the gel. PCR-SSCP analysis can be used as a screening tool for point mutations and small deletions and insertions.[15] However, it cannot detect the precise nucleotide change. This requires the use of an additional technique, such as DNA sequencing.

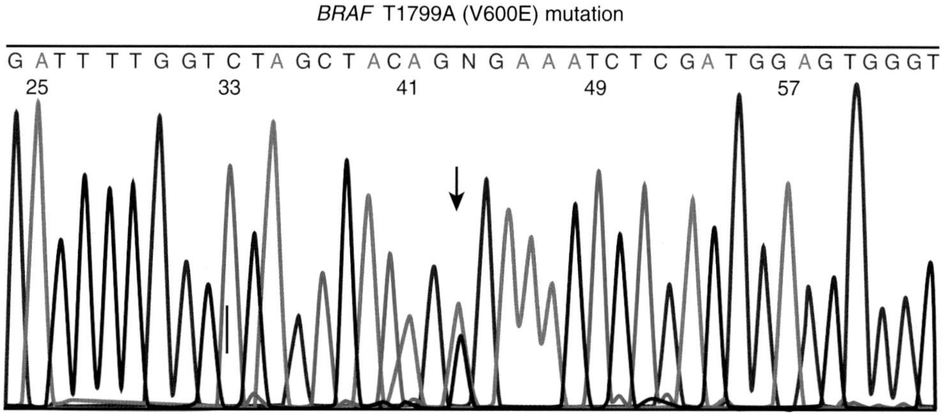

FIGURE 2.7 Sequence electropherogram of the PCR product of *BRAF* exon 15 showing two overlapping peaks at position 1799, which is diagnostic of a T→A mutation at this position.

Allele-Specific PCR and Allele-Specific Hybridization

Allele-specific PCR (AS-PCR) and allele-specific hybridization (ASH), also known as *dot-blot analysis,* are frequently used to detect point mutations and sequence polymorphisms. These methods are based on the fact that PCR amplification and PCR product detection by annealing of a probe are critically dependent on the perfect base pairing of primers or probes with template DNA. Under strict PCR conditions, even one nucleotide mismatch at the 3′ end of the primer will prevent PCR amplification. Similarly, strict hybridization conditions and certain design of an oligonucleotide probe will prevent annealing to the PCR product that differ by a single nucleotide. For AS-PCR, the amplification of target DNA is performed in two reactions. One reaction has primers complementary to a normal (wild-type) sequence, and another reaction has a forward primer complementary to a mutant sequence and a reverse primer complementary to a normal DNA sequence. Amplification is detected by gel electrophoresis or by real-time PCR. Normal DNA will show amplification with primers complementary to the normal sequence and no amplification with mutant-specific primer, whereas the mutant allele will show a reverse pattern of amplification. For ASH, the PCR products are directly spotted on the nylon membrane. After denaturing, the membrane is hybridized with the labeled oligonucleotide probe complementary to a mutant sequence. Both AS-PCR and ASH can be used to detect a specific nucleotide substitution located at a specific position, such as T to A transversion at nucleotide 1799 of *BRAF* [16] or several common point mutations at codons 12/13 of *KRAS*.[17] The methods are very sensitive and must be used with caution as they can detect small (<1%) subclones with mutation within a heterogeneous tumor sample.

DNA Sequencing Analysis

Sanger sequencing is the most common technique used in molecular laboratories to detect the exact nucleotide composition of PCR-amplified DNA fragments. It uses chain-terminating dideoxynucleoside triphosphates (ddNTPs), which terminate its elongation at a particular nucleotide upon incorporation into the growing DNA strand. This results in a mixture of DNA fragments of various lengths, with each fragment corresponding to one of four nucleotides positioned at a specific distance from the beginning of the sequence.[18] The mixture of labeled DNA fragments is separated by gel electrophoresis. The method is currently adopted for automated platforms and utilizes dideoxynucleotides labeled with different fluorescent dyes. An automated sequence analyzer (e.g., ABI 3730) detects the order of nucleotides and depicts them as a sequence electropherogram (Fig. 2.7). The automated sequencing analysis is easy to perform and is routinely used in molecular laboratories to detect various mutations.

Pyrosequencing is another and more recently developed sequencing technology.[19] It is based on the detection of the light emitted during synthesis of a complementary DNA strand for each added nucleotide. The incorporation of deoxynucleotide triphosphate nucleotide into the DNA strand causes the release of pyrophosphate (PPi) molecule in a quantity equimolar to the amount of incorporated nucleotide. The pyrophosphate molecule is then converted to ATP with production of light, which is detected by the instrument and converted to a peak in a pyrogram trace. Each light signal is proportional to the number of nucleotides incorporated. Pyrosequencing can be used to detect point mutations, such as *KRAS* codon 12/13, and methylated CpG islands.[20,21] It is a fast and accurate technique, although it can only analyze short DNA sequences.

Fluorescence *In Situ* Hybridization

Fluorescence *in situ* hybridization (FISH) is a common technique used to detect gene rearrangements, regions of chromosome deletion and amplification, and numerical chromosomal abnormalities. It utilizes fluorescently labeled DNA probes that bind to homologous chromosomal regions and can assay interphase nuclei. FISH can be performed on a variety of tissue specimens including frozen tissue or FFPE tissue sections, touch preparations from fresh or frozen tissue samples, cultured cells, and cytologic smears.

Optimal probe design is an essential part of the FISH technique. Most commercially available and homemade probes are prepared by selecting clones containing the inserted fragments of the DNA of interest. The most frequently used clones are cosmids, P1 artificial chromosomes (PACs), bacterial artificial chromosomes (BACs), and yeast artificial chromosomes (YACs). Some DNA probes can target the centromeric region of a chromosome, so they are ideal for detecting numerical chromosomal abnormalities such as the gain or loss of an entire chromosome. Other probes target the specific region of a chromosome and will detect gene rearrangement, deletion, or amplification. Finally, some probes are designed to hybridize to the full length of a chromosome and can be used to identify multiple regions of gain or loss on a particular chromosome.[22]

During the FISH procedure, DNA within cells placed on a slide and the fluorescently labeled probe of interest are denatured by incubation at high temperature. Then the probe is allowed to hybridize to the target DNA. The next step is a series of post-hybridization washes to remove the probe excess. Finally, after counterstaining the nuclei, the probe signal can be visualized under a fluorescent microscope.

The detection of numerical chromosome changes and regions of gene amplification or deletion typically employs a single probe and one-color FISH. The FISH assay for chromosomal translocations may utilize two strategies. One is a break-apart probe design, where a single probe spanning a gene of interest is used and will demonstrate a split signal in the presence of translocation. Another strategy is a fusion probe design, where two probes corresponding to the genes known to participate in the fusion are labeled with two different fluorochromes. Chromosomal rearrangement will manifest as a pair of fused signals.[23,24] The advantage of the break-apart design is that it can detect all possible translocations involving a particular gene (e.g., all types of translocation of the *EWSR1* gene in Ewing's sarcoma). However, it cannot identify the fusion partner. In contrast, the fusion probe can detect a specific type of rearrangement.

Comparative Genomic Hybridization

Comparative genomic hybridization (CGH) is a hybridization method used to identify gains or losses of a specific chromosomal region within the whole genome.[25-27] The procedure is based on simultaneous hybridization of fluorescently labeled tumor DNA and differently labeled normal reference DNA to the preparation of normal human metaphase chromosomes (standard CGH) or to the BAC library (array CGH). The ratio of fluorescent staining between the tumor and normal samples along the chromosomes is scored. The equal ratio will indicate the normal amount of tumor DNA in a given chromosomal region. The decrease in intensity of the tumor-specific fluorochrome will indicate the region of chromosomal loss, and the increase in intensity will label the regions of gain.

CGH analysis is used as a supplemental technique to conventional cytogenetics. It appears to be more sensitive than conventional cytogenetics and is capable of detecting chromosomal alterations down to 1 Mb in size. In addition, it can be performed using DNA isolated from FFPE specimens.[28]

DNA Microarrays

DNA microarrays can be used to determine expression of multiple genes in a single reaction.[29] They utilize a multiplex spotted microarray technology, where thousands of oligonucleotide probes corresponding to human genes are spotted on a solid surface (gene chip) or on microscopic beads. During the analysis, RNA isolated from a tumor sample is converted into cDNA, labeled, and hybridized to the chip or beads. After hybridization, the microarray is washed to eliminate non-specific binding and scanned to measure the amount of fluorescence from each spot. The intensity of signals is proportional to the abundance of specific cDNA sequences in a given specimen.

DNA microarrays may also be used for whole genome analysis of single nucleotide polymorphisms (SNPs) and for chromosome copy number change.[30]

DETECTION OF SMALL-SCALE MUTATIONS

There are a number of techniques available to detect point mutations and small deletions and insertions. In practice, the choice of method depends on mutation type, location (a known hot spot versus randomly distributed mutations), required sensitivity, specimen type, and test volume.

A variety of molecular techniques are available to detect point mutations at a specific hot spot (e.g., the *KRAS* mutation at codons 12 and 13 or the *BRAF* mutation at codon 600). These methods include real-time PCR amplification and post-PCR melting curve analysis, allele-specific PCR, direct DNA sequencing, pyrosequencing, and PCR-RFLP.[16,20,31-37] All of these methods demonstrate reliable detection of point mutations, such as the *KRAS* mutation in colorectal cancer or the *BRAF* mutation in thyroid cancer.

DNA sequencing analysis of PCR products is considered the gold standard for detection of point mutations. The automated sequencing analysis is typically used in molecular laboratories. For example, a heterozygous *KRAS* mutation in colon cancer will present as two overlapping peaks in the sequencing electropherogram (Fig. 2.8). The sensitivity of this method is in the range of 10% to 30%.

Real-time PCR-based detection methods are also frequently used in clinical molecular laboratories. They may be even more preferable because they are fast and run in a closed PCR system, which reduces the risk of contamination. To detect mutations, two probes complementary to wild-type sequences are designed so that one of the probes spans the known mutation site, such as codons 12 and 13 in the *KRAS* gene.[36] If no mutation

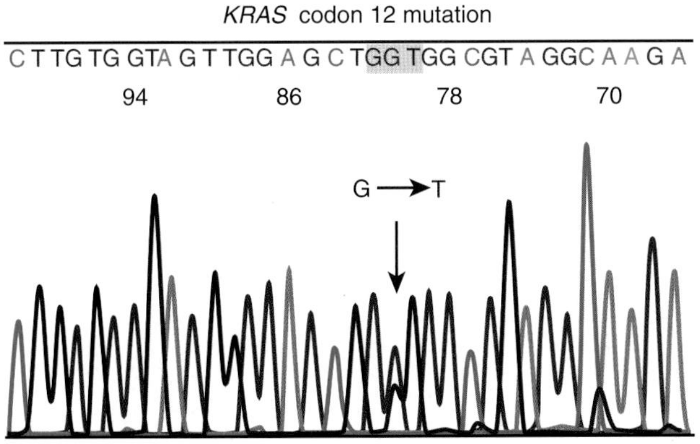

FIGURE 2.8 Detection of a *KRAS* mutation in a colon cancer sample using DNA sequencing. The electropherogram demonstrates a G→T mutation in codon 12.

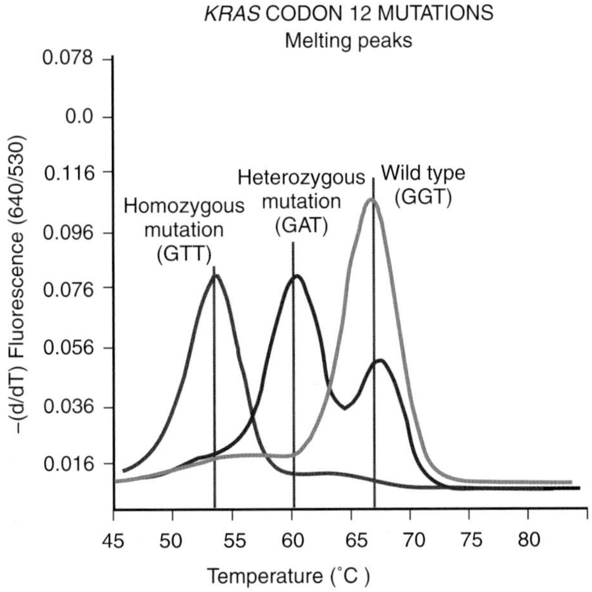

FIGURE 2.9 Detection of a *KRAS* mutation using real-time PCR and post-PCR melting curve analysis showing a single melting peak in the normal DNA sample (wild-type, GGT), two melting peaks in the DNA sample containing a heterozygous mutation (GAT), and a single lower T_m peak in DNA from a cell line containing a homozygous mutation (GTT).

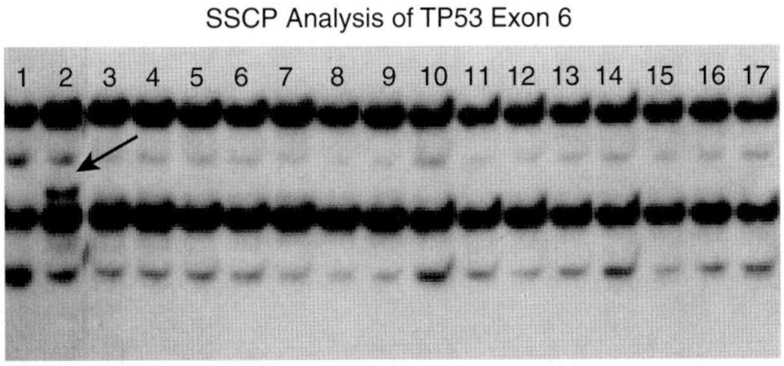

FIGURE 2.10 Detection of *TP53* exon 6 mutations using single-strand conformation polymorphism (SSCP) analysis. PCR products of seventeen tumor samples were amplified with a pair of primers flanking exon 6, with one primer being radioactively labeled, and electrophoresed in polyacrylamide gel. Sample 2 shows an additional abnormally migrating band *(arrow)*, which is indicative of a mutation.

is present, the probe will bind perfectly to the DNA sequence and show a single peak on post-PCR melting curve analysis (Fig. 2.9). In contrast, if a heterozygous mutation is present, the probe will bind to the mutant DNA with one nucleotide mismatch and will melt (dissociate) earlier, producing two melting peaks (a lower T_m for the mutant allele, and a higher T_m for the wild-type allele). Rarely, the mutation is homozygous, and it will present as a single melting peak at a lower T_m. The sensitivity of this method for detecting point mutations such as the *KRAS* mutation is generally similar to those of DNA sequencing.[36]

To detect point mutations with multiple hot spots, such as mutations in the *TP53* gene, DNA sequencing and SSCP analysis are most commonly used.[15] All exons known to harbor mutations are first amplified in several PCR reactions; then they are subjected to DNA sequencing and analyzed for the presence of a mutation. Alternatively, the SSCP analysis can be employed, and only those PCR products that show abnormal migration patterns in the SSCP gel (Fig. 2.10) can be selected for DNA sequencing.[38,39]

Small deletions and insertions can frequently be detected by DNA sequencing or gel electrophoresis of amplified PCR products.[40] For example, one can use PCR amplification followed by polyacrylamide gel electrophoresis to detect a small deletion (9 to 18 nt) in exon 19 of the *EGFR* gene, which is common in lung adenocarcinoma. In the presence of a heterozygous deletion, PCR will amplify an affected shorter allele and an intact wild-type allele. Since the shorter DNA sequence migrates at a higher speed, the gel will show two PCR bands. However, tumor samples negative for the deletion and normal DNA samples will demonstrate a single band of normal size.

DETECTION OF CHROMOSOMAL REARRANGEMENTS

FISH or RT-PCR are typically used to detect chromosomal rearrangements. FISH is the method of choice to detect gene rearrangements in FFPE samples, whereas RT-PCR is a reliable and sensitive technique to detect fusion transcripts in snap-frozen samples that can be performed as conventional or real-time RT-PCR.[24,41-43] Real-time RT-PCR has several significant advantages, as it is fast, is performed in a closed system with minimal risk of contamination, is more specific due to the addition of probes, and allows quantitation of the fusion transcript.

For example, *SYT/SSX* fusion (translocation t(X;18)) in synovial sarcoma can be reliably detected by FISH using a break-apart probe design (Fig. 2.11). The design employs a commercially available mixture of two DNA probes located close to each other and complementary to the *SYT* gene region. The probes are labeled with specific fluorophore (red and green). While normal interphase cells will show two fused signals (red/green or yellow), cells carrying the *SYT* rearrangement will demonstrate one fused signal and two split signals (one red and one green). Although this probe design

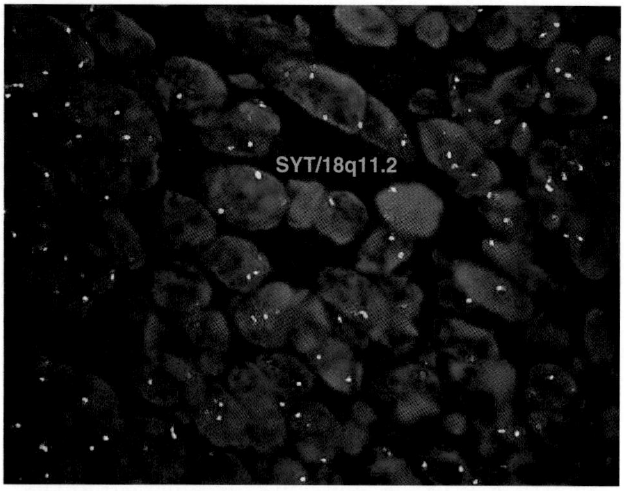

FIGURE 2.11 Detection of the *SYT* gene rearrangement in synovial sarcoma using fluorescence *in situ* hybridization (FISH). In the break-apart probe design, two probes adjacent to each other and spanning the *SYT* gene are labeled in red and green. In many cells in this tumor, the nuclei contain one yellow or green/red signal corresponding to the intact gene, and one green and one red signal on a distance corresponding to the rearranged gene.

can detect all types of rearrangements involving the *SYT* gene, it cannot identify the fusion partner (translocation type *SYT/SSX1*, *SYT/SSX2*, or other).

SYT/SSX translocation can also be detected by RT-PCR followed by a post-PCR detection technique or by real-time RT-PCR.[44] For example, one real-time RT-PCR design exploits the high similarity between *SSX1* and *SSX2* gene sequences in order to develop a pair of primers flanking the two most common fusion types (*SYT/SSX1* and *SYT/SSX2*) and a probe that is complementary to the *SSX1* sequence but has a two-nucleotide mismatch with the *SSX2* sequence (Fig. 2.12A). Such design allows simultaneous amplification of the two rearrangement types in the same reaction (Fig. 2.12B) but distinguishes them based on different melting peaks on post-PCR melting curve analysis (Fig. 2.12C). This method can be used to detect a specific type of *SYT/SSX* translocation in synovial sarcomas, but its best performance requires the input of high-quality RNA isolated from snap-frozen tissue.

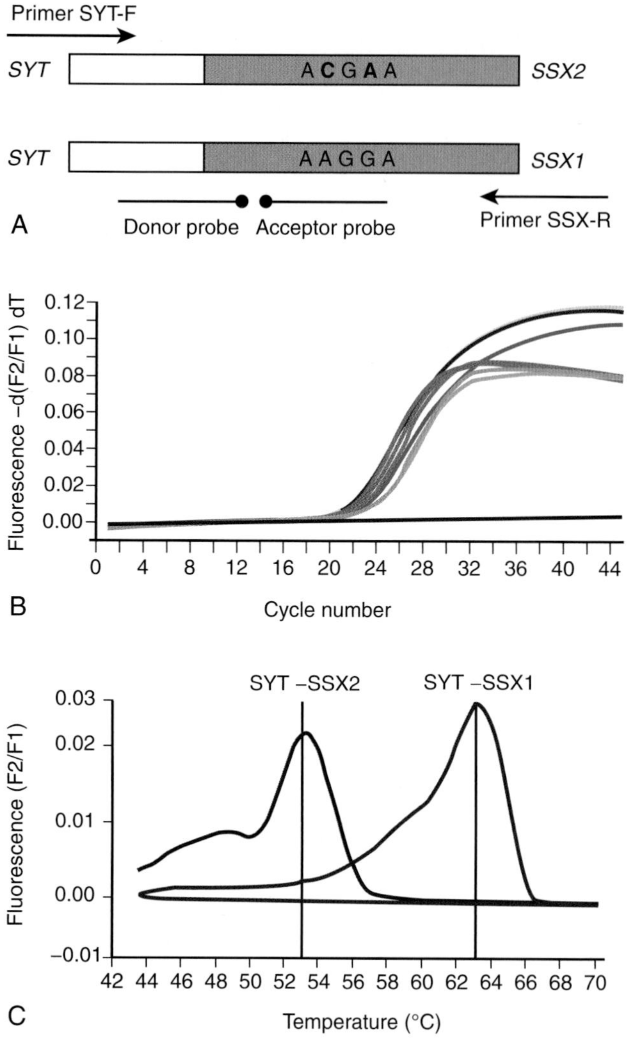

FIGURE 2.12 Detection of *SYT/SSX* rearrangement by real-time RT-PCR and post-PCR melting curve analysis followed by real-time RT-PCR. **(A)** The primers are designed to amplify both *SYT/SSX1* and *SYT/SSX2* fusion points; one probe is designed to be complementary to the *SSX1* sequence, but it has a two-nucleotide mismatch with the *SSX2* sequence. **(B)** All tumor samples carrying the *SYT/SSX* rearrangement are PCR amplified. **(C)** On post-PCR melting curve analysis, the difference in melting peaks distinguishes the *SYT/SSX1* and *SYT/SSX2* fusion types.

DETECTION OF CHROMOSOMAL DELETIONS/LOSS OF HETEROZYGOSITY ANALYSIS

Loss of heterozygosity (LOH) results from a deletion of small or large chromosomal regions and often correlates with the loss of important tumor suppressor genes located in these areas. LOH is typically detected by FISH or by PCR amplification of microsatellite loci followed by capillary gel electrophoresis.

The detection of a 1p deletion in oligodendroglioma by FISH is illustrated in Figure 2.13. A set of commercially available probes consists of two probes, one complementary to the frequently deleted chromosomal region on 1p36 and another differentially labeled control probe that targets the 1q25 region on the long arm of chromosome 1. When 1p deletion is present, the interphase nuclei will demonstrate two signals corresponding to the control probes and only one 1p36 signal.

An alternative PCR-based approach utilizes amplification of microsatellite repeats located in the area of 1p deletion. Loci of microsatellite repeats are highly polymorphic and therefore frequently have different numbers of repeats in the population. As a result, there is a high probability that in a given individual the maternal and paternal alleles are of different sizes. For LOH detection, two primers are designed to flank the microsatellite region (Fig. 2.14A). PCR amplification of tumor DNA and normal tissue DNA is performed, and PCR products are subjected to capillary gel electrophoresis (Fig. 2.14B). The PCR products from normal tissue are used

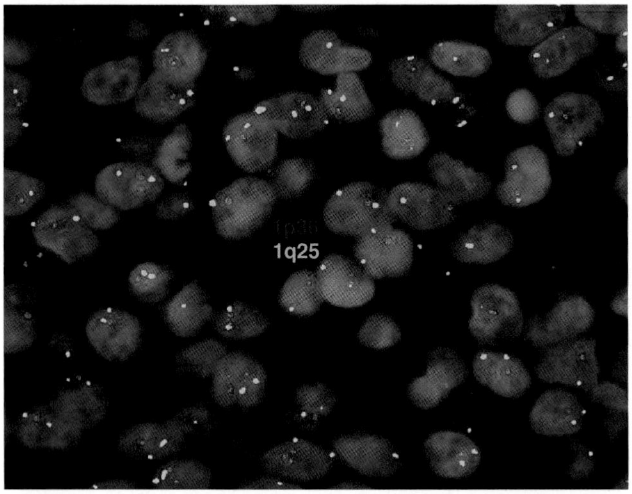

FIGURE 2.13 Detection of a 1p deletion in oligodendroglioma by FISH using a probe corresponding to the commonly deleted region on 1p36 labeled in red and a control probe for 1q25 region labeled in green. Many of the tumor cells show loss of one red signal and preservation of both green signals.

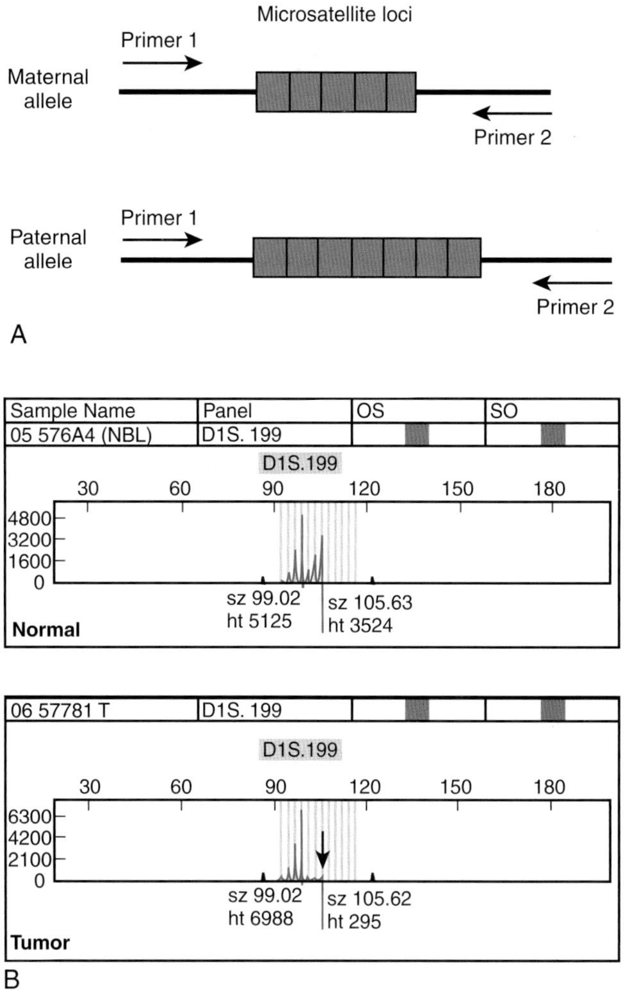

FIGURE 2.14 Detection of loss of heterozygosity (LOH) in a tumor sample. **(A)** PCR primers are designed to flank a region of microsatellite repeats that has a different number of repetitive units on the maternal and paternal alleles. The allele containing a smaller number of microsatellite repeats will yield a shorter PCR product, and the one with a larger number of repeats will yield a longer PCR product. **(B)** Capillary gel electropherograms demonstrating the amplification of two alleles in the normal tissue sample and the complete loss of the larger allele in the tumor sample.

to determine whether a given patient is heterozygous for this locus (i.e., has two alleles of different size) and therefore is informative for LOH analysis. If the locus is informative, the LOH can be determined as either complete absence or a significant decrease in amplification of one of the two alleles. A complete loss of one allele is rarely seen because some non-neoplastic cells are almost always present within the tumor. Therefore, LOH calculation is based on the difference in ratios of two allelic peaks in normal tissue as compared to the same peaks in tumor tissue. In most cases, an allele ratio within the range of <0.5 and >2.0 is considered as evidence of LOH.[45,46]

Both FISH and PCR-based detection of LOH can be achieved successfully in FFPE samples, and each method has its own limitations. FISH will show a false-negative result in the event of uniparental disomy (i.e., when cancer cells have lost one chromosome in the presence of duplication of another chromosomal allele). The PCR-based LOH analysis can detect the 1p loss in this situation. However, for optimal performance, the PCR-LOH analysis requires normal cells (isolated from normal tissue or blood) and must rely on amplification of several markers located in the same region because some of the microsatellite loci will be non-informative.

DETECTION OF MICROSATELLITE INSTABILITY

Microsatellite instability (MSI) is caused by defects in DNA mismatch repair proteins (MSH2, MLH1, PMS1, PMS2, MSH6, or MSH3). It manifests as an abnormal (increased or decreased) length of microsatellite repeats. The presence of microsatellite instability is a sign of DNA mismatch repair deficiency that can be inherited (e.g., caused by a germline mutation in the *MSH2* gene in hereditary nonpolyposis colon cancer syndrome) or sporadic (e.g., due to hypermethylation of the *MLH1* promoter in sporadic colorectal cancer).[47,48] Molecular testing for MSI is usually performed using PCR amplification of DNA regions containing microsatellite repeats followed by capillary gel electrophoresis. Typically, DNA isolated from normal and tumor tissue is separately amplified by PCR with fluorescent-labeled primers. The electrophoretic patterns of PCR products from the normal and tumor tissue are compared to identify insertions or deletions of repetitive units in the tumor sample. The National Cancer Institute guidelines for MSI testing recommend a panel of five microsatellite loci, including three dinucleotide repeat markers (D2S123, D5S346, D17S250) and two mononucleotide repeat markers (BAT 25 and BAT 26). This panel is known as the *Bethesda panel*.[47,48] High-frequency MSI (MSI-H) is defined as an instability in two or more of the five markers (Fig. 2.15), and low-frequency MSI (MSI-L) is

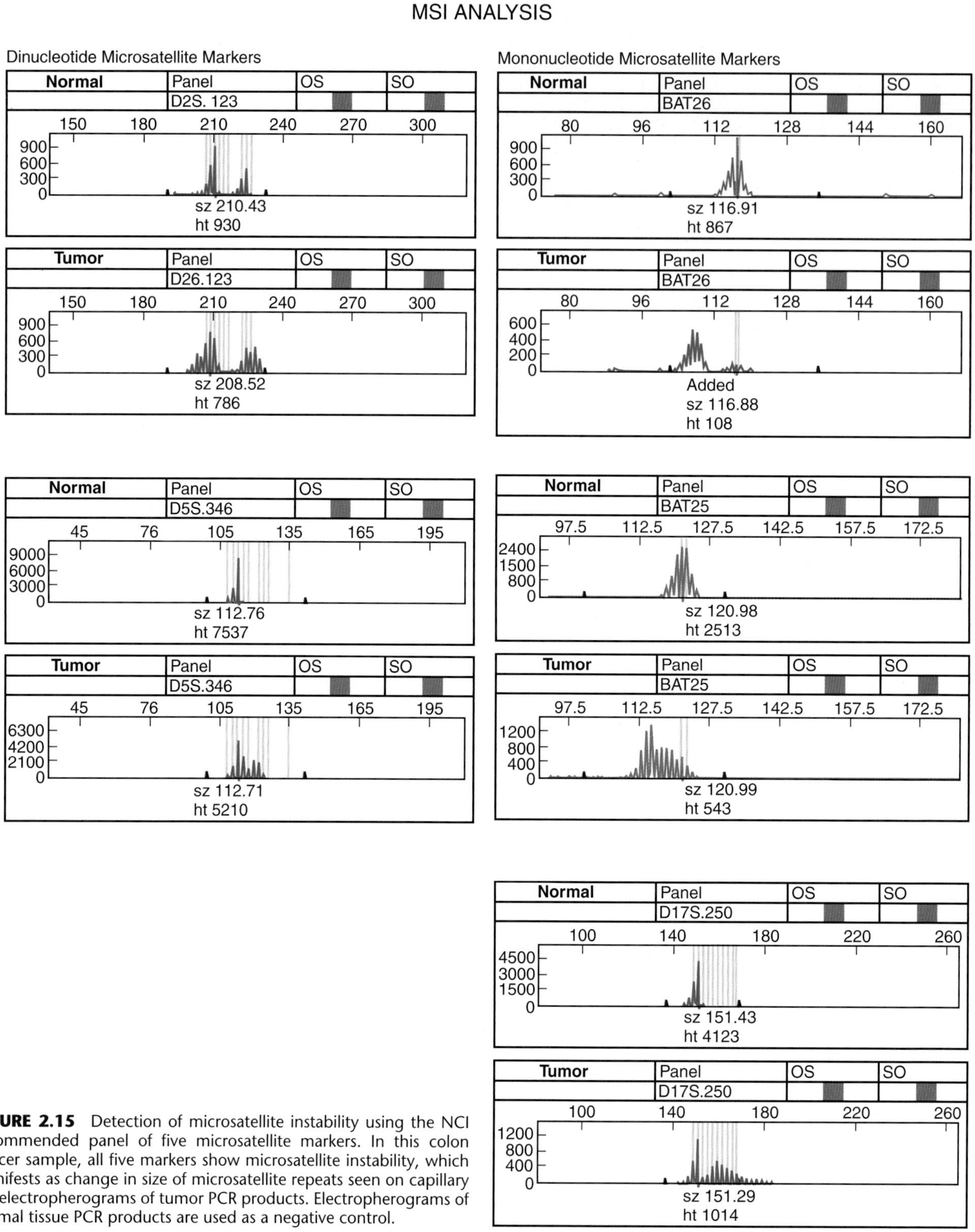

FIGURE 2.15 Detection of microsatellite instability using the NCI recommended panel of five microsatellite markers. In this colon cancer sample, all five markers show microsatellite instability, which manifests as change in size of microsatellite repeats seen on capillary gel electropherograms of tumor PCR products. Electropherograms of normal tissue PCR products are used as a negative control.

defined as an instability in one unstable marker. Microsatellite stable (MSS) status is established when none of the markers shows instability. The test can be performed using DNA isolated from either snap-frozen or FFPE tissue and provides a reliable and reproducible detection of MSI.

DNA-BASED TISSUE IDENTITY TESTING

In pathology practice, DNA-based tissue identity testing is typically used to detect tissue contaminants or "floaters" and for mislabeled specimens. It is particularly

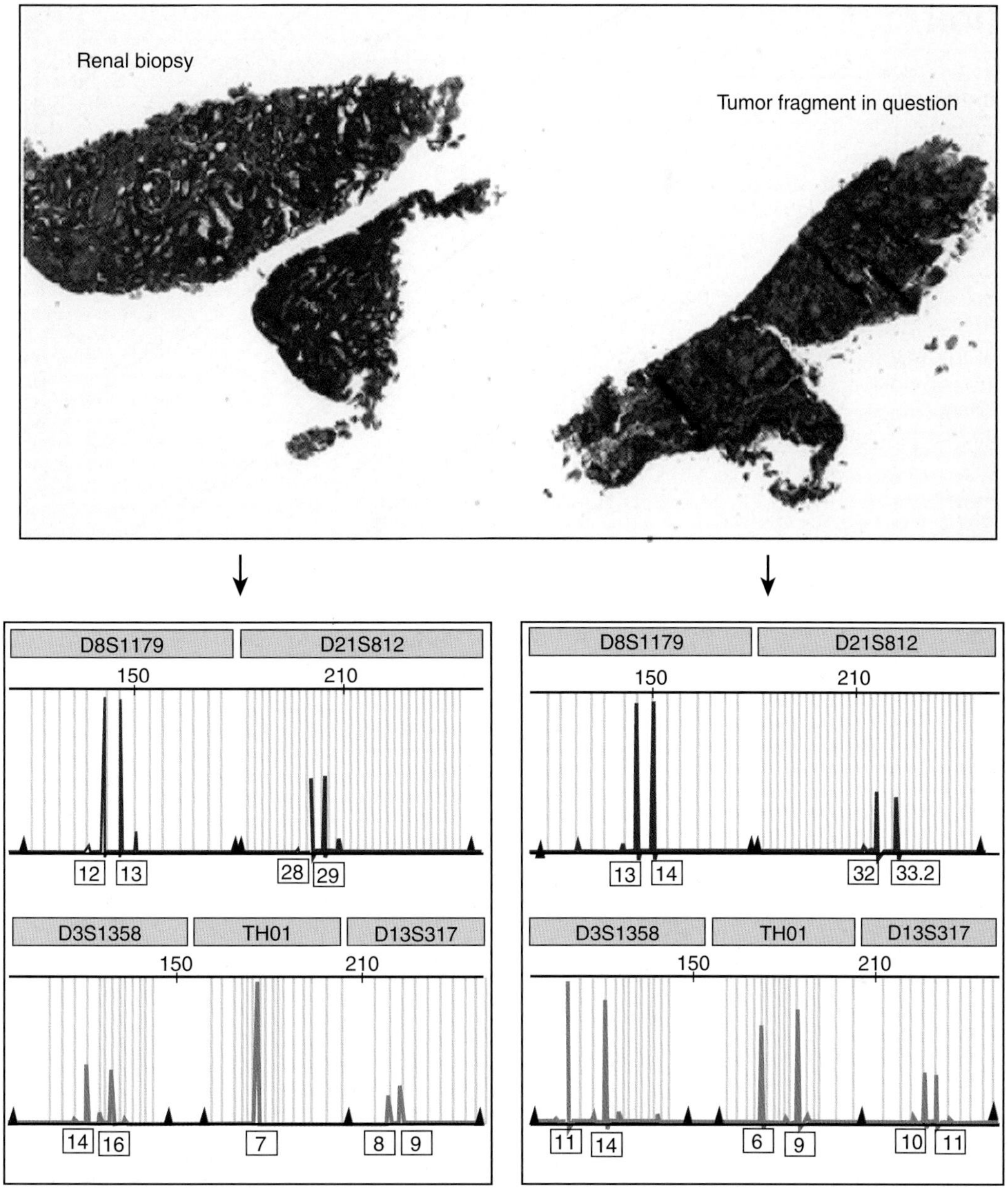

FIGURE 2.16 DNA-based tissue identity testing. In this case, H&E stained sections of a renal biopsy reveal a discrete fragment of tumor tissue, which was suspected to be a contaminant. Unstained sections were used to separately microdissect the renal biopsy tissue and the tumor fragment in question tissue for DNA extraction and PCR amplification for 16 polymorphic microsatellite loci. Capillary gel electropherograms show different size alleles for all tested markers, indicating that the two tissue fragments belong to different individuals and that the tissue fragment in question is indeed a contaminant.

important to detect tissue contaminants when no obvious distinction exists between the actual tissue sample and the tissue fragment in question based on microscopic or immunohistochemical characteristics. Tissue identity testing is performed using PCR amplification of DNA isolated from the obviously correct tissue fragment (or from the patient's blood) and from the fragment in question. It is based on comparison of the length of multiple hypervariable DNA regions, such as microsatellite repeats, between the two specimens.[49-51] Typically, multiplex PCR is performed and up to 16 different microsatellite loci are amplified in the same reaction. The most frequently used microsatellite loci are tetranucleotide repeats, which offer a larger difference in the allele size for ease of interpretation. Markers on chromosomes X and Y are included for gender determination. Multiple PCR products are amplified with primers labeled with different fluorophores and separated by capillary gel electrophoresis. The size of each PCR product is identified and compared between the two samples (Fig. 2.16). Since microsatellites are highly polymorphic in the population, the test is typically informative because it determines if two DNA profiles are identical or different (i.e., if they belong to the same or different patients).

The PCR-based tissue identity test requires a very small amount of DNA and can be successfully performed using FFPE tissue samples or hematoxylin and eosin-stained tissue fragments removed from glass slides.

CONCLUSION

In this chapter we provide the essential molecular tools for understanding the applications available in the molecular anatomic laboratory. These procedures are complementary to the IHC technique and can be very helpful in specific instances for diagnostic use in surgical pathology.

Each molecular tool has a specific indication for use, depending on the molecular abnormality under investigation. This is analogous to the use of reagents for specific diagnostic use in IHC.

A thorough understanding of the indications of these molecular tests provides an invaluable insight for diagnostic use and the understanding of molecular alterations in neoplastic tissues.

REFERENCES

1. Watson JD, Crick FH. Molecular structure of nucleic acids; a structure for deoxyribose nucleic acid. *Nature*. 1953;171: 737-738.
2. Lander ES, Linton LM, Birren B, et al. Initial sequencing and analysis of the human genome. *Nature*. 2001;409:860-921.
3. Chargaff E. Structure and function of nucleic acids as cell constituents. *Fed Proc*. 1951;10:654-659.
4. Shen LX, Cai Z, Tinoco Jr I. RNA structure at high resolution. *Faseb J*. 1995;9:1023-1033.
5. Sharp PA. Splicing of messenger RNA precursors. *Science*. 1987;235:766-771.
6. Bartel DP. MicroRNAs: genomics, biogenesis, mechanism, and function. *Cell*. 2004;116:281-297.
7. Ambros V. The functions of animal microRNAs. *Nature*. 2004;431:350-355.
8. Mullis KB, Faloona FA. Specific synthesis of DNA in vitro via a polymerase-catalyzed chain reaction. *Methods Enzymol*. 1987;155:335-350.
9. Freeman WM, Walker SJ, Vrana KE. Quantitative RT-PCR: pitfalls and potential. *Biotechniques*. 1999;26:112-122, 124-125.
10. Micke P, Ohshima M, Tahmasebpoor S, et al. Biobanking of fresh frozen tissue: RNA is stable in nonfixed surgical specimens. *Lab Invest*. 2006;86:202-211.
11. Ginzinger DG. Gene quantification using real-time quantitative PCR: an emerging technology hits the mainstream. *Exp Hematol*. 2002;30:503-512.
12. Krypuy M, Newnham GM, Thomas DM, et al. High resolution melting analysis for the rapid and sensitive detection of mutations in clinical samples: KRAS codon 12 and 13 mutations in non-small cell lung cancer. *BMC Cancer*. 2006;6:295.
13. Pryor RJ, Wittwer CT. Real-time polymerase chain reaction and melting curve analysis. *Methods Mol Biol*. 2006;336:19-32.
14. Dang GT, Cote GJ, Schultz PN, et al. A codon 891 exon 15 RET proto-oncogene mutation in familial medullary thyroid carcinoma: a detection strategy. *Mol Cell Probes*. 1999;13:77-79.
15. Nikiforov YE, Nikiforova MN, Gnepp DR, et al. Prevalence of mutations of ras and p53 in benign and malignant thyroid tumors from children exposed to radiation after the Chernobyl nuclear accident. *Oncogene*. 1996;13:687-693.
16. Jin L, Sebo TJ, Nakamura N, et al. BRAF mutation analysis in fine needle aspiration (FNA) cytology of the thyroid. *Diagn Mol Pathol*. 2006;15:136-143.
17. Bjorheim J, Lystad S, Lindblom A, et al. Mutation analyses of KRAS exon 1 comparing three different techniques: temporal temperature gradient electrophoresis, constant denaturant capillary electrophoresis and allele specific polymerase chain reaction. *Mutat Res*. 1998;403:103-112.
18. Sanger F, Nicklen S, Coulson AR. DNA sequencing with chain-terminating inhibitors. *Proc Natl Acad Sci U S A*. 1977;74: 5463-5467.
19. Ronaghi M. Pyrosequencing sheds light on DNA sequencing. *Genome Res*. 2001;11:3-11.
20. Ogino S, Kawasaki T, Brahmandam M, et al. Sensitive sequencing method for KRAS mutation detection by Pyrosequencing. *J Mol Diagn*. 2005;7:413-421.
21. Ogino S, Kawasaki T, Nosho K, et al. LINE-1 hypomethylation is inversely associated with microsatellite instability and CpG island methylator phenotype in colorectal cancer. *Int J Cancer*. 2008;122:2767-2773.
22. Tonnies H. Modern molecular cytogenetic techniques in genetic diagnostics. *Trends Mol Med*. 2002;8:246-250.
23. Nikiforova MN, Stringer JR, Blough R, et al. Proximity of chromosomal loci that participate in radiation-induced rearrangements in human cells. *Science*. 2000;290:138-141.
24. Zhu Z, Ciampi R, Nikiforova MN, et al. Prevalence of RET/PTC rearrangements in thyroid papillary carcinomas: effects of the detection methods and genetic heterogeneity. *J Clin Endocrinol Metab*. 2006;91:3603-3610.
25. Cowell JK, Wang YD, Head K, et al. Identification and characterization of constitutional chromosome abnormalities using arrays of bacterial artificial chromosomes. *Br J Cancer*. 2004;90: 860-865.
26. Forozan F, Karhu R, Kononen J, et al. Genome screening by comparative genomic hybridization. *Trends Genet*. 1997;13: 405-409.
27. Kallioniemi A, Kallioniemi OP, Sudar D, et al. Comparative genomic hybridization for molecular cytogenetic analysis of solid tumors. *Science*. 1992;258:818-821.
28. Johnson NA, Hamoudi RA, Ichimura K, et al. Application of array CGH on archival formalin-fixed paraffin-embedded tissues including small numbers of microdissected cells. *Lab Invest*. 2006;86:968-978.
29. Schulze A, Downward J. Navigating gene expression using microarrays—a technology review. *Nat Cell Biol*. 2001;3: E190-E195.
30. Bier FF, von Nickisch-Rosenegk M, Ehrentreich-Forster E, et al. DNA microarrays. *Adv Biochem Eng Biotechnol*. 2008;109: 433-453.
31. Sapio MR, Posca D, Troncone G, et al. Detection of BRAF mutation in thyroid papillary carcinomas by mutant allele-specific PCR amplification (MASA). *Eur J Endocrinol*. 2006;154: 341-348.
32. Rowe LR, Bentz BG, Bentz JS. Detection of BRAF V600E activating mutation in papillary thyroid carcinoma using PCR with allele-specific fluorescent probe melting curve analysis. *J Clin Pathol*. 2007;60:1211-1215.
33. Hayashida N, Namba H, Kumagai A, et al. A rapid and simple detection method for the BRAF(T1796A) mutation in fine-needle aspirated thyroid carcinoma cells. *Thyroid*. 2004;14:910-915.
34. Nikiforova MN, Kimura ET, Gandhi M, et al. BRAF mutations in thyroid tumors are restricted to papillary carcinomas and anaplastic or poorly differentiated carcinomas arising from papillary carcinomas. *J Clin Endocrinol Metab*. 2003;88:5399-5404.
35. Kimura ET, Nikiforova MN, Zhu Z, et al. High prevalence of BRAF mutations in thyroid cancer: genetic evidence for constitutive activation of the RET/PTC-RAS-BRAF signaling pathway in papillary thyroid carcinoma. *Cancer Res*. 2003;63:1454-1457.
36. Nikiforova MN, Lynch RA, Biddinger PW, et al. RAS point mutations and PAX8-PPAR gamma rearrangement in thyroid tumors: evidence for distinct molecular pathways in thyroid follicular carcinoma. *J Clin Endocrinol Metab*. 2003;88: 2318-2326.
37. van Krieken JH, Jung A, Kirchner T, et al. KRAS mutation testing for predicting response to anti-EGFR therapy for colorectal carcinoma: proposal for an European quality assurance program. *Virchows Arch*. 2008;453:417-431.
38. Kambouris M, Jackson CE, Feldman GL. Diagnosis of multiple endocrine neoplasia [MEN] 2A, 2B and familial medullary thyroid cancer [FMTC] by multiplex PCR and heteroduplex analyses of RET proto-oncogene mutations. *Hum Mutat*. 1996;8: 64-70.
39. Ceccherini I, Hofstra RM, Luo Y, et al. DNA polymorphisms and conditions for SSCP analysis of the 20 exons of the ret proto-oncogene. *Oncogene*. 1994;9:3025-3029.
40. Pan Q, Pao W, Ladanyi M. Rapid polymerase chain reaction-based detection of epidermal growth factor receptor gene mutations in lung adenocarcinomas. *J Mol Diagn*. 2005;7:396-403.

41. Nikiforova MN, Biddinger PW, Caudill CM, et al. PAX8-PPARgamma rearrangement in thyroid tumors: RT-PCR and immunohistochemical analyses. *Am J Surg Pathol.* 2002;26:1016-1023.
42. Nikiforova MN, Caudill CM, Biddinger P, et al. Prevalence of RET/PTC rearrangements in Hashimoto's thyroiditis and papillary thyroid carcinomas. *Int J Surg Pathol.* 2002;10:15-22.
43. Qian X, Jin L, Shearer BM, et al. Molecular diagnosis of Ewing's sarcoma/primitive neuroectodermal tumor in formalin-fixed paraffin-embedded tissues by RT-PCR and fluorescence in situ hybridization. *Diagn Mol Pathol.* 2005;14:23-28.
44. Nikiforova MN, Groen P, Mutema G, et al. Detection of SYT-SSX rearrangements in synovial sarcomas by real-time one-step RT-PCR. *Pediatr Dev Pathol.* 2005;8:162-167.
45. Johnson MD, Vnencak-Jones CL, Toms SA, et al. Allelic losses in oligodendroglial and oligodendroglioma-like neoplasms: analysis using microsatellite repeats and polymerase chain reaction. *Arch Pathol Lab Med.* 2003;127:1573-1579.
46. Marsh JW, Finkelstein SD, Demetris AJ, et al. Genotyping of hepatocellular carcinoma in liver transplant recipients adds predictive power for determining recurrence-free survival. *Liver Transpl.* 2003;9:664-671.
47. Boland CR, Thibodeau SN, Hamilton SR, et al. A National Cancer Institute Workshop on Microsatellite Instability for cancer detection and familial predisposition: development of international criteria for the determination of microsatellite instability in colorectal cancer. *Cancer Res.* 1998;58:5248-5257.
48. Umar A, Boland CR, Terdiman JP, et al. Revised Bethesda Guidelines for hereditary nonpolyposis colorectal cancer (Lynch syndrome) and microsatellite instability. *J Natl Cancer Inst.* 2004;96:261-268.
49. O'Briain DS, Sheils O, McElwaine S, et al. Sorting out mix-ups. The provenance of tissue sections may be confirmed by PCR using microsatellite markers. *Am J Clin Pathol.* 1996;106:758-764.
50. Kessis TD, Silberman MA, Sherman M, et al. Rapid identification of patient specimens with microsatellite DNA markers. *Mod Pathol.* 1996;9:183-188.
51. Hunt JL, Swalsky P, Sasatomi E, et al. A microdissection and molecular genotyping assay to confirm the identity of tissue floaters in paraffin-embedded tissue blocks. *Arch Pathol Lab Med.* 2003;127:213-217.

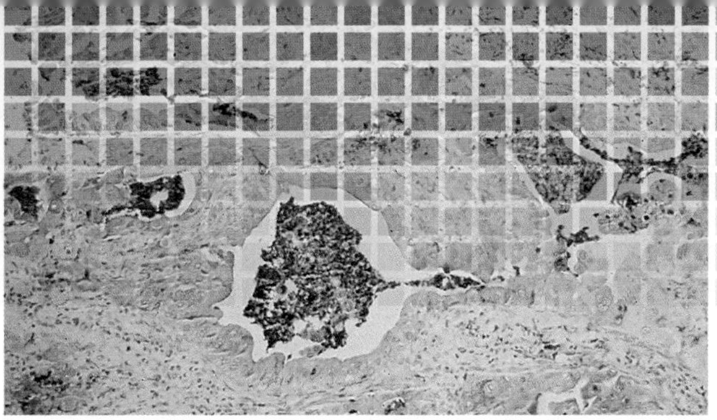

3

Immunohistology of Infectious Diseases

Eduardo J. Ezyaguirre • David H. Walker • Sherif R. Zaki

- Introduction 58
- Viral Infections 59
- Bacterial Infections 64
- Fungal Infections 67
- Protozoal Infections 68
- Emerging Infectious Diseases 69
- Pathologists, Immunohistochemistry, and Bioterrorism 70
- Beyond Immunohistology: Molecular Diagnostic Applications 72

INTRODUCTION

Since the 1980s, immunohistochemistry (IHC) has dramatically transformed the approach to histopathologic diagnosis, specifically in the diagnosis and classification of tumors, and more recently in the diagnosis of infectious diseases in tissue samples.[1]

Pathologists play an important role in recognizing infectious agents in tissue samples from patients, providing a rapid morphologic diagnosis, and facilitating clinical decisions in patient treatment. When fresh tissue is not available for culture, pathologists can provide a rapid morphologic diagnosis and facilitate clinical decisions in patient treatment.[2] In addition, pathologists have played a central role in identifying emerging and reemerging infectious agents, describing the pathogenetic processes of emerging diseases (e.g., hantavirus pulmonary syndrome, viral hemorrhagic fevers, leptospirosis, and rickettsial and ehrlichial infections), and diagnosing anthrax during the bioterrorist attack of 2001.[3-7]

Cultures and serologic assays are usually used for microbial identification in infectious diseases. However, fresh tissue is not always available, and culturing fastidious pathogens can be difficult and may take weeks or months to yield results. Moreover, culture alone cannot distinguish colonization from tissue invasion. In addition, serologic results can be difficult to interpret in the setting of immunosuppression or when only a single sample is available for evaluation. Some microorganisms have distinctive morphologic characteristics that allow their identification in formalin-fixed tissues using routine and special stains. Nevertheless, in many instances it is difficult or even impossible to identify an infectious agent specifically by conventional morphologic methods.

Immunohistochemistry is one of the most powerful techniques in surgical pathology. There has been an increasing interest in the use of specific antibodies to viral, bacterial, fungal, and parasitic antigens in the detection and identification of the causative agents in many infectious diseases. Coons and associates were the first to use a specific antibody to detect a microbial antigen to detect pneumococcal antigen in tissues.[8] The advantages of IHC over conventional staining methods (Table 3.1) and the contributions of IHC in infectious diseases (Table 3.2) are substantial. In many instances, IHC has shown high specificity, allowing the differentiation of morphologically similar microorganisms.[9] Immunohistochemistry is especially useful when microorganisms are difficult to identify by routine or special stains, are fastidious to grow, or exhibit atypical morphology (Table 3.3).[10-14] It is important to understand that there may be widespread occurrence of common antigens among bacteria and pathogenic fungi, and both monoclonal and polyclonal antibodies must be tested for possible cross-reactivity with other organisms.[15] Finally, it is important to emphasize that IHC has several steps, and that all of them can affect the final result; however, in general the only limitations are the availability of specific antibodies and the preservation of epitopes.[16]

Table 3.4 lists some commercially available antibodies for diagnostic use in surgical pathology.

TABLE 3.1	Advantages of IHC for the Diagnosis of Infectious Diseases
1.	Opportunity for rapid results
2.	Reduced risk of exposure to serious infectious diseases by performance on formalin-fixed, paraffin-embedded tissue
3.	High sensitivity allowing identification of infectious agents even before morphologic changes occur
4.	Opportunities for retrospective diagnosis of individual patients and for in-depth study of the disease
5.	Specific identification of infectious agents with many monoclonal antibodies and some polyclonal antibodies

TABLE 3.2	Contributions of IHC to the Diagnosis of Infectious Diseases
1.	Allows identification of new human pathogens
2.	Allows microbiological-morphological correlation establishing the pathogenic significance of microbiological results
3.	Provides a rapid morphologic diagnosis allowing early treatment of serious infectious diseases
4.	Contributes to understanding of the pathogenesis of infectious diseases
5.	Provides a diagnosis when fresh tissue is not available or when culture methods do not exist

TABLE 3.3	Applications of IHC in the Diagnosis of Infectious Diseases
1.	Identification of microorganisms that are difficult to detect by routine or special stains
2.	Detection of microorganisms that are present in low numbers
3.	Detection of microorganisms that stain poorly
4.	Identification of microorganisms that are fastidious to grow or noncultivable
5.	Identification of microorganisms that exhibit atypical morphology

VIRAL INFECTIONS

Immunohistochemistry has played an important role not only in the diagnosis of a large number of viral infections but also in the study of their pathogenesis and epidemiology. Conventionally, the diagnosis of viral infections has relied on cytopathic changes observed by routine histopathologic examination. Several viral pathogens produce characteristic intracellular inclusions, which allow pathologists to make a presumptive diagnosis of viral infection. However, for some viral infections the characteristic cytopathic changes are subtle and sparse, requiring a meticulous search.[17] Moreover, only 50% of known viral diseases are associated with characteristic intracellular inclusions.[18] In addition, formalin, which is the most commonly used fixative in histopathology, is a poor fixative for demonstrating the morphologic and tinctorial features of viral inclusions.[19] When viral inclusions are not detected in hematoxylin and eosin–stained sections or when the viral inclusions present cannot be differentiated from those of other viral diseases, immunohistochemical techniques offer a more reliable approach to reach a specific diagnosis.

Hepatitis B

Hepatitis B virus infection constitutes an important cause of chronic hepatitis in a significant proportion of patients. In many instances, the morphologic changes induced by hepatitis B virus in hepatocytes are not typical enough to render a presumptive diagnosis of hepatitis B viral infection. In other instances, there may be so little hepatitis B surface antigen (HBsAg) that it cannot be demonstrated by techniques such as orcein staining. In these cases, immunohistochemical techniques to detect HBsAg are more sensitive than histochemical methods and are helpful in reaching a diagnosis.[20] Immunostaining for HBsAg has been used in the diagnosis of hepatitis B and in the study of carrier states.[21,22] Eighty percent or more of cases with positive serologic results for HBsAg demonstrate cytoplasmic HBsAg using IHC.[23] By immunoperoxidase localization, hepatitis B core antigen (HBcAg) can be demonstrated within the nuclei or the cytoplasm of hepatocytes, or both. Cytoplasmic expression of HBcAg usually is associated with a higher grade of hepatitis activity,[23] and diffuse immunostaining of nuclei for HBcAg generally suggests uncontrolled viral replication in the setting of immunosuppression.[24] Immunostaining for HBsAg and HBcAg is useful in the diagnosis of recurrent hepatitis B infection in liver allografts, particularly when present with atypical histopathologic features.[25]

Herpesviruses

Histologically, the diagnosis of herpes simplex virus (HSV) infection involves the detection of multinucleated giant cells containing characteristic molded, ground glass–appearing nuclei and Cowdry's type A intranuclear inclusions. When abundant viral inclusions exist within infected cells, the diagnosis is usually straightforward. However, diagnosis can be difficult when the characteristic intranuclear inclusions or multinucleated cells, or both, are absent or when the amount of tissue in a biopsy specimen is small.[26] In these cases, IHC using either polyclonal or monoclonal antibodies against HSV antigens has proven to be a sensitive and specific technique used to diagnose HSV infections (Fig. 3.1).[27-30]

Although polyclonal antibodies against major HSV glycoprotein antigens are sensitive, they do not allow distinction between HSV-1 and HSV-2; this is because the two viruses are antigenically similar.[31] In addition, the histologic features of HSV infection are not specific and can also occur in patients with varicella-zoster (VZV) infection. Monoclonal antibodies against the VZV envelope glycoprotein gp1 are sufficiently sensitive

TABLE 3.4 Commercially Available Antibodies for Immunohistochemical Diagnosis of Infectious and Prion Diseases

Microorganism	Antibody/Clone	Dilution	Pretreatment	Source
Adenovirus	Mab/20/11 and 2/6	1:2000	Proteinase K	Chemicon
B. henselae	Mab	1:100	HIAR	Biocare Medical
BK virus	Mab/BK T.1	1:8000	Trypsin	Chemicon
C. albicans	Mab/1B12	1:400	HIAR	Chemicon
C. pneumoniae	Mab/RR402	1:200	HIAR	Accurate
Cryptosporidium	Mab/Mabc1	1:100	HIAR	Novocastra
CMV	Mab/DDG9/CCH2	1:50	HIAR	Novocastra
Clostridium spp.	Rabbit polyclonal	1:1000	None	Biodesign
G. intestinalis	Mab/9D5.3.1	1:50	HIAR	Novocastra
Hepatitis B core antigen	Rabbit polyclonal	1:2000	HIAR	Dako
Hepatitis B surface antigen	Mab/3E7	1:100	HIAR	Dako
Herpes simplex 1 and 2 viruses	Rabbit polyclonal	1:3200	HIAR	Dako
H. pylori	Rabbit polyclonal	1:40	Proteinase K	Dako
HHV 8	Mab/LNA-1	1:500	HIAR	Novocastra
K. pneumoniae	Rabbit polyclonal	1:200	Proteinase K	Biogenex
L. monocytogenes	Rabbit polyclonal	1:5000	Proteinase K	Difco
M. pneumoniae	Mab/1.B.432	1:25	HIAR	US Biological
Parvovirus B19	Mab/R92F6	1:500	HIAR	Novocastra
P. carinii	Mab/3F6	1:20	HIAR	Novocastra
P. falciparum	Mab/BDI400	1:1000	Proteinase K	Biodesign
Prion	Mab/3F4	1:200	Antigen retrieval	Dako
	Mab/12F10	1:1000	Proteinase K	Cayman Chemical
	Mab/KG9	1:1000	Proteinase K	TSE Resource Center
Respiratory syncytial virus	Mab/5H5N	1:200	HIAR	Novocastra
S. aureus	Rabbit polyclonal	1:500	Proteinase K	Biodesign
T. pallidum	Rabbit polyclonal		HIAR	Biodesign
T. gondii	Rabbit polyclonal	1:320	HIAR	Biogenex
West Nile virus	Mab/5H10	1:400	Proteinase K	Bioreliance

and specific to allow a clear-cut distinction between HSV and VZV infections.[27,32,33]

Immunohistochemistry has also been useful in demonstrating the association of human herpes virus 8 (HHV-8) with Kaposi's sarcoma, primary effusion lymphoma, and multicentric Castleman's disease.[34-38] Diagnosis of Kaposi's sarcoma may be problematic because of its broad morphologic spectrum and similar appearance to other benign and malignant neoplastic vascular lesions. Immunostaining of latent associated nuclear antigen-1 (LANA-1) is useful to confirm the diagnosis of Kaposi's sarcoma, particularly when difficult early lesions closely resemble the appearance of interstitial granuloma annulare and when the neoplasm presents in an unusual location. Immunostaining also allows distinction of Kaposi's sarcoma from several morphologically similar vasoproliferative lesions.[39-41] Immunostaining is restricted to the nuclei of spindle cells and endothelial cells of the slitlike vascular spaces (Fig. 3.2). Immunohistochemistry has also demonstrated expression of HHV-8 LANA-1 in mesothelial cells of HIV-associated recurrent pleural effusions.[42]

Cytomegalovirus (CMV) continues to be an important opportunistic pathogen in immunocompromised patients; it is estimated that 30% of transplant recipients experience CMV disease.[43] The range of organ involvement in post-transplant CMV disease is wide; hepatitis occurs in 40% of liver transplant recipients,[44] and pneumonitis is more frequently seen in heart and heart-lung transplant patients.[45] Other organs that are commonly affected are the gastrointestinal tract and the peripheral and central nervous systems. Histologic diagnosis of CMV in fixed tissues usually rests on identifying characteristic cytopathic effects including intranuclear inclusions, cytoplasmic inclusions, or both. However, histologic examination lacks sensitivity, and in some

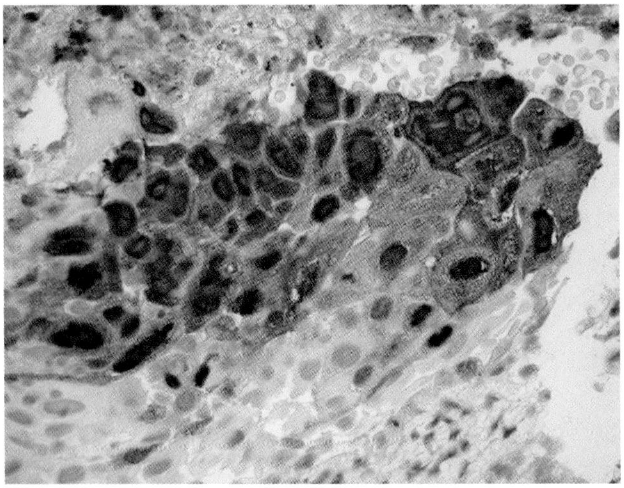

FIGURE 3.1 Photomicrograph of cervical biopsy from a patient with herpes simplex virus infection showing abundant nuclear and cytoplasmic antigen. (Immunoperoxidase staining with DAB and hematoxylin counterstain; ×400.)

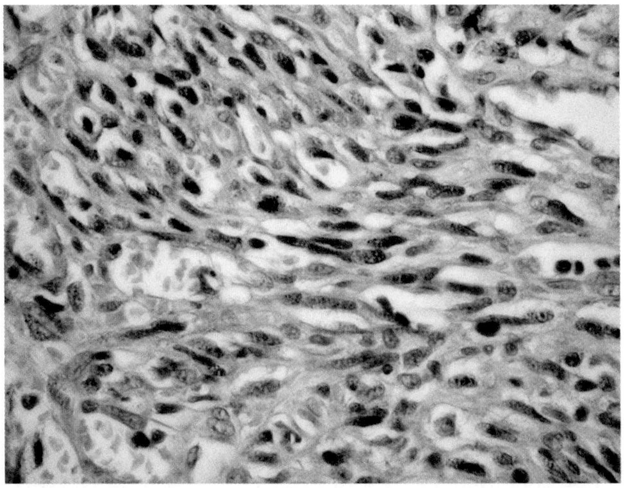

FIGURE 3.2 Lymph node biopsy from a patient with Kaposi's sarcoma. The spindle cells show strong nuclear staining for HHV-8 LANA-1 antigen. Endothelial cells of well formed vascular spaces are negative. (Immunoperoxidase staining with DAB and hematoxylin counterstain; ×400.)

cases atypical cytopathic features can be confused with reactive or degenerative changes.[46] Additionally, up to 38% of patients with gastrointestinal CMV disease fail to demonstrate any inclusions.[47] In these cases, IHC using monoclonal antibodies against early and late CMV antigens allows the detection of CMV antigens in the nucleus and cytoplasm of infected cells (Fig. 3.3). The sensitivity of IHC for detecting CMV infection ranges from 78% to 93%.[47,48] In addition, IHC may allow detection of CMV antigens early in the course of the disease when cytopathic changes have not yet developed.[49-54] For example, CMV early nuclear antigen is expressed 9 to 96 hours after cellular infection and indicates early active viral replication. Immunohistochemistry has been used to detect CMV infection in patients with steroid refractory ulcerative colitis, and the routine use of IHC for the detection of CMV in the evaluation of these patients is

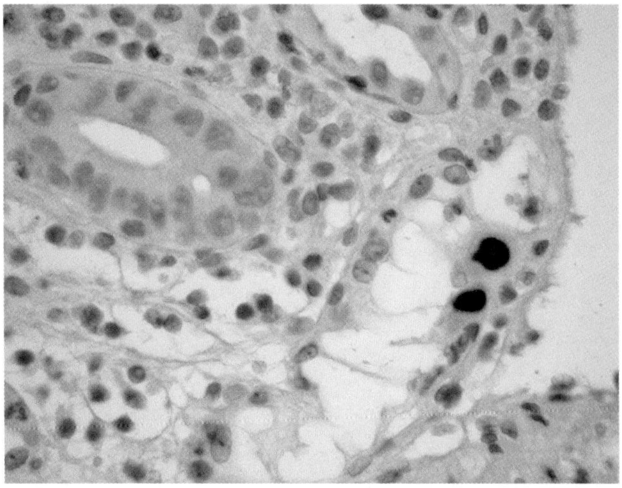

FIGURE 3.3 Colon biopsy of a patient with steroid-refractory ulcerative colitis. Rare epithelial cells show intranuclear CMV antigen. (Immunoperoxidase staining with DAB and hematoxylin counterstain; ×400.)

now recommended.[55,56] CMV immunostaining has been used to detect occult CMV infection of the central nervous system in liver transplant patients who develop neurologic complications.[57] It has also been used to demonstrate a high frequency of CMV antigens in tissues from first-trimester abortions.[58] CMV is the most common opportunistic organism found in liver biopsies from transplant patients; nonetheless, the incidence of CMV hepatitis appears to be decreasing owing to better prophylactic treatments.[59] Although CMV hepatitis presents with characteristic neutrophilic aggregates within the liver parenchyma, atypical features suggestive of acute rejection or changes indistinguishable from those of any other viral hepatitis are occasionally observed.[60] In addition, parenchymal neutrophilic microabscesses have been described in cases with no evidence of CMV infection.[61] In these cases, immunostaining for CMV antigens is most useful in determining the diagnosis of CMV infection.[62]

The sensitivity of IHC is better than light microscopic identification of viral inclusions and compares favorably with culture and *in situ* hybridization.[49,51,52,54,63] Additionally, immunohistochemical assays can be completed faster than the shell vial culture technique, allowing for rapid results that are important for early anti-CMV therapy.[54]

Other herpesvirus infections that have been diagnosed using immunohistochemical methods include human herpesvirus 6 infection[64] and Epstein-Barr viral infection.[65] Immunohistochemistry has been used to identify EBV latent membrane protein-1 in cases of Hodgkin's lymphoma and post-transplant lymphoproliferative disorder (Fig. 3.4).[66]

Adenoviruses

Adenovirus has been increasingly recognized as a cause of morbidity and mortality among immunocompromised patients owing to transplant and congenital immunodeficiency.[67,68] Rarely adenovirus infection has been described in HIV-infected patients.[69-71] Characteristic

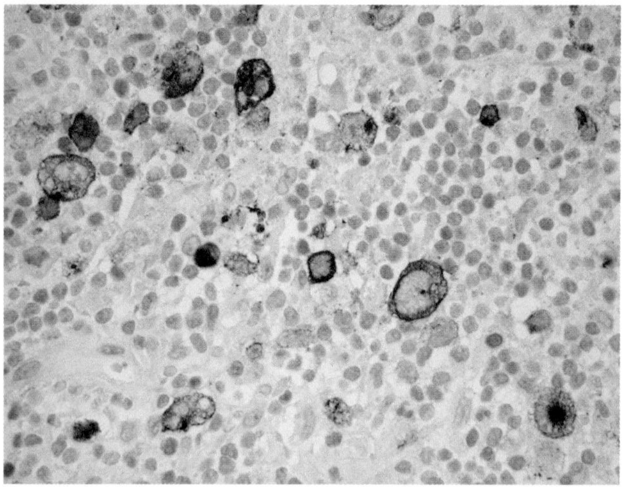

FIGURE 3.4 Epstein-Barr virus LMP-1 within cytoplasm of characteristic Reed-Sternberg cells in a case of Hodgkin's lymphoma. (Immunoperoxidase staining with DAB and hematoxylin counterstain; ×400.)

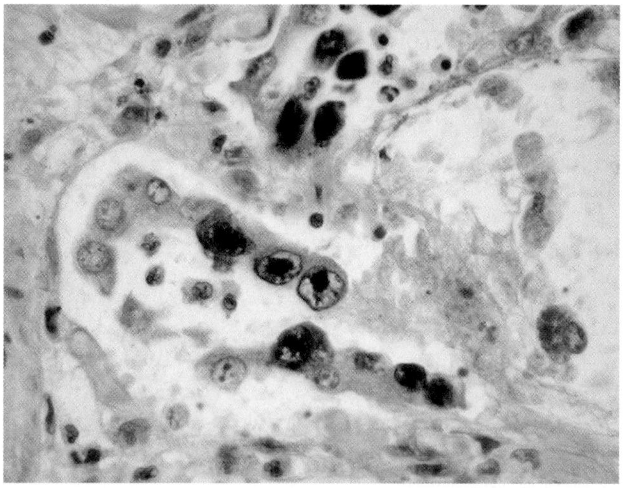

FIGURE 3.5 Adenovirus pneumonia in a heart transplant patient who developed ARDS and respiratory failure. Infected cells within necrotizing exudate show intranuclear reactivity with antibody to adenovirus antigen. Some cells show inclusions with a clear halo around them, making a differential diagnosis from CMV difficult on H&E stain. (Immunoperoxidase staining with DAB and hematoxylin counterstain; ×400.)

adenovirus inclusions are amphophilic, intranuclear, homogeneous, and glassy. However, in some cases, the infection may contain only rare cells showing the characteristic cytopathic effect.[70] In addition, other viral inclusions, including CMV, human papillomavirus (HPV), HSV, and VZV, can be mistaken for adenovirus inclusions and vice versa. In these circumstances, immunohistochemical assay may be necessary for a definitive diagnosis. A monoclonal antibody that is reactive with all 41 serotypes of adenovirus has been used in an immunohistochemical technique to demonstrate intranuclear adenoviral antigen in immunocompromised patients (Fig. 3.5).[70-74] Histologic diagnosis of adenovirus colitis is difficult, and it is usually underdiagnosed. Moreover, in immunosuppressed patients, the incidence

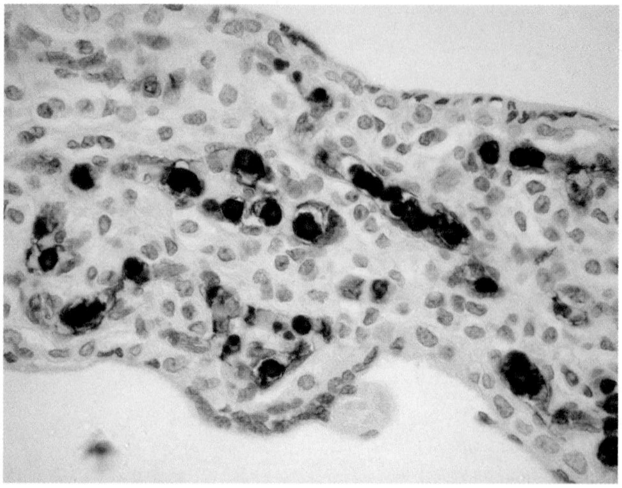

FIGURE 3.6 Hydrops fetalis caused by parvovirus B19 infection. Normoblasts within the villous capillaries show intranuclear viral antigen. (Immunoperoxidase staining with DAB and hematoxylin counterstain; ×400.)

of coinfection with other viruses is high, and the presence of adenovirus tends to be overlooked. Immunohistochemical staining has been of value in differentiating adenovirus colitis from CMV colitis.[70,75]

Parvovirus B19 Infection

Parvovirus B19 has been associated with asymptomatic infections, erythema infectiosum, acute arthropathy, aplastic crisis, hydrops fetalis, and chronic anemia and red cell aplasia. In addition, parvovirus B19 infection has been recognized as an important cause of severe anemia in immunocompromised leukemic patients receiving chemotherapy.[76]

The diagnosis of parvovirus infection can be achieved by identifying typical findings in bone marrow specimens, including decreased or absent red cell precursors, giant pronormoblasts, and eosinophilic or amphophilic intranuclear inclusions in erythroid cells.[77,78] Because intravenous immunoglobulin therapy is effective, a rapid and accurate diagnostic method is important. Immunohistochemistry with a monoclonal antibody against VP1 and VP2 capsid proteins has been used as a rapid and sensitive method to establish the diagnosis of parvovirus B19 infection in formalin-fixed, paraffin-embedded tissues.[79-82] Immunohistochemistry is of particular help in detecting parvovirus B19 antigen in cases with sparse inclusions, to study cases not initially identified by examination of routinely stained tissue sections, or in cases of hydrops fetalis with advanced cytolysis (Fig. 3.6).[79,83,84] Several studies have found a strong correlation among results obtained from morphologic, immunohistochemical, *in situ* hybridization (ISH), and polymerase chain reaction (PCR) methods.[78,79,82,84]

Viral Hemorrhagic Fevers

Since the 1980s, numerous emerging and reemerging agents of viral hemorrhagic fevers have attracted the attention of pathologists.[3-5] Investigators have played

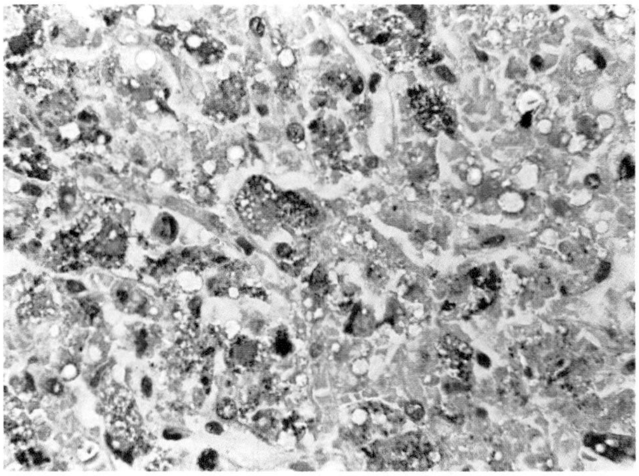

FIGURE 3.7 Yellow fever. Abundant yellow fever viral antigens are seen within hepatocytes and Kupffer cells. (Immunoperoxidase staining with AEC and hematoxylin counterstain; ×400.)

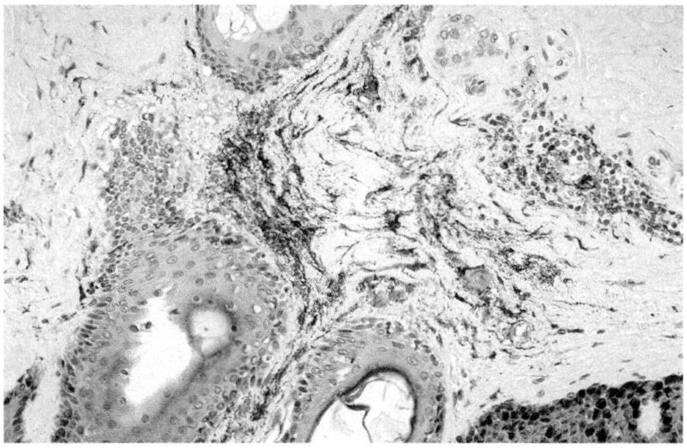

FIGURE 3.8 Extensive Ebola viral antigens are seen primarily within fibroblasts in the dermis of a skin specimen from a fatal case of Ebola hemorrhagic fever. (Immunoalkaline phosphatase with naphthol fast red substrate and hematoxylin counterstain; original magnification ×20.)

an important role in identifying these agents and in supporting epidemiologic, clinical, and pathogenetic studies of emerging viral hemorrhagic fevers.[4,5,7] Viral hemorrhagic fevers are often fatal. They are clinically difficult to diagnose (in the absence of bleeding or organ manifestations) and frequently require handling and testing of potentially dangerous biological specimens. In addition, histopathologic features are not pathognomonic, and they can resemble other viral, rickettsial, and bacterial (e.g., leptospirosis) infections. Immunohistochemistry is essential and has been successfully and safely applied to the diagnosis and study of the pathogenesis of these diseases.

Several studies have established the utility of IHC as a sensitive, safe, and rapid diagnostic method for the diagnosis of viral hemorrhagic fevers such as yellow fever (Fig. 3.7),[85-87] dengue hemorrhagic fever,[87,88] Crimean-Congo hemorrhagic fever,[89] Argentine hemorrhagic fever,[90] Venezuelan hemorrhagic fever,[91] and Marburg disease.[92] Additionally, a sensitive, specific, and safe immunostaining method has been developed to diagnose Ebola hemorrhagic fever in formalin-fixed skin biopsies (Fig. 3.8).[93] Immunohistochemistry demonstrated that Lassa virus targets primarily endothelial cells, mononuclear inflammatory cells, and hepatocytes (Fig. 3.9).[93-95]

Polyomaviruses

BK virus infections are frequent during infancy; in immunocompetent individuals the virus remains latent in the kidneys, central nervous system, and B lymphocytes. In immunocompromised patients, the infection reactivates and spreads to other organs. BK virus nephropathy is an important cause of graft failure in patients with a renal transplant,[96] with a prevalence varying from 2% to 4.5% in different transplant centers.[96,97] Since specific clinical signs and symptoms are lacking in BK virus nephropathy, the diagnosis can only be made histologically in a graft biopsy.[98] In the kidney, the infection is associated with mononuclear interstitial inflammatory infiltrates and tubular atrophy, findings that can be difficult to distinguish from acute rejection.[98] The cytopathic changes observed in BK virus infection are not pathognomonic and can be observed in other viral infections. Moreover, in early BK virus infection there are minimal or no histologic changes, although IHC can identify viral antigen.[99,100] In this setting, IHC with an antibody against the large T antigen of SV40 virus has been effective in demonstrating BK virus infection (Fig. 3.10).[96,99,101-103]

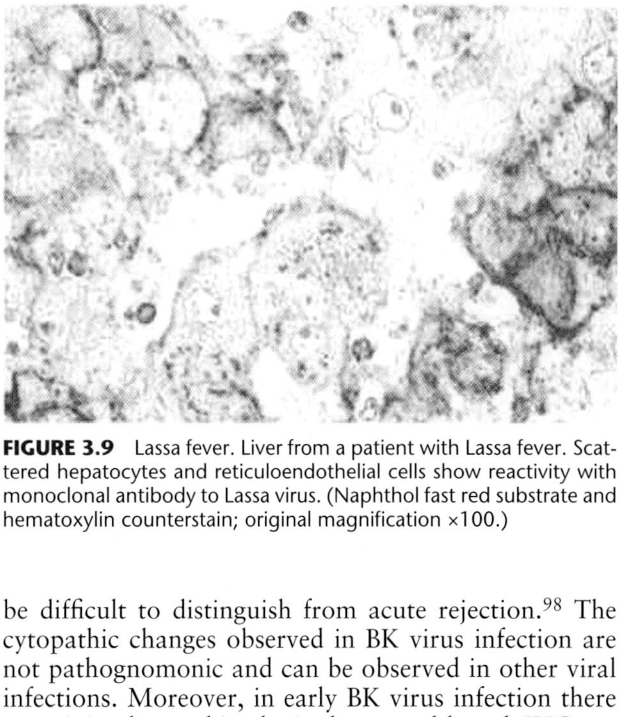

FIGURE 3.9 Lassa fever. Liver from a patient with Lassa fever. Scattered hepatocytes and reticuloendothelial cells show reactivity with monoclonal antibody to Lassa virus. (Naphthol fast red substrate and hematoxylin counterstain; original magnification ×100.)

The human polyomavirus JC is a double-stranded DNA virus that causes progressive multifocal leukoencephalopathy (PML). This fatal demyelinating disease is characterized by cytopathic changes in oligodendrocytes and bizarre giant astrocytes. In addition to detection by antibodies to SV40-T antigen, IHC using a polyclonal rabbit antiserum against the protein VP1 is a specific, sensitive, and rapid method used to confirm the diagnosis of PML.[104-107] JC virus antigen is usually seen within oligodendrocytes (Fig. 3.11) and occasional astrocytes, and antigen-bearing cells are more commonly seen in early lesions.

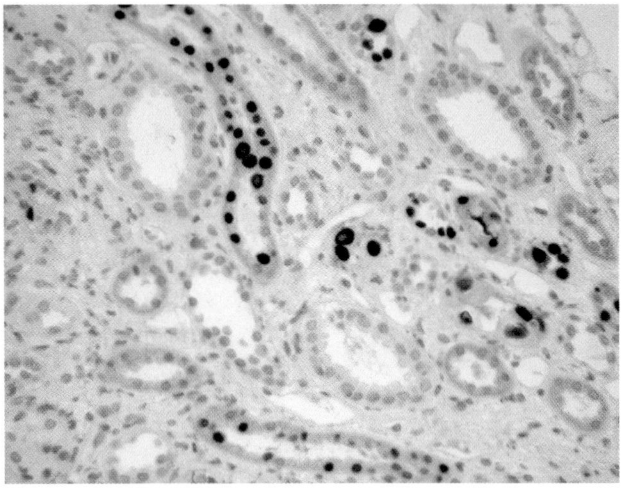

FIGURE 3.10 Immunohistochemical detection of SV40-T antigen in the nuclei of tubular cells in a renal transplant patient with BK virus–associated nephropathy. (Immunoperoxidase staining with DAB and hematoxylin counterstain; ×400.)

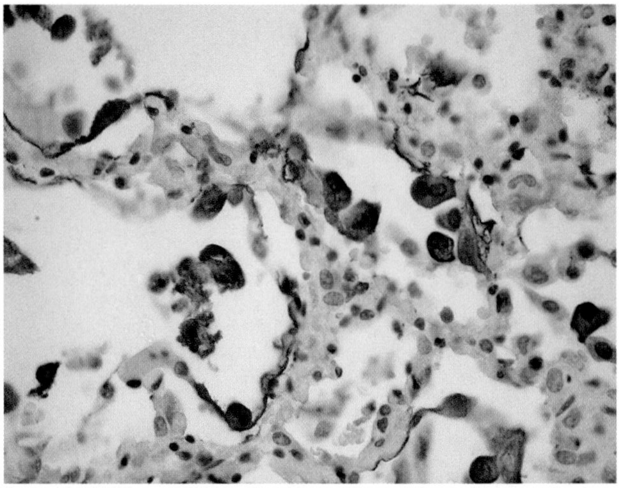

FIGURE 3.12 Immunostaining of RSV antigens in desquamated bronchial and alveolar lining cells using a monoclonal antibody. (Immunoperoxidase staining with DAB and hematoxylin counterstain; ×400.)

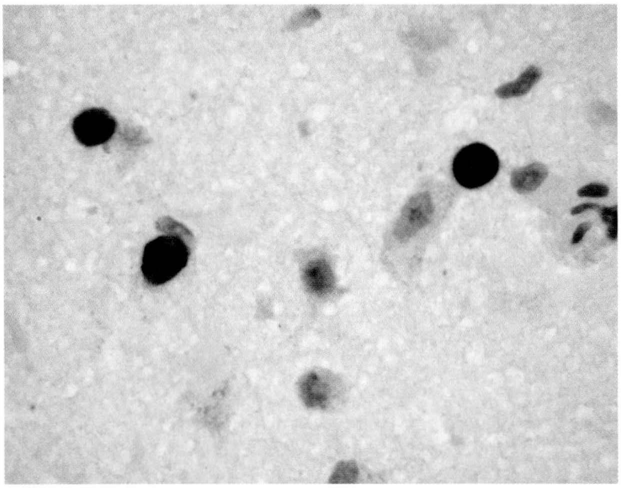

FIGURE 3.11 Progressive multifocal leukoencephalopathy: SV40-T antigen in the nuclei of enlarged oligodendrocytes in a patient with JC virus infection. (Immunoperoxidase staining with DAB and hematoxylin counterstain; ×400.)

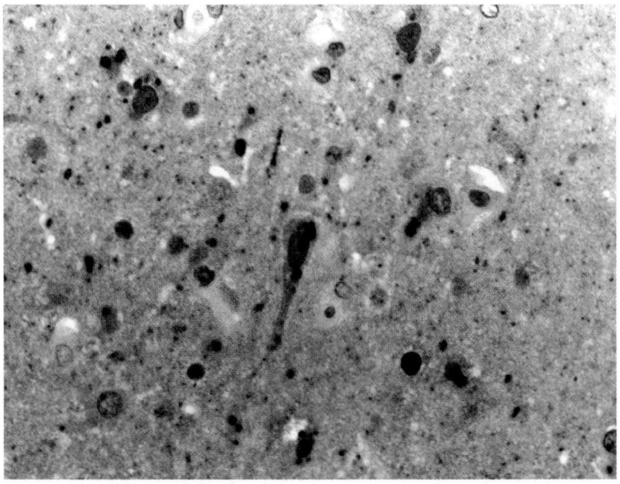

FIGURE 3.13 Immunostaining of rabies viral antigens in neurons of the CNS using a rabbit polyclonal antibody. Red precipitate corresponds to Negri inclusions by H&E staining. (Immunoalkaline phosphatase with naphthol fast red substrate and hematoxylin counterstain; original magnification ×40.)

Other Viral Infections

Immunohistochemistry has also been used to confirm the diagnosis of respiratory viral diseases such as influenza A virus and respiratory syncytial virus infections (Fig. 3.12) when cultures were not available.[108-111]

The diagnosis of rabies relies heavily on histopathologic examination of tissues to demonstrate its characteristic cytoplasmic inclusions (Negri bodies). In a significant percentage of cases, Negri bodies are inconspicuous and so few that confirming the diagnosis of rabies is extremely difficult.[112] Furthermore, in nonendemic areas the diagnosis of rabies usually is not suspected clinically, or the patient may present with ascending paralysis. In these settings, immunohistochemical staining is a very sensitive, specific, and safe diagnostic tool for rabies (Fig. 3.13).[112-116] Other viral agents that can be diagnosed using immunohistochemical methods include enteroviruses,[117-120] eastern equine encephalitis virus,[121-123] and rotavirus.[124-126]

Immunohistochemical staining has been used in the histopathologic diagnosis of viral hepatitis C; however, IHC for this virus is not as effective as serologic assays and detection of HCV RNA in serum.

BACTERIAL INFECTIONS

Among bacterial infections, the greatest number of immunohistochemical studies has been performed in the investigation of *Helicobacter pylori*. A few studies have evaluated the use of IHC for other bacterial, mycobacterial, rickettsial, and spirochetal infections.

Antigen retrieval is generally not required for the immunohistochemical demonstration of bacteria in

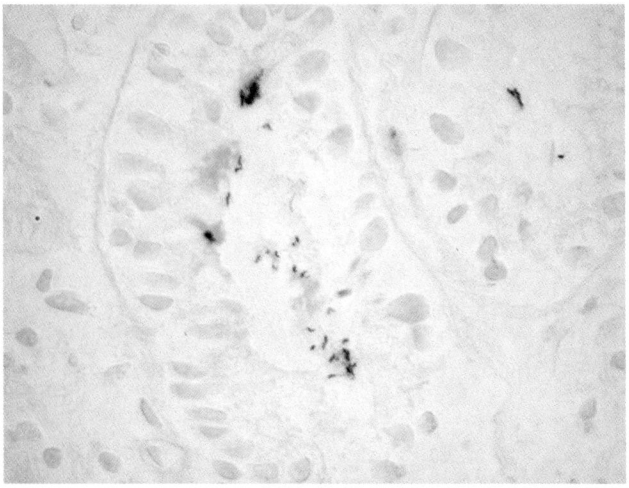

FIGURE 3.14 Numerous curved *H. pylori* in the superficial gastric mucus are clearly demonstrated by immunoperoxidase staining in this patient with chronic active gastritis. (Immunoperoxidase staining with DAB and hematoxylin counterstain; ×400.)

fixed tissue. However, interpreting the results can be complicated because many of these antibodies cross-react with other bacteria. Moreover, antibodies may react with only portions of the bacteria, and they may label remnants of bacteria or spirochetes when viable organisms are no longer present.

Helicobacter Pylori Infection

Gastric infection by *H. pylori* results in chronic active gastritis and is strongly associated with lymphoid hyperplasia, gastric lymphomas, and gastric adenocarcinoma. Heavy infections with numerous organisms are easily detected on routine hematoxylin and eosin–stained tissues; however, the detection rate is only 66% with many false-positive and false-negative results.[127,128] Conventional histochemical methods such as silver stains are more sensitive than hematoxylin and eosin in detecting *H. pylori*. Nonetheless, for detecting scant numbers of organisms, it has been proven that IHC has high specificity and sensitivity, is less expensive when all factors are considered, is superior to conventional histochemical methods, and has a low interobserver variation (Fig. 3.14).[127] Treatment for chronic active gastritis and *H. pylori* infection can change the shape of the microorganism. This can make it difficult to identify and differentiate the organism from extracellular debris or mucin globules. In these cases IHC improves the rate of successful identification of the bacteria, even when histologic examination and cultures are falsely negative.[129-132]

Whipple's Disease

Whipple's disease affects primarily the small bowel and mesenteric lymph nodes and less commonly other organs such as the heart and central nervous system. Numerous foamy macrophages characterize the disease, and the diagnosis usually relies on the demonstration of PAS-positive intracytoplasmic bacteria. Nevertheless, the presence of PAS-positive macrophages is not

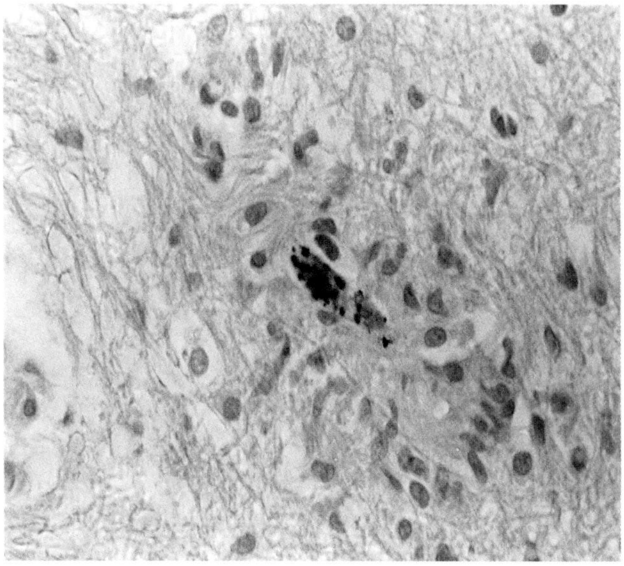

FIGURE 3.15 Immunohistologic demonstration of *R. rickettsii* within vascular endothelium in the pons of a patient with fatal Rocky Mountain spotted fever. (Immunoperoxidase staining with AEC and hematoxylin counterstain; ×600.)

pathognomonic; they can be observed in other diseases such as *Mycobacterium avium* infections, histoplasmosis, *Rhodococcus equi* infections, and macroglobulinemia. *Tropheryma whipplei* is a rare cause of endocarditis that shares many histologic features with other culture-negative endocarditides such as those caused by *Coxiella burnetii* and *Bartonella* sp.[133] The development of specific antibodies against these microorganisms has significantly enhanced the ability to detect them in the heart valves of patients with culture-negative endocarditis.[134] Immunohistochemical staining with rabbit polyclonal antibody provides a sensitive and specific method for the rapid diagnosis of intestinal and extraintestinal Whipple's disease and for follow-up of treatment response.[135-137]

Rocky Mountain Spotted Fever

Confirmation of Rocky Mountain spotted fever (RMSF) usually requires the use of serologic methods to detect antibodies to spotted fever group (SFG) Rickettsiae; however, most patients with RMSF lack diagnostic titers during the first week of disease. Immunohistochemistry has been successfully used to detect SFG Rickettsiae in formalin-fixed tissue sections, and it is superior to histochemical methods (Fig. 3.15).[138,139] Several studies illustrate the value of IHC in diagnosing suspected cases of RMSF using skin biopsies with high specificity and sensitivity, and in confirming fatal cases of seronegative RMSF.[10,140-144] *R. rickettsii* cannot be distinguished from other spotted fever group Rickettsiae such as *R. parkeri* or *R. conorii* because they cross-react.

Bartonella Infections

Bartonella are slow-growing, fastidious gram-negative, Warthin-Starry–stained bacteria associated with bacillary angiomatosis, peliosis hepatis, cat-scratch disease,

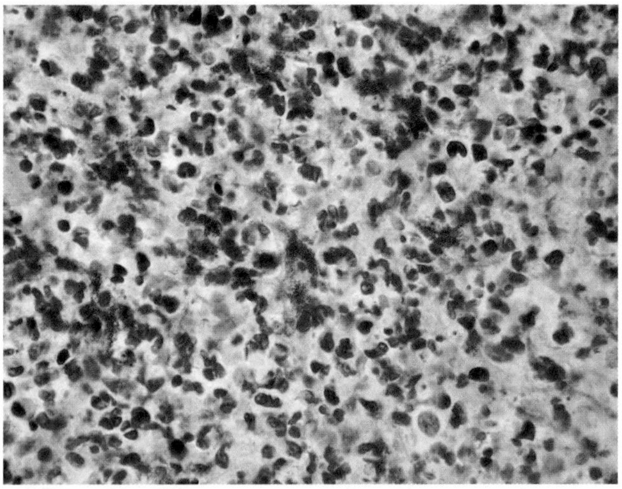

FIGURE 3.16 Photomicrograph of a lymph node biopsy from a patient with cat-scratch disease showing abundant extracellular, clumped coccobacilli of *B. henselae* in necrotic foci. (Immunoalkaline phosphatase with monoclonal antibody against *B. henselae,* naphthol fast red substrate and hematoxylin counterstain; ×200.) *Courtesy of Dr. Suimin Qiu, University of Texas Medical Branch.*

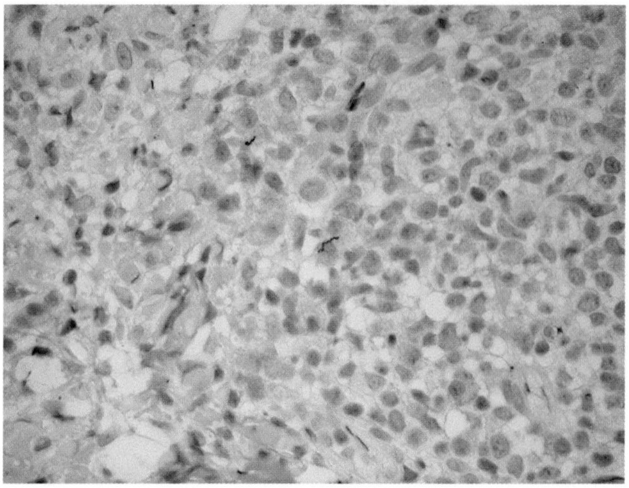

FIGURE 3.17 Syphilis. Skin biopsy from a patient with secondary syphilis. Scattered intact *T. pallidum* are easily visible with a rabbit polyclonal antibody against *T. pallidum*. (Immunoperoxidase staining with DAB and hematoxylin counterstain; ×400.)

trench fever, relapsing bacteremia, and disseminated granulomatous lesions of liver and spleen.[145] *Bartonella* are important agents of blood culture–negative endocarditis. Traditional techniques such as histology, electron microscopy, and serology have been employed to identify the agents of culture-negative endocarditis. However, *Bartonella* sp., *C. burnetii*, and *T. whipplei* endocarditis share many morphologic features that do not allow for a specific histologic diagnosis.[146] Besides, serologic tests for *Bartonella* sp. may show cross-reactivity with *C. burnetii* and *Chlamydia* sp.[147] Immunostaining has been successfully used to identify *Bartonella henselae* and *B. quintana* in the heart valves of patients with blood culture–negative endocarditis and has significantly enhanced the ability to establish a specific diagnosis in these cases.[148,149] A polyclonal rabbit antibody that does not differentiate between *B. henselae* and *B. quintana* has also been used to detect these microorganisms in cat-scratch disease (Fig. 3.16), bacillary angiomatosis, and peliosis hepatis.[150,151] A commercially available monoclonal antibody specific for *B. henselae* is also available and has been used to demonstrate the organism in a case of spontaneous splenic rupture caused by this bacterium.[152]

Syphilis

Syphilis continues to be a public health problem caused by *T. pallidum*, a fastidious organism that has not been cultivated.[153] The diagnosis of syphilis relies on serology and the identification of *T. pallidum* by dark-field microscopy. However, these methods have low sensitivity and specificity,[154] and serologic methods can be negative in early stages of the disease and in immunosuppressed patients such as those coinfected with human immunodeficiency virus (HIV).[155] In tissue sections, the usual method for detecting spirochetes is through silver impregnation stains (Warthin-Starry or Steiner). These stains, however, can be technically difficult to perform and interpret, are nonspecific, and frequently show marked background artifacts because silver stains also highlight melanin granules and reticulin fibers. Detection rates of spirochetes using silver stains vary from 33% to 71%.[156] It has been shown that immunostaining of biopsy specimens with anti–*T. pallidum* polyclonal antibody (Fig. 3.17) is more sensitive and specific than silver staining methods, with sensitivities ranging from 71% to 94%.[153,156,157]

Mycobacterium Tuberculosis Infection

Identification of *M. tuberculosis* is routinely achieved by acid-fast bacilli (AFB) staining, culture of biopsy specimens, or both. Nevertheless, AFB staining has a low sensitivity, and it is not specific because it does not differentiate mycobacterial species.[158] Furthermore, cultures may take several weeks, and sensitivity is low in paucibacillary lesions.[159] In the histologic diagnosis of mycobacterial infections, IHC with anti-BCG polyclonal antibody has shown better sensitivity than AFB staining. However, in paucibacillary lesions it is inferior to AFB staining and cannot differentiate between *M. tuberculosis* and other mycobacteria.[160] Recently a polyclonal antibody against the *M. tuberculosis*–secreted antigen MPT64 was used in cases of mycobacterial lymphadenitis. This method showed 90% sensitivity and 83% specificity and performed better than AFB staining in cases of paucibacillary disease and comparably to nested PCR.[161]

Other Bacterial Infections

Other bacterial diseases that can be identified by IHC in formalin-fixed tissue include leptospirosis, a zoonosis that usually presents as an acute febrile syndrome but occasionally can have unusual manifestations such as pulmonary hemorrhage with respiratory failure or abdominal pain.[162-164] Rabbit polyclonal antibodies

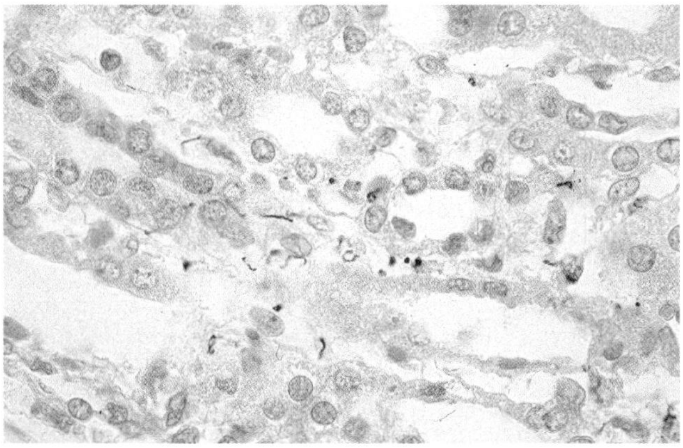

FIGURE 3.18 Leptospira. Immunostaining of intact leptospires and granular forms of leptospiral antigens in kidney of patient who died of pulmonary hemorrhage. (Immunoalkaline phosphatase with rabbit polyclonal antisera with naphthol fast red substrate and hematoxylin counterstain; original magnification ×63.)

have been used in IHC to detect leptospiral antigens in the gallbladder and lungs from patients with unusual presentations (Fig. 3.18).[162-165]

Lyme disease has protean clinical manifestations, and *Borrelia burgdoferi* is difficult to culture from tissues and fluids. In addition, cultures are rarely positive before 2 to 4 weeks of incubation. *Borrelia burgdorferi* can be identified in tissues by immunostaining with polyclonal or monoclonal antibodies. Although IHC is more specific than silver impregnation staining, the sensitivity of immunostaining is poor, and the microorganisms are difficult to detect owing to the low numbers present in tissue sections.[166,167]

Q fever is a zoonosis caused by *Coxiella burnetii* and is characterized by protean and non-specific manifestations. Acute Q fever can manifest as atypical pneumonia or granulomatous hepatitis, frequently with characteristic fibrin ring granulomas. This microorganism is recognized as one agent that causes blood culture–negative chronic endocarditis.[168] A monoclonal antibody has been used to specifically identify *C. burnetii* in cardiac valves of patients with chronic Q fever endocarditis.[12,169]

Recently IHC has been successfully used to identify *Streptococcus pneumoniae* in formalin-fixed organs with an overall sensitivity of 100% and a specificity of 71% when compared with cultures.[170] Immunohistochemical assays are used to identify *Clostridium* sp., *S. aureus,* and *S. pyogenes;*[171,172] *Haemophilus influenzae;*[173-175] *Chlamydia* species;[176-178] *Legionella pneumophila* and *L. dumoffii;*[179-181] *Listeria monocytogenes;*[182-184] *Salmonella;*[185,186] and rickettsial infections other than Rocky Mountain spotted fever such as boutonneuse fever, epidemic typhus, murine typhus,[187] rickettsialpox,[188,189] African tick bite fever,[138] and scrub typhus.[190]

FUNGAL INFECTIONS

The great majority of fungi are readily identified by hematoxylin and eosin staining alone or in combination with histochemical stains (e.g., periodic acid-Schiff [PAS], Gomori's methenamine silver [GMS]). However, these stains cannot distinguish morphologically similar fungi with potential differences in susceptibility to antimycotic drugs. In addition, several factors may influence the appearance of fungal elements, which may appear atypical in tissue sections because of steric orientation, age of the fungal lesion, effects of antifungal chemotherapy, type of infected tissue, and host immune response.[191] Currently the final identification of fungi relies on culture techniques; however, culture may take several days or longer to yield a definitive result, and surgical pathologists rarely have access to fresh tissue.

In past years, IHC has been used to identify various fungal elements in paraffin-embedded, formalin-fixed tissue.[192-194] Immunohistochemical methods have the advantage of providing rapid and specific identification of several fungi and allowing pathologists to identify unusual filamentous hyphal and yeast infections and to accurately distinguish them from confounding artifacts.[193,195] In addition, IHC allows pathologists to correlate microbiological and histologic findings of fungal infections and to distinguish them from harmless colonization. Immunohistochemistry can also be helpful when more than one fungus is present; in these cases dual immunostaining techniques can highlight the different fungal species present in the tissue.[196] An important limitation of IHC in the identification of fungi is the well-known, widespread occurrence of common antigens among pathogenic fungi that frequently results in cross-reactivity with polyclonal antibodies and even with some monoclonal antibodies.[193,195-197] Therefore, assessing cross-reactivity using a panel of fungi is a very important step in the evaluation of immunohistochemical methods.[193,194]

Candida species are often stained weakly with hematoxylin and eosin, and sometimes the yeast form may be difficult to differentiate from *Histoplasma capsulatum, Cryptococcus neoformans,* and even *Pneumocystis carinii.* Polyclonal and monoclonal antibodies against *Candida* genus antigens are sensitive and strongly reactive and do not show cross-reactivity with other fungi tested.[193,194,198,199] In particular, two monoclonal antibodies against *Candida albicans* mannoproteins show high sensitivity and specificity. Monoclonal antibody 3H8 recognizes primarily filamentous forms of *C. albicans,* whereas monoclonal antibody 1B12 highlights yeast forms.[199-203]

Identification of *Cryptococcus neoformans* usually is not a problem when the fungus produces a mucicarmine-positive capsule. However, infections by capsule-negative strains are more difficult to diagnose, and the disease can be confused with histoplasmosis, blastomycosis, or torulopsis. Also, in long-standing infections the yeast often appear atypical and fragmented. Polyclonal antibodies raised against *C. neoformans* yeast cells are sensitive and specific.[193,194] More recently, monoclonal antibodies have been produced that allow identification and differentiation of varieties of *C. neoformans* in formalin-fixed tissue. The antibodies are highly sensitive (97%) and specific (100%) and can differentiate *C. neoformans var. neoformans* from *C. neoformans var. gattii.*[204,205]

Sporothrix schenckii may be confused in tissue sections with *Blastomyces dermatitidis* and fungal agents of phaeohyphomycosis. In addition, yeast cells of *Sporothrix schenckii* may be sparsely present in tissues. Antibodies against yeast cells of *S. schenckii* are sensitive but demonstrate cross-reactivity with *Candida* species; however, after specific adsorption of the antibody with *Candida* yeast cells, the cross-reactivity of the antibodies is eliminated.[193,194]

Invasive aspergillosis is a frequent cause of fungal infection with high morbidity and mortality rates in immunocompromised patients.[206] The diagnosis is often difficult and relies heavily on histologic identification of invasive septate hyphae and culture confirmation. Nevertheless, several filamentous fungi such as *Fusarium* species, *Pseudallescheria boydii,* and *Scedosporium* species share similar morphology with *Aspergillus* species in hematoxylin and eosin–stained tissues.[207] A precise and rapid diagnosis of invasive aspergillosis is important because early diagnosis is associated with improved clinical response, and it allows planning of the correct duration and choice of antimycotic therapy. Researchers have shown that the yield of cultures in histologically proven cases is low, ranging from 25% to 50%.[206,208-211] Several polyclonal and monoclonal antibodies against *Aspergillus* antigens have been tested in formalin-fixed tissues with variable sensitivities, and most of them cross-react with other fungi.[197,212,213] More recently, monoclonal antibodies (WF-AF-1, 164G, and 611F) against *Aspergillus* galactomannan have shown high sensitivity and specificity in identifying *A. fumigatus, A. flavus,* and *A. niger* in formalin-fixed tissues without cross-reactivity with other filamentous fungi.[211,214,215]

Cysts and trophozoites of *Pneumocystis jirovecii* can be detected in bronchoalveolar lavage specimens using monoclonal antibodies that yield results that are slightly more sensitive than GMS, Giemsa, or Papanicolaou staining (Fig. 3.19).[194,216,217] Antibodies are most helpful in cases of extrapulmonary pneumocystosis or in the diagnosis of *P. jirovecii* pneumonia when atypical pathologic features are present (e.g., hyaline membranes or granulomatous pneumocystosis where microorganisms are usually very sparse).

Penicillium marneffei can cause a disseminated infection in immunocompromised patients.[218,219] Morphologically the organisms must be differentiated from *H. capsulatum, C. neoformans,* and *C. albicans*. The monoclonal antibody EBA-1 against the galactomannan of *Aspergillus* species cross-reacts with and detects *P. marneffei* in tissue sections.[209,220] Immunohistochemistry has also been used to detect *Blastomyces, Coccidioides,* and *Histoplasma*.[193,194,221] However, the antibodies have significant cross-reactivity with several other fungi.

PROTOZOAL INFECTIONS

Protozoa usually can be identified in tissue sections stained with hematoxylin and eosin or Giemsa stain; however, because of the small size of the organisms and the subtle distinguishing features, an unequivocal diagnosis cannot always be made. The role of IHC in the detection of protozoal infections has been particularly valuable in cases in which the morphology of the parasite is distorted by tissue necrosis or autolysis. In addition, in immunocompromised patients, toxoplasmosis can have an unusual disseminated presentation with numerous tachyzoites without bradyzoites (Fig. 3.20).[222,223] Immunohistochemistry has also been useful in cases with unusual presentation of the disease.[224]

The diagnosis of leishmaniasis in routine practice usually is not difficult; however, in certain circumstances pathologic diagnosis may be problematic, as is the case in chronic granulomatous leishmaniasis with small numbers of parasites, when the microorganism presents in unusual locations, or when necrosis distorts the morphologic appearance of the disease.[225] In these cases, immunohistochemical staining has been a valuable diagnostic tool.[225-228] The highly sensitive and specific monoclonal antibody p19-11 recognizes different

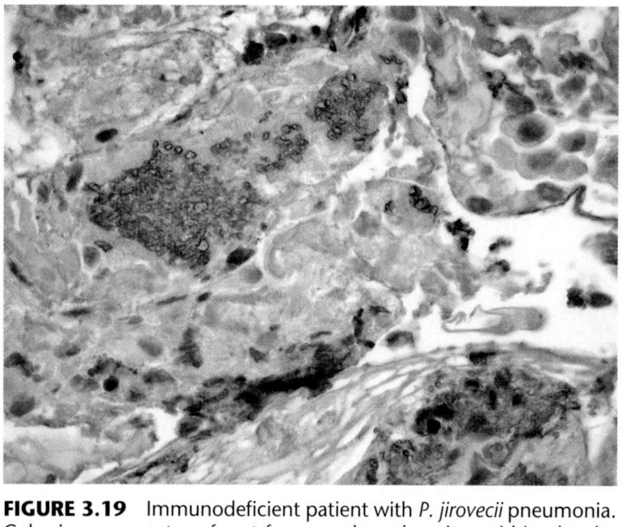

FIGURE 3.19 Immunodeficient patient with *P. jirovecii* pneumonia. Cohesive aggregates of cyst forms and trophozoites within alveolar spaces are demonstrated by a monoclonal antibody against pneumocystis with an immunoperoxidase technique. (Immunoperoxidase staining with DAB and hematoxylin counterstain; ×400.)

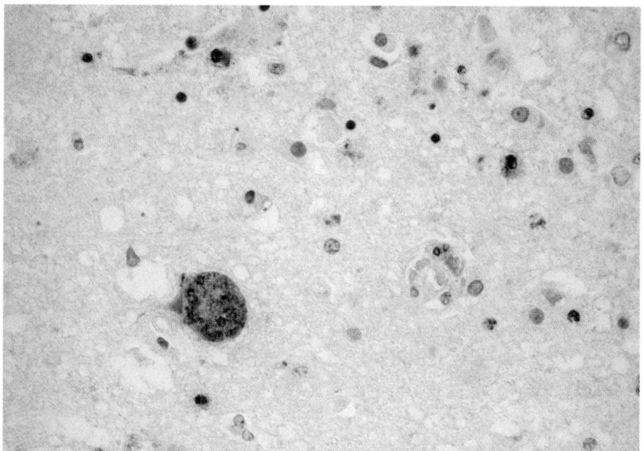

FIGURE 3.20 HIV-infected patient with toxoplasmic encephalitis. Immunoperoxidase staining highlights cyst forms and scattered tachyzoites. (DAB substrate with hematoxylin counterstain; ×400.)

species of *Leishmania* and allows differentiation from morphologically similar microorganisms (*Toxoplasma*, *Trypanosoma cruzi*, and *P. marneffei*).[225]

Immunohistochemical assays using polyclonal antibodies specific for *Balamuthia mandrillaris*, *Naegleria fowleri*, and *Acanthamoeba* sp. are used to demonstrate amebic trophozoites and cysts in areas of necrosis and can allow their differentiation from macrophages in cases of amebic meningoencephalitis.[229]

Immunohistochemistry has also been used to identify *Cryptosporidium*,[230] *Entamoeba histolytica*,[231] *Trypanosoma cruzi*,[232-234] babesia,[235] *Giardia lamblia*,[236] *Plasmodium falciparum*, and *P. vivax* in fatal cases of malaria[237] in formalin-fixed paraffin-embedded tissue samples.

EMERGING INFECTIOUS DISEASES

In 1992 the Institute of Medicine defined emerging infectious diseases (EIDs) as caused by new, previously unidentified microorganisms or those whose incidence in humans has increased within the previous two decades or threatens to increase in the near future.[238] The list of pathogens newly recognized since 1973 is long and continues to increase. Recognizing emerging infections is a challenge, and many new infectious agents remain undetected for years before emerging as an identified public health problem.[239] EIDs are a global phenomenon that requires a global response. The Centers for Disease Control and Prevention (CDC) has defined the strategy to prevent and detect EIDs.[239] The anatomic pathology laboratory plays a critical role in the initial and rapid detection of EIDs.[240,241] Besides assisting in the identification of new infectious agents, IHC has contributed to the understanding of the pathogenesis and epidemiology of EIDs.

Hantavirus Pulmonary Syndrome

In 1993 in the southwestern United States, several previously healthy individuals died of rapidly progressive pulmonary edema, respiratory insufficiency, and shock.[242,243] Immunohistochemistry played a central role in identifying the viral antigens of an unknown hantavirus,[244,245] detecting the occurrence of unrecognized cases of hantavirus pulmonary syndrome prior to 1993, and showing the distribution of viral antigen in endothelial cells of the microcirculation, particularly in the lung (Fig. 3.21).[244,246]

West Nile Virus Encephalitis

West Nile virus (WNV) was originally identified in Africa in 1937, and the first cases of WNV encephalitis in the United States were described in 1999. The clinical picture is variable and non-specific. It can range from subclinical infection to flaccid paralysis and encephalitis characterized morphologically by perivascular mononuclear cell inflammatory infiltrates, neuronal necrosis, edema, and microglial nodules, particularly prominent in the brainstem, cerebellum, and spinal cord.[247-251] The diagnosis of WNV encephalitis is usually established by identifying virus-specific IgM in CSF and/or serum and by demonstrating viral RNA in serum, CSF, or other tissue.[252] Immunostaining with monoclonal or polyclonal antibodies has been successfully used to diagnose WNV infection in immunocompromised patients with an inadequate antibody response (Fig. 3.22).[248]

Enterovirus 71 Encephalomyelitis

Enterovirus 71 (EV71) has been associated with hand, foot, and mouth disease; herpangina; aseptic meningitis; and poliomyelitis-like flaccid paralysis. More recently EV71 has been associated with unusual cases of fulminant encephalitis, pulmonary edema and hemorrhage, and heart failure.[253,254] Severe and extensive encephalomyelitis of the cerebral cortex, brainstem, and spinal cord has been described. Immunohistochemical staining with monoclonal antibody against EV71 has played a pivotal role in the linking of EV71 infection to fulminant encephalitis (Fig. 3.23). Viral antigen is observed within

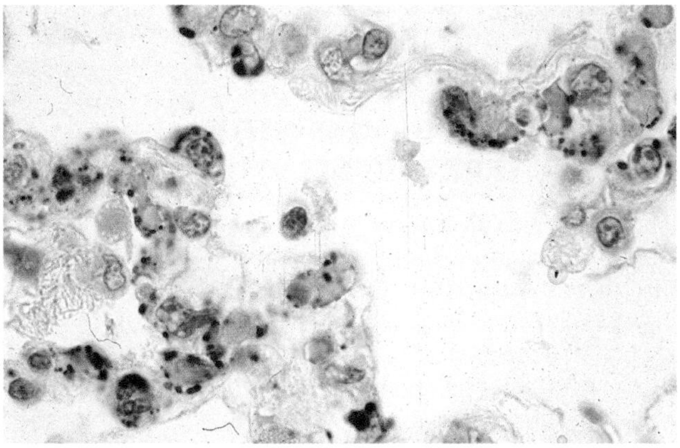

FIGURE 3.21 Hantavirus antigen–containing endothelial cells of the pulmonary microvasculature in the lung of an HPS patient as detected by immunohistochemistry using a mouse monoclonal antibody. (Immunoalkaline phosphatase with naphthol fast red substrate and hematoxylin counterstain; original magnification ×100.)

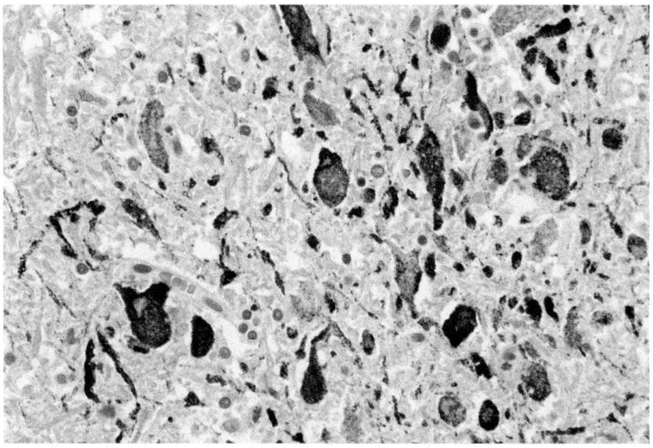

FIGURE 3.22 West Nile virus. Immunostaining of flaviviral antigens in neurons and neuronal processes in the central nervous system from an immunosuppressed patient who died of West Nile virus encephalitis. (Flavivirus-hyperimmune mouse ascitic fluid naphthol fast red substrate with hematoxylin counterstain; original magnification ×40.)

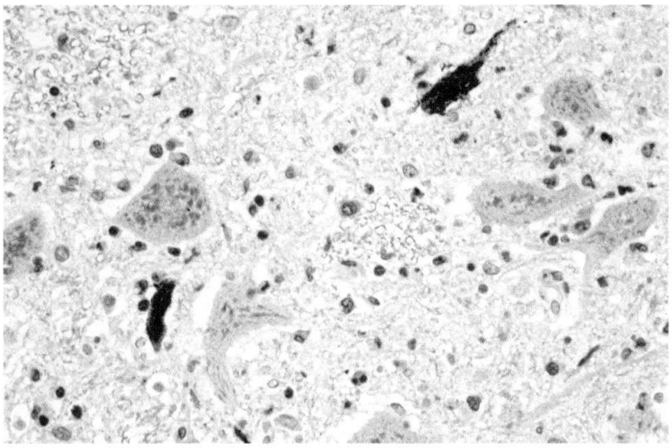

FIGURE 3.23 Enterovirus 71. Positive staining of EV71 viral antigens in neurons and neuronal processes of a fatal case of enterovirus encephalitis. (Immunoalkaline phosphatase with naphthol fast red substrate and hematoxylin counterstain; original magnification ×40.)

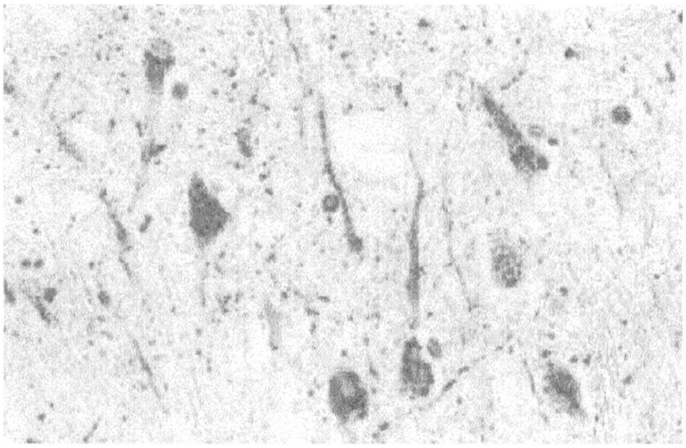

FIGURE 3.24 Nipah virus. Immunostaining of Nipah virus antigens in neurons and neuronal processes in CNS of a fatal case of Nipah virus encephalitis. (Immunoalkaline phosphatase with naphthol fast red substrate and hematoxylin counterstain; original magnification ×63.)

neurons, neuronal processes, and mononuclear inflammatory cells.[255-257]

Nipah Virus Infection

Nipah virus is a recently described paramyxovirus that causes an acute febrile encephalitic syndrome with a high mortality rate.[258-260] Pathology played a key role in identifying the causative agent. Histopathologic findings include vasculitis with thrombosis, microinfarctions, syncytial giant cells, and viral inclusions.[258,260] Although characteristic of this disease, syncytial giant endothelial cells are seen only in 25% of cases,[258] and viral inclusions of similar morphology can been seen in other paramyxoviral infections. Immunostaining provides a useful tool for unequivocal diagnosis of the disease, demonstrating viral antigen within neurons and endothelial cells of most organs (Fig. 3.24).[5,258]

Ehrlichioses

Tick-transmitted intracellular gram-negative bacteria belonging to the genera *Ehrlichia* and *Anaplasma* are the agents of human monocytotropic ehrlichiosis and human granulocytotropic anaplasmosis, respectively. The acute febrile illnesses usually present with cytopenias, myalgias, and mild to moderate hepatitis.[261-264]

Diagnosis of ehrlichiosis depends upon finding the characteristic monocytic and/or granulocytic cytoplasmic inclusions (morulae), PCR analysis of blood, and detection of specific antibodies in blood. However, morulae are rare and often missed on initial evaluation; hematoxylin and eosin–stained sections often fail to show organisms even when IHC reveals abundant ehrlichial antigen; and antibody titers may take several weeks to rise to diagnostic levels.[261,265] Additionally, immunocompromised patients may not develop anti-ehrlichial antibodies prior to death.[261,263] In these cases, immunostaining for *Ehrlichia* or *Anaplasma* is a sensitive and specific diagnostic method.[261,263,264,266]

Immunohistochemistry has been a very valuable tool used to identify and study several other EIDs such as Ebola hemorrhagic fever;[93-95] Hendra virus encephalitis;[5,267,268] leptospirosis;[163-165] emerging tick-borne rickettsioses such as *R. parkeri*[269] and *R. africae*;[270] and, recently, a new coronavirus associated with severe acute respiratory syndrome (SARS).[271,272] SARS was first recognized during a global outbreak of severe pneumonia that occurred in late 2002 in Guangdong Province, China, and then erupted in February 2003 with cases in more than two dozen countries in Asia, Europe, North America, and South America. Early in the investigation, clinical, pathologic, and laboratory studies focused on previously known agents of respiratory illness. Subsequently, a virus was isolated from the oropharynx of a SARS patient and identified by ultrastructural characteristics as belonging to the family Coronaviridae.[271,271] Various reports have described diffuse alveolar damage as the main histopathologic finding in SARS patients, and SARS-associated coronavirus (SARS-CoV) has been demonstrated in human and experimental animal tissues by immunohistochemical (Fig. 3.25) or ISH assays.[273-282]

PATHOLOGISTS, IMMUNOHISTOCHEMISTRY, AND BIOTERRORISM

There is increasing concern about the use of infectious agents as potential biological weapons. Biological warfare agents vary from rare exotic viruses to common bacterial agents, and the intentional use of biologic agents to cause disease can simulate naturally occurring outbreaks or may have unusual characteristics.[283] The CDC has issued recommendations for a complete public health response to a biological attack.[284-286] Two important components of this response plan include the rapid diagnosis and characterization of biological agents. Pathologists using newer diagnostic techniques such as IHC, ISH, and PCR will have a direct impact on the rapid detection and control of emerging infectious diseases from natural or intentional causes.[287] Immunohistochemistry provides a simple, safe, sensitive, and specific method for the rapid detection of biological threats (at the time of investigation or retrospectively), thereby facilitating the rapid implementation of effective public health responses.

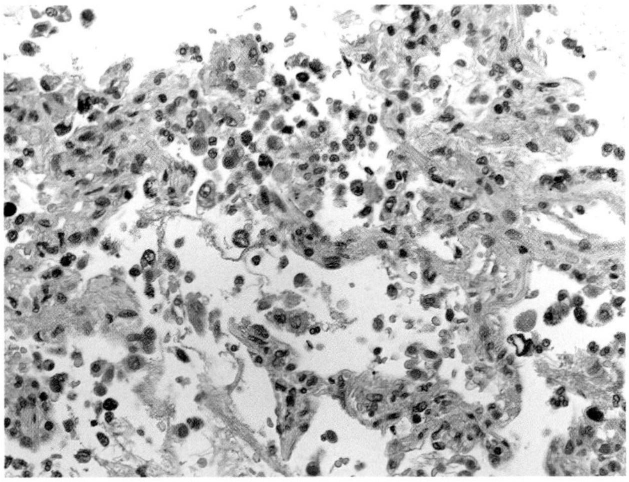

FIGURE 3.25 SARS. Coronavirus antigen–positive pneumocytes and macrophages in the lung of a SARS case. (Immunoalkaline phosphatase with naphthol fast red substrate and hematoxylin counterstain; original magnification ×63.)

Anthrax

Immunohistochemical staining of *Bacillus anthracis* with monoclonal antibodies against cell wall and capsule antigens has been successfully used in the recognition of bioterrorism-related anthrax cases and is an important step in early diagnosis and treatment (Fig. 3.26A-C).[5,288-292] Gram staining and culture isolation of *B. anthracis* are usually used to diagnose anthrax; however, previous antibiotic treatment will affect culture yield and Gram stain identification of the bacteria.[290] Immunohistochemistry has demonstrated high sensitivity and specificity for the detection of *B. anthracis* in skin biopsies, pleural biopsies, transbronchial biopsies, and pleural fluids (see Fig. 3.26).[289-291,293]

In addition, immunostaining has been very useful for determining the route of entry of the bacteria and identifying the mode of spread of the disease.[290,294]

Tularemia

Immunohistochemical staining is also valuable for rapid identification of *Francisella tularensis* in formalin-fixed tissue sections. Tularemia can have a variable clinical and pathologic presentation that can simulate other infectious diseases such as anthrax, plague, cat-scratch disease, or lymphogranuloma venereum. Moreover, the microorganisms are difficult to demonstrate in tissue sections, even with Gram stain or silver staining methods. A mouse monoclonal antibody against the

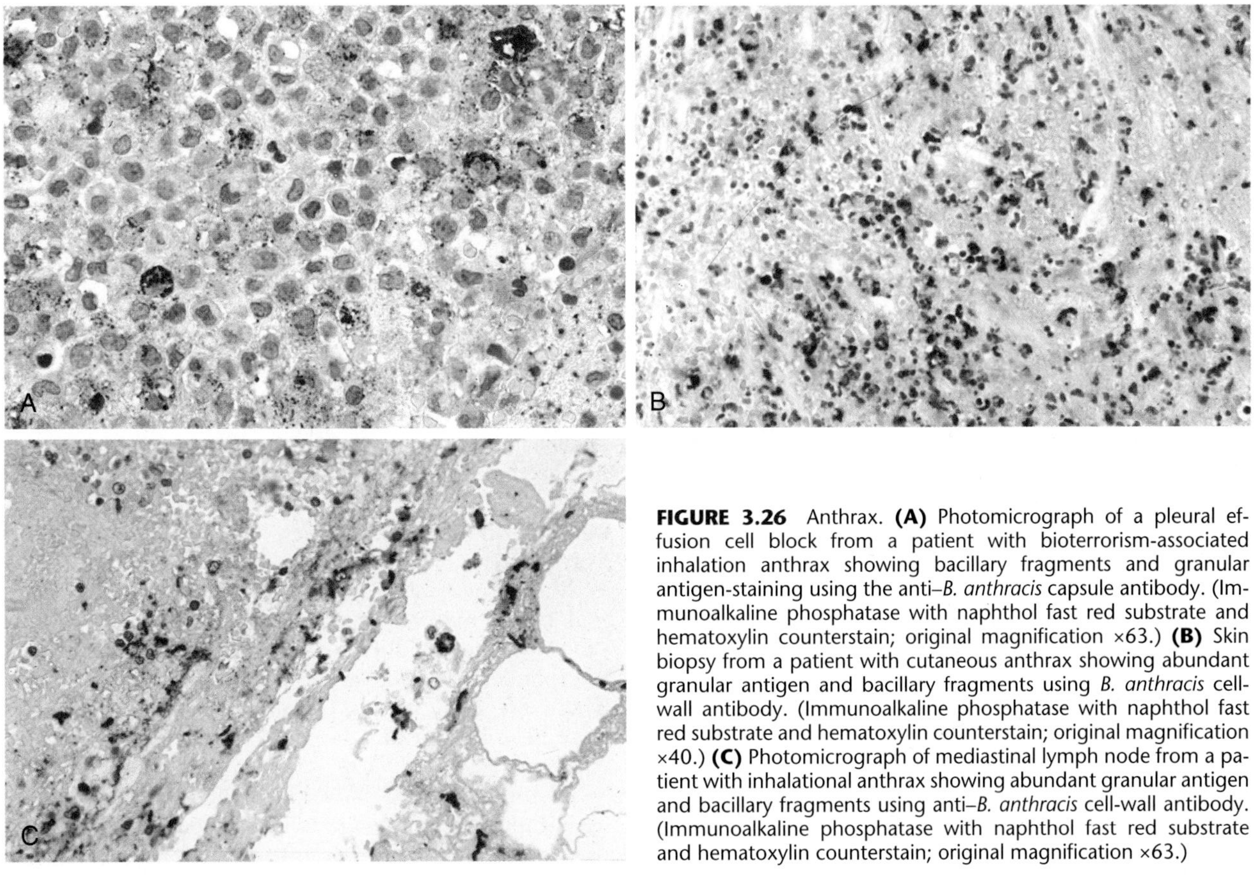

FIGURE 3.26 Anthrax. **(A)** Photomicrograph of a pleural effusion cell block from a patient with bioterrorism-associated inhalation anthrax showing bacillary fragments and granular antigen-staining using the anti–*B. anthracis* capsule antibody. (Immunoalkaline phosphatase with naphthol fast red substrate and hematoxylin counterstain; original magnification ×63.) **(B)** Skin biopsy from a patient with cutaneous anthrax showing abundant granular antigen and bacillary fragments using *B. anthracis* cell-wall antibody. (Immunoalkaline phosphatase with naphthol fast red substrate and hematoxylin counterstain; original magnification ×40.) **(C)** Photomicrograph of mediastinal lymph node from a patient with inhalational anthrax showing abundant granular antigen and bacillary fragments using anti–*B. anthracis* cell-wall antibody. (Immunoalkaline phosphatase with naphthol fast red substrate and hematoxylin counterstain; original magnification ×63.)

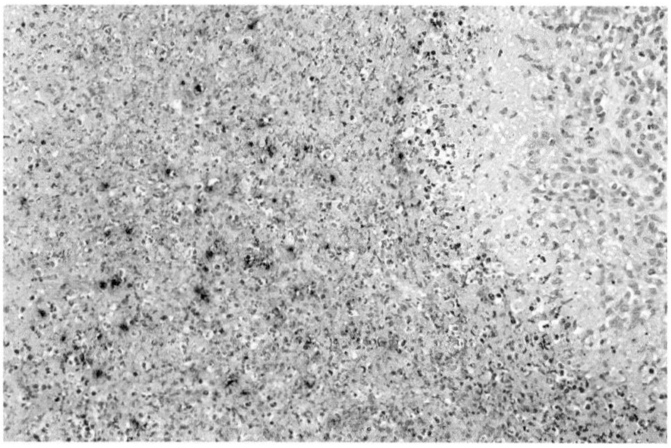

FIGURE 3.27 Tularemia. Immunohistochemistry of lymph node showing a stellate abscess with *F. tularensis* antigen-bearing macrophages in the central necrotic area using a mouse monoclonal antibody against the lipopolysaccharide of *F. tularensis*. (Immunoalkaline phosphatase with naphthol fast red substrate and hematoxylin counterstain; original magnification ×40.)

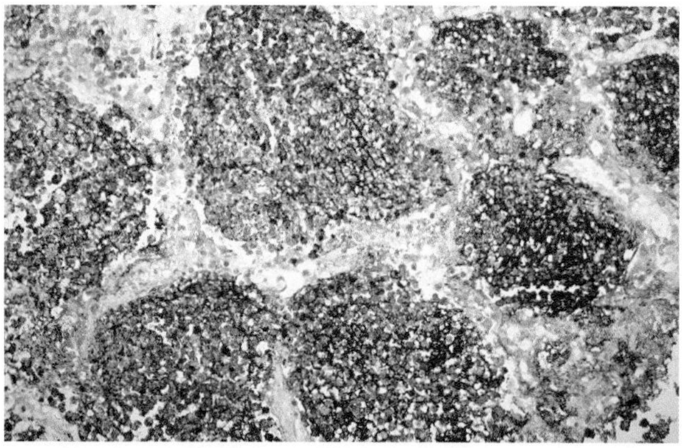

FIGURE 3.28 Immunohistochemical stain of lung containing abundant bacterial and granular *Yersinia pestis* antigen in the alveolar spaces using a mouse monoclonal antibody against F1 capsular antigen. (Immunoalkaline phosphatase with naphthol fast red substrate and hematoxylin counterstain; original magnification ×20.)

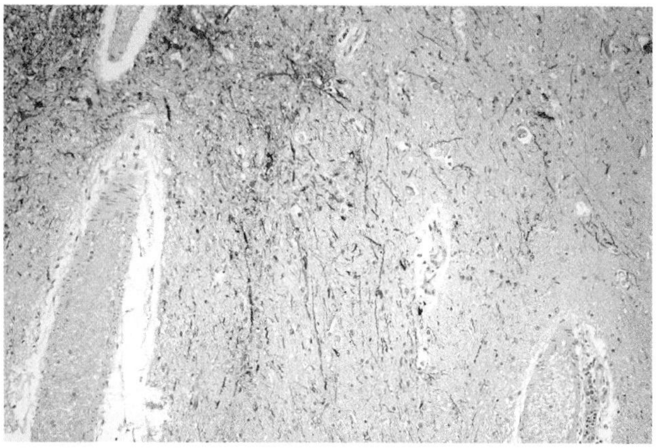

FIGURE 3.29 Immunostaining of viral antigens in neurons and neuronal processes in CNS using a mouse anti-eastern equine encephalitis virus antibody. (Immunoalkaline phosphatase with naphthol fast red substrate and hematoxylin counterstain; original magnification ×10.)

lipopolysaccharide of *F. tularensis* has been used with high sensitivity and specificity to demonstrate intact bacteria and granular bacterial antigen in the lungs, spleen, lymph nodes, and liver (Fig. 3.27).[295,296]

Plague

A mouse monoclonal antibody directed against the fraction 1 antigen of *Yersinia pestis* has been used to detect intracellular and extracellular bacteria in dermal blood vessels, lungs, lymph nodes, spleen, and liver (Fig. 3.28).[297-302] This technique is potentially useful for the rapid diagnosis of plague in formalin-fixed skin biopsies. In addition, IHC can differentiate primary and secondary pneumonic plague by identifying *Y. pestis* in different lung locations (e.g., alveoli vs. interstitium).[297]

Immunohistochemical methods using polyclonal or monoclonal antibodies have been used to identify several other potential biological terrorism agents, including the causative agents of brucellosis,[5] Q fever,[5,138,168,169] viral encephalitides (eastern equine encephalitis) (Fig. 3.29),[5,121-123] rickettsioses (typhus and Rocky Mountain spotted fever),[138-141,187] and viral hemorrhagic fevers (Ebola and Marburg hemorrhagic fever).[5,89-95]

BEYOND IMMUNOHISTOLOGY: MOLECULAR DIAGNOSTIC APPLICATIONS

Since the 1980s, an enormous advancement in molecular technology has dramatically influenced the diagnosis and study of infectious diseases. The application of molecular probes to the study and diagnosis of infectious diseases is a great adjunct to IHC as a diagnostic method and often allows for even more rapid and specific identification of organisms.[303-309] Along with rapid advances in molecular diagnostic techniques, there has been an increased interest in the use of paraffin-embedded specimens for nucleic acid hybridization assays. The two main hybridization formats used in the diagnostic pathology laboratory for the diagnosis of infectious diseases are ISH and PCR. *In situ* hybridization is analogous to IHC in that it allows the cellular identification and localization of microbial pathogens. Instead of microbial antigens, the targets of ISH are specific RNA or DNA sequences. Many viruses (Figs. 3.30-3.33), bacteria (Fig. 3.34), and other microorganisms can be localized in tissues by ISH; these include Epstein-Barr virus, HPV (Fig. 3.35), polyomaviruses (Fig. 3.36), *Mycobacterium leprae, Legionella, Haemophilus influenzae*, zygomycetes, and *Aspergillus*.[108,114,207,261,282,310-332] PCR has the advantage of increased sensitivity, minimal tissue requirements, and potential sequencing of the amplified product for specific identification of the microbial genotype or strain of the agent involved. There are PCR assays for most microorganisms that have been or can be adapted for use on formalin-fixed tissues.[11,124,172,293,333-345]

In summary, IHC, ISH, and PCR should be regarded as complementary diagnostic methods for use in the diagnostic pathology laboratory. The laboratory must

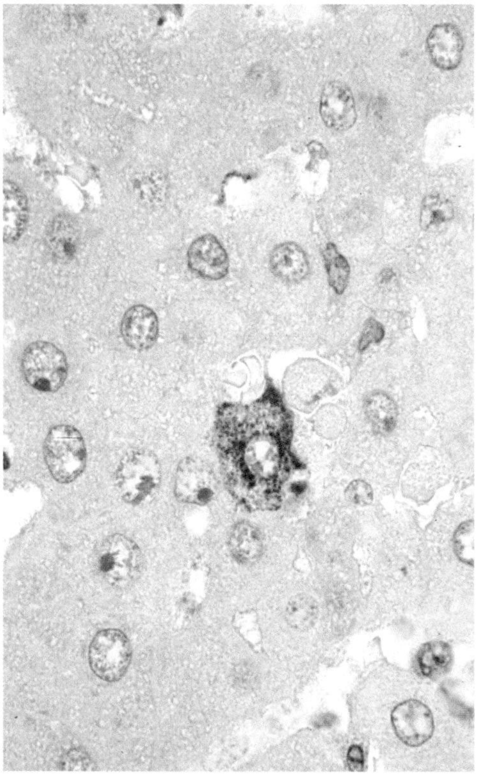

FIGURE 3.30 Crimean-Congo hemorrhagic fever (CCHF). Localization of CCHF viral RNA as seen in a single CCHF-infected hepatocyte. (Immunoalkaline phosphatase with naphthol fast red substrate and hematoxylin counterstain; original magnification ×250.)

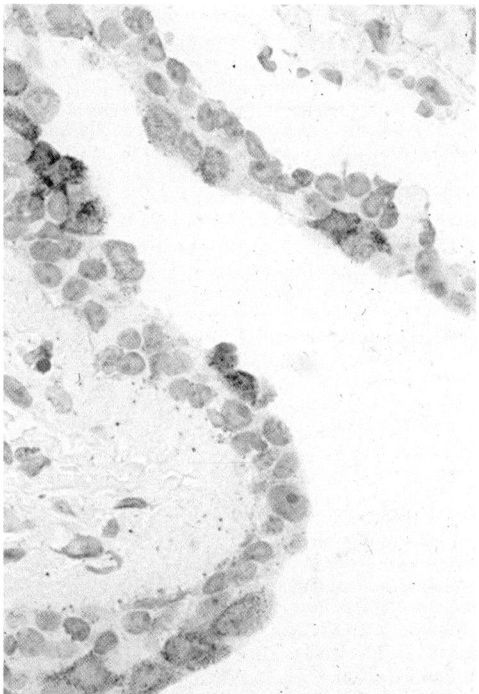

FIGURE 3.31 Influenza A. *In situ* hybridization showing localization of viral nucleic acids in bronchial epithelium using an influenza A hemagglutinin digoxigenin-labeled probe. (Immunoalkaline phosphatase with naphthol fast red substrate and hematoxylin counterstain; original magnification ×158.)

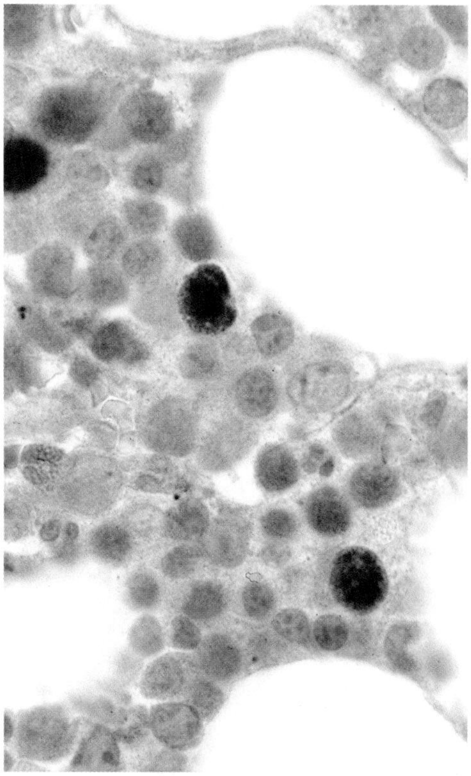

FIGURE 3.32 Parvovirus infection. Confirmation of B19-infected cells in bone marrow of an HIV-infected patient by using a digoxigenin-labeled B19 riboprobe and *in situ* hybridization. Staining is mainly nuclear and seen in multiple cells containing classic parvovirus inclusions. (Immunoalkaline phosphatase with naphthol fast red substrate and hematoxylin counterstain; original magnification ×250.)

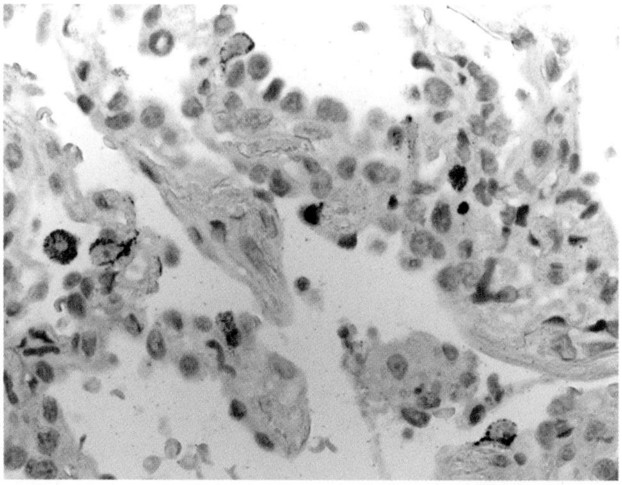

FIGURE 3.33 SARS. Lung showing diffuse alveolar damage and SARS-CoV nucleic acids primarily in pneumocytes as seen by colorimetric ISH. (Immunoalkaline phosphatase with naphthol fast red substrate and hematoxylin counterstain; original magnification ×158.)

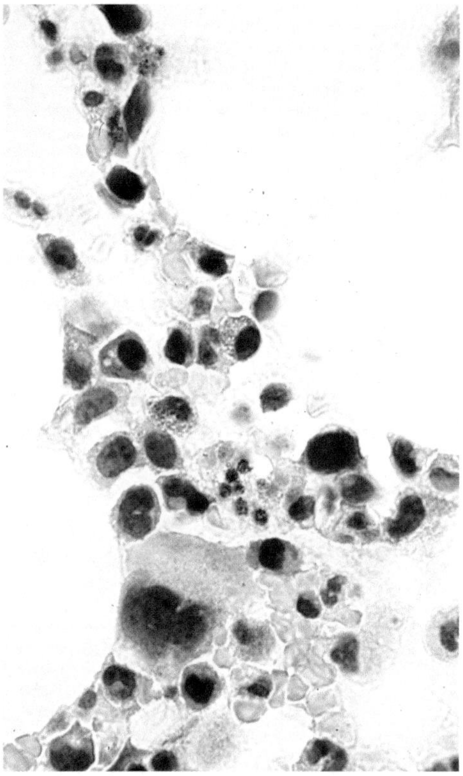

FIGURE 3.34 *Ehrlichia chaffeensis.* Organisms appear as red inclusions within monocytes by *in situ* hybridization. (Immunoalkaline phosphatase with naphthol fast red substrate and hematoxylin counterstain; original magnification ×250.)

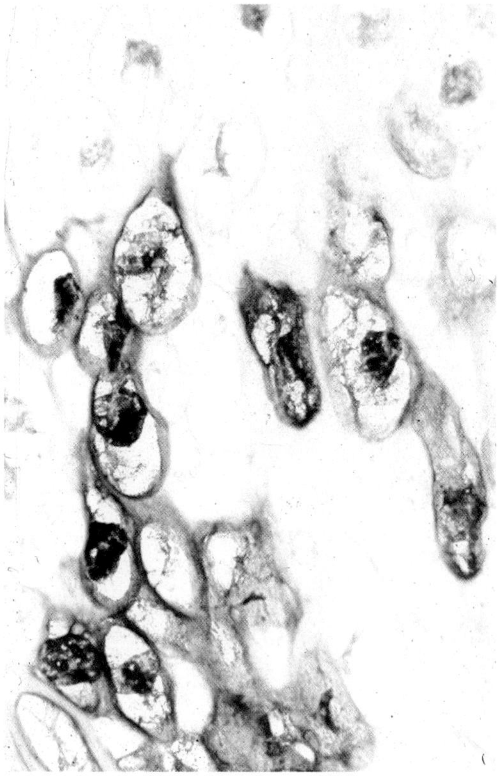

FIGURE 3.35 Human papillomavirus (HPV). *In situ* hybridization for HPV in a patient with a benign cervical lesion. HPV RNA is localized within nucleus and cytoplasm of koilocytotic cells. (Immunoalkaline phosphatase with naphthol fast red substrate and hematoxylin counterstain; original magnification ×250.)

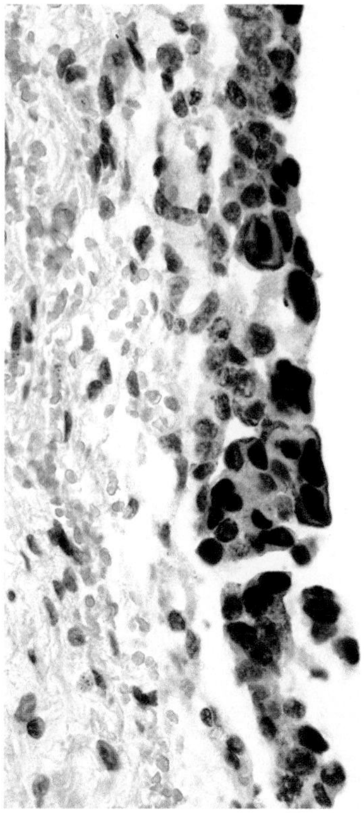

FIGURE 3.36 Polyomavirus (BK virus) infection. BK virus–infected cells in urothelium as seen by using a colorimetric ISH and a DNA probe. Staining is both nuclear and cytoplasmic and seen in multiple cells containing classic viral inclusions. (Immunoalkaline phosphatase with naphthol fast red substrate and hematoxylin counterstain; original magnification ×100.)

consider the advantages and limitations of each method and how they apply to each case and the common needs of the laboratory. This ever-expanding field behooves all pathologists interested in the field of infectious diseases to keep abreast of the changing technology and its ever-increasing application in the arena of diagnosis.

REFERENCES

1. Cartun RW. Use of immunohistochemistry in the surgical pathology laboratory for the diagnosis of infectious diseases. *Pathol Case Rev.* 1999;4:260-265.
2. Watts JC. Surgical pathology in the diagnosis of infectious diseases (Editorial). *Am J Clin Pathol.* 1994;102:711-712.
3. Schwartz DA, Bryan RT. Infectious disease pathology and emerging infections: Are we prepared? *Arch Pathol Lab Med.* 1996;120:117-124.
4. Schwartz DA. Emerging and reemerging infections: Progress and challenges in the subspecialty of infectious disease pathology. *Arch Pathol Lab Med.* 1997;121:776-784.
5. Zaki SR, Paddock CD. The emerging role of pathology in infectious diseases. In: Scheld WM, Armonstrong D, Hughes JM, eds. *Emerging Infections 3.* Washington, D.C.: ASM Press; 1999:181-200.
6. Medical Examiners, Coroners, and Biologic Terrorism: A Guidebook for Surveillance and Case Management. *MMWR Morbidity and Mortality Weekly Report.* 2004;53(RR-8):1-53.
7. Zaki SR, Peters CJ. Viral hemorrhagic fevers. In: Connor DH, Chandler FW, Schwartz DA, Manz HJ, Lack EE, eds. *Pathology of Infectious Diseases.* Stamford, CT: Appleton & Lange; 1997:347-364.

8. Coons AH, Creech HJ, Jone RN, et al. The demonstration of pneumococcal antigen in tissues by use of fluorescent antibodies. *J Immunol.* 1942;45:159-170.
9. Cohen PR. Tests for detecting herpes simplex virus and varicella-zoster virus infections. *Dermatol Clin.* 1994;12:51-68.
10. Procop GW, Burchette Jr JL, Howell DN, et al. Immunoperoxidase and immunofluorescent staining of Rickettsia rickettsii in skin biopsies. *Arch Pathol Lab Med.* 1997;121:894-899.
11. Guarner J, Greer PW, Whitney A, et al. Pathogenesis and diagnosis of human meningococcal disease using immunohistochemical and PCR assay. *Am J Clin Pathol.* 2004;122:754-764.
12. Lepidi H, Houpikina P, Liang Z, et al. Cardiac valves in patients with Q fever endocarditis: microbiological, molecular, and histologic studies. *J Infect Dis.* 2003;187:1097-1106.
13. Eyzaguirre EJ, Haque AK. Application of immunohistochemistry to infections. *Arch Pathol Lab Med.* 2008;132:424-431.
14. Lepidi H, Fenollar F, Dumler JS. Cardiac valves in patients with Whipple endocarditis: microbiological, molecular, quantitative histologic, and immunohistochemical studies of 5 patients. *J Infect Dis.* 2004;190:935-945.
15. Jeavons L, Hunt L, Hamilton A. Immunochemical studies of heat-shock protein 80 of Histoplasma capsulatum. *J Med Vet Mycol.* 1994;32:47-57.
16. Werner M, Chott A, Fabiano A, et al. Effect of formalin tissue fixation and processing on immunohistochemistry. *Am J Surg Pathol.* 2000;24:1016-1019.
17. Woods GL, Walker DH. Detection of infection or infectious agents by use of cytologic and histologic stains. *Clin Microbiol Rev.* 1996;9:382-404.
18. Chandler FW. Invasive microorganisms. In: Spicer SS, ed. *Histochemistry in Pathology Diagnosis.* New York, NY: Marcel Dekker; 1987:77-101.
19. Clausen PP, Thomsen P. Demonstration of hepatitis B surface antigen in liver biopsies. A comparative investigation of immunoperoxidase and orcein staining on identical sections on formalin-fixed, paraffin-embedded tissue. *Acta Pathol Microbiol Scand [A].* 1978;86A:383.
20. Thomsen P, Clausen PP. Occurrence of hepatitis B-surface antigen in a consecutive material of 1539 liver biopsies. *Acta Pathol Microbiol Immunol Scand [A].* 1983;91:71.
21. Al Adnani MS, Ali SM. Patterns of chronic liver disease in Kuwait with special reference to localization of hepatitis B surface antigen. *J Clin Pathol.* 1984;37:549.
22. Taylor C. Lung, pancreas, colon and rectum, stomach, liver. In: Taylor CR, Cote RJ, eds. *Immunomicroscopy: A Diagnostic Tool for the Surgical Pathologist.* 2nd ed. Philadelphia: Saunders; 1994:292-317.
23. Park YN, Han KH, Kim KS, et al. Cytoplasmic expression of hepatitis B core antigen in chronic hepatitis B virus infection: role of precore stop mutants. *Liver.* 1999;19:199-205.
24. McDonald JA, Harris S, Waters JA, et al. Effect of human immunodeficiency virus (HIV) infection on chronic hepatitis B hepatic viral display. *J Hepatol.* 1987;4:337-342.
25. Hubscher SG, Portmann BC. Transplantation pathology. In: Burt AD, Portmann BC, Ferrell LD, eds. *MacSween's Pathology of the Liver.* 5th ed. Philadelphia: Elsevier; 2007:815-879.
26. Feiden W, Borchard F, Burrig KF, et al. Herpes esophagitis: I. Light microscopical immunohistochemical investigations. *Virchows Arch [A].* 1984;404:167-176.
27. Nikkels AF, Delvenne P, Sadzot-Delvaux C, et al. Distribution of varicella zoster virus and herpes simplex virus in disseminated fatal infections. *J Clin Pathol.* 1996;49:243-248.
28. Greenson JK, Beschorner WE, Boitnott JK, et al. Prominent mononuclear cell infiltrate is characteristic of herpes esophagitis. *Hum Pathol.* 1991;22:541-549.
29. Wang JY, Montone KT. A rapid simple in situ hybridization method for herpes simplex virus employing a synthetic biotin-labeled oligonucleotide probe: a comparison with immunohistochemical methods for HSV detection. *J Clin Lab Anal.* 1994;8:105-115.
30. Kobayashi TK, Ueda M, Nishino T, et al. Brush cytology of herpes simplex virus infection in oral mucosa: use of the ThinPrep processor. *Diag Cytopath.* 1998;18:71-75.
31. Nicoll JAR, Love S, Burton PA, et al. Autopsy findings in two cases of neonatal herpes simplex virus infection: detection of virus by immunohistochemistry, in situ hybridization and the polymerase chain reaction. *Histopathology.* 1994;24:257-264.
32. Nikkels AF, Debrus S, Sadzot-Delvaux C, et al. Comparative immunohistochemical study of herpes simplex and varicella-zoster infections. *Virchows Archiv A Pathol Anat.* 1993;422:121-126.
33. Cohen PR. Tests for detecting herpes simplex virus and varicella-zoster virus infections. *Dermat Clin.* 1994;12:51-68.
34. Katano H, Sato Y, Kurata T, et al. Expression and localization of human herpesvirus 8-encoded proteins in primary effusion lymphoma, Kaposi's sarcoma, and multicentric Castleman's disease. *Virology.* 2000;269:335-344.
35. Katano H, Suda T, Morishita Y, et al. Human herpesvirus 8-associated solid lymphomas that occur in AIDS patients takes anaplastic large cell morphology. *Mod Pathol.* 2000;13:77-85.
36. Ely SA, Powers J, Lewis D, et al. Kaposi's sarcoma-associated herpesvirus-positive primary effusion lymphoma arising in the subarachnoid space. *Hum Pathol.* 1999;30:981-984.
37. Katano H, Sato Y, Kurata T, et al. High expression of HHV-8-encoded ORF73 protein in spindle-shape cells of Kaposi's sarcoma. *Am J Pathol.* 1999;155:47-52.
38. Said JW, Shintaku IP, Asou H, et al. Herpesvirus 8 inclusions in primary effusion lymphoma: report of a unique case with T-cell phenotype. *Archiv Pathol Lab Med.* 1999;123:257-260.
39. Cheuk W, Wong KO, Wong CS, et al. Immunostaining for human herpesvirus 8 latent nuclear antigen-1 helps distinguish Kaposi sarcoma from its mimickers. *Am J Clin Pathol.* 2004;121:335-342.
40. Robin YM, Guillou L, Michels JJ, et al. Human herpesvirus 8 immunostaining. A sensitive and specific method for diagnosing Kaposi sarcoma in paraffin-embedded sections. *Am J Clin Pathol.* 2004;121:330-334.
41. Wada DA, Perkins SL, Tripp S, et al. Human herpesvirus 8 and iron staining are useful in differentiating Kaposi sarcoma from interstitial granuloma annulare. *Am J Clin Pathol.* 2007;127:263-270.
42. Bryant-Greenwood P, Sorbara L, Filie AC, et al. Infection of mesothelial cells with human herpesvirus 8 in human immunodeficiency virus-infected patients with Kaposi sarcoma, Castleman disease, and recurrent pleural effusions. *Mod Pathol.* 2003;16:145-153.
43. de la Hoz RE, Stephens G, Sherlock C. Diagnosis and treatment approaches to CMV infections in adult patients. *J Clin Virol.* 2002;25(suppl 2):S1-S12.
44. Bronsther O, Makowka L, Jaffe R. The occurrence of cytomegalovirus hepatitis in liver transplant patients. *J Med Virol.* 1988;24:423-434.
45. Drummer JS, White LT, Ho M, et al. Morbidity of cytomegalovirus infection in recipients of heart or heart-lung transplant who receive cyclosporine. *J Infect Dis.* 1985;152:1182-1191.
46. Anwar F, Erice A, Jessurun J. Are there cytopathic features associated with cytomegalovirus infection predictive of resistance to antiviral therapy? *Ann Diag Pathol.* 1999;3:19-22.
47. Cote L, Drouet E, Bissuel F, et al. Diagnostic value of amplification of human cytomegalovirus DNA from gastrointestinal biopsies from human immunodeficiency virus-infected patients. *J Clin Microbiol.* 1993;31:2066-2069.
48. Rawlinson WD. Broadsheet number 50: Diagnosis of human cytomegalovirus infection and disease. *Pathology.* 1999;31:109-115.
49. Sheehan MM, Coker R, Coleman DV. Detection of cytomegalovirus (CMV) in HIV+ patients: comparison of cytomorphology, immunohistochemistry and in situ hybridization. *Cytopath.* 1998;9:29-37.
50. Kutza AS, Muhl E, Hackstein H, et al. High incidence of active cytomegalovirus infection among septic patients. *Clin Infect Dis.* 1998;26:1076-1082.
51. Saetta A, Agapitos E, Davaris PS. Determination of CMV placentitis: Diagnostic application of the polymerase chain reaction. *Virchows Arch.* 1998;432:159-162.
52. Solans EP, Yong S, Husain AN, et al. Bronchioloalveolar lavage in the diagnosis of CMV pneumonitis in lung transplant recipients: an immunocytochemical study. *Diagn Cytopath.* 1997;16:350-352.
53. Nebuloni M, Pellegrinelli A, Ferri A, et al. Etiology of microglial nodules in brains of patients with acquired immunodeficiency syndrome. *J Neurovirol.* 2000;6:46-50.

54. Rimsza LM, Vela EE, Frutiger YM, et al. Rapid automated combined in situ hybridization and immunohistochemistry for sensitive detection of cytomegalovirus in paraffin-embedded tissue biopsies. *Am J Clin Pathol.* 1996;106:544-548.
55. Kandiel A, Lashner B. Cytomegalovirus colitis complicating inflammatory bowel disease. *Am J Gastroenterol.* 2006;101:2857-2865.
56. Kambham N, Vij R, Cartwright CA, et al. Cytomegalovirus infection in steroid-refractory ulcerative colitis. A case-control study. *Am J Surg Pathol.* 2004;28:365-373.
57. Ribalta T, Martinez AJ, Jares P, et al. Presence of occult cytomegalovirus infection in the brain after orthotopic liver transplantation. An autopsy study of 83 cases. *Virchows Arch.* 2002;440:166-171.
58. Cruz-Spano L, Lima-Pereira FE, Gomes da Silva-Basso N, et al. Human cytomegalovirus infection and abortion: an immunohistochemical study. *Med Sci Monit.* 2002;8:BR230-BR235.
59. Seehofer D, Rayes N, Tullius SG, et al. CMV hepatitis after liver transplantation: incidence, clinical course, and long term follow-up. *Liver Transp.* 2002;8:1138-1146.
60. Lautenschlager I, Hockerstedt K, Taskinen E. Histologic findings associated with CMV infection in liver transplantation. *Transplant Proc.* 2003;35:819.
61. Lamps LW, Pinson CW, Raiford DS, et al. The significance of microabscesses in liver transplant biopsies: a clinicopathological study. *Hepatology.* 1998;28:1532-1537.
62. Barkholt LM, Ehrnst A, Veress B. Clinical use of immunohistopathologic methods for the diagnosis of cytomegalovirus hepatitis in human liver allograft biopsy specimens. *Scand J Gastroenterol.* 1994;29:553-560.
63. Colina F, Jucá NT, Moreno E, et al. Histological diagnosis of cytomegalovirus hepatitis in liver allografts. *J Clin Pathol.* 1995;48:351-357.
64. Lones MA, Shintaku IP, Weiss LM, et al. Posttransplant lymphoproliferative disorder in liver allograft biopsies: a comparison of three methods for the demonstration of Epstein Barr virus. *Hum Pathol.* 1997;28:533-539.
65. Challoner PB, Smith KT, Parker JD, et al. Plaque-associated expression of human herpesvirus 6 in multiple sclerosis. *Proc Natl Acad Sci U S A.* 1995;92:7440-7444.
66. Anderson J. Epstein-Barr virus and Hodgkin's lymphoma. *HERPES.* 2006;13:12-16.
67. Flomenberg P, Babbitt J, Drobyski WR, et al. Increasing incidence of adenovirus disease in bone marrow transplant recipients. *J Infect Dis.* 1994;169:775-781.
68. Strickler JG, Singleton TP, Copenhaver GM, et al. Adenovirus in the gastrointestinal tracts of immunosuppressed patients. *Am J Clin Pathol.* 1992;97:555-558.
69. Yi ES, Powell HC. Adenovirus infection of the duodenum in an AIDS patient: an ultrastructural study. *Ultrastruct Pathol.* 1994;18:549-551.
70. Yan Z, Nguyen S, Poles M, et al. Adenovirus colitis in human immunodeficiency virus infection: an underdiagnosed entity. *Am J Surg Pathol.* 1998;22:1101-1106.
71. Dombrowski F, Eis-Hubinger AM, Ackermann T, et al. Adenovirus-induced liver necrosis in a case of AIDS. *Virchows Archiv.* 1997;431:469-472.
72. Simsir A, Greenebaum E, Nuovo G, et al. Late fatal adenovirus pneumonitis in a lung transplant recipient. *Transplantation.* 1998;65:592-594.
73. Saad RS, Demetris AJ, Lee RG, et al. Adenovirus hepatitis in the adult allograft liver. *Transplantation.* 1997;64:1483-1485.
74. Ohori NP, Michaels MG, Jaffe R, et al. Adenovirus pneumonia in lung transplant recipients. *Hum Pathol.* 1995;26:1073-1079.
75. Marc J, Dieterich DT. The histopathology of 103 consecutive colonoscopy biopsies from 82 symptomatic patients with acquired immunodeficiency syndrome. *Arch Pathol Lab Med.* 2001;125:1042-1046.
76. El-Mahallawy HA, Mansour T, El-Din SE, et al. Parvovirus B19 infection as a cause of anemia in pediatric acute lymphoblastic leukaemia during maintenance chemotherapy. *J Pediatr Hematol Oncol.* 2004;26:403-406.
77. Brown KE, Young NS. Parvovirus B19 infection and hematopoiesis. *Blood Rev.* 1995;9:176-182.
78. Jordan JA, Penchansky L. Diagnosis of human parvovirus B19-induced anemia: correlation of bone marrow morphology with molecular diagnosis using PCR and immunohistochemistry. *Cell Vision.* 1995;2:279-282.
79. Morey AL, O'Neil HJ, Coyle PV, et al. Immunohistological detection of human parvovirus B19 in formalin-fixed, paraffin-embedded tissues. *J Pathol.* 1992;166:105-108.
80. Puvion-Dutilleul F, Puvion E. Human parvovirus B19 as a causative agent for rheumatoid arthritis. *Proc Nat Acad Sci U S A.* 1998;95:8227-8232.
81. Yufu Y, Matsumoto M, Miyamura T, et al. Parvovirus B19-associated haemophagocytic syndrome with lymphadenopathy resembling histiocytic necrotizing lymphadenitis (Kikuchi's disease). *Br J Haematol.* 1997;96:868-871.
82. Vadlamudi G, Rezuke N, Ross JW, et al. The use of monoclonal antibody R92F6 and polymerase chain reaction to confirm the presence of parvovirus B19 in bone marrow specimens of patients with acquired immunodeficiency syndrome. *Arch Pathol Lab Med.* 1999;123:768-773.
83. Wright C, Hinchliffe SA, Taylor C. Fetal pathology in intrauterine death due to parvovirus B19 infection. *Br J Obstet Gynaecol.* 1996;103:133-136.
84. Essary LR, Vnencak-Jones CL, Manning SS, et al. Frequency of parvovirus B19 infection in nonimmune hydrops fetalis and utility of three diagnostic methods. *Hum Pathol.* 1998;29:696-701.
85. Monath TP, Ballinger ME, Miller BR, et al. Detection of yellow fever viral RNA by nucleic acid hybridization and viral antigen by immunohistochemistry in fixed human liver. *Am J Trop Med Hyg.* 1989;40:663-668.
86. De Brito T, Siqueira SA, Santos RT, et al. Human fatal yellow fever. Immunohistochemical detection of viral antigens in the liver, kidney and heart. *Pathol Res Pract.* 1992;188:177-181.
87. Hall WC, Crowell TP, Watts DM, et al. Demonstration of yellow fever and dengue antigens in formalin-fixed paraffin-embedded human liver by immunohistochemical analysis. *Am J Trop Med Hyg.* 1991;45:408-417.
88. Ramos C, Sanchez G, Pando RH, et al. Dengue virus in the brain of a fatal case of hemorrhagic dengue fever. *J Neurovirol.* 1998;4:465-468.
89. Burt FJ, Swanepoel R, Shieh W-J, et al. Immunohistochemical and in situ localization of Crimean-Congo hemorrhagic fever (CCHF) virus in human tissues and implications for CCHF pathogenesis. *Arch Pathol Lab Med.* 1997;121:839-846.
90. Maiztegui JI, Laguens RP, Cossio PM, et al. Ultrastructural and immunohistochemical studies in five cases of Argentine hemorrhagic fever. *J Infect Dis.* 1975;132:35-53.
91. Hall WC, Geisbert TW, Huggins JW, et al. Experimental infection of guinea pigs with Venezuelan hemorrhagic fever virus (Guanarito): a model of human disease. *Am J Trop Med Hyg.* 1996;55:81-88.
92. Geisbert TW, Jaax NK. Marburg hemorrhagic fever: report of a case studied by immunohistochemistry and electron microscopy. *Ultrastruct Pathol.* 1998;22:3-17.
93. Zaki SR, Shieh W-J, Greer PW, et al. A novel immunohistochemical assay for the detection of Ebola virus in skin: implications for diagnosis, spread, and surveillance of Ebola hemorrhagic fever. *J Infect Dis.* 1999;179(suppl 1):S36-S37.
94. Ksiazek TG, Rollin PE, Williams AJ, et al. Clinical virology of Ebola hemorrhagic fever (EHF): virus, virus antigen, and IgG and IgM antibody findings among EHF patients in Kikwit, Democratic Republic of Congo. *J Infect Dis.* 1999;179:S177-S187.
95. Wyers M, Formenty P, Cherel Y, et al. Histopathological and immunohistochemical studies of lesions associated with Ebola virus in a naturally infected chimpanzee. *J Infect Dis.* 1999;179(suppl 1):S54-S59.
96. Nickeleit V, Hirsch HH, Zeiler M, et al. BK-virus nephropathy in renal transplants-tubular necrosis, MHC-class II expression and rejection in a puzzling game. *Nephrol Dial Transplant.* 2000;15:324-332.
97. White LH, Casian A, Hilton R, et al. BK virus nephropathy in renal transplant patients in London. *Transplantation.* 2008;85:1008-1015.
98. Drachenberg CB, Papadimitriou JC, Ramos E. Histologic versus molecular diagnosis of BK polyomavirus-associated nephropathy: a shifting paradigm? *Clin J Am Soc Nephrol.* 2006;1:374-379.

99. Vogler C, Wang Y, Brink DS, et al. Renal pathology in the pediatric transplant patient. *Adv Anat Pathol.* 2007;14:202-216.
100. Dall A, Hariharan S. BK virus nephritis after renal transplantation. *Clin J Am Soc Nephrol.* 2008;3(suppl 2):S68-S75.
101. Latif S, Zaman F, Veeramachaneni R, et al. BK polyomavirus in renal transplants: role of electron microscopy and immunostaining in detecting early infection. *Ultrastruct Pathol.* 2007;31:199-207.
102. Nebuloni M, Tosoni A, Boldorini R, et al. BK virus renal infection in a patient with the acquired immunodeficiency syndrome. *Arch Pathol Lab Med.* 1999;123:807-811.
103. Elli A, Banfi G, Battista-Fogazzi G, et al. BK polyomavirus interstitial nephritis in a renal transplant patient with no previous acute rejection episodes. *J Nephrol.* 2002;15:313-316.
104. Jochum W, Weber T, Frye S, et al. Detection of JC virus by anti-VP1 immunohistochemistry in brains with progressive multifocal leukoencephalopathy. *Acta Neuropathol.* 1997;94:226-231.
105. Chima SC, Agostini HT, Ryschlkeewitsch CF, et al. Progressive multifocal leukoencephalopathy and JC virus genotypes in West African patients with acquired immunodeficiency syndrome. A pathologic and DNA sequence analysis of 4 cases. *Arch Pathol Lab Med.* 1999;123:395-403.
106. Aoki N, Mori M, Kato K, et al. Antibody against synthetic multiple antigen peptides (MAP) of JC virus capsid protein (VP1) without cross reaction to BK virus: a diagnostic tool for progressive multifocal leukoencephalopathy. *Neurosci Lett.* 1996;205:111-114.
107. Silver SA, Arthur RR, Rozan YS, et al. Diagnosis of progressive multifocal leukoencephalopathy by stereotactic brain biopsy utilizing immunohistochemistry and the polymerase chain reaction. *Acta Cytol.* 1995;39:35-44.
108. Guarner J, Shieh WJ, Dawson J, et al. Immunohistochemical and in situ hybridization studies of influenza A virus infection in human lungs. *Am J Clin Pathol.* 2000;114:227-233.
109. Guarner J, Paddock CD, Shieh WJ, et al. Histopathologic and immunohistochemical features of fatal influenza virus infection in children during the 2003-2004 season. *Clin Infect Dis.* 2006;43:132-140.
110. Nielson KA, Yunis EJ. Demonstration of respiratory syncytial virus in an autopsy series. *Pediatr Pathol.* 1990;10:491-502.
111. Wright C, Oliver KC, Fenwick FI, et al. A monoclonal antibody pool for routine immunohistochemical detection of human respiratory syncytial virus antigens in formalin-fixed, paraffin-embedded tissue. *J Pathol.* 1997;182:238-244.
112. Jogai S, Radotra BD, Banerjee AK. Immunohistochemical study of human rabies. *Neuropathology.* 2000;20:197-203.
113. Jogai S, Radotra BD, Banerjee AK. Rabies viral antigen in extracranial organs: a postmortem study. *Neuropathol Appl Neurobiol.* 2002;28:334.
114. Warner CK, Zaki SR, Shieh WJ, et al. Laboratory investigation of humans from vampire bat rabies in Peru. *Am J Trop Med Hyg.* 1999;60:502-507.
115. Sinchaisri TA, Nagata T, Yoshikawa Y, et al. Immunohistochemical and histopathological study of experimental rabies infection in mice. *J Vet Med Sci.* 1992;54:409-416.
116. Jackson AC, Ye H, Phelan CC, et al. Extraneural organ involvement in human rabies. *Lab Invest.* 1999;79:945-951.
117. Yousef GE, Mann GF, Brown IN, et al. Clinical and research application of an enterovirus group-reactive monoclonal antibody. *Intervirol.* 1987;28:199-205.
118. Hohenadl C, Klingel K, Rieger P, et al. Investigation of the coxsackievirus B3 nonstructural proteins 2B, 2C, and 3AB: generation of specific polyclonal antisera and detection of replicating virus in infected tissue. *J Virol Methods.* 1994;47:279-295.
119. Zhang H, Li Y, Peng T, et al. Localization of enteroviral antigen in myocardium and other tissues from patients with heart muscle disease by an improved immunohistochemical technique. *J Histochem Cytochem.* 2000;48:579-584.
120. Li Y, Bourlet T, Andreoletti L, et al. Enteroviral capsid protein VP1 is present in myocardial tissues from some patients with myocarditis or dilated cardiomyopathy. *Circulation.* 2000;101:231-234.
121. Del Piero F, Wilkins PA, Dubovi EJ, et al. Clinical, pathologic, immunohistochemical, and virologic findings of eastern equine encephalitis in two horses. *Vet Pathol.* 2001;38:451-456.
122. Patterson JS, Maes RK, Mullaney TP, et al. Immunohistochemical diagnosis of eastern equine encephalomyelitis. *J Vet Diag Invest.* 1996;8:156-160.
123. Garen PD, Tsai TF, Powers JM. Human eastern equine encephalitis: immunohistochemistry and ultrastructure. *Mod Pathol.* 1999;12:646-652.
124. Tatti KM, Gentsch J, Shieh WJ, et al. Molecular and immunological methods to detect rotavirus in formalin-fixed tissue. *J Virol Methods.* 2002;105:305-319.
125. Morrison C, Gilson T, Nuovo GJ, et al. Histologic distribution of fatal rotaviral infection: an immunohistochemical and reverse transcriptase in situ polymerase chain reaction analysis. *Hum Pathol.* 2001;32:216-221.
126. Cioc AM, Nuovo GJ. Histologic and in situ viral findings in the myocardium in cases of sudden, unexpected death. *Mod Pathol.* 2001;15:914-922.
127. Toulaymant M, Marconi S, Garb J, et al. Endoscopic biopsy pathology of Helicobacter pylori gastritis. *Arch Pathol Lab Med.* 1999;123:778-781.
128. El-Zimaity HMT, Graham DY, Al-Assis MT, et al. Interobserver variation in the histopathological assessment of Helicobacter pylori gastritis. *Hum Pathol.* 1996;27:35-41.
129. Marcio L, Angelucci D, Grossi L, et al. Anti-Helicobacter pylori specific antibody immunohistochemistry improves the diagnostic accuracy of Helicobacter pylori in biopsy specimen from patients treated with triple therapy. *Am J Gastroenterol.* 1998;93:223-226.
130. Rotimi O, Cairns A, Gray S, et al. Histological identification of Helicobacter pylori: comparison of staining methods. *J Clin Pathol.* 2000;53:756-759.
131. Goldstein NS. Chronic inactive gastritis and coccoid Helicobacter pylori in patients treated for gastroesophageal reflux disease or with H. pylori eradication therapy. *Am J Clin Pathol.* 2002;118:719-726.
132. Eshun JK, Black DD, Casteel HB. Comparison of immunohistochemistry and silver stain for the diagnosis of pediatric Helicobacter pylori infection in urease-negative gastric biopsies. *Ped Devel Pathol.* 2001;4:82-88.
133. Lepidi H, Fenollar F, Dumler JS, et al. Cardiac valves in patients with Whipple endocarditis: microbiological, molecular, quantitative histologic, and immunohistochemical studies of 5 patients. *J Infect Dis.* 2004;190:935-945.
134. Houpikian P, Raoult D. Diagnostic methods: current best practices and guidelines for identification of difficult-to-culture pathogens in infective endocarditis. *Infect Dis Clin N Am.* 2007;16:377-392.
135. Baisden BL, Lepidi H, Raoult D, et al. Diagnosis of Whipple disease by immunohistochemical analysis. A sensitive and specific method for the detection of Tropheryma whipplei (the Whipple bacillus) in paraffin-embedded tissue. *Am J Clin Pathol.* 2002;118:742-748.
136. Lepidi H, Fenollar F, Gerolami R, et al. Whipple disease: Immunospecific and quantitative immunohistochemical study of intestinal biopsy specimens. *Hum Pathol.* 2003;34:589-596.
137. Lepidi H, Costedoat N, Piette JC, et al. Immunohistological detection of Tropheryma whipplei (Whipple bacillus) in lymph nodes. *Am J Med.* 2002;113:334-336.
138. Dumler JS, Walker DH. Diagnostic tests for Rocky Mountain spotted fever and other rickettsial diseases. *Dermat Clin.* 1994;12:25-36.
139. Parola P, Paddock CD, Raoult D. Tick-borne rickettsioses around the world: Emerging diseases challenging old concepts. *Clin Microbiol Rev.* 2005;18:719-756.
140. Walker DH, Burday MS, Folds JD. Laboratory diagnosis of Rocky Mountain spotted fever. *South Med J.* 1980;73:1443-1447.
141. Paddock CD, Greer PW, Ferebee TL, et al. Hidden mortality attributable to Rocky Mountain spotted fever: immunohistochemical detection of fatal, serologically unconfirmed disease. *J Infect Dis.* 1999;179:1469-1476.
142. Kaplowitz LG, Lange JV, Fischer JJ, Walker DH. Correlation of rickettsial titers, circulating endotoxin, and clinical features in Rocky Mountain spotted fever. *Arch Intern Med.* 1983;143:1149-1151.

143. Dumler JS, Gage WR, Pettis GL, et al. Rapid immunoperoxidase demonstration of Rickettsia rickettsii in fixed cutaneous specimens from patients with Rocky Mountain spotted fever. *Am J Clin Pathol.* 1990;93:410-414.
144. Chapman AS, Bakken JS, Folk SM, et al. Diagnosis and management of tickborne rickettsial diseases: Rocky Mountain spotted fever, ehrlichiosis, and anaplasmosis—United States: A practical guide for physicians and other health-care and public health professionals. *MMWR Recomm Rep.* 2006;55:1-27.
145. Spach DH, Koehler JE. Bartonella-associated infections. *Infect Dis Clin North Am.* 1998;12:137-155.
146. Lepidi H, Durack DT, Raoult D. Diagnostic methods: Current best practices and guidelines for histologic evaluation in infective endocarditis. *Infect Dis Clin North Am.* 2002;16:339-361.
147. Albrich WC, Kraft C, Fisk T, et al. A mechanic with a bad valve: Blood-culture-negative endocarditis. *Lancet Infect Dis.* 2004;4:777-784.
148. Lepidi H, Fournier PE, Raoult D. Quantitative analysis of valvular lesions during Bartonella endocarditis. *Am J Clin Pathol.* 2000;114:880-889.
149. Baorto E, Payne RM, Slater LN, et al. Culture-negative endocarditis caused by Bartonella henselae. *J Pediatr.* 1998;132:1051-1054.
150. Reed JA, Brigati DJ, Flynn SD, et al. Immunohistochemical identification of Rochalimaea henselae in bacillary (epithelioid) angiomatosis, parenchymal bacillary peliosis, and persistent fever with bacteremia. *Am J Surg Pathol.* 1992;16:650-657.
151. Min KW, Reed JA, Welch DF, et al. Morphologically variable bacilli of cat scratch disease are identified by immunohistochemical labeling with antibodies to Rochalimaea henselae. *Am J Clin Pathol.* 1994;101:607-610.
152. Daybell D, Paddock CD, Zaki SR, et al. Disseminated infection with Bartonella henselae as a cause of spontaneous splenic rupture. *Clin Infect Dis.* 2004;39:21-24.
153. Buffet M, Grange PA, Gerhardt P, et al. Diagnosing Treponema pallidum in secondary syphilis by PCR and immunohistochemistry. *J Invest Dermatol.* 2007;127:2345-2350.
154. Jethwa HS, Schmitz JL, Dallabetta G, et al. Comparison of molecular and microscopic techniques for detection of Treponema pallidum in genital ulcers. *J Clin Microbiol.* 1995;33:180-183.
155. Kingston AA, Vujevich J, Shapiro M, et al. Seronegative secondary syphilis in 2 patients coinfected with human immunodeficiency virus. *Arch Dermatol.* 2005;141:431-433.
156. Hoang MP, High WA, Molberg KH. Secondary syphilis: A histologic and immunohistochemical evaluation. *J Cutan Pathol.* 2004;31:595-599.
157. Guarner J, Greer PW, Bartlett J, et al. Congenital syphilis in a newborn: an immunopathologic study. *Mod Pathol.* 1999;12:82-87.
158. Ulrichs T, Lefmann K, Reich M, et al. Modified immunohistological staining allows detection of Ziehl-Neelsen-negative Mycobacterium tuberculosis organisms and their precise localization in human tissues. *J Pathol.* 2005;205:633-640.
159. Daniel TM. The rapid diagnosis of tuberculosis: A selective review. *J Lab Clin Med.* 1990;116:277-282.
160. Carabias E, Palenque R, Serrano JM, et al. Evaluation of an immunohistochemical test with polyclonal antibodies raised against mycobacteria used in formalin-fixed tissue compared with mycobacterial specific culture. *APMIS.* 1998;106:385-388.
161. Mustafa T, Hg Wiker, Mfinanga SGM, et al. Immunohistochemistry using a Mycobacterium tuberculosis complex specific antibody for improved diagnosis of tuberculosis lymphadenitis. *Mod Pathol.* 2006;19:1606-1614.
162. Zaki SR, Shieh WJ, and the Epidemic Working Group. Leptospirosis associated with an outbreak of acute febrile illness and pulmonary hemorrhage, Nicaragua 1995. *Lancet.* 1996;347:535-536.
163. Trevejo RT, Rigau-Pérez JG, Ashford DA, et al. Epidemic leptospirosis associated with pulmonary hemorrhage-Nicaragua. *J Infect Dis.* 1995;1998(178):1457-1463.
164. Guarner J, Shieh WJ, Morgan J, et al. Leptospirosis mimicking acute cholecystitis among athletes participating in a triathlon. *Hum Pathol.* 2001;32:750-752.
165. Nicodemo AC, Duarte MI, Alves VA, et al. Lung lesions in human leptospirosis: microscopic, immunohistochemical, and ultrastructural features related to thrombocytopenia. *Am J Trop Med Hyg.* 1997;56:181-187.
166. Lebech AM, Clemmensen O, Hansen K. Comparison of in vitro, immunohistochemical staining, and PCR for detection of Borrelia burgdorferi in tissue from experimentally infected animals. *J Clin Microbiol.* 1995;33:2328-2333.
167. Aberer E, Kersten A, Klade H, et al. Heterogeneity of Borrelia burgdorferi in the skin. *Am J Dermatopathol.* 1996;18:571-579.
168. Brouqui P, Raoult D. Endocarditis due to rare and fastidious bacteria. *Clin Microbiol Rev.* 2001;14:177-207.
169. Brouqui P, Dumler JS, Raoult D. Immunohistologic demonstration of Coxiella burnetii in the valves of patients with Q fever endocarditis. *Am J Med.* 1994;97:451-458.
170. Guarner J, Packard MM, Nolte KB, et al. Usefulness of immunohistochemical diagnosis of Streptococcus pneumoniae in formalin-fixed, paraffin-embedded specimens compared with culture and gram stain techniques. *Am J Clin Pathol.* 2007;127:617-618.
171. Guarner J, Bartlett J, Reagan S, et al. Immunohistochemical evidence of Clostridium sp, Staphylococcus aureus, and group A Streptococcus in severe soft tissue infections related to injection drug use. *Hum Pathol.* 2006;37:1482-1488.
172. Guarner J, Sumner J, Paddock CD, et al. Diagnosis of invasive group A streptococcal infections by using immunohistochemical and molecular assays. *Am J Clin Pathol.* 2006;126:148-155.
173. Terpstra WJ, Groeneveld K, Eijk PP, et al. Comparison of two nonculture techniques for detection of Hemophilus influenzae in sputum: In situ hybridization and immunoperoxidase staining with monoclonal antibodies. *Chest.* 1988;94:126S.
174. Groeneveld K, van Alphen L, van Ketel RJ, et al. Nonculture detection of Haemophilus influenzae in sputum with monoclonal antibodies specific for outer membrane lipoprotein P6. *J Clin Microbiol.* 1989;27:2263.
175. Forsgren J, Samuelson A, Borrelli S, et al. Persistence of nontypeable Haemophilus influenzae in adenoid macrophages: a putative colonization mechanism. *Act Oto-Laryngol.* 1996;116:766-773.
176. Shurbaji MS, Dumler JS, Gage WR, et al. Immunohistochemical detection of chlamydial antigens in association with cystitis. *Am J Pathol.* 1990;93:363.
177. Paukku M, Puolakkainen M, Paavonen T, et al. Plasma cell endometritis is associated with Chlamydia trachomatis infection. *Am J Clin Pathol.* 1999;112:211-215.
178. Naas J, Gnarpe JA. Demonstration of Chlamydia pneumoniae in tissue by immunohistochemistry. *APMIS.* 1999;107:882-886.
179. Suffin SC, Kaufmann AF, Whitaker B, et al. Legionella pneumophila. Identification in tissue sections by a new immunoenzymatic procedure. *Arch Pathol Lab Med.* 1980;104:283-286.
180. Maruta K, Miyamoto H, Hamada T, et al. Entry and intracellular growth of Legionella dumoffii in alveolar epithelial cells. *Am J Respir Crit Care Med.* 1998;157:1967-1974.
181. Fiore AE, Nuorti JP, Levine OS, et al. Epidemic Legionnaires' disease two decades later: Old sources, new diagnostic methods. *Clin Infect Dis.* 1998;26:426-433.
182. Parkash V, Morotti RA, Joshi V, et al. Immunohistochemical detection of Listeria antigens in the placenta in perinatal listeriosis. *Int J Gynecol Pathol.* 1998;17:343-350.
183. Chiba M, Fukushima T, Koganei K, et al. Listeria monocytogenes in the colon in a case of fulminant ulcerative colitis. *Scand J Gastroenterol.* 1998;33:778-782.
184. Weinstock D, Horton SB, Rowland PH. Rapid diagnosis of Listeria monocytogenes by immunohistochemistry in formalin-fixed brain tissue. *Vet Pathol.* 1995;32:193-195.
185. Pospischil A, Wood RL, Anderson TD. Peroxidase-antiperoxidase and immunogold labeling of Salmonella typhimurium and Salmonella cholerasuis var kunzendorf in tissues of experimentally infected swine. *Am J Vet Res.* 1990;51:619-624.
186. Thygesen P, Martinsen C, Hougen HP, et al. Histologic, cytologic, and bacteriologic examination of experimentally induced Salmonella typhimurium infection in Lewis rats. *Comp Med.* 2000;50:124-132.
187. Walker DH, Feng HM, Ladner S, et al. Immunohistochemical diagnosis of typhus rickettsioses using an anti-lipopolysaccharide monoclonal antibody. *Mod Pathol.* 1997;10:1038-1042.
188. Koss T, Carter EL, Grossman ME, et al. Increased detection of rickettsialpox in a New York City hospital following the anthrax outbreak of 2001: Use of immunohistochemistry for the rapid confirmation of cases in an era of bioterrorism. *Arch Dermatol.* 2003;139:1545-1552.

189. Walker DH, Hudnall SD, Szaniawski WK, et al. Monoclonal antibody-based immunohistochemical diagnosis of rickettsialpox: the macrophage is the principal target. *Mod Pathol.* 1999;12:529-533.
190. Moron CG, Popov VL, Feng HM, et al. Identification of the target cells of Orientia tsutsugamushi in human cases of scrub typhus. *Mod Pathol.* 2001;14:752-759.
191. Schwarz J. The diagnosis of deep mycoses by morphological methods. *Hum Pathol.* 1982;13:519-533.
192. Marques MEA, Coelho KIR, Bacchi CE. Comparison between histochemical and immunohistochemical methods for the diagnosis of sporotrichosis. *J Clin Pathol.* 1992;45:1089-1093.
193. Reed JA, Hemaan BA, Alexander JL, et al. Immunomycology: Rapid and specific immunocytochemical identification of fungi in formalin-fixed, paraffin-embedded material. *J Histochem Cytochem.* 1993;41:1217-1221.
194. Jensen HE, Schonheyder H, Hotchi M, et al. Diagnosis of systemic mycosis by specific immunohistochemical tests. *APMIS.* 1996;104:241-258.
195. Fukuzawa M, Inaba H, Hayama M, et al. Improved detection of medically important fungi by immunoperoxidase staining with polyclonal antibodies. *Virchows Arch.* 1995;427:407-414.
196. Kauffman L. Immunohistologic diagnosis of systemic mycosis: An update. *Eur J Epidemiol.* 1992;8:377-382.
197. Verweij PE, Smedts F, Poot T. Immunoperoxidase staining for identification of Aspergillus species in routinely processed tissue sections. *J Clin Pathol.* 1996;49:798-801.
198. Breier F, Oesterreicher C, Brugger S, et al. Immunohistochemistry with monoclonal antibody against Candida albicans mannan antigen demonstrates cutaneous Candida granulomas as evidence of Candida sepsis in an immunosuppressed host. *Dermatology.* 1997;194:293-296.
199. Marcilla A, Monteagudo C, Mormeneo S, et al. Monoclonal antibody 3H8: A useful tool in the diagnosis of candidiasis. *Microbiol.* 1999;145:695-701.
200. Monteagudo C, Marcilla A, Mormeneo S, et al. Specific immunohistochemical identification of Candida albicans in paraffin-embedded tissue with a new monoclonal antibody (1B12). *Am J Clin Pathol.* 1995;103:130-135.
201. Jarvensivu A, Hietanen J, Rautemaa R, et al. Candida yeast in chronic periodontitis tissues and subgingival microbial biofilms in vivo. *Oral Diseases.* 2004;10:106-112.
202. Williams DW, Jones HS, Allison RT. Immunohistochemical detection of Candida albicans in formalin fixed, paraffin embedded material. *J Clin Pathol.* 1998;51:857-859.
203. Jarvensivu A, Rautemaa R, Sorsa T, et al. Specificity of the monoclonal antibody 3H8 in the immunohistochemical identification of Candida species. *Oral Diseases.* 2006;12:428-433.
204. Kockenberger MB, Canfield PJ, Kozel TR, et al. An immunohistochemical method that differentiates Cryptococcus neoformans varieties and serotypes in formalin-fixed paraffin-embedded tissues. *Med Mycol.* 2001;39:523-533.
205. Tsunemi T, Kamata T, Fumimura Y, et al. Immunohistochemical diagnosis of Cryptococcus neoformans var. gatti infection in chronic meningoencephalitis: The first case in Japan. *Intern Med.* 2001;40:1241-1244.
206. Chamilos G, Luna M, Lewis RE, et al. Invasive fungal infections in patients with hematologic malignancies in a tertiary care cancer center: An autopsy study over a 15-year period (1989-2003). *Haematologica.* 2006;91:986-989.
207. Hayden RT, Isolato PA, Parrett T, et al. In situ hybridization for the differentiation of Aspergillus, Fusarium, and Pseudallescheria species in tissue sections. *Diagn Mol Pathol.* 2003;12:21-26.
208. Rickerts V, Mousset S, Lambrecht E, et al. Comparison of histopathological analysis, culture, and polymerase chain reaction assays to detect invasive mold infections from biopsy specimens. *Clin Infect Dis.* 2007;44:1078-1083.
209. Hope WW, Walsh TJ, Denning DW. Laboratory diagnosis of invasive aspergillosis. *Lancet Infect Dis.* 2005;5:609-622.
210. Tarrand JJ, Lichterfeld M, Warraich I, et al. Diagnosis of invasive septated mold infections. A correlation of microbiological culture and histologic or cytologic examination. *Am J Clin Pathol.* 2003;119:854-858.
211. Choi JK, Mauger J, McGowan KL. Immunohistochemical detection of Aspergillus species in pediatric tissue samples. *Am J Clin Pathol.* 2004;121:18-25.
212. Pierard GE, Arrese-Estrada J, Pierard-Franchimont C, et al. Immunohistochemical expression of galactomannan in the cytoplasm of phagocytic cells during invasive aspergillosis. *Am J Clin Pathol.* 1991;96:373-376.
213. Phillips P, Weiner MH. Invasive aspergillosis diagnosed by monoclonal and polyclonal reagents. *Hum Pathol.* 1987;18:1015-1024.
214. Fenelon LE, Hamilton AJ, Figueroa JI, et al. Production of specific monoclonal antibodies to Aspergillus species and their use in immunohistochemical identification of aspergillosis. *J Clin Microbiol.* 1999;37:1221-1223.
215. Jensen HE, Salonen J, Ekfors TO. The use of immunohistochemistry to improve sensitivity and specificity in the diagnosis of systemic mycoses in patients with haematological malignancies. *J Pathol.* 1997;181:100-105.
216. Wazir JE, Brown I, Martin-Bates E, et al. EB9, a new antibody for the detection of trophozoites of Pneumocystis carinii in bronchoalveolar lavage specimens in AIDS. *J Clin Pathol.* 1994;47:1108-1111.
217. Wazir JE, Macrorie SG, Coleman DV. Evaluation of the sensitivity, specificity, and predictive value of monoclonal antibody 3F6 for the detection of Pneumocystis carinii pneumonia in bronchoalveolar lavage specimens and induced sputum. *Cytopathol.* 1994;5:82-89.
218. Cooper CR, McGinnis MR. Pathology of Penicillium marneffei: An emerging acquired immunodeficiency syndrome-related pathogen. *Arch Lab Pathol Med.* 1997;121:798-804.
219. Chaiwun B, Khunamornpong S, Sirivanichai C, et al. Lymphadenopathy due to Penicillium marneffei infection: Diagnosis by fine needle aspiration cytology. *Mod Pathol.* 2002;15:939-943.
220. Arrese Estrada J, Stynen D, Van Cutsem J, et al. Immunohistochemical identification of Penicillium marneffei by monoclonal antibody. *Int J Dermatol.* 1992;31:410-412.
221. Burke DG, Emancipator SN, Smith MC, et al. Histoplasmosis and kidney disease in patients with AIDS. *Clin Infect Dis.* 1997;25:281-284.
222. Arnold SJ, Kinney MC, McCormick MS, et al. Disseminated toxoplasmosis: Unusual presentations in the immunocompromised host. *Arch Pathol Lab Med.* 1997;121:869-873.
223. Warnke C, Tuazon CU, Kovacs A, et al. Toxoplasma encephalitis in patients with acquired immunodeficiency syndrome: Diagnosis and response to therapy. *Am J Trop Med Hyg.* 1987;36:509.
224. Ganji M, Tan A, Maitar ML, et al. Gastric toxoplasmosis in a patient with acquired immunodeficiency syndrome. A case report and review of the literature. *Arch Pathol Lab Med.* 2003;127:732-734.
225. Hofman V, Brousset P, Mougneau E, et al. Immunostaining of visceral leishmaniasis caused by Leishmania infantum using monoclonal antibody (19-11) to the Leishmania homologue of receptors for activated C-kinase. *Am J Clin Pathol.* 2003;120:567-574.
226. Azadeh B, Sells PG, Ejeckman GC, et al. Localized Leishmania lymphadenitis immunohistochemical studies. *Am J Clin Pathol.* 1994;102:11-15.
227. Kenner JR, Aronson NE, Bratthauer GL, et al. Immunohistochemistry to identify Leishmania parasites in fixed tissues. *J Cutan Pathol.* 1999;26:130-136.
228. Amato VS, Duarte MIS, Nicodemo AC, et al. An evaluation of clinical, serologic, anatomopathologic and immunohistochemical findings for fifteen patients with mucosal leishmaniasis before and after treatment. *Rev Inst Med Trop S Paulo.* 1998;40:23-30.
229. Guarner J, Bartlett J, Shieh WJ, et al. Histopathologic spectrum and immunohistochemical diagnosis of amebic meningoencephalitis. *Mod Pathol.* 2007;20:1230-1237.
230. Bonnin A, Petrella T, Dubremetz JF, et al. Histopathologic methods for diagnosis of cryptosporidiosis using monoclonal antibodies. *Eur J Clin Microbiol Infect Dis.* 1990;9:664-665.
231. Perez de Suarez E, Perez-Schael I, Perozo-Ruggeri G, et al. Immunocytochemical detection of Entamoeba histolytica. *Trans R Soc Trop Med Hyg.* 1987;81:624-626.

232. Guarner J, Bartlett J, Zaki SR, et al. Mouse model for Chagas disease: Immunohistochemical distribution of different stages of Trypanosoma cruzi in tissues throughout infection. *Am J Trop Med Hyg.* 2001;65:152-158.
233. Anez N, Carrasco H, Parada H, et al. Myocardial parasite persistence in chronic chagasic patients. *Am J Trop Med Hyg.* 1999;60:726-732.
234. Reis MM, Higuchi Mde L, Benvenuti LA, et al. An in situ quantitative immunohistochemical study of cytokines and IL-2R+ in chronic human chagasic myocarditis: correlation with the presence of myocardial Trypanosoma cruzi antigens. *Clin Immunol Immunopathol.* 1997;83:165-172.
235. Torres-Velez FJ, Nace EK, Won KY, et al. Development of an immunohistochemical assay for the detection of babesiosis in formalin-fixed, paraffin-embedded tissue samples. *Am J Clin Pathol.* 2003;120:833-838.
236. Sanad MM, Darwish RA, Nasr ME, et al. Giardia lamblia and chronic gastritis. *J Egypt Soc Parasitol.* 1996;26:481-495.
237. Genrich GL, Guarner J, Paddock CD, et al. Fatal malaria infection in travelers: Novel immunohistochemical assays for the detection of Plasmodium falciparum in tissues and implications for pathogenesis. *Am J Trop Med Hyg.* 2007;76:251-259.
238. Institute of Medicine. *Emerging infections: microbial threats to health in the United States.* Washington, DC: National Academy Press; 1992.
239. CDC. Preventing Emerging Infectious Diseases: A Strategy for the 21st Century. Overview of the Updated CDC Plan. *MMWR Recomm Rep.* 1998;47:1-14.
240. Perkins BA, Flood JM, Danila R, et al. Unexplained deaths due to possibly infectious causes in the United States: Defining the problem and designing surveillance and laboratory approaches. *Emerg Infect Dis.* 1998;2:47-53.
241. Houpikina P, Raoult D. Traditional and molecular techniques for the study of emerging bacterial diseases: One laboratory's perspective. *Emerg Infect Dis.* 2002;8:122-131.
242. Khan AS, Khabbaz RF, Armstrong LR, et al. Hantavirus pulmonary syndrome: The first 100 US cases. *J Infect Dis.* 1996;173:1297-1303.
243. Moolenaar RL, Dalton C, Lipman HB, et al. Clinical features that differentiate hantavirus pulmonary syndrome from three other acute respiratory illnesses. *Clin Infect Dis.* 1995;21:643-649.
244. Nolte KB, Feddersen RM, Foucar K, et al. Hantavirus pulmonary syndrome in the United States: A pathological description of a disease caused by a new agent. *Hum Pathol.* 1995;26:110-120.
245. Zaki SR, Greer PW, Coffield LM, et al. Hantavirus pulmonary syndrome. Pathogenesis of an emerging infectious disease. *Am J Pathol.* 1995;146:552-579.
246. Zaki SR, Khan AS, Goodman RA, et al. Retrospective diagnosis of hantavirus pulmonary syndrome, 1978-1993. Implications for emerging infectious diseases. *Arch Pathol Lab Med.* 1996;120:134-139.
247. Shieh WJ, Guarner J, Layton M, et al. The role of pathology in an investigation of an outbreak of West Nile encephalitis in New York, 1999. *Emerg Infect Dis.* 2000;6:370-372.
248. Cushing MM, Brat DJ, Mosunjac MI, et al. Fatal West Nile virus encephalitis in a renal transplant recipient. *Am J Clin Pathol.* 2004;121:26-31.
249. Petersen RL, Roehrig JT, Hughes JM. West Nile virus encephalitis. *N Engl J Med.* 2002;347:1225-1226.
250. Sampson BA, Ambrosi C, Charlot A, et al. The pathology of human West Nile virus infection. *Hum Pathol.* 2000;31:527-532.
251. Guarner J, Shieh WJ, Hunter S, et al. Clinicopathologic study and laboratory diagnosis of 23 cases with West Nile virus encephalomyelitis. *Hum Pathol.* 2004;35:983-990.
252. Lanciotti RS, Kerst AJ, Nasci RS, et al. Rapid detection of West Nile virus from human clinical specimens, field-collected mosquitoes, and avian samples by a TaqMan reverse transcriptase PCR assay. *J Clin Microbiol.* 2000;38:4066-4071.
253. Ho M, Chen ER, Hsu KH, et al. An epidemic of enterovirus 71 infection in Taiwan. Taiwan enterovirus epidemic working group. *N Engl J Med.* 1999;341:929-935.
254. Chan LG, Parashar UD, Lye MS. Deaths of children during an outbreak of hand, foot, and mouth disease in Sarawak, Malaysia: Clinical and pathological characteristics of the disease. *Clin Infect Dis.* 2000;31:678-683.
255. Wong KT, Chua KB, Lam SK. Immunohistochemical detection of infected neurons as a rapid diagnosis of enterovirus 71 encephalomyelitis. *Ann Neurol.* 1999;45:271-272.
256. Yan JJ, Wang JR, Liu CC, et al. An outbreak of enterovirus 71 infection in Taiwan 1998: A comprehensive pathological, virological, and molecular study on a case of fulminant encephalitis. *J Clin Virol.* 2000;17:13-22.
257. Shieh WJ, Jung SM, Hsueh C, et al. Pathologic studies of fatal causes in outbreak of hand, foot, and mouth disease. *Taiwan. Emerg Infect Dis.* 2001;7:146-148.
258. Wong KT, Shieh WJ, Kumar S, et al. Nipah virus infection. Pathology and pathogenesis of an emerging paramyxoviral zoonosis. *Am J Pathol.* 2002;161:2153-2167.
259. Goh KJ, Tan CT, Chew NK, et al. Clinical features of Nipah virus encephalitis among pig farmers in Malaysia. *N Engl J Med.* 2000;342:1229-1235.
260. Chua KB, Bellini WJ, Rota PA, et al. Nipah virus: A recently emergent deadly paramyxovirus. *Science.* 2000;288:1432-1435.
261. Dawson JE, Paddock CD, Warner CK, et al. Tissue diagnosis of Ehrlichia chaffeensis in patients with fatal ehrlichiosis by use of immunohistochemistry, in situ hybridization, and polymerase chain reaction. *Am J Trop Med Hyg.* 2001;65:603-609.
262. Walker DH, Dumler JS. Human monocytic and granulocytic ehrlichiosis. Discovery and diagnosis of emerging tick-borne infections and the critical role of the pathologist. *Arch Pathol Lab Med.* 1997;121:785-791.
263. Paddock CD, Suchard DP, Grumbach KL, et al. Fatal seronegative ehrlichiosis in a patient with HIV infection. *N Engl J Med.* 1993;329:1164-1167.
264. Lepidi H, Bunnell JE, Martin ME, et al. Comparative pathology and immunohistology associated with clinical illness after Ehrlichia phagocytophila-group infections. *Am J Trop Med Hyg.* 2000;62:29-37.
265. Childs JE, Sumner JW, Nicholson WL, et al. Outcome of diagnostic tests using samples from patients with culture-proven human monocytic ehrlichiosis: Implications for surveillance. *J Clin Microbiol.* 1999;37:2997-3000.
266. Sehdev AE, Dumler JS. Hepatic pathology in human monocytic ehrlichiosis. Ehrlichia chaffeensis infection. *Am J Clin Pathol.* 2003;119:859-865.
267. Hooper PT, Russell GM, Selleck PW, et al. Immunohistochemistry in the identification of a number of new diseases in Australia. *Vet Microbiol.* 1999;68:89-93.
268. Williamson MM, Hooper PT, Selleck PW, et al. Experimental Hendra virus infection in pregnant guinea-pigs and fruit bats (Pteropus poliocephalus). *J Comp Pathol.* 2000;122: 201-207.
269. Paddock CD, Summer JW, Comer JA, et al. Rickettsia parkeri: A newly recognized cause of spotted fever rickettsiosis in the United States. *Clin Infect Dis.* 2004;38:805-811.
270. Lepidi H, Fournier PE, Raoult D. Histologic features and immunodetection of African tick-bite fever eschar. *Emerg Infect Dis.* 2006;12:1332-1337.
271. Ksiazek TG, Erdman D, Goldsmith CS, et al. A novel coronavirus associated with severe acute respiratory syndrome. *N Engl J Med.* 2003;348:1953-1966.
272. Peiris JS, Lai ST, Poon LL, et al. Coronavirus as a possible cause of severe acute respiratory syndrome. *Lancet.* 2003;361:1319-1325.
273. Nakajima N, Asahi-Ozaki Y, Nagata N, et al. SARS coronavirus-infected cells in lung detected by new in situ hybridization technique. *Jpn J Infect Dis.* 2003;56:139-141.
274. Kuiken T, Fouchier RA, Schutten M, et al. Newly discovered coronavirus as the primary cause of severe acute respiratory syndrome. *Lancet.* 2003;362:263-270.
275. Chong PY, Chui P, Ling AE, et al. Analysis of deaths during the severe acute respiratory syndrome (SARS) epidemic in Singapore: Challenges in determining a SARS diagnosis. *Arch Pathol Lab Med.* 2004;128:195-204.
276. McAuliffe J, Vogel L, Roberts A, et al. Replication of SARS coronavirus administered into the respiratory tract of African green, rhesus and cynomolgus monkeys. *Virology.* 2004;5: 8-15.
277. Roberts A, Vogel L, Guarner J, et al. SARS coronavirus infection of golden Syrian hamsters. *J Virol.* 2005;79:503-511.

278. Chen PC, Hsiao CH, Re: To KF, Tong JH, Chan PK, et al. Tissue and cellular tropism of the coronavirus associated with severe acute respiratory syndrome: An in-situ hybridization study of fatal cases. *J Pathol.* 2004;203:729-731.
279. Re: To KF, Tong JH, Chan PK, et al. Tissue and cellular tropism of the coronavirus associated with severe acute respiratory syndrome: An in-situ hybridization study of fatal cases. *J Pathol.* 2004;202:157-163.
280. Chow KC, Hsiao CH, Lin TY, et al. Detection of severe acute respiratory syndrome-associated coronavirus in pneumocytes of the lung. *Am J Clin Pathol.* 2004;121:574-580.
281. Ding Y, He L, Zhang Q, et al. Organ distribution of severe acute respiratory syndrome (SARS) associated coronavirus (SARS-CoV) in SARS patients: Implications for pathogenesis and virus transmission pathways. *J Pathol.* 2004;203:622-630.
282. Sheih WJ, Cheng-Hsiang H, Paddock CD, et al. Immunohistochemical, in situ hybridization, and ultrastructural localization of SARS-associated coronavirus in lung of a fatal case of severe acute respiratory syndrome in Taiwan. *Hum Pathol.* 2005;36:303-309.
283. Ashford DA, Kaiser RB, Bales ME, et al. Planning against biological terrorism: Lessons from outbreak investigations. *Emerg Infect Dis.* 2003;9:515-519.
284. Inglesby TV, O'Toole T, Henderson DA. Preventing the use of biological weapons: Improving response should prevention fail. *Clin Infect Dis.* 2000;30:926-929.
285. Lillibridge SR, Bell AJ, Roman RS. Thoughts for the new millennium: Bioterrorism. Centers for Disease Control and Prevention bioterrorism preparedness and response. *Am J Infect Control.* 1999;27:463-464.
286. Franz DR, Zajtchuk R. Biological terrorism: Understanding the threat, preparation, and medical response. *Dis Month.* 2000;46:125-190.
287. Guarner J, Zaki SR. Histopathology and immunohistochemistry in the diagnosis of bioterrorism agents. *J Histochem Cytochem.* 2006;54:3-11.
288. Ezzell JW, Abshire TG, Little SF, et al. Identification of Bacillus anthracis by using monoclonal antibodies to cell wall galactose-N-acetylglucosamine polysaccharide. *J Clin Microbiol.* 1990;28:223-231.
289. Shieh WJ, Guarner J, Paddock C, et al. The critical role of pathology in the investigation of bioterrorism-related cutaneous anthrax. *Am J Pathol.* 2003;163:1901-1910.
290. Guarner J, Jernigan JA, Shieh WJ, et al. Pathology and pathogenesis of bioterrorism-related inhalational anthrax. *Am J Pathol.* 2003;163:701-709.
291. Jernigan JA, Stephens DS, Ashford DA, et al. Bioterrorism-related inhalational anthrax: The first 10 cases reported in the United States. *Emerg Infect Dis.* 2001;7:933-944.
292. Jernigan DB, Raghunathan PL, Bell BP, et al. Investigation of bioterrorism-related anthrax, United States, 2001: Epidemiologic findings. *Emerg Infect Dis.* 2002;8:1019-1028.
293. Tatti KM, Greer P, White E, et al. Morphologic, immunologic, and molecular methods to detect Bacillus anthracis in formalin-fixed tissues. *Appl Immunohistochem Mol Morphol.* 2006;14:234-243.
294. Grinberg LM, Abramova FA, Yampolskaya OV, et al. Quantitative pathology of inhalational anthrax I: Quantitative microscopic findings. *Mod Pathol.* 2001;14:482-495.
295. Guarner J, Greer PW, Bartlett J, et al. Immunohistochemical detection of Francisella tularensis in formalin-fixed paraffin-embedded tissue. *Appl Immun Mol Morphol.* 1999;7:122-126.
296. DeBey BM, Andrews GA, Chard-Bergstrom C, et al. Immunohistochemical demonstration of Francisella tularensis in lesions of cats with tularaemia. *J Vet Diagn Invest.* 2002;14:162-164.
297. Guarner J, Shieh WJ, Greer PW, et al. Immunohistochemical detection of Yersinia pestis in formalin-fixed paraffin-embedded tissue. *Am J Clin Pathol.* 2002;117:205-209.
298. Davis KJ, Vogel P, Fritz DL, et al. Bacterial filamentation of Yersinia pestis by β-lactam antibiotics in experimentally infected mice. *Arch Pathol Lab Med.* 1997;121:865-868.
299. Davis KJ, Fritz DL, Pitt ML, et al. Pathology of experimental pneumonic plague produced by fraction 1-positive and fraction 1-negative Yersinia pestis in African green monkeys (Cercopithecus aethiops). *Arch Pathol Lab Med.* 1996;120:156-163.
300. Williams ES, Mills K, Kwiatkowski DR, et al. Plague in black-footed ferret (Mustela nigripes). *J Wild Dis.* 1994;30:581-585.
301. Gabastou JM, Proaño J, Vimos A, et al. An outbreak of plague including cases with probable pneumonic infection, Ecuador, 1998. *Trans R Soc Tro Med Hyg.* 2000;94:387-391.
302. Guarner J, Shieh WJ, Chu M, et al. Persistent Yersinia pestis antigens in ischemic tissues of a patient with septicemic plague. *Hum Pathol.* 2005;36:850-853.
303. Figueroa ME, Rasheed S. Molecular pathology and diagnosis of infectious diseases. *Am J Clin Pathol.* 1991;95:S8-S21.
304. Fredricks DN, Relman DA. Application of polymerase chain reaction to the diagnosis of infectious diseases. *Clin Infect Dis.* 1999;29:475-486;quiz 487-488.
305. McNicol AM, Farquharson MA. In situ hybridization and its diagnostic applications in pathology. *J Pathol.* 1997;182: 250-261.
306. Mothershed EA, Whitney AM. Nucleic acid-based methods for the detection of bacterial pathogens: Present and future considerations for the clinical laboratory. *Clin Chim Acta.* 2006;363:206-220.
307. Procop GW, Wilson M. Infectious disease pathology. *Clin Infect Dis.* 2001;32:1589-1601.
308. Sklar J. DNA hybridization in diagnostic pathology. *Hum Pathol.* 1985;16:654-658.
309. Tang YW, Procop GW, Persing DH. Molecular diagnostics of infectious diseases. *Clin Chem.* 1997;43:2021-2038.
310. Andrade ZR, Garippo AL, Saldiva PH, et al. Immunohistochemical and in situ detection of cytomegalovirus in lung autopsies of children immunocompromised by secondary interstitial pneumonia. *Pathol Res Pract.* 2004;200:25-32.
311. Burt FJ, Swanepoel R, Shieh WJ, et al. Immunohistochemical and in situ localization of Crimean-Congo hemorrhagic fever (CCHF) virus in human tissues and implications for CCHF pathogenesis. *Arch Pathol Lab Med.* 1997;121:839-846.
312. Fredricks DN, Relman DA. Localization of Tropheryma whippelii rRNA in tissues from patients with Whipple's disease. *J Infect Dis.* 2001;183:1229-1237.
313. Gentilomi G, Musiani M, Zerbini M, et al. Double in situ hybridization for detection of herpes simplex virus and cytomegalovirus DNA using non-radioactive probes. *J Histochem Cytochem.* 1992;40:421-425.
314. Gentilomi G, Zerbini M, Musiani M, et al. In situ detection of B19 DNA in bone marrow of immunodeficient patients using a digoxigenin-labelled probe. *Mol Cell Probes.* 1993;7:19-24.
315. Hayden RT, Qian X, Procop GW, et al. In situ hybridization for the identification of filamentous fungi in tissue section. *Diagn Mol Pathol.* 2002;11:119-126.
316. Hayden RT, Qian X, Roberts GD, et al. In situ hybridization for the identification of yeastlike organisms in tissue section. *Diagn Mol Pathol.* 2001;10:15-23.
317. Hulette CM, Downey BT, Burger PC. Progressive multifocal leukoencephalopathy. Diagnosis by in situ hybridization with a biotinylated JC virus DNA probe using an automated Histomatic Code-On slide stainer. *Am J Surg Pathol.* 1991;15: 791-797.
318. Krimmer V, Merkert H, von Eiff C, et al. Detection of Staphylococcus aureus and Staphylococcus epidermidis in clinical samples by 16S rRNA-directed in situ hybridization. *J Clin Microbiol.* 1999;37:2667-2673.
319. Matsuse T, Matsui H, Shu CY, et al. Adenovirus pulmonary infections identified by PCR and in situ hybridisation in bone marrow transplant recipients. *J Clin Pathol.* 1994;47:973-977.
320. Montone KT, Litzky LA. Rapid method for detection of Aspergillus 5S ribosomal RNA using a genus-specific oligonucleotide probe. *Am J Clin Pathol.* 1995;103:48-51.
321. Morey AL, Keeling JW, Porter HJ, et al. Clinical and histopathological features of parvovirus B19 infection in the human fetus. *Br J Obstet Gynaecol.* 1992;99:566-574.
322. Morey AL, Porter HJ, Keeling JW, et al. Non-isotopic in situ hybridisation and immunophenotyping of infected cells in the investigation of human fetal parvovirus infection. *J Clin Pathol.* 1992;45:673-678.
323. Moter A, Göbel UB. Fluorescence in situ hybridization (FISH) for direct visualization of microorganisms. *J Microbiol Methods.* 2000;41:85-112.

324. Musiani M, Zerbini M, Venturoli S, et al. Rapid diagnosis of cytomegalovirus encephalitis in patients with AIDS using in situ hybridisation. *J Clin Pathol.* 1994;47:886-891.
325. Naoumov NV, Daniels HM, Davison F, et al. Identification of hepatitis B virus-DNA in the liver by in situ hybridization using a biotinylated probe. Relation to HBcAg expression and histology. *J Hepatol.* 1993;19:204-210.
326. Porter HJ, Padfield CJ, Peres LC, et al. Adenovirus and intranuclear inclusions in appendices in intussusception. *J Clin Pathol.* 1993;46:154-158.
327. Schmidbauer M, Budka H, Ambros P. Herpes simplex virus (HSV) DNA in microglial nodular brainstem encephalitis. *J Neuropathol Exp Neurol.* 1989;48:645-652.
328. Schmidbauer M, Budka H, Pilz P, et al. Presence, distribution and spread of productive varicella zoster virus infection in nervous tissues. *Brain.* 1992;115(Pt 2):383-398.
329. Thompson CH, Biggs IM, de Zwart-Steffe RT. Detection of molluscum contagiosum virus DNA by in situ hybridization. *Pathology.* 1990;22:181-186.
330. Unger ER. In situ diagnosis of human papillomaviruses. *Clin Lab Med.* 2000;20:289-301.
331. Wu TC, Mann RB, Epstein JI, et al. Abundant expression of EBER1 small nuclear RNA in nasopharyngeal carcinoma. A morphologically distinctive target for detection of Epstein-Barr virus in formalin-fixed paraffin-embedded carcinoma specimens. *Am J Pathol.* 1991;138:1461-1469.
332. Zaki SR, Judd R, Coffield LM, et al. Human papillomavirus infection and anal carcinoma. Retrospective analysis by in situ hybridization and the polymerase chain reaction. *Am J Pathol.* 1992;140:1345-1355.
333. Akhtar N, Ni J, Langston C, et al. PCR diagnosis of viral pneumonitis from fixed-lung tissue in children. *Biochem Mol Med.* 1996;58:66-76.
334. Amaker BH, Chandler Jr FW, Huey LO, et al. Molecular detection of JC virus in embalmed, formalin-fixed, paraffin-embedded brain tissue. *J Forensic Sci.* 1997;42:1157-1159.
335. Beqaj SH, Flesher R, Walker GR, et al. Use of the real-time PCR assay in conjunction with MagNA Pure for the detection of mycobacterial DNA from fixed specimens. *Diagn Mol Pathol.* 2007;16:169-173.
336. Bhatnagar J, Guarner J, Paddock CD, et al. Detection of West Nile virus in formalin-fixed, paraffin-embedded human tissues by RT-PCR: A useful adjunct to conventional tissue-based diagnostic methods. *J Clin Virol.* 2007;38:106-111.
337. Clavel C, Binninger I, Polette M, et al. [Polymerase chain reaction (PCR) and pathology. Technical principles and application]. *Ann Pathol.* 1993;13:88-96.
338. Guarner J, Bhatnagar J, Shieh WJ, et al. Histopathologic, immunohistochemical, and polymerase chain reaction assays in the study of cases with fatal sporadic myocarditis. *Hum Pathol.* 2007;38:1412-1419.
339. Lamps LW, Madhusudhan KT, Greenson JK, et al. The role of Yersinia enterocolitica and Yersinia pseudotuberculosis in granulomatous appendicitis: A histologic and molecular study. *Am J Surg Pathol.* 2001;25:508-515.
340. Paddock CD, Sanden GN, Cherry JD, et al. Pathology and pathogenesis of fatal Bordetella pertussis infection in infants. *Clin Infect Dis.* 2008;47:328-338.
341. Qian X, Jin L, Hayden RT, et al. Diagnosis of cat scratch disease with Bartonella henselae infection in formalin-fixed paraffin-embedded tissues by two different PCR assays. *Diagn Mol Pathol.* 2005;14:146-151.
342. Schild M, Gianinazzi C, Gottstein B, et al. PCR-based diagnosis of Naegleria sp. infection in formalin-fixed and paraffin-embedded brain sections. *J Clin Microbiol.* 2007;45:564-567.
343. Singh HB, Katoch VM, Natrajan M, et al. Improved protocol for PCR detection of Mycobacterium leprae in buffered formalin-fixed skin biopsies. *Int J Lepr Other Mycobact Dis.* 2004;72:175-178.
344. Tatti KM, Wu KH, Sanden GN, et al. Molecular diagnosis of Bordetella pertussis infection by evaluation of formalin-fixed tissue specimens. *J Clin Microbiol.* 2006;44:1074-1076.
345. Wilson DA, Reischl U, Hall GS, et al. Use of partial 16S rRNA gene sequencing for identification of Legionella pneumophila and non-pneumophila Legionella spp. *J Clin Microbiol.* 2007;45:257-258.

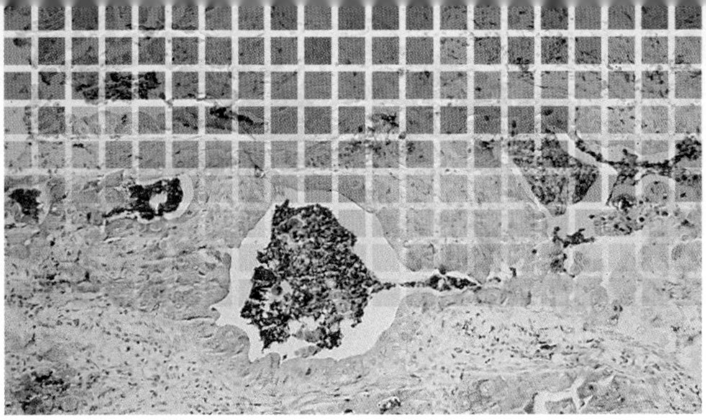

4

Immunohistology of Soft Tissue and Osseous Neoplasms

Mark R. Wick • Jason L. Hornick

Introduction 83
Biology of Antigens and Antibodies 83
Specific Soft Tissue Tumors 97

INTRODUCTION

Soft tissue and bone tumors are a diverse family, and its categorization continues to evolve as more insight is gained into the subtleties of their patterns of differentiation. As such, the classification of these neoplasms is an increasingly complex subject that requires at least a basic understanding of the biochemical attributes of the lesions in question. In this chapter we will present a practical summary of this topic; however, we do not purport it to be an encyclopedic or all-inclusive treatise. In particular, Chapter 13 considers the tumors that are most common in the skin and subcutis, and we have excluded lesions that are considered morphologically distinctive (i.e., they do not require immunohistology for diagnosis). In the same vein, we would like to emphasize that immunohistochemical evaluation of mesenchymal neoplasms is merely an adjunct to thorough histologic evaluation, not a substitute for it.

BIOLOGY OF ANTIGENS AND ANTIBODIES

Intermediate Filament Proteins

Intermediate filament proteins (IFPs) are structural components of all human cells, together with microfilaments and microtubules.[1,2] They are 7 to 10 nm in diameter and are often arranged in skeins or bundles in the cytoplasm. Parallel aggregation of IFPs often is observed in epithelial cells that are rich in high-molecular-weight keratins, yielding the structures known to electron microscopists as *tonofilaments* or *tonofibrils*.[3] Otherwise, the IFPs as a family are not morphologically distinguishable from one another at an ultrastructural level. Based on biochemical and functional grounds, they are composed of at least six distinct moieties: keratins, vimentin, desmin, neurofilament proteins (NFPs), glial fibrillary acidic protein (GFAP), and the lamins (nuclear envelope proteins).[4] In this chapter, we will discuss the first five of these entities, as they have been well characterized in diagnostic pathology.

All IFPs share structural homologies,[5] but their precise natures vary considerably. Their molecular weights vary between 40 and 200 kD. IFPs also have dissimilar isoelectric pH values, and, more important, characteristic distribution patterns in non-neoplastic cells and human tumors.[2] Two members of the IFP family—the keratins and NFPs—appear to be composed of heteropolymeric aggregations of two or more proteins, whereas the other members are homopolymers that contain only one protein isoform.[6] The IFPs are encoded by multiple genes on various chromosomes (e.g., chromosomes 12q and 17q for the keratins, chromosome 2q for desmin, chromosome 10p for vimentin, and chromosome 17q for GFAP),[7-10] a situation that is somewhat counterintuitive in light of their shared biochemical attributes.

In keeping with their proposed cytoskeletal nature, IFPs initially were thought to serve a purely structural role in muscle cells. It was hypothesized that the function of these proteins was to keep other cytoplasmic proteins in proper relationship to one another, as well as to anchor the cytoplasmic contractile apparatus to the cell membrane. However, subsequent developments in cell biology cast considerable doubt on this premise.[11] The intermediate filaments are now known to serve a nucleic acid–binding function; moreover, they are susceptible to processing by calcium-activated proteases and are substrates for cyclic adenosine monophosphate–dependent protein kinases. Thus, it has been proposed that all IFPs serve as modulators between extracellular influences governing calcium flux into the cell (and subsequent protease activation) and nuclear function at a transcriptional

TABLE 4.1 Cytokeratin Subclasses and Non-neoplastic Cell Types Expressing Them

Type II (Basic) Cytokeratins*			Type I (Acid) Cytokeratins*	
(Moll Catalog No.)	(Molecular Wt.)	Distribution	(Moll Catalog No.)	(Molecular Wt.)
–	–	Epidermis of palms and soles	CK9	64 kD
CK1	67 kD	Epidermis and keratinizing squamous epithelia in all other locations	CK10	56.5 kD
CK2	65 kD		CK11	56 kD
CK3	63 kD	Cornea	CK12	55 kD
CK4	59 kD	Nonkeratinizing epithelia of internal viscera	CK13	51 kD
CK5	58 kD	Basal cells of squamous and glandular epithelia, myoepithelial cells, and mesothelium	CK14	50 kD
CK6	56 kD	Squamous epithelia	CK16	48 kD
CK7	54 kD	Simple epithelia	–	–
–	–	Basal cells of glandular epithelia and myoepithelial cells	CK17	46 kD
CK8	52 kD	Simple epithelia	CK18	45 kD
–	–	Simple epithelia; most glandular and some squamous epithelial cells	CK19	40 kD
–	–	Simple epithelial cells of gastrointestinal tract; Merkel cells of skin	CK20	46 kD

*Cytokeratin pairs that typically are coexpressed together in the same cell types are shown on the same line.

or translational level.[12] Their morphologic associations with cell membranes and the perinuclear cytoplasm are consistent with this theory and relegate a cytoskeletal role to a secondary level. Present opinion favors the view that fibrils of the IFPs are formed to restrict the availability of their nucleic acid–binding domains in accord with cell cycle activity, not as cellular "buttresses." Although some of the IFPs insert into intercellular desmoplakin-containing desmosomes (which are responsible for maintaining tissue integrity), this does not necessarily assign a structural biological role to these filaments because intercellular junctions may be points of biochemical communication with the extracellular milieu.[13]

KERATINS

As the essential IFPs of epithelial cells and epithelial neoplasms, keratins have a high degree of specificity and sensitivity for the diagnosis of carcinoma among malignant tumors. Cytokeratins typically are expressed by any given cell type in pairs, representing an acidic (type I) and a basic (type II) keratin.[14] These vary in molecular weight from 40 to 67 kD and have been given catalog designations by Moll and colleagues such that they are numbered, within each respective type grouping, from lowest to highest molecular weight.[15] There are 12 type I keratins with acidic isoelectric points, and 8 type II proteins with basic biochemical attributes. As described by Miettinen, cytokeratins generally tend to pair themselves during cell development so that a type I keratin is associated with a type II keratin that is 7 to 9 kD larger.[14]

The particular keratin types that can be detected in given tissues or neoplasms follow predictable, known patterns of gene expression that serve, in part, to identify the cells composing them (Table 4.1). With particular reference to nonepithelial cells, selected cytokeratins (CK8, CK18, and occasionally CK19) are demonstrable in the physiologic state, but special techniques (e.g., acetone fixation, frozen section immunohistology, or amplified immunodetection methods) are usually necessary to preserve or detect extremely low densities of these IFPs. Selected mesenchymal neoplasms may likewise exhibit keratin reactivity, which is a bit broader in its scope. For example, CK1, CK7, CK8, CK13, CK14, CK18, and CK19 have all been observed in synovial sarcomas.[14,16] Other soft tissue or bone tumors that are regularly cytokeratin-reactive include epithelioid sarcoma (CK8, CK18, and CK19); chordoma (CK8, CK18, and CK19, with or without CK4 and CK5); myoepithelioma/myoepithelial carcinoma (including tumors previously known as parachordoma) (CK8, among others); and intraosseous adamantinoma (CK19).[14-19] Thus, together with synovial sarcoma, those neoplasms constitute a group of lesions that some authors have suggested are primary carcinosarcomas of soft tissue and bone.

In reference to still other mesenchymal neoplasms, experience since the 1990s has shown that under some circumstances, selected tumors that are typically devoid of keratins may synthesize those IFPs in an aberrant fashion (Table 4.2). Indeed, at this point, virtually all sarcoma morphotypes have been reported to show this potential. Nevertheless, we would like to emphasize that aberrant keratin reactivity is most common in a narrow spectrum of malignant mesenchymal neoplasms that are studied under usual diagnostic conditions, principally leiomyosarcoma (LMS), malignant peripheral

TABLE 4.2 Cytokeratin Subclasses Expressed Aberrantly in Mesenchymal Cells and Tumors

Moll Cytokeratin Catalog No.	Recognized by MoAb Clones	Potential Distribution
8	CAM5.2 (Becton-Dickinson) AE3 (PROGEN) KL1 (Serotec) F12-19 (Biogenesis) RCK102 (Biogenesis) DC10 (BioGenex) MAK-6 (Medac) 5D3 (Biogenesis) NCL-5D3 (Medac) 6D7/3F3 (Medac) 2A4 (Biohit) M20 (Accurate) KS8.7 (Paesel) NCL-CK8 (Novocastra) UCD/AB6.01 (ATCC) C22 (Biogenesis) 4.1.18 (BioGenex) H1 (Bioprobe) C51 (Neomarkers) 34BH11 (Enzo) Lu5 (Sera-Lab) C11 (Neomarkers)	Fetal fibroblasts; subserosal fibroblasts; myometrium; vascular smooth muscle; fetal myocardium; vascular endothelial cells; selected reticulum cells of lymphatic organs; neoplastic plasma cells and CD30+ lymphoid cells (very rarely); selected leiomyosarcomas, epithelioid hemangioendotheliomas, epithelioid angiosarcomas, primitive neuroectodermal tumors and Ewing's sarcomas, malignant peripheral nerve sheath tumors, and clear cell sarcomas
18	MFN116 (Axcel) PKK1 (LabSystems) CK18 (Novocastra) KS18.4 (Paesel) KS18.8 (Biotest) DC10 (BioGenex) K918.04 (Cymbus) KS-B17.2 (Sigma) 4B11 (Biohit) DA7 (Bioprobe) KS18.18 (Camon) 34BH11 (DiagBiosys) F12-19 (Biogenesis) C11 (Neomarkers) LP34 (Medac)	Fetal fibroblasts; myometrium; vascular smooth muscle; fetal myocardium; vascular endothelial cells; selected reticulum cells of lymphatic organs; some CD30+ lymphoid cells (rarely); selected leiomyosarcomas, epithelioid hemangioendotheliomas, epithelioid angiosarcomas, primitive neuroectodermal tumors and Ewing's sarcomas, malignant peripheral nerve sheath tumors, and clear cell sarcomas
19	AE1 (BM; ICN) PKK1 (LabSystems) CK19 (Novocastra) RCK108 (BioGenex) BA17 (Dako) KS19.1 (Serotec) F12-19 (Biogenesis) MAK-6 (Medac)	Myometrium; fetal myocardium; selected neoplastic myeloid cells; some leiomyosarcomas; rare primitive neuroectodermal tumors and Ewing's sarcomas

nerve sheath tumor (MPNST), epithelioid angiosarcoma, and, to a lesser degree, Ewing's sarcoma/primitive neuroectodermal tumor (ES/PNET).[20] In keeping with the comments mentioned earlier in this chapter, CK8, CK18, and CK19 are most often expected in this scenario. We would like to point out that aberrancy of IFP synthesis is not a frequent event overall. Many reports on this phenomenon actually represent idiosyncrasies or flaws in immunohistochemical technique, wherein antikeratin antibodies are used at inappropriately high concentration or with especially sensitive detection procedures. Inasmuch as IFPs are structurally interrelated,[21] we are not surprised that cross-labeling of vimentin, desmin, NFPs, or GFAP can be obtained spuriously with many antikeratin reagents. Using information on the interspecies relatedness of intermediate filaments and their similarities to one another, Geisler and Weber[22] outlined the following classes of monoclonal antibodies that may be raised against them:

- Tissue-specific (intermediate filament-discriminating) but broadly reactive across species
- Tissue-specific and species-specific
- Tissue–non-specific and species-specific
- Tissue–non-specific and species–non-specific

From a comparative biological point of view, all these reagents are of interest. However, only the first two categories have potential use as diagnostic discriminants in surgical pathology.

This brings our discussion to a crucial philosophical point regarding methodology. At this juncture, a large body of clinical literature exists on the IFP profiles of human neoplasms. To benefit from the value of its contents in a diagnostic setting, one must retain the techniques used in obtaining these data. Thus, in a practical sense, it is not advisable to substitute a new and improved immunodetection protocol for an old one without considering the effect the step has on the final interpretation. The diagnostic pathologist's goal should not be to identify every molecule of a particular IFP (no matter how sparse) in any given tumor, but rather to establish and maintain the windows of immunodetection to minimize the overlap between related moieties and maximize diagnostic utility. Regarding these maxims will lower the incidence of aberrant keratin expression in mesenchymal neoplasia when using routinely processed (paraffin-embedded) clinical substrates.

DESMIN

Desmin is a cytoplasmic IFP that is characteristically found in muscle cells and in the neoplasms associated with them.[23-25] In smooth muscle cells, it is seen with cytoplasmic dense bodies and subplasmalemmal dense plaques; in striated muscle, desmin filaments are linked to sarcomeric Z disks.

In 1977, Small and Sobieszek were first to recognize desmin as a distinct biochemical moiety.[26] They found that it represented a residual filamentous protein in muscle cells that had been depleted of actin and myosin *in vitro*, and they assigned the provisional designation skeletin to it. It was observed to have an isoelectric point of approximately 4 and to be heat stable and insoluble in salt-rich solutions. Amino acid analysis revealed a high concentration of glutamate and aspartate and a significant chemical homology with glial filaments and NFPs. A notable finding in this study was that muscle cells depleted of skeletin (desmin) were still able to contract in response to adenosine triphosphate and calcium. This point led the authors to conclude that the protein in question played no role in contractility but rather served to keep actin and myosin filaments in register and to anchor them to the plasmalemma.

These observations have been confirmed and expanded by others.[27-29] Desmin is now known to have a molecular weight of 53 kD, with a mass per unit of 36 to 37 kD/nm. It is composed of an N-terminal headpiece and a C-terminal tailpiece, both of which are nonhelical in conformation. These bracket an alpha helical middle domain of approximately 300 amino acid residues. The former are greatly variable in biochemical constitution from species to species, but the helical segment is highly conserved, meaning that interspecies homology in this domain is striking. Chicken and porcine desmin demonstrate less than a 9% biochemical divergence. In fact, this similarity supersedes that which is exhibited between different IFPs in the same species; nevertheless, all five IFPs show an amino acid sequence homology of approximately 30%.[29]

Like other intermediate filaments, desmin displays a 20 to 22 nm axial periodicity. Ip and Heuser showed that it forms heteropolymers that aggregate in a cross-linked, fibrillar, tetrameric fashion.[30] These are arranged side by side in a staggered half-unit register, such that the headpiece of one filament is associated with the middle domain of its neighbor. The helical segment composition of desmin allows it to form coiled coils with respect to the tertiary structure of the molecule; indeed, such a conformation would be predicted by biochemical models. Hydrophobic amino acid residues are thereby exposed, explaining the ability of desmin to associate with nuclear and plasmalemmal membranes, which are nonhydrophilic.

Desmin appears in developing striated muscle cells at the myotube-forming stage, in which myoblasts fuse with one another.[31] It replaces vimentin, at least in large measure, because the latter is the intermediate filament that is first expressed by virtually all embryonic mesenchymal cells. Desmin filaments are oriented in a longitudinal fashion initially, but as the muscle cell matures, they become concentrated around Z disks.[32] Fischman and Danto performed an analysis of desmin immunoreactivity in embryonic and adult muscle cells using monoclonal antibodies (D3 and D76).[33] D3 recognizes embryonic cellular desmin but does not react with adult cells; D76 displays the reverse of this pattern. These data suggest either that either desmin is biochemically altered during cellular development or that different epitopes are masked in fetal and adult cells.

Although desmin is most often expressed by myogenous cells, *in vitro* studies of chicken embryo and hamster kidney fibroblasts have also revealed its presence.[34] This finding is best explained by implicating a myofibroblastic nature for such cells. Other immunofluorescence assessments of intact myofibroblastic tissues have reportedly shown no desmin reactivity, however. Also, not all muscular cells contain desmin. For example, Schmid and colleagues documented three separate cell types in mammalian vascular (aortic) smooth muscle—those that display vimentin only, others that express vimentin and desmin concurrently, and a third group exhibiting only desmin.[35] Immunoelectron microscopic analyses have documented the binding of suitably specific antidesmins to the intermediate filaments of muscle cells and their neoplasms.[36] There should be no cross-reactivity of such reagents with associated contractile proteins, such as actin and myosin; this is particularly important because these three proteins appear to share some epitopes.

The three best-characterized monoclonal antibodies to desmin are designated D33, DER-11, and DEB-5. By the Western blot technique, they have been shown to recognize desmin epitopes between residues 324 and 415 and to have no cross-reactivity with other IFPs. These reagents show tissue-specificity but species–non-specificity.

In general, desmin is, as expected, a specific marker for myogenic differentiation among soft tissue tumors. As such, it is seen in the majority of rhabdomyomas, leiomyomas, rhabdomyosarcomas, and LMSs.[23-25,37-39] Because myofibromatoses also have a partially myogenous nature ultrastructurally, it is understandable that lesions such as desmoid tumors and myofibromas are likewise potentially desmin reactive.[40] Nonetheless, myoepithelial cells typically lack desmin. Desmin may also be coexpressed by neoplasms with divergent phenotypes, examples of which include desmoplastic small round cell tumors, epithelioid sarcomas, MPNSTs, and some malignant rhabdoid tumors.[41-45]

VIMENTIN

Vimentin is a 57-kD protein that was initially isolated from a mouse fibroblast culture.[2,46] Its name derives from the Latin vimentum, describing an array of flexible rods. This IFP is considered to be the primordial member of the intermediate filament family, because it is present in most, if not all, fetal cells early in development. Moreover, when two or more IFPs are coexpressed by a cell line or neoplasm, vimentin is virtually always one of them.[47] Accordingly, vimentin is not considered to be cell type-specific. From the perspective of mesenchymal tumor pathology, it is of interest that vimentin shows a greater amino acid homology to desmin, NFPs, and GFAP than it does to the keratins.[22,46]

The ubiquity of vimentin in soft tissues limits its diagnostic use in the setting of tumor pathology. However, it does serve a useful control marker function—to ensure that the tissue has been properly preserved and processed.[48] If vimentin cannot be easily detected in non-neoplastic endothelial cells, fibroblasts, and other mesenchymal elements that are routinely present in any tissue section, the reactivity or non-reactivity of accompanying neoplastic cells cannot be properly determined. Occasionally, the pattern of vimentin expression is also distinctive. For example, in malignant rhabdoid tumors of the soft tissues, the IFP usually assumes a densely globular cytoplasmic configuration, indenting the nuclei of the neoplastic cells.[45] Tables 4.3 to 4.7 list the characterized commercially available antibodies to vimentin, of which clones V9 are the most widely used.[47,49-54]

TABLE 4.3 Antibody Reagents Used by the Authors in the Study of Soft Tissue Tumors

Reagent	Source	Dilution	Protocol	Principal Diagnostic Use
Antikeratins (M)				
AE1/AE3	Boehringer-Mannheim	1:150	MWER	Recognition of epithelioid sarcoma, synovial sarcoma, and divergent epithelial differentiation in selected other soft tissue sarcomas
CAM5.2	Becton-Dickinson	1:200	MWER	
MAK-6	Medac	1:75	MWER	
DC10	BioGenex	1:50	MWER	
CK18	Novocastra	1:50	MWER	
CK19	Novocastra	1:50	MWER	
CK7	BioGenex	1:75	MWER	
Antidesmin (M)	BioGenex	1:2000	MWER	Recognition of smooth muscle and striated muscle tumors
Antivimentin (M)	BioGenex	1:2000	MWER	Ubiquitous intermediate filament in soft tissue neoplasms; serves as a positive specimen control
Anti-epithelial membrane antigen (M)	Dako	1:400	NT	Recognition of epithelioid sarcoma, synovial sarcoma, and selected peripheral nerve sheath tumors
Anti-muscle-specific actin (clone HHF-35) (M)	Enzo	1:8000	MWER	Recognition of smooth muscle and striated muscle tumors as well as myofibroblastic differentiation
Anti-alpha isoform actin (clone 1A4) (M)	Dako	1:200	MWER	Recognition of smooth muscle tumors and myofibroblastic differentiation
Antimyoglobin (P)	Dako	1:800	MWER	Recognition of striated muscle tumors
Anti-Myo-D1 (M)	Dako	1:10	MWER	Recognition of striated muscle tumors
Antimyogenin (M)	Novocastra	1:30	MWER	Recognition of striated muscle tumors
Anti-h-caldesmon (M)	Dako	1:200	MWER	Recognition of smooth muscle tumors
Anti-S-100 protein (P)	Dako	1:1000	NT	Recognition of melanocytic, schwannian, and cartilage neoplasms
Anti-CD57 (M)	Becton-Dickinson	1:20	MWER	Recognition of schwannian tumors
Anti-collagen type IV (M)	BioGenex	1:40	MWER	Recognition of synovial, myogenous, peripheral nerve sheath, and endothelial neoplasms
Antilaminin (M)	Sigma	1:20	MWER	Recognition of synovial, myogenous, peripheral nerve sheath, and endothelial neoplasms

Continued

TABLE 4.3 Antibody Reagents Used by the Authors in the Study of Soft Tissue Tumors, cont'd

Reagent	Source	Dilution	Protocol	Principal Diagnostic Use
Anti-factor VIII–related antigen (M)	Dako	1:20	MWER	Recognition of endothelial neoplasms
Anti-CD34 (M)	Dako	1:800	MWER	Recognition of endothelial tumors, dermatofibrosarcoma protuberans, solitary fibrous tumors, and selected peripheral nerve sheath tumors and epithelioid sarcomas
Anti-CD31 (M)	Dako	1:40	MWER	Recognition of endothelial tumors
Antithrombomodulin (M)	Dako	1:200	MWER	Recognition of endothelial tumors and mesotheliomas
Anti-*Ulex europaeus I* lectin (P)	Dako	1:4000	NT	Recognition of endothelial tumors via binding of *Ulex europaeus I* lectin
Ulex europaeus I (lectin)	Dako	1:1000	NT	Recognition of endothelial tumors
Anti-CD68	Dako	1:800	MWER	Putative marker of fibrohistiocytic tumors (see text)
Antiosteonectin (M)	BioDesign	1:100	MWER	Sensitive marker of possible osteoblastic differentiation
Antiosteocalcin (M)	Biogenesis	1:100	MWER	Specific marker of osteoblastic differentiation
Antisynaptophysin (M)	BioGenex	1:40	MWER	Detection of neuroectodermal differentiation
Anti-CD99 (M)	Dako	1:20	MWER	Recognition of virtually all primitive neuroectodermal tumors and Ewing's sarcomas; labels roughly 50% of synovial sarcomas and malignant peripheral nerve sheath tumors; also present in lymphoblastic lymphomas/leukemias presenting in soft tissue

M, monoclonal; MWER, microwave-enhanced epitope retrieval; NT, no pretreatment of tissue sections; P, polyclonal (heteroantiserum).

TABLE 4.4 Percentages of Positivity for Pertinent Immunoreactants in Malignant Small Round Cell Tumors of Soft Tissue and Bone*

Antigen/tumor	KER	EMA	VIM	DES	MSA	MYOGN	SYN	CD57	S-100P	CD45	CD99	OCN
RMS	<10[a]	<1[a]	93	94	96	92	0	17	7	0	19	0
ES/PNET	7	0	75	<1[b]	<1[b]	<1[b]	65	30	<10[a]	0	91	0
PSRCT	50[a]	30[a]	75[a]	50[a]	50[a]	50[a]	75[a]	30[a]	<10[a]	0	90[c]	0
MCS	<5[a]	0	98	0	0	0	0	58	97[d]	0	13	0
SCOS	<1[a]	0	100	<1	<5[a]	0	0	50[a]	33	0	35	73
ML/LEUK	0	0	75[a]	0	0	0	0	<5[a]	0	98	50[a]	0
SCSS	75[e]	75	100	0	0	0	0	90	30[a]	0	0	0

*All figures in this table represent percentages of immunoreactive cases in each tumor category. Unless otherwise specified, the source of these data is Frisman D. "Immunoquery," available at *http//www.immunoquery.com.*

[a]Data derived from authors' experience.

[b]Peripheral neuroectodermal tumors expressing DES, MSA, or MYOGN are classified as polyphenotypic small round cell tumors by many observers.

[c]Desmoplastic small round cell tumor variants of polyphenotypic small round cell tumors are generally negative for CD99.

[d]S-100 protein is seen only in the chondroid islands of mesenchymal chondrosarcoma.

[e]Keratins 7, 13, and 19 are seen in 45% to 50% of cases of small cell synovial sarcoma, but less than 10% of differential diagnostic alternatives.

KER, keratin, as detected with a mixture of antibodies CAM5.2, MAK-6, and AE1/AE3; EMA, epithelial membrane antigen; VIM, vimentin; DES, desmin; MSA, muscle-specific actin; MYOGN, myogenin; SYN, synaptophysin; S-100P, S-100 protein; OCN, osteocalcin; RMS, embryonal and alveolar rhabdomyosarcomas; ES/PNET, Ewing's sarcoma/primitive neuroectodermal tumor; PSRCT, polyphenotypic small round cell tumor; MCS, mesenchymal chondrosarcoma; SCOS, small cell osteosarcoma; ML/LEUK, malignant lymphoma/leukemia; SCSS, small cell poorly differentiated synovial sarcoma.

TABLE 4.5 Percentages of Positivity for Pertinent Immunoreactants in Malignant Spindle Cell Tumors of Soft Tissue and Bone*

Antigen/ tumor	KER	EMA	VIM	DES	MSA	SMA	CALD	S-100P	CD57	Collagen type IV	LM	CD34	CD31	UL	CD99	OCN
SCRMS	<10[a]	<1[a]	95	95	96	25	<1	7	17	98[a]	100	0	0	0	20	0
FS	0	0	100	0	0	<5[a]	0	2	0	0	0	0	0	0	0	0
LMS	<10[a]	0	91	75[a]	90	88	85	8	50	75	63	16	<1a	0	20	0
MPNST	<10[a]	25	100	11	18	<1	<1	63	43	83	80	9	0	0	50[a]	0
MSS	76	75	100	0	0	12	<1[a]	30[a]	90	100	95	0	0	0	50[a]	0
SCAS	<5[a]	0	100	0	<10[a]	<10[a]	<5[a]	<1[a]	0	10	55	80	80	70	0	0
KS	0	0	100	0	0	100	<5[a]	0	0	50[a]	50[a]	86	53	10	0	0
FOS	<1[a]	0[a]	100	<1[a]	<1[a]	<1[a]	<1[a]	10[a]	50[a]	0	0	0	0	0	0	80[a]

*All figures in this table represent percentages of immunoreactive cases in each tumor category. Unless otherwise specified, the source of these data is Frisman D. "Immunoquery," available at *http//www.immunoquery.com.*

[a]Data derived from authors' experience.

KER, keratin, detected by a mixture of CAM5.2, MAK-6, and AE1/AE3; EMA, epithelial membrane antigen; VIM, vimentin; DES, desmin; MSA, muscle-specific actin; SMA, smooth muscle (alpha isoform) actin; CALD, h-caldesmon; S-100P, S-100 protein; OCN, osteocalcin; LM, laminin; UL, *Ulex europaeus I* lectin binding; FS, fibrosarcoma; SCRMS, spindle cell rhabdomyosarcoma; LMS, leiomyosarcoma; MPNST, malignant peripheral nerve sheath tumor; MSS, monophasic spindle cell synovial sarcoma; SCAS, spindle cell angiosarcoma; KS, Kaposi's sarcoma; FOS, fibroblastic osteosarcoma.

TABLE 4.6 Percentages of Positivity for Pertinent Immunoreactants in Malignant Epithelioid Tumors of Soft Tissue and Bone*

Antigen/ tumor	KER	EMA	VIM	DES	MSA	SMA	CALD	S-100P	CD57	HMB-45	TY	M1	CD31	CD34	Collagen type IV	OCN
EPS	100	96	100	10	39	33	25[a]	<5[a]	0	0	0	0	<1[a]	52	50[a]	0
EPSS	95[a]	99[a]	100	0	0	0	0	10[a]	50[a]	0	0	0	0	0	100	0
EAS	10[a]	0	100	0	0	0	0	<1[a]	0	0	0	0	80	80	65[a]	0
EMPNST	<10[a]	20	100	11	18	<1	<1	63	43	<1[a]	<1[a]	<1[a]	0	9	83	0
CCS	<1[a]	0	100	0	30	0	0	90[a]	17	85	90[a]	70[a]	0	4	0	0
SEFS	<1[a]	0[a]	100[a]	0[a]	0[a]	0[a]	0[a]	0[a]	0[a]	0[a]	0[a]	0[a]	0[a]	0[a]	0[a]	0[a]
ELMS	<10[a]	0	90	75	90	85	75	8	50[a]	0	0	0	0[a]	16	75	0
ASPS	0	0	50[a]	20	<10[a]	0[a]	0	30	0	0	0	0	0	0	0	0
HMFH	<1[a]	0	100	<10[a]	17	18	<5[a]	<1[a]	0[a]	0	0	0	0	0	0	0
EOS	<1[a]	0[a]	100	<1[a]	<1[a]	<1[a]	0	<5[a]	50[a]	0	0	0	0	0	0	82

*All figures in this table represent percentages of immunoreactive cases in each tumor category. Unless otherwise specified, the source of these data is Frisman D. "Immunoquery," available at *http//www.immunoquery.com.*

[a]Data derived from authors' experience.

KER, keratin, as detected by a mixture of CAM5.2, MAK-6, and AE1/AE3; EMA, epithelial membrane antigen; VIM, vimentin; DES, desmin; MSA, muscle-specific actin; SMA, smooth muscle (alpha isoform) actin; CALD, h-caldesmon; S-100P, S-100 protein; TY, tyrosinase; M1, MART-1 (melan-A); OCN, osteocalcin; EPS, epithelioid sarcoma; EPSS, epithelioid synovial sarcoma; EAS, epithelioid angiosarcoma; EMPNST, epithelioid malignant peripheral nerve sheath tumor; CCS, clear cell sarcoma; SEFS, sclerosing epithelioid fibrosarcoma; ELMS, epithelioid leiomyosarcoma; ASPS, alveolar soft part sarcoma; HMFH, histiocytic malignant fibrous histiocytoma; EOS, epithelioid osteosarcoma.

NEUROFILAMENT PROTEINS

Neurofilament proteins are composed of three basic subunits with molecular weights of 68 kD, 150 kD, and 200 kD,[55,56] hence they are clearly larger than all other IFPs. Each NFP appears to be a separate gene product, rather than derivatives of the other two.[57] Expression of this family of IFPs is correlated with the differentiation of neurogenic blast cells into committed neurons in the developing embryo or in neoplasia.[58,59] Another peculiarity of NFPs that is not shared by other intermediate filament classes, except for GFAP, is that each of the three neurofilament isoforms may be either phosphorylated or nonphosphorylated *in vivo*.[60] Correspondingly, antibodies to the NFPs may be specific for only one of those two configurations.[61,62]

Practically speaking, NFPs are generally not well detected in formalin-fixed, paraffin-embedded tissue, even with modern immunohistochemical methods and commercial antibodies. Among these, our experience

TABLE 4.7 Percentages of Positivity for Pertinent Immunoreactants in Malignant Pleomorphic Tumors of Soft Tissue and Bone*

Antigen/ tumor	KER	EMA	VIM	DES	MSA	SMA	CALD	S-100P	CD57	Collagen type IV	LM	CD34	CD31	UL	CD99	OCN
PRMS	<10[a]	<1[a]	100	95	96	25	<1	7	17	98[a]	100	0	0	0	20	0[a]
PLPS/DLPS	0	0	100	0	<1[a]	<1[a]	<1[a]	70[b]	0	20[a]	10[a]	0	0	0	0	0[a]
PLMS/DLMS	<10[a]	0	91	75[a]	90	88	75	8	50	75	63	16	<1	0	20	0[a]
MPNST	<10[a]	20	100	11	18	<1	<1	63	43	83	80	9	0	0	10[a]	0[a]
MFH	76[b]	75[b]	100	0	0	12	<1[a]	30[a]	90[b]	100[b]	95[b]	0	0	0	50[b]	0[a]
DCHOR	<1[a]	0	100	<10[a]	17	18	<5[a]	<1[a]	0[a]	0	0	0	0	0	0	0[a]
DCHS	100[b]	94[b]	100	3	0	0	0	88[b]	32[b]	13	10	0	0	10[ab]	0	0[a]
POGS	<1[a]	0[a]	100	0	0	0	0	97[b]	58[b]	10[ab]	5[ab]	0	0	0	0	0[a]
	<1[a]	<1[a]	100	11	0	50	0	32[b]	50[b]	0	0	0	0	0	35	82

*All figures in this table represent percentages of immunoreactive cases in each tumor category. Unless otherwise specified, the source of these data is Frisman D. "Immunoquery," available at *http//www.immunoquery.com.*

[a]Data derived from authors' experience.

[b]Reactivity for specified determinants is focal only.

KER, keratin, detected by a mixture of CAM5.2, MAK-6, and AE1/AE3; EMA, epithelial membrane antigen; VIM, vimentin; DES, desmin; MSA, muscle-specific actin; SMA, smooth muscle (alpha isoform) actin; CALD, h-caldesmon; S-100P, S-100 protein; LM, laminin; UL, *Ulex europaeus* I lectin binding; OCN, osteocalcin; PRMS, pleomorphic rhabdomyosarcoma; PLPS/DLPS, pleomorphic and dedifferentiated liposarcoma; PLMS/DLMS, pleomorphic and dedifferentiated leiomyosarcoma; MPNST, pleomorphic malignant peripheral nerve sheath tumor; MFH, malignant fibrous histiocytoma; DCHOR, dedifferentiated chordoma; DCHS, dedifferentiated chondrosarcoma; POGS, pleomorphic osteosarcoma.

has been that the SMI series of monoclonal antibodies[63] is most consistently active against routinely processed surgical pathology specimens. It is known that among soft tissue neoplasms, neuroblastoma variants, ganglioneuromas, paragangliomas, and metastatic neuroendocrine carcinomas are the only lesions that are potentially labeled for NFPs.[64-67]

GLIAL FIBRILLARY ACIDIC PROTEIN

Among the IFPs, glial fibrillary acidic protein (GFAP) does not play a significant part in the diagnosis of soft tissue tumors. This 51-kD protein is the major component of astrocytes, ependymal cells, and retinal Müller cells and typically is not expressed by mature oligodendroglia.[67-69] Nonglial tissues with putative GFAP reactivity include Schwann cells, myoepithelial cells, Kupffer cells, and some chondrocytes.[69] It is therefore expected that selected neoplasms that include such elements (peripheral nerve sheath tumors and chondroid tumors)[70-75] may occasionally demonstrate immunolabeling for GFAP. As such, GFAP may be used as a second-line marker for malignant MPNSTs, although it is focally positive in only 30% of cases. In addition, GFAP may help support the diagnosis of soft tissue myoepithelioma, as discussed in the following section.

Epithelial-Related Markers

EPITHELIAL MEMBRANE ANTIGEN

Epithelial membrane antigen (EMA) is one of several human milk fat globule proteins (HMFGPs) that are derived from the mammary epithelium. The HMFGPs vary greatly in molecular weight (51 kD to >1000 kD). They are predominantly glycoproteinaceous[76] and compose part of the plasmalemma of epithelial cells in areas of the cell membrane overlying tight junctions.[77] In addition, because HMFGPs are packaged in the Golgi apparatus, globular labeling of this structure may be seen immunohistologically.[77] The function of HMFGPs, including EMA, is still not absolutely certain. It is thought that they serve a role in secretion or, alternatively, provide a protective function for the cell.[76]

The distribution of HMFGPs is such that many, but not all, non-neoplastic human epithelial cells express at least one member of this protein family. Exceptions include the gastrointestinal surface epithelium, endocervical epithelium, prostatic acinar epithelium, epididymis, germ cells, hepatocytes, adrenal cortical cells, rete testis, squamous cells of the epidermis, and thyroid follicular epithelium.[78]

The most well-characterized monoclonal antibody to EMA (which is the most widely used HMFGP) is E29. It labels a glycoprotein of approximately 450 kD. In specific reference to the soft tissues, the notochord, perineurial cells, and plasma cells are the only non-neoplastic elements capable of EMA positivity.[79-81] Nevertheless, neoplastic processes that may be EMA-immunoreactive are somewhat more numerous. Synovial sarcoma, epithelioid sarcoma, selected peripheral nerve sheath tumors (perineuriomas), chordomas, myoepitheliomas/myoepithelial carcinomas, and selected plasmacytomas are commonly labeled.[82] Note that true EMA reactivity (i.e., that which generally equates with epithelial differentiation) must be cell membrane based. Purely cytoplasmic labeling without a membrane component is a spurious pattern that should be ignored for diagnostic purposes.[83]

OTHER EPITHELIAL MARKERS

When stains for standard epithelial determinants (e.g., keratin and EMA) yield equivocal results, it may be desirable to assess additional potential indicators of epithelial differentiation, especially if morphologic features suggest aberrant reactivity. The best known among the adjunctive epithelial markers are desmoplakin, desmoglein, and E-cadherin. The first two are desmocollins or elements of desmosomal complexes, which represent specialized intercellular anchoring structures.[84,85] On the other hand, cadherins are calcium-dependent transmembranous intercellular adhesion molecules. They are divided into three subclasses (E-, P-, and N-cadherin), which have distinctive immunologic specificities and tissue distributions.[86,87] These molecules have subclass specificities in cell-cell binding and are involved in selective cellular adhesion. E-cadherin is typically associated with epithelial differentiation. Analysis of amino acid sequences, as deduced from the nucleotide sequences of cDNAs encoding cadherins, has demonstrated that they share common sequences and they are therefore regarded as a family of adhesion molecules with differential specificities. Although there are certainly exceptions, concurrent immunoreactivity for desmoplakin or desmoglein and E-cadherin is generally restricted to epithelial neoplasms and mesenchymal tumors with epithelial characteristics. These markers are not widely used in the diagnosis of soft tissue tumors.

Additional Myogenic Markers

ACTINS

Aside from desmin, the next most useful group of cytoplasmic determinants for the definition of myogenous differentiation is the protein family of the actins.[25,88] The six major isoforms of these microfilamentous contractile polypeptides are designated as: skeletal muscle–alpha; smooth muscle–alpha; smooth muscle–gamma; cardiac muscle–alpha; nonmyogenous beta; and nonmyogenous gamma.[88,89] Alpha and gamma muscle isoforms are seen in tissues with pure myogenic differentiation, but they are also demonstrable in cells with myofibroblastic or myoepithelial features.[90-93] The molecular weights of all these biochemical moieties cluster around 45 kD, and they may be labeled with antibodies that recognize conserved amino acid sequences or, alternatively, with isoform-selective reagents.[88-90] Obviously, from a diagnostic perspective, only the latter method is desirable. However, because of inevitable problems that arise in the immunohistologic detection of heteropolymeric proteins, even some of these antiactins are not truly specific for pure myogenous differentiation. This is particularly true of one commonly used commercial reagent, clone 1A4, which is widely known as *anti-(alpha) smooth muscle actin.*[91] In reality, it decorates some cell types besides smooth muscle, including myofibroblasts, myoepithelia, and others. In fact, nearly any neoplasm that shows spindle-cell morphology may express smooth muscle actin, including spindle cell (sarcomatoid) carcinomas. Another antibody designated HHF-35, or anti–muscle-specific actin, shows more muscle-restricted immunoreactivity in routinely processed specimens.[25,90]

OTHER SARCOMERIC CONTRACTILE PROTEINS

The contractile mechanism in skeletal muscle is effected by a complex of proteins that includes myosin II (molecular weight 460 kD), actin, tropomyosin (molecular weight 70 kD), and troponin. The troponin molecule has three subunits (troponin I, troponin T, and troponin C) with molecular weights between 18 kD and 35 kD.[94] Myosin is an actin-binding protein; it has two globular heads and an elongated tail. In particular, myosin II is composed of two heavy chains and four light (two phosphorylatable and two basic) chains. These combine with N-terminal portions of the myosin heavy chains to form globular heads, each of which has an actin-binding site and an enzymatic locus that hydrolyzes adenosine triphosphate. The heads of the myosin molecules form cross-bridges to actin.[95] Myosin molecules are configured in a symmetric fashion on either side of the center of the sarcomere. Sarcomeric thin filaments are polymers composed of two actin chains arranged in a double helix. Tropomyosin molecules, in turn, are situated in the groove between the two chains of actin. Troponins are interspersed along the tropomyosin.[96] Troponin T melds other troponin components with tropomyosin; troponin I inhibits the interaction of myosin and actin, and troponin C contains binding sites for calcium in the initiation of muscle contraction. Actinin, a 190-kD moiety, binds actin to the Z lines of the sarcomere. Another protein, titin, connects Z lines to M lines and provides the base on which thick filaments may form.[97] Because of their relatively poor sensitivity, the markers discussed in this section are used only in rare circumstances for diagnostic purposes.[98-103]

MYOGLOBIN

Myoglobin is a 17.8-kD protein that is found exclusively in skeletal muscle and that forms complexes with iron molecules.[104] The concentration of this molecule is highest in muscles that undergo sustained contraction. Because myoglobin appears relatively late in the maturational sequence of striated muscle, it is typically undetectable immunohistologically in embryonic neoplasms that show differentiation toward that tissue. Accordingly, pleomorphic adult-type rhabdomyosarcoma and rhabdomyoma are the soft tissue tumors in which myoglobin is identified most often.[98,99,101,105-111]

MYO-D1 AND MYOGENIN

A superfamily of transcription factors that regulates cell lineage–specific proliferation is represented in striated muscle by several moieties known as the *Myo-D family.*[112-114] They are encoded by genes that reside on chromosomes 1, 11, and 12 and are part of a polypeptide complex called the *basic helix-loop helix (BHLH) motif,* all of which are small proteins composed of 220 to 320 amino acids. Two members of this intranuclear protein group, Myo-D1 and myogenin, have been used since the 1990s as specific markers of striated muscle differentiation in human neoplasms.[112-115] They activate their own transcription and that of other BHLH proteins and, in concert with the retinoblastoma gene, govern exodus from the cell cycle and the initiation of striated muscle differentiation.

Because antibodies to Myo-D1 and myogenin must gain access to the nucleoplasm, they have been difficult to use in routine surgical specimens. However, modification of antigen retrieval solutions and utilization of heat-mediated epitope enhancement have allowed these reagents to enter diagnostic use.[114] It is important to note that Myo-D1 and myogenin are strictly localized to cellular nuclei, as are hormonal receptor proteins. Therefore, background cytoplasmic labeling (a consistent problem with antibodies to Myo-D1 especially) must be ignored as a spurious pattern of staining. In contrast, stains for myogenin do not generally show this problem.

CALDESMON

Caldesmon is a cytoplasmic protein with two isoform classes, one of which is found predominantly in smooth muscle cells and other cell types with partial myogenic differentiation. High-molecular-weight isoforms with molecular weights between 89 and 93 kD are capable of binding to actin, tropomyosin, calmodulin, myosin, and phospholipids, and they function to counteract actin-tropomyosin–activated myosin adenosine triphosphatase (ATPase). As such, they are mediators for the inhibition of calcium-dependent smooth muscle contraction.[116]

Commercial antibodies to caldesmon are now applied to diagnostic problems in surgical pathology. They appear to be relatively specific for smooth muscle differentiation and, as such, are useful adjuncts to desmin and actin immunostains.[116,117] Caldesmon is also expressed in the majority of gastrointestinal stromal tumors (GISTs), glomus tumors, and myopericytomas, and is therefore not entirely specific.[118,119]

Potential Markers of Schwannian Differentiation

S-100 PROTEIN

S-100 protein derives its name from the fact that it is soluble in saturated (100%) ammonium sulfate solution. It was first isolated from the central nervous system but is now known to have a wide distribution in human tissues, including glia, neurons, chondrocytes, Schwann cells, melanocytes, fixed phagocytic or antigen-presenting mononuclear cells, Langerhans' histiocytes, myoepithelial cells, notochord, and various epithelia (especially in the breast, salivary glands, sweat glands, and the female genital system).[120] S-100 protein is dimeric in nature, with alpha and beta subunits. Hence, it has three isoforms—S-100ao (alpha dimer); S-100a (alpha-beta isoform); and S-100b (beta dimer). Each of the two subunits of this protein has a molecular weight approximating 10.5 kD, and the function of S-100 protein is essentially that of a calcium flux regulator.[121]

Both monoclonal antibodies and heteroantisera to S100 protein are available for diagnostic use. Some of the former reagents are monospecific for the alpha or beta subunits, therefore they exhibit relatively narrower spectra of reactivity than seen with polyclonal antisera. For example, beta subunit–specific antibodies preferentially label glial cells and Schwann cells.[122] Beta subunit–specific antibodies have not enjoyed widespread use among clinically oriented pathologists, and hetero-antisera to S-100 protein are most commonly used in hospital practice. In the proper context, as part of panels of antibodies designed to evaluate several possible lineages of differentiation in a morphologically indeterminate neoplasm, reagents against S-100 protein are still valuable indicators of schwannian, melanocytic, or chondrocytic identity in tumors of the soft tissues and bone.[123-127]

CD56 AND CD57 (NEURAL CELL ADHESION MOLECULE/NKH1/LEU19 AND LEU7/HNK-1)

CD56 and CD57 are membrane antigens seen in peripheral blood mononuclear leukocytes, a proportion of which have natural killer activity. Their respective molecular weights are 140 kD and 95 kD. Antibodies in these cluster designations[128] also react with several neural molecules that have a variety of molecular weights.[129-132] Some of these moieties are associated with 5'-nucleotidase activity,[131] whereas others are the neural cell adhesion molecule and myelin-associated glycoproteins (MAGs).[129,132,133] The largest of the MAGs (MAG-72) is related structurally to the immunoglobulin superfamily gene products, as well as neural adhesion molecules and the autophosphorylation site of epidermal growth factor receptor. MAGs are integral cell membrane proteins that are found normally in oligodendroglia. It is believed that their function involves the mediation of interaxonal or axonal-glial interaction during myelination. As such, their additional association with Schwann cells and neural neoplasms should not be surprising. Nevertheless, HNK-1 reactivity has also been documented in perineurial (non-schwannian) peripheral nerve sheath lesions.[134] In general, CD56 and CD57 are used as potential markers not only of peripheral nerve sheath tumors but also of Ewing's sarcomas and PNETs, in which matrical proteins of neurosecretory granules and synaptic vesicles are thought to contain a target protein for the antibodies in question.[71,73,135-143]

It must be stressed that CD56 and CD57 are not restricted to nerve sheath cells or neuroectodermal elements among all soft tissue tumors, but rather are most often observed in those cell types. Synovial sarcomas, LMSs, and some metastatic carcinomas also may express the moieties in question.[135,144-147] Thus, inclusion of CD56 and CD57 antibodies in panels that are designed to detect myogenous, epithelial, and neural differentiation is the proper approach to their use. The most common settings in which such markers are valuable concern the differential diagnostic separation of fibrosarcoma versus MPNST, malignant fibrous histiocytoma (MFH) versus MPNST, and myxoid nerve sheath tumors (both benign and malignant) versus nonneural myxoid neoplasms.

COLLAGEN TYPE IV AND LAMININ

Volumetrically, collagen type IV is the predominant component of basement membranes, regardless of which cell types they invest. It is a triple helical molecule weighing 550 kD with globular end regions and two noncollagenous domains. One of the latter is located 330 nm from the carboxy end of the molecule, where there is a bending point that gives the moiety a hockey stick configuration overall.[148] Type IV collagen differs from other collagen types because it does not form fibrils, shows interruptions of its helical structure, and has a different amino acid constituency. Genes coding for the helical chains of this molecule are located on chromosome 13q.[149]

Laminin is another important component of basement membranes. It is a 1000-kD molecule, the three short forms and one long arm of which have globular end regions. Laminin binds to glycosaminoglycans, acting as a bridge for attachment of collagen type IV in basement membranes to the surrounding matrix.[150] The exact location of laminin in basement membranes has been contentious. Some investigators claim that it is part of the lamina densa, some suggest that it resides in the lamina lucida, and others believe that it is codistributed between these two compartments.[151] Beyond simple boundary and anchoring functions, laminin probably also influences intercellular interactions and contributes to alterations in cellular morphology.[152]

In soft tissues, complete basement membranes are formed around endothelial cells, smooth muscle cells, and Schwann cells.[153,154] Thus, reagents directed against collagen type IV and laminin are useful inclusions in antibody panels aimed at detecting those lineages. In particular, however, fibrosarcoma and MFH are often difficult to distinguish from MPNSTs, because not all MPNSTs are reactive for either S-100 protein or CD57. Immunoreactivity for either collagen type IV or laminin would greatly favor the interpretation of a peripheral nerve sheath tumor in these differential diagnoses. We use both markers most often in this specific setting, hence we have included them in this section as adjuvant neural determinants.

Endothelial Markers

Several determinants that are associated with endothelial cells have been applied to the recognition of vascular neoplasms of soft tissue. We will discuss the varying degrees of sensitivity and specificity of these determinants.

FACTOR VIII–RELATED ANTIGEN (VON WILLEBRAND FACTOR)

Factor VIII-related antigen, or von Willebrand factor (vWF), is a very large polymeric protein that is synthesized exclusively by endothelial cells and megakaryocytes. It consists of three multimeric subunits that are greater than 10,000 kD in molecular weight; physiologically, they undergo proteolysis to yield substantially smaller fragments that can be found in plasma.[155] The function of vWF is twofold. First, it forms circulating complexes with antihemophilic factor, also known as *factor VIII coagulant protein*. The latter moiety is a 265-kD protein that effects the activation of factor X in the intrinsic coagulation pathway; it is manufactured by hepatocytes. Second, vWF plays a crucial role in platelet aggregation so that patients with low levels or dysfunctional variants of this protein have the clinical bleeding diathesis known as von Willebrand syndrome.[156]

In the context of soft tissue pathology, vWF is used principally to distinguish vascular neoplasms from their morphologic simulants.[157-159] Because vWF is packaged within Weibel-Palade bodies (WPBs) in endothelial cells, it is logical to expect that immunoreactivity for that analyte would parallel the ultrastructural presence of such organelles. This is indeed the case, and because WPBs are rare in poorly differentiated neoplasms of the blood vessels, it explains why the sensitivity of vWF is as low as it is (approximately 10% to 15%) for the recognition of lesions such as high-grade angiosarcoma.[158,159] Accordingly, this marker has much more utility in the spectrum of benign and borderline endothelial tumors, such as hemangioma variants and the family of hemangioendotheliomas.[160]

CD34

CD34, or the human hematopoietic progenitor cell antigen, is recognized by several monoclonal antibodies including My10, QBEND-10, and BI-3C5.[161-164] It is a 110-kD protein that, as its name suggests, is expressed by embryonic cells of the hematopoietic system,[162,165] including lymphoid and myelogenous elements and also endothelial cells. Correspondingly, again in the setting of soft tissue tumors, CD34 is a potential indicator of vascular differentiation. It is highly sensitive for endothelial differentiation, regardless of tumor grade, and recognizes greater than 85% of angiosarcomas and Kaposi's sarcomas.[160-162,164] Nevertheless, the specificity of CD34 is a problem, inasmuch as it has been reported in some LMSs, peripheral nerve sheath tumors, and epithelioid sarcomas,[162,165,166] which could potentially simulate variants of angiosarcoma or hemangioendothelioma. In addition, CD34 is so commonly present in dermatofibrosarcoma protuberans (and its variants), spindle cell lipoma, and solitary fibrous tumor that it is regularly used as an adjunct to the diagnosis of these tumors.[167-169] Thus, as endothelial markers, antibodies to CD34 are best used in a panel of reagents that is designed to account for these other diagnostic possibilities.

CD31

The platelet–endothelial cell adhesion molecule-1 (PECAM-1) is also known as CD31.[170] It is a 130-kD transmembrane glycoprotein that is shared by vascular lining cells, megakaryocytes, platelets, and selected other hematopoietic elements, as recognized by monoclonal antibody JC/70A.[171] This marker is highly restricted to endothelial neoplasms among all tumors of the soft tissue, and its sensitivity is also excellent.[172] In our hands, virtually 100% of angiosarcomas are CD31+, regardless of grade or subtype, and the same statement applies to hemangioma and hemangioendothelioma variants.[173,174] It must be acknowledged, however, that KS is labeled more consistently for CD34 than for CD31,[174] the reasons being unknown. Since CD31 also commonly labels macrophages, which may be present in large numbers dispersed among tumor cells, this is a potential pitfall in interpretation.[175]

THROMBOMODULIN

Thrombomodulin (TMN;CD141) is a 75-kD cytoplasmic glycoprotein that is distributed among endothelial cells, mesothelial cells, osteoblasts, mononuclear phagocytic cells, and selected epithelia.[176-181] Its physiologic role is to convert thrombin from a coagulant protein to an anticoagulant.[178] Because of the potential presence of TMN in some metastatic carcinomas and most mesotheliomas[180,181] (both of which may be confused with epithelioid angiosarcomas), it cannot be used as a single marker for vascular neoplasms. Nevertheless, it has been proven that TMN is a sensitive indicator of endothelial differentiation, particularly in poorly differentiated vascular malignancies.[179,182]

KS is likewise immunoreactive for this determinant.[183] Thus its inclusion in antibody panels is certainly worthwhile.

ULEX EUROPAEUS I AGGLUTININ

Ulex europaeus I (UEAI) agglutinin is not an antibody reagent, but instead represents a lectin that is produced by the gorse plant. It recognizes the Fuc-alpha-1-2-Gal linkage in fucosylated oligosaccharides, which compose portions of various glycoproteins.[184] In particular, the H blood group antigen and carcinoembryonic antigen regularly bind to UEAI, as does a separate fucosylated protein that is expressed by endothelial cells.[159,179,184] Biotinylated *Ulex* may be used as a histochemical reagent in surgical pathology or, alternatively, unlabeled lectin can be used, with its binding to tissue subsequently detected by application of biotinylated anti-*Ulex* and avidin-biotin-peroxidase complex. Because of the nonspecificity of UEAI for endothelial differentiation, as mentioned earlier in this discussion, it is absolutely necessary to use this lectin as part of a histochemical/immunohistochemical panel. For example, epithelioid sarcoma and various metastatic carcinomas may also bind *Ulex,* in addition to vascular neoplasms.[185,186] However, the extremely high sensitivity of UEAI justifies its continued use as a potential endothelial determinant.

FLI-1

Human FLI-1 (Friend leukemia integration-1) is a member of a family of transcription factor proteins that share a conserved DNA-binding region, the ETS domain. That peptide sequence is 98 amino acid residues long, and bears a molecular resemblance to the helix-turn-helix motif of DNA-binding proteins.[187] FLI-1 is a sequence-specific transcriptional activator that is involved in cell proliferation. It recognizes the DNA sequence 5'-C(CA)GGAAGT-3', and is encoded by a gene on the long arm of chromosome 11 (11q24).[188]

In rodents, FLI-1 is a common region for viral nucleic acid integration, in virus-driven leukemogenesis.[189] In all vertebrates, this gene also appears to act at the top of the transcriptional network that governs the development of hematopoietic precursors and endothelial cells.[190] Landry and colleagues have shown that this effect occurs by regulation of the proximal promoter of the LMO2 gene in endothelia.[191]

The best-known association between FLI-1 and human tumors relates to its fusion with the EWS gene on chromosome 22 (22q12) in many examples of Ewing's sarcoma/primitive neuroectodermal tumor (PNET).[192] An associated fusion protein results from that event, which probably plays a role in the evasion of cellular senescence.[193]

Folpe and associates were the first to study FLI-1 immunoreactivity in human endothelial neoplasms.[188] They observed a 94% marker sensitivity in that specific context and found no labeling of nonvascular tumors. However, more recently, Mhawech-Fauceglia and colleagues have documented FLI-1 positivity in some carcinomas, lymphomas, and rhabdomyosarcomas as well.[195] In aggregate, these data support the use of FLI-1 as an adjuvant to the diagnoses of PNET or vascular neoplasms, but only in combination with other immunoreactants.

PODOPLANIN

Podoplanin (PPN) (also known as AGGRUS, gp36, M2A, and T1A-2) is recognized by antibody D2-40.[196] It is a transmembrane glycoprotein encoded by a gene on the short arm of chromosome 1 (1p36.21) and is expressed in various tissues. Breiteneder-Geleff and colleagues originally described this moiety in glomerular podocytes of the rat in 1997,[197] but it has since been observed in lymphatic endothelium, mesothelium, various epithelia, hematopoietic dendritic cells, follicular dendritic cells, and germ cells in several species, including humans. Tumors showing differentiation toward these cellular targets also may be PPN-positive.[198-211]

PPN is principally expressed during vertebrate development in lymphatic endothelial cells and is therefore thought to be a selective marker for them.[201] Overexpression of podoplanin significantly increases endothelial cell adhesion, migration, and vascular lumen formation.[198] In the particular context of soft tissue neoplasia, podoplanin is now increasingly utilized clinically as a semispecific determinant of lymphatic differentiation in the evaluation of vascular neoplasms.[206,209] Angiolymphatic invasion by carcinomas and melanomas is also well-delineated with PPN immunostains.[196]

WILMS' TUMOR-1

The Wilms' tumor-1 (WT1) gene is located on the short arm of chromosome 11 (11p13). It encodes a protein that is a critical determinant of urogenital development and is expressed in >80% of nephroblastomas.[212] With regard to osseous and soft tissue tumors, WT1 protein is not a specific marker and is potentially present in angiosarcoma, malignant peripheral nerve sheath tumor, synovial sarcoma, osteosarcoma, myxoid liposarcoma, and clear-cell sarcoma.[213] Nevertheless, it is most often utilized (in a structured panel with other immunodeterminants) as an adjunctive indicator of endothelial differentiation in diagnostic practice.[214]

VASCULAR ENDOTHELIAL GROWTH FACTOR RECEPTOR-3 (VEGFR3)

VEGFR3 is a transmembrane protein that is also known as tyrosine-protein kinase receptor FLT4; it is encoded by a gene at chromosomal locus 5q33-qter and is expressed exclusively by lymphatic endothelial cells.[215] In similarity to PPN, VEGFR3 is seen in non-neoplastic lymphatic vessels and in many vascular neoplasms.[216] However, it is more selective than PPN.

Fibrohistiocytic Markers

A variety of monoclonal antibodies and heteroantisera have been advanced since 1985 as histiocytic or fibrohistiocytic markers in paraffin sections. They are used to identify lesions such as benign or malignant fibrous histiocytomas, atypical fibroxanthomas, and histiocytomas of skin and soft tissue. The targets of these reagents include moieties such as alpha$_1$-antitrypsin, muramidase (lysozyme), alpha$_1$-antichymotrypsin, cathepsin B, CD68, CD163, factor XIIIa, and the HAM 56 antigen.[217-227]

Although it is true that a majority of fibrohistiocytic neoplasms do label for the specified determinants, the specificity of those markers is poor. Except for CD163,[227] carcinomas, melanomas, and other sarcoma morphotypes also potentially express them with relatively high frequency.[228,229] The current approach to the diagnosis of fibrohistiocytic tumors is ultimately one of exclusion because neoplasms of other lineages may demonstrate morphologic appearances that are strikingly similar to them. Thus, a putatively fibrohistiocytic lesion is interpretable as such only when epithelial, myogenous, neural, and endothelial differentiation has been excluded in a vimentin-reactive tumor by application of suitable immunostains or performance of electron microscopy. In that context, the application of additional antibodies to histiocytic markers is superfluous and may even be misleading. Therefore, we do not advocate their use.

Proposed Markers of Osteoblastic Differentiation

One of the greatest challenges in the realm of bone and soft tissue tumor pathology is the reliable recognition of osseous matrix production in malignant lesions. This is an important issue because the contextual presence of true osteoid equates with a diagnosis of osteosarcoma. Since the late 1990s, a number of putatively osteoblast-specific markers have been advanced in the pertinent literature, including bone morphogenetic protein, type I collagen, COL-I-C peptide, decorin, osteocalcin (OCN), osteonectin (ONN), osteopontin, proteoglycans I and II, bone sialoprotein, and bone glycoprotein 75.[230] Only two among these—ONN and OCN—have been associated with applicability to paraffin sections in diagnostic immunohistologic studies, but, frankly, we have not been impressed with their usefulness.

OSTEOCALCIN

Osteocalcin (OCN) is one of the most prevalent noncollagenous intraosseous proteins, and it is predominantly localized to osteoblasts. This 9-kD cytoplasmic protein contains abundant gamma carboxyglutamic acid residues. Its expression is down-regulated by helix-loop-helix–type transcription factors and up-regulated by vitamin D analogs such as 1,25 dihydroxyvitamin D2 and 24-epi-1,25 dihydroxyvitamin D2 in the final steps of osteoblastic differentiation and osteoid formation.[230-236]

Various heteroantisera and monoclonal antibodies to OCN have been used in reported immunohistochemical studies,[231-240] which indicate that polyclonal anti-OCN reagents are inferior to monoclonal antibodies for diagnostic work because of problems with specificity.[237] Although studies have shown that OCN has a reasonable level of sensitivity for osteoblastic differentiation (approximately 70%) and is, for practical purposes, apparently virtually completely specific for bone-forming cells,[239,240] it is rarely used in clinical practice.

OSTEONECTIN

Osteonectin (ONN) is a protein that is concerned with regulating the adhesion of osteoblasts and platelets to their extracellular matrix, as well as early stromal mineralization. ONN is modified differently at a post-translational level in bone cells and megakaryocytes to yield molecules with different oligosaccharide substructures; sequences of ONN-related genomic DNA, intranuclear RNA, and mRNA are identical in those two cell types.[230,239-245]

It would also appear that several other cells may synthesize ONN-associated epitopes; in one assessment, fibroblasts, vascular pericytes, endothelia, chondrocytes, selected epithelial cells, and nerves were also immunoreactive for this determinant.[240] Overall, a sensitivity of 90% and a specificity of 54% has been reported for ONN relative to the diagnosis of osteoblastic neoplasms.[239,240] Again, because of potential problems concerning cross-reactivity of available antisera to this marker,[240,246-248] monoclonal antibodies should be used diagnostically. Even then, since ONN does not demonstrate the selectivity of expression that is associated with OCN, it must be used only as part of a panel of reagents that are directed at several lineage-related proteins.

Genomic Applications of Other Markers of Interest in Soft Tissue and Bone Tumors

There are several other determinants that often figure into differential diagnosis in the sphere of soft tissue and bone tumor pathology. They include melanocyte-related markers such as melan-A (MART-1), tyrosinase, and HMB-45;[249-254] neuroendocrine and neuroectodermal products such as synaptophysin, neuron-specific (gamma dimer) enolase, protein gene product 9.5, and NB84;[255-261] and hematopoietic determinants such as CD1a, CD45, CD138, HLA-DR, and light-chain immunoglobulins.[262-269] We will simply mention these reactants here, as we will cover them in detail later in the book when we discuss the skin, endocrine organs, and the hematopoietic system. A bit more commentary is justified in reference to yet another lymphoreticular marker, CD99, which is also known as p30/32 glycoprotein or MIC2 protein.[270-272] It is a cell surface protein that is encoded by genes on the X and Y chromosomes.[273,274] CD99 is expressed in a membranous pattern by a high proportion of Ewing's sarcomas and PNETs, but it may be expressed in a less distinct pattern in lymphoblastic lymphomas, solitary fibrous tumors, and synovial sarcomas, as well as other mesenchymal neoplasms and selected epithelial lesions.[138,267,270,271,275-281] Available commercial monoclonal antibodies to this determinant include 12E7, O13, and HBA-71 (see Table 4.3).

Another marker of potential interest was likewise recognized originally in the sphere of hematopathology: namely, anaplastic lymphoma kinase-1 (ALK-1). It is a protein tyrosine kinase (also known as p80) that represents the translation of an abnormal ALK-NPM fusion gene—produced by a t(2;5)(p23;q35) chromosomal translocation—as seen in systemic anaplastic large-cell (Ki-1) lymphomas.[282] Unexpectedly, ALK-1 positivity is not restricted to hematopoietic lesions, however. In particular, it has been found in the neoplastic cells of approximately 50% of inflammatory myofibroblastic tumors (IMTs), formerly called inflammatory pseudotumors, probably because they often demonstrate abnormalities at the 2p23 chromosomal locus.[283,284] Despite initial enthusiasm that p80 might represent a specific marker of those lesions among all spindle-cell proliferations, it is now recognized that ALK-1 can also be seen in a subset of MPNSTs and rhabdomyosarcomas.[285] Thus, this determinant has limited differential diagnostic application. Its presence is probably best used to help exclude such lesions as nodular fasciitis, desmoid tumor, and infantile myofibromatosis, in the differential diagnosis with IMT.

The BCL-2 (B-cell lymphoma-2) proteins are anti-apoptotic polypeptides that are differentially expressed in some soft tissue lesions. Those that commonly label immunohistologically include solitary fibrous tumor, spindle-cell lipoma, Kaposi's sarcoma, and monophasic synovial sarcoma. In addition, a subset of fibrosarcomas and low-grade myxofibrosarcomas is BCL-2–positive. Given this wide distribution in soft tissue tumors, BCL-2 is of limited use in differential diagnosis.

Cyclin-dependent kinase-4 (CDK4) is one of the proteins involved with cell-cycle progression and is encoded by a gene at chromosome 12q13. CDK4 inhibits the retinoblastoma-1 (RB1) gene, and it is overexpressed in lipomatous tumors, often together with murine double-minute-type2 (MDM2) protein. This phenomenon reflects the common presence of ring or giant marker chromosomes that contain the q13-15 region of chromosome 12q, where both the CDK4 and MDM2 genes are located. The best diagnostic use of these determinants is in the recognition of dedifferentiated liposarcomas, as opposed to other high-grade tumors,[286-288] and in the distinction between benign lipomas and atypical lipomatous tumors (well-differentiated liposarcomas) [286,288,289] when the latter show very minimal atypical histologic features. Note that MDM2 protein is an intranuclear moiety, and cytoplasmic labeling for it is discounted interpretatively. A recent study suggested that p16 may also be used as a marker to distinguish atypical lipomatous tumor from deep benign lipoma.[290]

Human transducin–like enhancer of split (TLE) genes are analogues of others that are found in insects. They encode intranuclear proteins that are transcriptional repressors, acting through the *Wnt* pathway and playing a role in cell fate determination. Gene profiling studies have shown that nuclear TLE1 expression is particularly associated with synovial sarcomas, being present in >95% of these neoplasms. Important mimics of that tumor, such as MPNST and solitary fibrous tumor, lack TLE1 in the majority of cases.

Although alveolar soft part sarcoma (ASPS) is usually identifiable easily on morphologic grounds, it is characterized by a reproducible chromosomal translocation-der(17) t(X;17) (p11.q25). The transcription factor-3 (TFE3) gene at Xp11 is thereby apposed to the ASPL gene at 17q25, creating a fusion protein. Antibodies against the c-terminus of TFE3 recognize this polypeptide and are sensitive markers of ASPS.[291] Unfortunately, a potential diagnostic alternative in this setting—metastatic translocation-type renal cell carcinoma—is also TFE3-positive.[291,292]

KEY DIAGNOSTIC POINTS

Genomic Applications of Immunohistology

- CDK4 and MDM2 identify dedifferentiated liposarcoma. MDM2 overexpression is a sensitive indicator for liposarcoma versus sclerosing mesenteritis and retroperitoneal fibrosis. IHC overexpression can be confirmed by MDM2 FISH amplification (88% of cases in well differentiated liposarcoma).
- TLE1 expression is prominent in synovial sarcoma, but not mimics such as MPNST and SFT.
- TFE3 is found in ASPS and translocation-type renal carcinoma.

KEY DIAGNOSTIC POINTS

Soft Tissue Antigens and Antibodies

- Desmin is a specific marker for myogenic differentiation among soft tissue tumors, seen in almost all rhabdomyosarcomas/leiomyosarcomas, rhabdomyomas/leiomyomas.
- Desmin may be seen in the myofibromatoses and in polyphenotypic tumors.
- Vimentin is ubiquitous in soft tissue tumors, and is present in poorly differentiated sarcomas as the most primitive of cytoplasmic filaments.
- GFAP may be found in Schwann cells and chondrocytes.
- Keratins are regularly found in synovial sarcoma, chordoma, parachordoma, epithelioid sarcoma, and adamantinoma. They are seen less commonly in leiomyosarcoma, malignant peripheral nerve sheath tumors, epithelioid angiosarcoma, and polyphenotypic tumors such as PNET.
- EMA regularly decorates synovial sarcoma, epithelioid sarcoma, perineuriomas, neurothekeomas, chordoma/parachordoma, and plasmacytomas.
- (Alpha) smooth muscle actin is less specific for myogenous differentiation than h-caldesmon or HHF-35, muscle-specific actin.
- Myo-D1 and myogenin are nuclear transcription factors highly specific for striated muscle differentiation.
- Factor VIII–related antigen is found exclusively in endothelial cells and megakaryocytes.
- CD31 is highly restricted to endothelial neoplasms, with excellent sensitivity.
- Thrombomodulin reacts with mesothelial cells and carcinomas and is therefore not specific for vascular differentiation.
- CD34, while sensitive for detection of endothelial differentiation, lacks specificity as it reacts with a wide variety of mesenchymal cells.
- ALK-1 may be seen in leiomyosarcoma, rhabdomyosarcoma, and malignant fibrous histiocytoma, but is negative in nodular fasciitis, desmoid tumor, infantile myofibromatosis, and infantile fibrosarcoma.

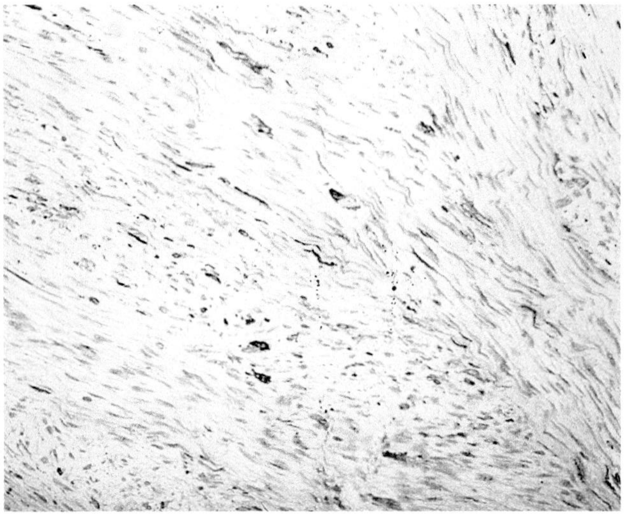

FIGURE 4.1 Desmoid tumor showing multifocal reactivity for desmin.

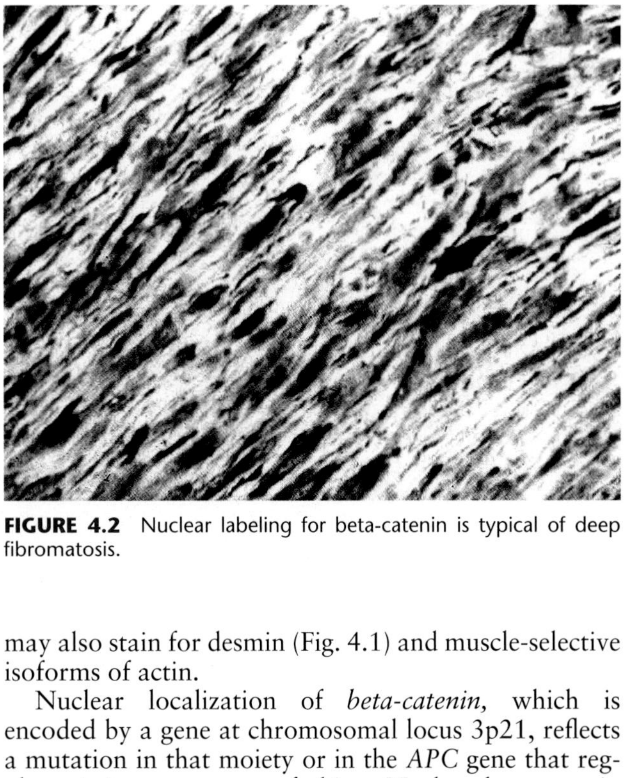

FIGURE 4.2 Nuclear labeling for beta-catenin is typical of deep fibromatosis.

SPECIFIC SOFT TISSUE TUMORS

Benign Tumors of Soft Tissue

FIBROMATOSES

Several forms of fibromatosis are currently recognized, including congenital myofibromatosis and several adult varieties (which differ mainly in location): abdominal, penile, plantar, and palmar. Other rare forms include hyaline, gingival, and digital fibromatoses. These lesions may appear histologically similar to hemangiopericytoma, leiomyoma, fibroma, and peripheral nerve sheath tumors. Separation of these entities continues to rely largely on the histopathologic and clinical impression (with one exception, which is discussed in the following paragraph), given that these fibroblastic entities do not harbor a unique immunophenotype. As expected, all show uniform strong vimentin positivity, but a subset may also stain for desmin (Fig. 4.1) and muscle-selective isoforms of actin.

Nuclear localization of *beta-catenin,* which is encoded by a gene at chromosomal locus 3p21, reflects a mutation in that moiety or in the *APC* gene that regulates it in an upstream fashion. Nuclear beta-catenin (NBC), as recognized by the 14/beta-catenin monoclonal antibody clone, functions as a transcriptional activator when complexed with members of the lymphocyte enhancer factor family of proteins.[286] It is present in most examples (>80%) of deep (desmoid-type) fibromatosis (Fig. 4.2), whereas potential differential diagnostic stimulants—such as low-grade fibromyxoid sarcoma, myofibrosarcoma, solitary fibrous tumor, low-grade fibrosarcoma, myofibroma, nodular fasciitis, and hypertrophic scars—demonstrate NBC in 25% of cases.[293-295] Reproducible reactivity for S-100 protein, CD56, or CD57 among peripheral nerve sheath tumors (neurofibroma, schwannoma) is useful to distinguish them from fibroblastic and myofibroblastic lesions.

Fibroma of tendon sheath and collagenous fibroma (desmoplastic fibroblastoma) are usually sufficiently distinct clinically and histologically to separate them from fibromatosis. They often react either diffusely or focally for muscle-specific actin[296] and smooth muscle actin[297] and may even show faint S-100 positivity.[298] Desmin, however, is not found.[296,298] In addition to sharing an immunophenotypic profile, fibroma of tendon sheath and collagenous fibroma have been observed to harbor the same abnormality of chromosome 11q12.[299]

PERIPHERAL NERVE SHEATH TUMORS

The most common peripheral nerve sheath tumors in both children and adults are neurofibromas and schwannomas. The differential diagnostic considerations differ somewhat between neurofibroma and schwannoma. Neurofibromas are commonly confused with myxomas, nonpigmented spindle cell or neurotizing melanocytic nevi, or cellular and organizing scar tissue, whereas schwannomas are more likely to be confused with leiomyomas. S-100 protein is extremely useful in this context, as it is strongly expressed by schwannomas and variably expressed by neurofibromas. The majority of peripheral nerve sheath tumors are also positive for the CD56 and CD57 antigens. Some diagnostic mimics, such as neurotized melanocytic nevi and leiomyomas, may also show reactivity for the same markers. In these instances, the presence of myogenic determinants, including desmin and muscle-associated actins, is useful for recognizing smooth muscle tumors. A potential pitfall in the use of HMB-45 to recognize melanocytic lesions is represented by psammomatous melanotic schwannoma, a tumor that arises in the gut, soft tissue, and bone and is composed of melanosome-laden cells that are otherwise typical of peripheral nerve sheath elements. Nearly all 31 examples in a series by Carney were HMB-45 reactive.[300] In difficult cases, the distinction between neurofibroma and melanocytic nevi is facilitated by the presence of factor XIIIa, which is found only in neurofibroma. In addition, the presence of scattered neurofilament protein (NFP)-positive axons is typical of neurofibroma, whereas axons are rare within schwannomas. Fine and colleagues have also found that calretinin is typically diffusely present in schwannomas, whereas neurofibromas lack that marker or are labeled only weakly for it.[301]

The perineurial cells in neurofibroma contain EMA, which may be detected immunohistochemically in a small population of cells in these tumors. EMA may also be of some value in the diagnosis of nerve sheath myxoma because of the existence of perineurial elements around most tumor lobules. Nerve sheath neoplasms are occasionally labeled by antibodies to GFAP, as are 50% of soft tissue myoepitheliomas, whereas other benign soft tissue tumors are not. Myelin basic protein may also be of some value in the diagnosis of schwannian tumors, although there has been some disagreement in the literature on this point.

KEY DIAGNOSTIC POINTS

Nerve Sheath Tumors

- Neurotized melanocytic nevi may be distinguished from neurofibroma: factor XIIIa is found in neurofibroma, not in melanocytic nevi.
- Nerve sheath tumors may occasionally have GFAP- and EMA-positive cells.

SPINDLE CELL LIPOMA

Although the diagnosis of spindle cell lipoma is usually straightforward, selected cases resemble other spindle cell proliferations. Spindle cell lipoma is strongly CD34-positive,[170,302] a feature shared by some of its histologic mimics, including solitary fibrous tumor, neurofibroma, dermatofibrosarcoma protuberans, giant cell fibroblastoma, giant cell angiofibroma (which is probably a morphologic variant of solitary fibrous tumor), and angiolipoma. Lack of S-100 protein staining in the spindle cells is useful for distinguishing it from neurofibroma. Additionally, strong BCL-2 reactivity is found in spindle cell lipoma, and this is also a feature of many cases of solitary fibrous tumor. Confident identification of spindle cell lipoma is usually possible using a panel of immunostains and close attention to the histologic features.

LEIOMYOMAS

Certain markers with specificity for muscle differentiation may be useful in recognizing leiomyomas, beyond desmin, caldesmon, and muscle-associated actins, but their application in diagnostic immunohistopathology is not generally considered routine. Smooth muscle myosin and Z-band protein have been advocated by some, particularly when either the histologic pattern is unusual (such as myxoid or hyalinized lesions) or the interpretation of a myogenous lesion is not corroborated by other stains.

GRANULAR CELL TUMOR

Granular cell tumor, a benign neoplasm with an only rarely seen clinicopathologic malignant counterpart, has been intensely studied by immunohistochemical means. In addition to resembling histiocytic lesions, granular change is a recognized variant of leiomyoma[303] and certain carcinomas such as renal cell carcinoma. Granular cell tumors of the adult type show consistent diffuse positivity for S-100 protein (nuclear and cytoplasmic), NSE, vimentin, alpha-inhibin, calretinin, and CD68.[304-308] A major subset is also reactive for CD57 or myelin basic protein, or both.[304]

A histologically identical lesion occurs almost exclusively in female newborns or infants along the alveolar ridge, designated *congenital granular cell tumor;* it differs from the adult variety by its complete lack of S-100 protein and NSE reactivity. Both the adult and congenital types share positivity for $alpha_1$-antitrypsin,

CD68, and vimentin. Although traditionally regarded as a histiocytic marker, CD68 positivity is related to the abundance of phagolysosomes, a distinctive feature of granular cell tumors. Therefore, it is not possible to distinguish true granular cell tumors from reactive histiocytic granular cell proliferations using only CD68, and CD163 must be employed for that purpose.

HEMANGIOMA

Benign vascular lesions showing a dense cellularity and relatively little overt canalization may prove diagnostically troublesome. Hobnail hemangioma and epithelioid hemangioma can be confused with low-grade angiosarcoma or epithelioid sarcoma, respectively. When the diagnosis of epithelioid sarcoma is under consideration, several endothelial markers should be applied concurrently. The absence of *factor VIII*–related antigen, podoplanin, FLI-1, and CD31 is typical of epithelioid sarcoma. Epithelial markers, which are characteristically positive in the latter tumor, are typically absent in benign vascular proliferations.

The potential of GLUT1 as a marker for juvenile hemangioma is interesting, but it is not a specific determinant; increased expression of GLUT1 has been reported in a variety of solid human tumors.[309-312] One study of vascular lesions found intense endothelial GLUT1-reactivity in 97% (139 of 143) of juvenile hemangiomas, and its absence in 66 vascular malformations.[311] To date, there are no substantiated immunohistochemical means of differentiating hemangiomas from histologically similar (minimal deviation) angiosarcomas.

As mentioned earlier in this discussion, FLI-1 is a relatively recently described endothelial determinant, and it is unique in this group because of its intranuclear localization. FLI-1 is a member of the ETS family of DNA-binding transcription factors and is involved in a diverse array of biological functions including cellular growth and differentiation as well as organ development. Several studies have shown consistent FLI-1 positivity in benign, intermediate, and malignant vascular neoplasms of various types.[187,194,313,314]

KEY DIAGNOSTIC POINTS

Vascular Tumors

- CD31 is highly specific and very sensitive for endothelium.
- FLI-1, a nuclear transcription factor, is consistently positive in benign, intermediate, and malignant vascular neoplasms. FLI-1 is consistently present in Ewing's/PNET and lymphoblastic lymphomas.

RHABDOMYOMA

Rhabdomyomas are benign tumors with striated muscle differentiation that may assume adult, juvenile, or fetal variants microscopically; the adult type shows abundant eosinophilic cytoplasm within tumor cells, whereas the fetal type consists of small, rather undifferentiated cells admixed with others having the appearance of fetal muscle. The juvenile form is a histologic hybrid of these patterns and may represent a lesion in transition. The differential diagnosis sometimes includes granular cell tumor, hibernoma, paraganglioma, and rhabdomyosarcoma.

In our experience, all forms of rhabdomyoma stain for vimentin, desmin, muscle-specific actin, myogenin, and, to varying degrees, myoglobin. Smooth muscle actin, vimentin, GFAP, CD56, CD57, CD68, cytokeratin, and EMA are generally absent, although one investigator noted rare SMA-reactive cells.[315-317] Focal CD56 positivity has also been observed.[318] Although S-100 protein has been seen in some cases of rhabdomyoma, its presence is focal and rare[315] and therefore not likely to be confused with the pattern of S-100 reactivity in paraganglioma and granular cell tumor. The presence of myogenic determinants and a lack of CD68 are also useful in the recognition of rhabdomyomas. As with vascular tumors, immunohistochemical distinction between benign skeletal muscle tumors and their malignant counterparts is impossible. In most cases, standard clinicopathologic evaluation is sufficient for their unequivocal separation.

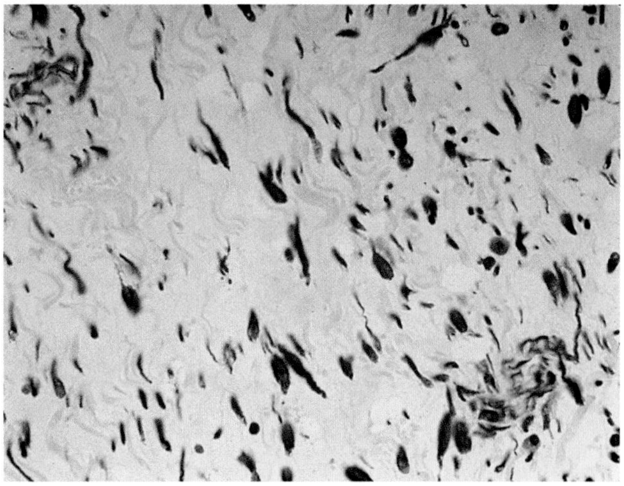

FIGURE 4.3 Desmin labeling in the spindle cells of angiomyofibroblastoma.

ANGIOMYOFIBROBLASTOMA

Angiomyofibroblastoma (AMF) is a distinctive lesion of the superficial soft tissues with a marked predilection for the vulvar region. This tumor shows reactivity for vimentin, desmin (Fig. 4.3), actin (Fig. 4.4), and estrogen receptor protein.[319,320] Some studies[321-323] have also elucidated a subset of cases with CD34 and progesterone receptor positivity.[321,322] There is no staining for factor XIIIa, keratin, S-100 protein, CD57, GFAP, or CD68.[321] These findings are shared with smooth muscle tumors, but not with most other myxoid tumors including myxoid liposarcoma, myxofibrosarcoma, myxoid neurofibroma, and myxoid MPNST.

Although the clinical features of angiomyofibroblastoma may overlap considerably with those of aggressive

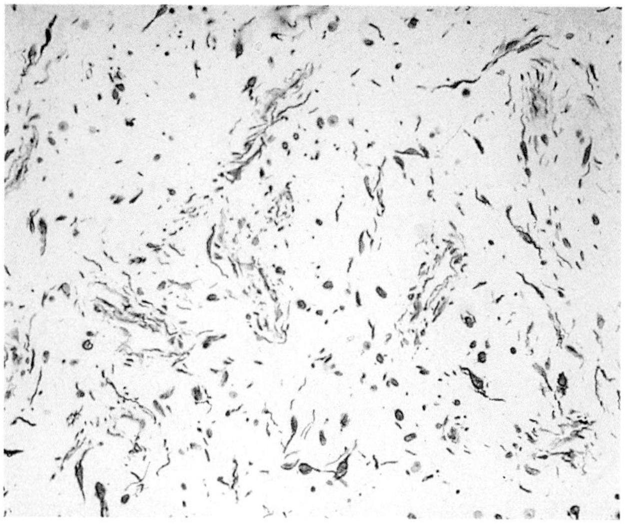

FIGURE 4.4 Alpha isoform (smooth muscle) actin is seen in the spindle cells and blood vessels of angiomyofibroblastoma.

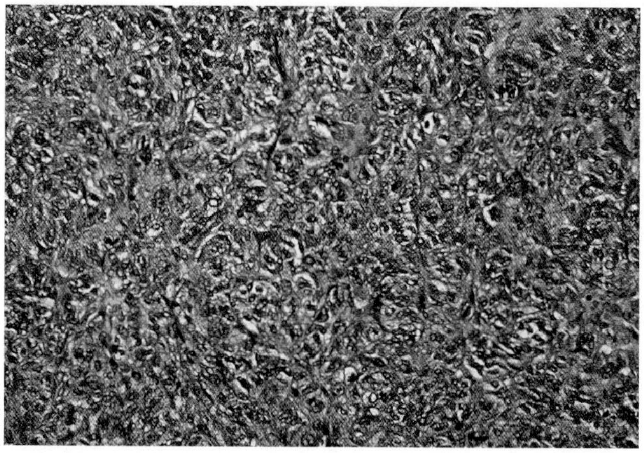

FIGURE 4.5 Hemangiopericytoma composed of ovoid tumor cells. This histologic image is potentially shared by a number of neoplasms of disparate lineages.

angiomyxoma, morphologic differences are usually sufficient for their separation. Angiomyofibroblastomas are smaller, well-circumscribed lesions, contrasting with the obviously infiltrative, more deeply seated aggressive angiomyxoma. The perivascular accentuation of stromal cells that is typical of angiomyofibroblastoma is not found in aggressive angiomyxoma. Desmin reactivity may be seen in both angiomyofibroblastomas and aggressive angiomyxomas, so immunohistochemistry is generally not helpful in this distinction, and it ultimately rests on conventional morphology. The separation of such lesions is important because aggressive angiomyxoma has a significant potential for recurrence that is not shared by angiomyofibroblastoma.

KEY DIAGNOSTIC POINTS

Angiomyofibroblastoma

- Angiomyofibroblastoma (AMF) is usually separated from aggressive angiomyxoma (AAM) on morphologic grounds, but desmin is usually positive in the perivascular cells of AMF and is not found in AAM.

Borderline Tumors of Soft Tissue

HEMANGIOPERICYTOMA

Hemangiopericytoma (HPC) is an uncommon neoplasm characterized by a dense, blunt spindle-cell proliferation with a richly vascular stroma. Supporting blood vessels often assume a staghorn configuration. The ovoid tumor cells of hemangiopericytomas are rather nondescript and may cause confusion with those of other soft tissue tumors (Fig. 4.5). The immunophenotype of these neoplasms is neither unique nor characteristic. In general, the diagnosis of hemangiopericytoma is one of histologic pattern recognition meshed with immunohistochemical exclusion of other possible interpretations. It should also be stated categorically that our presentation of HPC as a separate diagnostic entity is largely historical and almost certainly artificial. Solitary fibrous tumor (discussed in the next section) has been merged nosologically with HPC in current schemes of tumor classification.

The tumor cells in hemangiopericytoma consistently label for vimentin, although some variation in intensity is seen from tumor to tumor.[324] Factor XIIIa and HLA-DR are found in approximately 50% of hemangiopericytomas.[325-327] Factor XIIIa is also seen in some fibrohistiocytic proliferations, but it is consistently absent in meningiomas and glomus tumors, which likewise enter differential consideration with hemangiopericytoma. A few hemangiopericytomas have demonstrated focal reactivity for muscle-associated actins;[328] CD34 and CD57 are present in approximately 50% of cases. However, desmin, CD31, cytokeratin, and S-100 protein are uniformly lacking.[325,327]

Overexpression of insulin-like growth factor-II (IGF-II) is potentially found in hemangiopericytoma and is believed to play a major role in producing tumor-related hypoglycemia. The IGF-II peptide can be detected by immunohistochemical means in such cases, but this finding is not diagnostically discriminatory.

SOLITARY FIBROUS TUMOR

Although it was originally described in 1931 as a mesenchymal pleural lesion,[329] solitary fibrous tumor (SFT) was recognized increasingly in various extrapulmonary sites during the 1990s. Many reported cases of HPC likely represent solitary fibrous tumors that were previously unrecognized as such outside the thorax; indeed, as stated above, current nosological schemes have combined those entities. Other histologic differential diagnoses include synovial sarcoma, cellular angiofibroma, neurofibroma, and spindle cell lipoma. The neoplastic cells in solitary fibrous tumors are strongly positive for CD34 (Fig. 4.6) and vimentin, and frequently BCL-2 reactive as well. They are uniformly negative for cytokeratin and CD31,[169,330-332] but may show strong diffuse CD99 reactivity;[333] CD10 is present in approximately 65% of

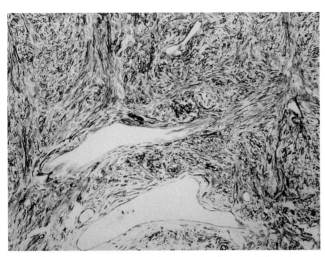

FIGURE 4.6 Solitary fibrous tumor, demonstrating uniform immunoreactivity for CD34.

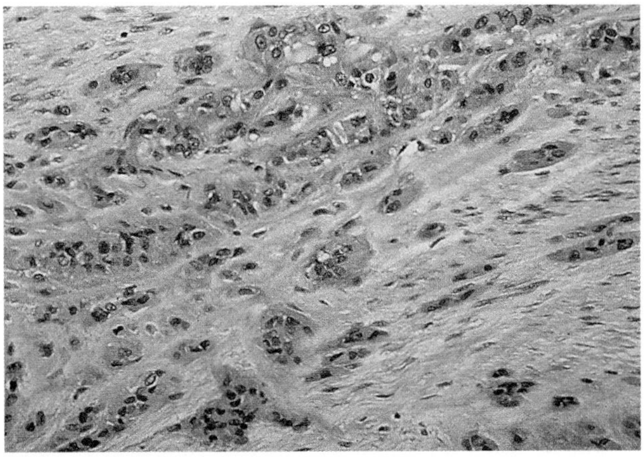

FIGURE 4.7 Epithelioid hemangioendothelioma composed of plump polygonal cells with bland cytologic features and intracellular lumen formation.

SFTs.[334] A panel of immunostains is typically necessary to exclude other spindle cell proliferations that may simulate the histologic image of solitary fibrous tumor. Neurofibromas may be reactive for BCL-2 and CD34, but they typically express S-100 protein, CD56, or CD57, or combinations thereof, unlike solitary fibrous tumors. BCL-2 reactivity is also common in synovial sarcoma,[331] but this neoplasm lacks CD34 and usually labels at least focally for epithelial antigens and TLE1, the latter of which is seen in <30% of solitary fibrous tumors. Spindle cell lipoma, another CD34-positive tumor, usually differs histologically from solitary fibrous tumor but may occasionally be very similar morphologically to the latter lesion. Reactivity for S-100 protein is seen in adipocytic elements of spindle cell lipoma, which usually can be found even in cellular variants of that tumor.

The myxoid variant of solitary fibrous tumor is potentially mistaken for other myxoid lesions such as low-grade fibromyxoid sarcoma, myxoid liposarcoma, and myxoid MPNST. Myxoid liposarcoma and low-grade fibromyxoid sarcoma are CD34-negative. Labeling for S-100 protein, CD56, or CD57 may assist in the recognition of myxoid MPNST; however, negativity for those markers is observed in roughly 25% of cases and does not necessarily exclude the latter diagnosis.

OSSIFYING FIBROMYXOID TUMOR OF SOFT PARTS

Ossifying fibromyxoid tumor (OFMT) of soft parts is a slowly growing mesenchymal lesion with a propensity to arise on the extremities, in the deep subcutis or skeletal muscles. Microscopically, this neoplasm is composed of lobulated nests of compact, cytologically bland round cells in a variably myxoid or densely hyalinized stroma. An incomplete shell of lamellar bone is a usual feature, but it may be absent in selected instances. The tumor cells of OFMT stain strongly and diffusely for S-100 protein and vimentin in most cases.[335-341] Occasional reactivity may also be seen for keratin, CD57, NSE,[335,339] synaptophysin,[335] and GFAP.[338,339,342] In addition, myogenous differentiation has been found in some examples, manifested by labeling for desmin and alpha smooth muscle actin.[335,336,341,342,343] EMA[337,338,341] and melanocytic markers[338] are consistently absent in OFMT.

EPITHELIOID HEMANGIOENDOTHELIOMA

Epithelioid hemangioendothelioma (EHE) is classified as a neoplasm with intermediate biological characteristics in the vascular tumor spectrum, falling between epithelioid hemangioma and epithelioid angiosarcoma. EHE is an angiocentric tumor showing primitive vascular differentiation, with a predilection for the liver, lungs, bone, and superficial soft tissue, in that order of frequency (Fig. 4.7). Obviously, an essential criterion for the diagnosis of EHE is clear evidence of endothelial differentiation. One can obtain this information with several vascular markers such as vWF, CD31, CD34, and FLI-1.[344,345] Podoplanin is absent in most examples of EHE.

Carcinomas may be confused with this tumor because the primitive intracellular vacuoles that typify EHE may mimic mucin-containing vacuoles as seen in adenocarcinoma. Several other sarcomas with an epithelioid appearance may likewise be considered, but perhaps the most troublesome mimic of EHE is epithelioid sarcoma. Both that neoplasm and EHE show a nodular growth pattern, plump eosinophilic tumor cells, and an arrangement in cords and nests. The presence of the keratin in EHE (as typically seen in epithelioid sarcoma) has been a point of debate. There are indeed convincing reports of coexpression of endothelial and epithelial markers in EHE.[346,347] In a study by Gray and associates, staining for keratin was observed in the majority of EHEs.[346] Another study of 30 cases from the skin and soft tissue documented keratin reactivity in 26% of cases.[348] These findings underscore the need to include several epithelial markers as well as endothelial determinants in immunohistologic evaluations of putative EHEs. A lack of EMA, E-cadherin, and desmoplakin is useful, especially together with concomitant reactivity for CD31, CD34, or both.

A recent study has shown that loss of nuclear labeling for INI1 (Snf5) is highly specific for epithelioid sarcoma in this differential diagnosis, since all evaluated cases of EHE showed retained nuclear staining for this ubiquitously expressed component of the SWI/SNF chromatin remodeling complex.[349]

EPITHELIOID SARCOMA-LIKE HEMANGIOENDOTHELIOMA

Billings and colleagues have described a peculiar tumor in this group that even more closely simulates the image of epithelioid sarcoma on conventional microscopy.[350] It has accordingly been named epithelioid sarcoma–like hemangioendothelioma (ESLH). Indeed, this entity shares immunoreactivity for keratin and vimentin with true epithelioid sarcoma (EPS), but ESLH paradoxically lacks CD34 (which is seen in EPS and most other hemangioendotheliomas) and additionally labels for CD31 and FLI-1.

KAPOSIFORM HEMANGIOENDOTHELIOMA

Kaposiform hemangioendothelioma (KHE) was first thought to arise exclusively in children and infants[351] but is now recognized as an unusual tumor that may also affect adults.[352] Many cases have been associated with lymphangiomatosis and Kasabach-Merritt syndrome (a consumption coagulopathy syndrome); in fact, the latter condition accounts for a great deal of the morbidity caused by KHEs.[353] These tumors show a micronodular pattern of spindle-cell growth that is reminiscent of Kaposi's sarcoma and spindle cell hemangioma, containing scattered nests of larger epithelioid cells with eosinophilic vacuolated cytoplasm; hemosiderin and hyaline droplets also may be seen.

The tumor cells of KHE manifest expression of several endothelial markers. CD34, PPN, and FLI-1 are generally found, but factor VIII–related antigen and UEAI are usually absent.[351,354] KS-associated herpesvirus (KSHV [HHV8])–related nucleic acid or proteins have not been found in KHE.[353] Vascular endothelial growth factor receptor-3 has been identified in this tumor, in common with other endothelial proliferations.[216]

AGGRESSIVE ANGIOMYXOMA

Aggressive angiomyxoma (AAM) is a peculiar neoplasm of the pelvic and perineal soft tissues that most commonly affects women. It is composed of loosely arranged, bland spindled to stellate cells embedded in a myxoid matrix punctuated by numerous venule- and capillary-sized blood vessels reminiscent of myxoid liposarcoma (Fig. 4.8). The vascular pattern of AAM lacks the arborizing appearance that is seen in some overtly malignant myxoid tumors. Some morphologic and immunophenotypic features of aggressive AAM also are shared in part by intramuscular myxoma.[355,356]

Immunohistochemical analyses of AAM have revealed reactivity for actin and often for desmin but not S-100 protein, suggesting a myogenic or myofibroblastic pattern of differentiation.[319] Ultrastructural studies[355] likewise support a fibroblastic/myofibroblastic phenotype in AAM.

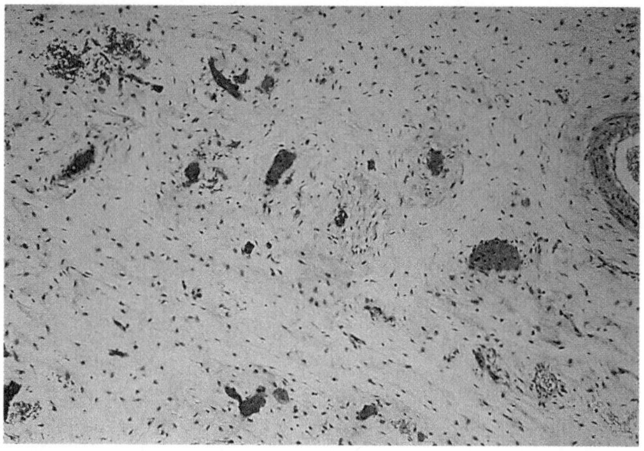

FIGURE 4.8 Aggressive angiomyxoma of pelvic soft tissues—a lesion for which differential diagnostic considerations include angiomyofibroblastoma, myxoid smooth muscle tumors, peripheral nerve sheath tumors, and myxoid liposarcoma. Immunohistology assists in eliminating only purely myogenous and neurogenic lesions.

Malignant Tumors of Soft Tissue

Sarcomas may be divided into four groups based on their primary histologic growth patterns. These categories include small round-cell tumors, epithelioid polygonal-cell tumors, spindle-cell neoplasms, and pleomorphic lesions. In each group, immunohistologic attributes lend themselves to an algorithm-based approach to interpretation.

SMALL ROUND CELL NEOPLASMS

The small round cell tumors of soft tissue (Fig. 4.9; see Table 4.4) compose a heterogeneous group of neoplasms that predominate in childhood and adolescence and share similar morphologic features. Rhabdomyosarcoma, PNET/ES, and lymphoma/leukemia are the prototypic members of this group. Another entity that may be confused with PNET is the intra-abdominal desmoplastic small round cell tumor.

RHABDOMYOSARCOMA

Embryonal rhabdomyosarcoma (E-RMS) accounts for more than half of all rhabdomyosarcomas and is the most problematic to recognize consistently. The morphologic image of E-RMS varies widely, depending on the degree of differentiation, cellularity, and pattern of growth. Strap cells, large eosinophilic myoblasts, and myxoid stroma may be seen focally in E-RMS but not in most of its microscopic mimics. A significant number of E-RMS cases consist only of densely apposed undifferentiated small cells (Fig. 4.10) that evoke a broad differential diagnostic list. Other considerations include neuroblastoma, ES, synovial sarcoma, melanoma, melanotic neuroectodermal tumor of infancy, granulocytic sarcoma, and malignant lymphoma. Furthermore, E-RMS may be confused

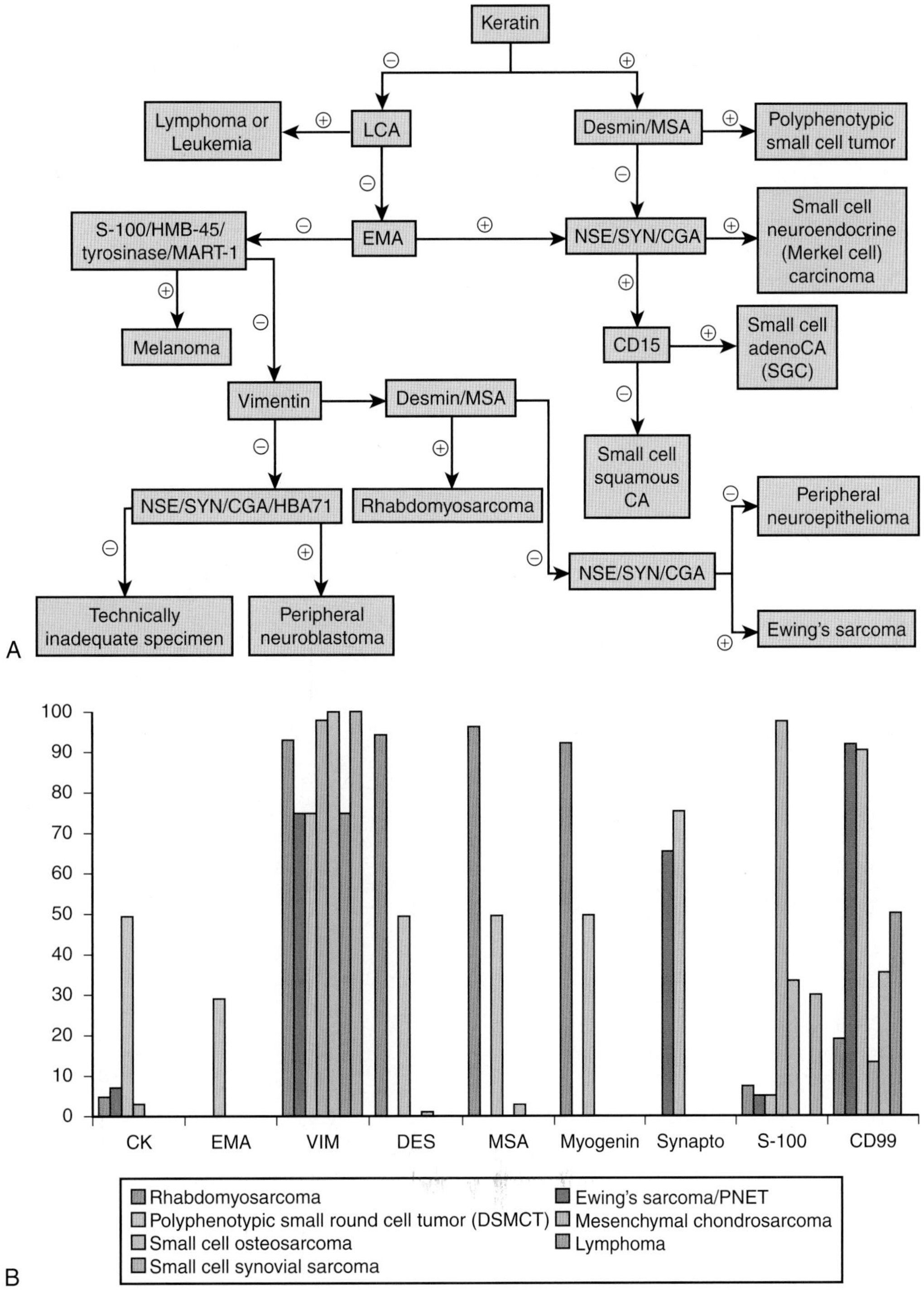

FIGURE 4.9 **(A)** Algorithmic immunohistologic diagnosis of malignant small round cell tumors. **(B)** Graphic representation of the frequency of reactivity for small round cell tumors against commonly used immunoreactants. CK, cytokeratin; EMA, epithelial membrane antigen; VIM, vimentin; DES, desmin; MSA, muscle-specific actin; Synapto, synaptophysin.

with the solid variant of alveolar rhabdomyosarcoma (Fig. 4.11), which has a significantly worse prognosis. In adult patients, small cell carcinoma and poorly differentiated small cell angiosarcoma also become considerations.

It is with the poorly differentiated variants of E-RMS that immunohistochemical analysis proves to be most helpful. Rhabdomyosarcoma expresses striated muscle markers in a cumulative and consistent sequence (vimentin, myogenin/Myo-D1, desmin, fast myosin, and myoglobin), recapitulating the pattern of normal myogenesis. Therefore, vimentin is uniformly present, although its diagnostic utility is minimal. Among myogenic markers, myogenin and desmin are the most consistently detectable in paraffin sections, showing appreciable staining in virtually all cases of E-RMS as well as in alveolar

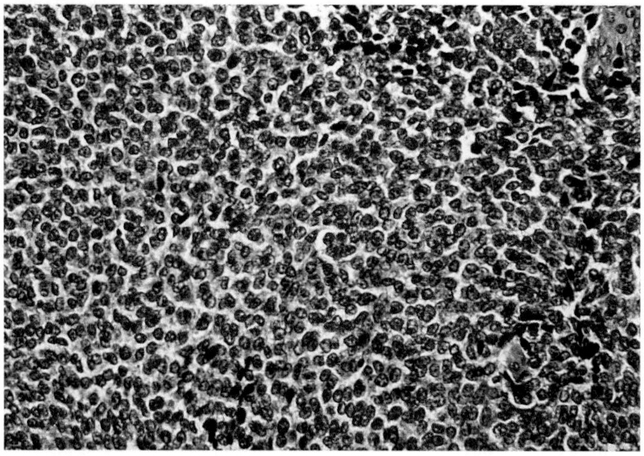

FIGURE 4.10 The solid form of primitive embryonal or alveolar rhabdomyosarcoma represents a prototypical small round cell malignancy for which several adjunctive studies are necessary.

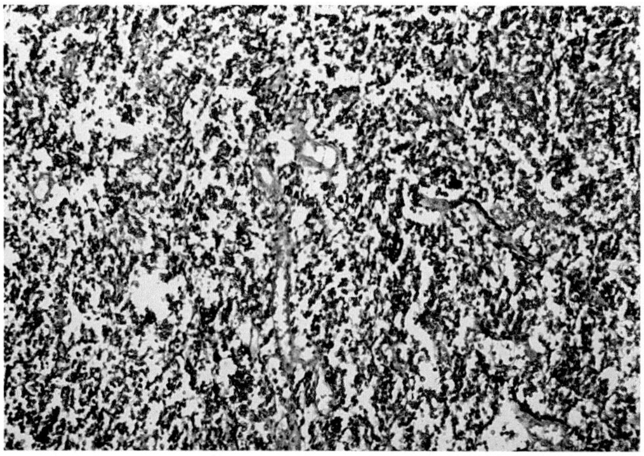

FIGURE 4.11 The typical image of alveolar rhabdomyosarcoma.

and pleomorphic subtypes of rhabdomyosarcoma (Fig. 4.12).[24] The extent of staining with myogenin is also helpful in subclassification, because the alveolar variant of rhabdomyosarcoma usually shows extensive labeling in nearly all neoplastic cells, whereas E-RMS shows more heterogeneous reactivity. Other small round cell tumors lack those determinants, with the notable exception of intra-abdominal desmoplastic small round cell tumors, which are usually positive for desmin, but not for myogenin.

Myo-D1 has been touted as highly specific and sensitive for rhabdomyosarcoma, showing nuclear expression in 82% to 100% of cases.[115,357-359] This myogenic marker is a DNA-binding nuclear regulatory protein that initiates myogenesis in mesenchymal stem cells. The staining pattern of Myo-D1 is heterogeneous among E-RMS cells;[358] nuclear labeling is most intense in small, primitive tumor cells, whereas larger cells with more obvious skeletal muscle differentiation generally are nonreactive.[115] On occasion, Myo-D1 cross-reacts with unknown *cytoplasmic* antigens in some small round cell tumors, showing variable fibrillary immunoreactivity in neuroblastoma and ES/PNET.[114,359] Among other muscle-related determinants, myogenin

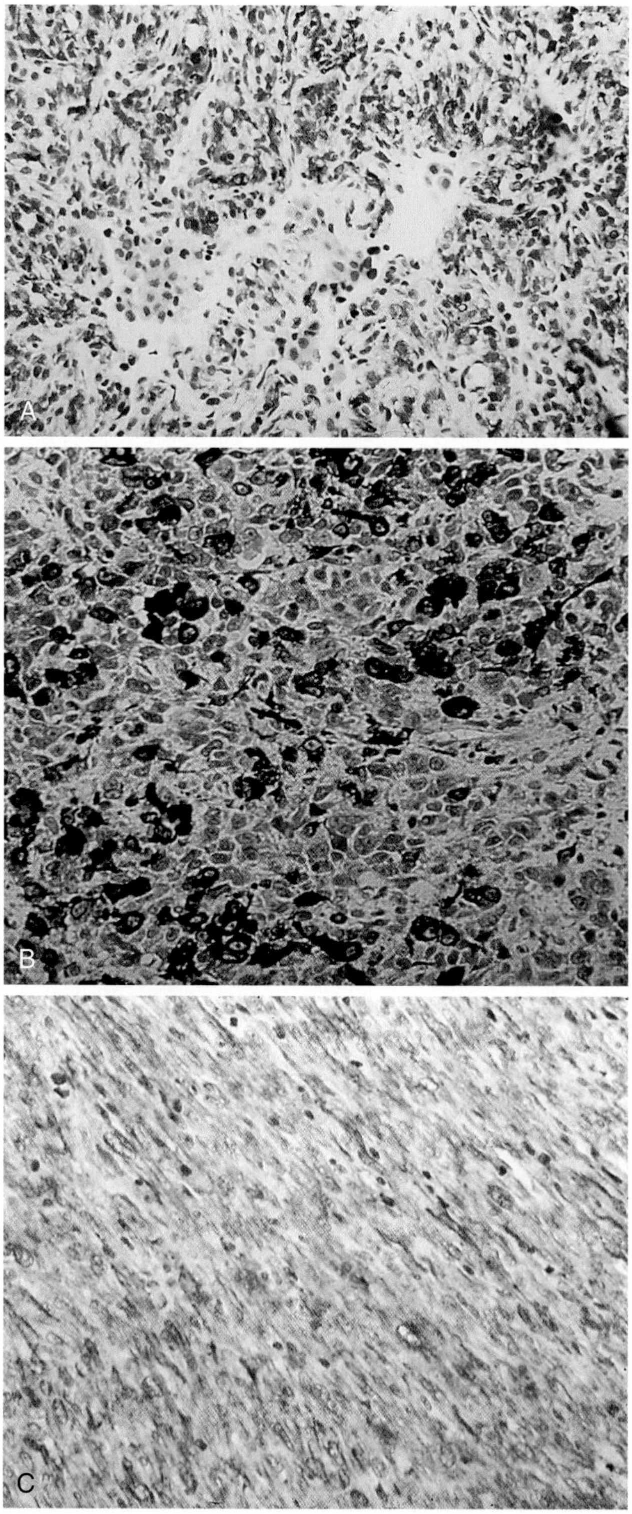

FIGURE 4.12 Desmin reactivity is a consistent feature in all histologic subtypes of rhabdomyosarcoma, including embryonal **(A)**; alveolar **(B)**; and pleomorphic **(C)** forms.

(MYG) is probably the most frequently detected in E-RMS. Nuclear labeling for myogenin is stronger than that seen with anti-Myo-D1.[115] In our experience, the sensitivity of MYG is comparable to that of desmin and muscle-associated actins with respect to rhabdomyosarcomas. ES/PNET typically lacks any MYG reactivity[115]

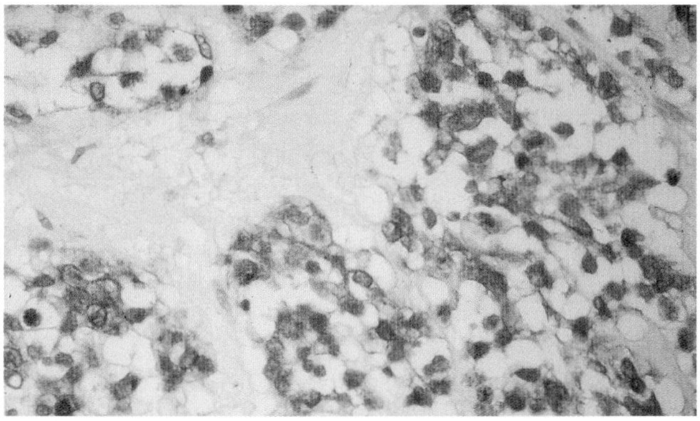

FIGURE 4.13 CD57 reactivity is infrequently observed in small cell rhabdomyosarcomas.

and may be reasonably excluded diagnostically if myogenin is present. This is true despite the fact that myogenin-related mRNA has been found in other childhood tumors using PCR-based techniques.[360]

The microfilament-associated protein vinculin is a major component of muscle tissue, in which it is believed to function in the alignment of sarcomeric myofibrils. Among the different histologic subtypes of rhabdomyosarcoma, vinculin expression is most prominent in differentiated tumors; only focal staining has been observed in E-RMS.[361] Vinculin immunoreactivity has also been observed in leiomyosarcoma.

Dystrophin, the protein product of the Duchenne muscular dystrophy locus, is a major cytoskeleton protein in skeletal muscle cells. There have been only limited studies on the use of this marker in the diagnosis of rhabdomyosarcoma.[362] Dystrophin was found in most cases of rhabdomyosarcoma in frozen sections, and was lacking in other small cell neoplasms including lymphoma, PNET, and Wilms' tumor.[362,363]

Undifferentiated rhabdomyosarcoma (defined as a small cell tumor lacking desmin but showing Myo-D1 or MYG reactivity) has been assessed with various other markers. Nestin is a filamentous protein expressed in immature skeletal muscle cells, endothelia, and some stromal cells adjacent to tumors.[364] Selected studies have suggested that nestin is also seen in undifferentiated rhabdomyosarcomas;[364] comparable assertions have been made in reference to insulin-like growth factor II (IGF-II). IGF-II expression has been inversely correlated with the degree of cellular differentiation in rhabdomyosarcomas by *in situ* hybridization.[365] The fetal form of the acetylcholine receptor may also be useful for identifying rhabdomyosarcomas with limited differentiation from other small cell tumors.[366] Fetal-type AChR is not expressed in mature striated muscle. Finally, the presence of CD56, CD57, and neurofilament isoforms has been noted in frozen sections of rhabdomyosarcoma and in selected paraffin sections of those lesions, and it does not militate against that diagnosis.[367]

Therapy often causes cytodifferentiation to occur in various neoplasms, and it decreases mitotic activity in all histologic categories of rhabdomyosarcoma. Indeed, unchanged or increased post-therapeutic proliferative activity, as assessed by Ki-67 immunostaining, has been equated with aggressive biological potential in E-RMS cases. Myogenous marker expression has not been found to change after therapy, other than detecting greater numbers of fast myosin-positive differentiated rhabdomyoblasts, correlating with the presence of more abundant brightly eosinophilic cytoplasm.[368] However, our personal experience has shown that divergent differentiation is more common in that context. In particular, reactivity for neuroectodermal determinants such as CD56, CD57, and synaptophysin is not uncommon in treated rhabdomyosarcomas.

The latter observation also recalls a notable pitfall in the diagnosis of E-RMS; namely, polyphenotypic small round cell tumors with partial myogenic differentiation. These lesions coexpress several markers of divergent cellular lineages. We will discuss them in greater detail later in this section (Fig. 4.13).

KEY DIAGNOSTIC POINTS

Rhabdomyosarcoma

- Striated muscle differentiation markers are expressed in a consistent sequence: vimentin, myogenin/Myo-D1, desmin, fast myosin, and myoglobin.

EWING'S SARCOMA AND PRIMITIVE NEUROECTODERMAL TUMOR

The Ewing family of tumors comprises small round cell neoplasms of bone and soft tissue that are, in part, defined by a particular chromosomal aberration [t(11;22)] and variants thereof. Over the past 15 years, it has become clear that ES and peripheral PNET are part of the same spectrum of neoplastic proliferations.[259,369,370] Besides the karyotypic marker just mentioned, both of those tumor types also show neuroectodermal features in tissue culture and similarities in proto-oncogene expression. As classically defined, ES was distinguished from PNET by an absence of pseudorosettes and the lack of ultrastructurally or immunohistochemically detectable neuroectodermal features. However, this diagnostic separation is now considered to be antiquated and has been abandoned.

The EWS and FLI-1 genes flank the translocation break point in ES/PNET. Reverse transcriptase (RT)-PCR methods have allowed for detection of chimeric mRNA transcripts produced by the fusion of those genes, which are present in roughly 75% of cases.[371,372-374] Such transcripts have not been detected in other small cell tumors. The Ewing's family of tumors is characterized by high MIC2/CD99 expression; that glycoprotein can be detected by various monoclonal antibodies, including HBA71, 12E7, RFB-1329, and 013 (see Table 4.3). It is diffusely present in nearly all cases of ES/PNET (>95%) with a cell-membranous pattern.[375-377] Although it was initially thought to be specific for ES/PNET, CD99 has since been identified in a variety of other tumors. In the small-cell group of pediatric neoplasms, lymphoblastic lymphoma and selected cases of alveolar

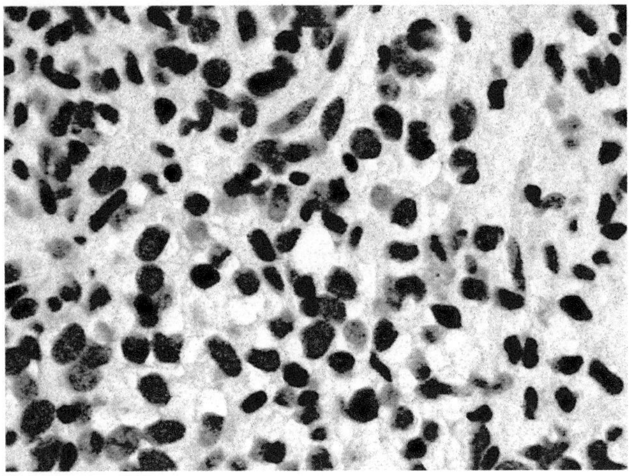

FIGURE 4.14 Nuclear staining for FLI-1 protein in primitive neuroectodermal tumor.

rhabdomyosarcoma represent the principal CD99-positive alternatives to ES/PNET. However, strong, diffuse membranous reactivity for CD99 favors ES/PNET over other diagnostic considerations. Obviously, MIC2 must be considered along with several other determinants in making a final diagnostic interpretation. In particular, concomitant nuclear labeling for FLI-1 is useful; the latter marker is seen in approximately 70% of ES/PNET cases (Fig. 4.14).[378]

Typical ES/PNET is nonreactive for chromogranin, cytokeratin, glial fibrillary protein, desmin, muscle-specific actin, myogenin, CD31, and CD45.[379,380] However, in studies of tumors that were confirmed by molecular identification of the t(11;22) translocation, immunoreactivity for cytokeratin has been present in 20% to 30% of ES/PNET cases.[381] Nonetheless, in our experience, keratin has been relatively focally expressed in these tumors when present. NB84 (a marker developed for recognition of neuroblastoma) is also apparent in roughly 20% of ES/PNETs.

Integrins are a large and heterogeneous family of cell membrane glycoproteins that show a complex pattern of expression. Subunits of integrins are variably seen among different small cell tumors of childhood. ES/PNET shows a beta 1+, alpha 1–, alpha 3–, alpha 5+, and alpha 6–pattern.[382] This profile overlaps considerably with that observed in rhabdomyosarcoma, but it is distinct from neuroblastoma, which is beta 1+, alpha 1+, alpha 3+, alpha 5–, and alpha 6–. ILK (beta 1– integrin-linked kinase) is a protein that interacts with the cytoplasmic domain of beta 1–integrin sequences. One study found ILK expression in all ES/PNET cases and in one-third of neuroblastomas.[383] In contrast, other small cell pediatric tumors did not label for this marker. Trk receptors are a tripartite family of proteins, again exhibiting differential expression in ES/PNET as compared with neuroblastoma. ES/PNET tends to manifest the presence of (A+/B–/C+) Trk A transcripts immunohistochemically, whereas neuroblastoma shows a (A–/B–/C+) phenotype. These markers are not used clinically in most laboratories.

MESENCHYMAL CHONDROSARCOMA

Mesenchymal chondrosarcoma (MCS) is an aggressive cartilaginous neoplasm that is seen most often in young adults, commonly in extraskeletal locations. It is typified by a small-cell population that is similar to that seen in classic ES, except that MCS is punctuated by islands of primitive cartilage that appear to arise from the small cells in a manner simulating embryonic chondrogenesis. Another salient feature of MCS is the presence of hemangiopericytoid vasculature.

Unlike other forms of chondrosarcoma, staining for S-100 protein is not diffuse in MCS. It is limited to the chondroblastic islands of that tumor and is lacking in the small cell component.[384,385] All elements potentially label for CD57, and most cases are also reactive for NSE.[384] Factor XIIIa has been documented in MCS as well, but that marker is non-specific.[385] Tumors of this type arising in the central nervous system are alleged to show cytokeratin and GFAP reactivity in 25% of cases,[386] but we are dubious of that contention based on our experience.

MCS typically does not express desmin, actin, cytokeratin, or EMA.[387] Unlike ES/PNET, MCS is nonreactive for synaptophysin[384] but both tumor types share CD99 positivity.[387,388]

KEY DIAGNOSTIC POINTS

PNET/Ewing

- Typically positive for FLI-1, CD99, NSE, synaptophysin
- Keratin+ in 20% of cases, focal distribution
- Differential panel includes muscle markers (negative)

POLYPHENOTYPIC SMALL ROUND-CELL TUMORS

There is clear evidence of divergent differentiation in a proportion of small round cell tumors in both adults and children. We have encountered approximately 25 examples of tumors that are phenotypically indistinct from classical ES/PNET but which nonetheless are concomitantly immunoreactive for epithelial, myogenous, and neuroectodermal markers. They are generally aggressive neoplasms, perhaps even more so than uncomplicated ES/PNETs. Other investigators have described pathologic variations on this basic theme by documenting histologic evidence of unusual divergent differentiation (including glandlike structures in PNET) or describing morphologic attributes that are peculiar to particular anatomic sites.[389-391]

The term *polyphenotypic small round cell tumor* seems most appropriate to describe the general attributes of these lesions. The desmoplastic small round cell tumor (DSRCT) is the best-recognized representative of this group. It is characterized by an EWS/WT1 chimeric transcript, and is a morphologically distinctive neoplasm that is characterized by reactive fibrosis surrounding discrete nests of tumor cells (Fig. 4.15). DSRCT has a relatively complicated immunoprofile,

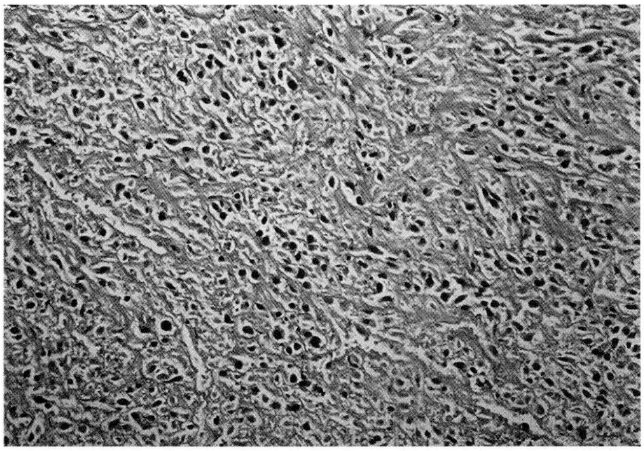

FIGURE 4.15 Desmoplastic small round cell tumor is a distinctive small round cell malignancy that manifests a densely fibrogenic stroma.

with frequent staining for keratin (86%), EMA (93%), NSE (81%), vimentin (97%), and desmin (90%).[392] Interestingly, CD99 reactivity is seen in only a small minority of cases; instead, WT1-immunoreactivity is frequently seen using a polyclonal antibody directed against the C-terminus of the protein, in contrast to the widely used monoclonal antibodies that recognize the N-terminus of the protein, which are useful for diagnosing malignant mesothelioma and serous adenocarcinoma.[41,392,393] Actin, myogenin, and chromogranin are generally absent in DSRCT, although there are exceptions to that statement.

KEY DIAGNOSTIC POINTS

DSRCT

- Typically positive for WT1, keratin 8/18, EMA, NSE, vimentin/desmin
- Rare CD99 or myogenin+

POORLY DIFFERENTIATED SMALL-CELL SYNOVIAL SARCOMA

The small-cell variant of poorly differentiated synovial sarcoma (PDSS) can easily be mistaken on morphologic grounds for other small round cell tumors such as ES/PNET, as well as high-grade malignant peripheral nerve sheath tumor (MPNST). To further complicate this situation, reports have been made of peripheral nerve-sheath tumors harboring the t(X;18) chromosomal translocation of synovial sarcoma.[394,395] However, that observation is controversial, and, for practical purposes, the specified karyotypic finding is currently regarded as synonymous with a diagnosis of synovial sarcoma. CD99 reactivity may further complicate the diagnostic interpretation if one is not aware of its frequent presence in PDSS.[396] Analysis of cytokeratin subsets may contribute to differential diagnosis in this setting; for example, CK7 has been reported in up to 50% of PDSS cases, but it is absent in PNET.[397] The TLE1 status of PNET and PDSS has not yet been assessed systematically to date, but FLI-1-reactivity favors the former of these lesions.

HEMATOLYMPHOID MALIGNANCIES

Hematopoietic neoplasms only rarely present as soft tissue masses, and this phenomenon is particularly unusual in pediatric patients in whom other forms of small round cell tumors are most common. Because of the virtually ubiquitous presence of CD45 in hematopoietic cells and its extremely high degree of specificity, that marker is very valuable in this context. Not all antibodies raised against CD45 identify determinants that survive routine tissue processing, but the monoclonal antibody cocktail PD7/26;2B11 (see Table 4.3) is indeed active in paraffin sections.

For practical purposes, reactivity for CD45 is diagnostic of a hematopoietic lineage; conversely, lymphomas and leukemias do not generally express markers of other lineages. With that having been said, it should be noted that lymphoblastic lymphomas commonly label for CD99 (as seen in ES/PNET), thereby presenting a potential pitfall in interpretation.[398-400] Concurrent reactivity for terminal deoxynucleotidyl transferase and CD10 are also present in lymphoblastic lymphoma; they are generally—but not always[401,402]—absent in other small round cell tumors. Lymphomas may present a variety of other unexpected morphologic images that simulate those of sarcomas, such as one featuring signet-ring cells,[403] another with myxoid stroma,[404] or the presence of a fibrillary matrix.[405]

SARCOMAS WITH A SPINDLE-CELL APPEARANCE

The spindle cell sarcomas of the deep soft tissues (Fig. 4.16) include fibrosarcoma, leiomyosarcoma (LMS), MPNST, monophasic spindle cell synovial sarcoma, and spindle cell angiosarcoma. Despite continuing advancements in immunohistochemistry, diagnostic distinctions among these tumor types remain challenging.

Fibrosarcoma

In the late 1960s, fibrosarcoma was perhaps the most common malignancy of soft tissue. However, the diagnostic criteria for that lesion have evolved considerably over time, now making it among the rarest of sarcomas. The recognition of other entities such as monophasic synovial sarcoma, MPNST, fibromatosis, and nodular fasciitis largely account for this change. Many tumors histologically indistinguishable from classical fibrosarcoma in fact represent fibrosarcomatous (higher-grade) variants of dermatofibrosarcoma protuberans (DFSP); when a fibrosarcoma-like lesion is encountered in superficial soft tissues, areas of conventional DFSP should be carefully sought. Fibrosarcoma most often presents as a slowly growing mass in middle adulthood, and it is widely distributed anatomically. This lesion may also be seen as a congenital tumor in infants, but is considered a separate entity in this setting.

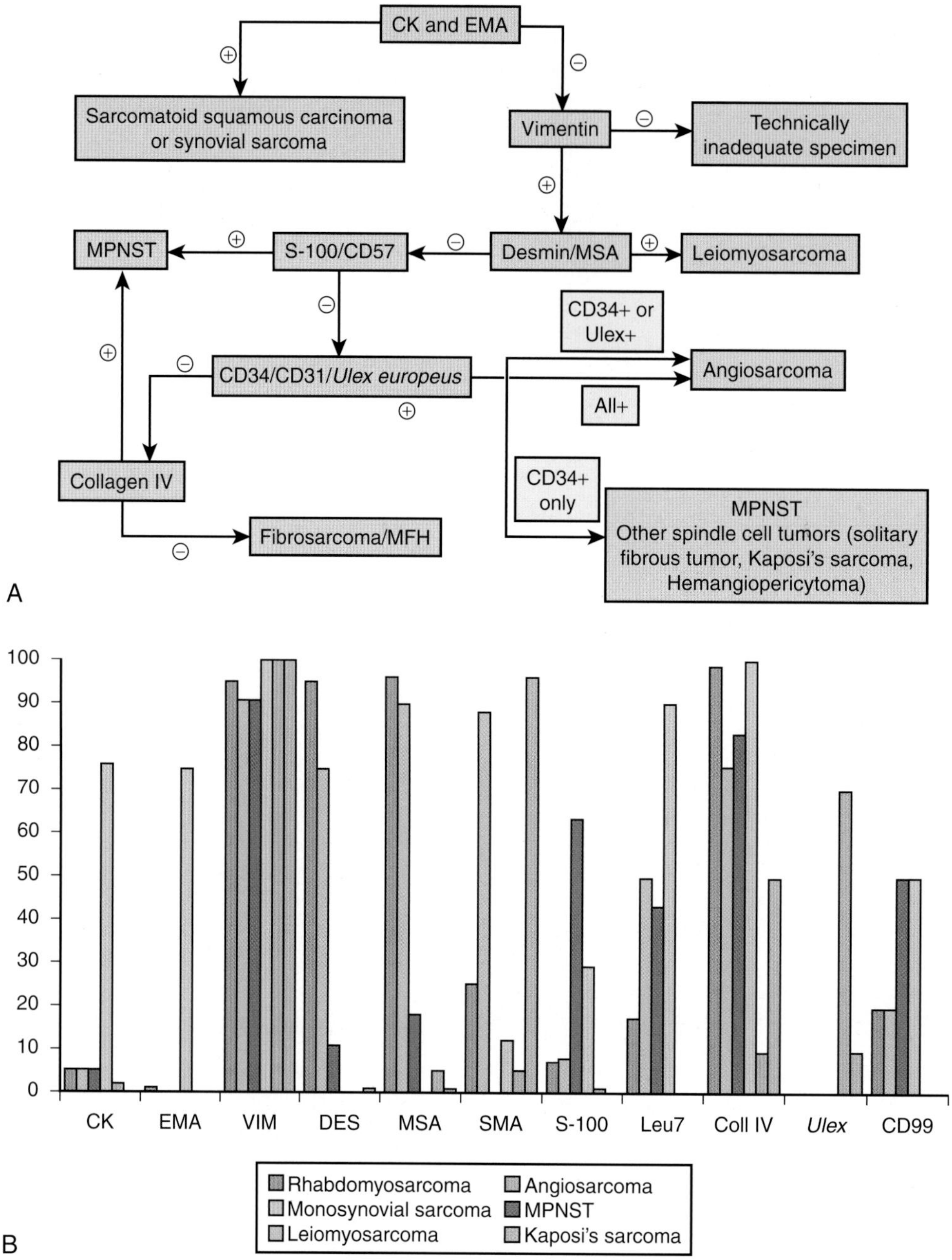

FIGURE 4.16 (A, B) Sarcomas with a spindled appearance.

The morphologic diagnosis of classical fibrosarcoma is predicated on finding a herringbone pattern of intersecting spindle-cell fascicles and a variably collagenized stroma, with no other specific signs of differentiation. As so defined, that lesion is reactive for vimentin but does not stain for any lineage-selective markers. In contrast, inflammatory fibrosarcoma of the mesentery and retroperitoneum shows evidence of myofibroblastic differentiation, with frequent actin positivity.[406] Inflammatory fibrosarcoma is currently widely believed to fall within the histologic spectrum of inflammatory myofibroblastic tumor.[407] Another variant of fibrosarcoma is the so-called sclerosing epithelioid subtype, and we will discuss it later in this chapter.

Leiomyosarcoma

Leiomyosarcomas are most commonly found in the retroperitoneum in adults. They uncommonly occur in the deep soft tissues of the extremities but may be seen in more superficial sites, particularly in the dermis and subcutis. The differential diagnosis of LMS traditionally includes other sarcomas composed of intersecting spindle-cell fascicles, including fibrosarcoma, MPNST, synovial sarcoma, and spindle cell rhabdomyosarcoma. Additional conditions such as IMT (inflammatory pseudotumor), neurofibroma, and hemangiopericytoma (see Fig. 4.5) are also considerations.

Currently, immunohistochemical confirmation of smooth muscle differentiation in LMS is based on the demonstration of desmin (see Fig. 4.16), alpha-smooth muscle actin, and h-caldesmon. Some studies have indicated that actin and caldesmon may be more sensitive than desmin in detecting myogenic differentiation in smooth muscle neoplasms. In our experience, however, the vast majority of LMS cases are indeed labeled for desmin. Examples of desmin-positive spindle cell rhabdomyosarcoma—a rare tumor—may be segregated from LMS by their negativity for caldesmon and smooth muscle actin, and their reactivity for myoglobin, MyoD1, and, especially, myogenin.

Partial immunophenotypic similarity to other soft tissue tumors is not uncommon in LMS; for example, labeling for S-100 protein and CD57 may be encountered in superficial smooth muscle tumors, as seen in cases of MPNST. Likewise, LMS may occasionally express so-called histiocytic markers such as CD68, and some may label for CD30 or CD34.[408] The potential presence of keratin and EMA in LMSs seems to be influenced by anatomic site, in our experience. Tumors arising in the pelvic soft tissue and pelvic viscera show aberrant epithelial immunophenotypes in 40% to 50% of cases, whereas lesions in other locations rarely do so. However, other authors have not reported this type of topographical variation in regard to this point.

Calponin is another smooth muscle-specific protein that is developmentally expressed in up to four isoforms and binds strongly to actin in a calcium-independent manner.[409] It is expressed in parenchymal and vascular smooth muscle cells and is also present in myofibroblasts, as well as myoepithelial cells, which limits its diagnostic utility.[409] Synovial sarcoma may also show calponin positivity,[118] making attention to other markers mandatory in separating this tumor from LMS.

LMS occasionally may show strong positivity for CD99, but with a dotlike cytoplasmic staining pattern.[410,411] In addition, smooth muscle sarcomas can demonstrate reactivity for estrogen and progesterone receptors, regardless of whether they arise in viscera or in the somatic soft tissues.[411,412]

Increased expression of the GLUT-1 protein has been reported in many human malignancies, including non–small cell lung cancer,[312] colorectal carcinoma,[309] angiosarcoma,[311] and thyroid carcinomas,[310] and GLUT1 overexpression has been associated with an adverse prognosis.[312] Some examples of soft-tissue LMS also show GLUT-1 immunopositivity, whereas leiomyomas are uniformly negative.[412] Although data on this point are still limited, they suggest that GLUT-1 labeling may correlate with a risk of distant metastases by LMS.[412]

Both benign and malignant smooth muscle tumors may be more common in persons who are infected with the human immunodeficiency virus (HIV). Such lesions in immunocompromised individuals occur in unusual locations and also show evidence of latent infection by clonal Epstein-Barr virus (EBV).[413] Several EBV antigens are expressed in HIV-related LMS, including latent antigen EBNA-1, immediate-early antigen BZFL1, and early antigen EA-D, as well as viral capsid antigen p160, gp125, and membrane antigen gp350.[414] These findings show that EBV is capable of lytic infection of selected mesenchymal cells and they support a role for EBV in smooth-muscle sarcomagenesis in the specified context. Interestingly, lesions of Kaposi's sarcoma in HIV-infected patients fail to show cellular EBV integration.[413]

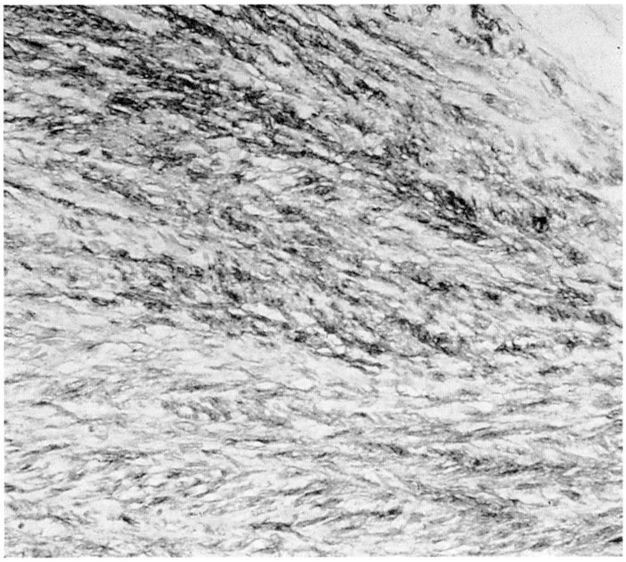

FIGURE 4.17 CD57 in malignant peripheral nerve sheath tumor (MPNST). Reactivity for S-100 protein, CD57, myelin basic protein, or collagen type IV is observed in greater than 85% of MPNSTs.

Malignant Peripheral Nerve Sheath Tumor

Malignant peripheral nerve sheath tumor (formerly also known as neurofibrosarcoma, malignant schwannoma, and neurogenic sarcoma) is a tumor with a highly variable histologic image. It may be indistinguishable from fibrosarcoma, or it may exhibit divergent differentiation with the presence of glandlike structures, or, more commonly, non-schwannian mesenchymal elements. However, many MPNSTs are indeed recognizable on morphologic grounds alone, especially if they show an anatomic association with large nerves.

Determinants associated with non-neoplastic Schwann cells and benign peripheral nerve sheath tumors are frequently detected in MPNSTs. They show reactivity for S-100 protein in 50% to 70% of cases, but usually with labeling of only a small proportion of tumor cells.[44] CD56 and CD57 are likewise observed in approximately 50% of MPNSTs (Fig. 4.17).[73] Myelin basic protein is much less frequently encountered. Note that none of these nerve sheath-associated determinants *by themselves* is definitive in the identification of MPNST. They are most helpful diagnostically when the only *other* marker present is vimentin. Roughly two-thirds of MPNSTs will label for S-100 protein, CD56, CD57, or myelin basic protein, taken together as a group.[44] *Conjoint* reactivity for at least two of these markers, however, is seen in no more than 35% of cases. Thus, it is apparent that strong immunohistologic support for a diagnosis of MPNST can be difficult to obtain in many instances. Moreover, nerve sheath malignancies have a potential for divergent differentiation—as mentioned earlier—and may be labeled in that circumstance for epithelial or myogenous determinants as well. To reiterate, LMS also has the potential for S-100 protein and CD57 reactivity, making it particularly important as a differential diagnostic alternative.[415,416] A recent study suggested that the neural crest transcription factor Sox-10 may be a more sensitive marker for MPNST than is S-100 protein; however, Sox10 is also detected in melanocytic lesions and must therefore be interpreted in context, similar to other markers.[417]

Another spindle cell tumor that shares immunophenotypic features with MPNST is monophasic synovial sarcoma (MSS). Roughly 40% of cases of MSS show S100 staining, and approximately 30% are CD57-positive.[418] Cytokeratin subset analysis may be useful in difficult cases, because most synovial sarcomas are reactive for CK7 or CK19, or both.[418] In contrast, MPNSTs typically lack those proteins. CD10-reactivity also favors a diagnosis of MPNST, whereas TLE1-positivity typifies MSS.

Reports of MPNSTs with angiosarcoma-like images have also been described.[419] Immunohistochemical analysis has confirmed the presence of endothelial differentiation in those cases.

One particularly difficult issue is the distinction of spindle-cell (sarcomatoid) malignant melanoma from MPNST, either in the skin or in metastatic sites.[420] There are several well-known embryologic associations between peripheral nerve sheath cells and melanocytes, as represented neoplastically by pigmented neurofibroma and melanotic schwannoma, neurotropic melanoma, epithelioid MPNST resembling melanoma, and the combined occurrence of epithelioid blue nevi and psammomatous melanotic schwannoma in Carney syndrome. As a practical approach, tumors with a histologic appearance that is similar to that of MPNST but with strong and diffuse S-100 protein reactivity generally should be considered as melanomas. This is especially true if concomitant positivity is obtained for HMB-45, HMB-50, tyrosinase, or MART-1, because the latter four markers are only rarely associated with nerve sheath tumors. Despite the production of collagen type IV by nerve sheath cells, the immunohistochemical detection of this marker has limited value in the diagnosis of schwannian neoplasms because cells with smooth muscle, endothelial, and myofibroblastic differentiation may also synthesize it.

KEY DIAGNOSTIC POINTS

Malignant Peripheral Nerve Sheath Tumors (MPNSTs)

- Two thirds are S-100 protein and CD56/CD57-positive, usually focal.
- S-100 is also positive in melanoma, and other melanoma markers are key diagnostic antibodies.
- MPNSTs are negative for CK7 (which is positive in synovial sarcoma).

Monophasic Spindle Cell Synovial Sarcoma

Monophasic spindle cell (so-called fibrous) synovial sarcomas represent one extreme of the morphologic spectrum of those neoplasms. Classic biphasic synovial sarcoma is not a diagnostic problem, whereas the image of MSS can simulate that of several other soft tissue neoplasms including fibrosarcoma, MPNST, hemangiopericytoma, solitary fibrous tumor, and LMS.

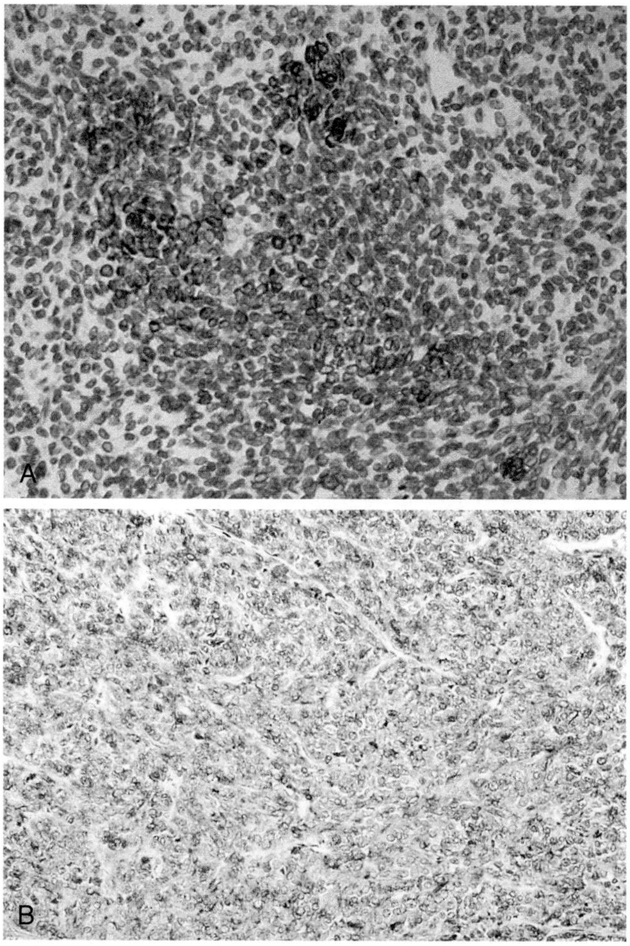

FIGURE 4.18 Synovial sarcoma showing immunoreactivity for keratin **(A)** and epithelial membrane antigen **(B)**.

The presence of EMA is typically observed in MSS (Fig. 4.18). Unlike its biphasic variant, spindle cell synovial sarcoma is only focally and inconsistently reactive for cytokeratin; in particular, it may show reactivity for CK7, CK8, CK18, and CK19.[396,421] Although carcinoembryonic antigen may occasionally be found in the epithelial components of biphasic synovial sarcomas, it is absent in spindle cells in all cases.[421] However, collagen type IV and E-cadherin may be diffusely expressed in MSS.[396]

CD99 is commonly present in MSS,[310,400,422] but this marker is also shared by a number of other spindle cell neoplasms. As mentioned earlier in this discussion, a minority of MSS cases also label for CD57 and S-100 protein.[36] Strong positivity for BCL-2 protein has been noted as well;[423,424] one study in which fluorescence *in situ* hybridization (FISH) analysis confirmed the presence of t(X;18), 79% of MSS cases were positive for BCL-2, whereas 20 LMSs, 4 MPNSTs, and 4 fibrosarcomas lacked this marker.[424] Nevertheless, BCL-2 reactivity has indeed been observed in a variety of other soft tissue tumors, such as spindle cell lipoma, Kaposi's sarcoma, solitary fibrous tumor, and gastrointestinal-type stromal tumors.[424] Interestingly, all of these lesions also typically express CD34, which is consistently absent in MSS and may therefore be a useful discriminant. Conversely, nuclear labeling for TLE1 supports the diagnosis of synovial sarcoma,[425] although its level of ultimate diagnostic specificity has yet to be defined.

Spindle Cell Angiosarcoma

A rare histologic manifestation of angiosarcoma is that of a spindle cell neoplasm.[426] Angiosarcomas of that type label with UEAI or FLI-1 in the great majority of cases, but <10% demonstrate vWF reactivity. CD31, CD34, and thrombomodulin are seen in combination with one another in virtually all instances. PPN-reactivity is variable.

Kaposi's Sarcoma

Kaposi's sarcoma (KS) occurs in four clinical forms—classical (Mediterranean), lymphadenopathic, transplantation-associated, and AIDS-related—but its microscopic features are the same in each of these settings. In its fully developed state, KS may be confused morphologically with spindle cell angiosarcoma as well as Kaposiform hemangioendothelioma. The tumor cells in each of these lesions are generally positive for CD34 and thrombomodulin, but only KS manifests nuclear reactivity for herpesvirus-type 8 latent nuclear antigen-1 among lesions that have its general histologic appearance.[427,428] PPN is also typically present in KS.

SARCOMAS WITH AN EPITHELIOID APPEARANCE

A number of soft tissue sarcomas (Fig. 4.19; see Table 4.6) are composed of large polygonal-shaped cells, yielding an appearance similar to that of carcinomas. These lesions include epithelioid sarcoma, epithelioid monophasic synovial sarcoma, clear cell sarcoma, alveolar soft part sarcoma, epithelioid LMS, epithelioid angiosarcoma, epithelioid MPNST, malignant granular cell tumor, and histiocytic MFH.

Epithelioid Sarcoma

Epithelioid sarcoma (EPS) has a characteristic histologic growth pattern, characterized by coalescing nodules with central necrosis. Its image may potentially simulate that of necrobiotic granuloma, melanoma, or metastatic carcinoma. The occasional presence of cytoplasmic vacuoles in EPS may also raise the diagnostic possibility of hemangioendothelioma or angiosarcoma.[429] Rare examples manifest unusual histologic findings such as a chondroid-like matrix[430] or a rhabdoid appearance.[431] The latter image is particularly common in proximal-type EPS.

A consistent immunophenotypic attribute of epithelioid sarcoma is an intense perinuclear zone of vimentin and keratin reactivity (Fig. 4.20). It is attributable to perinuclear collections of intermediate filaments that are seen at an ultrastructural level. The scope of cytokeratin labeling may be heterogeneous in any given tumor (Fig. 4.21); p63 protein, CK5, and CK6 tend to be absent in EPS, whereas histologically similar carcinomas often express those proteins.[431] CD34 positivity is seen in approximately 50% of EPS cases.[166,432] Isolated reports of neurofilament positivity have also been made.[433,434]

Epithelioid sarcomas share immunohistologic attributes with synovial sarcomas, in that both tumor types are reactive for cytokeratin and EMA. In addition, both types may occasionally show reactivity for carcinoembryonic antigen and S-100 protein.[435] Most cases of EPS and epithelioid synovial sarcoma also strongly express E-cadherin.[436,437]

Immunohistochemical studies are helpful in the diagnostic separation of EPS and isolated necrobiotic granulomas (e.g., deep granuloma annulare and cellular rheumatoid nodule). Granulomas manifest reactivity for CD45 and CD163, whereas the tumor cells of EPS do not; conversely, necrobiotic granulomas lack reactivity for EMA, cytokeratin,[438] and CD34.[439]

Because of the potential for epithelioid vascular tumors to demonstrate aberrant keratin reactivity, their confusion with epithelioid sarcomas is a real possibility. Indeed, as mentioned earlier in this discussion, one particular variant of hemangioendothelioma is particularly similar morphologically to EPS.[350] Reactivity for CD31 is strong evidence for true endothelial differentiation in this setting, as is labeling for FLI-1 protein. Obviously, however, because EPS is commonly CD34-positive, in similarity to the profile of vascular neoplasms, that marker cannot be used to separate those two tumor groups. Although keratin expression is not uncommon in epithelioid vascular tumors, EMA is very rarely detected. As mentioned above, expression of INI1 is retained in epithelioid vascular tumors, whereas it is lost in >90% of ES cases.[349]

An unexpected determinant was found in 91% of epithelioid sarcomas by Kato and colleagues; namely, CA125.[439] This marker is typically associated with Müllerian epithelial tumors, especially in the ovaries, and its presence in a mesenchymal neoplasm is inexplicable. All other polygonal-cell tumors of soft tissue in the series just cited were CA125-negative.[439]

Epithelioid Monophasic Synovial Sarcoma

Given the many clinicopathologic similarities between EPS (especially its proximal variant)[440] and the very rare purely epithelioid synovial sarcoma,[441] it would follow that they are difficult to separate by immunophenotypic analysis. A helpful discriminant between these neoplasms is CD34, which is present in EPS but not in epithelioid synovial sarcoma. Moreover, as cited above, Kato and associates found that nearly all EPS cases were immunoreactive for CA125,[439] whereas synovial sarcomas lacked that marker. As mentioned earlier in this discussion, monophasic spindle-cell synovial sarcoma is consistently reactive for nuclear TLE1 protein; however, that moiety has not been studied specifically in the monophasic epithelioid variant.

Epithelioid Angiosarcoma

Epithelioid variants of angiosarcoma are recognized as clinicopathologically distinct from epithelioid hemangioendothelioma, and they may involve the deep soft tissues. Other differential diagnostic considerations in such cases may include amelanotic melanoma, poorly

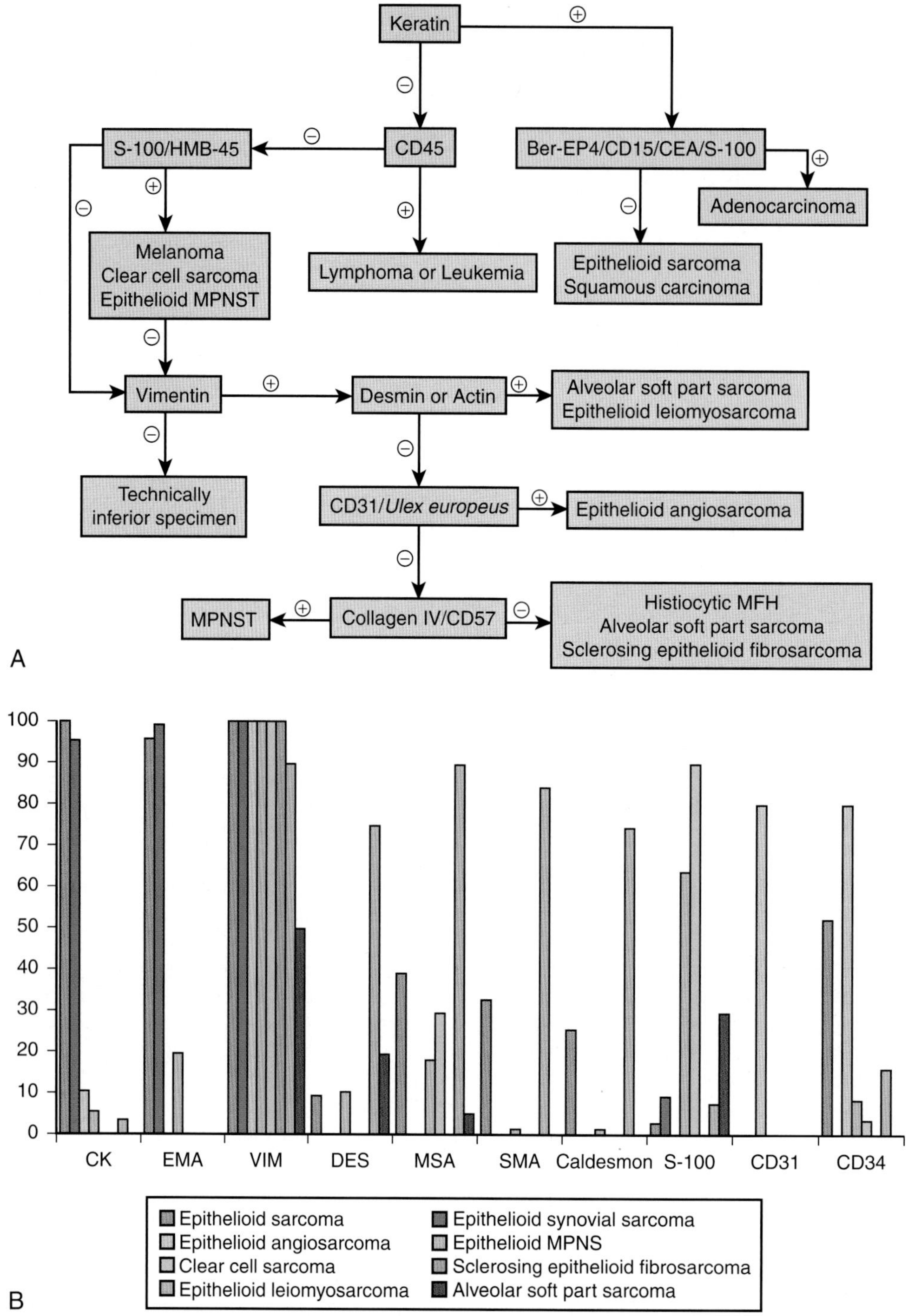

FIGURE 4.19 **(A)** Algorithmic immunohistochemical diagnosis of malignant epithelioid cell tumors. **(B)** Graphic representation of the frequency of reactivity for malignant spindle cell tumors against commonly used immunoreactants. MPNST, malignant peripheral nerve sheath tumor; MFH, malignant fibrous histiocytoma; CK, cytokeratin; EMA, epithelial membrane antigen; VIM, vimentin; DES, desmin; MSA, muscle-specific actin; SMA, smooth muscle actin.

differentiated carcinoma, and other polygonal-cell sarcomas (Fig. 4.22).

Immunoreactivity patterns may vary somewhat in epithelioid angiosarcoma as compared with classical forms of that tumor. In particular, keratin reactivity is much more often seen in the former group. However, CD31 and FLI-1 are sensitive and specific markers of epithelioid vascular malignancies as well as other endothelial proliferations (Fig. 4.23).[172,442,443] Podoplanin is also seen in a proportion of cases, as is WT1.[444]

The potential presence of CD34 in diverse polygonal-cell soft tissue tumors, including epithelioid LMS, epithelioid MPNST, clear cell sarcoma, and epithelioid sarcoma, has diminished its potential utility as an indicator of endothelial differentiation.[442] We also have observed that epithelioid angiosarcomas may be reactive

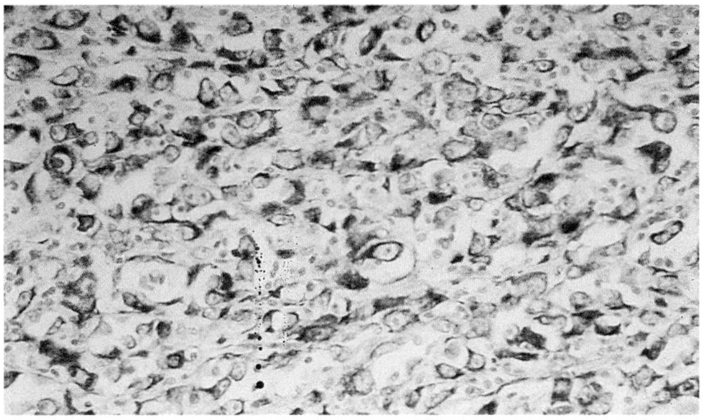

FIGURE 4.20 Epithelioid sarcoma showing intense immunoreactivity for vimentin, with perinuclear accentuation.

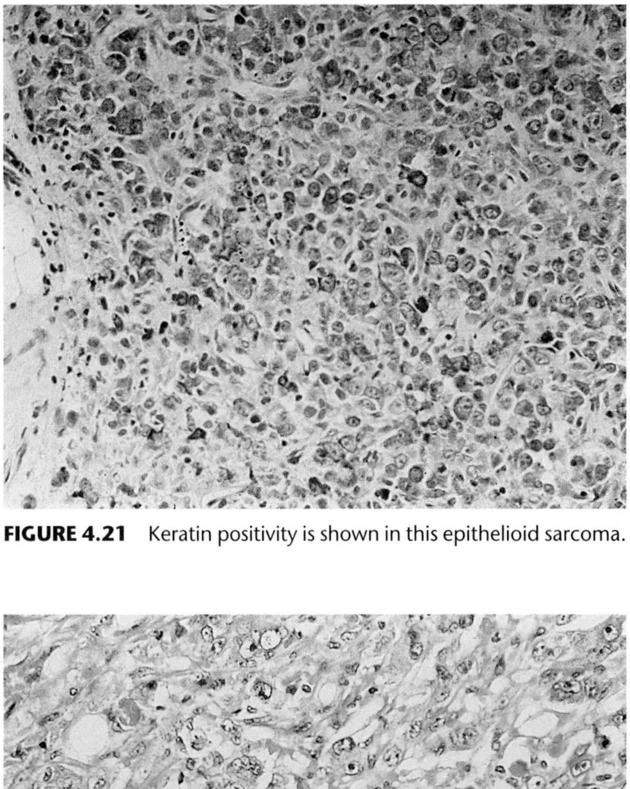

FIGURE 4.21 Keratin positivity is shown in this epithelioid sarcoma.

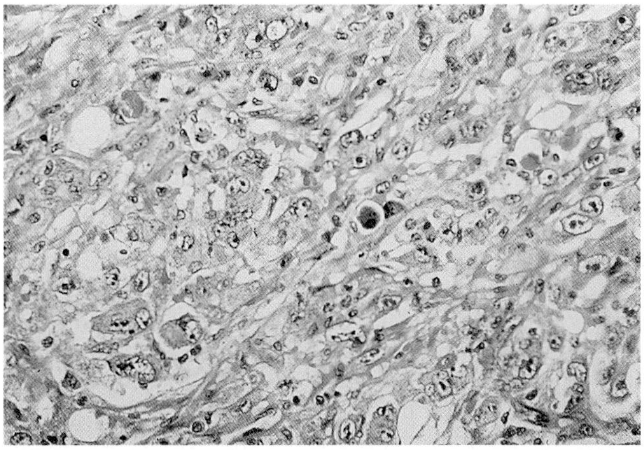

FIGURE 4.22 Epithelioid angiosarcoma is potentially confused diagnostically with metastatic malignant melanoma or poorly differentiated carcinoma in the soft tissues.

for CA72-4 (tumor-associated glycoprotein-72), a protein usually associated with glandular epithelium that is recognized by monoclonal antibody B72.3.[165] The biological significance of that observation is unclear, but it represents a possible diagnostic pitfall.

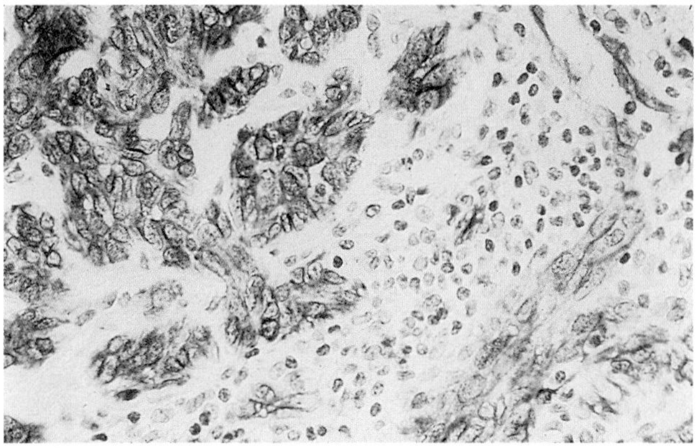

FIGURE 4.23 Reactivity with *Ulex europaeus I* agglutinin in epithelioid angiosarcoma.

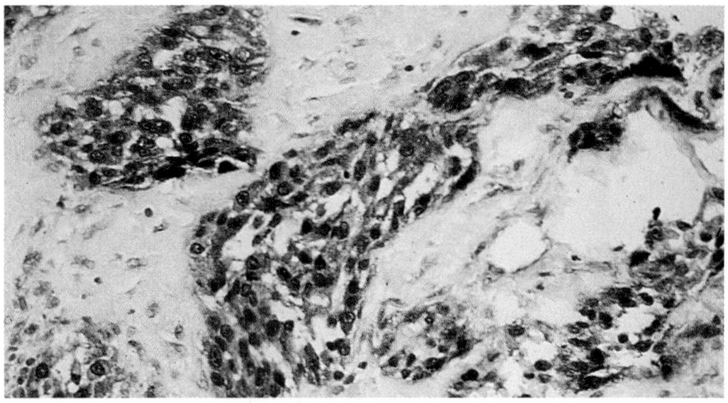

FIGURE 4.24 Clear cell sarcoma labels for S-100 protein in accord with the contention that it is a malignant melanoma of soft tissues.

KEY DIAGNOSTIC POINTS

Epithelioid Sarcoma/Synovial Sarcoma/ Angiosarcoma

- Keratin may be present in each entity.
- Angiosarcoma CD31+/FLI-1+; epithelioid sarcoma CD34+; synovial sarcoma negative for CD31/CD34/FLI-1.

Clear Cell Sarcoma

Clear cell sarcoma (CCS) was formerly thought to represent a primary soft tissue counterpart of cutaneous malignant melanoma. Nonetheless, it is now known that CCS exhibits a consistent and characteristic t(12;22) chromosomal translocation that is not shared by melanocytic lesions of the skin. This neoplasm is typified by an epithelioid and/or spindle cell constituency, with a delicate fibrovascular stroma and clear or lightly eosinophilic cytoplasm. Melanin pigmentation may or may not be observed.

The immunohistochemical attributes of CCS do largely mirror those of malignant melanoma. They include reactivity for vimentin, S-100 protein (Fig. 4.24), tyrosinase, MART-1, HMB-45, HMB-50, and microophthalmia transcription factor[445] (Fig. 4.25), together with the usual absence of EMA as well as

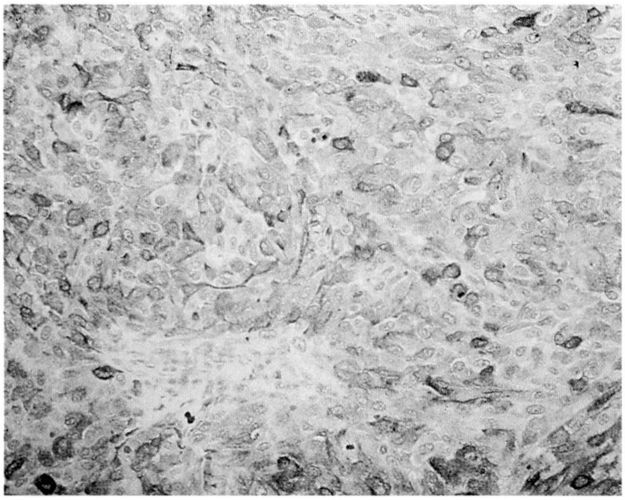

FIGURE 4.25 HMB-45 immunoreactivity in clear cell sarcoma.

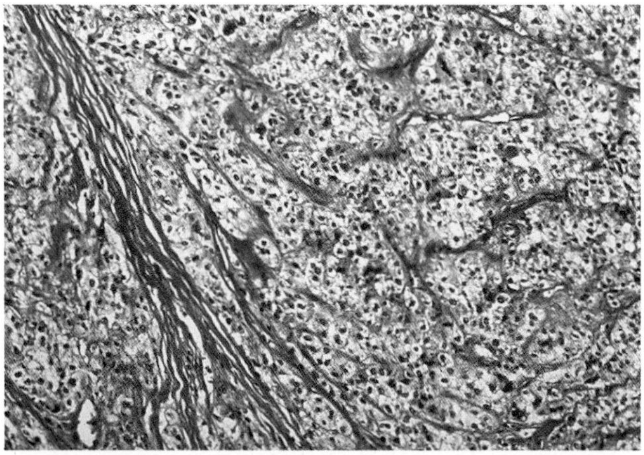

FIGURE 4.26 Epithelioid MPNST lacks distinguishing histologic features and requires intensive adjunctive study for proper diagnosis.

myogenous, neural, and endothelial markers. Generally, keratin is also lacking in CCSs, although one study reported that 29% were reactive for that marker.[446] Other reactants that are potentially seen in some CCS cases include CD56, CD57, synaptophysin, CD34, *HER2/neu* protein, CD117, and *c-met* protein.[447]

As stated, the t(12;22)(q13]2) translocation (yielding a hybrid EWS/ATF-1 gene) is characteristic of CCS.[448,449] Its presence can be evaluated by *in situ* hybridization methods as well as PCR-based technologies, providing a useful diagnostic adjunct to immunohistology.

Epithelioid Malignant Peripheral Nerve Sheath Tumors

Epithelioid MPNST is an extremely rare tumor variant that also has a histologic resemblance to melanoma, as well as metastatic carcinoma, CCS, and extrarenal rhabdoid tumor (Fig. 4.26). As a result, epithelioid MPNST is underrecognized as a diagnostic entity.

Labeling for S-100 protein is more frequently seen in epithelioid MPNSTs than in other forms of that tumor—at least 70% of cases, often with a strong and diffuse staining pattern.[450] The majority of these tumors are also reactive for NSE and protein gene product 9.5,[450,451] but CD56 and CD57 (Fig. 4.27) staining is less frequent. Despite their polygonal-cell appearance, cytokeratin and carcinoembryonic antigen are lacking in epithelioid MPNST; however, rare examples are positive for EMA. There is uniform nonreactivity for desmin, actin, UEAI, FLI-1, and CD31, allowing for exclusion of epithelioid leiomyosarcoma and angiosarcoma. Tyrosinase and HMB-45 staining is possible in a small minority of epithelioid MPNST cases, even if melanin pigmentation is absent.[452] However, the coexpression of CD56 or CD57 would argue against a diagnosis of CCS or melanoma in this setting. Another pertinent reactant in this differential diagnosis is PPN; Jokinen and colleagues have observed this marker in 75% of epithelioid MPNSTs, but not in melanomas.[453] INI1 is lost in 50% of epithelioid MPNST, whereas metastatic melanomas are consistently positive; this marker may be a useful diagnostic adjunct in a subset of cases.[349]

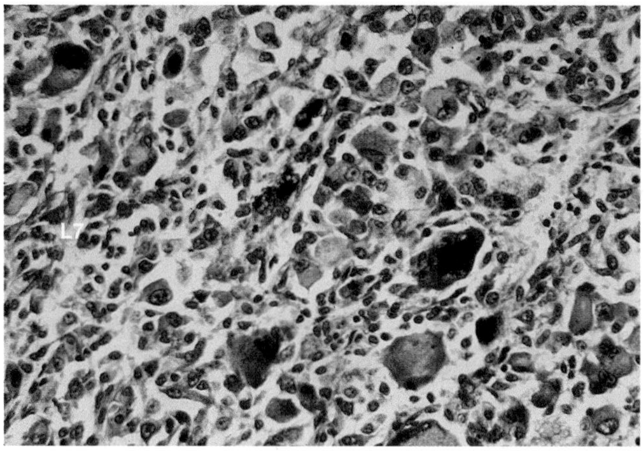

FIGURE 4.27 Reactivity for CD57 in epithelioid MPNST.

Sclerosing Epithelioid Fibrosarcoma

Sclerosing epithelioid fibrosarcoma (SEF) is a peculiar rare neoplasm that presents in deep soft tissue sites, and is intimately associated with fascial planes, the periosteum, or skeletal muscles.[454-456] It comprises small cords and nests of uniform small polygonal cells with clear cytoplasm, set in densely collagenized and hyalinized stroma that may have an osteoid-like configuration. SEFs also may contain areas that are morphologically characteristic of conventional fibrosarcomas, and some show storiform growth or myxoid zones as well. The differential diagnosis includes nodular fasciitis, myositis ossificans, desmoid tumors, hyalinized leiomyoma, sclerosing lymphoma, metastatic lobular breast carcinoma, ossifying fibromyxoid tumor, monophasic synovial sarcoma, clear cell sarcoma, extraosseous osteosarcoma, and extra-skeletal myxoid chondrosarcoma.

Immunohistochemical information on this entity is relatively limited.[454,457] Scattered tumor cells in roughly 50% of cases have stained weakly and focally for EMA. S-100 protein was found in 29% of cases, demonstrating a similarly focal pattern of immunoreactivity. Cytokeratin, NSE, CD45, HMB-45, CD68, and desmin were absent.[454] It is our estimation that the value of immunohistology in defining SEF is as yet unsettled.

Epithelioid Leiomyosarcoma

Epithelioid features are known to occur in smooth muscle tumors, usually as a focal finding but occasionally as the predominant pattern. Such tumors have previously been designated as *leiomyoblastomas,* but current information indicates that even relatively bland tumors in the soft tissue may have metastatic potential. Thus, the term *epithelioid LMS* is preferred for those lesions with any degree of mitotic activity and cellular atypia.

In our experience with 10 examples of epithelioid LMS, either muscle-specific actin or desmin was detected in each instance; however, only three of the lesions were reactive for both muscle-specific actin and desmin. This observation parallels the findings of other investigators[458] and probably reflects ultrastructural evidence of only poorly developed myofilamentous structures in many of these tumors. Epithelioid LMS is uniformly nonreactive for nonmyogenous markers; none has displayed reactivity for S-100 protein, cytokeratin, EMA, UEAI lectin, vWF, CD31, or carcinoembryonic antigen.[458,459] We have also observed staining for caldesmon, calponin, and alpha–smooth muscle actin among our cases. When an intra-abdominal lesion is encountered, the differential diagnosis with epithelioid GIST must be carefully considered because GIST is much more common than epithelioid LMS at that site.

Alveolar Soft Part Sarcoma

Controversy has existed over the line of cellular differentiation in alveolar soft part sarcoma (ASPS) ever since its seminal description in 1952. Despite attempts to prove a neuroectodermal or endocrine nature for this tumor, more recent studies have endorsed a myogenous phenotype.

The presence of immunoreactivity for several muscle-associated proteins such as desmin, actins, myosin, Z-band protein, and the MM isozyme of creatine kinase in ASPS provides compelling evidence that it demonstrates muscular differentiation. However, whether or not it is a form of rhabdomyosarcoma is still open to question.[25,105,460-462] In that specific regard, both alpha-sarcomeric actin and alpha–smooth muscle actin have been described in this lesion.[463-465]

Other studies of ASPS have evaluated the presence of Myo-D1 and myogenin.[464,466,467] Most analyses have found a complete absence of nuclear staining for Myo-D1.[468,469] Granular cytoplasmic reactivity with the Myo-D1 antibody 5.8A has been found in the majority of cases of ASPS but is regarded as a reproducible nonspecific artifact.

In our experience with ten cases, there has been no labeling for NSE, CD57, cytokeratin, chromogranin, S100 protein, EMA, vWF, CD31, UEAI, or carcinoembryonic antigen in ASPS. Melanocyte-specific markers are also absent in this neoplasm.[461]

As discussed above, a selective marker of the der (17) t(X;17) translocation of ASPS is now available; namely, nuclear TFE 3 protein.[470] Nonetheless, this determinant also may be encountered in metastatic translocation-type renal cell carcinoma and some PEComas.[471,472] Hence, caution is advisable against diagnostic overreliance on TFE3.

PLEOMORPHIC TUMORS OF SOFT TISSUE

Soft tissue sarcomas with a potentially pleomorphic histologic appearance (Fig. 4.28; see Table 4.7) include so-called MFH (undifferentiated pleomorphic sarcoma), pleomorphic rhabdomyosarcoma, pleomorphic or dedifferentiated liposarcoma, dedifferentiated LMS, and pleomorphic MPNST.

Malignant Fibrous Histiocytoma

In the past, malignant fibrous histiocytoma (MFH) has been defined by its histologic pattern with little reference to immunophenotype. Reactivity for various proteases (Fig. 4.29) and ferritin has been associated with the conclusion that MFH shows fibrohistiocytic differentiation, in accord with its original description; however, modern analyses have called this contention into serious question. Roholl and colleagues suggested that the immunophenotype of MFH was most closely allied to that of myofibroblasts.[473] Their observations have been supported by other analyses that identified subpopulations of muscle-specific actin-, and desmin-reactive cells in MFH,[474] together with ultrastructural data showing the presence of myofibroblast-like characteristics in neoplastic cells.[475]

If one chooses to continue using the term *MFH,* however, it is best defined tightly and immunophenotypically by the presence of vimentin in the absence of any lineage-specific markers.[476] It has become clear that MFH-like areas may evolve in tumors that are otherwise typical examples of neurogenic, myogenic, or lipoblastic lesions.[474,476] This observation gives credence to the suggestion that some examples of MFH reflect a common final pathway of clonal evolution (erroneously called *dedifferentiation*) in soft tissue sarcomas of other types.[477, 478] This hypothesis also has inverse support from cell culture studies and implantation of tumors into nude mice. Phenotypically uniform examples of MFH have developed other immunoprofiles once they were explanted; some exhibited a myogenic pattern, whereas others acquired neural or even epithelial characteristics.[479] Yet another contextual issue is whether or not the term *MFH* is preferable to pleomorphic high-grade sarcoma, not further specified, or pleomorphic (myo)fibrosarcoma.[476, 478, 480] The latter two designations are more supportable scientifically, but MFH still enjoys diagnostic usage nonetheless.

Pleomorphic Leiomyosarcoma

The previous discussion is especially apropos to the consideration of whether or not another tumor—pleomorphic leiomyosarcoma (PLMS)—can be defined as different from MFH. As described, PLMS is said to be immunoreactive for desmin or MSA or alpha-isoform actin,[481] all of which may be seen in myofibroblastic elements as well (as in MFH). For now, a working definition of PLMS might require that positivity for at least two smooth muscle markers be observed. However, this stipulation is still not absolutely exclusionary with

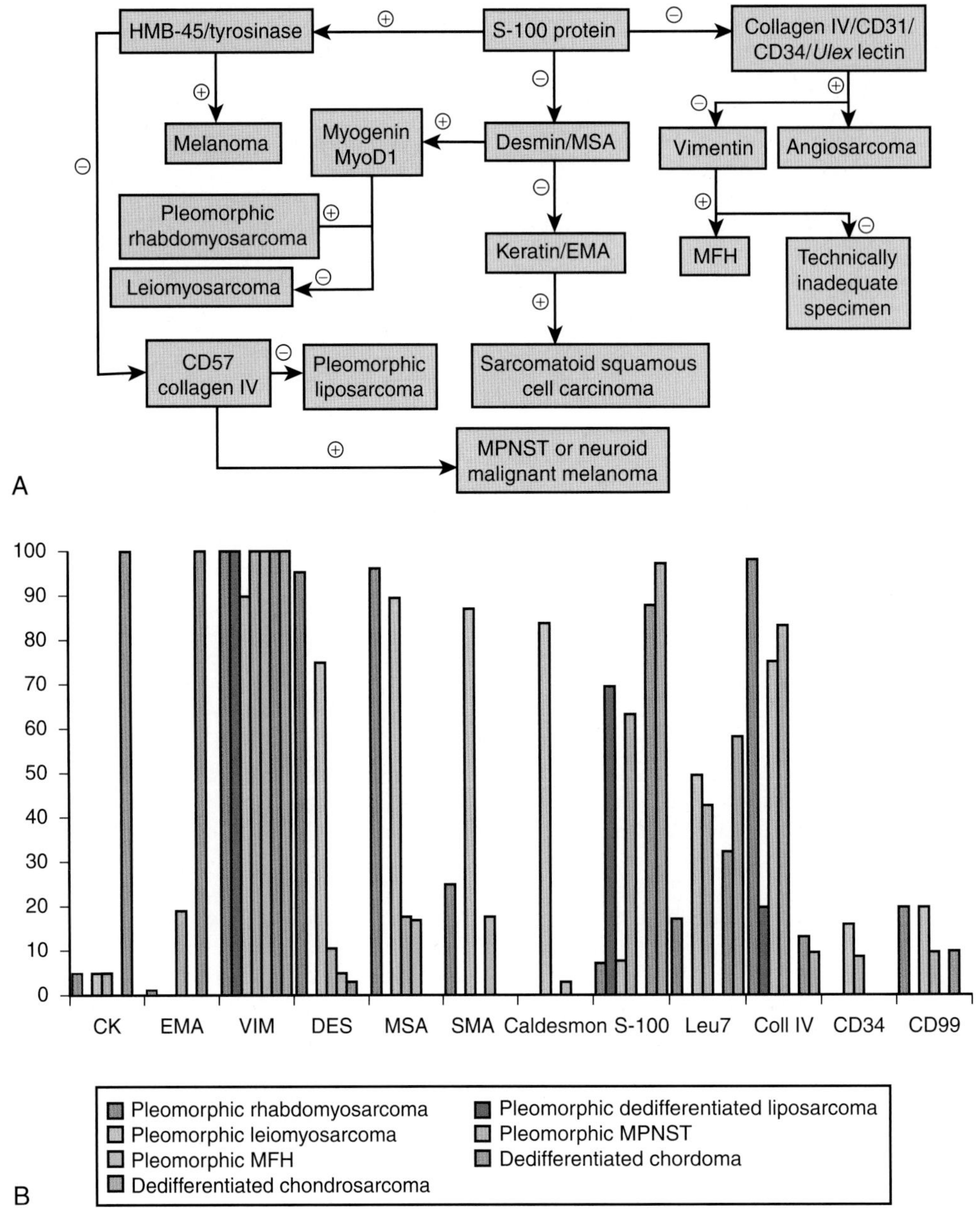

FIGURE 4.28 **(A)** Algorithmic immunohistologic diagnosis of malignant pleomorphic tumors. **(B)** Graphic representation of the frequency of reactivity for pleomorphic tumors against commonly used immunoreactants. MSA, muscle-specific actin; EMA, epithelial membrane antigen; MFH, malignant fibrous histiocytoma; MPNST, malignant peripheral nerve sheath tumor; CK, cytokeratin; VIM, vimentin; DES, desmin; SMA, smooth muscle actin.

regard to other diagnostic possibilities in the pleomorphic sarcoma group.

Pleomorphic Rhabdomyosarcoma

Among the various forms of rhabdomyosarcoma, the pleomorphic type is the most uncommon and is seen almost exclusively in adults (Fig. 4.30). This tumor is relatively easy to diagnose immunohistochemically because of the uniform presence of desmin, muscle-specific or sarcomeric actins, myosin, or myoglobin (Fig. 4.31).[482] These proteins can be detected in characteristic large strap cells in pleomorphic rhabdomyosarcoma (PRMS), and they are present in spindle-cell or epithelioid foci. Myogenin is typically positive in only scattered cells, unlike pediatric rhabdomyosarcomas, which generally show more extensive reactivity for this marker. PRMS lacks S-100 protein, CD56, CD57, and myelin basic protein. If present, any of these four markers would instead raise the possibility of pleomorphic MPNST.

Pleomorphic and Dedifferentiated Liposarcomas

Pleomorphic liposarcoma resembles MFH except for the regular interspersion of neoplastic lipoblasts, which may be of the mulberry or signet-ring cell type, but are commonly highly pleomorphic. The degree of lipoblastic differentiation in such tumors is highly variable. On the other hand, dedifferentiated liposarcoma has a composite histologic appearance in which pleomorphic MFH-like foci are juxtaposed to well-differentiated forms of liposarcoma. The dedifferentiated image is most often

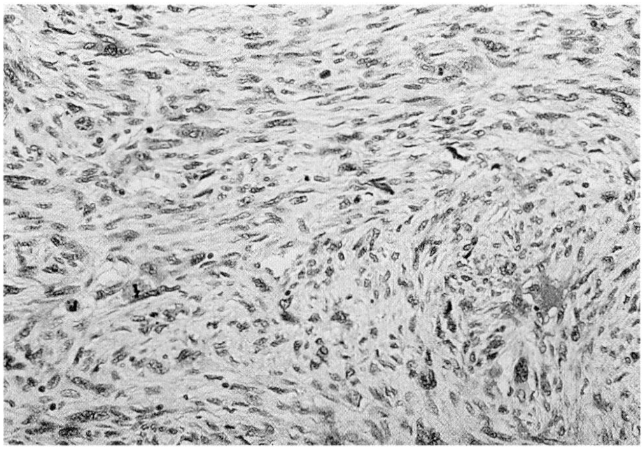

FIGURE 4.29 MFH labels for several determinants that are associated with mononuclear phagocytic cells, such as $alpha_1$-antichymotrypsin, as shown here. However, those markers are completely non-specific, and it is much more important to undertake systematic *elimination* of several lineage-related markers as the first step in the diagnosis of MFH.

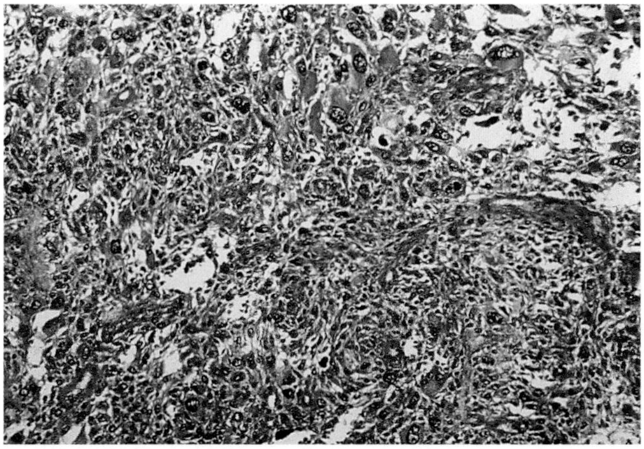

FIGURE 4.30 Pleomorphic rhabdomyosarcoma, shown here, is often indistinguishable from MFH on conventional morphologic studies.

seen in recurrences, reflecting overgrowth of the lesion by a secondary neoplastic clone of primitive mesenchymal cells. Along these lines, when a pleomorphic or heterogeneous sarcoma is seen in retroperitoneal or intra-abdominal locations, since dedifferentiated liposarcoma is overwhelmingly the most likely diagnosis, the tumor should be sampled (if needed, extensively) to identify a well-differentiated adipocytic component. It should not be unexpected that pleomorphic and dedifferentiated liposarcomas manifest immunoreactivity patterns like those of MFH.[230] Indeed, using data on MDM2 and CDK4 that were obtained from immunohistochemistry, *in situ* hybridization, and the polymerase chain reaction, Coindre and colleagues have concluded that inflammatory MFH and dedifferentiated liposarcoma are one and the same lesion.[483] Nevertheless, unlike MFH, pleomorphic liposarcomas may demonstrate focal labeling for S-100 protein in their lipoblastic elements.[484] As mentioned earlier in this discussion, dedifferentiated liposarcomas often show strong nuclear expression of MDM2, usually with CDK4.[485] The high mobility group A2

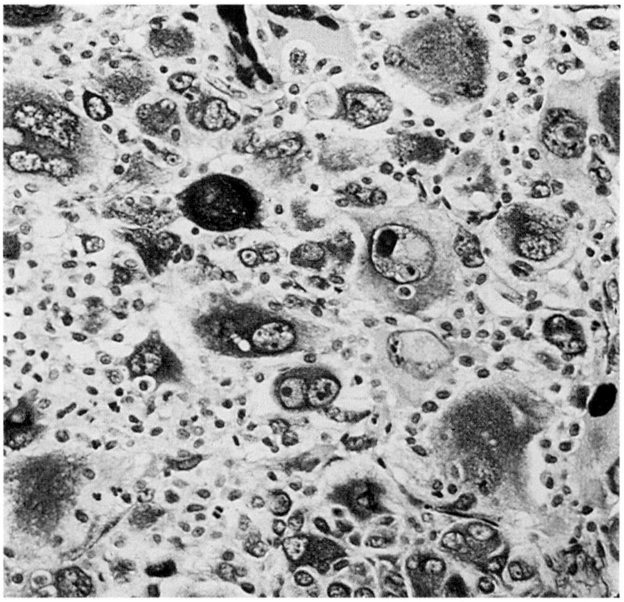

FIGURE 4.31 Reactivity for myoglobin in pleomorphic rhabdomyosarcoma.

(HMGA2) protein is another intranuclear architectural transcription factor that is also overexpressed in dedifferentiated liposarcoma, more often than CDK4.[486] Such tumors are typically nonreactive for epithelial, Schwann-cell related, and myogenic markers.

Pleomorphic Malignant Peripheral Nerve Sheath Tumor

Malignant peripheral nerve sheath tumor (MPNST) may likewise assume a pleomorphic appearance. In most instances, that tumor variant shows patterns of reactivity for S-100 protein, CD56, CD57, and collagen type IV that are superimposable with those of better differentiated (spindle cell) MPNSTs.[487] In the absence of focal S-100 protein expression and foci with conventional appearances, it is very difficult (if not impossible) to render this diagnosis with certainty. Unlike spindle cell variants of MPNST, pleomorphic subtypes have not been shown to be desmin-reactive.

Other Primary Neoplasms of Soft Tissue

Some primary tumors of the soft tissues do not fit neatly into one of the foregoing categories. Malignant extrarenal rhabdoid tumor, chordoma, extraosseous myxoid chondrosarcoma (chordoid sarcoma), extraskeletal osteosarcoma, and selected liposarcoma and angiosarcoma variants are included in this group.

GRANULAR CELL ANGIOSARCOMA

The granular cell variant of angiosarcoma is extremely rare (Fig. 4.32).[488] Immunohistochemical analysis demonstrates positivity for UEAI, CD31, FLI-1, and CD34 in this lesion, confirming its endothelial nature. CD68 positivity is also apparent, reflecting the lysosomal nature

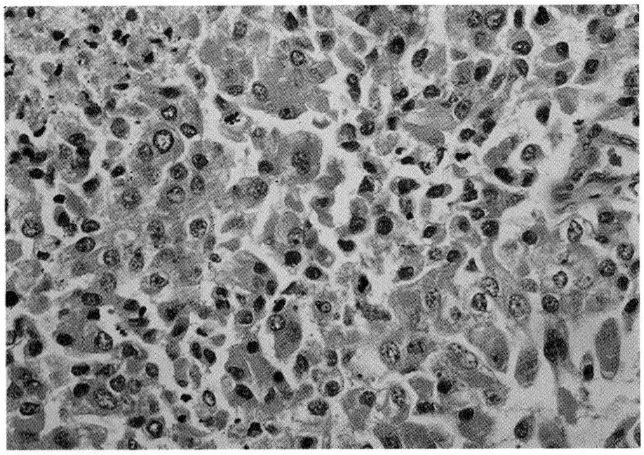

FIGURE 4.32 Granular cell angiosarcoma is an uncommon lesion with a differential diagnosis that includes granular cell tumor, metastatic melanoma, and epithelioid leiomyosarcoma.

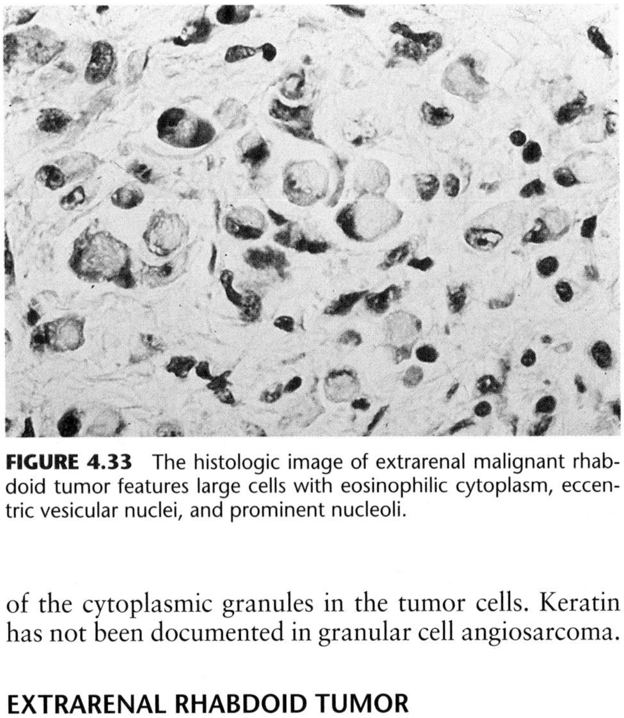

FIGURE 4.33 The histologic image of extrarenal malignant rhabdoid tumor features large cells with eosinophilic cytoplasm, eccentric vesicular nuclei, and prominent nucleoli.

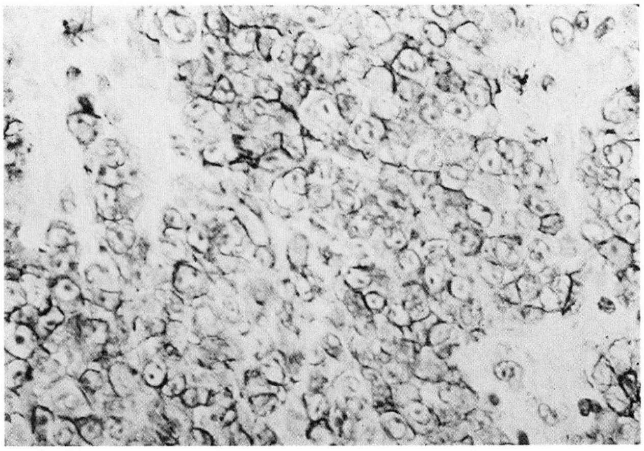

FIGURE 4.34 Epithelial membrane antigen may be seen in extrarenal rhabdoid tumor, potentially causing confusion with variants of epithelioid sarcoma or metastatic carcinoma.

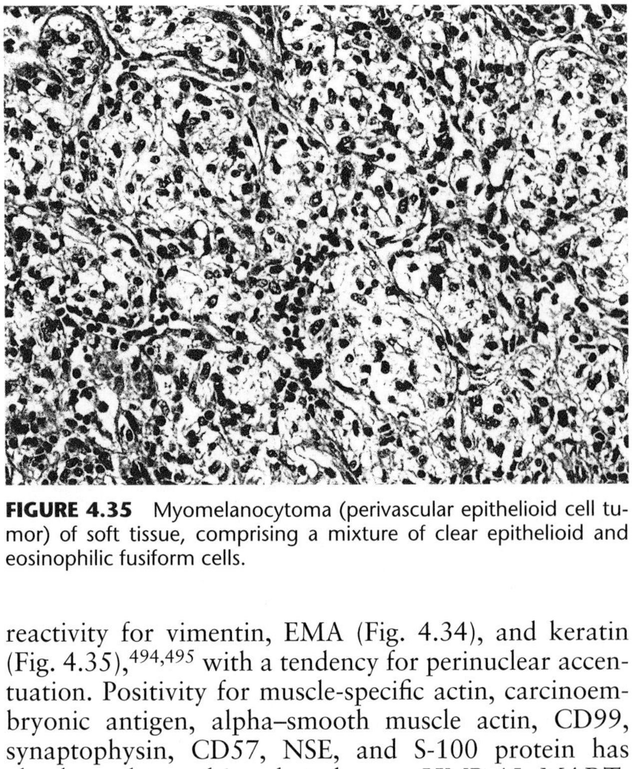

FIGURE 4.35 Myomelanocytoma (perivascular epithelioid cell tumor) of soft tissue, comprising a mixture of clear epithelioid and eosinophilic fusiform cells.

of the cytoplasmic granules in the tumor cells. Keratin has not been documented in granular cell angiosarcoma.

EXTRARENAL RHABDOID TUMOR

Tumors that are histologically identical to malignant rhabdoid tumor of the kidney in children may be encountered in a variety of extrarenal sites in adults, including the soft tissues.[489] The hallmarks of these neoplasms are hyaline paranuclear cytoplasmic eosinophilic inclusions; eccentric, rounded nuclei with vesicular chromatin; prominent nucleoli (Fig. 4.33); and a complex immunophenotype.

Extrarenal rhabdoid tumors (ERTs) often show epithelial differentiation, and some may be difficult—if not impossible—to separate diagnostically from such entities as proximal-type epithelioid sarcoma.[490-493] INI1, a protein encoded by a gene at chromosome 22q11.2, is involved in chromatin remodeling; it is usually absent in both ERT and proximal epithelioid sarcoma, as well as conventional (distal) epithelioid sarcoma.[349,492] The majority of tumors in each category also show reactivity for vimentin, EMA (Fig. 4.34), and keratin (Fig. 4.35),[494,495] with a tendency for perinuclear accentuation. Positivity for muscle-specific actin, carcinoembryonic antigen, alpha–smooth muscle actin, CD99, synaptophysin, CD57, NSE, and S-100 protein has also been detected in selected cases. HMB-45, MART-1, chromogranin, myoglobin, and CD34 are absent. On the other hand, a report by Izumi and colleagues suggested that dysadherin, a membrane glycoprotein concerned with intercellular adhesion, is present in epithelioid sarcoma but not in ERT.[496] Poorly differentiated malignant neoplasms of various types may on occasion show rhabdoid cytomorphology, including melanomas, mesotheliomas, and carcinomas. Although the immunophenotype of ERT overlaps those of other sarcomas and poorly differentiated carcinomas, the morphologic appearance of this tumor is generally sufficiently distinct for accurate diagnosis. Demonstrating loss of INI1 protein expression strongly supports ERT over metastatic carcinoma, although it does not distinguish the former from epithelioid sarcoma.

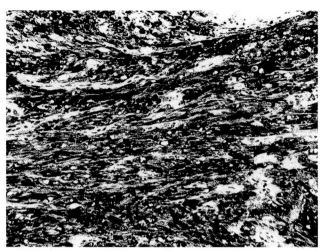

FIGURE 4.36 Diffuse immunoreactivity for HMB-45 in myomelanocytoma.

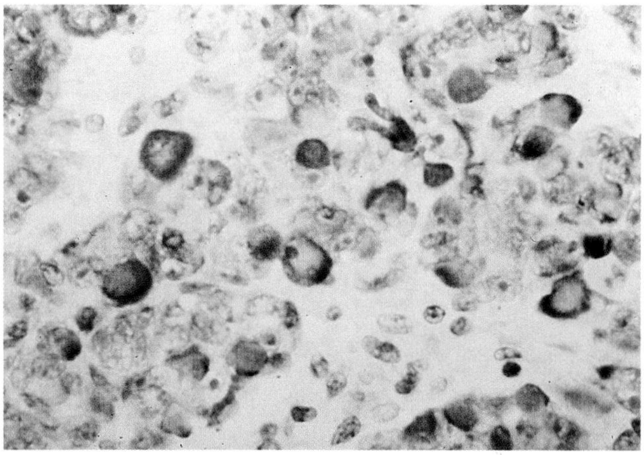

FIGURE 4.37 Keratin in rhabdoid tumor, raising diagnostic concern for another type of soft tissue sarcoma or metastatic carcinoma.

PERIVASCULAR EPITHELIOID-CELL TUMORS, MYOMELANOCYTOMAS, AND EPITHELIOID ANGIOMYOLIPOMAS

Perivascular epithelioid-cell tumors, myomelanocytomas, and epithelioid angiomyolipomas (PEComas) are a peculiar family of neoplasms with conjoint differentiation toward smooth muscle cells and melanocytes. They are represented by lesions in the lungs, kidneys, gynecological tract, liver, pancreas, gut, urinary tract, and soft tissue. They are variously called perivascular epithelioid-cell tumors, myomelanocytomas, or epithelioid angiomyolipomas (when involving the kidney or liver).[497] Clear to pale eosinophilic and granular epithelioid cells and eosinophilic spindle cells are admixed in such neoplasms, occasionally with adipocytes and multinucleated giant cells (Fig. 4.36). As such, differential diagnostic considerations may include pure smooth muscle tumors and clear-cell sarcomas, among others. PEComas commonly label for vimentin and CD1a,[498] as well as potential smooth muscle markers (alpha-isoform actin; muscle-specific actin; desmin; caldesmon; calponin; smooth-muscle myosin), together with indicators of melanocytic differentiation (HMB-45; MART-1; tyrosinase; microophthalmia transcription factor) (Fig. 4.37). S-100 protein expression is uncommon. Keratin, TFE3 protein, and CD117 also may be observed in some instances; CD34 is absent.[499] In the deep soft tissue, these lesions show a range of clinical behavior ranging from benign to very aggressive; minimal histologic criteria for malignancy are only beginning to be established.

LIPOSARCOMA VARIANTS

Liposarcoma is easily recognized by most pathologists in its prototypical differentiated forms. Nevertheless, myxoid and round cell variants of this neoplasm often contain few if any discernible lipoblasts and may therefore be difficult to identify.

Myxoid liposarcoma (MLPS) expresses vimentin and S-100 protein, with the latter usually confined to lipoblastic elements. In addition, a subset of tumors with the characteristic t(12;16) of MLPS may also express desmin, muscle-specific actin, and alpha–smooth muscle actin focally.[500] CD34 and CD56 are not detectable, but some examples of MLPS have expressed CD57 in our experience.

Round cell liposarcoma is a morphologic variant of high grade MLPS that may resemble extraskeletal chondrosarcoma, cellular peripheral nerve sheath tumors, or even metastatic poorly differentiated carcinomas. S-100 protein and vimentin are seen in all these tumor types. MPNSTs that are similar microscopically to round cell liposarcoma may express CD56 or myelin basic protein, unlike adipocytic lesions.

As mentioned earlier in this discussion, CDK4 and MDM2 immunostains can be utilized to help confirm the adipocytic nature of some problematic soft tissue tumors (namely, dedifferentiated liposarcoma). However, de Vreeze and colleagues have shown that MLPS and round-cell liposarcoma of the extremities typically lack these determinants immunohistochemically.[501] This reflects the fact that such lesions manifest karyotypic abnormalities that are different from well-differentiated and dedifferentiated liposarcomas.[502]

The type 1 TLS/CHOP chimeric transcript is a result of the above-mentioned t(12;16) and is a very sensitive and specific molecular alteration for the myxoid/round cell liposarcoma entity.[503] Oikawa and colleagues have developed a monoclonal antibody to this fusion transcript, which they claim is highly specific and sensitive with formalin-fixed paraffin-embedded tissue.[504] However, there is no literature on its use. As a diagnostic tool, this is a good example of a genomic application of IHC.

CHONDROID TUMORS OF SOFT TISSUE AND BONE

Chordoma

Chordoma is a malignant tumor with notochord-like differentiation that principally occurs in apposition to the axial skeleton; peripheral lesions are extremely rare.[505,506] Differential diagnosis includes metastatic

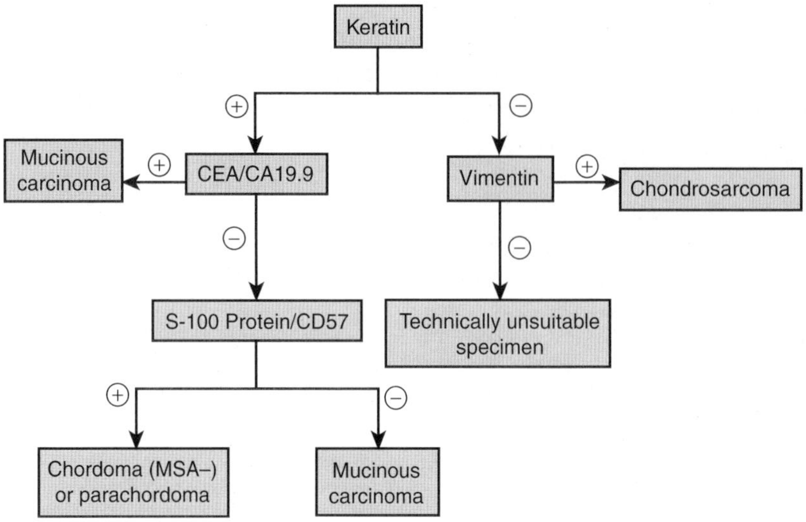

FIGURE 4.38 Algorithmic immunohistologic diagnosis of chordoid and mucomyxoid soft tissue tumors.

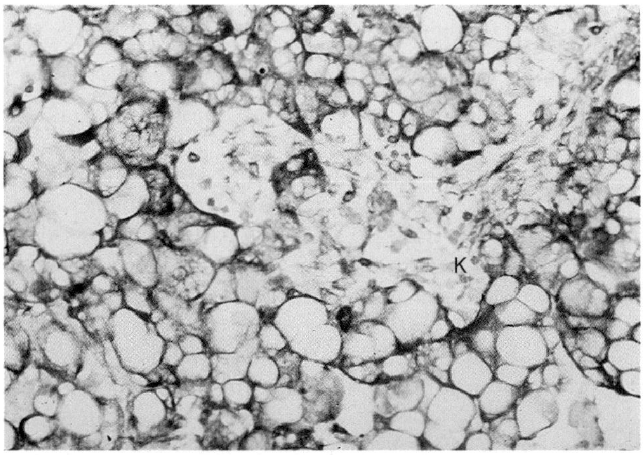

FIGURE 4.39 Reactivity for keratin+ in chordoma.

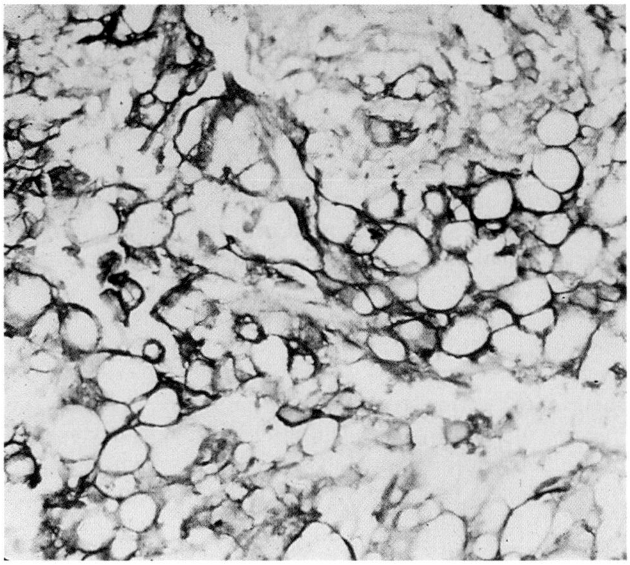

FIGURE 4.40 Immunoreactivity for epithelial membrane antigen in chordoma.

adenocarcinoma (especially renal cell carcinoma), chondrosarcoma, myxopapillary ependymoma, and hemangioendotheliomas.[507]

The uniform presence of keratin in chordoma confirms its epithelial nature. The subtypes of keratin proteins in this neoplasm potentially include CK1, CK5, CK8, CK10, CK14 to 16, CK18, and CK19, with CK5 predominating (Figs. 4.38, 4.39).[508]

With regard to differential diagnosis, chordoma also characteristically expresses EMA (Fig. 4.40)[509,510] as well as HBME-1, another glycoproteinaceous cell membrane antigen that is typically absent in metastatic renal cell carcinoma.[19] Chondrosarcoma is uniformly negative for epithelial markers, but it shares S-100 protein expression. Moreover, N-cadherin is virtually always expressed by chordoma but only rarely by chondrosarcoma. Conversely, Huse and associates have shown that low-grade chondroid lesions of the skull base are PPN-positive, whereas chordoma is not.[511] A recent study has demonstrated that brachyury, a transcription factor involved in notochord development, is uniformly expressed in chordomas, but not in cartilaginous neoplasms.[512] Some hemangioendotheliomas have the ability for cytokeratin synthesis, but they exhibit reactivity for CD31 and FLI-1 and lack S-100 protein. Finally, ependymomas are positive for GFAP,[507] unlike the other differential diagnostic possibilities discussed here.

In 1973, Heffelfinger and associates described a particular variant of chordoma with cartilaginous areas that simulated the appearance of chondrosarcoma.[513,514] They designated these lesions as *chondroid chordomas* and suggested that they had a better prognosis than that of conventional chordoma. Despite morphologic differences, the immunohistochemical staining pattern of chondroid chordoma is basically identical to that seen in classical forms of this tumor.[510,514-516]

In dedifferentiated chordoma (Fig. 4.41), a secondary anaplastic component emerges with the basic immunophenotype of MFH.[517,518] Nonetheless, occasional S-100 protein–positive cells may persist in the new clonal population; cytokeratin-positive constituents are

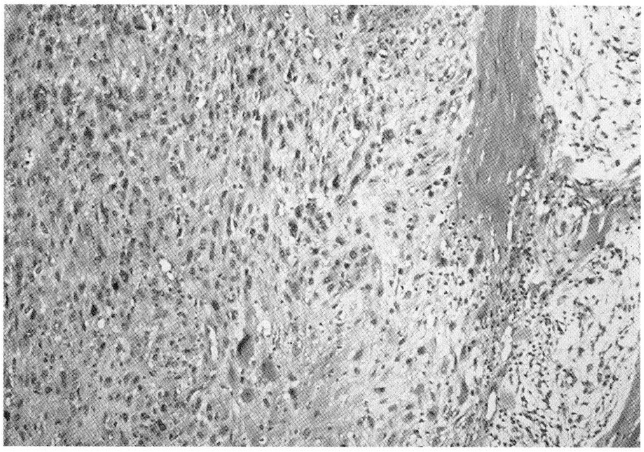

FIGURE 4.41 Rare examples of chordoma undergo anaplastic transformation (dedifferentiation), in which the undifferentiated foci acquire an immunophenotype that is closely similar to that of MFH.

less commonly retained in the dedifferentiated areas (Fig. 4.42). Divergent mesenchymal differentiation may also be encountered.[519]

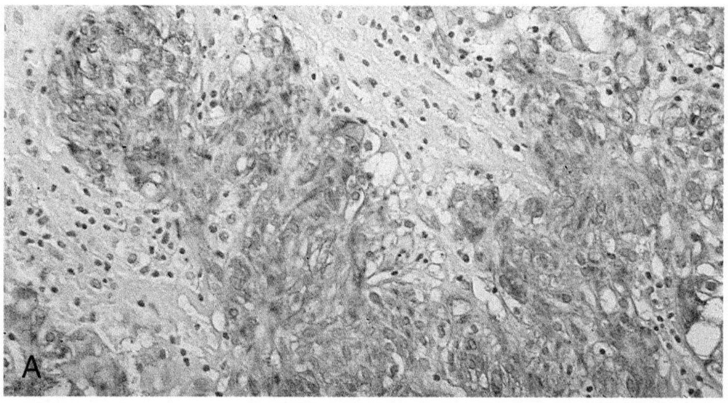

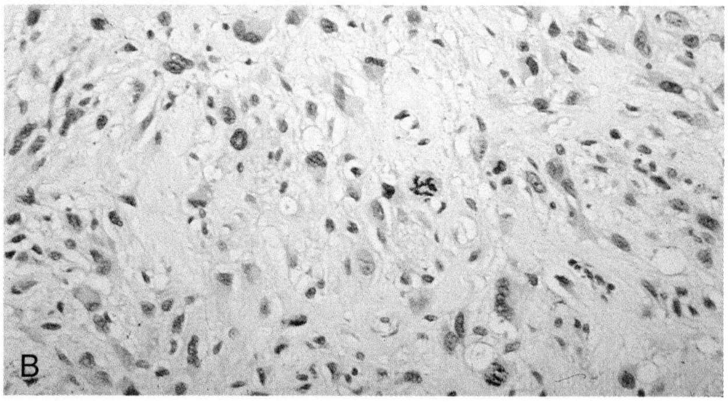

FIGURE 4.42 Reactivity for keratin in well-differentiated areas **(A)** of dedifferentiated chordoma, and negativity for the same marker **(B)** in anaplastic foci.

KEY DIAGNOSTIC POINTS

Chordoma

- Chordoma typically CK+, S-100+, HMBE-1+
- Differential diagnosis includes metastatic renal cell carcinoma (HBME-1–), chondrosarcoma (CK–), myxopapillary ependymoma (GFAP+), and hemangioendothelioma (CD31+/FLI-1+).

Myoepithelioma (Including Parachordoma and Related Tumors)

Soft tissue myoepitheliomas and their malignant counterparts (myoepithelial carcinomas) are uncommon tumors that usually arise in the extremities, either in subcutaneous or in deep soft tissues.[520,521] They characteristically exhibit a lobulated growth pattern, often contain myxoid stroma, and show a reticular, trabecular, or nested architecture. The constituent cells in myoepithelial tumors show the same range of morphologic features seen in their salivary gland counterparts (epithelioid, spindled, plasmacytoid/hyaline, or clear). Intratumoral heterogeneity in terms of both architecture and cytology is common. At one end of the morphologic spectrum is the rare lesion also known as *parachordoma,* which is composed of large epithelioid cells with abundant eosinophilic to clear, vacuolated cytoplasm.[17,18] The differential diagnosis for this group of lesions primarily centers on extraskeletal myxoid chondrosarcoma and the very rare peripheral chordoma (chordoma periphericum); however, chondroid lipoma, ossifying fibromyxoid tumor, and subcutaneous myxopapillary ependymoma may be considered as well. Myoepithelial tumors have a distinct immunoprofile that differs from that of extraskeletal myxoid chondrosarcoma. Myoepithelial tumors (including parachordoma) are typically positive for CK8 and CK18, EMA, S-100 protein, type IV collagen, and vimentin, and may express glial fibrillary acidic protein.[17,18,520-525] In contrast, extraskeletal myxoid chondrosarcoma lacks keratin 17 and is infrequently positive for S-100 protein and collagen type IV. Similar to myoepithelioma, ossifying fibromyxoid tumor usually shows reactivity for S-100 protein, but desmin expression, which is relatively common in the latter tumor type, is rare in myoepithelial tumors. Ossifying fibromyxoid tumor is generally negative for EMA and keratin.

On the other hand, myoepithelioma/parachordoma and peripheral chordoma may show considerable immunophenotypic overlap in reference to keratin subtypes, EMA, vimentin, S-100 protein, and collagen type IV. In fact, Scolyer and coworkers concluded that these tumor types could not always be separated from one another immunohistologically.[526] A recent study suggested that brachyury expression may distinguish chordoma from myoepithelial tumors.[527]

Chondroblastoma

Chondroblastoma is an infrequently encountered entity in the soft tissues.[528] It may be confused with giant cell reparative granulomas and giant cell tumors. Chondroblastoma is usually strongly reactive for vimentin, NSE, and S-100 protein, whereas its specified diagnostic alternatives lack the latter two markers.[529-531] In particular, the proliferating stromal cells in chondroblastomas show strong S-100 protein positivity, facilitating their distinction from giant cell tumor of bone and reparative granulomas.[531,532]

Aberrant cytokeratin expression is a potential feature of chondroblastoma.[531,533] Mononuclear chondroblastic tumor cells are negative for CD68.[530,534] A subset of chondroblastomas is said to show cytoplasmic muscle-specific actin positivity.[169]

Extraskeletal Myxoid Chondrosarcoma (Chordoid Sarcoma)

Although skeletal and extraskeletal myxoid chondrosarcomas share similar morphologic features, there are fundamental differences between these tumors at ultrastructural and molecular levels of analysis, which suggests that they represent distinct and separate entities. Extraskeletal myxoid chondrosarcoma (EMC) demonstrates a reciprocal t(9;22) chromosomal translocation that results in fusion of the EWS and CHN genes.[536-538] Immunohistochemically, it is at most only focally reactive for S-100 protein (in <20% of cases) and CD57, whereas skeletal chondrosarcomas of the myxoid type diffusely label for those determinants. Keratin is absent in both of those chondrosarcoma variants; E-cadherin and N-cadherin are also lacking.[86] An occasionally reported peculiarity in the immunophenotype of EMC is a putative tendency to show occult neuroendocrine differentiation, as represented by reactivity for synaptophysin or chromogranin.[539-541] The reasons for this finding are unknown.

Clear Cell Chondrosarcoma

Clear cell chondrosarcoma (CCC) is an uncommon subtype—especially in the soft tissues—with special clinicopathologic features and a relatively good prognosis.[542] The histologic pattern of this neoplasm features the presence of clear polygonal cells that are arranged in lobules with prominent zones of metaplastic ossification and scattered areas resembling the image of chondroblastoma. The tumor cells of CCC are reactive for S-100 protein, vimentin, CD57, and lysozyme.[537] Some examples also show strong ONN staining, unlike the profiles of conventional chondrosarcoma and mesenchymal chondrosarcoma.[543,544]

OTHER TUMORS SEEN IN SOFT TISSUE AND BONE

Osteosarcoma

Osteosarcoma is highly unusual outside the skeletal system. Like their intraosseous counterparts, extraskeletal osteosarcomas have a variety of histologic patterns, including fibroblastic, chondroblastic, small-cell, and telangiectatic images.

Immunohistochemical studies of these neoplasms have revealed few characteristic features and are used primarily to help exclude other lesions that are under pathologic consideration. Extraskeletal osteosarcomas are reactive for vimentin, and their matrical elements often label for CD57. Alpha-smooth muscle actin may be seen focally, and a subset of tumors is said to coexpress desmin,[545] perhaps representing myofibroblastic differentiation. S-100 protein is usually observed only in areas with overtly cartilaginous differentiation.[545] Epithelial markers are only exceptionally present.[545-547] GFAP and neurofilament proteins are absent.

Strong labeling for the osseous isozyme of alkaline phosphatase has been used in the past to distinguish extraskeletal osteosarcoma from other pleomorphic sarcomas. The major drawback of this marker is that it must be assessed using cryostat sections or imprint smears; paraffin sections are unsuitable for study.

The bone matrix proteins ONN and osteocalcin have generated much interest, but their efficacy in identifying osteosarcoma still needs further substantiation. Positive stains for ONN have been seen in the neoplastic components of osteosarcoma and osteoblastoma, but labeling of the mononuclear cells in giant cell tumors and chondroblastomas likewise has been observed.[248] Some pleomorphic and fibrosarcomatous osteosarcomas react focally for ONN as well.[548] The latter finding may relate to the fact that ONN production is an early event in osteoblastic differentiation. Overall, the reported specificity of immunoreactivity for ONN and OCN is roughly 40% and 95%, respectively, for the diagnosis of a bone-forming tumor.[241,242] Those two markers may be useful as part of a panel of immunostains to corroborate a diagnosis of extraskeletal osteosarcoma, but identification of osteoid matrix associated with the constituent malignant cells remains the sine qua non of diagnosis.

Giant Cell Tumors of Bone and Soft Tissue

Giant cell tumors of bone are potentially locally aggressive neoplasms that typically involve the epiphyses or proximal metaphyses of long tubular bones. Morphologically similar lesions may also arise rarely as primary lesions in the subcutis or deep soft tissue.[549,550] The terms *giant-cell tumor of soft parts*, *malignant giant-cell tumor of soft parts*, and *MFH of the giant cell type* have been used to refer to extraosseous giant cell neoplasms of the deep soft tissues, as distinguished from tenosynovial giant cell tumors (giant cell tumors of tendon sheath). Their immunohistochemical profiles, however, are comparable.

Immunohistochemical studies of these tumors have focused mainly on the nature of their constituent mononuclear-stromal and multinucleate giant cells. The osteoclast-like giant cells usually stain strongly for CD68[551-555]; however, mononuclear elements label much more weakly for that marker. The stromal cells also are potentially positive for alpha–smooth muscle actin, but they lack CD45, S-100 protein, desmin, and lysozyme.[551,553] Recent reports have suggested that p63 expression may distinguish these forms of giant cell tumor from some of their histologic mimics, in particular tenosynovial giant cell tumors (giant cell tumor of tendon sheath and diffuse-type giant cell tumor) and aneurysmal bone cyst.[556,557] The occurrence of vascular invasion in some giant cell tumors has prompted interest in their synthesis of matrix metalloproteinases (MMPs) and tissue inhibitors of metalloproteinases (TIMPs). It is thought that these molecules influence the invasiveness of tumor cells. MMP-9 (gelatinase B) is expressed in the multinucleated cells of giant cell tumors, but only focally in their mononuclear elements.[551,458,459] A relative increase in TIMP expression as compared with that of MMPs has been seen in recurrent and metastatic giant cell tumors in selected studies.[551,560]

Adamantinoma

Adamantinoma of long bones is a rare neoplasm that is principally seen in the mid-tibia in young adults. In classic form, it is part of a lesional continuum with a disorder known as osteofibrous dysplasia (Campanacci disease).[561,562] Nests of compact epithelioid or squamoid cells are seen, irregularly disposed throughout a cellular stroma (Fig. 4.43). This tumor has variously been considered as an endothelial proliferation or an epithelial lesion in the past, but it is now clear that the latter interpretation is correct. All examples of adamantinoma are reactive for cytokeratin, with keratin-14 and keratin-19 predominating (Fig. 4.44).[563-567] On the other hand, endothelial markers are consistently absent. Because of its morphologic appearance—which tends to be that of a biphasic epithelioid and spindle cell lesion—and its epithelial immunophenotype, there was speculation as to whether adamantinoma was the intraosseous counterpart of synovial sarcoma. However, these two neoplasms have completely dissimilar cytogenetic profiles[566-568] and are definitely separate examples of mesenchymal tumors that demonstrate epithelial differentiation.

From a pathologic perspective, some question may arise as to whether adamantinoma represents metastatic carcinoma rather than a primary bone tumor in biopsy specimens. To date, no systematic immunohistochemical comparisons of those two groups of lesions have been done. Nevertheless, the most straightforward approach to this problem is to review imaging studies of the lesion in question; adamantinoma has a distinctive radiographic appearance,[562] which differs markedly from that of metastatic carcinoma. The principal need for immunohistology in evaluating adamantinoma is restricted to lesions that are markedly sclerotic at the osteofibrous dysplasia pole of the tumoral spectrum. In such cases, the epithelial aggregates that define the tumor can be difficult to visualize with conventional stains alone.

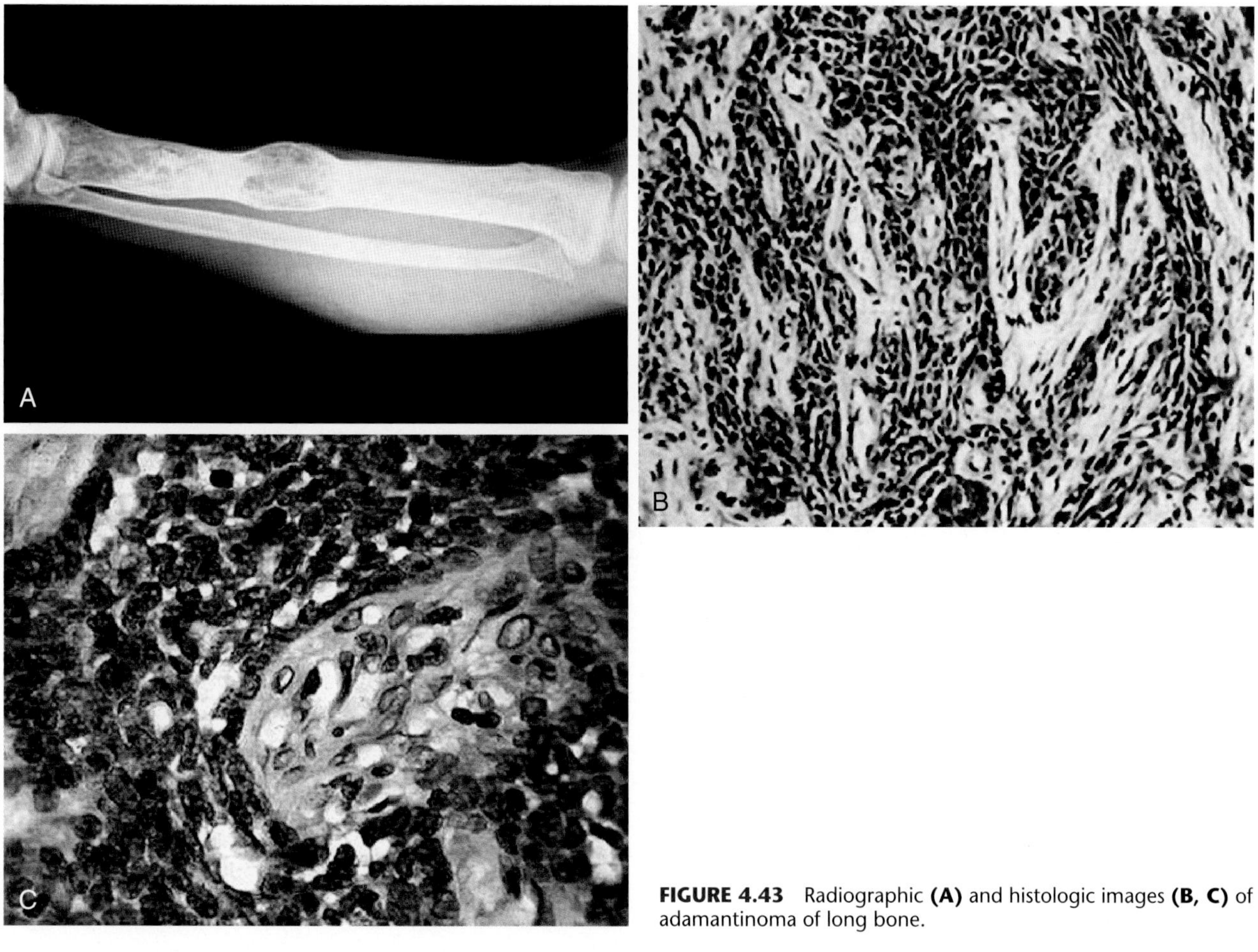

FIGURE 4.43 Radiographic **(A)** and histologic images **(B, C)** of adamantinoma of long bone.

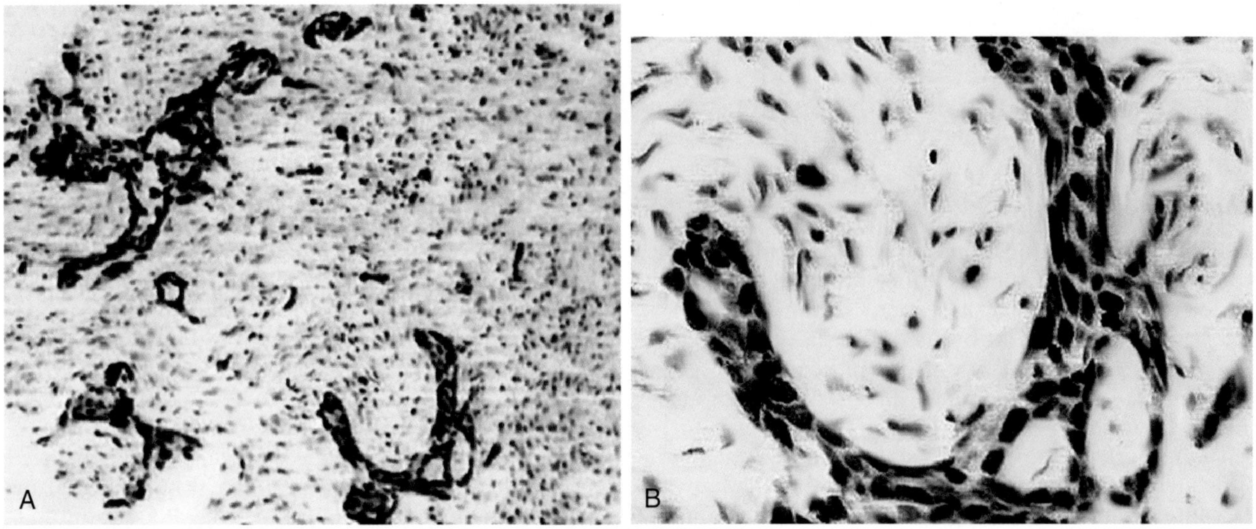

FIGURE 4.44 Immunohistochemical reactivity for cytokeratin 14 **(A)** and cytokeratin 19 **(B)** in adamantinoma of long bone.

REFERENCES

1. Denk H, Krepler R, Artlieb U, et al. Proteins of intermediate filaments: An immunohistochemical and biochemical approach to the classification of soft tissue tumors. *Am J Pathol.* 1983;110:193-208.
2. Lazarides E. Intermediate filaments: A chemically heterogeneous, developmentally regulated class of proteins. *Annu Rev Biochem.* 1982;51:219-250.
3. Erlandson RA. *Diagnostic transmission electron microscopy of tumors*. New York: Raven; 1994:165.
4. Osborn M, Weber K. Biology of disease: Tumor diagnosis by intermediate filament typing: A novel tool for surgical pathology. *Lab Invest.* 1983;48:372-394.
5. Anderton BH. Intermediate filaments: A family of homologous structures. *J Muscle Res Cell Motil.* 1981;2:141-166.
6. Hermann H, Aebi U. Intermediate filaments and their associates: Multitalented structural elements specifying cytoarchitecture and cytodynamics. *Curr Opin Cell Biol.* 2000;12:79-90.
7. Mischke D. The complexity of gene families involved in epithelial differentiation: Keratin genes and the epidermal differentiation complex. *Subcell Biochem.* 1998;31:71-104.
8. Saavedra-Matiz CA, Chapman NH, Wijsman EM, et al. Linkage of hereditary distal myopathy with desmin accumulation to 2q. *Hum Hered.* 2000;50:166-170.
9. Ferrari S, Cannizzaro LA, Battini R, et al. The gene encoding human vimentin is located on the short arm of chromosome 10. *Am J Hum Genet.* 1987;41:616-626.
10. Yoshime T, Maruno M, Kumura E, et al. Stochastic determination of the chromosomal region responsible for expression of human glial fibrillary acidic protein in astrocytic tumors. *Neurosci Lett.* 1998;247:29-32.
11. Goldman R, Goldman AE, Green K, et al. Intermediate filaments: Possible functions as cytoskeletal connecting links between the nucleus and the cell surface. *Ann NY Acad Sci.* 1985;455:1-17.
12. Osborn M. Summary: Intermediate filaments 1984. *Ann NY Acad Sci.* 1985;455:669-681.
13. Vandenburgh HH. Cell shape and growth regulation in skeletal muscle: Exogenous versus endogenous factors. *J Cell Physiol.* 1983;116:363-371.
14. Miettinen M. Keratin immunohistochemistry: Update of applications and pitfalls. *Pathol Annu.* 1993;28(Pt. 2):113-143.
15. Moll R, Franke WW, Schiller DL, et al. The catalogue of human cytokeratins: Patterns of expression in normal epithelia, tumors, and cultured cells. *Cell.* 1982;31:11-24.
16. Miettinen M, Limon J, Niezabitowski A, et al. Patterns of keratin polypeptides in 110 biphasic, monophasic, and poorly-differentiated synovial sarcomas. *Virchows Arch.* 2000;437:275-283.
17. Folpe AL, Agoff SN, Willis J, et al. Parachordoma is immunohistochemically and cytogenetically distinct from axial chordoma and extraskeletal myxoid chondrosarcoma. *Am J Surg Pathol.* 1999;23:1059-1067.
18. Fisher C, Miettinen M. Parachordoma: A clinicopathologic and immunohistochemical study of four cases of an unusual soft tissue neoplasm. *Ann Diagn Pathol.* 1997;1:3-10.
19. O'Hara BJ, Paetau A, Miettinen M. Keratin subsets and monoclonal antibodies HBME-1 in chordoma: Immunohistochemical differential diagnosis between tumors simulating chordoma. *Hum Pathol.* 1998;29:119-126.
20. Swanson PE, Dehner LP, Sirgi KE, et al. Cytokeratin immunoreactivity in malignant tumors of bone and soft tissue. *Appl Immunohistochem.* 1994;2:103-112.
21. Pruss RM, Mirsky R, Raff MC, et al. All classes of intermediate filaments share a common antigenic determinant defined by a monoclonal antibody. *Cell.* 1981;27:419-428.
22. Geisler N, Weber K. Comparison of the proteins of two immunologically distinct intermediate-sized filaments by amino acid sequence analysis: Desmin and vimentin. *Proc Natl Acad Sci USA.* 1981;78:4120-4123.
23. Wick MR. Antibodies to desmin in diagnostic pathology. In: Wick MR, Siegal GP, eds. *Monoclonal antibodies in diagnostic immunohistochemistry*. New York: Marcel Dekker; 1988:93-114.
24. Truong LD, Rangdaeng S, Cagle P, et al. The diagnostic utility of desmin: A study of 584 cases and review of the literature. *Am J Clin Pathol.* 1990;93:305-314.
25. Rangdaeng S, Truong LD. Comparative immunohistochemical staining for desmin and muscle specific actin: A study of 576 cases. *Am J Clin Pathol.* 1991;96:32-45.
26. Small JV, Sobieszek A. Studies on the function and composition of the 10-nm (100 A) filaments of vertebrate smooth muscle. *J Cell Sci.* 1977;23:243-268.
27. Geisler N, Weber K. Purification of smooth muscle desmin and a protein-chemical comparison of desmins from chicken gizzard and hog stomach. *Eur J Biochem.* 1980;111:425-433.
28. Lazarides E, Balzer Jr DR. Specificity of desmin to avian and mammalian muscle cells. *Cell.* 1978;14:429-438.
29. Geisler N, Weber K. The amino acid sequence of chicken muscle desmin provides a common structural model for intermediate filament proteins. *EMBO J.* 1982;1:1649-1656.
30. Ip W, Heuser JE. Subunit structure of desmin and vimentin protofilaments and how they assemble into intermediate filaments. *Ann NY Acad Sci.* 1985;455:185-199.
31. Ngai J, Capetanaki YG, Lazarides E. Expression of the genes encoding for the intermediate filament proteins vimentin and desmin. *Ann NY Acad Sci.* 1985;455:144-155.

32. Tokuyasu KT, Maher PA, Dutton AH, et al. Intermediate filaments in skeletal and cardiac muscle tissue in embryonic and adult chicken. *Ann NY Acad Sci.* 1985;455:200-212.
33. Fischman DA, Danto SI. Monoclonal antibodies to desmin: Evidence for stage-dependent intermediate filament immunoreactivity during cardiac and skeletal muscle development. *Ann NY Acad Sci.* 1985;455:167-184.
34. Tuszynski GP, Frank ED, Damsky CD, et al. The detection of smooth muscle desmin-like protein in BHK21/C13 fibroblasts. *J Biol Chem.* 1979;254:6138-6143.
35. Schmid E, Osborn M, Rungger-Brandle E, et al. Distribution of vimentin and desmin filaments in smooth muscle tissue of mammalian and avian aorta. *Exp Cell Res.* 1982;137:329-340.
36. Richardson FL, Stromer MH, Huiatt TW, et al. Immunoelectron and immunofluorescence localization of desmin in mature avian muscles. *Eur J Cell Biol.* 1981;26:91-101.
37. Daste G, Gioanni J, Lauque D, et al. GC12, marker of cells of mesodermal origin: Value and application to cytodiagnosis of serous effusions. *Arch Anat Cytol Pathol.* 1997;45:185-191.
38. Pollock L, Rampling D, Greenwald SE, et al. Desmin expression in forms: Influence of the desmin clone and immunohistochemical method. *J Clin Pathol.* 1995;48:535-538.
39. Chang TK, Li CY, Smithson WA. Immunocytochemical study of small round cell tumors in routinely processed specimens. *Arch Pathol Lab Med.* 1989;113:1343-1348.
40. Granter SR, Badizadegan K, Fletcher CDM. Myofibromatosis in adults, glomangiopericytoma, and myopericytoma: A spectrum of tumors showing perivascular myoid differentiation. *Am J Surg Pathol.* 1998;22:513-525.
41. Ordi J, de Alava E, Torne A, et al. Intraabdominal desmoplastic small round-cell tumor with EWS/ERG fusion transcripts. *Am J Surg Pathol.* 1998;22:1026-1032.
42. Parham DM, Dias P, Kelly DR, et al. Desmin positivity in primitive neuroectodermal tumors of childhood. *Am J Surg Pathol.* 1992;16:483-492.
43. Manivel JC, Wick MR, Dehner LP, et al. Epithelioid sarcoma: An immunohistochemical study. *Am J Clin Pathol.* 1987;87:319-326.
44. Wick MR, Swanson PE, Scheithauer BW, et al. Malignant peripheral nerve sheath tumor: An immunohistochemical study of 62 cases. *Am J Clin Pathol.* 1987;87:425-433.
45. Fanburg-Smith JC, Hengge M, Hengge UR, et al. Extrarenal rhabdoid tumors of soft tissue: A clinicopathologic and immunohistochemical study of 18 cases. *Ann Diagn Pathol.* 1998;2:351-362.
46. Geisler N, Plessmann U, Weber K. Amino acid sequence characterization of mammalian vimentin, the mesenchymal intermediate filament protein. *FEBS Lett.* 1983;163:22-24.
47. Gereben B, Leuheiber K, Rausch WD, et al. Inverse hierarchy of vimentin epitope expression in primary cultures of chicken and rat astrocytes: A double immunofluorescence study. *Neurobiology.* 1998;6:141-150.
48. Battifora H. Assessment of antigen damage in immunohistochemistry: The vimentin internal control. *Am J Clin Pathol.* 1991;96:669-671.
49. Gereben B, Gerics B, Galfi P, et al. Species specificity of glial vimentin, as revealed by immunocytochemical studies with the VIM3B4 and V9 monoclonal antibodies. *Neurobiology.* 1995;3:151-164.
50. Olah I, Glick B. Anti-vimentin monoclonal antibodies differentiate two resident cell populations in chicken spleen. *Dev Comp Immunol.* 1994;18:67-73.
51. Heatley M, Whiteside C, Maxwell P, et al. Vimentin expression in benign and malignant breast epithelium. *J Clin Pathol.* 1993;46:441-445.
52. Bohn W, Wiegers W, Beuttenmuller M, et al. Species-specific recognition patterns of monoclonal antibodies directed against vimentin. *Exp Cell Res.* 1992;201:1-7.
53. Carbone A, Gloghini A, Volpe R, et al. Anti-vimentin antibody reactivity with Reed-Sternberg cells of Hodgkin's disease. *Virchows Arch A.* 1990;417:43-48.
54. Meyer SA, Ingraham CA, McCarthy KD. Expression of vimentin by cultured astroglia and oligodendroglia. *J Neurosci Res.* 1989;24:251-259.
55. Dahl D. Immunohistochemical differences between neurofilaments in perikarya, dendrites, and axons: Immunofluorescence study with antisera raised to neurofilament polypeptides (200 kD, 150 kD, and 70 kD) isolated by anion exchange chromatography. *Exp Cell Res.* 1983;149:397-408.
56. Hickey WF, Lee V, Trojanowski JQ, et al. Immunohistochemical application of monoclonal antibodies against myelin basic protein and neurofilament triplet protein subunits: Advantage over antisera and technical limitations. *J Histochem Cytochem.* 1983;31:1126-1135.
57. Shaw G. Neurofilaments: Abundant but mysterious neuronal structures. *Bioessays.* 1986;4:161-166.
58. Tapscott SJ, Bennett GS, Toyama Y, et al. Intermediate filament proteins in the developing chick spinal cord. *Dev Biol.* 1981;86:40-54.
59. Tremblay GF, Lee VMY, Trojanowski JQ. Expression of vimentin, glial filament, and neurofilament proteins in primitive childhood brain tumors: A comparative immunoblot and immunoperoxidase study. *Acta Neuropathol.* 1985;68:239-244.
60. Lee VMY, Carden MJ, Trojanowski JQ. Novel monoclonal antibodies provide evidence for the in-situ existence of a non-phosphorylated form of the large neurofilament subunit. *J Neurosci.* 1986;6:850-858.
61. Brown A. Contiguous phosphorylated and non-phosphorylated domains along axonal neurofilaments. *J Cell Sci.* 1998;111:455-467.
62. Sternberger LA, Sternberger NH. Monoclonal antibodies distinguish phosphorylated and non-phosphorylated forms of neurofilaments in situ. *Proc Natl Acad Sci USA.* 1983;80:6126-6130.
63. Ulfig N, Nickel J, Bohl J. Monoclonal antibodies SMI311 and SMI312 as tools to investigate the maturation of nerve cells and axonal patterns in human fetal brain. *Cell Tissue Res.* 1998;291:433-443.
64. Trojanowski JQ, Lee VMY. Anti-neurofilament monoclonal antibodies: Reagents for the evaluation of human neoplasms. *Acta Neuropathol.* 1983;59:155-158.
65. Trojanowski JQ, Lee VMY, Schlaepfer WW. An immunohistochemical study of central and peripheral nervous system tumors with monoclonal antibodies against neurofilaments and glial filaments. *Hum Pathol.* 1984;15:248-257.
66. Trojanowski JQ, Lee VMY. Expression of neurofilament antigens by normal and neoplastic human adrenal chromaffin cells. *N Engl J Med.* 1985;313:101-104.
67. Osborn M, Altmannsberger M, Shaw G, et al. Various sympathetic derived human tumors differ in neurofilament expression: Use in diagnosis of neuroblastoma, ganglioneuroblastoma, and pheochromocytoma. *Virchows Arch B Cell Pathol.* 1982;40:141-156.
68. Shaw G, Weber K. The intermediate filament complement of the brain: A comparison between different mammalian species. *Eur J Cell Biol.* 1984;33:95-104.
69. Trojanowski JQ. Neurofilament and glial filament proteins. In: Wick MR, Siegal GP, eds. *Monoclonal antibodies in diagnostic immunohistochemistry.* New York: Marcel Dekker; 1988:115-146.
70. Dolman CL. Glial fibrillary acidic protein and cartilage. *Acta Neuropathol.* 1989;79:101-103.
71. Yasuda T, Sobue G, Ito T, et al. Human peripheral nerve sheath neoplasms: Expression of Schwann cell-related markers and their relation to malignant transformation. *Muscle Nerve.* 1991;14:812-819.
72. Lodding P, Kindblom LG, Angervall L, et al. A clinicopathologic study of 29 cases. *Virchows Arch A.* 1990;416:237-248.
73. Giangaspero F, Fratamico FC, Ceccarelli C, et al. Malignant peripheral nerve sheath tumors and spindle cell sarcomas: An immunohistochemical analysis of multiple markers. *Appl Pathol.* 1989;7:134-144.
74. Kawahara E, Oda Y, Ooi A, et al. Expression of glial fibrillary acidic protein (GFAP) in peripheral nerve sheath tumors: A comparative study of immunoreactivity of GFAP, vimentin, S100 protein, and neurofilament in 38 schwannomas and 18 neurofibromas. *Am J Surg Pathol.* 1988;12:115-120.

75. Memoli VA, Brown EF, Gould VE. Glial fibrillary acidic protein (GFAP) immunoreactivity in peripheral nerve sheath tumors. *Ultrastruct Pathol.* 1984;7:269-275.
76. Swanson PE. Monoclonal antibodies to human milk fat globule proteins. In: Wick MR, Siegal GP, eds. *Monoclonal antibodies in diagnostic immunohistochemistry.* New York: Marcel Dekker; 1988:227-283.
77. Petersen OW, VanDeuers B. Characterization of epithelial membrane antigen expression in human mammary epithelium by ultrastructural immunoperoxidase cytochemistry. *J Histochem Cytochem.* 1986;34:801-809.
78. Sloane JP, Ormerod MG. Distribution of epithelial membrane antigen in normal and neoplastic tissues and its value in diagnostic tumor pathology. *Cancer.* 1981;47:1786-1795.
79. Ormerod MG, Steele K, Westwood JH, et al. Epithelial membrane antigen: Partial purification, assay, and properties. *Br J Cancer.* 1983;48:533-541.
80. Heyderman E, Strudley I, Powell G, et al. A new monoclonal antibody to epithelial membrane antigen (EMA)-E29: A comparison of its immunocytochemical reactivity with polyclonal anti-EMA antibodies and another monoclonal antibody, HMFG-2. *Br J Cancer.* 1985;52:355-361.
81. Cordell J, Richardson TC, Pulford KAF, et al. Production of monoclonal antibodies against human epithelial membrane antigen for use in diagnostic immunocytochemistry. *Br J Cancer.* 1985;52:347-354.
82. Wick MR, Swanson PE, Manivel JC. Immunohistochemical analysis of soft tissue sarcomas: Comparisons with electron microscopy. *Appl Pathol.* 1988;6:169-196.
83. Swanson PE, Manivel JC, Scheithauer BW, et al. Epithelial membrane antigen in human sarcomas: An immunohistochemical study. *Surg Pathol.* 1989;2:313-322.
84. Franke WW, Moll R, Mueller H, et al. Immunocytochemical identification of epithelium-derived human tumors with antibodies to desmosomal plaque proteins. *Proc Natl Acad Sci USA.* 1983;80:543-547.
85. Arnemann J, Spurr NK, Magee AI, et al. The human gene (DSG2) coding for HDGC, a second member of the desmoglein subfamily of the desmosomal cadherins, is, like DSG1 coding for desmoglein DG1, assigned to chromosome 18. *Genomics.* 1992;13:484-486.
86. Laskin WB, Miettinen M. Epithelial-type and neural-type cadherin expression in malignant noncarcinomatous neoplasms with epithelioid features that involve the soft tissues. *Arch Pathol Lab Med.* 2002;126:425-431.
87. Sata H, Hasegawa T, Abe Y, et al. Expression of E-cadherin in bone and soft tissue sarcomas: A possible role in epithelial differentiation. *Hum Pathol.* 1999;30:1344-1349.
88. Miettinen M. Antibody specificity to muscle actins in the diagnosis and classification of soft tissue tumors. *Am J Pathol.* 1988;130:205-215.
89. Schurch W, Skalli O, Seemayer TA, et al. Intermediate filament proteins and actin isoforms as markers for soft tissue tumor differentiation and origin. I. Smooth muscle tumors. *Am J Pathol.* 1987;128:91-103.
90. Tsukada T, McNutt MA, Ross R, et al. HHF35, a muscle actin-specific monoclonal antibody. II. Reactivity in normal, reactive, and neoplastic human tissue. *Am J Pathol.* 1987;127:389-402.
91. Jones H, Steart PV, DuBoulay CE, et al. Alpha-smooth muscle actin as a marker for soft tissue tumors: A comparison with desmin. *J Pathol.* 1990;162:29-33.
92. Cintorino M, Vindigni C, DelVecchio MT, et al. Expression of actin isoforms and intermediate filament proteins in childhood orbital rhabdomyosarcomas. *J Submicrosc Cytol Pathol.* 1989;21:409-419.
93. Bussolati G, Papotti M, Foschini MP, et al. The interest of actin immunocytochemistry in diagnostic histopathology. *Basic Appl Histochem.* 1987;31:165-176.
94. Ogut O, Granzier H, Jin JP. Acidic and basic troponin-T isoforms in mature fast-twitch skeletal muscle and effect on contractility. *Am J Physiol.* 1999;276:C1162-C1170.
95. Lutz GJ, Lieber RL. Skeletal muscle myosin-II structure and function. *Exerc Sport Sci Rev.* 1999;27:63-77.
96. Lefevre G. Troponins: Biological and clinical aspects. *Ann Biol Clin.* 2000;58:39-48.
97. Atkinson RA, Joseph C, Dal Piaz F, et al. Binding of alpha-actinin to titin: Implications for Z-disk assembly. *Biochemistry.* 2000;39:5255-5264.
98. Dodd S, Malone M, McCulloch W. Rhabdomyosarcoma in children: A histological and immunohistochemical study of 59 cases. *J Pathol.* 1989;158:13-18.
99. Lai R, Tian Y, An J, et al. A comparative study on morphology and immunohistochemistry of rhabdomyosarcoma and embryonal skeletal muscles. *Chin Med J.* 1997;110:392-396.
100. Gruchala A, Niezabitowski A, Wasilewska A, et al. Rhabdomyosarcoma: Morphologic, immunohistochemical, and DNA study. *Gen Diagn Pathol.* 1997;142:175-184.
101. Carter RL, Jameson CF, Philp ER, et al. Comparative phenotypes in rhabdomyosarcoma and developing skeletal muscle. *Histopathology.* 1990;17:301-309.
102. Saku T, Tsuda N, Anami M, et al. Smooth and skeletal muscle myosins in spindle cell tumors of soft tissue: An immunohistochemical study. *Acta Pathol Jpn.* 1985;35:125-136.
103. Osborn M, Hill C, Altmannsberger M, et al. Monoclonal antibodies to titin in conjunction with antibodies to desmin separate rhabdomyosarcomas from other tumor types. *Lab Invest.* 1986;55:101-108.
104. Moczygemba C, Guidry J, Wittung-Stafshede P. Heme orientation affects holo-myoglobin folding and unfolding kinetics. *FEBS Lett.* 2000;470:203-206.
105. Parham DM, Webber B, Holt H, et al. Immunohistochemical study of childhood rhabdomyosarcomas and related neoplasms: Results of an Intergroup Rhabdomyosarcoma Study project. *Cancer.* 1991;67:3072-3080.
106. Carter RL, McCarthy KP, Machin LG, et al. Expression of desmin and myoglobin in rhabdomyosarcomas and in developing skeletal muscle. *Histopathology.* 1989;15:585-595.
107. Coindre JM, deMascarel A, Trojani M, et al. Immunohistochemical study of rhabdomyosarcoma: Unexpected staining with S100 protein and cytokeratin. *J Pathol.* 1988;155:127-132.
108. Seidal T, Kindblom LG, Angervall L. Myoglobin, desmin, and vimentin in ultrastructurally proven rhabdomyomas and rhabdomyosarcomas: An immunohistochemical study utilizing a series of monoclonal and polyclonal antibodies. *Appl Pathol.* 1987;5:201-219.
109. Brooks JJ. Immunohistochemistry of soft tissue tumors: Myoglobin as a tumor marker for rhabdomyosarcoma. *Cancer.* 1982;50:1757-1763.
110. Tsokos M, Howard R, Costa J. Immunohistochemical study of alveolar and embryonal rhabdomyosarcoma. *Lab Invest.* 1983;48:148-155.
111. Kraevsky NA. Use of immunohistochemical methods in the diagnosis of myogenous tumors. *Acta Histochem Suppl.* 1984;30:79-80.
112. Hosoi H, Sugimoto T, Hayashi Y, et al. Differential expression of myogenic regulatory genes, Myo-D1 and myogenin, in human rhabdomyosarcoma sublines. *Int J Cancer.* 1992;50:977-983.
113. Newsholme SJ, Zimmerman DM. Immunohistochemical evaluation of chemically induced rhabdomyosarcomas in rats: Diagnostic utility of Myo-D1. *Toxicol Pathol.* 1997;25:470-474.
114. Wang NP, Marx J, McNutt MA, et al. Expression of myogenic regulatory proteins (myogenin and Myo-D1) in small blue round cell tumors of childhood. *Am J Pathol.* 1995;147:1799-1810.
115. Cui S, Hano H, Harada T, et al. Evaluation of new monoclonal anti-Myo-D1 and anti-myogenin antibodies for the diagnosis of rhabdomyosarcoma. *Pathol Int.* 1999;49:62-68.
116. Dias P, Chen B, Dilday B, et al. Strong immunostaining for myogenin in rhabdomyosarcoma is significantly associated with tumors of the alveolar subclass. *Am J Pathol.* 2000;156:399-408.
117. Watanabe K, Kusakabe T, Hoshi N, et al. h-Caldesmon in leiomyosarcoma and tumors with smooth muscle-like differentiation: Its specific expression in the smooth muscle cell tumors. *Hum Pathol.* 1999;30:392-396.
118. Miettinen MM, Sarlomo-Rikala M, Kovatich AJ, et al. Calponin and h-caldesmon in soft tissue tumors: Consistent h-caldesmon immunoreactivity in gastrointestinal stromal tumors indicates traits of smooth muscle differentiation. *Mod Pathol.* 1999;12:756-762.

119. Mentzel T, Dei Tos AP, Sapi Z, et al. Myopericytoma of skin and soft tissues: Clinicopathologic and immunohistochemical study of 54 cases. *Am J Surg Pathol.* 2006;30:104-113.
120. Huber PA. *Caldesmon Int J Biochem Cell Biol.* 1997;29:1047-1051.
121. Shiro B, Siegal GP. The use of monoclonal antibodies to S100 protein in diagnostic immunohistochemistry. In: Wick MR, Siegal GP, eds. *Monoclonal antibodies in diagnostic immunohistochemistry.* New York: Marcel Dekker; 1988:455-503.
122. Fujii T, Machino K, Andoh H, et al. Calcium-dependent control of caldesmon-actin interaction by S100 protein. *J Biochem.* 1990;107:133-137.
123. Loeffel SC, Gillespie GY, Mirmiran SA, et al. Cellular immunolocalization of S100 protein within fixed tissue sections by monoclonal antibodies. *Arch Pathol Lab Med.* 1985;109:117-122.
124. Masui F, Ushigome S, Fujii K. Clear cell chondrosarcoma: A pathological and immunohistochemical study. *Histopathology.* 1999;34:447-452.
125. Abramovici LC, Steiner GC, Bonar F. Myxoid chondrosarcoma of soft tissue and bone: A retrospective study of 11 cases. *Hum Pathol.* 1995;26:1215-1220.
126. Swanson PE, Wick MR. Clear cell sarcoma: An immunohistochemical analysis of six cases and comparison with other epithelioid neoplasms of soft tissue. *Arch Pathol Lab Med.* 1989;113:55-60.
127. Kahn HJ, Marks A, Thom H, et al. Role of antibody to S100 protein in diagnostic pathology. *Am J Clin Pathol.* 1983;79:341-347.
128. Van den Berg LH, Sadiq SA, Thomas FP, et al. Characterization of HNK-1 bearing glycoproteins in human peripheral nerve myelin. *J Neurosci Res.* 1990;25:295-299.
129. Weiss SW, Langloss JM, Enzinger FM. Value of S100 protein in the diagnosis of soft tissue tumors, with particular reference to benign and malignant Schwann cell tumors. *Lab Invest.* 1983;49:299-308.
130. Hammer JA, O'Shannessy DJ, DeLeon M, et al. Immunoreactivity of PMP22, P0, and other 19 to 28 kD glycoproteins in peripheral nerve myelin of mammals and fish with HNK-1 and related antibodies. *J Neurosci Res.* 1993;35:546-558.
131. Merkouri E, Matsas R. Monoclonal antibody BM89 recognizes a novel cell surface glycoprotein of the L2/HNK-1 family in the developing mammalian nervous system. *Neuroscience.* 1992;50:53-68.
132. Vogel M, Kowalewski HJ, Zimmermann H, et al. Association of the HNK-1 epitope with 5-nucleotidase from Tomarmorata (electric ray) electric organ. *Biochem J.* 1991;278:199-202.
133. Lanier LL, Testi R, Bindl J, et al. Identity of Leu-19 (CD56) leukocyte differentiation antigen and neural cell adhesion molecule. *J Exp Med.* 1989;169:2233-2238.
134. Abo T, Balch CM. A differentiation antigen of human NK and killer cells, identified by a monoclonal antibody (HNK1). *J Immunol.* 1981;127:1024-1029.
135. Hirose T, Scheithauer BW, Sano T. Perineurial malignant peripheral nerve sheath tumor (MPNST): A clinicopathologic, immunohistochemical, and ultrastructural study of seven cases. *Am J Surg Pathol.* 1998;22:1368-1378.
136. Swanson PE, Manivel JC, Wick MR. Immunoreactivity for Leu7 in neurofibrosarcoma and other spindle cell sarcomas of soft tissue. *Am J Pathol.* 1987;126:546-560.
137. Michels S, Swanson PE, Robb JA, et al. Leu7 in small cell neoplasms: An immunohistochemical study. *Cancer.* 1987;60:2958-2964.
138. Amann G, Zoubek A, Salzer-Kuntschik M, et al. Relation of neurological marker expression and EWS gene fusion types in MIC2/CD99-positive tumors of the Ewing family. *Hum Pathol.* 1999;30:1058-1064.
139. Abe S, Imamura T, Park P, et al. Small round cell type of malignant peripheral nerve sheath tumor. *Mod Pathol.* 1998;11:747-753.
140. Gardner LJ, Polski JM, Fallon R, et al. Identification of CD56 and CD57 by flow cytometry in Ewing's sarcoma or primitive neuroectodermal tumor. *Virchows Arch A.* 1998;433:35-40.
141. Sangueza OP, Requena L. Neoplasms with neural differentiation: A review. Part II: Malignant neoplasms. *Am J Dermatopathol.* 1998;20:89-102.
142. Devaney K, Vinh TN, Sweet DE. Small cell osteosarcoma of bone: An immunohistochemical study with differential diagnostic considerations. *Hum Pathol.* 1993;24:1211-1225.
143. Pettinato G, Manivel JC, d'Amore ESG, et al. Melanotic neuroectodermal tumor of infancy: A reexamination of a histogenetic problem based on immunohistochemical, flow cytometric, and ultrastructural study of 10 cases. *Am J Surg Pathol.* 1991;15:233-245.
144. Miettinen M, Cupo W. Neural cell adhesion molecule distribution in soft tissue tumors. *Hum Pathol.* 1993;24:62-66.
145. Hartel PH, Fanburg-Smith JC, Frazier AA, et al. Primary pulmonary and mediastinal synovial sarcoma: A clinicopathologic study of 60 cases and comparison with five prior series. *Mod Pathol.* 2007;20:760-769.
146. Zevallos-Giampietri EA, Barrionuevo C. Proximal-type epithelioid sarcoma: report of two cases in the perineum: Differential diagnosis and review of soft tissue tumors with epithelioid and/or rhabdoid features. *Appl Immunohistochem Mol Morphol.* 2005;13:221-230.
147. Folpe AL, Schmidt RA, Chapman D, et al. Poorly differentiated synovial sarcoma: immunohistochemical distinction from primitive neuroectodermal tumors and high-grade malignant peripheral nerve sheath tumors. *Am J Surg Pathol.* 1998;22: 673-682.
148. Salzer JL, Holmes WP, Colman DR. The amino acid sequences of the myelin-associated glycoproteins: Homology to the immunoglobulin gene superfamily. *J Cell Biol.* 1987;104:959-965.
149. Dixit SN, Mainardi CL, Beachey EH, et al. 7S domain constitutes the amino-terminal end of type IV collagen: An immunohistochemical study. *Coll Rel Res.* 1983;3:263-273.
150. Griffin CA, Emanuel BS, Hansen JR, et al. Human collagen genes encoding basement membrane alpha-1 (IV) and alpha-2 (IV) chains map to the distal long arm of chromosome 13. *Proc Natl Acad Sci USA.* 1987;84:512-516.
151. Terranova VP, Rohrbach DH, Martin GR. Role of laminin in the attachment of PAM212 (epithelial) cells to basement membrane collagen. *Cell.* 1980;22:719-726.
152. Foidart JM, Bere EW, Yaar Jr M, et al. Distribution and immunoelectron microscopic localization of laminin, a non-collagenous basement membrane glycoprotein. *Lab Invest.* 1980;42:336-342.
153. McGarvey ML, Baron-Van Evercooren BV, Kleinman KH, et al. Synthesis and effects of basement membrane components in cultured rat Schwann cells. *Dev Biol.* 1984;105:18-28.
154. Nigar E, Dervan PA. Quantitative assessment of basement membranes in soft tissue tumors: Computerized image analysis of laminin and type IV collagen. *J Pathol.* 1998;185:184-187.
155. Ogawa K, Oguchi M, Yamabe H, et al. Distribution of collagen type IV in soft tissue tumors: An immunohistochemical study. *Cancer.* 1986;58:269-277.
156. d'Ardenne AJ, Kirkpatrick P, Sykes BC. Distribution of laminin, fibronectin, and interstitial collagen type III in soft tissue tumors. *J Clin Pathol.* 1984;37:895-904.
157. Fischer BE, Thomas KB, Schlokat U, et al. Triplet structure of human von Willebrand factor. *Biochem J.* 1998;331:483-488.
158. Kaufman RJ, Pipe SW. Regulation of factor VIII expression and activity by von Willebrand factor. *Thromb Haemost.* 1999;82:201-208.
159. Mukai K, Rosai J. Factor VIII-related antigen: An endothelial marker. In: DeLellis RA, ed. *Diagnostic immunohistochemistry.* New York: Masson; 1984:243-261.
160. Sehested M, Hou-Jensen K. Factor VIII-related antigen as an endothelial cell marker in benign and malignant diseases. *Virchows Arch A.* 1981;391:217-225.
161. Ordonez NG, Batsakis JG. Comparison of Ulex europaeus I lectin and factor VIII-related antigen in vascular lesions. *Arch Pathol Lab Med.* 1984;108:129-132.
162. Swanson PE, Wick MR. Immunohistochemical evaluation of vascular neoplasms. *Clin Dermatol.* 1991;9:243-253.
163. Ramani P, Bradley NJ, Fletcher CDM. QBEND10, a new monoclonal antibody to endothelium: Assessment of its diagnostic utility in paraffin sections. *Histopathology.* 1990;17:237-242.
164. Traweek ST, Kandalaft PL, Mehta P, et al. The human hematopoietic progenitor cell antigen (CD34) in vascular neoplasms. *Am J Clin Pathol.* 1991;96:25-31.

165. Sirgi KE, Wick MR, Swanson PE. B72.3 and CD34 immunoreactivity in malignant epithelioid soft tissue tumors: Adjuncts in the recognition of endothelial neoplasms. *Am J Surg Pathol.* 1993;17:179-185.
166. Miettinen M, Lindenmayer AE, Chanbal A. Endothelial cell markers CD31, CD34, and BNH9 antibody to H- and Y-antigens: Evaluation of their specificity and sensitivity in the diagnosis of vascular tumors and comparison with von Willebrand factor. *Mod Pathol.* 1994;7:82-90.
167. Natkunam Y, Rouse RV, Zhu S, et al. Immunoblot analysis of CD34 expression in histologically diverse neoplasms. *Am J Pathol.* 2000;156:21-27.
168. Arber DA, Kandalaft PL, Mehta P, et al. Vimentin-negative epithelioid sarcoma: The value of an immunohistochemical panel that includes CD34. *Am J Surg Pathol.* 1993;17:302-317.
169. Harvell JD, Kilpatrick SE, White WL. Histologic relations between giant cell fibroblastoma and dermatofibrosarcoma protuberans: CD34 staining showing the spectrum and a simulator. *Am J Dermatopathol.* 1998;20:339-345.
170. Templeton SF, Solomon Jr AR. Spindle cell lipoma is strongly CD34-positive: An immunohistochemical study. *J Cutan Pathol.* 1996;23:546-550.
171. Hasegawa T, Matsuno Y, Shimoda T, et al. Extrathoracic solitary fibrous tumors: Their histological variability and potentially aggressive behavior. *Hum Pathol.* 1999;30:1464-1473.
172. Metzelaar MJ, Korteweg J, Sizma JJ, et al. Biochemical characterization of PECAM-1 (CD31 antigen) on human platelets. *Thromb Haemost.* 1991;66:700-707.
173. Parums DV, Cordell JL, Michlein K, et al. JC70: A new monoclonal antibody that detects vascular endothelium associated antigen on routinely processed tissue sections. *J Clin Pathol.* 1990;43:752-757.
174. Ohsawa M, Naka N, Tomita Y, et al. Use of immunohistochemical procedures in diagnosing angiosarcomas: Evaluation of 98 cases. *Cancer.* 1995;75:2867-2874.
175. McKenney JK, Weiss SW, Folpe AL. CD31 expression in intratumoral macrophages: A potential diagnostic pitfall. *Am J Surg Pathol.* 2001;25:1167-1173.
176. DeYoung BR, Wick MR, Fitzgibbon JF, et al. CD31: An immunospecific marker for endothelial differentiation in human neoplasms. *Appl Immunohistochem.* 1993;1:97-100.
177. DeYoung BR, Swanson PE, Argenyi ZB, et al. CD31 immunoreactivity in mesenchymal neoplasms of the skin and subcutis. *J Cutan Pathol.* 1995;22:215-222.
178. Takahashi Y, Hosaka Y, Niina H, et al. Soluble thrombomodulin purified from human urine exhibits a potent anticoagulant effect in vitro and in vivo. *Thromb Haemost.* 1995;73:805-811.
179. Kurosawa S, Galvin JB, Esmon NC, et al. Proteolytic formation and properties of functional domains of thrombomodulin. *J Biol Chem.* 1987;262:2206-2212.
180. Karmochkine M, Boffa MC. Thrombomodulin: Physiology and clinical applications (excluding systemic diseases). *Rev Med Interne.* 1997;18:119-125.
181. Yonezawa S, Maruyama I, Sakae K, et al. Thrombomodulin as a marker for vascular tumors: Comparative study with factor VIII and Ulex europaeus I lectin. *Am J Clin Pathol.* 1987;88:405-411.
182. Kim SJ, Shiba E, Ishii H, et al. Thrombomodulin is a new biological and prognostic marker for breast cancer: An immunohistochemical study. *Anticancer Res.* 1997;17:2319-2323.
183. Ordonez NG. Value of thrombomodulin immunostaining in the diagnosis of mesothelioma. *Histopathology.* 1997;31:25-30.
184. Appleton MA, Attanoos RL, Jasani B. Thrombomodulin as a marker of vascular and lymphatic tumors. *Histopathology.* 1996;29:153-157.
185. Zhang YM, Bachmann S, Hemmer C, et al. Vascular origin of Kaposi's sarcoma: Expression of leukocytic adhesion molecule-1, thrombomodulin, and tissue factor. *Am J Pathol.* 1994;144:51-59.
186. Holthofer H, Virtanen I, Kariniemi AL, et al. Ulex europaeus I lectin as a marker for vascular endothelium in human tissues. *Lab Invest.* 1982;47:60-66.
187. Sato Y. Role of ETS family transcription factors in vascular development and angiogenesis. *Cell Struct Funct.* 2001;26:19-24.
188. Watson DK, Smyth FE, Thompson DM, et al. The ERGB/FLI-1 gene: Isolation and characterization of a new member of the family of human ETS transcription factors. *Cell Growth Differ.* 1992;3:705-713.
189. Torchia EC, Boyd K, Rehg JE, et al. EWS/FLI-1 induces rapid onset of myeloid/erythroid leukemia in mice. *Mol Cell Biol.* 2007;27:7918-7934.
190. Liu F, Walmsley M, Rodaway A, et al. FLI-1 acts at the top of the transcriptional network driving blood and endothelial development. *Curr Biol.* 2008;18:1234-1240.
191. Landry JR, Konston S, Knezevic K, et al. FLI-1, EFL1, and ETS1 regulate the proximal promoter of the LMO2 gene in endothelial cells. *Blood.* 2005;106:2680-2687.
192. Zwerner JP, Joo J, Warner KL, et al. The EWS/FLI1 oncogenic transcription factor deregulates GLI1. *Oncogene.* 2008;27:3282-3291.
193. Matsunobu T, Tanaka K, Nakamura T, et al. The possible role of EWS-FLI1 in evasion of senescence in Ewing family tumors. *Cancer Res.* 2006;66:803-811.
194. Folpe AL, Chand EM, Goldblum JR, et al. Expression of FLI-1, a nuclear transcription factor, distinguishes vascular neoplasms from potential mimics. *Am J Surg Pathol.* 2001;25:1061-1066.
195. Mhawech-Fauceglia P, Herrmann FR, Bshara W, et al. Friend leukemia integration-1 expression in malignant and benign tumors: A multiple tumor tissue microarray analysis using polyclonal antibody. *J Clin Pathol.* 2007;60:694-700.
196. Kahn HJ, Marks A. A new monoclonal antibody, D2-40, for detection of lymphatic invasion in primary tumors. *Lab Invest.* 2002;82:1255-1257.
197. Breiteneder-Geleff S, Matsui K, Soleiman A, et al. Podoplanin, novel 43 kD membrane protein of glomerular epithelial cells, is downregulated in puromycin nephrosis. *Am J Pathol.* 1997;151:1141-1152.
198. Raica M, Cimpean AM, Ribatti D. The role of podoplanin in tumor progression and metastasis. *Anticancer Res.* 2008;28:2997-3006.
199. Breiteneder-Geleff S, Soleiman A, Horvat R, et al. Podoplanin-a specific marker for lymphatic endothelium expressed in angiosarcoma. *Verh Dtsch Ges Pathol.* 1999;83:270-275.
200. Breiteneder-Geleff S, Soleiman A, Kowalski H, et al. Angiosarcomas express mixed endothelial phenotypes of blood and lymphatic capillaries: Podoplanin as a specific marker for lymphatic endothelium. *Am J Pathol.* 1999;154:385-394.
201. Makinen T, Norrmen C, Petrova TV. Molecular mechanisms of lymphatic vascular development. *Cell Mol Life Sci.* 2007;64:1915-1929.
202. Yu H, Pinkus GS, Hornick JL. Diffuse membranous immunoreactivity for podoplanin (D2-40) distinguishes primary and metastatic seminomas from other germ cell tumors and metastatic neoplasms. *Am J Clin Pathol.* 2007;128:767-775.
203. Kato Y, Kaneko M, Sata M, et al. Enhanced expression of Aggrus (T1-alpha/podoplanin), a platelet-aggregation-inducing factor in lung squamous cell carcinoma. *Tumour Biol.* 2005;26:195-200.
204. Sonne SB, Herlihy AS, Hoei-Hansen CE, et al. Identity of M2A (D2-40) antigen and gp36 (Aggrus, T1A-2, podoplanin) in human developing testis, testicular carcinoma in situ and germ-cell tumors. *Virchows Arch.* 2006 Aug;449:200-206.
205. Marks A, Sutherland DR, Bailey D, et al. Characterization and distribution of an oncofetal antigen (M2A antigen) expressed on testicular germ cell tumors. *Br J Cancer.* 1999;80:569-578.
206. Kahn HJ, Bailey D, Marks A. Monoclonal antibody D2-40, a new marker of lymphatic endothelium, reacts with Kaposi's sarcoma and a subset of angiosarcomas. *Mod Pathol.* 2002;15:434-440.
207. Kaiserling E. Immunohistochemical identification of lymph vessels with D2-40 in diagnostic pathology. *Pathologe.* 2004;25:362-374.
208. Chu AY, Litzky LA, Pasha TL, et al. Utility of D2-40, a novel mesothelial marker, in the diagnosis of malignant mesothelioma. *Mod Pathol.* 2005;18:105-110.
209. Fukunaga M. Expression of D2-40 in lymphatic endothelium of normal tissues and in vascular tumors. *Histopathology.* 2005;48:396-402.

210. Ordonez NG. D2-40 and podoplanin and highly specific and sensitive immunohistochemical markers of epithelioid malignant mesothelioma. *Hum Pathol.* 2005;36:372-380.
211. Yu H, Gibson JA, Pinkus GS, et al. Podoplanin (D2-40) is a novel marker for follicular dendritic cell tumors. *Am J Clin Pathol.* 2007;128:776-782.
212. Nakatsuka S, Oji Y, Horiuchi T, et al. Immunohistochemical detection of WT1 protein in a variety of cancer cells. *Mod Pathol.* 2006;19:804-814.
213. Lawley LP, Cerimele F, Weiss SW, et al. Expression of Wilms tumor 1 gene distinguishes vascular malformations from proliferative endothelial lesions. *Arch Dermatol.* 2005;141:1297-1300.
214. Timar J, Mezzaros L, Orosz Z, et al. WT1 expression in angiogenic tumors of the skin. *Histopathology.* 2005;47:67-73.
215. Iljin K, Karkkainen MJ, Lawrence EC, et al. VEGFR3 gene structure, regulatory region, and sequence polymorphisms. *FASEB J.* 2001;15:1028-1036.
216. Folpe AL, Veikkola T, Valtola R, et al. Vascular endothelial growth factor receptor-3 (VEGFR3): A marker of vascular tumors with presumed lymphatic differentiation, including Kaposi's sarcoma, kaposiform and Dabska-type hemangioendotheliomas, and a subset of angiosarcomas. *Mod Pathol.* 2000;13:180-185.
217. Leader M, Collins M, Patel J, et al. Staining for factor VIII-related antigen and Ulex europaeus I (UEA-I) in 230 tumors: An assessment of their specificity for angiosarcoma and Kaposi's sarcoma. *Histopathology.* 1986;10:1153-1162.
218. Wick MR, Manivel JC. Epithelioid sarcoma and epithelioid hemangioendothelioma: An immunohistochemical and lectin-histochemical comparison. *Virchows Arch A.* 1987;410:309-316.
219. DuBoulay CEH. Demonstration of alpha-1-antitrypsin and alpha-1-antichymotrypsin in fibrous histiocytomas using the immunoperoxidase technique. *Am J Surg Pathol.* 1982;6:559-564.
220. Kindblom LG, Jacobsen GK, Jacobsen M. Immunohistochemical investigations of tumors of supposed fibroblastic-histiocytic origin. *Hum Pathol.* 1982;13:834-840.
221. Meister P, Nathrath W. Immunohistochemical characterization of histiocytic tumors. *Diagn Histopathol.* 1981;4:79-87.
222. Pulford KAF, Rigney EM, Micklem KJ, et al. KP1: A new monoclonal antibody that detects a monocyte/macrophage-associated antigen in routinely processed tissue sections. *J Clin Pathol.* 1989;42:414-421.
223. Gloghini A, Volpe R, Carbone A. Ki-M6 immunostaining in routinely processed sections of reactive and neoplastic human lymphoid tissue. *Am J Clin Pathol.* 1990;94:734-741.
224. Gown AM, Tsukada T, Ross R. Human atherosclerosis. II: Immunocytochemical analysis of the cellular composition of human atherosclerotic lesions. *Am J Pathol.* 1986;125:191-207.
225. Takeya M, Yamashiro S, Yoshimura T, et al. Immunophenotypic and immunoelectron microscopic characterization of major constituent cells in malignant fibrous histiocytoma using human cell lines and their transplanted tumors in immunodeficient mice. *Lab Invest.* 1995;72:679-688.
226. Nemes Z, Thomazy V. Factor XIIIa and the classic histiocytic markers in malignant fibrous histiocytoma: A comparative immunohistochemical study. *Hum Pathol.* 1988;19:822-829.
227. Lau SK, Chu PG, Weiss LM. CD163: A specific marker of macrophages in paraffin-embedded tissue samples. *Am J Clin Pathol.* 2004;122:794-801.
228. Reid MB, Gray C, Fear JD, et al. Immunohistologic demonstration of factors XIIIa and XIIIs in reactive and neoplastic fibroblastic and fibrohistiocytic lesions. *Histopathology.* 1986;10:1171-1178.
229. Thewes M, Engst R, Boeck K, et al. Expression of cathepsins in dermal fibrous tumors: An immunohistochemical study. *Eur J Dermatol.* 1998;8:86-89.
230. Gloghini A, Rizzo A, Zanette I, et al. KP1/CD68 expression in malignant neoplasms including lymphomas, sarcomas, and carcinomas. *Am J Clin Pathol.* 1995;103:425-431.
231. Doussis IA, Gatter KC, Mason DY. CD68 reactivity of non-macrophage-derived tumors in cytological specimens. *J Clin Pathol.* 1993;46:334-336.
232. Schulz A, Loreth B, Battmann A, et al. Bone matrix production in osteosarcoma. *Verh Dtsch Ges Pathol.* 1998;82:144-153.
233. Park YK, Yang MH, Kim YW, et al. Osteocalcin expression in primary bone tumors: In situ hybridization and immunohistochemical study. *J Korean Med Sci.* 1995;10:263-268.
234. Lian JB, Stein GS. Development of the osteoblast phenotype: Molecular mechanisms mediating osteoblast growth and development. *Iowa Orthop J.* 1995;15:118-140.
235. Tamura T, Noda M. Identification of a DNA sequence involved in osteoblast-specific gene expression via interaction with helix-loop-helix (HLH)-type transcription factors. *J Cell Biol.* 1994;126:773-782.
236. Garnero P, Grimaux M, Seguin P, et al. Characterization of immunoreactive forms of human osteocalcin generated in vivo and in vitro. *J Bone Miner Res.* 1994;9:255-264.
237. Mahonen A, Jaaskelainen T, Maenpaa PH. A novel vitamin D analog with two double bonds in its side chain: A potent inducer of osteoblastic cell differentiation. *Biochem Pharmacol.* 1996;51:887-892.
238. Arbour NC, Darwish HM, DeLuca HF. Transcriptional control of the osteocalcin gene by 1/25 dihydroxyvitamin D-2 and its 24-epimer in rat osteosarcoma cells. *Biochim Biophys Acta.* 1995;1263:147-153.
239. Bradbeer JN, Virdi AS, Serre CM, et al. A number of osteocalcin antisera recognize epitopes on proteins other than osteocalcin in cultured skin fibroblasts: Implications for the identification of cells of the osteoblastic lineage in vitro. *J Bone Miner Res.* 1994;9:1221-1228.
240. Takada J, Ishii S, Ohta T, et al. Usefulness of a novel monoclonal antibody against human osteocalcin in immunohistochemical diagnosis. *Virchows Arch A.* 1992;420:507-511.
241. Fanburg JC, Rosenberg AE, Weaver DL, et al. Osteocalcin and osteonectin immunoreactivity in the diagnosis of osteosarcoma. *Am J Clin Pathol.* 1997;108:464-473.
242. Fanburg-Smith JC, Bratthauer GL, Miettinen M. Osteocalcin and osteonectin immunoreactivity in extraskeletal osteosarcoma: A study of 28 cases. *Hum Pathol.* 1999;30:32-38.
243. Naylor SL, Helin-Davies D, Charoenworawat P, et al. The human osteonectin gene (OSN) has Taq I and Msp I polymorphisms. *Nucleic Acids Res.* 1989;17:6753.
244. Rodan GA, Noda M. Gene expression in osteoblastic cells. *Crit Rev Eukaryot Gene Expr.* 1991;1:85-98.
245. Villarreal XC, Grant BW, Long GL. Demonstration of osteonectin mRNA in megakaryocytes: The use of the polymerase chain reaction. *Blood.* 1991;78:1216-1222.
246. Kelm Jr RJ, Hair GA, Mann KG, et al. Characterization of human osteoblast and megakaryocyte-derived osteonectin (SPARC). *Blood.* 1992;80:3112-3119.
247. Kamihagi K, Katayama M, Ouchi R, et al. Osteonectin/SPARC regulates cellular secretion rates of fibronectin and laminin extracellular matrix proteins. *Biochem Biophys Res Commun.* 1994;200:423-428.
248. Serra M, Morini MC, Scotlandi K, et al. Evaluation of osteonectin as a diagnostic marker of osteogenic bone tumors. *Hum Pathol.* 1992;23:1326-1331.
249. Wuisman P, Roessner A, Bosse A, et al. Osteonectin in osteosarcomas: A marker for differential diagnosis and/or prognosis? *Ann Oncol.* 1992;3(Suppl 2):S33-S35.
250. Bosse A, Vollmer E, Bocker W, et al. The impact of osteonectin for differential diagnosis of bone tumors: An immunohistochemical approach. *Pathol Res Pract.* 1990;186:651-657.
251. Fetsch PA, Marincola FM, Filie A, et al. Melanoma-associated antigen recognized by T-cells (MART-1): The advent of a preferred immunocytochemical antibody for the diagnosis of metastatic malignant melanoma with fine needle aspiration. *Cancer.* 1999;87:37-42.
252. Kaufmann O, Koch S, Burghardt J, et al. Tyrosinase, melan-A, and KBA62 as markers for the immunohistochemical identification of metastatic amelanotic melanomas in paraffin sections. *Mod Pathol.* 1998;11:740-746.
253. Zelger BG, Steiner H, Wambacher B, et al. Malignant melanomas simulating various types of soft tissue tumors. *Dermatol Surg.* 1997;23:1047-1054.
254. Fetsch JF, Michal M, Miettinen M. Pigmented (melanotic) neurofibroma: A clinicopathologic and immunohistochemical analysis of 19 lesions from 17 patients. *Am J Surg Pathol.* 2000;24:331-343.

255. Cangul IT, van Garderen E, Van der Poel HJ, et al. Tyrosinase gene expression in clear cell sarcoma indicates a melanocytic origin: Insight from the first reported canine case. *APMIS.* 1999;107:982-988.
256. Papas-Corden P, Zarbo RJ, Gown AM, et al. Immunohistochemical characterization of synovial, epithelioid, and clear cell sarcomas. *Surg Pathol.* 1989;2:43-58.
257. Gould VE, Wiedenmann B, Lee I, et al. Synaptophysin expression in neuroendocrine neoplasms as determined by immunocytochemistry. *Am J Pathol.* 1987;126:243-257.
258. Ladanyi M, Heinemann FS, Huvos AG, et al. Neural differentiation in small round cell tumors of bone and soft tissue with the translocation t(11;22)(q24]2): An immunohistochemical study of 11 cases. *Hum Pathol.* 1990;21:1245-1251.
259. Parham DM, Hijazi Y, Steinberg SM, et al. Neuroectodermal differentiation in Ewing's sarcoma family of tumors does not predict tumor behavior. *Hum Pathol.* 1999;30:911-918.
260. Roessner A, Jurgens H. Round cell tumors of bone. *Pathol Res Pract.* 1993;189:111-136.
261. Dierick AM, Roels H, Langlois M. The immunophenotype of Ewing's sarcoma: An immunohistochemical analysis. *Pathol Res Pract.* 1993;189:26-32.
262. Wang AR, May D, Bourne P, et al. PGP9.5: A marker for cellular neurothekeoma. *Am J Surg Pathol.* 1999;23:1401-1407.
263. Miettinen M, Chatten J, Paetau A, et al. Monoclonal antibody NB84 in the differential diagnosis of neuroblastoma and other small round cell tumors. *Am J Surg Pathol.* 1998;22:327-332.
264. Gerbig AW, Zala L, Hunziker T. Tumor-like eosinophilic granuloma of the skin. *Am J Dermatopathol.* 2000;22:75-78.
265. Stefanato CM, Andersen WK, Calonje E, et al. Langerhans cell histiocytosis in the elderly: A report of three cases. *J Am Acad Dermatol.* 1998;39:375-378.
266. Knowles II DM. Lymphoid cell markers: Their distribution and usefulness in the immunopathologic analysis of lymphoid neoplasms. *Am J Surg Pathol.* 1985;9(Suppl):85-108.
267. Weiss LM, Bindl JM, Picozzi VJ, et al. Lymphoblastic lymphoma: An immunophenotypic study of 26 cases with comparison to T-cell acute lymphoblastic leukemia. *Blood.* 1986;67:474-478.
268. Picker LJ, Weiss LM, Medeiros LJ, et al. Immunophenotypic criteria for the diagnosis of non-Hodgkin's lymphoma. *Am J Pathol.* 1987;128:181-201.
269. Orosz Z, Kopper L. Syndecan-1 expression in different soft tissue tumors. *Anticancer Res.* 2001;21:733-737.
270. Ozdemirli M, Fanburg-Smith JC, Hartmann DP, et al. Precursor B-lymphoblastic lymphoma presenting as a solitary bone tumor and mimicking Ewing's sarcoma: A report of four cases and review of the literature. *Am J Surg Pathol.* 1998;22:795-804.
271. Petruch UR, Horny HP, Kaiserling E. Frequent expression of hematopoietic and non-hematopoietic antigens by neoplastic plasma cells: An immunohistochemical study using formalin-fixed, paraffin-embedded tissue. *Histopathology.* 1992;20:35-40.
272. Robertson PB, Neiman RS, Worapongpaiboon S, et al. O13 (CD99) positivity in hematologic proliferations correlates with TdT positivity. *Mod Pathol.* 1997;10:277-282.
273. Soslow RA, Bhargava V, Warnke RA. MIC2, TdT, bcl-2, and CD34 expression in paraffin-embedded high-grade lymphoma/acute lymphoblastic leukemia distinguishes between distinct clinicopathologic entities. *Hum Pathol.* 1997;28:1158-1165.
274. Hibshoosh H, Lattes R. Immunohistochemical and molecular genetic approaches to soft tissue tumor diagnosis: A primer. *Semin Oncol.* 1997;24:515-525.
275. Smith MJ, Goodfellow PN. MIC2R: A transcribed MIC2-related sequence associated with a CpG island in the human pseudoautosomal region. *Hum Mol Genet.* 1994;3:1575-1582.
276. Smith MJ, Goodfellow PJ, Goodfellow PN. The genomic organization of the human pseudoautosomal gene MIC2 and the detection of a related locus. *Hum Mol Genet.* 1993;2:417-422.
277. Fellinger EJ, Garin-Chesa P, Su SL, et al. Biochemical and genetic characterization of the HBA-71 Ewing's sarcoma cell surface antigen. *Cancer Res.* 1991;51:336-340.
278. Renshaw AA. O13 (CD99) in spindle cell tumors: Reactivity with hemangiopericytoma, solitary fibrous tumor, synovial sarcoma, and meningioma, but rarely with sarcomatoid mesothelioma. *Appl Immunohistochem.* 1995;3:250-256.
279. Soslow RA, Wallace M, Goris J, et al. MIC2 gene expression in cutaneous neuroendocrine carcinoma (Merkel cell carcinoma). *Appl Immunohistochem.* 1996;4:235-240.
280. Lumadue JA, Askin FB, Perlman EJ. MIC2 analysis of small cell carcinoma. *Am J Clin Pathol.* 1994;102:692-694.
281. Nicholson SA, McDermott MB, Swanson PE, et al. CD99 and cytokeratin-20 in small-cell and basaloid tumors of the skin. *Appl Immunohistochem Mol Morphol.* 2000;8:37-41.
282. Shiota M, Fujimoto J, Semba T, et al. Hyperphosphorylation of a novel 80 kDa protein-tyrosine kinase similar to Ltk in a human Ki-lymphoma cell line, AMS3. *Oncogene.* 1994;9:1567-1574.
283. Cessna MH, Zhou H, Sanger WG, et al. Expression of ALK1 and p80 in inflammatory myofibroblastic tumor and its mesenchymal mimics: A study of 135 cases. *Mod Pathol.* 2002;15:931-938.
284. Sigel JE, Smith TA, Reith JD, et al. Immunohistochemical analysis of anaplastic lymphoma kinase expression in deep soft tissue calcifying fibrous pseudotumor: evidence of a late sclerosing stage of inflammatory myofibroblastic tumor? *Ann Diagn Pathol.* 2001;5:10-14.
285. Li XQ, Hisaoka M, Shi DR, et al. Expression of anaplastic lymphoma kinase in soft tissue tumors: An immunohistochemical and molecular study of 249 cases. *Hum Pathol.* 2004;35:711-721.
286. Binh MB, Sastre-Garau X, Guillou L, et al. MDM2 and CDK4 immunostainings are useful adjuncts in diagnosing well-differentiated and dedifferentiated liposarcoma subtypes: A comparative analysis of 559 soft tissue neoplasms with genetic data. *Am J Surg Pathol.* 2005;29:1340-1347.
287. Binh MB, Garau XS, Guillou L, et al. Reproducibility of MDM2 and CDK4 staining in soft tissue tumors. *Am J Clin Pathol.* 2006;125:693-697.
288. Sirvent N, Coindre JM, Maire G, et al. Detection of MDM2-CDK4 amplification by fluorescence in situ hybridization in 200 paraffin-embedded tumor samples: Utility in diagnosing adipocytic lesions and comparison with immunohistochemistry and real-time PCR. *Am J Surg Pathol.* 2007;31:1476-1489.
289. Dei Tos AP, Doglioni C, Piccinin S, et al. Coordinated expression and amplification of the MDM2, CDK4, and HMGI-C genes in atypical lipomatous tumours. *J Pathol.* 2000;190:531-536.
290. He M, Aisner S, Benevenia J, et al. p16 immunohistochemistry as an alternative marker to distinguish atypical lipomatous tumor from deep-seated lipoma. *Appl Immunohistochem Mol Morphol.* 2009;17:51-56.
291. Argani P, Lal P, Hutchinson B, et al. Aberrant nuclear immunoreactivity for TFE3 in neoplasms with TFE3 gene fusions: A sensitive and specific immunohistochemical assay. *Am J Surg Pathol.* 2003;27:750-761.
292. Argani P, Olgac S, Tickoo SK, et al. Xp11 translocation renal cell carcinoma in adults: expanded clinical, pathologic, and genetic spectrum. *Am J Surg Pathol.* 2007;31:1149-1160.
293. Carlson JW, Fletcher CDM. Immunohistochemistry for beta-catenin in the differential diagnosis of spindle-cell lesions: Analysis of a series and review of the literature. *Histopathology.* 2007;51:509-514.
294. Bhattacharya B, Dilworth HP, Iacobuzio-Donahue C, et al. Nuclear beta-catenin expression distinguishes deep fibromatosis from other benign and malignant fibroblastic and myofibroblastic lesions. *Am J Surg Pathol.* 2005;29:653-659.
295. Rakheja D, Molberg KH, Roberts CA, et al. Immunohistochemical expression of beta-catenin in solitary fibrous tumors. *Arch Pathol Lab Med.* 2005;129:776-779.
296. Eckert F, Schaich B. Tendon sheath fibroma: A case report with immunohistochemical studies. *Hautarzt.* 1992;43:92-96.
297. Ide F, Shimoyama T, Horie N, et al. Collagenous fibroma (desmoplastic fibroblastoma) presenting as a parotid mass. *J Oral Pathol Med.* 1999;28:465-468.
298. Neilsen GP, O'Connell JX, Dickersin GR, et al. Collagenous fibroma (desmoplastic fibroblastoma): A report of seven cases. *Mod Pathol.* 1996;9:781-785.
299. Sciot R, Samson I, van der Berghe H, et al. Collagenous fibroma (desmoplastic fibroblastoma): Genetic link with fibroma of tendon sheath? *Mod Pathol.* 1999;12:565-568.

300. Carney JA. Psammomatous melanotic schwannoma: A distinctive, heritable tumor with special associations, including cardiac myxoma and the Cushing syndrome. *Am J Surg Pathol.* 1990;14:206-222.
301. Fine SW, McClain SA, Li M. Immunohistochemical staining for calretinin is useful for differentiating schwannomas from neurofibromas. *Am J Clin Pathol.* 2004;122:552-559.
302. Suster S, Fisher C. Immunoreactivity for the human hematopoietic progenitor cell antigen (CD34) in lipomatous tumors. *Am J Surg Pathol.* 1997;21:195-200.
303. Shimokama T, Watanabe T. Leiomyoma exhibiting a marked granular change: Granular cell leiomyoma versus granular cell schwannoma. *Hum Pathol.* 1992;23:327-331.
304. Mazur MT, Shultz JJ, Myers JL. Granular cell tumor: Immunohistochemical analysis of 21 benign tumors and one malignant tumor. *Arch Pathol Lab Med.* 1990;114:692-696.
305. Cavaliere A, Sidoni A, Ferri I, et al. Granular cell tumor: An immunohistochemical study. *Tumori.* 1994;80:224-228.
306. Kurtin PJ, Bonin DM. Immunohistochemical demonstration of the lysosome-associated glycoprotein CD68 (KP-1) in granular cell tumors and schwannomas. *Hum Pathol.* 1994;25:1172-1178.
307. Filie AC, Lage JM, Azumi N. Immunoreactivity of S100 protein, alpha-1-antitrypsin, and CD68 in adult and congenital granular cell tumors. *Mod Pathol.* 1996;9:888-892.
308. Fine SW, Li M. Expression of calretinin and the alpha-subunit of inhibin in granular cell tumors. *Am J Clin Pathol.* 2003;119:259-264.
309. Younes M, Lechago LV, Lechago J. Overexpression of the human erythrocyte glucose transporter occurs as a late event in human colorectal carcinogenesis and is associated with an increased incidence of lymph node metastases. *Clin Cancer Res.* 1996;2:1151-1154.
310. Haber RS, Weiser KR, Pritsker A, et al. GLUT1 glucose transporter expression in benign and malignant thyroid nodules. *Thyroid.* 1997;7:363-367.
311. North PE, Waner M, Mizeracki A, et al. GLUT1: A newly discovered immunohistochemical marker for juvenile hemangiomas. *Hum Pathol.* 2000;31:11-22.
312. Younes M, Brown RW, Stephenson M, et al. Overexpression of Glut1 and Glut3 in stage I nonsmall cell lung cancer is associated with poor survival. *Cancer.* 1997;80:1046-1051.
313. Rossi S, Orvieto E, Furlanetto A, et al. Utility of the immunohistochemical detection of FLI-1 expression in round cell and vascular neoplasms using a monoclonal antibody. *Mod Pathol.* 2004;17:547-552.
314. Lelievre E, Lionneton F, Mattot V, et al. Ets-1 regulates FLI1 expression in endothelial cells: Identification of ETS binding sites in the FLI-1 gene promoter. *J Biol Chem.* 2002;277:25143-25151.
315. Kapadia SB, Meis JM, Frisman DM, et al. Fetal rhabdomyoma of the head and neck: A clinicopathological and immunophenotypic study of 24 cases. *Hum Pathol.* 1993;24:754-765.
316. Tanda F, Rocca PC, Bosincu L, et al. Rhabdomyoma of the tunica vaginalis of the testis: A histologic, immunohistochemical, and ultrastructural study. *Mod Pathol.* 1997;10:608-611.
317. Bastian BC, Brocker EB. Adult rhabdomyoma of the lip. *Am J Dermatopathol.* 1998;20:61-64.
318. Gibas Z, Miettinen M. Recurrent parapharyngeal rhabdomyoma: Evidence of neoplastic nature of the tumor from cytogenetic study. *Am J Surg Pathol.* 1192;16:721-728.
319. Ockner DM, Sayadi H, Swanson SE, et al. Genital angiomyofibroblastoma: Comparison with aggressive angiomyxoma and other myxoid neoplasms of skin and soft tissue. *Am J Clin Pathol.* 1997;107:36-44.
320. Fletcher CDM, Tsang WTW, Fisher C, et al. Angiomyofibroblastoma of the vulva: A benign neoplasm distinct from aggressive angiomyxoma. *Am J Surg Pathol.* 1992;16:373-382.
321. Neilsen GP, Rosenberg AE, Young RH, et al. Angiomyofibroblastoma of the vulva and vagina. *Mod Pathol.* 1996;9:284-291.
322. Granter SR, Nucci MR, Fletcher CD. Aggressive angiomyxoma: Reappraisal of its relationship to angiomyofibroblastoma in a series of 16 cases. *Histopathology.* 1997;30:3-10.
323. Laskin WB, Fetsch JF, Tavassoli FA. Angiomyofibroblastoma of the female genital tract: Analysis of 17 cases including a lipomatous variant. *Hum Pathol.* 1997;28:1046-1055.
324. Enzinger FM, Weiss SW. Fibrous tumors of infancy and childhood. In: Enzinger FM, Weiss SW, eds. *Soft tissue tumors.* 2nd ed. St Louis: Mosby-Year Book; 1995:722.
325. Nemes Z. Differentiation markers in hemangiopericytoma. *Cancer.* 1992;69:133-140.
326. Molnar P, Nemes Z. Hemangiopericytoma of the cerebellopontine angle: Diagnostic pitfalls and the diagnostic value of the subunit A of factor XIII as a tumor marker. *Clin Neuropathol.* 1995;14:19-24.
327. Catalano PJ, Brandwein M, Shah DK, et al. Sinonasal hemangiopericytomas: A clinicopathologic and immunohistochemical study of seven cases. *Head Neck.* 1996;18:42-53.
328. Middleton LP, Duray PH, Merino MJ. The histological spectrum of hemangiopericytoma: Application of immunohistochemical analysis including proliferative markers to facilitate diagnosis and predict prognosis. *Hum Pathol.* 1998;29:636-640.
329. Klemperer P, Rabin CB. Primary neoplasms of the pleura: A report of five cases. *Arch Pathol.* 1931;11:385-412.
330. Hanau CA, Miettinen M. Solitary fibrous tumor: Histological and immunohistochemical spectrum of benign and malignant variants presenting at different sites. *Hum Pathol.* 1995;26:440-449.
331. Hasegawa T, Matsuno Y, Shimoda T, et al. Frequent expression of bcl-2 protein in solitary fibrous tumors. *Jpn J Clin Oncol.* 1998;28:86-91.
332. Brunnemann RB, Ro JY, Ordonez NG, et al. Extrapleural solitary fibrous tumor: A clinicopathologic study of 24 cases. *Mod Pathol.* 1999;12:1034-1042.
333. de Saint Aubain Somerhausen N, Rubin BP, Fletcher CD. Myxoid solitary fibrous tumor: A study of seven cases with emphasis on differential diagnosis. *Mod Pathol.* 1999;12:463-471.
334. Bhargava R, Shia J, Hummer AJ, et al. Distinction of endometrial stromal sarcomas from "hemangiopericytomatous" tumors using a panel of immunohistochemical stains. *Mod Pathol.* 2005;18:40-47.
335. Matsumoto K, Yamamoto T, Min W, et al. Ossifying fibromyxoid tumor of soft parts: Clinicopathologic, immunohistochemical and ultrastructural study of four cases. *Pathol Int.* 1999;49:742-746.
336. Ekfors TO, Kulju T, Aaltonen M, et al. Ossifying fibromyxoid tumour of soft parts: Report of four cases including one mediastinal and one infantile. *APMIS.* 1998;106:1124-1130.
337. Yang P, Hirose T, Hasegawa T, et al. Ossifying fibromyxoid tumor of soft parts: A morphological and immunohistochemical study. *Pathol Int.* 1994;44:448-453.
338. Miettinen M. Ossifying fibromyxoid tumor of soft parts: Additional observations of a distinctive soft tissue tumor. *Am J Clin Pathol.* 1991;95:142-149.
339. Fukunaga M, Ushigome S, Ishikawa E. Ossifying subcutaneous tumor with myofibroblastic differentiation: A variant of ossifying fibromyxoid tumor of soft parts? *Pathol Int.* 1994;44:727-734.
340. Schofield JB, Krausz T, Stamp GW, et al. Ossifying fibromyxoid tumour of soft parts: Immunohistochemical and ultrastructural analysis. *Histopathology.* 1999;22:101-112.
341. Williams SB, Ellis GL, Meis JM, et al. Ossifying fibromyxoid tumour (of soft parts) of the head and neck: A clinicopathological and immunohistochemical study of nine cases. *J Laryngol Otol.* 1993;107:75-80.
342. Miettinen M, Finnell V, Fetsch JF. Ossifying fibromyxoid tumor of soft parts—a clinicopathologic and immunohistochemical study of 104 cases with long-term followup and a critical review of the literature. *Am J Surg Pathol.* 2008;32:996-1005.
343. Folpe AL, Weiss SW. Ossifying fibromyxoid tumor of soft parts: A clinicopathologic study of 70 cases with emphasis on atypical and malignant variants. *Am J Surg Pathol.* 2003;27:421-431.
344. Hamakawa H, Omori T, Sumida T, et al. Intraosseous epithelioid hemangioendothelioma of the mandible: A case report with an immunohistochemical study. *J Oral Pathol Med.* 1999;28:233-237.

345. Siddiqui MT, Evans HL, Ro JY, et al. Epithelioid haemangioendothelioma of the thyroid gland: A case report and review of literature. *Histopathology*. 1998;32:473-476.
346. Gray MH, Rosenberg AE, Dickerson GR, et al. Cytokeratin expression in epithelioid vascular neoplasms. *Hum Pathol.* 1990;21:212-217.
347. Van Haelst UJ, Pruszczynski M, ten Cate LN, et al. Ultrastructural and immunohistochemical study of epithelioid hemangioendothelioma of bone: Coexpression of epithelial and endothelial markers. *Ultrastruct Pathol.* 1990;14:141-149.
348. Mentzel T, Beham A, Calonje E, et al. Epithelioid hemangioendothelioma of skin and soft tissues: Clinicopathologic and immunohistochemical study of 30 cases. *Am J Surg Pathol.* 1997;21:363-374.
349. Hornick JL, Dal Cin P, Fletcher CDM. Loss of INI1 expression is characteristic of both conventional and proximal-type epithelioid sarcoma. *Am J Surg Pathol.* 2009, in press.
350. Billings SD, Folpe AL, Weiss SW. Epithelioid sarcoma-like hemangioendothelioma. *Am J Surg Pathol.* 2003;27:48-57.
351. Zukerberg LR, Nickoloff BJ, Weisee SW. Kaposiform hemangioendothelioma of infancy and childhood: An aggressive neoplasm associated with Kasaback-Merritt syndrome and lymphangiomatosis. *Am J Surg Pathol.* 1993;17:321-328.
352. Mentzel T, Mazzoleni G, Dei Tos AP, et al. Kaposiform hemangioendothelioma in adults. Clinicopathologic and immunohistochemical analysis of three cases. *Am J Clin Pathol.* 1997;108:450-455.
353. Lyons LL, North PE, MacMoune-Lai F, et al. Kaposiform hemangioendothelioma: A study of 33 cases emphasizing its pathologic, immunophenotypic, and biologic uniqueness from juvenile hemangioma. *Am J Surg Pathol.* 2004;28:559-568.
354. Arai E, Kuramochi A, Tsuchida T, et al. Usefulness of D2-40 immunohistochemistry for differentiation between kaposiform hemangioendothelioma and tufted angioma. *J Cutan Pathol.* 2006;33:492–407.
355. Begin LR, Clement PB, Kirk ME, et al. Aggressive angiomyxoma of pelvic soft parts: A clinicopathologic study of nine cases. *Hum Pathol.* 1985;16:621-628.
356. Sementa AR, Gambini C, Borgiani L, et al. Aggressive angiomyxoma of the pelvis and perineum: Report of a case with immunohistochemical and electron microscopic study. *Pathologica.* 1989;81:463-469.
357. Tsang WY, Chan JK, Lee KC, et al. Aggressive angiomyxoma: A report of four cases occurring in men. *Am J Surg Pathol.* 1992;16:1059-1065.
358. Tallini G, Parham DM, Dias P, et al. Myogenic regulatory protein expression in adult soft tissue sarcomas: A sensitive and specific marker of skeletal muscle differentiation. *Am J Pathol.* 1994;144:693-701.
359. Dias P, Parham DM, Shapiro DN, et al. Myogenic regulatory protein (MyoD1) expression in childhood solid tumors: Diagnostic utility in rhabdomyosarcoma. *Am J Pathol.* 1990;13:1283-1291.
360. Sorensen PH, Shimada H, Liu XF, et al. Biphenotypic sarcomas with myogenic and neural differentiation express the Ewing's sarcoma EWS/FLI1 fusion gene. *Cancer Res.* 1995;15:1385-1392.
361. Gattenlohner S, Muller-Hernelink HK, Marx A. Polymerase chain reaction-based diagnosis of rhabdomyosarcomas: Comparison of fetal type acetylcholine receptor subunits and myogenin. *Diagn Mol Pathol.* 1998;7:129-134.
362. Meyer T, Brinck U. Immunohistochemical detection of vinculin in human rhabdomyosarcomas. *Gen Diagn Pathol.* 1997;142:191-198.
363. Pinto A, Paslawski D, Sarnat HB, et al. Immunohistochemical evaluation of dystrophin expression in small round cell tumors of childhood. *Mod Pathol.* 1993;6:679-683.
364. Bowman F, Champigneulle J, Schmitt C, et al. Clear cell rhabdomyosarcoma. *Pediatr Pathol Lab Med.* 1996;16:951-959.
365. Kobayshi M, Sjoberg G, Soderhall S, et al. Pediatric rhabdomyosarcomas express the intermediate filament nestin. *Pediatr Res.* 1998;43:86-92.
366. Yun K. A new marker for rhabdomyosarcoma: Insulin-like growth factor II. *Lab Invest.* 1992;67:653-664.
367. Gattenlohner S, Vincent A, Leuschner I, et al. The fetal form of the acetylcholine receptor distinguished rhabdomyosarcomas from other childhood tumors. *Am J Pathol.* 1998;152:437-444.
368. Molenaar WM, Muntinghe FL. Expression of neural adhesion molecules and neurofilament protein isoforms in skeletal muscle tumors. *Hum Pathol.* 1998;29:1290-1293.
369. Coffin CM, Rulon J, Smith L, et al. Pathologic features of rhabdomyosarcoma before and after treatment: A clinicopathologic and immunohistochemical analysis. *Mod Pathol.* 1997;10:1175-1187.
370. Navarro S, Cavazzana AO, Llombart-Bosch A, et al. Comparison of Ewing's sarcoma of bone and peripheral neuroepithelioma: An immunocytochemical and ultrastructural analysis of two primitive neuroectodermal neoplasms. *Arch Pathol Lab Med.* 1994;118:608-615.
371. Lizard-Nacol S, Justrabo E, Mugneret F, et al. Immunocytologic study of light cell lines established in vitro from Ewing's sarcoma: Identification of neural markers. *C R Seances Soc Biol Fil.* 1988;182:118-125.
372. Lee CS, Southey MC, Waters K, et al. EWS/FLI-1 fusion transcript detection and MIC2 immunohistochemical staining in the detection of Ewing's sarcoma. *Pediatr Pathol Lab Med.* 1996;16:379-392.
373. Scotlandi K, Serra M, Manara MC, et al. Immunostaining of the p30/32MIC2 antigen and molecular detection of EWS rearrangements for the diagnosis of Ewing's sarcoma and peripheral neuroectodermal tumor. *Hum Pathol.* 1996;27:408-416.
374. de Alava E, Lozano MD, Sola I, et al. Molecular features in a biphenotypic small cell sarcoma with neuroectodermal and muscle differentiation. *Hum Pathol.* 1998;29:181-184.
375. Knezevich SR, Hendson G, Methers JA, et al. Absence of detectable EWS/FLI1 expression after therapy-induced neural differentiation in Ewing sarcoma. *Hum Pathol.* 1997;29:289-294.
376. Ambros IM, Ambros PF, Strehl S, et al. MIC2 is a specific marker for Ewing's sarcoma and peripheral primitive neuroectodermal tumors: Evidence for a common histogenesis of Ewing's sarcoma and peripheral primitive neuroectodermal tumors from MIC2 expression and specific chromosome aberration. *Cancer.* 1991;67:1886-1893.
377. Fellinger EJ, Garin-Chesa P, Triche TJ, et al. Immunohistochemical analysis of Ewing's sarcoma cell surface antigen p30/32MIC2. *Am J Pathol.* 1991;139:317-325.
378. Folpe AL, Hill CE, Parham DM, O'Shea PA, Weiss SW. Immunohistochemical detection of FLI-1 protein expression: A study of 132 round-cell tumors with emphasis on CD99-positive mimics of Ewing's sarcoma/primitive neuroectodermal tumor. *Am J Surg Pathol.* 2000;24:1657-1662.
379. Halliday BE, Slagel DD, Elsheikh TE, et al. Diagnostic utility of MIC-2 immunocytochemical staining in the differential diagnosis of small blue cell tumors. *Diagn Cytopathol.* 1998;19:410-416.
380. Miettinen M, Lehto VP, Virtanen J. Histogenesis of Ewing's sarcoma: An evaluation of intermediate filaments and endothelial cell markers. *Virchows Arch Cell Pathol.* 1988;41:277.
381. Navas-Palacios JJ, Aparicio-Duque R, Valdes MD. On the histogenesis of Ewing's sarcoma: An ultrastructural, immunohistochemical, and cytochemical study. *Cancer.* 1984;53:1882.
382. Gu M, Antonescu CR, Guiter G, et al. Cytokeratin immunoreactivity in Ewing's sarcoma: Prevalence in 50 cases confirmed by molecular diagnostic studies. *Am J Surg Pathol.* 1999;24:410-416.
383. Barth T, Moller P, Mechtersheimer G. Differential expression of beta 1, beta 3, beta 4 integrins in sarcomas of the small round blue cell category. *Virchows Arch.* 1995;426:19-25.
384. Chung DH, Lee JI, Kook MC, et al. ILK (beta1-integrin-linked protein kinase): A novel immunohistochemical marker for Ewing's sarcoma and primitive neuroectodermal tumour. *Virchows Arch.* 1998;433:113-117.
385. Swanson PE, Lillemoe TJ, Manivel JC, et al. Mesenchymal chondrosarcoma: An immunohistochemical study. *Arch Pathol Lab Med.* 1990;114:943-948.
386. Kurotaki H, Tateoka H, Takeuchi M, et al. Primary mesenchymal chondrosarcoma of the lung: A case report with immunohistochemical and ultrastructural features. *Acta Pathol Jpn.* 1992;42:364-371.

387. Rushing EJ, Armonda RA, Ansari Q, et al. Mesenchymal chondrosarcoma: A clinicopathologic and flow cytometric study of 13 cases presenting in the central nervous system. *Cancer.* 1996;77:1884-1891.
388. Brown RE, Boyle JL. Mesenchymal chondrosarcoma: Molecular characterization by a proteomic approach, with morphogenic and therapeutic implications. *Ann Clin Lab Sci.* 2003;33:131-141.
389. Granter SR, Renshaw AA, Fletcher CD, et al. CD99 reactivity in mesenchymal chondrosarcoma. *Hum Pathol.* 1996;27:1273-1276.
390. Lyon DB, Dortzbach RK, Gilbert-Barness E. Polyphenotypic small-cell orbitocranial tumor. *Arch Ophthalmol.* 1991;111:1402-1408.
391. Pearson JM, Harris M, Eyden BP, et al. Divergent differentiation in small round-cell tumours of the soft tissues with neural features—an analysis of 10 cases. *Histopathology.* 1993;23:1-9.
392. Frydman CP, Klein MJ, Abdelwahab IF, et al. Primitive multipotential primary sarcoma of bone: A case report and immunohistochemical study. *Mod Pathol.* 1991;4:768-772.
393. Gerald WL, Ladanyi M, de Alava E, et al. Clinical, pathologic, and molecular spectrum of tumors associated with t(11;22)(p13]2): Desmoplastic small round-cell tumor and its variants. *J Clin Oncol.* 1998;16:3028-3036.
394. Katz RL, Quezado M, Senderowicz AM, et al. An intra-abdominal small round cell neoplasm with features of primitive neuroectodermal and desmoplastic round cell tumor and a EWS/FLI-1 fusion transcript. *Hum Pathol.* 1997;28:502-509.
395. Noguera R, Navarro S, Cremades A, et al. Translocation (X:18) in a biphasic synovial sarcoma with morphologic features of neural differentiation. *Diagn Mol Pathol.* 1998;7:16-23.
396. Pelmus M, Guillou L, Hostein I, et al. Monophasic fibrous and poorly differentiated synovial sarcoma: Immunohistochemical reassessment of 60 t(X;18)(SYT-SSX)-positive cases. *Am J Surg Pathol.* 2002;26:1434-1440.
397. Masui F, Matsuno Y, Yokoyama R, et al. Synovial sarcoma, histologically mimicking primitive neuroectodermal tumor/Ewing's sarcoma at distant sites. *Jpn J Clin Oncol.* 1999;29:438-441.
398. Ozdemirli M, Fanburg-Smith JC, Hartmann DP, et al. Differentiating lymphoblastic lymphoma and Ewing's sarcoma: Lymphocyte markers and gene rearrangement. *Mod Pathol.* 2001;14:1175-1182.
399. Lucas DR, Bentley G, Dan ME, et al. Ewing sarcoma vs. lymphoblastic lymphoma: A comparative immunohistochemical study. *Am J Clin Pathol.* 2001;115:11-17.
400. Machen SK, Fisher C, Gautam RS, et al. Utility of cytokeratin subsets for distinguishing poorly differentiated synovial sarcoma from peripheral primitive neuroectodermal tumour. *Histopathology.* 1998;33:501-507.
401. Mathewson RC, Kjeldsberg CR, Perkins SL. Detection of terminal deoxynucleotidyl transferase (TdT) in non-hematopoietic small round cell tumors of children. *Pediatr Pathol Lab Med.* 1997;17:835-844.
402. Buresh CJ, Oliai BR, Miller RT. Reactivity with TdT in Merkel cell carcinoma: A potential diagnostic pitfall. *Am J Clin Pathol.* 2008;129:894-898.
403. Ramnani D, Lindberg G, Gokaslan ST, et al. Signet-ring cell variant of small lymphocytic lymphoma with a prominent sinusoidal pattern. *Ann Diagn Pathol.* 1999;3:220-226.
404. Tse CC, Chan JK, Yuen RW, et al. Malignant lymphoma with myxoid stroma: A new pattern in need of recognition. *Histopathology.* 1991;18:31-35.
405. Tsang WY, Chan JK, Tang SK, et al. Large cell lymphoma with a fibrillary matrix. *Histopathology.* 1992;29:80-82.
406. Meis JM, Enzinger FM. Inflammatory fibrosarcoma of the mesentery and retroperitoneum: A tumor closely simulating inflammatory pseudotumor. *Am J Surg Pathol.* 1991;15:1146-1156.
407. Gleason B, Hornick JL. Inflammatory myofibroblastic tumours: Where are we now? *J Clin Pathol.* 2008;61:428-437.
408. Mechtersheimer G, Moller P. Expression of Ki-1 antigen (CD30) in mesenchymal tumors. *Cancer.* 1990;66:1732-1737.
409. Winder SJ, Walsh MP. Calponin: Thin filament-linked regulation of smooth muscle contraction. *Cell Signal.* 1993;5:677-686.
410. Kaddu S, Baham A, Cerroni L, et al. Cutaneous leiomyosarcoma. *Am J Surg Pathol.* 1997;21:970-987.
411. Oliai BR, Tazelaar HD, Lloyd RV, et al. Leiomyosarcoma of the pulmonary veins. *Am J Surg Pathol.* 1999;23:1082-1088.
412. Rao UN, Finkelstein SD, Jones MW. Comparative immunohistochemical and molecular analysis of uterine and extrauterine leiomyosarcomas. *Mod Pathol.* 1999;1(2):1001-1009.
413. Bowman F, Gultekin H, Dickman PS. Latent Epstein-Barr virus infection demonstrated in low-grade leiomyosarcomas of adults with acquired immunodeficiency syndrome, but not in adjacent Kaposi's lesion or smooth muscle tumors in immunocompetent patients. *Arch Pathol Lab Med.* 1997;121:834-838.
414. Jenson HB, Montalvo EA, McClain KL, et al. Characterization of natural Epstein-Barr virus infection and replication in smooth muscle cells from a leiomyosarcoma. *J Med Virol.* 1999;57:36-46.
415. Swanson PE, Wick MR, Dehner LP. Leiomyosarcoma of somatic soft tissues in childhood: An immunohistochemical analysis of six cases with ultrastructural correlation. *Hum Pathol.* 1991;22:569-577.
416. Swanson PE, Stanley MW, Scheihauer BW, et al. Primary cutaneous leiomyosarcoma: A histological and immunohistochemical study of 9 cases, with ultrastructural correlation. *J Cutan Pathol.* 1988;15:129-141.
417. Nonaka D, Chiriboga L, Rubin BP. Sox10: A pan-schwannian and melanocytic marker. *Am J Surg Pathol.* 2008;32:1291-1298.
418. Smith TA, Machen SK, Fisher C, et al. Usefulness of cytokeratin subsets for distinguishing monophasic synovial sarcoma from malignant peripheral nerve sheath tumor. *Am J Clin Pathol.* 1999;112:641-648.
419. Morphopoulos GD, Banerjee SS, Ali HH, et al. Malignant peripheral nerve sheath tumour with vascular differentiation: A report of four cases. *Histopathology.* 1996;28:401-410.
420. King R, Busam K, Rosai J. Metastatic malignant melanoma resembling malignant peripheral nerve sheath tumor: Report of 16 cases. *Am J Surg Pathol.* 1999;23:1499-1505.
421. Lopes JM, Bjerkehagen B, Holm R, et al. Immunohistochemical profile of synovial sarcoma with emphasis on the epithelial-type differentiation: A study of 49 primary tumours, recurrences, and metastases. *Pathol Res Pract.* 1994;190:168-177.
422. Ordonez NG, Mahfouz SM, MacKay B. Synovial sarcoma: An immunohistochemical and ultrastructural study. *Hum Pathol.* 1990;21:733-749.
423. Nicholson AG, Goldstraw P, Fisher C. Synovial sarcoma of the pleura and its differentiation from other primary pleural tumours: A clinicopathological and immunohistochemical review of three cases. *Histopathology.* 1998;33:508-513.
424. Suster S, Fisher C, Moran CA. Expression of bcl-2 oncoprotein in benign and malignant spindle cell tumors of soft tissue, skin, serosal surfaces, and gastrointestinal tract. *Am J Surg Pathol.* 1998;22:863-872.
425. Terry J, Saito T, Subramanian S, et al. TLE1 as a diagnostic immunohistochemical marker for synovial sarcoma emerging from gene expression profiling studies. *Am J Surg Pathol.* 2007;31:240-246.
426. Morgan MB, Swann M, Somach S, et al. Cutaneous angiosarcoma: A case series with prognostic correlation. *J Am Acad Dermatol.* 2004;50:867-874.
427. Robin YM, Guillou L, Michels JJ, et al. Human herpesvirus 8 immunostaining: A sensitive and specific method for diagnosing Kaposi sarcoma in paraffin-embedded sections. *Am J Clin Pathol.* 2004;121:330-334.
428. Cheuk W, Wong KO, Wong CS, et al. Immunostaining for human herpesvirus 8 latent nuclear antigen-1 helps distinguish Kaposi sarcoma from its mimickers. *Am J Clin Pathol.* 2004;121:335-342.
429. Von Hochstetter AR, Meyer VE, Grant JW, et al. Epithelioid sarcoma mimicking angiosarcoma: The value of immunohistochemistry in the differential diagnosis. *Virchows Arch A Pathol Anat Histopathol.* 1991;418:271-278.
430. Chetty R, Slavin JL. Epithelioid sarcoma with extensive chondroid differentiation. *Histopathology.* 1994;24:400-401.
431. Laskin WB, Miettinen M. Epithelioid sarcoma: new insights based on an extended immunohistochemical analysis. *Arch Pathol Lab Med.* 2003;127:1161-1168.

432. Guillou L, Wadden C, Coindre JM, et al. "Proximal type" epithelioid sarcoma: A distinctive aggressive neoplasm showing rhabdoid feature: Clinicopathologic, immunohistochemical, and ultrastructural study of a series. *Am J Surg Pathol.* 1997;21:130-146.
433. Gerharz CD, Moll R, Meister P, et al. Cytoskeletal heterogeneity of an epithelioid sarcoma with expression of vimentin, cytokeratins, and neurofilaments. *Am J Surg Pathol.* 1990;14:274-283.
434. Domagala W, Weber K, Osborn M. Diagnostic significance of coexpression of intermediate filaments in fine needle aspiration. *Acta Cytol.* 1988;32:49-59.
435. Judkins AR, Montone KT, LiVolsi VA, et al. Sensitivity and specificity of antibodies on necrotic tumor tissue. *Am J Clin Pathol.* 1997;110:641-646.
436. Smith ME, Brown JI, Fisher C. Epithelioid sarcoma: Presence of vascular-endothelial cadherin and lack of epithelial cadherin. *Histopathology.* 1998;33:425-431.
437. Saito T, Oda Y, Itakura E, et al. Expression of intercellular adhesion molecules in epithelioid sarcoma and malignant rhabdoid tumor. *Pathol Int.* 2001;51:532-542.
438. Wick MR, Manivel JC. Epithelioid sarcoma and isolated necrobiotic granuloma: A comparative immunocytochemical study. *J Cutan Pathol.* 1986;13:253-260.
439. Kato H, Hatori M, Kokubun S, et al. CA125 expression in epithelioid sarcoma. *Jpn J Clin Oncol.* 2004;34:149-154.
440. Lee MW, Jee KJ, Ro JY, et al. Proximal-type epithelioid sarcoma: case report and results of comparative genomic hybridization. *J Cutan Pathol.* 2004;31:67-71.
441. Weidner N, Goldman R, Johnston J. Epithelioid monophasic synovial sarcoma. *Ultrastruct Pathol.* 1993;17:287-294.
442. Cerilli LA, Huffman HT, Anand A. Primary renal angiosarcoma: A case report with immunohistochemical, ultrastructural, and cytogenetic features and review of the literature. *Arch Pathol Lab Med.* 1998;122:929-935.
443. Poblet E, Gonzalez-Palacios F, Jimenez FJ. Different immunoreactivity of endothelial markers in well and poorly differentiated areas of angiosarcomas. *Virchows Arch.* 1996;428:217-221.
444. Ueda T, Oji Y, Naka N, et al. Overexpression of the Wilms' tumor gene WT1 in human bone and soft tissue sarcomas. *Cancer Sci.* 2003;94:271-276.
445. Meis-Kindblom JM. Clear cell sarcoma of tendons and aponeuroses: A historical perspective and tribute to the man behind the entity. *Adv Anat Pathol.* 2006;13:286-292.
446. Mooi WJ, Deenik W, Peterse JL, et al. Keratin immunoreactivity in melanoma of soft parts (clear cell sarcoma). *Histopathology.* 1995;27:61-65.
447. Hisaoka M, Ishida T, Kuo TT, et al. Clear cell sarcoma of soft tissue: A clinicopathologic, immunohistochemical, and molecular analysis of 33 cases. *Am J Surg Pathol.* 2008;32:452-460.
448. Hiraga H, Nojima T, Abe S, et al. Establishment of a new continuous clear cell sarcoma cell line: Morphological and cytogenetic characterization and detection of chimaeric EWS/ATF-1 transcripts. *Virchows Arch.* 1997;431:45-51.
449. Stenman G, Kindblom LG, Angervall L. Reciprocal translocation t(12;22)(q13]3) in clear-cell sarcoma of tendons and aponeuroses. *Genes Chromosomes Cancer.* 1992;4:122-127.
450. Laskin WB, Weiss SW, Bratthauer GL. Epithelioid variant of malignant peripheral nerve sheath tumor (malignant epithelioid schwannoma). *Am J Surg Pathol.* 1991;15:1136-1145.
451. Hoang MP, Sinkre P, Albores-Saavedra J. Expression of protein gene product 9.5 in epithelioid and conventional malignant peripheral nerve sheath tumors. *Arch Pathol Lab Med.* 2001;125:1321-1325.
452. Boyle JL, Haupt HM, Stern JB, et al. Tyrosinase expression in malignant melanoma, desmoplastic melanoma, and peripheral nerve sheath tumors. *Arch Pathol Lab Med.* 2002;126:816-822.
453. Jokinen CH, Dadras SS, Goldblum JR, et al. Diagnostic implications of podoplanin expression in peripheral nerve sheath neoplasms. *Am J Clin Pathol.* 2008;129:886-893.
454. Meis-Kindblom JM, Kindblom LG, Enzinger FM. Sclerosing epithelioid fibrosarcoma: A variant of fibrosarcoma simulating carcinoma. *Am J Surg Pathol.* 1995;19:979-993.
455. Hindermann W, Katenkamp D. Sclerosing epithelioid fibrosarcoma. *Pathologe.* 2003;24:103-108.
456. Antonescu CR, Rosenblum MK, Pereira P, et al. Sclerosing epithelioid fibrosarcoma: A study of 16 cases and confirmation of a clinicopathologically distinct tumor. *Am J Surg Pathol.* 2001;25:699-709.
457. Eyden BP, Manson C, Banerjee SS, et al. Sclerosing epithelioid fibrosarcoma: A study of five cases emphasizing diagnostic criteria. *Histopathology.* 1998;33:354-360.
458. Suster S. Epithelioid leiomyosarcoma of the skin and subcutaneous tissue: Clinicopathologic, immunohistochemical, and ultrastructural study of five cases. *Am J Surg Pathol.* 1994;18:232-240.
459. Lopez-Barea F, Rodriguez-Peralto JL, Sanchez-Herrera S, et al. Primary epithelioid leiomyosarcoma of bone: Case report and literature review. *Virchows Arch.* 1999;434:367-371.
460. Mukai M, Torikata C, Iri H, et al. Histogenesis of alveolar soft-part sarcoma: An immunohistochemical and biochemical study. *Am J Surg Pathol.* 1986;10:212-218.
461. Miettinen M, Ekfors T. Alveolar soft part sarcoma: Immunohistochemical evidence for muscle cell differentiation. *Am J Clin Pathol.* 1990;93:32-38.
462. Hurlimann J. Desmin and neural marker expression in mesothelial cells and mesotheliomas. *Hum Pathol.* 1994;25:753-757.
463. Foschini MP, Ceccarelli C, Eusebi V, et al. Alveolar soft-part sarcoma: Immunological evidence of rhabdomyoblastic differentiation. *Histopathology.* 1988;13:101-108.
464. Foschini MP, Eusein V. Alveolar soft part sarcoma: A new type of rhabdomyosarcoma? *Semin Diagn Pathol.* 1994;4:58-68.
465. Hirose T, Kudo E, Hasaegawa T, et al. Cytoskeletal properties of alveolar soft part sarcoma. *Hum Pathol.* 1990;21:204-211.
466. Menesce LP, Eyden BP, Edmondson D, et al. Immunophenotype and ultrastructure of alveolar soft part sarcoma. *J Submicrosc Cytol Pathol.* 1993;2593:377-387.
467. Rosai J, Dias P, Parham DM, et al. MyoD1 protein expression in alveolar soft part sarcoma as confirmatory evidence of its skeletal muscle nature. *Am J Surg Pathol.* 1991;15:974-981.
468. Nakano H, Tateishi A, Imamura T, et al. RT-PCR suggests human skeletal muscle origin of alveolar soft part sarcoma. *Oncology.* 2000;58:319-323.
469. Ordonez NG, Mackay B. Alveolar soft-part sarcoma: A review of the pathology and histogenesis. *Ultrastruct Pathol.* 1998;22:275-292.
470. Pang LJ, Chang B, Zou H, et al. Alveolar soft part sarcoma: A biomarker diagnostic strategy using TFE3 immunoassay and ASPL-TFE3 fusion transcripts in paraffin-embedded tumor tissues. *Diagn Mol Pathol.* 2008;17:245-252.
471. Wu A, Kunji LP, Cheng L, et al. Renal cell carcinoma in children and young adults: Analysis of clinicopathological, immunohistochemical, and molecular characteristics with an emphasis on the spectrum of Xp11.2 translocation-associated and unusual clear cell subtypes. *Histopathology.* 2008;53:533-544.
472. Cho HY, Chung DH, Khurana H, et al. The role of TFE3 in PEComa. *Histopathology.* 2008;53:236-249.
473. Roholl PJ, Prinsen I, Rademakers LP, et al. Two cell lines with epithelial cell-like characteristics established from malignant fibrous histiocytomas. *Cancer.* 1991;68:1963-1972.
474. Hasegawa T, Hasegawa F, Hirose T, et al. Expression of smooth muscle markers in so-called malignant fibrous histiocytomas. *J Clin Pathol.* 2003;56:666-671.
475. Nakanishi I, Katsuda S, Ooi A, et al. Diagnostic aspects of spindle-cell sarcomas by electron microscopy. *Acta Pathol Jpn.* 1983;33:425-437.
476. Hollowood K, Fletcher CDM. Malignant fibrous histiocytoma: Morphologic pattern or pathologic entity? *Semin Diagn Pathol.* 1995;12:210-220.
477. Brooks JJ. The significance of double phenotypic patterns and markers in human sarcomas: A new model of mesenchymal differentiation. *Am J Pathol.* 1986;125:113-123.
478. Lagace R, Aurias A. Does malignant fibrous histiocytoma exist? *Ann Pathol.* 2002;22:29-34.
479. Schneider P, Busch U, Meister H, et al. Malignant fibrous histiocytoma (MFH): A comparison of MFH in man and animals. A critical review. *Histol Histopathol.* 1999;14:845-860.

480. Erlandson RA, Antonescu CR. The rise and fall of malignant fibrous histiocytoma. *Ultrastruct Pathol.* 2004;28:283-289.
481. Oda Y, Miyajima K, Kawaguchi K, et al. Pleomorphic leiomyosarcoma: Clinicopathologic and immunohistochemical study with special emphasis on its distinction from ordinary leiomyosarcoma and malignant fibrous histiocytoma. *Am J Surg Pathol.* 2001;25:1030-1038.
482. Gaffney EF, Dervan PA, Fletcher CD. Pleomorphic rhabdomyosarcoma in adulthood: Analysis of 11 cases with definition of diagnostic criteria. *Am J Surg Pathol.* 1993;17:601-609.
483. Coindre JM, Hostein I, Maire G, et al. Inflammatory malignant fibrous histiocytomas and dedifferentiated liposarcomas: Histological review, genomic profile, and MDM2 and CDK4 status favor a single entity. *J Pathol.* 2004;203:822-830.
484. Gebhard S, Coindre JM, Michels JJ, et al. Pleomorphic liposarcoma: Clinicopathologic, immunohistochemical, and followup analysis of 63 cases. A study from the French Federation of Cancer Centers Sarcoma Group. *Am J Surg Pathol.* 2002;26:601-616.
485. Sandberg AA. Updates on the cytogenetics and molecular genetics of bone and soft tissue tumors: Liposarcoma. *Cancer Genet Cytogenet.* 2004;155:1-24.
486. Italiano A, Bianchini L, Keslair F, et al. HMGA2 is the partner of MDM2 in well-differentiated and dedifferentiated liposarcomas, whereas CDK4 belongs to a distinct inconsistent amplicon. *Int J Cancer.* 2008;122:2233-2241.
487. Fisher C, Carter RL, Ramachandra S, et al. Peripheral nerve sheath differentiation in malignant soft tissue tumours: An ultrastructural and immunohistochemical study. *Histopathology.* 1992;20:115-125.
488. Hitchcock MG, Hurt MA, Santa Cruz DJ. Cutaneous granular cell angiosarcoma. *J Cutan Pathol.* 1994;21:256-262.
489. Kodet R, Newton Jr WA, Sachs N, et al. Rhabdoid tumors of soft tissues: A clinicopathologic study of 26 cases enrolled on the Intergroup Rhabdomyosarcoma Study. *Hum Pathol.* 1991;22:674-684.
490. Shiratsuchi H, Oshiro Y, Saito T, et al. Cytokeratin subunits of inclusion bodies in rhabdoid cells: Immunohistochemical and clinicopathological study of malignant rhabdoid tumor and epithelioid sarcoma. *Int J Surg Pathol.* 2001;9:37-48.
491. Argenta PA, Thomas S, Chura JC. Proximal-type epithelioid sarcoma vs. malignant rhabdoid tumor of the vulva: A case report, review of the literature, and argument for consolidation. *Gynecol Oncol.* 2007;107:130-135.
492. Oda Y, Tsuneyoshi M. Extrarenal rhabdoid tumors of soft tissue: Clinicopathological and molecular genetic review and distinction from other soft-tissue sarcomas with rhabdoid features. *Pathol Int.* 2006;56:287-295.
493. Rekhi B, Gorad BD, Chinoy RF. Clinicopathological features with outcomes of a series of conventional and proximal-type epithelioid sarcomas, diagnosed over a period of 10 years at a tertiary cancer hospital in India. *Virchows Arch.* 2008;453:141-153.
494. Fanburg-Smith JC, Hengge M, Hengge UR, et al. Extrarenal rhabdoid tumors of soft tissue: A clinicopathologic and immunohistochemical study of 18 cases. *Ann Diagn Pathol.* 1998;2:351-362.
495. Perrone T, Swanson PE, Twiggs L, et al. Malignant rhabdoid tumor of the vulva: Is distinction from epithelioid sarcoma possible? A pathologic and immunohistochemical study. *Am J Surg Pathol.* 1989;13:848-858.
496. Izumi T, Oda Y, Hasegawa T, et al. Prognostic significance of dysadherin expression in epithelioid sarcoma and its diagnostic utility in distinguishing epithelioid sarcoma from malignant rhabdoid tumor. *Mod Pathol.* 2006;19:820-831.
497. Hornick JL, Fletcher CDM. PEComa: what do we know so far? *Histopathology.* 2006;48:75-82.
498. Fadare O, Liang SX. Epithelioid smooth muscle tumors of the uterus do not express CD1a: A potential immunohistochemical adjunct in their distinction from uterine perivascular epithelioid cell tumors. *Ann Diagn Pathol.* 2008;12:401-405.
499. Folpe AL, Mentzel T, Lehr HA, et al. Perivascular epithelioid cell neoplasms of soft tissue and gynecologic origin: A clinicopathologic study of 26 cases and review of the literature. *Am J Surg Pathol.* 2005;29:1558-1575.
500. Gibas Z, Miettinen M, Limon J, et al. Cytogenetic and immunohistochemical profile of myxoid liposarcoma. *Am J Clin Pathol.* 1995;103:20-26.
501. De Vreeze RS, de Jong D, Tielen IH, et al. Primary retroperitoneal myxoid/round cell liposarcoma is a nonexisting disease: An immunohistochemical and molecular biological analysis. *Mod Pathol.* 2008:E-pub.
502. Oda Y, Yamamoto H, Takahiira T, et al. Frequent alteration of p16 (INK4a/p14 (ARF) and p53 pathways in the round cell component of myxoid/round cell liposarcoma: p53 gene alterations and reduced p14 (ARF) expression both correlate with poor prognosis. *J Pathol.* 2005;207:410-421.
503. Hisaoka M, Tsuji S, Morimitsu Y, et al. Detection of TLS/FUS-CHOP fusion transcripts in myxoid and round cell liposarcomas by nested reverse RT-PCR using archival paraffin embedded tissue. *J Diagn Mol Pathol.* 1998;7:96-101.
504. Oikawa K, Ishida T, Imamura T, et al. Generation of the novel monoclonal antibody against TLS/EWS-CHOP chimeric oncoproteins that is applicable to one of the most sensitive assays for myxoid and round cell liposarcomas. *Am J Surg Pathol.* 2006;30:351-356.
505. Miettinen M, Gannon FH, Lackman R. Chordomalike soft tissue sarcoma in the leg: A light and electron microscopic and immunohistochemical study. *Ultrastruct Pathol.* 1992;16:577-586.
506. Tong G, Perle MA, Desai P, et al. Parachordoma or chordoma periphericum? *Diagn Cytopathol.* 2003;29:18-23.
507. Coffin CM, Swanson PE, Wick MR, et al. An immunohistochemical comparison of chordoma with renal cell carcinoma, colorectal adenocarcinoma, and myxopapillary ependymoma: A potential diagnostic dilemma in the diminutive biopsy. *Mod Pathol.* 1993;6:531-538.
508. Naka T, Iwamoto Y, Shinohara N, et al. Cytokeratin sub-typing in chordomas and the fetal notochord: An immunohistochemical analysis of aberrant expression. *Mod Pathol.* 1997;10:545-551.
509. Hu Y, Gao Y, Zhang X. A clinicopathological and immunohistochemical study of 34 cases of chordoma. *Chung Hua Ping li Hsueh Tsa Chih.* 1996;25:142-144.
510. Mi C. An immunohistochemical and ultrastructural study of 20 chordomas. *Chung Hua Ping li Hsueh Tsa Chih.* 1992;21:106-108.
511. Huse JT, Pasha TL, Zhang PJ. D2-40 functions as an effective chondroid marker distinguishing true chondroid tumors from chordoma. *Acta Neuropathol.* 2007;113:87-94.
512. Vujovic S, Henderson S, Presneau N, et al. Brachyury, a crucial regulator of notochordal development, is a novel biomarker for chordomas. *J Pathol.* 2006;209:157-165.
513. Heffelfinger MJ, Dahlin DC, MacCarty CS, et al. Chordomas and cartilaginous tumors at the skull base. *Cancer.* 1973;32:410-420.
514. Rosenberg AE, Brown GA, Bhan AK, et al. Chondroid chordoma—a variant of chordoma: A morphologic and immunohistochemical study. *Am J Clin Pathol.* 1994;101:36-41.
515. Wojno KJ, Hruban RH, Garin-Chesa P, et al. Chondroid chordomas and low-grade chondrosarcomas of the craniospinal axis: An immunohistochemical analysis of 17 cases. *Am J Surg Pathol.* 1992;16:1144-1152.
516. Ishida T, Dorfman HD. Chondroid chordoma versus low-grade chondrosarcoma of the base of the skull: Can immunohistochemistry resolve the controversy? *J Neurooncol.* 1994;18:199-206.
517. Meis JM, Raymond AK, Evans HL, et al. Dedifferentiated" chordoma: A clinicopathologic and immunohistochemical study of three cases. *Am J Surg Pathol.* 1987;11:516-525.
518. Crapanzano JP, Ali SZ, Ginsberg MS, et al. Chordoma: A cytologic study with histologic and radiologic correlation. *Cancer.* 2001;93:40-51.
519. Bisceglia M, D'Angelo VA, Guglielmi G, et al. Dedifferentiated chordoma of the thoracic spine with rhabdomyosarcomatous differentiation: Report of a case and review of the literature. *Ann Diagn Pathol.* 2007;11:262-272.
520. Hornick JL, Fletcher CDM. Myoepithelial tumors of soft tissue: A clinicopathologic and immunohistochemical study of 101 cases with evaluation of prognostic parameters. *Am J Surg Pathol.* 2003;27:1183-1196.
521. Gleason B, Hornick JL. Myoepithelial tumours of skin and soft tissue: An update. *Diagn Histopathol.* 2008;14:552-562.

522. Niezabitowski A, Limon J, Wasilewska A, et al. Parachordoma—a clinicopathologic, immunohistochemical, electron microscopic, flow cytometric, and cytogenetic study. *Gen Diagn Pathol.* 1995;141:49-55.
523. Wiebe BM, Jensen K, Laursen H. Parachordoma of the sacrococcygeal region—A neuroepithelial tumor. *Clin Neuropathol.* 1995;14:343-346.
524. Karabela-Bouropoulou V, Skourtas C, Liapi-Avgeri G, et al. Parachordoma: A case report of a very rare soft tissue tumor. *Pathol Res Pract.* 1996;192:972-978.
525. Ishida T, Oda H, Oka T, et al. Parachordoma: An ultrastructural and immunohistochemical study. *Virchows Arch A Pathol Anat Histopathol.* 1993;422:239-245.
526. Scolyer RA, Bonar SF, Palmer AA, et al. Parachordoma is not distinguishable from axial chordoma using immunohistochemistry. *Pathol Int.* 2004;54:364-370.
527. Tirabosco R, Mangham DC, Rosenberg AE, et al. Brachyury expression in extra-axial skeletal and soft tissue chordomas: A marker that distinguishes chordoma from mixed tumor/myoepithelioma/parachordoma in soft tissue. *Am J Surg Pathol.* 2008;32:572-580.
528. Granados R, Martin-Hita A, Rodriguez-Barbero JM, et al. Fineneedle aspiration cytology of chondroblastoma of soft parts. *Diagn Cytopathol.* 2003;28:76-81.
529. Nakamura Y, Becker LE, Marks A. S-100 protein in tumors of cartilage and bone: An immunohistochemical study. *Cancer.* 1983;52:1820-1824.
530. Posl M, Amling M, Ritzel H, et al. Morphologic characteristics of chondroblastoma: A retrospective study of 56 cases of the Hamburg bone tumor register. *Pathologe.* 1996;17:26-34.
531. Semmelink HJ, Pruszczynski M, Wiersma-van Tilburg A, et al. Cytokeratin expression in chondroblastomas. *Histopathology.* 1990;16:257-263.
532. Monda L, Wick MR. S-100 protein immunostaining in the differential diagnosis of chondroblastoma. *Hum Pathol.* 1985;16:287-293.
533. Edel G, Ueda Y, Nakanishi J, et al. Chondroblastoma of bone: A clinical, radiological, light and immunohistochemical study. *Virchows Arch A Pathol Anat Histopathol.* 1992;421:355-366.
534. Brecher ME, Simon MA. Chondroblastoma: An immunohistochemical study. *Hum Pathol.* 1988;19:1043-1047.
535. Povysil C, Tomanova R, Matejovsky Z. Muscle-specific actin expression in chondroblastoma. *Hum Pathol.* 1997;28:316-320.
536. Kilpatrick SE, Inwards CY, Fletcher CD, et al. Myxoid chondrosarcoma (chordoid sarcoma) of bone: A report of two cases and review of the literature. *Cancer.* 1997;79:1903-1910.
537. Antonescu CR, Argani P, Erlandson RA, et al. Skeletal and extraskeletal myxoid chondrosarcoma: A comparative clinicopathologic, ultrastructural, and molecular study. *Cancer.* 1998;83:1504-1521.
538. Orndal C, Carlen B, Akerman M, et al. Chromosomal abnormality t(9;22)(q22;q12) in an extraskeletal myxoid chondrosarcoma characterized by fine needle aspiration cytology, electron microscopy, immunohistochemistry and DNA flow cytometry. *Cytopathology.* 1991;2:261-270.
539. Domanski HA, Carlen B, Mertens F, et al. Extraskeletal myxoid chondrosarcoma with neuroendocrine differentiation: A case report with fine-needle aspiration biopsy, histopathology, electron microscopy, and cytogenetics. *Ultrastruct Pathol.* 2003;27:363-368.
540. Goh YW, Spagnolo DV, Platten M, et al. Extraskeletal myxoid chondrosarcoma: A light microscopic, immunohistochemical, ultrastructural, and immunoultrastructural study indicating neuroendocrine differentiation. *Histopathology.* 2001;39:514-524.
541. Algros MP, Collonge-Rame MA, Bedgejian I, et al. Neuroectodermal differentiation of extraskeletal myxoid chondrosarcoma: A classical feature? *Ann Pathol.* 2003;23:244-248.
542. Swanson PE. Clear cell tumors of bone. *Semin Diagn Pathol.* 1997;14:281-291.
543. Wang LT, Liu TC. Clear cell chondrosarcoma of bone: A report of three cases with immunohistochemical and affinity histochemical observations. *Pathol Res Pract.* 1993;189:411-415.
544. Bosse A, Ueda Y, Wuisman P, et al. Histogenesis of clear cell chondrosarcoma: An immunohistochemical study with osteonectin, a non-collagenous structure protein. *J Cancer Res Clin Oncol.* 1991;117:43-49.
545. Lidang Jensen LM, Schumacher B, Jensen MO, et al. Extraskeletal osteosarcomas: A clinicopathologic study of 25 cases. *Am J Surg Pathol.* 1998;22:588-594.
546. Dardick I, Schatz JE, Colgan TJ. Osteogenic sarcoma with epithelial differentiation. *Ultrastruct Pathol.* 1992;16:463-474.
547. Hasegawa T, Hirose T, Hizawa K, et al. Immunophenotypic heterogeneity in osteosarcomas. *Hum Pathol.* 1991;22:583-590.
548. Schulz Z, Jundt G, Berghauser KH, et al. Immunohistochemical study of osteonectin in various types of osteosarcoma. *Am J Pathol.* 1988;132:233-238.
549. Oliveira AM, Dei Tos AP, Fletcher CD, et al. Primary giant cell tumor of soft tissues: A study of 22 cases. *Am J Surg Pathol.* 2000;24:248-256.
550. O'Connell JX, Wehrli BM, Nielsen GP, et al. Giant cell tumors of soft tissue: A clinicopathologic study of 18 benign and malignant tumors. *Am J Surg Pathol.* 2000;24:386-395.
551. Masui F, Ushigome S, Fujii K. Giant cell tumor of bone: An immunohistochemical comparative study. *Pathol Int.* 1998;48:355-361.
552. Fornasier VL, Protzner K, Zhang I, et al. The prognostic significance of histomorphometry and immunohistochemistry in giant cell tumors of bone. *Hum Pathol.* 1996;27:754-760.
553. Watanabe K, Tajino T, Kusakabe T, et al. Giant cell tumor of bone: Frequent actin immunoreactivity in stromal tumor cells. *Pathol Int.* 1997;47:680-684.
554. Paulino AF, Spiro RH, O'Malley B, et al. Giant cell tumour of the retropharynx. *Histopathology.* 1998;33:344-348.
555. Folpe AL, Weiss SW, Fletcher CDM, et al. Tenosynovial giant cell tumors: evidence for a desmin-positive dendritic cell subpopulation. *Mod Pathol.* 1998;11:939-944.
556. Lee CH, Espinosa I, Jensen KC, et al. Gene expression profiling identifies p63 as a diagnostic marker for giant cell tumor of the bone. *Mod Pathol.* 2008;21:531-539.
557. Dickson BC, Li SQ, Wunder JS, et al. Giant cell tumor of bone express p63. *Mod Pathol.* 2008;21:369-375.
558. Ueda Y, Imai K, Tsuchiya H, et al. Matrix metalloproteinase 9 (gelatinase B) is expressed in multinucleated giant cells of human giant cell tumor of bone and is associated with vascular invasion. *Am J Pathol.* 1996;148:611-622.
559. Rao VH, Singh RK, Delimont DC, et al. Transcriptional regulation of MMP-9 expression in stromal cells of human giant cell tumor of bone by tumor necrosis factor-alpha. *Int J Oncol.* 1999;14:291-300.
560. Schoedel DE, Greco MA, Stetler-Stevenson WG, et al. Expression of metalloproteinases and tissue inhibitors of metalloproteinases in giant cell tumor of bone: An immunohistochemical study with clinical correlation. *Hum Pathol.* 1996;27:1144-1148.
561. Kahn LB. Adamantinoma, osteofibrous dysplasia, and differentiated adamantinoma. *Skeletal Radiol.* 2003;32:245-258.
562. Hazelbag HM, Hogendoorn PC. Adamantinoma of the long bones: An anatomicoclinical review of its relationship to osteofibrous dysplasia. *Ann Pathol.* 2001;21:499-511.
563. Kuruvilla G, Steiner GC. Osteofibrous dysplasia-like adamantinoma of bone: A report of five cases with immunohistochemical and ultrastructural studies. *Hum Pathol.* 1998;29:809-814.
564. Jundt G, Remberger K, Roessner A, et al. Adamantinoma of long bones: A histopathological and immunohistochemical study of 23 cases. *Pathol Res Pract.* 1995;191:112-120.
565. Benassi MS, Campanacci L, Gamberi G, et al. Cytokeratin expression and distribution in adamantinoma of the long bones and osteofibrous dysplasia of tibia and fibula: An immunohistochemical study correlated to histogenesis. *Histopathology.* 1994;25:71-76.
566. Ishida T, Iijima T, Kikuchi F, et al. A clinicopathological and immunohistochemical study of osteofibrous dysplasia, differentiated adamantinoma, and adamantinoma of long bones. *Skeletal Radiol.* 1992;21:493-502.
567. Knapp RH, Wick MR, Scheithauer BW, et al. Adamantinoma of bone: An electron microscopic and immunohistochemical study. *Virchows Arch A.* 1982;398:75-86.
568. Gleason BC, Liegl-Atzwanger B, Kozakewich HP, et al. Osteofibrous dysplasia and adamantinoma in children and adolescents: A clinicopathologic reappraisal. *Am J Surg Pathol.* 2008;32:363-376.

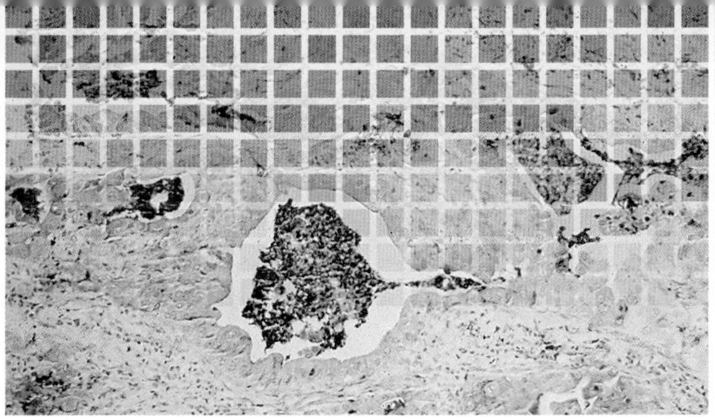

5

Immunohistology of Hodgkin Lymphoma

Parul Bhargava • Marshall E. Kadin

- Introduction 137
- Biology of Antigens 137
- Antibody Specifications 144
- Diagnostic Immunohistochemistry 146
- Molecular Anatomic Pathology 150
- Beyond Immunohistochemistry: Anatomic Molecular Diagnostic Applications 150
- Theranostic Applications 150
- Summary 151

INTRODUCTION

Hodgkin lymphoma (HL) is widely accepted to be a malignant clonal proliferation of B lymphocytes or, less often, T lymphocytes surrounded by variable numbers of inflammatory cells and fibrosis. The two major histologic types are classical Hodgkin lymphoma (CHL) and nodular lymphocyte predominance Hodgkin lymphoma (NLPHL). Classical Hodgkin lymphoma is further subdivided into four subtypes:

- Lymphocyte rich type
- Nodular sclerosis type
- Mixed cellularity type
- Lymphocyte depletion type (Figs. 5.1 and 5.2).[1-3]

NLPHL is a B-cell neoplasm derived from germinal center B cells that are continually undergoing somatic mutations of immunoglobulin genes.[3-5] CHL belongs to the group of germinal center/post–germinal center B-cell lymphomas in which the Hodgkin/Reed-Sternberg cells (H/RSCs) have undergone extensive somatic mutations of immunoglobulin genes.[6] Accordingly, these two major subtypes of HL express distinctive antigen profiles that can be used to distinguish NLPHL from the morphologically similar lymphocyte-rich variant of CHL. The German Hodgkin Study Group showed the importance of using an immunohistochemical approach for improving the diagnostic accuracy of nodular lymphocyte predominance Hodgkin lymphoma (NLPHL). Immunohistochemistry disproved the morphologic diagnosis of NLPHL by an expert panel in 25 of 104 cases, whereas 13 cases originally not confirmed as NLPHL showed an NLPHD-like immunophenotypic pattern with a significantly better survival than CHL.[7]

BIOLOGY OF ANTIGENS

Principal Antibodies (CD45, CD20, CD30, CD15)

The H/RSCs in NLPHL (also known as *popcorn cells* or *lymphocytic and histiocytic (L&H) cells* because of their distinctive morphology) generally express leukocyte common antigen (LCA) or CD45 (Fig. 5.3). In all cases of NLPHL and in a small number of CHL cases, there is an expression of B-cell antigen CD20 by the H/RSCs (Fig. 5.4).[8-11] CD45 is usually absent or weakly expressed in a minor subset of H/RSCs in CHL (Fig. 5.5).[12,13] In all cases of CHL and in a minor proportion of malignant cells in NLPHL, the tumor cells express CD30, a member of the tumor necrosis factor superfamily (Fig. 5.6).[14-16] Activation of CD30 signaling by native CD30L or Epstein-Barr virus latent membrane protein 1 (EBV-LMP1) results in activation of NF-κB transcription factor, which has an antiapoptotic effect, promotes cell proliferation, and causes up-regulation of cytokine production by H/RSCs.[17,18] H/RSCs in CHL, but not NLPHL, express CD15 detected by antibody LeuM1 in 60% to 85% of cases, with an average of 68% (Fig. 5.7).[19-22] The antigenic determinant for LeuM1 is a trisaccharide, 3-fucosyl-*N*-acetyllactosamine, which is formed by the 1-3 fucosylation of a type 2 blood group backbone chain (Gal1-4GlcNAc); the carbohydrate backbone is identical to that of Lewis X, also known as *X-hapten*.[23]

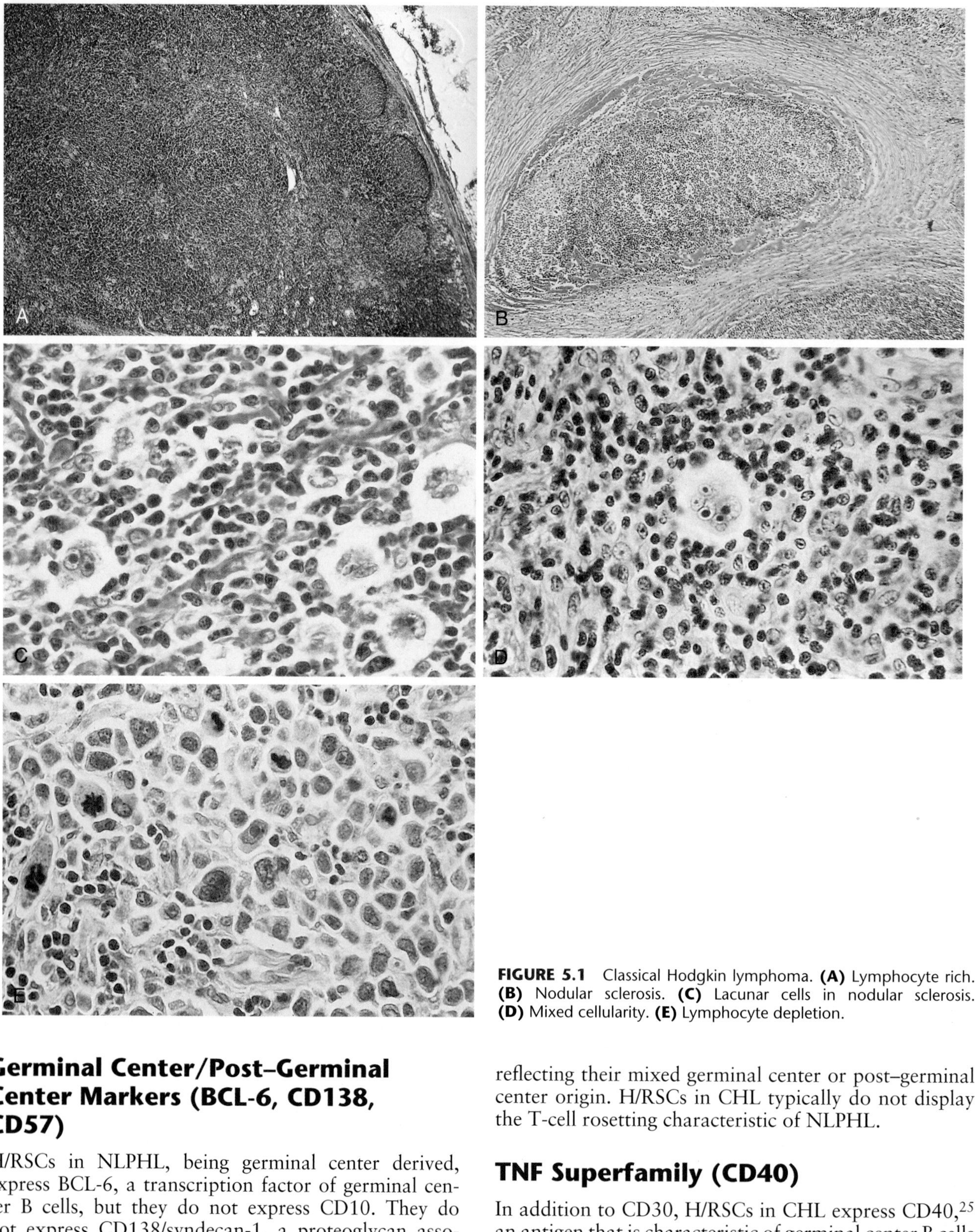

FIGURE 5.1 Classical Hodgkin lymphoma. **(A)** Lymphocyte rich. **(B)** Nodular sclerosis. **(C)** Lacunar cells in nodular sclerosis. **(D)** Mixed cellularity. **(E)** Lymphocyte depletion.

Germinal Center/Post–Germinal Center Markers (BCL-6, CD138, CD57)

H/RSCs in NLPHL, being germinal center derived, express BCL-6, a transcription factor of germinal center B cells, but they do not express CD10. They do not express CD138/syndecan-1, a proteoglycan associated with post–germinal center B cells.[24] H/RSCs in NLPHL often are surrounded by a population of activated helper-inducer memory T cells (CD4+, CD57+, CD45R+, CD45+), which are normally confined to the light zone of germinal centers of secondary follicles (Fig. 5.8).[4] Conversely, H/RSCs in CHL are heterogeneous with respect to expression of BCL-6 and CD138, reflecting their mixed germinal center or post–germinal center origin. H/RSCs in CHL typically do not display the T-cell rosetting characteristic of NLPHL.

TNF Superfamily (CD40)

In addition to CD30, H/RSCs in CHL express CD40,[25] an antigen that is characteristic of germinal center B cells and activation of which inhibits apoptosis (Fig. 5.9).[26]

Epithelial Membrane Antigen (EMA)

EMA is expressed in some cases of NLPHL, but it is not expressed in CHL. EMA is however commonly expressed by tumor cells in anaplastic large cell lymphoma

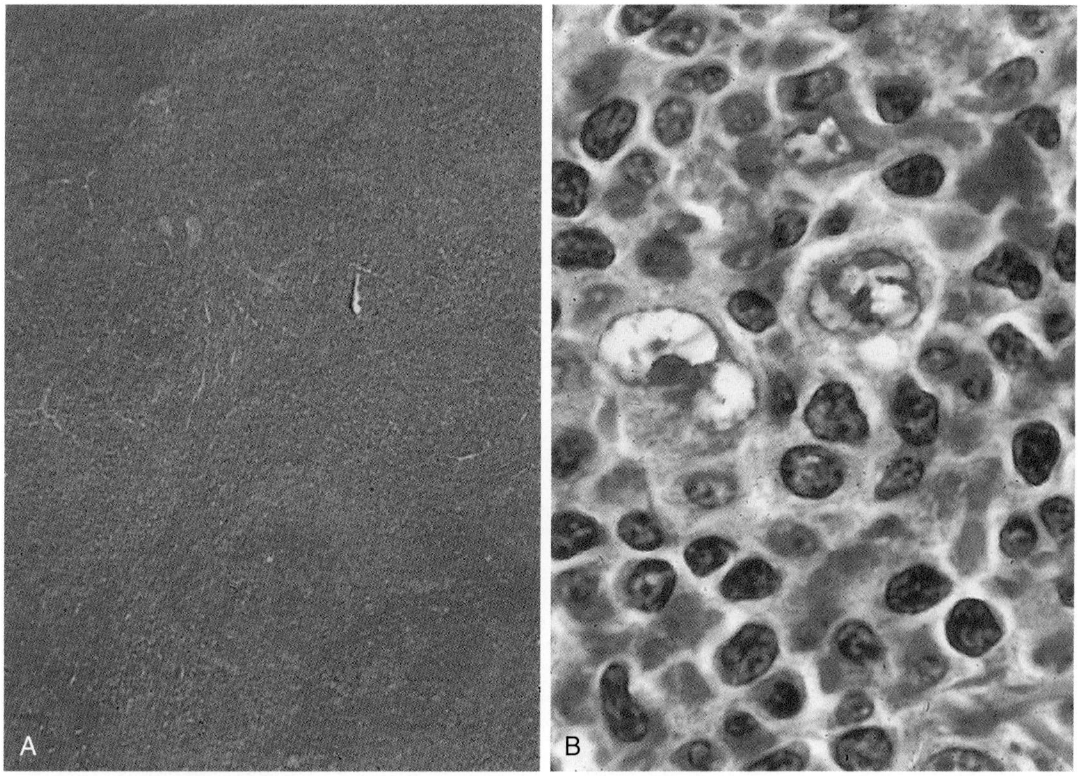

FIGURE 5.2 Nodular lymphocyte predominance Hodgkin lymphoma. **(A)** Low magnification showing nodular pattern. **(B)** Popcorn variants of Hodgkin/Reed-Sternberg cells.

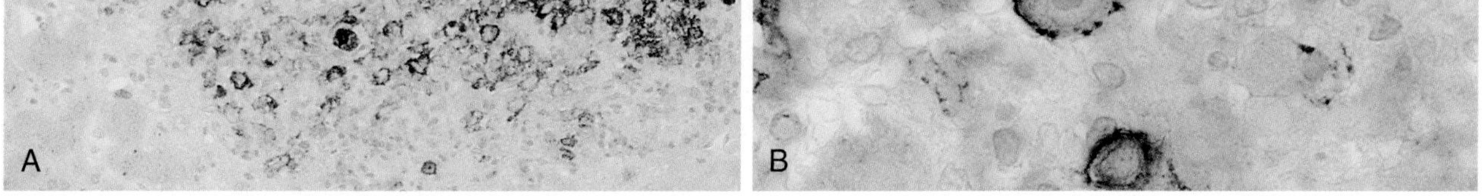

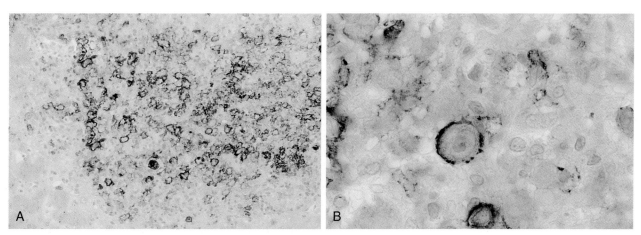

FIGURE 5.3 Expression of epithelial membrane antigen (EMA) in nodular lymphocyte predominance Hodgkin lymphoma. **(A)** Low magnification of nodule. **(B)** High magnification of individual Hodgkin/Reed-Sternberg cells.

(ALCL), which may be useful as a distinguishing feature between ALCL and CHL.

T-Cell and Cytotoxic Markers (CD2, CD3, CD5, CD4, CD8, Granzyme B, Perforin, TIA-1)

In 5% to 20% of CHL cases, H/RSCs appear to have variable expression of T-cell antigens (CD2, CD3, CD5, CD4, CD8) and antigens associated with cytotoxic molecules (granzyme B, perforin, and TIA-1) (Fig. 5.10).[27-33] In one study, a mean fraction of 40% of H/RSCs (from 20% to 100%) expressed the analyzed T-cell markers.[34] However, aberrant T-cell antigen expression was also detected in some CHLs with immunoglobulin gene rearrangements, presumably of B-cell derivation.[35] A T-cell derivation was proven for H/RSCs by polymerase chain reaction amplification of T-cell receptor genes from single picked H/RSCs in approximately 1% to 2% of CHL cases.[35-37]

EBV

EBV is associated with the etiology of HL, and EBV-LMP1 (or small RNAs of EBV known as *EBERs*) can be detected in about 50% of cases of CHL (Fig. 5.11).[38]

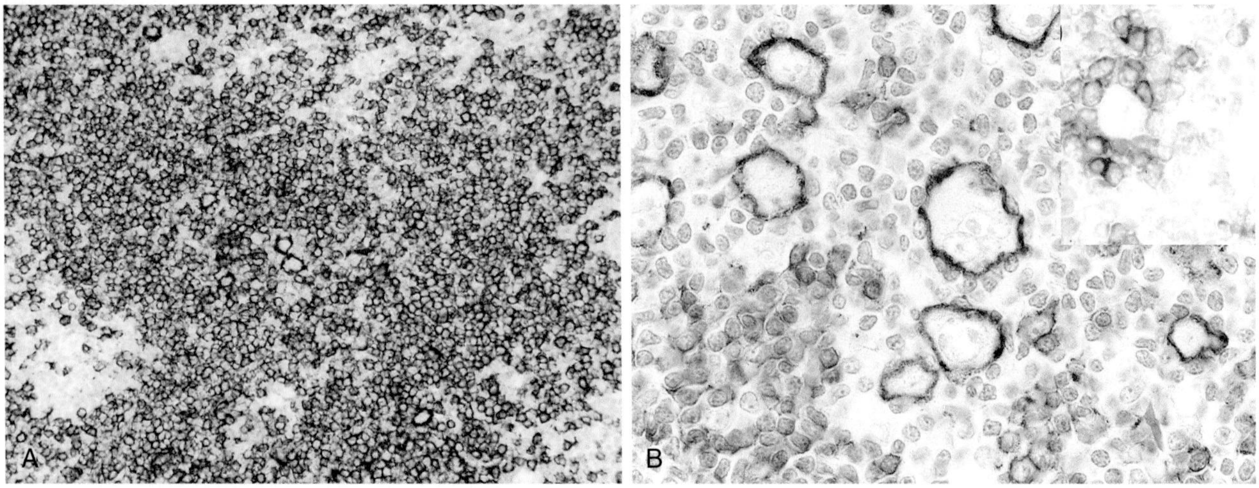

FIGURE 5.4 B-cell antigen expression in nodular lymphocyte predominance Hodgkin lymphoma. **(A)** Large Hodgkin/Reed-Sternberg cells in the center are surrounded by a nodule of smaller L26+ (CD20+) B lymphocytes. **(B)** CD20+ Hodgkin/Reed-Sternberg cells in lymphocyte predominance Hodgkin lymphoma.

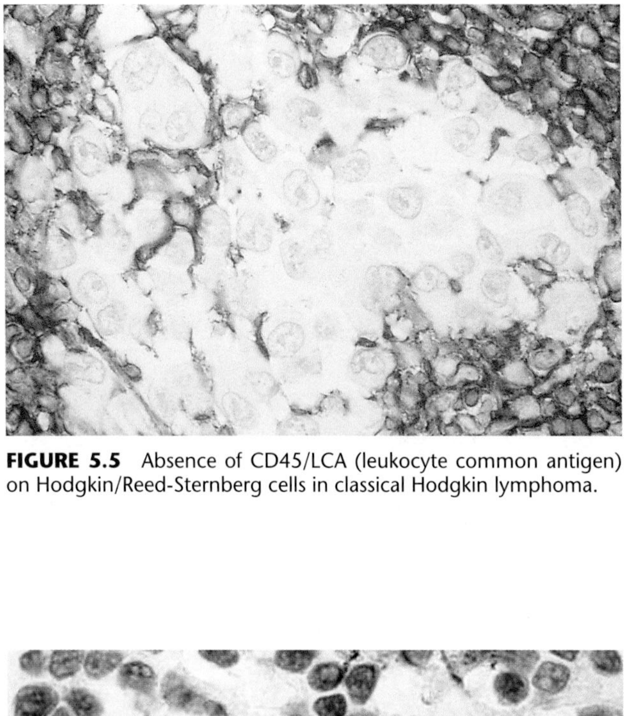

FIGURE 5.5 Absence of CD45/LCA (leukocyte common antigen) on Hodgkin/Reed-Sternberg cells in classical Hodgkin lymphoma.

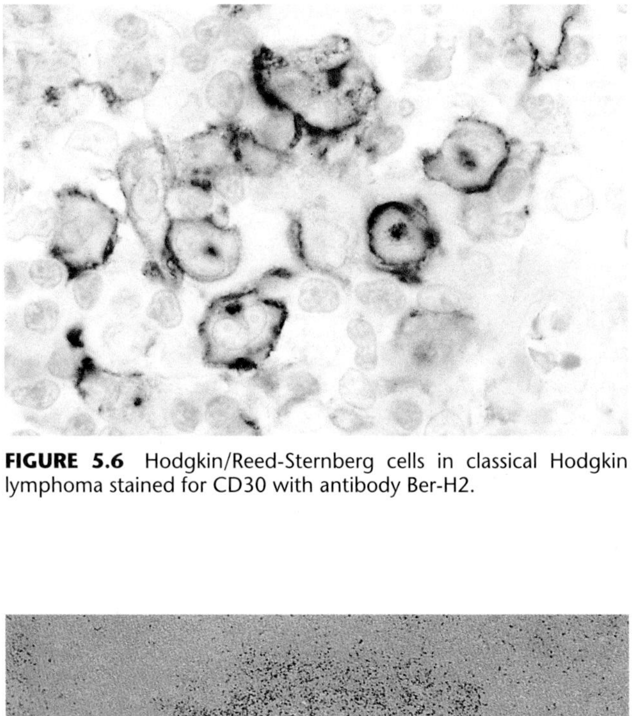

FIGURE 5.6 Hodgkin/Reed-Sternberg cells in classical Hodgkin lymphoma stained for CD30 with antibody Ber-H2.

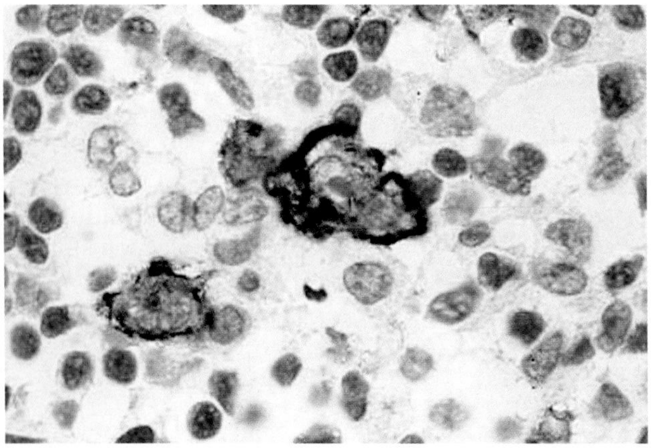

FIGURE 5.7 Hodgkin/Reed-Sternberg cells in classical Hodgkin lymphoma expressing CD15 detected by antibody LeuM1.

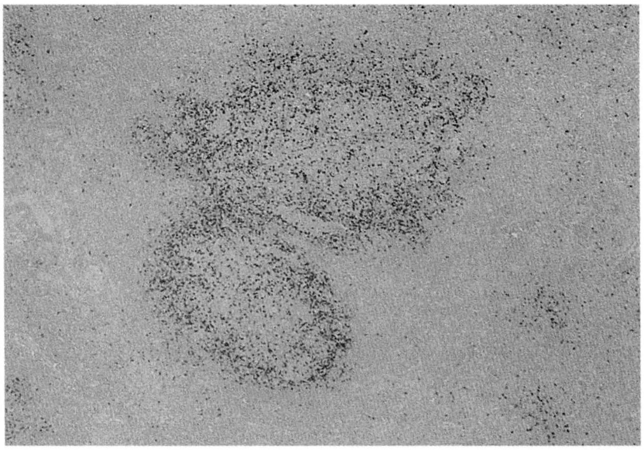

FIGURE 5.8 Leu7+ (CD57+) T lymphocytes surrounding Hodgkin/Reed-Sternberg cells in nodular lymphocyte predominance Hodgkin lymphoma.

H/RSCs commonly express the EBV gene product latent membrane protein 1 (LMP-1), a transforming protein that can confer a growth advantage on H/RSCs.[39,40] The frequency of EBV detection in HL is much higher in the mixed cellularity type and the lymphocyte depletion type than in the nodular sclerosis type.[40-42] EBV is frequently detected in CHL that occurs in immunocompromised patients, such as those infected with human immunodeficiency virus (HIV) and those with post-transplant immunoproliferative disorders.[43] EBV is also detected at higher frequency in HL patients in developing countries.[41,42]

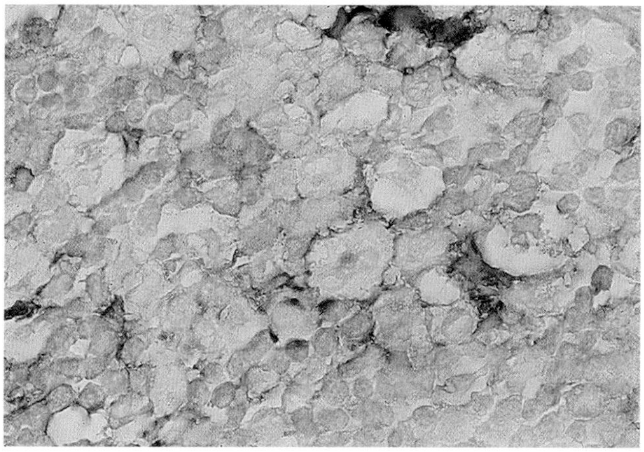

FIGURE 5.9 Hodgkin/Reed-Sternberg cells in CHL expressing CD40.

Dendritic or Antigen Presenting Cell Markers: Fascin

Fascin is a relatively new sensitive marker that has been described for H/RSCs in CHL.[44] Fascin is a 55-kD actin-bundling protein that is localized predominantly in dendritic cells in non-neoplastic tissues. The staining profile for fascin raises the possibility of a dendritic cell derivation (particularly an interdigitating reticulum cell) for the neoplastic cells of HL, notably in nodular sclerosis (Fig. 5.12). However, because fascin expression can be induced by EBV infection of B cells, the possibility of viral induction of fascin in lymphoid or other cell types must also be considered.[44] While fascin expression has been shown in all cases of CHL, giving it a high

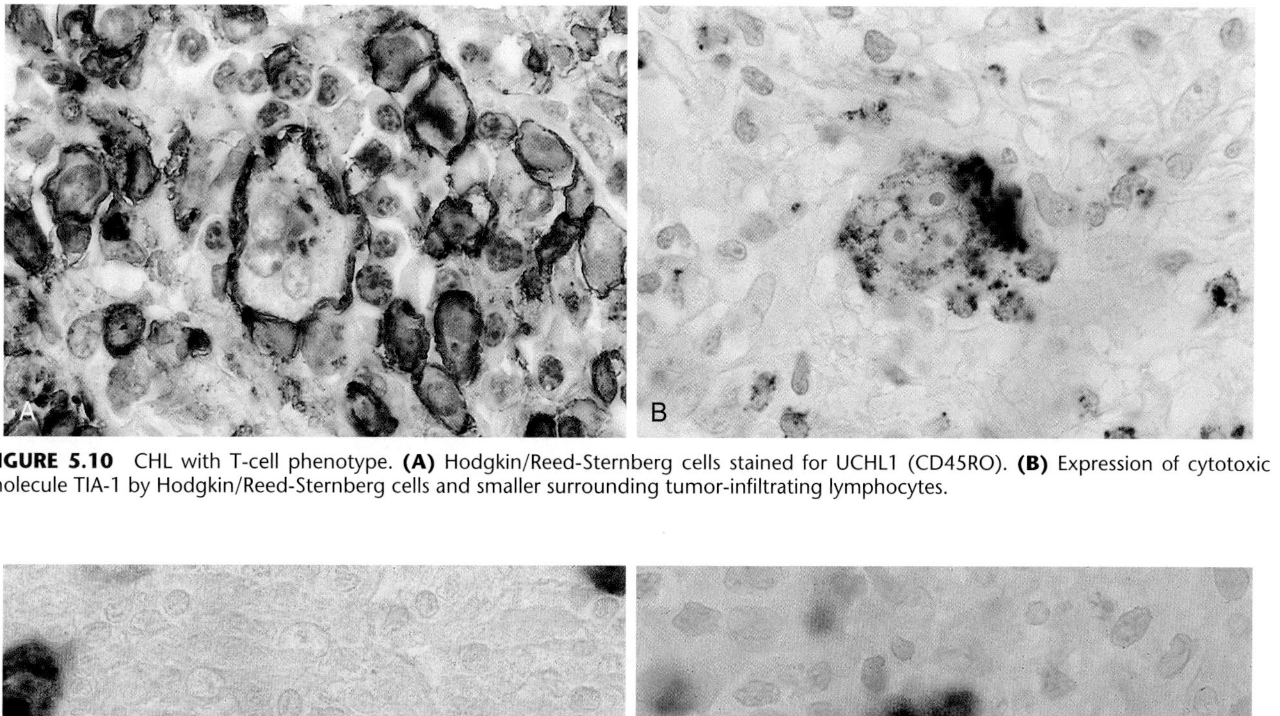

FIGURE 5.10 CHL with T-cell phenotype. **(A)** Hodgkin/Reed-Sternberg cells stained for UCHL1 (CD45RO). **(B)** Expression of cytotoxic molecule TIA-1 by Hodgkin/Reed-Sternberg cells and smaller surrounding tumor-infiltrating lymphocytes.

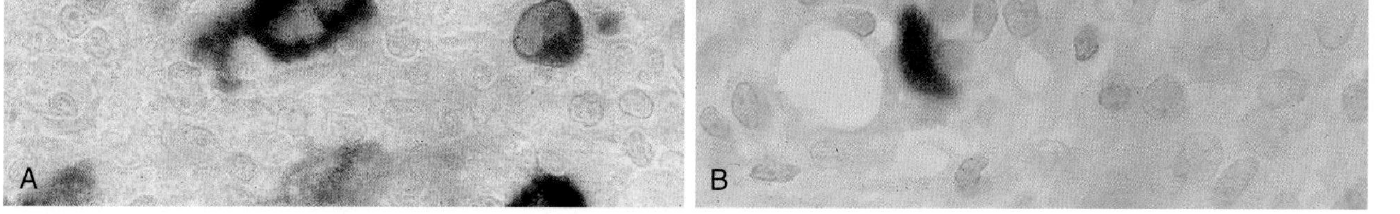

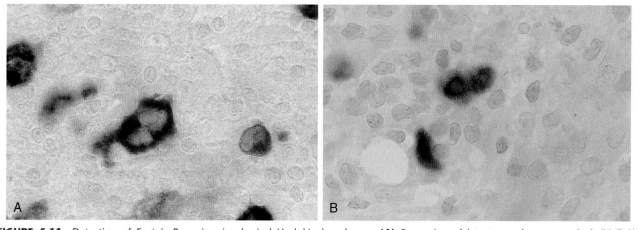

FIGURE 5.11 Detection of Epstein-Barr virus in classical Hodgkin lymphoma. **(A)** Expression of latent membrane protein-1 (LMP-1). **(B)** *In situ* hybridization studies for EBV encoded small RNAs known as EBER.

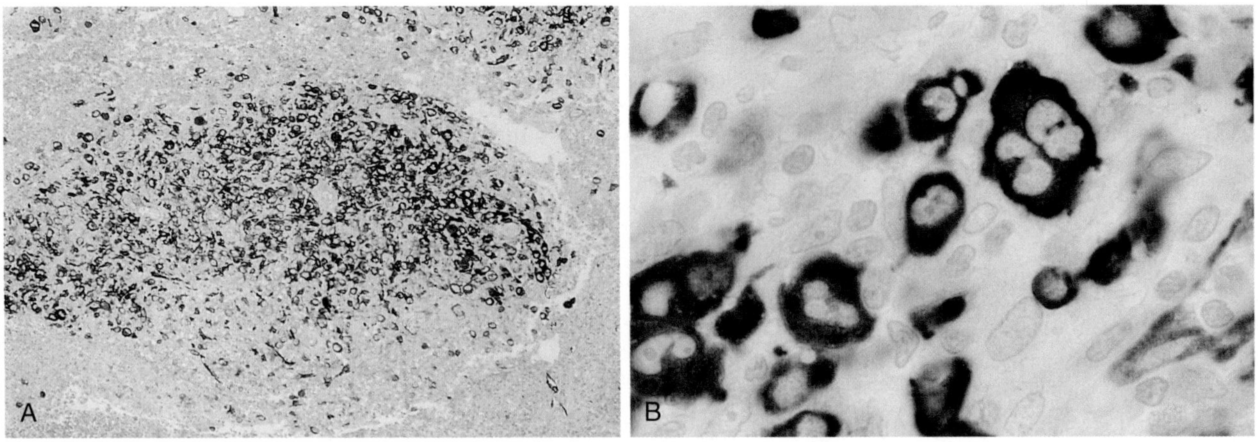

FIGURE 5.12 Fascin expression in nodular sclerosis HL. **(A)** Low magnification of nodule. **(B)** Staining of individual Hodgkin/Reed-Sternberg cells at high magnification.

negative predictive value, it is not specific for CHL. Fascin expression has also been described in a majority of cases of ALCL (50% to 70%),[45,46] which makes it less useful for this differential.

CLIP-170/Restin

H/RSCs of CHL strongly express CLIP-170/restin, which colocalizes with membranes of intermediate macropinocytic vesicles, assisting in the trafficking of macropinosomes to the cytoskeleton. This is a crucial step in antigen presentation. The strong expression of CLIP-170 restin in H/RSCs, dendritic cells, and activated B cells underscores their functional similarities, supporting a function-based concept of H/RSCs as professional antigen-presenting cells.[47]

B-Cell Markers (CD79a) and Transcription Factors (BSAP, Oct-2, BOB.1, JunB)

CD79 is a dimeric, transmembrane protein, which, along with surface immunoglobulin, is part of the B-cell receptor complex.[48] It is a pan B-cell marker expressed from the pre-B stage to the plasma cell stage of differentiation.[49] Like CD20, CD79 is generally expressed in all cases of NLPHL. However, H/RSCs of CHL are generally non-immunoreactive for CD79; in a minor subset (0% to 20%) of cases, a small proportion of the neoplastic cells may be positive.[11,50-52] Global loss of B-cell–specific gene expression is a distinctive feature of H/RSCs in CHL.[53] The loss may be due to aberrant expression of ID2, a suppressor of B-cell–specific gene expression in HL.[54]

B-cell–specific activator protein (BSAP) is a transcription factor expressed in B cells and B-cell–derived lymphomas. It is encoded by the PAX-5 gene and influences several B-cell functions such as B-cell antigen expression, Ig expression, and class switch. It is expressed in the majority of H/RSCs in CHL[55] as well as L&H cells of NLPHL,[56] further supporting their B-cell origin. In contrast, BSAP is not expressed in normal or malignant T cells, and thus is absent in T/null cell ALCLs.[55]

Oct-2 is a transcription factor, which, along with its co-activator BOB.1/OBF.1, binds to immunoglobulin gene octomer sites, thus inducing immunoglobulin synthesis.[57] Germinal center B cells normally demonstrate strong staining for Oct-2 and BOB.1. Because they are germinal center derived, L&H cells in NLPHL are consistently immunoreactive for both markers.[56] Conversely, the H/RSCs in CHL do not express both (80%) or express only one (20%) of the two proteins.[58,59] H/RSCs often do not express immunoglobulin (Ig), which is thought to be due to crippling mutations within Ig genes; absence of transcriptional activators such as Oct-2/BOB.1 may represent novel mechanisms for Ig dysregulation.[58] Although most T-cell lymphomas are Oct-2–negative, variable staining has been demonstrated in some peripheral T-cell lymphomas not otherwise specified (NOS) as well as a subset (~50%) of anaplastic lymphoma kinase (ALK)-positive ALCLs.[60]

JunB and c-Jun are part of the Activator Protein-1 (AP-1) family of transcription factors. AP-1 proteins are stimulated in a rapid and transient fashion by a number of extracellular signals that trigger growth factor pathways and/or stress signals (e.g., UV radiation). They promote mitogen-induced cell-cycle progression as well as regulate apoptosis. Recently it has been demonstrated that H/RSCs in CHL constitutively overexpress AP-1 proteins containing c-Jun and JunB (Fig. 5.13). Conversely, malignant cells in NLPHL had been shown to express neither c-Jun nor JunB.[61] However, in our experience,[60a] JunB is expressed in a minor subset of NLPHL cases. Additionally, JunB antibody stains scattered lymphocytes, particularly in areas of progressively transformed germinal centers. Most of the other B- and T-cell NHLs tested did not express or only weakly expressed JunB and/or c-Jun, with the exception of t(2;5) positive ALCLs (which showed strong expression).[61]

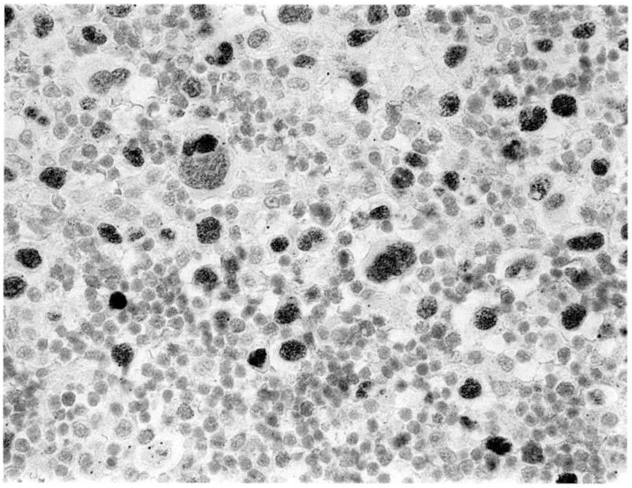

FIGURE 5.13 JunB expression in classical Hodgkin lymphoma.

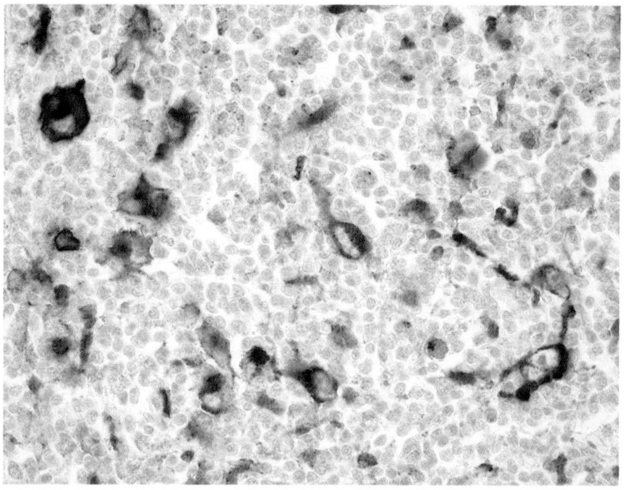

FIGURE 5.14 Hodgkin/Reed-Sternberg cells in classical Hodgkin lymphoma expressing CCR7.

Immunoglobulins (J Chain, IgD) J-chain

Immunoglobulins (J chain, IgD) J-chain is a 15-kD acidic protein synthesized by B cells and plasma cells that secrete polymeric immunoglobulins. J-chain expression has thus been observed in most H/RSCs in NLPHL, but not in H/RSCs of CHL with dysregulated Ig genes.[58,62,63] IgD expression in H/RSCs has been reported in a subset (27%)[64] of NLPHL cases with an extra-follicular distribution of L&H cells and a relatively T-cell–rich background. In contrast, IgD expression is rarely seen in T-cell–rich B-cell lymphoma (TCRBCL). Some studies demonstrated immunoreactivity for IgD in a minor subset of H/RSCs in CHL[65]; however, others were negative.[66]

CD74

CD74 functions as an MHC class II chaperone and is normally expressed by a variety of cell types including B cells, activated T cells, macrophages, activated endothelial cells, and epithelial cells. Although expressed by the H/RSCs of CHL, CD74 is not specific for this lymphoma; expression has been reported in a variety of non-Hodgkin lymphomas as well as in non-lymphoid epithelial malignancies.

Other Biological Markers in Hodgkin Lymphoma

It has been shown that expression of translation initiation factors eIF-4E and eIF-2alpha is increased in neoplastic cells of Hodgkin lymphoma, but not in surrounding lymphocytes.[67] An increase in eIF-4E expression may lead to constitutively high expression of NF-κB. H/RSCs have high expression of c-FLIP, which protects cells from apoptosis.[68] Tissue inhibitor of metalloproteinases (TIMP-1 and TIMP-2) are proteins with proteinase inhibition and cytokine properties. TIMP-1 is active primarily in B cells and B-cell lymphomas, whereas TIMP-2 is restricted to T cells. HL-derived cell lines express TIMP-1, with low expression of TIMP-2. TIMP-1 protein can be detected in frozen tissues of CHL lymph nodes, where it produces primarily a diffuse background staining and co-localization with CD30 in few H/RSCs.[69] Galectin-1 is an immunoregulatory glycan-finding protein that is expressed by H/RSCs. H/RS cell Gal-1 may contribute to the development and maintenance of an immunosuppressive Th2/Treg-skewed microenvironment in CHL and provide the molecular basis of selective Gal-1 expression in H/RSCs.[70] Programmed death-1 (PD-1) ligand (PD-L) signaling system is involved in the functional impairment of T cells such as in chronic viral infection or tumor immune evasion. PD-L expression is up-regulated in H/RSCs in tissues and cell lines as well as some T-cell lymphomas but not in B-cell lymphomas. PD-1 is elevated markedly in tumor-infiltrating T cells of HL and in peripheral blood T cells of HL patients.[71]

CYTOKINES IN HODGKIN LYMPHOMA

Clinical and histologic features of Hodgkin lymphoma have been associated with cytokine and chemokine production by tumor cells.[72,73] The majority of CHL cases are characterized by expression of tumor necrosis factor receptor (TNFR) family members and their ligands and an unbalanced production of Th2 cytokines and chemokines.[74] Chemokine receptor CCR7 is a lymphocyte homing receptor expressed in B, T, and activated dendritic cells and has been implicated in regulation of lymphocyte migration to secondary lymphoid organs. The promoter region of CCR7 has binding sites for both AP-1 and NF-κB. In line with the c-Jun/JunB overexpression seen in CHL but not in NLPHL, CCR7 is over-expressed in most H/RSCs of CHL (Fig. 5.14).[75] CD25 H/RSCs in CHL manifest variable expression of CD25 (Tac, p55), the alpha unit of the receptor for interleukin-2 (IL-2).[76,77] CD25 is not expressed by H/RSCs in NLPHL. Aggregation of TRAF adapter

TABLE 5.1	New Biological Markers of Hodgkin/Reed-Sternberg Cells			
Antigen	CHL	NLPHL	TCRBCL	ALCL
NF-κB	+	U	U*	–
JunB/c-Jun	+	S	U	+
CCR7	+	–	U	U
Oct-2/BOB.1	S**	+	+	S
J-chain	–	S	S	–
BSAP/PAX5	+ (weak)	+	+	–

+, Nearly all cases positive; S, sometimes positive; R, rare (<5%); –, negative; U, expression unknown.
*+/– in diffuse large B-cell lymphoma (DLBCL); not directly studied in TCRBCL.
**Both (80%); one (20%).

proteins TRAF2 and TRAF5 in H/RSCs is required for CD30 signaling and activation of NF-κB.[78] TGF-beta and basic fibroblast growth factor produced by HL cells are associated with the pathogenesis of nodular sclerosis.[79,80] IL-13 and IL-13 receptors are frequently expressed in H/RSCs and contribute to the production of TGF-beta 1–mediated fibrosis.[81,82] H/RSCs secrete IL-5, which stimulates production of eosinophils and eosinophilia.[83] H/RSCs also express eotaxin, which is a chemo-attractant for eosinophils.[84] Both neoplastic and reactive IL-10–producing cells are significantly more common in EBV+ HL cases. IL-10 is an immunosuppressive cytokine and can help H/RSCs to escape local immune surveillance.[85] STAT proteins (STATs) are a family of transcription factors responsible for signal transducers and activators of transcription. STAT 3, STAT5, and STAT6 are frequently constitutively activated in H/RSCs and can be demonstrated by immunohistochemistry. STAT5 appears to be activated by IL-21.[86] STAT 6 mediates signaling by IL-13, and antibody-mediated neutralization of IL-13 causes significant decreases in levels of HL cell proliferation and phosphorylated STAT6 in HL cell lines.[87]

Table 5.1 summarizes the expression pattern of some of the new biological markers in HL as well as other entities in the differential diagnosis of HL.

ANTIBODY SPECIFICATIONS

The antibodies most commonly used for diagnosing HL are Ber-H2 (CD30), LeuM1 (CD15), LCA (CD45), L26 (CD20), CD75 (LN1), CD74 (LN2), PAX5, CD3, UCHL1(CD45RO), ALK-1, fascin, and EBV-LMP1. EMA and CD57 can be used to recognize NLPHL. Monoclonal antibody LN1 reacts with H/RSCs in about one third of HL cases, most frequently in cases of NLPHD (>75% of cases).[10] Monoclonal antibody LN2, which recognizes the MHC class II-associated invariant chain, reacts with H/RSCs in approximately two thirds of HL cases.[10] All the antibodies mentioned previously can be used in formalin-fixed paraffin-embedded tissues. Additional antibodies that are useful

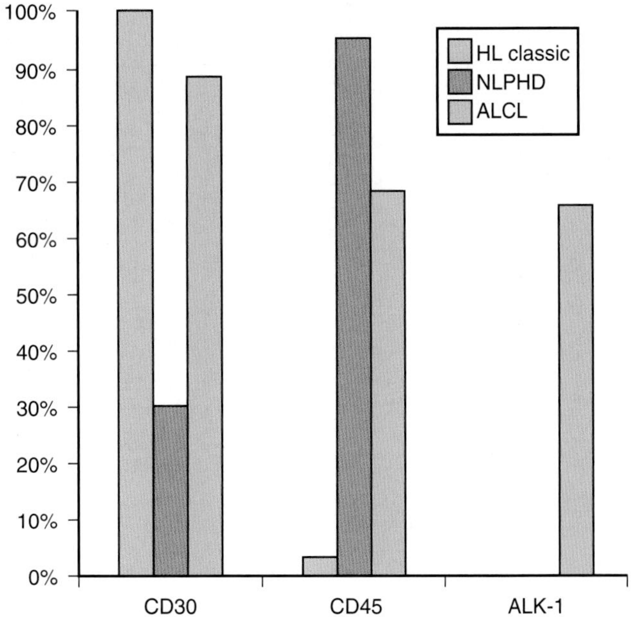

FIGURE 5.15 Frequency of antigens in classical Hodgkin lymphoma, nodular lymphocyte predominance Hodgkin lymphoma, and anaplastic large cell lymphoma.

in the diagnosis of difficult cases are BNH.9[88] and CBF.78 (Fig. 5.15 and Table 5.2).[89]

For antigen retrieval, we have replaced the use of a microwave oven with a steamer that heats the sections to 95°C to 98°C. The slides are immersed in Coplin jars containing citrate buffer (pH 6, 0.01 mol/L) and heated in the steamer for 20 minutes. Afterward, slides are cooled at room temperature for 30 minutes, rinsed in double-distilled water, and then transferred to phosphate-buffered saline, pH 7.4.

Immunostaining Pitfalls

CD15 ANTIGEN

When one relies on the demonstration of CD15 to make a diagnosis of HL, problems can arise because more than 30% of CHL cases will not express CD15 detected by LeuM1 antibody. A comparative study by Ree and coworkers, which we confirmed in our laboratory, showed that anti-Lewis-X (BG-7) (Signet Laboratories, Dedham, MA) is superior to LeuM1 for staining H/RSCs, yielding 87% versus 68.5% for LeuM1 (Fig. 5.16).[90] It is also important to identify the cells that express CD15 because granulocytes express high levels of CD15[19] and are often present in various tumors other than HL.

CD30 ANTIGEN

The use of monoclonal antibody Ber-H2 together with antigen retrieval methods has enabled sensitive detection of CD30 in formalin-fixed paraffin-embedded tissues. However, some hematopathologists prefer to use B5-fixed tissues, which afford excellent cytomorphology of lymphoid tissues. B5 is a mercuric chloride–containing

TABLE 5.2 Antibodies for Detection of Hodgkin Lymphoma–Associated Antigens

Antibody	Clone	Manufacturer	Dilution	Type of Antigen-Retrieval Method
CD30	Ber-H2	Dako	1:25	Steamer/citrate buffer pH 6, 20 min at 95°C to 98°C
CD15	LeuM1	Becton-Dickinson	1:25	Same as CD30
CD45 (LCA)	2B11	Dako	1:200	Same as CD30
CD20	L26	Dako	1:100	Same as CD30
CD45RO	UCHL1	Dako		Pepsin digest 10 min at 37°C
CD3	UCHT1	Dako		Steamer/citrate buffer pH 6, 20 min at 95°C to 98°C
CD40	MAB89	Immunotech	1:40	Same as CD3
ALK-1	ALK-1	Dako	1:25	Same as CD3
Fascin	55K-2	Dako	1:75	Same as CD3
Lewis-X type 2 chain (BG-7)	P12	Signet	1:40	Steamer/citrate buffer pH 8, 20 min at 95°C to 98°C
EBV-LMP1	CS1-4	Dako	1:50	Steamer/citrate buffer pH 6, 20 min at 95°C to 98°C
BCL-6	PG-B6p	Dako	1:10	Same as EBV-LMP1
CD57	Leu7	Dako	1:10	Same as EBV-LMP1
EMA	E29	Dako	1:50	Pepsin digest, 12 min at 37°C
CDw75	LN1	ICN Biomedicals	Undiluted	Steamer/citrate buffer pH 6, 20 min at 95°C to 98°C
CD74	LN2	ICN Biomedicals	Undiluted	Same as CDw75
NF-κB	P65C	Zymed Lab	1:200	Same as CDw75
CCR7	CCR7.6B3	eBioscience, San Diego, CA	1:200	Steam for 30 min in 1 mM EDTA pH 8.0[89a]
JunB	SC8051	Dako	1:75	HIER steamer/Target Retrieval Solution 30 min

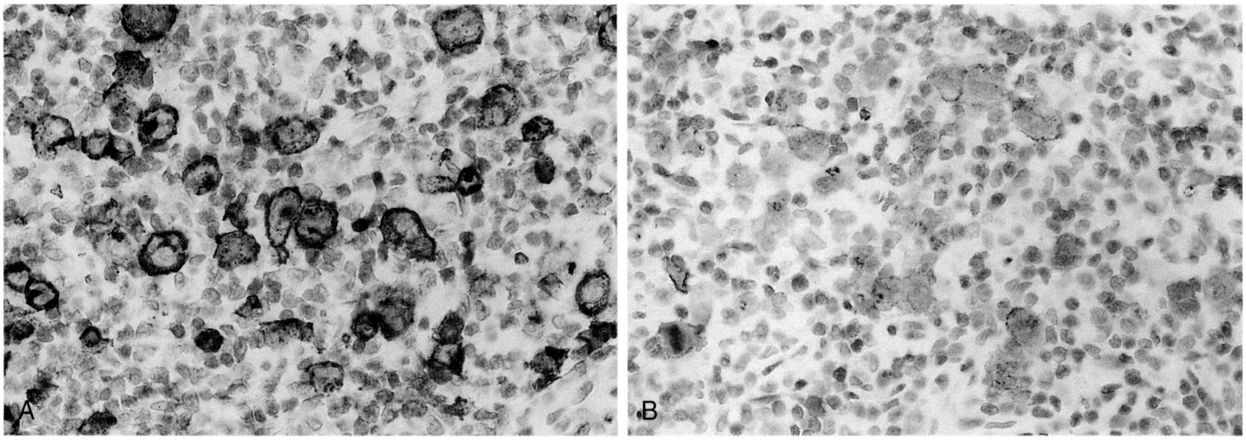

FIGURE 5.16 Comparative staining of Hodgkin/Reed-Sternberg cells for CD15 antigenic determinant with **(A)** anti-Lewis-X and **(B)** anti-LeuM1 antibodies in a case of lymphocyte depletion classical Hodgkin lymphoma shows increased sensitivity with anti-Lewis-X antibody.

fixative that requires removal of mercury before immunostaining. This is usually accomplished with Lugol's solution followed by sodium thiosulfate. A study by Facchetti and coworkers showed that omitting the Lugol's treatment is optimal for detection of CD30, even without wet heating with microwave or proteolytic predigestion of sections.[91]

CD45 (LCA)

It is often difficult to determine CD45 expression in tumor cells owing to strong immunoreactivity of surrounding cells in CHL. One should look for areas without adjacent cells to determine if the tumor cells are CD45 immunoreactive.

CD20 AND T-CELL ANTIGENS

With CD20 and T-cell antigen staining in CHL, similar difficulties can arise when interpreting the staining of tumor cells versus its surrounding cells.

DIAGNOSTIC IMMUNOHISTOCHEMISTRY

Although CHL and NLPHL have distinctive morphologic and immunophenotypic characteristics, it is important to note that an inconsistency of immunophenotype of H/RSCs has been reported in simultaneous and consecutive specimens from the same patients in paraffin sections. Chu and coworkers found that the immunophenotype of H/RSCs was identical in simultaneous biopsies in only 11 of 39 (28%) patients and remained constant in consecutive biopsies in only 4 of 21 (19%) patients.[92] Major differences were related to cell lineage–specific antigens, whereas minor differences involved mainly CD15 and CD74 antigens.

In most cases of CHL and NLPHL, an accurate diagnosis can be rendered with an adequate size biopsy, proper fixation, thorough morphologic review, and appropriate antibody selection. However, there are several caveats and differential diagnostic considerations that may cause confusion with HL. One of the major differential diagnoses includes non-Hodgkin lymphoma subtypes with an abundance of non-neoplastic reactive background inflammatory cells. We will now discuss these subtypes, as well as certain non-lymphoid malignancies and tumor-like non-neoplastic look-alikes.

Non-Hodgkin Lymphomas

ANAPLASTIC LARGE CELL LYMPHOMA

CD30 is displayed on the tumor cells of ALCL, which is a non-HL with a different natural history than HL.[14,93-96] The histologic features of ALCL, particularly cohesive growth pattern and lymph node sinus infiltration by tumor cells, were thought to be distinguishing characteristics of ALCL; however, experience has shown otherwise. Rare cases of cell-rich HL—particularly those classified as nodular sclerosis type II in the British National Investigation,[97] or the syncytial variant[98]—and some cases of lymphocyte-depletion HL can be confused with ALCL (Fig. 5.17).[99] In these cases, a panel of antibodies is used to make the distinction (Tables 5-1 and 5-3). Perhaps most useful is the monoclonal antibody ALK-1 directed against the ALK tyrosine kinase, which is most often activated by the translocation t(2;5)(p23; q35) and less frequently by other chromosomal rearrangements in ALCL (Fig. 5.18).[100,101] ALK is rarely, if ever, expressed in the malignant cells of HL.[99] Demonstration of a B-cell phenotype (as with subset CD20 expression or BSAP/PAX5) in H/RSCs in CHL is also useful in excluding T-ALCL.

LYMPHOEPITHELIOID CELL VARIANT OF PERIPHERAL T-CELL LYMPHOMA (LENNERT LYMPHOMA)

Lennert lymphoma is another T-cell lymphoma that can resemble CHL because of the presence of H/RS-like cells, eosinophils, and plasma cells. Small clusters of epithelioid histiocytes resembling granulomas are a distinctive feature. In Lennert lymphoma, the H/RS-like cells express a CD4+ T-cell phenotype.[102]

PRIMARY MEDIASTINAL B-CELL LYMPHOMA

Primary mediastinal B-cell lymphoma (PMBCL) can be confused with HL because it presents as a mass in the anterior mediastinum of young adults and often contains H/RS-like cells in a background of collagen sclerosis (Fig. 5.19).[103] Also, in one study, H/RS-like cells expressed CD30 in 35 of 51 (69%) cases.[104] However, PMBCL can be distinguished from HL by the strong, uniform expression of CD20, lack of CD15, absence of EBV (EBERs and LMP-1), and lack of inflammatory background, particularly eosinophils (which is characteristic of HL).

T-CELL–RICH B-CELL LYMPHOMA

T-cell–rich B-cell lymphoma was recognized as a non-Hodgkin lymphoma (NHL) usually occurring in patients older than 50 years with advanced (stage III or IV) disease. Response to commonly used chemotherapy regimens for HL is poor. Therefore, it is important to distinguish TCRBCL from HL, particularly NLPHD or LRCHL (Fig. 5.20).[104,105] The tumor cells in TCRBCL appear to be negative for CD30 and CD15, as well as for vimentin, all of which are expressed in H/RSCs in CHL. Furthermore, the reactive inflammatory infiltrate that is rich in TIA-1+ lymphocytes in TCRBCL and CHL is rarely encountered in NLPHD, whereas CD57+ lymphocytes characteristic of NLPHD are infrequent in TCRBCL.[106] NLPHL generally has at least one nodular area; the background cells in the nodules of NLPHL are B-cell rich in contrast to the T-cell–rich background of TCRBCL.

HODGKIN-LIKE POST-TRANSPLANT LYMPHOPROLIFERATIVE DISORDER (HL-PTLD)

HL-PTLD, with cells resembling H/RSCs (Fig. 5.21), has been reported in allograft recipients, post-methotrexate therapy patients, [107] and HIV-infected patients. CHL has also been reported in each of these conditions, and differential diagnosis is based on morphologic and immunophenotypic features.[108] The histopathologic features often show a mixed population of small- to intermediate-sized lymphocytes admixed with histiocytes, plasma cells, and rare eosinophils and neutrophils, as well as scattered large pleomorphic mononuclear and binucelated cells without sclerosis and no nodularity, resembling mixed cellularity or lymphocyte depletion Hodgkin lymphoma.[109] While H/RSCs in CHL characteristically express CD30 and CD15, HL-PTLD cells often have an activated B-cell phenotype (i.e., CD20+, CD30+, CD45+, but CD15−). The atypical cells in

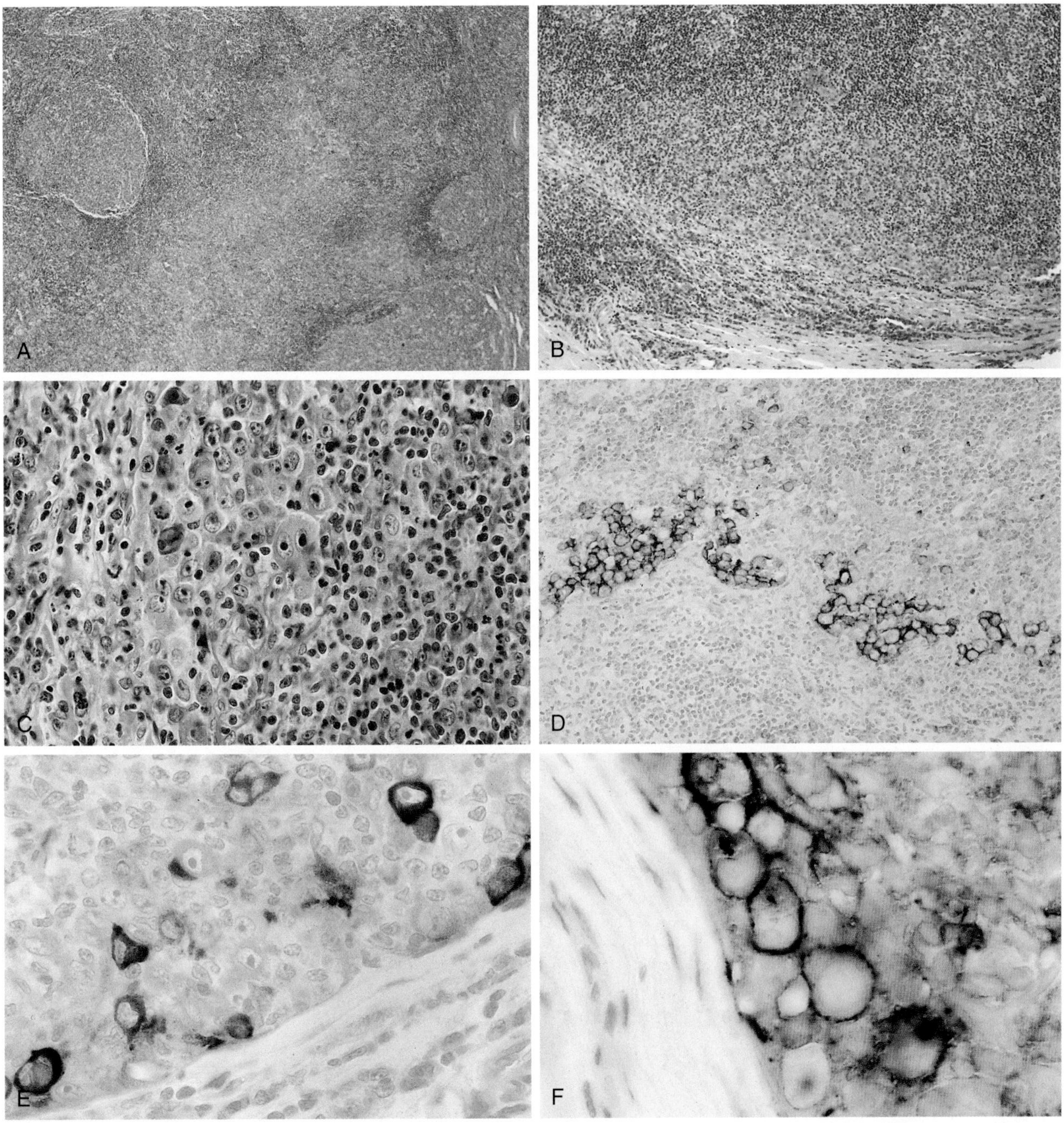

FIGURE 5.17 Cell-rich classical Hodgkin lymphoma with interfollicular and intrasinus distribution of tumor cells. **(A)** Low magnification of interfollicular pattern. **(B)** Low magnification of sinus infiltration. **(C)** High magnification of Hodgkin/Reed-Sternberg cells within sinus of lymph node. **(D)** Expression of CD30 by Hodgkin/Reed-Sternberg cells within sinus. **(E)** Expression of fascin by Hodgkin/Reed-Sternberg cells. **(F)** Expression of CD40 by Hodgkin/Reed-Sternberg cells within sinus.

HL-PTLD have been reported to express fascin, with a weak expression of BCL-2; CD45 is variably expressed. Virtually all cases of HL-PTLD are EBV-positive.

CHL IN CLL AND HODGKIN-LIKE CELLS IN CLL

Classical HL transformation is a rare form of Richter's transformation, which can occur in patients with B-chronic lymphocytic leukemia (B-CLL). H/RSCs are seen in a polymorphous background of inflammatory cells, and are morphologically and immunophenotypically indistinguishable from CHL. Such transformations have been variously reported to be clonally distinct[110-112] or clonally related[112,113] to B-CLL. Separately, H/RS-like cells may be seen (singly or clustered) in a background of B-CLL. Although RS-like cells in CLL are typically CD30-immunoreactive, with variable expression of CD20, CD15, and LMP1, the background is composed of monomorphous B-CLL cells and thus these cases are not thought to represent Richter's transformation.

TABLE 5.3 Antibody Panel for Differential Diagnosis of Hodgkin Lymphoma

Lymphoma Type	Classical Hodgkin Lymphoma	Nodular Lymphocyte Predominance Hodgkin Lymphoma	Anaplastic Large Cell Lymphoma	Primary Mediastinal Large B-Cell Lymphoma	T-Cell–Rich B-Cell Lymphoma
CD30	+	S	+	S	–
CD15	+	–	R	–	–
CD20	S	+	–	+	+
CD3	–	–	+	–	–
CD40	+	+	–	+	+
CD45	–	+	S	+	+
EBV-LMP-1	S	–	–	–	–
ALK	–	–	+	–	–
Fascin	+	–	–	–	–

+, Nearly all cases positive; S, sometimes positive; R, rare (<5%); –, negative.

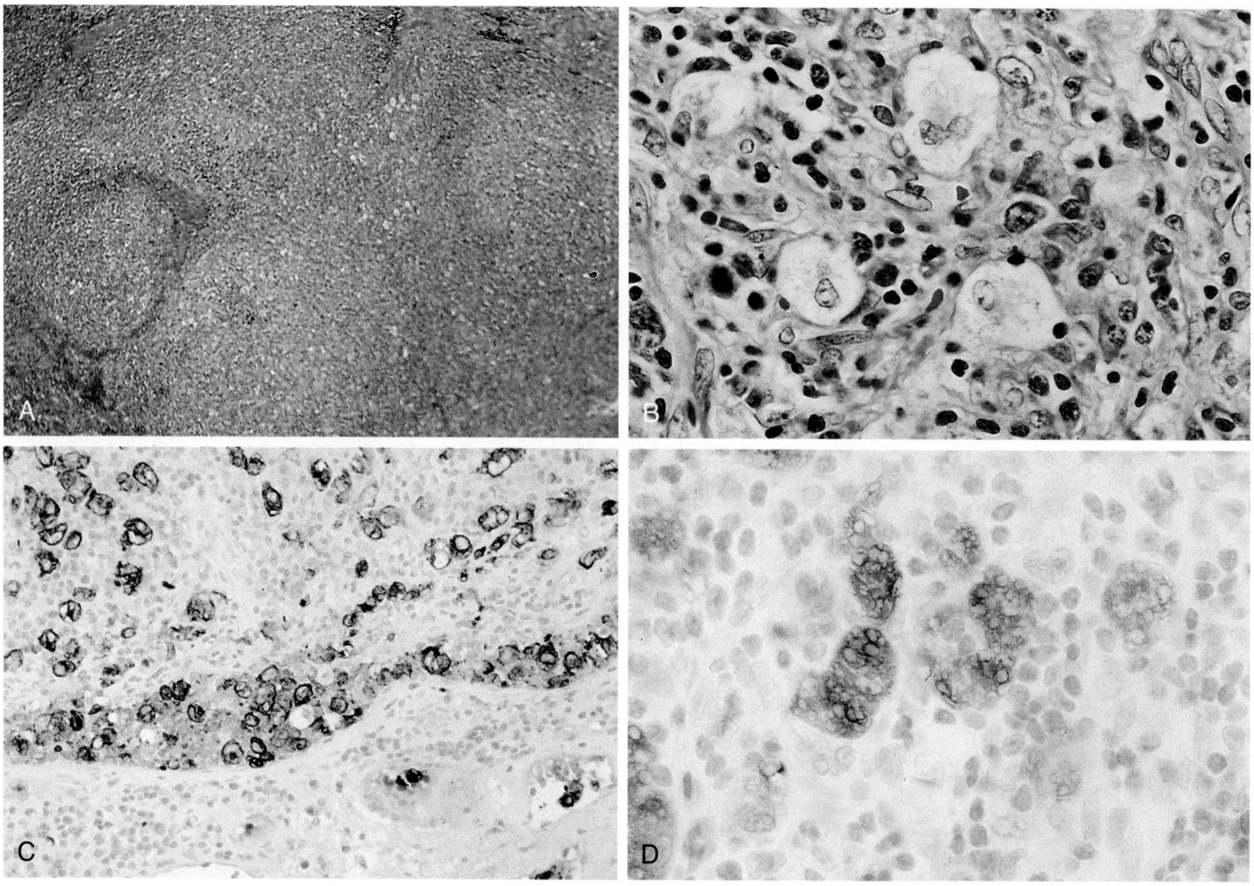

FIGURE 5.18 Hodgkin-like anaplastic large cell lymphoma with **(A)** nodular pattern and **(B)** lacunar cells. **(C)** CD30 staining of tumor cells within sinus. **(D)** Expression of p80NPM/ALK by tumor cells in lacunar spaces.

Nonlymphoid Tumors

CD30, the most consistent marker of H/RSCs, is readily detected in formalin-fixed, paraffin-embedded tissues.[14,114] However, tumor cells in some nonlymphoid malignancies, including embryonic carcinoma, melanoma, and pancreatic cancer, can also express CD30.[114,115] Because sinus infiltration of lymph nodes is characteristic of CD30+ ALCLs, there is potential for confusion of ALCLs with the few metastatic carcinomas that express CD30 antigen.[14] Moreover, because malignant

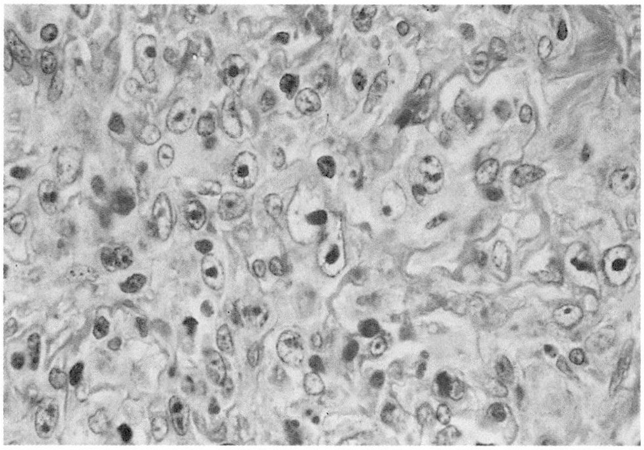

FIGURE 5.19 Hodgkin/Reed-Sternberg–like cells in primary mediastinal B-cell large cell lymphoma.

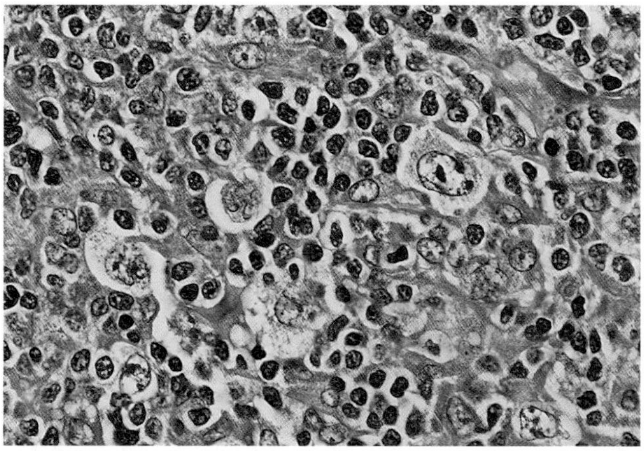

FIGURE 5.20 Hodgkin/Reed-Sternberg–like cells in T-cell–rich B-cell lymphoma.

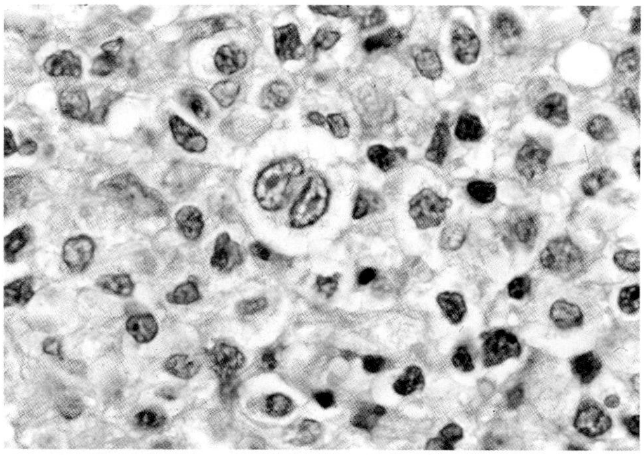

FIGURE 5.21 Hodgkin-like post-transplant lymphoproliferative disorder.

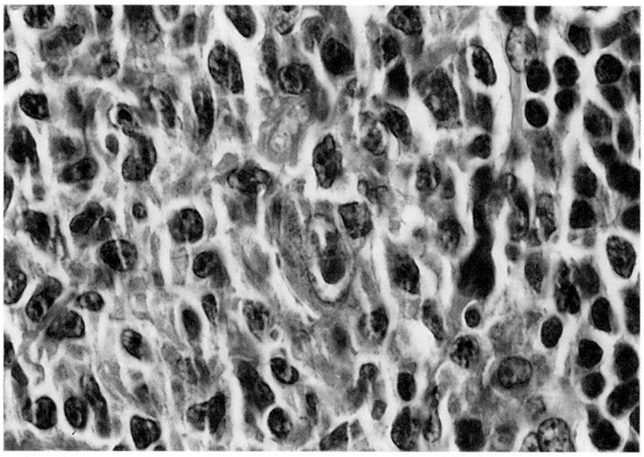

FIGURE 5.22 Hodgkin/Reed-Sternberg–like cells in lymph node infected by cytomegalovirus.

melanoma can express CD30, there is the possibility of mistaking an anaplastic melanoma for a primary CD30+ ALCL.[115]

CD15 expressed on H/RSCs is also associated with carcinomas.[116] Fortunately it is not common to encounter a carcinoma that could be clinically or histologically mistaken for HL. However, the cohesive growth pattern of tumor cells in the syncytial variant of nodular sclerosis HL might rarely be mistaken for metastatic carcinoma expressing CD15.

Pseudoneoplastic Look-alikes

INFECTIOUS MONONUCLEOSIS

H/RS-like cells in infectious mononucleosis are similar in most respects to their morphologic counterparts in HL with respect to expression of EBERs, EBV-LMP1, and CD30, and low expression of CD45.[117] However, the H/RS-like cells in infectious mononucleosis are CD15–.[118]

CYTOMEGALOVIRUS LYMPHADENITIS

Lymph nodes infected with cytomegalovirus contain H/RS-like cells that are caused by viral inclusions and are readily distinguished from HL by absence of CD15 and CD30 (Fig. 5.22).

INTERFOLLICULAR LYMPHADENITIS

Lymphadenitis mimicking Hodgkin disease has been described as a benign lymphadenopathy that can mimic interfollicular HL.[119,120] Cervical lymph nodes are affected most often. There is no progression to lymphoma. The lymph nodes show follicular hyperplasia with a mottled interfollicular zone with epithelioid histiocytes, lymphocytes, eosinophils, and immunoblasts. Some immunoblasts with prominent nucleoli resemble H/RSCs. However, their nucleoli are typically smaller and basophilic, in contrast to the eosinophilic nucleoli of H/RSCs. Immunohistochemistry distinguishes this disorder from interfollicular HL because

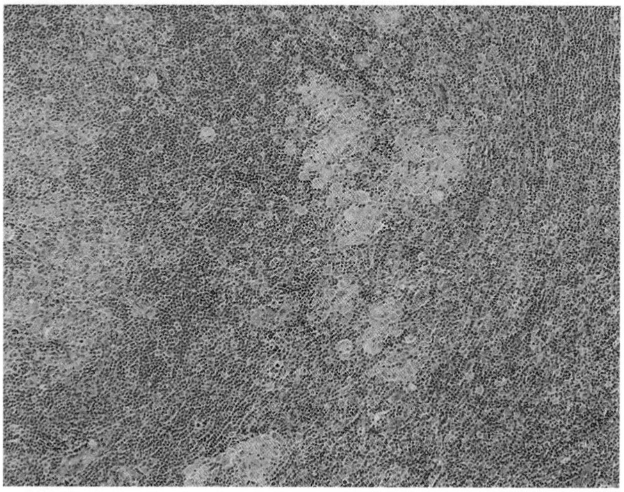

FIGURE 5.23 Granulomas in a lymph node involved by Hodgkin lymphoma.

the H/RS-like cells display B- or T-cell antigens and lack CD15.[120,121]

GRANULOMATOUS LYMPHADENITIS

The presence of non-caseating granulomas is a well-known histologic feature associated with several non-hematopoietic and hematopoietic malignancies, including HL (Fig 5.23). In HL, approximately 15% of patients have granulomas, which may be present in nodal and extranodal sites uninvolved by HL;[122] the presence of granulomas alone, in the absence of diagnostic H/RSCs, should not be interpreted as evidence of HL. Conversely, granulomatous reaction may be present in a site involved by HL and on occasion may be extremely florid, necessitating a thorough morphologic review to detect small foci of HL. H/RSCs in such areas have the classical immunophenotype (CD30+, CD15+, LCA–, CD20–) as opposed to reactive immunoblasts (LCA+, CD20+, CD30+, CD15–).

MOLECULAR ANATOMIC PATHOLOGY

In a majority of cases, the diagnosis of CHL and NLPHL is based on morphology and immunophenotyping, and molecular testing is rarely utilized. Polymerase chain reaction studies (PCR) for immunoglobulin heavy chain gene (IgH) rearrangements have been used to distinguish T-cell–rich large B-cell lymphoma from HL, with the former demonstrating clonal bands more frequently than the latter.[123] While demonstration of clonal IgH bands in CHL generally required special cell enrichment techniques and/or single cell microdissection, recent data suggest that detectable rearrangements without microdissection can be seen in a higher number of CHL cases using newer multiplex primers, making IgH analysis less useful in this context.[124]

Most T-HL (and a subset of B-HL) have TCR gamma rearrangements.[35] In one case of CHL, identical rearrangements of the TCR alpha chain were found in the HL lymph node and co-existent cutaneous T cell lymphoma.[125] In another case studied by single-cell PCR, identical TCR beta chain rearrangements were found in H/RSCs in a lymph node of mixed cellularity HL and skin lesions with CD30+ CD15+ H/RSCs.[37]

BEYOND IMMUNOHISTOCHEMISTRY: ANATOMIC MOLECULAR DIAGNOSTIC APPLICATIONS

The exact genomic alteration that drives lymphomagenesis in CHL and NLPHL is not completely understood. Nuclear factor of kappa light polypeptide gene enhancer in B cells 2 (NF-κB) is present in numerous cell types and is normally only transiently activated by stress, immune, and inflammatory signals. It has been shown that NF-κB is constitutively activated in cultured H/RSCs,[17] primarily owing to mutations and/or increased turnover of its natural inhibitor I-kappa B (IκB).[74] Constitutive NF-κB results in overexpressed anti-apoptotic genes that allow H/RSCs to escape apoptosis despite losing capability to produce Ig. Overexpression of NF-κB can be demonstrated immunohistochemically in CHL; however, it is not specific to this tumor type and can be seen in a variety of other malignancies, including mediastinal B-cell lymphoma.[126,127]

A tissue microarray study using immunohistochemistry and *in situ* hybridization to observe cell cycle and apoptosis regulating genes has shown multiple alterations in cell cycle checkpoints and major tumor suppressor pathways, some of which are linked to survival as well as EBV positivity.[128]

THERANOSTIC APPLICATIONS

Although newer therapeutic agents such as monoclonal antibodies are being evaluated, most are in early experimental stages. Nonetheless, accurate documentation of H/RSC expression of potential therapeutic targets would likely be beneficial when evaluating such biopsies.

CD20 and Monoclonal Antibody (Rituximab) Therapy

CD20 expression by a majority of L&H cells in NLPHL has been used as a basis for targeted monoclonal therapy.[129] Rituximab therapy is also being tried in CHL, not only targeting the minor CD20 expressing H/RSCs but also infiltrating background B-lymphocytes.[130]

CD40

CD40 is widely expressed on H/RSCs, and its ligand, CD40L, is expressed by many T cells surrounding H/RSCs. In B cells, CD40 regulates progression from immunoglobulin isotype switch to cytokine secretion and ultimately terminates in Fas-mediated apoptosis to terminate the immune response. CD40 signal transduction pathways result in activation of NF-κB; this in turn activates transcription of IL-2, IL-6, IL-8, TNF, and GM-CSF, thus affecting the proliferation and activation of many components of the immune system. CD40 activation of NF-κB is mediated by proteolysis of TRAF3, and a protease inhibitor has been used to block this pathway.[131]

CD30

Anti-CD30 monoclonal antibodies have been used in pre-clinical murine xenograft models of localized HL to demonstrate dose-dependent reduction in tumor mass. There is also a significant increase in survival of mice bearing disseminated HL treated with anti-CD30.[132] Anti-tumor activity of anti-CD30 has been enhanced by conjugation with monomethyl auristatin E, which induces G2/M growth arrest and cell death.[133] Trials using monoclonal anti-CD30 antibodies as well as bispecific molecules are also being conducted.[134,135]

Anti-EBV Therapy

In almost 40% of HL patients, H/RSCs express EBV-associated antigens. EBV-specific cytotoxic T lymphocytes expressing the anti-CD30ζ artificial chimeric T-cell receptor have been employed for immunotherapy of HL. Adoptive transfer of EBV-specific cytotoxic T lymphocytes (EBV-CTLs) have shown that these cells persist in patients with HL to produce complete tumor responses.[136] Treatment failure occurs if a subpopulation of malignant cells lacks or loses expression of EBV antigens. To overcome this limitation, investigators have prepared EBV-CTLs that retained antitumor activity conferred by their native receptor while expressing a chimeric antigen receptor specific for CD30.[137]

Interleukin-2 Receptor

Interleukin-2 receptor (CD25) has been used as a target for immunotherapy protocols to treat HL.[138] A pitfall of these protocols is that difficulty is sometimes encountered in demonstrating CD25 expression by H/RSCs against which the therapy is directed. Indeed, CD25 is often expressed on activated tumor-infiltrating lymphocytes (TILs) in HL, and it is important to distinguish them from H/RSCs. We found this possible in most cases when a biotinylated tyramine enhancement step[139] was applied to formalin-fixed paraffin-embedded tissues.[77]

CCR4

CCR4 is a chemokine receptor expressed on H/RSCs in 24% of patients with HL. A chimeric anti-CCR4 antibody KM2760, the Fc region of which is defucosylated to enhance antibody dependent cellular cytotoxicity, is being developed as a novel treatment for patients with CCR4+ HL.[140]

SUMMARY

The diagnosis of HL from routine H&E sections is often readily made. However, increasing recognition of new lymphoma types with overlapping morphologies dictates the use of immunohistochemistry to avoid incorrect diagnoses. Among the non-Hodgkin lymphomas that may be confused with HL are ALCL

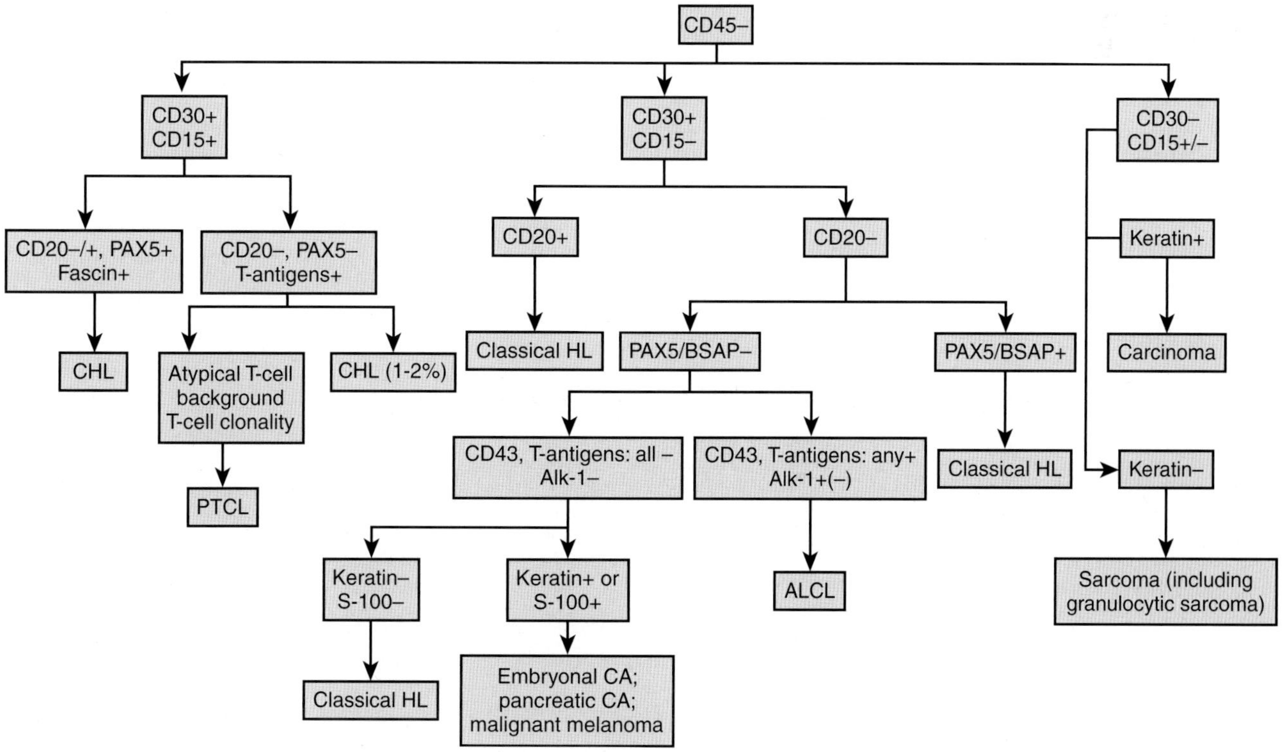

FIGURE 5.24 Diagnostic algorithm: Classical Hodgkin lymphoma.

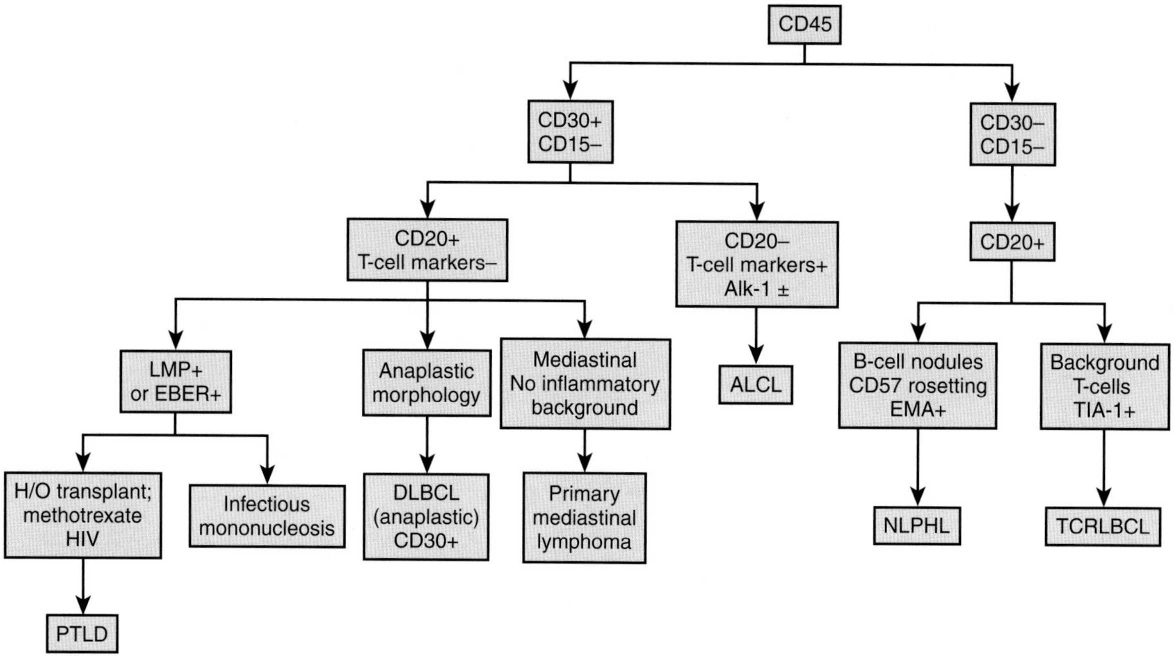

FIGURE 5.25 Diagnostic algorithm: B-cell lymphomas, NLPHL, and pseudoneoplastic lymphoproliferative disorders.

and T-cell–rich B-cell lymphoma. It is also important to distinguish NLPHL from lymphocyte-rich CHL by aid of immunohistochemistry. At the same time, one must be aware of antigens shared by H/RSCs and NHL cells. Recognition of certain antigens expressed or not expressed by H/RSCs informs us of the biology of these cells. The silencing of B-cell antigens by Id2 and possibly other mechanisms makes the diagnosis of HL difficult in some cases; however, it distinguishes H/RSCs from B cells in most NHLs. Finally, one must always be cognizant of pseudoneoplastic conditions that mimic HL, wherein immunohistochemistry is a useful aid to arrive at the correct diagnosis. Overall, immunohistochemistry contributes significantly to our knowledge of HL as well as better patient management. One possible immunohistologic approach to resolve differential diagnostic considerations is presented in the supplied diagnostic algorithm (Figs. 5.24, 5.25).

REFERENCES

1. Lukes RJ, Butler JJ. The pathology and nomenclature of Hodgkin's disease. *Cancer Res.* 1966;26:1063-1083.
2. Harris NL, Jaffe ES, Stein H, et al. A revised European-American classification of lymphoid neoplasms: A proposal from the International Lymphoma Study Group. *Blood.* 1994;84:1361-1392.
3. Mason DY, Banks PM, Chan J, et al. Nodular lymphocyte predominance Hodgkin's disease. A distinct clinicopathological entity. *Am J Surg Pathol.* 1994;18:526-530.
4. Poppema S. The nature of the lymphocytes surrounding Reed-Sternberg cells in nodular lymphocyte predominance and in other types of Hodgkin's disease. *Am J Pathol.* 1989;135:351-357.
5. Marafioti T, Hummel M, Anagnostopoulos I, et al. Origin of nodular lymphocyte-predominant Hodgkin's disease from a clonal expansion of highly mutated germinal-center B cells. *N Engl J Med.* 1997;337:453-458.
6. Kanzler H, Kuppers R, Hansmann ML, et al. Hodgkin and Reed-Sternberg cells in Hodgkin's disease represent the outgrowth of a dominant tumor clone derived from (crippled) germinal center B cells. *J Exp Med.* 1996;184:1495-1505.
7. von Wasielewski R, Werner M, Fischer R, et al. Lymphocyte-predominant Hodgkin's disease. An immunohistochemical analysis of 208 reviewed Hodgkin's disease cases from the German Hodgkin Study Group. *Am J Pathol.* 1997;150:793-803.
8. Pinkus GS, Said JW. Hodgkin's disease, lymphocyte predominance type, nodular—further evidence for a B cell derivation. L & H variants of Reed-Sternberg cells express L26, a pan B cell marker. *Am J Pathol.* 1988;133:211-217.
9. Epstein AL, Marder RJ, Winter JN, et al. Two new monoclonal antibodies (LN-1, LN-2) reactive in B5 formalin-fixed, paraffin-embedded tissues with follicular center and mantle zone human B lymphocytes and derived tumors. *J Immunol.* 1984;133:1028-1036.
10. Marder RJ, Variakojis D, Silver J, et al. Immunohistochemical analysis of human lymphomas with monoclonal antibodies to B cell and Ia antigens reactive in paraffin sections. *Lab Invest.* 1985;52:497-504.
11. Korkolopoulou P, Cordell J, Jones M, et al. The expression of the B-cell marker mb-1 (CD79a) in Hodgkin's disease. *Histopathology.* 1994;24:511-515.
12. Dorfman RF, Gatter KC, Pulford KA, et al. An evaluation of the utility of anti-granulocyte and anti-leukocyte monoclonal antibodies in the diagnosis of Hodgkin's disease. *Am J Pathol.* 1986;123:508-519.
13. Chittal SM, Caveriviere P, Schwarting R, et al. Monoclonal antibodies in the diagnosis of Hodgkin's disease. The search for a rational panel. *Am J Surg Pathol.* 1988;12:9-21.
14. Stein H, Mason DY, Gerdes J, et al. The expression of the Hodgkin's disease associated antigen Ki-1 in reactive and neoplastic lymphoid tissue: evidence that Reed-Sternberg cells and histiocytic malignancies are derived from activated lymphoid cells. *Blood.* 1985;66:848-858.
15. Durkop H, Latza U, Hummel M, et al. Molecular cloning and expression of a new member of the nerve growth factor receptor family that is characteristic for Hodgkin's disease. *Cell.* 1992;68:421-427.
16. Smith CA, Gruss HJ, Davis T, et al. CD30 antigen, a marker for Hodgkin's lymphoma, is a receptor whose ligand defines an emerging family of cytokines with homology to TNF. *Cell.* 1993;73:1349-1360.

17. Bargou RC, Leng C, Krappmann D, et al. High-level nuclear NF-kappa B and Oct-2 is a common feature of cultured Hodgkin/Reed-Sternberg cells. *Blood.* 1996;87:4340-4347.
18. Bargou RC, Emmerich F, Krappmann D, et al. Constitutive nuclear factor-kappaB-RelA activation is required for proliferation and survival of Hodgkin's disease tumor cells. *J Clin Invest.* 1997;100:2961-2969.
19. Stein H, Uchanska-Ziegler B, Gerdes J, et al. Hodgkin and Sternberg-Reed cells contain antigens specific to late cells of granulopoiesis. *Int J Cancer.* 1982;29:283-290.
20. Hsu SM, Jaffe ES. Leu M1 and peanut agglutinin stain the neoplastic cells of Hodgkin's disease. *Am J Clin Pathol.* 1984;82:29-32.
21. Pinkus GS, Thomas P, Said JW. Leu-M1—A marker for Reed-Sternberg cells in Hodgkin's disease. An immunoperoxidase study of paraffin-embedded tissues. *Am J Pathol.* 1985;119:244-252.
22. von Wasielewski R, Mengel M, Fischer R, et al. Classical Hodgkin's disease. Clinical impact of the immunophenotype. *Am J Pathol.* 1997;151:1123-1130.
23. Gooi HC, Feizi T, Kapadia A, et al. Stage-specific embryonic antigen involves alpha 1 goes to 3 fucosylated type 2 blood group chains. *Nature.* 1981;292:156-158.
24. Carbone A, Gloghini A, Gaidano G, et al. Expression status of BCL-6 and syndecan-1 identifies distinct histogenetic subtypes of Hodgkin's disease. *Blood.* 1998;92:2220-2228.
25. Carbone A, Gloghini A, Gattei V, et al. Expression of functional CD40 antigen on Reed-Sternberg cells and Hodgkin's disease cell lines. *Blood.* 1995;85:780-789.
26. Banchereau J, Bazan F, Blanchard D, et al. The CD40 antigen and its ligand. *Annu Rev Immunol.* 1994;12:881-922.
27. Kadin ME, Muramoto L, Said J. Expression of T-cell antigens on Reed-Sternberg cells in a subset of patients with nodular sclerosing and mixed cellularity Hodgkin's disease. *Am J Pathol.* 1988;130:345-353.
28. Casey TT, Olson SJ, Cousar JB, et al. Immunophenotypes of Reed-Sternberg cells: A study of 19 cases of Hodgkin's disease in plastic-embedded sections. *Blood.* 1989;74:2624-2628.
29. Dallenbach FE, Stein H. Expression of T-cell-receptor beta chain in Reed-Sternberg cells. *Lancet.* 1989;2:828-830.
30. Oka K, Mori N, Kojima M. Anti-Leu-3a antibody reactivity with Reed-Sternberg cells of Hodgkin's disease. *Arch Pathol Lab Med.* 1988;112:139-142.
31. Oudejans JJ, Kummer JA, Jiwa M, et al. Granzyme B expression in Reed-Sternberg cells of Hodgkin's disease. *Am J Pathol.* 1996;148:233-240.
32. Krenacs L, Wellmann A, Sorbara L, et al. Cytotoxic cell antigen expression in anaplastic large cell lymphomas of T- and null-cell type and Hodgkin's disease: Evidence for distinct cellular origin. *Blood.* 1997;89:980-989.
33. Felgar RE, Macon WR, Kinney MC, et al. TIA-1 expression in lymphoid neoplasms. Identification of subsets with cytotoxic T lymphocyte or natural killer cell differentiation. *Am J Pathol.* 1997;150:1893-1900.
34. Tzankov A, Zimpfer A, Went P, et al. Aberrant expression of cell cycle regulators in Hodgkin and Reed-Sternberg cells of classical Hodgkin's lymphoma. *Mod Pathol.* 2005;18:90-96.
35. Seitz V, Hummel M, Marafioti T, et al. Detection of clonal T-cell receptor gamma-chain gene rearrangements in Reed-Sternberg cells of classic Hodgkin disease. *Blood.* 2000;95:3020-3024.
36. Muschen M, Rajewsky K, Brauninger A, et al. Rare occurrence of classical Hodgkin's disease as a T cell lymphoma. *J Exp Med.* 2000;191:387-394.
37. Willenbrock K, Ichinohasama R, Kadin ME, et al. T-cell variant of classical Hodgkin's lymphoma with nodal and cutaneous manifestations demonstrated by single-cell polymerase chain reaction. *Lab Invest.* 2002;82:1103-1109.
38. Weiss LM, Movahed LA, Warnke RA, et al. Detection of Epstein-Barr viral genomes in Reed-Sternberg cells of Hodgkin's disease. *N Engl J Med.* 1989;320:502-506.
39. Wang D, Liebowitz D, Kieff E. An EBV membrane protein expressed in immortalized lymphocytes transforms established rodent cells. *Cell.* 1985;43:831-840.
40. Pallesen G, Hamilton-Dutoit SJ, Rowe M, et al. Expression of Epstein-Barr virus latent gene products in tumour cells of Hodgkin's disease. *Lancet.* 1991;337:320-322.
41. Ambinder RF, Browning PJ, Lorenzana I, et al. Epstein-Barr virus and childhood Hodgkin's disease in Honduras and the United States. *Blood.* 1993;81:462-467.
42. Gulley ML, Eagan PA, Quintanilla-Martinez L, et al. Epstein-Barr virus DNA is abundant and monoclonal in the Reed-Sternberg cells of Hodgkin's disease: Association with mixed cellularity subtype and Hispanic American ethnicity. *Blood.* 1994;83:1595-1602.
43. Herndier BG, Sanchez HC, Chang KL, et al. High prevalence of Epstein-Barr virus in the Reed-Sternberg cells of HIV-associated Hodgkin's disease. *Am J Pathol.* 1993;142:1073-1079.
44. Pinkus GS, Pinkus JL, Langhoff E, et al. Fascin, a sensitive new marker for Reed-Sternberg cells of Hodgkin's disease. Evidence for a dendritic or B cell derivation? *Am J Pathol.* 1997;150:543-562.
45. Bakshi NA, Finn WG, Schnitzer B, et al. Fascin expression in diffuse large B-cell lymphoma, anaplastic large cell lymphoma, and classical Hodgkin lymphoma. *Arch Pathol Lab Med.* 2007;131:742-747.
46. Fan G, Kotylo P, Neiman RS, et al. Comparison of fascin expression in anaplastic large cell lymphoma and Hodgkin disease. *Am J Clin Pathol.* 2003;119:199-204.
47. Sahin U, Neumann F, Tureci O, et al. Hodgkin and Reed-Sternberg cell-associated autoantigen CLIP-170/restin is a marker for dendritic cells and is involved in the trafficking of macropinosomes to the cytoskeleton, supporting a function-based concept of Hodgkin and Reed-Sternberg cells. *Blood.* 2002;100:4139-4145.
48. Kishimoto T, Goyert S, Kikutani H, et al. CD antigens. 1996. *Blood.* 1997;89:3502.
49. Mason DY, Cordell JL, Brown MH, et al. CD79a: A novel marker for B-cell neoplasms in routinely processed tissue samples. *Blood.* 1995;86:1453-1459.
50. Kuzu I, Delsol G, Jones M, et al. Expression of the Ig-associated heterodimer (mb-1 and B29) in Hodgkin's disease. *Histopathology.* 1993;22:141-144.
51. Browne P, Petrosyan K, Hernandez A, et al. The B-cell transcription factors BSAP, Oct-2, and BOB.1 and the pan-B-cell markers CD20, CD22, and CD79a are useful in the differential diagnosis of classic Hodgkin lymphoma. *Am J Clin Pathol.* 2003;120:767-777.
52. Tzankov A, Zimpfer A, Pehrs AC, et al. Expression of B-cell markers in classical Hodgkin lymphoma: A tissue microarray analysis of 330 cases. *Mod Pathol.* 2003;16:1141-1147.
53. Schwering I, Brauninger A, Klein U, et al. Loss of the B-lineage-specific gene expression program in Hodgkin and Reed-Sternberg cells of Hodgkin lymphoma. *Blood.* 2003;101:1505-1512.
54. Renne C, Martin-Subero JI, Eickernjager M, et al. Aberrant expression of ID2, a suppressor of B-cell-specific gene expression, in Hodgkin's lymphoma. *Am J Pathol.* 2006;169:655-664.
55. Foss HD, Reusch R, Demel G, et al. Frequent expression of the B-cell-specific activator protein in Reed-Sternberg cells of classical Hodgkin's disease provides further evidence for its B-cell origin. *Blood.* 1999;94:3108-3113.
56. Steimle-Grauer SA, Tinguely M, Seada L, et al. Expression patterns of transcription factors in progressively transformed germinal centers and Hodgkin lymphoma. *Virchows Arch.* 2003;442:284-293.
57. Laumen H, Nielsen PJ, Wirth T. The BOB.1 / OBF.1 co-activator is essential for octamer-dependent transcription in B cells. *Eur J Immunol.* 2000;30:458-469.
58. Stein H, Marafioti T, Foss HD, et al. Down-regulation of BOB.1/OBF.1 and Oct2 in classical Hodgkin disease but not in lymphocyte predominant Hodgkin disease correlates with immunoglobulin transcription. *Blood.* 2001;97:496-501.
59. Hertel CB, Zhou XG, Hamilton-Dutoit SJ, et al. Loss of B cell identity correlates with loss of B cell-specific transcription factors in Hodgkin/Reed-Sternberg cells of classical Hodgkin lymphoma. *Oncogene.* 2002;21:4908-4920.
60. Marafioti T, Ascani S, Pulford K, et al. Expression of B-lymphocyte-associated transcription factors in human T-cell neoplasms. *Am J Pathol.* 2003;162:861-871.
60a. Bhargava P, Pantanowitz L, Pinkus GS, et al. Utility of fascin and JunB in distinguishing nodular lymphocyte predominant from classical lymphocyte-rich Hodgkin lymphoma. *Appl Immunohistochem Mol Morphol.* Epub 22 Jun 2009.

61. Mathas S, Hinz M, Anagnostopoulos I, et al. Aberrantly expressed c-Jun and JunB are a hallmark of Hodgkin lymphoma cells, stimulate proliferation and synergize with NF-kappa B. *Embo J*. 2002;21:4104-4113.
62. Poppema S. The diversity of the immunohistological staining pattern of Sternberg-Reed cells. *J Histochem Cytochem*. 1980;28:788-791.
63. Stein H, Hansmann ML, Lennert K, et al. Reed-Sternberg and Hodgkin cells in lymphocyte-predominant Hodgkin's disease of nodular subtype contain J chain. *Am J Clin Pathol*. 1986;86:292-297.
64. Prakash S, Fountaine T, Raffeld M, et al. IgD positive L&H cells identify a unique subset of nodular lymphocyte predominant Hodgkin lymphoma. *Am J Surg Pathol*. 2006;30:585-592.
65. Payne SV, Wright DH, Jones KJ, et al. Macrophage origin of Reed-Sternberg cells: An immunohistochemical study. *J Clin Pathol*. 1982;35:159-166.
66. Mir R, Kahn LB. Immunohistochemistry of Hodgkin's disease. A study of 20 cases. *Cancer*. 1983;52:2064-2071.
67. Rosenwald IB, Koifman L, Savas L, et al. Expression of the translation initiation factors eIF-4E and eIF-2* is frequently increased in neoplastic cells of Hodgkin lymphoma. *Hum Pathol*. 2008;39:910-916.
68. Zheng B, Fiumara P, Li YV, et al. MEK/ERK pathway is aberrantly active in Hodgkin disease: A signaling pathway shared by CD30, CD40, and RANK that regulates cell proliferation and survival. *Blood*. 2003;102:1019-1027.
69. Oelmann E, Herbst H, Zuhlsdorf M, et al. Tissue inhibitor of metalloproteinases 1 is an autocrine and paracrine survival factor, with additional immune-regulatory functions, expressed by Hodgkin/Reed-Sternberg cells. *Blood*. 2002;99:258-267.
70. Juszczynski P, Ouyang J, Monti S, et al. The AP1-dependent secretion of galectin-1 by Reed Sternberg cells fosters immune privilege in classical Hodgkin lymphoma. *Proc Natl Acad Sci U S A*. 2007;104:13134-13139.
71. Yamamoto R, Nishikori M, Kitawaki T, et al. PD-1-PD-1 ligand interaction contributes to immunosuppressive microenvironment of Hodgkin lymphoma. *Blood*. 2008;111:3220-3224.
72. Kadin ME, Leibowitz D. Cytokines and cytokine receptors in Hodgkin's disease. In: Mauch P, ed. *Hodgkin's Disease*. Philadelphia: Lippincott Williams & Wilkins; 1999:139-157.
73. Gruss HJ, Kadin ME. Pathophysiology of Hodgkin's disease: Functional and molecular aspects. *Baillieres Clin Haematol*. 1996;9:417-446.
74. Skinnider BF, Mak TW. The role of cytokines in classical Hodgkin lymphoma. *Blood*. 2002;99:4283-4297.
75. Hopken UE, Foss HD, Meyer D, et al. Up-regulation of the chemokine receptor CCR7 in classical but not in lymphocyte-predominant Hodgkin disease correlates with distinct dissemination of neoplastic cells in lymphoid organs. *Blood*. 2002;99:1109-1116.
76. Hsu SM, Tseng CK, Hsu PL. Expression of p55 (Tac) interleukin-2 receptor (IL-2R), but not p75 IL-2R, in cultured H-RS cells and H-RS cells in tissues. *Am J Pathol*. 1990;136:735-744.
77. Levi E, Butmarc J, Kourea HP, et al. Detection of interleukin-2 receptors on tumor cells in formalin-fixed, paraffin-embedded tissues. *Appl Immunohistochem*. 1997;5:234.
78. Horie R, Watanabe T, Ito K, Morisita Y, et al. Cytoplasmic aggregation of TRAF2 and TRAF5 proteins in the Hodgkin-Reed-Sternberg cells. *Am J Pathol*. 2002;160:1647-1654.
79. Kadin ME, Agnarsson BA, Ellingsworth LR, et al. Immunohistochemical evidence of a role for transforming growth factor beta in the pathogenesis of nodular sclerosing Hodgkin's disease. *Am J Pathol*. 1990;136:1209-1214.
80. Ohshima K, Sugihara M, Suzumiya J, et al. Basic fibroblast growth factor and fibrosis in Hodgkin's disease. *Pathol Res Pract*. 1999;195:149-155.
81. Skinnider BF, Elia AJ, Gascoyne RD, et al. Interleukin 13 and interleukin 13 receptor are frequently expressed by Hodgkin and Reed-Sternberg cells of Hodgkin lymphoma. *Blood*. 2001;97:250-255.
82. Fichtner-Feigl S, Strober W, Kawakami K, et al. IL-13 signaling through the IL-13alpha2 receptor is involved in induction of TGF-beta1 production and fibrosis. *Nat Med*. 2006;12: 99-106.
83. Samoszuk M, Nansen L. Detection of interleukin-5 messenger RNA in Reed-Sternberg cells of Hodgkin's disease with eosinophilia. *Blood*. 1990;75:13-16.
84. Teruya-Feldstein J, Jaffe ES, Burd PR, et al. Differential chemokine expression in tissues involved by Hodgkin's disease: Direct correlation of eotaxin expression and tissue eosinophilia. *Blood*. 1999;93:2463-2470.
85. Dukers DF, Jaspars LH, Vos W, et al. Quantitative immunohistochemical analysis of cytokine profiles in Epstein-Barr virus-positive and -negative cases of Hodgkin's disease. *J Pathol*. 2000;190:143-149.
86. Scheeren FA, Diehl SA, Smit LA, et al. IL-21 is expressed in Hodgkin lymphoma and activates STAT5: Evidence that activated STAT5 is required for Hodgkin lymphomagenesis. *Blood*. 2008;111:4706-4715.
87. Skinnider BF, Elia AJ, Gascoyne RD, et al. Signal transducer and activator of transcription 6 is frequently activated in Hodgkin and Reed-Sternberg cells of Hodgkin lymphoma. *Blood*. 2002;99:618-626.
88. Delsol G, Blancher A, al Saati T, et al. Antibody BNH9 detects red blood cell-related antigens on anaplastic large cell (CD30+) lymphomas. *Br J Cancer*. 1991;64:321-326.
89. al Saati T, Tkaczuk J, Krissansen G, et al. A novel antigen detected by the CBF.78 antibody further distinguishes anaplastic large cell lymphoma from Hodgkin's disease. *Blood*. 1995;86:2741-2746.
89a. Fleming MD, Pinkus JL, Fournier MV, et al. Coincident expression of the chemokine receptors CCR6 and CCR7 by pathologic Langerhans cells in Langerhans cell histiocytosis. *Blood*. 2003;101(7):2473-2475.
90. Ree HJ, Teplitz C, Khan A. The Lewis X antigen. A new paraffin section marker for Reed-Sternberg cells. *Cancer*. 1991;67:1338-1346.
91. Facchetti F, Alebardi O, Vermi W. Omit iodine and CD30 will shine: A simple technical procedure to demonstrate the CD30 antigen on B5-fixed material. *Am J Surg Pathol*. 2000;24:320-322.
92. Chu WS, Abbondanzo SL, Frizzera G. Inconsistency of the immunophenotype of Reed-Sternberg cells in simultaneous and consecutive specimens from the same patients. A paraffin section evaluation in 56 patients. *Am J Pathol*. 1992;141:11-17.
93. Kadin ME, Sako D, Berliner N, et al. Childhood Ki-1 lymphoma presenting with skin lesions and peripheral lymphadenopathy. *Blood*. 1986;68:1042-1049.
94. Nakamura S, Takagi N, Kojima M, et al. Clinicopathologic study of large cell anaplastic lymphoma (Ki-1-positive large cell lymphoma) among the Japanese. *Cancer*. 1991;68:118-129.
95. Gascoyne RD, Aoun P, Wu D, et al. Prognostic significance of anaplastic lymphoma kinase (ALK) protein expression in adults with anaplastic large cell lymphoma. *Blood*. 1999;93:3913-3921.
96. Falini B, Pileri S, Zinzani PL, et al. ALK+ lymphoma: Clinico-pathological findings and outcome. *Blood*. 1999;93:2697-2706.
97. Haybittle JL, Hayhoe FG, Easterling MJ, et al. Review of British National Lymphoma Investigation studies of Hodgkin's disease and development of prognostic index. *Lancet*. 1985;1:967-972.
98. Strickler JG, Michie SA, Warnke RA, et al. The "syncytial variant" of nodular sclerosing Hodgkin's disease. *Am J Surg Pathol*. 1986;10:470-477.
99. Rudiger T, Jaffe ES, Delsol G, et al. Workshop report on Hodgkin's disease and related diseases ('grey zone' lymphoma). *Ann Oncol*. 1998;9(Suppl 5):S31-S38.
100. Shiota M, Fujimoto J, Takenaga M, et al. Diagnosis of t(2;5)(p23;q35)-associated Ki-1 lymphoma with immunohistochemistry. *Blood*. 1994;84:3648-3652.
101. Pulford K, Lamant L, Morris SW, et al. Detection of anaplastic lymphoma kinase (ALK) and nucleolar protein nucleophosmin (NPM)-ALK proteins in normal and neoplastic cells with the monoclonal antibody ALK1. *Blood*. 1997;89:1394-1404.
102. Suchi T, Lennert K, Tu LY, et al. Histopathology and immunohistochemistry of peripheral T cell lymphomas: a proposal for their classification. *J Clin Pathol*. 1987;40:995-1015.
103. Paulli M, Strater J, Gianelli U, et al. Mediastinal B-cell lymphoma: A study of its histomorphologic spectrum based on 109 cases. *Hum Pathol*. 1999;30:178-187.

104. Higgins JP, Warnke RA. CD30 expression is common in mediastinal large B-cell lymphoma. *Am J Clin Pathol.* 1999;112:241-247.
105. Chittal SM, Brousset P, Voigt JJ, et al. Large B-cell lymphoma rich in T-cells and simulating Hodgkin's disease. *Histopathology.* 1991;19:211-220.
106. Rudiger T, Ott G, Ott MM, et al. Differential diagnosis between classic Hodgkin's lymphoma, T-cell-rich B-cell lymphoma, and paragranuloma by paraffin immunohistochemistry. *Am J Surg Pathol.* 1998;22:1184-1191.
107. Chevrel G, Berger F, Miossec P, et al. Hodgkin's disease and B cell lymphoproliferation in rheumatoid arthritis patients treated with methotrexate: A kinetic study of lymph node changes. *Arthritis Rheum.* 1999;42:1773-1776.
108. Kamel OW, Weiss LM, van de Rijn M, et al. Hodgkin's disease and lymphoproliferations resembling Hodgkin's disease in patients receiving long-term low-dose methotrexate therapy. *Am J Surg Pathol.* 1996;20:1279-1287.
109. Pitman SD, Huang Q, Zuppan CW, et al. Hodgkin lymphoma-like posttransplant lymphoproliferative disorder (HL-like PTLD) simulates monomorphic B-cell PTLD both clinically and pathologically. *Am J Surg Pathol.* 2006;30:470-476.
110. Mao Z, Quintanilla-Martinez L, Raffeld M, et al. IgVH mutational status and clonality analysis of Richter's transformation: Diffuse large B-cell lymphoma and Hodgkin lymphoma in association with B-cell chronic lymphocytic leukemia (B-CLL) represent 2 different pathways of disease evolution. *Am J Surg Pathol.* 2007;31:1605-1614.
111. de Leval L, Vivario M, De Prijck B, et al. Distinct clonal origin in two cases of Hodgkin's lymphoma variant of Richter's syndrome associated With EBV infection. *Am J Surg Pathol.* 2004;28:679-686.
112. Fong D, Kaiser A, Spizzo G, et al. Hodgkin's disease variant of Richter's syndrome in chronic lymphocytic leukaemia patients previously treated with fludarabine. *Br J Haematol.* 2005;129:199-205.
113. Ohno T, Smir BN, Weisenburger DD, et al. Origin of the Hodgkin/Reed-Sternberg cells in chronic lymphocytic leukemia with "Hodgkin's transformation." *Blood.* 1998;91:1757-1761.
114. Schwarting R, Gerdes J, Durkop H, et al. BER-H2: A new anti-Ki-1 (CD30) monoclonal antibody directed at a formol-resistant epitope. *Blood.* 1989;74:1678-1689.
115. Polski JM, Janney CG. Ber-H2 (CD30) immunohistochemical staining in malignant melanoma. *Mod Pathol.* 1999;12:903-906.
116. Sheibani K, Battifora H, Burke JS, et al. Leu-M1 antigen in human neoplasms. An immunohistologic study of 400 cases. *Am J Surg Pathol.* 1986;10:227-236.
117. Strickler JG, Fedeli F, Horwitz CA, et al. Infectious mononucleosis in lymphoid tissue. Histopathology, in situ hybridization, and differential diagnosis. *Arch Pathol Lab Med.* 1993;117:269-278.
118. Reynolds DJ, Banks PM, Gulley ML. New characterization of infectious mononucleosis and a phenotypic comparison with Hodgkin's disease. *Am J Pathol.* 1995;146:379-388.
119. Fellbaum C, Hansmann ML, Lennert K. Lymphadenitis mimicking Hodgkin's disease. *Histopathology.* 1988;12:253-262.
120. Doggett RS, Colby TV, Dorfman RF. Interfollicular Hodgkin's disease. *Am J Surg Pathol.* 1983;7:145-149.
121. Chan JKC, Tsang WYW. Reactive lymphadenopathies. In: Weiss LM, ed. *Pathology of Lymph Nodes. Contemporary Issues in Surgical Pathology.* Philadelphia: Churchill Livingstone; 1996.
122. Kadin ME, Donaldson SS, Dorfman RF. Isolated granulomas in Hodgkin's disease. *N Engl J Med.* 1970;283:859-861.
123. Ohshima K, Kikuchi M, Shibata T, et al. Clonal analysis of Hodgkin's disease shows absence of TCR/Ig gene rearrangement, compared with T-cell-rich B-cell lymphoma and incipient adult T-cell leukemia/lymphoma. *Leuk Lymphoma.* 1994;15:469-479.
124. Chute DJ, Cousar JB, Mahadevan MS, et al. Detection of immunoglobulin heavy chain gene rearrangements in classic Hodgkin lymphoma using commercially available BIOMED-2 primers. *Diagn Mol Pathol.* 2008;17:65-72.
125. Davis TH, Morton CC, Miller-Cassman R, et al. Hodgkin's disease, lymphomatoid papulosis, and cutaneous T-cell lymphoma derived from a common T-cell clone. *N Engl J Med.* 1992;326:1115-1122.
126. Feuerhake F, Kutok JL, Monti S, et al. NFkappaB activity, function, and target-gene signatures in primary mediastinal large B-cell lymphoma and diffuse large B-cell lymphoma subtypes. *Blood.* 2005;106:1392-1399.
127. Savage KJ, Monti S, Kutok JL, et al. The molecular signature of mediastinal large B-cell lymphoma differs from that of other diffuse large B-cell lymphomas and shares features with classical Hodgkin lymphoma. *Blood.* 2003;102:3871-3879.
128. Garcia JF, Camacho FI, Morente M, et al. Hodgkin and Reed-Sternberg cells harbor alterations in the major tumor suppressor pathways and cell-cycle checkpoints: Analyses using tissue microarrays. *Blood.* 2003;101:681-689.
129. Schulz H, Rehwald U, Morschhauser F, et al. Rituximab in relapsed lymphocyte-predominant Hodgkin lymphoma: Long-term results of a phase 2 trial by the German Hodgkin Lymphoma Study Group (GHSG). *Blood.* 2008;111:109-111.
130. Younes A, Romaguera J, Hagemeister F, et al. A pilot study of rituximab in patients with recurrent, classic Hodgkin disease. *Cancer.* 2003;98:310-314.
131. Annunziata CM, Safiran YJ, Irving SG, et al. Hodgkin disease: Pharmacologic intervention of the CD40-NF kappa B pathway by a protease inhibitor. *Blood.* 2000;96:2841-2848.
132. Wahl AF, Klussman K, Thompson JD, et al. The anti-CD30 monoclonal antibody SGN-30 promotes growth arrest and DNA fragmentation in vitro and affects antitumor activity in models of Hodgkin's disease. *Cancer Res.* 2002;62:3736-3742.
133. Francisco JA, Cerveny CG, Meyer DL, et al. cAC10-vcMMAE, an anti-CD30-monomethyl auristatin E conjugate with potent and selective antitumor activity. *Blood.* 2003;102:1458-1465.
134. Falini B, Bolognesi A, Flenghi L, et al. Response of refractory Hodgkin's disease to monoclonal anti-CD30 immunotoxin. *Lancet.* 1992;339:1195-1196.
135. Borchmann P, Schnell R, Fuss I, et al. Phase 1 trial of the novel bispecific molecule H22xKi-4 in patients with refractory Hodgkin lymphoma. *Blood.* 2002;100:3101-3107.
136. Bollard CM, Aguilar L, Straathof KC, et al. Cytotoxic T lymphocyte therapy for Epstein-Barr virus+ Hodgkin's disease. *J Exp Med.* 2004;200:1623-1633.
137. Savoldo B, Rooney CM, Di Stasi A, et al. Epstein Barr virus specific cytotoxic T lymphocytes expressing the anti-CD30zeta artificial chimeric T-cell receptor for immunotherapy of Hodgkin disease. *Blood.* 2007;110:2620-2630.
138. Tepler I, Schwartz G, Parker K, et al. Phase I trial of an interleukin-2 fusion toxin (DAB486IL-2) in hematologic malignancies: Complete response in a patient with Hodgkin's disease refractory to chemotherapy. *Cancer.* 1994;73:1276-1285.
139. Merz H, Malisius R, Mannweiler S, et al. ImmunoMax. A maximized immunohistochemical method for the retrieval and enhancement of hidden antigens. *Lab Invest.* 1995;73:149-156.
140. Ishida T, Ishii T, Inagaki A, et al. The CCR4 as a novel-specific molecular target for immunotherapy in Hodgkin lymphoma. *Leukemia.* 2006;20:2162-2168.

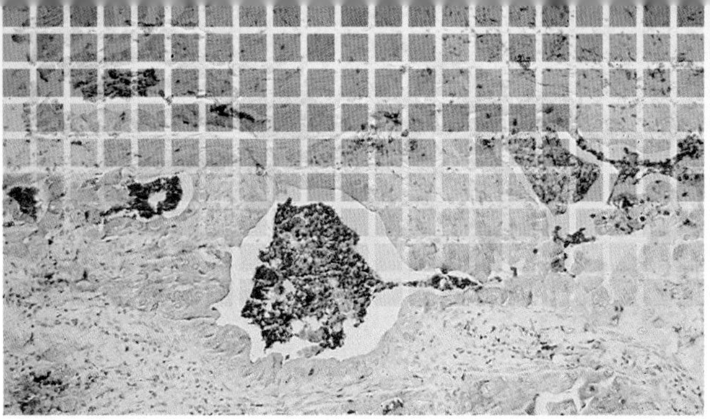

6

Immunohistology of Non-Hodgkin Lymphoma

Alvin W. Martin

- Introduction 156
- Biology of Antigens and Antibodies 157
- Non-Hodgkin Lymphoma and Reactive Conditions 168
- Non-Hodgkin Lymphoma and Other Malignancies 168
- Classification of Non-Hodgkin Lymphomas 169
- B-Cell Neoplasms 169
- T- and NK-Cell Neoplasms 178

INTRODUCTION

The development of immunohistochemistry as a diagnostic discipline has been intimately linked to the understanding of non-Hodgkin lymphomas. In part, this is attributable both to the lymphocyte's role as a producer of reagents for immunologic studies and to the ready availability of lymphocytes from humans and animals as targets of study. This interaction has been mutually reinforcing: understanding of lymphocyte development and lymphoma nosology has created a need for more diagnostic reagents, and the rapidly expanding pool of reagents has assisted with finer distinctions among non-Hodgkin lymphomas.

In the past decade, a number of changes have been made to the diagnostic schemas for non-Hodgkin lymphoma. The Kiel and Lukes-Collins classifications and a de facto classification, the Working Formulation, were replaced by the Revised European American Lymphoma (REAL) classification in 1994.[1] In this effort, an international group of expert hematopathologists compiled a list of recognizable disease entities in the area of lymphoid neoplasms. These diseases were defined on the basis of their morphologic, immunophenotypic, and genetic features, with occasional reference to clinical presentation. The contribution that each of these features makes to the diagnosis of a particular entity varies, so many lymphoid diseases can be recognized by morphology alone, whereas others require additional molecular or immunologic information. Although not without dissenters,[2-4] the REAL classification gained adherents as it demonstrated its clinical utility.[5,6]

In 2001 the World Health Organization (WHO) published a revision of the REAL Classification[7] in collaboration with the European Association for Hematopathology and the North American–based Society for Hematopathology. This WHO Classification of Tumors of Hematopoietic and Lymphoid Tissues is a listing of all recognized hematologic malignancies, with relatively minor modifications to the REAL lymphoma classification.[8,9] The most recent (2008) WHO classification of lymphomas is an attestation of the general acceptance of the WHO approach, which includes morphology, immunohistochemistry, flow cytometry, genetics, and clinical presentation in the classification scheme.

The use of antibody panels in immunohistochemistry is well accepted. This is particularly true in hematolymphoid diagnostics, where the combination of cytologic/histologic characteristics and a single antibody result may not be sufficient to distinguish benign from malignant or one form of lymphoma from another.[10,11] No single panel will suffice for all situations, but a number of proposed panels using a modest number of antibodies can often provide the needed information. As in other areas of pathology, lymphoma immunohistochemistry usually serves an adjunctive role to morphology. Hematopathologists also have at their disposal and need to judiciously employ a number of other aids to diagnosis such as molecular testing, flow cytometry, and cytogenetics. It must be emphasized that correlation of the patient's history with the laboratory data can be invaluable.

The terminology for lymphoma immunophenotyping differs slightly from that of many other tumor types. The cell surface antigens of leukocytes have been assigned cluster of differentiation (CD) designations, each of which may bind with any number of diagnostic antibodies.[12] To the average pathologist's chagrin, the CD nomenclature has not been organized by cell or tissue type; consequently, widely separated numbers may refer to similar cell types (e.g., B-cell restricted epitopes CD20 and CDw75). In addition to being designated by reference to their CD target, antibodies are also often given an arbitrary clone designation (e.g., 4C7) or one related to the place of origin (e.g., Ki-1 from Kiel, Germany).

Much of the early work in diagnostic hematopathology required frozen tissue or acetone-fixed frozen tissue because the available antibodies failed to recognize epitopes preserved by cross-linking fixatives. Because of the level of expertise involved in preparing and interpreting frozen section immunohistochemistry, few routine pathology laboratories offered such diagnostic services. However, there are now a large number of commercially available antibodies useful for tissue preserved with either formalin or mercuric fixatives. This chapter deals primarily with immunohistochemistry performed using antibodies effective on fixed, paraffin-embedded material. This technology is easily handled in most pathology laboratories and results in excellent cytologic evaluation not always obtainable with frozen sections. Partial digestion of proteins with enzymes provides better immunolabeling results for some antibodies.[13] A variety of antigen unmasking or retrieval procedures has also assisted in the move to fixed-tissue analysis.[14,15] Of course, snap frozen tissue may always be preserved and transferred to a reference laboratory for further study if necessary.

An understanding of the development, maturation, and migration of lymphocytes provides a rationale for lymphoma immunophenotyping because stages in lymphocyte maturation are defined, in part, by the macromolecules they produce. Reviews of the topic are provided in standard pathology texts,[16,17] and more detailed treatments are available.[18-21] Malignancies of lymphocytes certainly express antigen complements that bear a resemblance to different developmental stages. In fact, both the Lukes and Collins and Kiel classifications of lymphoma explicitly rely on the stages of normal lymphocyte differentiation as organizing principles.[22-24] Lymphomas are commonly thought of as being composed of cells arrested in development at certain stages.[25] This is a useful concept, although the many exceptions suggest that it is not a perfect representation of reality.

BIOLOGY OF ANTIGENS AND ANTIBODIES

B Cells

CD19

CD19 is a type-I transmembrane glycoprotein of 95 kDa that belongs to the immunoglobulin superfamily and is widely expressed on B cells throughout most stages of B-cell differentiation, though its expression is downregulated during their terminal differentiation to plasma cells. On B cells, CD19 associates with CD21, CD81, and CD225, forming a signal transduction complex. Expression of CD19 is found in the majority of B cell–derived malignancies, as well as on follicular dendritic cells. Antibodies have been developed to detect this antigen in formalin-fixed, paraffin-embedded material. The antibody is quite robust and has excellent correlation with flow cytometric determination of this antigen on both mature and immature B cell processes and performs well in decalcified bone marrow biopsy samples. CD19 is a potential target for monoclonal antibody therapy, and preliminary data have demonstrated its effectiveness in B-cell depletion, making this an attractive therapy for autoimmune disorders and treatment of malignant B-cell lymphomas.

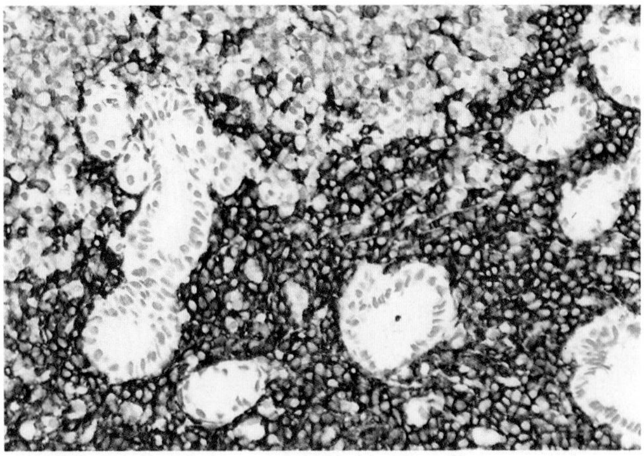

FIGURE 6.1 CD20 immunolabeling of marginal zone B-cell lymphoma of mucosa-associated lymphoid tissue type. Cytoplasmic staining of B cells infiltrating among gastric glands. Note the weaker or absent staining in the plasmacytic component toward the luminal surface *(top)*.

CD20

The CD20 epitope is acquired late in the pre–B-cell stage of maturation and remains on cells throughout most of their differentiation, although it is lost at the plasma cell stage. As recognized by the antibody L26, CD20 is strongly positive on approximately half of lymphoblastic lymphoma/leukemia, almost all mature B cell lymphomas (plasma cell lesions excepted), Reed-Sternberg cells in roughly one quarter of the cases of classical Hodgkin lymphoma, and almost no T-cell lymphomas (Fig. 6.1).

CD20 is the target for Rituxan, the anti-CD20 molecular targeted therapy for CD20 positive lymphomas. This is a common theranostic use for lymphoma patients, as well as for patients with rheumatoid arthritis.

A subset of precursor B leukemia/lymphomas may also express this antigen. The level of expression of CD20 ranges from very dim (in small cell lymphocytic lymphoma/chronic lymphocytic leukemia) to very bright in many of the other mature B-cell lymphomas. Though this characteristic dimness is helpful for classification purposes, it may produce problems in demonstrating this antigen successfully in formalin fixed paraffin embedded tissues. It is recommended that several cases of small cell lymphocytic lymphoma be included in the validation sequence for this antigen to ensure the methodology being evaluated is sensitive enough for

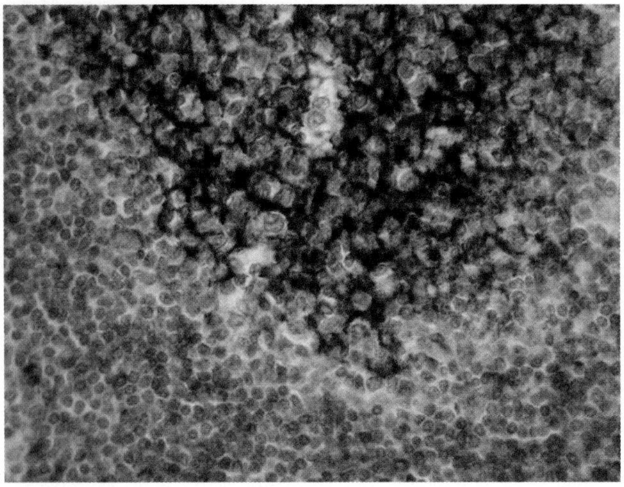

FIGURE 6.2 Immunohistochemical staining of a normal germinal center demonstrating CD23 expression on the dendritic reticulum cells (high-level expressor) and on the mantle zone B cells (low-level expressor).

adequate low-level detection. This antigen is sensitive to decalcification, and some difficulty may be noted in demonstrating this antigen in bone marrow biopsy samples. The addition of other pan B-cell markers such as PAX-5, CD19, or CD79 may be necessary. It should be noted that in patients treated with rituximab chemotherapy, CD20 expression may be lost and confirmation of B-cell lineage may necessitate the use of other B-cell markers such as PAX5, CD19, or CD79, the expression of which is not affected by this therapy.

CD21

The CD21 antibody cluster recognizes the receptor for complement component C3d, which mediates the phagocytosis of complement-coated particles. It is found on follicular dendritic cells and some B lymphocytes. It may be useful in outlining the follicular dendritic cell network in follicular lymphoma and helps identify the hyperplastic islands of dendritic cells in angioimmunoblastic T cell lymphoma.

CD21 is a useful marker to identify neoplasms of follicular dendritic cells. The antigen density on dendritic reticulum cells is fairly high; however, the same antigen is expressed at low levels on mantle zone B cells, which makes an excellent low-level control.

CD22

CD22 is a transmembrane molecule that inhibits signaling by the B-cell receptor, serving as a molecular switch that changes the fate of stimulated B cells from proliferation to apoptosis.[26] Its expression roughly parallels that of CD19. It is strongly expressed in hairy cell leukemia.

CD23

CD23 is the low-affinity receptor for IgE and is expressed on platelets, eosinophils, activated macrophages, follicular dendritic cells, and mature B cells. Though this antigen may be expressed on many B-cell lymphomas, its diagnostic utility is most helpful in separating small cell lymphocytic lymphoma from mantle cell lymphoma. Small cell lymphocytic lymphoma is characteristically positive for this antigen but is virtually absent from mantle cell lymphoma. It should be noted that rare cases of CD23 positive mantle cell lymphoma have been described. CD23 decorates dendritic reticulum cells intensely and mantle-zone B cells less intensely (Fig. 6.2). This antigen is being evaluated for targeted therapy.

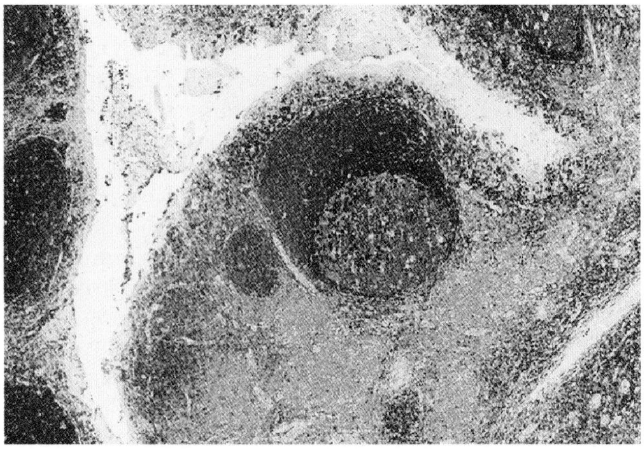

FIGURE 6.3 CD79a in a normal lymph node. The mantle lymphocytes, most germinal center cells, and scattered interfollicular B lymphocytes mark for this early B-cell antigen.

CD25

CD25 functions as a low-affinity interleukin-2 receptor and may be found on a number of cell types including activated T cells. This antigen is characteristically expressed on hairy cell leukemia, mast cell lesions, and certain T-cell malignancies but may be seen at low levels in certain B-cell lymphomas, particularly small cell lymphocytic lymphoma/chronic lymphocytic leukemia. Targeted therapy is available for this antigen (Ontak).

CD79

CD79 consist of two proteins, namely CD79a and CD79b. CD79a recognizes the Ig-alpha protein, and CD79b recognizes the Ig-beta protein of the B-cell antigen component of the B-lymphocyte antigen receptor.[27] The expression of CD79 precedes immunoglobulin (Ig) gene heavy-chain gene rearrangement and CD20 expression during B-cell ontogeny, making the detection of this antibody useful for determining B-cell lineage. CD79 is found in B-cell lymphomas, B-cell lines, the majority of acute leukemias of precursor B-cell type, and in some myelomas (Fig. 6.3). CD79 is an excellent marker for B-cell lineage, but it has been described as positive in a certain percentage of non–B-cell lesions. CD79a positivity has been reported in acute myeloid leukemias, megakaryocytes, and megakaryocytic lesions with an incidence of 0% to 90%. This positivity appears to be clone dependent. Clones 11E3 and JCB117 have the lowest incidence

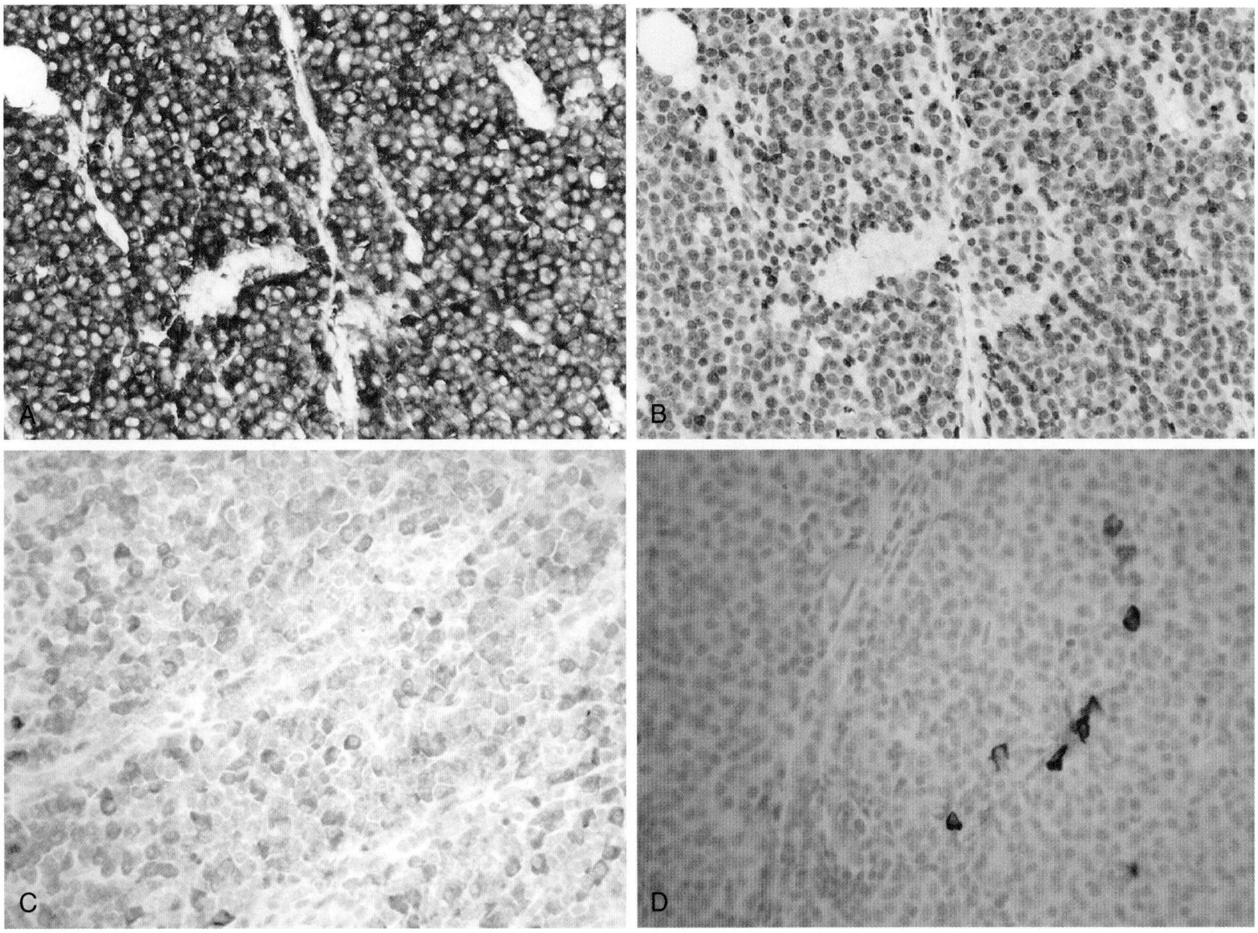

FIGURE 6.4 Lambda **(A)** and kappa **(B)** immunoglobulin light chain antibodies demonstrate the clear monotypia of the plasma cells in this multiple myeloma. Kappa light chain mRNA *in situ* hybrization **(C)** and lambda light chain mRNA **(D)**.

of non–B-cell positivity (virtually zero) with clones HM47/A9 and HM47/A9 having a positive rate in normal megakaryocytes and acute myeloid leukemias, which range from 67% to 86%. There has been an association with CD79b expression in chronic lymphocytic leukemia with the presence of trisomy 12 or atypical morphology, or both.

CD138

CD138 is a transmembrane (type I) heparan sulfate proteoglycan and a member of the syndecan proteoglycan family. It functions as an extracellular matrix receptor that assists in epithelial organization. This antigen is expressed on plasma cells and most benign and malignant epithelial lesions. Virtually no other hematopoietic lesions express CD138. It is highly recommended that a pan keratin antibody (such as AE1/3) be considered as part of the diagnostic panel grid using CD138.

DBA.44

DBA.44 is a B subset antibody that strongly stains the cytoplasm of most hairy cell leukemias (HCL). However, it is not specific for HCL because it is also found in some marginal zone lymphomas and large cell lymphomas.

IMMUNOGLOBULIN LIGHT CHAINS

Antibodies against the kappa and lambda immunoglobulin light chains are among the oldest immunologic diagnostic reagents in use. They are also among the most overused. (Fig. 6.4A and B).

Mature B cells produce and export immunoglobulin to the cell surface to serve as an antigen receptor. The immunoglobulin molecule, a heterodimer comprising one light chain and one heavy chain molecule, is unique in each cell. The gene rearrangement process that generates the immunoglobulin molecule results in either a productive kappa gene or a productive lambda gene. The mechanics of the rearrangement process normally produce approximately twice as many kappa-bearing cells as lambda.[28] This ratio is maintained in populations of normal or reactive B cells but is altered in malignant populations. Ranges of normal light chain ratios have been defined by flow cytometry,[29,30] but quantitative analysis is difficult to apply to histologic sections. The goal is identification of light chain restriction, or monotypia, in which one of the light chains is present on an abnormally large proportion of cells. Monotypia, although not synonymous with monoclonality, is generally assumed to be evidence of a malignant proliferation. In practice, whenever a B-cell or plasma cell population exceeds the normal 2:1 ratio by fourfold (i.e., >roughly 85% kappa-positive cells or roughly 65% lambda-positive cells), monotypia may be diagnosed safely. This is, admittedly, a subjective judgment.

Although most mature B cells and B-cell malignancies express one or the other of the light chains, paraffin section immunohistochemistry is frequently not sensitive enough to detect surface light chains on lymphocytes. Plasma cells, however, are more easily analyzed owing to the intracellular nature of the immunoglobulin and to its relative abundance. Light chain immunohistochemistry is also complicated by an elevated background owing to nonspecific uptake of immunoglobulin by a variety of cells or staining of extracellular serum or stromal immunoglobulin molecules. Immunoglobulin light chain antibodies must always be interpreted as a pair, with the absence or paucity of one antibody nearly as important as the excess of the other. Two situations are common: both antibodies staining most cells or neither antibody staining any cells. No interpretation should be rendered under either of these circumstances.

Immunoglobulin light chain immunohistochemistry challenges the pathologist with a system that is often low in signal and high in noise. Care should be directed as much to the decision to order light chain antibodies as to their interpretation. *In situ* hybridization for immunoglobulin light chain mRNA has been proposed as an alternative because of the absence of extracellular background.[31-34]

LIGHT CHAIN MESSENGER RIBONUCLEIC ACID

The detection of kappa or lambda messenger RNA via an *in situ* hybridization reaction provides an alternative to the immunohistochemical detection of cytoplasmic kappa or lambda light chain (Fig. 6.4C and D). This technique allows for a much cleaner reaction product because it is only demonstrated where there is mRNA for kappa and lambda and not protein. Several immunohistochemical standards now provide an automated platform for the performance of this *in situ* hybridization reaction. This allows for this technique to enter routine performance and can be accomplished in approximately 5 hours.

B-CELL TRANSCRIPTION FACTORS

Transcription factors are involved in the differentiation programs and in the activation processes of T lymphocytes and B lymphocytes in normal and neoplastic conditions. The availability of antibodies able to efficiently recognize these TFs in formalin-fixed paraffin embedded tissues represents a powerful tool in diagnostic hematopathology.

Most of the TFs are localized in the nucleus and are seen in all or most of the cells with the same differentiation program or functional status. The following are key diagnostic TFs for B-cell immunohistology. A summary of B-cell TFs is in Table 6.1.

TABLE 6.1 B-Cell Transcription Factors: Common Expression Patterns

	MUM1	PAX5	OCT-2/BOB.1
B-CLL	+(GC CELLS)	+	+
LPL	+	S	+
MZL	S	+	+
MCL	S	+	+
FCL	N(WEAK)	+	+
DLBCL	N	+	+
GC-like	+	+	+
PBML	S	+	+
PCNSL	N	+	+
GC-like	+	+	+
PCLBCL	N	+	+
GC-like	+	+	+
PTLD	S	+	+
DLBCL/ BL/BLL P-PTLD/IL	+	S	+
AIDS-L	+	S	+
IL	N	+	+
DLBCL	N	+	+
BL	+	+	+
PEL	+	S	+
LBL-B	N	+	N
MM	+	N	+
P-TCL	S	N	N
LBL-T	N	N	N
ALCL	+	N	N
PHL	N	+	+
CHL	+	+(WEAK)	+

AIDS-L, AIDS lymphoma; ALCL, anaplastic large cell lymphoma; BL, Burkitt lymphoma; BLL, Burkitt-like lymphoma; cHL, classical Hodgkin lymphoma; IL, immunoblastic lymphoma; LBL-B, lymphoblastic lymphoma precursor B-cell; LBL-T, lymphoblastic lymphoma precursor T-cell; LPL, lymphoplasmacytic lymphoma; MM, multiple myeloma; N, almost always negative; PCLBL, primary cutaneous large B-cell lymphoma; PEL, primary effusion lymphoma; pHL, lymphocyte predominance Hodgkin lymphoma; P-PTLD, polymorphic posttransplant lymphoproliferative disorders; P-TCL, peripheral T-cell lymphoma; PTLD, posttransplant lymphoproliferative disorders. S, sometimes positive; +, almost always strong and diffuse positive.

MUM1/IRF4

The multiple myeloma oncogene 1 (MUM1)/interferon regulatory factor 4 (IRF4) gene has been identified as a myeloma-associated oncogene, which is activated at the transcriptional level as a result of t(6;14)(p25;q32) chromosomal translocation. Mum1 protein is expressed in lymphoplasmacytic lymphoma, B-CLL, FCLs (grade III), MZLs, DLBCLs, primary effusion lymphomas, cHL, MM, ALCLs, and peripheral T-cell lymphoma (PTCL), generally with moderate to intense signal in more than

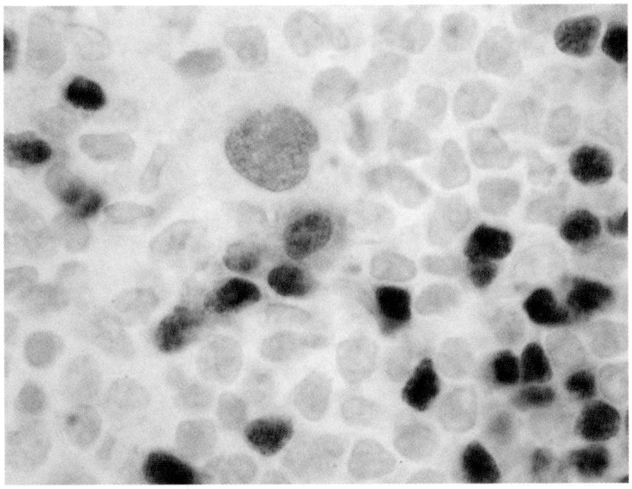

FIGURE 6.5 PAX5 shows weak nuclear expression in classic RS cells and more intense expression in normal B cells.

20% to 30% of the neoplastic cells. In low-grade FCLs (grade I to II) and in MCLs, the expression is weak and often restricted to a minority of cells.[35-37] MUM1 is a member of the interferon regulatory factor family of transcription factors. It is normally expressed in plasma cells, late B cells, and activated T cells and has been described in several B-cell malignancies. MUM1 is not helpful in separating different types of CD30-positive lymphoproliferative disorders.[38-41]

MUM1 is expressed in systemic ALCL and classical Hodgkin lymphoma.[41-43] L&H cells in LPHL are MUM1 negative, as well as CD138 and bcl-6 positive; in contrast, Reed-Sternberg cells in cHL are MUM1+, bcl-6, and partially CD138+.[44-48] MUM1 expression dichotomizes follicular lymphoma (FL) into low-grade FL of CD10+/Bcl-6+/MUM1-/Ki-67 low phenotype and high-grade FL of CD10+/–/Bcl-6+/weak/MUM1+/Ki-67 high phenotype.

PAX5

The PAX5 gene is a member of the paired box (PAX) family of TFs. The PAX5 gene encodes the B-cell lineage-specific activator protein (BSAP), a 52-kD molecule; in hematopoietic cells, PAX5 is detectable only in B lineage and at early, but not in late, stages of B-cell differentiation. In B-cell lineage PAX5 gene transcription is initiated in pro-B cells and is abundant at the pre–B-cell and mature B-cell differentiation stages, being absent in terminally differentiated plasma cells.[49-55] PAX5 expression has two distinctive characteristics: almost complete restriction for B-cell lineage and wide expression during B-cell differentiation. PAX5 has been reported to be an excellent pan B- and pan pre-B-cell marker because polyclonal and monoclonal antibodies against PAX5 protein are available for use in routinely processed histologic material. In normal lymphoid tissues, PAX5 is expressed in the nucleus of B lymphocytes and it is absent from plasma cells. In non-neoplastic/reactive lymphoid tissue, PAX5/BSAP nuclear reactivity is intense in mantle zones and weak to moderate in germinal center (GC) B cells.[56-58]

In Hodgkin lymphoma, PAX5 expression is prominent in both L&H cells and classic RS cells, but not as intensely staining as surrounding B cells (Fig. 6.5). Anaplastic large cell lymphomas are negative for PAX5. This antigen may also be detected in acute myeloid leukemias with the t(8:21), Merkel cell carcinoma, and small cell neuroendocrine carcinomas. The presence of PAX5 antigen in Hodgkin lymphoma cells can be of great value in separating this entity from anaplastic large cell lymphoma (a T-cell lymphoma). The density of PAX5 in Hodgkin lymphoma cells is very low, and careful attention must be paid to fixation and validation with cases of known Hodgkin lymphoma (may be used as a low-level control) to ensure adequate and reliable detection.

Oct-2 and BOB.1

Oct-2 is a transcription factor mainly restricted to B lymphocytes and is associated with the essential B cell transcriptional coactivator, BOB.1. Oct-2 encodes immunoglobulin genes including the CD20 and CD36 molecules.[59,60] It is believed that both Oct-2, as well as BOB.1, play an important role in controlling the expansion and/or the maintenance of mature B cells. Oct-2 expression is low in immature B-cell and T-cell lines, as well as myelomonocytic and epithelial cells, in contrast with the high levels of expression seen in mature B-cell lines.[61,62] Oct-2 expression is high in germinal center B cells, with a lesser degree of intensity in mantle zones.[56,63,64] A strong signal overlapping with germinal center B cells is observed in some monocytoid cells and in the splenic marginal zone. Nodal marginal zone displays a less intense signal.

In B-cell lymphomas, Oct-1 usually displays a weaker signal and highlights a fewer number of cells when it is compared with Oct-2 immunoreactivity. The highest expression levels for Oct-2, Oct-1, and BOB.1/OBF.1 are reported from independent studies in FCLs, DLBCLs, and Burkitt lymphomas,[56,65] whereas B-CLL, MALT-type, and MCLs score negative or display an heterogeneous/weaker reactivity.[64]

In T-cell lymphomas, Oct-1 is the most frequently represented molecule, followed by BOB.1/OBF.1. Oct-2 is relatively more prevalent within the angioimmunoblastic lymphoma group.[56] In classic Hodgkin lymphoma, data support the hypothesis that the absence of immunoglobulin expression in Reed-Sternberg cells may be due to a defect in the transcription machinery of immunoglobulin genes. It has been shown that Oct-2 and BOB.1/OBF.1 expression is down-regulated in Reed-Sternberg cells of cHL, with some exceptions,[64,66] and it has been proposed that this immunophenotypic profile, in the presence of PAX5 positivity, may be predictive of classical Hodgkin lymphoma.

T Cells

CD2

CD2, the E rosette receptor, is an extremely broad T-cell marker. Antibodies to it immunolabel the vast majority of T and natural killer cell malignancies but may require signal amplification by the Immunomax method for paraffin section use.[67] Some thymic B cells are also CD2 positive.

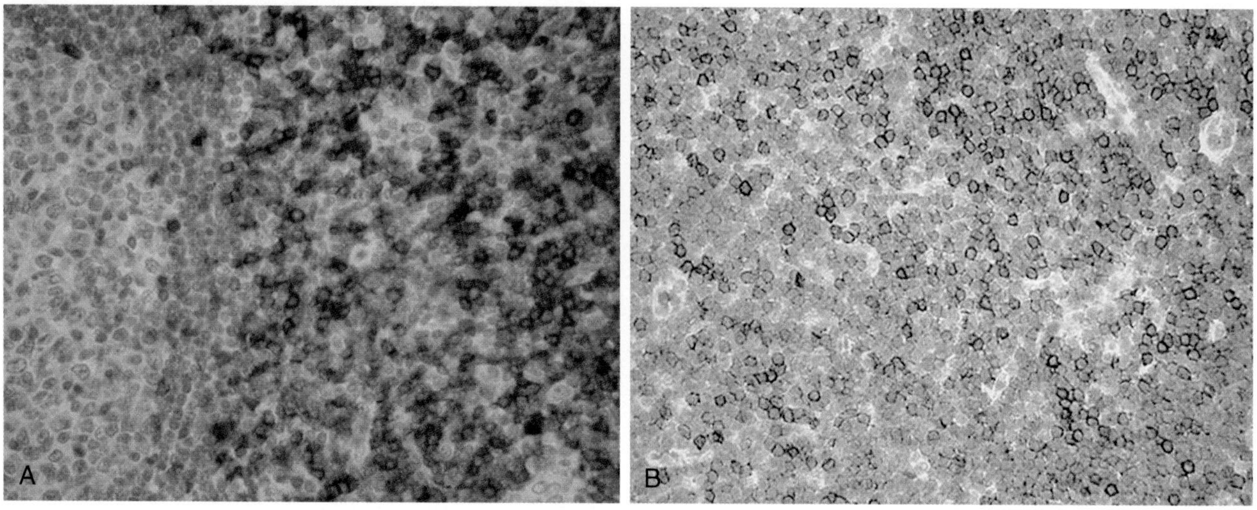

FIGURE 6.6 **A,** CD5 in normal germinal center. **B,** CD5 in small lymphocytic cell lymphoma.

CD3

The T-cell antigen receptor binds to the CD3 protein complex at the cell membrane. A commercially available anti-CD3 antibody is polyclonal and reacts with most T-cell lymphomas in fixed tissue, the exceptions being some anaplastic large cell lymphomas and natural killer leukemia/lymphomas. CD3 is specific for T-cell derivation.

CD4

The CD4 molecule interacts with HLA Class II during antigen recognition, and defines a helper/inducer subset of T cells. It is also found on a variety of monocyte-derived cells including Langerhans' and other dendritic cells. The CD4 epitope is absent from immature thymocytes and is expressed during T-cell development. Precursor T lymphoblastic lymphomas are therefore variable in their expression of CD4, but most mature T cell lymphomas are positive, with the exception of aggressive NK cell leukemia, extranodal NK cell lymphoma, γδ T-cell lymphoma, subcutaneous panniculitis-like T cell lymphoma, and enteropathy-type T-cell lymphoma. The antibody available for use on paraffin sections is not as sensitive as those for flow cytometry or frozen tissue.[68] Detection of TH1 and TH2 subsets has been reported with antibodies to CD134/CD69[69] and CD30/CD184,[70] respectively.

CD5

CD5 is a signal transduction molecule present on the surface of most thymocytes and immature peripheral T cells. It is also detectable on a small subset of circulating B cells, and its primary use in diagnostic immunohistochemistry is in the detection of malignancies derived from those cells: B-cell CLL/SLL and mantle cell lymphoma (Fig. 6.6A and B). Antigen retrieval is necessary.

CD7

CD7 has the distinction of being the most frequently lost T subset marker, particularly on mycosis fungoides.[71] It is also present on non–T-cell malignancies including NK tumors and acute myeloid leukemia. It is detectable on paraffin sections only with difficulty.

CD8

The CD8 antigen defines the suppressor/cytotoxic T-cell subset. It is expressed in concert with CD4 in thymocytes, but this state persists in only a small population of circulating cells. CD4/CD8 ratios are not analogous to immunoglobulin light chain ratios in B-cell malignancies; infectious and inflammatory conditions can markedly skew the normal 2:1 ratio. The beta chain of CD8 detected in fixed tissue has nearly the sensitivity of flow cytometry.

T-CELL TRANSCRIPTION FACTORS

T-BET

Naive T-helper (TH) cells differentiate into two subsets, TH1, committed to delayed hypersensitivity and to protection against viruses and intracellular pathogens, and TH2, directed to sustain B-cell antibody production and immune response against extracellular pathogens. TH1 and TH2 have distinct functions and specific cytokine profiles. "T-box expressed in T cells," or T-bet (also named Tbx21), is a TH1-specific T-box TF that controls the expression of the hallmark TH1 cytokine, interferon-gamma.[72] T-bet is also expressed in B lymphocytes, where it is involved in Ig class switch recombination. It represents a unique regulator of B-cell differentiation by participating in a T-independent-only activation pathway.[73]

T-bet expression has been studied in most subtypes of T-cell lymphomas. In particular, Dorfman and colleagues[74] demonstrated T-bet expression in 86% of

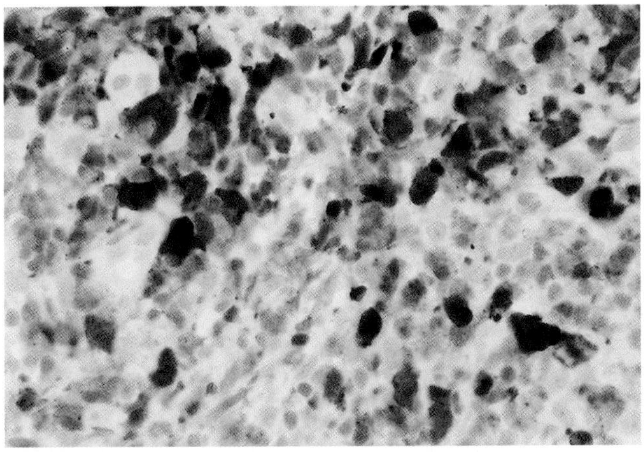

FIGURE 6.7 ALK antibody highlighting both cytoplasm and nuclei of malignant cells in lymphohistiocytic variant of anaplastic large cell lymphoma, T-cell, primary systemic type. Intervening small lymphs and histiocytes are negative.

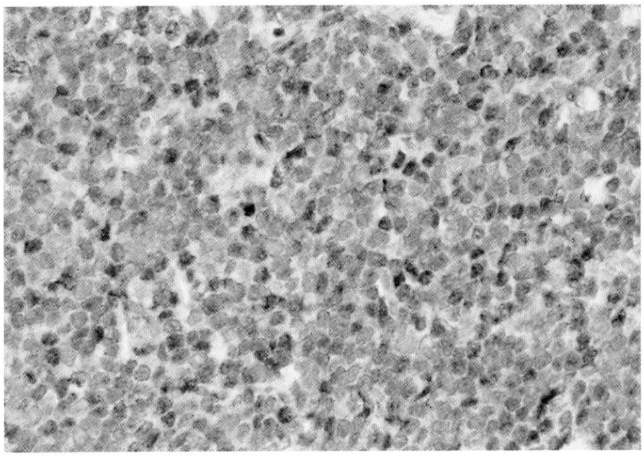

FIGURE 6.8 Cyclin D1 in a mantle cell lymphoma. Note nuclear positivity.

14 angioimmuno-blastic lymphoma, 5 out of 5 lymphoepithelioid lymphoma, 51% of 41 PTCL unspecified, and 25% of 36 ALCLs. T-bet was absent in all precursor T-ALLs. In enteropathy-associated T-cell lymphoma, T-bet was expressed only in those cases without anaplastic morphology.[75] Within B-cell lymphomas, T-bet expression has been detected in specific subgroups. Precursor B-ALL is consistently T-bet positive; most B-CLL, MZLs, and hairy cell leukemias were reported to be immunoreactive for T-bet in the paper of Dorfman and colleagues,[76] although with a variable proportion of stained cells and intensity.

Other Antibodies with Utility in Non-Hodgkin Lymphoma Diagnosis

ALK

ALK is the protein product of the anaplastic lymphoma kinase gene, first identified as a partner in the t(2;5) characteristic of anaplastic large cell lymphoma (ALCL). The protein is not normally detectable outside of the central nervous system. In ALCL, its expression is upregulated by fusion to the NPM gene, resulting in one of the few tumor-specific markers in hematopathology. Expression in lymphomas is limited to ALCL and rare diffuse large B-cell lymphomas.[77] Antibodies useful in fixed tissue localize both to the cytoplasm and to the nucleus of tumor cells.[78] Nearly all ALK positive tumors are also CD30 and EMA positive and CD115 negative (Fig. 6-7).

BCL-1 (CYCLIN D1)

PRAD1/Bcl-1 is a proto-oncogene first discovered in the PTH gene in a subset of parathyroid adenomas. It belongs to the cyclin family of proteins and resides on chromosome 11q13. The overexpression of its protein has been demonstrated in several epithelial tumors. Expression is more limited in lymphomas, particularly mantle cell lymphoma (Fig. 6.8), hairy cell leukemia, and a subset of multiple myeloma. Mantle cell lymphoma is characterized by a t (11;14)(q13;q32) translocation. This juxtaposes the bcl-1 locus to the immunoglobulin (Ig) gene sequences and leads to deregulation of cyclin D1. A similar translocation is present in a subset of multiple myeloma but is not present in hairy cell leukemia. The mechanism of overexpression of cyclin-D 1 in hairy cell leukemia is unknown. Detection of the expression of Bcl-1 is less helpful in establishing a diagnosis of mantle cell lymphoma. Several clones are available for the detection of this antigen in formalin fixed paraffin embedded material; however, rabbit monoclonal antibodies are the most robust. The level of cyclin-D 1 in mantle cell lymphomas, multiple myeloma, and hairy cell leukemia is much less than in epithelial tumors and even normal tissue and one must use cases of mantle cell lymphoma to successfully establish validation of your selected immunohistochemical platform.

BCL-2

BCL-2 was the first of the translocation-associated proteins to be identified in lymphoma. Approximately three quarters of follicular lymphomas (FLs) bear a t(14;18) translocation, which juxtaposes the BCL-2 gene to the immunoglobulin heavy chain gene, resulting in BCL-2 overexpression (Fig. 6.9). The protein is part of a heterodimeric complex that is regulated by binding with one of several partners and carries out a poorly understood "anti-apoptotic" function. BCL-2 is normally present in the cytoplasm of follicular mantle B lymphocytes, occasional germinal center cells, and many T lymphocytes. It is abundant in most lymphomas of small lymphocytes including approximately 80% of FLs. Its presence in other lymphomas is attributable to upregulation unrelated to t(14;18).

The normal expression or absence of BCL-2 staining can provide useful strategies in helping to separate benign from neoplastic lymphoproliferative lesions and can be quite useful in separating reactive germinal centers from follicular lymphomas. The B cells of normal germinal centers are negative for BCL-2, but the vast majority of follicular lymphomas are positive. Problems in interpretation may arise if many T cells are present

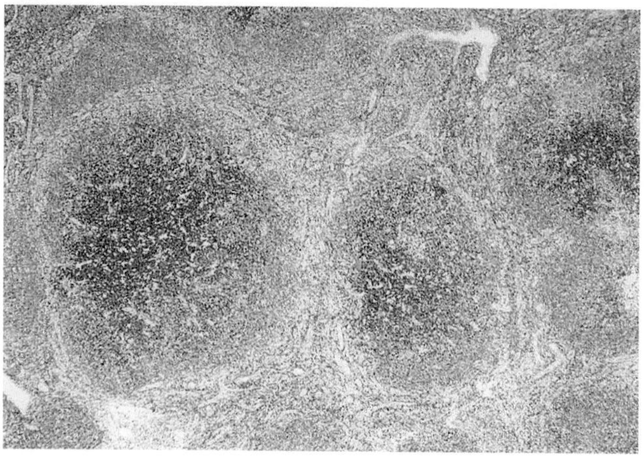

FIGURE 6.9 Bcl-2 In a follicular lymphoma. The malignant follicles stain with an antibody to bcl-2, whereas most surrounding lymphocytes are negative. The pattern is reversed in lymph nodes exhibiting follicular hyperplasia.

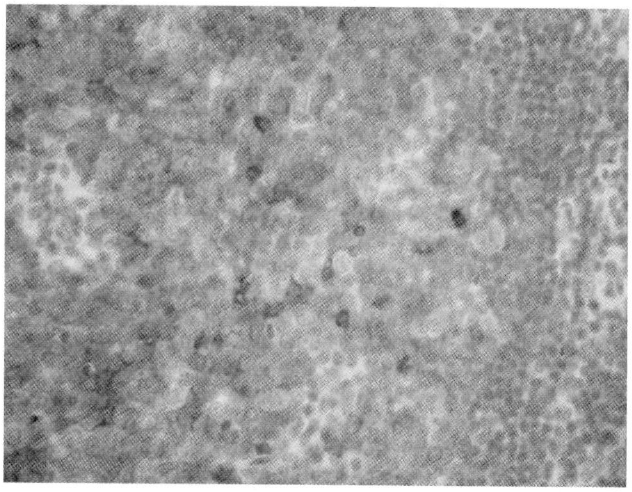

FIGURE 6.10 CD10 in normal germinal center.

in the reactive germinal centers, which may make interpretation difficult because the T cells will be positive. It should also be noted that the centroblasts in follicular lymphomas may be negative for BCL-2 and the grade 3 follicular lymphomas may be completely negative. However, careful attention to morphology usually allows the correct diagnosis to be made. BCL-2 is positive in many other lymphoproliferative lesions and so its utility for diagnostic purposes is limited.

BCL-6

BCL-6 protein is expressed normally in germinal center lymphocytes[79] and serves as a transcriptional regulatory protein. In the normal node it is distributed in a pattern reciprocal to that of BCL-2. Localized in the nucleus of tumor cells, it is expressed in a variety of B-cell neoplasms and is lost with follicular lymphoma progression. It is also detected in the L&H variants of nodular lymphocyte predominant Hodgkin disease. The bcl-6 protein is involved in control of germinal center formation and T-cell–dependent antigen response. In lymphoid tissues the bcl-6 protein is expressed in germinal center B cells in secondary follicles in both the dark (centroblast-rich) and light (centrocyte-rich) zones. Positivity for BCL6 gives evidence that the cell in question is germinal center in origin. It is also detectable in a few CD4+ T cells in the mantle, paracortical zones, and within germinal centers; and in large perifollicular CD30 positive lymphoid cells. Strong nuclear expression of bcl-6 occurs frequently in follicular lymphomas, paralleling the bcl-6 presence in germinal center cells, their normal counterpart. Expression of bcl-6 is also found in most Burkitt lymphomas and diffuse large B-cell lymphomas (DLBCLs).

CD1A

CD1a is a transmembrane antigen normally found on cortical thymocytes and Langerhans' cells. It is associated with beta 2 macroglobulin and may have a role in thymocyte development. It is found on a subset of precursor T lymphoblastic lymphoma/leukemia.

CD10 (CALLA)

Also known as the *common ALL antigen,* CD10 is a zinc metallopeptidase expressed in early lymphoid progenitors and normal germinal center cells. It is almost always present on the surface of precursor B lymphoblastic and Burkitt lymphomas, and much less frequently precursor T lymphoblastic leukemia/lymphoma. Many FLs and some diffuse large B-cell lymphomas, along with multiple myeloma, are positive. CD10 and BCL-6 are commonly considered markers of germinal center origin (Fig. 6.10).

The density of this antigen ranges from relatively abundant and bright in precursor B lymphoma/leukemias but is quite low or dim in immature lymphomas of follicle center cell origin. This antigen is reported to be detected in AILD-like T-cell lymphomas, though the rate of detection is quite variable between studies. A variety of nonhematopoietic tumors (in particular renal cell carcinomas and endometrial stromal sarcomas) express this antigen as well. The antigen density in nonhematopoietic tumors is relatively high and, if using CD10 expression to give support for a lymphoma a follicle center cell origin, care must be taken to ensure proper validation. Two separate titers and/or retrieval systems may be necessary to successfully demonstrate this antigen in hematopoietic and nonhematopoietic tumors. Germinal centers make an excellent low-level control for this antigen.

CD11C

CD11c is a type I transmembrane protein that is expressed on monocytes, granulocytes, a subset of B cells, dendritic cells, and macrophages and may be demonstrated on B-cell chronic lymphocytic leukemia, marginal zone lymphomas, and hairy cell leukemia. The amount of this antigen is varied with the antigen having dim to partial expression on chronic lymphocytic leukemia and a bright expression on hairy cell leukemia. CD11c is abundantly expressed in monocytes and macrophages. Paraffin reactive antibodies have been developed for this antigen and can certainly be used to give evidence for a histiocytic origin for lesion but make an excellent marker for hairy cell leukemia in paraffin-embedded tissue. Differences between paraffin reactivity and demonstration of this antigen by flow cytometry are noted in that marginal zone lymphomas may express CD11c by flow cytometry, but initial reports are not detected in formalin-fixed, paraffin-embedded material on the same lymphomas.

CD14

CD14 is expressed predominantly by monocytes (and to a much lesser extent on neutrophils) and makes an excellent marker for monocytes and macrophages. Paraffin-reactive antibodies have been developed for this antigen. It may be successfully demonstrated not only in formalin fixed material but also in decalcified bone marrow biopsies as well.

CD15

CD15, the X hapten or Lewis X antigen, can be identified with the LeuM1 antibody. Originally noted as a monocyte/myeloid cell marker, it was recognized as a marker for the Reed-Sternberg cells of classical Hodgkin lymphoma. It is negative in most non-Hodgkin lymphomas, with the exception of some primary cutaneous anaplastic large cell lymphomas and other peripheral T-cell lymphomas. The pattern of staining is typically membranous with a paranuclear, dotlike, Golgi localization. The surgical pathologist will note that this antibody is also used to stain adenocarcinomas.

CD25

The interleukin-2 receptor is designated CD25. Originally isolated from T lymphocytes, it is now known to be expressed on hairy cell leukemia and adult T-cell leukemia/lymphoma.

CD30

The CD30 antigen is part of the tumor necrosis factor-receptor superfamily and has pleiotropic effects on cells carrying it. An increase in soluble CD30 in a variety of diseases has been noted. In the surgical pathology laboratory, CD30 may be recognized in frozen tissue with the Ki-1 antibody or in paraffin sections with BerH2. The accepted staining pattern is membranous or paranuclear dotlike; cytoplasmic staining should be viewed skeptically (Fig. 6.11). Scattered large and small "activated" lymphs are positive in normal nodes and tonsils, particularly at the edge of germinal centers. Almost by definition, CD30 is present in ALCL and lymphomatoid papulosis and is seen in 95% of classical Hodgkin lymphoma cases in some (like CD15, not necessarily all) Reed-Sternberg cells. CD30 also marks sporadic nonanaplastic lymphoma cells. It has been noted in germ cell tumors (embryonal carcinomas) and some melanomas, and so is neither tumor specific nor lymphoma specific. CD30 has been proposed as either a marker of or a regulator of the TH2 T-cell subset.

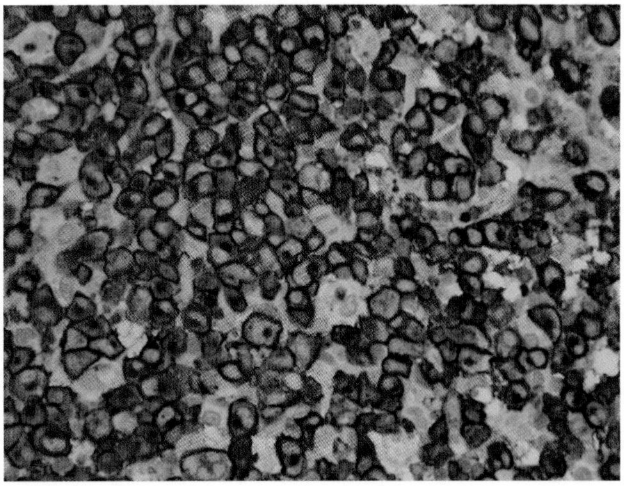

FIGURE 6.11 CD30 labeled with antibody Ber-H2 in an anaplastic large cell lymphoma, T-cell, primary cutaneous type. Some cells exhibit paranuclear Golgi staining (center) in addition to strong membrane positivity.

CD33

CD33 (a member of the immunoglobulin superfamily) is a transmembrane protein receptor expressed on the cell surface of myeloid and monocytic cells. Paraffin-reactive antibodies have been developed, and they demonstrate excellent correlation with flow cytometry in staining by immunohistochemistry of acute myeloid leukemias in formalin-fixed, paraffin-embedded, decalcified bone marrow biopsies. CD33 will also decorate lesions of monocytic/macrophages origin.

CD43

CD43 appears to function as an antiadhesion molecule, mediating repulsion among leukocytes. Also called *leukosialin,* the modified protein is expressed on the surface of all leukocytes except for some resting B cells. CD43 expression in lymphomas is highly correlated with CD5; thus most T-cell malignancies and a group of small lymphocyte B-cell malignancies (CLL/SLL, mantle cell lymphoma [MCL], prolymphocytic leukemia) are often positive, while FL is rarely positive. The broad expression pattern on most leukocytes makes CD43 less useful as a lineage marker but a sensitive indicator of aberrant B-cell populations. Coexpression with CD20 occurs with subsets of small lymphocytic lymphoma (Fig. 6.12 A and B).

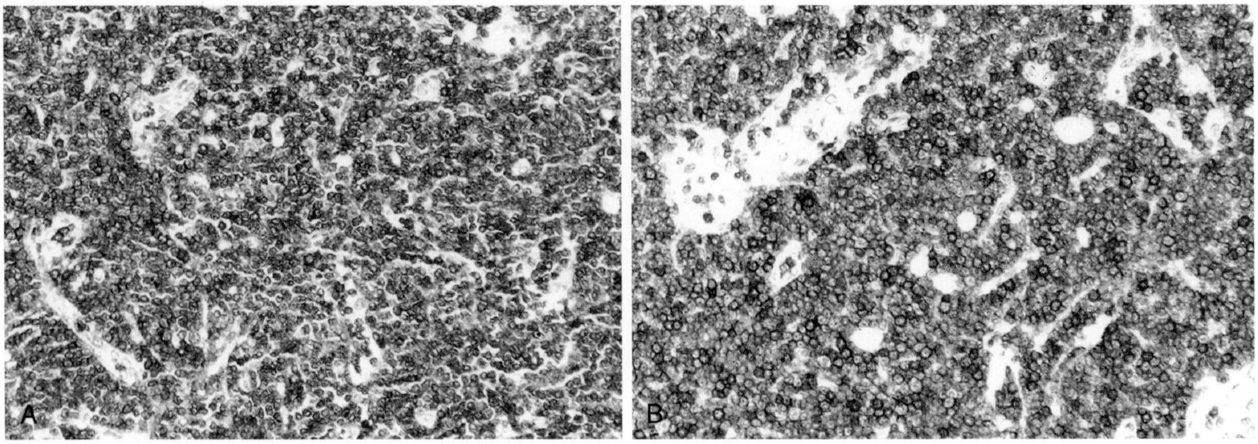

FIGURE 6.12 Coexpression of antibodies to CD43 **(A)** and CD20 **(B)** in a small lymphocytic lymphoma.

TABLE 6.2 Leukocyte Common Antigen Family

Isoform 5	Comments	Antibody Reactivity			
		CD45	CD45RA	CD45RB	CD45RO
ABC	Pre-B and B cells	+	+	+	–
AB	Naïve T cells	+	+	+	–
BC	T cells	+	–	+	+
B	Macrophages; T cells; plasma cell subset; marginal B cells	+	–	+	–
O	Macrophages, granulocytes, thymocytes, memory T cells, transformed B cells, pre-plasma cells	+	–	–	+

CD45

CD45 is a membrane protein tyrosine phosphatase found on all leukocytes in a number of isoforms. Alternate mRNA splicing leads to forms RA, RB, and RC, as well as a form without any of the spliced exons (RO). The RB form is widespread on cells, so antibodies to it are referred to as pan-leukocyte antibodies. CD45RA is present predominantly in B lymphocytes, whereas CD45RO is localized to myeloid and T cells. The antibody mixture 2B11/PD7, termed anti-LCA, is useful in identifying most lymphomas, excepting roughly 30% of ALCL and most Hodgkin disease. An anti-CD45RA antibody, 4KB5, is not quite as sensitive for B-cell lymphomas as CD20 and marks approximately 5% of T cell lymphoma cases. CD45RO antibodies (e.g., OPD4 and UCHL1) have roughly reciprocal specificity as compared with 4KB5. Immunoreactivity is summarized in Tables 6.2 and 6.3.

TABLE 6.3 Reactivity of CD45 Antibodies

	NHL	B	T	HD
CD45/45RB	95%	97%	89%	7%
CD45RA	60%	83%	6%	1%
CD45RO	36%	4%	77%	1%

CD52

CD52 is a protein present on a cell surface of the vast majority of all lymphoid cells and many other hematopoietic cells but not on stem cells. This antigen is a target for monoclonal antibody therapy (Campath). This antigen is currently not detectable in formalin-fixed, paraffin-embedded material but can be detected by flow cytometry. Virtually all mature T- and B-cell lymphomas express this antigen; however, its antigen density can be quite varied in other malignant lymphoreticular disorders. Because this antigen is present on so many hematopoietic cells, Campath therapy can lead to drastic cytopenias. Therefore its determination is recommended on the malignant tumor in question before therapy is given.

CD56

CD56 (also known as neural cell adhesion molecule) is expressed on the cell surface of a number of different tissues including natural killer cells, glial and neurons. This antigen may be demonstrated on monocytic and myeloid leukemias, plasma cell dyscrasias, natural killer cell lesions, neural and astrocytic tumors as well as tumors with neuroendocrine differentiation. Antigen density on hematopoietic tumors tends to be at a lower level than on non-hematopoietic lesions and the validation with flow cytometry determination for this antigen is recommended.

CD57

CD57 cluster antibodies also identify normal NK cells and a T-cell subset. CD57 is a member of the glucuronyltransferase gene family and is expressed on natural killer cells and nerves. CD57 may be used to give evidence for natural killer cell origin for both benign and malignant cells and is particularly useful in helping separate T-cell-rich B-cell lymphoma from lymphocyte-predominant Hodgkin lymphoma. A collaret of CD57–positive lymphocytes surrounds the variant cells in lymphocyte-predominant Hodgkin lymphoma but not in T-cell-rich B-cell lymphoma. CD57 may also be present in glial and neural tumors, as well as prostate carcinoma.

Thus malignancies that are CD57 positive include a minority of T-lymphoblastic leukemia/lymphomas, roughly three quarters of the indolent T-cell large granular lymphocytic leukemias, and a surprisingly small portion of NK cell lymphomas.[80] Thus a typical phenotype for an NK cell is CD3-, CD5-, CD56+, CD57–.[81]

CD61

CD61 recognizes platelet glycoprotein IIIa, which is localized to platelets and megakaryocytes and acute myeloid leukemias with megakaryocytic differentiation. This antigen can be destroyed by heat-induced epitope retrieval, so it is recommended to use enzyme digestion (Pronase) on formalin-fixed, paraffin-embedded material to enhance its detection. This antigen is sensitive to prolonged decalcification, a property that allows this marker to be used as an internal control to monitor for overdecalcification of bone marrow biopsies.

CD68

CD68 is a 110-kD glycoprotein that is expressed by macrophages and is associated with lysosomes. This antigen is expressed by many benign and malignant histiocytic lesions, but some clones have been known to stain malignant melanomas and have differential expression in acute myeloid leukemias. Microglial cells in normal brain may be used as a low-level control and normal node as a high-level control for validation purposes.

CD99

The MIC2 gene product is labeled CD99 and serves to regulate the interactions between intercellular adhesion molecules. It is found in many lymphoblastic leukemia/lymphomas, acute myeloid leukemias, some low-grade B-cell lymphomas, and a variety of solid tumors.

CD163

CD163 is a cell surface glycoprotein, a 175kD molecule, and is a member of the scavenger receptor family of proteins. CD163 is expressed by macrophages in most tissues and may be demonstrated in lesions of monocytic macrophage origin including atypical fibrous xanthoma and acute leukemias with monocytic differentiation. However, it is not expressed by immature monocytes, alveolar macrophages, or microglial cells.

EPSTEIN-BARR VIRUS LATENT MEMBRANE PROTEIN

The latent membrane protein (LMP-1) is a viral protein that protects infected cells from apoptosis through upregulation of BCL-2. As such, it serves as a marker of EBV infection. The correlation of LMP-1 by immunohistochemistry to EBV RNA by *in situ* hybridization is reportedly good for many diseases but is poor for NK/T cell lymphomas. This may be attributable to the latency state of the virus.

T-CELL–RESTRICTED INTRACELLULAR ANTIGEN

The T-cell–restricted intracellular antigen (TIA-1) is a cytotoxic granule-associated protein expressed in natural killer (NK) cells and cytotoxic T lymphocytes. It is expressed regardless of the state of activation of the cell. B-cell malignancies are uniformly negative, while NK cell and some T-cell lymphomas have a granular, cytoplasmic positivity.

PERFORIN/GRANZYME B

This pair of granule-associated proteins is also localized to cytotoxic T and NK cells. They are essential for both apoptosis and induced cell death of target cells via induction of perforated cell membranes. However, their expression is assumed to be evidence of an activated state. They mark subcutaneous panniculitis-like T-cell lymphoma, aggressive NK-cell leukemia, and extranodal NK/T cell lymphoma, nasal type.

KI-67

Ki-67 antibodies recognize a nuclear protein involved in the proliferative portion of the cell cycle. They can be used as a measure of the growth fraction by dividing the number of positive cells by all cells present. This index roughly correlates with tumor grade and is important in the differential diagnosis of some tumors (e.g., Burkitt lymphoma). Correlations between Ki-67 index

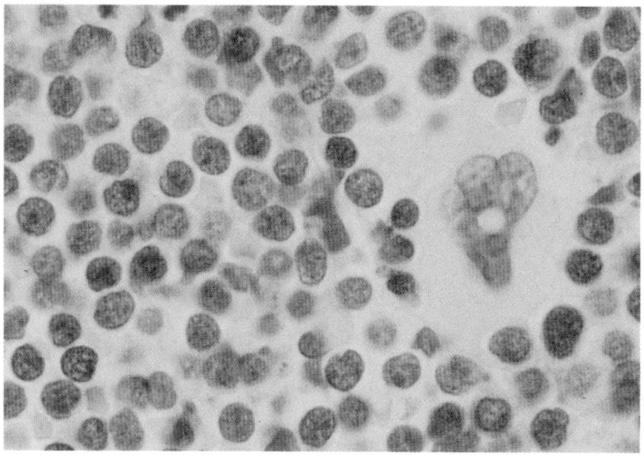

FIGURE 6.13 Antibody to terminal deoxynucleotidyl transfer (TdT) marking precursor B-lymphoblastic leukemia in a nuclear pattern.

and outcome have been made for MALT lymphomas and diffuse large cell lymphomas.

TERMINAL DEOXYNUCLEOTIDYL TRANSFERASE

Terminal deoxynucleotidyl transferase (TdT) is a DNA polymerase active during the process of immunoglobulin and T-cell receptor gene rearrangement early in a precursor B or T cell's life. Only normal early B and T lymphoblasts mark for TdT. The staining pattern is nuclear. TdT is a sensitive and specific antibody for lymphoblastic lymphoma/leukemia because only a small proportion of myeloid leukemia cases are positive (Fig. 6.13).

MYELOPEROXIDASE

Myeloperoxidase (MPO) is a lysosomal protein localized in the azurophilic granules of myeloid cells. Positivity for this antigen strongly supports a myeloid origin for the cell in question but may also be weakly expressed in cells of a monocytic origin. Detection of this antigen can be helpful in separating myeloid sarcoma from large cell lymphoma. Not all myeloid tumors will be positive for MPO and so consideration should be given for staining with CD33 and CD117.

NON-HODGKIN LYMPHOMA AND REACTIVE CONDITIONS

It is probably safe to say that no other area in hematopathology causes as much anxiety for pathologists as the distinction between an atypical reactive lymphoid process and lymphoma.[82] One of the most common dilemmas is a nodular process in a node, with a differential diagnosis of follicular lymphoma and marked follicular hyperplasia. When the usual morphologic clues have failed to resolve the issue, a small panel of antibodies may provide great assistance. BCL-2 is characteristically expressed in the cytoplasm of follicular lymphoma cells (74% to 97% of cases, depending on grade, according to one large study[83]) and is absent from the centrocytes and centroblasts of a hyperplastic follicle.[84] It should be cautioned that both normal mantle lymphocytes and many T cells express BCL-2 (although generally less intensely than follicular lymphoma cells), so occasional positive cells within reactive follicles are expected and should not be overinterpreted. Conversely, in some follicular lymphomas the large transformed cells may not mark with BCL-2 and this should not invalidate the diagnosis. CD10 and BCL-6 are positive in the paracortex and follicles of most follicular lymphomas but not hyperplasias.[85] Immunoglobulin light chain restriction is helpful as an indicator of malignancy[86]; unfortunately, this is relatively infrequent in follicular lymphomas studied by paraffin-section immunohistochemistry. Antibodies to CD45RA have been reported to separate follicular lymphoma from follicular hyperplasia with a distribution pattern similar to that of BCL-2.[87]

Interfollicular reactive processes are more frequently in the differential diagnosis of Hodgkin lymphoma, but some bear resemblance to non-Hodgkin lymphomas. Monocytoid cell aggregates or Langerhans' cell histiocytosis may occasionally raise concern for partial nodal involvement by marginal zone lymphoma. Again, BCL-2 positivity is an important guide because 79% of marginal zone lymphomas are positive and hyperplasias are not.[83] Malignant Langerhans' cells are typically S-100 and CD1a positive.[88] A florid paracortical immunoblastic proliferation as seen, for example, with infectious mononucleosis, may raise concern for a non-Hodgkin lymphoma and Hodgkin disease. Examination with pan B- and pan T-cell markers may be helpful, particularly if small sheets of B cells are identified.[11] Reactive processes typically show a mixture of B and T or a predominance of T immunoblasts. T-cell-rich B-cell lymphoma, a variant of diffuse large B-cell lymphoma, may be mistaken for a benign condition but can typically be properly diagnosed with a series of pan B-cell markers and immunoglobulin light chain antibodies.[89]

KEY DIAGNOSTIC POINTS

Follicular Lymphoma versus Reactive Hyperplasia

- BCL-2 positivity *in* enlarged follicles is seen in lymphoma; BCL-2 positivity *around* follicles is typical of hyperplasia.
- Immunoglobulin light chain staining is usually not helpful in distinguishing follicular processes.
- Beware BCL-2 positive benign, small, primary follicles and intrafollicular T cells.

NON-HODGKIN LYMPHOMA AND OTHER MALIGNANCIES

Non-Hodgkin lymphoma is sometimes part of the differential in poorly differentiated large cell malignancies. Most forms of lymphoma can be ruled in or out by the use of antibodies to CD45RB (leukocyte common antigen), S-100, and cytokeratin (e.g., the AE1/AE3 mixture or CAM5.2). Pitfalls to avoid pertain particularly to anaplastic large cell lymphoma (ALCL), which may mimic an epithelial malignancy in its sinusoidal distribution, apparent cohesive growth pattern, and cytology (especially when monomorphic). Leukocyte common antigen is frequently absent,[90,91] many cases are "null" cell (express neither T- nor B-cell epitopes),[91] and epithelial membrane antigen is present—albeit focally—in up to 80% of cases.[92] If the pathologist maintains an index of suspicion for ALCL, CD30 will typically resolve the issue. Vimentin is positive in a large variety of tissue types and, although useful as a control for antigen preservation,[93] it has little role in lymphoma diagnosis.

CLASSIFICATION OF NON-HODGKIN LYMPHOMAS

The initial distinction in the WHO classification separates lymphomas into B-cell, T-cell, and Hodgkin types. Although this separation is an immunologic one, it may not require immunohistochemistry or flow cytometry to be made. For example, follicular lymphomas are uniformly B-cell malignancies and generally do not require immunophenotyping for diagnosis. This is significant for both turn-around time and financial reasons because a large proportion of lymphomas in the United States are follicular lymphomas.[94] Other entities may be strongly suspected on the basis of routine morphologic study and require only confirmatory immunologic workup. It is a rare case that progresses sequentially through the immunohistochemistry laboratory from proof of lymphoid nature, through lineage assignment, to a final subclassification.

B-CELL NEOPLASMS

B- and T-cell neoplasms are divided into precursor disorders (lymphoblastic leukemias and lymphomas) with normal counterparts in the earliest bone marrow and thymus compartments, and mature, or "peripheral," malignancies akin to normal extrathymic, nodal, splenic, or circulating lymphocytes. Discussion is focused on those malignancies commonly diagnosed using immunohistochemistry (i.e., "solid" tumors).

Precursor B-Cell Neoplasms

PRECURSOR B-CELL LYMPHOBLASTIC LEUKEMIA/LYMPHOMA

Typical phenotype: CD19 +, CD79a +, CD20 –/+, CD22 +/–, CD10 +, TdT +, immunoglobulin –

Lymphoblastic lymphoma and acute lymphoblastic leukemia are morphologically and immunophenotypically the same disease and are distinguished on clinical grounds.[95] Although the majority of lymphoblastic leukemias are of B lineage, only approximately 20% of lymphoblastic lymphomas express B-cell markers.[96,97] Practically all cases of lymphoblastic leukemia/lymphoma produce an enzyme, terminal deoxynucleotidyl transferase (TdT), involved in gene rearrangement.[98-102] TdT marks the nucleus of lymphoblasts. CD19 is expressed in almost all lymphoblastic lymphomas but is not detectable in paraffin sections. CD20 is not reliably found,[99-101,103] nor is leukocyte common antigen (CD45RB).[104] Both CD74 (LN2)[105] and CD79a[100] antibodies are useful markers of B cell or pre–B-cell lymphoblastic lymphomas. Antibodies to CD43 are often thought of as T-cell markers, but their specificity is quite broad. Most examples of precursor B-cell lymphoblastic lymphoma/leukemia express CD43 but are CD3 negative.[100] The MIC2 gene product, CD99, parallels the expression distribution of TdT in lymphoblastic lymphomas,[106,107] although the antigen pattern is membranous rather than nuclear. Of course, other small round cell tumors, particularly in children, are also positive with anti-CD99. The majority of precursor B cell neoplasms are CD10 (CALLA) positive, but some precursor T cell tumors also express CD10.[108] Other antigens that are sometimes found in precursor B cell lymphoma include CD34,[102] cytokeratin,[99] the natural killer cell antigen CD56,[109] and the Fas ligand.[110] BCL-2 is frequently found in the cytoplasm and has been noted to assist in the differential diagnosis with Burkitt lymphoma/leukemia[111]; however, other "blastic" lymphoid neoplasms such as the blastoid variant of mantle cell lymphoma may also be BCL-2 positive.

> **KEY DIAGNOSTIC POINTS**
>
> ***Lymphoblastic Lymphoma/Leukemia***
>
> - CD20 and LCA may be negative in precursor B-cell lymphoblastic lymphoma/leukemia.
> - TdT is almost always present in the nucleus of lymphoblastic lymphoma cells (although it may also be found in biphenotypic and some myeloid leukemias).
> - CD10 and CD99 are usually present.

Mature B-Cell Neoplasms

B-CELL CHRONIC LYMPHOCYTIC LEUKEMIA/SMALL LYMPHOCYTIC LYMPHOMA

Typical phenotype: Positive: CD45, CD5, CD19, CD20, CD23, CD43, PAX5, BCL-2; Negative: CD10, CD11c, CD138, BCL-1

As with lymphoblastic leukemia/lymphoma, the immunophenotypes of B-cell CLL and SLL are practically indistinguishable. These malignancies of mature small B lymphocytes commonly have an indolent course. They are pan B-cell marker positive, although CD20 may have weaker cytoplasmic intensity than other B-cell lymphomas. An early study found expression of Leu 22 (CD43) in only 39% of cases,[86] but more recently authors have identified CD43 in 79% to 100% of cases.[112-114] With the advent of CD5 antibodies useful in fixed tissue (in particular, clone 4C7 used with antigen retrieval methods), most SLL could be shown to be positive, although some cases exhibited weak or incomplete staining of cells.[115,116] Although CD5 negativity by flow cytometry is often a cause for re-examining a diagnosis of B-CLL/SLL,[117] this is not yet true of paraffin immunohistochemistry. When present, CD23 (BU38) is useful in distinguishing from mantle cell lymphoma,[112,114,118-121] but it should be recalled that both follicular dendritic cells and follicular lymphomas may also express CD23. CD23 expression appears to be maintained even after large cell transformation of SLL.[122] BCL-2 is positive.[120] Pertinent negative findings in B-CLL/SLL include CD10,[112,123] cyclin D1,[120,124-127] and BCL-6.[128] Elevated levels of the oncoprotein p53, although infrequently encountered, have been associated with a poor clinical outcome.[129] Recently, the chemokine receptor CXCR3 was shown to be expressed in 37 of 39 cases of CLL/SLL and absent in mantle cell, follicular, and small noncleaved cell lymphomas.[130] Expression of ZAP-70, a nonreceptor tyrosine kinase, is found in a subset of B-cell CLL, normal and malignant T-cells, and infrequently in other B-cell malignancies. Both nuclear and cytoplasmic positivity is noted by immunohistochemistry.[131,132] Expression of ZAP-70 in CLL correlates with a decreased time to progression of disease and poorer survival.[133,134] The presence of this protein seems to be a superior marker of patient outcome compared with either the mutational status of the immunoglobulin heavy chain gene[133-136] or CD38 expression.[134]

Beyond Immunohistochemistry: Anatomic Molecular Diagnostic Applications

The genetic and molecular understanding of small cell lymphocytic lymphoma/chronic lymphocytic leukemia has advanced substantially in the past several years. This lymphoma has particularly low rates of growth and thus produces few if any abnormalities with standard cytogenetics. The application of FISH techniques, as well as molecular techniques to the study of this lymphoma, have revealed a more dynamic process than what was previously believed. This new knowledge was gained by the search for more potent prognostic indicators that had been previously developed such as clinical staging and pattern of bone marrow involvement (nondiffuse vs. diffuse).

INTERPHASE FISH Several recurrent genetic abnormalities identified in small cell lymphocytic lymphoma/chronic lymphocytic leukemia have had a direct relationship to disease progression. These abnormalities are:

- Trisomy 12
- Deletion 13q14.3
- Deletion 11q22-23 (ATM)
- Deletion 17p13 (p53)
- Deletion 6q
- Trisomy 8
- Trisomy 3

Of particular interest is the 17p deletion, which is thought to be associated with p53 deletion. This abnormality confers the worse prognosis of any of the above-listed abnormalities but also seems to indicate therapy selection. This abnormality confers fludarabine resistance and there is evidence to suggest that first-line therapy treatment with Campath would be indicated. These abnormalities may be detected in up to 80% of cases of small cell lymphocytic lymphoma.

Theranostic Applications

Traditional staging and prognostic parameters in this disorder have been able to demonstrate a minority of cases that behave in a more aggressive manner. However, 80% to 90% of cases of CLL end up in a low clinical stage. The understanding of the biology of SLL/CLL has greatly expanded, and a number of determinants are available to help guide clinicians in the behavior of SLL/CLL and are described as follows.

MUTATIONAL STATUS OF IGH V IGH V mutational status can be defined as mutated when there is 98% or greater homology to the germinal line sequence. Approximately 50% of cases of small cell lymphocytic lymphoma/chronic lymphocytic leukemia will demonstrate mutated IGH genes. The significance of this finding is that patients whose disease has mutated IGH three genes have a poorer prognosis than those that are not mutated. The techniques to demonstrate mutational status are complicated and labor intensive and do not lend themselves well to the clinical laboratory. Surrogate markers that have been suggested for this purpose are CD38 (>30% of cells) and to a greater extent ZAP-70 (>26% of cells expressing this antigen). The correlation for these markers is if the patient is CD38 and/or ZAP-70 positive, within the IGH V will be nonmutated, and if ZAP-70 negative, the IGH V will be mutated. Though the correlation of CD38 (in particular and) ZAP-70 with mutational status is imperfect and controversial, many studies have shown positivity for CD38 and ZAP-70 demonstrating poor prognosis. The determination of CD38 positivity is relatively straightforward and is easily demonstrated by flow cytometry. The level that CD38 is considered positive is when greater than 30% of cells demonstrate positivity as compared with isotype-matched control. ZAP-70 determination is somewhat more difficult. CD38 is a cell surface antigen and lends itself to study by flow cytometry quite well. Zap 70 is a cytoplasmic antigen, and fixation of the cells is necessary before flow cytometric determination may be made. When one is attempting to set negative for ZAP-70 so that positive can be determined, several factors have been suggested. ZAP-70 is not present on normal B cells but is seen on mature T cells and natural killer cells. One may use baseline positivity on the cells as a guide to set cursor placement for positive or negative; however, there is great variation among the levels of ZAP-70 in the cells and perhaps a better internal control would be normal B cells, which do not express ZAP-70 normally. This antigen may also be detected by immunohistochemistry in formalin-fixed, paraffin-embedded material.

CYTOGENETIC ABNORMALITIES In addition to IGH V mutational status, certain cytogenetic abnormalities offer prognostic information as well. These abnormalities are best detected by FISH testing because a low proliferative rate in this malignancy does not lend itself well to standard cytogenetic determination. The presence of the 13q deletion confers a good prognostic finding is present without an accompanying poor prognostic cytogenetic abnormality.

KEY DIAGNOSTIC POINTS

Mature B-Cell Lymphoma

- CD20 and BCL-2 mark mantle cell, follicular, and some marginal zone lymphomas along with B-CLL/SLL.
- B-CLL/SLL can be distinguished from mantle cell lymphoma by CD23 (present) and cyclin D1 (absent).
- B-CLL/SLL can be distinguished from follicular lymphoma by CD10 (absent) and CD5/CD43 (present).
- ZAP-70 predicts poor outcome in B-CLL.

B-CELL PROLYMPHOCYTIC LEUKEMIA

Typical phenotype: same as B-CLL/SLL, but maybe CD5, CD22+

B-cell prolymphocytic leukemia rarely presents as a diagnostic dilemma in a lymph node, and although splenic involvement may raise the possibility of a splenic lymphoma, the elevated white blood cell count and typical smear make this unlikely. B-PLL may be CD5 and CD23 negative[110] and is more likely to be CD22 positive than B-CLL/SLL.[137] Not surprisingly, measures of mitotic index—such as Ki-67[138]—are higher in B-PLL.

LYMPHOPLASMACYTIC LYMPHOMA

Typical phenotype: Positive: CD45, CD19, CD20, CD43+/, CD79, PAX5 (lymphoid component), CD138 (plasma cell component), BCL-2, Clonal Cytoplasmic Light chain with IgM; Negative: CD5, CD10, CD11c, BCL-1

This uncommon lymphoma morphologically consists of a mixture of lymphoid cells, plasma cells, and cells sharing the characteristics of both lymphocytes and plasma cells. Mast cells are quite prominent. Plasmacytoid features may take the form of Dutcher bodies, as well as Russell bodies, which may be enhanced by staining with PAS. The typical presentation for this lymphoma is bone marrow involvement with little nodal or spleen involvement. These lymphomas typically present with a monoclonal gammopathy of IgM and its associated hyperviscosity and/or cryoglobulinemia (Waldenstrom macroglobulinemia). An association with hepatitis C has been noted with this lymphoma.

This tumor of small lymphocytes and plasmacytoid lymphs is the pathologic correlate of the clinical syndrome Waldenstrom macroglobulinemia. As would be expected, immunoglobulin heavy chain in the cytoplasm of the more plasmacytic cells is typically of the IgM isotype.[139] Immunoglobulin light chain restriction is almost always demonstrable, again particularly in the more differentiated cells.[140,141] CD20 is positive, but CD23 and CD43 (present in only 20% to 40% of cases[113,114,123,142]) are far more frequently absent than in B-CLL/SLL. CD5 and CD10 are normally negative, but exceptions have been noted.[102] Interestingly, CD138 (syndecan, a marker of normal and malignant plasma cells) was absent from all 17 cases of B-PLL tested.[143] The Fas ligand is weakly expressed,[110] but Fas itself (CD95, a transmembrane receptor in the tumor necrosis factor receptor superfamily) is often present.[144] BCL-2 is reported to be positive in 80% of cases.[11]

Beyond Immunohistochemistry: Anatomic Molecular Diagnostic Applications

The majority of these lymphomas demonstrate clonal immunoglobulin gene rearrangements. The most common cytogenetic abnormality identified in this lymphoma is deletions in the long arm of chromosome 6 (del(6)(q21)) with a small number of these lymphomas demonstrating t(9;14)(p13;32). These translocations are not specific for lymphoplasmacytic lymphoma and have been demonstrated in other B-cell lymphomas.

SPLENIC MARGINAL ZONE B-CELL LYMPHOMA

Typical phenotype: Immunoglobulin –/+, B cell antigen +, CD5–, CD10–, CD23–, CD43 –/+, CD11c+/–

SMZL is one of the primary splenic lymphomas and may have a peripheral blood component of "villous" lymphocytes.[145] The cytoplasmic projections of these villous cells may lead to confusion with hairy cell leukemia, but the immunophenotypes are different. Mature B cell antigens are typically present (CD20, CD79a), but DBA.44 (CD72)—a B-cell marker found on a variety of low-grade, B-cell lymphoma cells and most closely associated with hairy cell leukemia—is found in the cytoplasm of only 30% of SMZL cases.[146] CD43 is rarely present.[83] CD11c is present in approximately half of the patients with SMZL[147-150] compared with nearly all cases of hairy cell leukemia, but antibodies are only effective for flow cytometry or frozen sections. Ki-67 is typically low.[151,152] BCL-2 is reportedly positive in most cases,[146,153,154] whereas cyclin D1 is uniformly negative.[126,152,155] An antibody that detects tartrate-resistant acid phosphatase in fixed tissues has been developed and is reportedly sensitive for hairy cell leukemia,[156,157] but only a few cases of SMZL, showing weak expression, have been published.[158]

Beyond Immunohistochemistry: Anatomic Molecular Diagnostic Applications

Two common genetic anomalies have been noted in splenic marginal zone lymphoma: del7q31-32 and trisomy 3. The range of detection of these anomalies is somewhat variable but has been reported in up to 40% of splenic marginal zone lymphomas for del7 and up to 20% for trisomy 3. Though these abnormalities are not diagnostic in isolation, the appropriate morphology and immunophenotype, along with positivity for del7 and/or trisomy 3 in the absence of 11;14 or 14;18 translocations, can be of great benefit in allowing appropriate disease classification. Rearrangement of the heavy and light chain genes have been reportedly demonstrated in the vast majority of cases of splenic marginal zone lymphoma.

HAIRY CELL LEUKEMIA

Typical phenotype: B-cell antigen +, CD5–, CD10–, CD23–, CD11c+ (strong), CD25+, PAX5+, CD79, CD19, DBA.44, annexin A1

Hairy cell leukemia is a chronic B-cell lymphoproliferative lesion that typically presents in a middle-aged man with pancytopenia and splenomegaly. Monocytopenia is invariably present. The hairy cells themselves have a characteristic appearance with a moderate amount of agranular cytoplasm, which may demonstrate cytoplasmic villi. These villi or cytoplasmic projections are seen around the entire circumference of the cell. The nucleus has a mature chromatin without nucleoli with an almost kidney bean–shaped outline.

The lack of white pulp involvement in the spleen of leukemic patients makes confusion with primary splenic lymphomas uncommon, but bone marrow involvement is constant and may be extensive. An aspirate is often unobtainable; the pathologist may be called on to discriminate between hairy cell leukemia and other low-grade, B-cell malignancies in the marrow trephine biopsy. Leukocyte common antigens, as well as most pan B-cell antigens, are present.[159] T-cell markers and CD43 are negative.[160,161] A marker such as CD20 may be useful in detecting minimal residual disease in the bone marrow.[162] As mentioned earlier, DBA.44 is frequently (50% to 100%) positive in hairy cell leukemia.[158,163,164] TRAP positivity by immunohistochemistry is also more frequent and more intense than in SMZL and MALT lymphomas (although one report notes that not all hairy cells in a given case stain[158]), and the combination of TRAP and DBA.44 positivity is reported to be specific for HCL.[158,165] Cyclin D1 is overexpressed in many cases of HCL, although at lower levels than in mantle cell lymphoma.[166,167] Some authors report weak immunoreactivity in most or all cases of HCL,[167] whereas others fail to detect cyclin D1.[126,127]

PLASMA CELL MYELOMA/PLASMACYTOMA

Typical phenotype: Cytoplasmic immunoglobulin + (strong), CD19–, CD20–, CD22–, CD79a+/–, CD45RB–/+, EMA –/+, CD43+/–, CD56+/– CD30+

Most myelomas and plasmacytomas do not present a diagnostic dilemma. They contain abundant intracellular immunoglobulin. Light chain antibodies will establish monotypia and separate them from reactive or infectious conditions, whereas the strong light chain positivity and absence of CD20 and (usually) leukocyte common antigen distinguish plasmacytoma/myeloma from large B-cell lymphoma. CD138 can provide support because it is quite sensitive and specific for plasmacytic differentiation.[143,168] CD138 is also positive in the vast majority of plasma cells.[169] BCL-2 is frequently present.[170]

KEY DIAGNOSTIC POINTS

B Cells and Plasma Cells

- Antigens such as CD45RB and CD20, commonly associated with mature B lymphocytes, are absent from many plasma cells.
- In immature or anaplastic myeloma, do not be misled by epithelial membrane antigen positivity.
- CD30 positivity (typically cytoplasmic rather than membranous or paranuclear) should not occasion a diagnosis of ALCL.

EXTRANODAL MARGINAL ZONE B-CELL LYMPHOMA OF MUCOSA-ASSOCIATED LYMPHOID TISSUE (MALT) TYPE

Typical phenotype: Immunoglobulin + (40%, may be either the lymphoid or plasma cell component, or both), CD20+, CD79a+, CD5–, CD10–, CD23–, CD43–/+, CD11c+/–

The extranodal marginal zone B-cell lymphoma or MALT-type lymphoma presents in adults with localized disease, most commonly in the gastrointestinal tract, less frequently in other mucosa-bearing sites such as the lacrimal gland, lung, and breast, and occasionally in nonmucosal sites like the skin and thyroid gland. It presents a heterogeneous cytologic picture, with abundant small marginal zone ("centrocyte-like") cells, monocytoid B cells with more abundant cytoplasm and reniform nuclei, and plasma cells. The small cells frequently infiltrate glandular epithelium to form lymphoepithelial lesions, which may be highlighted by a cytokeratin antibody. Immunostaining for light chains may provide assistance in distinguishing a reactive gastritis or similar condition, a common problem on small endoscopic biopsies. Light chain monotypia is reported in 40% or more of the cases[1,171]; cutaneous extranodal marginal zone lymphoma has been reported to be monotypic 70% of the time.[172] Both the small cell component and the plasma cell component should be examined for monotypia; lymphocyte staining may be weak, so careful comparison of the two antibodies and attention to the cytoplasm, not the surrounding interstitial staining, is necessary. The plasma cells are commonly found in a subepithelial location. In up to 40% of cases they are monotypic and are usually easier to diagnose than the small cell component.[1] Dutcher bodies may be present. In the balance of cases, plasma cells are reactive and do not demonstrate light chain monotypia.

The extranodal marginal zone lymphomas, with rare exception, do not express either CD5 or CD43[173,174]; those that do may exhibit more aggressive disease.[175] They can be discriminated from follicular lymphoma because they are CD10 negative.[174] Like other lymphomas comprising small lymphocytes, extranodal MZL is BCL-2 positive[176-180]; however, "high-grade" or MZL with areas of transformed large cells are much less often positive.[179] Conversely, p53 is more frequently overexpressed and proliferation-related antigens like Ki-67 are more abundant in the high-grade MALT lymphomas than in low-grade ones.[179,181,182] BCL-6, an oncoprotein regulator of lymphocyte differentiation found overexpressed in a subset of large cell lymphomas, can be identified in the large transformed lymphocytes of some high-grade MALT lymphomas.[181] Germinal centers are a common element in MALT lymphomas and may be made more apparent by immunostaining for CD21, particularly in cases of follicular colonization. The chemokine receptor CXCR3 is present in the monocytoid and plasmacytic cells of extranodal MZL.[130]

Immunoproliferative small intestinal disease (IPSID) is a disorder related to extranodal MALT lymphoma that is prevalent in populations living around the Mediterranean Sea. Although mucosal plasma cells expressing

TABLE 6.4 Recurrent Molecular and Genetic Findings in Malt Lymphoma

Translocation	Genes Involved	Additional Aberrations	Anatomic Sites
t(11;18)(q21;q21)*	API2-MALTI	None	Gastrointestinal tract, lung, head, and neck
t(14;18)(q32;q21)*	IgH-MALT1	Trisomy 3, 12, or 18	Lung, liver, ocular adnexa skin
t(1;14)(p22;q32)*	BCL10-IgH	None	Lung, stomach, skin
t(3;14)(p14;q32)	FOXPI-IgH	Trisomy 3	Thyroid, ocular adnexa, skin
t(1;2)(p22;p12)*	BCL10-IgLk	Trisomy 3	Lung, stomach, skin

*These abnormalities lead to overexpression or activation of the NF-κB pathway.

IgA without light chains predominate, at different stages IPSID has marginal zone lymphocytes or large transformed lymphs similar to non-Mediterranean cases of MALT lymphoma.[183]

Beyond Immunohistochemistry: Anatomic Molecular Diagnostic Applications

The majority of MALT-type lymphomas demonstrate immunoglobulin gene rearrangements, which can be helpful in separating this lymphoma from a reactive lymphocytic infiltrate. One must always keep in mind that false-negative results in lymphomas, as well as positive rearrangement studies in benign inflammatory disorders such as gastritis, have been reported. The results of gene rearrangement studies must always be placed in the clinical context and correlated with morphology. Somatic hypermutation of the immunoglobulin heavy chain genes, as well as extensive ongoing somatic mutation, had been demonstrated in these lymphomas and would suggest a late memory B-cell stage, which is in keeping with the morphologic appearance of chronic active inflammation and antigenic stimulation.

A detailed number of characteristic cytogenetic and molecular findings have been described in MALT lymphomas and are listed in Table 6.4. These abnormalities provide an insight into the anatomic site of involvement, clinical manifestations, and behavior of these lymphomas.

T(11;18)(Q21;Q21) This is the most common chromosomal abnormality in MALT lymphomas and is reported with the frequency of 10% to 35% and is quite specific for this type of lymphoma. This translocation results in a new fusion gene (API2-MALT1) and encodes for the api2-malt1 protein. It is postulated that this fusion leads to activation of the nuclear NF-κB pathway. Activation of this pathway is a common end result in the majority of translocations in these lymphomas. This translocation results in the nuclear expression of BCL10 protein. The consequences of this translocation result in decreased apoptosis and confer a growth advantage on this tumor. This translocation provides a growth mechanism for this lymphoma, which is independent from antigen stimulation/*Helicobacter pylori* infection. Thus the elimination of *Helicobacter pylori* infections will no longer provide effective therapy. Patients with this translocation present with more advanced stages of disease and may be *Helicobacter pylori* negative but tend not to have transformation to large cell lymphoma. Additional chromosome translocations are not described in this type of lymphoma.

T(14;18)(Q32;Q21) This chromosome abnormality occurs in approximately 20% of malt lymphomas and results in the MALT1 gene on chromosome 18q21 being joined with the IGH enhancer region on chromosome 14, which leads to overexpression of MALT1 leading to activation of the NF-κB pathway. Additional chromosome abnormalities consisting of trisomy 3, 12, and 18 have been described in MALT lymphomas with this translocation. Interestingly, this translocation seems to be much more prominent in nongastrointestinal MALT lymphomas.

T(3;14)(P14;Q32) This chromosome abnormality is detected in approximately 10% of MALT lymphomas. The translocation results in the Forkhead box protein P1(FOXP1) joining with the IGH enhancer region on chromosome 14. This translocation is more commonly seen in MALT lymphomas involving ocular adnexa, skin, and thyroid. The presence of trisomy 3 has also been noted in this subset of MALT lymphomas.

T(1;14)(P22;Q32) AND T(1;14)(P22;Q32) These translocations, though quite specific for MALT lymphomas, are only present in about 1% to 2% of cases. The translocation places the BCL10 and gene on chromosome 1p22 under the control of the IGH enhancer region on chromosome 14 or under regulation by IgLκ. Both translocations result in an overexpression of nuclear BCL10 and similarly resultant in activation of the NF-κB pathway, as does the t(11;18)(q21;q21).

Theranostic Applications

The t(11;18)(q21;q21) has been associated with high stage of disease at presentation and absence of *H. pylori* infection, though this translocation is not associated with large cell transformation. The t(3;14)(p14;q32) has been described in diffuse large B-cell lymphoma, and MALT lymphomas containing this translocation may be at risk for large cell transformation. Other abnormalities associated with large cell transformation include hypermethylation of p15 and p16, p16 deletions, and allelic loss and mutation of p53.

NODAL MARGINAL ZONE B-CELL LYMPHOMA

Typical phenotype: Immunoglobulin +, CD20+, CD79a+, CD45+, CD19+, CD20+, CD43+/–, CD5–, CD10–, CD23–, CD43–, CD11c+/–

The cytologic and immunophenotypic composition of nodal MZL is fundamentally the same as its extranodal counterpart, although some cases may be particularly rich in medium-sized monocytoid cells and relatively devoid of the smaller nodal marginal zone cells. As in the gastrointestinal tract, immunoglobulin light chain analysis is frequently productive, with approximately 30% of cases showing monotypia.[86,184,185] Monotypia can be particularly helpful in favoring a diagnosis of nodal MZL over a reactive follicular hyperplasia with monocytoid B cells. CD5, CD10, and CD23 are rarely positive,[117,123,186-189] excluding diagnoses of B-CLL/SLL and follicular lymphoma. Also, CD43 is expressed in 20% to 40% of the tumors.[75] The absence of cyclin D1[186,189] essentially excludes mantle cell lymphoma. As with MALT lymphoma, most nodal examples overexpress BCL-2 (79% in one large study[83]), albeit more weakly than follicular lymphoma, with which this entity may coexist.[190] Also as in the extranodal counterpart, p53 is immunohistochemically detectable in a small fraction of tumors (although point mutations in the gene are absent, indicating another mechanism of upregulation).[191] This is in contradistinction to splenic marginal zone lymphomas, which frequently harbor p53 mutations.[147,154] MZL has a phenotype similar to that of hairy cell leukemia, with the exception that DBA.44 is not expressed in most cases.[164]

FOLLICULAR LYMPHOMA

Typical phenotype: B-cell antigen +, CD10+, CD5−, CD23−/+, CD43−, CD11c−

Follicular lymphoma is the most common form of non-Hodgkin lymphoma in North America.[94] Fortunately, in most instances its characteristic morphology makes distinction from reactive conditions and other lymphomas straightforward. When small sample size or other limitations make diagnosis more difficult, the characteristic immunophenotype can resolve the issue. Pan B-cell antigens such as CD20 and CD79a are always present, and CD10 (CALLA) is expressed in 90% to 95% of cases using formalin-fixed tissue.[112,193] The latter is pertinent to the differential diagnosis of mantle cell and small lymphocytic lymphoma; also helpful is the infrequency (<5% of cases) of CD43 and CD5 positivity in follicular lymphoma.[86,112,113,116,117,186,194] Light chain monotypia has been noted in 28% of cases and is generally not helpful in distinguishing from other lymphomas.[86]

The BCL-2 protein was first isolated from follicular lymphomas and has played a large role in our understanding of non-Hodgkin lymphoma in general. BCL-2 has been pressed into service as a diagnostic tool for the disease. BCL-2 forms heterodimers with a number of related proteins including BCL-x; the BCL2 gene is on chromosome 18 and is involved in the translocation of chromosomes 14 and 18 characteristic of follicular lymphoma. The majority of tumors overexpress the BCL-2 protein as a result of the translocation, ranging from 97% of grade I neoplasms through 83% of grade II to 74% of grade III.[83,195-198] Interestingly, even FLs without an identifiable translocation overexpress BCL-2, although at a lower frequency,[199] suggesting another mechanism of upregulation. Staining is typically more intense in the small cleaved cells, and not all small cells may stain.[200] Even variant forms of follicular lymphoma mark with anti-BCL-2 antibodies.[201] Although BCL-2 status changes with grade, it has been shown not to predict clinical outcome.[202] Like normal follicle center cells,[128] most FLs also express BCL-6,[199,203] a regulator of gene transcription. Most other low-grade B-cell lymphomas do not.[128] Transformation of FLs to diffuse large B-cell lymphoma is accompanied by a decrease in BCL-6 expression.[204]

Cyclin D1, the hallmark of mantle cell lymphoma, is not found in FL.[125,126] Tumor suppressor gene products like p53,[196,198] RB (the Retinoblastoma protein),[198] and the p53 binding protein MDM2[200] are present in more high-grade FLs than low-grade FLs. Other points potentially useful in diagnosis include the rarity of CD57-positive T cells in FL (compared with nodular lymphocyte predominant Hodgkin disease[206]), the generally intact meshwork of follicular dendritic cells in FL as demonstrated by anti-CD21 antibodies,[207] the absence of CXCR3,[130] and the frequent presence of CD30-positive cells, particularly at the periphery of the follicles.[208,209] Finally, BCL-2 has been used as an indicator of minimal residual disease in the bone marrow of FL patients when staining is strong and uniform.[210]

KEY DIAGNOSTIC POINTS

Follicular Lymphomas

- BCL-2 expression is sensitive for follicular lymphoma, but not specific.
- The addition of CD43 or CD5, cyclin D1, BCL-6, and CD10 effectively separates the lymphomas of small lymphocytes.

MANTLE CELL LYMPHOMA

Typical phenotype: surface IgM/D+, B-cell antigen +, cyclin D1+, CD5+, CD10−/+, CD23−, CD43+, CD11c−

With the normal counterpart believed to arise from the lymphocytes found in the inner follicle mantle, it is no surprise that the usual mature B-cell markers (CD20, CD79a) are strongly positive (although DBA.44 may be present in only a minority of cases).[158] Immunoglobulin light chains can be detected in about 40% of the cases in paraffin.[86] CD23, found in a subset of activated B lymphocytes and follicular dendritic cells, is characteristically negative in mantle cell lymphoma, although approximately 5% to 10% of tumors are positive.[112,114,119-123,186,211-213] CD10 is infrequently present.[186,211,214] The most useful findings in paraffin-section immunohistochemistry are the presence in the nucleus of cyclin D1 protein (76% to 100% of cases) and in the cytoplasm of CD5 (73% to 100%, but some cases are weak).[112,117,120,124,126,127,186,211,213,215] As with other small lymphocyte lymphomas, CD43 is frequently coexpressed with CD5.[86,112-114,120] Uncommon forms of mantle cell lymphoma including the blastoid variant (characterized by larger cells with more dispersed chromatin) and tumors localized to the mucosa[212,214,216] express the same antigenic pattern as the standard type, permitting distinction from precursor B-cell lymphoblastic lymphoma [92,217] and transformed SLL.[117] In addition, TdT and CD99 are not found in the blastoid variant of mantle cell lymphoma but are in lymphoblastic lymphoma/leukemia.[107] Approximately 90% of tumors produce BCL-2, requiring the pathologist to be alert to the potential confusion with FL or SLL.[120,217] Mutation in the p53 gene may result in overexpression,[218] which may in turn correlate with a more aggressive course.[219-221] The Ki-67 index can be quite variable, ranging from 5% to 40%.[222]

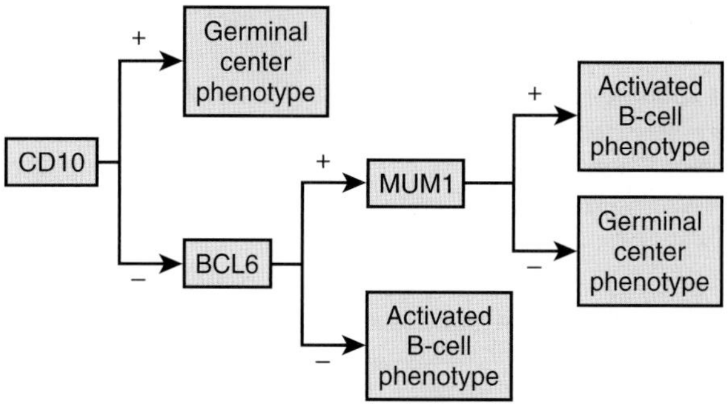

FIGURE 6.14 Strategic algorithm for the classification of diffuse large B-cell lymphoma.

KEY DIAGNOSTIC POINTS

Mantle Cell Lymphoma

- Cyclin D1 is only rarely expressed by lymphomas other than mantle cell.
- Mantle cell lymphomas are often not as intensely positive for cyclin D1 as parathyroid or breast control tissues.

DIFFUSE LARGE B-CELL LYMPHOMA

Typical phenotype: B-cell antigen +, CD45RB+, CD20+, PAX5+, CD19+, CD79+ (except for some anaplastic and mediastinal lymphomas), CD5–/+, CD10–/+

This group of lymphomas is the most common subtype of malignant lymphoma, accounting for 30% to 40% of all malignant lymphomas. These lymphomas for the most part have a common immunophenotype in that they are positive for CD45 and some combination of pan B-cell markers (CD20, CD19, CD79, and PAX5). These lymphomas express monotypic surface light chain in the vast majority of cases (90% to 95%); however, a small percentage will not be detectable by flow cytometry. Other antigens are heterogeneously expressed in diffuse large B-cell lymphoma, including CD10 (25% to 50%), BCL2 (50% to 60%) and BCL6 (40% to 90%). CD5 has been reported to be positive in a subset of diffuse large B-cell lymphomas; its presence should alert the pathologist to this representing a possible mantle cell lymphoma. There is some evidence to suggest that CD5-positive large B-cell lymphomas, not represented as mantle cell lymphoma, may behave in a more aggressive manner.

The vast majority of diffuse large B-cell lymphomas have clonal rearrangement of the immunoglobulin heavy chain genes. This is noted in cases that are negative for surface immunoglobulin, and its presence gives evidence for a clonal B-cell process even in the absence of clonal surface immunoglobulin. Other recurrent genetic abnormalities noted in this lymphoma are the presence of 3q27 abnormalities in approximately 30% of cases and t(14;18) seen in approximately 20% to 30% of cases. The second rearrangement is associated with positivity for BCL2 expression by immunohistochemistry and has been associated as a poor prognostic finding.

There are a variety of morphologic patterns to diffuse large B-cell lymphoma, and the immunophenotype is varied as well.[223,224] The following observations have been made on a wide range of different large cell lymphomas: CD5 is generally negative,[126] although there are exceptions that do not seem to derive from mantle cell lymphoma or SLL[225]; BCL-2 (24% to 74%) and BAX expression correlate with poor outcome,[199,225-229] as may CD44[230] and caspase[231]; CD43 is present in 15% to 30%[86,113] of typical B-cell antigen-positive cases, and DBA.44[158] and CD99 are identified in some.[107] The Ki-67 index is high relative to lymphomas of small lymphocytes.[232] BCL-6, the protein associated with development of follicle center cells and with transformation of FL,[128,203] is detectable in 70% to 80% of diffuse large B-cell lymphomas.[85,199] CD10 is present about half the time.[85] Cytokeratin has rarely been identified in large cell lymphoma.[233] CD30-positive large B-cell lymphomas, anaplastic or otherwise, are not currently distinguished from other DLBCL in the WHO classification because there is no proven prognostic significance.[234]

Theranostic Applications

Several studies have implicated a germinal center phenotype versus an activated B-cell phenotype to offer prognostic information that is independent of standard staging procedures and even the international prognostic index (IPI). This prognostic information was first gleaned from gene expression profiling studies, which suggested lymphomas with a germinal center phenotype had a better prognosis than those with an activated B-cell phenotype. Further studies have shown that immunohistochemical surrogate markers may accomplish this same separation into these two categories. The strategic algorithm is shown in Fig. 6.14.

T cell–rich B-cell lymphomas are not immunophenotypically distinct from other DLBCLs,[235] except that they may be epithelial membrane antigen positive.

Subtypes of Diffuse Large B-Cell Lymphoma

Several distinct subtypes of diffuse large B-cell lymphoma distinguish themselves clinically, morphologically, immunophenoptypically, and genetically and are listed as follows.

MEDIASTINAL LARGE B-CELL LYMPHOMA[236] This unique entity presents in the mediastinum and is currently believed to have, as a normal counterpart, thymic medullary B cells. These lymphomas are CD20 and CD22 positive but CD21 negative.[237-239] CD43 is not coexpressed.[237] Typically, CD20 immunolabeling is quite strong. CD30 is expressed in more than half of the cases[240]; staining may be diffuse cytoplasmic rather than punctate.

This lymphoma is one of the few lymphomas that has an increased incidence in females and typically presents as a mediastinal mass in younger to middle-aged women. Morphologically this lymphoma tends to have clear cytoplasm, somewhat lobulated nuclei, and a background of fibrosis that may cause some confusion with other tumors, particularly in small-needle biopsies. This lymphoma is a mature B-cell lymphoma, and in addition to CD45, expresses the pan B-cell antigens CD19, CD20, PAX5, and CD79. The B-cell transcription factors Oct-2 and BOB.1 are typically present. CD30 may be demonstrated in a majority of these lymphomas; however, it may be only weakly or focally positive. The strong positivity of CD30 seen for anaplastic large cell lymphoma is rarely encountered in this lymphoma. Many of these lymphomas do not express the surface immunoglobulin but do have clonal rearrangements of the heavy chain genes. BCL2 and MUM1 are expressed in a majority of cases with few cases expressing CD10 and less commonly CD5. Because the main differential diagnosis for this lymphoma is classic Hodgkin lymphoma, the strong positivity for CD45 and pan B-cell antigens even in the face of partial CD30 positivity is helpful in solving this dilemma.

The expression of a lipid raft protein (MAL) has been detected in approximately 50% of cases and is thought to be quite specific for this lymphoma. MAL expression is typically not seen in other diffuse large B-cell lymphomas. MAL expression appears to be limited to a minor subpopulation of thymic medullary B cells, which lends further support for the thymic B-cell origin for this lymphoma.

BEYOND IMMUNOHISTOCHEMISTRY: ANATOMIC MOLECULAR DIAGNOSTIC APPLICATIONS This lymphoma has a characteristic chromosome abnormality with a gain of chromosome 9p. This gain encompasses c-REL and JAK2 leading to the overexpression of c-REL. Rearrangements of c-MYC and BCL2 are not demonstrated. Immunoglobulin gene rearrangements are present. The presence of BCL6 mutations/rearrangements is somewhat controversial in this lymphoma. Studies have demonstrated hypermutation of BCL6 in up to 54% of cases of MLBCL, though the site of hypermutation of BCL6 appears to be different from those found in follicular lymphomas and diffuse large B-cell lymphomas. Epstein-Barr virus (EBV) genome is absent in this lymphoma.

Gene expression profiling of this lymphoma reveals a surprising similarity with classical Hodgkin lymphoma. A recent study has demonstrated greater than 30% of similarity of genes that were highly expressed in an MLBCL and classical Hodgkin lymphoma versus other diffuse large B-cell lymphomas.

PRIMARY EFFUSION LYMPHOMA[241] A neoplasm induced by human herpes virus 8 (Kaposi's sarcoma–associated herpesvirus), this large cell lymphoma is limited to the pleural, peritoneal, and pericardial spaces of immunosuppressed patients who are virally infected. Most cases fail to express either B- or T-cell markers and are frequently CD30 positive.[242,243]

INTRAVASCULAR LARGE B-CELL LYMPHOMA[244-246] The majority of cases express B-cell markers, although T cells have been reported. A variety of lymphocyte homing receptors have been discovered on the cell surface, allowing one to hypothesize about the mechanism of restriction of the lymphoma cells to the intravascular space.[245,247]

This is an uncommon subtype of large B-cell lymphoma. This lymphoma presents with exclusive localization of vascular spaces and does not form a tissue mass. The symptomatology associated with this lymphoma may be rather nonspecific, and the diagnosis may be made from such sites as skin biopsies for rashes or nerve biopsies for associated neurologic complaints. It is not uncommon for this lymphoma diagnosis to be made on autopsy. The immunophenotype of this lymphoma is positive for CD45; the pan B-cell antigens CD19, CD20, and CD79; and PAX5, with positivity for BCL2 and variable expression for CD10 and BCL6. Because this is such an uncommon lymphoma, recurrent genetic abnormalities have not been identified, but they do demonstrate rearranged immunoglobulin genes.

PRIMARY DIFFUSE LARGE B-CELL LYMPHOMA OF THE CENTRAL NERVOUS SYSTEM This is the most common lymphoma seen in the central nervous system and is more common in immunocompromised individuals. When this lymphoma develops in immunocompetent individuals, the age of presentation is higher than those who are immunocompromised. The diagnosis of this lymphoma can be challenging because large amounts of background necrosis are present in the biopsies, which may be quite small. These lymphomas characteristically have a perivascular localization. These lymphomas express CD45 along with the pan B-cell markers CD19 and CD20 and have variable expressions for BCL2 and BCL6. Recent studies have shown that these lymphomas typically have an activated B-cell phenotype with virtually all of these lymphomas expressing MUM1 with negativity for CD10. EBV is usually absent in lymphomas arising in immunocompetent individuals but may be expressed in immunosuppressed patients.

Several recurrent cytogenetic abnormalities have been reported in these lymphomas with abnormalities of 1q21, 6q, 7q, 12q, and 14q described. These lymphomas have clonal rearrangements of their immunoglobulin genes.

ALK-POSITIVE DIFFUSE LARGE B-CELL LYMPHOMA This is a rare and unusual subgroup of diffuse large B-cell lymphoma and has an unusual immunophenotype, which can lead to diagnostic confusion. Morphologically, the tumor cells have a resemblance to anaplastic large T-cell lymphoma cells. The tumor cells are positive for CD138, dim to partial CD45+, and epithelial membrane antigen and may also have expression of CD4 but are negative for the pan B-cell markers CD19, CD20, CD22, and CD79, as well as pan T-cell markers CD2, CD3, CD5, and CD7. These lymphomas are negative for CD8 and C30 with the negativity for CD30 assisting in the differential diagnosis of the anaplastic large cell lymphoma. As the name implies, these lymphomas are characteristically positive with ALK and the pattern of positivity is in a granular cytoplasmic pattern. Involvement of the clathrin gene at 17q23 has been shown to be involved in a translocation with the ALK gene(2p23) in many instances.

T-CELL/HISTIOCYTE-RICH B-CELL LYMPHOMA This subgroup of diffuse large B-cell lymphomas is composed of large tumor cells surrounded by a robust benign inflammatory infiltrate consisting of predominantly T cells and/or histiocytes, as the name implies. The differential diagnosis includes separation from a benign process or even lymphocyte-predominant Hodgkin lymphoma. The tumor cells are positive for CD45 and the pan B-cell markers CD19, CD20, CD79, and PAX5 and will have BCL6, BCL2, and CD10. The tumor cells are surrounded by large areas of reactive T cells.

PRIMARY CUTANEOUS LARGE B-CELL LYMPHOMA Two types of primary cutaneous large B-cell lymphomas are recognized.

Primary cutaneous large B-cell lymphoma, follicular center type presents as a subcutaneous mass in an area above the waist (trunk and head). Morphologically this lymphoma consists of a mixture of centrocytes and centroblasts with centroblast predominating and can have a follicular or diffuse growth pattern. The typical immunophenotype is positivity for CD45 and the pan B-cell antigens CD19, CD20, CD79, and PAX5, with variable positivity for CD10, BCL2, and BCL6 (giving rise to the follicular center cell phenotype) but usually negativity for MUM1 and BCL1. Translocations for c-myc, BCL2, and BCL6 are not present. Immunoglobulin gene rearrangement is present.

Primary cutaneous large B-cell lymphoma of the leg presents as a subcutaneous mass most commonly on the leg but may be seen in other locations. There is a slight female predominance for this lymphoma. Morphologically this lymphoma consists of sheets of centroblasts. Immunoblast may be noted, but there are few centrocytes, if any. The immunophenotype is positive for CD45 and the pan B-cell antigens CD19, CD20, CD79, and PAX5. BCL2, BCL6, and MUM1 are negative. Clonal rearrangements of immunoglobulin genes are present, and there may be translocations for myc, BCL6, and IgH genes. The BCL2/IGH rearrangement is not present in this lymphoma.

The importance of recognizing these two subtypes is in the difference in prognosis of these two lymphomas, with the primary cutaneous large B-cell lymphoma follicle center cell–type having an excellent prognosis with at least a 90% five-year survival rate versus a 55% five-year survival for primary cutaneous large B-cell lymphoma of the leg.

KEY DIAGNOSTIC POINTS
Diffuse Large B-Cell Lymphoma

- CD45RB and either CD20 or CD79a, along with S-100, cytokeratin, CD3, and CD30, form a useful panel for large cell neoplasms.
- CD30 positivity in large B-cell lymphomas is usually present in a minority of B cells, may be related to plasmacytic differentiation, and has no prognostic significance.
- Sheets of large B cells are unusual in reactive conditions and should raise strong concern for lymphoma.

BURKITT LYMPHOMA/LEUKEMIA

Typical phenotype: B-cell antigen +, CD10+/–, CD5–

Burkitt and Burkitt-like lymphoma are difficult to reproducibly categorize on morphology alone—although their natural histories may be distinctive—and have been collapsed into one category in the WHO classification.[7] CD19, CD20, and CD79a are all present and CD5 and CD23 are usually absent. In an important difference from lymphoblastic lymphoma/leukemia, TdT is not found in the nuclei of Burkitt cells.[249] Ki-67 is (not unexpectedly given the growth fraction) highly expressed, and Burkitt lymphoma has been defined as having a Ki-67 index of nearly 100%.[7] BCL-2 and CD10 have a roughly reciprocal relationship in the two variants of Burkitt lymphoma/leukemia: The incidence of CD10 positivity is high in Burkitt and low in Burkitt-like, whereas BCL-2 is high in Burkitt-like and low in Burkitt.[46] CD43 also serves to distinguish the two immunophenotypically: It is almost always present in Burkitt and present less than half the time in Burkitt-like.[113]

BEYOND IMMUNOHISTOCHEMISTRY: ANATOMIC MOLECULAR DIAGNOSTIC APPLICATIONS A common and unifying cytogenetic abnormality present in Burkitt lymphoma regardless of subtype is a translocation of myc (8q24) to the immunoglobulin heavy chain (14q32) and less commonly to one of the light chains (κ at 2p12 or γ at 22q11). The different subtypes of Burkitt lymphoma display differences in the breakpoints of myc. In sporadic Burkitt lymphoma the breakpoint is immediately 5′ to myc and predominantly involves the switch region of IGH. In the endemic Burkitt lymphoma, the breakpoint tends to be farther away from myc (>100 kb 5′) and involves predominantly the J region of the IGH. Burkitt lymphoma arising in immunocompromised individuals notably rearranges myc within the first exon/intron and involves predominantly the switch region of IGH.

Fortunately commercially available probes are available to flank the entire myc region, allowing for its detection in all of the previously mentioned translocations. Break-apart probes for FISH testing in formalin-fixed, paraffin-embedded tissue provide a powerful tool for the detection of myc rearrangement.

KEY DIAGNOSTIC POINTS

Burkitt Lymphoma

At times, Burkitt lymphoma may be difficult to separate from the following:
- Diffuse large B-cell lymphoma
- Precursor B or T lymphoblastic lymphoma/leukemia
- Blastic variant of mantle cell lymphoma

The blastic variant of mantle cell lymphoma can be separated from Burkitt lymphoma by the presence of CD5 and cyclin D1 positivity in mantle cell lymphoma.

Precursor B or T lymphoblastic lymphoma/leukemia has a similar overall cell size to Burkitt lymphoma but tends to have finer chromatin with inconspicuous nucleoli. These lymphomas have an immature phenotype and usually demonstrate positivity for TDT and/or CD34 with dim positivity for CD20 at best, and the absence of surface immunoglobulin allows a separation from Burkitt lymphoma.

The most problematic differential diagnosis occurs in the separation of diffuse large B-cell lymphoma from Burkitt lymphoma, which can be difficult on a small specimen. The morphology of diffuse large B-cell lymphoma is usually that of larger centroblasts, though more variable morphology can certainly be seen in Burkitt lymphoma. If the lymphoma has an MIB1 labeling index less than 95% and is positive for BCL2 and/or MUM1, then a diagnosis of diffuse large B-cell lymphoma is favored. If on the other hand the immunophenotype is that of the germinal center cell with CD10 and BCL6 positivity and negativity for BCL2 and MUM1, as well as a greater than 95% labeling index, the separation is more difficult. If the myc rearrangement is present, a diagnosis of Burkitt lymphoma is favored, but it must be remembered that rearrangement is not exclusive to Burkitt lymphoma and is seen in a small percentage of diffuse large B-cell lymphomas. The presence or absence of a BCL2 rearrangement may be helpful.

The distinction between Burkitt lymphoma and diffuse large B-cell lymphoma is not so necessarily clear-cut. Evidence suggests that some lymphomas have a double hit in that they are positive for both myc rearrangement and BCL2 rearrangement. These lymphomas have a higher proliferation fraction and may actually respond better to Burkitt lymphoma therapy than to standard diffuse large B-cell therapy.

LYMPHOMATOID GRANULOMATOSIS

Typical phenotype: B-cell antigen +, CD30+/−, CD15−, LMP+

Lymphomatoid granulomatosis is a lymphoproliferative disorder found in extranodal sites, particularly the lungs, of patients with either acquired or inherited immunodeficiency. EBV-transformed B cells are thought to spark a brisk T-cell response.[250] This leads to an angiocentric, infarctive process with a polymorphous lymphoid infiltrate and a range of appearances, from inflammatory to overt large cell lymphoma. Paraffin section immunohistochemistry is frequently crucial to the identification of the large, atypical B cells (CD20 positive) that are LMP positive amid a background of T cells. Although the large cells are cytologically atypical and may be CD30 positive, no true Reed-Sternberg cells are seen.

T- AND NK-CELL NEOPLASMS

Precursor T-Cell Neoplasms

PRECURSOR T-LYMPHOBLASTIC LEUKEMIA/LYMPHOMA

Typical phenotype: CD1a+/−, CD2+/−, CD3+ (always cytoplasmic CD3+), CD4/CD8 double positive or double negative, CD5+/−, CD7+, CD10−/+, TdT+, CD16−, CD57−, B antigen −

Lymphoblasts of this disease are morphologically indistinguishable from precursor B lymphoblastic lymphoma/leukemia and require immunologic analysis. TdT is uniformly expressed. In addition to the usual B and T lineage-specific antibodies, both the TAL-1 (SCL) protein and the c-kit receptor can be used to distinguish the nature of the malignancy. Antibodies to each of these proteins will detect approximately 40% to 50% of T lymphoblastic tumors and none of the B lineage cases.[251,252] The differential diagnosis with other blastic malignancies is usually straightforward: the blastoid variant of mantle cell lymphoma is TdT negative and marks as a mature B cell tumor, whereas granulocytic sarcomas are TdT negative and frequently myeloperoxidase or lysozyme positive. Note that CD43, in addition to identifying T-cell malignancies, also marks many myelogenous processes.[251] CD99 expression is almost universal in precursor T-cell ALL[107]; this fact must be borne in mind when considering the differential diagnosis of pediatric small cell tumors.

Mature T-Cell Neoplasms

Immunohistochemical analysis can be extremely helpful in the diagnosis and classification of the peripheral (or mature) T-cell neoplasms. Although there are no immunologic markers of T-cell clonality analogous to immunoglobulin light chains, there are aberrant patterns of antigen expression that are rarely if ever found in normal mature T cells.[39,253] Cells that are "double positive" for CD4 and CD8 (express both) or are "double negative" (express neither) are normally minor populations outside of the thymus. Similarly, loss of one or more pan T-cell antigens such as CD2, CD3, CD5, TCRαβ, or, most frequently, CD7, are supportive of a diagnosis of T-cell lymphoma. Of course, benign cases serve as exceptions to the rule. Most of these analyses can be carried out only on fresh or frozen tissue and are therefore of limited use in the average pathology laboratory. Flow cytometry or consultation with a reference laboratory may be necessary.

Several of the mature T-cell leukemias are so rarely seen in surgical pathology specimens that only their usual phenotypes are supplied.

T-CELL PROLYMPHOCYTIC LEUKEMIA

Typical phenotype: CD2+, CD3+, CD4+ (65%), CD5+, CD7+, CD4+, CD8+ (21%), CD25−

T-CELL LARGE GRANULAR LYMPHOCYTIC LEUKEMIA

Typical phenotype: CD2+, CD3+, CD4−, CD5−, CD7−, CD8+, TCRαβ+, CD16+, CD56−, CD57+/−, CD25−

AGGRESSIVE NK-CELL LEUKEMIA

Typical phenotype: CD2+, CD3−, CD4−, CD8+/−, TCRαβ−, CD16+, CD56+/−, CD57+/−

These leukemias may express the cytotoxic granule-associated protein TIA-1, which is normally found in natural killer cells and cytotoxic T lymphocytes regardless of their state of activation.[254] The tumor cells are commonly EBV infected.[255]

ADULT T-CELL LYMPHOMA/LEUKEMIA

Typical phenotype: CD2+, CD3+, CD4+ (most cases), CD5+, CD7−, CD25+

Another virally induced leukemia/lymphoma (this one attributable to HTLV1), ATLL commonly presents with an elevated white blood cell count but also has a pure lymphomatous form. In either case the diagnosis is most convincingly made by demonstration of clonal viral DNA in tumor cells by molecular biologic methods. The histologically heterogeneous pattern makes this tumor practically indistinguishable from unspecified peripheral T-cell lymphomas absent the characteristic clinical presentation.[256] CD25 expression is typically strong. A CD30-positive version of the malignancy accounting for approximately 20% of cases frequently presents extranodally and lacks leukemic manifestations but has similar survival as CD30-negative cases.[257]

EXTRANODAL NK/T-CELL LYMPHOMA, NASAL TYPE

Typical phenotype: CD2+, CD3−, CD4−/+, CD8−/+, CD5−/+, CD7−/+, CD56+, CD43+, TCRαβ−, EBV-LMP-1+/−

As with most of the T-cell lymphomas, the distinct clinical presentation (found more often in Asia, aggressive extranodal disease, often midfacial, with necrosis) is crucial to the diagnosis of this entity,[255] formerly known as *angiocentric lymphoma* or *lymphomatoid granulomatosis*. Angiocentricity and angioinvasiveness (leading to infarctive necrosis) are frequent, but not specific, features. This disease is intimately related to EBV infection (proven molecularly), and some cases may carry the EBV latent membrane protein (LMP-1) in tumor cells, demonstrable by paraffin section immunohistochemistry.[258-260] The expression of cytotoxic granule antigens (also detectable immunohistochemically) such as TIA-1, granzyme B, and perforin implies that this lymphoma is derived from an activated natural killer cell or, less commonly, cytotoxic T-cell precursor.[254,261-264] Pulmonary cases appear more convincingly to be B-cell large cell lymphomas.[250]

ENTEROPATHY-TYPE T-CELL LYMPHOMA

Typical phenotype: CD3+, CD4−, CD7+, CD8+/−, CD56−, CD103+

Intestinal T-cell lymphoma most often occurs in patients with gluten-sensitive enteropathy and presents with refractory, perforating ulcers in the jejunum. A mass may or may not be evident. The histology is heterogeneous, although a subset of cases comprises monomorphic medium-sized cells. Tropism for the epithelium is usually marked. Most of the intestinal lymphocytes exhibit a cytotoxic T-cell phenotype (TIA-1 and granzyme B positive) with CD56 expression relatively infrequent.[254,264,265] EBV infection as assessed either immunohistochemically or by *in situ* hybridization is infrequent.[266] ALCL involving the gastrointestinal tract has been described,[267] but it is not clear that these tumors belong to the enteropathy-type category. P53 is almost universally overexpressed.[268] CD103, an integrin alpha chain that is present on more than 90% of normal intestinal intraepithelial lymphocytes and likely plays a role in homing to epithelia, is present on all enteropathy-type T-cell lymphomas. The B-ly-7 antibody recognizing this epitope is not useful in fixed tissue.

HEPATOSPLENIC T-CELL LYMPHOMA

Typical phenotype: CD2+, CD3+, CD4−, CD5−, CD7+, CD8+/−, CD56+/−, TCRγδ+ (some TCRαβ+), EBV-LMP-1−

This rare primary hepatic lymphoma is composed of CD56+ T cells, most in a nonactivated state as assessed by the presence of TIA-1 and absence of perforin and granzyme B.[261,262,269] An unusual feature of these lymphomas is the expression of T-cell receptors of the γδ type, rather than the more common αβ heterodimer.[270] This can be determined on fixed, paraffin-embedded material now that satisfactory antibodies are available (βF1 and TCRγδ).

SUBCUTANEOUS PANNICULITIS-LIKE T-CELL LYMPHOMA

Typical phenotype: CD3+, CD4−, CD8+/− CD30−, CD43+, CD45RO+, CD56− TIA-1+, perforin +, granzyme B +, TCRαβ+

Subcutaneous panniculitis-like lymphoma, as the name indicates, has a distinct site of involvement and morphologic pattern. The epidermis is usually spared, the tumor cells surround the dermal fat cells but do not efface them, and there is often angioinvasion by lymphocytes but no substantial infarction. Most cases are of the CD8 type and generally do not express CD56.[271,272] All have an activated cytotoxic T-cell profile but, interestingly, CD30 is only infrequently identified.[272] Immunologic distinction from other T-cell lymphomas that may involve the panniculus such as nasal-type NK/T-cell lymphoma may be based in part on the absence of CD56 (although some cutaneous angiocentric lymphomas are CD56 negative and not EBV related[273]) and in part on the absence of an epidermal component or angiodestruction. Primary cutaneous anaplastic large cell lymphoma may extend to the subcutis and mimic SPTCL, but judicious interpretation of CD30 can assist in separating them.

MYCOSIS FUNGOIDES/SÉZARY SYNDROME

Typical phenotype: CD2+, CD3+, CD4+, CD5+, CD7−/+, CD8−, CD25−, TCRαβ+

Mycosis fungoides (MF) and its leukemic counterpart, Sézary syndrome, are nearly indistinguishable from one another immunophenotypically. Together, they form the bulk of T-cell lymphomas seen in the United States. The primary difficulty in diagnosing MF lies in the distinction from pseudo-lymphomas or reactive lesions of any etiology. In addition to the standard morphologic clues and molecular testing for T-cell gene rearrangements, immunohistochemistry can provide some guidance. MF frequently exhibits one or more aberrations in phenotype compared with normal T cells: CD7 is often lost,[274] approximately two thirds of cases lose another antigen (CD2, CD3, and/or CD5),[275] and βF1 and CD3 (normally coexpressed) may be discordant.[276] Admixtures of B cells and CD8-positive lymphocytes are also much more common in reactive conditions than in MF.[275] Characteristically, S-100 and CD1a-positive Langerhans' and interdigitating reticulum cells accompany the MF cells,[277] both in the dermis and in Pautrier's microabscesses. Large-cell transformation of MF may be correlated with p53 expression detected immunohistochemically.[278]

KEY DIAGNOSTIC POINTS

Mycosis Fungoides

- Pan–T-cell antigen loss may be demonstrable in many cases of mycosis fungoides, particularly if frozen section immunology is available.
- Abundant B cells or CD8+ T cells argue against MF.

PRIMARY CUTANEOUS CD30-POSITIVE T-CELL LYMPHOPROLIFERATIVE DISORDERS

Typical phenotype: CD3+, CD4+, CD8−, CD15+, CD30+, EMA−, ALK−

The presence of the CD30 molecule is crucial to the recognition of primary cutaneous anaplastic large cell lymphoma and the related CD30+ lymphoproliferative disorder, lymphomatoid papulosis.[279,280] The distinction is important for patient management because these proliferations do remarkably well with conservative therapy. The anaplastic cells may be monomorphous or polymorphous and range in number from few (in lymphomatoid papulosis type A) to numerous or sheetlike (in lymphomatoid papulosis type C and primary cutaneous ALCL). Although CD4 positive and CD8 negative, the lymphocytes have the phenotype of activated cytotoxic cells in their expression of TIA-1 and granzyme B.[281,282] EMA and ALK (anaplastic lymphoma kinase; the gene is involved in the t(2;5) translocation in roughly 40% to 80% of ALCL) may be found in cutaneous CD30-positive ALCL, but these are typically not primary cutaneous types and have a poorer prognosis.[92,283,284] CD30-negative large cell lymphoma also may not belong in the primary cutaneous ALCL disease category because it exhibits a poorer outcome.[285,286] EBV infection, as assessed by LMP-1, does not play a role in this disease.[287] The antibody HECA-452 detects an antigen on most normal skin-resident lymphocytes; the antigen is found on nearly half of primary cutaneous ALCL but no nodal ALCL.[92]

ANGIOIMMUNOBLASTIC T-CELL LYMPHOMA

Typical phenotype: CD2+, CD3+, CD4+, CD8−/+, CD21, and CD23+ (in proliferated follicular dendritic cells)

It is primarily the characteristic clinical features (prominent systemic symptoms, modest systemic lymphadenopathy, polyclonal gammopathy, and complications from autoantibodies and infections) that separate this entity from other peripheral T-cell lymphomas. Morphologically, there is a prominent, arborizing network of high endothelial vessels, a generalized paucity of lymphocytes, hyperplastic dendritic cell islands, and clusters of medium-sized lymphs with pale cytoplasm. The latter mark as CD4-positive T cells, with no evidence of cytotoxic differentiation.[254,262] The islands of proliferated follicular dendritic cells are characteristic of the entity and can be highlighted by antibodies to CD21 and CD23.[288] Large B cells may be found scattered through the node; these should not be mistaken for T-cell-rich B-cell lymphoma. Approximately two thirds of cases show LMP-1 positivity, with both B and T cells infected.[289] Data suggest that EBV infection is not causative but is related to the immunosuppression of the disorder; B-cell clones driven by EBV infection may explain the occasional B immunoblastic lymphoma that develops in these cases.[290]

PERIPHERAL T-CELL LYMPHOMA, UNSPECIFIED

Typical phenotype: T-cell antigens variable, CD4+ > CD8+ (may be double negative), rare B antigen +

A "wastebasket" category of post-thymic T-cell lymphomas,[256] this group is best defined by what it is not (i.e., one of the specific peripheral T-cell lymphomas).

Cytologically, there is a spectrum of T-cell sizes and sometimes an admixture of histiocytes or eosinophils. Distinction from a reactive process may be difficult immunohistochemically unless frozen tissue can be examined for antigenic loss or inappropriate expression characteristic of T-cell lymphoma.[76,276,291,292] TIA-1 is present in a minority of cases, particularly those in extranodal sites,[254] and LMP-1 expression is infrequent.[293]

ANAPLASTIC LARGE CELL LYMPHOMA

Typical phenotype: CD45RB+/–, CD3–/+, T-cell antigens variable, CD15–/+, CD21–, CD25+/–, CD30+, CD43–/+, CD45RO–/+, EMA+/–, CD68–, lysozyme–, ALK+/–

The systemic form of ALCL is one of the more common types of non-Hodgkin lymphoma, but because of its early sinusoidal localization in nodes and its pleomorphic cellular composition it may not be recognized as a lymphoma at all. The anaplastic lymphoma cells are large, with prominent nucleoli, convoluted, Reed-Sternberg-like nuclei, and a somewhat cohesive appearance. The phenotype is readily recognizable but may present some difficulty to the unwary.[90,294] LCA (CD45RB) is present in most cases; one review indicated a frequency of 70% to 80%, but paraffin-embedded tissue may yield a lower fraction.[295] The lineage is more frequently T cell than "null" cell (lacking both B- and T-cell markers). ALCL has a T lineage in 70% of cases, B lineage in 15% (these are considered diffuse large B-cell lymphomas), B and T in 5%, and null in 10%.[294] CD30 is by definition expressed in these tumors, with CD15 generally not seen.[91,296] CD30 decorates the cell membrane and marks the Golgi area in a paranuclear dotlike fashion; diffuse cytoplasmic positivity may represent nonspecific background staining or staining of benign large transformed cells. EMA is focal in many cases, and antibodies to cytokeratin are reported to stain the perinuclear area of rare cases.[296] As mentioned earlier, the cutaneous lymphocyte antibody HECA-452 marks less than 20% of primary systemic cases.[92] Detection of the latent membrane protein of EBV has been variable.[91,297] The small cell variant and lymphohistiocytic variant each have fewer large cells than prototypical cases, but the malignant cells maintain the expected phenotype.[298-300] The ALK protein is overexpressed in 43% to 75% of tumors; its presence correlates with EMA expression and increased patient survival.[301-304] Like many other mature T-cell lymphomas, primary systemic ALCL often exhibits a cytotoxic T-cell phenotype owing to its production of TIA-1 and granzyme B.[254,305-307] P53 is evident in the cytoplasm (>60% of cases), but mutations in the gene have not been isolated.[308,309] CD30 and EMA expression has been used as an immunohistochemical marker of minimal disease in the bone marrow.[310]

Hodgkin lymphoma is the most frequent differential in the diagnosis of systemic ALCL. Immunophenotyping can be invaluable if the typical LCA+/CD15–/T-cell marker +/EMA+/ALK+ picture is present. Borderline cases may be difficult to resolve even following molecular analysis. Carcinomas may be distinguished from ALCL by the presence of cytokeratins (rare in lymphoma) and absence of common and lineage-specific lymphocyte antigens. CD30 has been reported in germ cell tumors and melanoma. Melanoma, of course, may be excluded by its expression of S-100 and HMB45.

KEY DIAGNOSTIC POINTS

Anaplastic Large Cell Lymphoma

- Most cases of systemic ALCL are LCA+, CD3+, CD43+, and CD30+.
- Look for CD30 in a Golgi and cell membrane pattern.
- EMA and ALK positivity, along with T lineage markers, help to distinguish ALCL from Hodgkin lymphoma; fascin is usually negative in ALCL.

Summary

The diagnosis of NHL is complex. Immunohistology is but one part of the investigation process, which must also include clinical, morphologic, flow cytometric, and genetic information. All of these venues have greatly affected theranostic aspects of these diseases.

REFERENCES

1. Harris NL, Jaffe ES, Stein H, et al. A revised European-American classification of lymphoid neoplasms: a proposal from the International Lymphoma Study Group. *Blood.* 1994;84(5):1361-1392.
2. Poppema S. Lymphoma classification proposal. *Blood.* 1996; 87(1):412-413.
3. Meijer CJ, van der Valk P, de Bruin PC, et al. The revised European-American lymphoma (REAL) classification of non-Hodgkin's lymphoma: a missed opportunity? *Blood.* 1995; 85(7):1971-1972.
4. Rosenberg SA. Classification of lymphoid neoplasms. *Blood.* 1994;84(5):1359-1360.
5. Pittaluga S, Bijnens L, Teodorovic I, et al. Clinical analysis of 670 cases in two trials of the European Organization for the Research and Treatment of Cancer Lymphoma Cooperative Group subtyped according to the Revised European-American Classification of Lymphoid Neoplasms: a comparison with the Working Formulation. *Blood.* 1996;87(10):4358-4367.
6. A clinical evaluation of the International Lymphoma Study Group classification of non-Hodgkin's lymphoma. The Non-Hodgkin's Lymphoma Classification Project. *Blood.* 1997;89(11):3909-3918.
7. Jaffe ES, Harris NL, Stein H, et al. *Pathology and Genetics of Tumours of Haematopoietic and Lymphoid Tissues.* Lyon, France: IARC Press; 2001.
8. Jaffe ES, Harris NL, Diebold J, et al. World Health Organization Classification of lymphomas: a work in progress. *Ann Oncol.* 1998;9(Suppl 5):S25-S30.
9. Harris NL, Jaffe ES, Diebold J, et al. The World Health Organization classification of hematological malignancies report of the Clinical Advisory Committee Meeting, Airlie House, Virginia, November 1997 World Health Organization classification of neoplastic diseases of the hematopoietic and lymphoid tissues. A progress report. *Mod Pathol.* 2000;13(2):193-207.
10. Abbondanzo SL. Paraffin immunohistochemistry as an adjunct to hematopathology. *Ann Diagn Pathol.* 1999;3(5):318-327.
11. Chu PG, Chang KL, Arber DA, et al. Practical applications of immunohistochemistry in hematolymphoid neoplasms. *Ann Diagn Pathol.* 1999;3(2):104-133.

12. Leucocyte Typing VI , et al. White Cell Differentiation Antigens. In: Kishimoto T, Goyert S, Kikutani H, eds. *Sixth International Workshop and Conference; 1997*. Kobe, Japan: Garland Publishers; 1997.
13. Pileri SA, Roncador G, Ceccarelli C, et al. Antigen retrieval techniques in immunohistochemistry: comparison of different methods. *J Pathol*. 1997;183(1):116-123.
14. Shi SR, Cote RJ, Taylor CR. Antigen retrieval immunohistochemistry: past, present, and future. *J Histochem Cytochem*. 1997;45(3):327-343.
15. Shi SR, Key ME, Kalra KL. Antigen retrieval in formalin-fixed, paraffin-embedded tissues: an enhancement method for immunohistochemical staining based on microwave oven heating of tissue sections. *J Histochem Cytochem*. 1991;39(6):741-748.
16. Johnson K, Chensue S, Ward P. Immunopathology. In: Rubin E, Farber J, eds. *Pathology*. 3rd ed. Philadelphia: Lippincott-Raven; 1999:104-153.
17. Inghirami G, Knowles D. The immune system: structure and function. In: Knowles D, ed. *Neoplastic Hematopathology*. Baltimore: Williams & Wilkins; 1992:27-72.
18. Benoist C, Mathis D. T lymphocyte differentiation and biology. In: Paul W, ed. *Fundamental Immunology*. 4th ed. Philadelphia: Lippincott-Raven Publishers; 1999:367-410.
19. DeFranco AB. Lymphocyte activation. In: Paul W, ed. *Fundamental Immunology*. 4 ed. Philadelphia: Lippincott-Raven Publishers; 1999:225-261.
20. Melchers F, Rolink A. B-lymphocyte development and biology. In: Paul W, ed. *Fundamental Immunology*. 4th ed. Philadelphia: Lippincott-Raven Publishers; 1999:183-224.
21. Rudin CM, Thompson CB. B-cell development and maturation. *Semin Oncol*. 1998;25(4):435-446.
22. Lennert K, Feller A. *Histopathology of Non-Hodgkin's Lymphomas*. 2nd ed. Berlin: Springer-Verlag; 1992.
23. Lukes R, Collins R. A functional approach to the classification of malignant lymphoma. *Recent Results Cancer Res*. 1974;46:18-30.
24. Lukes RJ, Collins RD. Immunologic characterization of human malignant lymphomas. *Cancer*. 1974;34(4 Suppl):1488-1503.
25. Stetler-Stevenson M, Medieros L, Jaffe E. Immunophenotypic methods and findings in the diagnosis of lymphoproliferative diseases. In: Jaffe E, ed. *Surgical Pathology of the Lymph Nodes and Related Organs*. 2nd ed. Philadelphia: WB Saunders; 1995: 22-57.
26. Nitschke L, Tsubata T. Molecular interactions regulate BCR signal inhibition by CD22 and CD72. *Trends Immunol*. 2004;25(10):543-550.
27. Mason DY, Cordell JL, Brown MH, et al. CD79a: a novel marker for B-cell neoplasms in routinely processed tissue samples. *Blood*. 1995;86(4):1453-1459.
28. Dorshkind K. Chapter 8—B-Cell Development. In: Hoffman R, ed. *Hematology: basic principles and practice*. 3rd ed. New York: Churchill Livingstone; 2000:2584.
29. Chizuka A, Kanda Y, Nannya Y, et al. The diagnostic value of kappa/lambda ratios determined by flow cytometric analysis of biopsy specimens in B-cell lymphoma. *Clin Haematol*. 2002;24(1):33-36.
30. Samoszuk MK, Krailo M, Yan QH, et al. Limitations of numerical ratios for defining monoclonality of immunoglobulin light chains in B-cell lymphomas. *Diagn Immunol*. 1985;3(3):133-138.
31. Aguilera NS, Kapadia SB, Nalesnik MA, et al. Extramedullary plasmacytoma of the head and neck: use of paraffin sections to assess clonality with in situ hybridization, growth fraction, and the presence of Epstein-Barr virus. *Mod Pathol*. 1995;8(5):503-508.
32. Beck RC, Tubbs RR, Hussein M, et al. Automated colorimetric in situ hybridization (CISH) detection of immunoglobulin (Ig) light chain mRNA expression in plasma cell (PC) dyscrasias and non-Hodgkin lymphoma. *Diagn Mol Pathol*. 2003;12(1):14-20.
33. Lee LH, Cioc A, Nuovo GJ. Determination of light chain restriction in fine-needle aspiration-type preparations of B-cell lymphomas by mRNA in situ hybridization. *Appl Immunohistochem Mol Morphol*. 2004;12(3):252-258.
34. Pringle JH, Ruprai AK, Primrose L, et al. In situ hybridization of immunoglobulin light chain mRNA in paraffin sections using biotinylated or hapten-labelled oligonucleotide probes. *J Pathol*. 1990;162(3):197-207.
35. Iida S, Rao PH, Butler M, et al. Deregulation of MUM1/IRF4 by chromosomal translocation in multiple myeloma. *Nat Genet*. 1997;17:226-230.
36. Matsuyama T, Grossman A, Mittrucker H-W, et al. Molecular cloning of LSIRF, a lymphoid-specific member of the interferon regulatory factor family that binds the interferon-stimulated response element (ISRE). *Nucleic Acids Res*. 1995;23:2127-2136.
37. Grossman A, Mittrucker H-W, Nicholl J, et al. Cloning of human lymphocyte-specific interferon regulatory factor (hLSIRF-hIRF4) and mapping of the gene to 6p23-p25. *Genomics*. 1996:37229-37233.
38. Carbone A, Gloghini A, Larocca LM, et al. Expression profile of MUM1/IRF4, BCL-6, and CD138/syndecan-1 defines novel histogenetic subsets of human immunodeficiency virus-related lymphomas. *Blood*. 2001;97:744-751.
39. Gaidano G, Carbone A. MUM1: a step ahead toward the understanding of lymphoma histogenesis. *Leukemia*. 2000;14:563-566.
40. Tsuboi K, Iida S, Inagaki H, et al. MUM1/IRF4 expression as a frequent event in mature lymphoid malignancies. *Leukemia*. 2000;14:449-456.
41. Natkunam Y, Warnke RA, Montgomery K, et al. Analysis of MUM1/IRF4 protein expression using tissue microarrays and immunohistochemistry. *Mod Pathol*. 2001;14:686-694.
42. Dhodapkar MV, Abe E, Theus A, et al. Syndecan-1 is a multifunctional regulator of myeloma pathobiology: control of tumor cell survival, growth, and bone cell differentiation. *Blood*. 1998;91:2679-2688.
43. Falini B, Fizzotti M, Pucciarini A, et al. A monoclonal antibody (MUM1p) detects expression of the MUM1/IRF4 protein in a subset of germinal center B cells, plasma cells, and activated T cells. *Blood*. 2000;95:2084-2092. 1998;92:1011-1019.
44. Steimle-Grauer SA, Tinguely M, Seada L, et al. Expression patterns of transcription factors in progressively transformed germinal centers and Hodgkin lymphoma. *Virchows Arch*. 2003;442:284-293.
45. Buettner M, Greiner A, Avramidou A, et al. Evidence of abortive plasma cell differentiation in Hodgkin and Reed-Sternberg cell of classical Hodgkin lymphoma. *Hematol Oncol*. 2005;23:127-132.
46. Carbone A, Gloghini A, Aldinucci D, et al. Expression pattern of MUM1/IRF4 in the spectrum of pathology of Hodgkin's disease. *Br J Haematol*. 2002;117:366-372.
47. Bai M, Panoulas V, Papoudou-Bai A, et al. B-cell differentiation immunophenotypes in classical Hodgkin lymphomas. *Leuk Lymphoma*. 2006;47:495-501.
48. Pileri SA, Ascani S, Leoncini L, et al. Hodgkin's lymphoma: the pathologist's viewpoint. *J Clin Pathol*. 2002;55:162-176. *J Cutan Pathol*. 2005;32:647-674.
49. Barberis A, Widenhorn K, Vitelli L, et al. A novel B-cell lineage-specific transcription factor present at early but not late stages of differentiation. *Genes Dev*. 1990;4:849-859.
50. Dahl E, Koseki H, Balling R. Pax genes and organogenesis. *Bioessays*. 1997;19:755-765.
51. Muratovska A, Zhou C, He S, et al. Paired-box genes are frequently expressed in cancer and often required for cancer cell survival. *Oncogene*. 2003;22:7989-7997.
52. Urbanek P, Wang ZQ, Fetka I, et al. Complete block of early B cell differentiation and altered patterning of the posterior midbrain in mice lacking Pax5/BSAP. *Cell*. 1994;79:901-912.
53. Adams B, Dorfler P, Aguzzi A, et al. Pax-5 encodes the transcription factor BSAP and is expressed in B lymphocytes, the developing CNS, and adult testis. *Genes Dev*. 1992;6:1589-1607.
54. Horowitz MC, Xi Y, Pflugh DL, et al. Pax5-deficient mice exhibit early onset osteopenia with increased osteoclast progenitors. *J Immunol*. 2004;173:6583-6591.
55. Busslinger M. Transcriptional control of early B cell development. *Annu Rev Immunol*. 2004;22:55-79.
56. Krenacs L, Himmelmann AW, Quintanilla-Martinez L, et al. Transcription factor B cell specific activator protein is differentially expressed in B cells and in subsets of B cell lymphomas. *Blood*. 1998;92:1308-1316.
57. Torlakovic E, Torlakovic G, Nguyen PL, et al. The value of anti-pax5 immunostaining in routinely fixed and paraffin embedded sections: a novel pan-B and B-cell marker. *Am J Surg Pathol*. 2002;26:1343-1350.

58. Nagy M, Chapuis B, Matthes T. Expression of transcription factors Pu.1, Spi-B, Blimp-1, BSAP and oct-2 in normal human plasma cells and in multiple myeloma cells. *Br J Haematol.* 2002;116:429-435.
59. Thevenin C, Lucas BP, Kozlow EJ, et al. Cell type- and stage-specific expression of the CD20/B1 antigen correlates with the activity of a diverged octamer DNA motif present in its promoter. *J Biol Chem.* 1993;268:5949-5956.
60. Malone CS, Patrone L, Buchanan KL, et al. An upstream Oct-1 and Oct-2-binding silencer governs B29 (Ig beta) gene expression. *J Immunol.* 2000;164:2550-2556.
61. Staudt LM, Clerc RG, Singh H, et al. Cloning of a lymphoid-specific cDNA encoding a protein binding the regulatory octamer DNA motif. *Science.* 1988;241:577-580.
62. Sturm RA, Das G, Herr W. The ubiquitous octamer-binding protein Oct-1 contains a POU domain with a homeo box subdomain. *Genes Dev.* 1988;2:15. *Hum Pathol.* 2005;36:10-15.
63. Saez A-I, Artiga M-J, Sanchez-Beato M, et al. Analysis of octamer- binding transcription factors Oct2 and Oct1 and their coactivator BOB.1/OBF.1 in lymphomas. *Mod Pathol.* 2002;15:211-220. Diagnosis of classic Hodgkin lymphoma. *Am J Clin Pathol.* 2003;120:767-777.
64. Loddenkemper C, Anagnastopoulos I, Hummel M, et al. Differential Em enhancer activity and expression of BOB.1/OBF.1, Oct2, PU.1, and immunoglobulin in reactive B-cell populations, B-cell non-Hodgkin lymphomas, and Hodgkin lymphomas. *J Pathol.* 2004;202:60-69.
65. Greiner A, Müller KB, Hess J, et al. Up-regulation of BOB.1/ OBF.1 expression in normal germinal center B cells and germinal center-derived lymphomas. *Am J Pathol.* 2000;156:501-507.
66. Stein H, Marafioti T, Foss H-D, et al. Down-regulation of BOB.1/ OBF.1 and Oct2 in classical Hodgkin disease but not in lymphocyte predominant Hodgkin disease correlates with immuno- globulin transcription. *Blood.* 2001;97:496-501.
67. Malisius R, Merz H, Heinz B, et al. Constant detection of CD2, CD3, CD4, and CD5 in fixed and paraffin-embedded tissue using the peroxidase-mediated deposition of biotin-tyramide. *J Histochem Cytochem.* 1997;45(12):1665-1672.
68. Macon WR, Salhany KE. T-cell subset analysis of peripheral T-cell lymphomas by paraffin section immunohistology and correlation of CD4/CD8 results with flow cytometry. *Am J Clin Pathol.* 1998;109(5):610-617.
69. Dorfman DM, Shahsafaei A. CD69 expression correlates with expression of other markers of Th1 T cell differentiation in peripheral T cell lymphomas. *Hum Pathol.* 2002;33(3):330-334.
70. Weng AP, Shahsafaei A, Dorfman DM. CXCR4/CD184 immunoreactivity in T-cell non-Hodgkin lymphomas with an overall Th1- Th2+ immunophenotype. *Am J Clin Pathol.* 2003;119(3):424-430.
71. Picker LJ, Weiss LM, Medeiros LJ, et al. Immunophenotypic criteria for the diagnosis of non-Hodgkin's lymphoma. *Am J Pathol.* 1987;128(1):181-201.
72. Szabo SJ, Kim ST, Costa GL, et al. A novel transcription factor, T-bet, directs Th1 lineage commitment. *Cell.* 2000;100:655-669.
73. Peng SL, Szabo SJ, Glimcher LH. T-bet regulates IgG class switching and pathogenic autoantibody production. *Proc Natl Acad Sci U S A.* 2002;99:5545-5550.
74. Dorfman DM, van den Elzen P, Weng AP, et al. Differential expression of T-bet, a T-box transcription factor required for Th1 T-cell development, in peripheral T-cell lymphomas. *Am J Clin Pathol.* 2003;120:866-873.
75. Vermi W, Facchetti F, Riboldi E, et al. Role of dendritic cell- derived CXCL13 in the pathogenesis of Bartonella henselae B-rich granuloma. *Blood.* 2006;107:454-462.
76. Dorfman DM, Hwang ES, Shahsafaei A, et al. T-bet, a T-cell-associated transcription factor, is expressed in a subset of B-cell lymphoproliferative disorders. *Am J Clin Pathol.* 2004;122:92-297.
77. Delsol G, Lamant L, Mariame B, et al. A new subtype of large B-cell lymphoma expressing the ALK kinase and lacking the 2; 5 translocation. *Blood.* 1997;89(5):1483-1490.
78. Falini B, Bigerna B, Fizottii M, et al. ALK expression defines a distinct group of T/null lymphomas ("ALK lymphomas") with a wide morphological spectrum. *Am J Pathol.* 1998;153(3):875-886.
79. Falini B, Fizzotti M, Pileri S, et al. Bcl-6 protein expression in normal and neoplastic lymphoid tissues. *Ann Oncol.* 1997;8(Suppl 2):101-104.
80. Arber D, Weiss L. CD57: A review. *Appl Immunohistochem.* 1995;3:137-152.
81. Frizzera G, Wu CD, Inghirami G. The usefulness of immunophenotypic and genotypic studies in the diagnosis and classification of hematopoietic and lymphoid neoplasms. An update. *Am J Clin Pathol.* 1999;111(Suppl 1):S13-S39.
82. Troxel DB, Sabella JD. Problem areas in pathology practice. Uncovered by a review of malpractice claims. *Am J Surg Pathol.* 1994;18(8):821-831.
83. Lai R, Arber DA, Chang KL, et al. Frequency of bcl-2 expression in non-Hodgkin's lymphoma: a study of 778 cases with comparison of marginal zone lymphoma and monocytoid B-cell hyperplasia. *Mod Pathol.* 1998;11(9):864-869.
84. Wang T, Lasota J, Hanau CA, et al. Bcl-2 oncoprotein is widespread in lymphoid tissue and lymphomas but its differential expression in benign versus malignant follicles and monocytoid B-cell proliferations is of diagnostic value. *APMIS.* 1995;103(9):655-662.
85. Dogan A, Bagdi E, Munson P, et al. CD10 and BCL-6 expression in paraffin sections of normal lymphoid tissue and B-cell lymphomas. *Am J Surg Pathol.* 2000;24(6):846-852.
86. Gelb AB, Rouse RV, Dorfman RF, et al. Detection of immunophenotypic abnormalities in paraffin-embedded B-lineage non-Hodgkin's lymphomas. *Am J Clin Pathol.* 1994;102(6): 825-834.
87. Browne G, Tobin B, Carney DN, et al. Aberrant MT2 positivity distinguishes follicular lymphoma from reactive follicular hyperplasia in B5- and formalin-fixed paraffin sections. *Am J Clin Pathol.* 1991;96(1):90-94.
88. Emile JF, Wechsler J, Brousse N, et al. Langerhans' cell histiocytosis. Definitive diagnosis with the use of monoclonal antibody O10 on routinely paraffin-embedded samples. *Am J Surg Pathol.* 1995;19(6):636-641.
89. Ng CS, Chan JK, Hui PK, et al. Large B-cell lymphomas with a high content of reactive T cells. *Hum Pathol.* 1989;20(12):1145-1154.
90. Falini B, Pileri S, Stein H, et al. Variable expression of leucocyte-common (CD45) antigen in CD30 (Ki1)-positive anaplastic large-cell lymphoma: implications for the differential diagnosis between lymphoid and nonlymphoid malignancies. *Hum Pathol.* 1990;21(6):624-629.
91. Clavio M, Rossi E, Truini M, et al. Anaplastic large cell lymphoma: a clinicopathologic study of 53 patients. *Leuk Lymphoma.* 1996;22(3-4):319-327.
92. de Bruin PC, Beljaards RC, van Heerde P, et al. Differences in clinical behaviour and immunophenotype between primary cutaneous and primary nodal anaplastic large cell lymphoma of T-cell or null cell phenotype. *Histopathology.* 1993;23(2): 127-135.
93. Battifora H. Assessment of antigen damage in immunohistochemistry. The vimentin internal control. *Am J Clin Pathol.* 1991;96(5):669-671.
94. Anderson JR, Armitage JO, Weisenburger DD. Epidemiology of the non-Hodgkin's lymphomas: distributions of the major subtypes differ by geographic locations. Non-Hodgkin's Lymphoma Classification Project. *Ann Oncol.* 1998;9(7):717-720.
95. Medeiros LJ. Intermediate and high-grade diffuse non-Hodgkin's lymphomas in the Working Formulation. In: Jaffe E, ed. *Surgical Pathology of the Lymph Nodes and Related Organs.* 2 ed. Philadelphia: WB Saunders; 1995:283-343.
96. Weiss LM, Bindl JM, Picozzi VJ, et al. Lymphoblastic lymphoma: an immunophenotype study of 26 cases with comparison to T cell acute lymphoblastic leukemia. *Blood.* 1986;67(2):474-478.
97. Cossman J, Chused TM, Fisher RI, et al. Diversity of immunological phenotypes of lymphoblastic lymphoma. *Cancer Res.* 1983;43(9):4486-4490.
98. Braziel RM, Keneklis T, Donlon JA, et al. Terminal deoxynucleotidyl transferase in non-Hodgkin's lymphoma. *Am J Clin Pathol.* 1983;80(5):655-659.
99. Ozdemirli M, Fanburg-Smith JC, Hartmann DP, et al. Precursor B-Lymphoblastic lymphoma presenting as a solitary bone tumor and mimicking Ewing's sarcoma: a report of four cases and review of the literature. *Am J Surg Pathol.* 1998;22(7):795-804.

100. Iravani S, Singleton TP, Ross CW, et al. Precursor B lymphoblastic lymphoma presenting as lytic bone lesions. *Am J Clin Pathol.* 1999;112(6):836-843.
101. Chimenti S, Fink-Puches R, Peris K, et al. Cutaneous involvement in lymphoblastic lymphoma. *J Cutan Pathol.* 1999;26(8):379-385.
102. Soslow RA, Zukerberg LR, Harris NL, et al. BCL-1 (PRAD-1/cyclin D-1) overexpression distinguishes the blastoid variant of mantle cell lymphoma from B-lineage lymphoblastic lymphoma. *Mod Pathol.* 1997;10(8):810-817.
103. Soslow RA, Baergen RN, Warnke RA. B-lineage lymphoblastic lymphoma is a clinicopathologic entity distinct from other histologically similar aggressive lymphomas with blastic morphology. *Cancer.* 1999;85(12):2648-2654.
104. Van Eyken P, De Wolf-Peeters C, Van den Oord J, et al. Expression of leukocyte common antigen in lymphoblastic lymphoma and small noncleaved undifferentiated non-Burkitt's lymphoma: an immunohistochemical study. *J Pathol.* 1987;151(4):257-261.
105. Taubenberger JK, Cole DE, Raffeld M, et al. Immunophenotypic analysis of acute lymphoblastic leukemia using routinely processed bone marrow specimens. *Arch Pathol Lab Med.* 1991;115(4):338-342.
106. Robertson PB, Neiman RS, Worapongpaiboon S, et al. 013 (CD99) positivity in hematologic proliferations correlates with TdT positivity. *Mod Pathol.* 1997;10(4):277-282.
107. Riopel M, Dickman PS, Link MP, et al. MIC2 analysis in pediatric lymphomas and leukemias. *Hum Pathol.* 1994;25(4):396-399.
108. Sheibani K, Nathwani BN, Winberg CD, et al. Antigenically defined subgroups of lymphoblastic lymphoma. Relationship to clinical presentation and biologic behavior. *Cancer.* 1987;60(2):183-190.
109. Tsang WY, Chan JK, Ng CS, et al. Utility of a paraffin section-reactive CD56 antibody (123C3) for characterization and diagnosis of lymphomas. *Am J Surg Pathol.* 1996;20(2):202-210.
110. Mullauer L, Mosberger I, Chott A. Fas ligand expression in nodal non-Hodgkin's lymphoma. *Mod Pathol.* 1998;11(4):369-375.
111. Soslow RA, Bhargava V, Warnke RA. MIC2, TdT, bcl-2, and CD34 expression in paraffin-embedded high-grade lymphoma/acute lymphoblastic leukemia distinguishes between distinct clinicopathologic entities. *Hum Pathol.* 1997;28(10):1158-1165.
112. de Leon ED, Alkan S, Huang JC, et al. Usefulness of an immunohistochemical panel in paraffin-embedded tissues for the differentiation of B-cell non-Hodgkin's lymphomas of small lymphocytes. *Mod Pathol.* 1998;11(11):1046-1051.
113. Lai R, Weiss LM, Chang KL, et al. Frequency of CD43 expression in non-Hodgkin lymphoma. A survey of 742 cases and further characterization of rare CD43+ follicular lymphomas. *Am J Clin Pathol.* 1999;111(4):488-494.
114. Kumar S, Green GA, Teruya-Feldstein J, et al. Use of CD23 (BU38) on paraffin sections in the diagnosis of small lymphocytic lymphoma and mantle cell lymphoma. *Mod Pathol.* 1996;9(9):925-929.
115. Kaufmann O, Flath B, Spath-Schwalbe E, et al. Immunohistochemical detection of CD5 with monoclonal antibody 4C7 on paraffin sections. *Am J Clin Pathol.* 1997;108(6):669-673.
116. Dorfman DM, Shahsafaei A. Usefulness of a new CD5 antibody for the diagnosis of T-cell and B-cell lymphoproliferative disorders in paraffin sections. *Mod Pathol.* 1997;10(9):859-863.
117. Huang JC, Finn WG, Goolsby CL, et al. CD5- small B-cell leukemias are rarely classifiable as chronic lymphocytic leukemia. *Am J Clin Pathol.* 1999;111(1):123-130.
118. Orazi A, Cattoretti G, Polli N, et al. Distinct morphophenotypic features of chronic B-cell leukaemias identified with CD1c and CD23 antibodies. *Eur J Haematol.* 1991;47(1):28-35.
119. Singh N, Wright DH. The value of immunohistochemistry on paraffin wax embedded tissue sections in the differentiation of small lymphocytic and mantle cell lymphomas. *J Clin Pathol.* 1997;50(1):16-21.
120. Aguilera NS, Chu WS, Andriko JA, et al. Expression of CD44 (HCAM) in small lymphocytic and mantle cell lymphoma. *Hum Pathol.* 1998;29(10):1134-1139.
121. Dorfman DM, Pinkus GS. Distinction between small lymphocytic and mantle cell lymphoma by immunoreactivity for CD23. *Mod Pathol.* 1994;7(3):326-331.
122. Dunphy CH, Wheaton SE, Perkins SL. CD23 expression in transformed small lymphocytic lymphomas/chronic lymphocytic leukemias and blastic transformations of mantle cell lymphoma. *Mod Pathol.* 1997;10(8):818-822.
123. Watson P, Wood KM, Lodge A, et al. Monoclonal antibodies recognizing CD5, CD10 and CD23 in formalin-fixed, paraffin-embedded tissue: production and assessment of their value in the diagnosis of small B-cell lymphoma. *Histopathology.* 2000;36(2):145-150.
124. Swerdlow SH, Yang WI, Zukerberg LR, et al. Expression of cyclin D1 protein in centrocytic/mantle cell lymphomas with and without rearrangement of the BCL1/cyclin D1 gene. *Hum Pathol.* 1995;26(9):999-1004.
125. Yang WI, Zukerberg LR, Motokura T, et al. Cyclin D1 (Bcl-1, PRAD1) protein expression in low-grade B-cell lymphomas and reactive hyperplasia. *Am J Pathol.* 1994;145(1):86-96.
126. Vasef MA, Medeiros LJ, Koo C, et al. Cyclin D1 immunohistochemical staining is useful in distinguishing mantle cell lymphoma from other low-grade B-cell neoplasms in bone marrow. *Am J Clin Pathol.* 1997;108(3):302-307.
127. Zukerberg LR, Yang WI, Arnold A, et al. Cyclin D1 expression in non-Hodgkin's lmphomas. Detection by immunohistochemistry. *Am J Clin Pathol.* 1995;103(6):756-760.
128. Raible MD, Hsi ED, Alkan S. Bcl-6 protein expression by follicle center lymphomas. A marker for differentiating follicle center lymphomas from other low-grade lymphoproliferative disorders. *Am J Clin Pathol.* 1999;112(1):101-107.
129. Aguilar-Santelises M, Magnusson KP, Wiman KG, et al. Progressive B-cell chronic lymphocytic leukaemia frequently exhibits aberrant p53 expression. *Int J Cancer.* 1994;58(4):474-479.
130. Jones D, Benjamin RJ, Shahsafaei A, et al. The chemokine receptor CXCR3 is expressed in a subset of B-cell lymphomas and is a marker of B-cell chronic lymphocytic leukemia. *Blood.* 2000;95(2):627-632.
131. Admirand JH, Rassidakis GZ, Abruzzo LV, et al. Immunohistochemical detection of ZAP-70 in 341 cases of non-Hodgkin and Hodgkin lymphoma. *Mod Pathol.* 2004;17(8):954-961.
132. Sup SJ, Domiati-Saad R, Kelley TW, et al. ZAP-70 expression in B-cell hematologic malignancy is not limited to CLL/SLL. *Am J Clin Pathol.* 2004;122(4):582-587.
133. Crespo M, Bosch F, Villamor N, et al. ZAP-70 expression as a surrogate for immunoglobulin-variable-region mutations in chronic lymphocytic leukemia. *N Engl J Med.* 2003;348(18):1764-1775.
134. Wiestner A, Rosenwald A, Barry TS, et al. ZAP-70 expression identifies a chronic lymphocytic leukemia subtype with unmutated immunoglobulin genes, inferior clinical outcome, and distinct gene expression profile. *Blood.* 2003;101(12):4944-4951.
135. Rassenti LZ, Huynh L, Toy TL, et al. ZAP-70 compared with immunoglobulin heavy-chain gene mutation status as a predictor of disease progression in chronic lymphocytic leukemia. *N Engl J Med.* 2004;351(9):893-901.
136. Carreras J, Villamor N, Colomo L, et al. Immunohistochemical analysis of ZAP-70 expression in B-cell lymphoid neoplasms. *J Pathol.* 2005;205(4):507-513.
137. Bennett JM, Catovsky D, Daniel MT, et al. Proposals for the classification of chronic (mature) B and T lymphoid leukaemias. French-American-British (FAB) Cooperative Group. *J Clin Pathol.* 1989;42(6):567-584.
138. de Melo N, Matutes E, Cordone I, et al. Expression of Ki-67 nuclear antigen in B and T cell lymphoproliferative disorders. *J Clin Pathol.* 1992;45(8):660-663.
139. Harris NL, Bhan AK. B-cell neoplasms of the lymphocytic, lymphoplasmacytoid, and plasma cell types: immunohistologic analysis and clinical correlation. *Hum Pathol.* 1985;16(8):829-837.
140. Hall PA, D'Ardenne AJ, Richards MA, et al. Lymphoplasmacytoid lymphoma: an immunohistological study. *J Pathol.* 1987;153(3):213-223.
141. Zukerberg LR, Medeiros LJ, Ferry JA, et al. Diffuse low-grade B-cell lymphomas. Four clinically distinct subtypes defined by a combination of morphologic and immunophenotypic features. *Am J Clin Pathol.* 1993;100(4):373-385.

142. Tworek JA, Singleton TP, Schnitzer B, et al. Flow cytometric and immunohistochemical analysis of small lymphocytic lymphoma, mantle cell lymphoma, and plasmacytoid small lymphocytic lymphoma. *Am J Clin Pathol.* 1998;110(5):582-589.
143. Chilosi M, Adami F, Lestani M, et al. CD138/syndecan-1: a useful immunohistochemical marker of normal and neoplastic plasma cells on routine trephine bone marrow biopsies. *Mod Pathol.* 1999;12(12):1101-1106.
144. Nguyen PL, Harris NL, Ritz J, et al. Expression of CD95 antigen and Bcl-2 protein in non-Hodgkin's lymphomas and Hodgkin's disease. *Am J Pathol.* 1996;148(3):847-853.
145. Catovsky D, Matutes E. Splenic lymphoma with circulating villous lymphocytes/splenic marginal-zone lymphoma. *Semin Hematol.* 1999;36(2):148-154.
146. Hammer RD, Glick AD, Greer JP, et al. Splenic marginal zone lymphoma. A distinct B-cell neoplasm. *Am J Surg Pathol.* 1996;20(5):613-626.
147. Baldini L, Fracchiolla NS, Cro LM, et al. Frequent p53 gene involvement in splenic B-cell leukemia/lymphomas of possible marginal zone origin. *Blood.* 1994;84(1):270-278.
148. Matutes E, Morilla R, Owusu-Ankomah K, et al. The immunophenotype of hairy cell leukemia (HCL). Proposal for a scoring system to distinguish HCL from B-cell disorders with hairy or villous lymphocytes. *Leuk Lymphoma.* 1994;14(Suppl 1):57-61.
149. Matutes E, Morilla R, Owusu-Ankomah K, et al. The immunophenotype of splenic lymphoma with villous lymphocytes and its relevance to the differential diagnosis with other B-cell disorders. *Blood.* 1994;83(6):1558-1562.
150. Rosso R, Neiman RS, Paulli M, et al. Splenic marginal zone cell lymphoma: report of an indolent variant without massive splenomegaly presumably representing an early phase of the disease. *Hum Pathol.* 1995;26(1):39-46.
151. Piris MA, Mollejo M, Campo E, et al. A marginal zone pattern may be found in different varieties of non-Hodgkin's lymphoma: the morphology and immunohistology of splenic involvement by B-cell lymphomas simulating splenic marginal zone lymphoma. *Histopathology.* 1998;33(3):230-239.
152. Mollejo M, Lloret E, Menarguez J, et al. Lymph node involvement by splenic marginal zone lymphoma: morphological and immunohistochemical features. *Am J Surg Pathol.* 1997;21(7):772-780.
153. Wu CD, Jackson CL, Medeiros LJ. Splenic marginal zone cell lymphoma. An immunophenotypic and molecular study of five cases. *Am J Clin Pathol.* 1996;105(3):277-285.
154. Pawade J, Wilkins BS, Wright DH. Low-grade B-cell lymphomas of the splenic marginal zone: a clinicopathological and immunohistochemical study of 14 cases. *Histopathology.* 1995;27(2):129-137.
155. Savilo E, Campo E, Mollejo M, et al. Absence of cyclin D1 protein expression in splenic marginal zone lymphoma. *Mod Pathol.* 1998;11(7):601-606.
156. Janckila AJ, Cardwell EM, Yam LT, et al. Hairy cell identification by immunohistochemistry of tartrate-resistant acid phosphatase. *Blood.* 1995;85(10):2839-2844.
157. Janckila AJ, Lear SC, Martin AW, et al. Epitope enhancement for immunohistochemical demonstration of tartrate- resistant acid phosphatase. *J Histochem Cytochem.* 1996;44(3):235-244.
158. Hoyer JD, Li CY, Yam LT, et al. Immunohistochemical demonstration of acid phosphatase isoenzyme 5 (tartrate-resistant) in paraffin sections of hairy cell leukemia and other hematologic disorders. *Am J Clin Pathol.* 1997;108(3):308-315.
159. Stroup R, Sheibani K. Antigenic phenotypes of hairy cell leukemia and monocytoid B-cell lymphoma: an immunohistochemical evaluation of 66 cases. *Hum Pathol.* 1992;23(2):172-177.
160. Kreft A, Busche G, Bernhards J, et al. Immunophenotype of hairy-cell leukaemia after cold polymerization of methylmethacrylate embeddings from 50 diagnostic bone marrow biopsies. *Histopathology.* 1997;30(2):145-151.
161. Segal GH, Stoler MH, Fishleder AJ, et al. Reliable and cost-effective paraffin section immunohistology of lymphoproliferative disorders. *Am J Surg Pathol.* 1991;15(11):1034-1041.
162. Hakimian D, Tallman MS, Kiley C, et al. Detection of minimal residual disease by immunostaining of bone marrow biopsies after 2-chlorodeoxyadenosine for hairy cell leukemia. *Blood.* 1993;82(6):1798-1802.
163. Hounieu H, Chittal SM, al Saati T, et al. Hairy cell leukemia. Diagnosis of bone marrow involvement in paraffin-embedded sections with monoclonal antibody DBA.44. *Am J Clin Pathol.* 1992;98(1):26-33.
164. Ohsawa M, Kanno H, Machii T, et al. Immunoreactivity of neoplastic and non-neoplastic monocytoid B lymphocytes for DBA.44 and other antibodies. *J Clin Pathol.* 1994;47(10):928-932.
165. Yaziji H, Janckila AJ, Lear SC, et al. Immunohistochemical detection of tartrate-resistant acid phosphatase in non-hematopoietic human tissues. *Am J Clin Pathol.* 1995;104(4):397-402.
166. Bosch F, Campo E, Jares P, et al. Increased expression of the PRAD-1/CCND1 gene in hairy cell leukaemia. *Br J Haematol.* 1995;91(4):1025-1030.
167. de Boer CJ, Kluin-Nelemans JC, Dreef E, et al. Involvement of the CCND1 gene in hairy cell leukemia. *Ann Oncol.* 1996;7(3):251-256.
168. Costes V, Magen V, Legouffe E, et al. The Mi15 monoclonal antibody (anti-syndecan-1) is a reliable marker for quantifying plasma cells in paraffin-embedded bone marrow biopsy specimens. *Hum Pathol.* 1999;30(12):1405-1411.
169. Vallario A, Chilosi M, Adami F, et al. Human myeloma cells express the CD38 ligand CD31. *Br J Haematol.* 1999;105(2):441-444.
170. Hamilton MS, Barker HF, Ball J, et al. Normal and neoplastic human plasma cells express bcl-2 antigen. *Leukemia.* 1991;5(9):768-771.
171. Diss TC, Wotherspoon AC, Speight P, et al. B-cell monoclonality, Epstein Barr virus, and t(14;18) in myoepithelial sialadenitis and low-grade B-cell MALT lymphoma of the parotid gland. *Am J Surg Pathol.* 1995;19(5):531-536.
172. Baldassano MF, Bailey EM, Ferry JA, et al. Cutaneous lymphoid hyperplasia and cutaneous marginal zone lymphoma: comparison of morphologic and immunophenotypic features. *Am J Surg Pathol.* 1999;23(1):88-96.
173. Berger F, Felman P, Thieblemont C, et al. Non-MALT marginal zone B-cell lymphomas: a description of clinical presentation and outcome in 124 patients. *Blood.* 2000;95(6):1950-1956.
174. Arends JE, Bot FJ, Gisbertz IA, et al. Expression of CD10, CD75 and CD43 in MALT lymphoma and their usefulness in discriminating MALT lymphoma from follicular lymphoma and chronic gastritis. *Histopathology.* 1999;35(3):209-215.
175. Ferry JA, Yang WI, Zukerberg LR, et al. CD5+ extranodal marginal zone B-cell (MALT) lymphoma. A low grade neoplasm with a propensity for bone marrow involvement and relapse. *Am J Clin Pathol.* 1996;105(1):31-37.
176. Ashton-Key M, Biddolph SC, Stein H, et al. Heterogeneity of bcl-2 expression in MALT lymphoma. *Histopathology.* 1995;26(1):75-78.
177. Cerroni L, Signoretti S, Hofler G, et al. Primary cutaneous marginal zone B-cell lymphoma: a recently described entity of low-grade malignant cutaneous B-cell lymphoma. *Am J Surg Pathol.* 1997;21(11):1307-1315.
178. Chetty R, O'Leary JJ, Biddolph SC, et al. Immunohistochemical detection of p53 and Bcl-2 proteins in Hashimoto's thyroiditis and primary thyroid lymphomas. *J Clin Pathol.* 1995;48(3):239-241.
179. Nakamura S, Akazawa K, Kinukawa N, et al. Inverse correlation between the expression of bcl-2 and p53 proteins in primary gastric lymphoma. *Hum Pathol.* 1996;27(3):225-233.
180. Navratil E, Gaulard P, Kanavaros P, et al. Expression of the bcl-2 protein in B cell lymphomas arising from mucosa associated lymphoid tissue. *J Clin Pathol.* 1995;48(1):18-21.
181. Omonishi K, Yoshino T, Sakuma I, et al. bcl-6 protein is identified in high-grade but not low-grade mucosa-associated lymphoid tissue lymphomas of the stomach. *Mod Pathol.* 1998;11(2):181-185.
182. Nakamura S, Akazawa K, Yao T, et al. A clinicopathologic study of 233 cases with special reference to evaluation with the MIB-1 index. *Cancer.* 1995;76(8):1313-1324.
183. Isaacson PG. Gastrointestinal lymphomas of T- and B-cell types. *Mod Pathol.* 1999;12(2):151-158.
184. Davis GG, York JC, Glick AD, et al. Plasmacytic differentiation in parafollicular (monocytoid) B-cell lymphoma. A study of 12 cases. *Am J Surg Pathol.* 1992;16(11):1066-1074.

185. Nzze H, Cogliatti SB, von Schilling C, et al. Monocytoid B-cell lymphoma: morphological variants and relationship to low-grade B-cell lymphoma of the mucosa-associated lymphoid tissue. *Histopathology.* 1991;18(5):403-414.
186. Kurtin PJ, Hobday KS, Ziesmer S, et al. Demonstration of distinct antigenic profiles of small B-cell lymphomas by paraffin section immunohistochemistry. *Am J Clin Pathol.* 1999;112(3):319-329.
187. Ballesteros E, Osborne BM, Matsushima AY. CD5+ low-grade marginal zone B-cell lymphomas with localized presentation. *Am J Surg Pathol.* 1998;22(2):201-207.
188. Dierlamm J, Pittaluga S, Wlodarska I, et al. Marginal zone B-cell lymphomas of different sites share similar cytogenetic and morphologic features. *Blood.* 1996;87(1):299-307.
189. Campo E, Miquel R, Krenacs L, et al. Primary nodal marginal zone lymphomas of splenic and MALT type. *Am J Surg Pathol.* 1999;23(1):59-68.
190. Hernandez AM, Nathwani BN, Nguyen D, et al. Nodal benign and malignant monocytoid B cells with and without follicular lymphomas: a comparative study of follicular colonization, light chain restriction, bcl-2, and t(14;18) in 39 cases. *Hum Pathol.* 1995;26(6):625-632.
191. Levy V, Miller C, Koeffler HP, et al. p53 in lymphomas of mucosal-associated lymphoid tissues. *Mod Pathol.* 1996;9(3):245-248.
192. Baldini L, Guffanti A, Cro L, et al. Poor prognosis in non-villous splenic marginal zone cell lymphoma is associated with p53 mutations. *Br J Haematol.* 1997;99(2):375-378.
193. McIntosh GG, Lodge AJ, Watson P, et al. NCL-CD10-270: a new monoclonal antibody recognizing CD10 in paraffin-embedded tissue. *Am J Pathol.* 1999;154(1):77-82.
194. Contos MJ, Kornstein MJ, Innes DJ, et al. The utility of CD20 and CD43 in subclassification of low-grade B-cell lymphoma on paraffin sections. *Mod Pathol.* 1992;5(6):631-633.
195. Ashton-Key M, Diss TC, Isaacson PG, et al. A comparative study of the value of immunohistochemistry and the polymerase chain reaction in the diagnosis of follicular lymphoma. *Histopathology.* 1995;27(6):501-508.
196. Cooper K, Haffajee Z. bcl-2 and p53 protein expression in follicular lymphoma. *J Pathol.* 1997;182(3):307-310.
197. Gaulard P, d'Agay MF, Peuchmaur M, et al. Expression of the bcl-2 gene product in follicular lymphoma. *Am J Pathol.* 1992;140(5):1089-1095.
198. Nguyen PL, Zukerberg LR, Benedict WF, et al. Immunohistochemical detection of p53, bcl-2, and retinoblastoma proteins in follicular lymphoma. *Am J Clin Pathol.* 1996;105(5):538-543.
199. Skinnider BF, Horsman DE, Dupuis B, et al. Bcl-6 and Bcl-2 protein expression in diffuse large B-cell lymphoma and follicular lymphoma: correlation with 3q27 and 18q21 chromosomal abnormalities. *Hum Pathol.* 1999;30(7):803-808.
200. Logsdon MD, Meyn Jr RE, Besa PC, et al. Apoptosis and the Bcl-2 gene family—patterns of expression and prognostic value in stage I and II follicular center lymphoma. *Int J Radiat Oncol Biol Phys.* 1999;44(1):19-29.
201. Goates JJ, Kamel OW, LeBrun DP, et al. Floral variant of follicular lymphoma. Immunological and molecular studies support a neoplastic process. *Am J Surg Pathol.* 1994;18(1):37-47.
202. Pezzella F, Jones M, Ralfkiaer E, et al. Evaluation of bcl-2 protein expression and 14;18 translocation as prognostic markers in follicular lymphoma. *Br J Cancer.* 1992;65(1):87-89.
203. Cattoretti G, Chang CC, Cechova K, et al. BCL-6 protein is expressed in germinal-center B cells. *Blood.* 1995;86(1):45-53.
204. Szereday Z, Csernus B, Nagy M, et al. Somatic mutation of the 5' noncoding region of the BCL-6 gene is associated with intraclonal diversity and clonal selection in histological transformation of follicular lymphoma. *Am J Pathol.* 2000;156(3):1017-1024.
205. Moller MB, Nielsen O, Pedersen NT. Oncoprotein MDM2 overexpression is associated with poor prognosis in distinct non-Hodgkin's lymphoma entities. *Mod Pathol.* 1999;12(11):1010-1016.
206. Kamel OW, Gelb AB, Shibuya RB, et al. Leu 7 (CD57) reactivity distinguishes nodular lymphocyte predominance Hodgkin's disease from nodular sclerosing Hodgkin's disease, T-cell-rich B-cell lymphoma and follicular lymphoma. *Am J Pathol.* 1993;142(2):541-546.
207. Scoazec JY, Berger F, Magaud JP, et al. The dendritic reticulum cell pattern in B cell lymphomas of the small cleaved, mixed, and large cell types: an immunohistochemical study of 48 cases. *Hum Pathol.* 1989;20(2):124-131.
208. Miettinen M. CD30 distribution. Immunohistochemical study on formaldehyde-fixed, paraffin-embedded Hodgkin's and non-Hodgkin's lymphomas. *Arch Pathol Lab Med.* 1992;116(11):1197-1201.
209. Piris M, Gatter KC, Mason DY. CD30 expression in follicular lymphoma. *Histopathology.* 1991;18(1):25-29.
210. Chetty R, Echezarreta G, Comley M, et al. Immunohistochemistry in apparently normal bone marrow trephine specimens from patients with nodal follicular lymphoma. *J Clin Pathol.* 1995;48(11):1035-1038.
211. Kurtin PJ. Mantle cell lymphoma. *Adv Anat Pathol.* 1998;5(6):376-398.
212. Lavergne A, Brouland JP, Launay E, et al. Multiple lymphomatous polyposis of the gastrointestinal tract. An extensive histopathologic and immunohistochemical study of 12 cases. *Cancer.* 1994;74(11):3042-3050.
213. Pittaluga S, Wlodarska I, Stul MS, et al. Mantle cell lymphoma: a clinicopathological study of 55 cases. *Histopathology.* 1995;26(1):17-24.
214. Fraga M, Lloret E, Sanchez-Verde L, et al. Mucosal mantle cell (centrocytic) lymphomas. *Histopathology.* 1995;26(5):413-422.
215. Yatabe Y, Suzuki R, Tobinai K, et al. Significance of cyclin D1 overexpression for the diagnosis of mantle cell lymphoma: a clinicopathologic comparison of cyclin D1-positive MCL and cyclin D1-negative MCL-like B-cell lymphoma. *Blood.* 2000;95(7):2253-2261.
216. Kumar S, Krenacs L, Otsuki T, et al. bc1-1 rearrangement and cyclin D1 protein expression in multiple lymphomatous polyposis. *Am J Clin Pathol.* 1996;105(6):737-743.
217. Singleton TP, Anderson MM, Ross CW, et al. Leukemic phase of mantle cell lymphoma, blastoid variant. *Am J Clin Pathol.* 1999;111(4):495-500.
218. Gronbaek K, Nedergaard T, Andersen MK, et al. Concurrent disruption of cell cycle associated genes in mantle cell lymphoma: a genotypic and phenotypic study of cyclin D1, p16, p15, p53 and pRb. *Leukemia.* 1998;12(8):1266-1271.
219. Chang CC, Liu YC, Cleveland RP, et al. Expression of c-Myc and p53 correlates with clinical outcome in diffuse large B-cell lymphomas. *Am J Clin Pathol.* 2000;113(4):512-518.
220. Louie DC, Offit K, Jaslow R, et al. p53 overexpression as a marker of poor prognosis in mantle cell lymphomas with t(11;14)(q13;q32). *Blood.* 1995;86(8):2892-2899.
221. Hernandez L, Fest T, Cazorla M, et al. p53 gene mutations and protein overexpression are associated with aggressive variants of mantle cell lymphomas. *Blood.* 1996;87(8):3351-3359.
222. Fiel-Gan MD, Almeida LM, Rose DC, et al. Proliferative fraction, bcl-1 gene translocation, and p53 mutation status as markers in mantle cell lymphoma. *Int J Mol Med.* 1999;3(4):373-379.
223. Stein H, Lennert K, Feller AC, et al. Immunohistological analysis of human lymphoma: correlation of histological and immunological categories. *Adv Cancer Res.* 1984;42:67-147.
224. Doggett RS, Wood GS, Horning S, et al. The immunologic characterization of 95 nodal and extranodal diffuse large cell lymphomas in 89 patients. *Am J Pathol.* 1984;115(2):245-252.
225. Taniguchi M, Oka K, Hiasa A, et al. De novo CD5+ diffuse large B-cell lymphomas express VH genes with somatic mutation. *Blood.* 1998;91(4):1145-1151.
226. Fang JM, Finn WG, Hussong JW, et al. CD10 antigen expression correlates with the t(14;18)(q32;q21) major breakpoint region in diffuse large B-cell lymphoma. *Mod Pathol.* 1999;12(3):295-300.
227. Martinka M, Comeau T, Foyle A, et al. Prognostic significance of t(14;18) and bcl-2 gene expression in follicular small cleaved cell lymphoma and diffuse large cell lymphoma. *Clin Invest Med Clin Experiment.* 1997;20(6):364-370.
228. Gascoyne RD, Adomat SA, Krajewski S, et al. Prognostic significance of Bcl-2 protein expression and Bcl-2 gene rearrangement in diffuse aggressive non-Hodgkin's lymphoma. *Blood.* 1997;90(1):244-251.

229. Gascoyne RD, Krajewska M, Krajewski S, et al. Prognostic significance of Bax protein expression in diffuse aggressive non-Hodgkin's lymphoma. *Blood.* 1997;90(8):3173-3178.
230. Drillenburg P, Wielenga VJ, Kramer MH, et al. CD44 expression predicts disease outcome in localized large B cell lymphoma. *Leukemia.* 1999;13(9):1448-1455.
231. Donoghue S, Baden HS, Lauder I, et al. Immunohistochemical localization of caspase-3 correlates with clinical outcome in B-cell diffuse large-cell lymphoma. *Cancer Res.* 1999;59(20):5386-5391.
232. Weiss LM, Strickler JG, Medeiros LJ, et al. Proliferative rates of non-Hodgkin's lymphomas as assessed by Ki-67 antibody. *Hum Pathol.* 1987;18(11):1155-1159.
233. Frierson HFJ, Bellafiore FJ, Gaffey MJ, et al. Cytokeratin in anaplastic large cell lymphoma. *Mod Pathol.* 1994;7(3):317-321.
234. de Bruin PC, Gruss HJ, van der Valk P, et al. CD30 expression in normal and neoplastic lymphoid tissue: biological aspects and clinical implications. *Leukemia.* 1995;9(10):1620-1627.
235. Krishnan J, Wallberg K, Frizzera G. T-cell-rich large B-cell lymphoma. A study of 30 cases, supporting its histologic heterogeneity and lack of clinical distinctiveness. *Am J Surg Pathol.* 1994;18(5):455-465.
236. Suster S. Primary large-cell lymphomas of the mediastinum. *Semin Diagn Pathol.* 1999;16(1):51-64.
237. Davis RE, Dorfman RF, Warnke RA. Primary large-cell lymphoma of the thymus: a diffuse B-cell neoplasm presenting as primary mediastinal lymphoma. *Hum Pathol.* 1990;21(12):1262-1268.
238. Rodriguez J, Pugh WC, Romaguera JE, et al. Primary mediastinal large cell lymphoma. *Hematol Oncol.* 1994;12(4):175-184.
239. Rodriguez J, Pugh WC, Romaguera JE, et al. Primary mediastinal large cell lymphoma is characterized by an inverted pattern of large tumoral mass and low beta 2 microglobulin levels in serum and frequently elevated levels of serum lactate dehydrogenase. *Ann Oncol.* 1994;5(9):847-849.
240. Higgins JP, Warnke RA. CD30 expression is common in mediastinal large B-cell lymphoma. *Am J Clin Pathol.* 1999;112(2):241-247.
241. Knowles DM. Immunodeficiency-associated lymphoproliferative disorders. *Mod Pathol.* 1999;12(2):200-217.
242. Green I, Espiritu E, Ladanyi M, et al. Primary lymphomatous effusions in AIDS: a morphological, immunophenotypic, and molecular study. *Mod Pathol.* 1995;8(1):39-45.
243. Nador RG, Cesarman E, Chadburn A, et al. Primary effusion lymphoma: a distinct clinicopathologic entity associated with the Kaposi's sarcoma-associated herpes virus. *Blood.* 1996;88(2):645-656.
244. DiGiuseppe JA, Nelson WG, Seifter EJ, et al. Intravascular lymphomatosis: a clinicopathologic study of 10 cases and assessment of response to chemotherapy. *J Clin Oncol.* 1994;12(12):2573-2579.
245. Ferry JA, Harris NL, Picker LJ, et al. Intravascular lymphomatosis (malignant angioendotheliomatosis). A B- cell neoplasm expressing surface homing receptors. *Mod Pathol.* 1988;1(6):444-452.
246. Domizio P, Hall PA, Cotter F, et al. Angiotropic large cell lymphoma (ALCL): morphological, immunohistochemical and genotypic studies with analysis of previous reports. *Hematol Oncol.* 1989;7(3):195-206.
247. Kanda M, Suzumiya J, Ohshima K, et al. Intravascular large cell lymphoma: clinicopathological, immuno-histochemical and molecular genetic studies. *Leuk Lymphoma.* 1999;34(5-6):569-580.
248. Rudinger T, Ott G, Ott M, et al. Reply to: B-cell anaplastic large cell lymphoma—the forgotten entity. *Am J Surg Pathol.* 2000;24:159-160.
249. Suzumiya J, Ohshima K, Kikuchi M, et al. Terminal deoxynucleotidyl transferase staining of malignant lymphomas in paraffin sections: a useful method for the diagnosis of lymphoblastic lymphoma. *J Pathol.* 1997;182(1):86-91.
250. Guinee Jr D, Jaffe E, Kingma D, et al. Pulmonary lymphomatoid granulomatosis. Evidence for a proliferation of Epstein-Barr virus infected B-lymphocytes with a prominent T-cell component and vasculitis. *Am J Surg Pathol.* 1994;18(8):753-764.
251. Chetty R, Pulford K, Jones M, et al. An immunohistochemical study of TAL-1 protein expression in leukaemias and lymphomas with a novel monoclonal antibody, 2TL 242. *J Pathol.* 1996;178(3):311-315.
252. Sykora KW, Tomeczkowski J, Reiter A. C-kit receptors in childhood malignant lymphoblastic cells. *Leuk Lymphoma.* 1997;25(3-4):201-216.
253. Chan J, Tsang W. Reactive lymphadenopathies. In: Weiss L, ed. *Pathology of Lymph Nodes.* New York: Churchill Livingstone; 1996:81-167.
254. Chan AC, Ho JW, Chiang AK, et al. Phenotypic and cytotoxic characteristics of peripheral T-cell and NK-cell lymphomas in relation to Epstein-Barr virus association. *Histopathology.* 1999;34(1):16-24.
255. Chan JK, Sin VC, Wong KF, et al. Nonnasal lymphoma expressing the natural killer cell marker CD56: a clinicopathologic study of 49 cases of an uncommon aggressive neoplasm. *Blood.* 1997;89(12):4501-4513.
256. Chan JK. Peripheral T-cell and NK-cell neoplasms: an integrated approach to diagnosis. *Mod Pathol.* 1999;12(2):177-199.
257. Takeshita M, Akamatsu M, Ohshima K, et al. CD30 (Ki-1) expression in adult T-cell leukaemia/lymphoma is associated with distinctive immunohistological and clinical characteristics. *Histopathology.* 1995;26(6):539-546.
258. Tao Q, Ho FC, Loke SL, et al. Epstein-Barr virus is localized in the tumour cells of nasal lymphomas of NK, T or B cell type. *Int J Cancer.* 1995;60(3):315-320.
259. de Bruin PC, Jiwa M, Oudejans JJ, et al. Presence of Epstein-Barr virus in extranodal T-cell lymphomas: differences in relation to site. *Blood.* 1994;83(6):1612-1618.
260. Sabourin JC, Kanavaros P, Briere J, et al. Epstein-Barr virus (EBV) genomes and EBV-encoded latent membrane protein (LMP) in pulmonary lymphomas occurring in nonimmunocompromised patients. *Am J Surg Pathol.* 1993;17(10):995-1002.
261. Kanavaros P, Vlychou M, Stefanaki K, et al. Cytotoxic protein expression in non-Hodgkin's lymphomas and Hodgkin's disease. *Anticancer Res.* 1999;19(2A):1209-1216.
262. Boulland ML, Kanavaros P, Wechsler J, et al. Cytotoxic protein expression in natural killer cell lymphomas and in alpha beta and gamma delta peripheral T-cell lymphomas. *J Pathol.* 1997;183(4):432-439.
263. Macon WR, Williams ME, Greer JP, et al. Natural killer-like T-cell lymphomas: aggressive lymphomas of T-large granular lymphocytes. *Blood.* 1996;87(4):1474-1483.
264. Chott A, Vesely M, Simonitsch I, et al. Classification of intestinal T-cell neoplasms and their differential diagnosis. *Am J Clin Pathol.* 1999;111(1 Suppl 1):S68-S74.
265. de Bruin PC, Connolly CE, Oudejans JJ, et al. Enteropathy-associated T-cell lymphomas have a cytotoxic T-cell phenotype. *Histopathology.* 1997;31(4):313-317.
266. Ilyas M, Niedobitek G, Agathanggelou A, et al. Non-Hodgkin's lymphoma, coeliac disease, and Epstein-Barr virus: a study of 13 cases of enteropathy-associated T- and B-cell lymphoma. *J Pathol.* 1995;177(2):115-122.
267. Carey MJ, Medeiros LJ, Roepke JE, et al. Primary anaplastic large cell lymphoma of the small intestine. *Am J Clin Pathol.* 1999;112(5):696-701.
268. Murray A, Cuevas EC, Jones DB, et al. Study of the immunohistochemistry and T cell clonality of enteropathy-associated T cell lymphoma. *Am J Pathol.* 1995;146(2):509-519.
269. Wu H, Wasik MA, Przybylski G, et al. Hepatosplenic gamma-delta T-cell lymphoma as a late-onset posttransplant lymphoproliferative disorder in renal transplant recipients. *Am J Clin Pathol.* 2000;113(4):487-496.
270. Cooke CB, Krenacs L, Stetler-Stevenson M, et al. Hepatosplenic T-cell lymphoma: a distinct clinicopathologic entity of cytotoxic gamma delta T-cell origin. *Blood.* 1996;88(11):4265-4274.
271. Salhany KE, Macon WR, Choi JK, et al. Subcutaneous panniculitis-like T-cell lymphoma: clinicopathologic, immunophenotypic, and genotypic analysis of alpha/beta and gamma/delta subtypes. *Am J Surg Pathol.* 1998;22(7):881-893.
272. Kumar S, Krenacs L, Medeiros J, et al. Subcutaneous panniculitic T-cell lymphoma is a tumor of cytotoxic T lymphocytes. *Hum Pathol.* 1998;29(4):397-403.

273. Kinney MC. The role of morphologic features, phenotype, genotype, and anatomic site in defining extranodal T-cell or NK-cell neoplasms. *Am J Clin Pathol.* 1999;111(1 suppl 1): S104-S118.
274. Chang K, Weiss L. CD7: a review. *Appl Immunohistochem.* 1994;2:146-156.
275. Bakels V, van Oostveen JW, van der Putte SC, et al. Immunophenotyping and gene rearrangement analysis provide additional criteria to differentiate between cutaneous T-cell lymphomas and pseudo-T-cell lymphomas. *Am J Pathol.* 1997;150(6):1941-1949.
276. Picker LJ, Brenner MB, Weiss LM, et al. Discordant expression of CD3 and T-cell receptor beta-chain antigens in T-lineage lymphomas. *Am J Pathol.* 1987;129(3):434-440.
277. Bani D, Giannotti B. Differentiation of interdigitating reticulum cells and Langerhans cells in the human skin with T-lymphoid infiltrate. An immunocytochemical and ultrastructural study. *Arch Histol Cytol.* 1989;52(4):361-372.
278. Li G, Chooback L, Wolfe JT, et al. Overexpression of p53 protein in cutaneous T cell lymphoma: relationship to large cell transformation and disease progression. *J Invest Dermatol.* 1998;110(5):767-770.
279. Kempf W, Dummer R, Burg G. Approach to lymphoproliferative infiltrates of the skin. The difficult lesions. *Am J Clin Pathol.* 1999;111(1 Suppl 1):S84-S93.
280. Krishnan J, Tomaszewski MM, Kao GF. Primary cutaneous CD30-positive anaplastic large cell lymphoma. Report of 27 cases. *J Cutan Pathol.* 1993;20(3):193-202.
281. Kummer JA, Vermeer MH, Dukers D, et al. Most primary cutaneous CD30-positive lymphoproliferative disorders have a CD4-positive cytotoxic T-cell phenotype. *J Invest Dermatol.* 1997;109(5):636-640.
282. Boulland ML, Wechsler J, Bagot M, et al. Primary CD30-positive cutaneous T-cell lymphomas and lymphomatoid papulosis frequently express cytotoxic proteins. *Histopathology.* 2000;36(2):136-144.
283. Vergier B, Beylot-Barry M, Pulford K, et al. Statistical evaluation of diagnostic and prognostic features of CD30+ cutaneous lymphoproliferative disorders: a clinicopathologic study of 65 cases. *Am J Surg Pathol.* 1998;22(10):1192-1202.
284. Herbst H, Sander C, Tronnier M, et al. Absence of anaplastic lymphoma kinase (ALK) and Epstein-Barr virus gene products in primary cutaneous anaplastic large cell lymphoma and lymphomatoid papulosis. *Br J Dermatol.* 1997;137(5):680-686.
285. Beljaards RC, Kaudewitz P, Berti E, et al. Primary cutaneous CD30-positive large cell lymphoma: definition of a new type of cutaneous lymphoma with a favorable prognosis. A European Multicenter Study of 47 patients. *Cancer.* 1993;71(6):2097-2104.
286. Brice P, Cazals D, Mounier N, et al. Primary cutaneous large-cell lymphoma: analysis of 49 patients included in the LNH87 prospective trial of polychemotherapy for high-grade lymphomas. Groupe d'Etude des Lymphomes de l'Adulte. *Leukemia.* 1998;12(2):213-219.
287. Anagnostopoulos I, Hummel M, Kaudewitz P, et al. Low incidence of Epstein-Barr virus presence in primary cutaneous T-cell lymphoproliferations. *Br J Dermatol.* 1996;134(2):276-281.
288. Leung CY, Ho FC, Srivastava G, et al. Usefulness of follicular dendritic cell pattern in classification of peripheral T-cell lymphomas. *Histopathology.* 1993;23(5):433-437.
289. Anagnostopoulos I, Hummel M, Finn T, et al. Heterogeneous Epstein-Barr virus infection patterns in peripheral T-cell lymphoma of angioimmunoblastic lymphadenopathy type. *Blood.* 1992;80(7):1804-1812.
290. Nathwani B, Jaffe E. Angioimmunoblastic lymphadenopathy (AILD) and AILD-like T-cell lymphomas. In: Jaffe E, ed. *Surgical Pathology of the Lymph Nodes and Related Organs.* 2nd ed. Philadelphia: WB Saunders; 1995:390-412.
291. Borowitz MJ, Newby S, Brynes RK, et al. Multiinstitution study of non-Hodgkin's lymphomas using frozen section immunoperoxidase: the Southeastern Cancer Study Group experience. *Blood.* 1984;63(5):1147-1152.
292. Strickler JG, Weiss LM, Copenhaver CM, et al. Monoclonal antibodies reactive in routinely processed tissue sections of malignant lymphoma, with emphasis on T-cell lymphomas. *Hum Pathol.* 1987;18(8):808-814.
293. Hamilton-Dutoit SJ, Pallesen G. A survey of Epstein-Barr virus gene expression in sporadic non-Hodgkin's lymphomas. Detection of Epstein-Barr virus in a subset of peripheral T-cell lymphomas. *Am J Pathol.* 1992;140(6):1315-1325.
294. Kadin ME. Primary Ki-1-positive anaplastic large-cell lymphoma: a distinct clinicopathologic entity. *Ann Oncol.* 1994;5(Suppl 1): 25-30.
295. Perkins PL, Ross CW, Schnitzer B. CD30-positive, anaplastic large-cell lymphomas that express CD15 but lack CD45. A possible diagnostic pitfall. *Arch Pathol Lab Med.* 1992;116(11):1192-1196.
296. Biernat W. Ki-1-positive anaplastic large cell lymphoma: a morphologic and immunologic study of 14 cases. *Patol Pol.* 1994;45(1):39-44.
297. Brousset P, Rochaix P, Chittal S, et al. High incidence of Epstein-Barr virus detection in Hodgkin's disease and absence of detection in anaplastic large-cell lymphoma in children. *Histopathology.* 1993;23(2):189-191.
298. Bayle C, Charpentier A, Duchayne E, et al. Leukaemic presentation of small cell variant anaplastic large cell lymphoma: report of four cases. *Br J Haematol.* 1999;104(4):680-688.
299. Kinney MC, Collins RD, Greer JP, et al. A small-cell-predominant variant of primary Ki-1 (CD30)+ T-cell lymphoma. *Am J Surg Pathol.* 1993;17(9):859-868.
300. Piris M, Brown DC, Gatter KC, et al. CD30 expression in non-Hodgkin's lymphoma. *Histopathology.* 1990;17(3):211-218.
301. Gascoyne RD, Aoun P, Wu D, et al. Prognostic significance of anaplastic lymphoma kinase (ALK) protein expression in adults with anaplastic large cell lymphoma. *Blood.* 1999;93(11):3913-3921.
302. Hodges KB, Collins RD, Greer JP, et al. Transformation of the small cell variant Ki-1+ lymphoma to anaplastic large cell lymphoma: pathologic and clinical features. *Am J Surg Pathol.* 1999;23(1):49-58.
303. Nakagawa A, Nakamura S, Ito M, et al. CD30-positive anaplastic large cell lymphoma in childhood: expression of p80npm/alk and absence of Epstein-Barr virus. *Mod Pathol.* 1997;10(3):210-215.
304. Nakamura S, Shiota M, Nakagawa A, et al. Anaplastic large cell lymphoma: a distinct molecular pathologic entity: a reappraisal with special reference to p80(NPM/ALK) expression. *Am J Surg Pathol.* 1997;21(12):1420-1432.
305. Foss HD, Anagnostopoulos I, Araujo I, et al. Anaplastic large-cell lymphomas of T-cell and null-cell phenotype express cytotoxic molecules. *Blood.* 1996;88(10):4005-4011.
306. Foss HD, Demel G, Anagnostopoulos I, et al. Uniform expression of cytotoxic molecules in anaplastic large cell lymphoma of null/T cell phenotype and in cell lines derived from anaplastic large cell lymphoma. *Pathobiology.* 1997;65(2):83-90.
307. Krenacs L, Wellmann A, Sorbara L, et al. Cytotoxic cell antigen expression in anaplastic large cell lymphomas of T- and null-cell type and Hodgkin's disease: evidence for distinct cellular origin. *Blood.* 1997;89(3):980-989.
308. Cesarman E, Inghirami G, Chadburn A, et al. High levels of p53 protein expression do not correlate with p53 gene mutations in anaplastic large cell lymphoma. *Am J Pathol.* 1993;143(3):845-856.
309. Inghirami G, Macri L, Cesarman E, et al. Molecular characterization of CD30+ anaplastic large-cell lymphoma: high frequency of c-myc proto-oncogene activation. *Blood.* 1994;83(12):3581-3590.
310. Fraga M, Brousset P, Schlaifer, et al. Bone marrow involvement in anaplastic large cell lymphoma. Immunohistochemical detection of minimal disease and its prognostic significance. *Am J Clin Pathol.* 1995;103(1):82-89.

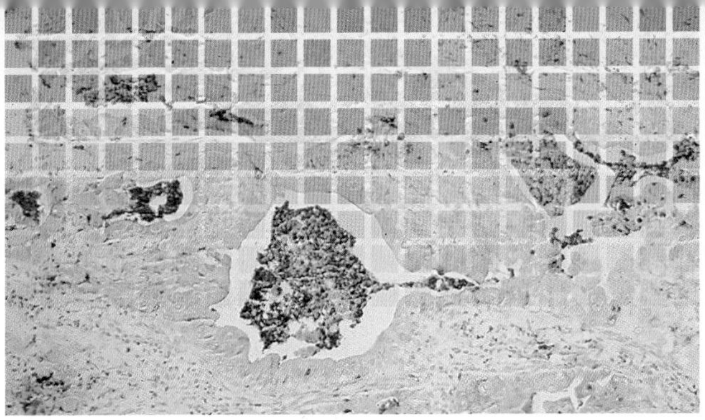

7

Immunohistology of Melanocytic Neoplasms

Mark R. Wick

- Introduction 189
- Biology of Antigens and Antibodies 189
- Neuroendocrine Markers in Melanocytic Lesions 196
- "Sentinel" Lymph Node Biopsies for Metastatic Melanoma 196
- Putatively Prognostic Markers for Melanoma 196

INTRODUCTION

Malignant melanoma (MM) continues to be one of the greatest diagnostic challenges in surgical pathology. Both as a primary lesion in the skin and in metastatic sites, this neoplasm is capable of assuming many different macroscopic and histologic guises. Recognized microscopic phenotypes of primary MM include superficial spreading, nodular, lentiginous, balloon (clear)-cell, pleomorphic-sarcomatoid, spindle-cell/desmoplastic/neuroid, small-cell (neuroendocrine-like), hemangiopericytoid, signet-ring-cell, myxoid, adenoid-pseudopapillary, metaplastic, rhabdoid, and "nevoid" forms (Figs. 7.1 to 7.3).[1-3] Because all of these images may be amelanotic in nature, the differential diagnostic considerations in such cases are truly protean. Accordingly, electron microscopy, immunohistology, and cytogenetic analysis have become exceedingly important in the accurate recognition of melanoma. This discussion focuses on the second of those investigative modalities and is directed principally at diagnostic questions concerning melanocytic tumors in general. However, brief consideration is also given to "prognostic" markers for MM.

BIOLOGY OF ANTIGENS AND ANTIBODIES

Filamentous Proteins in Melanocytic Neoplasms

Intermediate filament protein (IFP) analysis has been an important cornerstone of immunohistochemical evaluation for nearly 20 years. In general terms it can still be stated with accuracy that immunostains for keratins, vimentin, desmin, neurofilament proteins, and glial fibrillary acidic protein (GFAP) are broadly capable of distinguishing between histologically similar classes of neoplasms with dissimilar lineages.[4,5]

In specific regard to melanocytic neoplasms, nevi and MMs typically are labeled only for vimentin and lack the other four groups of IFP (Figs. 7.4 and 7.5).[5-7] Moreover, the *density* of vimentin in melanogenic tumors is high, yielding intense immunoreactivity for that marker in most instances. Using frozen tissue or specially (nonformalin)-fixed specimens, various authors have shown that MMs may, in fact, contain detectable amounts of keratin and other intermediate filaments.[2,8,9] However, in a cooperative interinstitutional study in which this author participated using paraffin sections and modern immunohistochemical methods, less than 3% of melanomas were keratin positive (Fig. 7.6), and lesions that expressed IFP generally did so in a focal fashion. Similarly, GFAP and desmin have been reported in a small minority (<1%) of MMs.[2] They have usually been tumors that demonstrated "metaplastic" sarcomatoid microscopic features or, conversely, desmoplastic and neuroid characteristics. For practical purposes, and in specific reference to studies of paraffin sections for IFPs, it is still true that more than 95% of melanocytic neoplasms are labeled *solely* for vimentin, even after application of current techniques such as heat-mediated epitope retrieval.

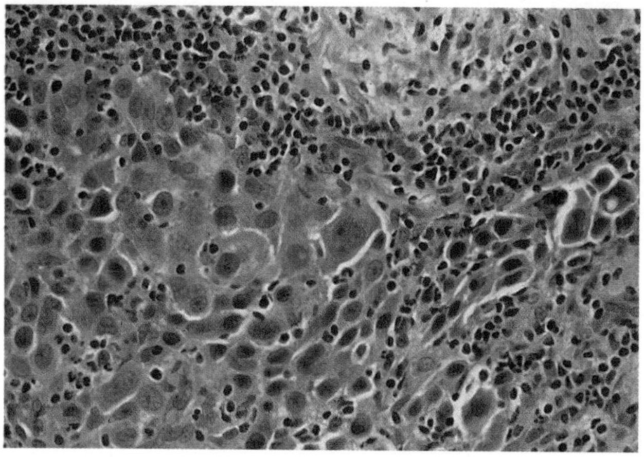

FIGURE 7.1 Large-cell epithelioid amelanotic malignant melanoma, the most commonly encountered histologic variant of that tumor.

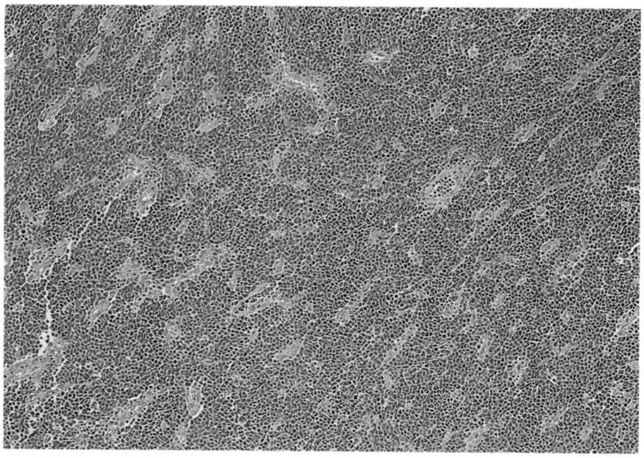

FIGURE 7.2 Small cell amelanotic melanoma, resembling neuroendocrine carcinoma.

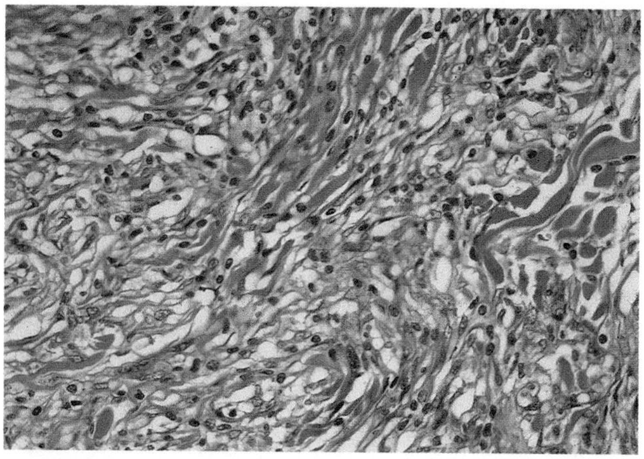

FIGURE 7.3 Sarcomatoid/desmoplastic amelanotic melanoma, simulating a sarcoma.

Because muscle-specific actin (recognized by monoclonal antibody HHF-35), alpha-isoform ("smooth muscle") actin (recognized by antibody 1A4), and caldesmon are also preferentially seen in nonepithelial, nonmelanocytic, nonglial tissues, those determinants would be unexpected in melanocytic neoplasms. Indeed,

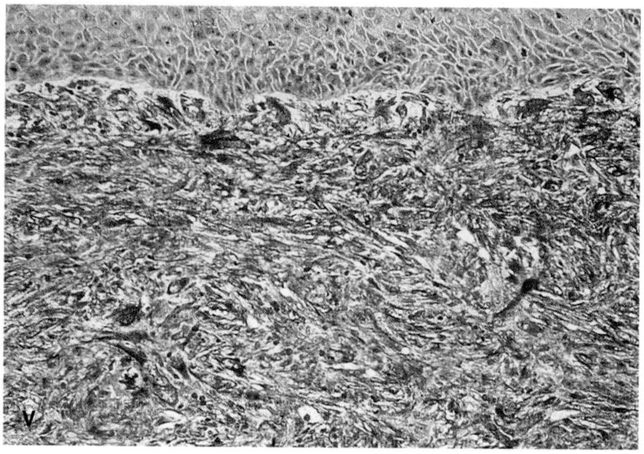

FIGURE 7.4 Intense vimentin *(V)* labeling is typically present in the cells of all malignant melanomas, as shown here.

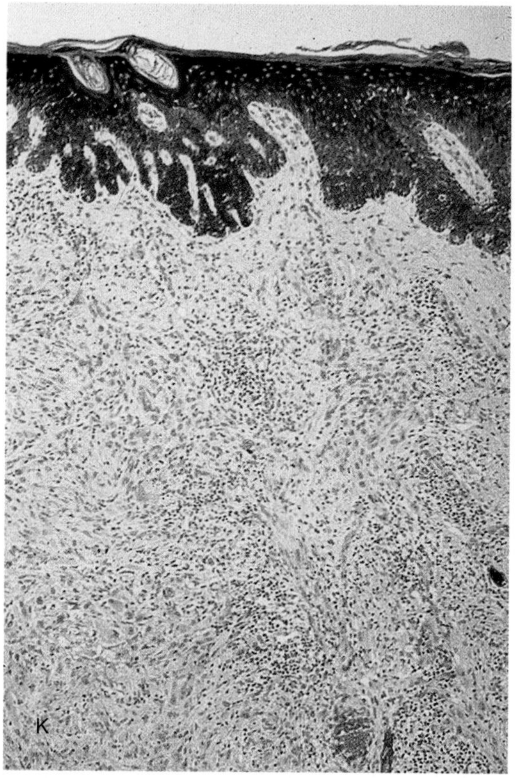

FIGURE 7.5 Keratin *(K)* is lacking in more than 97% of melanomas, in paraffin sections.

they are rarely detected in such lesions and, when observed, they are again restricted to spindle-cell melanomas that show evidence of divergent myofibroblastic differentiation.[2]

Cell-Membrane Proteins

A diversity of proteins that are associated with cell membranes come into play in relationship to the differential diagnosis of MM. Nonetheless, these fall into two broad categories: those associated with epithelial cells and those relating to hematopoietic elements.

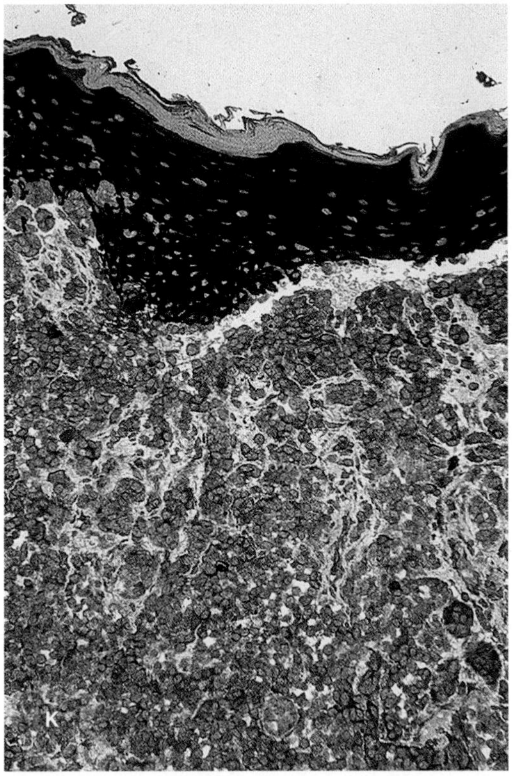

FIGURE 7.6 Only rare melanomas demonstrate keratin *(K)* reactivity (shown here) in routinely processed specimens.

EPITHELIAL DETERMINANTS

EPITHELIAL MEMBRANE ANTIGEN Epithelial membrane antigen (EMA), which is actually a family of glycoproteins that are related to the milk fat globule proteins, is expressed by a variety of epithelia and their neoplasms.[10] The principal exceptions in the latter group include germ cell tumors, adrenocortical proliferations, and hepatocellular neoplasms.[11,12] An EMA-like moiety also may be observed in selected lymphoid and plasmacellular tumors.[10,11] On the other hand, melanocytic proliferations are consistently nonreactive for this marker.[10-12] It may be observed with a tantalizingly spurious cell-membranous distribution in foci of melanomas that border zones of geographic necrosis; however, this pattern of labeling is artifactual and should be disregarded. Purely cytoplasmic reactivity for EMA is similarly discounted interpretatively.

CARCINOEMBRYONIC ANTIGEN Carcinoembryonic antigen (CEA) is also a family of glycoproteinaceous cell membrane constituents that are present mainly in tissues and neoplasms with endodermal derivation or differentiation. In the past, it has been contended that CEA may be observed in melanomas as well,[13] but on the basis of recent data,[14] that premise is felt to be a reflection of faulty technique and the use of unabsorbed heteroantisera in immunohistologic studies. Such reagents recognize several proteins other than CEA (e.g., nonspecific cross-reacting antigen; biliary glycoprotein), many of which are not restricted to epithelial cells. If monoclonal antibodies are employed with suitable specificity to restricted CEA epitopes, melanocytic neoplasms should demonstrate no labeling whatsoever.[15]

TUMOR-ASSOCIATED GLYCOPROTEIN-72/BER-EP4 ANTIGEN/MOC-31 ANTIGEN Tumor-associated glycoprotein (TAG72/CA72-4) (recognized by monoclonal antibody B72.3), BER-EP4, and MOC-31 are all cell-membrane glycoproteins that are most consistently synthesized by epithelial cells.[16] There are rare exceptions to that statement—for example, the presence of TAG72 in some epithelioid vascular tumors—but they do not include melanocytic neoplasms.[15] Therefore immunostains against this group of adjunctive epithelial markers are useful supplements to others for keratin, EMA, and CEA in helping to exclude epithelial neoplasms in the differential diagnosis of MMs. One can safely state that virtually all somatic carcinomas should be reactive for at least one of the membrane determinants cited earlier in this discussion, as well as keratin. In contrast, those rare melanomas that can be labeled for keratin lack similar corroborating evidence of epithelial differentiation.

PLACENTAL-LIKE ALKALINE PHOSPHATASE Placental-like alkaline phosphatase (PLAP) is an isozyme that is commonly synthesized by neoplastic germ cells, as well as selected somatic epithelial malignancies.[17] As such, it is a useful screening marker for gonadal tumors such as seminoma, embryonal carcinoma, and yolk sac carcinoma, all of which may enter the differential diagnosis of MM. In contrast, melanocytic proliferations are consistently nonreactive for PLAP. However, it must be remembered that this determinant is centered in cell membranes; therefore neoplasms that demonstrate only a cytoplasmic "blush" for PLAP in immunohistologic preparations (including melanomas) should not be regarded as truly positive for that marker.

"HEMATOPOIETIC" MARKERS

Selected cell-surface antigens that are typically associated with hematopoietic cells and neoplasms also are potentially seen in melanocytic cells and neoplasms. These include CD10, CD44, CD56, CD57, CD59, CD68, CD74, CD99, CD117 (c-*kit* protein), CD146, class II major histocompatibility antigens (MHC2A [HLA-DR, HLADP, HLA-DQ]), beta-2-microglobulin (B2M), and *bcl*-2 protein.[18-27] The author has observed all of those markers in selected examples of Spitz (epithelioid and spindle-cell) nevus, architecturally disordered ("dysplastic") nevus, and melanoma. Conversely, melanocytes uniformly lack other hematopoietic determinants that may enter into differential diagnostic evaluations of MM such as terminal deoxynucleotidyl transferase, factor XIIIa, myeloperoxidase, CD15, CD20, CD21, CD23, CD30, CD35, CD43, CD45, and CD138.[28,29]

The expression of MHC2A and B2M by melanocytic proliferations appears to be a property confined to inflamed banal nevi or architecturally disordered nevi, as well as MMs.[30] Clinicians interested in using immunotherapy for melanoma will often request that such a neoplasm be studied immunohistologically for its synthesis of those markers. Interestingly, MMs that "escape" immune surveillance have been noted to down-regulate their expression of B2M and histocompatibility antigens over time,[26] through mutations in the corresponding gene complexes and other mechanisms. Because of the immunophenotypic heterogeneity seen in melanocytic lesions (as well as other tumors) for MHC2A and B2M, such determinants should *not* be employed in a differential diagnostic capacity.

The ability of melanomas to be labeled for *bcl*-2 protein and CD10; CD68; CD56, CD57, and CD99; and CD117 creates the possibility that they may be confused with lymphomas, histiocytic lesions, primitive neuroectodermal and neuroendocrine neoplasms, and gastrointestinal stromal tumors, respectively. As usual, the application of carefully constructed panels of antibody reagents, tailored to specific diagnostic scenarios, should preclude those mistakes.

NB84

NB84 is a monoclonal antibody that was raised against a cell-membrane determinant found in neuroblastomas. It is active in paraffin sections and labels not only neuroblastic neoplasms but also a subset of primitive neuroectodermal tumors.[31] Melanocytic proliferations are nonreactive with this reagent. The latter fact is helpful in those circumstances where differential diagnosis centers around small cell melanoma *versus* a neuroblastic or neuroectodermal tumor arising in a large congenital nevus or neurocristic hamartoma.[32]

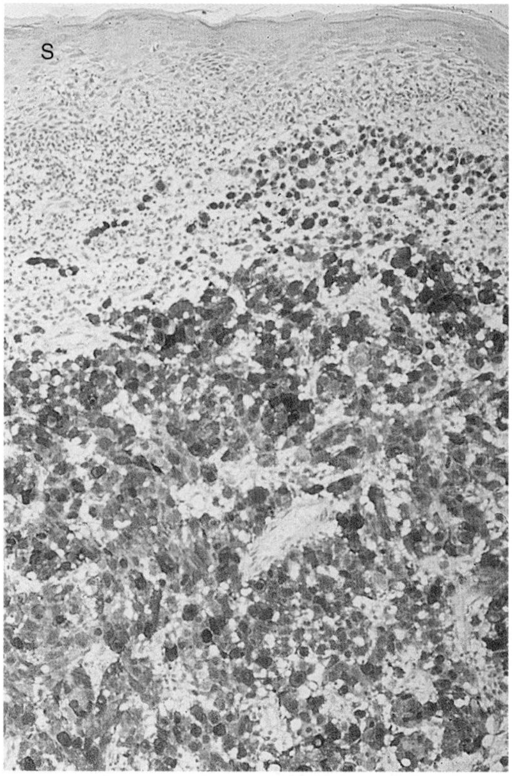

FIGURE 7.7 Intense nucleocytoplasmic immunoreactivity for S-100 protein *(S)* in primary cutaneous epithelioid melanoma.

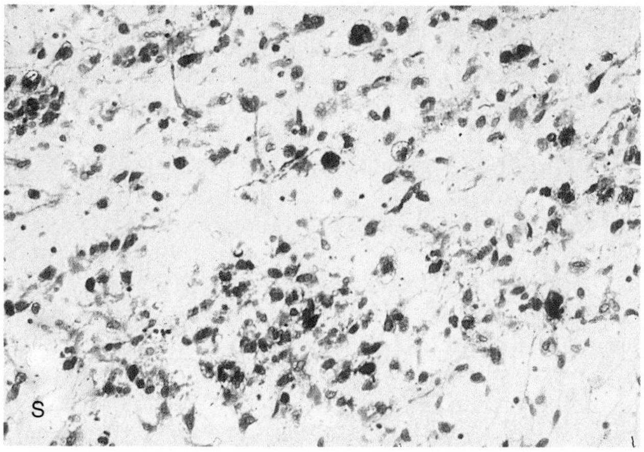

FIGURE 7.8 Nucleocytoplasmic labeling for S-100 protein *(S)* in myxoid/sarcomatoid melanoma.

Calcium-Binding Proteins

Several proteins that affect intracellular calcium metabolism including annexin VI, cap-g, annexin V, calmodulin, calretinin, and S-100 protein can be seen in melanocytic proliferations.[33] Only two of those have definite diagnostic importance and are discussed further here.

S-100 PROTEIN

One of the first, and one of the most enduring, markers for MM is S-100 protein (S100P). This 21 kD moiety was first detected in glial cells of the central nervous system, and it was given its name because of solubility in 100% saturated ammonium sulfate solution.[34] In 1981 Gaynor and colleagues[35] recognized the fact that S100P was present in human melanoma cells as well, leading to its widespread application as a diagnostic indicator for that tumor subsequently (Figs. 7.7 and 7.8).

The function of S100P has never been determined with precision; however, it is thought to function in intracellular calcium trafficking, or microtubular assembly, or both.[36,37] It has a loose physiologic relationship to calmodulin, another calcium flux protein.[33] There are two subunits to S100P—alpha and beta—yielding three possible dimeric forms: alpha-alpha; alpha-beta; and beta-beta.[38] Melanocytes synthesize only the first of those combinations. Immunoreactivity for S100P should be both nuclear and cytoplasmic in order to be regarded as valid. Immunoelectron microscopic studies have verified the presence of this protein in both intracellular compartments in normal and neoplastic melanocytes.[39]

At this point, many antibodies to S100P have been developed, some of which are dimer-specific monoclonal products.[40] In general practice, however, most clinical laboratories still use heteroantisera against this marker that recognize all three isotypes of the protein. This allows such reagents to be employed successfully as high-sensitivity screening tools. In that context the author's experience has been that more than 98% of MM cases can be labeled for S100P, regardless of histologic subtype. A redaction of the pertinent literature by

Smoller[41] yielded a slightly lower figure (97.4%). Other S100P-positive tumor types that enter into differential diagnostic consideration with melanocytic lesions include various poorly differentiated carcinomas, selected histiocytic proliferations, malignant gliomas, peripheral nerve sheath tumors, and Langerhans' cell proliferations.[39,41-45] It should be obvious, then, that S100P is most valuable in this setting as an initial screening reagent for melanocytic tumors, rather than being a specific marker for such neoplasms.

Recently, various isoforms of S100P (A2, A6, A8/A9, and A12) have also been considered diagnostically in regard to various melanocytic lesions. Ribe and McNutt[46] suggested that S100P-A6 was differentially expressed by Spitz nevi and melanomas. All Spitz tumors were A6 reactive, whereas only 33% of melanomas showed positivity. Moreover, differences in the scope of labeling were observed, with Spitz nevi being globally A6 reactive; in contrast, melanomas showed weak-patchy staining.

CALRETININ

Calretinin is a cytoplasmic 31 kD protein, which again was first isolated from central nervous system tissues.[47,48] It is also seen in peripheral nerves in the skin and elsewhere.[49] Otherwise, this polypeptide is rather restricted in distribution, having been detected thus far only in mesothelium,[48] germinal surface epithelium of the ovary,[48] and selected adenocarcinomas (most notably a subset in the colon and rectum).[50] Melanocytic tumors are not included in the list of neoplasms that show potential calretinin immunoreactivity.

Melanocyte-"Specific" Monoclonal Antibodies

Beginning in the early 1980s, the availability of monoclonal antibody technology was applied to a quest for a "melanoma-specific" reagent, which ideally would be suited not only for diagnostic but also for therapeutic utility.[51] This search continues almost 20 years later and has not yet come to ultimate fruition.

A variety of antimelanocyte hybridoma products have been described, only some of which are applicable to paraffin sections and routinely processed tissue specimens. They have been summarized previously by Smoller.[41] Those whose activity is restricted to frozen tissue substrates include PAL-M1, PAL-M2, 691-13-17, 691-15-Nu4B, and "MEL" series antibodies number 1 through number 4. In contrast, HMSA-2, 2-139-1, 6-26-3, KBA62, 1C11, 7H11, MEL-CAM, MEL-5, and SM5-1 do have immunoreactivity with formalin-fixed, paraffin-embedded specimens.[41,52,53] Generally speaking, the markers just listed have not entered or are no longer used in the sphere of diagnostic pathology because of special tissue processing requirements that are associated with them, an unavailability of commercial distribution, or a lack of sensitivity or specificity for malignant melanocytic lesions. Those that have been employed in a clinical context are considered in the following sections.

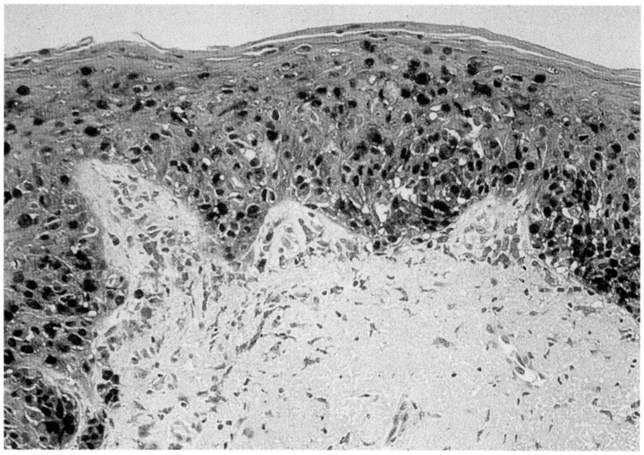

FIGURE 7.9 Global cytoplasmic immunoreactivity is seen in this primary superficial spreading melanoma, for MART-1/melan-A protein.

GP100/PMEL 17–RELATED MONOCLONAL ANTIBODIES

Several monoclonal antibodies have now been raised against a glycoproteinaceous antigenic group that is restricted to cells of melanocytic lineage. This group is designated "gp100," and corresponding cDNA to it has been cloned.[54,55] Two proteins are encoded by that nucleic acid sequence—gp100 itself (with a molecular weight of 100 kD) and gp10 (with a molecular weight of 10 kD).[55] The translational product related to gp100-C1 cDNA is closely homologous, but not identical, to yet another melanocytic protein termed PMel 17.[56] Both are localized to the inner membranes of types 1, 2, and 3 premelanosomes; they similarly serve as potential targets for cytotoxic T lymphocytes, probably in concert with MHC2A.[57] Indeed, one marker in this group—MART-1—was named specifically for that property (Melanoma Antigen Recognized by T-cells-1); it is recognized by two monoclonal antibodies, A103 and M2-7C10, and is also known as "melan-A" (Fig. 7.9).[58-69] Nucleotide sequence analysis performed by Adema and colleagues[55] has shown that the cDNAs for gp100 and PMel 17 emanate from a single gene, by alternative splicing. This conclusion gained further support by their observation that gp100 and PMel 17 are consistently expressed concomitantly by both non-neoplastic and neoplastic melanocytic populations.[70] Chiamenti and colleagues[71] conversely suggested that the protein target of HMB-45 was a unique premelanosome-related polypeptide, but that proposition has not been confirmed by other investigators.

Interestingly, gp100 *transcripts* are not specific for melanocytes and have been observed in a wide variety of tissue types.[54] Nonetheless, *translation* of the mRNA in question does occur only in melanocytic elements. This finding strongly suggests that immunohistology is the most practical technologic method for assessment of gp100 as a melanocyte marker, and that nucleic acid–based procedures (e.g., *in situ* hybridization; polymerase chain reaction) are likely to be associated with unacceptably low specificity of gp100 for pigment-producing cells.

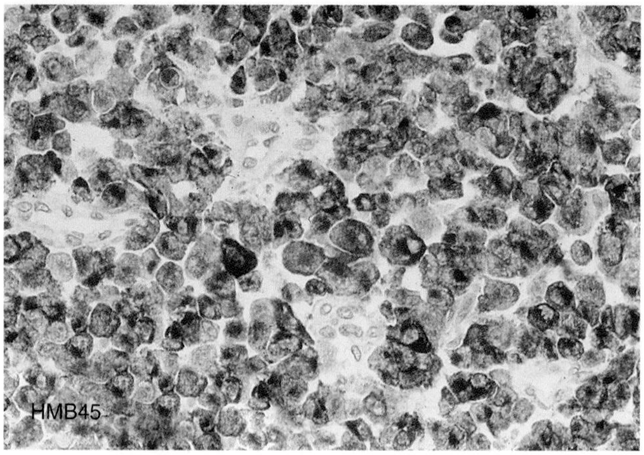

FIGURE 7.10 Intense cytoplasmic positivity with HMB-45 in epithelioid melanoma, metastatic to a lymph node.

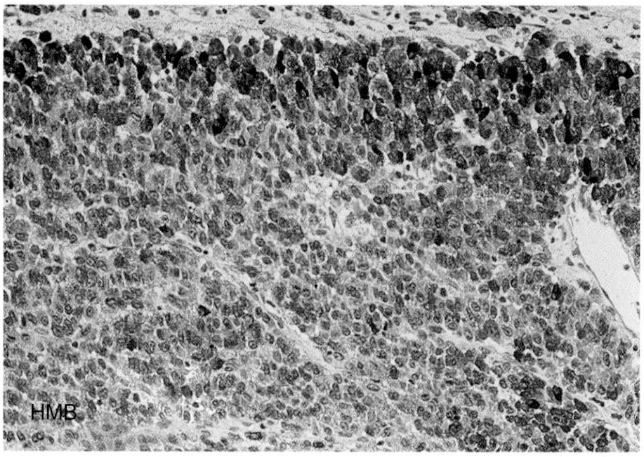

FIGURE 7.11 Heterogeneous cytoplasmic labeling with HMB-50 *(HMB)* in metastatic lymph nodal epithelioid melanoma.

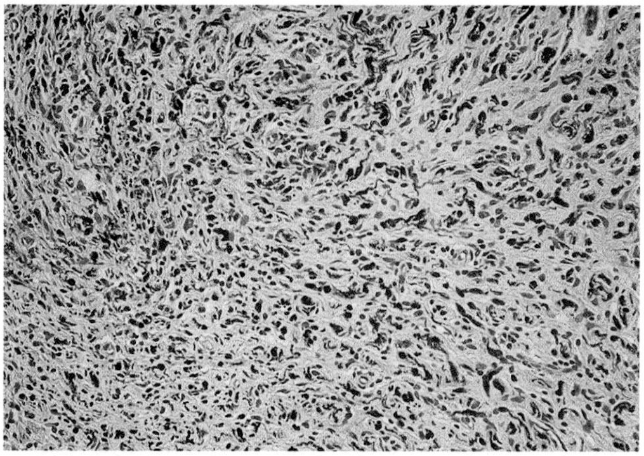

FIGURE 7.12 Multifocal immunoreactivity is apparent with HMB-45 in this spindle-cell–rich angiomyolipoma of the kidney.

Antibodies in the gp100/PMel 17 group include NKI-beteb, NKI/C3, HMB-45, HMB-50, and MART-1/melan-A (Figs 7.10 and 7.11).[55,56,58-70,72-90] These demonstrate variable levels of specificity and sensitivity for melanocytes, nevi, and melanomas, vis-à-vis other cell lineages and tumor types. In practice, HMB-45 and MART-1 have thus far enjoyed the greatest usage as agents to confirm the identity of S-100 protein-positive neoplasms as melanocytic in nature.

Unfortunate peculiarities exist that relate to the commercial distribution of HMB-45. The author had the opportunity to evaluate the original supernatant product from the HMB-45 clone, received as a generous gift from Dr. Allen Gown (one of the developers of the antibody) in the mid-1980s. In a published study that reflected this evaluation, our group found HMB-45 to be more than 95% sensitive for melanoma, and essentially 100% specific for that diagnosis among non–spindle-cell malignancies.[90] Afterward, HMB-45 was sold to a commercial firm that marketed an impure form of the hybridoma product. It showed a much lower degree of specificity and was seen to label a variety of tumors other than melanomas.[39,91-94] When other firms subsequently assumed distributorship of HMB-45, its specificity "recovered." Nevertheless, in a probable effort to maximize profits, many of those companies have now prediluted the "neat" antibody that is provided to users, and its overall sensitivity is now no better than 60% as a result of that manipulation.

Another observation relating to HMB-45, HMB-50, MART-1, and other gp100-related reagents has widely but quite erroneously been said to reflect "cross-reactivity" with non-melanocytic cells. This refers to the ability of the cited antibodies to label angiomyolipomas, lymphangioleiomyomatosis, "sugar" tumors (clear cell myomelanocytic tumors) of the lung and other organs, and other examples of proliferations showing epithelioid perivascular-cell features (Fig. 7.12).[95-101] These lesions do manifest ultrastructural evidence of premelanosome synthesis and therefore have at least partial melanocytic differentiation.[96,97] Hence gp100-related antibodies are not manifesting cross-reactivity in labeling such pathologic entities; that affinity is merely a biologic extension of their specificity for premelanosome-associated proteins.

One true exception to the last statement is represented by the ability of MART-1/melan-A (but not HMB-45, NKI-beteb, or HMB-50) to label the tumor cells of a subset of adrenocortical carcinomas and sex-cord tumors of the gonads (Fig. 7.13).[64,102] No evidence of true melanocytic differentiation has been seen in such neoplasms, and MART-1 antibodies are presumably recognizing an antigenic epitope in those steroidogenic proliferations, which is shared with the gp100/PMel 17 molecules.

As alluded to earlier, none of the antibodies considered in this section is effective at labeling more than a small fraction (<10%) of spindle-cell/desmoplastic/neuroid melanomas.[65,80,81] This "shortcoming" is likely a reflection of the fact that such neoplasms typically manifest clonal evolution from a melanocytic phenotype to a more fibroblastic or schwannian motif, losing, in the process, their ability to synthesize premelanosomes and proteins related to those organelles.

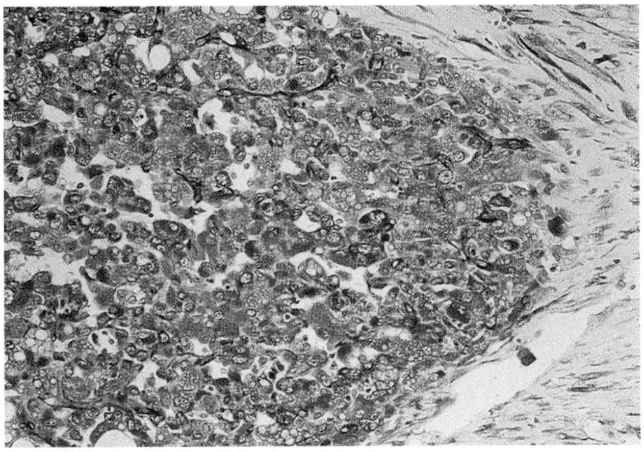

FIGURE 7.13 Diffuse labeling for MART-1/melan-A (with antibody clone A103) in adrenocortical carcinoma.

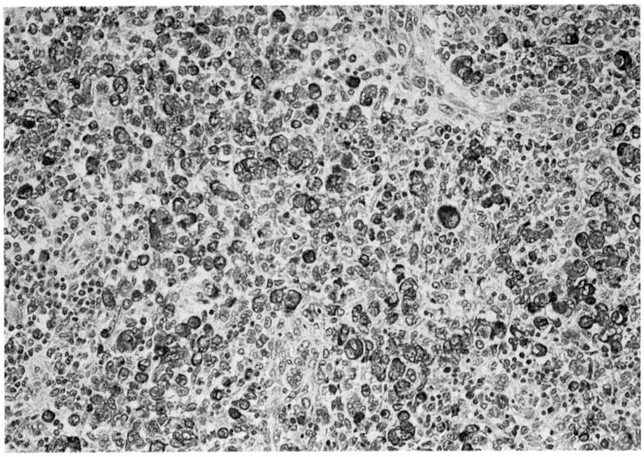

FIGURE 7.14 Multifocal intense positivity for tyrosinase in metastatic epithelioid melanoma in the liver.

KEY DIAGNOSTIC POINTS

Gp100 Antibodies

- HMB-45 and melan-A are highly specific for melanocytic cell types, with sensitivity in the 60% to 80% range.
- Gp100 antibodies regularly react with cells of angiomyolipoma and lesions of the PEComa group of neoplasms.
- Melan-A decorates adrenocortical carcinomas and sex-cord tumors of the ovary.
- A minority of desmoplastic/spindle melanomas show reactivity with the gp100 antibody group.

TYROSINASE-RELATED ANTIBODIES

In normal melaninogenesis, the amino acid tyrosine is hydroxylated to form 3,4-dihydroxyphenylalanine ("dopa"), which is then oxidized to dopa-quinone. The latter moiety is polymerized to form melanin, thereafter combining with melanoprotein to form a stable complex within premelanosomes and melanosomes.[103] Tyrosinase plays a central role in this process, by catalyzing the first step in the stated sequence.[104] As such, it is a specific marker for melanocytic differentiation. This premise has been affirmed by studies showing that tyrosinase gene transcripts are strictly confined to melanin-producing cells.[105]

T311 and MAT-1 are the two antityrosinase monoclonal antibodies that have been best analyzed in surgical pathology.[106-115] The second of them is an IgG reagent that was raised using a synthetic peptide corresponding to the carboxy terminus of human tyrosinase as an immunogen.[113] Both antibodies show a high level (>80%) of sensitivity and virtually absolute specificity for melanoma of the non-spindle-cell type, among all malignant tumors (Fig. 7.14). Interestingly, nevi are said to be nonreactive with MAT-1 in many instances, as are non-neoplastic melanocytes.[112] Hence the epitope it recognizes is presumably related to melanocytic maturation, as well as differentiation. In light of that finding, and because of the excellent specificity of antityrosinase antibodies, it would seem logical and permissible to use them diagnostically as mixtures (so-called "cocktails").

MICROPHTHALMIA TRANSCRIPTION FACTOR PROTEIN

The microphthalmia gene encodes a transcription factor that is necessary to the survival and development of melanocytes during embryogenesis.[116] Microphthalmia transcription factor protein (MTFP) is a nuclear basic helix-loop-helix leucine zipper moiety that, together with the PAX3 and MSG1 gene products, plays a role in controlling the activity of melanogenic enzymes by up-regulating the cyclic adenosine monophosphate pathway.[117-119] (Incidentally, another related gene, TFE, has similar properties and its transcription factor may emerge in the future as an additional melanocyte marker.[119])

Although data on the immunoreactivity of MTFP antibodies are relatively preliminary, these reagents appear to be sensitive and specific for the identification of melanocytic proliferations.[120-123] As is true of most other markers in this general category except for S100P, MTFP has typically labeled most non-sarcomatoid melanocytic lesions but a substantially lesser proportion of spindle-cell/desmoplastic melanomas.[120,121,123] In keeping with its known intracellular localization, MTFP should be regarded as truly present immunohistologically *only* if nuclear reactivity is observed.[122] Intriguingly, and in additional support for their partially melanocytic nature, angiomyolipoma, lymphangioleiomyomatosis, and "sugar" tumors share MTFP reactivity with MM.[124,125]

PNL2

In 2003, Rochaix and colleagues[126] described the clinical use of a new monoclonal antibody, PNL2, which had been raised against a fixative-resistant melanocyte antigen. In a study encompassing a spectrum of benign and malignant melanocytic lesions, those authors observed little if any labeling of banal nevocytes in the dermis, whereas junctional nevus cells were PNL2 positive.

Melanomas were also immunoreactive in all cases, except for tumors with a desmoplastic appearance. PNL2 has also been tested against non-melanocytic neoplasms,[127-129] and it appears to have adequate specificity to justify its use in clinical settings.

NEUROENDOCRINE MARKERS IN MELANOCYTIC LESIONS

Because of a conceptual association of both melanocytic and neuroendocrine proliferations with the neuroectoderm, it could be expected that these categories of neoplasia might demonstrate significant immunohistologic homologies. With the passage of time, however, it has become clear that there are both consistent similarities and differences between them.

Proteins that are restricted anatomically to neurosecretory granules and neurosynaptic vesicles such as chromogranins and synaptophysin are consistently absent in "pure" melanocytic tumors.[130-134] However, it is apparent that selected lesions that are basically neuroendocrine or non-melanocytic neuroectodermal neoplasms (e.g., neuroendocrine carcinomas, paragangliomas, primitive neuroectodermal tumors, peripheral nerve sheath tumors) may exhibit a variable degree of divergent melanocytic differentiation. This phenomenon yields such diagnostic entities as "pigmented carcinoid,"[135,136] "pigmented paraganglioma,"[137] "melanotic neuroectodermal tumor,"[138,139] and "melanotic schwannoma"[140] (both benign and malignant) (Fig. 7.15). In these lesions, "minor" melanocytic elements have the same immunophenotype as the cells of cutaneous nevi or MMs (i.e., S100P+, HMB-45+, MART-1+, tyrosinase+), but the remaining constituents are monodifferentiated epithelial, neural, or schwannian tissues. The latter cells lack melanocytic markers altogether, producing a dimorphic and mutually exclusive immunophenotype.

Other "neuroendocrine" determinants that may be seen in melanoma are, in fact, synthesized by a broad repertoire of cell types. They include, but are not limited to, melanocytes, neuroendocrine epithelial cells, neuroblasts, primitive mesenchymal neuroectodermal cells, and Schwann cells. The markers in question are principally represented by neuron-specific (*gamma* dimer) enolase, neural-cell adhesion molecule (CD56), CD57, and CD99 (MIC2 protein).[141-146] With the exception of CD99, they tend to be observed preferentially in melanocytic proliferations with neuroid features such as neurotized intradermal nevi and "neurotropic" melanomas.[144] Thus it is obvious that such markers cannot be used to distinguish between truly neuroendocrine and melanocytic neoplasms.

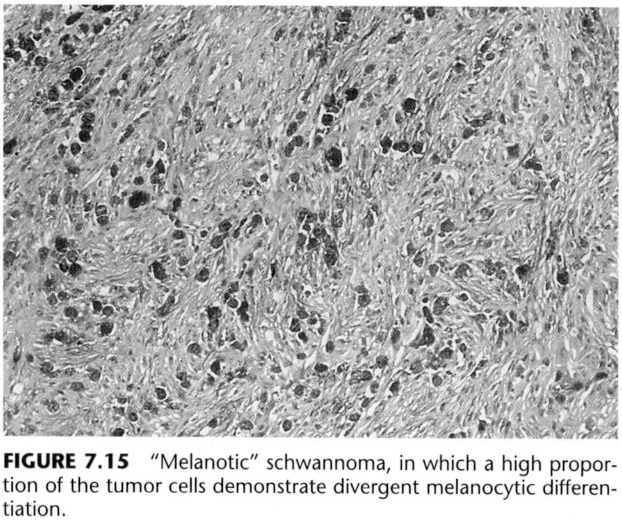

FIGURE 7.15 "Melanotic" schwannoma, in which a high proportion of the tumor cells demonstrate divergent melanocytic differentiation.

"SENTINEL" LYMPH NODE BIOPSIES FOR METASTATIC MELANOMA

Over the past decade, enthusiasm has grown among surgeons for the "sentinel" lymph node biopsy (SLNB) in assessing patients with melanoma for possible metastasis.[147] The basic precept underlying that technique is that the absence of melanoma in an SLNB obviates the need for regional lymphadenectomy, whereas metastasis—no matter how small it is—should prompt implementation of the latter procedure. This topic has relevance to our discussion here because pathology-oriented publications have suggested that extensive immunohistologic evaluation of SLNB specimens is necessary to detect all "micro"-metastases of melanoma.[148,149] Indeed, multiantibody "cocktails" have been devised for application to lymph nodes in that specific setting to maximize immunohistochemical sensitivity.[150]

The author has several conceptual problems with this practice,[151] as enumerated by Medalie and Ackerman[152] in their monograph on SLNB for melanoma. Overwhelmingly, the experience of several well-planned prospective randomized trials of lymphadenectomy for melanoma has shown that it does not improve overall survival. Moreover, there are currently no effective adjuvant treatments for that tumor. Thirdly, the prognostic value of a positive SLNB for melanoma—especially regarding "micro"-metastasis—is less than absolute in an individual, case-specific setting. Hence there is no practical reason to continue to use SLNB at all in this context, and the application of elaborate immunohistologic (or "molecular") methodology[149,153] is completely superfluous in the author's opinion. It follows that such procedures certainly should not be portrayed as representing "standard" practice.

PUTATIVELY PROGNOSTIC MARKERS FOR MELANOMA

Over the past decade, several publications have considered adjunctive morphologic pathologic procedures that have putative prognostic utility in MM. These include immunostaining for mutated p53 protein (a promoter of programmed cell death); Ki-67, proliferating cell nuclear antigen, and Ki-S5 (cell cycle-related indicators of proliferation); heat shock proteins (markers of replicating or "activated" cells); *bcl-2* protein (an inhibitor of apoptosis); VLA-4 and alpha-v/beta-3 integrins (intercellular adhesion molecules that correlate with entrance into the vertical growth phase of melanoma); CD26/dipeptidyl-aminopeptidase IV (a membrane-bound protease that assists tumor cell invasion); osteopontin (an adhesive matricellular glycoprotein that up-regulates metalloproteinase production); NM23 (a metastasis-suppressor gene product); Cdc42 and CXCR4 proteins (moieties influencing cellular motility); E-cadherin (a protein concerned with cell-matrix interaction); and cyclin-D1, cyclin-D3, *Trk-A*, and p16INK4-alpha (CDKN2A) gene products (cell cycle regulators).[154-164] Another proposed method uses immunostains for endothelial and lymphatic markers (e.g., von Willebrand factor, CD31, CD34, podoplanin)[165-167] to assess stromal vascularity in vertical growth-phase melanomas, with the premise that increased angiogenesis is correlated with an adverse prognosis.[168,169] In general, the afore-mentioned markers have not been embraced as clinically relevant tools yet because of disagreements on interpretative thresholds and methodologic issues attending them.

It is important to note that prognostically adverse results of the analytic techniques just cited appear to be intimately associated with acquisition of the vertical growth phase in melanomas. This reality probably reflects several biologic events that accompany the "malignant eclipse" from radial to vertical growth. They potentially include an increase in autocrine mitogenic growth factors in vertical growth melanomas (VGMs), decreased rates of apoptosis in VGM tumor cells, an acquired resistance to growth-inhibitory factors in the vertical growth phase, augmented angiogenesis by VGM cells, and loss of the *c-kit* (CD117) gene product (having tyrosine kinase activity).[170,171] On a cytogenetic level, it has been shown that the transition between radial and vertical growth phases is paralleled by gains in gene copy numbers on chromosomes 7, 8, 6p, 1q, 20, 17, and 2, in decreasing order of frequency.[172]

At present, non-morphologic techniques to evaluate the prognosis of MMs must be regarded as investigational and cannot yet be recommended for routine clinical application. All necessary pathologic data such as tumor location, size, depth, ulceration, mitotic activity, and growth phase can still be obtained by examination of standard microscopic preparations of melanoma as stained with hematoxylin and eosin.

Differential Diagnosis of Selected Lesions

MELANOMA VERSUS MELANOCYTIC NEVUS VARIANTS

Several papers have appeared on the use of immunohistology for the separation of benign and malignant melanocytic neoplasms of various types. In particular, the differential diagnosis of Spitz nevus versus melanoma has been discussed several times in reference to their relative expression of mutant p16 and p53 proteins, Ki-67, Ki-S5, S100P-A6, and other markers relating to cellular transformation or proliferation.[46,173-178] Although some general trends have emerged from such analyses, there is too much overlap in the immunophenotypes of melanocytic nevi and melanomas for those data to be used meaningfully in individual cases.

MELANOCYTIC NEOPLASMS VERSUS HISTIOCYTIC PROLIFERATIONS

In the skin and elsewhere, it may be histologically difficult to separate amelanotic melanocytic lesions from such histiocytic proliferations as epithelioid histiocytoma, foam-cell-poor xanthogranuloma, atypical fibroxanthoma, and reticulohistiocytoma(-sis).[179-181] Even though occasional histiocytic tumors may label for S100P, they are consistently non-reactive with HMB-45, HMB-50, MART-1, antityrosinase, and anti-MTFP. In contrast, histiocytomas and melanocytic neoplasms both may be reactive for factor XIIIa and CD68, which have been loosely (and mistakenly) advanced as "histiocytic markers."[23,182-184] In the author's experience, the only consistently reliable indicator of monocyte-macrophage differentiation is CD163,[185] which is lacking in melanocytic proliferations.[186]

RECOGNITION OF RHABDOID AND SARCOMATOID MALIGNANT MELANOMAS

Rhabdoid and sarcomatoid melanomas (including desmoplastic, myxoid, neurotropic, and osteochondroid subtypes) may be chosen for special discussion because they demonstrate antigenic deletion or aberrancy in a relatively substantial proportion of cases. Indeed, the first example of rhabdoid melanoma that the author encountered was a metastatic keratin-positive, S100P negative tumor in a patient who was known to have had melanoma in the past. That particular variant of melanocytic malignancy loses reactivity for S100P, HMB-45, MART-1, or tyrosinase in approximately 20% of cases in the author's experience and that of others[187] and acquires positivity for keratin or desmin in roughly 1% to 3%.[188-191] Obviously, an extended panel of reagents including essentially all of the available melanocytic markers must therefore be employed to recognize rhabdoid melanomas with accuracy.

Sarcomatoid melanomas are consistently S100P positive, but only 3% to 10% can be labeled for other, more specific melanocytic determinants (Fig. 7.16).[80,120,121,123,192] Because a proportion of such lesions becomes transmogrified into spindle-cell proliferations with divergent phenotypes, immunoreactivity for CD56, CD57, nerve growth factor receptor, desmin, and actin isoforms is potentially observed in them (Figs. 7.17 and 7.18).[2,141-146,187] Especially in the absence of a given history of melanoma, those immunophenotypic quirks represent distinct diagnostic pitfalls for the unwary.

AMELANOTIC MELANOMA VERSUS OTHER EPITHELIOID MALIGNANCIES

A classical differential diagnostic question posed by surgical pathologists is that of melanoma versus poorly differentiated carcinoma versus large cell non-Hodgkin

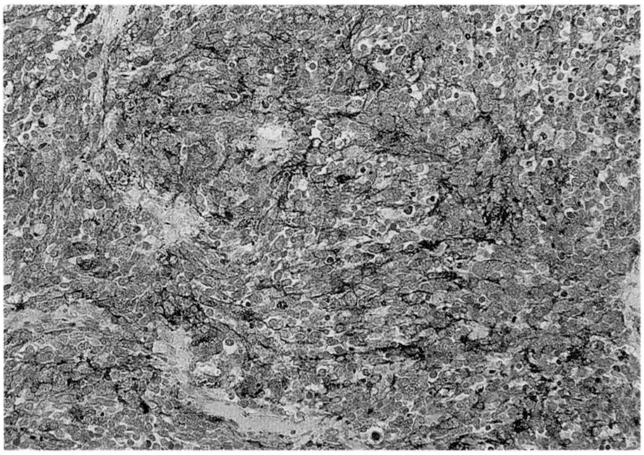

FIGURE 7.16 Immunolabeling for tyrosinase in sarcomatoid melanoma; less than 10% of examples of this tumor variant stain for melanocytic markers other than S-100 protein.

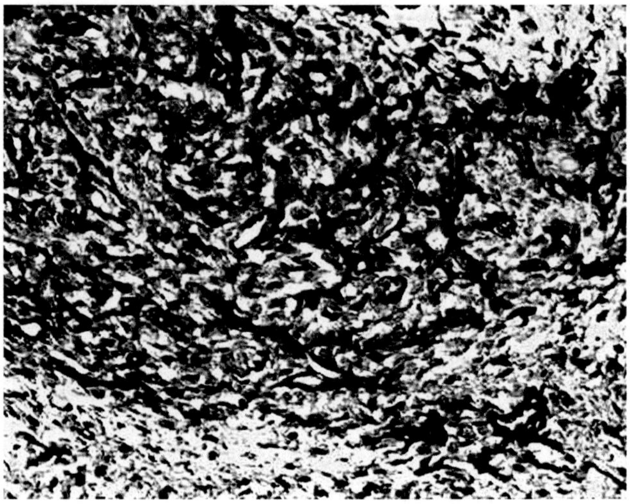

FIGURE 7.18 CD57 immunolabeling in a malignant peripheral nerve sheath tumor.

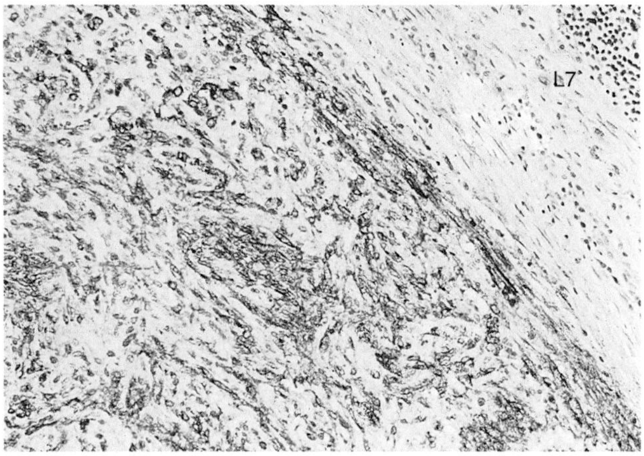

FIGURE 7.17 CD57/Leu 7 *(L7)* in sarcomatoid/desmoplastic malignant melanoma, likely reflecting neuroid differentiation in that tumor.

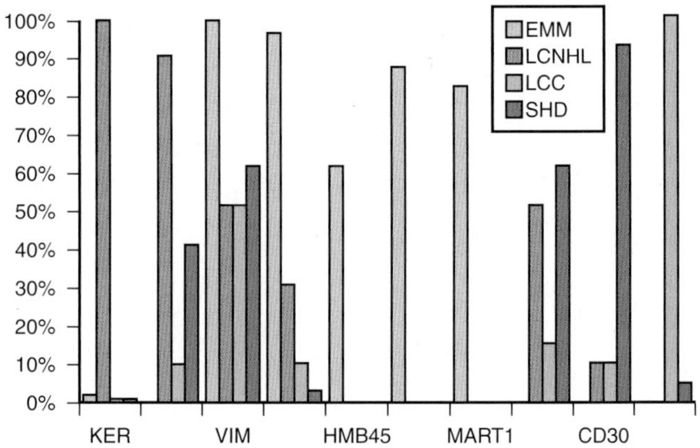

FIGURE 7.19 Immunoreactivity patterns in large cell undifferentiated malignancies.

lymphoma or "syncytial" Hodgkin disease.[192,193] This is particularly true of tumors presenting in lymph nodes, with no known history of a prior malignancy.

Under such circumstances, applicable antibody panels should include reagents to keratins, EMA, vimentin, S100P, HMB-45, tyrosinase, MART-1, CD15, CD30, and CD45. Expected results in the specified classes of tumor being considered are depicted in Figure 7.19.

The same basic approach may be used when the differential diagnosis is that of metastatic serosal melanoma versus malignant mesothelioma, except that antibodies to calretinin, thrombomodulin, and HBME-1 should be included. The great majority of mesotheliomas, if not all of them, will express at least one of the latter three determinants, whereas MM is non-reactive for all of them.[194-196]

Neuroendocrine carcinomas may be separated from MM by attention to keratin reactivity patterns and positivity for chromogranins and synaptophysin.[134] As stated earlier, melanocytic lesions lack the latter two markers consistently, whereas at least 50% of neuroendocrine epithelial tumors express at least one of them. Keratin often assumes a dotlike, perinuclear, globular intracytoplasmic pattern of labeling in neuroendocrine carcinomas,[197] but, in the small minority of MMs that show keratin expression, that configuration is not seen.

METASTATIC MELANOMA VERSUS MALIGNANT GLIOMA

In the central nervous system, metastatic amelanotic melanoma may imitate the microscopic appearance of a high-grade malignant glioma virtually perfectly. This resemblance is further complicated by the common reactivity seen in both lesions for S100P,[94,141,198,199] and the potential for a small minority of melanomas to express glial fibrillary acidic protein as well.[21] Hence other melanocytic markers such as HMB-45, anti-tyrosinase, and MART-1 are crucial to making this diagnostic distinction. All of those determinants are absent in pure glial neoplasms.[94,199]

In specific reference to the expression of melanocytic markers in metastatic tumors, Plaza and colleagues[200] have demonstrated that there is little if any antigenic "drift" as compared with primary melanoma.

MELANOMA VERSUS SOFT TISSUE SARCOMAS

The ability of melanoma to simulate the appearance of various soft tissue sarcomas is also well documented.[201] These include malignant peripheral nerve sheath tumors, gastrointestinal stromal tumors, epithelioid angiosarcoma, rhabdoid tumors, osteosarcomas, and primitive neuroectodermal tumors, to name a few.[202] The detailed immunophenotypic properties of those lesions are provided elsewhere in this book. However, none of them manifests reactivity for gp100-related melanocytic markers or tyrosinase, making those markers essential to the differential diagnostic process.

A notable exception to that statement is represented by clear cell sarcoma of soft tissue ("melanoma of soft parts"), which clearly does exhibit true melanocytic differentiation.[203-205] Because the immunohistologic profiles of that tumor and MM are superimposable,[205] other specialized studies are usually necessary to separate them in cases where clinical findings make the diagnosis uncertain. In particular, clear cell sarcoma regularly shows the presence of a t(12;22) chromosomal translocation, apposing the EWS and *ATF1* genes, which is not present in melanomas.[206-208]

Uncommonly, primitive neuroectodermal tumors may demonstrate divergent melanocytic differentiation and thereby imitate the appearance of small cell melanoma.[2,130,138,139] Furthermore, both lesions have the potential to express CD56, CD57, and CD99. Diffuse reactivity for S100P, gp100-related markers, or MTFP would argue strongly for an interpretation of melanoma in this setting. Conversely, immunopositivity for FLI-1 protein is restricted to primitive neuroectodermal tumors (PNETs).[209] Again, cytogenetic evaluation is advisable whenever possible in this particular situation, inasmuch as PNETs demonstrate a reproducible t(11;22) chromosomal translocation.[210]

The most difficult diagnostic distinction to make in this context is that of sarcomatoid MM versus superficial malignant peripheral nerve sheath tumor (SMPNST). Indeed, in many ways, the two are nearly identical.[211] Obviously, a history of previous melanoma would be important information to have in such a case, but if that is unavailable, the author generally restricts an interpretation of SMPNST to lesions that are clearly associated with a large nerve or preexisting neurofibroma, or which have occurred in patients with systemic neurofibromatosis.[212] As mentioned earlier in reference to small cell lesions, a useful immunohistochemical clue in the distinction between spindle-cell melanoma and SMPNST concerns the level of cellular labeling for S100 protein. If the neoplastic cells are only focally positive or negative for that marker, it is more likely that one is dealing with a peripheral nerve sheath tumor than a melanocytic one. Both of these neoplastic categories share potential reactivity for nestin, p16 (cINK4a) protein, CD10, CD99, bcl-2 protein, and WT-1.[213-218]

MELANOMA *IN SITU* VERSUS PIGMENTED ACTINIC KERATOSIS

A common problem for dermatopathologists is the separation of melanoma *in situ* (MIS) with relatively bland cytologic features from pigmented actinic keratosis (PAK). Shabrawi-Caelen and colleagues[219] have addressed this differential diagnosis specifically, using antibodies to S100P, HMB-45, MART-1, and tyrosinase. The results of that study suggested that immunohistology was indeed useful in making the specified distinction. However, it was also implied that MART-1 was *overly* sensitive in the context under discussion, yielding unwanted labeling of PAK cases. The author's experience has not paralleled that of Shabrawi-Caelen and associates regarding the latter point.[220] In fact, the author prefers MART-1 to all other reagents in separating MIS from PAK because of its high level of sensitivity and crispness of staining.

MELANOMA VERSUS CUTANEOUS GRANULAR CELL TUMOR

Melanoma is one of the lesions in the skin that may assume a granular-cell composition, along with cutaneous granular-cell tumor (CGCT), basal cell carcinoma, angiosarcoma, leiomyosarcoma, and others. Gleason and Nascimento[221] have compared S100 protein-positive CGCTs and melanomas with regard to their immunoreactivity for S100 protein, MART-1, HMB-45, and MITF. Of these markers, HMB45 was the best discriminator, followed closely by MART-1. On the other hand, MITF was commonly seen in both CGCT and melanoma.[221] Calretinin and inhibin represent additional determinants that are selective for CGCT in this specific setting.[222]

PROLIFERATIVE DERMAL NODULES IN CONGENITAL NEVI VERSUS MELANOMA

In large congenital compound nevi, proliferative melanocytic nodules (PNs) that assume a "clonal" appearance are sometimes encountered in the dermis and thereby raise considerable alarm over the possibility of secondary melanoma. Herron and colleagues[223] have systematically examined a series of congenital nevi containing PNs, finding that the tumor cells in those foci paradoxically expressed putatively mutant p53 protein and *bcl*-2 protein (both of which are antiapoptotic) with *Bax* protein (a proapoptotic mediator). CD117 was also usually retained in PNs, as opposed to its common absence in melanomas. The specified immunoprofile may therefore prove to be helpful in distinguishing PNs in congenital nevi from malignant melanocytic lesions.

PRIMARY VERSUS SECONDARY INTRACUTANEOUS MELANOMA

Cutaneous melanoma has a well-known ability to metastasize *back* to the skin, and, when it does so, that tumor may even demonstrate apparent junctional dermo-epidermal growth and intraepidermal "pagetoid" spread.

As such, there are no reliable morphological features that can distinguish primary from secondary "epidermotropic" melanoma. Guerriere-Kovach and colleagues[224] assessed a group of cases in which both of the latter possibilities were represented, using antibodies to *bcl*-2 protein, mutant p53 protein, Ki-67, proliferating cell nuclear antigen (PCNA), alpha-isoform actin, and CD117 (c-kit protein). Although some trends were observed toward greater labeling of metastatic melanomas for mutant p53 protein and Ki-67, but with diminution of CD117 reactivity, that pattern was not consistent. Thus at the present time, no immunohistologic solution to this specific problem can be offered with confidence.

REFERENCES

1. Nakhleh RE, Wick MR, Rocamora A, et al. Morphologic diversity in malignant melanomas. *Am J Clin Pathol.* 1990;93:731-740.
2. Banerjee SS, Harris M. Morphologic and immunophenotypic variation in malignant melanoma. *Histopathology.* 2000;36:387-402.
3. Reed RJ, Martin P. Variants of melanoma. *Semin Cutan Med Surg.* 1997;16:137-158.
4. Battifora H. Clinical application of the immunohistochemistry of filamentous proteins. *Am J Surg Pathol.* 1988;12(Suppl):24-42.
5. Osborn M. Intermediate filaments as histologic markers: an overview. *J Invest Dermatol.* 1983;81(Suppl 1):104s-109s.
6. Ramaekers FCS, Puts JJ, Moesker O, et al. Intermediate filaments in malignant melanomas: identification and use as a marker in surgical pathology. *J Clin Invest.* 1983;71:635-643.
7. Caselitz J, Janner M, Breitbart E, et al. Malignant melanomas contain only the vimentin type of intermediate filaments. *Virchows Arch A.* 1983;400:43-51.
8. Zarbo RJ, Gown AM, Nagle RB, et al. Anomalous cytokeratin expression in malignant melanoma: one- and two-dimensional Western blot analysis and immunohistochemical survey of 100 melanomas. *Mod Pathol.* 1990;3:494-502.
9. Miettinen M, Franssila K. Immunohistochemical spectrum of malignant melanoma: the common presence of keratins. *Lab Invest.* 1989;61:623-628.
10. Swanson PE. Monoclonal antibodies to human milk fat globule proteins. In: Wick MR, Siegal GP, eds. *Monoclonal antibodies in diagnostic immunohistochemistry.* New York: Dekker; 1988:227-284.
11. Pinkus GS, Kurtin PJ. Epithelial membrane antigen—a diagnostic discriminant in surgical pathology. *Hum Pathol.* 1985;16:929-940.
12. Sloane JP, Ormerod MG. Distribution of epithelial membrane antigen in normal and neoplastic tissues and its value in diagnostic tumor pathology. *Cancer.* 1981;47:1786-1795.
13. Selby WL, Nance KV, Park KH. Carcinoembryonic antigen—immunoreactivity in metastatic malignant melanoma. *Mod Pathol.* 1992;5:415-419.
14. Ravindranath MH, Shen P, Habal N, et al. Does human melanoma express carcinoembryonic antigen? *Anticancer Res.* 2000;20:3083-3092.
15. Ben-Izhak B, Levy R, Weill S, et al. Anorectal malignant melanoma: a clinicopathology study, including immunohistochemistry and DNA flow cytometry. *Cancer.* 1997;79:18-25.
16. Muraro R, Kuroki M, Wunderlich D, et al. Generation and characterization of B72.3 second generation monoclonal antibodies reactive with the tumor associated glycoprotein72 antigen. *Cancer Res.* 1988;48:4588-4596.
17. Wick MR, Swanson PE, Manivel JC. Placental alkaline phosphatase-like reactivity in human tumors: an immunohistochemical study of 520 cases. *Hum Pathol.* 1987;18:946-954.
18. Chorvath B, Hunakova L, Turzova M, et al. Monoclonal antibodies to two adhesive cell surface antigens (CD43 and CD59) with different distribution on hematopoietic and non-hematopoietic tumor cell lines. *Neoplasma.* 1992;39:325-329.
19. Radka SF, Charron DJ, Brodsky FM. Class II molecules of the major histocompatibility complex considered as differentiation markers. *Hum Immunol.* 1986;16:390-400.
20. Carrel S, Schmidt-Kessen A, Mach JP, et al. Expression of common acute lymphoblastic leukemia antigen (CALLA) on human malignant melanoma cell lines. *J Immunol.* 1983;130:2456-2460.
21. Herbold KW, Zhou J, Haggerty JG, et al. CD44 expression on epidermal melanocytes. *J Invest Dermatol.* 1996;106:1230-1235.
22. Sarlomo-Rikala M, Kovatich AJ, Barusevicius A, et al. CD117: a sensitive marker for gastrointestinal stromal tumors that is more specific than CD34. *Mod Pathol.* 1998;11:728-734.
23. Pernick NL, DaSilva M, Gangi MD, et al. "Histiocytic" markers in melanoma. *Mod Pathol.* 1999;12:1072-1077.
24. Tang NE, Luyten GP, Mooy CM, et al. HNK-1 antigens on uveal and cutaneous melanoma cell lines. *Melanoma Res.* 1996;6:411-418.
25. Weidner N, Tjoe J. Immunohistochemical profile of monoclonal antibody O13. *Am J Surg Pathol.* 1994;18:486-494.
26. Tron VA, Krajewski S, Klein-Parker H, et al. Immunohistochemical analysis of bcl-2 protein regulation in cutaneous melanoma. *Am J Pathol.* 1995;146:643-650.
27. Wilkerson AE, Glasgow MA, Hiatt KM. Immunoreactivity for CD99 in invasive malignant melanoma. *J Cutan Pathol.* 2006;33:663-666.
28. Chu PG, Arber DA, Weiss LM. Expression of T/NK-cell and plasma-cell antigens in nonhematopoietic epithelioid neoplasms: an immunohistochemical study of 447 cases. *Am J Clin Pathol.* 2003;120:64-70.
29. Sagi A, Yun SS, Yu GH, et al. Utility of CD138 (syndecan-1) in distinguishing carcinomas from mesotheliomas. *Diagn Cytopathol.* 2005;33:65-70.
30. Ruiter DJ, Bhan AK, Harrist TJ, et al. Major histocompatibility antigens and mononuclear inflammatory infiltrate in benign nevomelanocytic proliferations and malignant melanoma. *J Immunol.* 1982;129:2808-2815.
31. Miettinen M, Chatten J, Paetan A, et al. Monoclonal antibody NB84 in the differential diagnosis of neuroblastoma and other small round cell tumors. *Am J Surg Pathol.* 1998;22:327-332.
32. Mezebish D, Smith K, Williams J, et al. Neurocristic cutaneous hamartoma: a distinctive dermal melanocytosis with an unknown malignant potential. *Mod Pathol.* 1998;11:573-578.
33. Van Ginkel PR, Gee RL, Walker TM, et al. The identification and differential expression of calcium-binding proteins associated with ocular melanoma. *Biochim Biophys Acta.* 1998;1448:290-297.
34. Ludwin SK, Kosek JC, Eng LF. The topographical distribution of S100 protein and GFA protein in the adult rat brain: an immunohistochemical study using horseradish peroxidase-labeled antibodies. *J Comp Neurol.* 1976;165:197-208.
35. Gaynor R, Irie R, Morton D, et al. S100 protein: a marker for human malignant melanomas? *Lancet.* 1981;1:869-871.
36. Baudier J, Briving C, Deinum J, et al. Effect of S100 protein and calmodulin on calcium-induced disassembly of brain microtubule proteins in vitro. *FEBS Lett.* 1982;147:165-168.
37. Stefansson K, Wollmann R, Jerkovic M. S100 protein in soft tissue tumors derived from Schwann cells and melanocytes. *Am J Pathol.* 1982;106:261-268.
38. Takahashi K, Isobe T, Ohtsuki Y, et al. Immunohistochemical study on the distribution of alpha and beta subunits of S100 protein in human normal and neoplastic tissues. *Virchows Arch B.* 1984;45:385-396.
39. Herrera GA, Pena JR, Turbat-Herrera EA, et al. The diagnosis of melanoma: current approaches addressing tumor differentiation. *Pathol Annu.* 1994;29(Part 1):233-260.
40. Loeffel SC, Gillespie GY, Mirmiram SA, et al. Cellular immunolocalization of S100 protein within fixed tissue sections by monoclonal antibodies. *Arch Pathol Lab Med.* 1985;109:117-122.
41. Smoller BR. Immunohistochemistry in the diagnosis of melanocytic neoplasms. *Pathol State Art Rev.* 1994;2:371-383.
42. Kindblom LG, Lodding P, Rosengren L, et al. S100 protein in melanocytic tumors. *Acta Pathol Microbiol Scand.* 1984;92:219-230.

43. Nakajima T, Watanabe S, Sato Y, et al. An immunoperoxidase study of S100 protein distribution in normal and neoplastic tissues. *Am J Surg Pathol.* 1982;7:715-727.
44. Cochran AJ, Lu HF, Li PX, et al. S100 protein remains a practical marker for melanocytic and other tumors. *Melanoma Res.* 1993;3:325-330.
45. Swanson PE, Wick MR. Immunohistochemistry of cutaneous tumors. In: *Applied immunohistochemistry for the surgical pathologist.* Cambridge, UK: Edward Arnold; 1993:269-308.
46. Ribe A, McNutt NS. S100A6 protein expression is different in Spitz nevi and melanomas. *Mod Pathol.* 2003;16:505-511.
47. Rogers J, Khan M, Ellis J. Calretinin and other calcium binding proteins in the nervous system. *Adv Exp Med Biol.* 1990;269:195-203.
48. Tos AP, Doglioni C. Calretinin: a novel tool for diagnostic immunohistochemistry. *Adv Anat Pathol.* 1998;5:61-66.
49. Schulze E, Witt M, Fink T, et al. Immunohistochemical detection of human skin nerve fibers. *Acta Histochem.* 1997;99: 301-309.
50. Gotzos V, Wintergerst ES, Musy JP, et al. Selective distribution of calretinin in adenocarcinomas of the human colon and adjacent tissues. *Am J Surg Pathol.* 1999;23:701-711.
51. Nance KV, Siegal GP. The use of monoclonal antibodies in the search for tumor-specific antigens. In: Wick MR, Siegal GP, eds. *Monoclonal Antibodies in Diagnostic Immunohistochemistry.* New York: Dekker; 1988:593-622.
52. Shih IM, Nesbit M, Herlyn M, et al. A new MEL-CAM (CD146)-specific monoclonal antibody, MN-4, on paraffin-embedded tissue. *Mod Pathol.* 1998;11:1098-1106.
53. Trefzer U, Rietz N, Chen Y, et al. SM5-1: a new monoclonal antibody which is highly sensitive and specific for melanocytic lesions. *Arch Dermatol Res.* 2000;292:583-589.
54. Brouwenstijn N, Slager EH, Bakker AB, et al. Transcription of the gene encoding melanoma-associated antigen gp10 tissues and cell lines other than those of the melanocytic lineage. *Br J Cancer.* 1997;76:1562-1566.
55. Adema GJ, deBoer AJ, Vogel AM, et al. Molecular characterization of the melanocyte lineage-specific antigen gp100. *J Biol Chem.* 1994;269:20126-20133.
56. Adema GJ, Bakker AB, deBoer J, et al. PMel17 is recognized by monoclonal antibodies NKI-beteb, HMB-45, HMB-50, and by anti-melanoma cytotoxic T-cells. *Br J Cancer.* 1996;73: 1044-1048.
57. Kawakami Y, Nishimura MI, Restifo NP, et al. T-cell recognition of human melanoma antigens. *J Immunother.* 1993;14: 88-93.
58. Chen YT, Stockert E, Jungbluth A, et al. Serological analysis of Melan-A (MART-1), a melanocyte-specific protein homogeneously expressed in human melanomas. *Proc Natl Acad Sci USA.* 1996;93:5916-5919.
59. Kawakami Y, Battles JK, Kobayashi T, et al. Production of recombinant MART-1 proteins and specific anti-MART-1 polyclonal and monoclonal antibodies: use in the characterization of the human melanoma antigen MART-1. *J Immunol Methods.* 1997;202:13-25.
60. Kageshita T, Kawakami Y, Hirai S, et al. Differential expression of MART-1 in primary and metastatic melanoma lesions. *J Immunother.* 1997;20:460-465.
61. Nicotra MR, Nistico P, Mangoni A, et al. Melan-A/MART-1 antigen expression in cutaneous and ocular melanomas. *J Immunother.* 1997;20:466-469.
62. Pierard-Franchimont C, Letawe C, Nikkels AF, et al. Patterns of the immunohistochemical expression of melanoma-associated antigens and density of CD45R0+ activated T-lymphocytes and L1-protein-positive macrophages in primary cutaneous melanomas. *Int J Mol Med.* 1998;2:721-724.
63. Fetsch PA, Marincola FM, Filie A, et al. Melanoma-associated antigen recognized by T-cells (MART-1): the advent of a preferred immunocytochemical antibody for the diagnosis of metastatic malignant melanoma with fine needle aspiration. *Cancer.* 1999;87:37-42.
64. Busam KJ, Jungbluth AA. Melan-A, a new melanocytic differentiation marker. *Adv Anat Pathol.* 1999;6:12-18.
65. Orosz Z. Melan-A/MART-1 expression in various melanocytic lesions and in non-melanocytic soft tissue tumors. *Histopathology.* 1999;34:517-525.
66. Yu LL, Flotte TJ, Tanabe KK, et al. Detection of microscopic melanoma metastases in sentinel lymph nodes. *Cancer.* 1999;86:617-627.
67. Anichini A, Molla A, Mortarini R, et al. An expanded peripheral T-cell population to a cytotoxic T-lymphocyte (CTL)-defined, melanocyte-specific antigen in metastatic melanoma patients impacts on generation of peptide-specific CTLs but does not overcome tumor escape from immune surveillance in metastatic lesions. *J Exp Med.* 1999;190:651-667.
68. Bergman R, Azzam H, Sprecher E, et al. A comparative immunohistochemical study of MART-1 expression in Spitz nevi, ordinary melanocytic nevi, and malignant melanomas. *J Am Acad Dermatol.* 2000;42:496-500.
69. Heegaard S, Jensen OA, Prause JU. Immunohistochemical diagnosis of malignant melanoma of the conjunctiva and uvea: comparison of the novel antibody against Melan-A with S100 protein and HMB-45. *Melanoma Res.* 2000;10:350-354.
70. Adema GJ, deBoer AJ, VantHullenaar R, et al. Melanocyte lineage-specific antigens recognized by monoclonal antibodies NKI-beteb, HMB-50, and HMB-45 are encoded by a single cDNA. *Am J Pathol.* 1993;143:1579-1585.
71. Chiamenti AM, Vella F, Bonetti F, et al. Anti-melanoma monoclonal antibody HMB-45 on enhanced chemi-luminescence-Western blotting recognizes a 30-35 kDa melanosome-associated sialated glycoprotein. *Melanoma Res.* 1996;6:291-298.
72. Esclamado RM, Gown AM, Vogel AM. Unique proteins defined by monoclonal antibodies specific for human melanoma. *Am J Surg.* 1986;152:376-385.
73. Gown AM, Vogel AM, Hoak DH, et al. Monoclonal antibodies specific for melanocytic tumors distinguish subpopulations of melanocytes. *Am J Pathol.* 1986;123:195-203.
74. Schaumburg-Lever G, Metzler G, Kaiserling E. Ultrastructural localization of HMB-45 binding sites. *J Cutan Pathol.* 1991;18:432-435.
75. Palazzo JP, Duray PH. Congenital agminated Spitz nevi: immunoreactivity with a melanoma-associated monoclonal antibody. *J Cutan Pathol.* 1988;15:166-170.
76. Smoller BR, McNutt NS, Hsu A. HMB-45 staining of dysplastic nevi: support for a spectrum of progression toward melanoma. *Am J Surg Pathol.* 1989;13:680-684.
77. Skelton III HG, Smith KJ, Barrett TL, et al. HMB-45 staining in benign and malignant melanocytic lesions: a reflection of cellular activation. *Am J Dermatopathol.* 1991;131:543-550.
78. Wick MR. HMB-45: a clue to the biology of malignant melanoma? *J Cutan Pathol.* 1991;18:307-308.
79. Smoller BR, Hsu A, Krueger J. HMB-45 monoclonal antibody recognizes an inducible and reversible melanocyte cytoplasmic protein. *J Cutan Pathol.* 1991;18:315-322.
80. Wick MR, Swanson PE, Rocamora A. Recognition of malignant melanoma by monoclonal antibody HMB-45: an immunohistochemical study of 200 paraffin-embedded cutaneous tumors. *J Cutan Pathol.* 1988;15:201-207.
81. Blessing K, Sanders DS, Grant JJ. Comparison of immunohistochemical staining of the novel antibody melan-A with S100 protein and HMB-45 in malignant melanoma and melanoma variants. *Histopathology.* 1998;32:139-146.
82. Vogel AM, Esclamado RM. Identification of a secreted Mr 95,000 glycoprotein in human melanocytes and melanomas by a melanocyte specific monoclonal antibody. *Cancer Res.* 1988;48:1286-1294.
83. Kim RY, Wistow GJ. The cDNA RPE1 and monoclonal antibody HMB-50 define gene products preferentially expressed in retinal pigment epithelium. *Exp Eye Res.* 1992;55:657-662.
84. Bar H, Schlote W. Malignant melanoma in the CNS: subtyping and immunocytochemistry. *Clin Neuropathol.* 1997;16: 337-345.
85. Barrett AW, Bennett JH, Speight PM. A clinicopathological and immunohistochemical analysis of primary oral mucosal melanoma. *Eur J Cancer B Oral Oncol.* 1995;31B:100-105.
86. Fernando SS, Johnson S, Bate J. Immunohistochemical analysis of cutaneous malignant melanoma: comparison of S100 protein, HMB-45 monoclonal antibody, and NKI/C3 monoclonal antibody. *Pathology.* 1994;26:16-19.
87. Bishop PW, Menasce LP, Yates AJ, et al. An immunophenotypic survey of malignant melanomas. *Histopathology.* 1993;23: 159-166.

88. Mackie RM, Campbell I, Turbitt M. Use of NKI/C3 monoclonal antibody in the assessment of benign and malignant melanocytic lesions. *J Clin Pathol.* 1984;37:367-372.
89. Yaziji H, Gown AM. Immunohistochemical markers of melanocytic tumors. *Int J Surg Pathol.* 2003;11:11-15.
90. Mangini J, Li N, Bhawan J. Immunohistochemical markers of melanocytic lesions: a review of their diagnostic usefulness. *Am J Dermatopathol.* 2002;24:270-281.
91. Friedman HD, Tatum AH. HMB-45 positive malignant lymphoma: a case report with literature review of aberrant HMB-45 reactivity. *Arch Pathol Lab Med.* 1991;115:826-830.
92. Hancock C, Allen BC, Herrera GA. HMB-45 detection in adenocarcinomas. *Arch Pathol Lab Med.* 1991;115:886-890.
93. Unger PD, Hoffman K, Thung SN, et al. HMB-45 reactivity in adrenal pheochromocytomas. *Arch Pathol Lab Med.* 1992;116:151-153.
94. Zimmer CM, Gottschalk J, Goebel S, et al. Melanoma-associated antigens in tumors of the nervous system: an immunohistochemical study with the monoclonal antibody HMB-45. *Virchows Arch A.* 1992;420:121-126.
95. Eble JN, Amin MB, Young RH. Epithelioid angiomyolipoma of the kidney: a report of five cases with prominent and diagnostically confusing epithelioid smooth muscle component. *Am J Surg Pathol.* 1997;21:1123-1130.
96. Fetsch PA, Fetsch JF, Marincola FM, et al. Comparison of melanoma antigen recognized by T-cells (MART-1) to HMB-45: additional evidence to support a common lineage for angiomyolipoma, lymphangiomyomatosis, and clear cell sugar tumor. *Mod Pathol.* 1998;11:699-703.
97. Ribalta T, Lloreta J, Munne A, et al. Malignant pigmented clear cell epithelioid tumor of the kidney: clear cell ("sugar") tumor versus malignant melanoma. *Hum Pathol.* 2000;31:516-519.
98. Zamboni G, Pea M, Martignoni G, et al. Clear cell "sugar" tumor of the pancreas: a novel member of the family of lesions characterized by the presence of perivascular epithelioid cells. *Am J Surg Pathol.* 1996;20:722-730.
99. Bonetti F, Pea M, Martignoni G, et al. Clear cell ("sugar") tumor of the lung is a lesion strictly related to angiomyolipoma—the concept of a family of lesions characterized by the presence of the perivascular epithelioid cells (PEC). *Pathology.* 1994;26:230-236.
100. Tanaka Y, Ijiri R, Kato K, et al. HMB-45/Melan-A and smooth muscle actin-positive clear-cell epithelioid tumor arising in the ligamentum teres hepatis: additional example of clear-cell "sugar" tumors. *Am J Surg Pathol.* 2000;24:1295-1299.
101. Gaffey MJ, Mills SE, Zarbo RJ, et al. Clear cell tumor of the lung: immunohistochemical and ultrastructural evidence of melanogenesis. *Am J Surg Pathol.* 1991;15:644-653.
102. Busam KJ, Iversen K, Coplan KA, et al. Immunoreactivity for A103, an antibody to melan-A (MART-1) in adrenocortical and other steroid tumors. *Am J Surg Pathol.* 1998;22:57-63.
103. Lerner AB, Fitzpatrick TB. Biochemistry of melanin formation. *Physiol Rev.* 1950;30:91-126.
104. Fitzpatrick TB, Miyomato M, Iskikawa K. The evolution of concepts of melanin biology. *Arch Dermatol.* 1967;96:305-323.
105. Pellegrino D, Bellina CR, Manca G, et al. Detection of melanoma cells in peripheral blood and sentinel lymph nodes by RT-PCR analysis: a comparative study with immunohistochemistry. *Tumori.* 2000;86:336-338.
106. Orchard GE. Comparison of immunohistochemical labeling of melanocyte differentiation antibodies melan-A, tyrosinase, and HMB-45 with NKI/C3 and S100 protein in the evaluation of benign nevi and malignant melanoma. *Histochem J.* 2000;32: 475-481.
107. Jungbluth AA, Iversen K, Coplan K, et al. T311—an anti-tyrosinase monoclonal antibody for the detection of melanocytic lesions in paraffin embedded tissues. *Pathol Res Pract.* 2000;196:235-242.
108. DeVries TJ, Trancikova D, Ruiter DJ, et al. High expression of immunotherapy candidate proteins gp100, MART-1, tyrosinase, and TRP-1 in uveal melanoma. *Br J Cancer.* 1998;78:1156-1161.
109. Kaufmann O, Koch S, Burghardt J, et al. Tyrosinase, melan-A, and KBA62 as markers for the immunohistochemical identification of metastatic amelanotic melanomas on paraffin sections. *Mod Pathol.* 1998;11:740-746.
110. Blaheta HJ, Schittek B, Breuninger H, et al. Lymph node micrometastases of cutaneous melanoma: increased sensitivity of molecular diagnosis in comparison to immunohistochemistry. *Int J Cancer.* 1998;79:318-323.
111. Cormier JN, Abati A, Fetsch P, et al. Comparative analysis of the in vivo expression of tyrosinase, MART-1/Melan-A, and gp100 in metastatic melanoma lesions: implications for immunotherapy. *J Immunother.* 1998;21:27-31.
112. Sato N, Suzuki S, Takimoto H, et al. Monoclonal antibody MAT-1 against human tyrosinase can detect melanogenic cells on formalin-fixed paraffin-embedded sections. *Pigment Cell Res.* 1996;9:72-76.
113. Takimoto H, Suzuki S, Masui S, et al. MAT-1, a monoclonal antibody that specifically recognizes human tyrosinase. *J Invest Dermatol.* 1995;105:764-768.
114. Chen YT, Stockert E, Tsang S, et al. Immunophenotyping of melanomas for tyrosinase: implications for vaccine development. *Proc Natl Acad Sci U S A.* 1995;92:8125-8129.
115. Clarkson KS, Sturdgess IC, Molyneux AJ. The usefulness of tyrosinase in the immunohistochemical assessment of melanocytic lesions: comparison of the novel T311 antibody (anti-tyrosinase) with S100, HMB-45, and A103 (MART-1; Melan-A). *J Clin Pathol.* 2001;54:196-200.
116. Takeda K, Yasumoto K, Takada R, et al. Induction of melanocyte-specific microphthalmia-associated transcription factor by Wnt-3a. *J Biol Chem.* 2000;275:14013-14016.
117. Vachtenheim J, Novotna H. Expression of genes for microphthalmia isoforms, Pax3 and MSG1, in human melanomas. *Cell Mol Biol.* 1999;45:1075-1082.
118. Galibert MD, Yavuzer U, Dexter TJ, et al. Pax3 and regulation of the melanocyte-specific tyrosinase-related protein-1 promoter. *J Biol Chem.* 1999;274:26894-26900.
119. Verastegui C, Bertolotto C, Bille K, et al. TFE3, a transcription factor homologous to microphthalmia, is a potential transcriptional activator of tyrosinase and TyrpI genes. *Mol Endocrinol.* 2000;14:449-456.
120. Koch MB, Shih IM, Weiss SW, et al. Microphthalmia transcription factor and melanoma cell adhesion molecule expression distinguish desmoplastic/spindle-cell melanoma from morphologic mimics. *Am J Surg Pathol.* 2001;25:58-64.
121. King R, Googe PB, Weilbaecher KN, et al. Microphthalmia transcription factor expression in cutaneous benign and malignant melanocytic, and nonmelanocytic tumors. *Am J Surg Pathol.* 2001;25:51-57.
122. King R, Weilbaecher KN, McGill G, et al. Microphthalmia transcription factor: a sensitive and specific melanocyte marker for melanoma diagnosis. *Am J Pathol.* 1999;155:731-738.
123. Miettinen M, Fernandez M, Franssila K, et al. Microphthalmia transcription factor in the immunohistochemical diagnosis of metastatic melanoma: comparison with four other melanoma markers. *Am J Surg Pathol.* 2001;25:205-211.
124. Zavala-Pompa A, Folpe AL, Jimenez RE, et al. Immunohistochemical study of microphthalmia transcription factor and tyrosinase in angiomyolipoma of the kidney, renal cell carcinoma, and retroperitoneal sarcomas: comparative evaluation with traditional diagnostic markers. *Am J Surg Pathol.* 2001;25: 65-70.
125. Folpe AL, Goodman ZD, Ishak KG, et al. Clear cell myomelanocytic tumor of the falciform ligament/ligamentum teres: a novel member of the perivascular epithelioid cell family of tumors with a predilection for children and young adults. *Am J Surg Pathol.* 2000;24:1239-1246.
126. Rochaix P, Lacroix-Triki M, Lamant L, et al. PNL2, a new monoclonal antibody directed against a fixative-resistant melanocyte antigen. *Mod Pathol.* 2003;16:481-490.
127. Busam KJ. The use and application of special techniques in assessing melanocytic tumors. *Pathology.* 2004;36:462-469.
128. Busam KJ, Kucukgol D, Sato E, et al. Immunohistochemical analysis of novel monoclonal antibody PNL2 and comparison with other melanocyte differentiation markers. *Am J Surg Pathol.* 2005;29:400-406.
129. Ohsie SJ, Sarantopoulos GP, Cochran AJ, Binder SW. Immunohistochemical characteristics of melanoma. *J Cutan Pathol.* 2008;35:433-444.

130. Wick MR, Stanley SJ, Swanson PE. Immunohistochemical diagnosis of sinonasal melanoma, carcinoma, and neuroblastoma with monoclonal antibodies HMB-45 and antisynaptophysin. *Arch Pathol Lab Med*. 1988;112:616-620.
131. Franquemont DW, Mills SE. Sinonasal malignant melanoma: a clinicopathologic and immunohistochemical study of 14 cases. *Am J Clin Pathol*. 1991;96:689-697.
132. Wiedenmann B, Franke WW, Kuhn C, et al. Synaptophysin: a marker protein for neuroendocrine cells and neoplasms. *Proc Natl Acad Sci U S A*. 1986;83:3500-3504.
133. Lloyd RV, Wilson BS. Specific endocrine tissue marker defined by a monoclonal antibody. *Science*. 1983;222:628-630.
134. Kontochristopoulos GJ, Stavropoulos PG, Krasagakis K, et al. Differentiation between Merkel cell carcinoma and malignant melanoma: an immunohistochemical study. *Dermatology*. 2000;201:123-126.
135. Klemm KM, Moran CA, Suster S. Pigmented thymic carcinoids: a clinicopathological and immunohistochemical study of two cases. *Mod Pathol*. 1999;12:946-948.
136. Gal AA, Koss MN, Hochholzer L, et al. Pigmented pulmonary carcinoid tumor: an immunohistochemical and ultrastructural study. *Arch Pathol Lab Med*. 1993;117:832-836.
137. Moran CA, Albores-Saavedra J, Wenig BM, et al. Pigmented extraadrenal paragangliomas: a clinicopathologic and immunohistochemical study of five cases. *Cancer*. 1997;79:398-402.
138. Pettinato G, Manivel JC, d'Amore ESG, et al. Melanotic neuroectodermal tumor of infancy: a reexamination of a histogenetic problem based on immunohistochemical, flow cytometric, and ultrastructural study of 10 cases. *Am J Surg Pathol*. 1991;15:233-245.
139. Kapadia SB, Frisman DM, Hitchcock CL, et al. Melanotic neuroectodermal tumor of infancy: clinicopathological, immunohistochemical, and flow cytometric study. *Am J Surg Pathol*. 1993;17:566-573.
140. Mennemeyer RP, Hallman KO, Hammar SP, et al. Melanotic schwannoma: clinical and ultrastructural studies of three cases with evidence of intracellular melanin synthesis. *Am J Surg Pathol*. 1979;3:3-10.
141. Orchard GE, Wilson-Jones E. Immunocytochemistry in the diagnosis of malignant melanoma. *Br J Biomed Sci*. 1994;51:44-56.
142. Springall DR, Gu J, Cocchia D, et al. The value of S100 immunostaining as a diagnostic tool in human malignant melanomas: a comparison using S100 and neuron-specific enolase antibodies. *Virchows Arch A*. 1983;400:331-343.
143. Dhillon AP, Rode J, Leathem A. Neuron-specific enolase: an aid to the diagnosis of melanoma and neuroblastoma. *Histopathology*. 1982;6:81-92.
144. Reed JA, Finnerty B, Albino AP. Divergent cellular differentiation pathways during the invasive stage of cutaneous malignant melanoma progression. *Am J Pathol*. 1999;155:549-555.
145. Sangueza OP, Requena L. Neoplasms with neural differentiation: a review. Part II: Malignant neoplasms. *Am J Dermatopathol*. 1998;20:89-102.
146. Mooy CM, Luyten GP, DeJong PT, et al. Neural cell adhesion molecule distribution in primary and metastatic uveal melanomas. *Hum Pathol*. 1995;26:1185-1190.
147. Cochran AJ, Roberts A, Wen DR, et al. Update on lymphatic mapping and sentinel node biopsy in the management of patients with melanocytic tumors. *Pathology*. 2004;36:478-484.
148. Prieto VG, Clark SH. Processing of sentinel lymph nodes for detection of metastatic melanoma. *Ann Diagn Pathol*. 2002;6:257-264.
149. Spanknebel K, Coit DG, Bieligk SC, et al. Characterization of micrometastatic disease in melanoma sentinel lymph nodes by enhanced pathology: recommendations for standardizing pathologic analysis. *Am J Surg Pathol*. 2005;29:305-317.
150. Shidham VB, Komorowski R, Macias V, et al. Optimization of an immunostaining protocol for the rapid intraoperative evaluation of melanoma sentinel lymph node imprint smears with the "MCW melanoma cocktail". *Cytojournal*. 2004;1:2.
151. Wick MR. Principles of evidence-based medicine as applied to "sentinel" lymph node biopsies. *Pathol Case Rev*. 2008;13:102-108.
152. Medalie N, Ackerman AB. *Sentinel lymph node biopsy has no benefit for patients with primary cutaneous melanoma: an assertion based on comprehensive, critical analysis*. 2nd ed. New York: Ardor Scribendi Press; 2004:1-95.
153. Abrahamsen HN, Hamilton-Dutoit SJ, Larsen J, et al. Sentinel lymph nodes in malignant melanoma: extended histopathologic evaluation improves diagnostic precision. *Cancer*. 2004;100:1683-1691.
154. Wick MR. Prognostic factors for cutaneous melanoma. *Am J Clin Pathol*. 1998;110:713-718.
155. Moretti S, Spallanzani A, Chiarugi A, et al. Correlation of Ki-67 expression in cutaneous primary melanoma with prognosis in a prospective study: different correlation according to thickness. *J Am Acad Dermatol*. 2001;44:188-192.
156. Florenes VA, Faye RS, Maelandsmo GM, et al. Levels of cyclin D1 and D3 in malignant melanoma: deregulated cyclin expression is associated with poor clinical outcome in superficial melanomas. *Clin Cancer Res*. 2000;6:3614-3620.
157. Straume O, Sviland L, Akslen LA. Loss of nuclear p16 protein expression correlates with increased tumor proliferation (Ki-67) and poor prognosis in patients with vertical growth phase melanoma. *Clin Cancer Res*. 2000;6:1845-1853.
158. Kaleem Z, Lind AC, Humphrey PA, et al. Concurrent Ki-67 and p53 immunolabeling in cutaneous melanocytic neoplasms: an adjunct for recognition of the vertical growth phase in malignant melanomas? *Mod Pathol*. 2000;13:217-222.
159. Henrique R, Azevedo R, Bento MJ, et al. Prognostic value of Ki-67 expression in localized cutaneous malignant melanoma. *J Am Acad Dermatol*. 2000;43:991-1000.
160. Florenes VA, Maelandsmo GM, Holm R, et al. Expression of activated Trk-A protein in melanocytic tumors: relationship to cell proliferation and clinical outcome. *Am J Clin Pathol*. 2004;122:412-420.
161. Rangaswami H, Kundu GC. Osteopontin stimulates melanoma growth and lung metastasis through NIK-MeKK1-dependent MMP-9 activation pathways. *Oncol Rep*. 2007;18:909-915.
162. Rangel J, Nosrati M, Torabian S, et al. Osteopontin as a molecular prognostic marker for melanoma. *Cancer*. 2008;112:144-150.
163. Ferrari D, Lombardi M, Ricci R, et al. Dermatopathological indicators of poor melanoma prognosis are significantly inversely correlated with the expression of NM23 protein in primary cutaneous melanoma. *J Cutan Pathol*. 2007;34:705-712.
164. Tucci MG, Lucarini G, Brancorsini D, et al. Involvement of E-cadherin, beta-catenin, Cdc42, and CXCR4 in the progression and prognosis of cutaneous melanoma. *Br J Dermatol*. 2007;157:1212-1216.
165. Xu X, Gimotty PA, Guerry D, et al. Lymphatic invasion revealed by multispectral imaging is common in primary melanomas and associates with prognosis. *Hum Pathol*. 2008;39:901-909.
166. Straume O, Jackson DG, Akslen LA. Independent prognostic impact of lymphatic vessel density and presence of low-grade lymphangiogenesis in cutaneous melanoma. *Clin Cancer Res*. 2003;9:250-256.
167. Cassarino DS, Cabral ES, Kartha RV, Swetter SM. Primary dermal melanoma: distinct immunohistochemical findings and clinical outcome compared with nodular and metastatic melanoma. *Arch Dermatol*. 2008;144:49-56.
168. Graham CH, Rivers J, Kerbel RS, et al. Extent of vascularization as a prognostic indicator in thin (<0.76 mm) malignant melanomas. *Am J Pathol*. 1994;145:510-514.
169. Vlaykova T, Talve L, Hahka-Kemppinen M, et al. MIB-1 immunoreactivity correlates with blood vessel density and survival in disseminated malignant melanoma. *Oncology*. 1999;57:242-252.
170. Kerbel RS, Kobayashi H, Graham CH, et al. Analysis and significance of the malignant "eclipse" during the progression of primary cutaneous human melanomas. *J Invest Dermatol Symp Proc*. 1996;1:183-187.
171. Gutman M, Singh RK, Radinsky R, et al. Intertumoral heterogeneity of receptor-tyrosinase kinase expression in human melanoma cell lines with metastatic capabilities. *Anticancer Res*. 1994;14:1759-1765.
172. Elder D. Tumor progression, early diagnosis, and prognosis of melanoma. *Acta Oncol*. 1999;38:535-547.

173. Nagasaka T, Lai R, Medeiros LJ, et al. Cyclin D1 overexpression in Spitz nevi: an immunohistochemical study. *Am J Dermatopathol.* 1999;21:115-120.
174. Kanter-Lewensohn L, Hedblad MA, Wedje J, et al. Immunohistochemical markers for distinguishing Spitz nevi from malignant melanomas. *Mod Pathol.* 1997;10:917-920.
175. Bergman R, Shemer A, Levy R, et al. Immunohistochemical study of p53 protein expression in Spitz nevi as compared with other melanocytic tumors. *Am J Dermatopathol.* 1995;17:547-550.
176. Penneys NS, Seigfried E, Nahass G, et al. Expression of proliferating cell nuclear antigen in Spitz nevus. *J Am Acad Dermatol.* 1995;32:964-967.
177. Takahashi H, Maeda K, Maeda K, et al. Immunohistochemical characterization of Spitz's nevus: differentiation from common melanocytic nevi, dysplastic melanocytic nevus, and malignant melanoma. *J Dermatol.* 1987;14:533-541.
178. Nasr MR, El-Zammar O. Comparison of pHH3, Ki-67, and survivin immunoreactivity in benign and malignant melanocytic lesions. *Am J Dermatopathol.* 2008;30:117-122.
179. Glusac EJ, McNiff JM. Epithelioid cell histiocytoma: a simulant of vascular and melanocytic neoplasms. *Am J Dermatopathol.* 1999;21:1-7.
180. Busam KJ, Granter SR, Iversen K, et al. Immunohistochemical distinction of epithelioid histiocytic proliferations from epithelioid melanocytic nevi. *Am J Dermatopathol.* 2000;22:237-241.
181. Busam KJ, Rosai J, Iversen K, et al. Xanthogranulomas with inconspicuous foam cells and giant cells mimicking malignant melanoma: a clinical, histologic, and immunohistochemical study of three cases. *Am J Surg Pathol.* 2000;24:864-869.
182. Ma CK, Zarbo RJ, Gown AM. Immunohistochemical characterization of atypical fibroxanthoma and dermatofibrosarcoma protuberans. *Am J Clin Pathol.* 1992;97:478-483.
183. Diaz-Cascajo C, Borghi S, Bonczkowitz M. Pigmented atypical fibroxanthoma. *Histopathology.* 1998;33:537-541.
184. Gloghini A, Rizzo A, Zanette I, et al. KP1/CD68 expression in malignant neoplasms including lymphomas, sarcomas, and carcinomas. *Am J Clin Pathol.* 1995;103:425-431.
185. Miettinen M, Fetsch JF. Reticulohistiocytoma (solitary epithelioid histiocytoma): a clinicopathologic and immunohistochemical study of 44 cases. *Am J Surg Pathol.* 2006;30:521-528.
186. Lau SK, Chu PG, Weiss LM. CD163: a specific marker of macrophages in paraffin-embedded tissue samples. *Am J Clin Pathol.* 2004;122:794-801.
187. Banerjee SS, Eyden B. Divergent differentiation in malignant melanomas: a review. *Histopathology.* 2008;52:119-129.
188. Suster S. Tumors of the skin composed of large cells with abundant eosinophilic cytoplasm. *Semin Diagn Pathol.* 1999;16:162-177.
189. Borek BT, McKee PH, Freeman JA, et al. Primary malignant melanoma with rhabdoid features: a histologic and immunocytochemical study of two cases. *Am J Dermatopathol.* 1998;20:123-127.
190. Laskin WB, Knittel DR, Frame JN. S100 protein and HMB-45-negative "rhabdoid" malignant melanoma: a totally dedifferentiated malignant melanoma? *Am J Clin Pathol.* 1995;103:772-773.
191. Anstey A, Cerio R, Ramnarain N, et al. Desmoplastic malignant melanoma: an immunocytochemical study of 25 cases. *Am J Dermatopathol.* 1994;16:14-22.
192. Gatter KC, Alcock K, Heryet A, et al. The differential diagnosis of routinely-processed anaplastic tumors using monoclonal antibodies. *Am J Clin Pathol.* 1984;82:33-43.
193. Strickler JG, Michie SA, Warnke RA, et al. The "syncytial" variant of nodular sclerosing Hodgkin's disease. *Am J Surg Pathol.* 1986;10:470-477.
194. Ritter JH, Mills SE, Gaffey MJ, et al. Clear cell tumors of the alimentary tract and abdominal cavity. *Semin Diagn Pathol.* 1997;14:213-219.
195. Ordonez NG. Role of immunohistochemistry in differentiating epithelial mesothelioma from adenocarcinoma. *Am J Clin Pathol.* 1999;112:75-89.
196. Mizutani H, Ohyanagi S, Hayashi T, et al. Functional thrombomodulin expression on epithelial skin tumors as a differentiation marker for suprabasal keratinocytes. *Br J Dermatol.* 1996;135:187-193.
197. Battifora H, Silva EG. The use of antikeratin antibodies in the immunohistochemical distinction between neuroendocrine (Merkel cell) carcinoma of the skin, lymphoma, and oat cell carcinoma. *Cancer.* 1986;58:1040-1046.
198. Clark HB. Immunohistochemistry of nervous system antigens: diagnostic applications in surgical neuropathology. *Semin Diagn Pathol.* 1984;1:309-316.
199. Gottschalk J, Jautzke G, Schreiner C. Epithelial and melanoma antigens in gliosarcoma: an immunohistochemical study. *Pathol Res Pract.* 1992;188:182-190.
200. Plaza JA, Suster S, Perez-Montiel D. Expression of immunohistochemical markers in primary and metastatic malignant melanoma: a comparative study in 70 patients using a tissue microarray technique. *Appl Immunohistochem Mol Morphol.* 2007;15:421-425.
201. Lodding P, Kindblom LG, Angervall L. Metastases of malignant melanoma simulating soft tissue sarcoma: a clinicopathological, light- and electron microscopic and immunohistochemical study of 21 cases. *Virchows Arch A.* 1990;417:377-388.
202. Banerjee SS, Coyne JD, Menasce LP, et al. Diagnostic lessons of mucosal melanoma with osteocartilaginous differentiation. *Histopathology.* 1998;33:255-260.
203. Swanson PE, Wick MR. Clear cell sarcoma: an immunohistochemical analysis of six cases and comparison with other epithelioid neoplasms of soft tissue. *Arch Pathol Lab Med.* 1989;113:55-60.
204. Mechtersheimer G, Tilgen W, Klar E, et al. Clear cell sarcoma of tendons and aponeuroses: case presentation with special reference to immunohistochemical findings. *Hum Pathol.* 1989;20:914-917.
205. Almeida MM, Nunes AM, Frable WJ. Malignant melanoma of soft tissue: a report of three cases with diagnosis by fine needle aspiration cytology. *Acta Cytol.* 1994;38:241-246.
206. Stenman G, Kindblom LG, Angervall L. Reciprocal translocation t(12;22)(q13;q13) in clear-cell sarcoma of tendons and aponeuroses. *Genes Chromosomes Cancer.* 1992;4:122-127.
207. Langezaal SM, Graadt van Roggen JF, et al. Malignant melanoma is genetically distinct from clear cell sarcoma of tendons and aponeuroses (malignant melanoma of soft parts). *Br J Cancer.* 2001;84:535-538.
208. Curry CV, Dishop MK, Hicks MJ, et al. Clear cell sarcoma of soft tissue: diagnostic utility of fluorescence in-situ hybridization and reverse transcriptase polymerase chain reaction. *J Cutan Pathol.* 2008;35:411-417.
209. Folpe AL, Hill CE, Parham DM, et al. Immunohistochemical detection of FLI-1 protein expression: a study of 132 round cell tumors with emphasis on mimics of Ewing's sarcoma/primitive neuroectodermal tumor. *Am J Surg Pathol.* 2000;24:1657-1662.
210. Winters JL, Geil JD, O'Connor WN. Immunohistology, cytogenetics, and molecular studies of small round cell tumors of childhood: a review. *Ann Clin Lab Sci.* 1995;25:66-78.
211. Swanson PE, Scheithauer BW, Wick MR. Peripheral nerve sheath neoplasms: clinicopathologic and immunochemical observations. *Pathol Annu.* 1995;30(Pt. 2):1-82.
212. Wick MR. Malignant peripheral nerve sheath tumors of the skin. *Mayo Clin Proc.* 1990;65:279-282.
213. Suster S, Fisher C, Moran CA. Expression of bcl-2 oncoprotein in benign and malignant spindle-cell tumors of soft tissue, skin, serosal surfaces, and gastrointestinal tract. *Am J Surg Pathol.* 1998;22:863-872.
214. Kanitakis J, Bourchany D, Claudy A. Expression of the CD10 antigen (neutral endopeptidase) by mesenchymal tumors of the skin. *Anticancer Res.* 2000;20:3539-3544.
215. Olsen SH, Thomas DG, Lucas DR. Cluster analysis of immunohistochemical profiles in synovial sarcoma, malignant peripheral nerve sheath tumor, and Ewing sarcoma. *Mod Pathol.* 2006;19:659-668.
216. Shimada S, Tsuzuki T, Kuroda M, et al. Nestin expression as a new marker in malignant peripheral nerve sheath tumors. *Pathol Int.* 2007;57:60-67.
217. Yoo J, Park SY, Kang SJ, et al. Altered expression of G1 regulatory proteins in human soft tissue sarcomas. *Arch Pathol Lab Med.* 2002;126:567-573.

218. Brychtova S, Fluraskova M, Hlovilkova A, et al. Nestin expression in cutaneous melanomas and melanocytic nevi. *J Cutan Pathol.* 2007;34:370-375.
219. Shabrawi-Caelen LE, Kerl H, Cerroni L. Melan-A: not a helpful marker in distinction between melanoma in-situ on sun-damaged skin and pigmented actinic keratosis. *Am J Dermatopathol.* 2004;26:364-366.
220. Wiltz KL, Qureshi H, Patterson JW, et al. Immunostaining for MART-1 in the interpretation of problematic intraepidermal pigmented lesions. *J Cutan Pathol.* 2007;34:601-605.
221. Gleason BC, Nascimento AF. HMB-45 and Melan-A are useful in the differential diagnosis between granular cell tumor and malignant melanoma. *Am J Dermatopathol.* 2007;29:22-27.
222. Ray S, Jukic DM. Cutaneous granular cell tumor with epidermal involvement: a potential mimic of melanocytic neoplasia. *J Cutan Pathol.* 2007;34:188-194.
223. Herron MD, Vanderhoof SL, Smock K, et al. Proliferative nodules in congenital melanocytic nevi: a clinicopathologic and immunohistochemical analysis. *Am J Surg Pathol.* 2004;28:1017-1025.
224. Guerriere-Kovach PM, Hunt EL, Patterson JW, et al. Primary melanoma of the skin and cutaneous melanomatous metastases: comparative histologic features and immunophenotypes. *Am J Clin Pathol.* 2004;122:70-77.

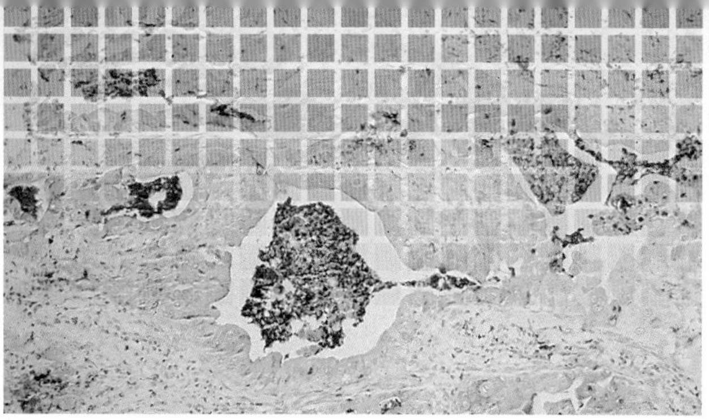

8

Immunohistology of Metastatic Carcinomas of Unknown Primary

Rohit Bhargava • David J. Dabbs

Introduction 206

CUPS: Clinical Aspects and Economic Considerations 206

Diagnostic Approach to the Study of CUPS: Specimen Preparation 208

Determining Site of Origin: A Stepwise Approach 209

Combined Antibody (Panel) Approach to Solving Diagnostic Problems 237

Special Clinical Presentations 237

Beyond Immunohistochemistry: Anatomic Molecular Diagnostic Applications 242

Summary 244

INTRODUCTION

The impact of diagnostic immunohistochemistry (IHC) for the surgical pathologist is legendary, and it is best appreciated when studying malignancies of unknown primary site. A cost-effective tool, IHC is performed in most hospital laboratories, is often automated, and provides for a rapid turnaround time, all desirable qualities for the pathologist. The number of antibodies that are available for diagnostic use rises exponentially each year, which attests to the importance of ongoing research in this field. Since the first edition of this book, there has been a substantial addition of important antibodies that are especially useful in the workup for patients with metastatic malignancy of unknown primary. Even with the larger armamentarium of antibodies, there remains a paucity of specific antibodies that allow for "100% unequivocal, definitive diagnosis" in every case. Indeed, it has been said that "it may be dangerous to base any distinction in tumor pathology primarily on the basis of the pattern of immunoreactivity of a given marker, no matter how specific it is purported to be."[1] This statement echoes the importance of histopathologic morphology, which is the basis of diagnosis in surgical pathology. The standard tissue section is the starting point for raising questions that need to be answered for the patient when morphology alone is not enough, and IHC is perhaps the best method to obtain more information from the paraffin section.

Even the most specific antibodies (e.g., TTF1, WT1, or prostate-specific antigen [PSA]) are not entirely site specific, and we therefore resort to panels of antibodies that give statistical power to our morphologic diagnoses. Relevant diagnostic panels of antibodies change rapidly on the basis of information from immunohistochemical studies, and we can expect this constant infusion of new data on antibody sensitivity and specificity to impart an uncomfortable state of chronic flux on the discipline of IHC. Nevertheless, change is often incremental in IHC, and the basics of separating the category of metastatic malignancy of unknown primary into the categories of carcinoma, melanoma, lymphoma, germ cell neoplasia, and sarcoma have stood the test of time.

Although the term *cancer of unknown primary site* (CUPS) is sometimes used interchangeably with carcinoma (cancers of epithelial differentiation) of unknown primary site, not all cancers of unknown primary site are epithelial in origin. This chapter will review the triage and evaluation of all types of cancers, but the main focus will remain on the carcinomas, which form the predominant category (~90% to 95% cases) of CUPS.[2-4]

CUPS: CLINICAL ASPECTS AND ECONOMIC CONSIDERATIONS

Patients who present with CUPS by definition have no obvious identifiable primary site, despite a careful clinical history, physical examination, radiologic imaging, and biochemical or histologic investigations. Studies of patients with malignancies have shown that CUPS accounts for 5% to 15% of all patients who present with a malignancy.[3,5-7] The impact of recent improvements in radiologic imaging has reduced this percentage of patients to 3% to 7% of patients who present with a CUPS diagnosis.[2,8,9]

The clinical presentation in CUPS cases depends on a number of factors including age, gender, sites of involvement, and line of differentiation (e.g., epithelial, mesenchymal, lymphoid, germ cell, melanocytic). The tumors that present as CUPS are apparently biologically and clinically different from the known primary tumors that metastasize several years after diagnosis. CUPS patients fail to show any symptoms related to the primary tumor and demonstrate an unpredictable pattern of spread (i.e., difference in frequency of involvement of a particular site than would be expected of a known primary tumor). The majority of CUPS cases present with multiple sites of involvement with a few presenting with only one or two sites of involvement. On the basis of sites of involvement, several clinico-pathologic entities have been characterized as helpful in identifying the primary site.

The liver is one of the single largest repositories for metastatic malignancies of all types, especially for carcinomas. The most common malignancies metastatic to the liver are from the gastrointestinal tract, with colorectal carcinomas leading this group. Lung and breast carcinomas also commonly metastasize to the liver, as do pancreaticobiliary carcinomas. This entire group of adenocarcinomas may appear similar to primary cholangiocarcinoma of the liver and may simulate some hepatocellular carcinomas, particularly the less-differentiated hepatocellular carcinomas. Prostate carcinoma, although unusual, does metastasize to the liver and can be confused with cholangiocarcinoma. Thus for hepatic metastases of unknown primary in women, colorectal, breast, and lung carcinomas are of primary consideration, whereas in men, colorectal, lung, and prostate carcinomas top the list. Malignant melanoma metastatic to the liver is not uncommon, with the highest frequency of liver metastases seen with primary eye melanomas.[5] Pisharodi and associates, in a fine-needle biopsy study of 200 malignant aspirates of the liver, found that 32% were hepatocellular carcinomas, 49.5% were readily diagnosed as metastatic carcinomas, and 18.5% were problematic.[10] Of this latter group, IHC contributed to definitive diagnosis in half of the cases.

Along with the liver, the lung is a major repository for metastatic carcinomas, especially adenocarcinomas. Identification of the origin of an adenocarcinoma in the lung is a frequent, difficult, and challenging process for the surgical pathologist because adenocarcinomas are not only the most frequent primary lung tumor but also the most common metastatic tumor found in the lung. Distinction among these tumor types can be especially challenging on scant biopsy materials such as transbronchial biopsy or fine-needle aspiration biopsy (FNAB). It is important to identify those carcinomas that can be treated by chemotherapy or hormonal manipulation, or both, especially metastatic breast or prostate carcinomas.

In the brain, distinguishing metastatic adenocarcinoma or poorly differentiated carcinoma from a glial tumor is straightforward, although determining the source of the metastasis may be problematic, especially when the occult primary is unknown.[11,12] Lung carcinomas are the most likely primary to be discovered subsequent to central nervous system (CNS) presentation, and other common primaries include breast, kidney, thyroid, and gastrointestinal tract.[11-13] Patients with other adenocarcinomas such as ovarian, prostatic, and pancreaticobiliary rarely present with brain metastases because there is almost always evidence of widespread dissemination of these tumors before the occurrence of cerebral metastases. The site of origin of carcinoma remains unknown in up to 5% of patients.[14] The survival of most patients with carcinomatous brain metastases is in the range of 3 to 11 months.[15-17]

Patients presenting with skeletal metastases often have primary carcinomas in the lung, breast, kidney, or urogenital region, and imaging studies have been particularly useful in elucidating the primary tumor.[18]

For patients who present with pleural effusions, the breast is the most common primary site for women, with the lung being the most common site for a primary tumor in men.[19] Malignant lymphomas are seen in both sexes.

In women who present with malignant abdominal effusions (malignant ascites), common abdominal sites include ovaries, endometrium, and cervix, whereas men with malignant ascites typically have primary tumor sites in the gastrointestinal tract, predominantly in the colon, rectum, or stomach.[20] Patients with peritoneal carcinomatosis of nongynecologic origin most often have origins in the stomach, colon, or pancreas and have a median survival of 3 months.[21]

For patients who present with primary lymph node metastases, there may be clues to the primary site of the tumor on the basis of tumor morphology (adenocarcinoma, squamous cell carcinoma, or undifferentiated carcinoma) and the anatomic site of lymph node involvement.

In women presenting with adenocarcinoma in the axilla, the primary tumor is most often found in the ipsilateral breast. For the patient who presents with metastatic adenocarcinoma in the neck, the metastatic workup will begin in the lung (males) or breast (females), although gastrointestinal and prostate adenocarcinomas both show a predilection for the left side of the neck.[22]

Undifferentiated carcinomas of the head and neck are the most common primary source for metastatic tumors in head and neck lymph nodes,[6] and the majority of these are of squamous mucosal derivation. The prognosis for this group of patients rests largely on the nodal status, with patients having stage N3 lesions carrying a poor prognosis.[23] For a squamous cell carcinoma involving the upper and midcervical lymph nodes, a thorough examination of the oropharynx, hypopharynx, nasopharynx, larynx, and upper esophagus by direct vision and fiberoptic nasopharyngolaryngoscopy, with biopsy of any suspicious areas, is more valuable than further pathologic examination. Advanced diagnostic techniques such as computed tomography (CT) and positron emission tomography (PET) are helpful in determining the primary site.[24-26] Occasionally, systematic random biopsies of mucosal sites such as nasopharynx, base of tongue, pyriform sinus, and tonsils may reveal an occult tumor.[27] Metastatic squamous cell carcinoma involving lower cervical lymph nodes or at any other site except inguinal nodes is highly suspicious for a lung primary.[28] Occasionally, esophageal squamous cell carcinomas may preferentially involve the lower cervical lymph nodes.[29] The vast majority of patients with squamous cell carcinoma involving the inguinal nodes generally have detectable primary tumor in the anogenital area.[30] Therefore all women must undergo a thorough evaluation of the vulva, vagina, and cervix, and all men should undergo careful inspection of the penis. Both sexes must also have examination of the anorectal region.

The current clinical approach is an attempt to identify favorable prognostic groups in patients with unknown primary tumors so that they can be managed appropriately.[31-35] This group of tumors includes leukemia/lymphoma, germ cell tumors, small cell carcinoma of the lung, and carcinomas of the breast, ovary, endometrium, adrenal gland, thyroid, and prostate.[5,36,37] When possible, it is useful to separate regional from distant metastases because localized disease is more amenable to treatment.[5,38] Other favorable clinical features that have been described include location of tumor in the retroperitoneum or peripheral lymph nodes, tumor limited to one or two metastatic sites, a negative smoking history, and young age.[5] Kirsten and colleagues[36] studied 286 patients with CUPS and concluded that the factors that predicted survival were lymph node presentation, good performance status, and body weight loss of less than 10%. Using a panel of antibodies to determine differentiation of tumors in 41 patients with CUPS, Van der Gaast and associates concluded that the immunohistochemical panel approach to uncover tumor origin is useful for selecting appropriate treatment of patients, especially those who may benefit from combination chemotherapy.[32,39] Other immunohistochemical studies of CUPS have elucidated the origin of tumors in as low as 5% to as high as 70% of patients.[40] However, most investigators have arrived at the same conclusion: for individual patient therapy, knowledge of site of origin improves patient survival.[41] Furthermore, with the advent of targeted therapy (still in its infancy), the benefit of identifying the site of origin may be manifold.[42-44]

The appropriate workup for identifying a primary tumor depends on the patient's clinical symptoms, age, history, and gender and the likelihood of finding the primary tumor. Patients with CUPS do poorly as a group, with a median survival of 6 to 11 months, and the importance of establishing the origin of the primary site guides therapeutic interventions of hormonal manipulation, chemotherapy, and radiation.[45-47] The clinician must also take into account the economics of an extensive clinical workup, as well as the inconvenience and discomfort to which the patient is subjected.[48]

The economic considerations of clinical workup in these patients have not been extensively studied. Few data are available on the cost-effectiveness of IHC in surgical pathology. Schapira and Jerrett[7] analyzed the clinical workups in a group of 199 patients and concluded that the search for a primary neoplasm incurred an average cost of $17,973, with only 19.6% of patients surviving for more than 1 year. As a matter of fact, IHC is probably undervalued and is likely a cost-effective maneuver in the study of CUPS. Radiologic studies themselves have limited value in the management of these patients, and prognosis is not affected.[49,50] Even autopsies on some of these patients may not detect the primary site of tumor because of small size, extensive dissemination, or regression due to therapy.[51] In 1988 Le Chevalier and coworkers[52] studied 302 autopsy specimens from patients who presented with CUPS. The primary tumor site was located premortem in 27% of patients, was determined at autopsy in 50% of patients, and remained unidentified in 16% of patients.[52] The most common primary tumor sites in this study included pancreas, lung, kidney, and colon/rectum, a list that includes the two malignancies with the highest incidence in both men and women.

DIAGNOSTIC APPROACH TO THE STUDY OF CUPS: SPECIMEN PREPARATION

The goal of the surgical pathologist is to identify the line of differentiation of the tumor and identify those tumors that are within the "treatable" group of tumors, namely, carcinomas of breast, prostate, ovary, and endometrium, thyroid, and adrenal, as well as germ cell tumors and neuroendocrine carcinomas.[32] Hormonal and antihormonal therapies are useful for patients with breast, prostate, and adrenal carcinomas. Neuroendocrine, thyroid, and germ cell tumors may be responsive to suppression by chemical agents. The therapeutic response of other carcinomas is less certain,[53] but the identity of the carcinoma, if available, is useful to determine more useful therapeutic regimens for these patients prospectively.[32,47,52,54] Recent studies on patients with CUPS demonstrate that up to one third respond to taxane-based therapies.[55,56]

Tissue procurement is the first step in the workup for tumors of unknown primary origin. It is a common practice to obtain tissue by fine-needle aspiration biopsy (FNAB) or core tissue biopsy. The sensitivity of FNAB for metastatic carcinoma in a series of 266 superficial lymph nodes was 96.5%, with no false-positive results and nine false-negative results.[57] Tissue from both FNAB and core biopsies can be triaged for ancillary studies in the same manner. There is also great value in the immunocytochemical study of malignant effusions, and often these are the first samples available by virtue of therapeutic evacuation.[58-64] Whatever the method of obtaining tissue, it is ideal to be able to monitor the process so that adequate tissue may be obtained to triage the patient's problem appropriately, namely, triage of the specimen for immunohistology, electron microscopy, flow cytometry, and molecular-cytogenetic studies. If there is not enough tissue available, our recommendation would be to freeze at least some tumor sample after tissue has been collected for morphologic analysis because fresh frozen tissue is the best sample for molecular analysis.[65]

Monitoring the tissue procurement process can be performed with frozen sections, immediate interpretation of FNAB, or tissue imprints. In addition to tissue procurement, the pathologist must define the problem by taking into account the patient's age, gender, known risk factors, duration of symptoms, and clinical and radiologic findings. On the basis of this information and the morphologic appearance of the tumor, the quest for the study of tumor origin begins.

In surgical pathology and cytopathology, poorly differentiated carcinomas can be broadly classified as large cell undifferentiated, small cell undifferentiated, and spindle cell. The starting point for diagnostic interpretation is the standard hematoxylin and eosin or Papanicolaou-stained slide. The importance of the histologic morphology should not be underestimated in arriving at a definitive diagnosis. Morphology is the foundation on which the interpretation of all immunohistochemical studies rests.

In this chapter the role of diagnostic IHC in diagnosing CUPS is emphasized, especially as it relates to adenocarcinoma/poorly differentiated carcinoma of unknown primary site and germ cell tumors, which account for more than 90% cases of CUPS. Specific tables that aid in the differential diagnosis of tumors in specific anatomic sites are presented. The role of molecular studies in combination with IHC for patients with CUPS has been discussed.

DETERMINING SITE OF ORIGIN: A STEPWISE APPROACH

Carcinomas form the predominant category (~90% to 95% cases) of CUPS[2-4] and will therefore remain the main focus of this chapter. Because virtually all carcinomas show significant positivity for cytokeratins (CK), carcinomatous differentiation becomes readily apparent when the tumor is diffusely CK positive. The simple and broad-spectrum CKs are the initial antibodies of choice for detecting carcinomatous differentiation. More specific subcategorization of the tumor origin is then possible using a variety of site-specific CKs, as well as antibodies directed against various cellular products. It is a combination of these cellular antigens that may yield a cost-effective approach to tumor categorization.

The approach to definitive diagnosis of the patient with CUPS effectively follows five sequential steps:

1. Determine the cell line of differentiation using major lineage markers including keratins, lymphoid, melanoma, germ cell, and sarcoma markers.
2. Determine the CK type or types of distribution in the tumor cells because some subsets of CKs are unique to certain tumor types.
3. Determine if there is coexpression of vimentin.
4. Determine if there is expression of supplemental antigens of epithelial or germ cell derivation, that is, carcinoembryonic antigen (CEA), epithelial membrane antigen (EMA), or placental alkaline phosphatase (PLAP).
5. Determine if there is expression of cell-specific products, cell-specific structures, and transcription factors or receptors that are unique identifiers of cell types (e.g., neuroendocrine granules, peptide hormones, thyroglobulin, PSA, prostate-specific membrane antigen, inhibin, gross cystic disease fluid protein [GCDFP], villin, uroplakin, thyroid transcription factor-1 [TTF-1] or transcription factor CDX-2).

Step 1: Screening Immunohistochemistry

An abbreviated first-line panel to determine the line of differentiation should be composed of epithelial markers (pankeratin AE1/3 and CAM5.2, both used together), mesenchymal marker (vimentin), lymphoid marker (leukocyte common antigen or LCA), and melanocytic marker (S100). Although vimentin is included in the panel, it is generally the least helpful. It should be interpreted with caution. Vimentin is considered a mesenchymal marker[66] but may be expressed quite diffusely in many poorly differentiated carcinomas.[67] In fact, vimentin coexpression in a carcinoma may point toward a specific primary site. Except for vimentin, a diffuse strong expression of any of the abovementioned markers is generally suggestive of a particular line of differentiation.

LINE OF DIFFERENTIATION: LYMPHOID

The first-line panel generally leads to a more extensive workup. At this point, if the tumor is strongly positive for LCA and negative for keratins, further workup is directed toward classifying the lymphoma using pan-B, pan T-cell (CD20, CD79a, and CD3), and other markers.[68,69] If LCA is ±; pan-B, pan-T cell markers are negative; and the morphology is still suggestive of lymphoid neoplasm, it is not unreasonable to think about a myeloid neoplasm and perform myeloid markers for granulocytic sarcoma. This is one diagnosis, which may be missed even after an expensive and extended immunohistologic evaluation.[70-72] The stains that are helpful in demonstrating myeloid lineage are myeloperoxidase, chloracetate esterase, lysozyme stains, and CD117 (also known as C-kit or stem cell marker).[73-75] CD43 and CD68 stains are also positive in granulocytic sarcomas.[71,76,77]

LINE OF DIFFERENTIATION: MELANOCYTIC

A diffuse strong staining with S100, negative for CK in a tumor of unknown origin, is good evidence that it may be a melanoma.[78-80] However, this still needs to be confirmed by additional melanoma markers such as HMB-45, Melan A, tyrosinase, or NKI/C3. This is because

S100 is not a specific (although very sensitive) marker for melanoma. S100 is also expressed by some carcinomas[81,82] and sarcomas (liposarcoma, chondrosarcoma, neural tumors).[83,84] Although the typical variants of these sarcomas are easy to diagnose on hematoxylin and eosin (H&E) stain alone, the unusual variants such as de-differentiated liposarcoma, mesenchymal chondrosarcoma, or a malignant peripheral nerve sheath tumor (MPNST) may pose a challenge to distinguish from melanomas. Therefore additional melanoma markers should be performed for definitive diagnosis. Similarly, a pathologist should also be careful in distinguishing melanoma from carcinoma on the basis of only a limited number of immunostains. As mentioned earlier, some carcinomas may show strong S100 expression; an additional pitfall is that some melanomas may show polyclonal CEA and/or focal CAM5.2 keratin immunoreactivity.[85-87] Caution is thus advised when the diagnosis is heavily based on immunohistochemical expression of markers.

LINE OF DIFFERENTIATION: MESENCHYMAL

Strong vimentin expression in a nonmelanocytic, nonlymphoid neoplasm is generally an indication of its being a sarcoma. Most, but not all, sarcomas are negative for epithelial markers. Epithelioid sarcomas, as the name suggests, show some epithelial differentiation, and synovial sarcoma may have a well-defined biphasic pattern that shows strong staining for epithelial markers in the glandlike component.[88-91] The sarcomas that need to be considered in a CUPS case are the ones that do not demonstrate a particular line of differentiation on morphology alone. These sarcomas may have small round blue-cell tumor morphology (Ewing's sarcoma, desmoplastic small round cell tumor, and rhabdomyosarcoma); spindle and epithelioid cells (synovial sarcoma, clear cell sarcoma, angiosarcoma); and pure epithelioid cells (epithelioid sarcoma). Although a number of immunohistochemical stains are available to further classify a sarcoma into a defined category, many stains are not specific enough to provide a definitive diagnosis.[92] Occasionally a high index of suspicion is required to make the correct diagnosis (Fig. 8.1). However, IHC may be performed to narrow down the differential diagnosis and streamline the molecular tests that need to be ordered.[93,94] For example, a small round blue-cell tumor positive for CD99 and PAS in a child or young adult should be evaluated for EWS-FLI1 fusion transcript (Fig. 8.2). As mentioned earlier, fresh frozen tissue is the best sample for molecular testing; reverse transcriptase–polymerase chain reaction assays can also be performed on formalin-fixed paraffin-embedded (FFPE) tissue.[95,96] Triage for suspected sarcoma cases can be performed, as shown in Table 8.1.

LINE OF DIFFERENTIATION: EPITHELIAL

Carcinoma comprises approximately 90% cases of CUPS. Within the carcinoma category, the overwhelming majority of tumors are adenocarcinomas (~70%).[97] The poorly differentiated carcinoma group comprises approximately 15% to 20%. The remainder of tumors represent either squamous cell carcinoma (5%) or neuroendocrine carcinomas (5%). Cytokeratin stains are an excellent marker of epithelial differentiation and are strongly and diffusely expressed in carcinomas.[98] However, examples of keratin positivity have been described in almost all tumor types including sarcomas, melanomas, and even lymphomas.[99-106] Despite these disturbing reports, when an epithelioid tumor is overwhelmingly positive for pankeratin stains, a diagnosis of carcinoma must be seriously evaluated. The cytokeratins are further discussed in Step 2, as follows.

Step 2: The Cytokeratins, an Overview

The soft epithelial keratin intermediate filaments comprise approximately 20 different keratin polypeptides.[107-109] The polypeptides, numbered 1 through 20, comprise type II (basic) keratins and type I (acidic) keratins (Table 8.2). This family of intermediate filaments is crucial in diagnostic IHC for the identification of carcinomatous differentiation and for identification of specific carcinoma subtypes.

Keratin filaments are formed by tetrameric heteropolymers of two different keratins, two from type I and two from type II, to maintain cellular electrical neutrality. The vast majority of keratins are paired together as acidic and basic types, with rare exception. The classification and numbering system of the keratins is based on the catalog of Moll and associates.[110]

Twelve keratins with more acidic isoelectric points form type I (acidic) keratins, and eight keratins with more basic isoelectric points compose the type II (basic-neutral) keratins.[111] The keratins are products of two gene families: Most genes for type II keratins are localized on chromosome 12, and the genes for type I keratins are localized on chromosome 17.[112-114] Within each group, the CKs are numbered consecutively, from highest to lowest molecular weight in each group. Most low-molecular-weight (LMW) keratins are typically found in all epithelia except squamous epithelium, whereas high-molecular-weight (HMW) keratins are typical of squamous epithelium.[110]

The original methods for identification of the different keratin types in tissues relied on tedious biochemical methods, chiefly performed by Franke and Moll and their associates.[110,115] More recently, the problem of keratin subtyping has been expedited by the development of numerous monoclonal keratin-specific antibodies.[108-110,116] This development was crucial for the ease of keratin subtyping, which is now indispensable to the surgical pathologist.

The detection of keratin, and therefore carcinomatous differentiation, is possible in tumors with extensive necrosis. Judkins and colleagues[117] studied a small number of tumors with necrotic areas—including carcinomas, melanomas, and sarcomas—with a panel of antibodies and found that 78% of carcinomas stained with at least one antikeratin antibody in necrotic areas with 100% specificity.

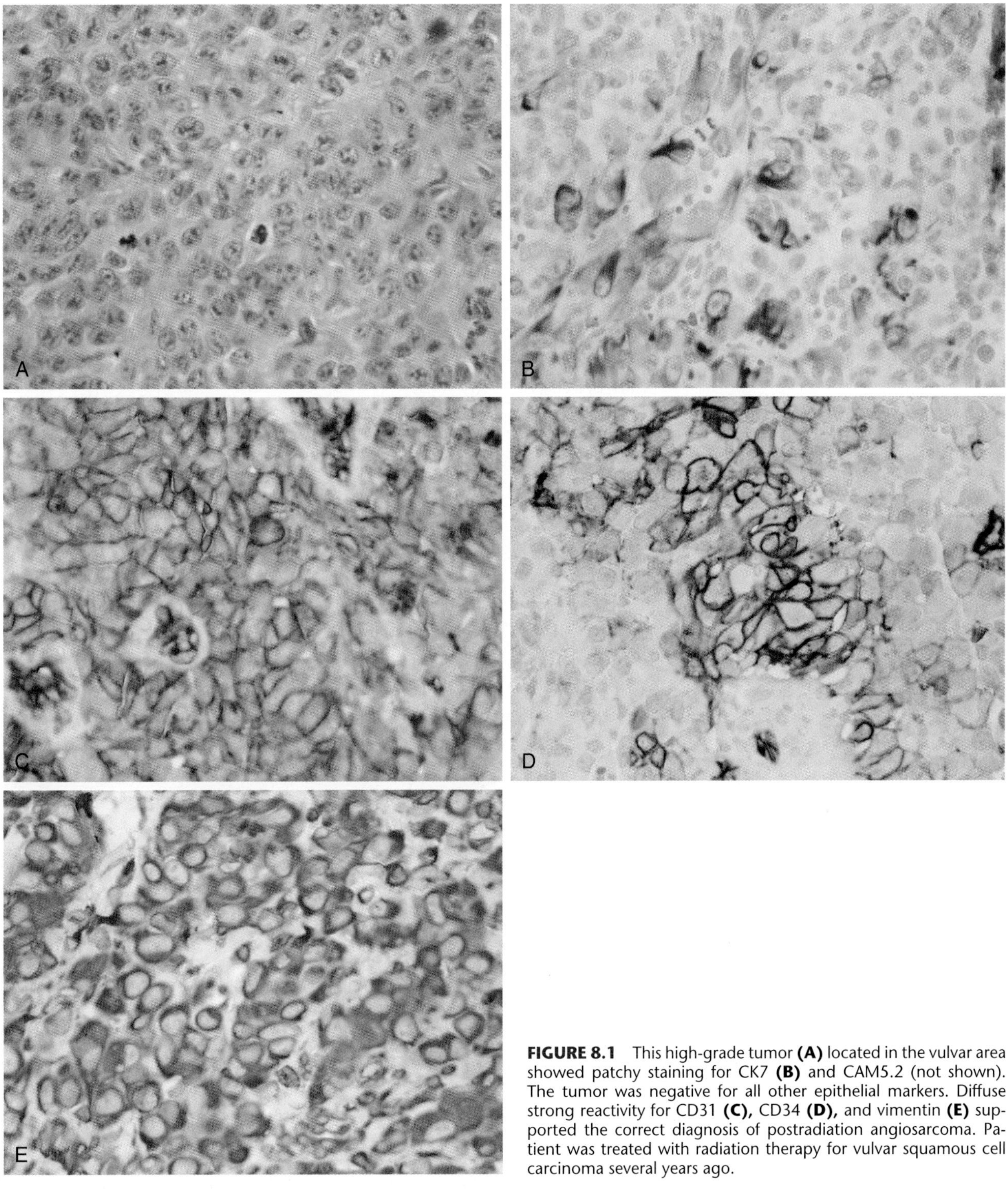

FIGURE 8.1 This high-grade tumor **(A)** located in the vulvar area showed patchy staining for CK7 **(B)** and CAM5.2 (not shown). The tumor was negative for all other epithelial markers. Diffuse strong reactivity for CD31 **(C)**, CD34 **(D)**, and vimentin **(E)** supported the correct diagnosis of postradiation angiosarcoma. Patient was treated with radiation therapy for vulvar squamous cell carcinoma several years ago.

DISTRIBUTION OF KERATIN ANTIGENS IN TISSUES

Simple Epithelial Keratins

Simple epithelial keratins are the first keratins to appear in embryonic development because they are expressed in virtually all simple (nonstratified), ductal, and pseudostratified epithelial tissues.[109,110] Because these keratins are widespread, they may be useful for the identification of epithelial differentiation. Almost all mesotheliomas and carcinomas,[109,110] except squamous cell carcinomas, contain the simple keratins 8 and 18. A few visceral organs such as liver contain only keratins 8 and 18.

Although identified by many keratin antibodies that recognize a cocktail of keratin peptides (e.g., pankeratin

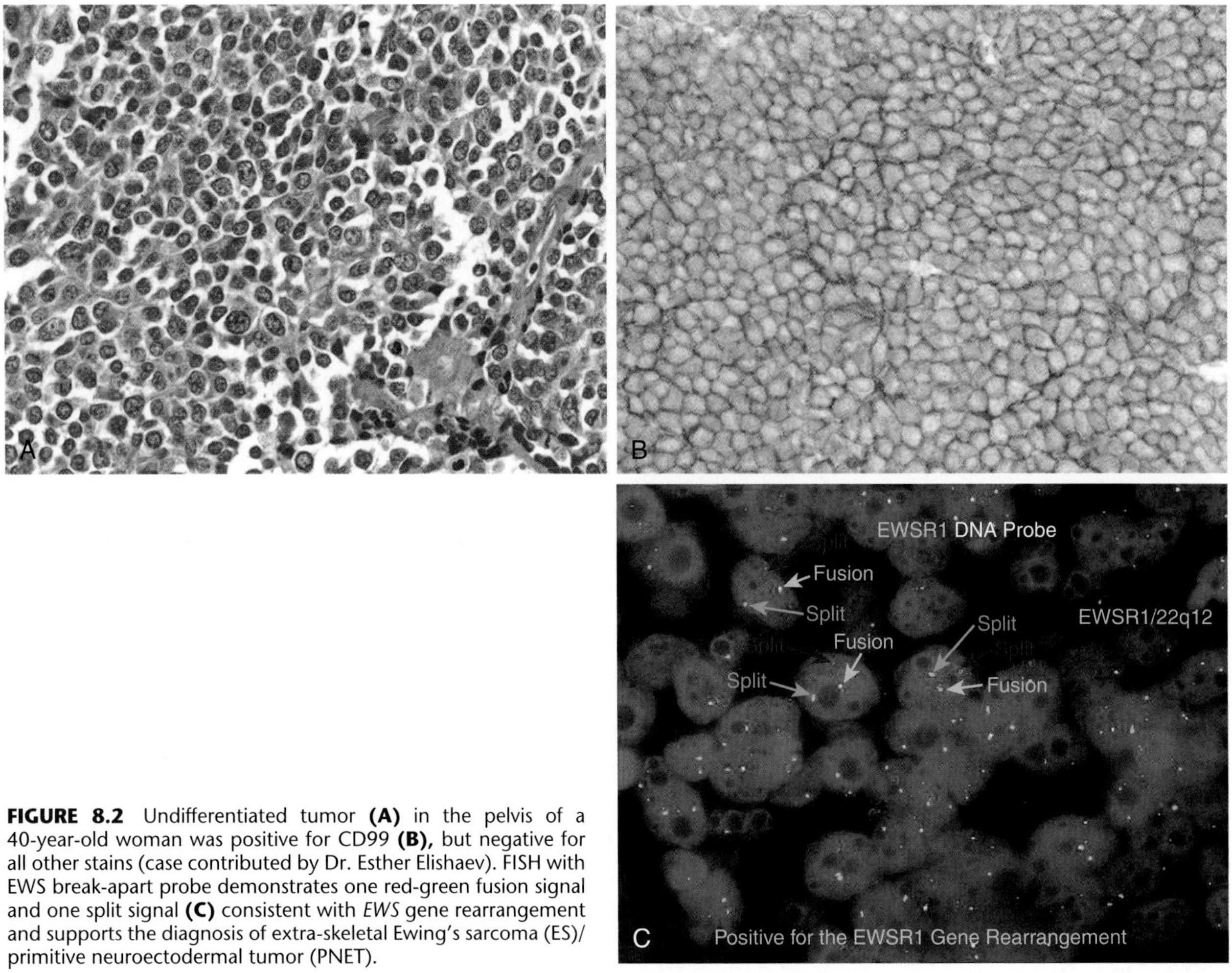

FIGURE 8.2 Undifferentiated tumor **(A)** in the pelvis of a 40-year-old woman was positive for CD99 **(B),** but negative for all other stains (case contributed by Dr. Esther Elishaev). FISH with EWS break-apart probe demonstrates one red-green fusion signal and one split signal **(C)** consistent with *EWS* gene rearrangement and supports the diagnosis of extra-skeletal Ewing's sarcoma (ES)/ primitive neuroectodermal tumor (PNET).

AE1 and AE3 antibodies), CAM5.2 and 35BH11 recognize keratins 8 and 18 almost exclusively (Fig. 8.3). This group of antibodies is perhaps the most commonly used to demonstrate the simple keratins in surgical pathology. Because simple keratins are widely distributed in most carcinomas, these antibodies are particularly useful in the initial approach to investigation for carcinomatous differentiation (Table 8.3; see also Table 8.2).

CYTOKERATIN 19 The lowest molecular weight of the keratin group, CK19 is a simple keratin that has a distribution similar to keratins 8 and 18 and is also present in the basal layer of the squamous epithelium of mucosal surfaces and may be seen in epidermal basal cells.[118] CK19 is a good screening marker for epithelial neoplasms because of its wide distribution in simple epithelia and in many squamous tissues. The monoclonal antibody AE1 (Boehringer-Mannheim, Indianapolis, Ind) reacts with CK19, as does the AE1/ AE3 cocktail (Boehringer-Mannheim). Also reacting in formalin-fixed tissues is a monoclonal antibody to CK19-RCK108 (DAKO, Carpinteria, Calif).[119] CK19 is mostly negative and rarely seen focally in hepatocellular carcinoma.[119]

CYTOKERATIN 7 CK7 is a 54-kD type II simple keratin that has a restricted distribution compared with keratins 8 and 18. Its presence in many simple, pseudostratified, and ductal epithelia and mesothelia is similar in distribution to that of keratins 8 and 18. Much of the data in the literature on CK7 are based on the reactivity patterns of antibody OV-TL 12/30 (DAKO, Carpinteria, Calif) in formalin-fixed, paraffin-embedded tissues. The OV-TL 12/30 antibody parallels the CK7 immunoreactivity with RCK 105, an antibody for use on frozen sections.[120-122] Predigestion with protease or heat-induced epitope retrieval (HIER) is required for OV-TL 12/30. The lack or extreme paucity of CK7 distribution in tissues such as colonic epithelium, hepatocytes, and prostatic acinar tissue is used to diagnostic advantage.[120-124] This antibody identifies transitional cell epithelium (Fig. 8.4A) but is predominantly negative in most squamous epithelia. The restricted topography of CK7 makes it especially useful in evaluating the origin of adenocarcinomas because this keratin is present in most breast, lung, ovarian, pancreaticobiliary, and transitional cell carcinomas, but it is either absent or present in only rare cells in colorectal, renal, and prostatic carcinomas (Tables 8.4 and 8.5).[116,120,121,125-132] Cytokeratin 7 stains squamous cell carcinoma and squamous dysplasias of the cervix.[116] A diagnostic pitfall in the interpretation

TABLE 8.1 Sarcomas That Can Present as CUPS

Sarcoma Type	Age/Site	Morphology	Special Stains/IHC	Ancillary Techniques for Confirmation of Diagnosis
ES/PNET	Usually < 30 yr. Chest wall, extremities, retroperitoneum, pelvis. Metastases to lungs and bone.	Small round blue cell tumor	PAS+, CD99+, FLI1+	RT-PCR for EWS-FLI1, EWS-ERG, EWS-ETV1, EWS-E1AF, EWS-FEV. EWS translocation can also be shown by FISH with EWS break-apart probe.
Rhabdomyosarcoma (RMS)—alveolar (A), embryonal (E), and pleomorphic (P)	A-RMS: 10-20 yr. Extremities and perineum. E-RMS: 3-10 yr. Prostate, paratesticular, orbit, nasal cavity. P-RMS: 50+ yr. Abdomen, retroperitoneum, chest wall, testes, extremities.	Small round blue cells with alveolar growth pattern in alveolar RMS; round and spindle cells in embryonal; round, spindle and pleomorphic cells in pleomorphic RMS	Muscle specific actin (MSA)+, desmin+, myoglobin+, myogenin (most specific)+, myoD1+	RT-PCR for PAX3-FKHR and PAX7-FKHR in alveolar RMS only
Desmoplastic small round cell tumor	Young adults, often adolescent boys. Abdomen and pelvis, peritoneal implants.	Round/oval cells in desmoplastic stroma in classic cases, other cases with variable morphology	Vimentin+, cytokeratin+, EMA+, desmin+, WT1+	RT-PCR for EWS-WT1
Synovial sarcoma	Young adults. Extremities around large joints. Now described in various locations including lung and pleura.	Spindle cell or biphasic glandular and spindle cell pattern; small round cells in poorly differentiated tumor	EMA+, keratin+ (biphasic tumors), CD99+, bcl2+; recently TLE1+	RT-PCR for SYT-SSX1 and SYT-SSX2
Clear cell sarcoma (melanoma of soft parts)	Young adults. Deep soft tissue with nodal and lung metastases.	Mixed epithelioid and spindle cells in nested growth pattern	S100+, HMB45+, melanA+	RT-PCR for EWS-ATF1 (not seen in cutaneous melanoma)
Alveolar soft part sarcoma	Young adults—often females. Deep soft tissue. Lung metastases common.	Large polygonal cells, granular cytoplasm, prominent nucleoli, rare mitoses	PASD+, TFE3+	Membrane bound rhomboidal crystals by electron microscopy (EM); RT-PCR for ASPL-TFE3
PEComas	40-50 yr—usually females. Various visceral organs and soft tissue.	Epithelioid and spindle cells with perivascular arrangement, clear to granular cytoplasm	HMB45+, melan-A+, but S100 negative	EM: glycogen, pre-melanosomes, occasional dense bodies
Epithelioid sarcoma	Young adults. Deep soft tissue of extremities. Metastases to lung, lymph node, & skin.	Epithelioid tumor cells, granuloma-like growth pattern	Keratin+, EMA+, vimentin+, CD34+, CK5/6–, p63–	Nothing specific; EM may be helpful
Vascular tumors	Adults. Soft tissue and various visceral organs.	Angiosarcoma: epithelioid and spindle cell tumor, vasoformative areas; epithelioid in hemangioendothelioma	FVIII+, CD31+, CD34+, FLI1+, thrombomodulin+, patchy keratin+	EM to identify endothelial cells rarely required
Leiomyosarcoma	Adults. Abdomen, pelvis, and various other locations.	Spindle or epithelioid cells with areas of smooth muscle differentiation	SMA+, HHF35+, desmin+, caldesmon+, patchy keratin+	EM: smooth muscle differentiation

Continued

TABLE 8.1 Sarcomas That Can Present as CUPS—cont'd

Malignant peripheral nerve sheath tumor	Adults. NF1 patients (50%). Deep soft tissue in association with major nerve.	Spindle cells with neural differentiation, abundant mitosis, necrosis±; rarely epithelioid	S100+ (weak, patchy), CD56+, CD57+, PGP9.5+, CD99+; negative for melanoma and vascular markers	Negative for SYT-SSX1 and SYT-SSX2 EM: neural differentiation
Chordoma	Adults, usually males. Sacro-coccygeal, thoraco-lumbar spine.	Physaliferous cells, vacuolated cytoplasm, mucoid stroma	S100+, keratin+, but CK7−/CK20−, EMA+	EM rarely required
Extraskeletal myxoid chondrosarcoma	Adults. Deep soft tissues of extremities. Metastases may be confused with myoepithelial-type carcinomas.	Cords of spindle and epithelioid cells in myxoid stroma	S100+, NSE+, synaptophysin±, keratin−, chromogranin−	RT-PCR for EWS-CHN and TAF2N-CHN
Endometrial stromal sarcoma	Adult females. Abdominopelvic region. Distant metastases to lungs.	Oval/round to spindle cells; vague resemblance to proliferative pattern endometrial stroma	CD10+, ER+, bcl2−, CD34−, SMA and desmin positivity with smooth muscle differentiation	FISH for 7p15 translocation better than RT-PCR for JAZF1-JJAZ fusion
Gastrointestinal stromal tumor	Adults. GI tract. Abdominopelvic region. Metastases often to the liver.	Spindle or epithelioid cells	CD117+, CD34+, often negative for S100, actin, and desmin	KIT activating mutations

EM, extramammary; EWS, Ewing's sarcoma; FISH, fluorescent *in situ* hybridization; GI, gastrointestinal; IHC, immunohistochemistry; PNET, primitive neuroectodermal tumor.

of CK7 is that CK7 stains subsets of endothelial cells of normal soft tissues, as well as endothelial cells in venules and lymphatics in intestinal mucosa, uterine exocervix, and lymphoid tissue.

Diagnostic Utility of Cytokeratin 7

The specific diagnostic utility of CK7 lies in the fact that there are three dominant patterns[116] of immunostaining:

1. Tumors that are characteristically strongly and diffusely positive include those of the salivary glands, lung, breast, ovary, endometrium, bladder, and thymus, as well as mesotheliomas, neuroendocrine tumors, pancreaticobiliary adenocarcinomas, and the fibrolamellar variant of hepatocellular carcinoma.[133] CK7 is also typically expressed in tumor cells of mammary and extramammary Paget disease.[134]
2. CK7 variably stains the tumor cells in biliary and gastric tumors.
3. Carcinomas that are almost invariably negative but may occasionally show rare CK7-positive cells include hepatocellular carcinomas, duodenal ampullary carcinomas, colon carcinomas, renal (clear cell type), prostate, and adrenal cortical tumors.

Strong diffuse CK7 immunostaining is a valuable marker in the diagnostic workup of a carcinoma and may be used as a starting point for further immunohistochemical study. Metastatic carcinomas in lung that are CK7 positive must be differentiated from a primary lung carcinoma with a panel of antibodies, and the IHC workup will be dependent on the patient's age, gender, and presenting findings. It is important to remember that CK7 may be expressed infrequently in certain tumors (see Table 8.5).[135] In general, there is high fidelity of CK7 expression between primary and metastatic carcinomas.[135]

CYTOKERATIN 20 CK20 is a 46-kD LMW keratin that was discovered by Moll and associates.[136] The tissue distribution of CK20 is limited predominantly to gastrointestinal epithelium and its tumors, mucinous tumors of the ovary, and Merkel cell neoplasms.[127,130,131,137-139] The limited distribution of CK20 in colorectal, pancreatic, and gallbladder carcinomas; Merkel cell carcinomas; and transitional cell carcinomas (Fig. 8.4B) is useful in the identification of this group of tumors in primary or even metastatic sites.[63,138,140] When combined with the specific tissue distribution of other keratins such as CK7, it is possible to identify colon cancer metastases in the lung, distinguish pulmonary small cell carcinoma from Merkel cell carcinoma,[141,142] and distinguish transitional cell carcinoma from other squamous cell carcinomas and poorly differentiated carcinomas. It is important to recognize that CK20 in this subgroup of tumors is most often distributed strongly and diffusely. Rare CK20+ cells may be seen in some other neoplasms. Up to 10% of primary pulmonary adenocarcinomas not otherwise specified (NOS) and up to 25% of mucinous bronchioloalveolar types may show CK20+ cells.[143,144] In addition, the controversial primary mucinous carcinoma of the lung ("colloid carcinoma," goblet cell variant) shows CK20 immunostaining in about 50% of

TABLE 8.2 Most Common Keratins and Their Distribution

Type II (Basic) Keratin	Molecular Wt (kD)	Typical Distribution in Normal Tissue	Type I (Acidic) Keratin	Molecular Wt (kD)
CK1	67	Epidermis of palms and soles	CK9	64
			CK10	56.5
CK2	65	Epithelia, all locations	CK11	56
CK3	63	Cornea	CK12	55
CK4	59	Nonkeratinizing squamous epithelia	CK13	51
CK5	58	Basal cells of squamous and glandular epithelia, myoepithelial, mesothelium	CK14	50
			CK15	50
CK6	56	Squamous epithelia, especially hyperproliferative	CK16	48
CK7	54	Simple epithelia	CK17	46
CK8	52	Basal cells of glandular epithelia, myoepithelial	CK18	45
		Simple epithelia, most glandular and squamous epithelia (basal)	CK19	40
		Simple epithelia of intestines and stomach, Merkel cells	CK20	46

From Quinlan RA, Schiller DL, Hatzfeld M, et al. Patterns of expression and organization of cytokeratin intermediate filaments. *Ann N Y Acad Sci.* 1985;455:282-306.

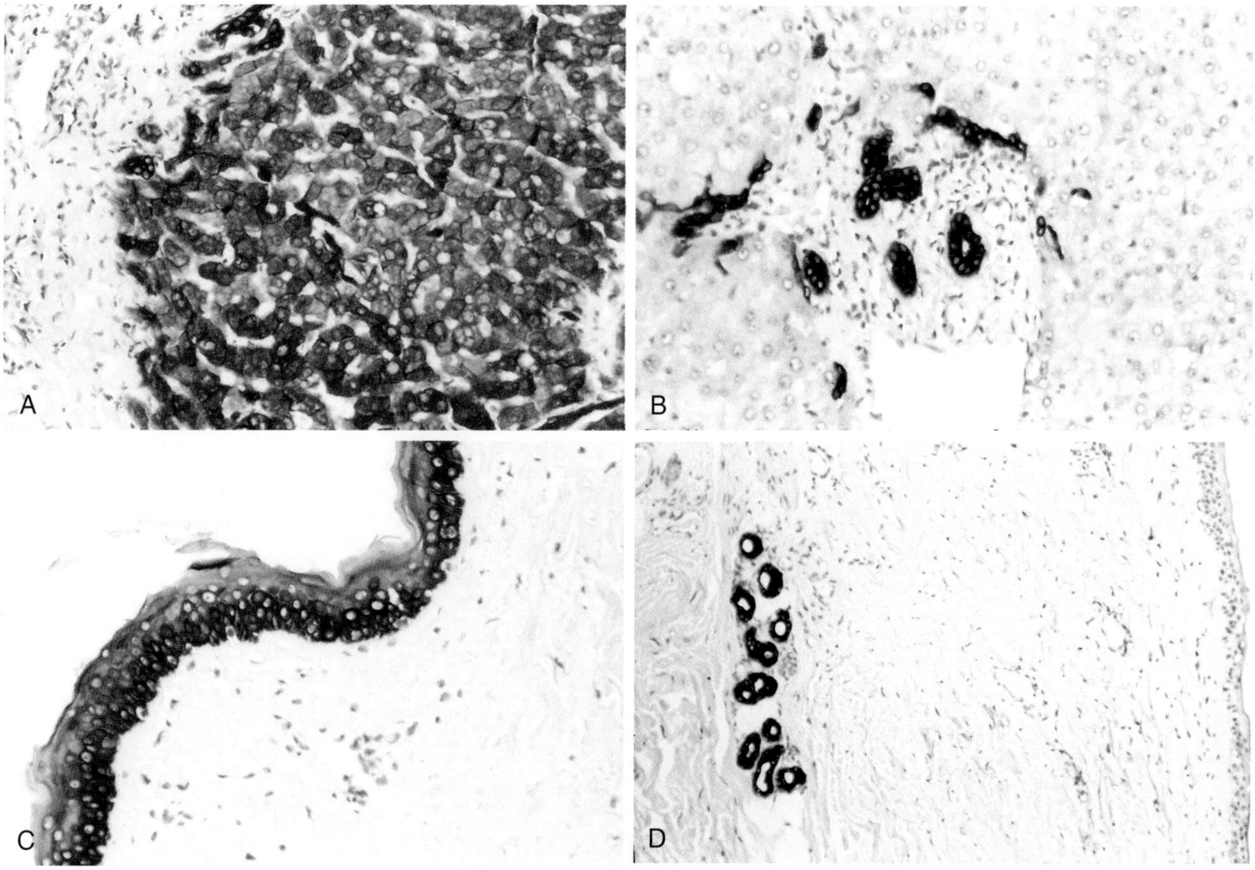

FIGURE 8.3 CAM5.2 stains liver and adjacent bile ducts **(A)**, whereas keratin 34βE12 (K903) stains bile ducts **(B)** and stratum corneum of skin **(C)**. CAM 5.2 and 35BH11 stain only eccrine coils and not epidermis **(D)**.

cases, along with nuclear positivity for CDX2, a gut-specific marker.[145] A small percentage of breast carcinomas may also show CK20 positivity.[146]

Cholangiocarcinomas of liver, whether of central or peripheral origin, are nearly always strongly and diffusely positive, whereas central (large duct) carcinomas are more likely to have a high labeling index for CK20 in addition to CK7.[147] The positive predictive value using the combination of CK7 and CK20 to predict the presence of metastatic carcinomas of colorectal or pancreaticobiliary

TABLE 8.3 Keratin Antigens and Antibodies

CK Antigen	Antibody	Notes
CK8	35BH11	Carcinomas of simple epithelium
CK8	CAM5.2	Carcinoma of simple epithelium
Pankeratin	AE1/AE3	Carcinomas of simple and complex epithelium
CK1/10	34B4	Squamous cell carcinoma
CK7	OV-TL 12/30	Non–gastrointestinally derived carcinomas
CK20	K20	Most gastrointestinal carcinomas; mucinous ovarian, biliary, transitional, and Merkel cell carcinoma
CK19	RCK 108	Most carcinomas; many carcinomas with squamous component; myoepithelial cells
CK1/5/10/14	34betaE12	Basal cells of prostate; most duct-derived carcinomas
CK18/19	PKK1	Most carcinomas
CK10/11/13/14/15/16/19	AE1	Most squamous lesions and many carcinomas
CK8/14/15/16/18/19	MAK-6	Most carcinomas

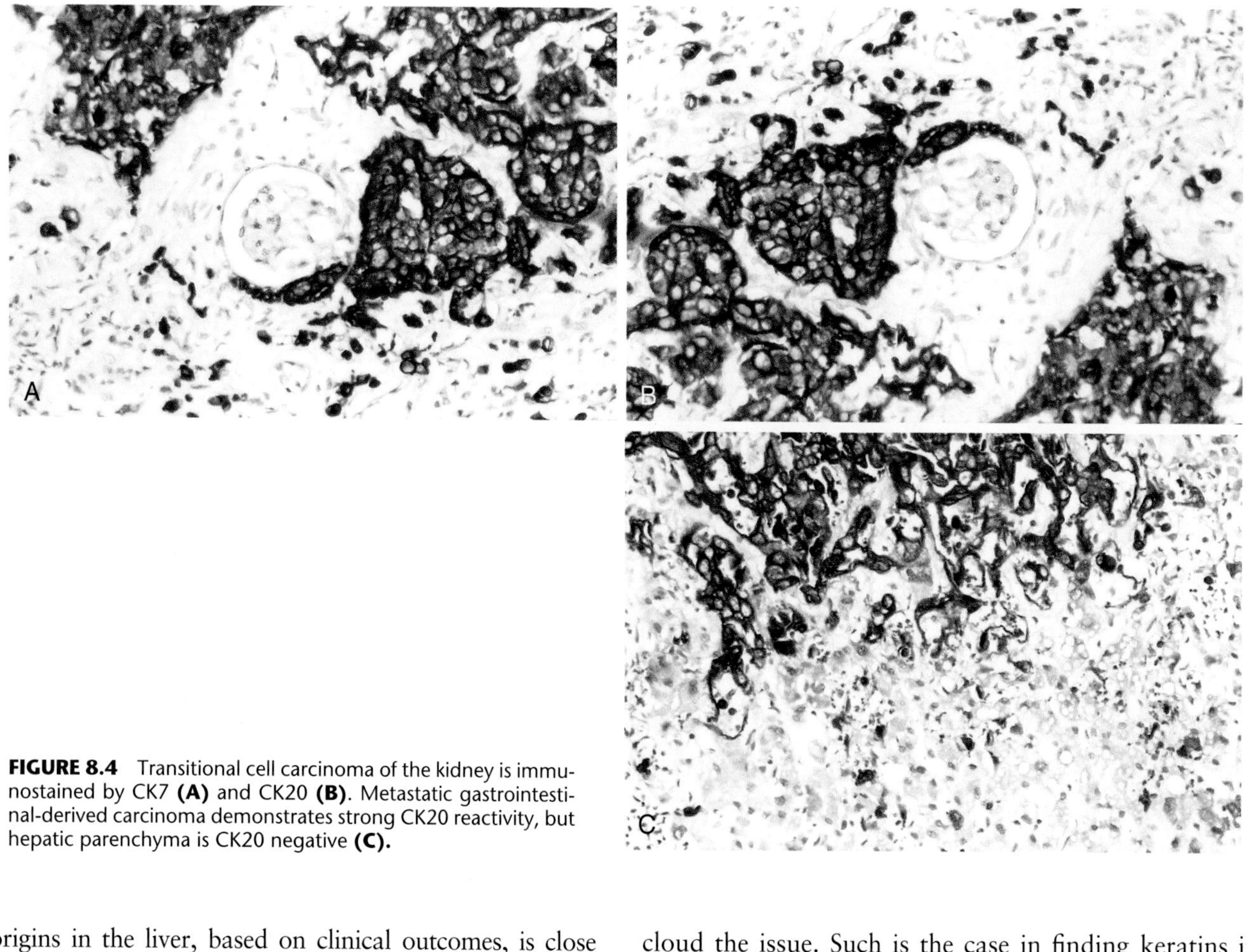

FIGURE 8.4 Transitional cell carcinoma of the kidney is immunostained by CK7 **(A)** and CK20 **(B)**. Metastatic gastrointestinal-derived carcinoma demonstrates strong CK20 reactivity, but hepatic parenchyma is CK20 negative **(C)**.

origins in the liver, based on clinical outcomes, is close to 0.9.[148] It is important to remember that CK20 may be expressed infrequently in certain tumors (Table 8.6).[135,149] In general, there is high fidelity of CK20 expression between primary and metastatic carcinomas (Fig. 8.4C).[135]

Although the prominent expression of CKs is the essential element of epithelial differentiation, on occasion expression of other lineage-specific markers may cloud the issue. Such is the case in finding keratins in nonepithelial tissues (see later), as well as the rare observation of leukocyte common antigen (CD45) in some undifferentiated or neuroendocrine carcinomas[150] and CD30 in embryonal carcinomas. The use of a panel of antibodies and the pattern and intensity of immunostaining is critically important in these confounding situations.

TABLE 8.4 Dominant CK7/CK20 Immunoprofiles in Select Neoplasms

CK7+/CK20+
Transitional cell carcinoma
Pancreatic carcinoma
Ovarian mucinous carcinoma
CK7+/CK20−
Non–small cell carcinoma of lung
Small cell carcinoma of lung
Breast carcinoma, ductal and lobular
Nonmucinous ovarian carcinoma
Endometrial adenocarcinoma
Mesothelioma
Squamous cell carcinoma of cervix
CK7−/CK20+
Colorectal adenocarcinoma
Merkel cell carcinoma
CK7−/CK20−
Squamous cell carcinoma, lung
Prostate adenocarcinoma
Renal cell carcinoma
Hepatocellular carcinoma
Adrenocortical carcinoma
Some thymic carcinoma

From Wang MP, Zee S, Zarbo RJ, et al. Coordinate expression of cytokeratin 7 and 20 defines unique subsets of carcinomas. *Appl Immunohistochem.* 1995;3:99-107; and Chu P, Wu E, Weiss L. Cytokeratin 7 and cytokeratin 20 expression in epithelial neoplasms: A survey of 435 cases. *Mod Pathol.* 2000;13:962-972.

TABLE 8.5 Cytokeratin 7: Percentage of Tumors with Expression

Tumor	Percentage Expression
Lung, adenocarcinoma	100
Lung, small cell carcinoma	43
Ovary, adenocarcinoma	100
Salivary gland, all tumors	100
Uterus, endometrium	100
Thyroid, all tumors	98
Breast, ductal/lobular	96
Liver, cholangiocarcinoma	93
Pancreas, adenocarcinoma	92
Bladder, transitional cell	88
Cervix, squamous cell	87
Mesothelioma	65
Neuroendocrine carcinoma	56
Stomach, adenocarcinoma	38
Head and neck, squamous cell	27
Esophagus, squamous cell	21
Kidney, adenocarcinoma	11
Germ cell, carcinoma	7
Colon, adenocarcinoma	5
Adrenal, carcinoma	0
Prostate, carcinoma	0
Thymus, thymoma	0

Data from Chu P, Wu E, Weiss L. Cytokeratin 7 and cytokeratin 20 expression in epithelial neoplasms: A survey of 435 cases. *Mod Pathol.* 2000; 13:962-972.

KEY DIAGNOSTIC POINTS

Simple Cytokeratins

- CAM5.2 and AE1/AE3: broad coverage for detection of carcinomatous differentiation. Both should be used together for screening.
- CK7 (+): adenocarcinomas of breast, lung, ovary, endometrium, and pancreas; mesothelioma, urothelial carcinomas, thymic carcinomas; and fibrolamellar variant of hepatocellular carcinomas.
- CK7 (negative/rare positive): renal, prostate, adrenocortical, squamous (except uterine cervix), small cell carcinomas, and hepatocellular carcinomas.
- CK20 (+): colorectal, pancreas, mucinous ovarian, Merkel cell, and urothelial carcinomas.
- CK20 (negative/rare positive): most breast, lung, and salivary gland carcinomas; hepatocellular, renal, prostate, adrenocortical, squamous, and small cell carcinomas.
- See Table 8.4 for CK7/CK20 immunoprofile of various carcinomas.

Keratins of Stratified Epithelia: Complex Keratins

Keratins of high molecular weight (HMW) are observed in stratified epithelia and are generally not present in the simple visceral-type epithelia. Basal cells of prostate and myoepithelial cell populations of ducts and glandular tissue also contain an abundance of HMW type II keratins and LMW type I keratins. The antibody 34bE12 or (catalog number) keratin 903 (K903)[151-153] identifies a cocktail of keratins including Moll types I, II, V, X, XI, and XIV/XV. The practical diagnostic use of this pattern of expression is to identify basal and myoepithelial cells in their respective organs (Fig. 8.5). For example, the staining of myoepithelial cells around ductal carcinoma in situ or sclerosing adenosis can confirm a noninvasive lesion. This keratin of stratified type is also typically present in squamous epithelium and, using antibody K903, is a good antibody for detecting squamous differentiation in an otherwise poorly differentiated carcinoma.

These HMW structural keratins are also commonly seen in duct-derived epithelium (breast, pancreas, biliary tract, lung) and in transitional, ovarian, and mesothelial tissues.[151-153] The degree of immunostaining of these tissues with HMW keratin antibodies is typically strong and diffuse, a feature that is helpful diagnostically because HMW keratin immunostaining is seen only focally in visceral epithelial tissues such as colon, stomach, kidney, and liver.

KEY DIAGNOSTIC POINTS

Antibodies to Complex Keratins

- Confirms the presence of basal cells of prostate (see Fig. 8.5)
- Confirms the presence of myoepithelial cells
- Present in basal cell layer of stratified and squamous epithelium
- Strong and diffuse in tumors of squamous epithelial differentiation
- Present in a wide variety of duct-derived carcinomas and mesotheliomas, as well as most neoplasms that demonstrate tonofilaments ultrastructurally

CYTOKERATIN 5 AND CYTOKERATIN 5/6 CK5 and CK6 are basic (type II) polypeptides with molecular weight of 58 kDa and 56 kDa, respectively. Most studies have been performed using antibodies to CK5/6 and have been found useful in the differential diagnosis of metastatic carcinoma in the pleura versus epithelial mesothelioma. Epithelial mesotheliomas are strongly positive in all cases (Fig. 8.6), but up to 30% of pulmonary adenocarcinomas will show focal variable immunostaining.[154]

Almost all squamous cell carcinomas, half of transitional cell carcinomas, and many undifferentiated large cell carcinomas immunostain with CK5/6 (Table 8.7).[155-157] CK5/6 has excellent sensitivity and specificity for the detection of squamous differentiation in poorly differentiated carcinomas.[155-157] p63 is also seen with high frequency in squamous and transitional carcinomas, and when used with the CK5/6 antibody affords high sensitivity and specificity for squamous differentiation.[155,158]

Myoepithelial cells of the breast, glandular epithelium, and basal cells of the prostate are express CK5/6.[157] Some carcinomas of ovarian origin may display CK5/6.[157]

Hyperplastic mesothelial cells can be seen on occasion in the sinuses of lymph nodes from the chest or cervical chain.[159] The differential diagnosis in this instance is metastatic carcinoma. The presence of strong, diffuse CK5/6 in the cells of these nests should aid in identifying them as mesothelial in origin.

Renewed interest in these antibodies has occurred because both CK5 and CK5/6 are also used to identify the basal-like molecular class of breast cancer. We have recently shown that CK5 (clone XM26) is superior to CK5/6 (clone D5/16B4) antibody in identifying the basal-like phenotype of breast carcinoma with high sensitivity and specificity.[160] Whether CK5 is superior

TABLE 8.6 Cytokeratin 20: Percentage of Tumors with Expression

Tumor	Percentage Expression
Colon, adenocarcinoma	100
Skin, Merkel cell	78
Pancreas, adenocarcinoma	62
Stomach, adenocarcinoma	50
Liver, cholangiocarcinoma	43
Bladder, transitional cell	29
Lung, adenocarcinoma	10
Liver, hepatoma	9
Gut, carcinoid	6
Lung, adenocarcinoma	10
Head and neck, squamous cell	6
Ovary, adenocarcinoma	4
Adrenal, carcinoma	0
Breast, ductal/lobular	0
Cervix, squamous cell	0
Esophagus, squamous cell	0
Germ cell, carcinoma	0
Kidney, carcinoma	0
Mesothelioma	0
Prostate, adenocarcinoma	0
Salivary gland, all tumors	0
Thyroid, all tumors	0
Thymus, thymoma	0
Uterus, endometrium	0
Lung, carcinoid	0
Lung, small cell	0
Lung, squamous cell	0

Data from Chu P, Wu E, Weiss L. Cytokeratin 7 and cytokeratin 20 expression in epithelial neoplasms: A survey of 435 cases. *Mod Pathol.* 2000;13:962-972.

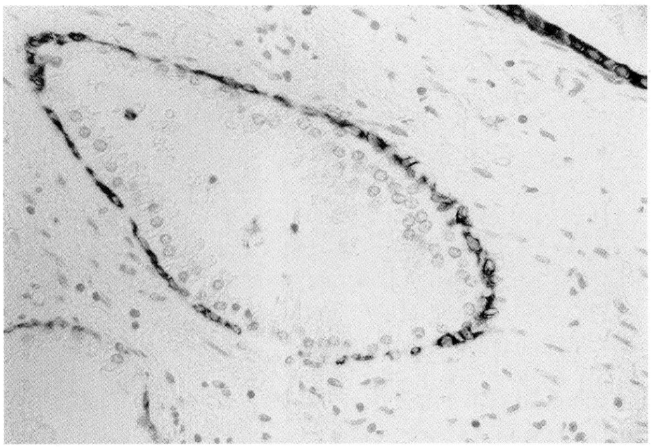

FIGURE 8.5 Basal cells in this prostate section are seen with K903. Myoepithelial cells in the breast can also be seen with K903.

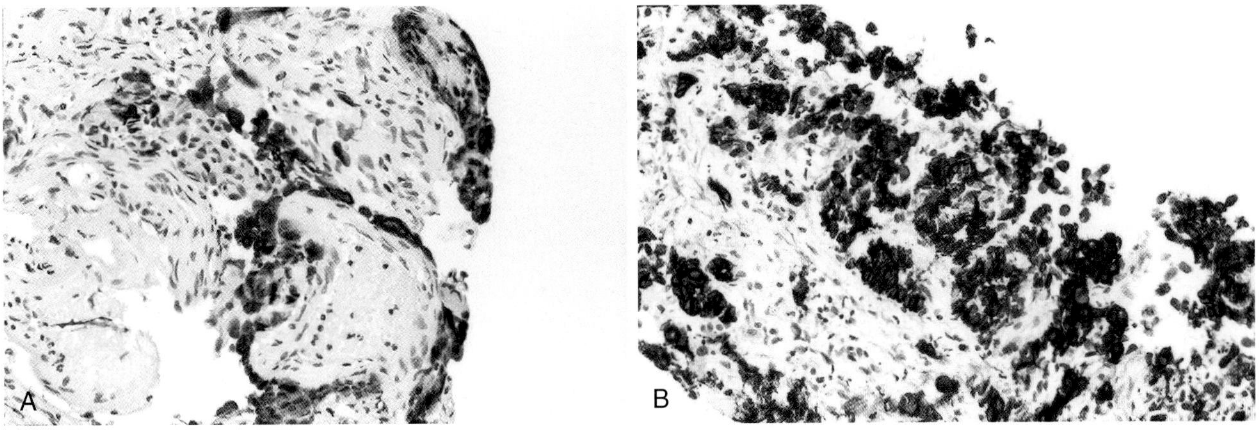

FIGURE 8.6 Antibodies to CK5/CK6 strongly immunostain reactive mesothelial cells in a pleural biopsy **(A)** and epithelial mesothelioma cells **(B)**.

to CK5/6 in other distinctions (mesothelioma versus carcinoma; or in identifying squamous differentiation) needs to be investigated.

KEY DIAGNOSTIC POINTS

CK5 and CK5/6

- Good indicator of squamous and transitional cell differentiation
- Good discriminator of mesothelial differentiation versus adenocarcinoma in lung
- Positive in myoepithelial cells of breast and prostate basal cells
- Sensitive and specific markers of basal-like phenotype of breast carcinoma
- CK5 best to identify basal-like carcinoma of the breast

Keratins in Nonepithelial Cells

Keratins have been documented by IHC,[107,161-164] dot immunoblot,[87] and polymerase chain reaction[105] in several types of tumors in which there is no morphologic evidence of epithelial differentiation. This type of keratin immunostaining has been referred to as anomalous, aberrant, spurious, and unexpected.[165]

The keratins most often found in these nonepithelial mesenchymal tissues or melanocytic lesions are keratins 8 and 18 and, less commonly, keratin 19. Antibodies that detect these LMW keratins have demonstrated positive immunostaining in a variety of formalin-fixed, paraffin-embedded (FFPE) mesenchymal tumors including leiomyosarcomas (21%-25%), fibrosarcoma (4%), liposarcoma (21%), rhabdomyosarcoma, malignant peripheral nerve sheath tumors (5%), some malignant fibrous histiocytomas (5%), gastrointestinal stromal tumors (50%), rare solitary fibrous tumors of pleura, angiosarcoma (33%), endometrial stromal sarcoma, and primitive neuroectodermal tumors (50%).[100,166-180] Keratin usually stains scattered cells in this group of tumors

TABLE 8.7 Cytokeratin 5/6: Percentage of Tumors with Expression

Tumor	Percentage Expression
Skin, squamous cell	100
Skin, basal cell	100
Thymus, thymoma	100
Salivary gland, all tumors	93
Mesothelioma	76
Bladder, transitional cell	62
Uterus, endometrium	50
Pancreas, carcinoma	38
Breast, carcinoma	31
Ovary, carcinoma	25
Liver, cholangiocarcinoma	14
Gut, carcinoid	10
Lung, adenocarcinoma	5
Liver, hepatoma	4
Adrenal, carcinoma	0
Colon, adenocarcinoma	0
Germ cell, carcinoma	0
Kidney, carcinoma	0
Prostate, carcinoma	0
Stomach, adenocarcinoma	0
Thyroid, all tumors	0

Data from Chu P, Weiss LM. Expression of CK 5/6 in epithelial neoplasms: An immunohistochemical study of 509 cases. *Mod Pathol.* 2002;6:6-10.

in traditional FFPE tissue, whereas carcinomas and sarcomatoid carcinomas are heavily and diffusely stained (Fig. 8.7).[181] In addition, keratin-positive soft tissue and bone tumors with partial epithelial differentiation are variably stained with keratin in the epithelial areas as

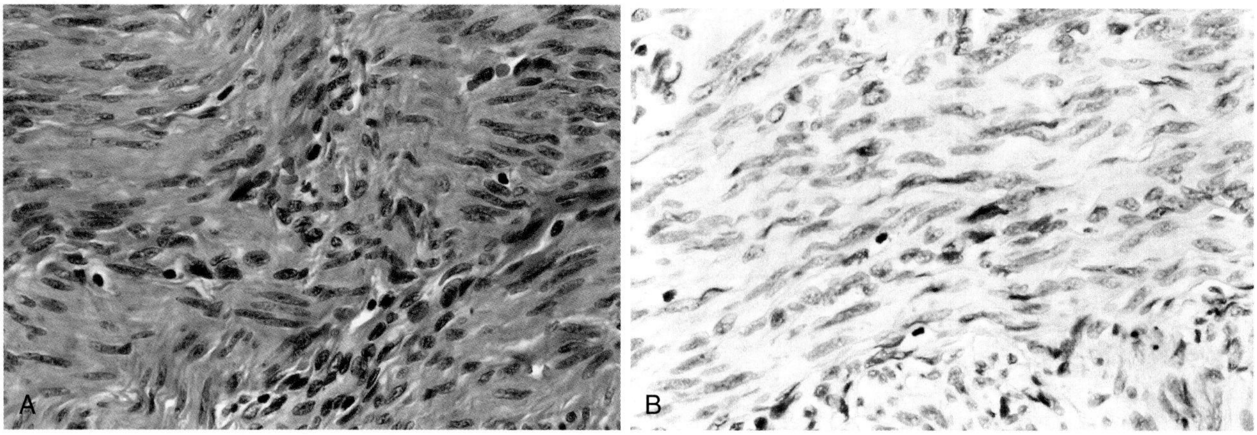

FIGURE 8.7 Smooth muscle neoplasm **(A)** shows scattered CAM5.2-positive cells **(B)**, a typical focal pattern of immunostaining for keratin seen in a variety of mesenchymal tumors.

expected. This group includes synovial sarcomas, epithelioid sarcoma, chordoma, malignant peripheral nerve sheath tumor, and adamantinoma of long bones.[182-187] Although some of the soft tissue tumors may mimic metastatic carcinoma morphologically, the finding of sporadic cell immunostaining is unlike the strong, diffuse immunostaining seen in carcinomas, especially when using the broad-coverage antibodies. Frozen tissues fixed in acetone or alcohol, including alcohol-fixed cytologic specimens, yield far more keratin-positive cells, and this can be confusing diagnostically, especially with cytologic specimens for which alcohol is a standard fixative for needle aspiration specimens.

Malignant melanoma also demonstrates immunostaining for keratins 8 and 18, but in formalin-fixed, paraffin-embedded tissues the prevalence is around 1% of cases, with focal tumor cell staining.[85,188-190] Frozen sections and alcohol-fixed melanomas show substantially more positive tumor cells than do formalin-fixed specimens, and it is important to recognize this to avoid misdiagnosing melanoma as a carcinoma, especially in alcohol-fixed cytologic preparations. The consensus regarding keratin immunostaining of nonepithelioid sarcomas and melanomas is that although the presence of keratin is real as measured by molecular techniques and more sensitive immunohistologic methods (frozen sections, alcohol fixation), the observed nonexpression of keratin staining in these tumors in formalin-fixed tissue is desirable because of its diagnostic usefulness.

Truly "spurious" keratin immunoreactivity has been described in human glial tissue and in some human astrocytomas, especially with antibodies AE1 and 34BE12.[191] In addition, the cocktail AE1/AE3 may cross-react with both normal and neoplastic astrocytes.[192] The spurious keratin immunoreactivity is probably due to cross-reaction with glial cells containing glial fibrillary acidic proteins.[191] This is an obvious pitfall for the misdiagnosis of metastatic carcinoma in the brain. The antibody CAM5.2 does not react with astroglial cells and thus is best used to detect carcinomatous differentiation in the CNS.

Meningiomas, especially the "secretory variant," may express keratin in up to one third of cases.[193-196]

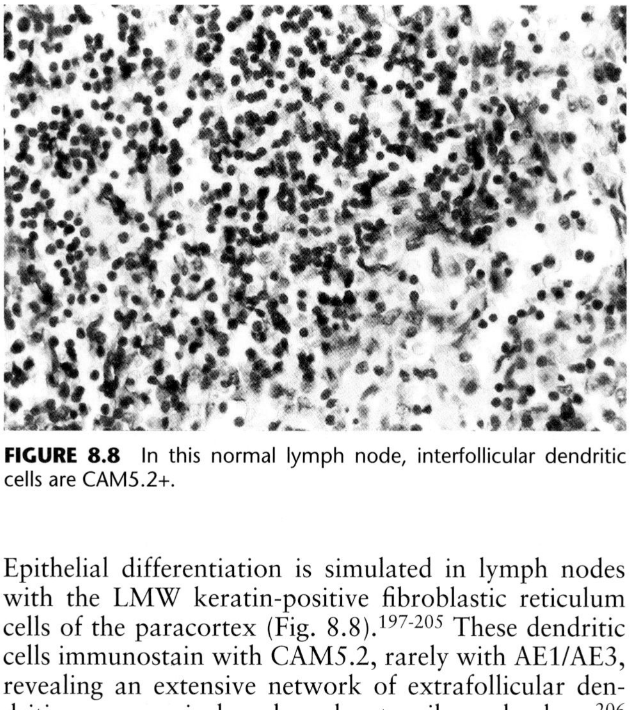

FIGURE 8.8 In this normal lymph node, interfollicular dendritic cells are CAM5.2+.

Epithelial differentiation is simulated in lymph nodes with the LMW keratin-positive fibroblastic reticulum cells of the paracortex (Fig. 8.8).[197-205] These dendritic cells immunostain with CAM5.2, rarely with AE1/AE3, revealing an extensive network of extrafollicular dendritic processes in lymph nodes, tonsils, and spleen.[206] These keratin-positive cells are a pitfall for the diagnosis of metastatic carcinoma because the conventional wisdom had been that keratin-positive cells in a lymph node equated with metastatic carcinoma. The pitfall is twofold. When searching for keratin-positive micrometastases in patients with breast carcinoma, one must distinguish the dendritic processes from carcinoma cells that cluster in the subcapsular sinus. Also, needle aspirates and touch imprints of lymph nodes may contain keratin-positive cells without containing metastatic carcinoma; one must be aware of the morphologic features of the keratin-positive cells.

Keratin positivity has been described in plasma cells, plasmacytoma, and anaplastic large cell lymphoma.[206-211] For anaplastic large cell lymphoma, keratins may be detected in up to 30% of cases and, along with some EMA-positive anaplastic lymphoma cells, the definitive diagnosis can be confusing. However, adherence to a broad-spectrum antibody for keratin immunoreactivity will show only focal rare staining at most in these lymphomas. Plasmacytomas likewise should be studied with broad-coverage antibodies in a panel that includes antibodies to CD138 and kappa/lambda light chains.

The majority of keratin immunostaining is performed on FFPE tissues. The duration of formalin fixation is a key factor when trying to optimize the technical performance of keratin immunoperoxidase stains. The fixation time is closely related to the time required for enzymatic predigestion.[212] Generally, tissue fixed in 10% formalin for more than 2 days requires greater antigen retrieval, with less time required for tissues fixed briefly (hours) in 10% formalin. Most, if not all, keratin antibodies require epitope retrieval (depending on antibody and fixation duration) for optimal keratin antibody performance.

KEY DIAGNOSTIC POINTS

Keratin in Nonepithelial Tumors

- Focal presence in many sarcomas (see text)
- Focal rare presence in melanoma mainly with CAM5.2
- Plasma cells common; other lymphoid neoplasms rare
- Common in dendritic cells of lymph nodes mainly with CAM5.2
- Antibody AE1/AE3 may give spurious positive keratin result in astrocytic neoplasms

Step 3: Carcinoma Subsets with Frequent Vimentin Coexpression

Mesenchymal and endothelial cells regularly immunostain with vimentin, and this immunostaining generally provides a measure of internal quality control for immunoreactivity.[213] If there is no immunostaining of blood vessels or stromal cells by vimentin, it denotes significant damage to tissue antigens or other failure of the staining procedure.

Carcinomas in effusion specimens are universally positive for vimentin (presumably an *in vivo* fluid effect) and thus have no diagnostic utility.[214]

Initially thought to be an intermediate filament restricted to mesenchymal cells, vimentin has been found in a diverse number of neoplasms including a variety of carcinomas (Table 8.8). Vimentin stains virtually all spindle cell neoplasms—mesenchymal spindle cell neoplasms and sarcomatoid carcinomas included. However, vimentin stains a subset of carcinomas regularly and to a significant degree, and this may be useful in the context of a panel of antibodies to narrow a differential diagnosis. The cellular vimentin immunostaining pattern is often a perinuclear band of reactivity, particularly for endometrioid adenocarcinomas. Carcinomas with frequent (>50% to 60%) and strong (>25% of cells) vimentin coexpression include spindle cell carcinomas, renal cell carcinomas (except the chromophobe variant), endometrial endometrioid adenocarcinomas and malignant mixed müllerian tumors, serous ovarian carcinomas, pleomorphic salivary gland tumors, "basal-like" breast carcinomas, and follicular thyroid carcinomas.[215-217] Epithelial and sarcomatoid mesotheliomas also regularly demonstrate vimentin. Certain carcinomas may immunostain with vimentin but with lesser frequency (10% to 20%) and with far less intensity (<10% of cells). This group includes adenocarcinomas of colorectum, lung, breast, and prostate and nonserous ovarian carcinomas.

TABLE 8.8 Major Patterns of Coexpression of Cytokeratin/Vimentin in Carcinomas

Coexpression Common (>50%)	Coexpression Uncommon (<10%)
Endometrial adenocarcinoma	Endocervical adenocarcinoma
Renal cell carcinoma	Colorectal adenocarcinoma
Salivary gland carcinoma	Breast ductal-lobular carcinoma
Spindle cell carcinoma	Lung non–small cell carcinoma
Thyroid follicular carcinoma	Prostate adenocarcinoma

Therefore the finding of substantial coexpression of vimentin in a metastatic carcinoma may aid in narrowing the differential diagnosis and adds value to the rest of the antibody panel (Fig. 8.9).

Vimentin coexpression is especially useful in differentiating endometrial endometrioid carcinomas in uterine curettage specimens from endocervical adenocarcinomas including the endometrioid variant of endocervical adenocarcinoma. Endometrial endometrioid carcinomas immunostain strongly for vimentin, but endocervical carcinomas rarely stain (weak focal staining in up to 13% of endocervical carcinomas).[218,219] However, with the current antigen retrieval techniques, moderate to occasionally strong vimentin expression may be seen in endocervical carcinomas, and a panel approach is more useful in this distinction.[220]

KEY DIAGNOSTIC POINTS

Vimentin Coexpression in Carcinomas

- Common in renal, endometrial, ovarian serous, salivary gland, follicular thyroid, and sarcomatoid (spindle cell) carcinomas, "basal-like" breast carcinomas, as well as in the epithelial and stromal components of malignant mixed müllerian tumors
- May be seen in few cells in 10% to 20% of colorectal, lung, breast, prostate, and nonserous ovarian adenocarcinomas
- Not diagnostically useful in body cavity effusion specimens
- Epithelial and sarcomatoid mesotheliomas are usually vimentin positive
- Important internal quality measure for antigen assessment in any tissue

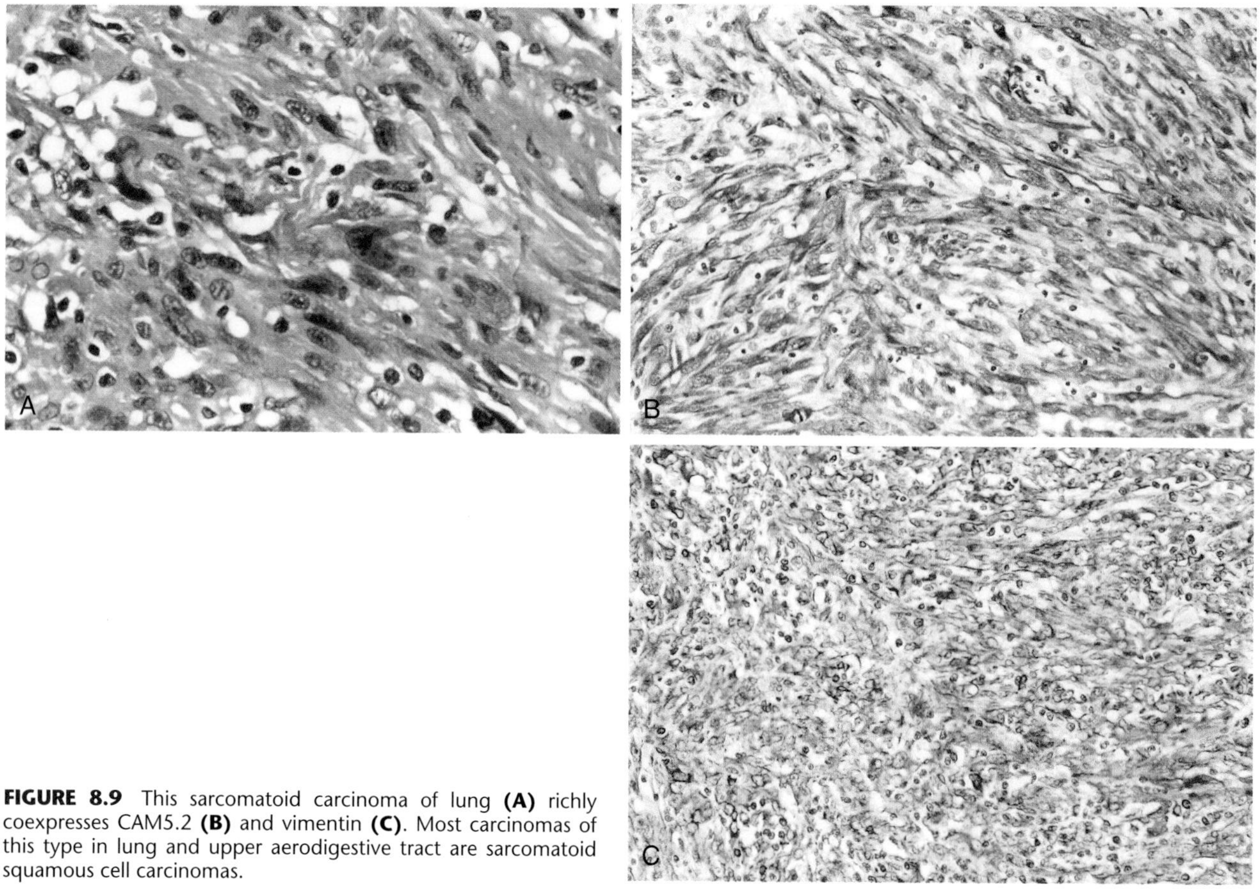

FIGURE 8.9 This sarcomatoid carcinoma of lung **(A)** richly coexpresses CAM5.2 **(B)** and vimentin **(C)**. Most carcinomas of this type in lung and upper aerodigestive tract are sarcomatoid squamous cell carcinomas.

Step 4: Supplemental Epithelial Markers

Although not specific for tissue lineage, these epithelial markers demonstrate characteristic immunostaining patterns for certain tissue types and therefore are useful in corroborating a diagnosis when used as part of a panel of antibodies.

CARCINOEMBRYONIC ANTIGEN

CEA is a 180-kD glycoprotein that is 50% carbohydrate. Many CEA antibodies are available to a variety of CEA epitopes. The polyclonal antibodies commonly cross-react with tissue-nonspecific cross-reacting antigen and biliary glycoprotein I.[221-223] Although CEA is a sensitive marker, adenocarcinomas of colorectal origin cannot be distinguished from lung adenocarcinomas or ductal carcinomas of the breast because of the low specificity of CEA.

Primary adenocarcinomas of the lung are typically CK7+, CK20−, and CEA+, whereas colorectal carcinomas are CK7−, CK20+, and CEA+; ductal and lobular breast carcinomas are CK7+, CK20−, and often CEA+; and ovarian carcinomas are CK7+, CK20±, and CEA−.[121,125-129,224-227] Neoplasms that typically are strongly positive for most CEA antibodies include adenocarcinomas of the lung, colon, stomach, biliary tree, pancreas, urinary bladder, endocervix, paranasal sinuses, sweat glands, and breast (Table 8.9).[228] The usefulness of CEA when used with keratins is to corroborate expected staining for CEA, whether positive or negative.

TABLE 8.9 Carcinoembryonic Antigen Immunostaining of Adenocarcinoma

Carcinoembryonic Antigen (+)	Carcinoembryonic Antigen (−)
Paranasal sinuses	Prostate
Lung	Kidney
Colon	Adrenal
Stomach	Endometrium
Biliary	Serous ovarian
Pancreas	
Sweat glands	
Breast	

Neoplasms that are essentially negative with most CEA antibodies include adenocarcinomas of prostate, kidney, adrenal gland, and endometrium,[220] along with serous ovarian tumors and mesotheliomas. Liver cell-derived tumors are nonreactive with the monoclonal CEA antibodies but do react with the polyclonal antibodies

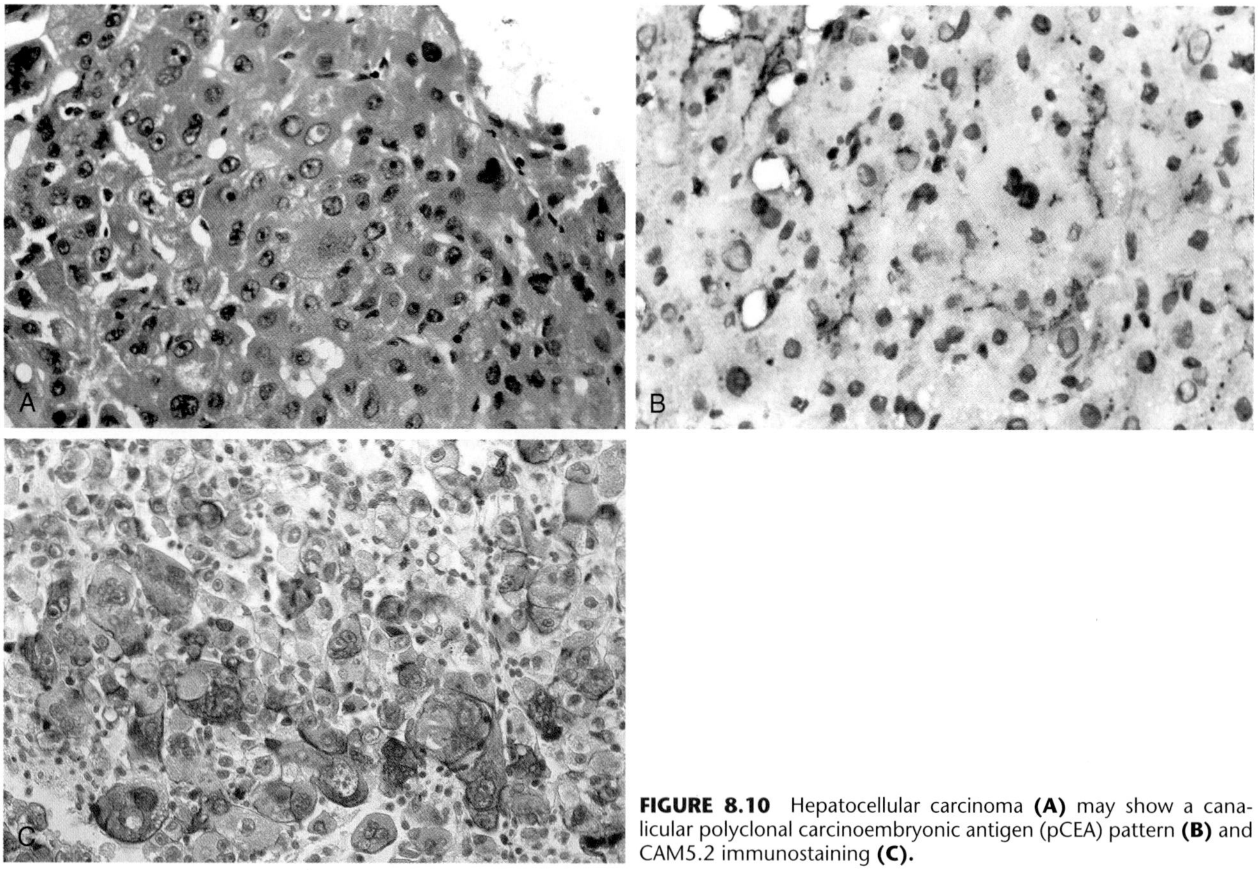

FIGURE 8.10 Hepatocellular carcinoma **(A)** may show a canalicular polyclonal carcinoembryonic antigen (pCEA) pattern **(B)** and CAM5.2 immunostaining **(C)**.

in a distinct pattern of pericanalicular staining (Fig. 8.10) because the polyclonal antibodies cross-react with the hepatic bile canalicular biliary glycoprotein-1.[229,230] Adenocarcinomas of pulmonary, gastrointestinal, thymic, endocervical, and pancreaticobiliary origin typically show strong, although variable, cytoplasmic immunostaining for CEA antibodies.

KEY DIAGNOSTIC POINTS

Carcinoembryonic Antigen

- CEA+ tumor (pericanalicular pattern): hepatocellular carcinoma
- Other CEA+ tumors: gastrointestinal, lung, breast, thymus, endocervical, primary cholangiocarcinoma
- CEA– tumors: prostate, renal, endometrial, adrenal, and serous ovarian tumors and mesothelioma
- Epithelioid hemangioendothelioma of liver (mimicker of hepatocellular carcinoma): CEA negative but positive for vascular markers

Immunostaining patterns of CEA in the liver are particularly useful. The epithelioid hemangioendothelioma (EH) of liver can mimic carcinoma to perfection. Demonstration of positive CD31/CD34 and factor VIII with variable (usually focal, sometimes diffuse) keratin and lack of CEA will separate this entity from hepatocellular carcinoma.[231] However, it is important to remember that unlike normal liver, neoplastic liver sinusoids demonstrate the presence of immunoreactive CD34. This may be confused with EH but is useful in the differential diagnosis of primary liver neoplasm versus metastatic carcinoma and non-neoplastic liver, especially on small biopsy samples (Fig. 8.11).[232]

EPITHELIAL MEMBRANE ANTIGEN

Encoded by the MUC1 gene on chromosome 1 and a derivative human antigen, EMA is a transmembrane glycoprotein of the breast mucin complex, and its expression is increased in carcinomas.[233,234] Unlike normal breast, in which EMA is present on the apical cell membrane, neoplasms demonstrate EMA on the entire circumference of the cell membrane.[234] Increased amounts of the large glycoprotein interfere with cell-to-cell and cell-to-matrix adhesion in neoplastic cells.[235]

The utility of EMA antibody is in the detection of epithelial differentiation, as a supplement to the cytokeratins. Spindle cell, small cell, and large cell neoplasms may on rare occasion be stained with EMA but may be only focally positive for cytokeratins.[236,237]

Several EMA antibodies, each of which reacts to different epitopes of the large glycoprotein antigen, are available, including MAM-6, episialin, polymorphic epithelial mucin, CA15-3, DF3 antigen, and breast epithelial mucin.[238-244] The EMA antibodies stain skin

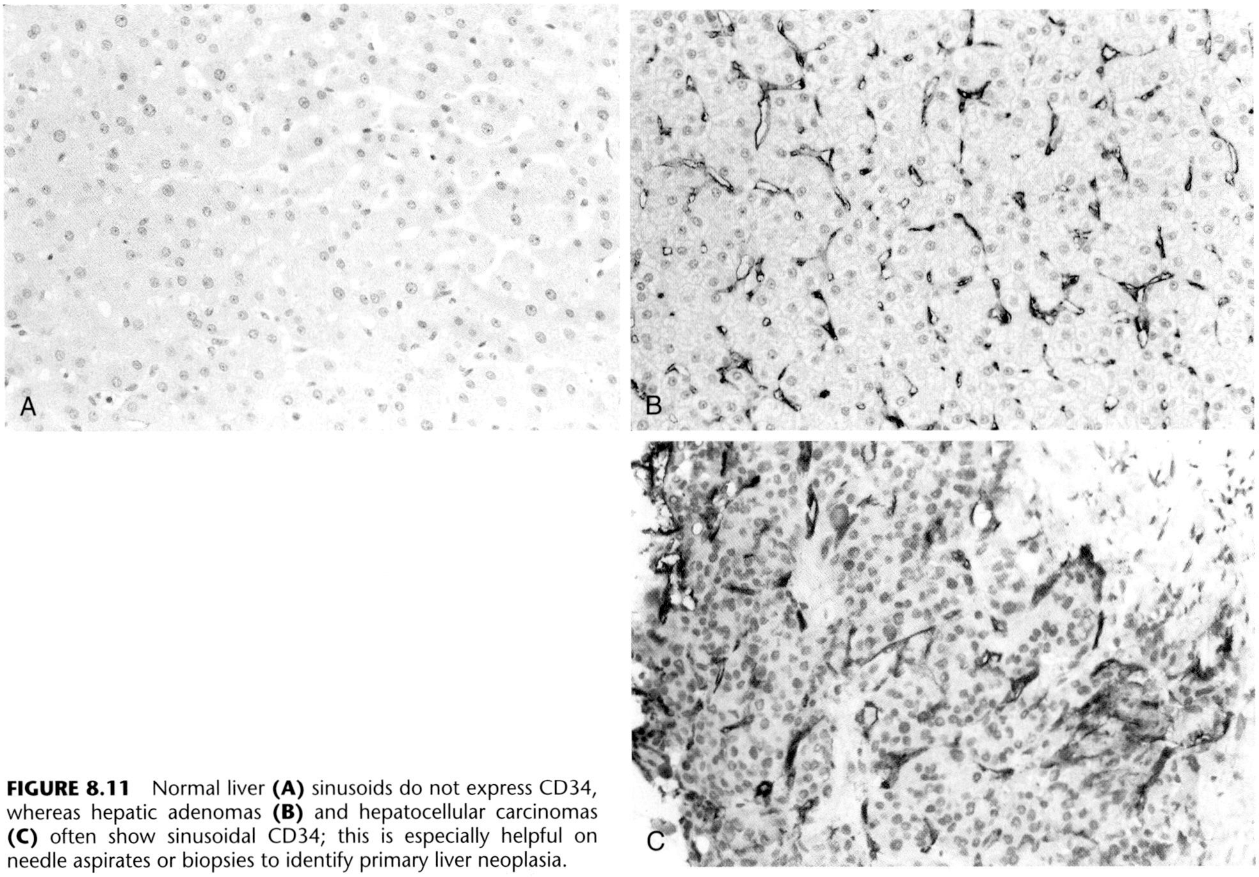

FIGURE 8.11 Normal liver **(A)** sinusoids do not express CD34, whereas hepatic adenomas **(B)** and hepatocellular carcinomas **(C)** often show sinusoidal CD34; this is especially helpful on needle aspirates or biopsies to identify primary liver neoplasia.

and adnexa, breast, lung, bile ducts, pancreas, salivary gland, urothelium, endometrium and endocervix, prostate ducts, thyroid, mesothelium, and neoplasms of these tissues (Table 8.10). Many sarcomatoid carcinomas and epithelial and sarcomatoid mesotheliomas are positive. Reactive mesothelium may stain weakly compared with thick membranous staining of mesothelioma.[245,246] Many types of adenocarcinomas immunostain with EMA and must be distinguished from mesothelial cells in effusions by using a panel of immunostains that includes CK5/CK6, CEA, LeuM1, and BER-EP4.[59,154,247]

Subsets of normal and neoplastic hematopoietic cells express EMA, including plasma cells and erythroblasts and neoplastic cells as well as the lymphocytic and histiocytic (L&H) cells (60% of cases) of lymphocyte-predominant Hodgkin lymphoma, 5% of B-cell lymphomas, 18% of T-cell lymphomas, and about 60% of anaplastic large cell lymphomas.[208,248-257] The EMA antibodies do not have absolute sensitivity and specificity for carcinomas and therefore should always be used with a panel of cytokeratins and other corroborating antibodies such as leukocyte common antigen.[258]

In addition to epithelial neoplasms, a number of sarcomas, CNS tumors, small round cell tumors, and a few germ cell tumors may be positive with EMA. These tumors include malignant nerve sheath tumors, synovial sarcoma, leiomyosarcoma, malignant fibrous histiocytoma, epithelioid sarcoma, and chordoma. With the exception of the last two tumors mentioned, EMA immunostaining is focal.

TABLE 8.10 Epithelial Membrane Antigen in Carcinomas and Nonepithelial Tissues

Typically Positive	**Carcinomas:** Skin and adnexa, breast, bile ducts, lung, pancreas, salivary gland, urothelium, endometrium, endocervix, prostate, thyroid
	Noncarcinomatous lesions: Meningioma, mesotheliomas
Focal/Patchy Positive	**Carcinomas:** Sarcomatoid carcinomas
	Noncarcinomatous lesions: Plasma cell tumors, L&H cells of Hodgkin lymphoma, few cells of non-Hodgkin lymphoma, anaplastic large cell lymphoma, malignant peripheral nerve sheath tumors, synovial sarcoma, leiomyosarcoma
Mostly Negative	Germ cell tumors except choriocarcinoma, ovarian sex cord stromal tumors

Choroid plexus neoplasms and meningiomas show strong membranous EMA immunostaining. Germ cell tumors are largely negative[259] except for variable EMA immunostaining in choriocarcinoma and teratoma, whereas the epithelial small round cell tumors of nephroblastoma and hepatoblastoma immunostain with EMA in the majority of cases.

KEY DIAGNOSTIC POINTS

Epithelial Membrane Antigen (EMA)

- Used as a supplement to detect epithelial neoplasms because CKs may rarely be focally positive or negative in undifferentiated carcinomas
- EMA immunostaining may be membranous or cytoplasmic, or both
- Negative in malignant melanoma
- Negative in germ cell neoplasms except choriocarcinoma and teratoma
- EMA stains plasma cells, 60% of anaplastic large cell lymphomas, L&H cells of Hodgkin lymphoma and a few T- and B-cell lymphomas
- Strongly positive in malignant mesothelioma and some reactive mesothelial proliferations, and weak or negative immunostaining for normal mesothelial cells

BER-EP4, BG8, AND MOC-31

These are markers of epithelial differentiation. These stains are most often used to distinguish adenocarcinomas from mesothelial proliferations (Fig. 8.12).[260-262] BER-EP4 and MOC-31 antibodies are directed against the epitope on glycoproteins present on the surface of glandular epithelial cells of endodermal derivation. Squamous epithelium of ectodermal derivation virtually never expresses BER-EP4.[263] The characteristic staining with BER-EP4 and MOC-31 is membranous. Bg8 antibody is directed against the Lewis Y antigen and shows cytoplasmic staining in carcinomas. When BER-EP4, Bg8, and MOC-31 are combined with calretinin (nuclear and cytoplasmic staining in mesotheliomas), the combination provides the best sensitivity and specificity for distinguishing adenocarcinoma from mesothelioma.[264] MOC-31 is also useful in distinguishing metastatic tumors from primary hepatocellular carcinoma when used in a panel format. Along with HepPar-1 and pCEA, MOC-31 permits distinction of metastatic carcinomas in liver from hepatocellular carcinoma 99% of the time.[265-267]

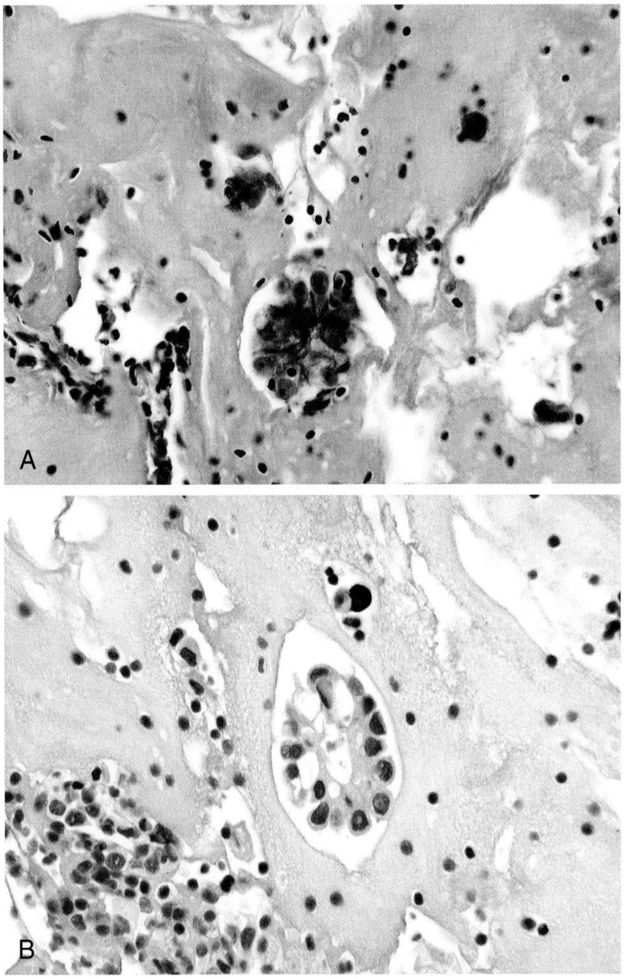

FIGURE 8.12 This ovarian carcinoma in a pelvic wash is positive for BER-EP4 **(A)** and negative for calretinin **(B)**.

KEY DIAGNOSTIC POINTS

BER-EP4, Bg8, MOC-31

- Best epithelial markers to distinguish adenocarcinomas from mesothelioma.
- Membranous reactivity is seen for BER-EP4 and MOC-31 and cytoplasmic reactivity for Bg8.
- Squamous cell carcinomas almost never express BER-EP4.
- MOC-31 is especially useful in distinguishing between primary liver carcinoma versus metastatic tumor.

Step 5: Focusing on Tumor Differentiation: Cell-Specific Products

Even though the tissue of origin of most metastases can be ascertained with the panel approach of CKs, CEA, EMA, and vimentin, there remains a subset of neoplasms that do not readily lend themselves to definitive identification. The use of additional antibodies to cell-specific products in most instances has a high specificity for certain tissues, enabling the pathologist to "fine focus" the search for the origin of a metastasis.

The antibodies discussed here include neuroendocrine markers, thyroglobulin, TTF-1, calretinin, WT1, GCDFP-15, mammaglobin, hormone receptors, villin, CDX2, Hep Par1, DPC4, prostate carcinoma antigens, uroplakin III, thrombomodulin, RCC, CD10, PAX2, melan-A, inhibin, adrenal binding protein, germ cell tumor markers, and CD5.

NEUROENDOCRINE ANTIBODIES

Antibodies to neuroendocrine cell components are usually used in the context of trying to distinguish tumor cell types in specific organs such as lung, thyroid, colon, and adrenal gland. The antibodies are not typically used in the initial screening panel of the workup of an undifferentiated tumor, and there is little literature that deals with this topic.[268] It is critically important to use the following antibody immunostains together as a panel because no single antibody has perfect specificity and sensitivity.

It is well known that a few "neuroendocrine cells" can be seen with IHC in a wide variety of carcinomas. This is not to be equated with a diagnosis of neuroendocrine carcinoma. Only after a complete account of the clinical findings, imaging studies, histologic studies, and immunohistochemical findings should a diagnosis be rendered.

Chromogranins

The chromogranins (types A, B, and C) are a group of monomeric proteins that compose the major portion of the soluble protein extract of the neurosecretory granules of neuroendocrine cells; chromogranin A, with a molecular weight of 75 kD, is the most abundantly distributed. There is a strong correlation between the chromogranin cellular immunostaining quantity and the number of neuroendocrine-type secretory granules seen at the level of electron microscopy.[269]

The LK2H10 clone is a monoclonal antibody with abundant representation in the literature.[269-272] Immunostaining intensity decreases with poor differentiation. The specificity of LK2H10 is close to 100%, but sensitivity is closer to 75%.

Synaptophysin

Synaptophysin is a glycoprotein that is an integral part of the neuroendocrine secretory granule membrane[268,273] and is recognized by monoclonal antibody (SY38) in a variety of neuroendocrine tumors. Synaptophysin is a broad-spectrum neuroendocrine marker,[274] with higher sensitivity but lower specificity than antibody to chromogranin. Immunostaining for SY38 has also been documented to be most effective in identifying metastases of neuroendocrine type.[268] Synaptophysin immunostaining alone is insufficient grounds for labeling a neoplasm "neuroendocrine." When used in the context of appropriate morphology, synaptophysin is useful to identify neuroendocrine features.

Large cell undifferentiated neuroendocrine carcinoma (LCNEC) can present as CUPS, and it is easy to miss the diagnosis without applying the appropriate neuroendocrine markers. The correct diagnosis of LCNEC is an important distinction because it carries the same dismal prognosis as does small cell carcinoma, whether in the lung or gastrointestinal tract.[275,276] Synaptophysin may be the most frequent positive marker in LCNEC.[275]

In one study, small cell lung carcinomas were stained by synaptophysin in up to 79% of cases, whereas chromogranin was positive in 47% to 60% of cases, bombesin was positive in 45% of cases, and NSE was seen in 33% to 60% of cases.[277] Synaptophysin may be seen in 8% of non–small cell carcinomas.[278]

Leu 7

The CD57 antigen of a human T-cell line generated a monoclonal antibody (HNK-1). The differentiation antigen of the T-cell line is indicative of a natural killer cell activity.[279] The CD57 antibody also recognizes antigen of myelin-associated glycoprotein in the myelin of the central and peripheral nervous systems. CD57 reactivity has also been found in enterochromaffin cells, pancreatic islet cells, islet cell tumors, carcinoid tumors, pheochromocytomas, and small cell carcinoma of the lung.[280-283] CD57 lacks the high sensitivity and specificity of chromogranin and synaptophysin and therefore should be used as part of a panel that includes these antibodies.

Neuron-Specific Enolase

The enolase enzymes comprise five different forms, each of which is composed of three homodimers and two hybrids. Neuron-specific enolase (NSE) is found in a variety of normal and neoplastic neuroendocrine cells and predominates in the brain.[284-287] Originally believed to be a specific marker for neuroendocrine differentiation, it has subsequently been observed that NSE can be found in virtually any type of neoplasm. Because of this, it is a poor antibody to use to screen for neuroendocrine differentiation. Overall a poor marker for detection of neuroendocrine differentiation because of its lack of specificity, NSE may be useful in combination with other more specific antibodies such as chromogranin and synaptophysin for the appropriate neuroendocrine morphologic identification and documentation of immunostaining.

Peptide Hormones

Peptide hormones are present in unique, sequestered tissues in the normal state and generally recapitulate the same hormone production in neoplasms. Endocrine neoplasms, with few exceptions, show a characteristic histologic pattern, and therefore the study of hormone production is often of academic interest only.

Poorly differentiated endocrine neoplasms, depending on the site of origin, may produce characteristic peptide hormones. The group of poorly differentiated neuroendocrine tumors and their hormone production include islet cell tumors (insulin, glucagon, somatostatin, gastrin), pulmonary small cell carcinoma (bombesin in 45% of cases),[277] and medullary thyroid carcinoma (calcitonin).

Cytokeratin Profile of Neuroendocrine Carcinoma

The CK profile of neuroendocrine carcinomas is somewhat distinctive in that virtually all are positive to some degree for cytokeratins 8 and 18 (e.g., CAM5.2), sometimes positive for CK7, and negative with CK20 and HMW keratin (e.g., K903). Merkel cell carcinomas are characteristically positive for cytokeratin 20 (67% of cases)[288] and negative for cytokeratin 7, which is the reverse for immunostaining of small cell carcinomas of lung (CK7+, CK20-).

KEY DIAGNOSTIC POINTS

Neuroendocrine Differentiation

- Typical neuroendocrine keratin profile is CAM5.2+ and CK7+.
- Chromogranin and synaptophysin complement each other as part of a diagnostic panel.
- Specific peptide (bombesin, glucagon, etc.) may supplement the preceding studies.
- Subsets of peripheral neuroendocrine carcinomas may be TTF-1+ (see text).
- Subsets of neuroendocrine carcinomas of gastrointestinal tract may be CDX-2+ (see text).

THYROGLOBULIN

Thyroglobulin, a 670-kD heavily glycosylated protein, provides iodination sites for the production of thyroid hormones and is unique to the thyroid follicular epithelium. The great majority of thyroid carcinomas show immunostaining with thyroglobulin, although most of the positive cases are readily interpreted as follicular or papillary carcinomas. The undifferentiated anaplastic carcinomas are generally negative for thyroglobulin. Thyroid carcinomas are almost always negative with monoclonal CEA antibody, which is a helpful feature in differential diagnosis. Thyroglobulin may be seen as scattered positive cells in medullary carcinoma and, conversely, calcitonin-positive cells may be seen in poorly differentiated follicular carcinomas.[289-291] Thyroglobulin may be seen in 10% to 25% of cases of leukemic blast cells in bone marrow.[292]

KEY DIAGNOSTIC POINTS

Thyroglobulin

- Positive in almost all thyroid carcinomas, with reduced immunostaining of poorly differentiated carcinoma to complete absence in anaplastic types
- Highly specific for thyroid carcinomas, with rare positivity in some leukemic blast cells

THYROID TRANSCRIPTION FACTOR-1

Thyroid transcription factor-1 (TTF-1), a nuclear tissue-specific protein transcription factor, is found in thyroid and thyroid tumors regardless of histologic type (except anaplastic type), as well as in lung carcinomas including adenocarcinomas (75%), non–small cell carcinomas (63%), neuroendocrine and small cell carcinomas (>90%), and squamous cell carcinomas (10%).[293-298] Selectively expressed during embryogenesis in the thyroid, the diencephalon of the brain, and in respiratory epithelium, TTF-1 binds to and activates factors for surfactant protein derived from Clara cells.[299] TTF-1 is rarely seen in carcinomas outside of the lung or thyroid (Fig. 8.13).[300-302] Neuroendocrine tumors of the lung including typical and atypical carcinoids and large cell neuroendocrine carcinomas are almost always positive with TTF-1, demonstrating a kinship with small cell carcinomas.[300] Small cell and large cell neuroendocrine carcinomas from origins other than the lung are also frequently TTF-1 positive.[303] These sites include prostate, bladder, cervix, GI tract, thyroid, and breast.[303,304] However, Merkel cell carcinomas are TTF-1 negative.[303,305]

The utility of TTF-1 becomes readily apparent in the differential diagnosis of primary versus metastatic carcinomas, especially in the lung or in effusions.[306,307] CK7 and CK20, along with TTF-1 and CEA, are the antibodies that best discriminate primary lung carcinoma from carcinomas metastatic to the lung. In a study by Roh, the sensitivity of TTF-1 for metastatic lung carcinoma in lymph nodes was 69%.[308]

The specificity of TTF-1 for pulmonary lesions was confirmed by Chang and colleagues.[309] TTF-1 demonstrates cytoplasmic immunostaining of hepatocellular carcinomas in 71% of cases, but no nuclear immunostaining.[310]

Some recent reports have challenged the specificity of TTF-1. Kubba and colleagues[311] and Siami and colleagues[312] (both from M.D. Anderson Cancer Center) have shown TTF-1 (clone 8G7G3/1) reactivity in tumors of the endocervix, endometrium, and ovary; however, the majority of the cases in their study showed only rare and focal staining.

KEY DIAGNOSTIC POINTS

Thyroid Transcription Factor-1

- Nuclear immunostaining in all carcinomas of thyroid origin (except anaplastic type)
- Nuclear immunostaining of the vast majority of carcinomas of the lung—adenocarcinomas (66%), large cell neuroendocrine and small cell (95%)
- Small cell carcinomas of other sites (gastrointestinal tract, bladder, cervix, prostate) frequently TTF-1+, although they are rare
- Merkel cell carcinomas negative for TTF-1
- Recent reports of focal TTF-1 expression in gynecologic tract tumors

CALRETININ AND WILMS' TUMOR PROTEIN-1

Calretinin and Wilms' tumor (WT1) protein are two positive mesothelial markers. Calretinin is a 29-kD intracellular calcium-binding protein that has been described in a variety of cells including neurons, steroid-producing cells, renal convoluted tubules, eccrine glands, thymic keratinized cells, and mesothelial cells.[313,314] There has been a difference in immunostaining results depending on the antibody used, with the greater specificity seen with the Zymed clone.[315] Calretinin may be expressed in 8% of lung adenocarcinomas, but the expression is

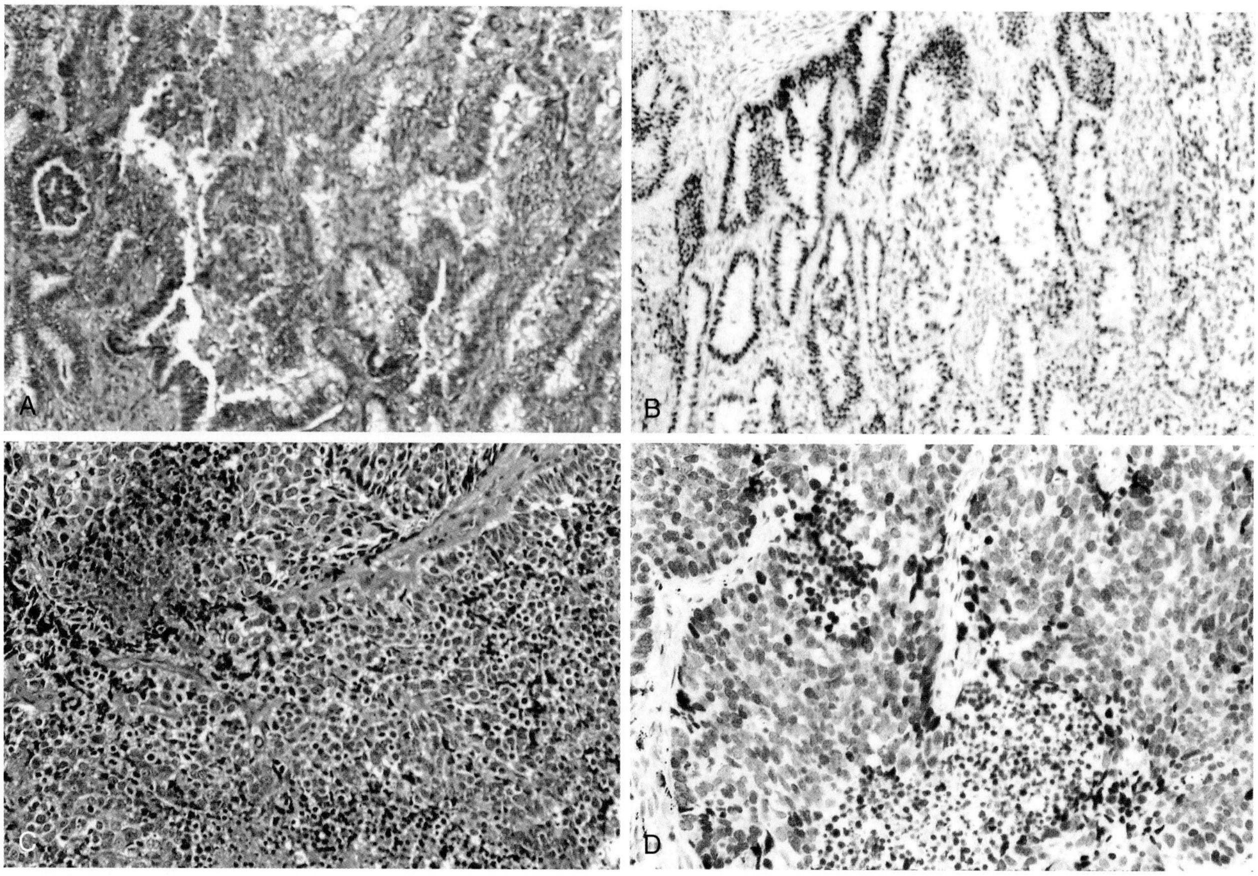

FIGURE 8.13 Thyroid transcription factor 1 (TTF-1) antibody identifies 60% to 70% of pulmonary adenocarcinomas **(A, B)** and 95% of pulmonary small cell carcinomas **(C, D).**

generally focal and weak.[316] Focal weak expression may also be seen in carcinoma from other sites.

Wilms' tumor (WT1) protein is expressed at high levels in kidney glomeruli, gonadal ridge of developing gonads, Sertoli cells of the testis, and both epithelial and granulosa cells of the ovary, suggesting a developmental role in both the genital system and kidney.[317] WT1 nuclear expression is seen in normal mesothelium and mesothelioma, Wilms' tumor (hence its name), desmoplastic small round cell tumor (with antibody to the carboxy-terminal end), and most notably in müllerian epithelial neoplasms (especially ovarian serous carcinoma; Fig. 8.14).[318,319] The literature regarding endometrial serous carcinoma is contradictory, but it appears that strong nuclear expression may be seen in approximately 20% of endometrial serous carcinomas.[320-325] WT1 expression is not seen in endometrioid-type tumors. Recently, Domfeh and colleagues[326] have shown weak to moderate WT1 expression in 64% of pure mucinous carcinomas of the breast and in 29% of breast mucinous carcinomas mixed with other subtypes.

KEY DIAGNOSTIC POINTS

Calretinin and WT1

- Calretinin and WT1 are two most sensitive mesothelial markers with high specificity.
- Calretinin may be expressed in up to 8% of adenocarcinomas from various sites.
- Ovarian serous carcinomas demonstrate diffuse strong WT1 nuclear expression.
- The majority of endometrial serous carcinomas are negative for WT1; positive cases generally show patchy staining.
- Pure and mixed mucinous breast carcinomas may be WT1+; however, staining is rarely intense compared with serous ovarian carcinomas.

GROSS CYSTIC DISEASE FLUID PROTEIN AND MAMMAGLOBIN

Originally described by Pearlman and colleagues[327] and Haagensen and associates,[328] the prolactin-inducing protein identified by Murphy and coworkers[329] has the same amino acid sequence as GCDFP-15 and is found in abundance in breast cystic fluid and any cell type that has apocrine features.[330,331] The latter, in addition to breast, includes acinar structures in salivary glands, apocrine glands, sweat glands, and Paget disease of skin, vulva, and prostate.[332-336] Aside from these immunoreactivities, most other carcinomas show no appreciable immunostaining.

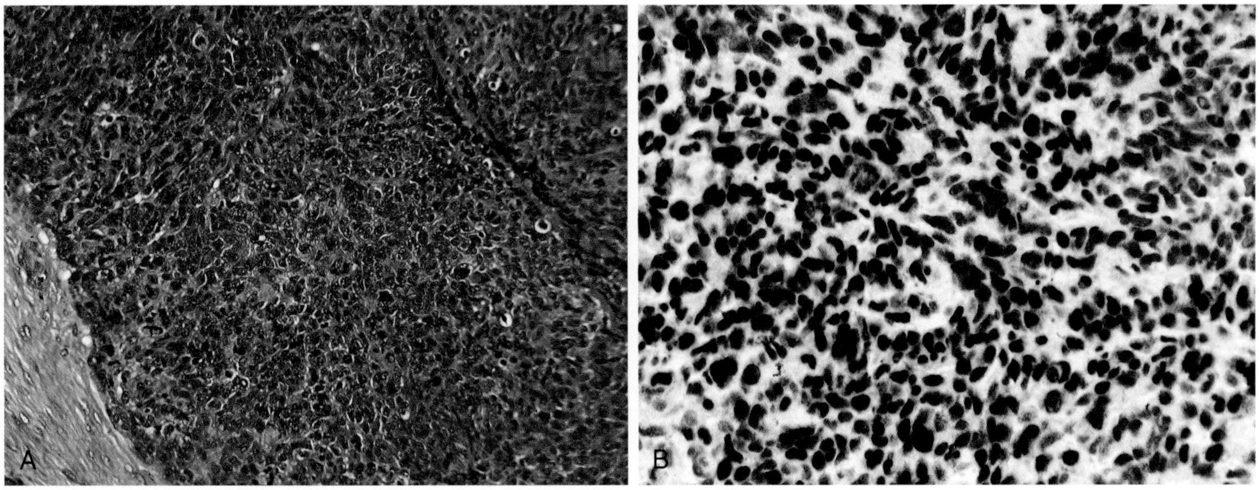

FIGURE 8.14 Solid carcinoma of unknown origin **(A)** invading the bowel wall in an elderly female. WT-1 positivity **(B)** confirms ovarian origin (also positive for CK7 and BER-EP4; not shown).

The positive predictive value and specificity of GCDFP-15 are both reported to be 99%.[336] The sensitivity for the monoclonal antibody clone D6 (Cambridge Research Laboratories, Cambridge, Mass) has been reported to be as high as 74%,[336] but the experience of others has been closer to 40% to 50%[333] and even lower.[337] Similar results are obtained with the use of antibody BRST-2 (Signet Laboratories, Inc., Dedham, Mass).

Because the specificity of GCDFP antibodies for breast carcinoma is so high, it is often used in a screening panel in the appropriate clinical situation, which often turns out to be the presentation of a woman with CUPS or a new lung mass in a patient with a history of breast cancer. Others have demonstrated the utility and specificity of GCDFP-15 antibodies in the distinction of breast carcinoma metastatic in the lung.[338,339]

Recently, the absolute specificity of GCDFP-15 has also been challenged. Striebel and colleagues[340] reported GCDFP-15 immunoreactivity in 5.2% (11/211) of pulmonary adenocarcinomas. These tumors were characteristically of mixed acinar and papillary types with abundant extracellular mucin production. However, 81% percent of these tumors co-expressed TTF-1, which would be helpful in their distinction from breast carcinomas.

The mammaglobin gene encodes a 93 amino acid protein that is largely confined to breast tissue. Han and colleagues[341] developed antibodies to mammaglobin and found high sensitivity (84.3%) and specificity (85%) for the discrimination of breast carcinoma in lymph nodes. In contrast, the sensitivity and specificity for GCDFP-15 (BRST-2) expression in their study was 44.3% and 97.9%. Among non–breast carcinomas, convincing mammaglobin expression is seen in endometrioid carcinomas (~40% cases) and sweat and salivary gland tumors.[337,341-343] This nonspecificity of mammaglobin expression in endometrioid adenocarcinomas could be used diagnostically.[344] Caution is advised in interpreting weak/equivocal immunoreactivity with mammaglobin because this pattern of staining can be seen in several nonbreast, nonendometrial carcinomas. With respect to breast carcinoma, mammaglobin is a more sensitive marker than GCDFP-15 (Fig. 8.15).[337]

KEY DIAGNOSTIC POINTS

GCDFP-15 and Mammaglobin

- GCDFP-15 has greater than 90% specificity but much lower sensitivity for breast carcinoma.
- Mammaglobin has high sensitivity (~60%) for breast carcinoma, but the specificity is lower.
- Both GCDFP-15 and mammaglobin should be included in the panel for diagnosing breast carcinoma (GCDFP-15+, mammaglobin+, CK7+/CK20 negative, ER/PR+, CEA+).
- Mammaglobin expression in endometrioid carcinomas could be useful diagnostically.

HORMONE RECEPTORS (ESTROGEN AND PROGESTERONE)

Intuitively, it would seem as though the estrogen receptor/progesterone receptor (ER/PR) would be confined to hormone-responsive tissues such as breast, but even the recent literature on this topic is controversial. Although some authors conclude that ER/PR is found only in subsets of breast carcinomas and carcinomas of the ovary and endometrium,[339] others have observed mostly ER, and rarely PR, in carcinomas of the lung,[345-348] stomach, and thyroid.

Vargas and colleagues[349] demonstrated the estrogen-related protein p29 in 98% of non–small cell lung cancers by IHC, suggesting that the estrogen axis may be important in this group of malignancies. In the study by Vargas

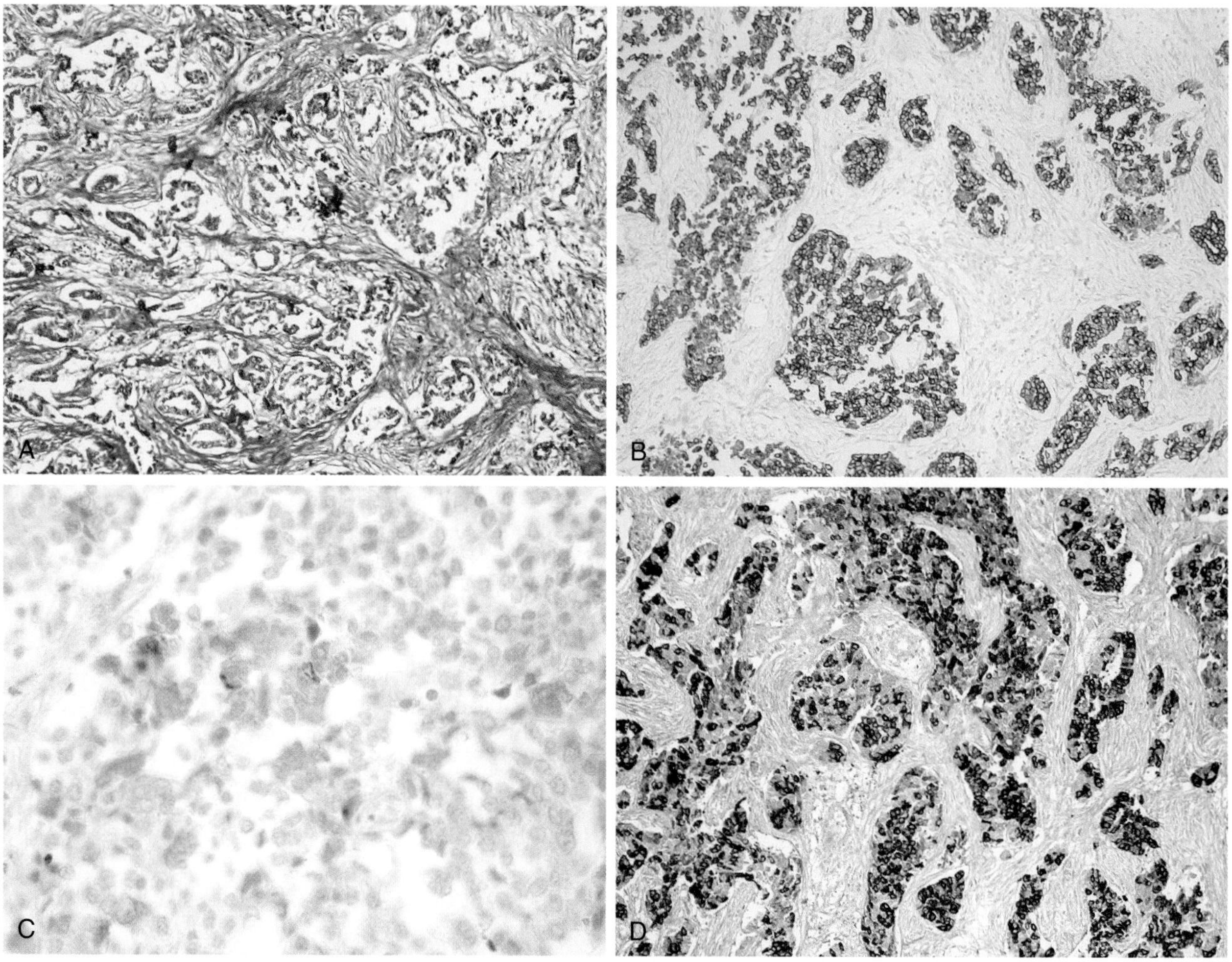

FIGURE 8.15 Adenocarcinoma involving abdominal wall **(A).** The tumor cells are strongly and diffusely positive for CK7 **(B),** patchy positive for GCDFP-15 **(C),** and show diffuse strong staining for mammaglobin **(D).** Despite negative receptor status, the morphology and IHC profile was consistent with the patient's known history of breast carcinoma from several years ago.

and associates, these same tumors were all negative with the commercially available antibody ER1D5 (DAKO, Carpinteria, Calif). Survival of this group of patients differed for men versus women, suggesting some gender-specific p29-associated factor influence.

Dabbs and colleagues[350] observed ER in pulmonary adenocarcinomas using antibody clone 6F11 (Ventana, Tucson, Ariz) with heat-induced epitope retrieval (HIER). Nuclear estrogen receptor was observed in 67% of lung adenocarcinomas including the bronchioloalveolar variants but was not seen with antibody clone ER1D5 (DAKO, Carpinteria, Calif). As a result of these findings, the authors are reluctant to use the presence of ER in an adenocarcinoma of lung as definitive evidence of a metastatic breast carcinoma with antibody ER6F11. Other investigators have arrived at the same conclusion regarding the low specificity of ER when used alone in the study of CUPS. However, diffuse strong staining for ER (clone 1D5 or rabbit monoclonal SP1) in the right clinical context and appropriate cytokeratin expression profile (CK7+/CK20−) is highly indicative of a breast or gynecologic primary tumor.[351]

KEY DIAGNOSTIC POINTS

Hormone Receptors (ER and PR)

- Diffuse strong expression is indicative of breast or gynecologic primary tumor.
- Weak/moderate expression should be judged more carefully, taking into account the clinical presentation and results of other immunohistochemical stains.
- ER antibody clone 6F11 gives more false-positive results compared with other clones.

VILLIN

Villin is a calcium-dependent actin-binding cytoskeletal protein that is found in the brush border of the intestine and in the proximal renal tubular epithelium. A brush border is characteristic of colorectal carcinomas and is recognized at the ultrastructural level by the presence of microvilli with a dense core of microfilaments, core rootlets, and surface glycocalyx. Up to 33% of pulmonary adenocarcinomas may demonstrate microvillus rootlets by ultrastructure, and their presence correlates closely with villin immunostaining.[352-355] Antibodies to villin are useful for identifying its molecular presence, which is in almost all colorectal carcinomas and in more than 90% of lung carcinomas that have microvillus rootlets. CKs are a necessary part of a diagnostic panel to distinguish lung and colon carcinomas, and 90% of lung adenocarcinomas are CK20−, whereas colorectal carcinomas are CK20+. Villin may stain hepatocellular neoplasms in a canalicular pattern similar to polyclonal CEA.[356]

CDX2

CDX2 is a homeobox gene that encodes a transcription protein factor that guides development of intestinal epithelial cells from the region of the duodenum to the rectum.[357] Discovered in 1983, the homeobox gene encodes proteins called homeodomains, which are important in developmental processes of many multicellular organisms. The homeobox is a conserved DNA motif that encodes proteins that act as transcription factors, controlling the actions of other genes by binding to segments of DNA. The absence of CDX2 is a lethal event in utero, and heterozygotes have gastrointestinal developmental abnormalities.[358-361]

Barbareschi and colleagues, using clone CDX2-88, found a high sensitivity and specificity for detection of colorectal carcinomas, with some CDX2 expression in other adenocarcinomas of the gastrointestinal tract and in ovarian mucinous tumors.[362] Useful in both paraffin tissue and cytology specimens, they concluded that CDX2 was highly sensitive and specific for intestinal differentiation (Table 8.11). Other studies have confirmed the high specificity of CDX2 for intestinally derived adenocarcinomas including the stomach and duodenum and the gastroesophageal, pancreatic, and biliary tree.[363,364] Colorectal and duodenal adenocarcinomas tend to have a diffuse distribution of nuclear staining in a majority of cells, whereas adenocarcinomas from other intestinal sites tend to have staining in a minority of cells. CDX2 expression decreases dramatically in the subset of colon carcinomas that are "minimally differentiated" and are usually associated with mutations of the DNA mismatch repair genes.[365]

Neuroendocrine carcinomas of intestinal derivation showed a focal pattern of nuclear immunostaining in only 42% of cases in one study.[364] In the study by Babareschi and colleagues,[366] well-differentiated neuroendocrine carcinomas of the ileum/appendix showed greatest expression, and rectal and upper gastrointestinal tract tumors showed lower expression. In addition, 39% of neuroendocrine tumors from sites outside the gastrointestinal tract, including the bladder, breast, uterus, salivary gland, prostate, and lung, showed low expression.[366]

Not surprisingly, urinary bladder adenocarcinomas, derived from the intestinal urachus, are often CDX2+, as are urachal cysts in the bladder (Fig. 8.16). Wang and colleagues[367] studied the immunohistochemical distinction between primary adenocarcinomas of the bladder and secondary involvement of the bladder by colorectal adenocarcinoma. The key antibodies that permitted discrimination of these tumors were beta-catenin (clone 14, Transduction Labs, Lexington, Ken), CK7, and thrombomodulin. All

TABLE 8.11 Percentage of Adenocarcinomas by Site with CDX2 and Villin Immunostaining (2-3+)

Carcinoma	CDX2	Villin
Colorectal	99	82
Duodenal	100	100
Gastric	70	42
Esophagus	67	78
Pancreas	32	40
Biliary	25	60
Mucinous ovary	64	64
Urinary bladder	100	100
Thyroid	4	0
Prostate	4	0

Data from Werling RW, Yaziji H, Bacchi CE, Gown AM. CDX2, a highly sensitive and specific marker of adenocarcinomas of intestinal origin: An immunohistochemical survey of 476 primary and metastatic carcinomas. *Am J Surg Pathol.* 2003;27(3):303-310.

colorectal tumors showed nuclear beta-catenin (bladder negative), were CK7 negative, and were negative for thrombomodulin. Bladder adenocarcinomas were all thrombomodulin positive and variably positive for CK7.

Importantly, other mucinous neoplasms with morphologic intestinal features, the "colloid" carcinoma of the lung[145] with goblet cells (100%), and a subset of ovarian mucinous carcinomas (64%) are CDX2 positive.[364] The majority of the colloid lung tumors are TTF-1 positive, a feature that allows distinction from metastatic colorectal mucinous carcinoma. Ovarian mucinous carcinomas may be separated from gastrointestinal mucinous carcinomas by virtue of typical immunostaining for CK7 in the ovarian tumors.

A prior study has reported uterine cervical adenocarcinomas with intestinal features to be negative for both CDX2 and CK20,[368] but a few recent studies have shown nuclear CDX2 immunoreactivity in up to 30% of cervical adenocarcinomas.[369-371] This immunoreactivity is seen not only with müllerian mucinous or intestinal mucinous differentiation but also in endometrioid tumors of the uterine cervix.[371] However, dominant CK7 reactivity is useful in determining gynecologic origin.[370]

CDX2 immunostaining may rarely be seen focally in prostate or thyroid carcinomas.[364] Concomitant use of villin antibody adds specificity for intestinal differentiation. Though some CDX2 may be seen in nonintestinal carcinomas, villin is negative in these tumors.[364] CDX2 does not immunostain liver, hepatocellular carcinoma, or carcinomas of kidney, breast, lung, or salivary gland.[368] The specificity of CDX2 for metastatic colorectal carcinoma in the liver is enhanced by the concomitant use of a CK20+/CK7- profile because CDX2 may be positive in upper gastrointestinal carcinomas.[372] Endometrioid carcinomas of the uterus or ovary may mimic colorectal carcinomas and may demonstrate nuclear CDX2, in which case a panel of antibodies that includes CK7, CK20, villin, vimentin, and estrogen receptor would be necessary to discriminate from colorectal carcinomas (Fig. 8.17).

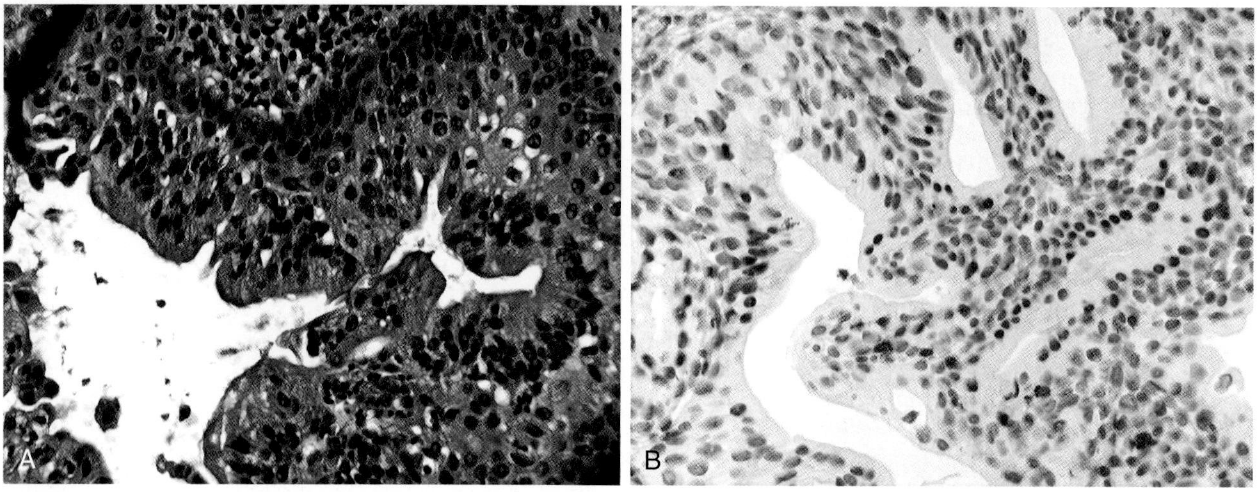

FIGURE 8.16 Urachal cyst (hematoxylin and eosin stain) **(A).** CDX2 positive nuclei in this urachal remnant **(B)** from the dome of the bladder confirm the gastrointestinal origin of this cyst.

KEY DIAGNOSTIC POINTS

Villin and CDX2

- Villin is positive in colorectal and pulmonary adenocarcinomas.
- Canalicular villin expression occurs in hepatocellular carcinoma.
- CDX2 is highly sensitive and specific for intestinal differentiation.
- Adenocarcinomas of urinary bladder (urachal origin) are CDX2+ but are also positive for thrombomodulin and CK7, whereas colorectal carcinomas are negative with thrombomodulin and CK7 and have nuclear beta-catenin expression.
- Adenocarcinomas of the uterine cervix have been reported to be CDX2+ in 30% of cases.
- Endometrioid adenocarcinomas of the ovary and the uterus are CDX2+ in up to 25% of cases.
- Other CDX2+ tumors include colloid lung carcinomas (also positive for TTF-1) and ovarian mucinous carcinomas (CK7+ with CK20 expression weaker than CK7).

HEP PAR1

Hepatocyte paraffin1 (Hep Par1) is the most sensitive and highly specific marker of hepatocytic differentiation in paraffin embedded tissue. The antibody is directed against a mitochondrial antigen present within hepatocytes and shows a characteristic granular cytoplasmic staining (Fig. 8.18). The antibody HepPar-1 is 79% specific for hepatic differentiation, and sensitivity is high.[265,356,373] However, just like any other so-called specific marker, staining is also observed in a limited number of other tumors.[374-376] True hepatocellular carcinoma differentiation (polyclonal CEA+, HepPar-1+, sinusoidal cell CD34+) has been described on rare occasions as a component of some adenocarcinomas from urinary bladder and stomach.[377,378] Hepatoid carcinomas as components of ovarian tumors regularly express significant HepPar-1.[379]

Signet ring cell carcinomas (SRCC) of the stomach usually show diffuse cytoplasmic staining, unlike breast or colorectal SRCC, which are negative for HepPar-1.[380] Antibody MOC-31 (DAKO, Carpinteria, Calif) detects a cell surface glycoprotein that is found largely on epithelial cells and carcinomas. Morrison and colleagues demonstrated that along with HepPar-1 and pCEA, MOC-31 permitted distinction of metastatic carcinomas in liver from hepatocellular carcinoma 99% of the time.[265-267]

DPC4

Deleted in pancreatic carcinoma, Locus-4 (DPC4) is a tumor suppressor gene[381] whose expression is lost in approximately 45% to 50% of pancreatic adenocarcinomas. DPC4 protein expression is retained in many of the malignancies that enter into the differential diagnosis of metastatic mucinous carcinomas with diffuse peritoneal involvement.[382] A positive staining by IHC is therefore noninformative. A negative staining (which should always be interpreted with caution) is suggestive of a pancreatic primary tumor. However, some nonpancreatic tumors (such as from the ampulla, small intestine, and gallbladder) have also been shown to lack DPC4 expression.[383-385]

KEY DIAGNOSTIC POINTS

Hep Par1 and DPC4

- Hep Par1: specific marker of hepatocellular differentiation and shows characteristic cytoplasmic granular staining
- Other Hep Par1+ tumors: signet ring cell carcinoma of stomach, and hepatoid differentiation in carcinomas from other sites (e.g., ovary)
- DPC4: Lack of staining is specific for pancreatic primary; however, should be interpreted with caution with appropriate controls
- Other rare tumors sometimes negative for DPC4: ampullary and gallbladder carcinoma

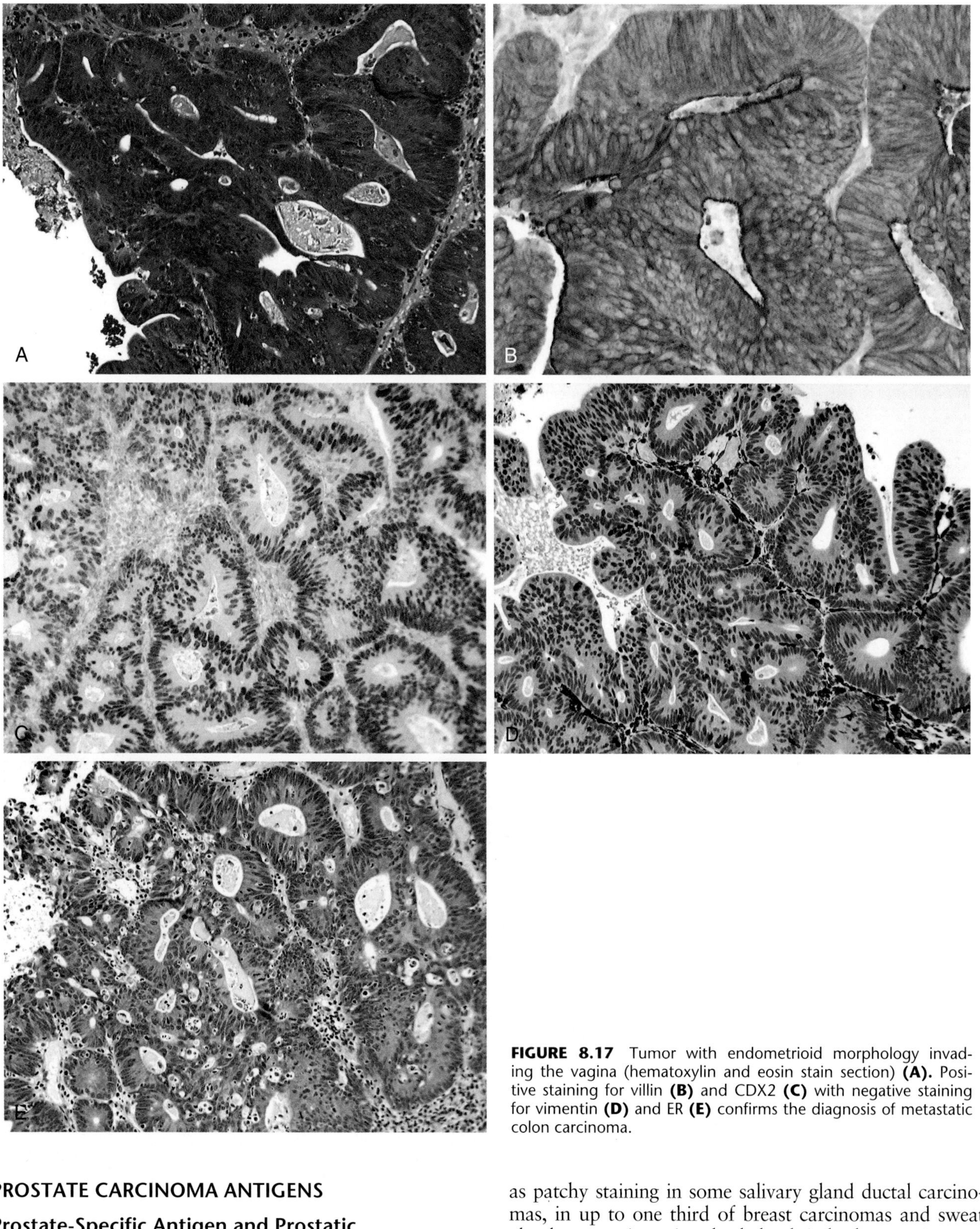

FIGURE 8.17 Tumor with endometrioid morphology invading the vagina (hematoxylin and eosin stain section) **(A).** Positive staining for villin **(B)** and CDX2 **(C)** with negative staining for vimentin **(D)** and ER **(E)** confirms the diagnosis of metastatic colon carcinoma.

PROSTATE CARCINOMA ANTIGENS

Prostate-Specific Antigen and Prostatic Acid Phosphatase

Together, antibodies to PSA and prostatic acid phosphatase (PAP) will stain more than 95% of prostate carcinomas, but there are some caveats. The immunostaining of tumor cells falls off with increasing Gleason grade with both antibodies, and PAP is found in a wide variety of other tumors including hindgut carcinoid tumors.[386] PSA has been found as patchy staining in some salivary gland ductal carcinomas, in up to one third of breast carcinomas and sweat gland tumors, in periurethral glands in both sexes, in cystitis glandularis of the bladder, in urachal remnants, and in some anal glands.[387-394] Nevertheless, PSA is highly specific for prostate tissue because it functions as a serine protease of the seminal fluid[395,396] and it stains the histologic subtypes of tumors including mucinous, signet ring, and endometrioid carcinomas.[397-399] Metastatic prostate carcinoma may be immunostained to a variable degree in metastatic

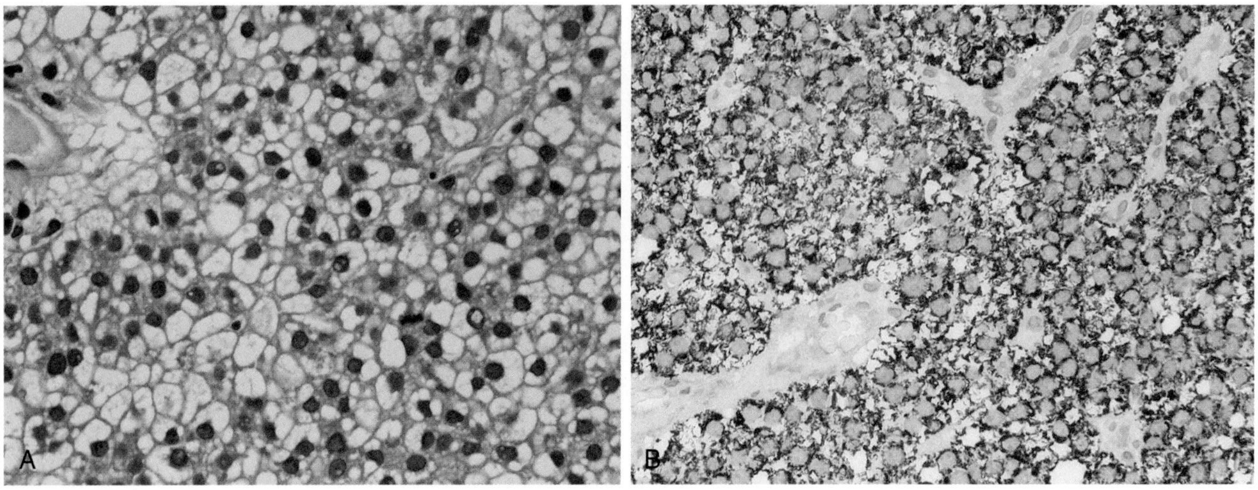

FIGURE 8.18 Hepatocellular carcinoma with clear cell features **(A)** showing granular cytoplasmic positivity for HepPar1 **(B)**.

sites, including lymph nodes.[400,401] Immunoreactivity is not diminished by brief decalcification procedures.

PSA has been found to stain scattered tumor cells from cutaneous malignant melanoma and its metastases.[402] This should not create a diagnostic dilemma because prostate cancers are strongly and diffusely positive with LMW keratin antibodies such as CAM5.2, which is another illustration of the necessity of examining tumors with a panel of antibodies.

Salivary gland ductal carcinomas are commonly positive in a patchy distribution for both PSA and PAP and immunostain strongly for androgen receptors (AR).[403] Close clinical correlation with a PSA+, PAP+, AR+ profile becomes mandatory.

Pro-PSA (pPSA), an antibody to the PSA precursor, is present in benign, preneoplastic, and malignant prostate epithelium with no diminution of staining in high-grade carcinomas. The antibody, PS2P446 (Beckman Coulter, San Diego, Calif), shows promise for the detection of high-grade prostate in metastatic sites.[404,405]

Prostate-Specific Membrane Antigen

Prostate-specific membrane antigen (PSMA), which has a partial homologous structure with the transferrin receptor, is highly specific for prostate cells.[406-408] Unlike PAP, PSMA is upregulated in prostate carcinoma so that stronger staining is seen in higher-grade carcinomas.[408,409] Extraprostatic expression of PSMA has been documented.[408] The antibodies that have been cited in the literature are 7E11-C5.3[409,410] and 3F5.4G6.[411] PSMA in a tumor of unknown primary is highly specific for prostate carcinoma.

Alpha-Methylacyl-CoA Racemase

This mitochondrial peroxisome enzyme, alpha-methylacyl-CoA racemase (AMACR) (encoded by the gene P504S) catalyzes the racemization of alpha-methyl branched carboxylic coenzyme A thioesters and is present in prostate tissue and a wide variety of carcinomas (colorectal, ovarian, breast, bladder, lung, renal cell), melanoma, and lymphoma.[412] AMACR is useful in prostate needle biopsies when the differential diagnosis is carcinoma versus benign prostatic tissue, but it is not specific for prostate carcinoma in metastatic sites. Zhou and colleagues,[412] using a polyclonal antibody, found AMACR positive in the majority of prostate carcinomas (83%). Jiang and colleagues,[413] using a monoclonal antibody (clone 13H4) to P504S, found AMACR immunoreactivity in 100% of prostatic carcinomas. Although a positive staining with AMACR in a case of CUPS is of no diagnostic use, a negative staining would make the diagnosis of prostate carcinoma unlikely.

KEY DIAGNOSTIC POINTS

Prostate Carcinoma Antigens

- Prostate-specific membrane antigen, prostate-specific antigen (PSA), and prostatic acid phosphatase used together provide a sensitive and specific panel for diagnosis of prostatic carcinoma at metastatic site.
- Extraprostatic expression for all prostate carcinoma antigens has been described (breast—rare in males, salivary gland tumors, pancreas, and anal glands). Rare PSA expression occurs in melanomas.
- AMACR is useful in distinguishing prostatic carcinoma from benign prostatic tissue but has limited utility in a case of CUPS.

UROPLAKIN III AND THROMBOMODULIN

The asymmetric unit membrane that is unique to the umbrella cells of urinary tract transitional epithelium contains a transmembrane protein that is unique to urothelium. In studies performed thus far, the uroplakins are highly specific for transitional epithelium, with moderate sensitivity,[414,415] and are not seen in squamous epithelial tissue.

The study by Parker and colleagues[416] demonstrated a sensitivity of 57% for uroplakin III (UROIII) and a nearly perfect specificity.

Unlike uroplakin, thrombomodulin (TM) is a highly sensitive but unspecific marker of urothelial

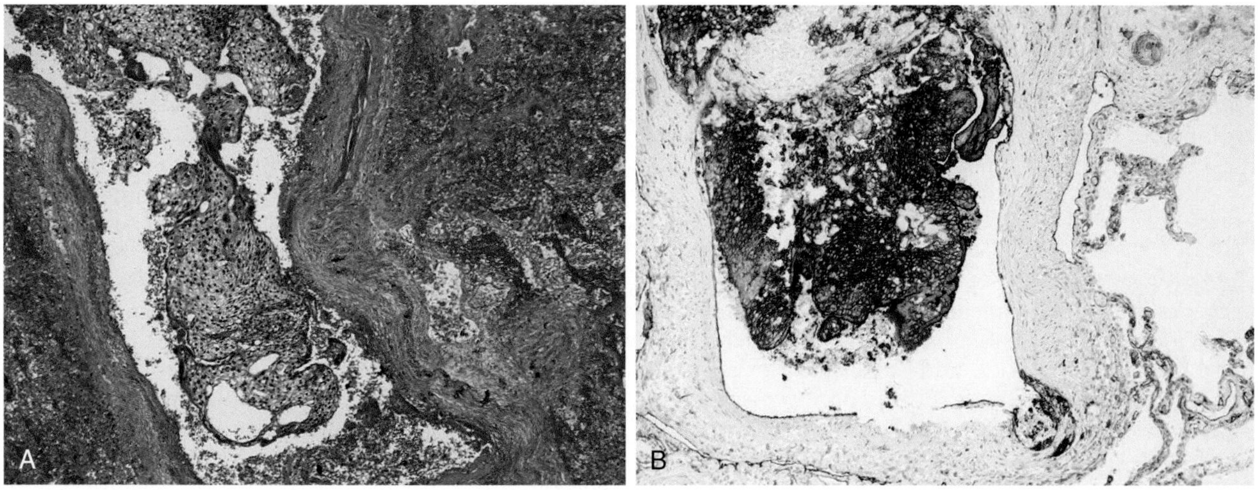

FIGURE 8.19 Metastatic carcinoma in a lung vascular space **(A)**. The tumor cells were diffusely and strongly positive for thrombomodulin **(B)** and showed only focal weak staining with uroplakin III (not shown), confirming urothelial differentiation of the tumor cells.

differentiation (Fig. 8.19). Thrombomodulin is an endothelial cell surface glycoprotein that forms a 1:1 complex with thrombin. Therefore thrombomodulin is expressed in vascular tumors composed of endothelial cells.[417,418] Thrombomodulin expression is also seen in squamous carcinomas.[419] In addition, it is a sensitive marker for mesotheliomas and is useful in the distinction of mesothelioma versus adenocarcinoma.[420]

Given the moderate sensitivity of UROIII and lack of specificity of TM, it is usually necessary to employ a panel of antibodies to increase the probability that one is dealing with a urothelial cell carcinoma. The best antibody panel to use to differentiate urothelial carcinoma in pelvic organs when the differential diagnosis is colorectal carcinoma, prostate carcinoma, renal cell carcinoma, or ovarian transitional cell carcinoma includes UROIII, TM, p63, CK5/6, 34βE12, and CK7/20.[416,421-423] The highest sensitivities for urothelial carcinoma detection are p63 (96%), 34βE12 (88%), TM (70% to 90%), and CK20 (48%).[416,423]

Transitional cell components of ovarian carcinomas differ immunohistologically from urothelial carcinomas.[424] Thrombomodulin (18%) and UROIII (6%) are rarely and focally expressed in ovarian transitional cell carcinomas, which also express WT1 (82%) and CK7 but not CK20, whereas urothelial carcinomas are WT1–, CK7+/20+ (50%), TM+ (76%), and UROIII+ (50%).[424-426] Brenner tumors of the ovary have an immunoprofile similar to urothelial tumors.

KEY DIAGNOSTIC POINTS

Local Pelvic Tumors

- Urothelial carcinoma: UROIII+, TM+, p63+, CK5/6+, CK7+/20+, WT1–
- Ovarian transitional cell carcinoma: WT1+, CK7+, CK20–, UROIII–, TM–, p63–
- Prostate carcinoma: PSA+, PAP+, CK7–/20–, UROIII–, TM–, p63–
- Colorectal carcinoma: CDX2+, CK20+, CK7–, UROIII–, WT1–, TM–, p63–

RENAL CELL CARCINOMA ANTIGEN

Renal cell carcinoma (RCC) antigen is a 200-kD glycoprotein known as gp200 and is present on the surface and cytoplasm of various normal tissues including the brush border of renal proximal tubules, the surface of breast acini, epididymis, parathyroid, and thyroid tissue.[427] McGregor and colleagues[428] surveyed a number of nonrenal tumors and found that 29% of breast tumors, 28% of embryonal carcinomas, and all parathyroid adenomas were positive with RCC. Eighty percent of primary renal cell carcinomas were positive (clear cell 84%, papillary 96%, chromophobe 45%, sarcomatoid 25%, and collecting duct 0%) with greater than 10% of cells positive in 93% of cases. No other primary renal tumors were positive, including oncocytomas. Only 67% of metastatic renal carcinomas were positive with RCC antibody. Only 2% of nonrenal metastases were positive with RCC (mostly metastatic breast carcinomas). Bakshi and colleagues[429] recently showed that RCC may not be a specific marker because 76 of 362 nonrenal tumor samples demonstrated either focal or diffuse expression for RCC. These tumors included adrenocortical neoplasms (37/170; 22%), colonic (11/29; 37.5%), breast (9/27; 33%), prostate (5/18; 27.7%), ovary (2/17; 11.7%), melanoma (3/18; 16.6%), lung (3/21; 14.2%), and parathyroid (3/3; 100%).[429] RCC antibody has a moderate degree of specificity and relatively low sensitivity for renal cell carcinoma, especially for small biopsies when only few tumor cells may show immunostaining.

CD10

CD10 is a marker of early lymphoid progenitor and normal germinal center cells. However, in the nonhematopoietic arena, it reacts mainly against proteins of the epithelium of the renal proximal tubule. It is considered a sensitive marker for renal cell carcinoma and endometrial stromal sarcomas. CD10 stains some other tumors as well (transitional cell carcinoma, prostatic carcinoma, schwannomas, melanomas, rhabdomyosarcomas, leiomyosarcomas, hemangiopericytoma, solitary fibrous tumors, and hepatomas [in a canalicular pattern]); however; given the right clinical context, it could be a specific marker of renal cell carcinoma.[430]

PAX2

Paired box gene 2 or PAX2 gene expression is required for the normal development of the kidney. Using *in-situ* hybridization technique on formalin-fixed human embryonic tissue, Tellier and colleagues[431] demonstrated PAX2 expression in mesonephros, metanephros, adrenals, spinal cord, optic and otic vesicle, retina, semicircular canals of the inner ear, and hindbrain. Although the immunohistochemical studies of PAX2 on human tumors are rather limited, so far the PAX2 protein expression is concordant with the findings of Tellier and colleagues. PAX2 expression is mainly seen in renal tumors (positive in up to 88% of renal clear cell carcinomas) and ovarian tumors (~65% of serous carcinoma).[432-434] A preliminary (unpublished) study at our institution has demonstrated PAX2 reactivity in ovarian clear cell carcinoma (36% positive), uterine endometrioid (28%), and uterine serous carcinomas (63%). All bladder urothelial carcinomas (11 cases) and breast carcinomas (89 cases) were negative for PAX2.

KEY DIAGNOSTIC POINTS

Renal Cell Carcinoma Markers

- Common renal clear cell carcinoma profile: CK7–, CK20–, EMA+, CAM5.2+, CD10+, RCC+, PAX2+, vimentin+
- Of the positive markers, none is specific; therefore panel approach preferred
- Other CD10 positive carcinomas: transitional cell and prostate carcinoma
- Other RCC positive carcinoma: breast, colon, adrenocortical, prostate
- Other PAX2 positive carcinomas: gynecologic tumors (serous, clear cell and endometrioid types), but breast and transitional cell carcinomas negative

Clear cell carcinomas in metastatic sites are always problematic. The differential diagnosis of site of origin in most cases includes clear cell carcinomas of kidney, adrenal, lung, liver, and ovary. Metastatic clear cell carcinomas to pleura are also problematic. The antibody panels that are most likely to yield a separation among these tumors with a high degree of certainty are PAX2, RCC, A103, CD10, CKs, inhibin, vimentin, and HepPar-1.[435-439]

MELAN-A AND INHIBIN IN ADRENOCORTICAL TUMORS

Alpha inhibin is a dimeric glycoprotein functionally similar to TGF-beta and has been found in ovaries (granulosa cells), testes (Sertoli cells), adrenal cortex, placenta, and pituitary.[440] Useful in the diagnosis of sex cord–stromal ovarian tumors, alpha inhibin is also useful to differentiate adrenal cortical adenomas and carcinomas from renal cell carcinomas and metastases to the adrenal with high specificity and sensitivity.

Melan-A, a product of the MART-1 gene, is an antigen recognized by antibody A103, and although its primary utility is in the identification of melanoma cells, it also identifies more than half of adrenocortical neoplasms, especially carcinomas.[441-445] Tumors other than adrenal cortical neoplasms and malignant melanoma are rarely positive for A103, rendering the antibody useful for the discrimination of adrenal cortical neoplasm from renal neoplasm and metastatic carcinoma.[446,447] Like inhibin, it also reacts with some sex cord–stromal tumors. The A103 antibody is more specific for adrenocortical tumors because it does not react with other carcinomas, whereas inhibin is more sensitive.[445] However, if melanoma is excluded as a diagnostic possibility, a positive A103 immunostain is strong evidence in favor of an adrenocortical carcinoma.[441]

Transcription factor adrenal 4 binding protein (Ad4BP), also known as steroid factor-1, is a transcription factor that is positive in virtually all adrenal cortical carcinomas, being negative in renal carcinoma, hepatocellular carcinoma, and pheochromocytoma. Ad4BP is a marker of adrenocortical malignancy.[448,449]

KEY DIAGNOSTIC POINTS

Renal Clear Cell Carcinoma Versus Other "Clear Cell"

- Renal clear cell: PAX2+, RCC+, CAM5.2+, vimentin+, CD10+, CK7 (rare to negative), inhibin–, A103–, HepPar-1–
- Adrenocortical: AD4BP+, A103+, vimentin+, inhibin+, CK7 (rare to negative), CAM5.2 (rare to negative), RCC–/+, CD10–, HepPar-1–
- Lung: TTF-1+, CK7+, RCC–/+, CD10–, inhibin–, A103–, HepPar-1–
- Ovarian clear cell: CK7+, ER+ (patchy), PAX2+ (~1/3), WT1–/+, RCC (rare), CD10–, inhibin–, A103–, HepPar-1–
- Hepatic clear cell carcinoma: HepPar-1+, CD10+ (canalicular), RCC–, A103–, vimentin–, inhibin–, CK7–
- Mesothelioma: Calretinin+, mesothelin+, WT1+, CK5/6+, CK7+, CD10+, RCC–, MOC-31–

GERM CELL TUMOR MARKERS

It is important to be able to diagnose germ cell neoplasms correctly because they are highly amenable to treatment, even in advanced stages.[5,7] They may present as carcinoma of unknown primary including seminoma and its variants, embryonal carcinoma, yolk sac tumor, and choriocarcinoma. A combination of antibodies to simple CKs, EMA, PLAP, CD117 (c-KIT), OCT3/4, CD30, alpha-fetoprotein, and human chorionic gonadotropin (hCG) can be used to arrive at the correct diagnosis in most cases.

Germ cell tumors are diffusely positive for CAM5.2, except seminoma, which is largely negative in most cases but may demonstrate rare focal staining.[450] More than focal keratin staining should raise the suspicion of an embryonal carcinoma component arising in a seminoma.

The PLAP antibodies database from the literature includes M2A, 43-9F, and TRA-1-60.[451-453] The PLAP is strongly positive with crisp membranous and cytoplasmic staining in classic seminoma, negative in the spermatocytic variant,[454,455] and variably positive in embryonal carcinoma and yolk sac tumors and in choriocarcinomas.[455-460] The PLAP is not 100% specific for germ cell tumors because 10% to 15% of non–germ cell carcinomas will be positive, and this group includes müllerian carcinomas, gastrointestinal, lung, and rare breast and renal carcinomas.[461] However, these carcinomas are EMA positive, whereas germ cell tumors are negative. The EMA is negative in all these tumors except choriocarcinoma, in which it stains about 50% of cases.[450,455,462]

Alpha-fetoprotein is present in most yolk sac tumors in patchy distribution, but only focally in some cases of embryonal carcinoma.[450,455,462-464] Hepatoid differentiation in germ cell tumors, especially with yolk sac tumors, typically immunostains with alpha-fetoprotein and does not show the immunoprofile of true hepatocytic differentiation, that is, the biliary pattern of immunostaining with polyclonal CEA.

OCT3/4 is a transcription factor encoded by the POU5F1 gene and is involved in the initiation, maintenance, and differentiation of pluripotent and germline cells. OCT3/4 is a highly sensitive and specific antibody that detects seminoma/dysgerminoma and embryonal carcinoma.[465-467] Immunostaining for OCT3/4 is nuclear and typically stains 90% of nuclei in seminoma/dysgerminoma and embryonal carcinoma. Mixed germ cell tumors with components of seminoma are positive.

Although the previously mentioned markers are helpful in distinguishing between different germ cell tumors, they are not entirely specific. CD117 or c-kit is a marker of interstitial cell of Cajal (and therefore stains gastrointestinal stromal tumors), mast cells, and melanocytes in addition to germ cells.[468,469] CD30 (+ in embryonal carcinoma) is an activation marker, often seen in Hodgkin and anaplastic large cell lymphoma.[470] AFP can be positive in hepatocytic or hepatoid tumors, and HCG-positive cells have been described in several carcinomas.[471]

KEY DIAGNOSTIC POINTS

Germ Cell Tumor Markers

- Seminoma: CAM5.2 (rare to negative), PLAP+, OCT3/4+, CD117+, EMA–
- Embryonal carcinoma: CAM5.2+, PLAP+, OCT3/4+, EMA–, alpha-fetoprotein (rare to negative), CD30+
- Yolk sac tumor: CAM 5.2+, PLAP+, EMA–, alpha-fetoprotein+, OCT3/4–
- Choriocarcinoma: CAM5.2+, PLAP+/–, EMA +, HCG+, OCT3/4–
- PLAP immunostains 10% to 15% of non–germ cell carcinomas, but they are also EMA positive

CD5

CD5 is a 67-kD glycoprotein receptor that may be present on a variety of T lymphocytes and mantle zone lymphocytes. Hishima and colleagues[472] found CD5 expression in thymic carcinoma, and subsequent reports verified and expanded those findings. In the studies published, the clones of antibodies used include NCL-CD5 (CD5/54/B4),[339,473] with sensitivities of 29% to 67% for immunostaining of thymic carcinomas[474,475]; for clone NCL-CD5-4C7, sensitivities of 62% to 100% are reported.[475,476] For mediastinal carcinomas, the usual differential diagnosis includes metastatic squamous carcinoma and other poorly differentiated metastatic lung carcinomas and germ cell tumors, none of which immunostains with clone NCL-CD5-4C7.[476] Although some normal epithelia and carcinomas of gastrointestinal, breast, and urologic sites react with this clone, this fact is largely irrelevant to the focused study on the mediastinum.[476] A positive CD5 mediastinal tumor is strong evidence for thymic carcinoma, although some atypical thymomas and thymic carcinomas arising in a thymoma are also positive.[476,477] Spindle cell carcinomas have been nonreactive with CD5 antibody.[478]

KEY DIAGNOSTIC POINTS

CD5

- Positive in the majority of thymic carcinomas of most histologic types
- Negative in spindle cell thymic carcinoma
- Lung carcinomas largely negative for CD5

COMBINED ANTIBODY (PANEL) APPROACH TO SOLVING DIAGNOSTIC PROBLEMS

When antibodies to CK7, CK20, CK5, or other keratins are combined in panels with various antibodies to other intermediate filaments (e.g., vimentin), antibodies to supplemental epithelial antigens (e.g., CEA, EMA), or antibodies to specific cell products or transcription factors (e.g., neuroendocrine granules, TTF1, WT1), a more specific identification of cell type may be rendered. An algorithmic approach as shown in Fig. 8.20 may be used in arriving at the correct diagnosis.

SPECIAL CLINICAL PRESENTATIONS

Determination of tumor site of origin in certain special circumstances is discussed next.

Metastatic Carcinoma in the Pleura versus Epithelial Mesothelioma

As discussed in the opening of this chapter, the anatomic site of metastasis of a neoplasm is the prime starting point in determining the origin of the neoplasm. Neoplasms metastatic to the pleura are most often due to primary lung carcinomas but may be due to carcinomas originating in other anatomic sites. Metastasis to the pleura from distant sites is more common because patients are living longer with their disease. Therefore the differential diagnosis of a malignant epithelial neoplasm in the pleura includes metastatic lung carcinoma, metastatic nonpulmonary carcinoma, and malignant mesothelioma.

The single best antibody to use to make the distinction between lung carcinoma and mesothelioma is TTF-1, which has a high sensitivity and high specificity for lung carcinomas, especially adenocarcinoma, and small cell carcinoma.[296,297] In addition, CK5/6, which is largely restricted to mesothelial cells, may stain squamous cell carcinomas, lung carcinomas, and nonpulmonary carcinomas to a focal degree. A panel approach is generally used to arrive at the correct diagnosis. Most tumors can be reliably identified as mesothelioma or adenocarcinoma on the basis of clinical history and available IHC markers (Table 8.12). Electron microscopy is still a useful "accessory" technique that may be helpful for equivocal cases, including mesothelioma variants.[479]

KEY DIAGNOSTIC POINTS

Metastatic Carcinoma in Pleura/Abdomen versus Epithelial Mesothelioma

- Positive mesothelioma markers: calretinin, WT1, CK5/6, thrombomodulin, mesothelin
- Negative mesothelioma markers: MOC-31, BG8, BER-EP4, B72.3, CEA, CD15
- Pitfall: CK5/6+ in squamous and transitional cell carcinomas; WT1+ in ovarian papillary serous carcinoma
- Lung carcinoma: TTF1+, CEA+ thyroglobulin–, CK7+/CK20–
- Breast carcinoma: GCDFP-15+, mammaglobin+, CEA+, ER/PR+, CK7+/CK20–
- Thyroid carcinoma: TTF-1+, thyroglobulin+, CEA– (except medullary type), CK7+/CK20–

Mediastinal Tumors: Type and Site of Origin

Tumors that may be confused with CUPS within the mediastinum include thymic neoplasm (thymoma, thymic carcinoid, or thymic carcinoma), thyroid tumors, lymphomas, paragangliomas, and germ cell tumors. Thymomas are generally easy to recognize owing to their characteristic admixture of neoplastic thymic epithelial cells with non-neoplastic lymphocytes. The neoplastic thymic epithelial cells are positive for keratins, but the expression profile may vary according to thymoma subtype.[480] They are also positive for CEA and EMA.[481,482] The thymic lymphocytes in a thymoma are of T-cell derivation but do not stain with markers of mature (peripheral) T cells. Instead they are positive for TdT, CD1a, and CD99.[483,484] In contrast, the thymic carcinomas rarely resemble a thymoma and are morphologically more similar to carcinoma types in other organs. The microscopic types of thymic carcinoma recognized by WHO are epidermoid keratinizing and nonkeratinizing carcinoma (constitutes 90% of all thymic carcinomas) and lymphoepithelioma-like, sarcomatoid, clear cell, basaloid, mucoepidermoid, papillary, mucinous, small cell, and undifferentiated carcinomas. Therefore their identification as thymic neoplasms is difficult or sometimes impossible. One stain that is specific to thymic carcinoma is CD5, which is present in most thymic carcinomas but absent in thymomas and carcinomas of nonthymic origin.[472,474,475]

Tumors of thyroid origin may occur in the mediastinum as primary tumors owing to the presence of the retrosternal location of the thyroid gland. The major subtypes of thyroid carcinomas are papillary, follicular, Hürthle cell, poorly differentiated, anaplastic, and medullary. All carcinomas are generally positive for pankeratin stains. The usual profile is CK7+/CK20–. The two stains that are most helpful in determining site of origin are thyroglobulin and TTF-1.[485] All carcinoma subtypes are positive for TTF-1 except anaplastic carcinoma. All carcinomas are positive for thyroglobulin except anaplastic and medullary types. Because medullary carcinomas are endocrine tumors, they also express other endocrine markers such as chromogranin, synaptophysin, and the specific product of C cells (i.e., calcitonin). Another feature of medullary thyroid carcinoma is the consistent positivity for CEA. As far as the anaplastic carcinoma is concerned, it is difficult to prove not only the site of origin but also that it is a carcinoma and not a sarcoma. Keratin stains are generally helpful in this regard. Vimentin positivity is the rule in the spindle cell component, and EMA and CEA reactivity may be identified, particularly in the squamoid component.[486] Recently, Nonaka and colleagues[487] reported the diagnostic utility of PAX8 antibody, which stained 79% (22 of 28 cases) of anaplastic thyroid carcinoma but was negative in all lung carcinomas tested (147 cases). PAX8 was also expressed in renal tubules, fallopian tubes, ovarian inclusion cysts, and lymphoid follicles as well as in renal carcinoma, nephroblastoma, seminoma, and ovarian carcinoma but was not expressed in normal tissue and carcinomas of the lung. PAX8 could be a useful marker of anaplastic thyroid carcinoma if the differential diagnosis includes lung carcinoma.[487] Mediastinal germ cells tumors are often primary in this location, likely arising from extragonadal germ cells. Although the possibility of metastasis from the gonads should always be considered, the presence of a single lesion in the mediastinum without retroperitoneal involvement argues against a gonadal primary. All varieties of germ cell tumors can be seen within the mediastinum. Dysgerminomas are practically never seen in females, and other tumors (seminoma, embryonal carcinoma, yolk

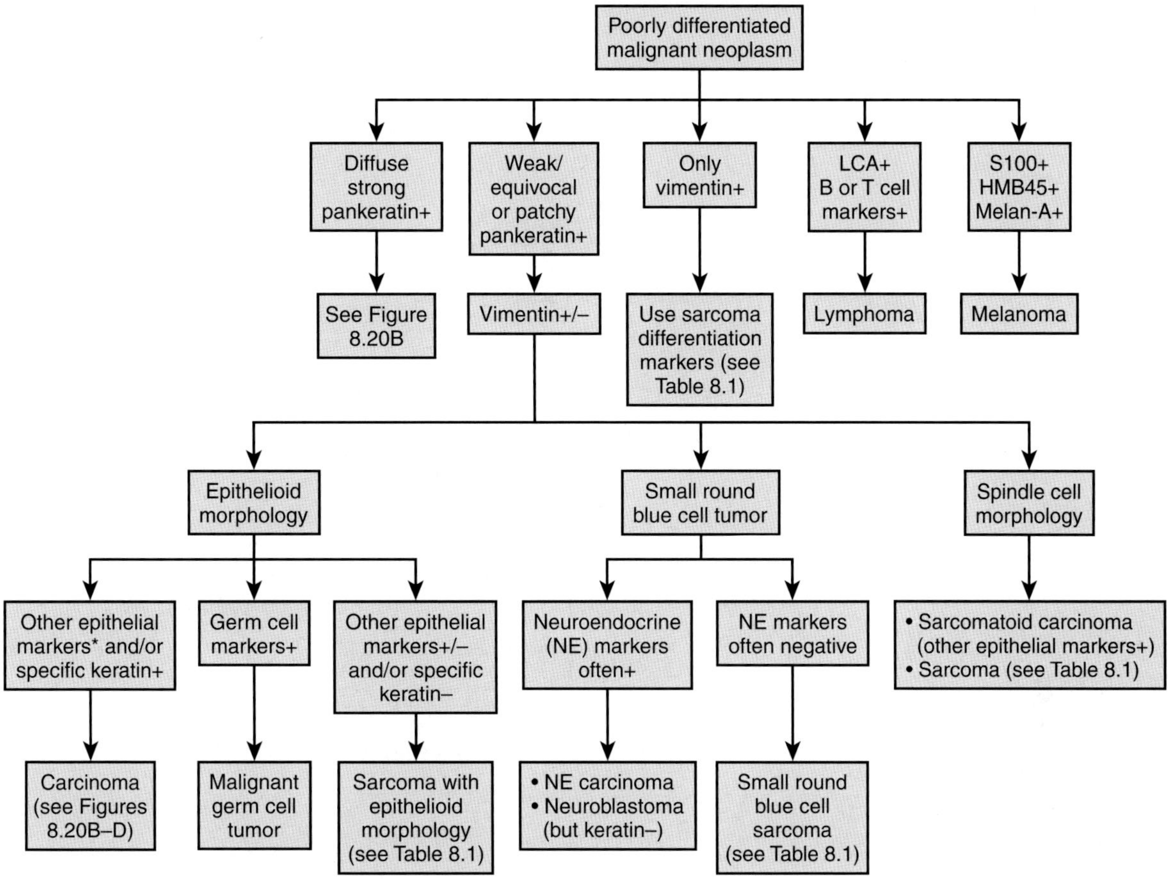

*Other epithelial markers: EMA, CEA, BER-EP4, B72.3.

A Specific keratins: CK7, CK20, CK5/6, CK14, CK17.

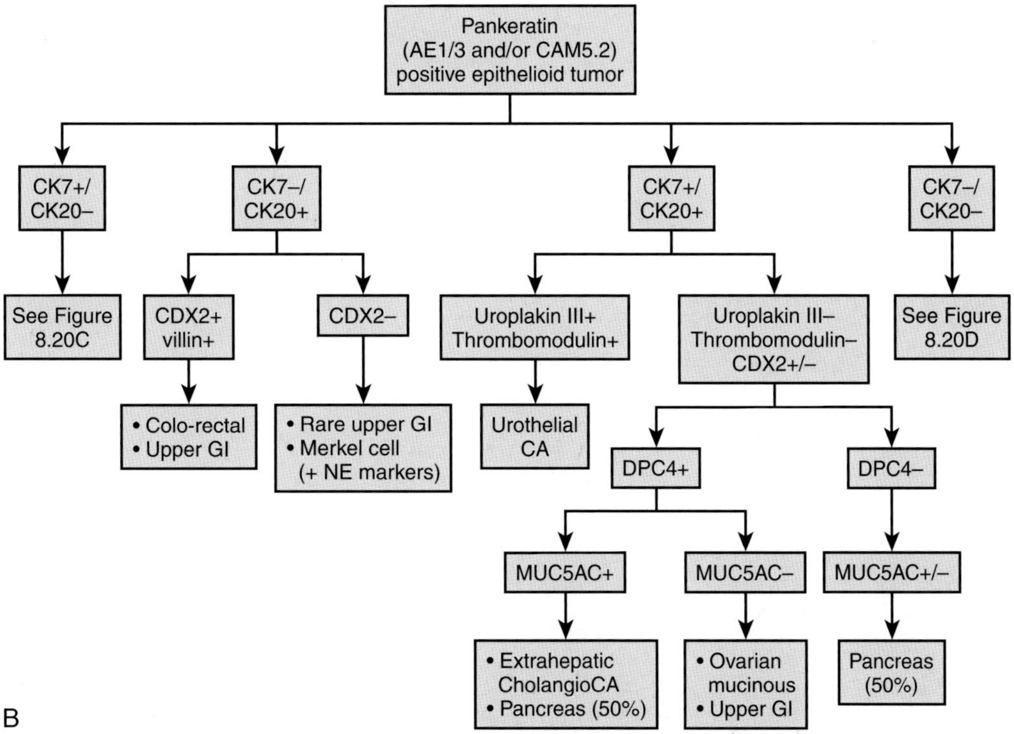

B

FIGURE 8.20 Algorithmic approach to determine line of differentiation in a poorly differentiated malignant neoplasm **(A).** Algorithmic approach to determine site of origin in an adenocarcinoma or a poorly differentiated carcinoma **(B).**

Continued

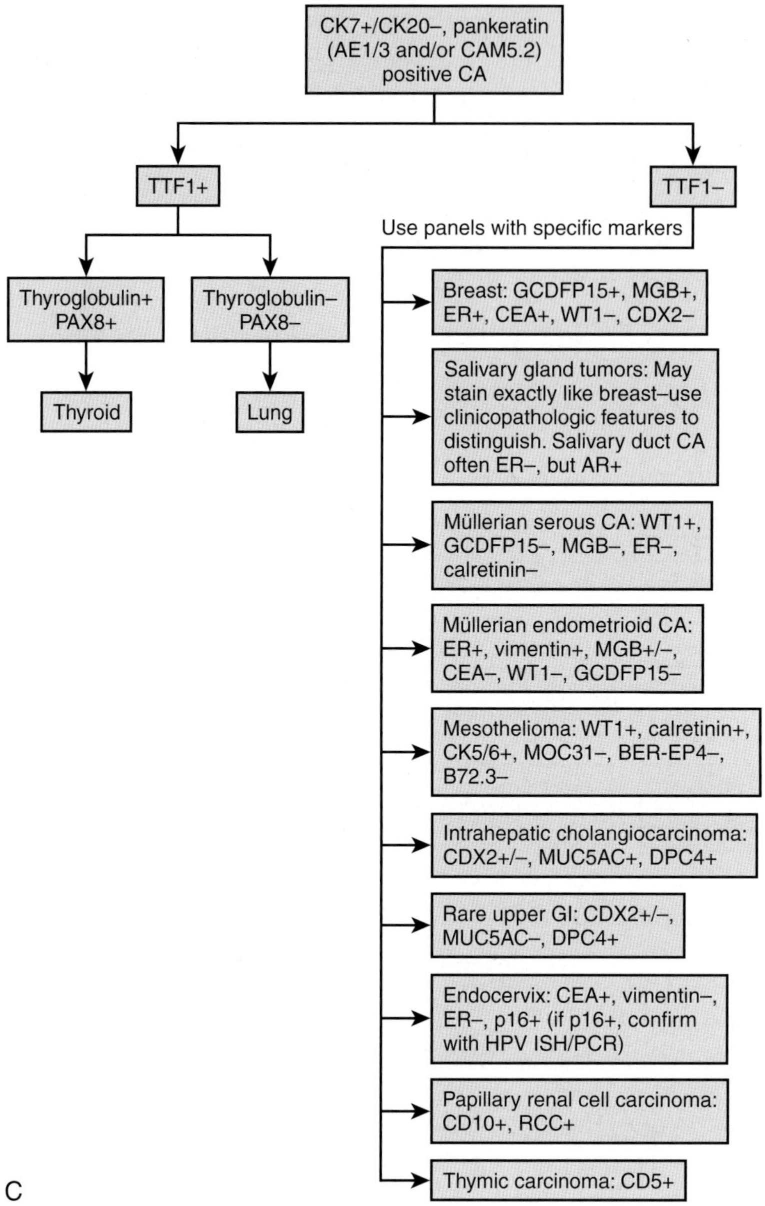

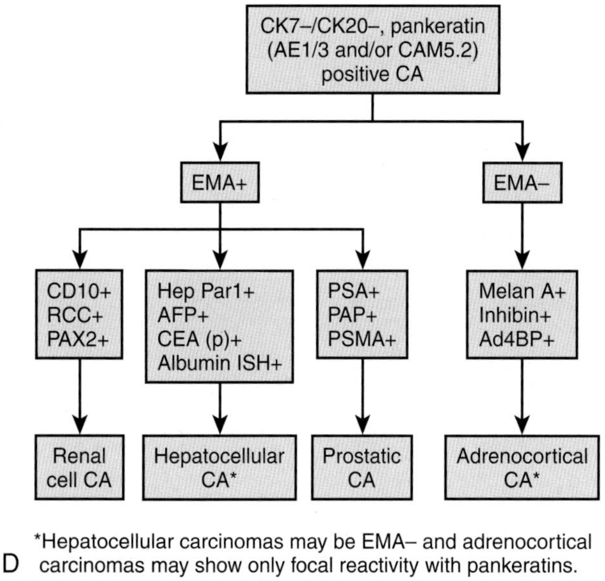

FIGURE 8.20, cont'd Further workup of a CK7+/CK20– tumor **(C).** Further workup of a CK7–/CK20– tumor **(D).**

TABLE 8.12 Antibody Panels: Mesothelioma versus Lung Carcinoma

	Mesothelioma	Carcinoma
Calretinin	+	R
WT-1	+	N
Mesothelin	+	N
CK5	+	S
Bg8	N	+
BER-Ep4	N	+
MOC-31	N	+

+, Positive; S, sometimes positive; R, rare cells show staining; N, negative.

sac tumor, choriocarcinoma, teratocarcinoma) show high male predilection.[488] Mature cystic teratomas are seen with equal frequency in both males and females. The immunohistochemical profile is generally similar to the gonadal tumors with some occasional differences.[489] Seminoma is often positive for PLAP, OCT3/4, CD117, and CD57 and generally negative for keratins. Although focal reactivity for CAM5.2 may be seen in seminomas, it is often negative for AE1/3.[490-492] In contrast, embryonal carcinomas often show AE1/3 reactivity and are also positive for CD30. Embryonal carcinomas are positive for OCT3/4 and may show reactivity for PLAP.[493,494] Yolk sac tumors are positive for AFP and choriocarcinomas show reactivity for HCG.[464] However, it is important to note that immunostains for AFP and HCG often show high background and should be interpreted with caution and in the right context. Serum elevation of AFP and HCG is commonly associated with nonseminomatous germ cell neoplasms, and therefore measuring serum levels is another alternative to IHC in confirming the diagnosis. Another important feature of all germ cell tumors, regardless of origin or microscopic type, is the presence of a cytogenetic aberration isochromosome 12p [i(12p)].[495] This results in gain of 12p, which can be identified by routine cytogenetic techniques even in formalin-fixed paraffin-embedded material.[496] Finally, an attempt should be made to classify a tumor as germ cell before rendering a diagnosis of undifferentiated malignant neoplasm.

PERITONEAL CARCINOMATOSIS

It is not uncommon to receive a biopsy from a patient with tumor extensively involving the abdomen and peritoneum without a known primary. In a female patient, serous papillary morphology is most suggestive of an ovarian primary. In the absence of ovarian/tube/endometrial involvement, it is considered to be a primary peritoneal serous carcinoma (PPSC). The immunohistochemical profile of PPSC is identical to an ovarian primary tumor. The differential diagnosis is more challenging when the tumor shows a mucinous morphology. The source of metastases in a mucinous carcinoma (in both males and females) is often gastrointestinal, and it is worth looking at appendix, bowel, pancreas, and stomach clinically or radiographically. In a female patient, mucinous carcinoma involving bilateral ovaries may also be metastatic from the uterine cervix.[497] A combination of CK7, CK20, CDX2, DPC4, MUC stains, p16, and vimentin may be helpful in arriving at the correct diagnosis.[498] When the morphology is unrevealing, the differential diagnosis should include not only carcinomas but also mesothelioma, and in females it should include ovarian stromal tumors. The ovarian stromal tumors may show keratin positivity but are almost always EMA negative. They are positive for inhibin, calretinin, and CD99.[499-501]

PAGET DISEASE

Paget disease occurs in mammary and extramammary (EM) forms. Paget disease of the breast is almost always indicative of an underlying breast carcinoma,[502-504] whereas EM Paget disease may be an indicator of metastatic carcinoma.

Paget disease of the breast manifests as CK7+ malignant cells infiltrating the epidermis of the nipple. Tumor cells are conspicuous by their infiltrative "shotgun" pattern, large size, abundant cytoplasm, signet-ring forms, and, sometimes, mucin positivity. Epidermal keratinocytes are negative with CK7, while most Paget cells are CK7+, GCDFP-15+, and CEA+ (Fig. 8.21). Toker cells are CK7+ and may be present in the skin of the normal nipple, but generally they are inconspicuous compared with Paget cells[505] and should not cause diagnostic problems because they are bland cytologically and difficult to find in the normal epithelium.

The presence of CK7+ cells in the nipple epidermis does not equate with Paget disease, including those circumstances in which there is a benign nipple lesion such as nipple adenoma. The presence of benign-appearing CK7+ cells in the epidermis may be a manifestation of the extension of cells from the lactiferous ducts or benign nipple epithelial proliferations into the epidermis.[506]

The Paget cells may be assessed for ER[507] or the neu-oncoprotein.[508] However, HER2 is a better marker of Paget disease because the underlying carcinoma is often a high-grade ductal carcinoma *in situ* with comedonecrosis, which is generally ER negative and HER2 positive.

The differential diagnosis for Paget disease includes melanoma and Bowen's disease (squamous cell carcinoma), for which appropriate IHC stains could be used. For diagnosing melanoma, at least two melanoma markers should be used because S100 staining can be seen in up to 18% of breast carcinoma cases.

The EM forms of Paget disease occur predominantly in females as vulvar or perianal disease but may also occur in males and at other sites.

Primary vulvar Paget disease is a localized carcinoma of sweat duct origin that may be *in situ* or invasive; histologically, it is composed of large cells with voluminous cytoplasm containing mucin that are universally CK7+ and GCDFP-15+.[329]

The extravulvar form of the disease presents in the perianal areas as metastatic disease from sites that may include the rectum, cervix, or urinary bladder. Therefore the diagnostic problem inherent with a histologic diagnosis of extravulvar Paget disease is the differential diagnosis of adnexal skin neoplasm versus metastatic carcinoma from rectum, cervix, or urinary bladder. Colorectal carcinomas presenting as Paget disease are often mucin positive with signet-ring forms and intraluminal "dirty" necrosis[333]; they are GCDFP-15 negative, CEA+, and strongly positive for CK20, and although they are largely CK7 negative they may be focally or weakly positive for CK7.[329,331-333,335] Transitional cell carcinomas are typically strongly positive for both CK7 and CK20; they are GCDFP-15 negative and they lack signet cells or mucin and may immunostain with uroplakin antibody.

KEY DIAGNOSTIC POINTS

Paget Disease

- Mammary Paget disease: CK7+, GCDFP-15+, CEA+, HER2+
- Pagetoid squamous carcinoma: p63+, CK5+, CK7−
- Vulvar Paget disease, primary adnexal carcinoma: CK7+, GCDFP-15+, CEA+
- Metastatic colorectal carcinoma presenting as perianal-vulvar Paget disease: CK7 (negative), CK20+, CDX2+, CEA+, GCDFP-15 (negative)
- Metastatic transitional carcinoma presenting as perianal-vulvar Paget disease: CK7+, CK20+, GCDFP-15 (negative), CEA+, uroplakin+

BEYOND IMMUNOHISTOCHEMISTRY: ANATOMIC MOLECULAR DIAGNOSTIC APPLICATIONS

Several different types of molecular techniques can be applied for identifying tumor of unknown origin. These could range from identifying a single molecular event to transcriptional profiling that examines expression of hundreds and thousands of genes. The examples of the former are summarized in Table 8.13. Molecular assays determining a single fusion transcript or identifying a virus by polymerase chain reaction have been in diagnostic use for a number of years; however, with recent technologic advancements, gene expression profiling technology has also come to the forefront of diagnostic testing. Both cDNA and oligonucleotide microarrays are now used extensively for a variety of different applications.

For the first time in 2001, Ramaswamy and colleagues provided a proof of principle that gene expression analysis could be used in identifying tumor site of origin.[509] They subjected 218 tumors of 14 different morphologic types and 90 normal tissue samples to

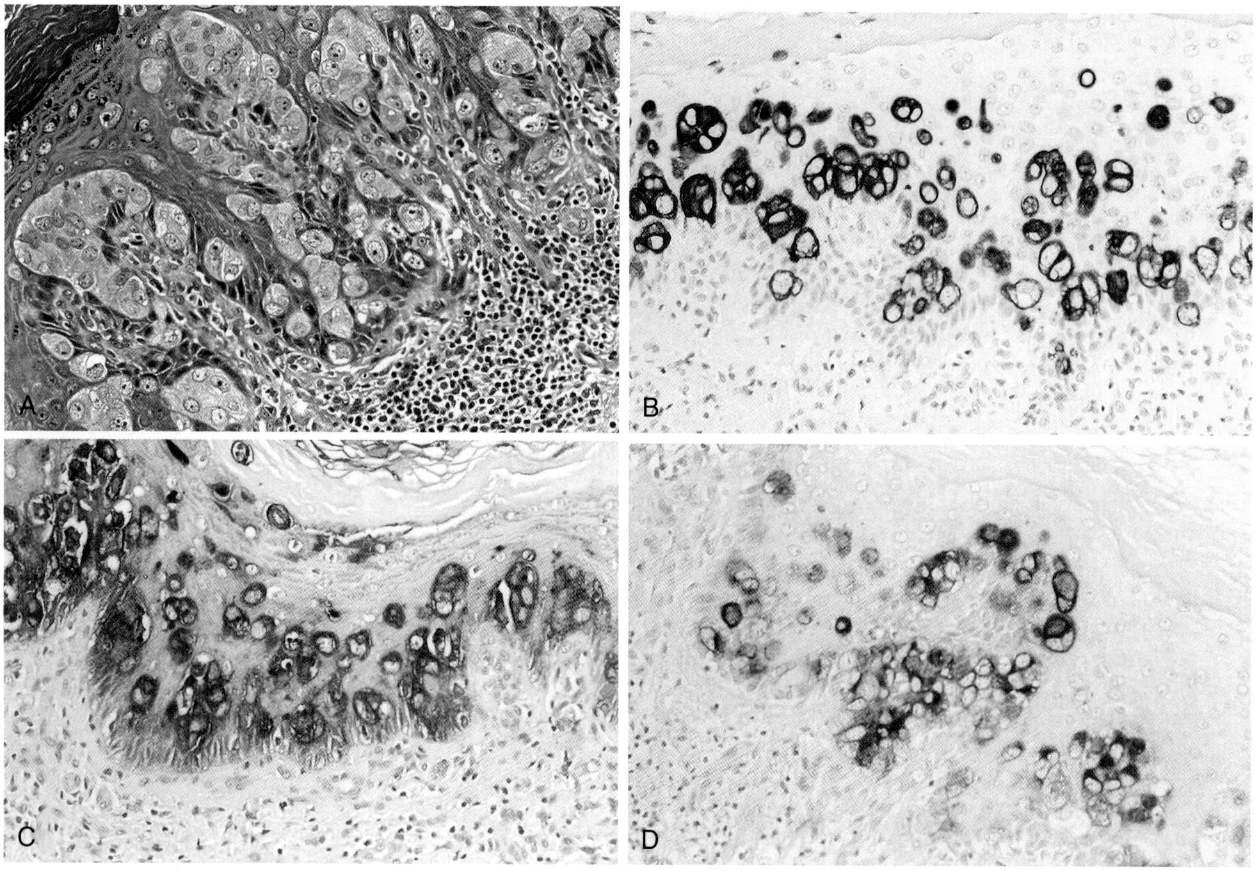

FIGURE 8.21 A typical case of primary perineal Paget disease **(A)**, which is CK7+ **(B)**, CEA+ **(C)**, and GCDFP-15+ **(D)**.

TABLE 8.13 Molecular (Single Gene/Event) Assays for Determining Site of Origin

Technique	Determinant	Tumor Type/Site
RT-PCR	Fusion transcripts	Various sarcomas (see Table 8.1)
PCR	HPV	Uterine cervix and some head and neck tumors
ISH	HPV	Uterine cervix and some head and neck tumors
ISH	Albumin	Hepatocellular carcinoma
ISH	EBV	Nasopharyngeal carcinomas, lymphomas (Burkitt, Hodgkin, some T-cell lymphomas), subset of gastric cancers, immunodeficiency associated tumors
FISH	Isochromosome 12p [i(12p)]	Germ cell tumors
Mutation Analysis	*KIT* gene	Gastrointestinal stromal tumors

EBV, Epstein-Barr virus; FISH, fluorescence *in situ* hybridization; HPV, human papilloma virus; ISH, *in situ* hybridization; PCR, polymerase chain reaction; RT, reverse transcriptase.

TABLE 8.14 Multigene Expression Assays for Determining Site of Origin

	CancerTYPE ID	CupPrint	Tissue of Origin
Company	bioTheranostics, San Diego, Calif	Agendia BV, Amsterdam, Netherlands	Pathwork Diagnostics, Sunnyvale, Calif
Technique	RT-PCR	cDNA microarray	Oligonucleotide array
Platform used	TaqMan, Applied Biosystems	Agilent	Affymetrix
Number of genes analyzed	92	495	>1500
Specimen requirement	FFPE	FFPE	Fresh/frozen
Number of tumor types/ subtypes identified	32	49 subtypes of approximately 30 tumor types/sites	15
Classification accuracy	87%	88%	84%
In-house testing requirement	None	Specimen preparation	Specimen processing required
FDA approval	No	No	Yes

bioTheranostics was formerly AviaraDx (originally Arcturus Bioscience, Inc.) and has provided licenses to U.S. laboratories (through LabCorp) and Quest Diagnostics to perform tests for identifying tumor types.

gene expression analysis.[509] Expression levels of more than 16,000 genes were used to test the accuracy of a multiclass classifier on the basis of a support vector machine algorithm. An overall classification accuracy of 78% was achieved. They were also able to correctly classify metastatic samples, which indicated that cancers retain their tissue of origin identity throughout metastatic evolution. Prediction is driven by cancer-intrinsic gene expression patterns and not by the gene expression signature of contaminating nonmalignant tissue. However, Ramaswamy and colleagues were unable to classify the majority of poorly differentiated carcinomas correctly. Several smaller studies that followed showed somewhat similar results but were unable to provide a test that could be useful practically and lacked a broad coverage of all tumor types.[510-514] Subsequently, Ma and colleagues translated their microarray findings in designing a 92-gene reverse transcriptase polymerase chain reaction (RT-PCR) assay for determining tumor site of origin.[515] They achieved an overall success rate of 87% in classifying 32 different tumor classes in the validation set of 119 FFPE tumor samples. This RT-PCR–based assay for tumor of unknown origin is now offered by two large commercial laboratories in the United States.

A gene expression–based assay to determine site of origin in a centralized format is offered by Agendia BV, Netherlands. This test uses cDNA microarrays for 495 genes to determine 49 tumor subtypes using "k-nearest neighbor" bioinformatics strategy. The test has been reported to have 88% overall accuracy for determining site of origin.[516] Recently, another gene expression–based test in a decentralized format has become available (Pathwork Diagnostics, Sunnyvale, Calif). The test measures the expression of more than 1500 genes to identify 15 different tumor types representing 60 different morphologies. The 15 tumor types identified in this assay are carcinomas (bladder, breast, colorectal, gastric, hepatocellular, kidney, non–small cell lung, ovarian, pancreatic, prostate, thyroid), germ cell neoplasms, melanoma, non-Hodgkin lymphoma, and soft tissue sarcomas. The test requires specimen processing to be performed in a CLIA-certified laboratory using a standardized protocol and a proprietary microarray chip. The chip is then scanned and the data file is submitted via the Internet to the company, where fully automated software generates a report. The report contains a similarity score (ranging from 0 to 100) for each of the 15 tumor types, and the final interpretation is performed by the molecular pathologist who initiated the testing. In a clinical validation study of 487 metastatic, poorly differentiated, and undifferentiated tumors that had been identified as one of the 15 tumor types on the panel using existing methods, the test demonstrated 89% positive percent agreement (sensitivity) and 99% negative percent agreement (specificity) with available diagnoses.[517] Another study examining the Pathwork tissue of origin test has shown high reproducibility among different laboratories despite numerous sources of variability.[518] The multigene molecular assays available to predict primary tumor site are summarized in Table 8.14.

Another recent approach in identifying tissue of origin is by using microRNA (miRNA) based methodology. MiRNAs are non-coding regulatory RNAs that are considered to be highly tissue specific biomarkers based on the current knowledge.[519] They have a role in cellular differentiation during tissue development and have also been thought to play a role in development of specific malignancies.[520] Ronsenfeld and colleagues recently demonstrated the enormous potential of miRNA in identifying tissue of origin.[521] Using a decision-tree–based classification, Rosenfeld et al. used 48 miRNA markers to achieve an overall accuracy of 89% among 22 different tumor tissues of origin. This study was performed using FFPE tissues, and the technique has the potential for incorporation into diagnostic pathology in dealing with challenging cases.

All of these molecular assays have been designed using robust techniques, but it is useful to remember that these have been compared with the existing technologies (i.e., clinical suspicion, radiographic evaluation, morphology, immunohistochemistry, and possibly autopsy findings) for validation. Therefore these molecular tests will complement our current diagnostic tools but are unlikely to replace the existing method of evaluation for CUPS. Another prohibitive factor for using these molecular tests in routine practice is their high cost, which is generally $3000 or more.

SUMMARY

By working closely with the clinician who performs a careful clinical history and assessment, the pathologist should develop a working differential diagnosis on the basis of the tumor location or radiologic assessment of the tumor, or both. This information is key to using IHC and other ancillary techniques as a cost-effective tool in patient care.

REFERENCES

1. Rosai J. Cytokeratin expression in cauda equina paragangliomas. Author's response to letter. *Am J Surg Pathol.* 1999;23:491.
2. Blaszyk H, Hartmann A, Bjornsson J. Cancer of unknown primary: clinicopathologic correlations. *APMIS.* 2003;111:1089-1094.
3. Greco FA, Burris 3rd HA, Erland JB, et al. Carcinoma of unknown primary site. *Cancer.* 2000;89:2655-2660.
4. Yakushiji S, Ando M, Yonemori K, et al. Cancer of unknown primary site: review of consecutive cases at the National Cancer Center Hospital of Japan. *Int J Clin Oncol.* 2006;11:421-425.
5. Haskell CM, Cochran AJ, Barsky SH, Steckel RJ. Metastasis of unknown origin. *Curr Probl Cancer.* 1988;12:5-58.
6. Krementz ET, Cerise EJ, Foster DS, Morgan Jr LR. Metastases of undetermined source. *Curr Probl Cancer.* 1979;4:4-37.
7. Schapira DV, Jarrett AR. The need to consider survival, outcome, and expense when evaluating and treating patients with unknown primary carcinoma. *Arch Intern Med.* 1995;155:2050-2054.
8. Pavlidis N, Briasoulis E, Hainsworth J, Greco FA. Diagnostic and therapeutic management of cancer of an unknown primary. *Eur J Cancer.* 2003;39:1990-2005.
9. van de Wouw AJ, Jansen RL, Griffioen AW, Hillen HF. Clinical and immunohistochemical analysis of patients with unknown primary tumour. A search for prognostic factors in UPT. *Anticancer Res.* 2004;24:297-301.
10. Pisharodi LR, Lavoie R, Bedrossian CW. Differential diagnostic dilemmas in malignant fine-needle aspirates of liver: a practical approach to final diagnosis. *Diagn Cytopathol.* 1995;12:364-370; discussion 370-371.
11. Debevec M. Management of patients with brain metastases of unknown origin. *Neoplasma.* 1990;37:601-606.
12. Merchut MP. Brain metastases from undiagnosed systemic neoplasms. *Arch Intern Med.* 1989;149:1076-1080.
13. Nussbaum ES, Djalilian HR, Cho KH, Hall WA. Brain metastases. Histology, multiplicity, surgery, and survival. *Cancer.* 1996;78:1781-1788.
14. Bartelt S, Lutterbach J. Brain metastases in patients with cancer of unknown primary. *J Neurooncol.* 2003;64:249-253.
15. Kambhu SA, Kelsen DP, Fiore J, et al. Metastatic adenocarcinomas of unknown primary site. Prognostic variables and treatment results. *Am J Clin Oncol.* 1990;13:55-60.
16. Lagerwaard FJ, Levendag PC, Nowak PJ, et al. Identification of prognostic factors in patients with brain metastases: a review of 1292 patients. *Int J Radiat Oncol Biol Phys.* 1999;43:795-803.
17. Nguyen LN, Maor MH, Oswald MJ. Brain metastases as the only manifestation of an undetected primary tumor. *Cancer.* 1998;83:2181-2184.
18. Rougraff BT, Kneisl JS, Simon MA. Skeletal metastases of unknown origin. A prospective study of a diagnostic strategy. *J Bone Joint Surg Am.* 1993;75:1276-1281.
19. Sears D, Hajdu SI. The cytologic diagnosis of malignant neoplasms in pleural and peritoneal effusions. *Acta Cytol.* 1987;31:85-97.
20. Ringenberg QS, Doll DC, Loy TS, Yarbro JW. Malignant ascites of unknown origin. *Cancer.* 1989;64:753-755.
21. Sadeghi B, Arvieux C, Glehen O, et al. Peritoneal carcinomatosis from non-gynecologic malignancies: results of the EVOCAPE 1 multicentric prospective study. *Cancer.* 2000;88:358-363.
22. Cho KR, Epstein JI. Metastatic prostatic carcinoma to supradiaphragmatic lymph nodes. A clinicopathologic and immunohistochemical study. *Am J Surg Pathol.* 1987;11:457-463.
23. Nguyen C, Shenouda G, Black MJ, et al. Metastatic squamous cell carcinoma to cervical lymph nodes from unknown primary mucosal sites. *Head Neck.* 1994;16:58-63.
24. Conessa C, Clement P, Foehrenbach H, Poncet JL. [Positron emission tomography in head and neck squamous cell carcinomas]. *Ann Otolaryngol Chir Cervicofac.* 2006;123:227-239.
25. Schmalbach CE, Miller FR. Occult primary head and neck carcinoma. *Curr Oncol Rep.* 2007;9:139-146.
26. Silva P, Hulse P, Sykes AJ, et al. Should FDG-PET scanning be routinely used for patients with an unknown head and neck squamous primary? *J Laryngol Otol.* 2007;121:149-153.
27. Gluckman JL, Robbins KT, Fried MP. Cervical metastatic squamous carcinoma of unknown or occult primary source. *Head Neck.* 1990;12:440-443.
28. Jereczek-Fossa BA, Jassem J, Orecchia R. Cervical lymph node metastases of squamous cell carcinoma from an unknown primary. *Cancer Treat Rev.* 2004;30:153-164.
29. Calabrese L, Jereczek-Fossa BA, Jassem J, et al. Diagnosis and management of neck metastases from an unknown primary. *Acta Otorhinolaryngol Ital.* 2005;25:2-12.

30. Zaren HA, Copeland 3rd EM. Inguinal node metastases. *Cancer*. 1978;41:919-923.
31. Ayoub JP, Hess KR, Abbruzzese MC, et al. Unknown primary tumors metastatic to liver. *J Clin Oncol*. 1998;16:2105-2112.
32. Greco FA, Hainsworth JD. The management of patients with adenocarcinoma and poorly differentiated carcinoma of unknown primary site. *Semin Oncol*. 1989;16:116-122.
33. Guthrie Jr TH. Treatable carcinoma of unknown origin. *Am J Med Sci*. 1989;298:74-78.
34. Hainsworth JD, Greco FA. Managing carcinomas of unknown primary site. *Oncology (Williston Park)*. 1988;2:43-49.
35. Lenzi R, Hess KR, Abbruzzese MC, et al. Poorly differentiated carcinoma and poorly differentiated adenocarcinoma of unknown origin: favorable subsets of patients with unknown-primary carcinoma? *J Clin Oncol*. 1997;15:2056-2066.
36. Kirsten F, Chi CH, Leary JA, et al. Metastatic adeno or undifferentiated carcinoma from an unknown primary site—natural history and guidelines for identification of treatable subsets. *Q J Med*. 1987;62:143-161.
37. Perchalski JE, Hall KL, Dewar MA. Metastasis of unknown origin. *Prim Care*. 1992;19:747-757.
38. Jakobsen JH, Johansen J, Jorgensen KE. [Neck lymph node metastases from an unknown primary tumor]. *Ugeskr Laeger*. 1991;153:428-430.
39. van der Gaast A, Verwij J, Planting AS, et al. The value of immunohistochemistry in patients with poorly differentiated adenocarcinomas and undifferentiated carcinomas of unknown primary. *J Cancer Res Clin Oncol*. 1996;122:181-185.
40. Matthews P, Ellis IO. Use of immunocytochemistry in the diagnosis of metastatic carcinoma. *Ann Med*. 1996;28:297-300.
41. Abbruzzese JL, Abbruzzese MC, Lenzi R, et al. Analysis of a diagnostic strategy for patients with suspected tumors of unknown origin. *J Clin Oncol*. 1995;13:2094-2103.
42. Bartsch R, Wenzel C, Zielinski CC, Steger GG. HER-2-positive breast cancer: hope beyond trastuzumab. *BioDrugs*. 2007;21:69-77.
43. Molina JR, Adjei AA, Jett JR. Advances in chemotherapy of non-small cell lung cancer. *Chest*. 2006;130:1211-1219.
44. Ramalingam S, Belani CP. Recent advances in targeted therapy for non-small cell lung cancer. *Expert Opin Ther Targets*. 2007;11:245-257.
45. Hess KR, Abbruzzese MC, Lenzi R, et al. Classification and regression tree analysis of 1000 consecutive patients with unknown primary carcinoma. *Clin Cancer Res*. 1999;5:3403-3410.
46. Osteen RT, Kopf G, Wilson RE. In pursuit of the unknown primary. *Am J Surg*. 1978;135:494-497.
47. Song SY, Kim WS, Lee HR, et al. Adenocarcinoma of unknown primary site. *Korean J Intern Med*. 2002;17:234-239.
48. Mackay B, Ordonez NG. Pathological evaluation of neoplasms with unknown primary tumor site. *Semin Oncol*. 1993;20:206-228.
49. Kagan AR, Steckel RJ. The limited role of radiologic imaging in patients with unknown tumor primary. *Semin Oncol*. 1991;18:170-173.
50. Steckel RJ, Kagan AR. Metastatic tumors of unknown origin. *Cancer*. 1991;67:1242-1244.
51. Jonk A, Kroon BB, Rumke P, et al. Lymph node metastasis from melanoma with an unknown primary site. *Br J Surg*. 1990;77:665-668.
52. Le Chevalier T, Cvitkovic E, Caille P, et al. Early metastatic cancer of unknown primary origin at presentation. A clinical study of 302 consecutive autopsied patients. *Arch Intern Med*. 1988;148:2035-2039.
53. Hainsworth JD, Wright EP, Johnson DH, et al. Poorly differentiated carcinoma of unknown primary site: clinical usefulness of immunoperoxidase staining. *J Clin Oncol*. 1991;9:1931-1938.
54. Hainsworth JD, Greco FA. Poorly differentiated carcinoma and poorly differentiated adenocarcinoma of unknown primary tumor site. *Semin Oncol*. 1993;20:279-286.
55. Greco FA, Gray J, Burris 3rd HA, et al. Taxane-based chemotherapy for patients with carcinoma of unknown primary site. *Cancer J*. 2001;7:203-212.
56. Mukai H, Watanabe T, Ando M, Katsumata N. Unknown primary carcinoma: a feasibility assessment of combination chemotherapy with cisplatin and docetaxel. *Int J Clin Oncol*. 2003;8:23-25.
57. Martelli G, Pilotti S, Lepera P, et al. Fine needle aspiration cytology in superficial lymph nodes: an analysis of 266 cases. *Eur J Surg Oncol*. 1989;15:13-16.
58. Ascoli V, Taccogna S, Scalzo CC, Nardi F. Utility of cytokeratin 20 in identifying the origin of metastatic carcinomas in effusions. *Diagn Cytopathol*. 1995;12:303-308.
59. Bedrossian CW. Special stains, the old and the new: the impact of immunocytochemistry in effusion cytology. *Diagn Cytopathol*. 1998;18:141-149.
60. Bonnefoi H, Smith IE. How should cancer presenting as a malignant pleural effusion be managed? *Br J Cancer*. 1996;74:832-835.
61. DiBonito L, Falconieri G, Colautti I, et al. The positive peritoneal effusion. A retrospective study of cytopathologic diagnoses with autopsy confirmation. *Acta Cytol*. 1993;37:483-488.
62. Lai CR, Pan CC, Tsay SH. Contribution of immunocytochemistry in routine diagnostic cytology. *Diagn Cytopathol*. 1996;14:221-225.
63. Lidang Jensen M, Johansen P. Immunocytochemical staining of serous effusions: an additional method in the routine cytology practice? *Cytopathology*. 1994;5:93-103.
64. Longatto Filho A, Bisi H, Alves VA, et al. Adenocarcinoma in females detected in serous effusions. Cytomorphologic aspects and immunocytochemical reactivity to cytokeratins 7 and 20. *Acta Cytol*. 1997;41:961-971.
65. Frayling IM. Methods of molecular analysis: mutation detection in solid tumours. *Mol Pathol*. 2002;55:73-79.
66. Leader M, Collins M, Patel J, Henry K. Vimentin: an evaluation of its role as a tumour marker. *Histopathology*. 1987;11:63-72.
67. Azumi N, Battifora H. The distribution of vimentin and keratin in epithelial and nonepithelial neoplasms. A comprehensive immunohistochemical study on formalin- and alcohol-fixed tumors. *Am J Clin Pathol*. 1987;88:286-296.
68. Kurtin PJ, Pinkus GS. Leukocyte common antigen—a diagnostic discriminant between hematopoietic and nonhematopoietic neoplasms in paraffin sections using monoclonal antibodies: correlation with immunologic studies and ultrastructural localization. *Hum Pathol*. 1985;16:353-365.
69. Ries S, Barr R, LeBoit P, McCalmont T, Waldman J. Cutaneous sarcomatoid B-cell lymphoma. *Am J Dermatopathol*. 2007;29:96-98.
70. Colella G, Tirelli A, Capone R, et al. Myeloid sarcoma occurring in the maxillary gingiva: a case without leukemic manifestations. *Int J Hematol*. 2005;81:138-141.
71. Menasce LP, Banerjee SS, Beckett E, Harris M. Extra-medullary myeloid tumour (granulocytic sarcoma) is often misdiagnosed: a study of 26 cases. *Histopathology*. 1999;34:391-398.
72. Sadahira Y, Sugihara T, Yawata Y, Manabe T. Cutaneous granulocytic sarcoma mimicking immunoblastic large cell lymphoma. *Pathol Int*. 1999;49:347-353.
73. Chen J, Yanuck 3rd RR, Abbondanzo SL, et al. c-Kit (CD117) reactivity in extramedullary myeloid tumor/granulocytic sarcoma. *Arch Pathol Lab Med*. 2001;125:1448-1452.
74. Palomino-Portilla EA, Valbuena JR, Quinones-Avila Mdel P, Medeiros LJ. Myeloid sarcoma of appendix mimicking acute appendicitis. *Arch Pathol Lab Med*. 2005;129:1027-1031.
75. Roth MJ, Medeiros LJ, Elenitoba-Johnson K, et al. Extramedullary myeloid cell tumors. An immunohistochemical study of 29 cases using routinely fixed and processed paraffin-embedded tissue sections. *Arch Pathol Lab Med*. 1995;119:790-798.
76. Hudock J, Chatten J, Miettinen M. Immunohistochemical evaluation of myeloid leukemia infiltrates (granulocytic sarcomas) in formaldehyde-fixed, paraffin-embedded tissue. *Am J Clin Pathol*. 1994;102:55-60.
77. Traweek ST, Arber DA, Rappaport H, Brynes RK. Extramedullary myeloid cell tumors. An immunohistochemical and morphologic study of 28 cases. *Am J Surg Pathol*. 1993;17:1011-1019.
78. Blessing K, Sanders DS, Grant JJ. Comparison of immunohistochemical staining of the novel antibody melan-A with S100 protein and HMB-45 in malignant melanoma and melanoma variants. *Histopathology*. 1998;32:139-146.
79. DeYoung BR, Wick MR. Immunohistologic evaluation of metastatic carcinomas of unknown origin: an algorithmic approach. *Semin Diagn Pathol*. 2000;17:184-193.

80. Drlicek M, Bodenteich A, Urbanits S, Grisold W. Immunohistochemical panel of antibodies in the diagnosis of brain metastases of the unknown primary. *Pathol Res Pract.* 2004;200:727-734.
81. Drier JK, Swanson PE, Cherwitz DL, Wick MR. S100 protein immunoreactivity in poorly differentiated carcinomas. Immunohistochemical comparison with malignant melanoma. *Arch Pathol Lab Med.* 1987;111:447-452.
82. Stroup RM, Pinkus GS. S-100 immunoreactivity in primary and metastatic carcinoma of the breast: a potential source of error in immunodiagnosis. *Hum Pathol.* 1988;19:949-953.
83. Hashimoto H, Daimaru Y, Enjoji M. S-100 protein distribution in liposarcoma. An immunoperoxidase study with special reference to the distinction of liposarcoma from myxoid malignant fibrous histiocytoma. *Virchows Arch A Pathol Anat Histopathol.* 1984;405:1-10.
84. Nakajima T, Watanabe S, Sato Y, et al. An immunoperoxidase study of S-100 protein distribution in normal and neoplastic tissues. *Am J Surg Pathol.* 1982;6:715-727.
85. Miettinen M, Franssila K. Immunohistochemical spectrum of malignant melanoma. The common presence of keratins. *Lab Invest.* 1989;61:623-628.
86. Selby WL, Nance KV, Park HK. CEA immunoreactivity in metastatic malignant melanoma. *Mod Pathol.* 1992;5:415-419.
87. Zarbo RJ, Gown AM, Nagle RB, et al. Anomalous cytokeratin expression in malignant melanoma: one- and two-dimensional western blot analysis and immunohistochemical survey of 100 melanomas. *Mod Pathol.* 1990;3:494-501.
88. Laskin WB, Miettinen M. Epithelioid sarcoma: new insights based on an extended immunohistochemical analysis. *Arch Pathol Lab Med.* 2003;127:1161-1168.
89. Machen SK, Fisher C, Gautam RS, et al. Utility of cytokeratin subsets for distinguishing poorly differentiated synovial sarcoma from peripheral primitive neuroectodermal tumour. *Histopathology.* 1998;33:501-507.
90. Olsen SH, Thomas DG, Lucas DR. Cluster analysis of immunohistochemical profiles in synovial sarcoma, malignant peripheral nerve sheath tumor, and Ewing sarcoma. *Mod Pathol.* 2006;19:659-668.
91. Ordonez NG, Mahfouz SM, Mackay B. Synovial sarcoma: an immunohistochemical and ultrastructural study. *Hum Pathol.* 1990;21:733-749.
92. Sebire NJ, Gibson S, Rampling D, et al. Immunohistochemical findings in embryonal small round cell tumors with molecular diagnostic confirmation. *Appl Immunohistochem Mol Morphol.* 2005;13:1-5.
93. Folpe AL, Goldblum JR, Rubin BP, et al. Morphologic and immunophenotypic diversity in Ewing family tumors: a study of 66 genetically confirmed cases. *Am J Surg Pathol.* 2005;29:1025-1033.
94. Lazar A, Abruzzo LV, Pollock RE, et al. Molecular diagnosis of sarcomas: chromosomal translocations in sarcomas. *Arch Pathol Lab Med.* 2006;130:1199-1207.
95. Fritsch MK, Bridge JA, Schuster AE, et al. Performance characteristics of a reverse transcriptase-polymerase chain reaction assay for the detection of tumor-specific fusion transcripts from archival tissue. *Pediatr Dev Pathol.* 2003;6:43-53.
96. Scicchitano MS, Dalmas DA, Bertiaux MA, et al. Preliminary comparison of quantity, quality, and microarray performance of RNA extracted from formalin-fixed, paraffin-embedded, and unfixed frozen tissue samples. *J Histochem Cytochem.* 2006;54:1229-1237.
97. Hammar SP. Metastatic adenocarcinoma of unknown primary origin. *Hum Pathol.* 1998;29:1393-1402.
98. Spagnolo DV, Michie SA, Crabtree GS, et al. Monoclonal antikeratin (AE1) reactivity in routinely processed tissue from 166 human neoplasms. *Am J Clin Pathol.* 1985;84:697-704.
99. Al-Abbadi MA, Almasri NM, Al-Quran S, Wilkinson EJ. Cytokeratin and epithelial membrane antigen expression in angiosarcomas: an immunohistochemical study of 33 cases. *Arch Pathol Lab Med.* 2007;131:288-292.
100. Bhargava R, Shia J, Hummer AJ, et al. Distinction of endometrial stromal sarcomas from "hemangiopericytomatous" tumors using a panel of immunohistochemical stains. *Mod Pathol.* 2005;18:40-47.
101. Fuchs U, Kivela T, Summanen P, et al. An immunohistochemical and prognostic analysis of cytokeratin expression in malignant uveal melanoma. *Am J Pathol.* 1992;141:169-181.
102. Gustmann C, Altmannsberger M, Osborn M, et al. Cytokeratin expression and vimentin content in large cell anaplastic lymphomas and other non-Hodgkin's lymphomas. *Am J Pathol.* 1991;138:1413-1422.
103. Korabiowska M, Fischer G, Steinacker A, et al. Cytokeratin positivity in paraffin-embedded malignant melanomas: comparative study of KL1, A4 and Lu5 antibodies. *Anticancer Res.* 2004;24:3203-3207.
104. Srivastava A, Rosenberg AE, Selig M, et al. Keratin-positive Ewing's sarcoma: an ultrastructural study of 12 cases. *Int J Surg Pathol.* 2005;13:43-50.
105. Traweek ST, Liu J, Battifora H. Keratin gene expression in non-epithelial tissues. Detection with polymerase chain reaction. *Am J Pathol.* 1993;142:1111-1118.
106. Vakar-Lopez F, Ayala AG, Raymond AK, Czerniak B. Epithelial phenotype in Ewing's sarcoma/primitive neuroectodermal tumor. *Int J Surg Pathol.* 2000;8:59-65.
107. Miettinen M. Keratin immunohistochemistry: update of applications and pitfalls. *Pathol Annu.* 1993;28(Pt 2):113-143.
108. Moll R. Cytokeratins in the histological diagnosis of malignant tumors. *Int J Biol Markers.* 1994;9:63-69.
109. Quinlan RA, Schiller DL, Hatzfeld M, et al. Patterns of expression and organization of cytokeratin intermediate filaments. *Ann N Y Acad Sci.* 1985;455:282-306.
110. Moll R, Franke WW, Schiller DL, et al. The catalog of human cytokeratins: patterns of expression in normal epithelia, tumors and cultured cells. *Cell.* 1982;31:11-24.
111. Schaafsma HE, Ramaekers FC. Cytokeratin subtyping in normal and neoplastic epithelium: basic principles and diagnostic applications. *Pathol Annu.* 1994;29(Pt 1):21-62.
112. Romano V, Bosco P, Rocchi M, et al. Chromosomal assignments of human type I and type II cytokeratin genes to different chromosomes. *Cytogenet Cell Genet.* 1988;48:148-151.
113. Rosenberg M, Fuchs E, Le Beau MM, et al. Three epidermal and one simple epithelial type II keratin genes map to human chromosome 12. *Cytogenet Cell Genet.* 1991;57:33-38.
114. Rosenberg M, RayChaudhury A, Shows TB, et al. A group of type I keratin genes on human chromosome 17: characterization and expression. *Mol Cell Biol.* 1988;8:722-736.
115. Franke WW, Schmid E, Schiller DL, et al. Differentiation-related patterns of expression of proteins of intermediate-size filaments in tissues and cultured cells. *Cold Spring Harb Symp Quant Biol.* 1982;46(Pt 1):431-453.
116. Chu P, Wu E, Weiss LM. Cytokeratin 7 and cytokeratin 20 expression in epithelial neoplasms: a survey of 435 cases. *Mod Pathol.* 2000;13:962-972.
117. Judkins AR, Montone KT, LiVolsi VA, van de Rijn M. Sensitivity and specificity of antibodies on necrotic tumor tissue. *Am J Clin Pathol.* 1998;110:641-646.
118. Stasiak PC, Purkis PE, Leigh IM, Lane EB. Keratin 19: predicted amino acid sequence and broad tissue distribution suggest it evolved from keratinocyte keratins. *J Invest Dermatol.* 1989;92:707-716.
119. Bartek J, Bartkova J, Taylor-Papadimitriou J, et al. Differential expression of keratin 19 in normal human epithelial tissues revealed by monospecific monoclonal antibodies. *Histochem J.* 1986;18:565-575.
120. Ramaekers F, Huysmans A, Schaart G, et al. Tissue distribution of keratin 7 as monitored by a monoclonal antibody. *Exp Cell Res.* 1987;170:235-249.
121. Ramaekers F, van Niekerk C, Poels L, et al. Use of monoclonal antibodies to keratin 7 in the differential diagnosis of adenocarcinomas. *Am J Pathol.* 1990;136:641-655.
122. van Niekerk CC, Jap PH, Ramaekers FC, et al. Immunohistochemical demonstration of keratin 7 in routinely fixed paraffin-embedded human tissues. *J Pathol.* 1991;165:145-152.
123. Loy TS, Calaluce RD. Utility of cytokeratin immunostaining in separating pulmonary adenocarcinomas from colonic adenocarcinomas. *Am J Clin Pathol.* 1994;102:764-767.
124. van de Molengraft FJ, van Niekerk CC, Jap PH, Poels LG. OV-TL 12/30 (keratin 7 antibody) is a marker of glandular differentiation in lung cancer. *Histopathology.* 1993;22:35-38.
125. Berezowski K, Stastny JF, Kornstein MJ. Cytokeratins 7 and 20 and carcinoembryonic antigen in ovarian and colonic carcinoma. *Mod Pathol.* 1996;9:426-429.

126. Guerrieri C, Franlund B, Boeryd B. Expression of cytokeratin 7 in simultaneous mucinous tumors of the ovary and appendix. *Mod Pathol.* 1995;8:573-576.
127. Loy TS, Calaluce RD, Keeney GL. Cytokeratin immunostaining in differentiating primary ovarian carcinoma from metastatic colonic adenocarcinoma. *Mod Pathol.* 1996;9:1040-1044.
128. Osborn M, van Lessen G, Weber K, et al. Differential diagnosis of gastrointestinal carcinomas by using monoclonal antibodies specific for individual keratin polypeptides. *Lab Invest.* 1986;55:497-504.
129. Prayson RA, Hart WR, Petras RE. Pseudomyxoma peritonei. A clinicopathologic study of 19 cases with emphasis on site of origin and nature of associated ovarian tumors. *Am J Surg Pathol.* 1994;18:591-603.
130. Ronnett BM, Kurman RJ, Shmookler BM, et al. The morphologic spectrum of ovarian metastases of appendiceal adenocarcinomas: a clinicopathologic and immunohistochemical analysis of tumors often misinterpreted as primary ovarian tumors or metastatic tumors from other gastrointestinal sites. *Am J Surg Pathol.* 1997;21:1144-1155.
131. Ronnett BM, Shmookler BM, Diener-West M, et al. Immunohistochemical evidence supporting the appendiceal origin of pseudomyxoma peritonei in women. *Int J Gynecol Pathol.* 1997;16:1-9.
132. Ueda G, Sawada M, Ogawa H, et al. Immunohistochemical study of cytokeratin 7 for the differential diagnosis of adenocarcinomas in the ovary. *Gynecol Oncol.* 1993;51:219-223.
133. Van Eyken P, Sciot R, Brock P, et al. Abundant expression of cytokeratin 7 in fibrolamellar carcinoma of the liver. *Histopathology.* 1990;17:101-107.
134. Ramalingam P, Hart WR, Goldblum JR. Cytokeratin subset immunostaining in rectal adenocarcinoma and normal anal glands. *Arch Pathol Lab Med.* 2001;125:1074-1077.
135. Cytokeratins Tot T. 20 and 7 as biomarkers: usefulness in discriminating primary from metastatic adenocarcinoma. *Eur J Cancer.* 2002;38:758-763.
136. Moll R, Schiller DL, Franke WW. Identification of protein IT of the intestinal cytoskeleton as a novel type I cytokeratin with unusual properties and expression patterns. *J Cell Biol.* 1990;111:567-580.
137. Miettinen M. Keratinv 20: immunohistochemical marker for gastrointestinal, urothelial, and Merkel cell carcinomas. *Mod Pathol.* 1995;8:384-388.
138. Moll R, Lowe A, Laufer J, Franke WW. Cytokeratin 20 in human carcinomas. A new histodiagnostic marker detected by monoclonal antibodies. *Am J Pathol.* 1992;140:427-447.
139. Moll R, Zimbelmann R, Goldschmidt MD, et al. The human gene encoding cytokeratin 20 and its expression during fetal development and in gastrointestinal carcinomas. *Differentiation.* 1993;53:75-93.
140. Tot T. Adenocarcinomas metastatic to the liver: the value of cytokeratins 20 and 7 in the search for unknown primary tumors. *Cancer.* 1999;85:171-177.
141. Chan JK, Suster S, Wenig BM, et al. Cytokeratin 20 immunoreactivity distinguishes Merkel cell (primary cutaneous neuroendocrine) carcinomas and salivary gland small cell carcinomas from small cell carcinomas of various sites. *Am J Surg Pathol.* 1997;21:226-234.
142. Moll I, Kuhn C, Moll R. Cytokeratin 20 is a general marker of cutaneous Merkel cells while certain neuronal proteins are absent. *J Invest Dermatol.* 1995;104:910-915.
143. Goldstein NS, Thomas M. Mucinous and nonmucinous bronchioloalveolar adenocarcinomas have distinct staining patterns with thyroid transcription factor and cytokeratin 20 antibodies. *Am J Clin Pathol.* 2001;116:319-325.
144. Lau SK, Desrochers MJ, Luthringer DJ. Expression of thyroid transcription factor-1, cytokeratin 7, and cytokeratin 20 in bronchioloalveolar carcinomas: an immunohistochemical evaluation of 67 cases. *Mod Pathol.* 2002;15:538-542.
145. Rossi G, Murer B, Cavazza A, et al. Primary mucinous (so-called colloid) carcinomas of the lung: a clinicopathologic and immunohistochemical study with special reference to CDX-2 homeobox gene and MUC2 expression. *Am J Surg Pathol.* 2004;28:442-452.
146. Tot T. Patterns of distribution of cytokeratins 20 and 7 in special types of invasive breast carcinoma: a study of 123 cases. *Ann Diagn Pathol.* 1999;3:350-356.
147. Rullier A, Le Bail B, Fawaz R, et al. Cytokeratin 7 and 20 expression in cholangiocarcinomas varies along the biliary tract but still differs from that in colorectal carcinoma metastasis. *Am J Surg Pathol.* 2000;24:870-876.
148. Tot T, Samii S. The clinical relevance of cytokeratin phenotyping in needle biopsy of liver metastasis. *APMIS.* 2003;111:1075-1082.
149. Nikitakis NG, Tosios KI, Papanikolaou VS, et al. Immunohistochemical expression of cytokeratins 7 and 20 in malignant salivary gland tumors. *Mod Pathol.* 2004;17:407-415.
150. Nandedkar MA, Palazzo J, Abbondanzo SL, et al. CD45 (leukocyte common antigen) immunoreactivity in metastatic undifferentiated and neuroendocrine carcinoma: a potential diagnostic pitfall. *Mod Pathol.* 1998;11:1204-1210.
151. Gown AM, Vogel AM. Monoclonal antibodies to human intermediate filament proteins. II. Distribution of filament proteins in normal human tissues. *Am J Pathol.* 1984;114:309-321.
152. Gown AM, Vogel AM. Anti-intermediate filament monoclonal antibodies: tissue-specific tools in tumor diagnosis. *Surv Synth Pathol Res.* 1984;3:369-385.
153. Gown AM, Vogel AM. Monoclonal antibodies to human intermediate filament proteins. III. Analysis of tumors. *Am J Clin Pathol.* 1985;84:413-424.
154. Clover J, Oates J, Edwards C. Anti-cytokeratin 5/6: a positive marker for epithelioid mesothelioma. *Histopathology.* 1997;31:140-143.
155. Kaufmann O, Fietze E, Mengs J, Dietel M. Value of p63 and cytokeratin 5/6 as immunohistochemical markers for the differential diagnosis of poorly differentiated and undifferentiated carcinomas. *Am J Clin Pathol.* 2001;116:823-830.
156. Ordonez NG. Value of cytokeratin 5/6 immunostaining in distinguishing epithelial mesothelioma of the pleura from lung adenocarcinoma. *Am J Surg Pathol.* 1998;22:1215-1221.
157. Reis-Filho JS, Simpson PT, Martins A, et al. Distribution of p63, cytokeratins 5/6 and cytokeratin 14 in 51 normal and 400 neoplastic human tissue samples using TARP-4 multi-tumor tissue microarray. *Virchows Arch.* 2003;443:122-132.
158. Chu PG, Weiss LM. Expression of cytokeratin 5/6 in epithelial neoplasms: an immunohistochemical study of 509 cases. *Mod Pathol.* 2002;15:6-10.
159. Argani P, Rosai J. Hyperplastic mesothelial cells in lymph nodes: report of six cases of a benign process that can stimulate metastatic involvement by mesothelioma or carcinoma. *Hum Pathol.* 1998;29:339-346.
160. Bhargava R, Beriwal S, McManus K, Dabbs DJ. CK5 is more sensitive than CK5/6 in identifying "basal-like" phenotype of breast carcinoma. *Am J Clin Pathol.* 2008;130:724-730.
161. Litzky LA, Brooks JJ. Cytokeratin immunoreactivity in malignant fibrous histiocytoma and spindle cell tumors: comparison between frozen and paraffin-embedded tissues. *Mod Pathol.* 1992;5:30-34.
162. Miettinen M. Immunoreactivity for cytokeratin and epithelial membrane antigen in leiomyosarcoma. *Arch Pathol Lab Med.* 1988;112:637-640.
163. Miettinen M. Keratin subsets in spindle cell sarcomas. Keratins are widespread but synovial sarcoma contains a distinctive keratin polypeptide pattern and desmoplakins. *Am J Pathol.* 1991;138:505-513.
164. Rosenberg AE, O'Connell JX, Dickersin GR, Bhan AK. Expression of epithelial markers in malignant fibrous histiocytoma of the musculoskeletal system: an immunohistochemical and electron microscopic study. *Hum Pathol.* 1993;24:284-293.
165. Swanson PE. Heffalumps, jagulars, and Cheshire cats. A commentary on cytokeratins and soft tissue sarcomas. *Am J Clin Pathol.* 1991;95:S2-S7.
166. Aubry MC, Myers JL, Colby TV, et al. Endometrial stromal sarcoma metastatic to the lung: a detailed analysis of 16 patients. *Am J Surg Pathol.* 2002;26:440-449.
167. Brown DC, Theaker JM, Banks PM, et al. Cytokeratin expression in smooth muscle and smooth muscle tumours. *Histopathology.* 1987;11:477-486.

168. Eusebi V, Carcangiu ML, Dina R, Rosai J. Keratin-positive epithelioid angiosarcoma of thyroid. A report of four cases. *Am J Surg Pathol.* 1990;14:737-747.
169. Fletcher CD, Beham A, Bekir S, et al. Epithelioid angiosarcoma of deep soft tissue: a distinctive tumor readily mistaken for an epithelial neoplasm. *Am J Surg Pathol.* 1991;15:915-924.
170. Goldblum JR, Rice TW. Epithelioid angiosarcoma of the pulmonary artery. *Hum Pathol.* 1995;26:1275-1277.
171. Gown AM, Boyd HC, Chang Y, et al. Smooth muscle cells can express cytokeratins of "simple" epithelium. Immunocytochemical and biochemical studies in vitro and in vivo. *Am J Pathol.* 1988;132:223-232.
172. Hasegawa T, Fujii Y, Seki K, et al. Epithelioid angiosarcoma of bone. *Hum Pathol.* 1997;28:985-989.
173. Hirose T, Kudo E, Hasegawa T, et al. Expression of intermediate filaments in malignant fibrous histiocytomas. *Hum Pathol.* 1989;20:871-877.
174. Jochum W, Schroder S, Risti B, et al. [Cytokeratin-positive angiosarcoma of the adrenal gland]. *Pathologe.* 1994;15:181-186.
175. Knapp AC, Franke WW. Spontaneous losses of control of cytokeratin gene expression in transformed, non-epithelial human cells occurring at different levels of regulation. *Cell.* 1989;59:67-79.
176. Kwaspen FH, Smedts FM, Broos A, et al. Reproducible and highly sensitive detection of the broad spectrum epithelial marker keratin 19 in routine cancer diagnosis. *Histopathology.* 1997;31:503-516.
177. McCluggage WG, Clarke R, Toner PG. Cutaneous epithelioid angiosarcoma exhibiting cytokeratin positivity. *Histopathology.* 1995;27:291-294.
178. Meis-Kindblom JM, Kindblom LG. Angiosarcoma of soft tissue: a study of 80 cases. *Am J Surg Pathol.* 1998;22:683-697.
179. Miettinen M, Rapola J. Immunohistochemical spectrum of rhabdomyosarcoma and rhabdomyosarcoma-like tumors. Expression of cytokeratin and the 68-kD neurofilament protein. *Am J Surg Pathol.* 1989;13:120-132.
180. Rizeq MN, van de Rijn M, Hendrickson MR, Rouse RV. A comparative immunohistochemical study of uterine smooth muscle neoplasms with emphasis on the epithelioid variant. *Hum Pathol.* 1994;25:671-677.
181. Frisman DM, McCarthy WF, Schleiff P, et al. Immunocytochemistry in the differential diagnosis of effusions: use of logistic regression to select a panel of antibodies to distinguish adenocarcinomas from mesothelial proliferations. *Mod Pathol.* 1993;6:179-184.
182. Banks ER, Jansen JF, Oberle E, Davey DD. Cytokeratin positivity in fine-needle aspirates of melanomas and sarcomas. *Diagn Cytopathol.* 1995;12:230-233.
183. Gerharz CD, Moll R, Meister P, et al. Cytoskeletal heterogeneity of an epithelioid sarcoma with expression of vimentin, cytokeratins, and neurofilaments. *Am J Surg Pathol.* 1990;14:274-283.
184. Heikinheimo K, Persson S, Kindblom LG, et al. Expression of different cytokeratin subclasses in human chordoma. *J Pathol.* 1991;164:145-150.
185. Ordonez NG, Tornos C. Malignant peripheral nerve sheath tumor of the pleura with epithelial and rhabdomyoblastic differentiation: report of a case clinically simulating mesothelioma. *Am J Surg Pathol.* 1997;21:1515-1521.
186. Rosai J, Pinkus GS. Immunohistochemical demonstration of epithelial differentiation in adamantinoma of the tibia. *Am J Surg Pathol.* 1982;6:427-434.
187. Smith KJ, Skelton 3rd HG, Morgan AM, et al. Spindle cell neoplasms coexpressing cytokeratin and vimentin (metaplastic squamous cell carcinoma). *J Cutan Pathol.* 1992;19:286-293.
188. Ben-Izhak O, Stark P, Levy R, et al. Epithelial markers in malignant melanoma. A study of primary lesions and their metastases. *Am J Dermatopathol.* 1994;16:241-246.
189. Gatter KC, Ralfkiaer E, Skinner J, et al. An immunocytochemical study of malignant melanoma and its differential diagnosis from other malignant tumours. *J Clin Pathol.* 1985;38:1353-1357.
190. Mooi WJ, Deenik W, Peterse JL, Hogendoorn PC. Keratin immunoreactivity in melanoma of soft parts (clear cell sarcoma). *Histopathology.* 1995;27:61-65.
191. Kriho VK, Yang HY, Moskal JR, Skalli O. Keratin expression in astrocytomas: an immunofluorescent and biochemical reassessment. *Virchows Arch.* 1997;431:139-147.
192. Cosgrove M, Fitzgibbons PL, Sherrod A, et al. Intermediate filament expression in astrocytic neoplasms. *Am J Surg Pathol.* 1989;13:141-145.
193. Artlich A, Schmidt D. Immunohistochemical profile of meningiomas and their histological subtypes. *Hum Pathol.* 1990;21:843-849.
194. Meis JM, Ordonez NG, BrunerMeningiomas JM. An immunohistochemical study of 50 cases. *Arch Pathol Lab Med.* 1986;110:934-937.
195. Probst-Cousin S, Villagran-Lillo R, Lahl R, et al. Secretory meningioma: clinical, histologic, and immunohistochemical findings in 31 cases. *Cancer.* 1997;79:2003-2015.
196. Radley MG, di Sant'Agnese PA, Eskin TA, Wilbur DC. Epithelial differentiation in meningiomas. An immunohistochemical, histochemical, and ultrastructural study—with review of the literature. *Am J Clin Pathol.* 1989;92:266-272.
197. Carbone A, Manconi R, Poletti A, Volpe R. Heterogeneous immunostaining patterns of follicular dendritic reticulum cells in human lymphoid tissue with selected antibodies reactive with different cell lineages. *Hum Pathol.* 1988;19:51-56.
198. Cho J, Gong G, Choe G, et al. Extrafollicular reticulum cells in pathologic lymph nodes. *J Korean Med Sci.* 1994;9:9-15.
199. Doglioni C, Dell'Orto P, Zanetti G, et al. Cytokeratin-immunoreactive cells of human lymph nodes and spleen in normal and pathological conditions. An immunocytochemical study. *Virchows Arch A Pathol Anat Histopathol.* 1990;416:479-490.
200. Franke WW, Moll R. Cytoskeletal components of lymphoid organs. I. Synthesis of cytokeratins 8 and 18 and desmin in subpopulations of extrafollicular reticulum cells of human lymph nodes, tonsils, and spleen. *Differentiation.* 1987;36:145-163.
201. Gould VE, Bloom KJ, Franke WW, et al. Increased numbers of cytokeratin-positive interstitial reticulum cells (CIRC) in reactive, inflammatory and neoplastic lymphadenopathies: hyperplasia or induced expression? *Virchows Arch.* 1995;425:617-629.
202. Iuzzolino P, Bontempini L, Doglioni C, Zanetti G. Keratin immunoreactivity in extrafollicular reticular cells of the lymph node. *Am J Clin Pathol.* 1989;91:239-240.
203. Lasota J, Hyjek E, Koo CH, et al. Cytokeratin-positive large-cell lymphomas of B-cell lineage. A study of five phenotypically unusual cases verified by polymerase chain reaction. *Am J Surg Pathol.* 1996;20:346-354.
204. Ramaekers F, Haag D, Jap P, Vooijs PG. Immunochemical demonstration of keratin and vimentin in cytologic aspirates. *Acta Cytol.* 1984;28:385-392.
205. Zoltowska A. Immunohistochemical comparative investigations of lymphatic tissue in reactive processes, myasthenic thymuses and Hodgkin's disease. *Arch Immunol Ther Exp (Warsz).* 1995;43:15-22.
206. Xu X, Roberts SA, Pasha TL, Zhang PJ. Undesirable cytokeratin immunoreactivity of native nonepithelial cells in sentinel lymph nodes from patients with breast carcinoma. *Arch Pathol Lab Med.* 2000;124:1310-1313.
207. Battifora H, Kopinski M. The influence of protease digestion and duration of fixation on the immunostaining of keratins. A comparison of formalin and ethanol fixation. *J Histochem Cytochem.* 1986;34:1095-1100.
208. Delsol G, Al Saati T, Gatter KC, et al. Coexpression of epithelial membrane antigen (EMA), Ki-1, and interleukin-2 receptor by anaplastic large cell lymphomas. Diagnostic value in so-called malignant histiocytosis. *Am J Pathol.* 1988;130:59-70.
209. Frierson Jr HF, Bellafiore FJ, Gaffey MJ, et al. Cytokeratin in anaplastic large cell lymphoma. *Mod Pathol.* 1994;7:317-321.
210. Petruch UR, Horny HP, Kaiserling E. Frequent expression of haemopoietic and non-haemopoietic antigens by neoplastic plasma cells: an immunohistochemical study using formalin-fixed, paraffin-embedded tissue. *Histopathology.* 1992;20:35-40.
211. Wotherspoon AC, Norton AJ, Isaacson PG. Immunoreactive cytokeratins in plasmacytomas. *Histopathology.* 1989;14:141-150.

212. Miettinen M. Immunostaining of intermediate filament proteins in paraffin sections. Evaluation of optimal protease treatment to improve the immunoreactivity. *Pathol Res Pract.* 1989;184:431-436.
213. Battifora H. Assessment of antigen damage in immunohistochemistry. The vimentin internal control. *Am J Clin Pathol.* 1991;96:669-671.
214. Ramaekers FC, Haag D, Kant A, et al. Coexpression of keratin- and vimentin-type intermediate filaments in human metastatic carcinoma cells. *Proc Natl Acad Sci U S A.* 1983;80:2618-2622.
215. Geisinger KR, Dabbs DJ, Marshall RB. Malignant mixed müllerian tumors. An ultrastructural and immunohistochemical analysis with histogenetic considerations. *Cancer.* 1987;59:1781-1790.
216. Livasy CA, Karaca G, Nanda R, et al. Phenotypic evaluation of the basal-like subtype of invasive breast carcinoma. *Mod Pathol.* 2006;19:264-271.
217. McNutt MA, Bolen JW, Gown AM, et al. Coexpression of intermediate filaments in human epithelial neoplasms. *Ultrastruct Pathol.* 1985;9:31-43.
218. Dabbs DJ, Geisinger KR, Norris HT. Intermediate filaments in endometrial and endocervical carcinomas. The diagnostic utility of vimentin patterns. *Am J Surg Pathol.* 1986;10:568-576.
219. Dabbs DJ, Sturtz K, Zaino RJ. The immunohistochemical discrimination of endometrioid adenocarcinomas. *Hum Pathol.* 1996;27:172-177.
220. Jones MW, Onisko A, Dabbs DJ, et al. The value of immunohistochemistry in distinction between endocervical adenocarcinoma and adenocarcinoma of endometrium, endometrioid type. A comparative tissue microarray study of 76 cases. International Academy of Pathology. 2008; XXVII International Congress:Abstract.
221. Buchegger F, Schreyer M, Carrel S, Mach JP. Monoclonal antibodies identify a CEA crossreacting antigen of 95 kD (NCA-95) distinct in antigenicity and tissue distribution from the previously described NCA of 55 kD. *Int J Cancer.* 1984;33:643-649.
222. Nagura H, Tsutsumi Y, Watanabe K, et al. Immunohistochemistry of carcinoembryonic antigen, secretory component and lysozyme in benign and malignant common bile duct tissues. *Virchows Arch A Pathol Anat Histopathol.* 1984;403:271-280.
223. Svenberg T. Carcinoembryonic antigen-like substances of human bile. Isolation and partial characterization. *Int J Cancer.* 1976;17:588-596.
224. Chedid A, Chejfec G, Eichorst M, et al. Antigenic markers of hepatocellular carcinoma. *Cancer.* 1990;65:84-87.
225. Ferrandez-Izquierdo A, Llombart-Bosch A. Immunohistochemical characterization of 130 cases of primary hepatic carcinomas. *Pathol Res Pract.* 1987;182:783-791.
226. Maeda T, Kajiyama K, Adachi E, et al. The expression of cytokeratins 7, 19, and 20 in primary and metastatic carcinomas of the liver. *Mod Pathol.* 1996;9:901-909.
227. Ronnett BM, Kurman RJ, Zahn CM, et al. Pseudomyxoma peritonei in women: a clinicopathologic analysis of 30 cases with emphasis on site of origin, prognosis, and relationship to ovarian mucinous tumors of low malignant potential. *Hum Pathol.* 1995;26:509-524.
228. Sheahan K, O'Brien MJ, Burke B, et al. Differential reactivities of carcinoembryonic antigen (CEA) and CEA-related monoclonal and polyclonal antibodies in common epithelial malignancies. *Am J Clin Pathol.* 1990;94:157-164.
229. Balaton AJ, Nehama-Sibony M, Gotheil C, et al. Distinction between hepatocellular carcinoma, cholangiocarcinoma, and metastatic carcinoma based on immunohistochemical staining for carcinoembryonic antigen and for cytokeratin 19 on paraffin sections. *J Pathol.* 1988;156:305-310.
230. Ma CK, Zarbo RJ, Frierson Jr HF, Lee MW. Comparative immunohistochemical study of primary and metastatic carcinomas of the liver. *Am J Clin Pathol.* 1993;99:551-557.
231. Van Eyken P, Sciot R, Paterson A, et al. Cytokeratin expression in hepatocellular carcinoma: an immunohistochemical study. *Hum Pathol.* 1988;19:562-568.
232. Cui S, Hano H, Sakata A, et al. Enhanced CD34 expression of sinusoid-like vascular endothelial cells in hepatocellular carcinoma. *Pathol Int.* 1996;46:751-756.
233. Hilkens J, Buijs F, Hilgers J, et al. Monoclonal antibodies against human milk-fat globule membranes detecting differentiation antigens of the mammary gland and its tumors. *Int J Cancer.* 1984;34:197-206.
234. McGuckin MA, Walsh MD, Hohn BG, et al. Prognostic significance of MUC1 epithelial mucin expression in breast cancer. *Hum Pathol.* 1995;26:432-439.
235. Hilkens J, Ligtenberg MJ, Vos HL, Litvinov SV. Cell membrane-associated mucins and their adhesion-modulating property. *Trends Biochem Sci.* 1992;17:359-363.
236. Gatter KC, Alcock C, Heryet A, Mason DY. Clinical importance of analysing malignant tumours of uncertain origin with immunohistological techniques. *Lancet.* 1985;1:1302-1305.
237. Pinkus GS, Etheridge CL, O'Connor EM. Are keratin proteins a better tumor marker than epithelial membrane antigen? A comparative immunohistochemical study of various paraffin-embedded neoplasms using monoclonal and polyclonal antibodies. *Am J Clin Pathol.* 1986;85:269-277.
238. Gendler S, Taylor-Papadimitriou J, Duhig T, et al. A highly immunogenic region of a human polymorphic epithelial mucin expressed by carcinomas is made up of tandem repeats. *J Biol Chem.* 1988;263:12820-12823.
239. Hayes DF, Zurawski Jr VR, Kufe DW. Comparison of circulating CA15-3 and carcinoembryonic antigen levels in patients with breast cancer. *J Clin Oncol.* 1986;4:1542-1550.
240. Hilkens J, Buijs F. Biosynthesis of MAM-6, an epithelial sialomucin. Evidence for involvement of a rare proteolytic cleavage step in the endoplasmic reticulum. *J Biol Chem.* 1988;263:4215-4222.
241. Hilkens J, Buijs F, Ligtenberg M. Complexity of MAM-6, an epithelial sialomucin associated with carcinomas. *Cancer Res.* 1989;49:786-793.
242. Kufe D, Inghirami G, Abe M, et al. Differential reactivity of a novel monoclonal antibody (DF3) with human malignant versus benign breast tumors. *Hybridoma.* 1984;3:223-232.
243. Peterson JA, Couto JR, Taylor MR, Ceriani RL. Selection of tumor-specific epitopes on target antigens for radioimmunotherapy of breast cancer. *Cancer Res.* 1995;55:5847s-5851s.
244. Peterson JA, Zava DT, Duwe AK, et al. Biochemical and histological characterization of antigens preferentially expressed on the surface and cytoplasm of breast carcinoma cells identified by monoclonal antibodies against the human milk fat globule. *Hybridoma.* 1990;9:221-235.
245. al-Nafussi A, Carder PJ. Monoclonal antibodies in the cytodiagnosis of serous effusions. *Cytopathology.* 1990;1:119-128.
246. Leong AS, Parkinson R, Milios J. "Thick" cell membranes revealed by immunocytochemical staining: a clue to the diagnosis of mesothelioma. *Diagn Cytopathol.* 1990;6:9-13.
247. Singh HK, Silverman JF, Berns L, et al. Significance of epithelial membrane antigen in the work-up of problematic serous effusions. *Diagn Cytopathol.* 1995;13:3-7.
248. Al Saati T, Caveriviere P, Gorguet B, et al. Epithelial membrane antigen in hematopoietic neoplasms. *Hum Pathol.* 1986;17:533-534.
249. Chittal SM, Caveriviere P, Schwarting R, et al. Monoclonal antibodies in the diagnosis of Hodgkin's disease. The search for a rational panel. *Am J Surg Pathol.* 1988;12:9-21.
250. Chittal SM, Delsol G. The interface of Hodgkin's disease and anaplastic large cell lymphoma. *Cancer Surv.* 1997;30:87-105.
251. Delsol G, Gatter KC, Stein H, et al. Human lymphoid cells express epithelial membrane antigen. Implications for diagnosis of human neoplasms. *Lancet.* 1984;2:1124-1129.
252. Fujimoto J, Hata J, Ishii E, et al. Ki-1 lymphomas in childhood: immunohistochemical analysis and the significance of epithelial membrane antigen (EMA) as a new marker. *Virchows Arch A Pathol Anat Histopathol.* 1988;412:307-314.
253. Gatter KC, Abdulaziz Z, Beverley P, et al. Use of monoclonal antibodies for the histopathological diagnosis of human malignancy. *J Clin Pathol.* 1982;35:1253-1267.
254. Hall PA, d'Ardenne AJ, Stansfeld AG. Paraffin section immunohistochemistry. I. Non-Hodgkin's lymphoma. *Histopathology.* 1988;13:149-160.
255. Sarker AB, Akagi T, Yoshino T, et al. Expression of vimentin and epithelial membrane antigen in human malignant lymphomas. *Acta Pathol Jpn.* 1990;40:581-587.

256. Stein H, Hansmann ML, Lennert K, et al. Reed-Sternberg and Hodgkin cells in lymphocyte-predominant Hodgkin's disease of nodular subtype contain J chain. *Am J Clin Pathol.* 1986;86:292-297.
257. Strickler JG, Weiss LM, Copenhaver CM, et al. Monoclonal antibodies reactive in routinely processed tissue sections of malignant lymphoma, with emphasis on T-cell lymphomas. *Hum Pathol.* 1987;18:808-814.
258. Thomas P, Battifora H. Keratins versus epithelial membrane antigen in tumor diagnosis: an immunohistochemical comparison of five monoclonal antibodies. *Hum Pathol.* 1987;18:728-734.
259. Shek TW, Yuen ST, Luk IS, Wong MP. Germ cell tumour as a diagnostic pitfall of metastatic carcinoma. *J Clin Pathol.* 1996;49:223-225.
260. Ordonez NG. Value of the MOC-31 monoclonal antibody in differentiating epithelial pleural mesothelioma from lung adenocarcinoma. *Hum Pathol.* 1998;29:166-169.
261. Ordonez NG. Value of the Ber-EP4 antibody in differentiating epithelial pleural mesothelioma from adenocarcinoma. The M.D. Anderson experience and a critical review of the literature. *Am J Clin Pathol.* 1998;109:85-89.
262. Riera JR, Astengo-Osuna C, Longmate JA, Battifora H. The immunohistochemical diagnostic panel for epithelial mesothelioma: a reevaluation after heat-induced epitope retrieval. *Am J Surg Pathol.* 1997;21:1409-1419.
263. Rossen K, Thomsen HK. Ber-EP4 immunoreactivity depends on the germ layer origin and maturity of the squamous epithelium. *Histopathology.* 2001;39:386-389.
264. Yaziji H, Battifora H, Barry TS, et al. Evaluation of 12 antibodies for distinguishing epithelioid mesothelioma from adenocarcinoma: identification of a three-antibody immunohistochemical panel with maximal sensitivity and specificity. *Mod Pathol.* 2006;19:514-523.
265. Morrison C, Marsh Jr W, Frankel WL. A comparison of CD10 to pCEA, MOC-31, and hepatocyte for the distinction of malignant tumors in the liver. *Mod Pathol.* 2002;15:1279-1287.
266. Porcell AI, De Young BR, Proca DM, Frankel WL. Immunohistochemical analysis of hepatocellular and adenocarcinoma in the liver: MOC31 compares favorably with other putative markers. *Mod Pathol.* 2000;13:773-778.
267. Siddiqui MT, Saboorian MH, Gokaslan ST, Ashfaq R. Diagnostic utility of the HepPar1 antibody to differentiate hepatocellular carcinoma from metastatic carcinoma in fine-needle aspiration samples. *Cancer.* 2002;96:49-52.
268. Wiedenmann B, Kuhn C, Schwechheimer K, et al. Synaptophysin identified in metastases of neuroendocrine tumors by immunocytochemistry and immunoblotting. *Am J Clin Pathol.* 1987;88:560-569.
269. Wilson BS, Lloyd RV. Detection of chromogranin in neuroendocrine cells with a monoclonal antibody. *Am J Pathol.* 1984;115:458-468.
270. DeStephano DB, Lloyd RV, Pike AM, Wilson BS. Pituitary adenomas. An immunohistochemical study of hormone production and chromogranin localization. *Am J Pathol.* 1984;116:464-472.
271. Lloyd RV, Mervak T, Schmidt K, et al. Immunohistochemical detection of chromogranin and neuron-specific enolase in pancreatic endocrine neoplasms. *Am J Surg Pathol.* 1984;8:607-614.
272. Lloyd RV, Wilson BS. Specific endocrine tissue marker defined by a monoclonal antibody. *Science.* 1983;222:628-630.
273. Wiedenmann B, Franke WW. Identification and localization of synaptophysin, an integral membrane glycoprotein of Mr 38,000 characteristic of presynaptic vesicles. *Cell.* 1985;41:1017-1028.
274. Thomas L, Hartung K, Langosch D, et al. Identification of synaptophysin as a hexameric channel protein of the synaptic vesicle membrane. *Science.* 1988;242:1050-1053.
275. Piehl MR, Gould VE, Warren WH, et al. Immunohistochemical identification of exocrine and neuroendocrine subsets of large cell lung carcinomas. *Pathol Res Pract.* 1988;183:675-682.
276. Staren ED, Gould VE, Warren WH, et al. Neuroendocrine carcinomas of the colon and rectum: a clinicopathologic evaluation. *Surgery.* 1988;104:1080-1089.
277. Guinee Jr DG, Fishback NF, Koss MN, et al. The spectrum of immunohistochemical staining of small-cell lung carcinoma in specimens from transbronchial and open-lung biopsies. *Am J Clin Pathol.* 1994;102:406-414.
278. Kayser K, Schmid W, Ebert W, Wiedenmann B. Expression of neuroendocrine markers (neuronspecific enolase, synaptophysin and bombesin) in carcinoma of the lung. *Pathol Res Pract.* 1988;183:412-417.
279. Abo T, Balch CM. A differentiation antigen of human NK and K cells identified by a monoclonal antibody (HNK-1). *J Immunol.* 1981;127:1024-1029.
280. Baylin SB, Jackson RD, Goodwin G, Gazdar AF. Neuroendocrine-related biochemistry in the spectrum of human lung cancers. *Exp Lung Res.* 1982;3:209-223.
281. Caillaud JM, Benjelloun S, Bosq J, et al. HNK-1-defined antigen detected in paraffin-embedded neuroectoderm tumors and those derived from cells of the amine precursor uptake and decarboxylation system. *Cancer Res.* 1984;44:4432-4439.
282. Cole SP, Mirski S, McGarry RC, et al. Differential expression of the Leu-7 antigen on human lung tumor cells. *Cancer Res.* 1985;45:4285-4290.
283. Shioda Y, Nagura H, Tsutsumi Y, et al. Distribution of Leu 7 (HNK-1) antigen in human digestive organs: an immunohistochemical study with monoclonal antibody. *Histochem J.* 1984;16:843-854.
284. Battifora H, Silva EG. The use of antikeratin antibodies in the immunohistochemical distinction between neuroendocrine (Merkel cell) carcinoma of the skin, lymphoma, and oat cell carcinoma. *Cancer.* 1986;58:1040-1046.
285. Osborn M, Dirk T, Kaser H, et al. Immunohistochemical localization of neurofilaments and neuron-specific enolase in 29 cases of neuroblastoma. *Am J Pathol.* 1986;122:433-442.
286. Tsokos M, Linnoila RI, Chandra RS, Triche TJ. Neuron-specific enolase in the diagnosis of neuroblastoma and other small, round-cell tumors in children. *Hum Pathol.* 1984;15:575-584.
287. Vinores SA, Bonnin JM, Rubinstein LJ, Marangos PJ. Immunohistochemical demonstration of neuron-specific enolase in neoplasms of the CNS and other tissues. *Arch Pathol Lab Med.* 1984;108:536-540.
288. Nicholson SA, McDermott MB, Swanson PE, Wick MR. CD99 and cytokeratin-20 in small-cell and basaloid tumors of the skin. *Appl Immunohistochem Mol Morphol.* 2000;8:37-41.
289. Jiang C, Tan Y, Li E. [Histopathological and immunohistochemical studies on medullary thyroid carcinoma]. *Zhonghua Bing Li Xue Za Zhi.* 1996;25:332-335.
290. Kargi A, Yorukoglu Aktas S, et al. Neuroendocrine differentiation in non-neuroendocrine thyroid carcinoma. *Thyroid.* 1996;6:207-210.
291. Kovacs CS, Mase RM, Kovacs K, et al. Thyroid medullary carcinoma with thyroglobulin immunoreactivity in sporadic multiple endocrine neoplasia type 2-B. *Cancer.* 1994;74:928-932.
292. Ruck P, Horny HP, Greschniok A, et al. Nonspecific immunostaining of blast cells of acute leukemia by antibodies against nonhemopoietic antigens. *Hematol Pathol.* 1995;9:49-56.
293. Bejarano PA, Baughman RP, Biddinger PW, et al. Surfactant proteins and thyroid transcription factor-1 in pulmonary and breast carcinomas. *Mod Pathol.* 1996;9:445-452.
294. Di Loreto C, Di Lauro V, Puglisi F, et al. Immunocytochemical expression of tissue specific transcription factor-1 in lung carcinoma. *J Clin Pathol.* 1997;50:30-32.
295. Di Loreto C, Puglisi F, Di Lauro V, et al. TTF-1 protein expression in pleural malignant mesotheliomas and adenocarcinomas of the lung. *Cancer Lett.* 1998;124:73-78.
296. Fabbro D, Di Loreto C, Stamerra O, et al. TTF-1 gene expression in human lung tumours. *Eur J Cancer.* 1996;32A:512-517.
297. Lazzaro D, Price M, de Felice M, Di Lauro R. The transcription factor TTF-1 is expressed at the onset of thyroid and lung morphogenesis and in restricted regions of the foetal brain. *Development.* 1991;113:1093-1104.
298. Stahlman MT, Gray ME, Whitsett JA. Expression of thyroid transcription factor-1(TTF-1) in fetal and neonatal human lung. *J Histochem Cytochem.* 1996;44:673-678.
299. Guazzi S, Price M, De Felice M, et al. Thyroid nuclear factor 1 (TTF-1) contains a homeodomain and displays a novel DNA binding specificity. *Embo J.* 1990;9:3631-3639.
300. Folpe AL, Gown AM, Lamps LW, et al. Thyroid transcription factor-1: immunohistochemical evaluation in pulmonary neuroendocrine tumors. *Mod Pathol.* 1999;12:5-8.

301. Holzinger A, Dingle S, Bejarano PA, et al. Monoclonal antibody to thyroid transcription factor-1: production, characterization, and usefulness in tumor diagnosis. *Hybridoma*. 1996;15:49-53.
302. Khoor A, Whitsett JA, Stahlman MT, et al. Utility of surfactant protein B precursor and thyroid transcription factor 1 in differentiating adenocarcinoma of the lung from malignant mesothelioma. *Hum Pathol*. 1999;30:695-700.
303. Kaufmann O, Dietel M. Expression of thyroid transcription factor-1 in pulmonary and extrapulmonary small cell carcinomas and other neuroendocrine carcinomas of various primary sites. *Histopathology*. 2000;36:415-420.
304. Ordonez NG. Value of thyroid transcription factor-1 immunostaining in distinguishing small cell lung carcinomas from other small cell carcinomas. *Am J Surg Pathol*. 2000;24:1217-1223.
305. Agoff SN, Lamps LW, Philip AT, et al. Thyroid transcription factor-1 is expressed in extrapulmonary small cell carcinomas but not in other extrapulmonary neuroendocrine tumors. *Mod Pathol*. 2000;13:238-242.
306. Afify AM, al-Khafaji BM. Diagnostic utility of thyroid transcription factor-1 expression in adenocarcinomas presenting in serous fluids. *Acta Cytol*. 2002;46:675-678.
307. Jang KY, Kang MJ, Lee DG, Chung MJ. Utility of thyroid transcription factor-1 and cytokeratin 7 and 20 immunostaining in the identification of origin in malignant effusions. *Anal Quant Cytol Histol*. 2001;23:400-404.
308. Roh MS, Hong SH. Utility of thyroid transcription factor-1 and cytokeratin 20 in identifying the origin of metastatic carcinomas of cervical lymph nodes. *J Korean Med Sci*. 2002;17:512-517.
309. Chang YL, Lee YC, Liao WY, Wu CT. The utility and limitation of thyroid transcription factor-1 protein in primary and metastatic pulmonary neoplasms. *Lung Cancer*. 2004;44:149-157.
310. Wieczorek TJ, Pinkus JL, Glickman JN, Pinkus GS. Comparison of thyroid transcription factor-1 and hepatocyte antigen immunohistochemical analysis in the differential diagnosis of hepatocellular carcinoma, metastatic adenocarcinoma, renal cell carcinoma, and adrenal cortical carcinoma. *Am J Clin Pathol*. 2002;118:911-921.
311. Kubba LA, McCluggage WG, Liu J, et al. Thyroid transcription factor-1 expression in ovarian epithelial neoplasms. *Mod Pathol*. 2008;21:485-490.
312. Siami K, McCluggage WG, Ordonez NG, et al. Thyroid transcription factor-1 expression in endometrial and endocervical adenocarcinomas. *Am J Surg Pathol*. 2007;31:1759-1763.
313. Andressen C, Blumcke I, Celio MR. Calcium-binding proteins: selective markers of nerve cells. *Cell Tissue Res*. 1993;271:181-208.
314. Doglioni C, Tos AP, Laurino L, et al. Calretinin: a novel immunocytochemical marker for mesothelioma. *Am J Surg Pathol*. 1996;20:1037-1046.
315. Ordonez NG. Value of calretinin immunostaining in differentiating epithelial mesothelioma from lung adenocarcinoma. *Mod Pathol*. 1998;11:929-933.
316. Ordonez NG. The immunohistochemical diagnosis of mesothelioma: a comparative study of epithelioid mesothelioma and lung adenocarcinoma. *Am J Surg Pathol*. 2003;27:1031-1051.
317. Pritchard-Jones K, Fleming S, Davidson D, et al. The candidate Wilms' tumour gene is involved in genitourinary development. *Nature*. 1990;346:194-197.
318. Shimizu M, Toki T, Takagi Y, et al. Immunohistochemical detection of the Wilms' tumor gene (WT1) in epithelial ovarian tumors. *Int J Gynecol Pathol*. 2000;19:158-163.
319. Waldstrom M, Grove A. Immunohistochemical expression of wilms tumor gene protein in different histologic subtypes of ovarian carcinomas. *Arch Pathol Lab Med*. 2005;129:85-88.
320. Acs G, Pasha T, Zhang PJ. WT1 is differentially expressed in serous, endometrioid, clear cell, and mucinous carcinomas of the peritoneum, fallopian tube, ovary, and endometrium. *Int J Gynecol Pathol*. 2004;23:110-118.
321. Al-Hussaini M, Stockman A, Foster H, McCluggage WG. WT-1 assists in distinguishing ovarian from uterine serous carcinoma and in distinguishing between serous and endometrioid ovarian carcinoma. *Histopathology*. 2004;44:109-115.
322. Dupont J, Wang X, Marshall DS, et al. Wilms Tumor Gene (WT1) and p53 expression in endometrial carcinomas: a study of 130 cases using a tissue microarray. *Gynecol Oncol*. 2004;94:449-455.
323. Egan JA, Ionescu MC, Eapen E, et al. Differential expression of WT1 and p53 in serous and endometrioid carcinomas of the endometrium. *Int J Gynecol Pathol*. 2004;23:119-122.
324. Goldstein NS, Uzieblo A. WT1 immunoreactivity in uterine papillary serous carcinomas is different from ovarian serous carcinomas. *Am J Clin Pathol*. 2002;117:541-545.
325. Hashi A, Yuminamochi T, Murata S, et al. Wilms tumor gene immunoreactivity in primary serous carcinomas of the fallopian tube, ovary, endometrium, and peritoneum. *Int J Gynecol Pathol*. 2003;22:374-377.
326. Domfeh AB, Carley AL, Striebel JM, et al. WT1 immunoreactivity in breast carcinoma: selective expression in pure and mixed mucinous subtypes. *Mod Pathol*. 2008;21:1217-1223.
327. Pearlman WH, Gueriguian JL, Sawyer ME. A specific progesterone-binding component of human breast cyst fluid. *J Biol Chem*. 1973;248:5736-5741.
328. Haagensen Jr DE, Mazoujian G, Holder Jr WD, et al. Evaluation of a breast cyst fluid protein detectable in the plasma of breast carcinoma patients. *Ann Surg*. 1977;185:279-285.
329. Murphy LC, Lee-Wing M, Goldenberg GJ, Shiu RP. Expression of the gene encoding a prolactin-inducible protein by human breast cancers in vivo: correlation with steroid receptor status. *Cancer Res*. 1987;47:4160-4164.
330. Eusebi V, Magalhaes F, Azzopardi JG. Pleomorphic lobular carcinoma of the breast: an aggressive tumor showing apocrine differentiation. *Hum Pathol*. 1992;23:655-662.
331. Mazoujian G, Parish TH, Haagensen Jr DE. Immunoperoxidase localization of GCDFP-15 with mouse monoclonal antibodies versus rabbit antiserum. *J Histochem Cytochem*. 1988;36:377-382.
332. Mazoujian G, Margolis R. Immunohistochemistry of gross cystic disease fluid protein (GCDFP-15) in 65 benign sweat gland tumors of the skin. *Am J Dermatopathol*. 1988;10:28-35.
333. Mazoujian G, Pinkus GS, Davis S, Haagensen Jr DE. Immunohistochemistry of a gross cystic disease fluid protein (GCDFP-15) of the breast. A marker of apocrine epithelium and breast carcinomas with apocrine features. *Am J Pathol*. 1983;110:105-112.
334. Swanson PE, Pettinato G, Lillemoe TJ, Wick MR. Gross cystic disease fluid protein-15 in salivary gland tumors. *Arch Pathol Lab Med*. 1991;115:158-163.
335. Viacava P, Naccarato AG, Bevilacqua G. Spectrum of GCDFP-15 expression in human fetal and adult normal tissues. *Virchows Arch*. 1998;432:255-260.
336. Wick MR, Lillemoe TJ, Copland GT, et al. Gross cystic disease fluid protein-15 as a marker for breast cancer: immunohistochemical analysis of 690 human neoplasms and comparison with alpha-lactalbumin. *Hum Pathol*. 1989;20:281-287.
337. Bhargava R, Beriwal S, Dabbs DJ. Mammaglobin vs GCDFP-15: an immunohistologic validation survey for sensitivity and specificity. *Am J Clin Pathol*. 2007;127:103-113.
338. Kaufmann O, Deidesheimer T, Muehlenberg M, et al. Immunohistochemical differentiation of metastatic breast carcinomas from metastatic adenocarcinomas of other common primary sites. *Histopathology*. 1996;29:233-240.
339. Raab SS, Berg LC, Swanson PE, Wick MR. Adenocarcinoma in the lung in patients with breast cancer. A prospective analysis of the discriminatory value of immunohistology. *Am J Clin Pathol*. 1993;100:27-35.
340. Striebel JM, Dacic S, Yousem SA. Gross cystic disease fluid protein-(GCDFP-15): expression in primary lung adenocarcinoma. *Am J Surg Pathol*. 2008;32:426-432.
341. Han JH, Kang Y, Shin HC, et al. Mammaglobin expression in lymph nodes is an important marker of metastatic breast carcinoma. *Arch Pathol Lab Med*. 2003;127:1330-1334.
342. Ciampa A, Fanger G, Khan A, et al. Mammaglobin and CRxA-01 in pleural effusion cytology: potential utility of distinguishing metastatic breast carcinomas from other cytokeratin 7-positive/cytokeratin 20-negative carcinomas. *Cancer*. 2004;102:368-372.
343. Sasaki E, Tsunoda N, Hatanaka Y, et al. Breast-specific expression of MGB1/mammaglobin: an examination of 480 tumors from various organs and clinicopathological analysis of MGB1-positive breast cancers. *Mod Pathol*. 2007;20:208-214.

344. Onuma K, Dabbs DJ, Bhargava R. Mammaglobin expression in the female genital tract: immunohistochemical analysis in benign and neoplastic endocervix and endometrium. *Int J Gynecol Pathol.* 2008;27:418-425.
345. Beattie CW, Hansen NW, Thomas PA. Steroid receptors in human lung cancer. *Cancer Res.* 1985;45:4206-4214.
346. Cagle PT, Mody DR, Schwartz MR. Estrogen and progesterone receptors in bronchogenic carcinoma. *Cancer Res.* 1990;50:6632-6635.
347. Kaiser U, Hofmann J, Schilli M, et al. Steroid-hormone receptors in cell lines and tumor biopsies of human lung cancer. *Int J Cancer.* 1996;67:357-364.
348. Su JM, Hsu HK, Chang H, et al. Expression of estrogen and progesterone receptors in non-small-cell lung cancer: immunohistochemical study. *Anticancer Res.* 1996;16:3803-3806.
349. Vargas SO, Leslie KO, Vacek PM, et al. Estrogen-receptor-related protein p29 in primary nonsmall cell lung carcinoma: pathologic and prognostic correlations. *Cancer.* 1998;82:1495-1500.
350. Dabbs DJ, Landreneau RJ, Liu Y, et al. Detection of estrogen receptor by immunohistochemistry in pulmonary adenocarcinoma. *Ann Thorac Surg.* 2002;73:403-405; discussion 406.
351. Tot T. The role of cytokeratins 20 and 7 and estrogen receptor analysis in separation of metastatic lobular carcinoma of the breast and metastatic signet ring cell carcinoma of the gastrointestinal tract. *APMIS.* 2000;108:467-472.
352. Bacchi CE, Gown AM. Distribution and pattern of expression of villin, a gastrointestinal-associated cytoskeletal protein, in human carcinomas: a study employing paraffin-embedded tissue. *Lab Invest.* 1991;64:418-424.
353. Nambu Y, Iannettoni MD, Orringer MB, Beer DG. Unique expression patterns and alterations in the intestinal protein villin in primary and metastatic pulmonary adenocarcinomas. *Mol Carcinog.* 1998;23:234-242.
354. Sharma S, Tan J, Sidhu G, et al. Lung adenocarcinomas metastatic to the brain with and without ultrastructural evidence of rootlets: an electron microscopic and immunohistochemical study using cytokeratins 7 and 20 and villin. *Ultrastruct Pathol.* 1998;22:385-391.
355. Tan J, Sidhu G, Greco MA, et al. Villin, cytokeratin 7, and cytokeratin 20 expression in pulmonary adenocarcinoma with ultrastructural evidence of microvilli with rootlets. *Hum Pathol.* 1998;29:390-396.
356. Lau SK, Prakash S, Geller SA, Alsabeh R. Comparative immunohistochemical profile of hepatocellular carcinoma, cholangiocarcinoma, and metastatic adenocarcinoma. *Hum Pathol.* 2002;33:1175-1181.
357. Drummond F, Putt W, Fox M, Edwards YH. Cloning and chromosome assignment of the human CDX2 gene. *Ann Hum Genet.* 1997;61:393-400.
358. Beck F, Chawengsaksophak K, Waring P, et al. Reprogramming of intestinal differentiation and intercalary regeneration in Cdx2 mutant mice. *Proc Natl Acad Sci U S A.* 1999;96:7318-7323.
359. Chawengsaksophak K, James R, Hammond VE, et al. Homeosis and intestinal tumours in Cdx2 mutant mice. *Nature.* 1997;386:84-87.
360. Mallo GV, Rechreche H, Frigerio JM, et al. Molecular cloning, sequencing and expression of the mRNA encoding human Cdx1 and Cdx2 homeobox. Down-regulation of Cdx1 and Cdx2 mRNA expression during colorectal carcinogenesis. *Int J Cancer.* 1997;74:35-44.
361. Tamai Y, Nakajima R, Ishikawa T, et al. Colonic hamartoma development by anomalous duplication in Cdx2 knockout mice. *Cancer Res.* 1999;59:2965-2970.
362. Barbareschi M, Murer B, Colby TV, et al. CDX-2 homeobox gene expression is a reliable marker of colorectal adenocarcinoma metastases to the lungs. *Am J Surg Pathol.* 2003;27:141-149.
363. Bai YQ, Yamamoto H, Akiyama Y, et al. Ectopic expression of homeodomain protein CDX2 in intestinal metaplasia and carcinomas of the stomach. *Cancer Lett.* 2002;176:47-55.
364. Werling RW, Yaziji H, Bacchi CE, Gown AM. CDX2, a highly sensitive and specific marker of adenocarcinomas of intestinal origin: an immunohistochemical survey of 476 primary and metastatic carcinomas. *Am J Surg Pathol.* 2003;27:303-310.
365. Hinoi T, Tani M, Lucas PC, et al. Loss of CDX2 expression and microsatellite instability are prominent features of large cell minimally differentiated carcinomas of the colon. *Am J Pathol.* 2001;159:2239-2248.
366. Barbareschi M, Roldo C, Zamboni G, et al. CDX-2 homeobox gene product expression in neuroendocrine tumors: its role as a marker of intestinal neuroendocrine tumors. *Am J Surg Pathol.* 2004;28:1169-1176.
367. Wang HL, Lu DW, Yerian LM, et al. Immunohistochemical distinction between primary adenocarcinoma of the bladder and secondary colorectal adenocarcinoma. *Am J Surg Pathol.* 2001;25:1380-1387.
368. Raspollini MR, Baroni G, Taddei A, Taddei GL. Primary cervical adenocarcinoma with intestinal differentiation and colonic carcinoma metastatic to cervix: an investigation using Cdx-2 and a limited immunohistochemical panel. *Arch Pathol Lab Med.* 2003;127:1586-1590.
369. McCluggage WG, Shah R, Connolly LE, McBride HA. Intestinal-type cervical adenocarcinoma in situ and adenocarcinoma exhibit a partial enteric immunophenotype with consistent expression of CDX2. *Int J Gynecol Pathol.* 2008;27:92-100.
370. Park KJ, Bramlage MP, Ellenson LH, Pirog EC. Immunoprofile of adenocarcinomas of the endometrium, endocervix, and ovary with mucinous differentiation. *Appl Immunohistochem Mol Morphol.* 2008.
371. Sullivan LM, Smolkin ME, Frierson Jr HF, Galgano MT. Comprehensive evaluation of CDX2 in invasive cervical adenocarcinomas: immunopositivity in the absence of overt colorectal morphology. *Am J Surg Pathol.* 2008; 32:1715-1720.
372. Tot T. Identifying colorectal metastases in liver biopsies: the novel CDX2 antibody is less specific than the cytokeratin 20+/7-phenotype. *Med Sci Monit.* 2004;10:BR139-BR143.
373. Wennerberg AE, Nalesnik MA, Coleman WB. Hepatocyte paraffin 1: a monoclonal antibody that reacts with hepatocytes and can be used for differential diagnosis of hepatic tumors. *Am J Pathol.* 1993;143:1050-1054.
374. Chu PG, Ishizawa S, Wu E, Weiss LM. Hepatocyte antigen as a marker of hepatocellular carcinoma: an immunohistochemical comparison to carcinoembryonic antigen, CD10, and alpha-fetoprotein. *Am J Surg Pathol.* 2002;26:978-988.
375. Fan Z, van de Rijn M, Montgomery K, Rouse RV. Hep par 1 antibody stain for the differential diagnosis of hepatocellular carcinoma: 676 tumors tested using tissue microarrays and conventional tissue sections. *Mod Pathol.* 2003;16:137-144.
376. Kakar S, Muir T, Murphy LM, et al. Immunoreactivity of Hep Par 1 in hepatic and extrahepatic tumors and its correlation with albumin in situ hybridization in hepatocellular carcinoma. *Am J Clin Pathol.* 2003;119:361-366.
377. Ishikura H, Fukasawa Y, Ogasawara K, et al. An AFP-producing gastric carcinoma with features of hepatic differentiation. A case report. *Cancer.* 1985;56:840-848.
378. Sinard J, Macleay Jr L, Melamed J. Hepatoid adenocarcinoma in the urinary bladder. Unusual localization of a newly recognized tumor type. *Cancer.* 1994;73:1919-1925.
379. Pitman MB, Triratanachat S, Young RH, Oliva E. Hepatocyte paraffin 1 antibody does not distinguish primary ovarian tumors with hepatoid differentiation from metastatic hepatocellular carcinoma. *Int J Gynecol Pathol.* 2004;23:58-64.
380. Chu PG, Weiss LM. Immunohistochemical characterization of signet-ring cell carcinomas of the stomach, breast, and colon. *Am J Clin Pathol.* 2004;121:884-892.
381. Hahn SA, Schutte M, Hoque AT, et al. DPC4, a candidate tumor suppressor gene at human chromosome 18q21.1. *Science.* 1996;271:350-353.
382. Ji H, Isacson C, Seidman JD, et al. Cytokeratins 7 and 20, Dpc4, and MUC5AC in the distinction of metastatic mucinous carcinomas in the ovary from primary ovarian mucinous tumors: Dpc4 assists in identifying metastatic pancreatic carcinomas. *Int J Gynecol Pathol.* 2002;21:391-400.
383. McCarthy DM, Hruban RH, Argani P, et al. Role of the DPC4 tumor suppressor gene in adenocarcinoma of the ampulla of Vater: analysis of 140 cases. *Mod Pathol.* 2003;16:272-278.
384. Parwani AV, Geradts J, Caspers E, et al. Immunohistochemical and genetic analysis of non-small cell and small cell gallbladder carcinoma and their precursor lesions. *Mod Pathol.* 2003;16:299-308.

385. Svrcek M, Jourdan F, Sebbagh N, et al. Immunohistochemical analysis of adenocarcinoma of the small intestine: a tissue microarray study. *J Clin Pathol.* 2003;56:898-903.
386. Lowe FC, Trauzzi SJ. Prostatic acid phosphatase in 1993. Its limited clinical utility. *Urol Clin North Am.* 1993;20:589-595.
387. Alanen KA, Kuopio T, Koskinen PJ, Nevalainen TJ. Immunohistochemical labelling for prostate specific antigen in nonprostatic tissues. *Pathol Res Pract.* 1996;192:233-237.
388. Bostwick DG. Prostate-specific antigen. Current role in diagnostic pathology of prostate cancer. *Am J Clin Pathol.* 1994;102:S31-S37.
389. Elgamal AA, Van de Voorde W, Van Poppel H, et al. Immunohistochemical localization of prostate-specific markers within the accessory male sex glands of Cowper, Littre, and Morgagni. *Urology.* 1994;44:84-90.
390. Frazier HA, Humphrey PA, Burchette JL, Paulson DF. Immunoreactive prostatic specific antigen in male periurethral glands. *J Urol.* 1992;147:246-248.
391. Golz R, Schubert GE. Prostatic specific antigen: immunoreactivity in urachal remnants. *J Urol.* 1989;141:1480-1482.
392. Kamoshida S, Tsutsumi Y. Extraprostatic localization of prostatic acid phosphatase and prostate-specific antigen: distribution in cloacogenic glandular epithelium and sex-dependent expression in human anal gland. *Hum Pathol.* 1990;21:1108-1111.
393. Nowels K, Kent E, Rinsho K, Oyasu R. Prostate specific antigen and acid phosphatase-reactive cells in cystitis cystica and glandularis. *Arch Pathol Lab Med.* 1988;112:734-737.
394. van Krieken JH. Prostate marker immunoreactivity in salivary gland neoplasms. A rare pitfall in immunohistochemistry. *Am J Surg Pathol.* 1993;17:410-414.
395. Kuriyama M, Wang MC, Lee CL, et al. Multiple marker evaluation in human prostate cancer with the use of tissue-specific antigens. *J Natl Cancer Inst.* 1982;68:99-105.
396. Nadji M, Tabei SZ, Castro A, et al. Prostatic origin of tumors. An immunohistochemical study. *Am J Clin Pathol.* 1980;73:735-739.
397. Lee SS. Endometrioid adenocarcinoma of the prostate: a clinicopathologic and immunohistochemical study. *J Surg Oncol.* 1994;55:235-238.
398. Leong FJ, Leong AS, Swift J. Signet-ring carcinoma of the prostate. *Pathol Res Pract.* 1996;192:1232-1238; discussion 1239–1241.
399. Millar EK, Sharma NK, Lessells AM. Ductal (endometrioid) adenocarcinoma of the prostate: a clinicopathological study of 16 cases. *Histopathology.* 1996;29:11-19.
400. Esteban JM, Battifora H. Tumor immunophenotype: comparison between primary neoplasm and its metastases. *Mod Pathol.* 1990;3:192-197.
401. Kramer SA, Farnham R, Glenn JF, Paulson DF. Comparative morphology of primary and secondary deposits of prostatic adenocarcinoma. *Cancer.* 1981;48:271-273.
402. Bodey B, Bodey Jr B, Kaiser HE. Immunocytochemical detection of prostate specific antigen expression in human primary and metastatic melanomas. *Anticancer Res.* 1997;17:2343-2346.
403. Fan CY, Wang J, Barnes EL. Expression of androgen receptor and prostatic specific markers in salivary duct carcinoma: an immunohistochemical analysis of 13 cases and review of the literature. *Am J Surg Pathol.* 2000;24:579-586.
404. Beach R, Gown AM, De Peralta-Venturina MN, et al. P504S immunohistochemical detection in 405 prostatic specimens including 376 18-gauge needle biopsies. *Am J Surg Pathol.* 2002;26:1588-1596.
405. Chan TY, Mikolajczyk SD, Lecksell K, et al. Immunohistochemical staining of prostate cancer with monoclonal antibodies to the precursor of prostate-specific antigen. *Urology.* 2003;62:177-181.
406. Horoszewicz JS, Kawinski E, Murphy GP. Monoclonal antibodies to a new antigenic marker in epithelial prostatic cells and serum of prostatic cancer patients. *Anticancer Res.* 1987;7:927-935.
407. Murphy GP, Elgamal AA, Su SL, et al. Current evaluation of the tissue localization and diagnostic utility of prostate specific membrane antigen. *Cancer.* 1998;83:2259-2269.
408. Silver DA, Pellicer I, Fair WR, et al. Prostate-specific membrane antigen expression in normal and malignant human tissues. *Clin Cancer Res.* 1997;3:81-85.
409. Murphy GP, Barren RJ, Erickson SJ, et al. Evaluation and comparison of two new prostate carcinoma markers. Free-prostate specific antigen and prostate specific membrane antigen. *Cancer.* 1996;78:809-818.
410. Troyer JK, Beckett ML, Wright Jr GL. Location of prostate-specific membrane antigen in the LNCaP prostate carcinoma cell line. *Prostate.* 1997;30:232-242.
411. Murphy GP, Tino WT, Holmes EH, et al. Measurement of prostate-specific membrane antigen in the serum with a new antibody. *Prostate.* 1996;28:266-271.
412. Zhou M, Chinnaiyan AM, Kleer CG, et al. Alpha-Methylacyl-CoA racemase: a novel tumor marker over-expressed in several human cancers and their precursor lesions. *Am J Surg Pathol.* 2002;26:926-931.
413. Jiang Z, Fanger GR, Woda BA, et al. Expression of alpha-methylacyl-CoA racemase (P504s) in various malignant neoplasms and normal tissues: astudy of 761 cases. *Hum Pathol.* 2003;34:792-796.
414. Moll R, Wu XR, Lin JH, Sun TT. Uroplakins, specific membrane proteins of urothelial umbrella cells, as histological markers of metastatic transitional cell carcinomas. *Am J Pathol.* 1995;147:1383-1397.
415. Wu RL, Osman I, Wu XR, et al. Uroplakin II gene is expressed in transitional cell carcinoma but not in bilharzial bladder squamous cell carcinoma: alternative pathways of bladder epithelial differentiation and tumor formation. *Cancer Res.* 1998;58:1291-1297.
416. Parker DC, Folpe AL, Bell J, et al. Potential utility of uroplakin III, thrombomodulin, high molecular weight cytokeratin, and cytokeratin 20 in noninvasive, invasive, and metastatic urothelial (transitional cell) carcinomas. *Am J Surg Pathol.* 2003;27:1-10.
417. Appleton MA, Attanoos RL, Jasani B. Thrombomodulin as a marker of vascular and lymphatic tumours. *Histopathology.* 1996;29:153-157.
418. Yonezawa S, Maruyama I, Sakae K, et al. Thrombomodulin as a marker for vascular tumors. Comparative study with factor VIII and Ulex europaeus I lectin. *Am J Clin Pathol.* 1987;88:405-411.
419. Lager DJ, Callaghan EJ, Worth SF, et al. Cellular localization of thrombomodulin in human epithelium and squamous malignancies. *Am J Pathol.* 1995;146:933-943.
420. Kushitani K, Takeshima Y, Amatya VJ, et al. Immunohistochemical marker panels for distinguishing between epithelioid mesothelioma and lung adenocarcinoma. *Pathol Int.* 2007;57:190-199.
421. Jiang J, Ulbright TM, Younger C, et al. Cytokeratin 7 and cytokeratin 20 in primary urinary bladder carcinoma and matched lymph node metastasis. *Arch Pathol Lab Med.* 2001;125:921-923.
422. Langner C, Ratschek M, Tsybrovskyy O, et al. P63 immunoreactivity distinguishes upper urinary tract transitional-cell carcinoma and renal-cell carcinoma even in poorly differentiated tumors. *J Histochem Cytochem.* 2003;51:1097-1099.
423. Ordonez NG. Value of thrombomodulin immunostaining in the diagnosis of mesothelioma. *Histopathology.* 1997;31:25-30.
424. Logani S, Oliva E, Amin MB, et al. Immunoprofile of ovarian tumors with putative transitional cell (urothelial) differentiation using novel urothelial markers: histogenetic and diagnostic implications. *Am J Surg Pathol.* 2003;27:1434-1441.
425. Mhawech P, Uchida T, Pelte MF. Immunohistochemical profile of high-grade urothelial bladder carcinoma and prostate adenocarcinoma. *Hum Pathol.* 2002;33:1136-1140.
426. Ordonez NG. Transitional cell carcinomas of the ovary and bladder are immunophenotypically different. *Histopathology.* 2000;36:433-438.
427. Yoshida SO, Imam A. Monoclonal antibody to a proximal nephrogenic renal antigen: immunohistochemical analysis of formalin-fixed, paraffin-embedded human renal cell carcinomas. *Cancer Res.* 1989;49:1802-1809.
428. McGregor DK, Khurana KK, Cao C, et al. Diagnosing primary and metastatic renal cell carcinoma: the use of the monoclonal antibody "Renal Cell Carcinoma Marker." *Am J Surg Pathol.* 2001;25:1485-1492.
429. Bakshi N, Kunju LP, Giordano T, Shah RB. Expression of renal cell carcinoma antigen (RCC) in renal epithelial and nonrenal tumors: diagnostic implications. *Appl Immunohistochem Mol Morphol.* 2007;15:310-315.
430. Chu P, Arber DA. Paraffin-section detection of CD10 in 505 nonhematopoietic neoplasms. Frequent expression in renal cell carcinoma and endometrial stromal sarcoma. *Am J Clin Pathol.* 2000;113:374-382.

431. Tellier AL, Amiel J, Delezoide AL, et al. Expression of the PAX2 gene in human embryos and exclusion in the CHARGE syndrome. *Am J Med Genet.* 2000;93:85-88.
432. Mazal PR, Stichenwirth M, Koller A, et al. Expression of aquaporins and PAX-2 compared to CD10 and cytokeratin 7 in renal neoplasms: a tissue microarray study. *Mod Pathol.* 2005;18:535-540.
433. Memeo L, Jhang J, Assaad AM, et al. Immunohistochemical analysis for cytokeratin 7, KIT, and PAX2: value in the differential diagnosis of chromophobe cell carcinoma. *Am J Clin Pathol.* 2007;127:225-229.
434. Tong GX, Chiriboga L, Hamele-Bena D, Borczuk AC. Expression of PAX2 in papillary serous carcinoma of the ovary: immunohistochemical evidence of fallopian tube or secondary Müllerian system origin? *Mod Pathol.* 2007;20:856-863.
435. Avery AK, Beckstead J, Renshaw AA, Corless CL. Use of antibodies to RCC and CD10 in the differential diagnosis of renal neoplasms. *Am J Surg Pathol.* 2000;24:203-210.
436. Cameron RI, Ashe P, O'Rourke DM, et al. A panel of immunohistochemical stains assists in the distinction between ovarian and renal clear cell carcinoma. *Int J Gynecol Pathol.* 2003;22:272-276.
437. Fetsch PA, Powers CN, Zakowski MF, Abati A. Anti-alpha-inhibin: marker of choice for the consistent distinction between adrenocortical carcinoma and renal cell carcinoma in fine-needle aspiration. *Cancer.* 1999;87:168-172.
438. Ghorab Z, Jorda M, Ganjei P, Nadji M, Melan A. (A103) is expressed in adrenocortical neoplasms but not in renal cell and hepatocellular carcinomas. *Appl Immunohistochem Mol Morphol.* 2003;11:330-333.
439. Murakata LA, Ishak KG, Nzeako UC. Clear cell carcinoma of the liver: a comparative immunohistochemical study with renal clear cell carcinoma. *Mod Pathol.* 2000;13:874-881.
440. Meunier H, Rivier C, Evans RM, Vale W. Gonadal and extragonadal expression of inhibin alpha, beta A, and beta B subunits in various tissues predicts diverse functions. *Proc Natl Acad Sci U S A.* 1988;85:247-251.
441. Busam KJ, Iversen K, Coplan KA, et al. Immunoreactivity for A103, an antibody to melan-A (Mart-1), in adrenocortical and other steroid tumors. *Am J Surg Pathol.* 1998;22:57-63.
442. Busam KJ, Jungbluth AA. Melan-A, a new melanocytic differentiation marker. *Adv Anat Pathol.* 1999;6:12-18.
443. Hofbauer GF, Kamarashev J, Geertsen R, et al. Melan A/MART-1 immunoreactivity in formalin-fixed paraffin-embedded primary and metastatic melanoma: frequency and distribution. *Melanoma Res.* 1998;8:337-343.
444. Jungbluth AA, Busam KJ, Gerald WL, et al. A103: An anti-melan-a monoclonal antibody for the detection of malignant melanoma in paraffin-embedded tissues. *Am J Surg Pathol.* 1998;22:595-602.
445. Renshaw AA, Granter SR. A comparison of A103 and inhibin reactivity in adrenal cortical tumors: distinction from hepatocellular carcinoma and renal tumors. *Mod Pathol.* 1998;11:1160-1164.
446. Loy TS, Phillips RW, Linder CL. A103 immunostaining in the diagnosis of adrenal cortical tumors: an immunohistochemical study of 316 cases. *Arch Pathol Lab Med.* 2002;126:170-172.
447. Shin SJ, Hoda RS, Ying L, DeLellis RA. Diagnostic utility of the monoclonal antibody A103 in fine-needle aspiration biopsies of the adrenal. *Am J Clin Pathol.* 2000;113:295-302.
448. Sasano H, Shizawa S, Suzuki T, et al. Transcription factor adrenal 4 binding protein as a marker of adrenocortical malignancy. *Hum Pathol.* 1995;26:1154-1156.
449. Sasano H, Suzuki T, Moriya T. Recent advances in histopathology and immunohistochemistry of adrenocortical carcinoma. *Endocr Pathol.* 2006;17:345-354.
450. Fogel M, Lifschitz-Mercer B, Moll R, et al. Heterogeneity of intermediate filament expression in human testicular seminomas. *Differentiation.* 1990;45:242-249.
451. Giwercman A, Andrews PW, Jorgensen N, et al. Immunohistochemical expression of embryonal marker TRA-1-60 in carcinoma in situ and germ cell tumors of the testis. *Cancer.* 1993;72:1308-1314.
452. Giwercman A, Marks A, Bailey D, et al. A monoclonal antibody as a marker for carcinoma in situ germ cells of the human adult testis. *APMIS.* 1988;96:667-670.
453. Jacobsen GK, Norgaard-Pedersen B. Placental alkaline phosphatase in testicular germ cell tumours and in carcinoma-in-situ of the testis. An immunohistochemical study. *Acta Pathol Microbiol Immunol Scand [A].* 1984;92:323-329.
454. Burke AP, Mostofi FK. Placental alkaline phosphatase immunohistochemistry of intratubular malignant germ cells and associated testicular germ cell tumors. *Hum Pathol.* 1988;19:663-670.
455. Cummings OW, Ulbright TM, Eble JN, Roth LM. Spermatocytic seminoma: an immunohistochemical study. *Hum Pathol.* 1994;25:54-59.
456. Bailey D, Marks A, Stratis M, Baumal R. Immunohistochemical staining of germ cell tumors and intratubular malignant germ cells of the testis using antibody to placental alkaline phosphatase and a monoclonal anti-seminoma antibody. *Mod Pathol.* 1991;4:167-171.
457. Hustin J, Collette J, Franchimont P. Immunohistochemical demonstration of placental alkaline phosphatase in various states of testicular development and in germ cell tumours. *Int J Androl.* 1987;10:29-35.
458. Niehans GA, Manivel JC, Copland GT, et al. Immunohistochemistry of germ cell and trophoblastic neoplasms. *Cancer.* 1988;62:1113-1123.
459. Uchida T, Shimoda T, Miyata H, et al. Immunoperoxidase study of alkaline phosphatase in testicular tumor. *Cancer.* 1981;48:1455-1462.
460. Wick MR, Swanson PE, Manivel JC. Placental-like alkaline phosphatase reactivity in human tumors: an immunohistochemical study of 520 cases. *Hum Pathol.* 1987;18:946-954.
461. Watanabe H, Tokuyama H, Ohta H, et al. Expression of placental alkaline phosphatase in gastric and colorectal cancers. An immunohistochemical study using the prepared monoclonal antibody. *Cancer.* 1990;66:2575-2582.
462. Mostofi FK, Sesterhenn IA, Davis Jr CJ. Immunopathology of germ cell tumors of the testis. *Semin Diagn Pathol.* 1987;4:320-341.
463. Eglen DE, Ulbright TM. The differential diagnosis of yolk sac tumor and seminoma. Usefulness of cytokeratin, alpha-fetoprotein, and alpha-1-antitrypsin immunoperoxidase reactions. *Am J Clin Pathol.* 1987;88:328-332.
464. Jacobsen GK, Jacobsen M. Alpha-fetoprotein (AFP) and human chorionic gonadotropin (HCG) in testicular germ cell tumours. A prospective immunohistochemical study. *Acta Pathol Microbiol Immunol Scand [A].* 1983;91:165-176.
465. Cheng L, Thomas A, Roth LM, et al. OCT4: a novel biomarker for dysgerminoma of the ovary. *Am J Surg Pathol.* 2004;28:1341-1346.
466. Hattab EM, Tu PH, Wilson JD, Cheng L. OCT4 immunohistochemistry is superior to placental alkaline phosphatase (PLAP) in the diagnosis of central nervous system germinoma. *Am J Surg Pathol.* 2005;29:368-371.
467. Jones TD, Ulbright TM, Eble JN, et al. OCT4 staining in testicular tumors: a sensitive and specific marker for seminoma and embryonal carcinoma. *Am J Surg Pathol.* 2004;28:935-940.
468. Miettinen M, Lasota JKIT. (CD117): a review on expression in normal and neoplastic tissues, and mutations and their clinicopathologic correlation. *Appl Immunohistochem Mol Morphol.* 2005;13:205-220.
469. Miettinen M, Sobin LH, Sarlomo-Rikala M. Immunohistochemical spectrum of GISTs at different sites and their differential diagnosis with a reference to CD117 (KIT). *Mod Pathol.* 2000;13:1134-1142.
470. Al-Shamkhani A. The role of CD30 in the pathogenesis of haematopoietic malignancies. *Curr Opin Pharmacol.* 2004;4:355-359.
471. Grammatico D, Grignon DJ, Eberwein P, et al. Transitional cell carcinoma of the renal pelvis with choriocarcinomatous differentiation. Immunohistochemical and immunoelectron microscopic assessment of human chorionic gonadotropin production by transitional cell carcinoma of the urinary bladder. *Cancer.* 1993;71:1835-1841.
472. Hishima T, Fukayama M, Fujisawa M, et al. CD5 expression in thymic carcinoma. *Am J Pathol.* 1994;145:268-275.
473. Berezowski K, Grimes MM, Gal A, Kornstein MJ. CD5 immunoreactivity of epithelial cells in thymic carcinoma and CASTLE using paraffin-embedded tissue. *Am J Clin Pathol.* 1996;106:483-486.

474. Dorfman DM, Shahsafaei A, Chan JK. Thymic carcinomas, but not thymomas and carcinomas of other sites, show CD5 immunoreactivity. *Am J Surg Pathol.* 1997;21:936-940.
475. Kornstein MJ, Rosai J. CD5 labeling of thymic carcinomas and other nonlymphoid neoplasms. *Am J Clin Pathol.* 1998;109:722-726.
476. Tateyama H, Eimoto T, Tada T, et al. Immunoreactivity of a new CD5 antibody with normal epithelium and malignant tumors including thymic carcinoma. *Am J Clin Pathol.* 1999;111:235-240.
477. Kuo TT, Chan JK. Thymic carcinoma arising in thymoma is associated with alterations in immunohistochemical profile. *Am J Surg Pathol.* 1998;22:1474-1481.
478. Suster S, Moran CA. Spindle cell thymic carcinoma: clinicopathologic and immunohistochemical study of a distinctive variant of primary thymic epithelial neoplasm. *Am J Surg Pathol.* 1999;23:691-700.
479. Hammar SP. Macroscopic, histologic, histochemical, immunohistochemical, and ultrastructural features of mesothelioma. *Ultrastruct Pathol.* 2006;30:3-17.
480. Kodama T, Watanabe S, Sato Y, et al. An immunohistochemical study of thymic epithelial tumors. I. Epithelial component. *Am J Surg Pathol.* 1986;10:26-33.
481. Fukai I, Masaoka A, Hashimoto T, et al. The distribution of epithelial membrane antigen in thymic epithelial neoplasms. *Cancer.* 1992;70:2077-2081.
482. Truong LD, Mody DR, Cagle PT, et al. Thymic carcinoma. A clinicopathologic study of 13 cases. *Am J Surg Pathol.* 1990;14:151-166.
483. Chan JK, Tsang WY, Seneviratne S, Pau MY. The MIC2 antibody 013. Practical application for the study of thymic epithelial tumors. *Am J Surg Pathol.* 1995;19:1115-1123.
484. Pomplun S, Wotherspoon AC, Shah G, et al. Immunohistochemical markers in the differentiation of thymic and pulmonary neoplasms. *Histopathology.* 2002;40:152-158.
485. Bejarano PA, Nikiforov YE, Swenson ES, Biddinger PW. Thyroid transcription factor-1, thyroglobulin, cytokeratin 7, and cytokeratin 20 in thyroid neoplasms. *Appl Immunohistochem Mol Morphol.* 2000;8:189-194.
486. Ordonez NG, El-Naggar AK, Hickey RC, Samaan NA. Anaplastic thyroid carcinoma. Immunocytochemical study of 32 cases. *Am J Clin Pathol.* 1991;96:15-24.
487. Nonaka D, Tang Y, Chiriboga L, et al. Diagnostic utility of thyroid transcription factors Pax8 and TTF-2 (FoxE1) in thyroid epithelial neoplasms. *Mod Pathol.* 2008;21:192-200.
488. Weidner N. Germ-cell tumors of the mediastinum. *Semin Diagn Pathol.* 1999;16:42-50.
489. Suster S, Moran CA. Applications and limitations of immunohistochemistry in the diagnosis of malignant mesothelioma. *Adv Anat Pathol.* 2006;13:316-329.
490. Cossu-Rocca P, Jones TD, Roth LM, et al. Cytokeratin and CD30 expression in dysgerminoma. *Hum Pathol.* 2006;37:1015-1021.
491. Moran CA, Suster S, Przygodzki RM, Koss MN. Primary germ cell tumors of the mediastinum: II. Mediastinal seminomas—a clinicopathologic and immunohistochemical study of 120 cases. *Cancer.* 1997;80:691-698.
492. Ulbright TM. Germ cell tumors of the gonads: a selective review emphasizing problems in differential diagnosis, newly appreciated, and controversial issues. *Mod Pathol.* 2005;18(Suppl 2):S61-S79.
493. Cheng L. Establishing a germ cell origin for metastatic tumors using OCT4 immunohistochemistry. *Cancer.* 2004;101:2006-2010.
494. Sung MT, Jones TD, Beck SD, et al. OCT4 is superior to CD30 in the diagnosis of metastatic embryonal carcinomas after chemotherapy. *Hum Pathol.* 2006;37:662-667.
495. Bosl GJ, Ilson DH, Rodriguez E, et al. Clinical relevance of the i(12p) marker chromosome in germ cell tumors. *J Natl Cancer Inst.* 1994;86:349-355.
496. Kernek KM, Brunelli M, Ulbright TM, et al. Fluorescence in situ hybridization analysis of chromosome 12p in paraffin-embedded tissue is useful for establishing germ cell origin of metastatic tumors. *Mod Pathol.* 2004;17:1309-1313.
497. Elishaev E, Gilks CB, Miller D, et al. Synchronous and metachronous endocervical and ovarian neoplasms: evidence supporting interpretation of the ovarian neoplasms as metastatic endocervical adenocarcinomas simulating primary ovarian surface epithelial neoplasms. *Am J Surg Pathol.* 2005;29:281-294.
498. Nonaka D, Kusamura S, Baratti D, et al. CDX-2 expression in pseudomyxoma peritonei: a clinicopathological study of 42 cases. *Histopathology.* 2006;49:381-387.
499. Baker PM, Oliva E. Immunohistochemistry as a tool in the differential diagnosis of ovarian tumors: an update. *Int J Gynecol Pathol.* 2005;24:39-55.
500. Deavers MT, Malpica A, Liu J, et al. Ovarian sex cord-stromal tumors: an immunohistochemical study including a comparison of calretinin and inhibin. *Mod Pathol.* 2003;16:584-590.
501. McCluggage WG, Young RH. Immunohistochemistry as a diagnostic aid in the evaluation of ovarian tumors. *Semin Diagn Pathol.* 2005;22:3-32.
502. Ashikari R, Park K, Huvos AG, Urban JA. Paget disease of the breast. *Cancer.* 1970;26:680-685.
503. Kister SJ, Haagensen CD. Paget disease of the breast. *Am J Surg.* 1970;119:606-609.
504. Salvadori B, Fariselli G, Saccozzi R. Analysis of 100 cases of Paget disease of the breast. *Tumori.* 1976;62:529-535.
505. Lundquist K, Kohler S, Rouse RV. Intraepidermal cytokeratin 7 expression is not restricted to Paget cells but is also seen in Toker cells and Merkel cells. *Am J Surg Pathol.* 1999;23:212-219.
506. Yao DX, Hoda SA, Chiu A, et al. Intraepidermal cytokeratin 7 immunoreactive cells in the non-neoplastic nipple may represent interepithelial extension of lactiferous duct cells. *Histopathology.* 2002;40:230-236.
507. Tani EM, Skoog L. Immunocytochemical detection of estrogen receptors in mammary Paget cells. *Acta Cytol.* 1988;32:825-828.
508. Meissner K, Riviere A, Haupt G, Loning T. Study of neu-protein expression in mammary Paget disease with and without underlying breast carcinoma and in extramammary Paget disease. *Am J Pathol.* 1990;137:1305-1309.
509. Ramaswamy S, Tamayo P, Rifkin R, et al. Multiclass cancer diagnosis using tumor gene expression signatures. *Proc Natl Acad Sci U S A.* 2001;98:15149-15154.
510. Bloom G, Yang IV, Boulware D, et al. Multi-platform, multi-site, microarray-based human tumor classification. *Am J Pathol.* 2004;164:9-16.
511. Buckhaults P, Zhang Z, Chen YC, et al. Identifying tumor origin using a gene expression-based classification map. *Cancer Res.* 2003;63:4144-4149.
512. Shedden KA, Taylor JM, Giordano TJ, et al. Accurate molecular classification of human cancers based on gene expression using a simple classifier with a pathological tree-based framework. *Am J Pathol.* 2003;163:1985-1995.
513. Talantov D, Baden J, Jatkoe T, et al. A quantitative reverse transcriptase-polymerase chain reaction assay to identify metastatic carcinoma tissue of origin. *J Mol Diagn.* 2006;8:320-329.
514. Tothill RW, Kowalczyk A, Rischin D, et al. An expression-based site of origin diagnostic method designed for clinical application to cancer of unknown origin. *Cancer Res.* 2005;65:4031-4040.
515. Ma XJ, Patel R, Wang X, et al. Molecular classification of human cancers using a 92-gene real-time quantitative polymerase chain reaction assay. *Arch Pathol Lab Med.* 2006;130:465-473.
516. Horlings HM, Warmoes MO, Kerst JM, et al. Successful classification of metastatic carcinoma of known primary using the CUPPRINT. *J Clin Oncol (Meeting Abstracts).* 2006;24:20028.
517. Monzon FA, Dumur CI, Lyons-Weiler M, et al. Validation of a gene expression-based tissue of origin test applied to poorly differentiated and undifferentiated cancers. *Association for Molecular Pathology.* 2007; Annual Meeting:Abstract.
518. Dumur CI, Lyons-Weiler M, Sciulli C, et al. Interlaboratory performance of a microarray-based gene expression test to determine tissue of origin in poorly differentiated and undifferentiated cancers. *J Mol Diagn.* 2008;10:67-77.
519. Landgraf P, Rusu M, Sheridan R, et al. A mammalian microRNA expression atlas based on small RNA library sequencing. *Cell.* 2007;129:1401-1414.
520. Lu J, Getz G, Miska EA, et al. MircoRNA expression profiles classify human cancers. *Nature.* 2005;435:834-838.
521. Rosenfeld N, Aharonov R, Meiri E, et al. MicroRNAs accurately identify cancer tissue origin. *Nat Biotechnol.* 2008;26:426-469.

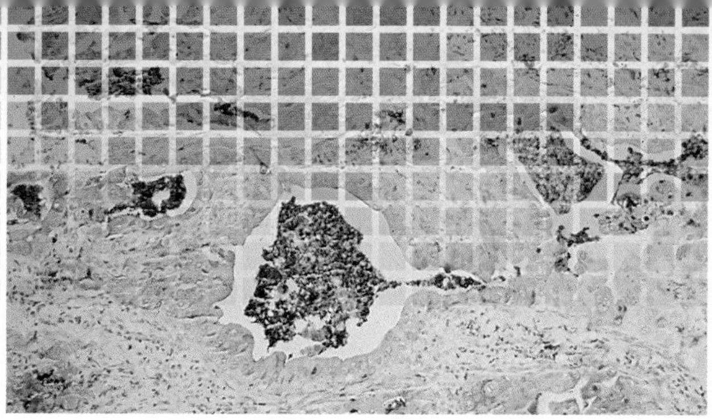

9

Immunohistology of Head and Neck Neoplasms

Jennifer L. Hunt

- Introduction 256
- Biology of Antigens and Antibodies 256
- Squamoproliferative Lesions 256
- Nasal Cavity and Paranasal Sinuses 262
- Nasopharynx 270
- Oral Cavity and Oropharynx 271
- Larynx/Hypopharynx 271
- Salivary Glands 273
- Ear/Temporal Bone 280
- Paragangliomas and Malignant Paragangliomas 282
- Metastatic Tumors 283
- Summary 284

INTRODUCTION

The head and neck, arbitrarily defined as the area between the clavicles at the inferior aspect and the sella turcica at the superior extent, is an anatomically complex region composed of a heterogeneous array of tissues and organs. Among the various tissues are epithelia of the mucosal surfaces, soft tissues, peripheral and sometimes central nervous system components, bone, cartilage, salivary glands, lymphoid tissue, the odontogenic apparatus, paraganglia, endocrine organs, and skin.

Because many of the neoplasms derived from these tissues are discussed elsewhere in this book, this chapter includes only lesions that either are commonly encountered in the head and neck or are unique to this region. The discussion focuses heavily on lesions in which immunohistochemistry and molecular workup may be useful for establishing the diagnosis or for providing additional prognostic-predictive information. It is not intended to be a compendium of all head and neck neoplasms. Tumors that can be recognized by routine hematoxylin and eosin-stained slides without adjunctive immunohistochemistry or molecular analysis are not covered.

BIOLOGY OF ANTIGENS AND ANTIBODIES

The pathology of the head and neck encompasses nearly every type of tumor that can occur throughout the body, and therefore there is a broad spectrum of antigens/antibodies that are in diagnostic use in this area (Table 9.1). For example, mucosal melanomas are unique tumors, but S100, HMB45, tyrosinase, and melan-A are used in the same manner as they are in the skin. These general antibodies are not discussed in detail in this introduction. The most commonly used antibodies in the head and neck are cytokeratin stains. Again, these parallel their use in other organ systems. Several antibodies are particularly important in head and neck tumors and deserve special mention. One antibody that has become increasingly useful in the head and neck is p63. p63 is a group of different isotypes of a protein that is a homologue for p53. This protein product will immunostain squamous epithelium within the head and neck but is also an excellent marker for myoepithelial cells. Androgen receptor is another important marker, particularly for salivary duct carcinoma. This antibody recognizes the androgen receptor, which also stains positive in prostate carcinoma. The remainder of the antibodies discussed in this chapter is not specific for the head and neck and has been discussed elsewhere.

SQUAMOPROLIFERATIVE LESIONS

Reactive Changes

The squamous mucosa withstands substantial environmental pressure and physical trauma from enzymatic secretions, mastication, dentures, and inhaled

TABLE 9.1 Antibodies Used in the Evaluation of Head and Neck Specimens

Antibody	Source	Dilution	Antibody	Source	Dilution
Androgen receptor	Biogenex	1:2000	CK19	Novocastro	1:50
Bcl-2	Dako	1:200	CK20	Dako	1:40
β-Catenin	BD Transduction Laboratories		CK903	Sigma	1:20
			Ki-67	AMAC	1:200
Calponin	Dako	1:200	Laminin	Sigma	1:20
Calretinin	Zymed	1:750	LCA	Dako	1:20
CD31	Dako	1:40	Melan-A	Novocastro	1:40
CD34	Dako	1:800	Microphthalmic transcription factor	Neomarkers	1:40
CD99	Dako	1:20			
CD x 2	Bio Genex	1:50			
CEA	Boehringer-Mannheim	1:4000	Muscle-specific actin (HHF-35)	Enzo	1:8000
Chromogranin	Boehringer-Mannheim	1:4000	MUC2	Novocastro	1:100
Desmin	Biogenex	1:2000	MUC5	Novocastro	1:150
EMA	Dako	1:400	Myogenin	Novocastro	1:30
FLI-1	Santa Cruz	1:40	Neuron-specific enolase	Bio Genes	1:450
GFAP	Dako	1:300			
HER2/neu	Dako	1:100	Pit-1	Santa Cruz	
HMB-45	Biogenex	1:60	p53	Oncogene	1:160
AE1/3	Boehringer-Mannheim	1:100	p63	Neomarkers	1:200
			S-100 protein	Dako	1:1000
CAM5.2	Becton-Dickinson	1:200	Smooth muscle actin	Dako	1:80
CK4	Novocastra	1:100			
CK5/6	Roche	1:20	Synaptophysin	Boehringer-Mannheim	1:40
CK7	Biogenex	1:800			
CK8	Novocastro	1:60	Thyroid transcription factor	Neomarkers	1:50
CK10	Novocastro	1:50			
CK13	Dako	1:100	Tyrosinase	Novocastro	1:20
CK14	Novocastro	1:40	Vimentin	Biogenex	1:20

or chemical toxins, primarily in the form of tobacco and alcohol. Local trauma is commonly blamed for reactive alterations and the toxins are considered to be the most common cause of neoplastic changes in the squamous epithelium.

Reactive epithelial changes can have a variety of histologic patterns. Nuclear and cytologic atypia are characteristically seen, but nuclear hyperchromasia, atypical mitotic figures, or nuclear irregularities typical of dysplastic changes generally are not seen. The nuclei in reactive changes can have nucleoli, are often vesicular, and are well spaced and not overcrowded. Architecturally, there is relatively normal maturation toward the surface of the epithelium. No immunohistochemical stains exist to help identify or classify reactive cytologic changes.

One specialized type of reactive change is pseudoepitheliomatous hyperplasia. This type of reaction can be found overlying a granular cell tumor but can also occur in response to local trauma. Granular cell tumors are important to recognize and diagnose because they can recur if the lesion is incompletely excised. Granular cell tumors are characteristically positive for S100, as well as showing PAS-positive cytoplasmic granules.[1] The etiology for the epithelial proliferative hyperplasia is not well understood, though it is not thought to be neoplastic.[2] There is some suggestion that the proliferation overlying granular cell tumors may be related to growth factors or other agents secreted by the tumor cells.[3]

Dysplasia and Conventional Squamous Cell Carcinoma

Squamous cell carcinoma (SCC) is the most common malignancy that arises in the head and neck.[4,5] Carcinogenesis is directly related to tobacco and alcohol in the vast majority of cases.[6-8] Invasive SCC tends to occur in the sixth decade or later and generally has a male predominance.

Tumorigenesis in SCC is most commonly related to exposure to the toxins in tobacco. Many studies have shown that exposure of the mucosa in the upper aerodigestive tract to chemical toxins can induce not only the morphologic evidence of early neoplasia, but also molecular mutational changes characteristic of neoplasia. Smokeless tobacco and other chewed tobacco-containing products such as Betel-nut-quid are also etiologic agents in the development of SCC, particularly in lesions of the oral cavity.[9,10]

Viral etiology for head and neck SCC has been a controversial topic. Epstein-Barr virus (EBV) is certainly related to some tumors (see "Nasopharynx" later). Recent evidence has shown fairly strong association between human papillomavirus (HPV) and some types of squamoproliferative lesions of the head and neck including some SCCs. This is discussed in context of the variants of SCC.[11-15] In the uterine cervix, HPV-infected dysplastic cells also tend to express p16ink4a as a surrogate marker of HPV presence in the genome.[16-18] This has also been seen in studies of HPV-related head and neck SCCs.[19,20] However, in the head and neck, the p16 gene may also function as a tumor suppressor gene, and therefore altered expression does not completely correlate with the presence of HPV.[21]

Despite the growing evidence that suggests an etiologic role for HPV in some types of head and neck SCC, there remains controversy about the true incidence. The variability in detection rates is probably related to which technique is used for detection.[15] Immunohistochemical stains for HPV are not very sensitive to detect the presence of the organism. *In situ* hybridization detects integrated HPV genomic material, which is considered to be important to suggest a causative relationship.[12] PCR-based assays only detect the presence of the HPV DNA in general; this technique is highly sensitive (perhaps overly sensitive), but information about the cellular localization is lost when PCR is used.[22]

Dysplastic and neoplastic transformation of the squamous mucosa is typically classified into one of four basic categories: low-grade dysplasia, moderate dysplasia, severe dysplasia (or carcinoma *in situ*), and invasive carcinoma. The cytologic and architectural features of dysplasia are fairly characteristic. Cells in dysplasia often show nuclear hyperchromasia and enlargement, a basaloid appearance, nuclear irregularities and pleomorphism, and increased or atypical mitoses. Architecturally, dysplastic epithelium shows crowding, disorganization, and lack of maturation, and mitoses may be aberrantly located above the basal layer.

The definitions for the categories of head and neck dysplasia are not as well established as in the uterine cervix, but most pathologists apply similar criteria when grading head and neck epithelial dysplasia. Low-grade dysplasia shows nuclear and architectural changes that are limited to the lower one third of the epithelial thickness; moderate dysplasia shows changes into the middle third, and severe dysplasia/carcinoma *in situ* (CIS) shows changes in the upper third.[4,23-25]

Transformation from dysplasia to SCC is not well understood but involves a number of cellular pathways. Inactivating mutations in tumor suppressor genes and activating events in tumor oncogenes represent the most common genetic changes.[26,27] Many of these tumorigenic pathways have identifiable protein products, and therefore a multitude of studies describe immunohistochemical staining in squamous cell carcinomas. However, no diagnostic immunohistochemical stains are currently used in common practice for squamous dysplasias. Some studies have suggested that p53 and ki-67 can be used as adjunctive markers to help grade dyplasias.[28]

Conventional SCC usually has fairly diagnostic histologic features, and in well-differentiated tumors no additional stains are generally necessary. In poorly differentiated tumors, particularly in metastatic sites, cytokeratin stains may be helpful. Typically, head and neck SCCs are positive for cytokeratin cocktails, AE1-3, and pancytokeratin. Cytoplasmic expression of keratins CK5, CK5/6, CK14, and CK17 are also frequently found in SCCs, along with nuclear p63 expression.

Detection of metastatic disease may occasionally require the use of immunohistochemical stains in challenging specimens such as postradiation lymph nodes. Subtle post-treatment residual tumors can be detected clinically using PET/CT scans, but histologically these isolated foci may show only granulomatous or necrotic tissue without viable tumor. In these cases, cytokeratin stains can be helpful to identify the etiology of the necrotic deposits. Sentinel lymph node examinations are occasionally used in head and neck surgery. Currently no standard practice for using immunohistochemistry to examine the sentinel lymph nodes exists, and indeed the procedure is fairly unreliable for mucosally based tumors.

KEY DIAGNOSTIC POINTS

Conventional Squamous Cell Carcinoma

- Squamous carcinomas are nearly always positive for cytokeratin.
- Common cytokeratin expression in squamous carcinomas includes AE1/AE3, CK5, CK5/6, CK14, and CK17.
- Nuclear p63 expression is common in squamous carcinomas but is not completely specific for squamous tumors.
- Cytokeratin stains can help detect subtle metastatic foci, particularly in the post-treatment setting in lymph nodes.

Basaloid Squamous Cell Carcinoma

Basaloid squamous cell carcinoma (BSCC) is an uncommon, histologically distinct variant of SCC. In the upper aerodigestive tract, it occurs frequently in the base of the tongue, tonsils, hypopharynx, and larynx but has also been described in many other locations such as the palate, buccal mucosa, floor of mouth, nasopharynx, nasal cavity, and trachea.[29-31] This is one of the subtypes of squamous carcinoma that can present with large neck node metastases and an unknown primary tumor.[32]

TABLE 9.2 Differentiating Basaloid Squamous Cell Carcinoma from Adenoid Cystic and Small Cell Neuroendocrine Carcinoma

	Tumor Type		
Antibody Marker	Basaloid Squamous Cell Carcinoma	Adenoid Cystic Carcinoma	Small Cell Neuroendocrine Carcinoma
Cytokeratin	+	+	+
Chromogranin	N	N	+
S-100	S	+ (peripheral, myoepithelial)	N
p53	+	S	+
Ki-67	High	Low	High
C-*kit*	S	+	+
p63	+ (diffuse and strong)	+ (peripheral, myoepithelial)	S

+, almost always positive; N, negative; S, sometimes positive.

BSCC has a male predominance (82%), and the mean age at diagnosis is about 63 years (range 27 to 88 years).[33] Symptoms vary according to site of origin but most commonly include dysphagia, hoarseness, pain, otalgia, cough, hemoptysis, neck mass, or weight loss.[34] Several studies have suggested the BSCC has a worse prognosis than conventional SCC, especially with a higher risk of lymph node metastases in BSCC.[35]

Tobacco and alcohol are probably key etiologic agents for BSCC, with the majority of patients having been heavy smokers and consumers of alcoholic beverages. However, many recent studies have also highlighted the probable relationship between HPV and BSCC. These studies demonstrate a high rate of HPV positivity in tumors with both basaloid and nonkeratinizing morphology, particularly when they occur in the tonsillar and tongue base regions.[11,12,36-39] This relationship has begun to be exploited diagnostically, both in the workup of metastatic disease with an unknown primary tumor and in the primary tumor themselves.[40,41] Detection of HPV does appear to have some clinical utility, primarily because HPV-related tumors may have a different response rate to radiation therapy and there may also be a lower risk of second tumors.[42] HPV can be detected using a variety of techniques including immunohistochemistry, *in situ* hybridization, and PCR-based techniques. The hybrid-capture techniques that are available for liquid-based cytology may also be potentially modified for clinical use in tissue or paraffin embedded tissue samples.[43,44]

Histologically, BSCC has a biphasic appearance, where the basaloid component usually dominates. The second component of a conventional SCC is usually only minor and can even be quite focal.[45] BSCC usually grows in smooth contoured lobules, large nests, or trabecular cordlike arrangements of small clusters or even single cells. The lobules often contain central comedo-type necrosis. Cystic spaces and even abortive ductal differentiation can be present in a minority of the tumors. Very rarely the tumor can have deposition of basement membrane type material with a cribriform growth pattern that can mimic adenoid cystic carcinoma.

Cytologically, the cells of BSCC are round to oval and have hyperchromatic nuclei with a high nuclear-to-cytoplasmic ratio. The nuclei may demonstrate peripheral palisading around the lobules. There are often prominent mitoses and apoptotic bodies in the basaloid component.[33,46,47] The conventional SCC component can be invasive or *in situ*, and it can be found in separate foci or merge with the basaloid component.

The differential diagnosis for BSCC can be broad, especially in small biopsies where it can be difficult to appreciate all of the histologic features. Included in the differential diagnosis are the two most important mimickers: adenoid cystic carcinoma and small cell neuroendocrine carcinoma.[33] Immunohistochemical stains are particularly useful in resolving this differential diagnosis (Table 9.2).

Several studies have examined the staining patterns in BSCCs.[48-51] Most of the tumors are positive for AE1/AE3 and epithelial membrane antigen (EMA), 53% are positive for CEA, and 39% are positive for S-100 protein.[48,50,52] Diffuse, weak staining for neuron-specific enolase can be seen in up to 75% of BSCC, but they are generally negative for chromogranin, synaptophysin, muscle-specific actin, and glial fibrillary acidic protein. These immunostains will help to differentiate BSCC from neuroendocrine carcinomas. C-*kit*, which is positive in the majority of adenoid cystic carcinomas,[53] is probably not a useful marker in this differential because some BSCCs can also express C-*kit*.[54] The most useful marker in differentiating BSCC from adenoid cystic carcinoma is p63, which is strongly and diffusely positive in BSCC. The staining pattern of adenoid cystic carcinoma for p63 depends on the growth pattern (see salivary gland tumor section) but will usually show a peripheral staining pattern as it marks the myoepithelial component of that tumor.[55-57] P53 may also be a useful marker because BSCCs are often strongly positive for p53. Adenoid cystic carcinomas with high grade transformation and less commonly solid type adenoid cystic carcinoma can also show p53 staining.[36,52,58-61]

KEY DIAGNOSTIC POINTS

Basaloid Squamous Cell Carcinoma

- The differential diagnosis for basaloid squamous cell carcinoma (BSCC) includes adenoid cystic carcinoma and small cell neuroendocrine carcinoma.
- The best markers to differentiate these are p63 and neuroendocrine markers: BSCC will be positive for cytokeratin and p63 and negative for most neuroendocrine markers.

Verrucous Carcinoma and Papillary Squamous Cell Carcinoma

Verrucous carcinoma (VC) and papillary squamous cell carcinoma (PSCC) are exophytic tumors that occur most commonly in the oral cavity and larynx. VC is a locally aggressive, nonmetastasizing variant of SCC, whereas PSCC is an invasive tumor that has metastatic potential. Tobacco is the main etiologic agent of these tumors, though poor oral hygiene and HPV have also been implicated.[62]

Verrucous carcinomas show markedly thickened epithelium that can have a papillary or exophytic surface and minimal atypia or displasia. The leading edge at the tumor-stroma interface shows a characteristic pushing border, with bulbous rete pegs.[63] Cytologic atypia in the epithelium should raise the possibility of a combined verrucous and conventional SCC (hybrid type) or PSCC.[64] PSCCs have papillary-frond–like growth, with true fibrovascular cores.[65] The cells lining the papillary fronds show cytologic evidence of dysplastic epithelium.[66] The invasive component can appear as a conventional SCC underlying the papillary surface component or as invasive SCC dropping off of the base of the PSCC.[67]

The differential among benign papillary proliferative lesions, VC carcinoma, and PSCC can be extremely challenging, particularly in small biopsies. Some evidence indicates that HPV may also be involved in the pathogenesis of VC and possibly PSCC.[68,69] However, these markers are not used diagnostically or prognostically. The histologic features remain paramount in both VC and PSCC, and there are no immunostains that will aid in this differential diagnosis.

KEY DIAGNOSTIC POINTS

Verrucous Carcinoma and Papillary Squamous Cell Carcinoma

- Verrucous carcinoma (VC) and papillary squamous cell carcinoma (PSCC) have a similar gross appearance, but VC has a pushing leading edge and no atypia, whereas PSCC shows cytologic atypia and more typical invasion.
- No diagnostic immunohistochemical markers can be used to identify VC or PSCC.

Spindle Cell Carcinoma

Spindle cell carcinoma (SPCC) is another rare variant of SCC that has had many different names over the years including "pseudocarcinoma," "sarcomatoid carcinoma," and "carcinosarcoma." The average age is 64 years (range 31 to 88 years), and there is a strong male predominance. Common primary locations of tumors include the glottis and hypopharynx, though they have been reported in numerous other head and neck locations. Tobacco and alcohol are the leading risk factors.[70]

Grossly, these tumors are often polypoid and can grow rapidly.[71] Histologically, SPCC can be quite difficult to diagnose, particularly on small biopsies. The majority of the tumor tends to be composed of the spindle component, and this can range from bland to highly atypical, with cellularity ranging from sparse to dense. To make the diagnosis, it is helpful to identify squamous neoplasia, either as overlying dysplastic or more rarely as an invasive SCC component. A typical invasive SCC component is seen in less than 50% of SPCCs.

Immunohistochemical stains are nearly always necessary but may not be specific or sensitive. The spindle cell component is uniformly and strongly positive for vimentin. Proving the epithelial origin can be difficult because there is highly variable staining for cytokeratins (Figs. 9.1 and 9.2).[70,72,73] Cytokeratins are positive in the spindle cell component in approximately 70% of tumors, but the staining is patchy and the examination of multiple keratin antibodies may be necessary. p63 and CK5/6 can be useful markers to detect the epithelial nature of SPCC (Fig. 9.3). However, in up to 36% of SPCCs keratin staining can be completely absent.[70,74] Other mesenchymal markers such as smooth muscle actin, muscle specific actin, and desmin may have some minor reactivity (ranging from ~1% to 30%) in the spindle component.

The major differential diagnosis for SPCC includes reactive and benign neoplastic stromal proliferations and rare primary sarcomas of mucosal sites. Benign entities can include granulation tissue, pyogenic granuloma, leiomyoma, fibromatosis, and other benign stromal lesions. Malignant tumors can include synovial sarcoma and other phenotypic sarcomas. Immunohistochemistry can be helpful in differentiating SPCC from some of these lesions, but because of overlapping histologic and immunophenotypes, the final diagnosis will rest on the histologic features and a compatible immunoprofile. Some investigators have suggested the possibility that the lack of immunohistochemical staining for epithelial markers may be an adverse prognostic indicator.[71]

The molecular mutational profile of SPCC is not well understood, though it is presumed to be similar to other tobacco-induced squamous cell carcinomas. One recent study did not find any evidence of KRAS mutations,

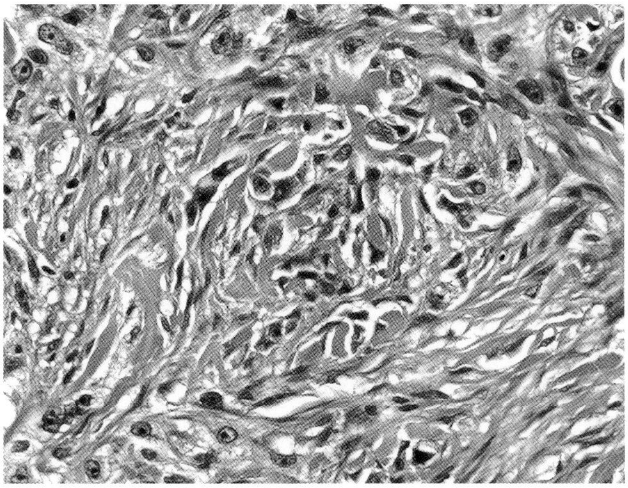

FIGURE 9.1 Spindle cell carcinoma demonstrating striking spindle cell morphology. (H&E, ×200 original magnification.)

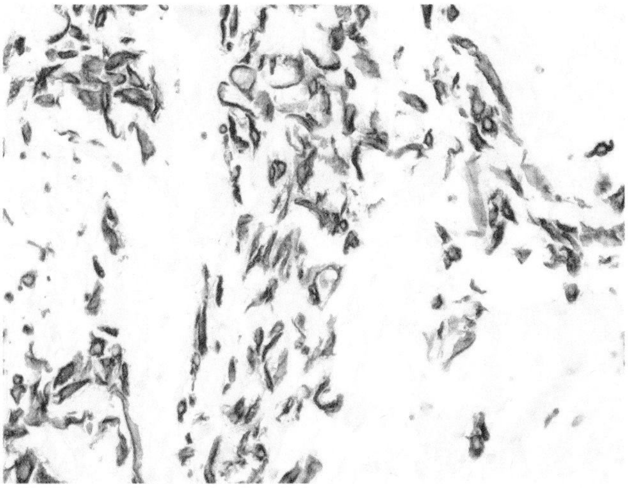

FIGURE 9.2 CAM5.2 stain of spindle cell carcinoma demonstrating strong cytoplasmic immunostain. (CAM5.2, ×200 original magnification.)

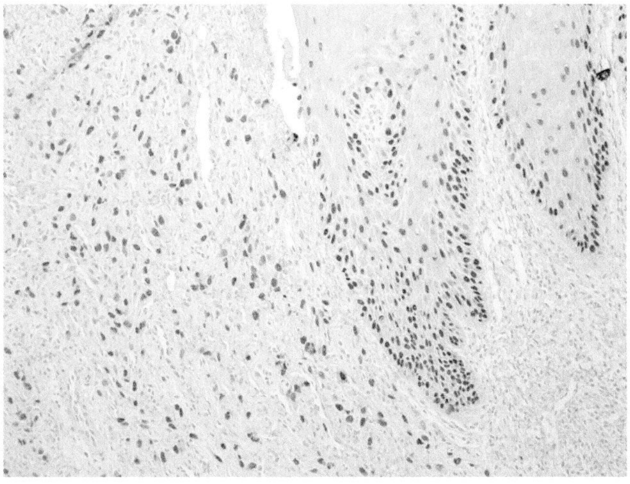

FIGURE 9.3 p63 nuclear expression of spindle cell. Note expression in overlying squamous epithelium. (p63, ×200 original magnification.)

KEY DIAGNOSTIC POINTS

Spindle Cell Carcinoma

- The diagnosis of spindle cell carcinoma (SPCC) requires the identification of a component of squamous neoplasia or epithelial differentiation of the spindle cells.
- Multiple cytokeratin and epithelial markers may be necessary to show positive staining in the spindle cells, but up to 30% of SPCCs will not stain for cytokeratin in the spindle cell component.

which is consistent with typical SCC of the head and neck.[74,75]

Theranostic Applications

Although many markers for SCC are related to underlying genomic changes, none has proven to have clinical value, either for diagnostic, prognostic, or theranostic purposes.

VIRUSES

The detection of viruses in tumors including HPV and EBV does have a role in head and neck pathology. Both viruses are associated with specific subtypes of SCCs. HPV has been highly associated with BSCC and oropharyngeal carcinomas, particularly those arising in the tonsil and tongue base.[38,76-78] There are valid clinical reasons to identify tumors with HPV, but there also may be a role in the workup of neck metastases in patients with unknown primary tumors.[40] EBV has a strong association with lymphoepithelial carcinoma, particularly in the nasopharynx in endemic locations such as Southeast Asia.[79,80]

Many SCCs of the head and neck are treated surgically with primary resection and possibly neck dissection.[81-83] Some patients can present with metastatic SCC in the neck, but despite careful clinical and radiologic workup, a primary tumor cannot be found. In these cases, HPV analysis, particularly using an *in situ* hybridization approach, can be useful. In several series, HPV-associated tumors are largely restricted to the tonsil and tongue base area.[15,68,76] When HPV is positive in the neck nodes from a patient with an unknown primary tumor, the clinical management can be directed toward these high-risk areas.

EPIDERMAL GROWTH FACTOR RECEPTOR

Epidermal growth factor receptor (EGFR) has become an important biomarker for several different tumor types, mainly because there are several FDA-approved compounds that use this receptor for targeted drug therapy.[84] The main tumor types that have been examined for efficacy of anti-EGFR drugs are lung cancer, head and neck cancer, and colon cancer.[85-91] Recent evidence in lung cancer suggests that certain mutations found at

TABLE 9.3 Immunohistochemical Staining of Round Cell Tumors of the Sinonasal Tract

Tumor	CK	EMA	LCA	Synaptophysin	HMB-45	Desmin	Vimentin	CD99
SNUC	+	+	N	N	N	N	N	N
ONB	S	N	N	+	N	N	N	N
NPC	+	+	N	N	N	N	N	N
Lymphoma	N	N	+	N	N	N	+	S
Melanoma	N	N	N	N	+	N	+	N
Rhabdomyosarcoma	N	N	N	N	N	+	+	N
Small cell carcinoma	+	+	N	+	N	N	N	N
ES/PNET	N	N	N	+	N	N	+	+

CK, cytokeratin; EMA, epithelial membrane antigen; LCA, leukocyte common antigen; NPC, nasopharyngeal carcinoma; ONB, olfactory neuroblastoma; ES/PNET, Ewing's sarcoma/peripheral neuroectodermal tumor; SNUC, sinonasal undifferentiated carcinoma.
+, almost always positive; S, sometimes positive; N, negative.

the DNA level may improve response to therapy, but partial response can also be seen in patients whose tumors do not harbor these mutations.[92-94] Somatic mutations are not prevalent in other types of carcinoma,[95] though overexpression of EGFR is found in many different types of tumors.

In head and neck SCC, EGFR overexpression by immunohistochemistry has been identified.[91] Anti-EGFR therapies are being currently used in the head and neck and have met with some success.[91,96-98] However, there does not appear to be a role for testing EGFR expression before therapy because the protein expression does not correlate with response to therapy.[99]

p53

Mutations and overexpression of the p53 gene are common in head and neck SCC, with approximately 50% to 60% of tumors showing aberrant p53.[100,101] The p53 gene has been extensively studied for prognostic significance, both at the protein product level and the genomic level, with conflicting results.[102] In several studies p53 overexpression has been associated with a poor prognosis, whereas other studies have shown no correlation.[103] Additional evidence is now also suggesting that p53 status may be linked to response to chemotherapy and radiation therapy in SCCs.[104]

p53 protein expression may also have a role for detecting dysplasia, especially in conjunction with the proliferative marker ki-67.[105-108] Because the detection and grading of dysplasia is so controversial, the use of staining may have the potential to improve our ability to objectively identify dysplastic lesions with consistency. p53 mutational analysis has also been described for assessment of margins, but this has only been in the research setting.[102,109,110] The presence of p53 alterations in margins does correlate with recurrence, which suggests that DNA alterations can precede histologic alterations and also supports the concept of the field effect, which is so important in tobacco-induced neoplasia.

Currently, there are no diagnostic molecular mutation markers that are in use for the workup of routine SCC.

NASAL CAVITY AND PARANASAL SINUSES

Many of the tumors of the nasal cavity and paranasal sinuses fall under the category of "round cell neoplasms."[111-114] Among these are olfactory neuroblastoma, sinonasal undifferentiated carcinoma, malignant melanoma, neuroendocrine carcinoma–small cell neuroendocrine carcinoma, malignant lymphoma, extramedullary plasmacytoma, invasive-ectopic pituitary adenoma, rhabdomyosarcoma, and Ewing's sarcoma (ES)–peripheral neuroectodermal tumor (ES/PNET). But there is also a host of other epithelial lesions that are unique to the sinonasal tract.

Respiratory Epithelial Adenomatoid Hamartoma

Respiratory epithelial adenomatoid hamartoma (REAH) is a benign lesion of the nasal cavity and sinuses. They often arise from the posterior nasal septum.[115] In practice, these lesions are often associated with histologic and clinical evidence of chronic sinusitis.[116] Occasionally, areas of REAH-like changes are seen in a background of nasal polyposis and chronic sinusitis as well. The etiology of REAH is not well understood. For years, it has been considered to be a hamartoma. But recent evidence at the molecular level has suggested that it may actually be a benign neoplasm.[117]

Histologically, REAH is characteristically composed of hyperplastic glands located deep in the stroma.[116] The glands can vary from relatively closely packed to more loosely spaced. They are usually lined by respiratory type of epithelium with abundant cilia on the luminal surface. The epithelium lining these glands is not thickened or hyperplastic. A thickened basement membrane or densely hyalinized stroma is characteristically seen surrounding the deep glands. The stroma between the glands can vary from cellular to fibrotic and can be well vascularized or edematous.

The immunohistochemical staining profile of REAH is fairly straightforward. The epithelial cells lining the

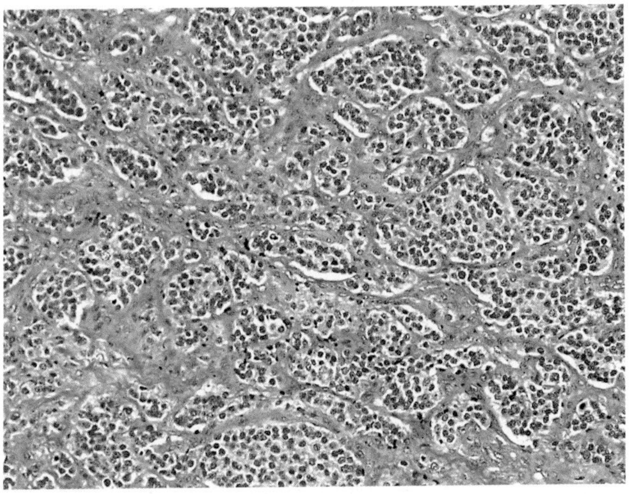

FIGURE 9.4 Olfactory neuroblastoma highlighting the nested pattern of growth and the neuroendocrine nuclear features. (H&E, ×100 original magnification.)

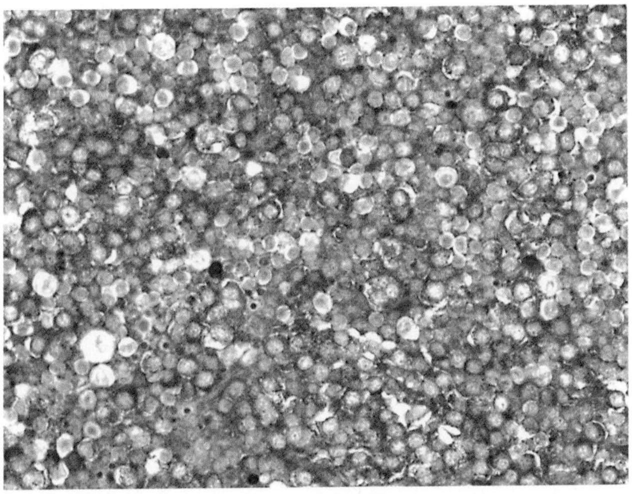

FIGURE 9.5 Synaptophysin strong cytoplasmic immunostain of olfactory neuroblastoma. (Synaptophysin, ×200 original magnification.)

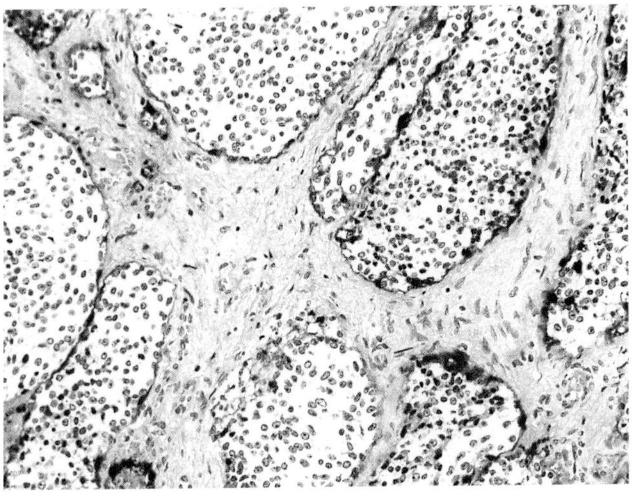

FIGURE 9.6 S100 protein with red chromogen decorating the sustentacular cells of neuroblastoma. (S-100, ×100 original magnification.)

deep glands stain positive for CK7. The glands are surrounded by intact basal-type cells that are positive for p63 and 34βE12 but negative for calponin, smooth muscle actin (SMA), and S100.[118]

Olfactory Neuroblastoma

Olfactory neuroblastoma (ONB) is the prototypic "round cell tumor" of the sinonasal tract. It occurs over a broad age range (average 40 to 45 years) and affects both sexes equally. The tumor most commonly arises high in the nasal cavity and has its primary attachment or origin at the cribriform plate. Rare cases will have origins in other locations within the sinonasal cavity. The tumor is frequently polypoid. Clinically, patients with ONB can present with nonspecific sinonasal symptoms such as obstruction and nasal congestion, and they might also have epistaxis.[119,120]

ONB is composed of cells with poorly defined cytoplasm and prominent, uniformly round nuclei with barely discernible nucleoli. The tumor cells are usually quite bland, with minimal pleomorphism. ONB tumor cells have neuroendocrine-type chromatin with minimal hyperchromasia. The cells grow in a lobular, diffuse, or mixed lobular-diffuse pattern (Fig. 9.4). Rosettes, especially Homer Wright and exceptionally Flexner-Wintersteiner, may be seen. Necrosis and mitoses are uncommon. The stroma is highly vascular and, at times, neurofibrillary.

Immunohistochemical staining is fairly consistent and straightforward in ONB. The tumor cells are positive for synaptophysin and neuron-specific enolase and, occasionally, for chromogranin (Fig. 9.5). Up to 30% of cases may be positive for CAM 5.2. However, ONBs are uniformly negative for epithelial membrane antigen, muscle markers, and CD 99 (MIC-2). Elongated cells often observed at the periphery of the lobules, so-called sustentacular cells, are positive for S-100 protein and glial fibrillary acidic protein (Fig. 9.6, Tables 9.4 and 9.5).

Rare cases of ONB can have divergent differentiation. The reported secondary components have included true gland formation, rhabdomyosarcoma, and other types of rare tumors.[121-123] When present, areas with divergent differentiation will stain as expected for the specific tumor type.

Recent studies have begun to examine the molecular profiles of ONB and have demonstrated both chromosomal gains and losses at some conserved regions.[124] To date, however, there are no defined diagnostic or clinically relevant markers.

KEY DIAGNOSTIC POINTS

Olfactory Neuroblastoma

- Olfactory neuroblastoma (ONB) is composed of small round blue cells that grow in a lobular or diffuse pattern.
- The tumor cells are positive for neuroendocrine markers, and up to 30% can be positive for cytokeratin.
- Sustentacular cells surrounding the lobules of ONB stain for S-100.

Sinonasal Undifferentiated Carcinoma

Sinonasal undifferentiated carcinoma (SNUC) is an aggressive tumor that is two to three times more common in men and occurs over a broad age range (average 55 to 60 years). The tumor commonly arises primarily in the nasal cavity but also can originate from the sinuses. Widespread invasion of the nasal cavity and paranasal sinuses is often present at the time of presentation. The tumor may also invade into the adjacent structures including the orbit or even into the cranial cavity.

Microscopically, SNUCs have highly variable growth patterns and cytologic features. They usually have small- to medium-sized polygonal cells that grow in sheets, nests, wide trabeculae, and/or ribbons. The nuclei are round to oval and hyperchromatic and show mild to moderate pleomorphism. Nucleoli vary from inconspicuous to prominent. Mitoses, angiolymphatic invasion, and necrosis are prominent (Fig. 9.7).

SNUCs are almost always strongly positive for cytokeratin (CK), especially when a panel of antibodies is used (Fig. 9.8). More specifically, they are uniformly positive for CK 8 and about half will stain for CK 7 and CK 19. They are often negative for CK 4, 5/6, 10, 13, and 14 (see Table 9.5).[125] Less than half the cases are positive for EMA, NSE, and p53.[126] It is uncommon for the tumors to have neuroendocrine differentiation, and some authors have argued that, by definition, the diagnosis of SNUC should be reserved for truly undifferentiated tumors. A few tumors have been reported to be positive for CD99, but in these instances the staining is cytoplasmic rather than membranous (see Tables 9.3 through 9.7).[126] In some Asian series, SNUCs have been reported to be occasionally positive for EBV.[126,127] It may be difficult, however, to differentiate these tumors from endemic type lymphoepithelial carcinoma or nasopharyngeal carcinoma that is secondarily involving the sinonasal tract.

TABLE 9.4 Olfactory Neuroblastoma (ONB) versus Sinonasal Undifferentiated Carcinoma (SNUC)

Feature	ONB	SNUC
Age (average)	40-45	58
Site	Roof of nasal cavity	Multiple sites
Prognosis/survival	60%-80% 5 yr	18-mo median
Ocular-cranial nerve	Occasional	Common
Anaplasia	Occasional	Common
Mitoses	Variable	Numerous
Necrosis	Occasional	Prominent
Vascular invasion	Occasional	Prominent
Neurofibrillary stroma	Common	Absent
Homer Wright rosettes	Common	Absent
Keratin	25%-35%	90%
EMA	0%	65%
NSE	80%-100%	50%
S-100	60%	0%-15%
Synaptophysin	100%	0%
Neurosecretory granules	Numerous	Rare

ONB is typically negative but may infrequently focally express low-molecular-weight cytokeratin.

KEY DIAGNOSTIC POINTS

Sinonasal Undifferentiated Carcinoma

- Sinonasal undifferentiated carcinoma is composed of high-grade, small- to medium-sized cells with prominent mitoses and necrosis.
- The tumor cells are positive for cytokeratin and may be positive for EMA.
- Neuroendocrine markers are rarely positive; when they are, staining should be only focal.

Malignant Melanoma

Malignant melanomas (MMs) of the sinonasal tract are uncommon and typically occur in patients older than 50 years of age. Most arise intranasally from the anterior nasal septum or lateral wall in the vicinity of the inferior or middle turbinates. Although they may originate in a sinus, the sinuses are most often involved secondarily from a nasal primary.

MMs of the sinonasal tract often undergo hemorrhagic necrosis and ulceration, and as a result, junctional

TABLE 9.5 Cytokeratin Expression in Sinonasal Tumors

Tumor	4	5/6	7	8	10	13	14	19
SCC (*N* = 10)	30%	90%	60%	90%	—	90%	80%	90%
NKSCC (*N* = 10)	—	90%	—	90%	—	80%	80%	90%
NPTC (*N* = 5)	—	80%	—	80%	—	80%	—	100%
SNUC (*N* = 6)	—	—	50%	100%	—	—	—	50%

NKSCC, nonkeratinizing squamous cell carcinoma; NPTC, nasopharyngeal-type undifferentiated carcinoma; SCC, squamous cell carcinoma; SNUC, sinonasal undifferentiated carcinoma.

From Franchi A, Moroni M, Massi D, et al. Sinonasal undifferentiated carcinoma, nasopharyngeal-type undifferentiated carcinoma, and keratinizing and nonkeratinizing squamous cell carcinoma express different cytokeratin patterns. *Am J Surg Pathol.* 2002; 26:1597-1604.

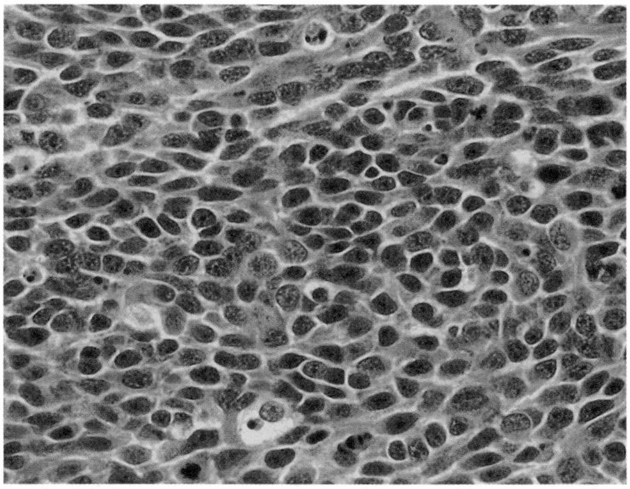

FIGURE 9.7 Sinonasal undifferentiated carcinoma. (H&E, ×200 original magnification.)

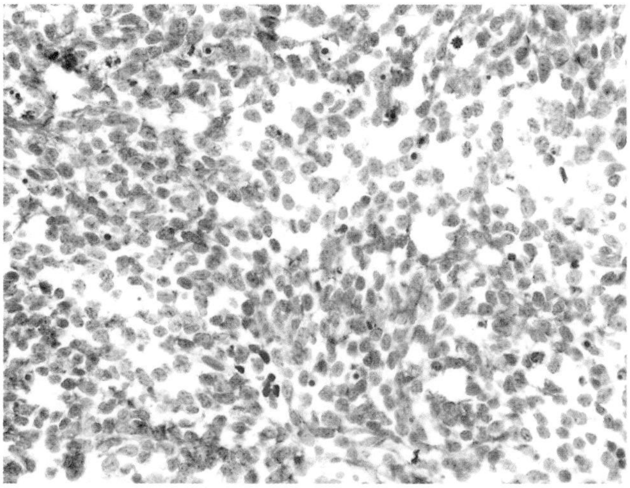

FIGURE 9.8 CAM5.2 staining in sinonasal undifferentiated carcinoma. (CAM5.2, ×200 original magnification.)

activity may not be apparent and is not essential for diagnosis. However, in its absence, one must have a high index of suspicion when dealing with this neoplasm.[128,129] The diagnosis may be especially problematic in tumors that are amelanotic or display alternative cell types (epithelioid, spindled, plasmacytoid, rhabdoid, undifferentiated) and patterns of growth (alveolar, papillary, peritheliomatous, solid) (Fig. 9.9).

The standard immunohistochemical markers, which are known to be positive in cutaneous melanoma, are also usually positive in melanoma of the sinonasal tract. S-100 has been positive in 91% to 95% of cases, HMB-45 in 76% to 98%, tyrosinase in 78% to 100%, melan-A in 65% to 100%, and microphthalmic transcription factor (MITF) in 57% to 91% (Figs. 9.10 and 9.11).[129,130] For spindle cell or desmoplastic MMs, S-100 and tyrosinase may be more sensitive than the other antibodies.

TABLE 9.6 Sinonasal Undifferentiated Carcinoma (SNUC) versus Small Cell Neuroendocrine Carcinoma (SCNEC)

Feature	SNUC	SCNEC
Spindle cells	N	+
Nucleoli	S	N
Nuclear molding	N	+
DNA coating	N	+
Dysplasia—CIS	S	N
Synaptophysin	N	S
Thyroid transcription factor	N	S
Dotlike keratin positivity	N	S

+, almost always positive; N, negative; S, sometimes positive.

TABLE 9.7 Sinonasal Undifferentiated Carcinoma versus Undifferentiated Nasopharyngeal Carcinoma (UNPC)

Feature	SNUC	UNPC
Location	Sinonasal tract	Nasopharynx
Clinical	Large primary, ± cervical lymph nodes	Small primary, positive cervical lymph nodes
X-ray	Marked destruction and spread beyond site of origin	Little destruction or spread beyond site of origin
Growth	Trabeculae, nests, sheets	Syncytial
Cells	Hyperchromatic to vesicular nuclei with or without nucleoli	Large, vesicular nuclei with prominent nucleoli
Mitoses	Very prominent	Not prominent
Necrosis	Very prominent	Not prominent
Vascular invasion	Very prominent	Not prominent
Lymphocytes	Absent to mild	Heavy infiltrate
Epstein-Barr virus (USA)	Negative	Positive
CK5/6 & 13	Negative	Positive
CK7	±	Negative

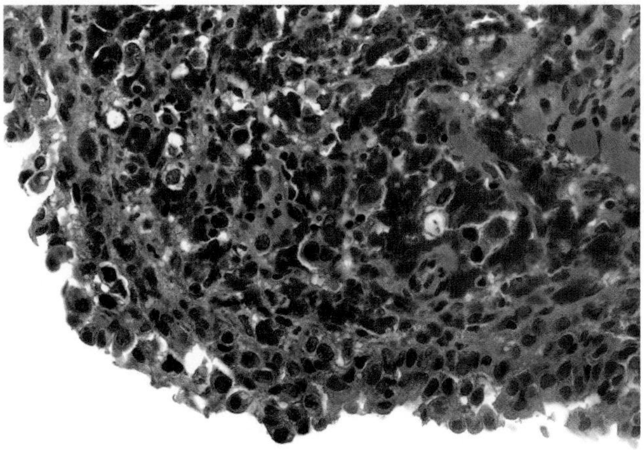

FIGURE 9.9 Mucosal malignant melanoma with heavy pigmentation. (H&E, ×200 original magnification.)

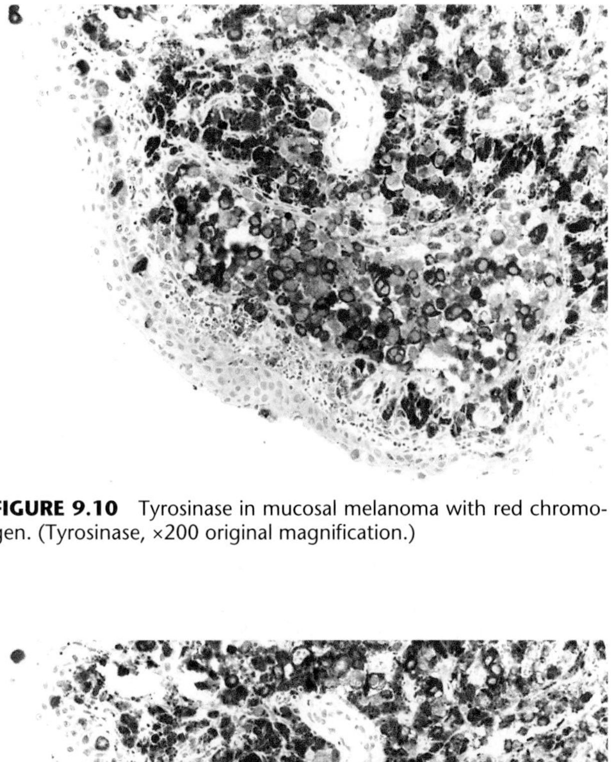

FIGURE 9.10 Tyrosinase in mucosal melanoma with red chromogen. (Tyrosinase, ×200 original magnification.)

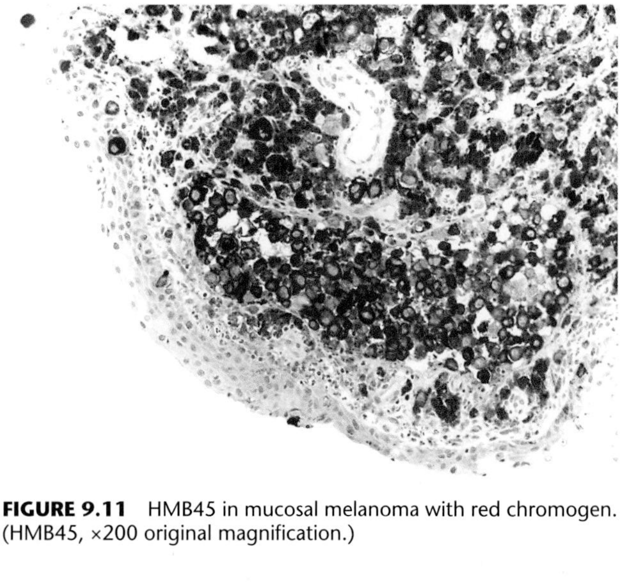

FIGURE 9.11 HMB45 in mucosal melanoma with red chromogen. (HMB45, ×200 original magnification.)

MMs are invariably positive for vimentin, which may be a pitfall in dealing with amelanotic spindle cell MMs. As a general rule, in diagnosing a spindle cell lesion of the sinonasal tract one must consider MM, spindle cell carcinoma, and a malignant myoepithelioma before soft tissue sarcomas. Rare MMs may also be focally positive for CAM 5.2 and EMA,[131] which poses a problem when dealing with an epithelioid MM.

KEY DIAGNOSTIC POINTS

Malignant Melanoma

- Mucosal melanomas stain with similar panels of markers to their cutaneous counterparts (S-100, HMB45, tyrosinase).
- Rare cases of mucosal melanomas have been reported to be positive for CAM5.2.

Small Cell Neuroendocrine Carcinoma and Neuroendocrine Carcinoma

The differential diagnosis for neuroendocrine tumors in the sinonasal tract will include olfactory neuroblastoma, small cell neuroendocrine carcinoma, carcinoid, atypical carcinoid, paraganglioma, and possibly even sinonasal undifferentiated carcinoma. Once these more specific neuroendocrine entities have been excluded, there remains a small group of tumors that cannot be further classified. These should be referred to as "neuroendocrine carcinoma, not otherwise specified." These tumors can be graded using standard morphologic features.

Small cell neuroendocrine carcinomas similar to those seen in the lung are exceptionally rare in the nasal cavity and paranasal sinuses. They affect both sexes equally and occur over a broad age range (38 to 68 years in one study).[132] They may arise either in the nasal cavity or in the paranasal sinuses, especially the ethmoid and maxilla. Though some tumors will remain localized to the site of origin, higher grade tumors are likely to invade into adjacent structures such as the orbit, cribriform plate, or cranial cavity.

Microscopically, small cell neuroendocrine carcinomas are identical to their pulmonary counterparts and, as such, are composed primarily of round to short spindle cells with sparse, poorly defined cytoplasm and hyperchromatic nuclei without nucleoli. Nuclear molding, frequent mitoses, necrosis, and single-cell apoptosis are common.

Neuroendocrine carcinomas and small cell neuroendocrine carcinomas are almost invariably positive for cytokeratins (such as CAM 5.2 and AE 1/3), synaptophysin, chromogranin, and neuron-specific enolase. A dotlike pattern of positivity may be seen in cytokeratin stains. They are negative for cytokeratin 20, S-100, and neurofilament.[132,133] About half of small cell neuroendocrine carcinomas are positive for thyroid transcription factor (TTF-1) and at least one has been reported to be positive for CD 99 (see Tables 9.3, 9.6).[132,133] Rarely they may also express ectopic hormones (calcitonin, adrenocortical hormone, beta melanocyte stimulating hormone, serotonin, parathyroid hormone).[134] A metastasis from a pulmonary SCNEC should always be considered in the differential diagnosis.

KEY DIAGNOSTIC POINTS

Small Cell Neuroendocrine Carcinoma

Neuroendocrine carcinomas are positive for cytokeratins and for typical neuroendocrine markers, such as chromogranin and synaptophysin.

Invasive-Ectopic Pituitary Adenoma

Pituitary adenomas presenting in the nasal cavity, paranasal sinuses, and nasopharynx are distinctly unusual and can be divided into two types: invasive and ectopic.[135-137] Invasive sinonasal pituitary adenomas are secondary to downward proliferation of a primary sellar tumor. This event occurs in about 2% of all sellar tumors.[136] Ectopic adenomas are those that arise from aberrant embryogenesis of the pituitary gland.

Pathologically these adenomas are identical to the "usual" type, but because biopsies are frequently small and distorted, a high index of suspicion and knowledge of the clinical history and laboratory and physical findings are helpful in recognizing these tumors in unusual sites.

The tumors are positive for synaptophysin, chromogranin, and neuron-specific enolase and may express a variety of hormones (growth hormone, prolactin, TSH, ACTH, and FSH). A few are hormone negative and are designated as *null-cell adenomas.* Almost all are positive for CAM 5.2, either focally or diffusely, and about half are positive for AE 1/3.[138] They are negative for cytokeratin 7, 19, and 20, as well as S-100 protein. Pituitary transcription factor-1 is selectively expressed in tumors that express growth hormone, prolactin, and TSH.[139] No diagnostic molecular markers are currently in use for sporadic pituitary lesions.[140]

The differential diagnosis might include olfactory neuroblastoma, paraganglioma, and carcinoid. Table 9.8 shows features that might be helpful in distinguishing these tumors.

KEY DIAGNOSTIC POINTS

Invasive-Ectopic Pituitary Adenoma

- Pituitary lesions can present in the sinonasal tract, either as invasive adenomas or as ectopic tumors.
- Functional pituitary adenomas can be found to express a variety of hormones, such as growth hormone, prolactin, thyroid-stimulating hormone, adrenocorticotropic hormone, or follicle-stimulating hormone.

Rhabdomyosarcoma

Rhabdomyosarcoma (RMS) is the most common soft tissue sarcoma of children and, in this age group, approximately one third of all RMSs occur in the head and neck, particularly involving the orbit, middle ear-mastoid, nasopharynx, and sinonasal tract.[141,142] In contrast, RMS is uncommon in adults, especially in the head and neck.[143,144] When the tumor does involve the head and neck in adults, the most common site is the sinonasal tract. The tumor is discussed in detail in Chapter 17.

Although a variety of immunomarkers to identify RMS exist, desmin and myogenin remain the most sensitive and specific. Cytoplasmic desmin intermediate filaments will be present in almost 80% of all RMSs. Myogenin nuclear expression is highly sensitive for RMS. In the study of Cessma and colleagues, all 32 RMSs tested were positive for this marker (Figs. 9.12 and 9.13).[145] In general, however, alveolar RMS stains more strongly than embryonal RMS. Myogenin, like desmin, may rarely stain (usually focally) a few other soft tissue neoplasms. Among these are desmoid, infantile myofibromatosis, infantile fibrosarcoma, and synovial sarcoma.[145]

KEY DIAGNOSTIC POINTS

Rhabdomyosarcoma

- Rhabdomyosarcoma can rarely arise in the sinonasal tract.
- This tumor stains similar to soft tissue counterparts, with desmin and myogenin positivity.

TABLE 9.8 Differential Diagnosis of Invasive-Ectopic Pituitary Adenoma

Feature	Pituitary Adenoma	Olfactory Neuroblastoma	Paraganglioma	Carcinoid
Synaptophysin	+	+	+	+
CAM 5.2	+	S	N	S
S-100 (sustentacular cells)	N	+	+	R
Hormones	+	N	N	S
Pit-1	+	unknown	unknown	unknown

+, almost always positive; N, negative; R, rare, and focally positive; S, sometimes positive.

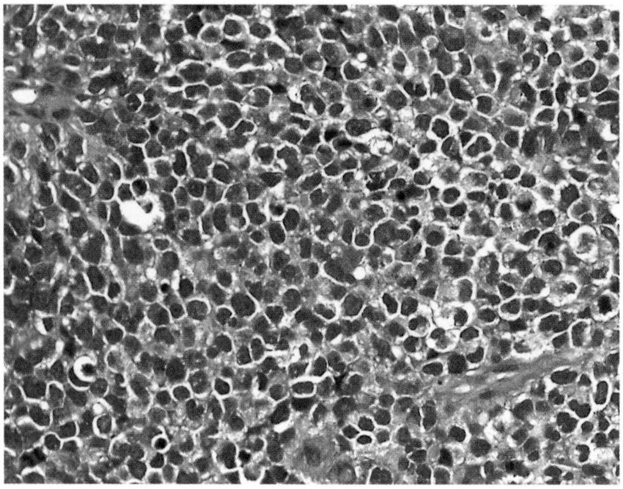

FIGURE 9.12 Rhabdomyosarcoma of sinonasal tract. (H&E, ×100 original magnification.)

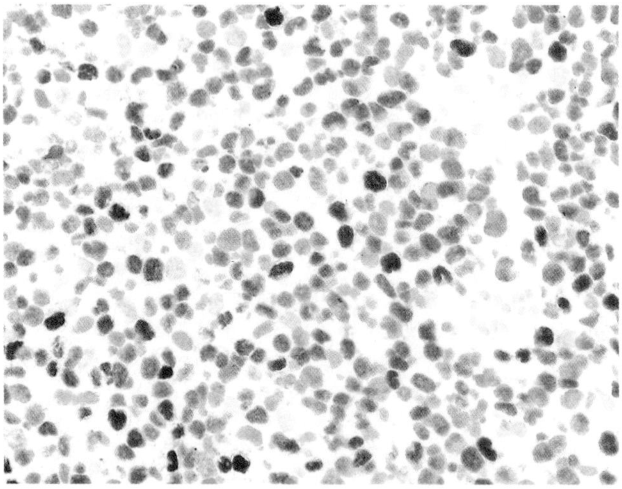

FIGURE 9.13 Myogenin nuclear expression in rhabdomyosarcoma of sinonasal tract. (Myogenin, ×100 original magnification.)

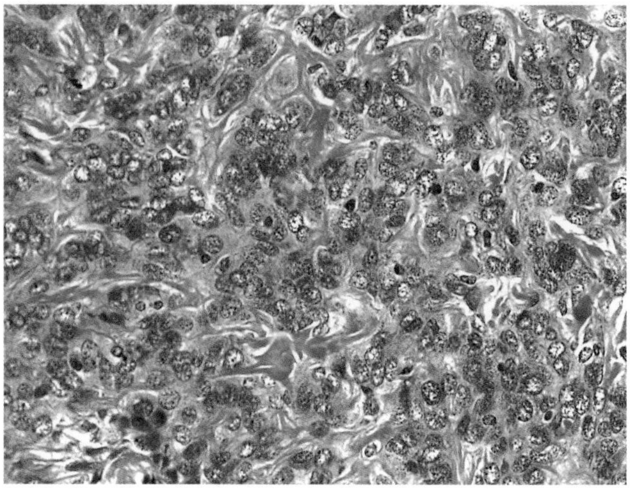

FIGURE 9.14 Ewing's sarcoma of sinonasal tract. (H&E, ×200 original magnification.)

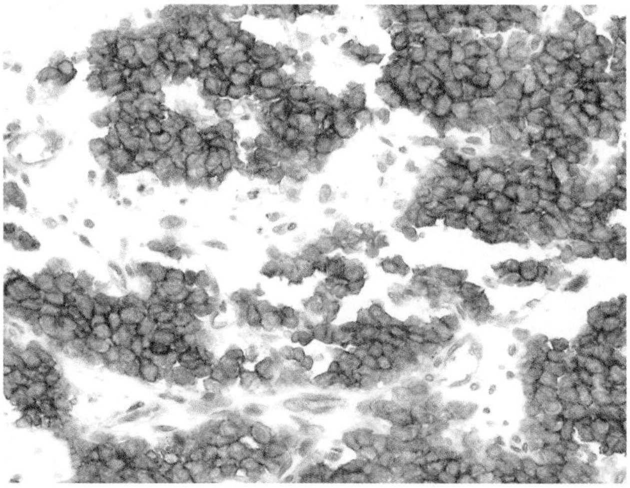

FIGURE 9.15 CD99 staining in Ewing's sarcoma of sinonasal tract. (CD99, ×200 original magnification.)

Ewing's Sarcoma and Peripheral Neuroectodermal Tumor

Although the peripheral neuroectodermal tumor (PNET) and ES were first described, respectively, by Stout in 1918 and Ewing in 1921, it has only recently been established through immunohistochemical and genetic-molecular studies that the two are not only related but also belong to the same family of tumors. ES/PNET may be found in bone, soft tissue, and various parenchymal organs (lung, pancreas, kidney), as well as the head and neck.

The majority of patients are adolescents or young adults, usually younger than 30 years of age. Occurrences in older individuals, however, have been documented. When all sites are considered, they are slightly more common in males (male-to-female ratio = 1.4:1). Only 2% to 10% of ES/PNETs occur in the head and neck.[146,147]

By light microscopy, ES/PNETs are composed of uniform round cells, which often grow in a lobular configuration (Fig 9.14). The nuclei have finely dispersed chromatin, sometimes with barely discernible nucleoli. The cytoplasm is scanty, poorly defined, and frequently pale owing to an abundance of glycogen. Homer Wright rosettes may be seen, as well as rare Flexner-Wintersteiner rosettes. Mitoses are highly variable.

ES/PNETs are positive for glycogen (PAS stain), vimentin, and CD 99 (Fig. 9.15). Some may also express synaptophysin, chromogranin, neuron-specific enolase, Leu-7, PGP 9.5, and NB-84. Up to 20% may also be positive, either focally or diffusely, for cytokeratin AE 1/3 and/or CAM 5.2.[148] Rarely, desmin may be focally positive.

KEY DIAGNOSTIC POINTS

Ewing's Sarcoma and Peripheral Neuroectodermal Tumor

- Ewing's sarcoma/peripheral neuroectodermal tumor is composed of uniform round cells with a lobular configuration.
- The tumor cells are positive for vimentin and CD99.

TABLE 9.9 Intestinal-type Adenocarcinoma versus Metastatic Adenocarcinoma of Colon

	CK7	CK20	CEA	CDX-2	Chromogranin	MUC2	MUC5
ITAC	S	+	S	+	S	+	R-N
Colon	R	+	+	+	R	+	R-N

+, almost always positive; N, negative; R, rare, and focally positive; S, sometimes positive.

Intestinal-Type Adenocarcinoma

Intestinal-type adenocarcinomas (ITACs) are rare tumors of the sinonasal tract that bear a remarkable histologic resemblance to tumors arising in the intestines.[149] Rare cases can even resemble normal small intestinal mucosa. There is an epidemiologic linkage to occupational exposure to wood dust, particularly the hard woods, as found in furniture making. ITAC is more common in males by a ratio of 4:1 and occurs over a broad age range, with an average of 58 years.[149]

Among several different classification schemes, all focus on morphologic features. Five histologic growth patterns are recognized: papillary, colonic, mucinous, solid, and mixed. One of the major dilemmas in ITAC is differentiating them from metastatic adenocarcinoma of the colon. Though subtle features may help in making this distinction (Table 9.9), clinical history is the most important variable.[150-155]

ITACs have features of a sinonasal-derived tumor but also share some immunohistochemical markers seen in the colorectal tumors that they resemble. For example, most ITACs will stain positive for CK7, which is the typical epithelial marker of the Schneiderian membrane.[118,156] They are also usually positive for CK20 and CDX2, which are typical of intestinal-derived malignancies.[156-158] Villin and MUC2 have also been described in ITACs.[157,159]

KEY DIAGNOSTIC POINTS

Intestinal-Type Adenocarcinoma

- Intestinal-type adenocarcinomas resemble colorectal carcinomas at the histologic level.
- ITACs usually stain positive with CK7, CK20, and CDX2.

Glomangiopericytoma (Sinonasal-Type Hemangiopericytoma)

Glomangiopericytoma was originally designated *sinonasal-type hemangiopericytoma.* Its relationship to the soft tissue hemangiopericytoma has been the subject of ongoing debate. Recent evidence suggests that the sinonasal lesions may be related to glomus tumors and this relationship is why new terminology has been applied, with the diagnostic entity being renamed as "glomangiopericytoma."[129,160-162] Glomangiopericytoma is an uncommon tumor that occurs more often in the nasal cavity than the sinuses. It is slightly more common in males and occurs over a broad age range with an average of 63 years.[129] Microscopically, it is composed of short spindled or epithelioid cells with hyperchromatic nuclei and clear to eosinophilic cytoplasm. A prominent vascularity is seen, resembling the staghorn vessels that are characteristic of their soft tissue counterparts.

In a review of 104 glomangiopericytomas, Thompson and colleagues[129] observed that 98% were positive for vimentin, 92% for smooth muscle actin, 78% for factor XIIIa, 77% for muscle specific actin, 52% for laminin, 8% for CD34, 3% for S-100 protein, and 3% for bcl-2. All were negative for desmin.

Although data indicate that extrasinonasal soft tissue hemangiopericytomas and solitary fibrous tumors are related and represent a spectrum of a single entity, glomangiopericytomas are unlikely to be related to solitary fibrous tissue. Glomangiopericytoma is rarely positive for CD34, bcl-2, or CD99.

KEY DIAGNOSTIC POINTS

Glomangiopericytoma

- Glomangiopericytomas are unique lesions that occur exclusively within the sinonasal tract.
- They are strongly positive for SMA and vimentin, but less commonly for CD34.

Theranostic Applications

Few molecular markers have diagnostic, prognostic, or theranostic value for lesions of the head and neck. The exceptions are SNUC and melanoma.

A recent study of SNUCs at the molecular level has revealed an interesting mutation in a subset of these tumors. Approximately 20% of undifferentiated tumors of the upper aerodigestive tract (including some in the sinonasal tract) were positive for the *NUT-BRD4* translocation.[163] These tumors tended to have an unusual morphologic appearance with abrupt keratinization and often had p63 positivity. This translocation was previously seen only in what were termed "central lethal carcinomas." The diagnostic and potential therapeutic applications of testing for the translocation are not well understood at this point.

In cutaneous MM, *BRAF* gene mutations are relatively common and have begun to be targeted for the therapeutic interventions.[164,165] Mucosal melanomas, however, do not appear to harbor significant numbers of *BRAF* mutations.[166] Interestingly, however, approximately a third of mucosal melanomas will have *KIT* mutations, similar to those seen in gastrointestinal stromal tumors.[167] This gene may also become a potential therapeutic target in mucosal melanomas.[168] From the diagnostic perspective, it appears that overexpression of KIT by immunohistochemistry correlates with the presence of the mutation, and thus this may become a useful marker in mucosal melanomas.[169]

Beyond Immunohistochemistry: Anatomic Molecular Diagnostic Applications

The sarcomas that arise in the sinonasal tract are similar to sarcomas in other locations and harbor molecular mutations that can be used diagnostically. At the molecular level, alveolar rhabdomyosarcomas are often positive for a specific translocation, PAX-FKHR.[144,170] There are diagnostic assays available for this translocation using fluorescence *in situ* hybridization or RT-PCR. ES/PNETs are associated with two characteristic chromosomal translocations resulting in fusion of the EWS gene with a member of the ETS family of transcription factors. The most common translocation t (11; 22) (q 24:q 12) is seen in about 85% to 90% of all tumors and involves a fusion of the EWS gene on chromosome 22 with the FLI-1 gene on chromosome 11, creating the chimeric gene product EWS-FLI-1.[171] The second translocation t (21; 22)(q 22; q 12) is seen in 5% to 10% of all ES/PNETs. Commercial antibodies are available for FLI1.[172,173] Immunohistochemistry that shows overexpression of FLI1 has been shown to correlate fairly well with the presence of the translocation.[172,173] According to Folpe and colleagues,[174] it is relatively sensitive (71%) and highly specific (92%) for ES/PNET in the setting of appropriate morphology.

NASOPHARYNX

Nasopharyngeal Carcinoma

Nasopharyngeal carcinoma (NPC) is defined by the World Health Organization as "a carcinoma arising in the nasopharyngeal mucosa that shows light or ultrastructural evidence of squamous differentiation. It encompasses squamous cell carcinoma, nonkeratinizing carcinoma (including differentiated and undifferentiated types), and BSCC. Adenocarcinomas and salivary gland–type carcinoma are excluded."[175]

The tumor occurs worldwide but has a distinct ethnic and geographic distribution. It is especially common in Southeast Asia and North Africa and among Eskimos. All age groups are affected, and it is two to three times more common in males. The etiology of NPC is multifactorial and relates to the interaction of race (particularly the Chinese), genetics, the environment, and the EBV.

The World Health Organization divides NPC into three categories (Table 9.10). The term "squamous cell carcinoma" is used for those tumors that show

TABLE 9.10 World Health Organization Classification of Nasopharyngeal Carcinoma

1. Squamous cell carcinoma
2. Nonkeratinization carcinoma A. Differentiated nonkeratinizing carcinoma B. Undifferentiated carcinoma
3. Basaloid squamous cell carcinoma

From Barnes L, Eveson JW, Reichart PA. Pathology and Genetics of Head and Neck Tumours. World Health Organization, 2005.

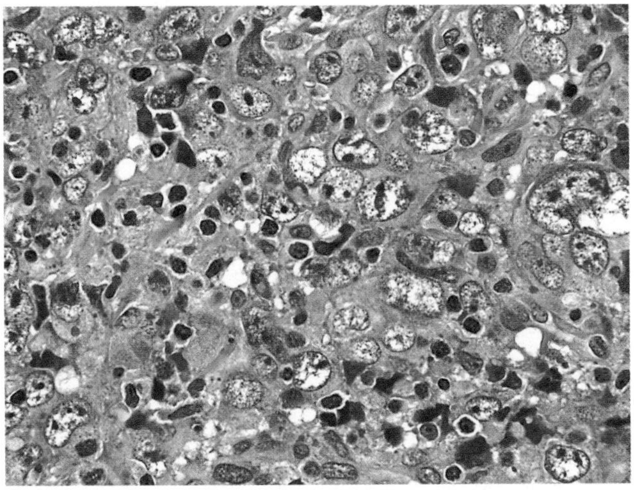

FIGURE 9.16 Lymphoepithelial carcinoma demonstrating syncytial sheets, vesicular nuclei, and infiltrating lymphocytes. (H&E, ×200 original magnification.)

definite evidence of squamous differentiation (intercellular bridges, keratinization) over most of its extent and is associated with a desmoplastic reaction. It can be graded as well, moderately, or poorly differentiated, has a weak relationship to EBV, tends to remain localized, and has a variable response to irradiation. It rarely occurs in individuals younger than 40 years of age.

The differentiated nonkeratinizing carcinoma, as the name implies, shows no evidence of keratinization. The cells are stratified and have an appearance similar to that of transitional cell carcinoma of the urinary bladder. The cell margins are distinct, and the junction between stroma and epithelium is sharp. This type tends to disseminate from its site of origin, and has a variable but usually good response to irradiation.

Undifferentiated carcinoma (also known as *lymphoepithelial carcinoma* and *lymphoepithelioma*) is composed of cells with indistinct margins and round to oval nuclei with prominent, round nucleoli (Fig. 9.16). The cells tend to grow in a syncytium rather than having a stratified or pavemented appearance. In some instances the tumor grows in well-defined epithelial aggregates (Regaud pattern) that are easily recognizable as carcinoma. In other instances, it grows as ill-defined sheets, small clusters, or individual cells admixed with lymphocytes (Schmincke pattern) simulating a malignant

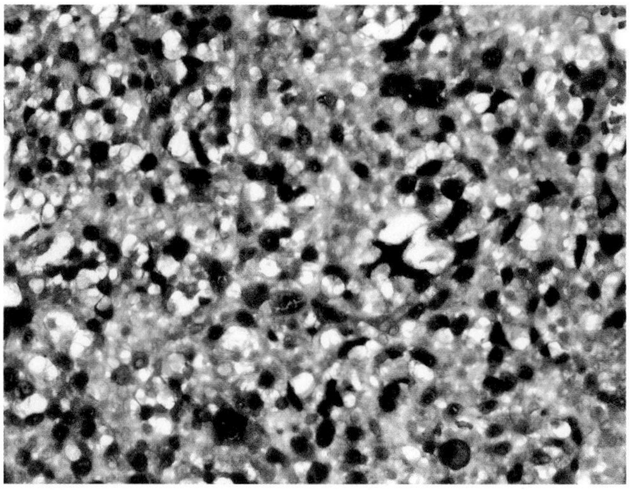

FIGURE 9.17 Epstein-Barr encoded RNA (EBER) *in situ* hybridization in lymphoepithelial carcinoma. (EBER *in situ* hybridization, ×200 original magnification.)

lymphoma. The lymphoid element, however, is not malignant and is rarely, if ever, observed in sites of metastasis. The undifferentiated carcinoma is the type most often found in children. It has a strong correlation with EBV (Fig. 9.17), tends to disseminate, and has a good response to irradiation.

Tumors identical to the undifferentiated type of NPC may originate in sites other than the nasopharynx, especially the sinonasal tract, oropharynx, larynx, and salivary gland.[176,177] They are distinguished from NPC only by location and observing the nasopharynx to be free of tumor. Likewise, the presence of EBV in a tumor is not unique to NPC. The virus has been found in a variety of histologically diverse tumors of the nasopharynx in patients from Southeast Asia.[178]

BSCCs of the nasopharynx are rare and only a few cases have been documented, mainly from Hong Kong. Some of these have been associated with EBV.

The undifferentiated NPC is strongly positive for pankeratin and cytokeratins 5/6, 8, 13, and 19. It is negative for cytokeratins 4, 7, 10, and 14 (see Table 9.5).[125] NPC is also generally positive for p53, occasionally positive for C-*kit*, and negative for HER 2 and leukocyte common antigen (LCA).[179,180] The lymphocytes are a mixture of T and B cells, and the interspersed plasma cells are polyclonal. S-100 protein-positive dendritic cells may also be apparent.

Diagnostic problems may arise with the differential diagnosis. The keratinizing NPC (SCC) is easily recognized and resembles SCC anywhere else in the body. The nonkeratinizing variants, on the other hand, may be more problematic and can be confused with a myriad of other small round cell tumors of the sinonasal tract including malignant lymphoma, malignant melanoma, olfactory neuroblastoma, extramedullary plasmacytoma, and rhabdomyosarcoma (see Table 9.3). Sinonasal undifferentiated carcinoma (SNUC), especially, is often confused with the undifferentiated NPC. Features that are useful in separating these two neoplasms are shown in Table 9.7. The other small round cell tumors can usually be excluded with an appropriate panel of immunostains (e.g., leukocyte common antigen, S-100 protein, HMB-45, synaptophysin, IgG, lambda and kappa light chains, myogenin) (see Table 9.3).

Nasopharyngeal Angiofibroma

Nasopharyngeal angiofibroma (NAF) is a highly vascular, histologically benign, but sometimes locally aggressive tumor of the nasopharynx that occurs almost exclusively in males, usually between 10 and 20 years of age. They are composed of two components: blood vessels and a fibrous stroma. The blood vessels are characteristically large and stellate, often with a "staghorn" appearance. Others range from smaller capillaries to sinusoids. The blood vessels are typically devoid of smooth muscle, although NAFs have vessels with an uneven layer of smooth muscle. The stroma is dense and fibrous. The stromal cells are predominantly fibroblasts and rarely myofibroblasts. Cellularity can vary.

The stromal cells are strongly positive for vimentin and negative for CD 34.[181,182] A few cells may be focally positive for smooth muscle actin. Beta-catenin has also been observed in the nuclei of fibroblasts but not in endothelial cells of most NAFs.[183]

The frequency of finding hormonal receptors, especially estrogen receptors, is controversial. Hwang and colleagues[184] studied 24 NAFs for androgen receptors (AR), estrogen receptors (ER), and progesterone receptors (PR) using immunochemistry. Eighteen (75%) of these cases were positive for AR and two (8.3%) were positive for PR. The receptors were observed in both stromal and endothelial cells. None of the cases were positive for ER. More recently, Montag and colleagues[185] studied 10 NAFs for AR, ER, and PR. Four (40%) of these cases were positive for AR in stromal cells only, and one (10%) was positive for PR, also only in stromal cells. All 10 (100%) of their cases were positive for ER-beta in both stromal and endothelial cells, while all cases were negative for ER-alpha. They suggested that the discrepancies in ER expression in various studies might be related to the character of the antibody.

ORAL CAVITY AND OROPHARYNX

Granular Cell Tumor

The granular cell tumor (GCT) is an uncommon tumor of Schwann cell origin with a predilection for skin and mucosal surfaces, especially the tongue. Most are benign, but a few are malignant. The tumor is positive for S-100 protein, neuron specific enolase, alpha-1-antitrypsin, CD 68, vimentin, inhibin-alpha, protein gene product 9.5, calretinin, and occasionally CD 57.[186-189] It is negative for keratin, MAC 387, smooth muscle actin, muscle-specific actin, and desmin.

LARYNX/HYPOPHARYNX

Both benign and malignant tumors can arise in the larynx and hypopharynx. By far the most common malignancy is SCC and its variants. Salivary gland–type

TABLE 9.11 Immunohistochemical Staining Pattern for Tumors in the Differential Diagnosis for Paragangliomas

Stain	Carcinoid Tumor	Paraganglioma	Medullary	Melanoma	Renal Cell	Metastatic (Thyroid CA, Carcinoma, or Lung Carcinoma)
Chromogranin	+	+	+	N	N	+
Synaptophysin	+	+	S	N	N	+
Cytokeratin 7	S	N	N	N	S	+
Cytokeratin 20	S	N	N	N	N	+
CEA	S	Unk	+	N	S	+
S-100	N	+ (sustentacular)	N	+	S	N
Calcitonin	N	N	+	N	N	N
TTF-1	N	N	+	N	N	+

+, almost always positive; N, negative; S, sometimes positive.

tumors may also arise from the mucoserous glands of the larynx (as well as stromal tumors). Benign lesions that are unique to the larynx and hypopharynx include vocal cord nodules and respiratory papillomatosis. Neuroendocrine tumors are relatively common in the larynx.

Vocal Cord Nodule

Vocal cord nodules are almost always associated with vocal abuse. They are confined to the true vocal cord, usually occurring on the free edge. There are five different histologic types of vocal cord nodules: myxoid, fibrinous, vascular, fibrous, and mixed. The vocal cord nodule will not stain with any specific immunohistochemical markers. Staining is only necessary to distinguish this lesion from other benign entities in the differential diagnosis. One example would be the use of an S100 stain to differentiate the fibrous type of vocal cord nodule from a neurofibroma.

Respiratory Papillomatosis

Respiratory papillomatosis is a disease that has a bimodal distribution, "juvenile-onset" and "adult-onset." These lesions are unequivocally related to HPV infection, which can be detected using immunohistochemical stains or *in situ* hybridization. HPV types 6 and 11 are found most frequently.[190]

Neuroendocrine Carcinoma Spectrum

The classification of neuroendocrine tumors of the head and neck has been controversial.[191] The WHO classification has divided the tumors into four categories: typical carcinoid, atypical carcinoid, small cell neuroendocrine carcinoma, and paraganglioma. Each of these tumor types is discussed separately. Immunohistochemical stains will not easily separate the four types of neuroendocrine carcinomas but will aid in differentiating this spectrum of diseases from the other tumor types in the differential diagnosis. The diagnostic algorithm is described in Table 9.11. Paragangliomas of the larynx are discussed later under "Paragangliomas and Malignant Paragangliomas."[192]

TYPICAL CARCINOID

These tumors in the larynx are rare, representing less than 3% of all neuroendocrine carcinomas of the larynx.[193] Histologically, the small, uniform cells can grow in a variety of patterns including small nests, cords, large sheets, glands, or pseudorosettes. The nuclei have typical features of neuroendocrine cells, with finely stippled chromatin. The stroma is highly vascular but can also exhibit some degree of fibrosis or hyalinization. Mitoses are rare to absent and necrosis is not seen.

ATYPICAL CARCINOID

This tumor is the most common neuroendocrine neoplasm of the larynx and accounts for approximately 54% of all tumors.[194] It occurs most frequently in the supraglottic larynx and has a male predominance. Atypical carcinoids have an infiltrative growth and can have variety of morphologic patterns. The cells differ from those of a typical carcinoid in that they are larger and show nucleoli and occasional mitoses. Furthermore, they may exhibit necrosis and vascular or perineural invasion.

SMALL CELL NEUROENDOCRINE CARCINOMA

Small cell neuroendocrine carcinoma (SCNEC) of the larynx is rare, representing less than 1% of all laryngeal carcinomas.[195] These tumors have been categorized in a similar fashion to lung tumors, into oat cell type, intermediate, and combined. The first two tumor types have typical neuroendocrine differentiation and show similar histologic features to those seen in lung carcinomas. They have small- to intermediate-sized cells with prominent necrosis, apoptosis, nuclear molding, and vascular and perineural invasion. The combined type shows conventional SCC or adenocarcinoma in addition to the neuroendocrine carcinoma.

These three neuroendocrine tumors of the larynx all display positivity for typical neuroendocrine markers such as chromogranin, synaptophysin, and neuron-specific enolase.[196] They may also be positive for carcinoembryonic antigen (CEA) or epithelial membrane antigen (EMA). Atypical carcinoid and SCNEC can also express other neuroendocrine markers such as serotonin, calcitonin, and somatostatin.[197] TTF-1 is probably not a useful marker to distinguish metastatic pulmonary small cell carcinoma from primary tumors in the head and neck because up to 50% of extrapulmonary small cell carcinomas are positive for TTR-1.[198]

The differential diagnosis of carcinoid and atypical carcinoid tumors of the larynx includes paraganglioma, melanoma, and medullary thyroid carcinoma. Paragangliomas are rarely always negative for cytokeratins and also exhibit the characteristic sustentacular cell pattern with S100 protein. Thyroid transcription factor-1 (TTF1) is positive in medullary thyroid carcinoma, as are calcitonin and CEA. Melanomas will typically stain with HMB45 and tyrosinase, both of which are negative in neuroendocrine carcinomas.

SCNEC must also be differentiated from BSCC, malignant lymphoma, and metastatic carcinomas from the lung. BSCC does not usually exhibit neuroendocrine staining. Malignant lymphoma can be detected using typical markers for hematopoietic cells such as CD20, CD3, CD43, and LCA. The primary head and neck neuroendocrine tumors and metastatic disease from the lung can be difficult because the staining patterns for CK7, CK20, and rarely TTF-1 can overlap; clinical and radiographic correlation is essential.

KEY DIAGNOSTIC POINTS

Neuroendocrine Tumors

- The three categories of neuroendocrine tumors (carcinoid, atypical carcinoid, and small cell neuroendocrine carcinoma) are distinguished from one another mainly on the basis of histologic appearance.
- The immunophenotype of these tumors includes positivity for neuroendocrine markers and for cytokeratins.
- TTF-1 may be positive in these extrapulmonary neuroendocrine/small cell carcinomas.

SALIVARY GLANDS

The majority of salivary gland tumors can be diagnosed by routine hematoxylin- and eosin-stained slides. Immunohistochemistry may play a role in the diagnosis of some tumors, especially to identify myoepithelial cells to highlight perineural and angiolymphatic invasion or to assess the proliferative rate of a tumor.

Pleomorphic Adenoma (Benign Mixed Tumor)

Pleomorphic adenoma (PA) is the most common salivary gland tumor. It occurs in all age groups, affects females more often than males, and may arise in either a major or a minor salivary gland location. When it originates in a major salivary gland, it is always encapsulated. Those of minor salivary gland origin are not encapsulated.

Microscopically, PAs are composed of varying proportions of epithelial and myoepithelial cells and a stroma that ranges from myxoid to hyaline to chondromyxoid. Although the tumor is usually easily recognized when excised intact, it may be difficult to separate from other tumors, especially polymorphous low-grade adenocarcinomas and adenoid cystic carcinomas, on small biopsies. Features that may be helpful are shown in Table 9.12.[54,199-202]

Myoepithelioma

Although myoepithelial cells are a significant component of several salivary neoplasms, tumors composed exclusively of myoepithelial cells are uncommon and are designated as myoepitheliomas.[203,204] Because they are rare and tend to be morphologically diverse, myoepitheliomas are likely to be underrecognized. Myoepitheliomas affect both sexes equally and occur over a broad age range including children, with an average age of 40 to 50 years.[205] They may arise in either a major or minor salivary gland, but encapsulation is usually only seen in the major glands. Myoepithelial cells have a variety of morphologic appearances including plasmacytoid (hyaline), spindle cells, and clear or epithelioid cells. Myoepitheliomas can be composed of a single cell type or can show mixed features. They are usually classified by the predominant cell type (e.g., spindle cell myoepithelioma, clear cell myoepithelioma). (Fig. 9.18). These morphologic variations do not have prognostic significance, but they do alter the considerations for the differential diagnosis.

Paralleling their histologic diversity, myoepitheliomas may also exhibit disparities in their immunoprofile. Numerous antibodies have been proposed to identify myoepithelial cells, all of which differ in their sensitivity and specificity (Table 9.13). One should therefore never rely on one marker for a suspected myoepithelioma; instead, a panel of immunohistochemical stains should be used. A broad panel that has good sensitivity and specificity includes p63, calponin, CK5, CK5/6, SMA, vimentin, and S-100 (Fig. 9.19).

Myoepitheliomas should be distinguished from pleomorphic adenomas and other salivary gland neoplasms. But the differential diagnosis may also include non–salivary gland lesions, depending on the predominant cell type in the myoepithelioma. For example, spindle cell myoepitheliomas should be differentiated from leiomyomas, schwannomas, and other spindle cell lesions.

TABLE 9.12 Differential Diagnosis of Pleomorphic Adenoma (PA), Polymorphous Low-Grade Adenocarcinoma (PLGA), and Adenoid Cystic Carcinoma (ACC)

Feature	PA	PLGA	ACC
Site	Major or minor salivary gland	Predominantly intraoral, especially palate	Major or minor salivary gland
Capsule	S	N	N
Cartilage	S	N	N
Perineural	N	S	+
Ki-67	<5%	<5%	>20%
S-100 protein	Strong	Strong	Strong
Bcl-2	Weak-moderate	Weak-moderate	Strong
GFAP	+	R	R
Smooth muscle actin	+	R-N	+
Myoepithelial cells	+	R	+
C-*kit*	19%	25%	94%

+, almost always positive; N, negative; R, rare, and focally positive; S, sometimes positive.

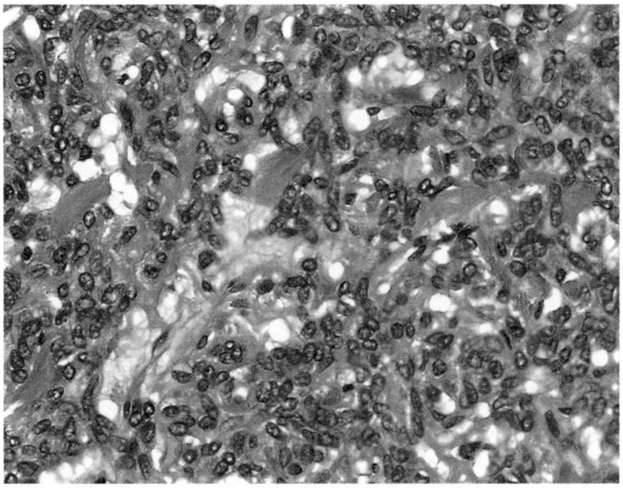

FIGURE 9.18 Myoepithelioma with spindle cell morphology. (H&E, ×200 original magnification.)

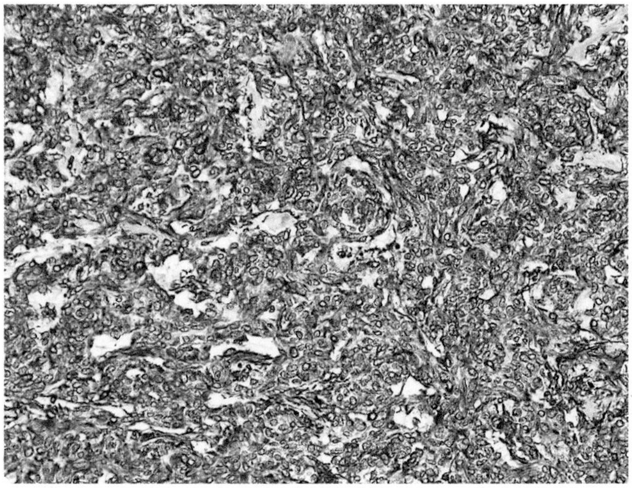

FIGURE 9.19 Vimentin staining in myoepithelioma. (Vimentin, ×200 original magnification.)

TABLE 9.13 Immunohistochemical Stains Used to Identify Myoepitheliomas

AE1/3	S-100 protein	CD10
CAM5.2	Calponin*	Maspin
CK5/6*	Smooth muscle actin	Metallothionein
CK14	Smooth muscle myosin heavy*	GFAP
34βE12	p63*	

*Best current sensitive and specific markers.
GFAP, glial fibrillary acidic protein.

The plasmacytoid variant may be mistaken for an extramedullary plasmacytoma. Clear cell myoepithelioma can be distinguished from an epithelial-myoepithelial carcinoma by the absence of ducts in myoepithelioma. Other clear cell tumors that might enter the differential diagnosis include clear cell carcinoma and metastatic renal cell carcinoma. These entities can be differentiated from myoepithelioma by morphologic and immunohistochemical clues.

Although the majority of myoepitheliomas are benign, rare myoepithelial carcinomas do exist. Myoepithelial carcinoma can be *de novo* or may arise from a pleomorphic adenoma as a form of carcinoma ex pleomorphic adenoma. Myoepithelial carcinomas generally show typical features of malignancy—invasion, pleomorphism, necrosis, and increased or atypical mitoses. Nagao and colleagues[206] indicate that tumors that exhibit greater than 7 mitoses/10 high power fields, a ki-67 index of greater than 10%, and strong expression of p53 are likely to be malignant. In a review of 25 myoepithelial carcinomas, Savera and colleagues[207] observed that 100% were positive for AE 1/3, 53% for CK 14, 100% for calponin, 50% for smooth muscle actin, and 31% for GFAP.

Mucoepidermoid Carcinoma

Mucoepidermoid carcinoma (MEC) is the most common salivary gland malignancy; it represents between 2% and 16% of all salivary gland tumors and up to one third of malignant salivary gland tumors.[208] About 50% of MECs occur in the major salivary glands, with the minor salivary glands in the palate being the most common secondary site.[209] Other unusual sites can also be affected (retromolar area, floor of mouth, buccal mucosa, lip, and tongue).[210,211] This is the most common malignant salivary gland tumor in children.[212-214] Rare tumors are thought to arise primarily within the bone.[215]

Histologically, MEC carcinoma has three cellular components: mucus cells, epidermoid cells, and intermediate cells. Mucus cells can be either clear cells that contain glycogen or mucin[208] or goblet-like cells that are columnar and contain abundant mucin, which can be prominent in low-grade tumors. Epidermoid cells have eosinophilic cytoplasm. Keratin production should be sparse. Intermediate cells can be either basal cells or larger cells that have a transitional appearance between squamous and mucin secreting cells. Clear cells, columnar cells, and reserve cells make up minor components of MEC.[209] Occasionally, MECs can be oncocytic, and these are referred to as *oncocytic variant of MEC*.[216,217]

Grading is extremely important in MEC because it correlates with prognosis in almost every study that has been done. The grading systems have varied over time. The first grading system only measured the amount of cyst content. Tumors with more than 90% cyst content were considered to be low grade and those with less than 90% were considered to be high grade.[218,219] Later grading systems converted to a three-tiered system, with low-, intermediate-, and high-grade tumors.[220] The three-tiered grading system has been validated by several additional series that consistently show correlation between tumor grade and prognosis.[221-224] The histologic features for grading these tumors have become more complex than the earlier systems of just examining cyst content. Auclair and colleagues[225] developed a system for grading MECs with a point system to assess prognostic features, and this was modified by Brandwein with additional features.[208]

Immunohistochemistry has not been useful in the diagnosis of MEC because there are no specific markers for this tumor. However, p63 will stain the epidermoid component, and this can potentially be diagnostically useful.

KEY DIAGNOSTIC POINTS

Mucoepidermoid Carcinoma

- Three cell populations can generally be seen in mucoepidermoid carcinoma (MEC): epidermoid cells, mucous cells, and intermediate cells.
- No immunohistochemical stains are sensitive or specific for MEC in routine diagnostic use.
- p63 nuclear expression resides in the epidermoid component.

Polymorphous Low-Grade Adenocarcinoma

Polymorphous low-grade adenocarcinoma (PLGA) was first described independently and almost simultaneously in 1983 by Freedman and Lumerman and Batsakis and colleagues.[226,227] As the name implies, it is a low-grade, slowly growing tumor that arises almost exclusively from the minor salivary glands of the oral cavity, especially the palate. Exceptionally, it may arise in the parotid gland, either *de novo* or in a pleomorphic adenoma (PLGA ex pleomorphic adenoma) or from other nonoral minor mucoserous glands. It is two times more common in females and occurs over a broad age range (23 to 94 years), with an average age of about 55 to 60 years.[201]

The histologic hallmarks of PLGA are its many morphologic (polymorphic) patterns of growth, cytologic uniformity, and infiltrative growth. The growth patterns include solid (lobular), glandular, cribriform, trabecular, cystic, fascicular, or papillary configuration. The cells have scant to moderate amounts of eosinophilic to amphophilic cytoplasm and uniform, round to oval nuclei with typically vesicular chromatin. The nuclei can even have a "ground glass" appearance, like those seen in papillary carcinoma of the thyroid. Nucleoli are inconspicuous to absent, mitoses are few, and necrosis is not generally seen. Cells with clear or oxyphilic cytoplasm are focally present in some tumors. Myoepithelial cells are sparse to absent. The stroma varies from mucoid to hyaline to fibrovascular, but chondroid stroma is not seen. Occasionally glands may contain luminal mucin, but intracytoplasmic mucin is uncommon. Intratubular psammoma body–like calcifications are identified in some tumors. PLGAs are nonencapsulated and infiltrate adjacent tissues. Perineural invasion is common and characteristically involves the nerve in a "targetoid" fashion.

The differential diagnosis includes pleomorphic adenoma and adenoid cystic carcinoma (ACC). An immunohistochemical stain for GFAP may be helpful in separating PLGA from PA. According to Gnepp and el-Mofty,[200] the stromal and sometimes the epithelial components of PA are typically positive for GFAP, whereas in PLGA, these cells are usually negative.

Few specific and sensitive immunohistochemical stains will be useful to distinguish PLGA from ACC. Both tumors can be positive for bcl-2 and C-*kit*,[228-230] and both tumors can be positive for S100. PLGA, however, is often diffusely and strongly positive for S100, whereas ACC will show only peripheral myoepithelial type staining with S100.[231] EMA may also be useful because more than 90% of the tumor cells in PLGA are

KEY DIAGNOSTIC POINTS

Polymorphous Low-Grade Adenocarcinoma

- Polymorphous low-grade adenocarcinoma (PLGA) is predominantly a tumor of minor salivary glands of the oral cavity.
- Myoepithelial cells are sparse or absent in PLGA, but S-100 protein is usually diffusely positive.

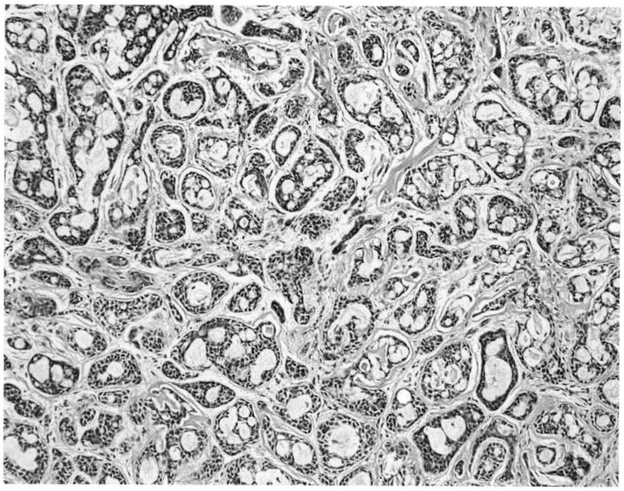

FIGURE 9.20 Adenoid cystic carcinoma demonstrating characteristic tubular and cribriform growth patterns. (H&E, ×200 original magnification.)

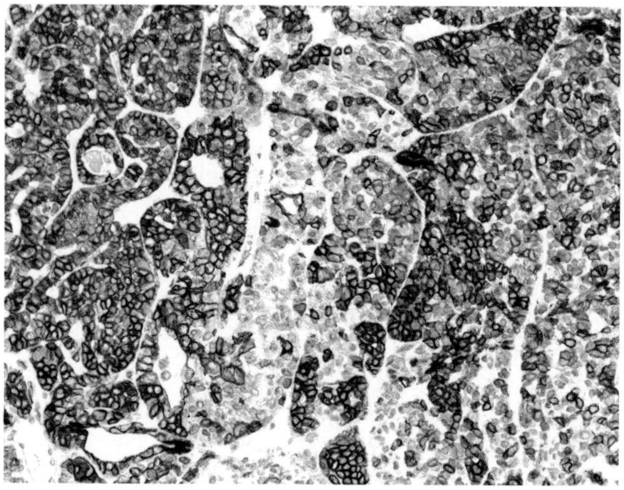

FIGURE 9.21 C-*kit* membrane immunostaining in adenoid cystic carcinoma. (C-*kit*, ×200 original magnification.)

positive for EMA, whereas it will stain only those cells lining true lumina (not the nonluminal tumor cells) in ACC.[232] Other features that are helpful in differentiating these neoplasms are shown in Table 9.12.

Adenoid Cystic Carcinoma

Adenoid cystic carcinoma (ACC), with few exceptions, is a low-grade tumor with a relentless clinical course, characterized by repeated local recurrences, late metastasis, and ultimate death over a course of 5 to 15 years. It is more common in females and occurs over a broad age range, though it is uncommon in individuals younger than 20 years of age.

Pathologically, it consists of two populations of cells—epithelial and myoepithelial—arranged in a tubular, cribriform, and/or solid pattern (Fig. 9.20). Stromal deposits are usually either myxoid or hyaline material that is deposited with the lumens of cribriform spaces. The epithelial cells stain with a variety of cytokeratins (AE 1/3, 1, 5, 7, 8, 10, 14, 18, and 19).[61,202] The myoepithelial cells are characteristically small, dark, and angulated and stain with a variety of "myoepithelial" markers (see Table 9.13).

Initially, it was thought that C-*kit* expression was unique to ACC and could be used to distinguish it from other "look-alike" salivary tumors on small biopsies. With experience, it has become apparent that C-*kit* can be found in other salivary tumors such as polymorphous low-grade adenocarcinoma and basal cell adenocarcinoma.[54] Nevertheless, the extent and intensity of staining of C-*kit* in ACC usually exceeds these other tumors and, accordingly, it may have some diagnostic significance (Fig. 9.21). The stain highlights only the epithelial cells in ACC, with myoepithelial cells being negative.

ACC is usually not difficult to recognize when totally excised. However, small biopsies, especially from the palate, may pose problems in diagnosis (see Table 9.12). Rare cases of ACC will undergo high-grade transformation, or dedifferentiation.[60] These tumors exhibit high-grade morphologic features including cytologic pleomorphism, necrosis, and vascular invasion.[60] In the areas of high-grade transformation, the cells take on a purely epithelial phenotype, with total loss of the myoepithelial component. The immunohistochemical stains will parallel the histology. Furthermore, these high-grade tumors will often overexpress p53.[60,61]

KEY DIAGNOSTIC POINTS

Adenoid Cystic Carcinoma

- Adenoid cystic carcinoma has three growth patterns: cribriform, tubular, and solid.
- These tumors are composed of both an epithelial cell component and a myoepithelial component, and immunohistochemical stains can be used to identify each.
- High-grade transformation is accompanied by a change to pure epithelial cells and a complete loss of myoepithelial cells. These tumors are often p53 positive.

Epithelial-Myoepithelial Carcinoma

Epithelial-myoepithelial carcinoma (EMC) is a low-grade, malignant biphasic salivary tumor of probable intercalated duct origin that comprises 1% to 2% of all salivary neoplasms. Donath and coworkers[233] are usually credited with calling attention to this tumor in 1972. It occurs most often in the parotid gland but may also arise from minor salivary glands.[234] It is slightly more common in women (1.5 females-to-1 male) and occurs in patients averaging 60 years of age (range 13 to 83 years).[234,235]

The tumors are either partially encapsulated or nonencapsulated. On low-power magnification, EMC tends to grow in a diffuse or multinodular pattern. The tumors are composed of small ducts composed of cuboidal cells with pink cytoplasm and centrally or basally located round nuclei. This epithelial cell component

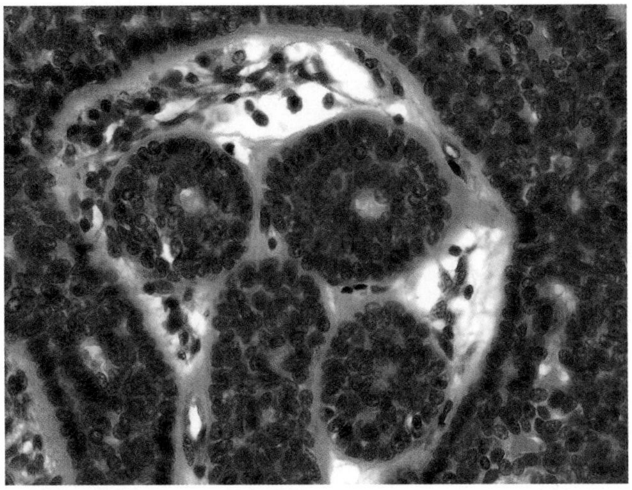

FIGURE 9.22 Epithelial-myoepithelial carcinoma demonstrating two cell populations and dense surrounding basement membrane. (H&E, ×200 original magnification.)

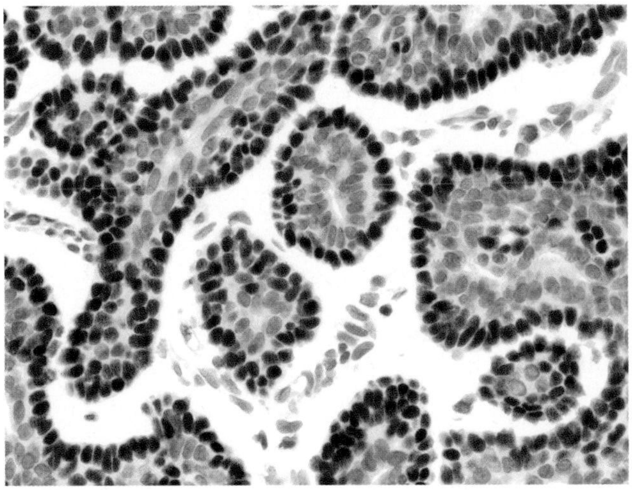

FIGURE 9.23 p63 in epithelial-myoepithelial carcinoma highlighting the myoepithelial cells. (p63, ×200 original magnification.)

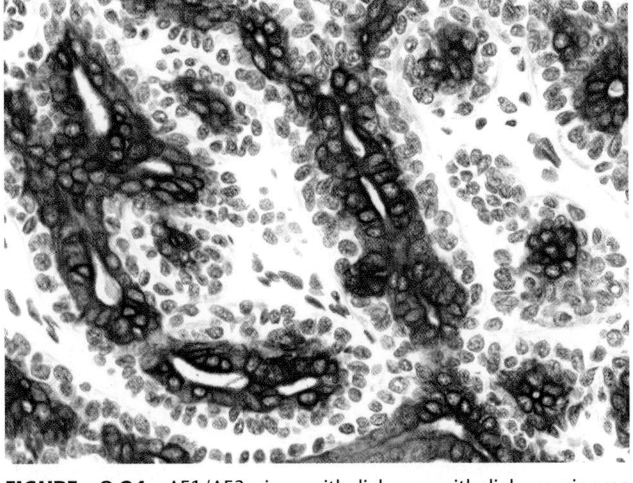

FIGURE 9.24 AE1/AE3 in epithelial-myoepithelial carcinoma highlighting the epithelial luminal cells. (AE1-3, ×200 original magnification.)

is surrounded by one or more layers of myoepithelial cells. These myoepithelial cells are often cleared and vary from cuboidal, to ovoid, to spindled, with vesicular to mildly hyperchromatic nuclei. Surrounding these biphasic ducts, there is often a deposition of dense, eosinophilic basement membrane–type material (Fig. 9.22). Some ducts contain eosinophilic secretory material that may stain for mucin; intracytoplasmic mucin, however, is not seen. The clear cells contain abundant glycogen.

The histologic appearance varies not only between tumors but also within the same neoplasm. Some areas of the tumor may be composed primarily of clear cells with only few widely scattered ducts, whereas other areas may be composed primarily of ducts. Sebaceous differentiation is also possible, as are other types of cellular differentiation such as oncocytic changes.[236,237] These tumors can occasionally undergo dedifferentiation in a similar manner to adenoid cystic carcinoma.[238] On immunostaining, the ductal cells are strongly positive for cytokeratins such as AE1-3 and CAM5.2. The myoepithelial component is usually strongly positive for typical myoepithelial cell markers such as p63, SMA, and calponin (see Table 9.13, Figs. 9.23 and 9.24).

Results of proliferating nuclear antigen immunohistochemical studies indicate that the myoepithelial cell, rather than the epithelial cell, is the predominant proliferating element in EMC.[239] There is no overexpression of HER-2/neu oncogene and, from initial studies, determination of DNA ploidy offers no additional prognostic information.[235,240]

KEY DIAGNOSTIC POINTS

Epithelial-Myoepithelial Carcinoma

- Epithelial-myoepithelial carcinoma is a biphasic tumor, composed of well-organized epithelial cells growing in ducts and tubules and surrounded by myoepithelial cells; these are often encircled by dense hyalinized stroma.
- Both the epithelial and the myoepithelial cell components can be identified with immunohistochemical stains.

Clear Cell Carcinoma

Many salivary and nonsalivary tumors contain clear cells. Among these are mucoepidermoid carcinoma, acinic cell carcinoma, oncocytoma, renal cell carcinoma, and clear cell odontogenic carcinoma.[241,242] Though most of these can be distinguished by their morphology and staining profile, a group of these tumors cannot be further categorized and are referred to as *clear cell carcinomas*.

Clear cell carcinomas, also known as *hyalinizing clear cell carcinomas,* arise primarily from minor salivary glands in the oral cavity and oropharynx. Of 60 cases reviewed by Ellis and Auclair, 28% occurred in the parotid gland and 12% in the submandibular gland; the remaining 60% were of minor salivary gland origin.[243]

TABLE 9.14 Staining Pattern in the Differential Diagnosis for Clear Cell Tumors

Stain	Renal Cell Carcinoma	Oncocytoma	Hyalinizing Clear Cell Carcinoma	Clear Cell Myoepithelioma
EMA	+	N	+	+
CD10	+	N	Unk	S
Vimentin	+	+	Unk	+
RCC	S	N	Unk	Unk
CEA	N	Unk	+	N
S-100	S	Unk	N	+
SMA	N	Unk	N	+
GFAP	N	Unk	N	+

+, almost always positive; N, negative; S, sometimes positive.

There is a female predilection of 1.6:1, and the median age is 53 years (range 1 to 86 years).[244] Most present as a submucosal, painless mass between 0.5 and 3.5 cm.

Clear cell carcinomas are composed of round to polygonal cells with centrally placed relatively uniform nuclei and inconspicuous nucleoli. The cytoplasm is clear as a result of glycogen accumulation. There is generally no significant pleomorphism and mitoses are rare to absent. The tumor cells grow in solid nests, cords, and/or trabeculae, frequently separated by bands of hyalinized connective tissue. Perineural invasion is common. The cells are negative for mucin. They are positive for cytokeratin, EMA, and, exceptionally, for CEA. They are negative for myoepithelial markers (e.g., S-100 protein, actin, GFAP, P63) (Table 9.14).

Clear cell carcinoma can be distinguished from clear cell myoepithelioma/carcinoma and epithelial-myoepithelial carcinoma by the fact that the latter two entities contain myoepithelial cells, which are absent in clear cell carcinoma.[244,245] Renal cell carcinomas may be positive for renal cell carcinoma antigen and usually positive for vimentin and negative for high-molecular-weight cytokeratin 903 (specific for cytokeratins 1, 5, 10, and 11).[246] Clear cell carcinomas, in turn, are positive for EMA and negative for vimentin and renal cell carcinoma antigen.

Salivary Duct Carcinoma

Salivary duct carcinoma (SDC) is a relatively uncommon, clinically aggressive adenocarcinoma of salivary origin that is histologically similar to carcinoma of the breast. In a review of 104 cases in 1994, Barnes and colleagues[247] noted that the tumor was three times more common in men and occurred primarily in patients older than the age of 50 years (range 22 to 91 years). The tumor occurs mainly in the parotid gland (88% of all cases), infrequently in the submandibular gland (8% of all cases), and rarely in the minor salivary glands (4% of all cases). The tumor may arise *de novo* or from a pleomorphic adenoma (carcinoma ex pleomorphic adenoma).

Microscopically, SDCs are characterized by both intraductal and infiltrating ductal carcinoma. The tumor grows in papillary, cribriform, and/or solid patterns, with central (comedo) necrosis (Fig. 9.25). In other instances the infiltrating tumor forms small ducts or cords of cells with a desmoplastic stromal resection such as seen in some forms of breast carcinoma. The tumor cells have amphophilic to pink cytoplasm and large, pleomorphic, vesicular nuclei with prominent nucleoli. Some have an apocrine appearance and can even demonstrate apical snouts. Mitoses, lymphatic, vascular, and perineural invasion are common. Dystrophic calcification may also be seen, sometimes even on radiographs, and may masquerade as calculi.

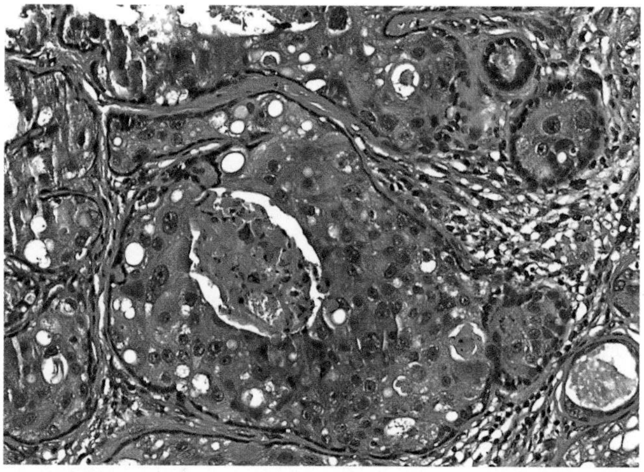

FIGURE 9.25 Salivary duct carcinoma showing central comedo-type necrosis. (H&E, ×200 original magnification.)

The presence of a uniform layer of cells around tumor islands that are positive for myoepithelial markers such as p63 is useful in identifying an *in situ* (intraductal) component of the tumor. Lewis and colleagues[248] studied 25 cases and observed that 100% were positive for EMA, 88% for AE 1/3, 76% for GCDFP, and 72% for CEA. In contrast to breast carcinomas, which are frequently positive for estrogen and progesterone receptors, SDCs, with rare exceptions, are negative for these receptors. More than 90% of SDCs, however, are positive for androgen receptor (Fig 9.26).[249] Rare cases may also stain with prostate-specific antigen (PSA) and/or prostatic acid phosphatase (PA), which together with a positive androgen receptor may result in confusion with a metastatic prostatic carcinoma.[250]

HER2/neu (C-erb B-2) overexpression has been found in 25% to 88% of SDCs (Fig. 9.27).[251] Whether it has prognostic significance, however, is controversial. In one study of HER 2-neu and SDC, Skalova and colleagues[252] observed that 8 of 11 cases showed strong distinct membrane staining for this marker (score 3+) with immunohistochemistry, while the remaining three cases were inconclusive with scores of 1+ to 2+. Using FISH, they observed that 4 of the 10 cases that were analyzed showed HER2/neu gene amplification. They, however, observed no differences in prognosis between amplified and nonamplified tumors. p53 positivity was found in 58% of SDCs studied by Felix and colleagues[251] but did not correlate with the clinical course.

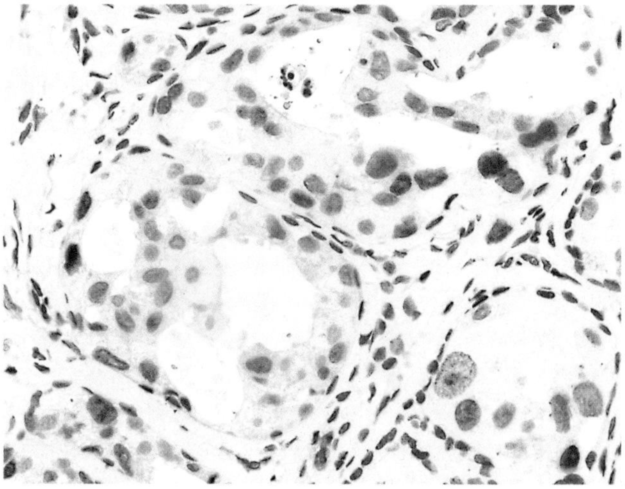

FIGURE 9.26 Androgen receptor in salivary duct carcinoma. (Androgen receptor, ×200 original magnification.)

KEY DIAGNOSTIC POINTS

Salivary Duct Carcinoma

- Salivary duct carcinoma (SDC) resembles some breast carcinomas histologically.
- SDC is positive for androgen receptor and HER2/neu; HER2/neu is often amplified by FISH.

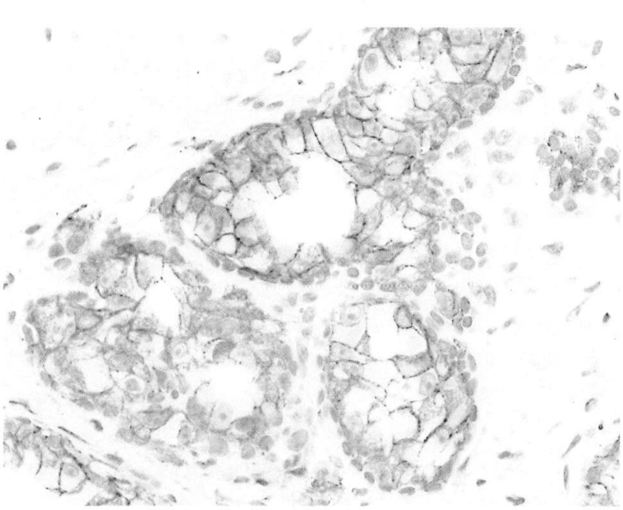

FIGURE 9.27 HER2/neu staining in salivary duct carcinoma showing a membranous pattern. (HER2/neu, ×100 original magnification.)

Low-Grade Cribriform Cystadenocarcinoma

A relatively newly described entity that has gone under several different names is low-grade cribriform cystadenocarcinoma. It has been also called *low-grade salivary duct carcinoma*[253] and *low-grade intraductal carcinoma*.[254]

Low-grade cribriform cystadenocarcinoma has a variety of growth patterns including cribriform, papillary and micropapillary, and Roman bridge formation (Fig. 9.28).[255] Cytologically, the tumor cells may be apocrine and can even have apocrine snouts. Other features are distinctive microvesicles, and these have been described as containing refractile pigment.

The immunohistochemical staining profile of low-grade cystadenocarcinoma can be helpful in the workup of these rare lesions. The lesion will be strongly and diffusely positive for S-100 (Fig. 9.29). Importantly, a myoepithelial cell layer will be preserved around the periphery of the nests of tumor cells. It has been claimed that this tumor should be considered to be an *in situ* tumor because a myoepithelial layer is preserved (Fig. 9.30).[254] The tumors are usually negative for androgen receptor and for HER2/Neu.[256]

Some low-grade cribriform cystadenocarcinomas have been reported in conjunction with salivary duct carcinoma. Others have been described as having minimal stromal invasive components and these areas do lose their myoepithelial cells.[256] However, in pure low-grade cribriform cystadenocarcinoma lesions, the prognosis is excellent. No recurrences were seen in two separate series, with a mean follow-up of 32 months in one series and 2 to 12 years in the second series.[256,257]

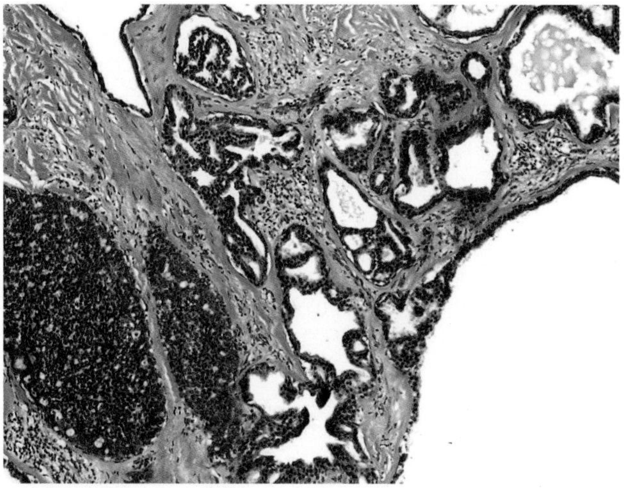

FIGURE 9.28 Low-grade cribriform cystadenocarcinoma, demonstrating several different morphologic patterns that can be seen in this lesion. (H&E, ×100 original magnification.)

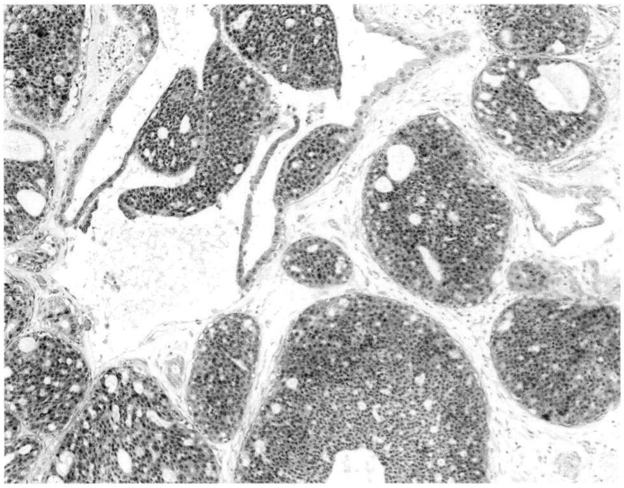

FIGURE 9.29 Low-grade cribriform cystadenocarcinoma showing typical strong and diffuse immunostaining with S-100. (S-100, ×100 original magnification.)

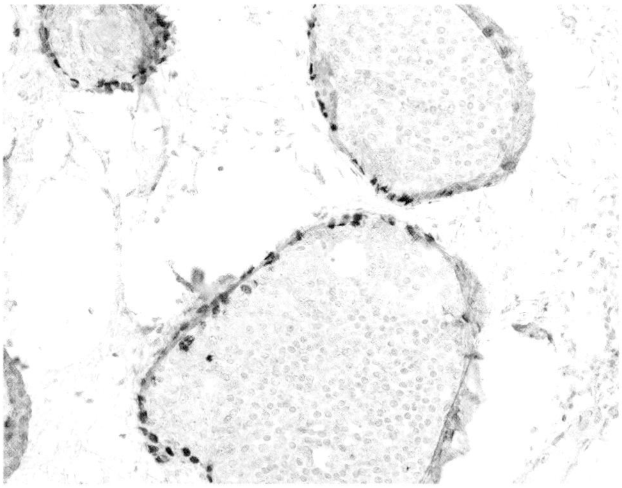

FIGURE 9.30 Low-grade cribriform cystadenocarcinoma showing layer of p63 positive myoepithelial cells around the lobules of tumor cells. (p63, ×400 original magnification.)

KEY DIAGNOSTIC POINTS

Low-Grade Cribriform Cystadenocarcinoma

- Low-grade cribriform cystadenocarcinoma is a rare tumor that grows in a variety of patterns.
- This tumor is positive for S-100 in a strong and diffuse manner.
- Because it is an *in situ* carcinoma, the nests of tumor cells are surrounded by a well-defined myoepithelial cell layer that can be detected with typical myoepithelial cell immunohistochemical markers.

Theranostic Applications

Although C-*kit* is typically positive in ACC, these tumors do not harbor mutations in the KIT gene, and therefore the Gleevec has shown little effectiveness against ACC.[53,258,259] No other genomic alterations recognized by IHC in salivary gland tumors have potential therapeutic value to date.

Beyond Immunohistochemistry: Anatomic Molecular Diagnostic Applications

The molecular events that contribute to the development of other salivary gland tumors such as MEC are beginning to be discovered. An interesting discovery in MEC was the identification of the translocation t(11;19)(q21-22;p13) between *WAMTP1*(*MECT*) and *MAML2* that disrupts the Notch signaling pathway.[260-263] Recent evidence suggests that this translocation may have prognostic relevance because it is seen almost exclusively in low- and intermediate-grade MEC and not in high-grade tumors.[261]

EAR/TEMPORAL BONE

Ectopic Neuroglial Tissue

Islands of neuroglial tissue occurring outside the central nervous system (CNS) are uncommon but have been described in a variety of sites in the head and neck. Two of the most common sites are the nose ("nasal glioma") and middle ear–temporal bone.[264-266] Ectopic neuroglial tissue (ENGT) should not be confused with an encephalocele. An encephalocele retains a connection to the CNS, whereas ENGT does not.

ENGT appears gray and may be localized, diffuse, or totally unexpected in the tissue specimen submitted to the laboratory. Often it is associated with a cholesteatoma or granulation tissue.

ENGT may or may not appear inflamed and/or fibrotic but often exhibits gliosis. Meninges are usually absent. Microscopically, it can be difficult to distinguish from granulation tissue. This can, however, be easily accomplished with a glial fibrillary acidic protein stain (GFAP). ENGT is positive for GFAP and granulation tissue is negative.

Middle Ear Adenoma

Middle ear adenomas (MEAs, also known as *carcinoid tumors* and *neuroendocrine adenomas*) are distinctly uncommon tumors that affect both sexes equally and occur over a broad age range (14 to 80 years) with an average of about 40 to 45 years.[267,268] The most common complaints are unilateral hearing loss, tinnitus, and fullness in the ear. Otorrhea and pain are uncommon. On imaging, the tumor is always extraosseous with no evidence of bone destruction.

Grossly the tumors are white, gray, red, brown, or yellow and may be localized or fill the entire middle ear, often encasing the ossicles. Microscopically, MEAs are characterized by architectural diversity and cytologic uniformity. Some are composed of well-formed glands, sheets of cells, small cells/or clusters, short trabeculae, or a combination of these patterns (Fig. 9.31). Individual cells vary from round or cuboidal to columnar

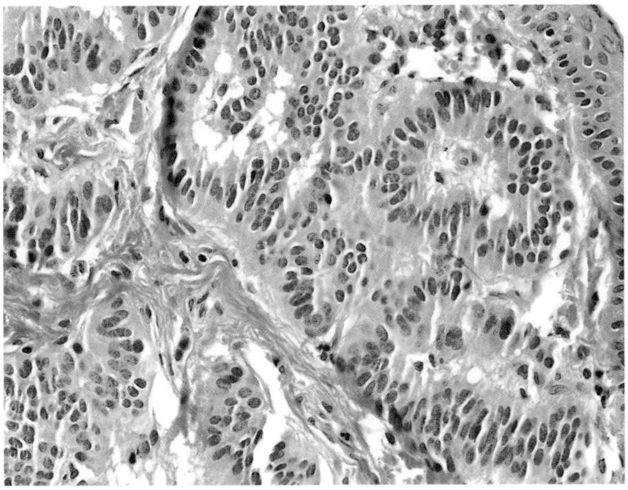

FIGURE 9.31 Middle ear adenoma. (H&E, ×100 original magnification.)

and contain a single central to eccentric nucleus. The cytoplasm is pink to amphophilic. Mitoses and necrosis are not seen. The stroma is vascular and varies from loose and edematous to fibrous. Inflammatory cells are inconspicuous.

In a study of 48 cases, Torske and colleagues observed 90% to be positive for AE 1/AE3, 90% for CK 7, 6% for CK 20, 81% for CAM 5.2, 88% for chromogranin, 31% for synaptophysin, 25% for serotonin, 84% for human pancreatic polypeptide, and 100% for vimentin.[268]

Whether the MEA and carcinoid tumor are separate or related entities continues to be debated. The current opinion is that they represent the same tumor but with different degrees of neuroendocrine differentiation.

The differential diagnosis includes otitis media with glandular differentiation (OMGD), ceruminous adenoma, jugulotympanic paraganglioma (JTPG), endolymphatic sac tumor (ELST), and a metastasis to the temporal bone. In contrast to MEA, the glands in OMGD are not densely concentrated but rather loosely arranged in an inflammatory background. Moreover, the glands are negative for neuroendocrine markers. A ceruminous adenoma can be excluded almost by history alone. It occurs only in the external auditory canal and not the middle ear. Ceruminous adenomas have a ductal epithelial component and an outer myoepithelial component by immunohistochemistry, and they are also negative for neuroendocrine markers.[269] The JTPG is devoid of glands, exhibits a "Zellballen" growth, and is negative for cytokeratin. The ELST has a characteristic papillary configuration that is not seen in MEA. Carcinomas of the breast, lung, and kidney are the most common tumors to metastasize to the temporal bone. The metastases are hematogenous and are found within bone, whereas the MEA is always extraosseous. In addition, metastatic tumors generally show cellular pleomorphism and abnormal mitoses. Metastatic tumors are often negative for neuroendocrine markers, which are generally observed in MEAs.

Endolymphatic Sac Tumor

Endolymphatic sac tumors (ELST, aggressive papillary middle ear tumor, papillary adenoma, low-grade papillary adenocarcinomas, Heffner's tumor) are rare, slowly growing, locally aggressive tumors of endolymphatic sac origin that characteristically involve the middle ear–temporal bone and cerebellopontine angle.[270,271]

As with middle ear adenomas, ELSTs occur over a broad age range (average ≈ 40 years) and affect both sexes equally. Unilateral hearing loss, tinnitus, and vertigo are the usual presenting symptoms, occasionally associated with facial nerve paralysis.

Physical examination may be normal or show a blue or red mass behind the tympanic membrane. There is no significant lateralization to either ear. Bilateral lesions, either synchronous or asynchronous, have been described but are exceptional and should always arouse suspicion of Von-Hippel-Lindau disease (VHLD). Preliminary data indicate that at least 15% of all ELSTs are associated with VHLD and that the ELST is just another expanding list of lesions associated with this syndrome.[272]

Histologically, the tumor is composed of papillary-cystic components. The papillae are well vascularized and covered by a single layer of cuboidal cells that have clear to pink cytoplasm and uniform round nuclei. Cellular pleomorphism and mitoses are absent. The cystic spaces characteristically contain pink colloid-like material imparting a thyroid-like appearance. The secretory material is strongly positive with the periodic acid-Schiff stain and negative with mucicarmine. Areas of closely packed glands, fibrosis, hemorrhage, and cholesterol clefts may also be seen. The epithelial cells contain glycogen but no intracytoplasmic mucin. In contrast to the middle ear adenoma, which does not invade bone, the ELST often shows this feature.

Because of its rarity, the immunoprofile of the ELST is still evolving.[271,273,274] Preliminary evidence indicates that about 100% are positive for cytokeratin (AE 1/3, CAM 5.2), 100% for vimentin, 86% for neuron specific enolase, 61% for S-100 protein, and 0% to 20% for GFAP.[273] It is negative for transthyretin (pre-albumen) and thyroglobulin.

ELST is most often confused with metastatic papillary thyroid carcinoma (PTC) and chorioid plexus papilloma (CPP). PTC is positive for thyroglobulin, whereas ELST is not. CPPs are positive for transthyretin and GFAP; the ELST is usually negative for both of these markers.[273,275]

Ectopic Meningioma

Meningiomas occurring outside the cranial cavity (ectopic or extracranial meningiomas) are uncommon. When they do occur, they are usually in the middle ear–mastoid and sinonasal tract–nasopharynx. When found, a primary intracranial meningioma with secondary involvement of the head and neck should be excluded.

True ectopic meningiomas of the ear-mastoid are more common in females by a ratio of 2:1 and have

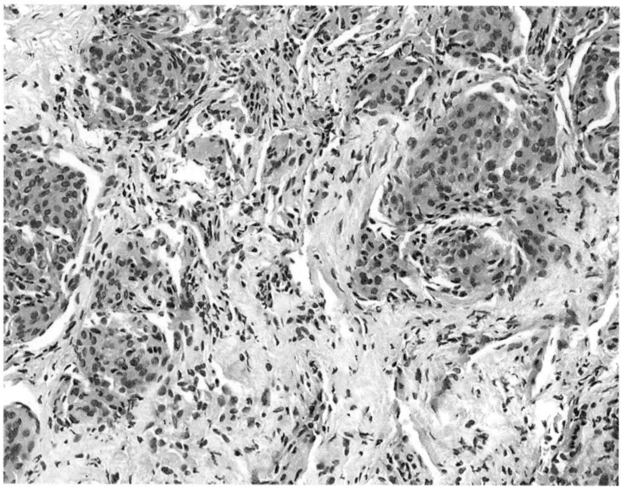

FIGURE 9.32 Meningioma of the mastoid. (H&E, ×100 original magnification.)

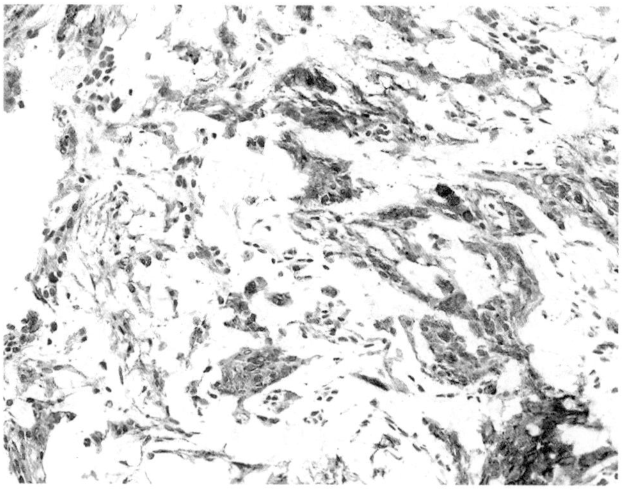

FIGURE 9.33 EMA immunostaining in mastoid meningioma. (EMA, ×200 original magnification.)

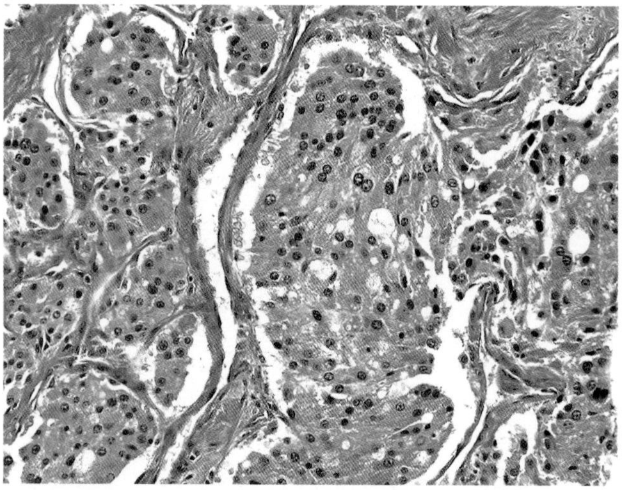

FIGURE 9.34 Paraganglioma. (H&E, ×100 original magnification.)

been found in patients from 10 to 80 years of age (average 50 years).[276] Occasionally they are incidental findings in a patient with a cholesteatoma and/or otitis and are more consistent with a "meningothelial rest" than a tumor. Others, however, are larger (≤4.5 cm) and may result in hearing loss, headaches, dizziness, vertigo, tinnitus, or otalgia.

In a review of 36 cases, Thompson and colleagues[276] observed that 25 were found in the middle ear, 4 in the external auditory canal, and 2 in the temporal bone (intraosseous). Five involved multiple sites.

Histologically, they resemble their intracranial counterpart, and on immunostaining they are uniformly positive for vimentin and generally positive, either weakly or focally, for EMA and progesterone receptor (Figs. 9.32 and 9.33).

PARAGANGLIOMAS AND MALIGNANT PARAGANGLIOMAS

Paragangliomas of the head and neck can occur in many locations. The most common is the neck, usually related to the carotid or vagal bodies, or the middle ear (jugulotympanic paraganglioma).[277,278] Paragangliomas can rarely occur in other locations as well such as the larynx, nasal cavity and paranasal sinuses, and oral cavity.[197,277] The symptoms of these tumors depend on the anatomic location, but patients may present with a pulsatile mass lesion. Paragangliomas in all of these locations have similar histologic and immunophenotypic appearance.

Malignant paraganglioma is a difficult diagnosis to make because the diagnosis rests almost entirely on finding metastatic lesions.[279] Although some histologic and cytologic features are thought to correlate with malignancy, none of these are absolute indicators of poor prognosis.

Histologically, paragangliomas are composed of variably sized cells that grow in a variety of patterns including nests (Zellballen), trabeculae, and rarely spindle cell morphology (Fig. 9.34).[280] The cytoplasm varies from clear to eosinophilic and granular to basophilic. The nuclei are usually bland and small but can exhibit bizarre pleomorphism. Mitoses are rare, and necrosis is not prominent. One important exception is the tumor with a large geographic area of necrosis after preoperative embolization.

Necrosis and increased mitoses are all features that raise the suspicion of possible malignancy. Evidence of capsular, vascular, and perineural invasion are not indicative of malignancy because these features can be seen in benign lesions as well.[281]

The staining pattern of paraganglioma is characteristic, with nearly all tumors being positive for chromogranin and synaptophysin, and other neuroendocrine markers such as NSE and Leu-7.[280] The tumor cells are negative for cytokeratin stains. The supporting cells that surround the tumor cell nests are called sustentacular cells, and these are uniquely positive for S-100 and GFAP (Fig. 9.35).[282] When using S-100 diagnostically, it must be shown to be positive peripheral to the cell

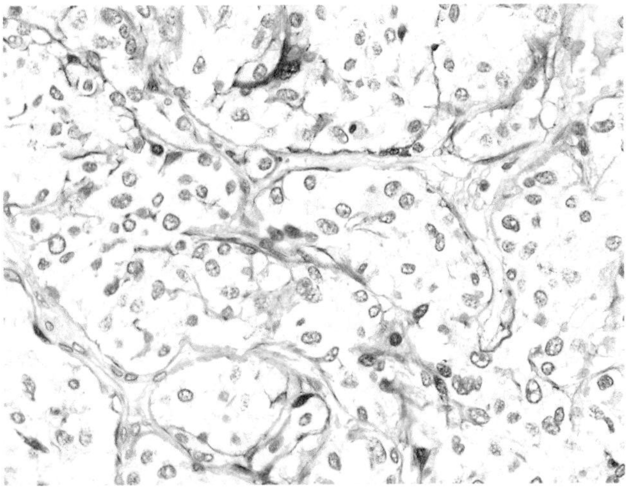

FIGURE 9.35 S-100 in paraganglioma highlighting the sustentacular cells. (S-100, ×200 original magnification.)

nests, in the fibrovascular supporting network where the sustentacular cells are located. Some studies have suggested that malignant paragangliomas will have either absent or decreased S-100 staining sustentacular cells.[283,284]

The differential diagnosis of paraganglioma will vary by anatomic location. The differential diagnosis of jugulotympanic paragangliomas will include middle ear adenoma, carcinoid tumor, and meningioma.[268,276,285] The histologic features can usually differentiate between these entities, but a directed immunohistochemical stain panel will also help. Middle ear adenoma may stain for neuroendocrine markers but will also stain for cytokeratins. Carcinoid tumors will show positive staining with the same neuroendocrine markers but will not have the sustentacular pattern of staining for S-100.[285,286] Meningiomas are often EMA positive and are negative for neuroendocrine markers.[276]

Paragangliomas located in the usual or unusual locations in the neck must be differentiated from other epithelial neuroendocrine tumors such as carcinoids, atypical carcinoids, small cell neuroendocrine carcinoma, and medullary thyroid carcinoma.[197] The staining panel that will differentiate these tumors is discussed in the neuroendocrine tumor section (see Table 9.11).

KEY DIAGNOSTIC POINTS

Paragangliomas

- Paragangliomas of the head and neck can occur in rather specific locations.
- The tumor cells are positive for chromogranin and synaptophysin and negative for cytokeratin.
- The sustentacular, supporting cells are positive for S-100.
- Malignancy cannot be predicted by histologic features alone; only metastasis identifies a tumor as being malignant.

METASTATIC TUMORS

Any type of tumor can metastasize to the head and neck, and all sites should be considered in the differential diagnosis of a tumor with unknown primary site. Certainly, it is most common for tumors from head and neck sites to involve the cervical lymph nodes.

Metastatic Prostatic Adenocarcinoma

An infrequent but important tumor to recognize in metastatic lesions in the head and neck is prostatic adenocarcinoma.[287] These tumors can have a variety of histologic appearances but usually have prominent nucleoli typical of prostatic adenocarcinoma. The diagnosis of metastatic prostatic adenocarcinoma in the head and neck can precede the diagnosis of the primary tumor. The immunostaining pattern of these tumors is similar to that of primary prostatic adenocarcinoma, though some poorly differentiated tumors can lose staining with PSA.[287] It can be difficult to differentiate metastatic adenocarcinoma from salivary duct carcinoma (see section on salivary gland tumors) owing to possibly overlapping PSA, AR, and PSAP staining profiles. Clinical and radiographic correlation will be essential.

Metastatic Renal Cell Carcinoma

Metastatic renal cell carcinoma can also present with no history of a primary renal cell carcinoma.[288] Histologically, these tumors usually exhibit clear and oncocytic cells with the fine vascular network of typical renal cell carcinoma. The differential diagnosis depends on the anatomic location but includes oncocytic tumors and tumors with clear cell differentiation such as clear cell hyalinizing carcinoma and clear cell myoepithelioma. Again, the immunostaining panel can help to differentiate these entities.

Lung Carcinoma

Rare cases of lung carcinoma can metastasize to the head and neck, particularly to the low cervical lymph nodes. These tumors usually carry the same immunophenotype as the primary lung tumor. Typical stains that are used to aid in this differential diagnosis will include cytokeratin 7, cytokeratin 20, and thyroid transcription factor-1 (TTF-1).

Unfortunately, most SCCs of the lung will be negative for TTF-1, as will their head and neck counterparts. Therefore when the pathologist encounters metastatic SCC in the neck with an unknown primary, the differential diagnosis should include the most common source, head and neck SCC, and the more remote possibility of metastatic lung carcinoma. Clinical and radiologic evaluation will often be the only way to make this distinction.

KEY DIAGNOSTIC POINTS

Metastatic Tumors

- Metastatic tumors are most commonly attributed to head and neck primary tumors, but sites below the clavicle are also possible.
- A histologically guided immunohistochemical staining panel can often help to identify the tumor type.
- Determining the source of a metastatic carcinoma in the head and neck can be difficult or impossible, even with immunohistochemical stains, and will often require clinical and radiologic correlation.

SUMMARY

A plethora of tumors can arise as a primary in the head and neck region, and this region may also serve as a repository of metastatic tumors. The differential diagnosis by light microscopy, in concert with the immunostaining insight supplied here, should help resolve the majority of diagnostic problems. At this time there are no genomic findings translatable to IHC for diagnostic use, nor are there any specific IHC theranostic applications.

REFERENCES

1. Simons JP, Hunt JL, Johnson JT. Pathology quiz case. Granular cell tumor of the tongue, with extensive overlying pseudoepitheliomatous hyperplasia. *Arch Otolaryngol Head Neck Surg.* 2003;129(1):127-128.
2. Lassaletta L, Alonso S, Granell J, et al. Synchronous glottic granular cell tumor and subglottic spindle cell carcinoma. *Arch Otolaryngol Head Neck Surg.* 1998;124(9):1031-1034.
3. Barkan GA, Paulino AF. Are epidermal growth factor and transforming growth factor responsible for pseudoepitheliomatous hyperplasia associated with granular cell tumors? *Ann Diagn Pathol.* 2003;7(2):73-77.
4. Wenig BM. Squamous cell carcinoma of the upper aerodigestive tract: precursor and problematic variants. *Modern Pathol.* 2002;15(3):229-254.
5. van Oijen MG, Leppers Vd Straat FG, Tilanus MG, Slootweg OJ. The origins of multiple squamous cell carcinomas in the aerodigestive tract. *Cancer.* 2000;88(4):884-893.
6. Sturgis EM, Wei Q. Genetic susceptibility-molecular epidemiology of head and neck cancer. *Curr Opin Oncol.* 2002;14(3):310-317.
7. Crowe DL, Hacia JG, Hsieh CL, et al. Molecular pathology of head and neck cancer. *Histol Histopathol.* 2002;17(3):909-914.
8. van Oijen MG, Slootweg PJ. Oral field cancerization: carcinogen-induced independent events or micrometastatic deposits? *Cancer Epidemiol Biomark Prev.* 2000;9(3):249-256.
9. Jacob BJ, Straif K, Thomas G, et al. Betel quid without tobacco as a risk factor for oral precancers. *Oral Oncol.* 2004;40(7):697-704.
10. Richardson CM, Sharma RA, Cox G, et al. Epidermal growth factor receptors and cyclooxygenase-2 in the pathogenesis of non-small cell lung cancer: potential targets for chemoprevention and systemic therapy. *Lung Cancer.* 2003;39(1):1-13.
11. Herrero R, Castellsaque X, Pawlita M, et al. Human papillomavirus and oral cancer: the International Agency for Research on Cancer multicenter study. *J Natl Cancer Inst.* 2003;95(23):1772-1783.
12. Hafkamp HC, Speel EJ, Haesevoets A, et al. A subset of head and neck squamous cell carcinomas exhibits integration of HPV 16/18 DNA and overexpression of p16INK4A and p53 in the absence of mutations in p53 exons 5-8. *Int J Cancer.* 2003;107(3):394-400.
13. Ha PK, Pai SI, Westra WH, et al. Real-time quantitative PCR demonstrates low prevalence of human papillomavirus type 16 in premalignant and malignant lesions of the oral cavity. *Clin Cancer Res.* 2002;8(5):1203-1209.
14. Gillison ML, Shah KV. Human papillomavirus-associated head and neck squamous cell carcinoma: mounting evidence for an etiologic role for human papillomavirus in a subset of head and neck cancers. *Curr Opin Oncol.* 2001;13(3):183-188.
15. Hobbs CG, Sterne JA, Bailey M, et al. Human papillomavirus and head and neck cancer: a systematic review and meta-analysis. *Clin Otolaryngol.* 2006;31(4):259-266.
16. Mulvany NJ, Allen DG, Wilson SM. Diagnostic utility of p16INK4a: a reappraisal of its use in cervical biopsies. *Pathology.* 2008;40(4):335-344.
17. Benevolo M, Vocaturo A, Mottolese M, et al. Clinical role of p16INK4a expression in liquid-based cervical cytology: correlation with HPV testing and histologic diagnosis. *Am J Clin Pathol.* 2008;129(4):606-612.
18. Bernard JE, Butler MO, Sandweiss L, Weidner N. Anal intraepithelial neoplasia: correlation of grade with p16INK4a immunohistochemistry and HPV *in situ* hybridization. *Appl Immunohistochem Mol Morphol.* 2008;16(3):215-220.
19. O'Regan EM, Toner ME, Finn SP, et al. p16(INK4A) genetic and epigenetic profiles differ in relation to age and site in head and neck squamous cell carcinomas. *Hum Pathol.* 2008;39(3):452-458.
20. Slebos RJ, Yi Y, Ely K, et al. Gene expression differences associated with human papillomavirus status in head and neck squamous cell carcinoma. *Clin Cancer Res.* 2006;12(3 Pt 1):701-709.
21. Paradiso A, Ranieri G, Stea B, et al. Altered p16INK4a and Fhit expression in carcinogenesis and progression of human oral cancer. *Int J Oncol.* 2004;24(2):249-255.
22. Hesselink AT, van den Brule AJ, Brink AA, et al. Comparison of hybrid capture 2 with *in situ* hybridization for the detection of high-risk human papillomavirus in liquid-based cervical samples. *Cancer.* 2004;102(1):11-18.
23. McGregor F, Muntoni A, Fleming J, et al. Molecular changes associated with oral dysplasia progression and acquisition of immortality: potential for its reversal by 5-azacytidine. *Cancer Research.* 2002;62(16):4757-4766.
24. Sudbo J, Lippman SM, Lee JJ, et al. The influence of resection and aneuploidy on mortality in oral leukoplakia [see comment]. *N Engl J Med.* 2004;350(14):1405-1413.
25. Lydiatt WM, Anderson PE, Bazzana T, et al. Molecular support for field cancerization in the head and neck. *Cancer.* 1998;82(7):1376-1380.
26. Saunders Jr JR. The genetic basis of head and neck carcinoma. *Am J Surg.* 1997;174(5):459-461.
27. Fiedler W, Hoppe C, Schimmel B, et al. Molecular characterization of head and neck tumors by analysis of telomerase activity and a panel of microsatellite markers. *Int J Mol Med.* 2002;9(4):417-423.
28. Wayne S, Robinson RA. Upper aerodigestive tract squamous dysplasia: correlation with p16, p53, pRb, and Ki-67 expression. *Arch Pathol Lab Med.* 2006;130(9):1309-1314.
29. Paulino AF, Singh B, Shah JP, et al. Basaloid squamous cell carcinoma of the head and neck. *Laryngoscope.* 2000;110(9):1479-1482.
30. Erdamar B, Suoglu Y, Sirin M, et al. Basaloid squamous cell carcinoma of the supraglottic larynx. *Eur Arch Oto-Rhino-Laryngol.* 2000;257(3):154-157.
31. Winzenburg SM, Niehans GA, George E, et al. Basaloid squamous carcinoma: a clinical comparison of two histologic types with poorly differentiated squamous cell carcinoma. *Otolaryngol Head Neck Surg.* 1998;119(5):471-475.
32. Thompson LD, Heffner DK. The clinical importance of cystic squamous cell carcinomas in the neck: a study of 136 cases. *Cancer.* 1998;82(5):944-956.
33. Barnes L, Ferlito A, Altavilla G, et al. Basaloid squamous cell carcinoma of the head and neck: clinicopathological features and differential diagnosis. *Ann Otol Rhinol Laryngol.* 1996;105(1):75-82.
34. Ferlito A, Altavilla G, Rinaldo A, et al. Basaloid squamous cell carcinoma of the larynx and hypopharynx. *Ann Otol Rhinol Laryngol.* 1997;106(12):1024-1035.

35. Soriano E, Faure C, Lantuejoul S, et al. Course and prognosis of basaloid squamous cell carcinoma of the head and neck: a case-control study of 62 patients. *Eur J Cancer*. 2008;44(2):244-250.
36. Poetsch M, Lorenz G, Bankau A, et al. Basaloid in contrast to nonbasaloid head and neck squamous cell carcinomas display aberrations especially in cell cycle control genes. *Head Neck*. 2003;25(11):904-910.
37. Gillison ML, Koch WM, Capone RB, et al. Evidence for a causal association between human papillomavirus and a subset of head and neck cancers. *J Natl Cancer Inst*. 2000;92(9):709-720.
38. Begum S, Westra WH. Basaloid squamous cell carcinoma of the head and neck is a mixed variant that can be further resolved by HPV status. *Am J Surg Pathol*. 2008;32(7):1044-1050.
39. Szentirmay Z, Polus K, Tamas L, et al. Human papillomavirus in head and neck cancer: molecular biology and clinicopathological correlations. *Cancer Metastasis Rev*. 2005;24(1):19-34.
40. Zhang MQ, El-Mofty SK, Davila RM. Detection of human papillomavirus-related squamous cell carcinoma cytologically and by *in situ* hybridization in fine-needle aspiration biopsies of cervical metastasis: a tool for identifying the site of an occult head and neck primary. *Cancer*. 2008;114(2):118-123.
41. El-Mofty SK, Lu DW. Prevalence of high-risk human papillomavirus DNA in nonkeratinizing (cylindrical cell) carcinoma of the sinonasal tract: a distinct clinicopathologic and molecular disease entity. *Am J Surg Pathol*. 2005;29(10):1367-1372.
42. Worden FP, Kumar B, Lee JS, et al. Chemoselection as a strategy for organ preservation in advanced oropharynx cancer: response and survival positively associated with HPV16 copy number. *J Clin Oncol*. 2008;26(19):3138-3146.
43. Guvenc MG, Midilli K, Ozdogan A, et al. Detection of HHV-8 and HPV in laryngeal carcinoma. *Auris Nasus Larynx*. 2008;35(3):357-362.
44. Nonogaki S, Wakamatsu A, Filho AL, et al. Molecular strategies for identifying human papillomavirus infection in routinely processed samples: focus on paraffin sections. *J Low Genit Tract Dis*. 2005;9(4):219-224.
45. Muller S, Barnes EL. Basaloid squamous cell carcinoma of the head and neck with a spindle cell component. An unusual histologic variant. *Arch Pathol Lab Med*. 1995;119:181-182.
46. Ide F, Shimoyama T, Horie N, et al. Basaloid squamous cell carcinoma of the oral mucosa: a new case and review of 45 cases in the literature. *Oral Oncol*. 2002;38(1):120-124.
47. Raslan WF, Barnes L, Krause JR, et al. Basaloid squamous cell carcinoma of the head and neck: a clinicopathologic and flow cytometric study of 10 new cases with review of the English literature. *Am J Otolaryngol*. 1994;15(3):204-211.
48. Klijanienko J, el-Naggar A, Ponzio-Prion A, et al. Basaloid squamous carcinoma of the head and neck. Immunohistochemical comparison with adenoid cystic carcinoma and squamous cell carcinoma. *Arch Otolaryngol Head Neck Surg*. 1993;119(8):887-890.
49. Coletta RD, Cotrim P, Almeida OP, et al. Basaloid squamous carcinoma of oral cavity: a histologic and immunohistochemical study. *Oral Oncol*. 2002;38(7):723-729.
50. Banks ER, Frierson Jr HF, Mills SE, et al. Basaloid squamous cell carcinoma of the head and neck. A clinicopathologic and immunohistochemical study of 40 cases. *Am J Surg Pathol*. 1992;16(10):939-946.
51. Morice WG, Ferreiro JA. Distinction of basaloid squamous cell carcinoma from adenoid cystic and small cell undifferentiated carcinoma by immunohistochemistry. *Human Pathol*. 1998;29:609-612.
52. Tsubochi H, Suzuki T, Suzuki S, et al. Immunohistochemical study of basaloid squamous cell carcinoma, adenoid cystic and mucoepidermoid carcinoma in the upper aerodigestive tract. *Anticancer Research*. 2000;20(2B):1205-1211.
53. Holst VA, Marshall CE, Moskaluk CA, et al. KIT protein expression and analysis of c-kit gene mutation in adenoid cystic carcinoma. *Mod Pathol*. 1999;12(10):956-960.
54. Mino M, Pilch BZ, Faquin WC. Expression of KIT (CD117) in neoplasms of the head and neck: an ancillary marker for adenoid cystic carcinoma. *Mod Pathol*. 2004;16(12):1224-1231.
55. Emanuel P, Wang B, Wu M, et al. p63 Immunohistochemistry in the distinction of adenoid cystic carcinoma from basaloid squamous cell carcinoma. *Mod Pathol*. 2005;18(5):645-650.
56. Serrano MF, el-Mofty SK, Gnepp DR, et al. Utility of high molecular weight cytokeratins, but not p63, in the differential diagnosis of neuroendocrine and basaloid carcinomas of the head and neck. *Hum Pathol*. 2008;39(4):591-598.
57. Bilal H, Handra-Luca A, Bertrand JC, et al. p63 is expressed in basal and myoepithelial cells of human normal and tumor salivary gland tissues. *J Histochem Cytochem*. 2003;51(2):133-139.
58. Kiyoshima T, Shima K, Kobayashi I, et al. Expression of p53 tumor suppressor gene in adenoid cystic and mucoepidermoid carcinomas of the salivary glands. *Oral Oncol*. 2001;37(3):315-322.
59. Owonikoko T, Loberg C, Gabbert HE, et al. Comparative analysis of basaloid and typical squamous cell carcinoma of the oesophagus: a molecular biological and immunohistochemical study. *J Pathol*. 2001;193(2):155-161.
60. Seethala RR, Hunt JL, Baloch ZW, et al. Adenoid cystic carcinoma with high-grade transformation: a report of 11 cases and a review of the literature. *Am J Surg Pathol*. 2007;31(11): 1683-1694.
61. Nagao T, Gaffey TA, Serizawa H, et al. Dedifferentiated adenoid cystic carcinoma: a clinicopathologic study of 6 cases. *Mod Pathol*. 2003;16(12):1265-1272.
62. Kroch BB, Trask DK, Hoffman HT. National survey of head and neck verrucous carcinoma: Patterns of presentation, care and outcome. *Cancer*. 2001;92:110-120.
63. Barnes EL, Hunt JL. Squamous cell carcinoma of the oral cavity and oropharynx: A review of current data. *Sel Readings Oral Maxillofac Surg*. 2003;3(11):1-40.
64. Medina JE, Dichtel W, Luna MA. Verrucous-squamous carcinomas of the oral cavity. A clinicopathologic study of 104 cases. *Arch Otolaryngol*. 1984;110(7):437-440.
65. Ishiyama A, Eversole LR, Ross DA, et al. Papillary squamous neoplasms of the head and neck. *Laryngoscope*. 1994;104(12):1446-1452.
66. Suarez PA, Adler-Storthz K, Luna MA, et al. Papillary squamous cell carcinomas of the upper aerodigestive tract: a clinicopathologic and molecular study. *Head Neck*. 2000;22(4):360-368.
67. Thompson LD, Wenig BM, Heffner DK, et al. Exophytic and papillary squamous cell carcinomas of the larynx: A clinicopathologic series of 104 cases. *Otolaryngol Head Neck Surg*. 1999;120(5):718-724.
68. Cobo F, Talavera P, Concha A. Review article: relationship of human papillomavirus with papillary squamous cell carcinoma of the upper aerodigestive tract: a review. *Int J Surg Pathol*. 2008;16(2):127-136.
69. Fujita S, Senba M, Kumatori A, et al. Human papillomavirus infection in oral verrucous carcinoma: genotyping analysis and inverse correlation with p53 expression. *Pathobiology*. 2008;75(4):257-264.
70. Thompson LD, Wieneke JA, Miettinen M, et al. Spindle cell (sarcomatoid) carcinomas of the larynx: a clinicopathologic study of 187 cases. *Am J Surg Pathol*. 2002;26(2):153-170.
71. Olsen KD, Lewis JE, Suman VJ. Spindle cell carcinoma of the larynx and hypopharynx. *Otolaryngol Head Neck Surg*. 1997;116(1):47-52.
72. Lewis JE, Olsen KD, Sebo TJ. Spindle cell carcinoma of the larynx: review of 26 cases including DNA content and immunohistochemistry. *Hum Pathol*. 1997;28(6):664-673.
73. Thompson LD. Diagnostically challenging lesions in head and neck pathology. *Eur Arch Oto-Rhino-Laryngol*. 1997;254(8):357-366.
74. Gupta R, Singh S, Hedau S, et al. Spindle cell carcinoma of head and neck: an immunohistochemical and molecular approach to its pathogenesis. *J Clin Pathol*. 2007;60(5):472-475.
75. Weber A, Langhanki L, Sommerer F, et al. Mutations of the BRAF gene in squamous cell carcinoma of the head and neck. *Oncogene*. 2003;22(30):4757-4759.
76. Pintos J, Black MJ, Sadeghi N, et al. Human papillomavirus infection and oral cancer: A case-control study in Montreal, Canada. *Oral Oncol*. 2008;44(3):242-250.
77. Koyama K, Uobe K, Tanaka A. Highly sensitive detection of HPV-DNA in paraffin sections of human oral carcinomas. *J Oral Pathol Med*. 2007;36(1):18-24.
78. da Silva CE, da Silva ID, Cerri A, et al. Prevalence of human papillomavirus in squamous cell carcinoma of the tongue. *Oral Surg Oral Med Oral Pathol Oral Radiol Endod*. 2007;104(4): 497-500.

79. Yang XR, Diehl S, Pfeiffer R, et al. Evaluation of risk factors for nasopharyngeal carcinoma in high-risk nasopharyngeal carcinoma families in Taiwan. *Cancer Epidemiol Biomarkers Prev.* 2005;14(4):900-905.
80. Spano JP, Busson P, Atlan D, et al. Nasopharyngeal carcinomas: an update. *Eur J Cancer.* 2003;39(15):2121-2135.
81. Vartanian JG, Pontes E, Agra IM, et al. Distribution of metastatic lymph nodes in oropharyngeal carcinoma and its implications for the elective treatment of the neck. *Arch Otolaryngol Head Neck Surg.* 2003;129(7):729-732.
82. Slootweg PJ, Hordijk GJ, Schade Y, et al. Treatment failure and margin status in head and neck cancer. A critical view on the potential value of molecular pathology. *Oral Oncol.* 2002;38(5):500-503.
83. Hoffman HT. Surgical treatment of cervical node metastases from squamous cell carcinoma of the upper aerodigestive tract: evaluation of the evidence for modifications of neck dissection. *Head Neck.* 2001;23:907-915.
84. Khalil MY, Grandis JR, Shin DM. Targeting epidermal growth factor receptor: novel therapeutics in the management of cancer. *Expert Rev Anticancer Ther.* 2003;3(3):367-380.
85. Iqbal S, Lenz HJ. Integration of novel agents in the treatment of colorectal cancer. *Cancer Chemother Pharmacol.* 2004(1):54.
86. Diaz-Rubio E. New chemotherapeutic advances in pancreatic, colorectal, and gastric cancers. *Oncologist.* 2004;9(3):282-294.
87. Resnick MB, Routhier J, Konkin T, et al. Epidermal growth factor receptor, c-MET, beta-catenin, and p53 expression as prognostic indicators in stage II colon cancer: a tissue microarray study. *Clin Cancer Res.* 2004;10(9):3069-3075.
88. Kondo Y, Hollingsworth EF, Kondo S. Molecular targeting for malignant gliomas (Review). *Int J Oncol.* 2004;24(5):1101-1109.
89. Li B, Chang CM, Yuan M, et al. Resistance to small molecule inhibitors of epidermal growth factor receptor in malignant gliomas. *Cancer Res.* 2003;63(21):7443-7450.
90. Nadal A, Cardesa A. Molecular biology of laryngeal squamous cell carcinoma. *Virchows Arch.* 2003;442(1):1-7.
91. Ford AC, Grandis JR. Targeting epidermal growth factor receptor in head and neck cancer. *Head Neck.* 2003;25(1):67-73.
92. Paez JG, Janne PA, Lee JC, et al. EGFR mutations in lung cancer: correlation with clinical response to gefitinib therapy [see comment]. *Science.* 2004;304(5676):1497-1500.
93. Lynch TJ, Bell DW, Sordella R, et al. Activating mutations in the epidermal growth factor receptor underlying responsiveness of non-small-cell lung cancer to gefitinib [see comment]. *N Engl J Med.* 2004;350(21):2129-2139.
94. Yaziji H, Gown AM. Testing for epidermal growth factor receptor in lung cancer: have we learned anything from HER-2 testing?[comment]. *J Clin Oncol.* 2004;22(17):3646-3648.
95. Lee JW, Soung YH, Kim SY, et al. Absence of EGFR mutation in the kinase domain in common human cancers besides non-small cell lung cancer. *Int J Cancer.* 2005;113(3):510-511.
96. Brockstein B, Lacouture M, Agulnik M. The role of inhibitors of the epidermal growth factor in management of head and neck cancer. *J Natl Compr Canc Netw.* 2008;6(7):696-706.
97. Loeffler-Ragg J, Schwentner I, Sprinzl GM, et al. EGFR inhibition as a therapy for head and neck squamous cell carcinoma. *Expert Opin Investig Drugs.* 2008;17(10):1517-1531.
98. Egloff AM, Grandis JR. Targeting epidermal growth factor receptor and SRC pathways in head and neck cancer. *Semin Oncol.* 2008;35(3):286-297.
99. Yamatodani T, Ekblad L, Kjellen E, et al. Epidermal growth factor receptor status and persistent activation of Akt and p44/42 MAPK pathways correlate with the effect of cetuximab in head and neck and colon cancer cell lines. *J Cancer Res Clin Oncol.* 2009;135(3):395-402.
100. Gasco M, Crook T. The p53 network in head and neck cancer. *Oral Oncol.* 2003;39(3):222-231.
101. Blons H, Laurent-Puig P. TP53 and head and neck neoplasms. *Hum Mutat.* 2003;21(3):252-257.
102. van Houten VM, Tabor MP, van den Brekel MW, et al. Mutated p53 as a molecular marker for the diagnosis of head and neck cancer. *J Pathol.* 2002;198(4):476-486.
103. Vielba R, Bilbao J, Ispizua A, et al. p53 and cyclin D1 as prognostic factors in squamous cell carcinoma of the larynx. *Laryngoscope.* 2003;113(1):167-172.
104. Smith BD, Haffty BG. Molecular markers as prognostic factors for local recurrence and radioresistance in head and neck squamous cell carcinoma. *Radiat Oncol Investig.* 1999;7(3):125-144.
105. Fregonesi PA. P16INK4A immunohistochemical overexpression in premalignant and malignant oral lesions infected with human papillomavirus. *J Histochem Cytochem.* 2003;51:1291-1297.
106. Namazie A, Alavi S, Olopade OI, et al. Cyclin D1 amplification and p16(MTS1/CDK4I) deletion correlate with poor prognosis in head and neck tumors. *Laryngoscope.* 2002;112(3):472-481.
107. Schoelch ML, Regezi JA, Dekker NP, et al. Cell cycle proteins and the development of oral squamous cell carcinoma. *Oral Oncol.* 1999;35(3):333-342.
108. Oliver RJ, MacDonald DG, Felix DH. Aspects of cell proliferation in oral epithelial dysplastic lesions. *J Oral Pathol Med.* 2000;29(2):49-55.
109. Nathan CA, Amirghahri N, Rice C, et al. Molecular analysis of surgical margins in head and neck squamous cell carcinoma patients. *Laryngoscope.* 2002;112(12):2129-2140.
110. Tabor MP, Brakenhoff RH, van Houten VM, et al. Persistence of genetically altered fields in head and neck cancer patients: biological and clinical implications. *Clin Cancer Res.* 2001;7(6):1523-1532.
111. Mills SE, Fechner RE. "Undifferentiated" neoplasms of the sinonasal region: differential diagnosis based on clinical, light microscopic, immunohistochemical, and ultrastructural features. *Semin Diagn Pathol.* 1989;6(4):316-328.
112. Devaney K, Wenig BM, Abbondanzo SL. Olfactory neuroblastoma and other round cell lesions of the sinonasal region. *Mod Pathol.* 1996;9(6):658-663.
113. Meis-Kindblom JM, Stenman G, Kindblom LG. Differential diagnosis of small round cell tumors. *Semin Diagn Pathol.* 1996;13(3):213-241.
114. Devoe K, Weidner N. Immunohistochemistry of small round-cell tumors. *Semin Diagn Pathol.* 2000;17(3):216-224.
115. Kessler HP, Unterman B. Respiratory epithelial adenomatoid hamartoma of the maxillary sinus presenting as a periapical radiolucency: a case report and review of the literature. *Oral Surg Oral Med Oral Pathol Oral Radiol Endodont.* 2004;97(5):607-612.
116. Sangoi AR, Berry G. Respiratory epithelial adenomatoid hamartoma: diagnostic pitfalls with emphasis on differential diagnosis. *Adv Anat Pathol.* 2007;14(1):11-16.
117. Ozolek JA, Hunt JL. Tumor suppressor gene alterations in respiratory epithelial adenomatoid hamartoma (REAH): comparison to sinonasal adenocarcinoma and inflamed sinonasal mucosa. *Am J Surg Pathol.* 2006;30(12):1576-1580.
118. Ozolek JA, Barnes EL, Hunt JL. Basal/myoepithelial cells in chronic sinusitis, respiratory epithelial adenomatoid hamartoma, inverted papilloma, and intestinal-type and nonintestinal-type sinonasal adenocarcinoma: an immunohistochemical study. *Arch Pathol Lab Med.* 2007;131(4):530-537.
119. Broich G, Pagliari A, Ottaviani F. Esthesioneuroblastoma: a general review of the cases published since the discovery of the tumour in 1924. *Anticancer Res.* 1997;17(4A):2683-2706.
120. Dulguerov P, Allal AS, Calcaterra TC. Esthesioneuroblastoma: a meta-analysis and review. *Lancet Oncol.* 2001;2(11):683-690.
121. Slootweg PJ, Lubsen H. Rhabdomyoblasts in olfactory neuroblastoma. *Histopathology.* 1991;19(2):182-184.
122. Miyagami M, Katayama Y, Kinukawa N, et al. An ultrastructural and immunohistochemical study of olfactory neuroepithelioma with rhabdomyoblasts. *Med Electron Microscopy.* 2002;35(3):160-166.
123. Silva EG, Butler JJ, Mackay B, et al. Neuroblastomas and neuroendocrine carcinomas of the nasal cavity: a proposed new classification. *Cancer.* 1982;50(11):2388-2405.
124. Guled M, Myllykangas S, Frierson Jr HF, et al. Array comparative genomic hybridization analysis of olfactory neuroblastoma. *Mod Pathol.* 2008;21(6):770-778.
125. Franchi A, Moroni M, Massi D, et al. Sinonasal undifferentiated carcinoma, nasopharyngeal-type undifferentiated carcinoma, and keratinizing and nonkeratinizing squamous cell carcinoma express different cytokeratin patterns. *Am J Surg Pathol.* 2002;26(12):1597-1604.
126. Cerilli LA, Holst VA, Brandwein MS, et al. Sinonasal undifferentiated carcinoma: immunohistochemical profile and lack of EBV association. *Am J Surg Pathol.* 2001;25(2):156-163.

127. Lopategui JR, Gaffey MJ, Frierson Jr HF, et al. Detection of Epstein-Barr viral RNA in sinonasal undifferentiated carcinoma from Western and Asian patients. *Am J Surg Pathol.* 1994;18(4):391-398.
128. Nakhleh RE, Wick MR, Rocamora A, et al. Morphologic diversity in malignant melanomas [see comment]. *Am J Clin Pathol.* 1990;93(6):731-740.
129. Thompson LD, Miettinen M, Wenig BM. Sinonasal-type hemangiopericytoma: a clinicopathologic and immunophenotypic analysis of 104 cases showing perivascular myoid differentiation. *Am J Surg Pathol.* 2003;27(6):737-749.
130. Prasad ML, Jungbluth AA, Iversen K, et al. Expression of melanocytic differentiation markers in malignant melanomas of the oral and sinonasal mucosa. *Am J Surg Pathol.* 2001;25(6):782-787.
131. Franquemont DW, Mills SE. Sinonasal malignant melanoma. A clinicopathologic and immunohistochemical study of 14 cases. *Am J Clin Pathol.* 1991;96(6):689-697.
132. Perez-Ordonez B, Caruana SM, Huvos AG, et al. Small cell neuroendocrine carcinoma of the nasal cavity and paranasal sinuses. *Hum Pathol.* 1998;29(8):826-832.
133. Cheuk W, Kwan MY, Suster S, et al. Immunostaining for thyroid transcription factor 1 and cytokeratin 20 aids the distinction of small cell carcinoma from Merkel cell carcinoma, but not pulmonary from extrapulmonary small cell carcinomas. *Arch Pathol Lab Med.* 2001;125(2):228-231.
134. Mineta H, Miura K, Takebayashi S, et al. Immunohistochemical analysis of small cell carcinoma of the head and neck: a report of four patients and a review of sixteen patients in the literature with ectopic hormone production. *Ann Otol Rhinol Laryngol.* 2001;110(1):76-82.
135. Lloyd RV, Chandler WF, Kovacs K, et al. Ectopic pituitary adenomas with normal anterior pituitary glands. *Am J Surg Pathol.* 1986;10(8):546-552.
136. van der May AG, van Seters AP, van Krieken JH, et al. Large pituitary adenomas with extension into the nasopharynx. Report of three cases with a review of the literature. *Ann Otol Rhinol Laryngol.* 1989;98(8 Pt 1):618-624.
137. Luk IS, Chan JK, Chow SM, et al. Pituitary adenoma presenting as sinonasal tumor: pitfalls in diagnosis. *Hum Pathol.* 1996;27(6):605-609.
138. O'Hara BJ, Paetau A, Miettinen M. Keratin subsets and monoclonal antibody HBME-1 in chordoma: immunohistochemical differential diagnosis between tumors simulating chordoma. *Hum Pathol.* 1998;29(2):119-126.
139. Asa SL, Puy LA, Lew AM, et al. Cell type-specific expression of the pituitary transcription activator pit-1 in the human pituitary and pituitary adenomas. *J Clin Endocrinol Metab.* 1275; 77(5):1275–1280.
140. Keil MF, Stratakis CA. Pituitary tumors in childhood: update of diagnosis, treatment and molecular genetics. *Expert Rev Neurother.* 2008;8(4):563-574.
141. Ahmed AA, Tsokos M. Sinonasal rhabdomyosarcoma in children and young adults. *Int J Surg Pathol.* 2007;15(2):160-165.
142. Mauer HM, Beltangady M, Gehan EA, et al. The Intergroup Rhabdomyosarcoma Study-I. A final report. *Cancer.* 1988;61(2):209-220.
143. Callender TA, Weber RS, Janjan N, et al. Rhabdomyosarcoma of the nose and paranasal sinuses in adults and children. *Otolaryngol Head Neck Surg.* 1995;112(2):252-257.
144. Montone KT, LiVolsi V. Alveolar rhabdomyosarcomas of the sinonasal tract. *Head Neck*, in press.
145. Cessna MH, Zhou, H, Perkins, SL, et al. Are myogenin and myoD1 expression specific for rhabdomyosarcoma? A study of 150 cases, with emphasis on spindle cell mimics. *Am J Surg Pathol* 1150;25(9):1150–1157.
146. Jones JE, and McGill T. Peripheral primitive neuroectodermal tumors of the head and neck. *Arch Otolaryngol Head Neck Surg.* 1392;121(12): 1392–1395.
147. Nikitakis NG, Salama AR, O'Malley Jr BW, et al. Malignant peripheral primitive neuroectodermal tumor-peripheral neuroepithelioma of the head and neck: a clinicopathologic study of five cases and review of the literature. *Head Neck.* 2003;25(6):488-498.
148. Gu M, Antonescu CR, Guiter G, et al. Cytokeratin immunoreactivity in Ewing's sarcoma: prevalence in 50 cases confirmed by molecular diagnostic studies [see comment]. *Am J Surg Pathol.* 2000;24(3):410-416.
149. Barnes L. Intestinal-type adenocarcinoma of the nasal cavity and paranasal sinuses. *Am J Surg Pathol.* 1986;10(3):192-202.
150. McKinney CD, Mills SE, Franquemont DW. Sinonasal intestinal-type adenocarcinoma: immunohistochemical profile and comparison with colonic adenocarcinoma. *Mod Pathol.* 1995;8(4):421-426.
151. Krane JF, O'Connel JT, Pilch BZ. Sinonasal adenocarcinoma: Evidence for histogenetic divergence of the enteric and nonenteric phenotypes. *Mod Pathol.* 2000;17:139A (Abstract).
152. Choi HR, Sturgis EM, Rashid A, et al. Sinonasal adenocarcinoma: evidence for histogenetic divergence of the enteric and nonenteric phenotypes. *Hum Pathol.* 1101;34(11): 1101-1107.
153. Bashir AA, Robinson RA, Benda JA, et al. Sinonasal adenocarcinoma: immunohistochemical marking and expression of oncoproteins. *Head Neck.* 2003;25(9):763-771.
154. Franchi A, Massi D, Baroni G, et al. CDX-2 homeobox gene expression [comment]. *Am J Surg Pathol.* 1390;27(10):1390–1391.
155. Amre R, Ghali V, Elmberger GEA. Sinonasal "intestinal-type" adenocarcinomas (SNITAC): An immunohistochemical (IHC) study of 22 cases. *Mod Pathol.* 2004;17:221A (Abstract).
156. Abecasis J, Viana G, Pissarra C, et al. Adenocarcinomas of the nasal cavity and paranasal sinuses: a clinicopathological and immunohistochemical study of 14 cases. *Histopathology.* 2004;45(3):254-259.
157. Resto VA, Krane JF, Faquin WC, et al. Immunohistochemical distinction of intestinal-type sinonasal adenocarcinoma from metastatic adenocarcinoma of intestinal origin. *Ann Otol Rhinol Laryngol.* 2006;115(1):59-64.
158. Franchi A, Massi D, Palomba A, et al. CDX-2, cytokeratin 7 and cytokeratin 20 immunohistochemical expression in the differential diagnosis of primary adenocarcinomas of the sinonasal tract. *Virchows Arch.* 2004;445(1):63-67.
159. Kennedy MT, Jordan RC, Berean KW, et al. Expression pattern of CK7, CK20, CDX-2, and villin in intestinal-type sinonasal adenocarcinoma. *J Clin Pathol.* 2004;57(9):932-937.
160. Chu PG, Chang KL, Wu AY, et al. Nasal glomus tumors: report of two cases with emphasis on immunohistochemical features and differential diagnosis. *Hum Pathol.* 1259;30(10):1259-1261.
161. Watanabe K, Saito A, Suzuki M, et al. True hemangiopericytoma of the nasal cavity. *Arch Pathol Lab Med.* 2001;125(5):686-690.
162. Tse LL, Chan JK. Sinonasal haemangiopericytoma-like tumour: a sinonasal glomus tumour or a haemangiopericytoma? *Histopathology.* 2002;40(6):510-517.
163. Stelow EB, Bellizzi AM, Taneja K, et al. NUT rearrangement in undifferentiated carcinomas of the upper aerodigestive tract. *Am J Surg Pathol.* 2008;32(6):828-834.
164. Kalinsky K, Haluska FG. Novel inhibitors in the treatment of metastatic melanoma. *Expert Rev Anticancer Ther.* 2007;7(5):715-724.
165. Brose MS, Volpe P, Feldman M, et al. BRAF and RAS mutations in human lung cancer and melanoma. *Cancer Res.* 2002;62(23):6997-7000.
166. Wong CW, Fan YS, Chan TL, et al. BRAF and NRAS mutations are uncommon in melanomas arising in diverse internal organs. *J Clin Pathol.* 2005;58(6):640-644.
167. Curtin JA, Busam K, Pinkel D, et al. Somatic activation of KIT in distinct subtypes of melanoma. *J Clin Oncol.* 2006;24(26):4340-4346.
168. Lutzky J, Bauer J, Bastian BC. Dose-dependent, complete response to imatinib of a metastatic mucosal melanoma with a K642E KIT mutation. *Pigment Cell Melanoma Res.* 2008;21(4):492-493.
169. Rivera RS, Nagatsuka H, Gunduz M, et al. C-kit protein expression correlated with activating mutations in KIT gene in oral mucosal melanoma. *Virchows Arch.* 2008;452(1):27-32.
170. Mercado GE, Barr FG. Fusions involving PAX and FOX genes in the molecular pathogenesis of alveolar rhabdomyosarcoma: recent advances. *Curr Mol Med.* 2007;7(1):47-61.
171. de Alava E, Gerald WL. Molecular biology of the Ewing's sarcoma/primitive neuroectodermal tumor family. *J Clin Oncol.* 2000;18(1):204-213.

172. Nilsson G, Wang M, Wejde J, et al. Detection of EWS/FLI-1 by immunostaining. An adjunctive tool in diagnosis of Ewing's sarcoma and primitive neuroectodermal tumour on cytological samples and paraffin-embedded archival material. *Sarcoma.* 1999;3(1):25-32.
173. Mhawech-Fauceglia P, Herrmann F, Penetrante R, et al. Diagnostic utility of FLI-1 monoclonal antibody and dual-colour, break-apart probe fluorescence *in situ* (FISH) analysis in Ewing's sarcoma/primitive neuroectodermal tumour (EWS/PNET). A comparative study with CD99 and FLI-1 polyclonal antibodies. *Histopathology.* 2006;49(6):569-575.
174. Folpe AL, Hill CE, Parham DM, et al. Immunohistochemical detection of FLI-1 protein expression: a study of 132 round cell tumors with emphasis on CD99-positive mimics of Ewing's sarcoma/primitive neuroectodermal tumor. *Am J Surg Pathol.* 1657;24(12):1657–1662.
175. Barnes L, Eveson JW, Reichert PA, et al. Pathology and Genetics of Head and Neck Tumours. In: Kleihues P, Sobin LH, eds. World Health Organization Classification of Tumours. Lyon, France: IARC Press; 2005.
176. Dubey P, Ha CS, Ang KK, et al. Nonnasopharyngeal lymphoepithelioma of the head and neck. *Cancer.* 1556;82(8): 1556–1562.
177. Jeng YM, Sung MT, Fang CL, et al. Sinonasal undifferentiated carcinoma and nasopharyngeal-type undifferentiated carcinoma: two clinically, biologically, and histopathologically distinct entities. *Am J Surg Pathol.* 2002;26(3):371-376.
178. Leung SY, Yuen ST, Chung LP, et al. Epstein-Barr virus is present in a wide histological spectrum of sinonasal carcinomas. *Am J Surg Pathol.* 1995;19(9):994-1001.
179. Sheu LF, Chen A, Tseng HH, et al. Assessment of p53 expression in nasopharyngeal carcinoma. *Hum Pathol.* 1995;26(4):380-386.
180. Bar-Sela G, Kuten A, Ben-Eliezer S, et al. Expression of HER2 and C-KIT in nasopharyngeal carcinoma: implications for a new therapeutic approach. *Mod Pathol.* 2003;16(10):1035-1040.
181. Beham A, Kainz J, Stammberger H, et al. Immunohistochemical and electron microscopical characterization of stromal cells in nasopharyngeal angiofibromas. *Eur Arch Oto Rhino Laryngol.* 1997;254(4):196-199.
182. Beham A, Regauer S, Beham-Schmid C, et al. Expression of CD34-antigen in nasopharyngeal angiofibromas. *Int J Pediatr Otorhinolaryngol.* 1998;44(3):245-250.
183. Abraham SC, Montgomery EA, Giardiello FM, et al. Frequent beta-catenin mutations in juvenile nasopharyngeal angiofibromas. *Am J Pathol.* 1073;158(3):1073–1078.
184. Hwang HC, Mills SE, Patterson K, et al. Expression of androgen receptors in nasopharyngeal angiofibroma: an immunohistochemical study of 24 cases. *Mod Pathol.* 1122;11(11): 1122–1126.
185. Montag AG, Richardson MS, Tretiakova M. Nasopharyngeal angiofibromas: Consistent expression of estrogen receptor beta. *Mod Pathol.* 2004;17:228A(Abstract).
186. Filie AC, Lage JM, Azumi N. Immunoreactivity of S100 protein, alpha-1-antitrypsin, and CD68 in adult and congenital granular cell tumors. *Mod Pathol.* 1996;9(9):888-892.
187. Fanburg-Smith JC, Meis-Kindblom JM, Fante R, et al. Malignant granular cell tumor of soft tissue: diagnostic criteria and clinicopathologic correlation [erratum appears in *Am J Surg Pathol* 1999 Jan;23(1):136]. *Am J Surg Pathol.* 1998;22(7):779–794.
188. Fine SW, Li M. Expression of calretinin and the alpha-subunit of inhibin in granular cell tumors. *Am J Clin Pathol.* 2003;119(2):259-264.
189. Le BH, Boyer PJ, Lewis JE, et al. Granular cell tumor: immunohistochemical assessment of inhibin-alpha, protein gene product 9.5, S100 protein, CD68, and Ki-67 proliferative index with clinical correlation. *Arch Pathol Lab Med.* 2004;128(7):771-775.
190. Steinberg BM, DiLorenzo TP. A possible role for human papillomaviruses in head and neck cancer. *Cancer Metastasis Rev.* 1996;15(1):91-112.
191. Mills SE. Neuroectodermal neoplasms of the head and neck with emphasis on neuroendocrine carcinomas. *Mod Pathol.* 2002;15(3):264-278.
192. Barnes EL. Paraganglioma of the larynx: A critical review of the literature. *ORL.* 1991;53:220-234.
193. el Naggar A, Batsakis JG. Carcinoid tumors of the larynx. A critical review of the literature. *ORL.* 1991;53:185-187.
194. Woodruff JM, Senie RT. Atypical carcinoid tumor of the larynx. *ORL.* 1991;53:194-209.
195. Gnepp DR. Small cell neuroendocrine carcinoma of the larynx: A critical review of the literature. *ORL.* 1991;53:210-219.
196. Milroy CM, Ferlito A. Immunohistochemical markers in the diagnosis of neuroendocrine neoplasms of the head and neck. *Ann Otol Rhinol Laryngol.* 1995;104(5):413-418.
197. Woodruff JM, Huvos AG, Erlandson RA, et al. Neuroendocrine carcinomas of the larynx. A study of two types, one of which mimics thyroid medullary carcinoma. *Am J Surg Pathol.* 1985;9(11):771-790.
198. Oliveira AM, Tazelaar HD, Myers JL, et al. Thyroid transcription factor-1 distinguishes metastatic pulmonary from well-differentiated neuroendocrine tumors of other sites. *Am J Surg Pathol.* 2001;25(6):815-819.
199. Vargas V, Sudilovsky D, Kaplan MJ. Mixed tumor, polymorphous low-grade adenocarcinoma and adenoid cystic carcinoma of the salivary gland: pathogenic implications and differential diagnosis by Ki-67 (Mib 1), Bcl 2 and S-100 immunohistochemistry. *Appl Immunohistochem.* 1997;5:8-16.
200. Gnepp DR, el-Mofty S. Polymorphous low-grade adenocarcinoma: glial fibrillary acidic protein staining in the differential diagnosis with cellular mixed tumors. *Oral Surg Oral Med Oral Pathol Oral Radiol Endod.* 1997;83(6):691-695.
201. Castle JT, Thompson LD, Frommelt RA, et al. Polymorphous low grade adenocarcinoma: a clinicopathologic study of 164 cases. *Cancer.* 1999;86(2):207-219.
202. Darling MR, Schneider JW, Phillips VM. Polymorphous low-grade adenocarcinoma and adenoid cystic carcinoma: a review and comparison of immunohistochemical markers. *Oral Oncol.* 2002;38(7):641-645.
203. Prasad AR, Savera AT, Gown AM, et al. The myoepithelial immunophenotype in 135 benign and malignant salivary gland tumors other than pleomorphic adenoma. *Arch Pathol Lab Med.* 1999;123(9):801-806.
204. Savera AT, Zarbo RJ. Defining the role of myoepithelium in salivary gland neoplasia. *Adv Anat Pathol.* 2004;11(2):69-85.
205. Barnes L, Appel BN, Perez H, et al. Myoepithelioma of the head and neck: case report and review. *J Surg Oncol.* 1985;28(1): 21-28.
206. Nagao T, Sugano I, Ishida Y, et al. Salivary gland malignant myoepithelioma: a clinicopathologic and immunohistochemical study of ten cases. *Cancer.* 1998;83(7):1292-1299.
207. Savera AT, Sloman A, Huvos AG, et al. Myoepithelial carcinoma of the salivary glands: a clinicopathologic study of 25 patients. *Am J Surg Pathol.* 2000;24(6):761-774.
208. Brandwein M, Ivanov K, Wallace DC, et al. Mucoepidermoid carcinoma: A clinicopathologic study of 80 patients with special reference to histologic grading. *Am J Surg Pathol.* 2001;25(7):835-845.
209. Luna MA. Salivary mucoepidermoid carcinoma: revisited. *Adv Anat Pathol.* 2006;13(6):293-307.
210. Ferlito A, Recher G, Bottin R. Mucoepidermoid carcinoma of the larynx. A clinicopathological study of 11 cases with review of the literature. *ORL J Otorhinolaryngol Relat Spec.* 1981;43(5):280-299.
211. Yang CS, Kuo KT, Chou TY, et al. Mucoepidermoid tumors of the lung: analysis of 11 cases. *J Chin Med Assoc.* 2004;67(11):565-570.
212. Vedrine PO, Coffinet L, Temam S, et al. Mucoepidermoid carcinoma of salivary glands in the pediatric age group: 18 clinical cases, including 11 second malignant neoplasms. *Head Neck.* 2006;28(9):827-833.
213. Rahbar R, Grimmer JF, Vargas SO, et al. Mucoepidermoid carcinoma of the parotid gland in children: A 10-year experience. *Arch Otolaryngol Head Neck Surg.* 2006;132(4):375-380.
214. Shapiro NL, Bhattacharyya N. Clinical characteristics and survival for major salivary gland malignancies in children. *Otolaryngol Head Neck Surg.* 2006;134(4):631-634.
215. Martinez-Madrigal F, Pineda-Daboin K, Casiraghi O, et al. Salivary gland tumors of the mandible. *Ann Diagn Pathol.* 2000;4(6):347-353.

216. Jahan-Parwar B, Huberman RM, Donovan DT, et al. Oncocytic mucoepidermoid carcinoma of the salivary gland. *Am J Surg Pathol*. 1999;23(5):523-529.
217. Weinreb I, Seethala RR, Hoschar AP, et al. Oncocytic mucoepidermoid carcinoma of salivary gland origin. *Am J Surg Pathol*, in press.
218. Jakobsson PA, Blanck C, Eneroth CM. Mucoepidermoid carcinoma of the parotid gland. *Cancer*. 1968;22(1):111-124.
219. Evans HL. Mucoepidermoid carcinoma of salivary glands: a study of 69 cases with special attention to histologic grading. *Am J Clin Pathol*. 1984;81(6):696-701.
220. Batsakis JG. Staging of salivary gland neoplasms: role of histopathologic and molecular factors. *Am J Surg*. 1994;168(5):386-390.
221. Guzzo M, Andreola S, Sirizzotti G, et al. Mucoepidermoid carcinoma of the salivary glands: clinicopathologic review of 108 patients treated at the National Cancer Institute of Milan. *Ann Surg Oncol*. 2002;9(7):688-695.
222. Plambeck K, Friedrich RE, Bahlo M, et al. TNM staging, histopathological grading, and tumor-associated antigens in patients with a history of mucoepidermoid carcinoma of the salivary glands. *Anticancer Res*. 1999;19(4A):2397-2404.
223. Goode RK, Auclair PL, Ellis GL. Mucoepidermoid carcinoma of the major salivary glands: clinical and histopathologic analysis of 234 cases with evaluation of grading criteria. *Cancer*. 1998;82(7):1217-1224.
224. Hicks MJ, el-Naggar AK, Flaitz CM, et al. Histocytologic grading of mucoepidermoid carcinoma of major salivary glands in prognosis and survival: a clinicopathologic and flow cytometric investigation. *Head Neck*. 1995;17(2):89-95.
225. Auclair PL, Goode RK, Ellis GL. Mucoepidermoid carcinoma of intraoral salivary glands. Evaluation and application of grading criteria in 143 cases. *Cancer*. 1992;69(8):2021-2030.
226. Freedman PD, Lumerman H. Lobular carcinoma of intraoral minor salivary gland origin. Report of twelve cases. *Oral Surg Oral Med Oral Pathol*. 1983;56(2):157-166.
227. Batsakis JG, Pinkston GR, Luna MA, et al. Adenocarcinomas of the oral cavity: a clinicopathologic study of terminal duct carcinomas. *J Laryngol Otol*. 1983;97(9):825-835.
228. Beltran D, Faquin WC, Gallagher G, et al. Selective immunohistochemical comparison of polymorphous low-grade adenocarcinoma and adenoid cystic carcinoma. *J Oral Maxillofac Surg*. 2006;64(3):415-423.
229. Andreadis D, Epivatianos A, Poulopoulos A, et al. Detection of C-KIT (CD117) molecule in benign and malignant salivary gland tumours. *Oral Oncol*. 2006;42(1):57-65.
230. Toida M, Shimokawa K, Makita H, et al. Intraoral minor salivary gland tumors: a clinicopathological study of 82 cases. *Int J Oral Maxillofac Surg*. 2005;34(5):528-532.
231. Perez-Ordonez B, Linkov I, Huvos AG. Polymorphous low-grade adenocarcinoma of minor salivary glands: a study of 17 cases with emphasis on cell differentiation. *Histopathology*. 1998;32(6):521-529.
232. Gnepp DR, Chen JC, Warren C. Polymorphous low-grade adenocarcinoma of minor salivary gland. An immunohistochemical and clinicopathologic study. *Am J Surg Pathol*. 1988;12(6): 461-468.
233. Donath K, Seifert G, Schmitz R. [Diagnosis and ultrastructure of the tubular carcinoma of salivary gland ducts. Epithelial-myoepithelial carcinoma of the intercalated ducts]. *Virch Arch A: Pathol Pathologische Anat*. 1972;356(1):16-31.
234. Seethala RR, Barnes EL, Hunt JL. Epithelial-myoepithelial carcinoma: a review of the clinicopathologic spectrum and immunophenotypic characteristics in 61 tumors of the salivary glands and upper aerodigestive tract. *Am J Surg Pathol*. 2007;31(1): 44-57.
235. Cho KJ, el-Naggar AK, Ordonez NG, et al. Epithelial-myoepithelial carcinoma of salivary glands. A clinicopathologic, DNA flow cytometric, and immunohistochemical study of Ki-67 and HER-2/neu oncogene. *Am J Clin Pathol*. 1995;103(4):432-437.
236. Shinozaki A, Nagao T, Endo H, et al. Sebaceous epithelial-myoepithelial carcinoma of the salivary gland: clinicopathologic and immunohistochemical analysis of 6 cases of a new histologic variant. *Am J Surg Pathol*. 2008;32(6):913-923.
237. Antic T, Venkataraman G, Oshima K. Oncocytic epithelial-myoepithelial carcinoma: an evolving new variant with comparative immunohistochemistry. *Pathology*. 2008;40(4):415-418.
238. Kusafuka K, Takizawa Y, Ueno T, et al. Dedifferentiated epithelial-myoepithelial carcinoma of the parotid gland: a rare case report of immunohistochemical analysis and review of the literature. *Oral Surg Oral Med Oral Pathol Oral Radiol Endod*. 2008;106(1):909-915.
239. Fronseca I, Soares J. Proliferating cell nuclear antigen immunohistochemistry in epithelial-myoepithelial carcinoma of the salivary glands. *Arch Pathol Lab Med*. 1993;117(10):993-995.
240. Rosa JC, Felix A, Fonseca I, et al. Immunoexpression of c-erbB-2 and p53 in benign and malignant salivary neoplasms with myoepithelial differentiation. *J Clin Pathol*. 1997;50(8):661-663.
241. Seifert G. Classification and differential diagnosis of clear and basal cell tumors of the salivary glands. *Semin Diagn Pathol*. 1996;13(2):95-103.
242. Ellis GL. Clear cell neoplasms in salivary glands: clearly a diagnostic challenge. *Ann Diagn Pathol*. 1998;2(1):61-78.
243. Ellis GL, Auclair PL. Clear cell carcinoma in Surgical Pathology of the Salivary Glands. In: Ellis GL, Auclair PL, Gnepp DR, eds. Philadelphia: WB Saunders; 1991:379-389.
244. Wang B, Brandwein M, Gordon R, et al. Primary salivary clear cell tumors—a diagnostic approach: a clinicopathologic and immunohistochemical study of 20 patients with clear cell carcinoma, clear cell myoepithelial carcinoma, and epithelial-myoepithelial carcinoma [see comment]. *Arch Pathol Lab Med*. 2002;126(6):676-685.
245. Michal M, Skalova A, Simpson RH, et al. Clear cell malignant myoepithelioma of the salivary glands. *Histopathology*. 1996;28(4):309-315.
246. Rezende RB, Drachenberg CB, Kumar D, et al. Differential diagnosis between monomorphic clear cell adenocarcinoma of salivary glands and renal (clear) cell carcinoma. *Am J Surg Pathol*. 1532;23(12):1532-1538.
247. Barnes L, Rao U, Krause J, et al. Salivary duct carcinoma. Part I. A clinicopathologic evaluation and DNA image analysis of 13 cases with review of the literature. *Oral Surg Oral Med Oral Pathol*. 1994;78(1):64-73.
248. Lewis JE, McKinney BC, Weiland LH, et al. Salivary duct carcinoma. Clinicopathologic and immunohistochemical review of 26 cases. *Cancer*. 1996;77(2):223-230.
249. Kapadia SB, Barnes L. Expression of androgen receptor, gross cystic disease fluid protein, and CD44 in salivary duct carcinoma. *Mod Pathol* 1033;11(11):1033–1038.
250. Fan CY, Wang J, Barnes EL. Expression of androgen receptor and prostatic specific markers in salivary duct carcinoma: an immunohistochemical analysis of 13 cases and review of the literature. *Am J Surg Pathol*. 2000;24(4):579-586.
251. Felix A, El-Naggar AK, Press MF, et al. Prognostic significance of biomarkers (c-erbB-2, p53, proliferating cell nuclear antigen, and DNA content) in salivary duct carcinoma. *Hum Pathol*. 1996;27(6):561-566.
252. Skalova A, Starek I, Vanecek T, et al. Expression of HER-2/neu gene and protein in salivary duct carcinomas of parotid gland as revealed by fluorescence in-situ hybridization and immunohistochemistry [see comment]. *Histopathology*. 2003;42(4):348-356.
253. Guzzo M, Di Palma S, Grandi C, et al. Salivary duct carcinoma: clinical characteristics and treatment strategies. *Head Neck*. 1997;19(2):126-133.
254. Weinreb I, Tabanda-Lichauco R, van der Kwast T, et al. Low-grade intraductal carcinoma of salivary gland: report of 3 cases with marked apocrine differentiation. *Am J Surg Pathol*. 2006;30(8):1014-1021.
255. Brandwein MS, Jagirdar J, Patil J, et al. Salivary duct carcinoma (cribriform salivary carcinoma of excretory ducts). A clinicopathologic and immunohistochemical study of 12 cases. *Cancer*. 1990;65(10):2307-2314.
256. Brandwein-Gensler M, Hille J, Wang BY, et al. Low-grade salivary duct carcinoma: description of 16 cases. *Am J Surg Pathol*. 2004;28(8):1040-1044.
257. Delgado R, Klimstra D, Albores-Saavedra J. Low grade salivary duct carcinoma. A distinctive variant with a low grade histology and a predominant intraductal growth pattern. *Cancer*. 1996;78(5):958-967.
258. Hotte SJ, Winquist EW, Lamont E, et al. Imatinib mesylate in patients with adenoid cystic cancers of the salivary glands expressing c-kit: a Princess Margaret Hospital phase II consortium study. *J Clin Oncol*. 2005;23(3):585-590.

259. Alcedo JC, Fabrega JM, Arosemena JR, et al. Imatinib mesylate as treatment for adenoid cystic carcinoma of the salivary glands: report of two successfully treated cases. *Head Neck*. 2004;26(9):829-831.
260. Tonon G, Modi S, Wu L, et al. t(11;19)(q21;p13) translocation in mucoepidermoid carcinoma creates a novel fusion product that disrupts Notch signaling pathway. *Nature Genet*. 2003;33:208-213.
261. Okabe M, Miyabe S, Nagatsuka H, et al. MECT1-MAML2 fusion transcript defines a favorable subset of mucoepidermoid carcinoma. *Clin Cancer Res*. 2006;12(13):3902-3907.
262. Behboudi A, Enlund F, Winnes M, et al. Molecular classification of mucoepidermoid carcinomas—prognostic significance of the MECT1-MAML2 fusion oncogene. *Genes Chromosomes Cancer*. 2006;45(5):470-481.
263. Martins C, Cavaco B, Tonon G, et al. A study of MECT1-MAML2 in mucoepidermoid carcinoma and Warthin's tumor of salivary glands. *J Mol Diagn*. 2004;6(3):205-210.
264. Tashiro Y, Sueishi K, Nakao K. Nasal glioma: an immunohistochemical and ultrastructural study. *Pathol Int*. 1995;45(5): 393-398.
265. Francis HW, Nager GT, Holliday MJEA. Association of heterotropic neuroglial tissue with an arachnoid cyst in the internal auditory canal. *Skull Base Surg*. 1995;5:37-49.
266. Glasscock III ME, Dickins JR, Jackson CG, et al. Surgical management of brain tissue herniation into the middle ear and mastoid. *Laryngoscope*. 1979;89(11):1743-1754.
267. Mills SE, Fechner RE. Middle ear adenoma. A cytologically uniform neoplasm displaying a variety of architectural patterns. *Am J Surg Pathol*. 1984;8(9):677-685.
268. Torske KR, Thompson LD. Adenoma versus carcinoid tumor of the middle ear: a study of 48 cases and review of the literature. *Mod Pathol*. 2002;15(5):543-555.
269. Thompson LD, Nelson BL, Barnes EL. Ceruminous adenomas: a clinicopathologic study of 41 cases with a review of the literature. *Am J Surg Pathol*. 2004;28(3):308-318.
270. Gaffey MJ, Mills SE, Fechner RE, et al. Aggressive papillary middle-ear tumor. A clinicopathologic entity distinct from middle-ear adenoma [see comment]. *Am J Surg Pathol*. 1988;12(10):790-797.
271. Heffner DK. Low-grade adenocarcinoma of probable endolymphatic sac origin A clinicopathologic study of 20 cases. *Cancer*. 1989;64(11):2292-2302.
272. Gaffey MJ, Mills SE, Boyd JC Aggressive papillary tumor of middle ear/temporal bone and adnexal papillary cystadenoma. Manifestations of von Hippel-Lindau disease. *Am J Surg Pathol*. 1254;18(12):1254-1260.
273. Megerian CA, Pilch BZ, Bhan AK, et al. Differential expression of transthyretin in papillary tumors of the endolymphatic sac and choroid plexus. *Laryngoscope*. 1997;107(2):216-221.
274. Horiguchi H, Sano T, Toi H, et al. Endolymphatic sac tumor associated with a von Hippel-Lindau disease patient: an immunohistochemical study. *Mod Pathol*. 2001;14(7):727-732.
275. Gyure KA, Morrison AL. Cytokeratin 7 and 20 expression in choroid plexus tumors: utility in differentiating these neoplasms from metastatic carcinomas. *Mod Pathol*. 2000;13(6): 638-643.
276. Thompson LD, Bouffard JP, Sandberg GD, et al. Primary ear and temporal bone meningiomas: a clinicopathologic study of 36 cases with a review of the literature. *Mod Pathol*. 2003;16(3):236-245.
277. Erickson D, Kudva YC, Ebersold MJ, et al. Benign paragangliomas: clinical presentation and treatment outcomes in 236 patients. *J Clin Endocrinol Metab*. 2001;86(11):5210-5216.
278. Sennaroglu L, Sungur A. Histopathology of paragangliomas. *Otol Neurotol*. 2002;23(1):104-105.
279. Lam KY, Lo CY, Wat NM, et al. The clinicopathological features and importance of p53, Rb, and mdm2 expression in phaeochromocytomas and paragangliomas. *J Clin Pathol*. 2001;54(6):443-448.
280. Martinez-Madrigal F, Bosq J, Micheau C, et al. Paragangliomas of the head and neck. Immunohistochemical analysis of 16 cases in comparison with neuro-endocrine carcinomas. *Pathol Res Pract*. 1991;187(7):814-823.
281. Barnes EL, Taylor S. Carotid body paragangliomas: a clinicopathologic and DNA analysis of 13 tumors. *Arch Otolaryngol*. 1991;116:447-453.
282. Min KW. Diagnostic usefulness of sustentacular cells in paragangliomas: immunocytochemical and ultrastructural investigation. *Ultrastruct Pathol*. 1998;22(5):369-376.
283. Achilles E, Padberg BC, Holl K, et al. Immunocytochemistry of paragangliomas—value of staining for S100 protein and glial fibrillary acidic protein in diagnosis and prognosis. *Histopathology*. 1991;18:458.
284. Kliewer KE, Wen DR, Cancilla PA. Paragangliomas: assessment of prognosis by histologic, immunohistochemical, and ultrastructural techniques. *Hum Pathol*. 1989;20:29-39.
285. Mooney EE, Dodd LG, Oury TD, et al. Middle ear carcinoid: an indolent tumor with metastatic potential. *Head Neck*. 1999;21(1):72-77.
286. Mandigers CM, van Gils AP, Derksen J, et al. Carcinoid tumor of the jugulo-tympanic region. *J Nucl Med*. 1996;37(2): 270-272.
287. Hunt JL, Tomaszewski JE, Montone KT. Prostatic adenocarcinoma metastatic to the head and neck and the workup of an unknown epithelioid neoplasm. *Head Neck*. 2004;26(2):171-178.
288. Ozolek JA, Bastacky S, Myers E, et al. Immunohistochemical staining characteristics of oncocytomas of major salivary glands: comparison to conventional renal cell carcinoma. *Laryngoscope*. In press.

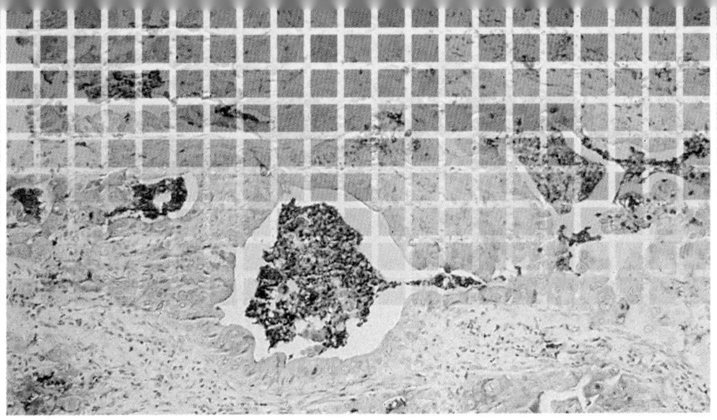

10

Immunohistology of Endocrine Tumors

Ronald A. DeLellis • Sandra J. Shin • Diana O. Treaba

- Introduction 291
- Biology of Antigens and Antibodies 291
- Tumors of Specific Sites 295
- Summary 329

INTRODUCTION

Immunohistochemical methods have had a profound impact on the understanding of the endocrine system and its changes in a wide variety of disease states.[1] In particular, these methods have led to the development of a series of functional classifications of endocrine tumors that have supplemented and, in some cases, replaced traditional morphologic classifications. The use of immunohistochemistry in endocrine pathology has been critical for the recognition of new tumor entities, the identification of sites of origin of metastatic tumors, and prognostic assessments on the basis of patterns of hormone expression and the presence of various other markers. Moreover, these methods have played a key role both in the identification of precursors of endocrine tumors and in elucidating the steps in the hyperplasia-neoplasia sequence. The goals of this chapter are to review the major classes of immunohistochemical markers currently used in the assessment of endocrine tumors, to review the diagnostic approaches of these methods for endocrine tumors of specific sites, to highlight advances in the molecular diagnosis of these tumors, and to review selected theranostic approaches on the basis of these studies.

BIOLOGY OF ANTIGENS AND ANTIBODIES

Hormones

An important approach to the diagnosis and classification of endocrine tumors relies on the demonstration of their hormonal content.[1,2] This can be accomplished by the use of antibodies directed against the mature hormones and hormone precursors. An additional approach involves the use of *in situ* hybridization (hybridization histochemistry) for the demonstration of specific hormonal messenger RNAs (mRNAs). The latter approach is discussed in detail in several reviews.[3,4] Virtually all classes of hormones (small peptides, large polypeptide hormones, steroids, amines) and hormone receptors can be visualized in immunohistochemical formats.[2,5] With the advent of microwave-based antigen retrieval methods, the vast majority of these products can be demonstrated in formalin-fixed, paraffin-embedded samples. However, hormonal products by themselves cannot be used as lineage-specific markers.[6] For example, somatostatin is present in the D cells of the pancreatic islets, gastrointestinal and bronchopulmonary endocrine cells, thymic endocrine cells, thyroid C cells, and in their corresponding tumors. Therefore the presence of immunoreactive somatostatin by itself does not provide evidence of the site of origin of a metastatic lesion. The discussion of individual hormones is addressed in sections on specific endocrine cell types and their corresponding tumors.

Enzymes

Enzymes that are active in the biosynthesis and processing of hormones are important markers of endocrine cells.[6] Immunoreactivity for aromatic L-amino acid decarboxylase, for example, is widely distributed in neuroendocrine (NE) cells.[7] Tyrosine hydroxylase, dopamine β-hydroxylase, and phenylethanolamine *N*-methyl transferase, in contrast, have a more limited tissue distribution and are confined to known sites of catecholamine biosynthesis.[8] Immunolocalization of these enzymes permits catecholamine-synthesizing abilities to be deduced from paraffin sections. The presence of immunoreactive enzyme, however, does not necessarily imply that the enzyme is present in a functional form.

A variety of endopeptidases and carboxypeptidases that are required for the formation of biologically active peptides from precursor molecules are present in the trans-Golgi region and secretory granules of NE cells. They include the prohormone convertases PC1/PC3 and PC2 and carboxypeptidases H and E.[9,10] The proconvertases are widely distributed in NE cells and their corresponding tumors, whereas other types of endocrine cells (thyroid follicular cells, parathyroid chief cells, adrenal cortical cells, and testis) are negative.[10] NE cells with a neural phenotype (e.g., adrenal medullary cells) contain a predominance of PC2, whereas epithelial NE cells contain a predominance of PC1/PC3. With the exception of parathyroid cells, the presence of PC2 and PC3 correlates with the presence of chromogranins and secretogranins. PC2 and PC1/PC3 are present in normal pituitaries and in pituitary adenomas, with adrenocorticotropic hormone (ACTH)-producing adenomas containing a predominance of PC1/PC3 and other adenomas expressing a predominance of PC2.[9] Both peptidylglycine alpha-amidating monooxygenase and peptidylamidoglycolate lyase are present in NE secretory granules.[11] These enzymes are responsible for the alpha-amidation of the C-terminal regions of peptide hormones. This function is critical for biologic activity of the peptides.

Neuron-specific enolase (NSE) is an additional enzyme that has been studied extensively in NE cells.[12] The staining of NE tumors is unrelated to the cellular content of secretory granules, and even degranulated cells are NSE positive. This enzyme is the most acidic isoenzyme of the glycolytic enzyme enolase and is present in both neurons and NE cells.[12] The enolases are products of three genetic loci that have been designated alpha, beta, and gamma. Non-neuronal enolase (alpha-alpha) is present in fetal tissues of different types, glial cells, and many non-NE tissues in the adult. Muscle enolase is of the beta-beta type, whereas the neuronal form of enolase has been designated gamma-gamma. Hybrid enolases are present in megakaryocytes and a variety of other cell types. NSE (gamma-gamma) replaces non-neuronal enolase during the migration and differentiation of neurons, and the appearance of this isoenzyme heralds the formation of synapses and electrical excitability. Although many earlier studies employed NSE as a marker of NE cells, more recent studies have indicated that the utility of this marker is limited by its lack of specificity.[13,14]

The protein gene product 9.5 (PGP9.5) is a ubiquitin carboxyterminal hydrolase that plays a role in the catalytic degradation of abnormal denatured proteins.[15-17] PGP9.5 is present in neurons and nerve fibers and in a variety of NE cells, with the possible exception of those in the normal gastrointestinal tract. In contrast, gastrointestinal endocrine tumors (GI-ETs) and a variety of other NE tumors contain PGP9.5. The patterns of staining for NSE and PGP9.5 are generally similar in that positive cells show diffuse cytoplasmic reactivity that is unrelated to the type of hormone produced or the degree of cellular differentiation.[18] Comparative studies, however, have demonstrated that some NE tumors may be positive for PGP9.5 and negative for NSE, whereas others may be positive for NSE and negative for PGP9.5. Antibodies to PGP9.5 are particularly useful for the demonstration of neurons and cells with neuronal differentiation. It should be recognized that some non-NE tumors such as those of the exocrine pancreas may also be positive for PGP9.5.[19]

Histaminase (diamine oxidase) has been used as a marker for some NE cells and their tumors. This enzyme is present in high concentrations in medullary thyroid carcinomas and has been reported in small cell carcinomas of the lung and other NE neoplasms.[20] High serum levels of histaminase also occur in pregnancy, and immunohistochemical studies have revealed the presence of this enzyme in decidual cells.

Enzymes of the biosynthetic pathway of steroid hormones can also be demonstrated effectively in immunohistochemical formats. Among the enzymes that have been localized are $P450_{scc}$ (cholesterol side chain cleavage), 3β-hydroxysteroid dehydrogenase, 21-hydroxylase, 17α-hydroxylase, and 11β-hydroxylase.[21-23] To date, however, there have been relatively few studies evaluating antibodies to these enzymes as diagnostic reagents.

Chromogranins, Secretogranins, and Other Granule Proteins

The chromogranins and secretogranins represent the major constituents of NE secretory granules.[24-28] Three major chromogranin proteins have been identified and categorized and have been designated chromogranin A, chromogranin B, and secretogranin II. Additional granins that have been characterized include secretogranins III, IV, and V. The chromogranin and secretogranin proteins contain multiple dibasic residues that are sites for endogenous proteolytic processing to smaller peptides.[29] For example, chromogranin A contains 439 amino acids with 10 pairs of amino acids that represent potential cleavage sites by proteases such as the prohormone convertases. Resultant peptides include chromostatin, pancreastatin, parastatin, and vasostatin. Functional roles for these smaller peptides include intracellular hormone binding functions, inhibitory effects on the secretion of other hormones, and antibacterial and antifungal effects. Many NE cells contain all major granins, whereas others show distinctive patterns of chromogranin distribution.

The monoclonal antibody LK2H10, developed by Lloyd and Wilson, is directed against chromogranin A and is currently the most commonly used chromogranin antibody in general practice.[24] Chromogranins are present within the matrices of secretory granules of NE cells. As a result, tumors with abundant secretory granules demonstrate intense chromogranin immunoreactivity, whereas those with fewer granules are less intensely stained. Numerous studies have demonstrated that chromogranin A represents the single most specific marker of NE differentiation in general use. Antibodies to chromogranin B and secretogranin II are available but are not in general use.

Tissue-specific patterns and ratios of the chromogranin proteins are typically maintained in NE tumors.

For example, chromogranin A is the major granin expressed by gastric ETs and serotonin-producing ETs of the appendix and ileum. In contrast, strong immunoreactivity for chromogranin B and secretogranin II is typical of rectal ETs (carcinoids and small cell carcinomas) and of prolactinomas, which lack chromogranin A.[30,31]

NE secretory protein-55 (NESP-55) is a 241 amino acid polypeptide that is a member of the chromogranin family.[32] It is expressed exclusively in endocrine and neuronal tissue but has a less wide distribution than chromogranin A in human tissues. The reactivity of NESP-55 appears to be restricted to endocrine tumors of the pancreas and adrenal medulla, and several studies have indicated that it may be useful in the identification of sites of origin of metastatic endocrine tumors.[33,34]

Synaptophysin and Other Synaptic Vesicle Proteins

Synaptophysin is a calcium-binding glycoprotein (38,000 kD), which is the most abundant integral membrane protein constituent of synaptic vesicles of neurons.[35] It is also present in a wide spectrum of NE cells and in many of their corresponding tumors. Typically, synaptophysin reactivity is present in a punctate pattern in synaptic regions of neurons and is present diffusely throughout the cytoplasm of NE cells. Ultrastructurally, synaptophysin is present in micro-vesicles, whereas chromogranin is present in secretory granules.[35] These differences indicate that chromogranins and synaptophysin are complementary generic NE markers. Synaptophysin immunoreactivity, however, is not specific to NE cells because it is also present in adrenal cortical cells and their tumors.[36]

Synaptic vesicle protein 2 (SV2) is present in the central and peripheral nervous systems and in a wide variety of NE cell types. Comparative studies of the distribution of SV2, synaptophysin, and chromogranin A in NE tumors have shown excellent agreement with the exception of hindgut ETs, which showed weak synaptophysin immunoreactivity, no staining for chromogranin A, but strong staining for SV2.[37] Gastrointestinal stromal tumors also express SV2, suggesting that these tumors may have an NE phenotype.[38]

Vesicular monoamine transporters (VMATs) mediate the transport of amines into vesicles of neurons and endocrine cells. VMAT1 and VMAT2 are differentially expressed by gastrointestinal endocrine tumors with patterns specific for each tumor type.[39] For example, serotonin-producing endocrine tumors expressed VMAT1 predominantly while histamine-producing endocrine tumors (gastric ETs) expressed VMAT2 almost exclusively. Peptide hormone–producing gastrointestinal tumors (rectal ETs) and pancreatic endocrine tumors, on the other hand, contained few VMAT1 or 2 positive cells.[39]

Synaptotagmins (p65), which form a large calcium-binding family, are implicated in neurotransmitter release, although synaptotagmin I is the only isoform demonstrated to have a role in vesicle fusion. In the pancreatic islets, synaptotagmins have been co-localized with insulin, but the roles of this family of proteins have not been fully explored as markers of NE tumors.[40,41]

The vesicle-associated membrane proteins (VAMP or synaptobrevin) occur in three isoforms and are proteins that are anchored to the cytoplasmic portion of synaptic membrane vesicles and secretory granules. VAMP2 and 3 are present in pancreatic beta cells, but the roles of this family of proteins have not been widely studied as markers of NE tumors.[42] In contrast to synaptophysin and other synaptic vesicle proteins, SNAP-25 (synaptosomal protein of 25 KD) and syntaxin are present in the plasma membranes. At present, there are few studies on the application of these markers in diagnostic pathology.[43]

CD57

The CD57 antigen is present on subsets of T cells and natural killer cells.[44-46] Antibodies to CD57 also react with Schwann cells, oligodendroglial cells, and a variety of NE cells of both neural and epithelial types. Additionally, CD57 positivity is present in prostatic, renal, and cortical thymic epithelial cells. Antibodies to CD57 react with varying proportions of neural tumors including schwannomas, neurofibromas, neuromas, and granular cell tumors. Among endocrine tumors, CD57 has been used most commonly as a marker for NE tumors. For example, CD57 is present in 100% of pheochromocytomas, 85% of extra-adrenal paragangliomas and ETs of diverse origins, and 50% of small cell bronchogenic carcinomas. However, CD57 is not restricted in its distribution to NE tumors because reactivity is present in more than 95% of papillary thyroid carcinomas and approximately 70% of follicular carcinomas.[47] Nonendocrine tumors that are frequently CD57 positive include prostatic carcinomas, thymomas, and a variety of small, round, blue cell tumors. These results indicate that the use of CD57 antibodies alone is unreliable for the specific identification of NE tumors.

Neural Cell Adhesion Molecule (CD56)

The neural cell adhesion molecules (NCAMs) comprise a family of glycoproteins that play critical roles in cell binding, migration, and differentiation.[48] The NCAM family includes three principal moieties that are generated from alternative splicing of RNA from a gene that is a member of the immunoglobulin supergene family. The molecules are modified post-translationally by phosphorylation, glycosylation, and sulfation. The homophilic binding properties of NCAMs are modulated by the differential expression of polysialic acid. Although initial studies indicated that NCAM was restricted in its distribution to the nervous system, more recent studies indicate a considerably wider distribution including the adrenal medulla and cortex (zona glomerulosa), cardiac muscle, thyroid follicular epithelium, proximal renal tubular epithelium, hepatocytes, gastric parietal cells, and islets of Langerhans. Among tumors, follicular and papillary thyroid carcinomas, as well as renal cell carcinomas and hepatocellular carcinomas, are NCAM+.[49] The Leu7 antigen, recognized by the HNK-1 monoclonal antibody, has now been identified as a carbohydrate epitope present on NCAM and a number of other adhesion molecules. Most NE cells and tumors with neurosecretory granules contain both NCAM mRNA and NCAM protein.[50] Antibodies to a long chain form of polysialic acid (polySia) found on NCAM have been used in studies of normal and neoplastic C cells and NE tumors of the lung.[51,52]

Intermediate Filaments

Cytokeratins are the major intermediate filaments of endocrine cells with the exception of steroid-producing cells. These proteins are members of the intermediate filament (10 nm) superfamily of cytoskeletal proteins.[53] They differ from other cytoskeletal filaments on the basis of size and other physical and chemical properties. Microfilaments (5 to 15 nm) contain actin, whereas the 25-nm microtubules contain tubulin. Other types of intermediate filaments that are present in endocrine cells and their supporting elements include vimentin, glial fibrillary acidic protein (GFAP), and the neurofilament proteins. The cytokeratins are the largest and most complex group of intermediate filaments and include a family of at least 30 proteins with molecular weights ranging from 40 to 68 kD. The type II keratins are basic and include eight epithelial proteins (CK1 to CK8). The type II keratins are more acidic and include 11 epithelial keratins that are designated CK9 to CK20. Pairs of basic and acidic keratins are expressed differentially in epithelial cells at different stages of development and differentiation. They can be identified immunohistochemically using pancytokeratin antibodies that react with epitopes on multiple different molecular weight cytokeratin species or with chain-specific monoclonal antibodies that recognize one specific cytokeratin type. The cytokeratins are distributed in tissue-specific patterns, and primary tumors tend to recapitulate the cytokeratin profiles of the cells from which they are derived.[54,55] In some cases, cytokeratin expression patterns tend to be simple, whereas in other cases, complex patterns of cytokeratin expression are apparent. Vimentin (57 kD) is also expressed together with cytokeratins in many normal and neoplastic endocrine cell types. In steroid-producing cells, vimentin is the major intermediate filament protein.

The neurofilaments are composed of heteropolymers of three different subunits with molecular weights of 70, 170, and 195 kD, corresponding to low (L), medium (M), and high (H) molecular weight subunits.[56] All three neurofilament subunits are phosphorylated in proportion to the molecular weight of each subunit. The neurofilaments represent the major intermediate filaments of mature and developing neurons, paraganglionic cells, and certain normal NE cells. These intermediate filaments are expressed in tumors with evidence of neuronal differentiation and are also present to varying degrees in NE tumors of epithelial type, which also express cytokeratins. Normal epithelial NE-type cells (pancreatic islets, Merkel cells) most commonly lack neurofilament immunoreactivity, whereas their corresponding neoplasms are commonly positive for this marker. Moreover, the pattern of staining in a dotlike area corresponding to the Golgi region is typical of NE neoplasms. The studies of Perez and coworkers[57] have suggested that the differential expression of neurofilament subtypes is related to tumor site. Glial fibrillary acidic protein (GFAP) (50 kD) is the major intermediate filament type of fibrous and protoplasmic astrocytes. GFAP is also present in nonmyelinated Schwann cells, supporting cells of the anterior pituitary and paraganglia, and various carcinomas. Immunoreactive GFAP is also present in mixed tumors of the skin and salivary glands, nerve sheath tumors, and chordomas.

Transcription Factors

Transcription factors are proteins that bind to the upstream regulatory elements of genes in the promoter and enhancer regions of DNA and stimulate or inhibit gene expression and protein synthesis.[1,58] They play critical roles in embryogenesis and development. Transcription factors may be tissue specific or may be present in a variety of different tissue types. Many of the so-called tissue-specific transcription factors, however, are not restricted to a single tissue type. For example, thyroid transcription factor-1 (TTF-1) is present both in thyroid follicular cells and in lung, whereas the adrenal 4 site/steroidogenic factor (ad4BP/SF-1) is present in steroid-producing cells and in certain anterior pituitary cell types. The pituitary transcription factor, Pit-1, is present in certain cells of the adenohypophysis and is also present in the placenta. Additional transcription factors that have been used in immunohistochemical formats include mammalian achete scute homolog (MASH-1), TTF, PAX-2 PAX-8, PDX-2, and Isl1. Applications of transcription factor localization in the endocrine system are discussed in subsequent sections.

Somatostatin Receptors

Somatostatin acts via specific receptors, which belong to the seven transmembrane G-protein coupled superfamily.[59] Somatostatin receptors (sst) are categorized into five major subtypes designated sst 1-5. The inhibitory action of somatostatin on hormone secretion is mediated by sst2, whereas suppression of cell growth is mediated by sst 1, 2, and 5. The effects of somatostatin on apoptosis are mediated by ssts 2 and 3. Immunohistochemical analysis of ssts has been used to gauge the responsiveness of NE tumors to somatostatin analogs.[59]

Cell Cycle Markers

Antibodies to cell cycle markers have been used in endocrine pathology primarily as an adjunct for the distinction of benign and malignant tumors.[60-62] In general, malignant tumors have a higher labeling index than benign tumors, as assessed with antibodies to Ki-67 (MIB-1). However, there may be considerable overlap in proliferative indices between benign and malignant endocrine tumors. The cyclin-dependent kinase inhibitor, p27, is

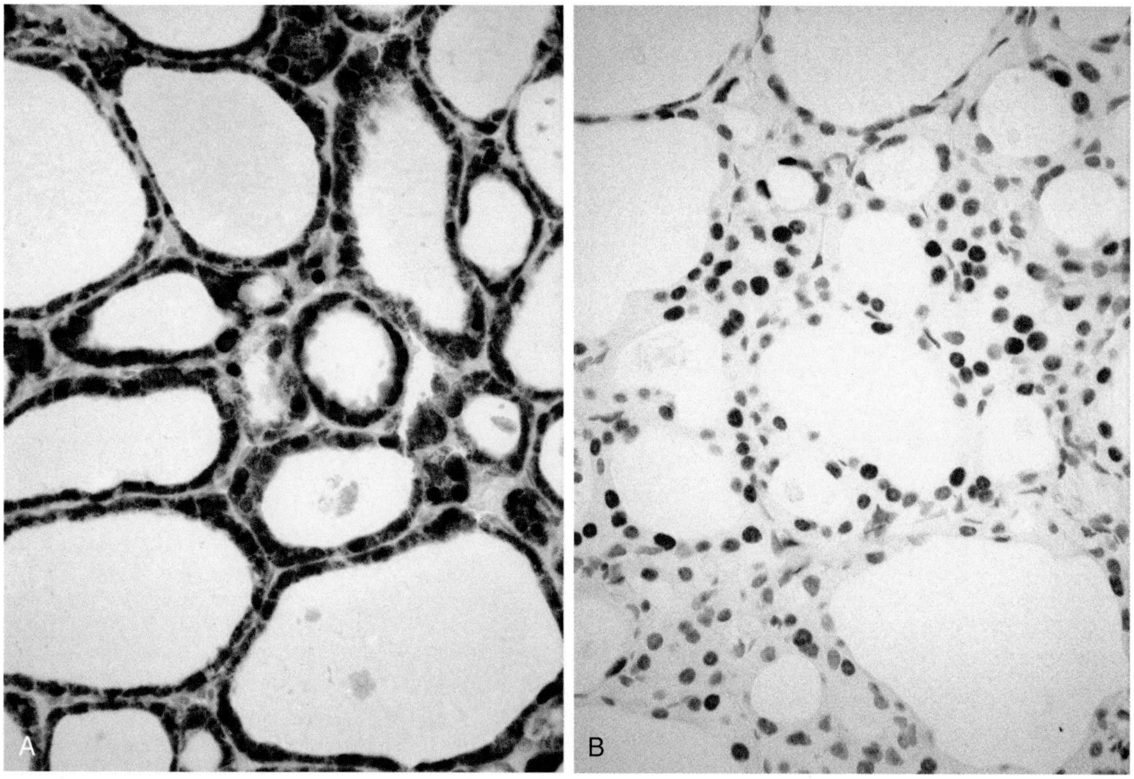

FIGURE 10.1 Normal human thyroid gland stained for TTF-1. **A,** Streptavidin biotin peroxidase technique with incomplete blocking of endogenous biotin. Both the nuclei and cytoplasm are stained positively. **B,** Polymer-based (En Vision +) technique. Positive staining is restricted to nuclei.

decreased in many malignant endocrine tumors as compared with their benign counterparts. In some instances the combined use of Ki-67 and p27 is more effective than the use of either antibody alone.[60]

Pitfalls of Immunohistochemistry of Endocrine Tumors

Many endocrine cells including thyroid follicular and adrenal cortical cells contain high levels of biotin-like activity, which is enhanced following heat-induced epitope retrieval (Fig. 10.1). Because endogenous biotin is often incompletely blocked following standard blocking procedures, the use of polymer based detection systems is recommended for all studies of endocrine cells and tumors.[63] The use of the latter system essentially circumvents nonspecific background staining observed with avidin or streptavidin-based systems.

TUMORS OF SPECIFIC SITES

Adenohypophysis

The cell types of the adenohypophysis were categorized originally on the basis of their reactivities with hematoxylin and eosin (H&E) as acidophils, basophils, and chromophobes. With more sophisticated histochemical staining sequences, the three cell types were subdivided further. For example, acidophils were further differentiated into the orange G-positive prolactin-positive cells and the erythrosin-positive growth hormone–producing cells, whereas basophils could be demonstrated by their periodic acid Schiff positivity. The subsequent development of immunohistochemical methods allowed the distinction of cell types on the basis of their contents of specific hormones.[64] The major cell types and their corresponding products include somatotrophs (growth hormone); lactotrophs (prolactin); mammosomatotrophs (growth hormone, prolactin); thyrotrophs (thyroid-stimulating hormone); corticotrophs (adrenocorticotropin, beta-endorphin, melanocyte-stimulating hormone); and gonadotrophs (follicle-stimulating hormone, luteinizing hormone). The somatotrophs are present predominantly in the lateral wings and account for approximately 50% of the cells of the adenohypophysis. Lactotrophs predominate at the posterolateral edges of the gland and account for 15% to 25% of the cells. The corticotrophs are present primarily in the central mucoid wedge and account for 15% to 20% of the cells. Thyrotrophs account for 5% of the cells and are located in the anteromedial regions of the gland. The gonadotrophs compose approximately 5% of the cell populations and are scattered throughout the anterior lobe.

In addition to the hormone-producing cells, a second cell population (folliculostellate cells) is also present in the normal gland.[65] The latter cells have a dendritic shape and typically encircle the hormone-positive cells. The folliculostellate cells are positive for S-100 protein and are variably positive for GFAP.

Pituitary adenomas are currently classified according to their content of specific hormones as summarized in

TABLE 10.1 Classification and Immunohistochemistry of Pituitary Adenomas

Type	Frequency (%)	Immunohistochemistry
Sparsely granulated prolactin	27	PRL (paranuclear); α-su, (rare); pit-1; focal ER positivity
Densely granulated prolactin cell adenoma	0.4	PRL (diffuse); pit-1
Sparsely granulated growth hormone cell adenomas	7.6	GH (weak); α-su (weak); pit-1
Densely granulated growth hormone cell adenoma	7.1	GH (strong); α-su (~50%); pit-1
Mixed growth hormone cell and prolactin cell adenomas	3.5	GH and PRL in different cells
Mammosomatotroph cell adenoma	1.2	GH and PRL in same cells; pit-1; focal ER positivity
Corticotroph cell adenoma	9.6	ACTH; β-end; β-LPH; neuro D1; pit-1
Thyrotroph cell adenoma	1.1	β-TSH; α-su (variable)
Gonadotroph cell adenoma	9.8	β-FSH; β-LH; α-su; SF-1
Silent corticotroph cell adenoma (subtype1)	2.0	ACTH; β-end (β-end>ACTH)
Silent corticotroph cell adenoma (subtype 2)	1.5	ACTH (focal); β-end (β-end>ACTH)
Silent adenoma (subtype 3)	1.4	GH; PRL; α-su
Null cell adenoma	12.4	Usually negative for hormones, but some cases are positive for β-FSH and α-su; SF-1
Oncocytoma	13.4	Similar to null cell
Unclassified	8.8	

ACTH, adrenocorticotropin; α-su, alpha subunit; β-end, beta-endorphin; β-FSH, beta follicle stimulating hormone; β-LH, beta luteinizing hormone; β-LPH, beta lipotropin; β-TSH, beta thyroid stimulating hormone, ER, estrogen receptor; GH, growth hormone.

Table 10.1 and Figs. 10.2 and 10.3. The tumors also have distinctive patterns of reactivity with antibodies to transcription factors and cytokeratins. More than 90% of adenomas contain CK8, and in sparsely granulated growth hormone cell adenomas, the staining is globular, corresponding to the presence of fibrous bodies. Perinuclear staining is typical of densely granulated growth hormone cell and mammosomatotroph adenomas, whereas corticotroph cell adenomas exhibit more diffuse cytoplasmic staining for CK8. Approximately 50% of adenomas exhibit keratin immunoreactivity with the AE1/AE3 antibody cocktail, whereas 7% and 10% are reactive with CKs 19 and 7, respectively (Fig. 10.4).[54]

Pituitary adenomas are typically positive for NE markers including chromogranin (100%), synaptophysin (92%), and NSE (80%).[1,32,66] The hormonal content of these tumors can be demonstrated with monoclonal antibodies to specific anterior pituitary hormones and hormone precursor fragments (Table 10.1). In contrast to their presence in the normal anterior pituitary, S-100 protein-positive folliculostellate cells are generally absent from pituitary adenomas.[67]

Pituitary carcinomas are rare, and their diagnosis rests on the demonstration of metastases. These tumors are typically positive for generic NE markers and for one or more anterior pituitary hormones.[68] The most frequently synthesized hormones are prolactin and ACTH, and the production of growth hormone, thyroid-stimulating hormone (TSH), and follicle-stimulating hormone/luteinizing hormone (FSH/LH) is rare.[68] The distinction of adenomas from carcinomas in the absence of metastases is difficult, if not impossible. There are significant differences in MIB-1 labeling indices among adenomas, invasive adenomas, and carcinomas, but overlaps in these indices exist and in some carcinomas, the labeling index is in the range of adenomas.[69] Thappar and coworkers[70] have reported p53 in 0%, 15%, and 100% of adenomas, atypical adenomas, and carcinomas, respectively, but exceptions to these generalizations exist.

BEYOND IMMUNOHISTOCHEMISTRY: MOLECULAR DIAGNOSTIC APPLICATIONS

Relatively few studies have focused on the diagnostic molecular aspects of pituitary tumors.[71] The distinction of benign and malignant pituitary tumors is difficult, if not impossible, by standard histopathological criteria. In a study of prolactin-producing tumors using molecular and immunohistochemical approaches, Wierinckx and colleagues[72] identified nine genes implicated in invasion, proliferation, and differentiation, which were differentially expressed in noninvasive, invasive, and invasive/aggressive tumors. By routine histology and immunohistochemistry, the presence of four markers of differentiation (mitoses, Ki-67, pituitary tumor transforming gene [PTTG], p53) and a marker of invasion (polysialic acid of NCAM) demonstrated that no single marker could distinguish invasive from noninvasive tumors. However, mitoses and Ki-67 labeling were statistically different in five invasive tumors, while p53 and PTTG nuclear labeling was also statistically different. The five invasive tumors with high Ki-67 indices and nuclear labeling of PTTG and p53 were classified as aggressive-invasive tumors, corresponding to so-called "atypical

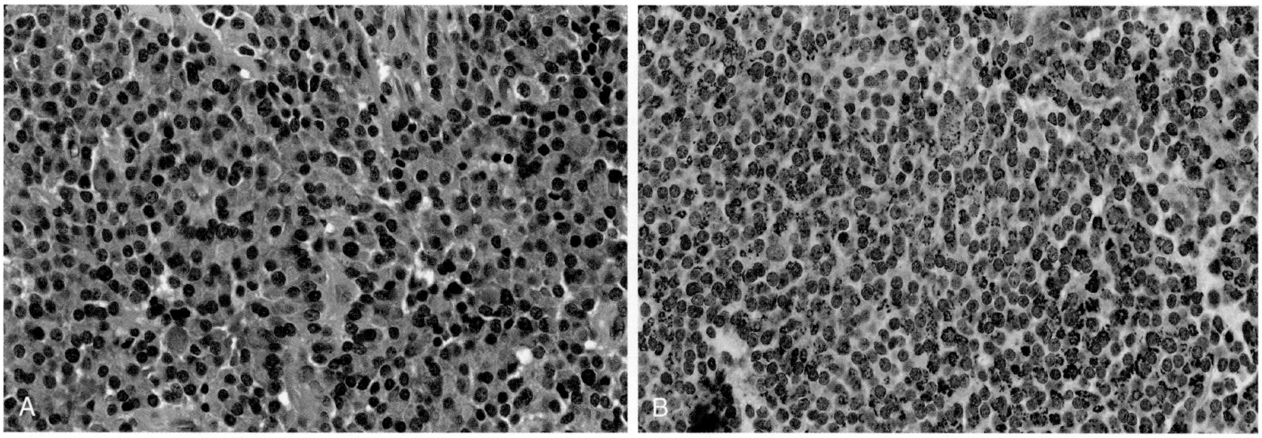

FIGURE 10.2 **A,** Pituitary adenoma (H&E stain). **B,** Immunoperoxidase stain for prolactin. The cells show weak granular cytoplasmic positivity (sparsely granulated prolactinoma).

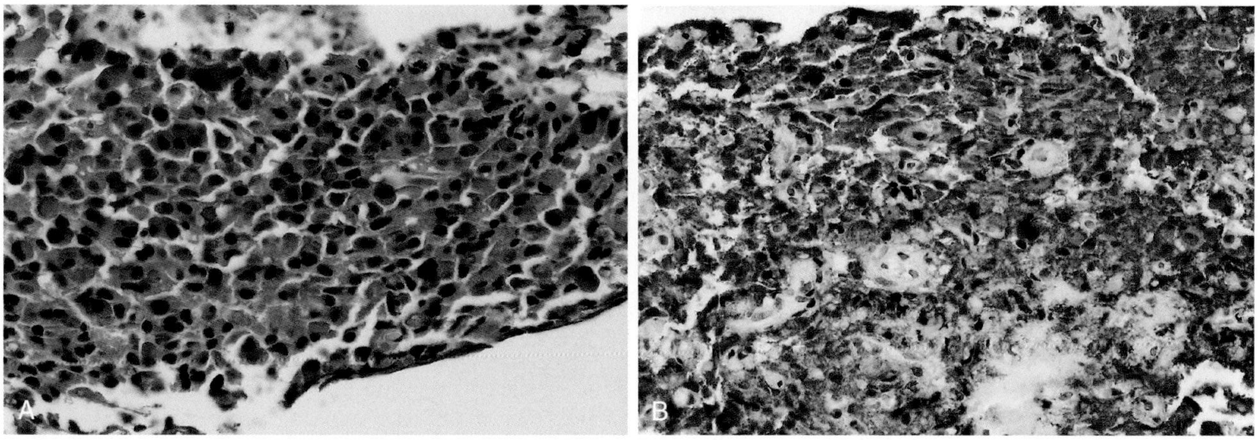

FIGURE 10.3 **A,** Pituitary adenoma (H&E stain). **B,** Immunoperoxidase stain for growth hormone. All the cells contain immunoreactive growth hormone.

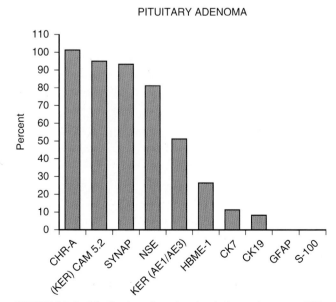

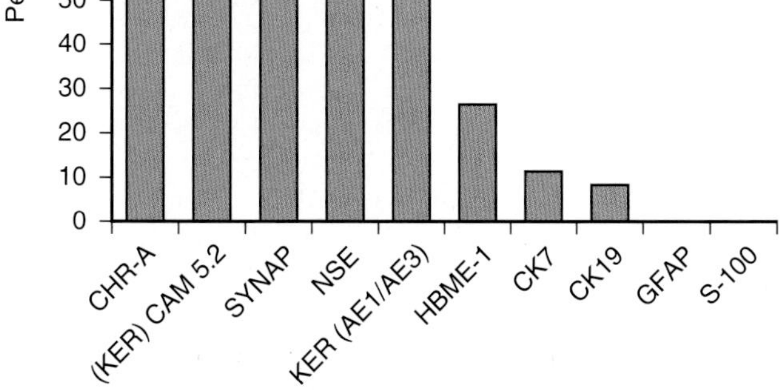

FIGURE 10.4 Distribution of markers in pituitary adenomas. CHR-A, chromogranin A; KER (CAM5.2), keratins detected with monoclonal antibody CAM5.2; SYNAP, synaptophysin; NSE, neuron-specific enolase; KER (AE1/AE3), keratins detected with antibodies AE1 and AE3; HBME-1; CK7, cytokeratin 7; CK19, cytokeratin 19; GFAP, glial fibrillary acid protein.

adenomas." PTTG expression was restricted to the cytoplasm in noninvasive and invasive tumors, whereas it was present in both the nucleus and cytoplasm of the invasive/aggressive tumors.[72] Galectin-3 may also play a role in pituitary tumor progression.[73]

As noted by Asa, the best predictive marker for pituitary tumors is the classification based on hormone content and cell structure.[74] For example, the response to long-acting somatostatin analogs in acromegalic patients who fail surgical resection is best determined by the classification of tumors into sparsely and densely granulated types. Responders to octreotide are more likely to have densely granulated adenomas that typically have a weak perinuclear pattern of cytokeratin immunoreactivity with CAM 5.2. Sparsely granulated adenomas, on the other hand, have a characteristic globular juxtanuclear fibrous body. Additionally, silent corticotroph adenomas will recur more often and more aggressively than silent gonadotroph adenomas.

Pineal Gland

Tumors of the pineal gland include parenchymal neoplasms (pineocytomas, pineoblastoma, and pineal parenchymal tumor of intermediate differentiation),

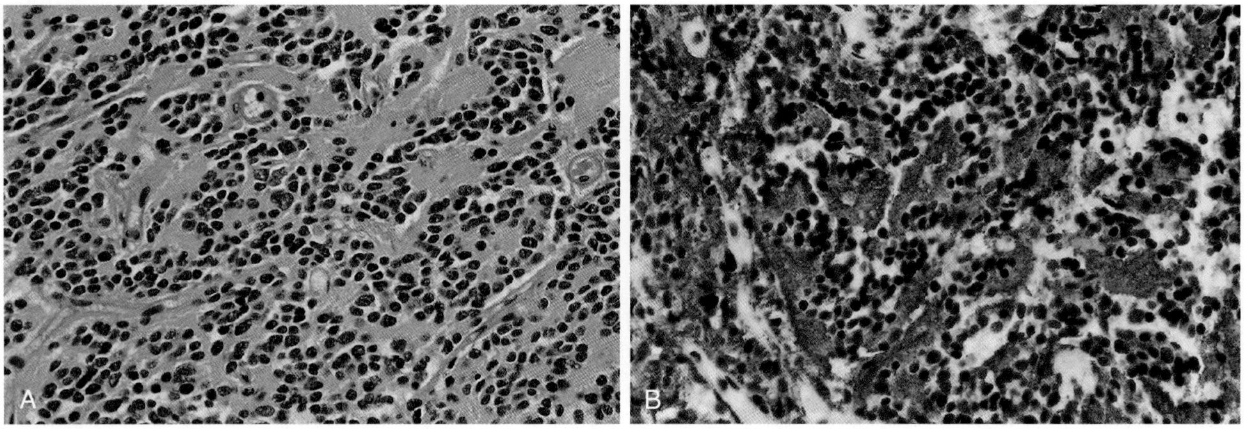

FIGURE 10.5 **A,** Pineocytoma (H&E stain). **B,** Immunoperoxidase stain for synaptophysin. The cell processes show strong reactivity for synaptophysin.

germ cell neoplasms, gliomas, meningeal tumors, and various other tumor types such as lymphomas and lipomatous tumors. Parenchymal tumors comprise a spectrum of lesions ranging from the most immature (pineoblastoma) to the well-differentiated pineocytoma. Tumors with intermediate features are classified as pineal parenchymal tumors of intermediate differentiation (PPT-ID).[75]

Most primary tumors of the pineal gland originate from pineocytes, which represent modified neurons similar to retinal photoreceptor cells.[75] Pineocytomas are typically positive for NSE, synaptophysin, neurofilament proteins, tau protein, and microtubule-associated protein-2 (MAP2) (Fig. 10.5).[75-77] GFAP and S-100 protein are present in 75% and 83% of cases, respectively. S-antigen, a protein localized in photoreceptor cells, has been demonstrated in 28% of pineocytomas and 50% of pineoblastomas.[78,79] Most pineoblastomas are negative for neurofilament proteins but are typically positive for synaptophysin. In general, neurofilament positivity indicates a better prognosis in pineal parenchymal tumors while the MIB-1 labeling index is 1.58, 16.1, and 23.5 in pineocytomas, PPT-IDs, and pineoblastomas, respectively.[80] In contrast to germ cell tumors, pineocytomas are negative for placental alkaline phosphatase, human chorionic gonadotropin (hCG), and alpha-fetoprotein.[75]

Thyroid Gland

The epithelial components of the thyroid gland include follicular cells and C cells. Follicular cells contain thyroglobulin (TGB), thyroxine (T_4), and triiodothyronine (T_3), which can be demonstrated in frozen sections and formalin-fixed, paraffin-embedded sections, whereas the major product of the C cell is calcitonin.

FOLLICULAR CELLS AND THEIR NEOPLASMS

Thyroglobulin, T3, T4, TTF-1, and TTF-2

Thyroglobulin (TGB) is a 660-kD glycoprotein with a sedimentation constant of 19S. Iodoproteins of higher and lower sedimentation constants have also been localized immunohistochemically.[81] Considerable variation occurs in TGB staining intensity in normal thyroid glands. The cuboidal to columnar cells of the normal gland consistently exhibit greater degrees of TGB immunoreactivity than the flattened (atrophic) cells of follicles that are distended with colloid. Variation in the staining of colloid is also apparent. Hyperplastic cells are typically strongly stained for TGB, whereas cells lining involuted follicles are weakly reactive or negative. Follicular cells both in Graves' disease and in the hyperplastic phase of Hashimoto's disease are moderately to strongly reactive for TGB.

Follicular adenomas are positive for TGB but also show considerable variability in staining intensity on the basis of the functional status of their component cells.[81] As would be expected, hyperfunctional adenomas exhibit strong positivity for TGB, whereas the cells of macrofollicular adenomas have considerably less reactivity and may be negative. Normofollicular adenomas demonstrate moderate immunoreactivity for TGB, whereas adenomas of solid and oncocytic types contain smaller amounts of TGB in the component cells.

Hyalinizing trabecular tumors are typically positive for TGB and may occasionally exhibit positivity for some NE markers including chromogranin A and hormonal peptides (neurotensin, endorphins).[82] These tumors have plasma membrane patterns of staining with the monoclonal antibody MIB-1[83]; however, this pattern of reactivity occurs only when staining is performed at room temperature rather than at 37° C (Fig. 10.6).[84] The most likely explanation for the plasma membrane pattern of reactivity is that the antibody cross-reacts with an epitope present in the plasma membrane under these conditions.[84]

The frequency of TGB positivity in thyroid carcinomas is dependent on the degree of differentiation and the histologic subtype. Generally, poorly differentiated carcinomas contain less TGB than do better-differentiated tumors. The levels of TGB mRNA are also correspondingly lower in poorly differentiated than in well-differentiated thyroid carcinomas.[85] TGB immunoreactivity is present in more than 95% of papillary carcinomas (Figs. 10.7 and 10.8) and follicular tumors. Because TGB is also expressed in metastatic lesions, stains for this marker are particularly valuable in

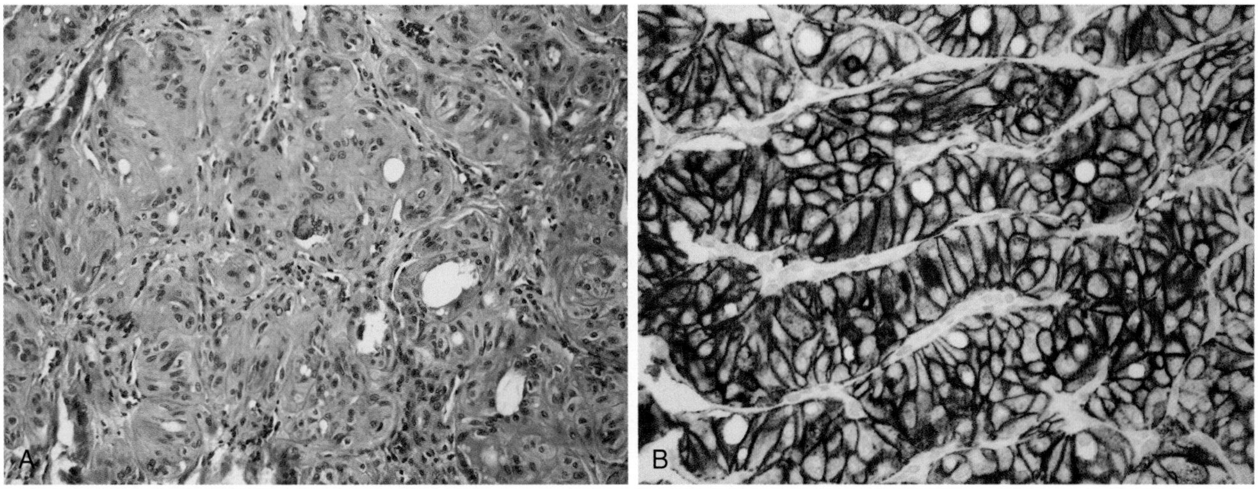

FIGURE 10.6 **A,** Hyalinizing trabecular tumor of thyroid (H&E stain). **B,** Immunoperoxidase stain for MIB-1 performed at room temperature. There is prominent staining of the plasma membranes of tumor cells.

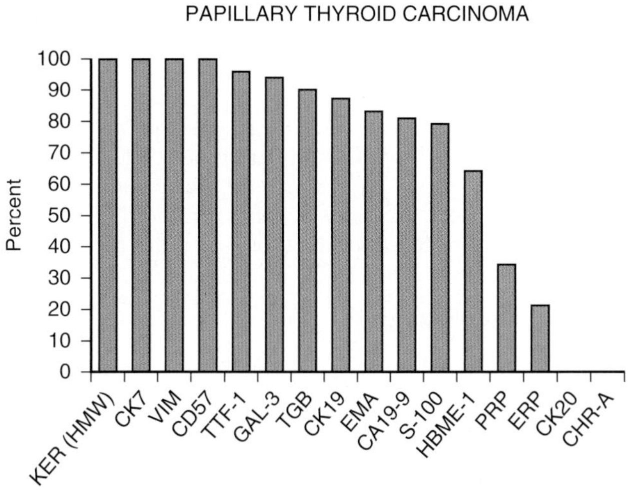

FIGURE 10.7 Distribution of markers in papillary thyroid carcinoma. KER (HMW), high-molecular-weight cytokeratins; CK7, cytokeratin 7; VIM, vimentin; CD57; TTF-1, thyroid transcription factor-1; GAL-3, galectin-3; TGB, thyroglobulin; CK19, cytokeratin 19; EMA, epithelial membrane antigen; CA19-9; S-100; HBME-1; PRP, progesterone receptor protein; ERP, estrogen receptor protein; CK20, cytokeratin 20; CHR-A, chromogranin A.

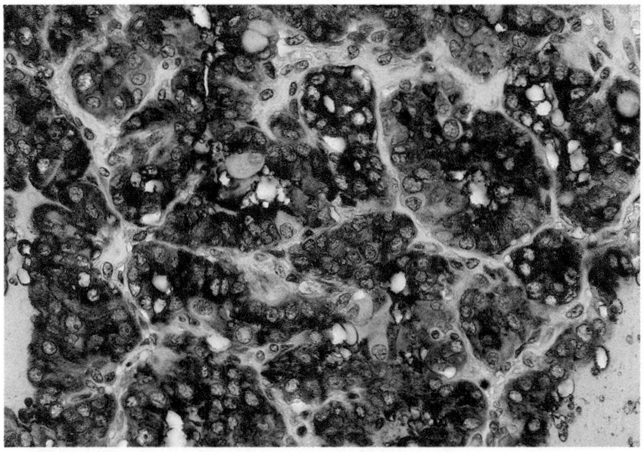

FIGURE 10.8 Papillary thyroid carcinoma. The cells in this well-differentiated tumor reveal uniform reactivity for thyroglobulin. (Immunoperoxidase stain for thyroglobulin.)

establishing the origins of metastatic tumors of unknown origin. Immunoreactivity for TGB in differentiated follicular and papillary tumors is generally present in a patchy distribution. Although some cells exhibit diffuse and uniform staining, others have focal apical or basal positivity. Some tumor cells may be completely unreactive, and for this reason the absence of TGB in a small biopsy sample does not completely exclude the possibility of a thyroid origin in a metastatic site. Rarely, TGB immunoreactivity, as demonstrated both with monoclonal antibodies and polyclonal antisera, has been reported in nonthyroid malignancies.[86]

Poorly differentiated thyroid carcinomas of the insular type are usually TGB positive, although the extent of cellular staining is generally weak and focal.[87] Undifferentiated (anaplastic) thyroid carcinomas are most commonly negative for TGB. In the series reported by Ordonez and coworkers,[88] 5 of 32 (15.6%) cases of anaplastic carcinoma exhibited TGB immunoreactivity in a small number of cells using both monoclonal antibodies and polyclonal antisera. In this series, positivity was present in 3 of 8 giant cell, 1 of 4 spindle cell, and none of 6 squamoid or 13 mixed variants. Examination of serial sections in these cases failed to reveal evidence of entrapped normal follicular cells or foci of differentiated thyroid carcinoma. Other authors, however, have failed to demonstrate any TGB immunoreactivity in anaplastic carcinomas except in foci of residual differentiated tumor.[89]

Antibodies to T_3 and T_4 have been used less extensively than TGB in studies of thyroid carcinoma. Kawaoi and coworkers[90] reported T_4 positivity in 95% of papillary carcinomas and 54% of follicular carcinomas but in no cases of anaplastic thyroid carcinoma. T_3 was present in 66% of papillary carcinomas, 81% of follicular carcinomas, and 45% of anaplastic carcinomas.[90] The significance of T_3 staining in the absence of T_4 immunoreactivity, however, is unknown. In addition to thyroglobulin, T_3, and T_4, thyroid peroxidase has also been used for studies of thyroid tumors.[91]

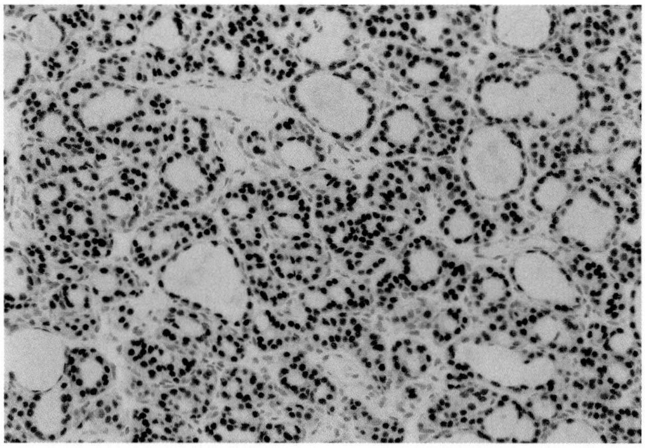

FIGURE 10.9 Well-differentiated follicular thyroid carcinoma. Immunoperoxidase stain for thyroid transcription factor-1 shows the typical nuclear positivity.

TTF-1 is a homeodomain-containing transcription factor that is expressed in the thyroid, diencephalon, and lung. TTF-1 regulates the expression of thyroperoxidase and TGB genes in the thyroid. In the lung TTF-1 plays a key role in the specific expression of surfactant proteins A, B, and C and Clara cell secretory protein.[92,93] TTF-1 immunoreactivity has been reported in 96% of papillary, 100% of follicular, 20% of Hurthle cell, 100% of insular, and 90% of medullary carcinomas (Fig. 10.9).[93] In general the intensity of TTF-1 staining in C-cell tumors is less than that observed in follicular cell tumors. Undifferentiated (anaplastic) carcinomas, on the other hand, have been negative. In the lung, this marker has been reported in 72.5% of adenocarcinomas, 10% of squamous carcinomas, 26% of large cell carcinomas, 75% of large cell NE carcinomas, more than 90% of small cell carcinomas, and 100% of alveolar adenomas. In contrast, only 2 of 286 adenocarcinomas of nonpulmonary and nonthyroid types exhibited TTF-1 immunoreactivity.

In their study of thyroid and pulmonary carcinomas, Kaufmann and Dietel[94] demonstrated reactivity for surfactant protein A in 3 of 7 thyroid carcinomas in a focal pattern. Byrd-Gloster and coworkers[95] reported that TTF-1 is useful in the distinction of pulmonary small cell carcinomas from Merkel cell carcinomas. In their study, 97% of small cell bronchogenic carcinomas were TTF-1 positive, whereas none of 21 Merkel cell tumors exhibited positivity. However, TTF-1 has been reported in some nonpulmonary small cell carcinomas including those arising in the prostate, urinary bladder, and uterine cervix (see Table 10.6).[96]

Thyroid transcription factor-2 (TTF-2) and PAX-8, which are essential for thyroid organogenesis and differentiation, have also been studied in thyroid tumors.[97] TTF-1, TTF-2, and PAX-8 were expressed in differentiated and poorly differentiated thyroid carcinomas, whereas TTF-1 and TTF-2 were expressed in 18% and 7% of anaplastic carcinomas, respectively. PAX-8, on the other hand, was present in 79% of anaplastic carcinomas.[97] TTF-2 was negative in all other neoplastic and non-neoplastic tissues including those of pulmonary origin. Although PAX-8 was present in a variety of normal and neoplastic tissues, it was not expressed in pulmonary tumors or normal pulmonary tissue. These findings suggest that PAX-8 may be a useful marker for the diagnosis of anaplastic thyroid carcinoma, particularly when the differential diagnosis includes pulmonary carcinoma.[97]

TABLE 10.2 Cytokeratin Distribution in Papillary Carcinomas and Follicular Tumors

Cytokeratin Type	Papillary (%)	Follicular (%)
8	100	100
18	100	100
7	100	100
19	98*	84*
1, 5, 10, 11/14	97	22
5,6	68	8
17	40	15
13	30	0
20	26	12
14	11	10
4	2.4	0

*Although CK19 is present in papillary carcinoma and in follicular tumors, the extent of staining is consistently higher in papillary carcinoma.

Intermediate Filaments

The body of literature on the distribution of intermediate filaments in normal and neoplastic follicular cells is extensive (Table 10.2).[98-109] Broad-spectrum keratin antibodies react with normal and hyperplastic follicular cells, follicular cells in chronic thyroiditis, and virtually all thyroid epithelial malignancies. Antibodies to high-molecular-weight keratins, in contrast, have been reported to react with some follicular cells in 8% of normal thyroids, 44% of hyperplastic glands, and all cases of thyroiditis. High-molecular-weight keratins were present in 100% of papillary carcinomas, 6% of follicular carcinomas, and 20% of anaplastic carcinomas in one study.[99] Studies reported by Schelfhout and coworkers[101] have demonstrated uniform reactivity for CK19 in 100% of papillary carcinomas (Fig. 10.10). Focal reactivity for CK19 (in < 5% of the tumor cells) was present in 80% of follicular carcinomas and 90% of follicular adenomas, whereas 90% of colloid nodules demonstrated more diffuse positivity in less than 50% of the cells. These data were largely confirmed by Raphael and associates.[102]

More recent studies have demonstrated that normal thyroid strongly expresses the simple epithelial cytokeratins CK7 and CK18 and, to a lesser extent, CK8 and CK19 but not stratified epithelial cytokeratins.[103] The same patterns of staining were present in lymphocytic thyroiditis, but reactivity for CK19 was more intense. Immunoreactivity for CK7, CK8, CK18, and CK19 was present in both papillary and follicular carcinomas, although the extent and intensity of CK19 staining

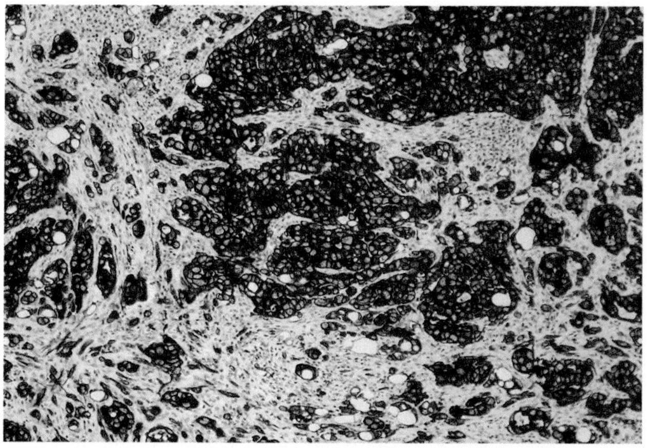

FIGURE 10.10 Papillary thyroid carcinoma. Immunoperoxidase stain for CK19 demonstrates intense cytoplasmic reactivity.

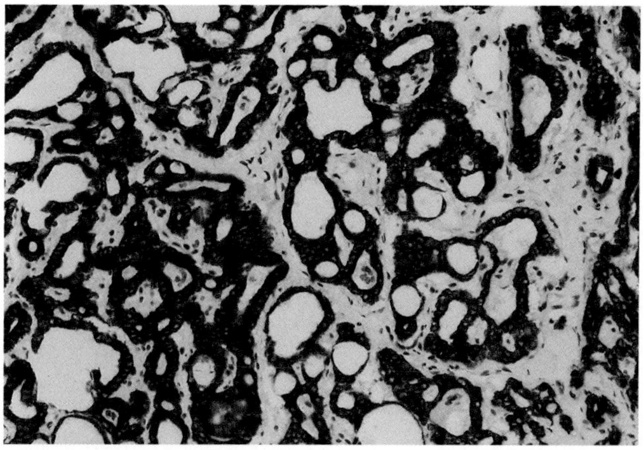

FIGURE 10.11 Papillary thyroid carcinoma, follicular variant. Immunoperoxidase stain for CK19 demonstrates intense cytoplasmic reactivity.

was greater in papillary carcinomas. However, CK19 was present in all cases of follicular carcinoma at least focally.[103] The stratified epithelial keratins (CK5/CK6 and CK13) were present in 27 of 41 (66%) and 14 of 41 (34%) papillary carcinomas, respectively, but these keratins were absent from other tumor types. Miettinen and associates[104] observed CK19 in all papillary carcinomas and in approximately 50% of follicular carcinomas, whereas CK5/CK6 was present focally in papillary carcinomas. Kragsterman and coworkers[105] concluded that CK19 is of limited value as a marker for routine histopathologic diagnosis but that the presence of this marker should raise the suspicion of papillary carcinoma.

Baloch and coworkers[106] examined a large series of papillary carcinomas of both usual types and follicular variants for a spectrum of cytokeratins including CK5/CK6/CK18, CK18, CK10/CK13, CK20, CK17, and CK19. In this series, all cases of papillary carcinoma including the follicular variant were positive for CK19 (Fig. 10.11). The follicular variants showed strong immunoreactivity in areas with nuclear features of papillary carcinoma, whereas the remaining areas had moderate to strong staining. Normal thyroid parenchyma immediately adjacent to the follicular variants was also positive, but normal thyroid tissue adjacent to the conventional papillary carcinomas was negative. Follicular adenomas, follicular carcinomas, and hyperplastic nodules were negative for CK19. The reasons for the discrepancies in CK19 immunoreactivity in follicular tumors between this and other series are unknown.

There is considerable controversy with respect to the presence of CK19 in hyalinizing trabecular tumors of the thyroid. Fonseca and coworkers[107] reported CK19 in all cases of hyalinizing trabecular tumors and suggested that this tumor represented a peculiar encapsulated variant of papillary carcinoma. Hirokawa and colleagues,[108] in contrast, found no or minimal CK19 in their series of cases.

Liberman and Weidner[109] studied the distribution of high-molecular-weight cytokeratins as demonstrated with the monoclonal antibody 34βE12 (CK1, CK5, CK10, and CK14) and antibodies to involucrin, a structural protein of the stratum corneum, in a series of papillary and follicular carcinomas. Antibodies to high-molecular-weight cytokeratins reacted with 91% of papillary carcinomas including the follicular variant and 20% of follicular neoplasms (adenomas and carcinomas). In general, the staining pattern in papillary carcinomas was strong and patchy, whereas follicular neoplasms stained weakly. Involucrin was positive in 72.5% of papillary carcinomas and 29% of follicular tumors. It has been suggested that the pattern of staining with 34βE12 might be best explained by the presence of an epitope on CK1 or by an epitope that is not recognized by other monoclonal antibodies to CK5, CK10, and CK14.[109]

Cytokeratins are demonstrable in 70% to 75% of anaplastic carcinomas using antibodies AE1/AE3, 34βH11, and CAM5.2, while approximately 30% exhibit reactivity with 34βE12 (Fig. 10.12).[87,88] Poorly differentiated carcinomas exhibit positivity in 100% of cases with broad-spectrum cytokeratin antibodies.[1]

Vimentin is coexpressed with cytokeratins in the vast majority of normal and neoplastic thyroids. In the series of Miettinen and colleagues, follicular and papillary tumors expressed vimentin in more than 50% of the tumor cells. Immunoreactivity for vimentin was generally present in the basal portions of the cells in contrast to the more diffuse cytoplasmic reactivity for cytokeratins.[99] Vimentin immunoreactivity has been reported in 94% of anaplastic thyroid carcinomas.

Oncogenes and Tumor Suppressor Genes

The distribution of p53 has been examined in cases of thyroid carcinoma. In the series reported by Soares and coworkers,[110] p53 was absent from 14 cases of goiter and adenoma and from 12 cases of papillary carcinoma. p53 was present in 20% of follicular carcinomas (predominantly of the widely invasive type), 16% of poorly differentiated carcinomas, and 67% of undifferentiated carcinomas. In the series reported by Holm and Nesland, 6 of 32 (19%) papillary carcinomas, 5 of 29 (17%) follicular carcinomas, and 18 of 24 (75%) undifferentiated carcinomas were p53+. In contrast, the RB gene product was present in all thyroid carcinomas, suggesting that it does not play a major role in thyroid carcinogenesis.[111]

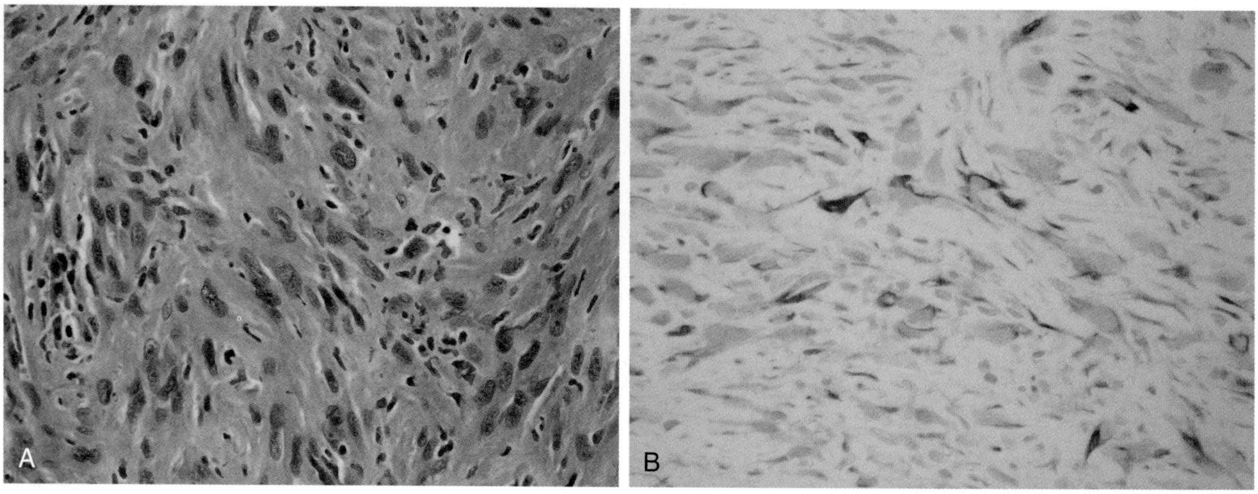

FIGURE 10.12 **A,** Anaplastic (undifferentiated) thyroid carcinoma (H&E stain). **B,** Immunoperoxidase stain for broad-spectrum cytokeratins (AE1/AE3) shows cytoplasmic staining.

The *ret* oncogene protein has been demonstrated by immunohistochemistry both in papillary carcinomas and in a subset of hyalinizing trabecular tumors.[112-114] However, additional studies are required to ascertain the sensitivity and specificity of currently available *ret* antibodies in immunohistochemical formats for the identification of papillary carcinomas.[115]

The *t*(2;3)(q13; p25) translocation, found in a subset of thyroid follicular carcinomas, results in fusion of the DNA binding domains of the thyroid transcription factor PAX-8 to domains A-F of the peroxisome proliferation-activated receptor (PPAR) γ 1 (Fig. 10.13).[116] Studies using PCR and immunohistochemistry demonstrated that most follicular carcinomas positive for PPAR γ were widely invasive while tumors lacking the rearrangement were PPAR γ negative.[117] Papillary carcinomas and Hürthle cell tumors were negative. Other studies, however, have reported positivity both in follicular carcinomas and adenomas.[118,119]

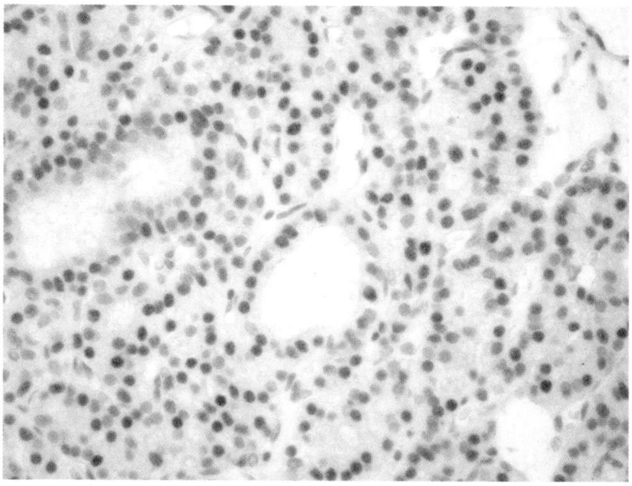

FIGURE 10.13 Well-differentiated follicular carcinoma stained for PAX-8-PPARγ. Positive staining is confined to the nuclei of the tumor cells. *(Courtesy of Dr. Yuri Nikiforov.)*

HBME-1

The monoclonal antibody HBME-1 recognizes an uncharacterized antigen in the microvilli of mesothelial cells, tracheal epithelium, and adenocarcinomas of the pancreas, lung, and breast. It has also been assessed for its efficacy in differentiating benign and malignant thyroid lesions both in aspirates (direct smears and cell blocks) and in tissue sections.[120] Miettinen and Karkkainen[121] demonstrated positivity for HBME-1 in 100% of papillary (145/145) and follicular (27/27) carcinomas, and benign lesions either were negative or showed focal positivity in approximately 30% of the cases (Table 10.3). In a more recent series, Mase and colleagues[122] demonstrated positivity in 13% of adenomatous goiters, 27% of adenomas, 84% of follicular carcinomas, and 97% of papillary carcinomas (Fig. 10.14). Among follicular neoplasms, the sensitivity for the detection of carcinomas was 84.6%, while specificity, positive predictive value, and overall accuracy were 72.6%, 66%, and 77.2%, respectively.[122] Sack and colleagues[120] have concluded that a positive result for HBME-1 on FNA is supportive evidence that the lesion is a carcinoma but that a negative result does not exclude the diagnosis of malignancy. This marker has been considered a useful discriminant for the distinction of papillary hyperplasia and papillary carcinoma; however, a positive finding does not guarantee a diagnosis of malignancy.[123] Generally, oncocytic neoplasms of both papillary and follicular types are less commonly positive for HBME-1 than their nononcocytic counterparts.[124-126] Up to 90% of poorly differentiated thyroid carcinomas and approximately 20% of undifferentiated thyroid carcinomas are positive for HBME-1.[125]

Galectin-3

Galectin-3 is a beta galactoside binding lectin that is expressed in a large number of normal and neoplastic tissues.[127] In 1995 Xu and coworkers[127] examined the expression of galectin-1 and galectin-3 in a small series of thyroid tumors and found expression of these lectins in papillary and follicular carcinomas but not

TABLE 10.3 Marker Expression in Benign and Malignant Thyroid Lesions*

Diagnosis	CK19 (%)	HBME-1 (%)	GAL (%)	CITED (%)	FN-1 (%)	CD44 v 6 (%)
Nodular hyperplasia	20	0-10	20-55	20-25	5-10	40
Follicular adenoma	10	5-25	10	10-15	5-10	30-40
Papillary thyroid carcinoma	80-90	60-100	60-100	85-90	80-90	70-90
Follicular carcinoma	35	35-100	45-95	10-50	50	80-90
Poorly differentiated thyroid carcinoma	50	65-90	60-70	—	—	50
Undifferentiated (anaplastic carcinoma)	60-70	10-50	90-100	—	100	40

*The expression of most of the markers is generally highest in papillary carcinoma followed by follicular carcinomas. The extent of staining in cases of nodular (adenomatous) hyperplasia and follicular adenomas is considerably less than that observed in papillary and follicular carcinomas. *Follicular tumors of uncertain malignant potential often have intermediate patterns of staining. The percentage in this table represents averages from multiple reported series.*

CK19, cytokeratin 19; HBME-1, Hector Battifora mesothelial cell-1; GAL, galectin-3; CITED, Cbp/p300-interacting transactivator-1; FN-1, fibronectin-1.

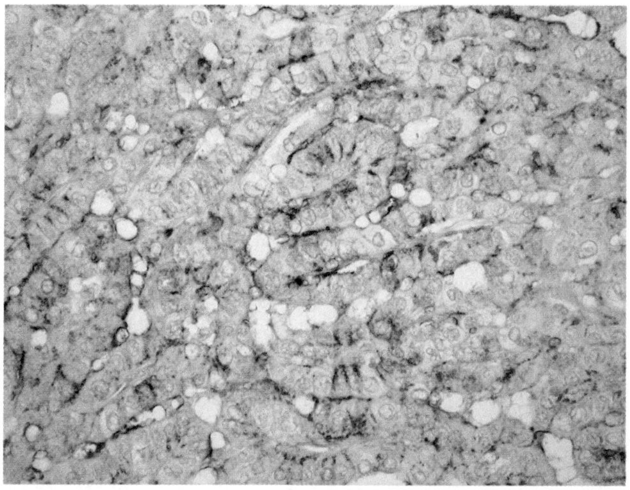

FIGURE 10.14 Papillary thyroid carcinoma. Immunoperoxidase stain for HBME-1 demonstrates positive staining of plasma membranes of tumor cells.

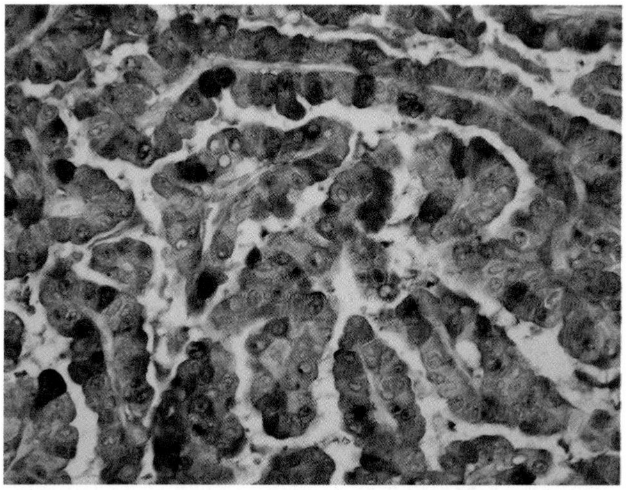

FIGURE 10.15 Papillary thyroid carcinoma. Immunoperoxidase stain demonstrates cytoplasmic and nuclear positivity for galectin 3.

in adenomas, nodular goiter, or normal thyroid tissue. On the basis of these studies, they concluded that the galectins could be useful in the distinction of benign and malignant thyroid tumors. Generally similar results were reported in a number of other studies (Fig. 10.15).[128-130]

Bartolazzi and colleagues[131] performed a large retrospective and prospective study of galectin-3 expression in more than 1000 benign and malignant thyroid lesions. The sensitivity, specificity, positive predictive value, and diagnostic accuracy for the discrimination of benign and malignant tumors were 99%, 98%, 92%, and 99%, respectively. These findings suggest that galectin-3 is a useful marker for the diagnosis of low-grade thyroid carcinomas. It should be noted, however, that in a recent study comparing galectin-3 expression in a series of cases of papillary carcinoma and papillary hyperplasia, there was considerable overlap in the frequency of expression of this marker.[123] Both galectin-3 and HBME-1 have also been analyzed concurrently.[132] The sensitivity of galectin-3 for oncocytic carcinomas and oncocytic variants of papillary carcinoma was 95%, whereas that for HBME-1 was 53%. The combination of the two markers increased the sensitivity to 99%; however, the specificity was 88% for both markers.[132] Galectin-3 is present in approximately 60% of poorly differentiated thyroid carcinomas and in up to 90% of undifferentiated carcinomas.[131]

Other Markers and Marker Panels

Numerous other proteins have been explored as potential markers for different types of thyroid malignancies (Table 10.3).[133,134] Cbp/p300-interacting transactivator 1 (CITED1) is a nuclear protein that is involved in the coregulation of transcription factors. This protein is present in a variety of different cell types and is overexpressed in papillary thyroid carcinomas (87% to 93%).[136] However, CITED1 immunoreactivity is also expressed in up to 50% of follicular carcinomas, 16% of follicular adenomas, and 24% of nodular goiters.

Fibronectin-1 (FN-1) is upregulated in thyroid carcinomas as compared with normal thyroid tissue.[136] In the study of Prasad and colleagues,[137] FN was present in

91% of papillary carcinomas, 50% of follicular carcinomas, 100% of anaplastic carcinomas, 5% of follicular adenomas, and 7% of nodular goiters.

Studies of multiple markers (galectin-3, FN-1, CITED-1, CK19, HBME-1) have demonstrated a significant association of expression with malignancy.[137] Expression of galectin-3, FN1, and/or HBME-1 was seen in 100% of carcinomas and 24% of adenomas. Coexpression of multiple proteins was present in 95% of carcinomas and in only 5% of adenomas ($p < 0.0001$). Among non-neoplastic thyroid tissues, adenomatous hyperplasia frequently expressed galectin-3, CK19, and CITED1, but their expression was frequently focal. Sconamiglio and colleagues[138] found that galectin-3, CK19, HBME-1, and CITED1 were more highly expressed in papillary carcinomas than in follicular adenomas. In this study, HBME-1 was the most specific and CK19 the most sensitive marker of malignancy. The expression of CK19 and HBME-1 was 100% specific for malignancy. A group of follicular lesions with questionable features of PTC (follicular tumors of uncertain malignant potential) most often had intermediate patterns of staining.

The cadherins are an important class of adhesion molecules whose expression has also been studied in thyroid tumors. Expression of E-cadherin mRNA is high in normal thyroid cells and becomes variably reduced in differentiated thyroid carcinomas and is lost in undifferentiated carcinomas.[139] These changes are reflected at the protein level, suggesting that the loss of E-cadherin is associated with the process of thyroid tumor dedifferentiation. Beta-catenin also plays a role in cell adhesion and Wnt signaling. Typically, membrane β-catenin is reduced in follicular cell adenomas and carcinomas (Fig. 10.16) with further loss of membrane expression correlating with loss of differentiation.[140] These studies indicate that low membrane β-catenin expression, as well as its nuclear localization or CTNNB1 mutations, is significantly associated with poor prognosis, independent of conventional prognostic indicators. Decreased expression of E-cadherin and β-catenin have also been observed by Wiseman and coworkers during anaplastic transformation.[141] These studies also demonstrated that transformation was characterized by decreased expression of thyroglobulin, bcl-2, and VEGF with increased expression of p53, MIB-1, and topoisomerase II-α.[141]

Carcinoembryonic antigen (CEA) is generally absent from nonmedullary thyroid carcinomas. Using six different monoclonal CEA antibodies, Dasovic-Knezevic and colleagues[142] found that 10 papillary, 10 follicular, and 8 anaplastic carcinomas were negative for CEA. Ordonez and coworkers, in contrast, reported CEA immunoreactivity in 9% of anaplastic thyroid carcinomas using a monoclonal antibody.[88]

CD15 is present in approximately 30% of papillary carcinomas and its expression is more likely to occur in tumors at advanced stages.[143] Thus CD15 has been considered a prognostic marker for these tumors. Ghali and coworkers[47] reported strong positive staining for CD57 in 100% of papillary and follicular carcinomas, whereas focal positive staining was present in 25% of colloid goiters and 21% of follicular adenomas. Other authors, however, have questioned the specificity of CD57 as a marker of malignancy in thyroid tumors.[144,145]

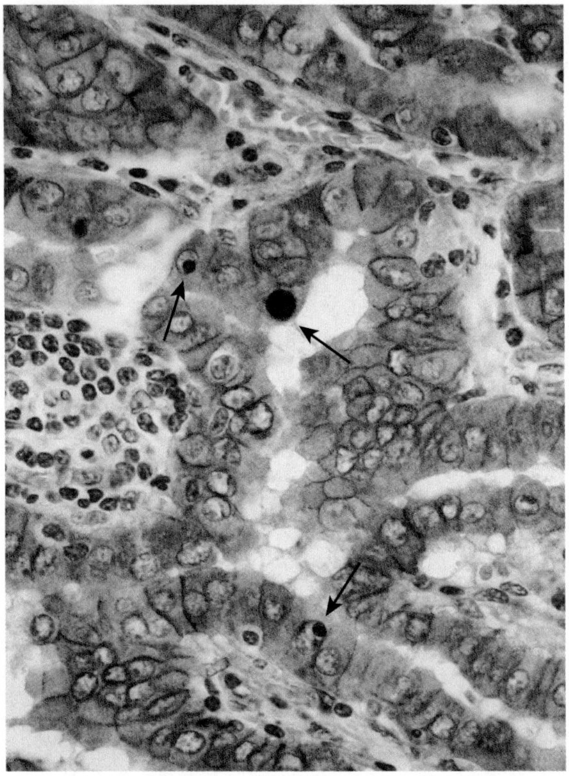

FIGURE 10.16 Beta-catenin stain of papillary thyroid carcinoma. The tumor cells exhibit prominent staining of their plasma membranes and moderate cytoplasmic positivity. Intranuclear pseudoinclusions are positively stained *(arrows)*.

CA 15-3 and CA 19-9 are variably expressed in thyroid follicular tumors. Both follicular and papillary carcinomas reveal CA 15-3 positivity in 100% of cases, whereas CA 19-9 is present in 70% of papillary tumors but in no follicular carcinomas.[146] CA 125 immunoreactivity has been reported in approximately 40% of papillary carcinomas.[86] The distribution of mucin-related antigens (MUC) has also been analyzed in thyroid tumors.[147] These studies have demonstrated that MUC1 plays a key role in the glycosylation of well-differentiated thyroid carcinomas. However, there are no consistent differences between papillary and follicular carcinomas with respect to the expression of mucins.

Cyclo-oxygenase-1 and cyclo-oxygenase-2 (COX-1, COX-2) have been investigated in thyroid tumors using both immunohistochemistry and *in situ* hybridization.[148] These studies have demonstrated that the expression of COX-1 mRNA and its corresponding protein is similar and weak in normal and neoplastic thyroid tissue. COX-2 mRNA and its corresponding protein, on the other hand, are strongly expressed in well-differentiated thyroid carcinomas, as compared with normal thyroid tissue and follicular adenomas. COX-2 appears to be upregulated, particularly in papillary microcarcinomas, whereas larger and more advanced tumors have reduced expression.[149,150]

CD44v6 (heparan sulfate proteoglycan) mediates cell-to-cell and cell-to-matrix interactions. Typically

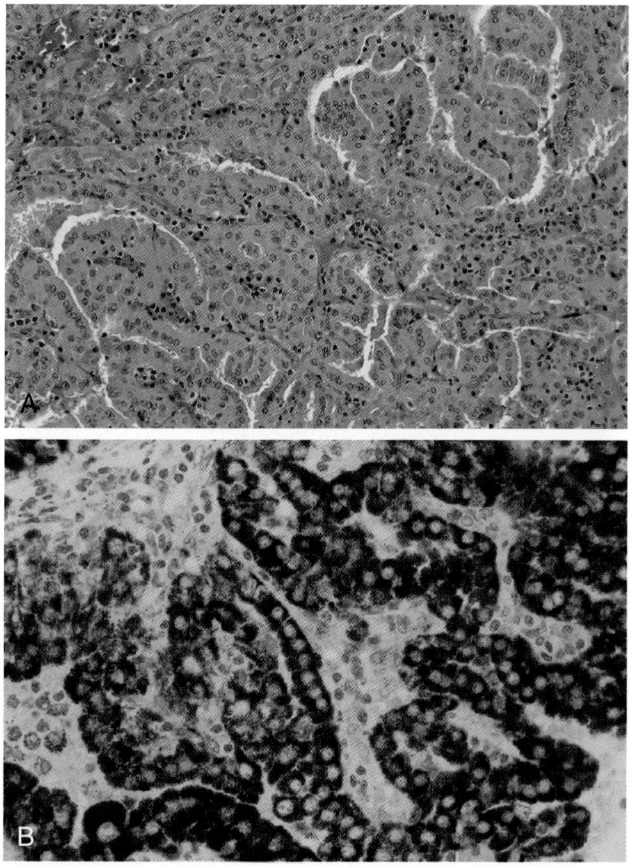

FIGURE 10.17 **A,** Papillary thyroid carcinoma, oncocytic type (H&E stain). **B,** Immunoperoxidase stain for mitochondria using the antibody MITO-113 demonstrates intense granular cytoplasmic staining.

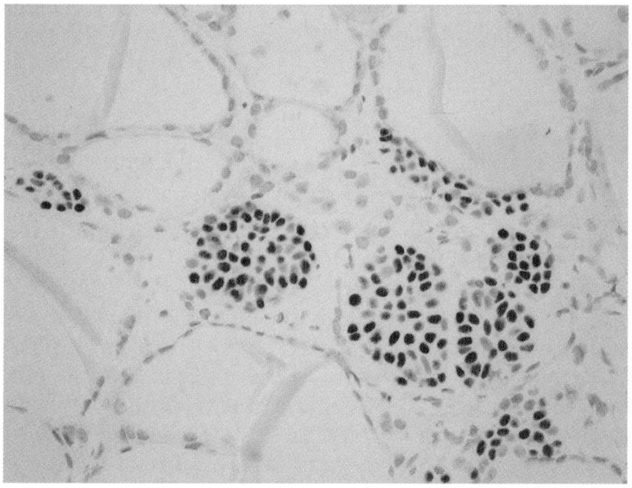

FIGURE 10.18 Normal thyroid stained for p63. Positive nuclear staining is confined to the cells of the solid cell nest.

papillary and follicular carcinomas strongly express CD44v6[131]; however, a significant proportion of benign thyroid lesions are also positive.

Steroid hormone receptors (estrogen, progesterone, androgen) are variably expressed in thyroid tumors. Bur and associates[151] reported estrogen receptor positivity in 8 of 39 (21%) papillary carcinomas, while follicular carcinomas of conventional and oncocytic types were negative. Progesterone receptor positivity was present in 13 of 39 (33%) papillary carcinomas, 2 of 5 (40%) follicular tumors (one third were adenomas and one half were carcinomas), and 8 of 15 (53%) oncocytic tumors. There was no significant correlation between gender, age, or pathologic findings associated with aggressive behavior and the estrogen/progesterone receptor status of the tumors.

S-100 protein has also been studied in neoplastic lesions of the thyroid gland. McLaren and Cossar reported positivity in 100% of papillary carcinomas, 75% of follicular carcinomas, 37.5% of follicular adenomas, and 28.5% of papillary hyperplasias.[152]

Antibodies to mitochondrial antigens are of value in the identification of thyroid tumors with oncocytic (Hürthle cell) features.[153] Positive cells typically exhibit intense cytoplasmic positivity corresponding to the distribution of mitochondria (Fig. 10.17).

p63, a homolog of p53, is expressed in a variety of cells including basal cells of squamous epithelium, myoepithelial cells of breast and salivary glands and basal cells of the prostate. In the thyroid, it is expressed selectively in solid cell nests which represent remnants of the ultimobranchial bodies (Fig. 10.18).[154] In thyroid tumors, p63 is expressed in sclerosing mucoepidermoid carcinomas with eosinophilia, which are thought to be derived from remnants of the ultimobranchial bodies.[155] Papillary and anaplastic carcinomas are uncommonly positive for p63.

KEY DIAGNOSTIC POINTS
Thyroid Carcinomas

- TGB, TTF-1, and TTF-2 are present in benign thyroid lesions and in more than 95% of differentiated thyroid carcinomas.
- HBME-2 and galectin-3 are useful, although not completely specific, markers for differentiated thyroid carcinomas.
- Cytokeratin (CK)19 is usually expressed in papillary carcinomas but may also be present in other thyroid malignancies and in some benign thyroid tumors.
- Marker panels including CK19, HBME-1, and galectin-3 are usually positive in the follicular variant of papillary carcinomas.
- Follicular tumors with questionable features of papillary carcinoma (follicular tumors of uncertain malignant potential) often demonstrate intermediate and/or irregular patterns of staining for CK19, HBME-1, and galectin-3.
- Undifferentiated thyroid carcinomas are typically negative for TGB, TTF-1, and TTF-2 but commonly express vimentin and/or cytokeratins.

C CELLS AND MEDULLARY THYROID CARCINOMA

C cells, the second major endocrine cell population of the thyroid gland, are the primary sites of synthesis and storage of calcitonin. These cells also synthesize a variety

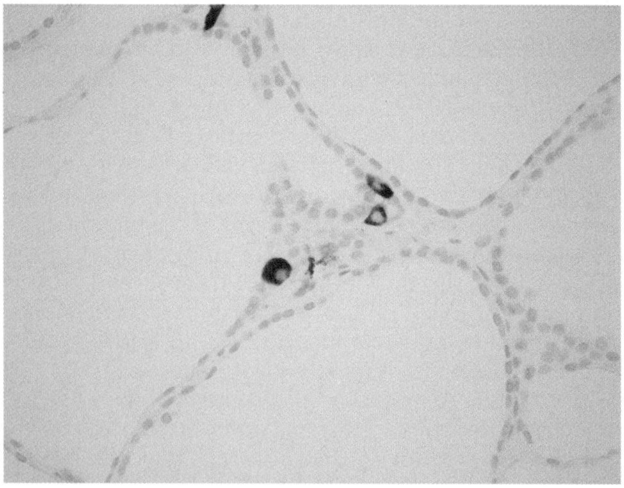

FIGURE 10.19 Normal thyroid C cells. Immunoperoxidase stain for calcitonin demonstrates the intrafollicular topography of the normal C cells.

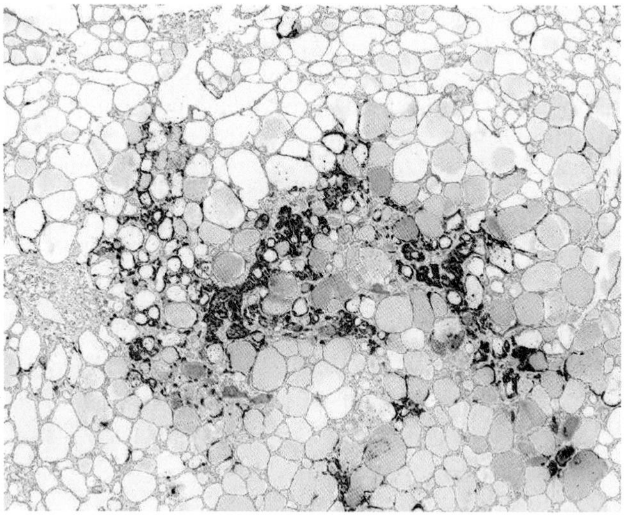

FIGURE 10.20 C-cell hyperplasia from a patient with multiple endocrine neoplasia 2A. This immunoperoxidase stain for calcitonin is strongly positive in the C cells, whereas the follicular cells are negative.

of other regulatory products including somatostatin and gastrin-releasing peptide and amines.[156,157] They can be distinguished from the follicular cells on the basis of their content of calcitonin and the presence of generic NE markers including chromogranin A and synaptophysin.

C cells in normal glands have an exclusive intrafollicular topography and are concentrated at the junctions of the upper and middle thirds of the lobes (Fig. 10.19).[156] In patients with multiple endocrine neoplasia, type 2 (MEN2), C-cell hyperplasia has been recognized as the precursor of medullary thyroid carcinoma. Detailed immunohistochemical studies have shown that C-cell hyperplasia is characterized by increased numbers of C cells within the follicles in the same regions of the gland where C cells normally predominate (Fig. 10.20). These relationships are maintained in areas of more advanced C-cell hyperplasia, where C cells often completely encircle and displace the follicular epithelium centrally. Nodular hyperplasia is characterized by the complete obliteration

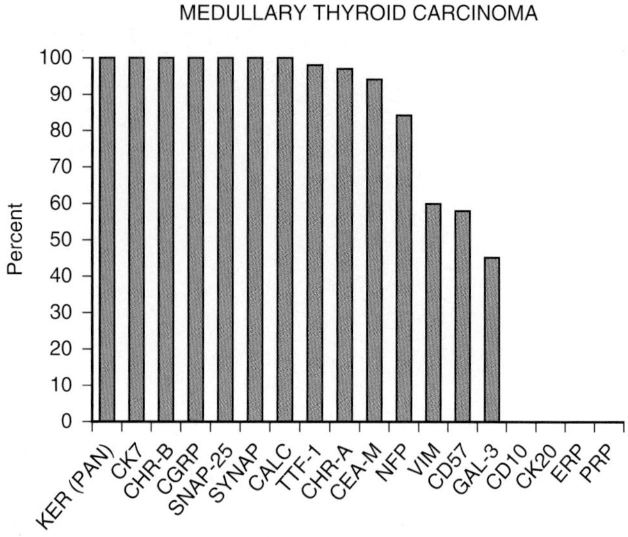

FIGURE 10.21 Distribution of markers in medullary thyroid carcinoma. KER(PAN), pancytokeratin; CK7, cytokeratin 7; CHR-B, chromogranin B; CGRP, calcitonin gene–related protein; SNAP-25, synaptosomal associated protein-25; CALC, calcitonin; TTF-1, thyroid transcription factor-1; CHR-A, chromogranin A; CEA-M, monoclonal CEA; NFP, neurofilament protein; VIM, vimentin; CD57; GAL-3, galectin 3; CD10; CK20, cytokeratin 20; ERP, estrogen receptor protein; PRP, progesterone receptor protein.

of the follicular space by proliferating C cells. The earliest phases of medullary carcinoma are characterized by invasion of C cells through the follicular basement membrane. In addition to its occurrence in patients with MEN2, C-cell hyperplasia may occur in patients with hypercalcemia or hypergastrinemia and around follicular or papillary neoplasms. These types of C-cell hyperplasia have been termed *secondary* or *physiologic hyperplasia* in contrast to the hyperplasia occurring in patients with MEN2 (primary or "neoplastic" hyperplasia).[158]

Medullary thyroid carcinomas are positive for calcitonin in more than 95% of cases (Figs. 10.21 and 10.22).[157,159,160] In rare cases negative for calcitonin peptide, calcitonin mRNA may be demonstrated by *in situ* hybridization.[161] Rarely, small cell carcinomas resembling oat cell carcinomas may occur within the thyroid and have been reported to be negative for calcitonin peptide and the corresponding mRNA.[162] Several studies have suggested that the patterns of calcitonin staining in these tumors may have prognostic significance and that tumors with low levels of calcitonin may behave more aggressively. Franc and coworkers[163] have demonstrated in univariate analyses that patients with tumors containing fewer than 50% calcitonin immunoreactive cells had less favorable survival patterns than did patients whose tumors contained more than 50% immunoreactive cells. In addition to calcitonin, normal and neoplastic C cells contain the calcitonin gene-related peptide (CGRP).[164] CGRP results from alternate splicing of the primary transcript of the calcitonin gene. The normal thyroid expresses calcitonin predominantly, whereas CGRP is found primarily in the central and peripheral nervous system. In medullary carcinomas, calcitonin and CGRP are produced in a concordant manner.[164]

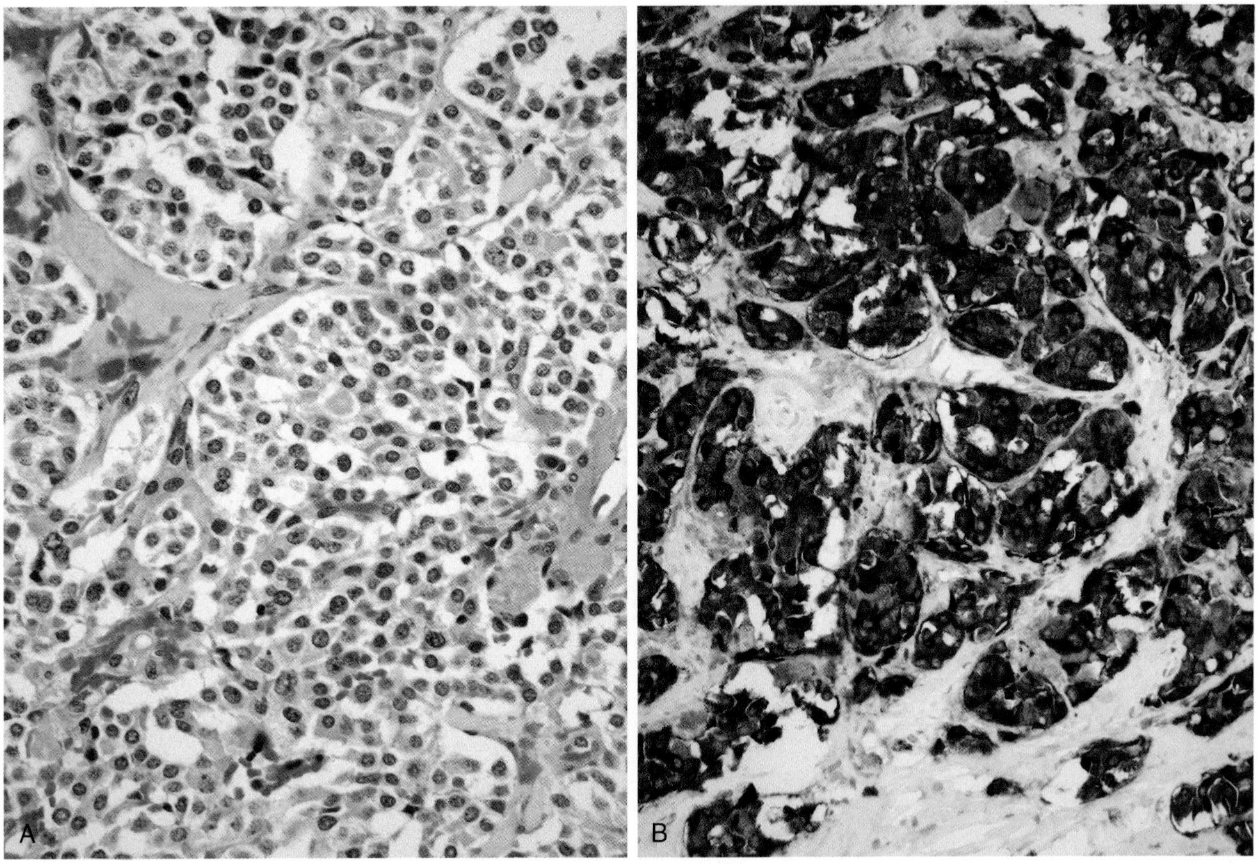

FIGURE 10.22 **A,** Medullary thyroid carcinoma (H&E stain). **B,** Immunoperoxidase stain for calcitonin. The tumor cells are strongly positive for calcitonin.

A variety of other peptides have been demonstrated by immunohistochemistry, and their presence has been confirmed by correlative radioimmunoassays of tumor extracts. Somatostatin and gastrin-releasing peptide are found commonly in medullary thyroid carcinomas.[165,166] Scopsi and coworkers[165] used antisera raised against four different regions of the prosomatostatin molecule and demonstrated positive staining in 100% (33 of 33) of cases. Most, but not all, of the somatostatin-positive cells were also positive for calcitonin. Somatostatin immunoreactive cells are generally present singly or in small groups, representing less than 5% of the entire tumor cell population. The somatostatin-positive cells have a dendritic shape with branching cell processes extending between adjacent tumor cells. Gastrin-releasing peptide is present in approximately 30% of medullary carcinomas.[166] Other peptide products that are present in these tumors include ACTH and pro-opio melanocortin peptides, neurotensin, substance P, and vasoactive intestinal peptide (VIP).[159] The alpha chain of hCG has been demonstrated in 46% (17 of 37) of cases.[167]

Both catecholamines and serotonin are present in medullary thyroid carcinomas. Uribe and coworkers[160] demonstrated serotonin immunoreactivity in 70% (14 of 20) of cases. Serotonin immunoreactivity in these tumors is generally present in cells with a dendritic morphology, similar to that of the somatostatin-positive cells.

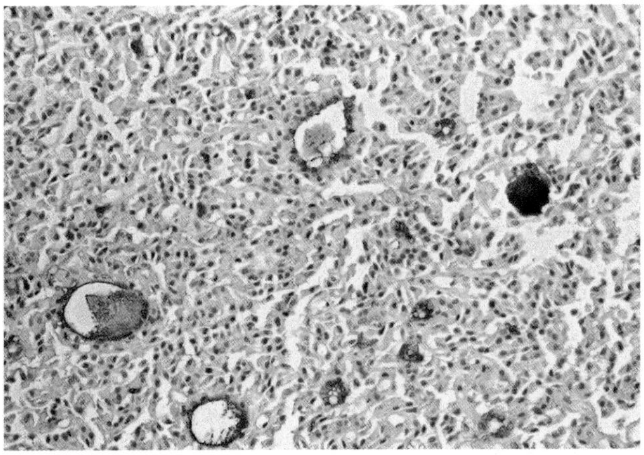

FIGURE 10.23 Medullary thyroid carcinoma. Immunoperoxidase stain for thyroglobulin demonstrates positive staining in entrapped follicles.

Medullary thyroid carcinomas are typically positive for TTF-1, although the staining intensity is often less than that seen in follicular cells.[93] TGB may occur in these tumors as entrapped follicles, single follicular cells, or extracellular deposits (Fig. 10.23). This phenomenon is most likely to occur at the junction of the tumor and the adjacent thyroid parenchyma or along vascular septa. In one series, TGB immunoreactivity was present in approximately 60% of primary thyroid tumors but in no case of metastatic medullary thyroid

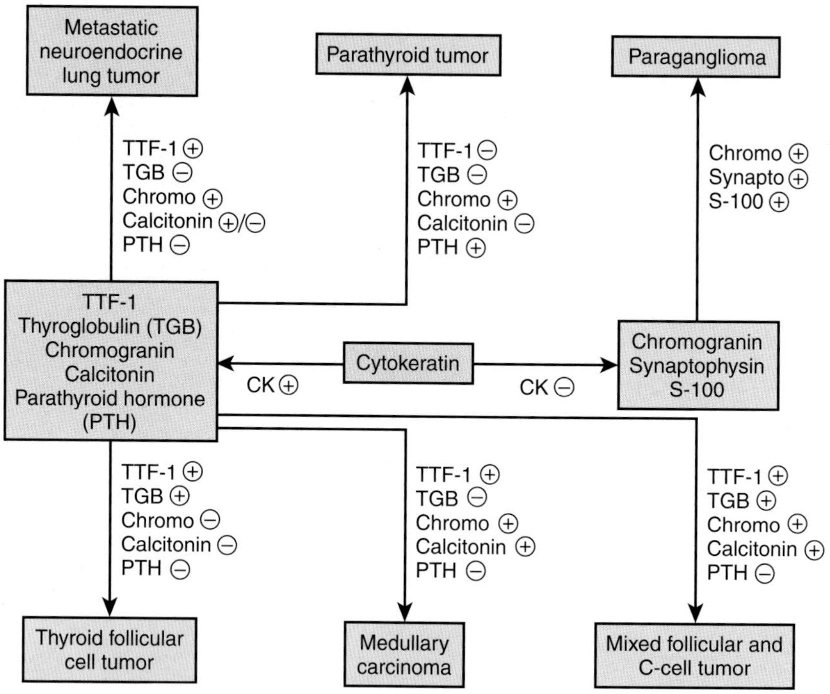

FIGURE 10.24 Algorithm of head and neck endocrine tumors.

carcinoma.[168] True mixed tumors with C-cell and follicular features have also been reported. These tumors are composed of cells that contain calcitonin or other peptides and TGB (Fig. 10.24).[169,170] The existence of such tumors may explain the rare cases of medullary thyroid carcinoma that have the capacity for radioactive iodine uptake.

The proposed origin of tumors with mixed medullary and follicular features has been controversial. Volante and coworkers[171] have proposed an origin from two different progenitors. According to their hypothesis, neoplastic transformation of C cells leads to the development of medullary thyroid carcinoma with entrapped normal follicles. Stimulation of the entrapped follicular cells results in hyperplasia and ultimately follicular (or papillary) neoplasia (hostage hypothesis). Neoplastic C cells and follicular cells would have the capacity to metastasize and could explain the presence of both components in distant sites.

Medullary carcinomas are typically positive for the entire battery of generic NE markers including NSE, the chromogranin proteins, synaptophysin, and histaminase (Fig. 10.21).[156,159] Because NSE is also expressed in a variety of non-C-cell neoplasms, it should never be used as the sole marker to distinguish medullary carcinomas from other thyroid tumor types. In addition to chromogranin A, medullary carcinomas also consistently express chromogranin B and secretogranin II.[172] The calcium-binding protein calbindin-D_{28K}, which is also regarded as a general NE marker, has been found in 95% (18 of 19) of medullary carcinomas.[173]

Polysialic acid of NCAM is consistently expressed in medullary carcinomas. Komminoth and coworkers[51] demonstrated that 100% (33 of 33) of medullary carcinomas were positive, whereas other thyroid tumor types were consistently negative. Strong polySia immunoreactivity occurred in all cases of primary C-cell hyperplasia, whereas normal C cells and C cells in cases of secondary C-cell hyperplasia were negative in most cases.

Bcl-2 immunoreactivity is present in 79% (26 of 33) of cases of medullary carcinoma.[174] In the study reported by Viale and associates,[151] lack of bcl-2 immunoreactivity correlated significantly with shorter survival (p = .0001). In multivariate analyses, lack of bcl-2 was an independent predictor of poor prognosis. Viale and colleagues[174] also demonstrated that p53 immunoreactivity was present in 12% (4 of 33) of medullary carcinomas. Holm and Nesland reported p53 immunoreactivity in 13% (6 of 46) of medullary carcinomas.[111]

CEA as detected by both monoclonal antibodies and polyclonal antisera is present in the vast majority of medullary carcinomas.[175] Monoclonal antibodies that are specific to CEA react with approximately 75% of cases of medullary carcinoma but not with other tumor types.[176] Antibodies that react with epitopes present on CEA and the nonspecific cross-reacting antigens react with almost 90% of medullary carcinomas but also give positive reactions with other thyroid tumor types. Several groups have demonstrated that some medullary thyroid carcinomas may lose their ability to synthesize and secrete calcitonin while maintaining their capacity for CEA production and that such tumors may have an aggressive course.[177] Franc and coworkers[163] demonstrated that patients with medullary carcinomas containing more than 50% CEA-positive cells and less than 50% calcitonin-positive cells had a poorer prognosis compared with other groups.

Medullary carcinomas are typically positive for low-molecular-weight cytokeratins. Vimentin immunoreactivity is present in approximately 60% of cases; whereas neurofilament proteins have been reported in 85%

(10 of 12) cases.[178] Normal C cells have been reported to lack neurofilament proteins but are typically positive for low-molecular-weight cytokeratins and are variably positive for vimentin.

KEY DIAGNOSTIC POINTS

Medullary Thyroid Carcinoma

- Normal C cells have an intrafollicular topography and can be identified by their positivity for calcitonin.
- Ninety-five percent of medullary carcinomas are positive for calcitonin, and a variety of other peptides may also be present.
- Generic neuroendocrine markers, including chromogranins A and B and secretogranin II, are present in medullary carcinomas.
- CEA is present in most medullary carcinomas.
- Medullary carcinomas are variably positive for TTF-1 and TTF-2 but are negative for TGB.
- True mixed C-cell and follicular tumors are rare.
- Familial forms of medullary carcinoma are preceded in their development by C-cell hyperplasia.

TABLE 10.4 Genetic Alterations in Thyroid Cancer

	Papillary (%)	Follicular (%)	Poorly Differentiated (%)	Anaplastic (%)
BRAF	39	0	13	14
RAS	15	35	35	53
RET/PTC	28	0	9	0
PAX8-PAXγ	1	34	0	0
p53	5	7	24	59
β-catenin	0	0	16	66

Modified from Nikiforov Y. Genetic alterations involved in the transition from well to poorly differentiated and anaplastic carcinoma. *Endocr Pathol.* 2004;15:319-328.
The percentages represent means from several different series.

BEYOND IMMUNOHISTOCHEMISTRY: MOLECULAR DIAGNOSTIC APPLICATIONS

Papillary Carcinoma

A variety of different genetic alterations including rearrangements (RET and TRK) and point mutations (BRAF and RAS) have been implicated in the development of PTC (Table 10.4).[179-183] Although radiation exposure has been linked to the development of rearrangements, the origin of point mutations remains unknown. The various mutations and rearrangements result in the activation of the mitogen activated protein kinase (MAPK) pathway, which is involved in signaling from a variety of growth factors and cell surface receptors. Together, these genetic alterations are present in approximately 70% of PTCs and they rarely overlap in the same tumor.

The RET proto-oncogene encodes a tyrosine kinase (TK) receptor consisting of an extracellular domain with a ligand binding site, a transmembrane domain, and an intracellular TK domain. Ligand binding results in receptor dimerization leading to the autophosphorylation of tyrosine residues and initiation of the signaling cascade. RET/PTC results from rearrangement of the 3' area of RET with the 5' area of several genes that are expressed in normal follicular cells.[184] RET/PTC1 and RET/PTC3 are the most common rearrangements and result from paracentric inversion of the long arm of chromosome 10, whereas RET/PTC2 results from a 10;17 reciprocal translocation involving R1α on 17q23. Additional rearrangements have been described in radiation-induced tumors but their frequencies are low. RET/PTC1 and RET/PTC3 account for 60% to 70% and 20% to 30% of the cases, respectively, whereas RET/PTC2 is responsible for approximately 10%. RET rearrangements are common in pediatric patients and in individuals exposed to accidental or therapeutic irradiation. RET/PTC1 is more common in classic PTCs, micro PTCs, and the diffuse sclerosing variant than in other types, whereas RET/PTC3 has been associated with the solid variant.[185] RET rearrangements are less common in the follicular variant than in PTCs of conventional type. Interestingly, RET rearrangements are associated with PTCs that lack evidence of progression to poorly differentiated or undifferentiated thyroid carcinomas.

The neurotrophic receptor tyrosine kinase (NTRK1) on chromosome 1q22 encodes the receptor for nerve growth factor. Rearrangements of NTRK are considerably less common than RET rearrangements in PTCs.[186]

BRAF is a serine/threonine protein kinase, which is a potent activator of the MAPK pathway. Mutations in this gene have been found in approximately two thirds of malignant melanomas and in a similar proportion of ovarian and colonic adenocarcinomas. The most common mutation results in a thymidine-to-adenine transversion at nucleotide position 1799 and a valine to glutamate substitution at residue 600 (V600E). An identical substitution has been identified in 40% to 70% of papillary carcinomas.[187,188] There is no evidence of similar mutations in other thyroid tumor types. BRAF mutations have been associated with conventional PTCs, tall cell and oncocytic variants, and microcarcinomas. In contrast, BRAF mutations are uncommon in the follicular variants.[189]

Approximately 15% of poorly differentiated thyroid carcinomas and a significantly higher proportion of undifferentiated/anaplastic carcinomas are positive for BRAF mutations.[189] Moreover, the mutations occur more commonly in those poorly differentiated and undifferentiated carcinomas with a papillary component. These findings suggest that the high-grade tumors progress from BRAF-positive papillary carcinomas.

RAS mutations are uncommon in papillary carcinomas of the conventional type, in contrast to the follicular variant, in which they are considerably more common.[190]

Follicular Adenoma and Carcinoma

RAS mutations are present in approximately 50% of follicular carcinomas and 20% to 40% of follicular adenomas (Table 10.4).[191] Among RAS-positive carcinomas, N-RAS codon 61 mutations are present in approximately 80% of cases and H-RAS codon 61 mutations are present in almost 20%. Identical mutations are present at lower frequencies in follicular adenomas. RAS mutations also occur in approximately 25% of oncocytic carcinomas and in up to 5% of oncocytic adenomas.

PAX8-PPARγ rearrangements in follicular tumors occur as a result of a recurrent translocation t(2;3)(q13;p25) leading to fusion of the PAX8 and the PPARγ genes.[116,117] This rearrangement occurs in approximately 35% of conventional follicular carcinomas and in up to 10% of follicular adenomas. Similar rearrangements have also been noted in a small proportion of follicular carcinomas of oncocytic type. As noted in a previous section, the rearrangement results in overexpression of the PPARγ protein, which can be detected by immunohistochemistry. It should be noted, however, that only strong nuclear staining correlates with the presence of the rearrangement and that rearrangements may occur in benign thyroid tumors.[118,119] Follicular carcinomas harboring the PAX8- PPARγ rearrangement typically occur at a younger age than those without the rearrangement, and they tend to be smaller in size and more likely to be angioinvasive.

Deletions and point mutations involving mitochondrial DNA are common in follicular neoplasms of oncocytic type, but the role of these mutations in the genesis of the tumors is unknown.[192] Mutations of the GRIM-19 gene, which is involved in the mitochondrial respiratory chain and in apoptosis, have been found in 15% of oncocytic carcinomas but do not occur in other thyroid tumor types.[193]

Poorly Differentiated and Undifferentiated Thyroid Carcinoma

Point mutations of RAS genes occur in approximately 20% of poorly differentiated and 50% of undifferentiated thyroid carcinomas, and BRAF mutations occur in 15% to 20% of these tumors (Table 10.4).[194] The PTEN and P1K3CA genes are mutated in 15% to 20% of the cases, respectively.[194]

p53 mutations are present in 15% to 30% of poorly differentiated thyroid carcinomas and 60% to 80% of undifferentiated carcinomas.[110] In contrast, relatively few (<2%) differentiated thyroid carcinomas harbor mutations of p53. These findings suggested that progressive loss of differentiation in thyroid tumors occurs as a result of mutations of this gene.

The CTNNB1 gene encodes β-catenin, which is an important intermediary in the Wnt signaling pathway.[140,141] Point mutations of CTNNB1 occur in 25% and 66% of poorly differentiated and undifferentiated thyroid carcinomas, respectively. As discussed in a previous section, most tumors with mutations have a nuclear pattern of localization, in contrast to the usual plasma membrane staining pattern of differentiated tumors.

Medullary Thyroid Carcinoma

Germline mutations of the RET gene are present in virtually all patients with familial forms of medullary thyroid carcinoma including MEN2A, MEN2B, and FMTC.[195] Codon 634 mutations occur in a high proportion of patients with MEN2A and FMTC, whereas codon 918 mutations predominate in patients with MEN2B. Somatic mutations of RET codon 918 occur in 20% to 80% of cases of sporadic MTC, and their distribution both within the primary tumors and metastases is heterogeneous.

Microarray Gene Profiling

Alterations in gene expression of papillary thyroid carcinomas have been studied using cDNA microarrays. The findings have shown that the gene expression profiles of these tumors are different from those of follicular carcinomas and other thyroid tumor types.[136,196] However, distinct sets of differently expressed genes have been found in classic papillary carcinoma, in the follicular variant, and possibly in other variants (such as tall cell variant), supporting the histopathologic and biologic differences between these tumor variants.[196,197] The results of gene expression array studies have confirmed the overexpression of a number of genes previously known to be upregulated in papillary carcinoma, such as MET, LGALS3 (galectin-3), and KRT19 (cytokeratin 19). Several additional overexpressed genes such as CITED1 were discovered using this approach and are now being explored in possible immunohistochemical diagnostic markers, as discussed previously.[136] In addition, variations in gene expression profiles between papillary carcinomas carrying BRAF, RAS, RET/PTC, and TRK mutations have been detected, providing a molecular basis for distinct phenotypic and biologic features associated with each mutation type.[197,198]

THERANOSTIC APPLICATIONS

Molecular targeted therapies have considerable potential for treatment of poorly differentiated, undifferentiated, and medullary carcinomas, each of which has diminished or absent ability to incorporate radioactive iodine.[179,180] An agent that has considerable clinical promise is ZD6474 (Zactima), a tyrosine kinase inhibitor, which is a potent inhibitor of the vascular endothelial growth factor receptor-2 (VEGR-2) and which effectively blocks RET tyrosine kinase.[199] Multikinase inhibitors with potent activity against RAF, VEGFR-2, VEGFR-3, PDGFRβ, FLT3, and c-kit are also being evaluated for therapeutic effects in patients with advanced thyroid tumors. The challenges for investigators are the assessment of the effects to which the various tyrosine kinases are being inhibited and then correlating these findings with a variety of biomarkers that are indicative of disease status and outcome data.

Parathyroid Glands

Both normal and adenomatous glands are positive for CK8, CK18, and CK19 while vimentin is restricted to stromal cells (Fig. 10.25).[200] The chief cells of normal

KEY DIAGNOSTIC POINTS

Molecular Aspects of Thyroid Carcinoma

- Genetic rearrangements (RET and TRK) and mutations (BRAF and RAS) are responsible for the development of the majority (70%) of papillary carcinomas.
- RAS mutations are considerably more common in the follicular variant of papillary carcinoma than in papillary carcinomas of the conventional type.
- The various rearrangements and mutations result in the activation of the mitogen-activated protein kinase pathway and rarely overlap in the same tumor.
- RAS mutations are present in approximately 50% of follicular carcinomas and in 20% to 40% of follicular adenomas.
- PAX-8-PPARγ rearrangements occur in approximately 35% of follicular carcinomas and in 10% of follicular adenomas.
- Deletions and point mutations involving mitochondrial DNA are common in follicular tumors of oncocytic type, and mutations of the GRIM-1 gene occur in 15% of these tumors.
- Common sites of mutation in poorly differentiated and undifferentiated thyroid carcinomas include RAS, PTEN, PIK3CA, p53, and CTNNB1 genes.
- Germline mutations of RET are present in familial forms of medullary thyroid carcinoma, while somatic mutations of RET are common in sporadic forms of medullary carcinoma.
- Gene expression profiles of thyroid carcinomas differ according to the major histopathologic classifications of these tumors.

glands are negative for neurofilaments, whereas 33% of adenomas contain some neurofilament positive cells and are also positive for cytokeratins. In contrast to thyroid follicular cells, which are positive for thyroglobulin and TTF-1, normal and neoplastic chief cells are negative for these markers.

In the past, the immunohistochemical analysis of parathyroid hormone (PTH) was difficult because of both the lack of suitable antibodies and the low level of hormone storage within the chief cells.[201] Antigen retrieval methods, however, have greatly assisted the localization of PTH in formalin-fixed, paraffin-embedded sections (Fig. 10.26).[202] PTH and chromogranin A are demonstrable in the vast majority of normal, hyperplastic, and neoplastic parathyroid glands (Fig. 10.25). In normal glands, chief cells stain more intensely for PTH and chromogranin A than do oncocytes. Hyperplastic glands generally stain less intensely than do normal glands. The intensity of staining for PTH and chromogranin A is less intense in adenomas than in normal and hyperplastic glands. Generally, however, staining of the rim of adjacent normal parathyroid *tissue* is more intense than that of the adenomas.[202] A similar pattern of reactivity has been observed in *in situ* hybridization formats with probes for parathyroid mRNA.[203] In a single case of parathyroid carcinoma, Tomita reported

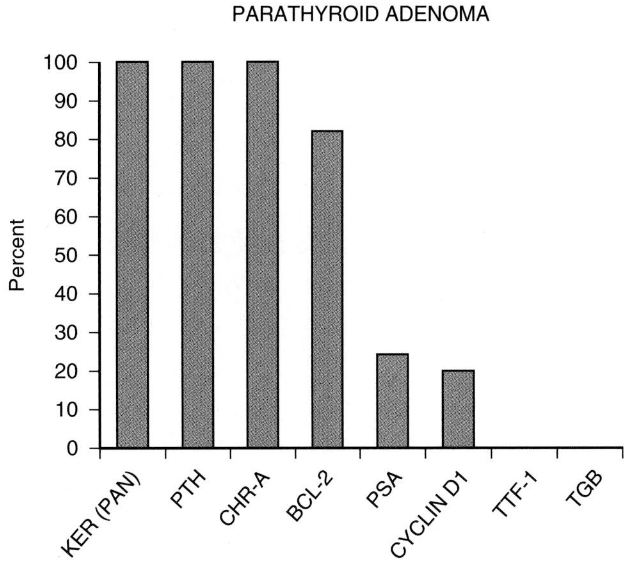

FIGURE 10.25 Distribution of markers in parathyroid adenomas. KER(PAN), pancytokeratin; PTH, parathyroid hormone; CHR-A, chromogranin A; BCL-2; PSA, prostatic specific antigen; cyclin D1; TTF-1, thyroid transcription factor-1; TGB, thyroglobulin.

positive staining for PTH but no significant reaction for chromogranin A.[202] Patterns of PTH reactivity generally correspond to the levels of extractable PTH, with the highest levels being present in normal glands and the lowest in adenomatous glands.[204] In addition to PTH, PTH-related protein has also been demonstrated by immunohistochemistry.[205]

Schmid and coworkers reported that 14% (12 of 86) of hyperplastic parathyroid glands demonstrated focal reactivity for chromogranin B and that in 10 of 12 of these cases calcitonin was co-localized with chromogranin B.[206] CGRP was found in a small proportion of the calcitonin cells in 4 of 10 of the cases. These observations were confirmed by the demonstration of mRNAs for calcitonin and CGRP. The results of this study indicate that calcitonin and CGRP may be synthesized and stored in hyperplastic parathyroid chief cells. These results have also been confirmed in other studies.[207]

CD4 immunoreactivity is present both in normal and abnormal parathyroid glands.[208] Positive staining is restricted to chief cells, whereas oncocytic cells are nonreactive. Normal, hyperplastic, and neoplastic cells demonstrate positive staining primarily on cell surfaces. In contrast, parathyroid carcinomas demonstrated primarily cytoplasmic staining. Although the functional significance of CD4-like immunoreactivity in the parathyroid is unknown, this moiety may play a role in calcium-regulated PTH release. The renal cell carcinoma antigen (RCC) is commonly expressed in parathyroid tumors,[209,210] and some may also be positive for PAX-2.[211]

The distribution of cyclin D1 has also been examined in normal and neoplastic parathyroid tissue.[212] In normal glands, cyclin D1 was present in 6% of cases. In contrast, cyclin D1 was present in 10 of 11 (91%) parathyroid carcinomas, 11 of 38 (39%) parathyroid

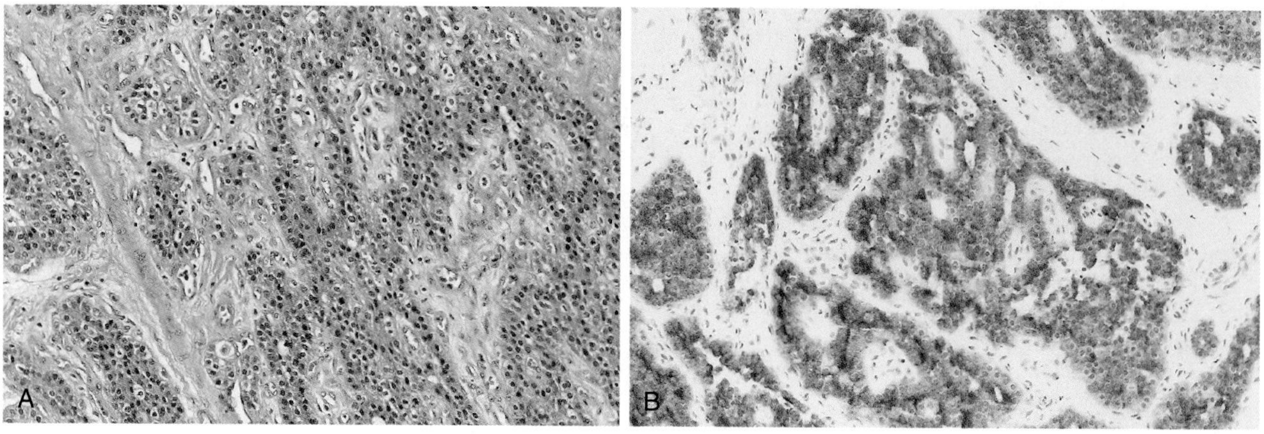

FIGURE 10.26 **A,** Intrathyroidal parathyroid adenoma. **B,** Immunoperoxidase stain for parathyroid hormone shows strong cytoplasmic positivity in chief cells.

adenomas, and 11 of 18 (61%) hyperplastic parathyroid glands. These studies confirm the high frequency of cyclin D1 expression in adenomas and carcinomas, but they also indicate that high levels of expression may occur in cases of hyperplasia.[212]

The distinction between parathyroid adenomas and carcinomas is, on occasion, extremely difficult. Several studies have used MIB-1 to aid in the differential diagnosis. Abbona and coworkers[213] reported a significant difference between carcinomas (aggressive and nonaggressive) and adenomas with respect to MIB-1 scores. There were no significant differences, however, between nonaggressive carcinomas and adenomas. Conversely, mitotic rates and MIB-1 scores of clinically aggressive carcinomas were significantly higher than adenomas. Vargas and coworkers[214] reported that a MIB-1 fraction in excess of 40 positive signals per 1000 cells correlated strongly with malignancy. p27 (Kip 1) has also been examined in parathyroid hyperplasia, adenoma, and carcinoma.[60] The p27 labeling index was 56.8 ± 3.4 for adenomas and 13.9 ± 2.6 for carcinomas, whereas the MIB-1 labeling index was significantly higher in carcinomas than in adenomas. These findings suggest that both p27 and MIB-1 may be helpful when used together for the distinction of parathyroid adenomas and carcinomas.

Another approach to the distinction of parathyroid adenomas and carcinomas involves the use of antibodies to the retinoblastoma (RB) protein. Cryns and coworkers[215] reported the absence of RB protein in a small series of carcinomas, whereas this protein was present in adenomas. However, Vargas and coworkers[214] demonstrated positive staining for RB in 100% of adenomas and 80% of carcinomas. Farnebo and coworkers[216] also demonstrated the lack of utility of RB immunoreactivity for the distinction of adenomas and carcinomas.

p53 has also been examined in normal, hyperplastic, and neoplastic parathyroid tissues. In the study reported by Kayath and colleagues,[217] p53 was present in 36% (10 of 28) of adenomas, 42% (5 of 12) of cases of primary hyperplasia, 72% (13 of 18) of cases of diffuse hyperplasia, 44% (17 of 39) of cases of nodular hyperplasia, and 40% (2 of 5) of carcinomas. These results indicate that the analysis of p53 by immunohistochemistry is not useful in the distinction of the various proliferative states of the parathyroid.

Beyond Immunohistochemistry: Anatomic Molecular Diagnostic Applications

Several groups have demonstrated LOH on chromosome 13q, a region that includes *RB* and *BRCA2,* in parathyroid carcinomas. In the series reported by Cryns and colleagues,[215] 11 of 11 specimens from patients with parathyroid carcinoma and 1 of 19 adenomas lacked an *RB* allele. *BRCA2* has also been suggested as a potential suppressor gene in these tumors.[218] However, the contribution of both *RB* and *BRCA2* to the development of carcinomas has been controversial. In a recent study by Cetani and colleagues,[219] LOH for the least one marker of the *RBI* locus was found in 6 of 6 carcinomas, whereas LOH for *BRCA2* was found in 3 of 5 cases. In the same series, LOH for *RB* and *BRCA2* was demonstrated in 28.8% and 17.4%, respectively, of adenomas.

Shattuck and colleagues[220] recently performed direct sequencing of parathyroid carcinomas that demonstrated lesions of RB or *BRCA2* and were unable to find microdeletions, insertions, or point mutations of either gene. They concluded that neither *RB* nor *BRCA2* was likely to act as a tumor suppressor gene in carcinomas. However, these results do not exclude the possibility that the decreased *RB* function in carcinomas, whether secondary or because of epigenetic effects, may play a role in tumor development. It is also possible that other genes on chromosome 13 may be implicated in the development of parathyroid carcinomas.

Studies of heritable tumor syndromes have provided considerable insight into the molecular basis of the corresponding sporadic tumors. Mutations of the HRPT2 gene are responsible for the development of the hyperparathyroidism-jaw tumor (HPT-JT) syndrome, which is inherited as an autosomal dominant trait.[221] The commonest manifestations of this syndrome include primary hyperparathyroidism, fibro-osseous lesions of the mandible and maxilla, and a variety of renal lesions.[222] In this syndrome, hyperparathyroidism occurs as a result of neoplasms of one or more parathyroid glands, which

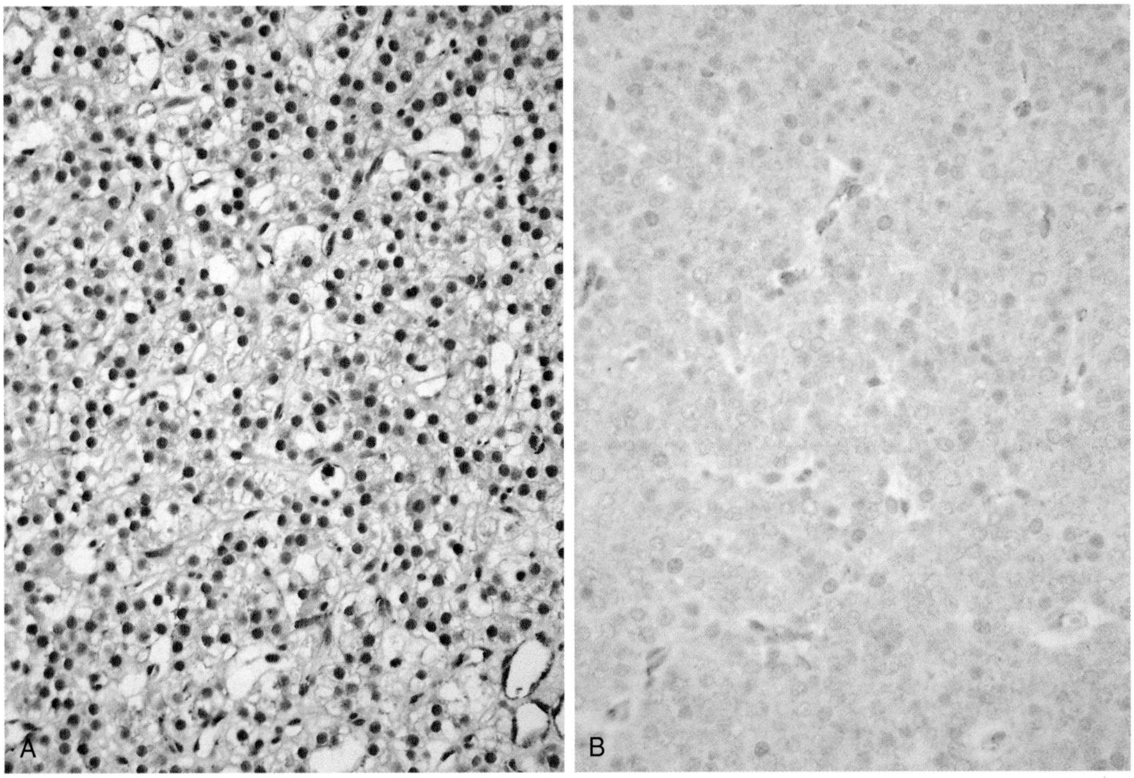

FIGURE 10.27 Parafibromin stain of parathyroid adenoma **(A)** and parathyroid carcinoma **(B)**. **A,** There is intense nuclear staining in the adenoma. **B,** In this area of the carcinoma, there is no staining of tumor cell nuclei. Other areas of the carcinoma, however, exhibited foci of positive staining.

frequently show cystic change. Importantly, parathyroid carcinomas occur in 10% to 15% of patients with this syndrome.

The role of the HRPT2 gene in the pathogenesis of sporadic parathyroid carcinomas was first demonstrated by Howell and colleagues[223] in 2003. Subsequent studies by Shattuck and coworkers[224] demonstrate that parathyroid carcinomas from 10 of 15 patients had HRPT2 mutations that were predicted to inactivate the encoded parafibromin protein. Importantly, the HRPT2 mutations in three of the parathyroid carcinomas of these patients were identified as germline mutations. The latter finding suggests that a subset of patients with apparent sporadic parathyroid carcinomas carry germline mutations in the HRPT2 gene and may, in fact, have the HPT-JT syndrome or a variant of that syndrome. These findings suggest that all patients with parathyroid carcinoma should have jaw and renal imaging studies and patients with parathyroid carcinoma should be tested for germline HRPT2 mutations.

Loss of parafibromin was first reported as a molecular marker for parathyroid carcinoma by Tan and colleagues (Fig. 10.27).[225] These workers noted that loss of parafibromin nuclear staining had a 96% sensitivity and 99% specificity for the definitive diagnosis of parathyroid carcinoma. In addition to parafibromin loss in carcinomas, this protein was also absent from HPT-JT–associated adenomas. Generally, similar results have been reported by other groups, although the different studies employed somewhat different scoring systems.[226-228]

Juhlin and colleagues[229] have demonstrated that 68% of unequivocal carcinomas exhibited reduced expression of parafibromin and 100% of adenomas were positive. Moreover, three of six carcinomas with known HRPT2 mutations showed reduced expression of parafibromin. They conclude that parafibromin immunohistochemistry could be used as an additional marker for parathyroid tumor classification with parafibromin-positive cases having a low risk of malignancy and cases with reduced protein expression representing either carcinomas or adenomas with HRPT2 mutations.[229] Of particular interest is the observation that four of five metastatic parathyroid carcinomas observed in patients with chronic renal failure were positive for parafibromin. This finding suggests that genetic events other than HRPT2 mutations may be of significance in the genesis of different subsets of parathyroid carcinoma.[230]

In our own experience,[231,232] loss of parafibromin staining has been noted in a subset of adenomas unassociated with the HPT-JT syndrome, whereas some carcinomas have shown positive staining. These observations emphasize the need for the use of well-characterized parafibromin antibodies, as well as standardized fixation and retrieval conditions, staining protocols, and scoring systems before this approach becomes the standard of practice. Although parafibromin immunohistochemistry represents an important step in the ability to diagnose parathyroid carcinoma, additional studies will be required to test the validity of this approach and to determine the roles of other genes in the development of these tumors.

KEY DIAGNOSTIC POINTS

Parathyroid Tumors

- Normal parathyroid chief cells and hyperplastic and neoplastic parathyroids are positive for parathyroid hormone and a variety of neuroendocrine markers including synaptophysin and chromogranin A.
- Low levels of expression of MIB-1 and high levels of p27 are characteristic of parathyroid adenomas, whereas carcinomas have high levels of MIB-1 and low levels of p27.
- Parafibromin is uniformly expressed in parathyroid adenomas, whereas its expression is often reduced and/or heterogeneous in carcinomas.

Adrenal Cortex

Markers that have been used for the identification of adrenal cortical cells include steroidogenic enzymes, the monoclonal antibody D11, adrenal 4 binding protein (Ad4BP), A103 (melan A), calretinin, and inhibin A (Fig. 10.28). Studies reported by Sasano and coworkers[21-23] demonstrated strong staining for $P450_{17\alpha}$ in the fasciculata and reticularis zones of patients with Cushing's disease. Cortical adenomas associated with cortisol overproduction demonstrated strong staining for this enzyme, whereas the adjacent zona reticularis showed weak staining, consistent with suppression of the normal gland.

The monoclonal antibody D11 recognizes several 59kD proteins capable of binding apolipoprotein E.[233,234] Approximately 80% of adrenal cortical tumors have positive nuclear staining for D11; however, 100% of hepatocellular carcinomas, 60% of lung carcinomas, and occasional renal carcinomas have been reported to show cytoplasmic staining for this marker.[235] Ad4BP, which is also known as steroid factor (SF)-1, is a transcription factor that regulates steroidogenic cytochrome P450 gene expression. Ad4BP has been reported in 100% of adrenal cortical carcinomas, whereas no cases of renal cell carcinoma, hepatocellular carcinoma, or other tumor types (including pheochromocytoma) exhibited positivity.[236]

The monoclonal antibody A103 (melan A) has been used primarily for the identification of malignant melanoma (Fig. 10.29). This antibody cross-reacts with an epitope, which is present in steroid-producing cells including those of the adrenal cortex.[237] Busam and coworkers[237] reported A103 immunoreactivity in 100% of adrenal cortical carcinomas but in no cases of renal cell carcinoma, hepatocellular carcinoma, pheochromocytoma, or other types of epithelial tumors. In a smaller series, Renshaw and Granter[238] reported positive staining in two of four adrenal cortical carcinomas. Loy and coworkers reported a more extensive study of A103 immunoreactivity in a wide array of tumors which would be considered in the differential diagnosis of adrenocortical tumors.[239] They found that although all 21 adrenal cortical tumors were positive, none of 16 metastatic carcinomas from the lung, kidney, breast, liver, and esophagus or 10 pheochromocytomas showed immunoreactivity. Additionally, these authors also studied 269 extra-adrenal carcinomas from various sites

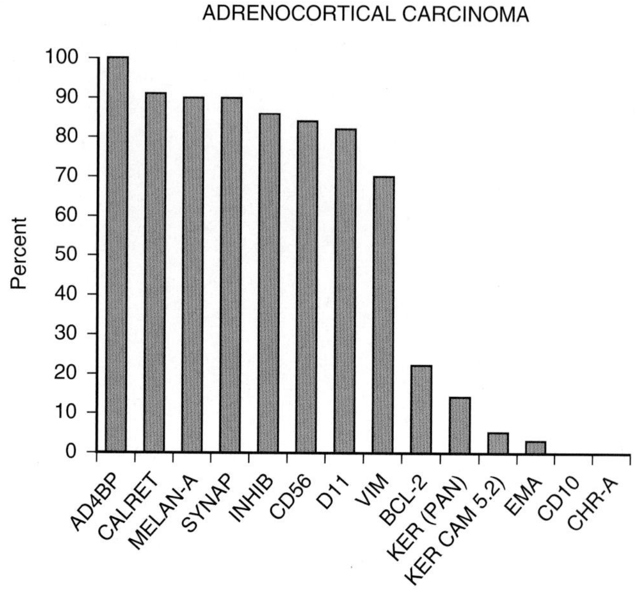

FIGURE 10.28 Distribution of markers in adrenocortical tumors. AD4BP, adrenal 4 binding protein; calret, calretinin; melan-A (A103); synap, synaptophysin; inhib, inhibin; CD56; D11; VIM, vimentin; BCL-2; KER(PAN), pancytokeratin; EMA, epithelial membrane antigen; CD10; CHR-A, chromogranin-A.

including lung, breast, kidney, pancreas, liver, esophagus, stomach, ovary, colon, biliary tract, bladder, larynx, and gallbladder and all but one case of ovarian serous carcinoma was A103 negative.[239] Another study by Ghorab and colleagues[240] found 31 of 32 adrenocortical neoplasms (21 adenomas, 11 carcinomas) were A103 positive. With the exception of one clear cell renal cell carcinoma, all 86 renal cell carcinomas (67 clear cell, 10 papillary, 4 chromophobe, 4 sarcomatoid, 1 collecting duct) and 57 hepatocellular (25 well differentiated, 25 moderately differentiated, 7 poorly differentiated) carcinomas were negative for A103.[240] These studies underscore the utility of A103 in identifying primary adrenal cortical neoplasms and distinguishing them from tumors of other sites including the adrenal medulla.[241]

The inhibin A antibody is also useful for the identification of steroid-producing cells.[242] Fetsch and coworkers[243] used this antibody for the identification of adrenal cortical tumors in cytologic preparations. They reported positive staining in 100% of adrenal cortical tumors but in no cases of renal cell carcinoma. Renshaw and Granter[238] have demonstrated that inhibin A and A103 are useful in the immunohistochemical identification of adrenal cortical neoplasms and that A103 is marginally more specific and inhibin A slightly more sensitive for the identification of cortical tumors.

Subsequent studies have reported similar results. Overall, the range of positivity for inhibin A in adrenal cortical neoplasms has been 71% to 100% and 75% to 100% in adenomas and carcinomas, respectively, whereas immunoreactivity in metastatic carcinomas such as renal cell carcinomas (0% to 20%), hepatocellular carcinomas (0% to 4%), and pheochromocytomas (0% to 14%) is considerably less frequent.[244-249]

The distinction of benign and malignant adrenocortical tumors is often problematic by standard histopathologic

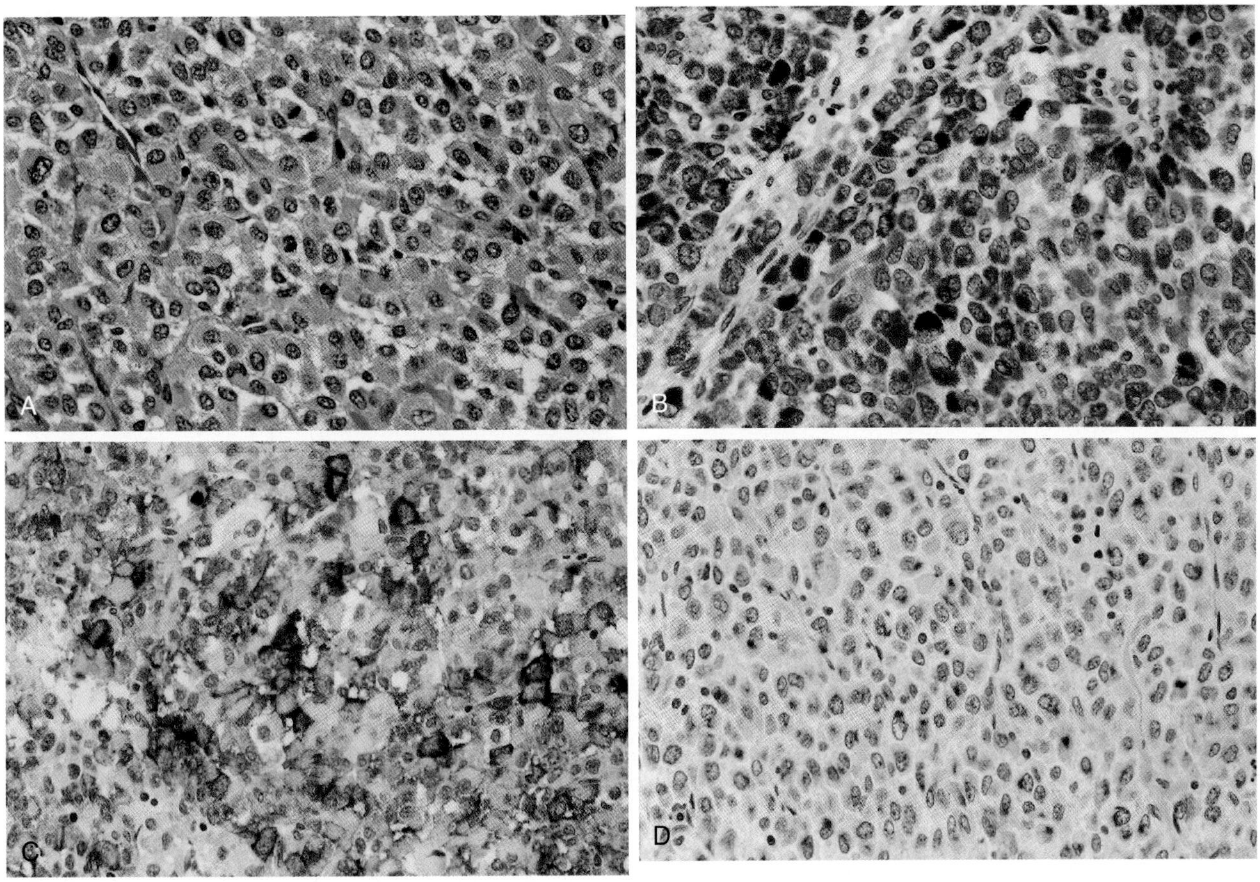

FIGURE 10.29 **A,** Adrenal cortical carcinoma (H&E stain). **B,** Immunoperoxidase stain for melan A (A103) shows granular positivity. **C,** Immunoperoxidase stain for synaptophysin shows prominent cytoplasmic reactivity. **D,** Immunoperoxidase stain for cytokeratins (CAM5.2) shows focal cytoplasmic reactivity.

criteria. Vargas and colleagues[250] demonstrated that the mean proliferative fraction, as assessed by counting the proportion of MIB-1 positive cells, was 1.49% in adenomas, 20.8% in carcinomas, and 16.6% in recurrent or metastatic tumors. None of 20 benign lesions had a score that exceeded 8%, whereas only 1 of 20 carcinomas had a score of less than 8%. Moreover, 45% of the carcinomas were positive for p53 and none of the carcinomas was p53 positive.[250] The expression of RB, on the other hand, did not discriminate benign and malignant cortical tumors. Schmitt and coworkers[251] have confirmed the value of the MIB-1 labeling index for the distinction of adenomas and carcinomas and further demonstrated that the carcinomas commonly overexpressed IGF2 and cyclin dependent kinase 4.

The main difficulties lie in the differentiation of adrenal cortical tumors from adrenal medullary tumors, namely, pheochromocytomas, and the differentiation of adrenal tumors from extra-adrenal tumors (i.e., metastatic carcinomas or primary carcinomas of neighboring structures such as the kidney or liver) (Fig. 10.30).

Adrenal cortical carcinomas may show evidence of NE differentiation, as manifested by immunoreactivity for synaptophysin, neurofilament proteins, and NSE (Fig. 10.29C).[36,252] In contrast to pheochromocytomas, however, adrenal cortical carcinomas are typically negative for the chromogranin proteins. In one series, 60% of cortical carcinomas were positive for the low-molecular-weight neurofilament protein, 80% were positive for synaptophysin, and 60% were positive for NSE.[252] The significance of these findings with respect to the histogenesis of cortical carcinomas is unknown. In addition to chromogranin as a distinguishing characteristic, pheochromocytomas are known to be negative for keratins, although some studies have reported positivity in up to 29% of cases.[178,253]

More recent studies have directed attention to other markers such as bcl-2 and calretinin to assist in this distinction. Bcl-2 is typically present in all cell layers of the normal adrenal cortex but is consistently absent from the medulla. Fogt and coworkers[254] demonstrated bcl-2 immunoreactivity in 23 of 23 cortical adenomas and carcinomas but in only 1 of 11 pheochromocytomas. This study suggests that bcl-2 may be helpful in the differential diagnosis of adrenal cortical and medullary tumors. However, a more recent study by Zhang and colleagues[255] did not demonstrate similar staining trends using bcl-2. In their study, only a minority of adrenal cortical neoplasms (2/15 [13%] of adenomas and 3/10 [30%] of carcinomas) showed positive staining and surprisingly, the majority of pheochromocytomas (12/14 or 86%) were bcl-2 positive. The authors concluded that these seemingly conflicting results may be related to different antigen retrieval methodologies.

Calretinin, a calcium-binding protein, is typically used as a marker for neural, mesothelial, or ovarian sex-cord stromal tumors but was recently found to be expressed in 73% of adrenal cortical tumors.[256] These findings were confirmed by Zhang and colleagues,[255] who found all 16 of 16 (100%) and 11 of 12 (92%) adrenal cortical adenomas and carcinomas, respectively, were calretinin positive while none of 20 pheochromocytomas showed staining.

The differentiation of adrenal cortical carcinomas from metastatic carcinomas to the adrenal gland may be difficult. This distinction may be assisted by studies of the distribution of intermediate filaments, particularly cytokeratins and vimentin. Normal and neoplastic adrenal cortical cells are typically vimentin-positive but exhibit considerable differences in patterns of cytokeratin immunoreactivity depending on factors such as tissue preparation (fixed versus frozen) and the reactivities of the cytokeratin antibodies.[257,258] With fresh frozen tissues and with formalin-fixed, paraffin-embedded tissues subjected to microwave antigen retrieval, cytokeratin immunoreactivity may be present focally in up to 60% of adrenal cortical neoplasms, particularly with CAM5.2 (see Fig. 10.29D). The typical intermediate filament profile for cortical carcinomas is, therefore, vimentin-positive with variable and generally weak cytokeratin immunoreactivity.[259,260] Metastases to the adrenal gland, in contrast, are more likely to exhibit intense cytokeratin staining and are also usually positive for CEA, CD15, and epithelial membrane antigen (EMA), whereas adrenal cortical carcinomas are negative for these markers. It should be remembered that some markers such as RCC may also be expressed in adrenocortical tumors.[210]

S-100 may be part of a panel when considering a metastatic malignant melanoma; however, sustentacular cells in the adrenal medulla are also positive for this marker. Additionally, HMB-45, which is known to be positive in malignant melanomas, is occasionally positive in pheochromocytomas.[261,262]

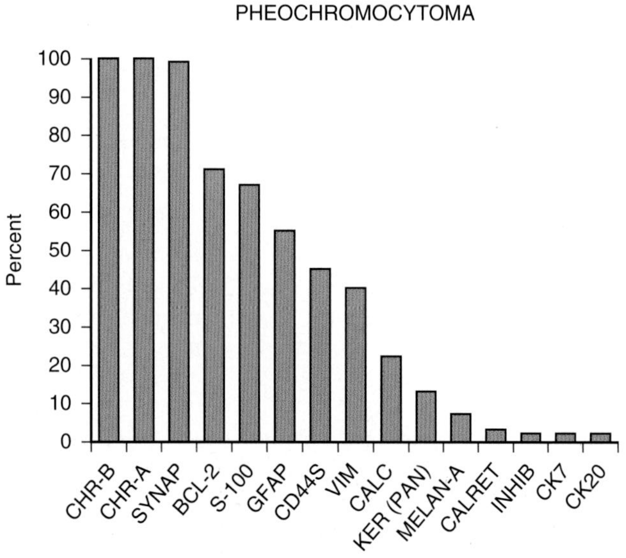

FIGURE 10.30 Distribution of markers in pheochromocytoma. CHR-B, chromogranin B; CHR-A, chromogranin A; synap, synaptophysin; BCL-2; S-100; GFAP, glial fibrillary acidic protein; CD44S; VIM, vimentin; CALC, calcitonin; KER(PAN), pancytokeratin; melan-A (A103); calret, calretinin; inhib, inhibin; CK7, cytokeratin7; CK20, cytokeratin 20.

BEYOND IMMUNOHISTOCHEMISTRY: MOLECULAR DIAGNOSTIC AND THERANOSTIC APPLICATIONS

Over the past decade, there have been considerable advances in the understanding of both sporadic and heritable adrenocortical tumors at the molecular level. Genetic alterations present in familial tumors include mutations of p53 (Li-Fraumeni syndrome), menin (MEN1) PRKARIA (Carney complex) and p57kip2 (CDNKIC), KCNQIOT, H19, and IGF-II overexpression in Beckwith-Weidemann.[263]

Gene expression profiling studies have demonstrated that the most significantly upregulated genes in cortical carcinomas include ubiquitin specific protease 4 (*USP4*) and ubiquitin degradation 1-like *(UFD1L)*.[264,265] Additional upregulated genes include members of the insulin-like growth factor (IGF) family such as *IGF2*, *IGF2R*, *IGFBP3*, and *IGFBP6*. Giordano and coworkers also demonstrated increased expression of IGF2 in adrenal cortical carcinomas. Down-regulated genes in carcinomas include the chemokine (C-X-C motif) ligand 10 (*CXCL10*), the retinoic acid receptor responder 2, the aldehyde dehydrogenase family member A1 (*ALD1f1A1*), cytochrome b reductase 1, and glutathione S-transferase A4.

Similar patterns of gene expression occur in pediatric adrenal cortical tumors with a consistent marked decrease in the expression of all histocompatibility class II genes in carcinomas as compared with adenomas.[266] These results parallel the observations by Marx and colleagues[267] that prenatal and postnatal adrenals do not express MHC class II antigens in contrast to adult adrenals, which express these antigens.

Adrenocortical carcinomas are generally resistant to chemotherapy because the tumor cells express high levels of multidrug resistance protein (MDR1) or P-glycoprotein. Clinical trials with the MDR1 efflux pump inhibitor (Tariquidar), epidermal growth factor inhibitor (Gefitinib), antivascular endothelial growth factor (Bevacizumab), and tyrosine kinase inhibitor (Sunitinib) are currently in progress.[268] Treatment of patients whose tumors were positive for c-kit and PDGF-R did not appear to benefit from treatment with imatinib mesylate (Gleevec).

KEY DIAGNOSTIC POINTS

Adrenocortical Tumors

- Adrenocortical tumors are positive for vimentin and are variably positive for cytokeratins.
- Melan A (A103), inhibin, and calretinin are useful for the distinction of adrenocortical tumors from other tumor types.
- Adrenocortical tumors are often positive for synaptophysin and neurofilaments.
- Adrenocortical carcinomas have a proliferative index (assessed with MIB-1) in excess of 8% and are positive for p53 in approximately 45% of cases.
- Adrenocortical tumors generally overexpress IGF-2 and cyclin-dependent kinase 4.

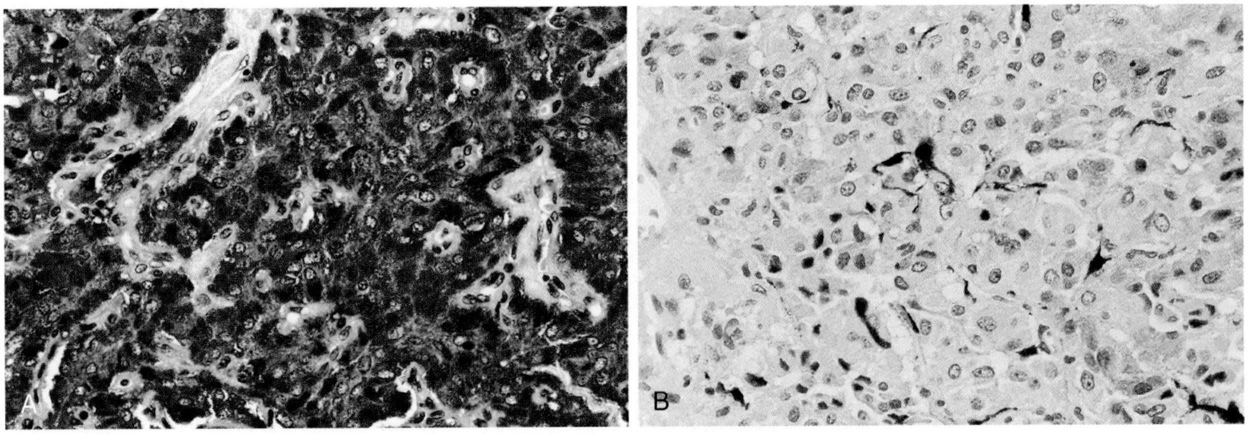

FIGURE 10.31 **A,** Adrenal pheochromocytoma. Immunoperoxidase stain for chromogranin A shows strong cytoplasmic staining. **B,** Immunoperoxidase stain for S-100 protein demonstrates positivity in sustentacular cells.

Adrenal Medulla and Extra-adrenal Paraganglia

The major cell types of the adrenal medulla and extra-adrenal paraganglia include the catecholamine-synthesizing cells and the supporting or sustentacular cells.[269,270] Both catecholamines and catecholamine-synthesizing enzymes have been demonstrated in the former cells with immunofluorescent techniques in frozen sections and immunoperoxidase techniques in paraffin-embedded material.[8,269-271] The catecholamine-synthesizing cells typically exhibit positivity for a variety of generic NE markers and are variably positive for certain peptide hormones. Sustentacular cells, in contrast, are positive for S-100 protein.[269]

The adrenal medullary cells and extra-adrenal paraganglionic cells and their tumors typically exhibit a neurofilament- and vimentin-positive phenotype (Fig. 10.30).[56,257,272] The presence of cytokeratin immunoreactivity in these tumors has been controversial. Kimura and coworkers[178] reported cytokeratin immunoreactivity in almost 30% of pheochromocytomas using a broad-spectrum cytokeratin antibody. Cytokeratin immunoreactivity was generally sparse, but positive cells were sometimes present in small groups or clusters. In contrast to the cytokeratin positivity in pheochromocytomas, extra-adrenal paragangliomas in Kimura and associates' study were cytokeratin-negative.[178] Other authors, however, have failed to demonstrate cytokeratins in pheochromocytomas and extra-adrenal paragangliomas. Chetty and colleagues[253] examined 18 extra-adrenal paragangliomas and 7 pheochromocytomas for cytokeratins using the antibodies AE1/AE3, CAM5.2, and 34βE12 after microwave antigen retrieval. Reactivity with AE1/AE3 and CAM5.2 was present in three extra-adrenal paragangliomas (cauda equina, intravagal, and orbital). However, none of the pheochromocytomas was positive. Other epithelial markers such as EMA are typically negative in pheochromocytomas and paragangliomas.

NSE is present in virtually all pheochromocytomas and paragangliomas.[269,273] Synaptophysin is present in 100% of cases, whereas chromogranin A is expressed in more than 95%.[269,273,274] Generally, chromogranin immunoreactivity is more intense in normal than in neoplastic cells of paraganglionic tissue (Fig. 10.31A). Chromogranin immunoreactivity appears in a distinctive granular pattern, whereas NSE immunoreactivity appears diffusely within the cytoplasm. Another generic NE marker that has been analyzed in these tumors is PGP9.5, which is present in approximately 80% of reported cases.[275] S-100 protein is present only in the sustentacular cells (Fig. 10.31B).

In the normal adrenal gland, CD56 is present in the medulla and the zona glomerulosa.[49] Pheochromocytomas are typically strongly positive for CD56. Komminoth and associates[36] used a monoclonal antibody that binds specifically to a long chain form of polysialic acid (polySia) found on NCAM and demonstrated staining restricted to the medulla of normal human glands. All pheochromocytomas were diffusely polySia-positive, whereas 8 of 28 (28%) cortical carcinomas exhibited focal positivity.

In addition to catecholamines, serotonin immunoreactivity has been demonstrated in approximately 80% of pheochromocytomas.[273] Both pheochromocytomas and extra-adrenal paragangliomas may also contain peptide hormones including neuropeptide Y (64%), substance P (36%), calcitonin (21%), and leu- and met-enkephalin (70%).[273,275] Several studies have indicated that determination of circulating levels of neuropeptide Y may be useful in the diagnosis and monitoring of patients with these tumors. Helman and coworkers[276] demonstrated that neuropeptide Y mRNA is present in all benign pheochromocytomas but in only 30% of malignant pheochromocytomas.

Although alpha inhibin is considered to be a specific marker for cortical neoplasms, Pelkey and coworkers[242] reported immunoreactivity in 2 of 19 pheochromocytomas.

Clarke and coworkers[277] used a variety of markers to aid in the distinction of benign and malignant pheochromocytomas. In their study, an MIB-1 labeling index of greater than 3% yielded a specificity of 100% and

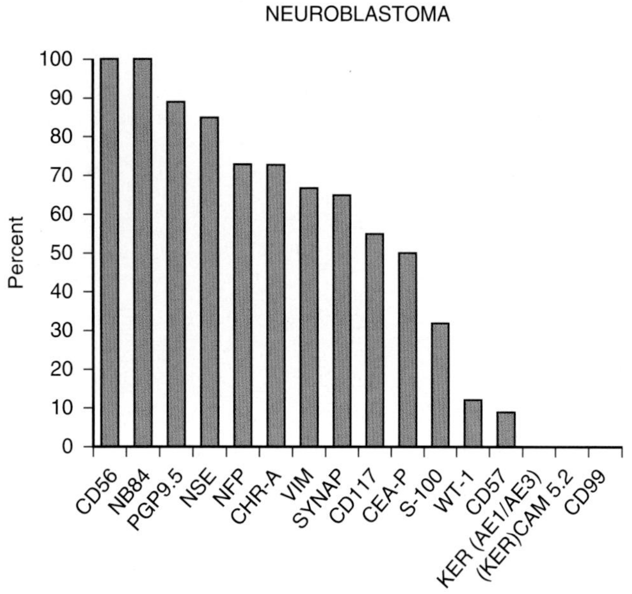

FIGURE 10.32 Distribution of markers in neuroblastoma. CD56; NB84; PGP 9.5, protein gene product 9.4; NSE, neuron-specific enolase; NFP, neurofilament protein; CHR-A, chromogranin A; VIM, vimentin; synap, synaptophysin; CD117; CEA-P, polyclonal CEA; S-100; WT-1, Wilms' tumor; CD57; Ker(AE1/AE3), keratin detected with monoclonal antibodies AE1 and AE3; KER(CAM5.2), keratin detected with CAM 5.2; CD99.

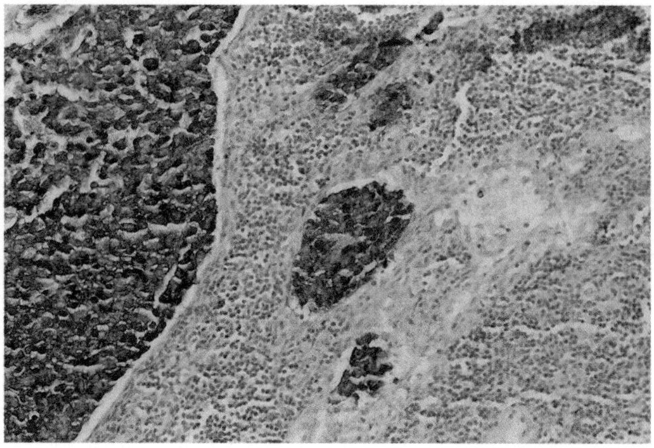

FIGURE 10.33 Metastatic neuroblastoma involving a lymph node. Immunoperoxidase stain for neuron-specific enolase is restricted to tumor cells.

a sensitivity of 50% for predicting malignant behavior in these tumors. August and coworkers[278] reported that the presence of more than 5% MIB-1 positive cells was associated with malignant behavior in 85% of the cases in their series. These authors also noted that tumors were more likely to metastasize when CD44-S was negative in the tumors. As indicated in prior studies, S-100 positivity had a significant ($p = 0.02$) but nonlinear association with benign tumors and the absence of S-100 correlated with greater tumor weight. Cathepsin B, cathepsin D, and type IV collagenase were present in both benign and malignant tumors, as were c-met, bcl-2, and basic fibroblast growth factor.

NEUROBLASTOMA

Neuroblastomas are small, round, blue cell tumors that may arise in the adrenal gland and a variety of extra-adrenal sites. The differential diagnosis is wide and includes rhabdomyosarcoma, Ewing's sarcoma-primitive neuroectodermal tumor (ES-PNET), medulloblastoma, small cell osteosarcoma, lymphoblastic lymphoma, blastematous Wilms' tumor, and small cell desmoplastic tumor. Numerous markers have been used for the diagnosis of neuroblastomas including NE markers, cytoskeletal proteins, catecholamine-synthesizing enzymes, and neuroblastoma-"specific" antibodies (Fig. 10.32).[279-285] Many of these markers lack specificity or sensitivity, or both, as individual reagents and must be used as panels.

NSE is present in 85% to 100% of cases of neuroblastoma, and a similarly high level of positivity has been reported for PGP9.5 (Fig. 10.33).[283] However, both of these markers may also be present in other small, round, blue cell tumors. Wirnsberger and colleagues[283] reported that among antibodies directed against chromogranins and related proteins, HISL-19 was present in 100% of neuroblastomas, followed by chromogranin A (52%) and chromogranin A and B (45%) (Fig. 10.34A). Neurofilament protein was present in 80% and was localized primarily in cell processes or nerve fibers, whereas synaptophysin was present in 75% of cases. Dopamine β-hydroxylase was present in 75% of cases. In general, reactivity for these markers was greater in well-differentiated than in poorly differentiated neuroblastomas.[283] Among peptide hormones, VIP was present in 30% and neuropeptide Y was present in 10%. CD57 was not found in any neuroblastoma but was demonstrable in seven of seven ganglioneuromas.[283] Microtubule associated protein-1 (MAP1) and MAP2 and beta-tubulin are present in 100% of cases, but the number of cases studied to date has been small.[284,285] S-100 protein is restricted in its distribution to the sustentacular (stromal) cells (see Fig. 10.34B).

CD99 is a useful marker for the distinction of neuroblastomas from other small, round, blue cell tumors.[286-290] More than 100 cases of neuroblastoma have now been studied for CD99, and all have been negative. In contrast, nearly 100% of cases of Ewing's sarcoma–primitive neuroectodermal tumor (ES-PNET) are CD99-positive. Anti-β_2-microglobulin is another marker that is negative in neuroblastoma but positive in approximately 75% of ES-PNET.[291]

Worthy of note is an immunohistochemical marker, NB84, that is a monoclonal antibody raised to neuroblastoma cells.[291] Miettinen and coworkers[292] studied 22 cases of undifferentiated neuroblastomas and 83 cases of differentiated neuroblastomas (total of 105 cases) and found that 95.5% of the former and 100% of the latter were positive for NB84. In addition, 4 of 5 (80%) of ES-PNETs and 3 of 3 (100%) of desmoplastic small, round cell tumors also showed positive staining. In contrast, 7 of 39 (17.9%) of ES and 1 of

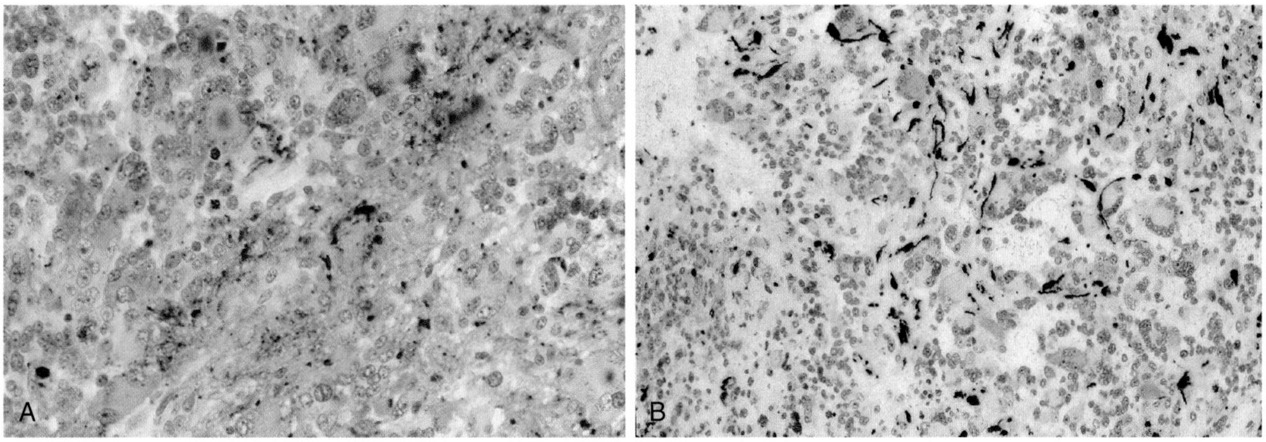

FIGURE 10.34 **A,** Extra-adrenal neuroblastoma. Immunoperoxidase stain for chromogranin A reveals a granular staining pattern in areas of process formation. **B,** Extra-adrenal neuroblastoma. Immunoperoxidase stain for S-100 protein shows positivity restricted to sustentacular cells.

14 (7.1%) cases of blastomatous Wilms' tumors were NB84-positive. Alveolar and embryonal rhabdomyosarcomas, lymphoblastic lymphomas, and pulmonary small cell carcinomas were negative.[292] However, Folpe and coworkers[293] reported NB84 immunoreactivity in 3 of 13 rhabdomyosarcomas, 10 of 11 medulloblastomas, 1 of 9 esthesioneuroblastomas, and 2 of 3 small cell osteosarcomas. A panel of antibodies including NB84, CD99, cytokeratins, lymphoid, and muscle-specific markers should be used in rendering a diagnosis of neuroblastoma.

BEYOND IMMUNOHISTOCHEMISTRY: MOLECULAR DIAGNOSTIC APPLICATIONS

The molecular aspects of meuroblastomas are covered in Chapter 20. Heritable conditions associated with the development of pheochromocytomas and paragangliomas include multiple endocrine neoplasia (MEN2A, MEN2B), von Hippel Lindau disease (VHL), and neurofibromatosis type 1 (NF1).[294] These syndromes result from mutations of the RET proto-oncogene (MEN2A and 2B), the VHL gene (VHL syndrome), and the NF1 gene (neurofibromatosis 1 gene). More recently, the familial paraganglioma (PGL) syndromes have been identified as resulting from mutations in the succinic dehydrogenase (SDH) genes SDHD (PGL1), ADHC (PGL3), and SDHB (PGL4). Approximately 50% of tumors with SDHB mutations are malignant, whereas approximately 5% or less of the other mutations are associated with malignancy. Expression profiling studies have demonstrated different clusters of markers in tumors with specific genetic background and in subsets of sporadic tumors. For example, chromogranin B is more highly expressed in MEN2-associated tumors than in VHL-associated pheochromocytomas.[295]

Gene profiling studies of benign and malignant pheochromocytomas have demonstrated that almost 90% of the differentially expressed genes are underexpressed in malignant versus benign tumors.[296,297] These features are consistent with a less differentiated biochemical pathway in the malignant tumors characterized by a lack of production of epinephrine and relatively high production of dopamine compared with norepinephrine.[296]

KEY DIAGNOSTIC POINTS

Adrenal Medullary Tumors

- Neuroblastomas and pheochromocytomas are positive for a wide spectrum of neuroendocrine markers.
- Both tumor types may also contain peptide hormones.
- Pheochromocytomas are positive for chromogranins and synaptophysin, while the expression of synaptophysin is characteristic of adrenocortical tumors.
- Malignant pheochromocytomas have a higher MIB-1 proliferative index than benign pheochromocytomas.
- Gene-profiling studies have demonstrated that almost 90% of the differentially expressed genes are underexpressed in malignant pheochromocytomas as compared with their benign counterparts.

Several of the downregulated genes include peptidylglycine α-amidating mono-oxygenase and glutaminylpeptide cyclotransferase.[297]

Gastrointestinal Endocrine Cells

Endocrine tumors (carcinoids) of the gastrointestinal tract (GI-ETs) have been divided into three major groups on the basis of their origins from foregut, midgut, and hindgut derivatives. There is a strong correlation between their sites of origin and the distribution patterns of peptide hormones and amines. For example, serotonin is present in 89% of midgut, 30% of foregut, and 13% of hindgut GI-ETs (Table 10.5).[298]

GI-ETs are typically positive for cytokeratins, with 100% exhibiting positivity for CAM5.2, 80% exhibiting positivity with other pancytokeratin antibodies, and approximately 40% exhibiting positivity for CK20.[299-301] Approximately 25% are positive for vimentin, and neurofilament proteins are present in a variable proportion of cases. GI-ETs are positive for a wide variety of generic NE markers. NSE is present in nearly 80% of cases, whereas PGP9.5 is present in approximately 90%.[15] Synaptophysin is present in 100% of cases at all sites. The

TABLE 10.5 Hormonal Profiles of Gastrointestinal Endocrine Tumors

Product	Foregut (%+)	Midgut (%+)	Hindgut (%+)
Serotonin	30	89	13
Somatostatin	80	4	63
Substance P	10	41	0
Pancreatic polypeptide	0	0	88
Glucagon	10	0	50
Calcitonin	0	11	0
Adrenocorticotrophic hormone	20	4	0
Gastrin	30	0	0

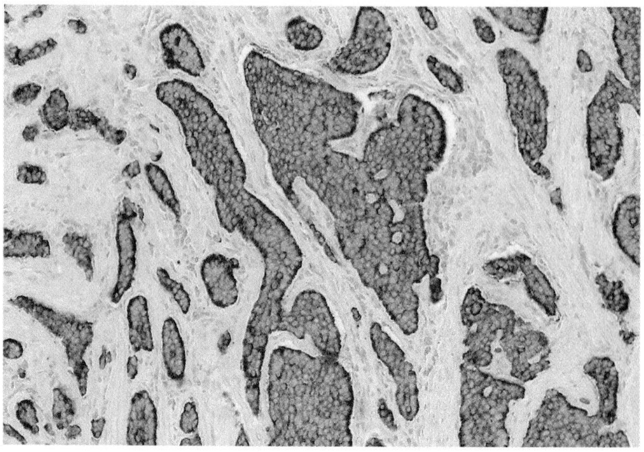

FIGURE 10.35 Ileal carcinoid tumor. Immunoperoxidase stain for chromogranin A reveals positivity in tumor cell nests.

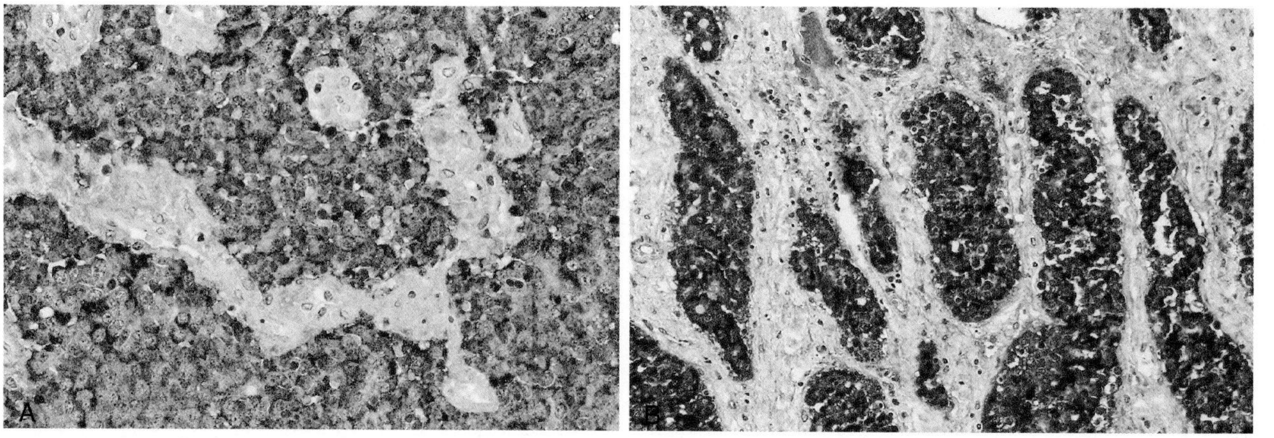

FIGURE 10.36 **A,** Metastatic carcinoid involving the liver. Immunoperoxidase stain for chromogranin A shows strong positivity in tumor cells. **B,** Metastatic carcinoid involving the liver. Immunoperoxidase stain for serotonin shows strong positivity in tumor cells.

reactivity of other NE markers differs according to the site of origin.[302] Chromogranin A is present in 88% to 100% of foregut, 100% of midgut, and 24% to 40% of hindgut GI-ETs (Figs. 10.35 and 10.36). Chromogranin B, in contrast, is present in 100% of hindgut NETs.[30,303] NESP-55, a member of the chromogranin family, is present in approximately 10% of rectal GI-ETs and is absent from GI-ETs from other sites in the GI tract; however, approximately 40% of pancreatic endocrine tumors (PETs) are positive for this marker.[33,34]

Peptidylglycine alpha-amidating enzyme has been reported in 14% of gastric, 100% of ileal, and 100% of rectal GI-ETs,[303] while NCAM is present in 76% of foregut, 58% of midgut, and 20% of hindgut tumors. Antibodies to NCAM stain both tumor cells and sustentacular elements.[303] The S-100 protein is present in 41% of foregut and 50% of midgut and hindgut tumors. The pattern of staining for S-100 is generally similar to that observed for NCAM, with reactivities present in both tumor cells and sustentacular elements.

CEA is present in approximately 40% of GI-ETs with polyclonal antisera or monoclonal antibodies, whereas CD15 is present in 30% of these tumors.[304-306] The monoclonal antibody CA15.3, which identifies both carbohydrate and peptide determinants (MUC1-type mucin), reacts with 75% of GI-ETs, whereas CA 19.9, which reacts with sialylated Lewis antigen, is negative.[146]

CDX2 has also been demonstrated in variable proportions of gastrointestinal NE tumors depending on their sites of origin (Fig. 10.37). In the study of Moskaluk and coworkers,[307] 73% of midgut and 44% of hindgut GI-ETs showed the most extensive staining for CDX2. Srivastava and coworkers reported CDX2 positivity in nearly 100% of ileal and appendiceal GI-ETs but in no gastroduodenal or rectal GI-ETs.[33] Homeobox factor-1 (PDX-1) was present in 70% of gastroduodenal, 50% of appendical, and 17% of rectal GI-ETs.[33] In addition, PDX-1 was present in almost 30% of PETs.[34]

Prostatic acid phosphatase (PAP) may be present in some GI-ET tumors. In a study of 33 GI-ETs of foregut, midgut, and hindgut origins, PAP was present in five of five hindgut tumors, whereas other cases were negative.[308] Prostate-specific antigen, in contrast, is typically negative in these tumors. The alpha chain of hCG is also present to varying extents in GI-ET tumors. Heitz and coworkers[167] reported staining for the alpha chain in 46% of foregut, 25% of hindgut, but in none of 35 midgut GI-ETs. Calbindin, a 28,000-kD calcium-binding protein has been localized to subpopulations of central and peripheral nervous system neurons, distal tubular

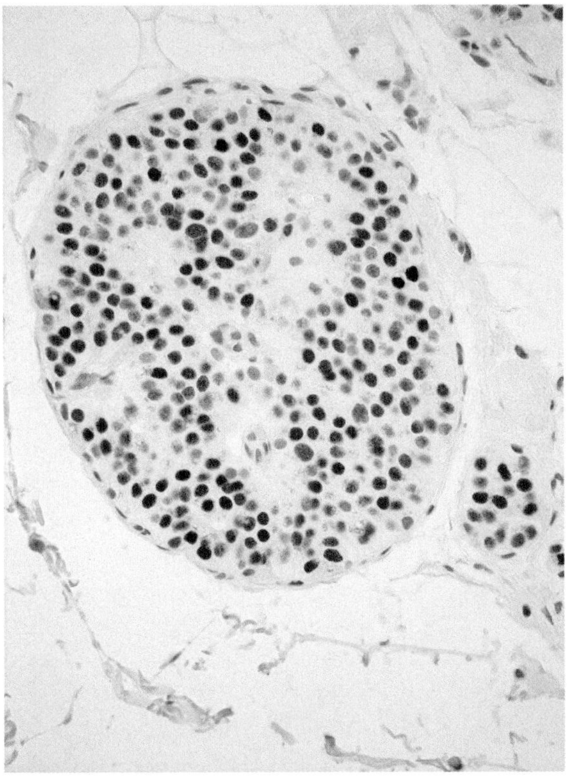

FIGURE 10.37 Ileal carcinoid tumor stained for CDX2. The nuclei of the tumor cells are strongly positive.

cells of the kidney, and enteric NE cells. Immunohistochemical studies have demonstrated that calbindin is present in a small number of NE cells, predominantly in the appendix and small intestine, and in 100% of midgut and foregut GI-ETs.[173] In contrast, calbindin immunoreactivity was absent from a single case of rectal ET.

BEYOND IMMUNOHISTOCHEMISTRY: DIAGNOSTIC MOLECULAR APPLICATIONS

Few studies have been done on the molecular features of gastrointestinal endocrine tumors. Allelic loss of 11q has been detected in GI endocrine tumors associated with MEN1, and LOH of 11q is also present in a subset of sporadic GI endocrine tumors.[309] Mutations of the MEN1 gene are present in approximately 30% of sporadic gastrinomas and in occasional midgut and hindgut endocrine tumors. In contrast to pancreatic endocrine tumors, the CpG island methylator phenotype is frequent in GI endocrine tumors. Beta-catenin exon 3 mutations are relatively common (38%) in these tumors, and up to 80% of the tumors show nuclear and cytoplasmic localization of the corresponding protein.[310] Other studies, however, reported absence of exon 3 mutations, but nuclear β-catenin was found in 30% of cases.[311] In contrast, extra-GI endocrine tumors were negative for nuclear β-catenin.

Pancreatic Endocrine Cells

Cytokeratin immunoreactivity is present in normal pancreatic endocrine cells and in approximately 90% of pancreatic endocrine tumors (PETs), whereas CK20

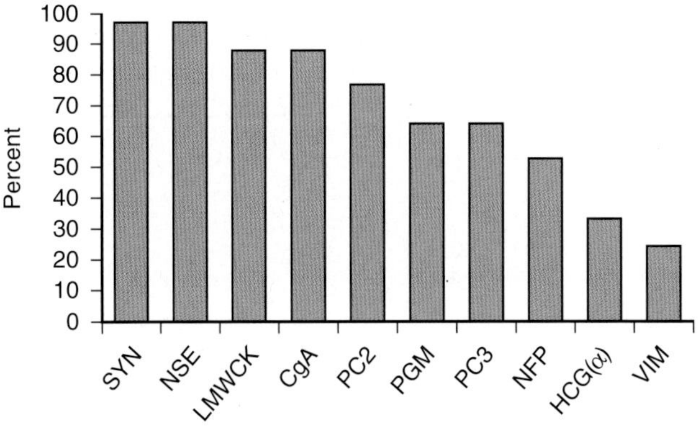

FIGURE 10.38 Distribution of markers in pancreatic endocrine tumors. SYN, synaptophysin; NSE, neuron-specific enolase; LMWCK, low-molecular-weight cytokeratin; CgA, chromogranin A; PC2, proconvertase 2; PGM, peptidylglycine alpha-amidating enzyme; PC3, proconvertase 3; NFP, neurofilament protein; HCG(α), human chorionic gonadotropin alpha; VIM, vimentin.

is present in 12.5% of cases (Fig. 10.38).[54,57,178,301,312] Vimentin has variable reactivity with approximately 25% of cases demonstrating cytoplasmic staining. Neurofilament immunoreactivity occurs in up to 50% of cases. Among NE markers, NSE and synaptophysin are present in all normal pancreatic endocrine cells and in virtually all PETs.[313] Chromogranin A is present in approximately 75% of all PETs and generally, the extent of staining correlates with the degree of granularity, as compared with sections stained for peptide hormones.[313] Calbindin and MIC2 (CD99) are expressed in a subset of PETs.[173,288]

The normal islets of Langerhans contain four major cell types.[314] The insulin-producing beta cells comprise 60% to 70% of the cells in the main part of the pancreas and 20% to 30% of the cells in the posterior head of the gland. Glucagon-producing alpha cells constitute 15% to 20% of the cells in the main portion of the gland and less than 5% of the cells in the posterior head. Somatostatin positive cells comprise 5% to 10% of the cells in the main portion of the gland and approximately 5% of the islet cell population in the posterior portion of the gland. Pancreatic polypeptide (PP) cells represent 70% of the islet cells in the posterior portion gland and 2% to 5% of the cells in the remaining islets. Approximately 10% of pancreatic endocrine cells are present in extrainsular sites, where they are distributed among ductal cells or paraductular acinar cells. Occasional serotonin-producing cells are present in large ducts and are the most likely cells of origin of true carcinoid tumors of the pancreas.

Insulinomas are typically positive for insulin and proinsulin including cases that are negative by standard histochemical stains.[314,315] Approximately 50% of insulinomas are multihormonal and may contain cells that are positive for glucagon, somatostatin, PP, gastrin, ACTH, or calcitonin. There is often considerable variation in the staining intensity for insulin, with cells containing the most abundant granules ultrastructurally giving the most intense immunoreactivity. Glucagonomas are identified on the basis of reactivity for the corresponding peptide. Both glicentin and glucagon-like

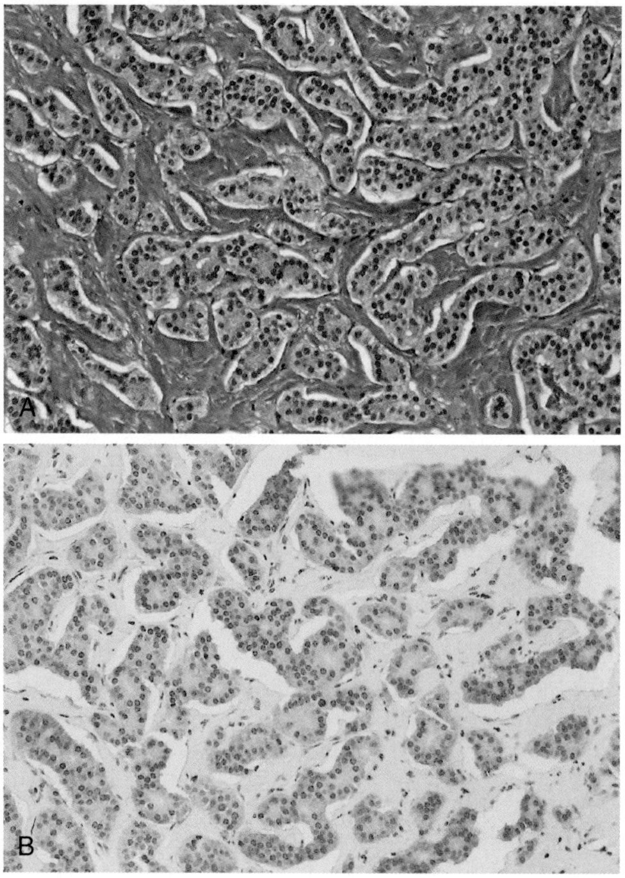

FIGURE 10.39 **A,** Pancreatic gastrinoma (H&E stain). **B,** Immunoperoxidase stain for gastrin shows weak cytoplasmic staining.

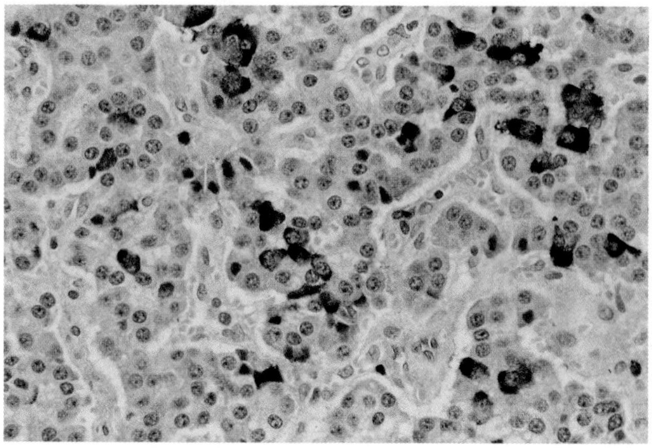

FIGURE 10.40 Nonfunctional pancreatic endocrine tumor. Immunoperoxidase stain for pancreatic polypeptide shows positivity in scattered individual tumor cells.

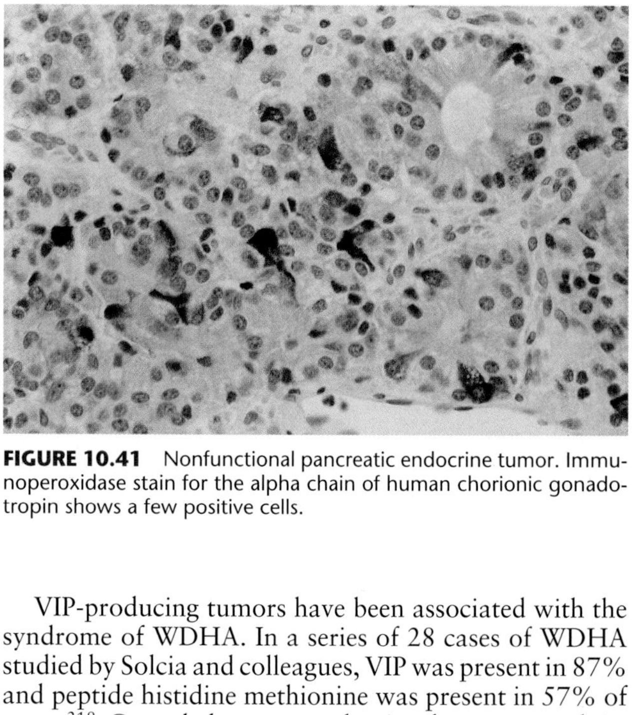

FIGURE 10.41 Nonfunctional pancreatic endocrine tumor. Immunoperoxidase stain for the alpha chain of human chorionic gonadotropin shows a few positive cells.

peptides are typically present as well. Glucagonomas may also contain peptides unrelated to proglucagon including somatostatin and insulin.

Somatostatinomas are identified on the basis of their reactivity with antibodies to somatostatin.[314] These tumors may also contain calcitonin, ACTH, and gastrin. Tumors of identical morphology and immunohistochemical profiles also occur within the duodenum. PP-producing tumors are generally classified among nonfunctional tumors, although rarely these tumors may be associated with the syndrome of watery diarrhea, hypokalemia, and achlorhydria (WDHA). In addition to their content of PP, these tumors may contain scattered cells with other hormonal peptides.

Gastrinomas are characterized by varying degrees of immunoreactivity for gastrin; however, some of these tumors may be nonreactive (Fig. 10.39).[314,315] In the latter instance, antibodies to different regions of the N- and C-terminal portions of the gastrin molecule may be positive. Some gastrinomas that may be entirely negative for gastrin may give positive signals for gastrin mRNA in *in situ* hybridization formats.[316] Gastrinomas, similar to other pancreatic endocrine tumors, may contain scattered cells positive for glucagon, PP, insulin, somatostatin, serotonin, or ACTH.[317] Gastrinomas may also occur in a variety of extrapancreatic sites including the duodenum.[314]

VIP-producing tumors have been associated with the syndrome of WDHA. In a series of 28 cases of WDHA studied by Solcia and colleagues, VIP was present in 87% and peptide histidine methionine was present in 57% of cases.[318] Growth hormone–releasing hormone and PP were present in 50% and 53% of cases, respectively.[318] In addition to pancreatic endocrine tumors, ganglioneuromas and ganglioneuroblastomas have been associated with the syndrome of WDHA.

Rare examples of serotonin-producing endocrine tumors may occur within the pancreas. Other tumors occurring as primary pancreatic endocrine tumors may produce growth hormone–releasing hormone (acromegaly), ACTH (Cushing's syndrome), and PTH or PTH-like peptide (hypercalcemia). Nonfunctional pancreatic endocrine tumors may contain scattered cells positive for a variety of hormones, most commonly PP and glucagon (Fig. 10.40).

The alpha chain of hCG has been regarded as a marker of malignancy in pancreatic endocrine tumors and occurs in approximately 70% of cases (Fig. 10.41).[319] More recent studies, however, have also demonstrated immunoreactivity for this marker in benign endocrine pancreatic tumors.[320] Progesterone receptor protein is present in a significant proportion of pancreatic endocrine tumors.[321]

The MIB-1 labeling index has been used as a predictor of survival in several studies of pancreatic endocrine tumors and has been included as a criterion in the WHO Classification of these tumors.[322,323] Positive staining for CK19 has also been regarded as a marker of malignancy in pancreatic endocrine tumors. In a study of MIB-1 and CK19 in a series of PETs, Deshpande and coworkers[324] demonstrated that the expression of each marker was significant prognostically by univariate analysis. However, by multivariate analysis, only the expression of CK19 was significant. Loss of CD99 expression has also been associated with a poor prognosis in PETs.[325] In a correlative study of the expression of a variety of markers and the 2004 WHO criteria, Schmitt and colleagues[326] demonstrated that CK19 was a useful prognostic marker independent of the WHO criteria. However, there was no prognostic significance of COX2, p27, or CD99 expression. Most recently, LaRosa and coworkers[327] demonstrated that CK19 expression correlated with patient survival only when detected with the RCK108 antibody and mainly in insulinomas. Moreover, they demonstrated that the MIB-1 index and the presence of metastases were the only two independent predictors of survival.

The expression of neuro D1 and mammalian achaete-scute complex-like protein (MASH) have been assessed in gastroenteropancreatic (GEP) tumors.[328] These studies have demonstrated that MASH-1 is highly expressed in poorly differentiated GEP tumors, whereas neuroD1 is present in all well-differentiated carcinomas and tumors. Interestingly, low levels of neuroD1 expression were seen in approximately one third of poorly differentiated GEP carcinomas and this feature was associated with a significantly shorter overall survival.

BEYOND IMMUNOHISTOCHEMISTRY: MOLECULAR DIAGNOSTIC APPLICATIONS

Pancreatic endocrine tumors (PETs) occur with increased frequency in patients with MEN1 and VHL and are considerably less common in association with NF1 or tuberous sclerosis.[329] However, the vast majority of these tumors are sporadic. There are relatively few expression array studies of these tumors. Couvelard and coworkers demonstrated 71 upregulated and 51 downregulated genes in malignant PETs including genes related to (1) angiogenesis and remodeling (CD34, cadherin-5, E-selectin, semaphorin-E, fibrillin); (2) signal transduction via tyrosine kinase (tyrosine kinase-2, PDGF-RB, MKK4, discoidin domain receptor-1); (3) calcium-dependent cell signaling (transient receptor potential cation channel-1, calcium channel voltage dependent beta-2, neurocalcium delta, GABA-A receptor gamma-2); and (4) responses to drugs (MDR1 and CEA related cell adhesion molecule).[329] By using tissue arrays, the authors confirmed the differential expression of CD34, E-selectin, MKK4, and MDR1 in metastatic versus nonmetastatic tumors.

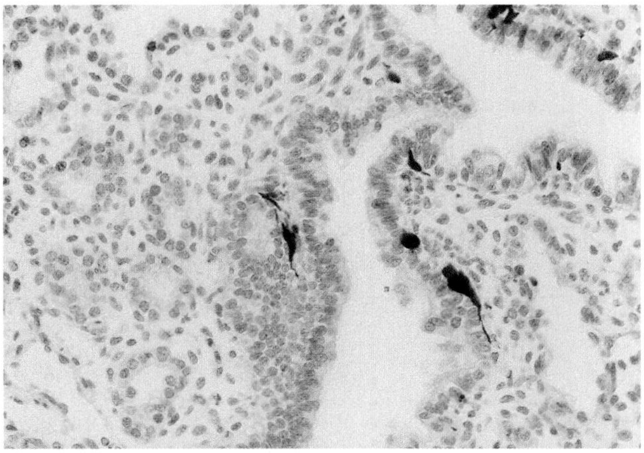

FIGURE 10-42 Fetal lung. Immunoperoxidase stain for gastrin-releasing peptide shows positivity in single cells.

Almost all PETs in MEN1 demonstrate allelic loss of the MEN1 gene, whereas somatic mutations of MEN1 occur in approximately 20% of sporadic PETs.[330] Mutations are present in approximately 10% of insulinomas and nonfunctioning tumors but are more common in gastrinomas, glucagonomas, and VIPomas. In contrast, almost 70% of PETs demonstrate losses at 11q13. This suggests that there might be haploinsufficiency of the MEN1 gene or that the other allele might be inactivated by epigenetic mechanisms. CpG island methylation in the MEN1 promoter, however, has not been identified. An alternative explanation is that this region of chromosome 11 might contain other tumor suppressor genes. Mutations of the VHL gene are uncommon in PETs despite the relatively high rates of LOH of 3p25. Moreover, p16, PTEN, k-RAS, p53, and DPC4 are only occasionally mutated in these tumors.[330]

Pulmonary Endocrine Cells

The NE cells of the lung are present as single cells and as small cell clusters that have been termed *neuroepithelial bodies.*[331] Neuroepithelial bodies may have a chemoreceptor function, in which single NE cells may act as paracrine elements. A variety of regulatory products including serotonin, gastrin-releasing peptide, and calcitonin are present both in single NE cells and in neuroepithelial bodies, while leu-enkephalin is present only in single NE cells (Fig. 10.42).[331] Pulmonary NE cells may undergo a series of hyperplastic changes in response to irritation or after exposure to carcinogens. Generally, hyperplastic NE cells retain the patterns of expression of regulatory products characteristic of their normal counterparts. More severe forms of hyperplasia and dysplasia are accompanied by the production of ectopic products including VIP and different molecular forms of ACTH.

NE tumors of the lung include four major entities that can be distinguished on the basis of morphology and immunohistochemistry.[332] The tumor types include typical carcinoids, atypical carcinoids, small cell carcinomas, and large cell NE carcinomas. The marker profiles for these tumors are summarized in Figures 10.43 through 10.46. Occasional pulmonary NE tumors may contain peptides such as calcitonin (Fig. 10-47). Approximately

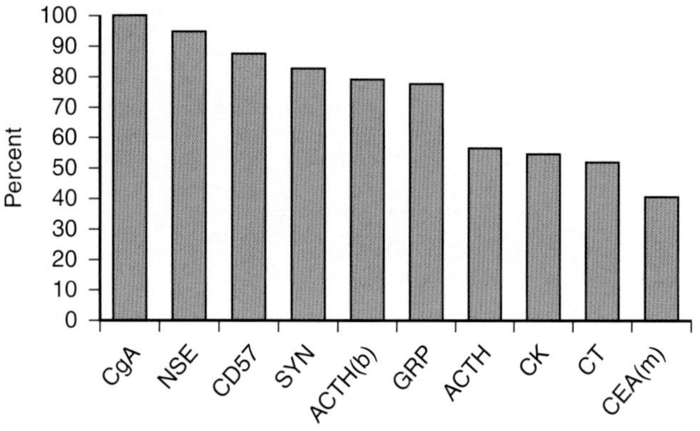

FIGURE 10.43 Distribution of markers in typical lung carcinoid. CgA, chromogranin A; NSE, neuron-specific enolase; SYN, synaptophysin; ACTH (b), big adrenocorticotropic hormone; GRP, gastrin-releasing peptide; CK, cytokeratin; CT, calcitonin; CEA(m), monoclonal carcinoembryonic antigen.

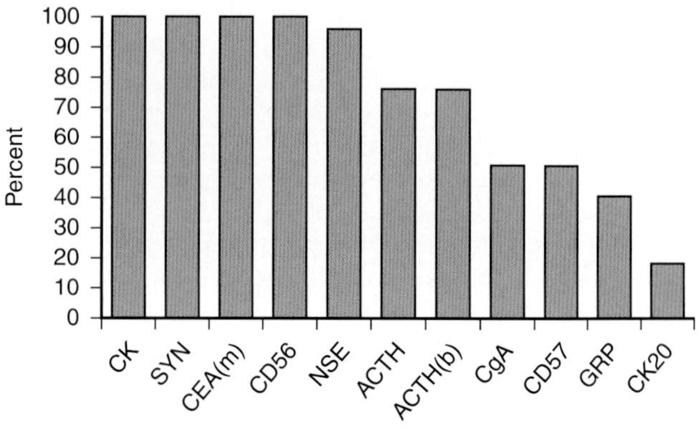

FIGURE 10.45 Distribution of markers in small cell carcinoma. CK, cytokeratin; SYN, synaptophysin; CEA(m), monoclonal carcinoembryonic antigen; NSE, neuron-specific enolase; ACTH (b), big adrenocorticotropic hormone; CgA, chromogranin A; GRP, gastrin-releasing peptide.

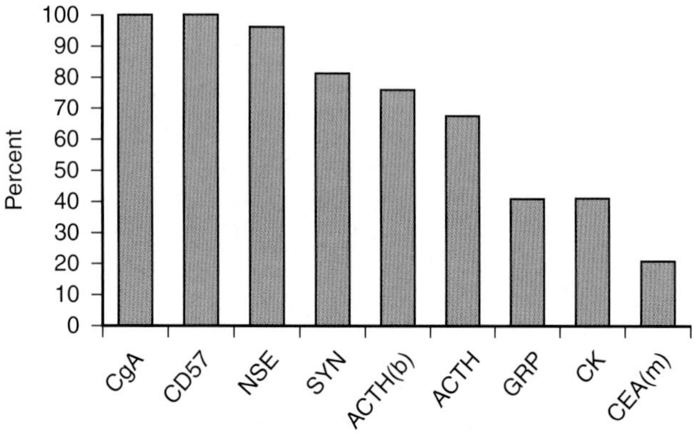

FIGURE 10.44 Distribution of markers in atypical lung carcinoid. CgA, chromogranin A; NSE, neuron-specific enolase; SYN, synaptophysin; ACTH (b), big adrenocorticotropic hormone; GRP, gastrin-releasing peptide; CK, cytokeratin; CEA(m), monoclonal carcinoembryonic antigen.

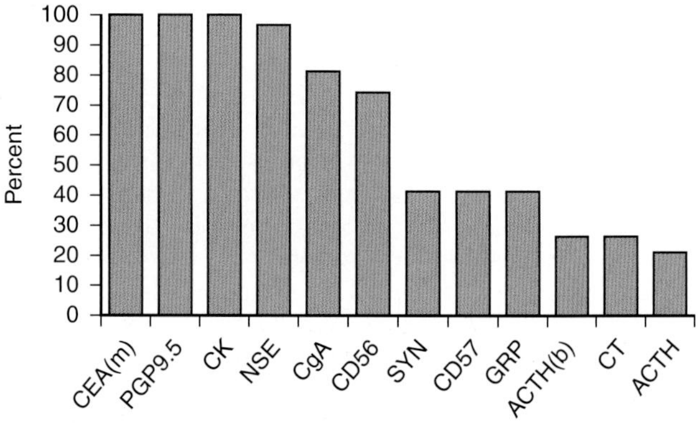

FIGURE 10.46 Distribution of markers in large cell NE carcinoma. CEA(m), monoclonal carcinoembryonic antigen; PGP, protein gene product 9.5; CK, cytokeratin; NSE, neuron-specific enolase; CgA, chromogranin A; SYN, synaptophysin; GRP, gastrin-releasing peptide; ACTH (b), big adrenocorticotropic hormone; CT, calcitonin.

85% of pulmonary NE tumors are reactive with antibodies to low-molecular-weight cytokeratins.[332,333] In the series reported by Travis and associates,[332] reactivity with broad-spectrum keratin antibodies (AE1/AE3) was present in 56% of typical carcinoids, 40% of atypical carcinoids, and 100% of small cell carcinomas and large cell NE carcinomas. Eighty-two percent of small cell carcinomas were negative for CK7 and CK20.[55]

TTF-1 is present in normal pulmonary NE cells and is a useful marker for the identification of pulmonary NE tumors. However, TTF-1 is present in small cell carcinomas arising in a variety of extrapulmonary sites (Table 10.6). Most studies report TTF-1 positivity in more than 90% of pulmonary small cell NE carcinomas. In the study of Oliveira and colleagues,[334] TTF-1 was present in 19 of 20 (95%) well-differentiated pulmonary NE tumors (including typical and atypical carcinoids) and in 8 of 10 (80%) metastases of these tumors. On the other hand, Du and colleagues[335] reported TTF-1 positivity in 28%, 29%, and 37% of typical carcinoids, atypical carcinoids, and large cell NE carcinomas, respectively. Interestingly, TTF-1 positivity was more commonly present in peripheral carcinoids of spindle cell type than in central carcinoids.[335] Rarely, TTF-1 may be present in gastrointestinal and pancreatic NE tumors.[336]

Chromogranin A is present in 100% of typical and atypical carcinoids, in 80% of large cell NE carcinomas, and in up to 50% of small cell carcinomas, depending on the antigen retrieval method and sensitivity of the detection method.[332] Synaptophysin is present in 84% of typical carcinoids, 80% of atypical carcinoids, 40% of large cell NE carcinomas, and 100% of small cell carcinomas. CD57 immunoreactivity is present in 89% of typical carcinoids, 100% of atypical carcinoids, and 40% and 50% of large cell NE carcinomas and small cell carcinomas, respectively. Pulmonary tumorlets are also positive for CD57 (Fig. 10.48). CEA (monoclonal) is present in 100% of large cell NE carcinomas and small cell carcinomas, 42% of typical carcinoids, and 20% of atypical carcinoids. Jiang and colleagues[337] also studied large cell NE carcinomas and confirmed the findings of Travis and coworkers.[332] In addition, Jiang and coworkers[337] reported positivity for PGP9.5 in 100% of the cases and positivity for TuJ1 (neuron-specific class III beta-tubulin) in 82%. NCAM positivity was present in 73%.[337]

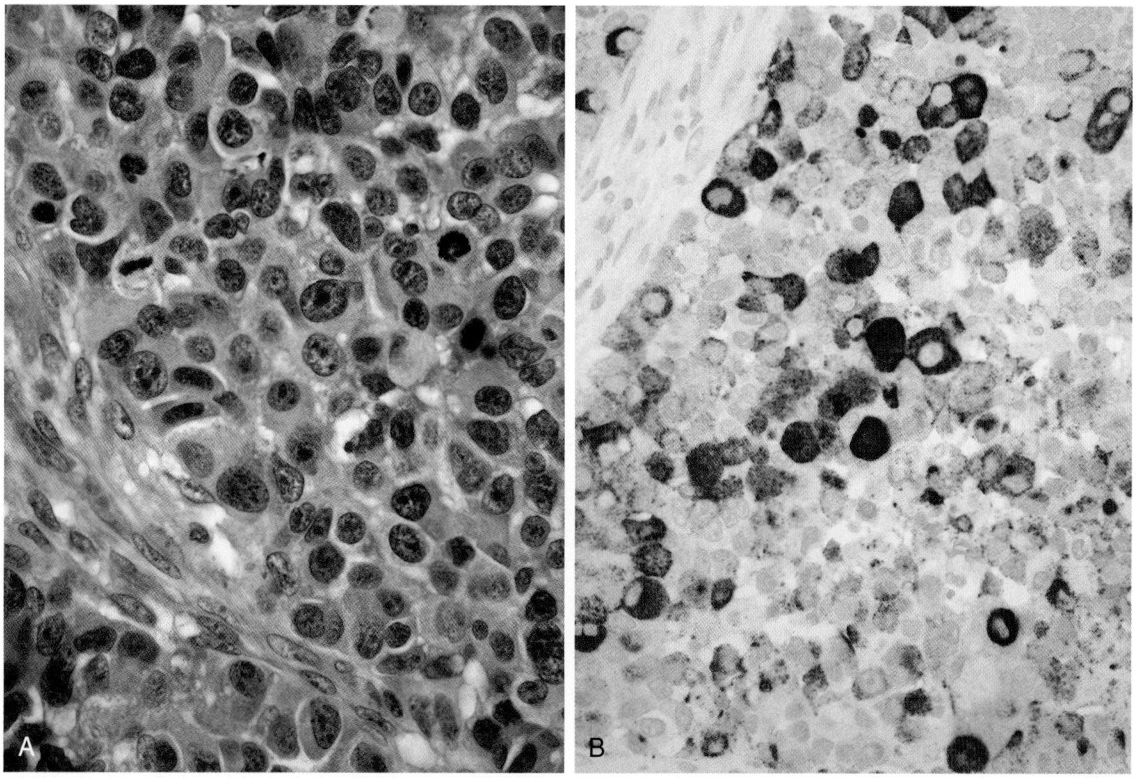

FIGURE 10.47 Pulmonary large cell NE carcinoma. **A,** H&E. **B,** Immunoperoxidase stain for calcitonin. Many of the tumor cells are strongly positive.

TABLE 10.6 Immunohistochemical Profile of Small Cell Carcinoma of Various Sites*

Anatomic Site/Origin	TTF-1	CK7	CK20	ER/PR	PSA	PAP
Lung	+	S	S	–	–	–
Prostate	+	S	S	–	S	S
Bladder	S	–	–	–	–	–
Breast	S	+	–	S	–	–
Gastrointestinal	S	?	–	–	–	–
Salivary gland	–	?	S	–	–	–
Cervix	S	?	S	?	–	–
Skin (Merkel cell)	–	–	+	–	–	–

+, almost always positive; S, sometimes positive; –, negative.
*Neuroendocrine-specific markers such as chromogranin and synaptophysin are variably positive in all tumors regardless of site and are therefore not useful for this purpose.
TTF-1, thyroid transcription factor-1; CK, cytokeratin; ER, estrogen receptor, PR, progesterone receptor; PSA, prostate-specific antigen; PAP, prostatic acid phosphatase.

BEYOND IMMUNOHISTOCHEMISTRY: MOLECULAR DIAGNOSTIC APPLICATIONS

Xu and colleagues[338] suggested the use of antibodies to KOC (K-homology domain containing protein overexpressed in cancer), a member of the insulin growth factor messenger RNA-binding protein family, in the diagnosis of high-grade NE carcinomas of the lung and their distinction from carcinoids.[338] In their study, all high-grade NE carcinomas of the lung had diffuse or focal cytoplasmic positivity for KOC and the typical and atypical carcinoids were largely negative (a single atypical carcinoid with oncocytic cells showed weak cytoplasmic staining). In addition, high-grade NE carcinomas were more likely to express c-kit and bcl-2 when compared with carcinoid tumors. LaPoint and colleagues[339] found that all high-grade NE carcinomas (small cell carcinomas and large cell NE carcinomas of the lung) coexpressed c-kit and bcl-2, while all atypical and typical carcinoids were negative for c-kit and only 6.3% of typical carcinoids and 16.7% of atypical carcinoids were positive for bcl-2. These findings suggest a future possible therapeutic role in targeting of these two molecules in patients with high-grade NE carcinomas of the lung.

Collapsin response mediator proteins (CRMPs) include a family of five members that are involved in

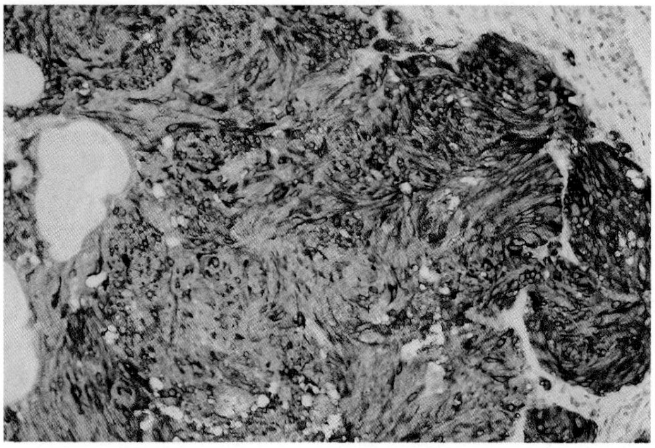

FIGURE 10.48 Pulmonary tumorlet. Immunoperoxidase stain for CD57 shows positivity in lesional cells.

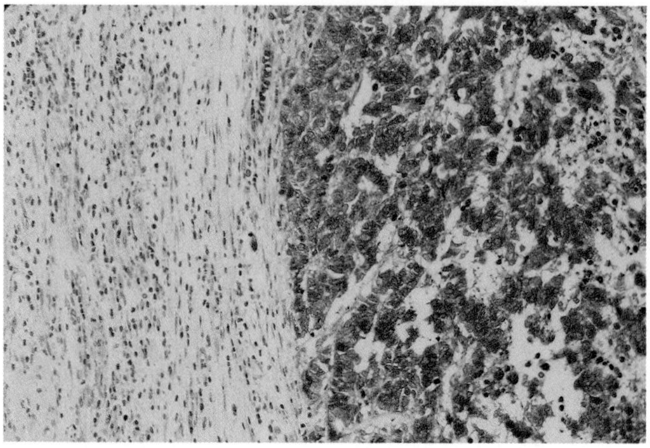

FIGURE 10.49 Large cell (neuroendocrine) carcinoma of the cervix. Immunoperoxidase stain for neuron-specific enolase shows positivity in tumor cells.

the semaphorin signaling pathway during neurogenesis. CRMP5 is involved in the development of neural tissue, and antibodies to CRMP5 have been used as serologic markers of SCLC in the setting of paraneoplastic neurologic disorders.[340] CRMP5 is expressed strongly and extensively in 98% of high-grade pulmonary NE tumors including small and large cell NE tumors but not in adenocarcinomas or squamous carcinomas. In contrast to the high frequency of strong positivity in high-grade pulmonary NE carcinomas, most pulmonary carcinoids and atypical carcinoids were negative or weakly reactive for this marker.

Endocrine Tumors in Other Sites

CERVIX

Carcinoids, atypical carcinoids, small cell carcinomas, and large cell NE carcinomas have been reported as primary cervical tumors.[341-343] All small cell cervical carcinomas studied to date have been cytokeratin-positive, and more than 90% have been positive for EMA. Reactivity for CEA with polyclonal antisera occurs in 77%. Small cell cervical carcinomas are positive for CK20 or TTF-1 in 14.3% and 20% of cases, respectively.[96,344,345] With respect to NE markers, NSE is present in 95%, synaptophysin in 46%, chromogranin A in 43%, and CD57 in 37%. Similar frequencies of positivity for NE markers have been reported in more recent studies.[346-348] These tumors may also contain peptide and amine hormones including serotonin (31%), ACTH (23%), and somatostatin (8%).

Chromogranin A immunoreactivity has been reported in all large cell NE cervical carcinomas.[239] In this study, synaptophysin staining was present in 66% of cases and NSE occurred in 50% (Fig. 10.49). Occasional serotonin-positive cells were present in 50% of cases, whereas somatostatin-positive cells were present in 37%. Seventy-five percent of cases contained CEA, as demonstrated with a monoclonal antibody.

Stoler and associates[349] demonstrated human papillomavirus 18 (HPV18) in 78% of small cell cervical carcinomas with NE differentiation. The presence of this papilloma subtype was five times more frequent than HPV-16 in the 20 cases studied. Ishida and coworkers[350] found that of 10 small cell NE carcinomas of the cervix, HPV-18 was detected in all three pure cases and in five of seven mixed tumors (mixed small cell and adenocarcinomas). No other HPV types were detected even though types 6, 11, 16, 31, 33, 42, 52, and 58 were also investigated. Other studies have confirmed the high frequency of HPV-18 in these tumors.[347,351]

Unlike small cell carcinomas, large cell NE carcinomas of the uterine cervix appear to be associated with HPV-16 infection.[352,353] In addition, overexpression of p16, a cyclin-dependent kinase inhibitor associated with HPV infection, has been noted in almost all cases.[347,351]

Effective treatment options for primary cervical NE tumors are lacking and despite multiple studies, reliable prognostic and predictive factors have not been identified.[357,354] Tangitgamol and colleagues[355] only found expression of HER2/neu to be significantly associated with survival of patients with cervical small cell carcinomas and large cell NE carcinomas. Patients whose tumors lacked HER2/neu expression had significantly shorter survival than those with HER2/neu-positive tumors. Immunostains for epidermal growth factor receptor, vascular endothelial growth factor, cyclooxygenase-2, estrogen receptor, and progesterone receptor did not show consistent expression related to survival in these patients. In contrast, Straughn and coworkers[346] did not find any HER2/neu expression in any of their series of cervical small cell NE carcinomas studied. Zarka and coworkers studied four cases of cervical small cell carcinomas by immunohistochemistry and found that all tumors exhibited a unique profile with E-cadherin, P-cadherin, N-cadherin, bcl-2, and p53.[356] The only commonality among these tumors was the absence of N-cadherin immunoreactivity. The authors suggested that because 65% of small cell carcinomas from other sites reportedly exhibit expression for N-cadherin, this differential staining pattern could be used to distinguish primary small cell carcinoma of the cervix from metastatic disease.

PROSTATE

Normal prostatic epithelium contains subpopulations of NE cells that can be identified on the basis of their contents of NSE, chromogranin, peptide hormones, and

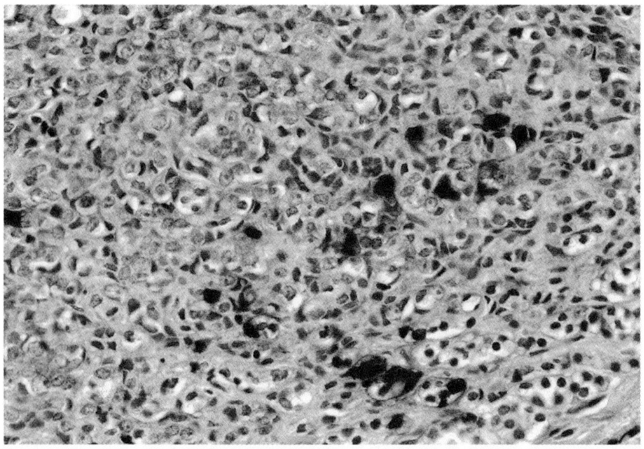

FIGURE 10.50 Metastatic prostatic adenocarcinoma with neuroendocrine cells. Immunoperoxidase stain for chromogranin A shows positivity in a few tumor cells.

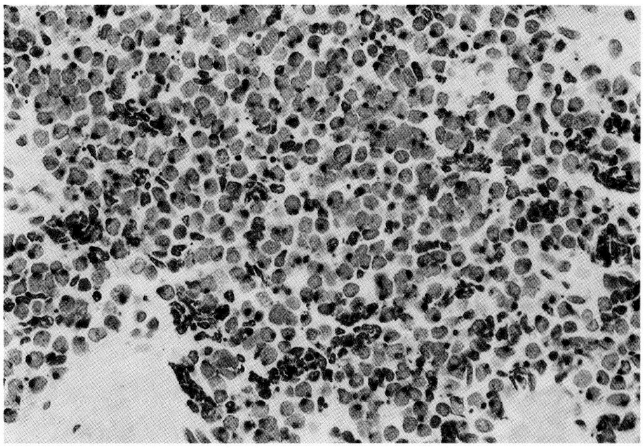

FIGURE 10.51 Merkel cell carcinoma. Immunoperoxidase stain for cytokeratin 20 shows a dotlike pattern of staining.

serotonin.[357-359] These cells are involved in regulating epithelial cell growth and differentiation in an androgen-independent manner.[360] Prostatic neoplasms with NE differentiation include carcinoids, small cell carcinomas, and "usual" adenocarcinomas with subpopulations of NE cells. "Pure" NE neoplasms such as carcinoids and small cell carcinomas are rare and comprise less than 5% of all prostatic malignancies.[345,361-367] Small cell carcinomas of the prostate are TTF-1 positive in approximately 50% of cases (Table 10.6),[96,345] whereas more than 200 conventional prostatic adenocarcinomas with high Gleason scores were negative for this marker.[364] CD44 appears to be a useful marker to discriminate prostatic small cell NE carcinomas from Gleason 5 pattern adenocarcinomas and small cell carcinomas of other origins.[368] The origin of prostatic carcinomas with NE cells remains unclear, although some studies support the concept that they arise from multipotential prostatic stem cells as evidenced by the coexpression of both NE and prostate-specific markers.[362,365,366] Moreover, NE cells from normal and hyperplastic prostates express BCL-2. There is a positive correlation between the expression of BCL-2 and NE markers in prostatic carcinomas with NE differentiation. In addition, α-methylacyl-CoA racemase (AMACR) is expressed in the NE components of carcinomas with NE cells but not in normal NE cells.[360]

NE differentiation in conventional prostatic carcinomas occurs in approximately 10% of cases in which, at least focally, prominent collections of neoplastic NE cells may be evident.[361] The presence of NE differentiation may be more prognostically significant in androgen-independent tumors and metastatic tumors than in hormone-sensitive and locally recurrent tumors.[358] Androgen withdrawal contributes to increased NE differentiation in prostatic carcinomas. In adenocarcinomas with NE cells, 54% contain serotonin, 46% are positive for NSE, 65% are positive for chromogranin (Fig. 10.50), and 22% are positive for hCG. Somatostatin, calcitonin, and ACTH are present in less than 5% of cases.[367] Schmid and coworkers[359] demonstrated that the pattern of chromogranin distribution is correlated with tumor grade. Grade I tumors show positive reactions for chromogranins A and B and secretogranin II, with colocalization of all three products in the majority of NE cells. In grade II and grade III tumors, in contrast, chromogranin B is the predominant granin.

Scattered NE cells have been demonstrated in up to 88% of cases of high-grade prostatic intraepithelial neoplasia.[367] The highest proportion of cases is immunoreactive for serotonin (73%), NSE (67%), chromogranin (62%), and hCG (30%).

The results of molecular studies have demonstrated identical allelic profiles in NE and nonendocrine cells of prostatic carcinomas.[369] These findings support the concept of trans-differentiation of exocrine tumor cells to cells with an NE phenotype. Activation of the ERK/MAPK pathway appears to be one of the major mechanisms for the transdifferentiation of prostatic carcinoma cells into cells with NE differentiation.

SKIN

Merkel cell (NE) carcinoma of the skin is an uncommon entity that was first described as trabecular carcinoma.[370] These tumors are uniformly positive for broad-spectrum cytokeratins and stain positively for CK20 in 97% of cases, with a dotlike pattern of reactivity (Fig. 10.51, Table 10.5).[301,344] This high frequency of CK20 immunoreactivity has been confirmed in many other studies.[371-374] Other small cell malignancies that may exhibit CK20 positivity include pulmonary small cell carcinomas (2%), small cell cervical carcinomas (9%), and small cell carcinomas of salivary gland origin (60%). Nagao and coworkers[375] recently reported that 11 of 15 (73%) cases of small cell carcinomas originating in the salivary gland were CK20 positive, and almost all had a paranuclear dotlike pattern of reactivity. Cheuk and coworkers[372] reported lack of CK20 immunoreactivity in small cell carcinomas from various sites including gastrointestinal, pancreas, prostate, bladder, thymus, and orbit with the exception of two cases originating in the cervix/vagina. Cytokeratin 7 has been reported to be positive in 25% of cases of Merkel cell carcinoma, but none of the cases was positive for CK5/6 or CK17.[376] Seventy-eight percent of Merkel cell carcinomas are positive for EMA.[377] Microtubule-associated protein is also

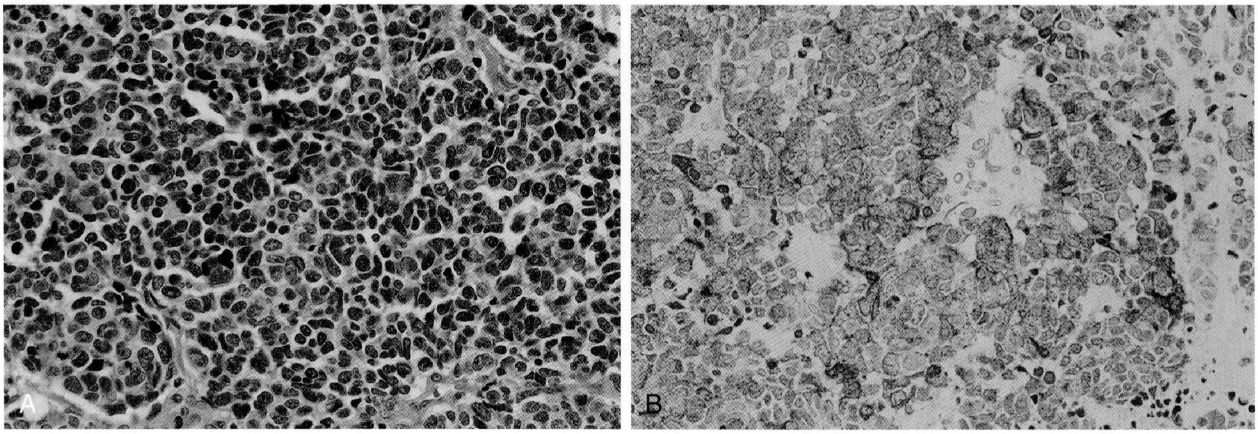

FIGURE 10.52 **A,** Small cell (neuroendocrine) carcinoma of the breast (H&E). **B,** Immunoperoxidase stain for chromogranin A shows moderately intense cytoplasmic staining.

present in these tumors,[378] but TTF-1 is typically negative.[96] Virtually all Merkel cell carcinomas are positive for NSE, whereas chromogranins B and A are found in 100% and 72% of the tumors, respectively.[379] CD56 is also highly expressed in these tumors.[380] Secretoneurin, which is derived from secretogranin II, is present in 22% of cases, while synaptophysin is present in 39%.[381] Merkel cell tumors are variably positive for CD99, and in the series reported by Nicholson and associates, 12 of 30 cases (40%) were positive for this marker.[374] In nine cases that were consistent with Merkel cell carcinoma clinically, CD99 was positive and CK20 was negative.[374] Several studies have reported the expression of terminal deoxynucleotidyl transferase (TdT) in up to 70% of Merkel cell carcinomas.[382,383] In addition to TdT, PAX-5, a B-cell specific activation protein, is commonly expressed in these tumors.[384]

Some studies have shown c-kit positivity in up to 95% of cases.[385-387] Pulmonary small cell carcinomas may also be positive for c-kit.[385] Nuclear localization of E-cadherin immunoreactivity has been reported in Merkel cell carcinomas and may have diagnostic utility for this entity.[388,389]

An additional approach to the distinction of Merkel cell tumors from small cell pulmonary carcinomas involves the use of antibodies to the mammalian achaete-scute complex-like protein (MASH). Although more than 80% of small cell pulmonary carcinomas are MASH positive, only 1 of 30 Merkel cell carcinomas was positive for this marker.[390] Merkel cell carcinomas also express the K homology domain containing protein (KOC), similar to other high-grade NE malignancies.[391]

Molecular alterations underlying the development and progression of Merkel cell carcinomas are poorly understood. Recently, Feng and coworkers[392] reported the identification of a fifth human polyoma virus that was designated Merkel cell polyomavirus on the basis of its detection in Merkel cell carcinomas. A subsequent study by Kassem and colleagues[393] analyzed 39 Merkel cell carcinomas and found the presence of Merkel cell polyomavirus DNA in 77% of cases. This study was limited in that the use of formalin-fixed paraffin tissues prevented the investigators from testing whether the viral DNA was integrated or not. However, their findings together with the above-reported findings of 80% Merkel cell polyomavirus DNA-positive Merkel cell carcinomas with clonal integration suggest Merkel cell polyomavirus as a putative etiologic agent in the development of these tumors.

C-kit positivity in these tumors has led to investigations of the efficacy of imatinib, a specific inhibitor of tyrosine kinases.[394] This agent has been shown to decrease proliferation of Merkel cell carcinomas cells *in vitro*.[395]

BREAST

NE tumors of the breast include carcinoids and NE carcinomas of small cell type (Fig. 10.52).[396-399] These tumors, as well as breast carcinomas with focal NE differentiation, are thought by some to arise from NE cells that form a small, intrinsic component of the normal breast epithelium, whereas others claim that there are no such indigenous cell types in the breast.[400,401] Primary mammary NE carcinoma is now recognized as a distinct entity and has been added to the World Health Organization (WHO) Classification of Tumors (2003) under the category of NE tumors.[402] This category includes solid NE carcinoma, small cell/oat cell carcinoma, and large-cell NE carcinoma. Small cell carcinomas are typically positive for cytokeratins including AE1/AE3 (91%), CAM5.2 (82%), CK7 (78%), and CK19 (78%), whereas stains for CK20 are negative (Table 10.6).[403] These tumors may not exhibit a typical NE phenotype, and immunoreactivity for various markers has been reported as variable. It should be stressed, however, that the diagnosis of mammary small-cell carcinoma is not contingent on the demonstration of NE differentiation by immunohistochemistry, as is true for small cell carcinomas of other sites such as the lung.[403] Among NE markers, NSE is present in 90%, whereas synaptophysin and chromogranin occur in 56% and 41% of cases, respectively (see Fig. 10.52B). CD56 and CD57 have been noted in 78% and 43% of cases, respectively.

Immunoreactivity for calcitonin occurs in 27% of cases, whereas stains for gastrin-releasing peptide and serotonin have been reported in 39% and 14%, of cases, respectively. Estrogen and progesterone receptor positivity have been reported in 54%, and 45%, respectively. Bcl-2 is consistently positive, but stains for HER-2/neu are negative.[403] CD 99 has been reported in 3 of 3 cases of small cell carcinomas and cell membrane immunoreactivity for E-cadherin in 11 of 12 (92%) of reported cases.[404-406]

Weigelt and colleagues[407] analyzed 113 special types of breast cancer including NE carcinomas by gene expression profiling including hierarchical clustering analysis in an attempt to refine breast cancer classification and improve patient stratification. Results from this study included the identification of a family of cancers with endocrine/NE features existing within the larger group of "luminal" cancers. The "luminal" type is part of three major subtypes (the other being basal-like and HER2+) that comprise a widely applied molecular classification of breast cancers by gene expression profiling that are distinct in their transcriptomic features and patient outcomes.[407-409] The results of Weigelt and colleagues suggest that the panel of subtypes as defined by WHO criteria can be condensed and thus simplified on the basis of their molecular profiles. Ideally, this would lead to refinement in prognostication and development of tailored therapies for breast cancer patients.[407,410]

THYMUS

Thymic NE tumors include carcinoids, atypical carcinoids, and small cell carcinomas. Morphologically, individual tumors often show admixtures of these growth patterns.[411-413] They are typically positive for cytokeratins (AE1/AE3 and CAM5.2)[411-413] and express a wide variety of NE markers including NSE (100%), synaptophysin (81%), chromogranins (75%), and CD57 (67.5%). They may also be positive for glycoprotein and peptide hormones and amines including alpha HCG (100%), beta HCG (37.5%), somatostatin (36%), ACTH (32%), cholecystokinin (18%), calcitonin (11%), serotonin (5%), and CGRP (25%).[303,413-417] In contrast to pulmonary NE tumors, thymic NE tumors are negative for TTF-1 (Table 10.6).[334,335]

Few studies have investigated the molecular profiles of thymic NE tumors. Using comparative genomic hybridization, Pan and colleagues[418] studied 11 tumors (10 sporadic; 1 MEN1 associated). Genomic alterations were identified in nine cases with gains in chromosomes X, 8, 18, and 20p and losses in chromosomes 6,13q, 13p 9q, and 11q.

The chromosomal aberrations detected in the single MEN1 associated case were dissimilar from those of the sporadic cases. Additionally, there was no evidence of 11q13 deletion, the locus of the MEN1 gene. This is in marked contrast to the high frequency of allelic losses on 11q in both sporadic and MEN-associated NE tumors in other (foregut) sites (2). These findings support the fundamental molecular divergence between thymic and other foregut NE tumors. Theoretically, molecular characterization could be used in a diagnostic setting to distinguish a primary thymic NE tumor from a metastasis of a nonthymic foregut primary.

Rieker and coworkers[419] evaluated 10 thymic NE tumors (5 atypical carcinoids, 4 typical carcinoids, 1 spindle cell carcinoid) by immunohistochemistry and comparative genomic hybridization. Chromosomal imbalances were detected in 8 of 10 cases with the most frequent gains on chromosome Xp and 7p, 7q, 11q, 12q, and 20q. Losses were most frequently found in 6q, 6p, 4q, 3p, 10q, 11q, and 13q. These results demonstrated a degree of overlap, with chromosomal imbalances commonly observed in advanced thymomas, suggesting a genetic/evolutionary relationship between thymic NE and non-NE tumors.

SUMMARY

Even though the range of NE neoplasms in various sites has common themes, the immunohistologic profiles tend to be unique to the various anatomic sites. The challenge remains to recognize tumors by standard histologic stains along with clinical data and apply appropriate panels of immunohistochemistry as described earlier to arrive at a correct diagnosis. Genomic and theranostic applications of NE tumors are taking on a new, important role in patient management, and molecular data may be extremely useful to enhance diagnostic accuracy and prognostic assessment.

ACKNOWLEDGMENTS

The authors wish to acknowledge the assistance of Path/Iq ImmunoQuery for some of the data provided in the bar graphs.

The authors also thank Ms. Joanne Harker for her help in the preparation of this manuscript.

REFERENCES

1. Erickson LA, Lloyd RV. Practical markers used in the diagnosis of endocrine tumors. *Adv Anat Pathol.* 2004;11:175-189.
2. DeLellis RA. Endocrine tumors. In: Colvin RB, Bhan AK, McCluskey RT, eds. *Diagnostic Immunopathology.* New York: Raven Press; 1995:551-578.
3. DeLellis RA, Wolfe HJ. Analysis of gene expression in endocrine cells. In: Fenoglio-Preiser CM, Williman CL, eds. *Molecular Diagnostics in Pathology.* Baltimore: Williams & Wilkins; 1991:299-323.
4. Lloyd RV. Practical markers used in the diagnosis of NE tumors. *Endocr Pathol.* 2003;14:293-301.
5. Portela-Gomes GM, Stridsberg M, Grimelius L, et al. Expression of five different somatostatin receptor subtypes in endocrine cells of the pancreas. *Appl Immunohistochem.* 2000;8:126-132.
6. DeLellis RA, Tischler AS. The dispersed NE cell system. In: Kovacs K, Asa SL, eds. *Functional Endocrine Pathology.* Oxford: Blackwell Science; 1998:529-549.
7. Lauweryns JM, Van Ranst L. Immunocytochemical localization of aromatic l-amino acid decarboxylase in human, rat and mouse bronchopulmonary and gastrointestinal endocrine cells. *J Histochem Cytochem.* 1988;36:1181-1186.
8. Lloyd RV, Sisson JC, Shapiro B, Verhofstad AA. Immunohistochemical localization of epinephrine, norepinephrine, catecholamine-synthesizing enzymes and chromogranin in NE cells and tumors. *Am J Pathol.* 1986;125:45-54.
9. Lloyd RV, Jin L, Qian X, et al. Analysis of the chromogranin A post-translational cleavage product pancreastatin and the prohormone convertases PC2 and PC3 in normal and neoplastic human pituitaries. *Am J Pathol.* 1995;146:1188-1198.

10. Scopsi L, Gullo M, Rilke F, et al. Proprotein convertases (PC1/PC3 and PC2) in normal and neoplastic tissues: Their use as markers of NE differentiation. *J Clin Endocrinol Metab.* 1995;80:294-301.
11. Scopsi L, Lee R, Gullo M, et al. Peptidylglycine, α-amidating monooxygenase in NE tumors: Its identification, characterization, quantification and relation to the grade of morphologic differentiation, amidated peptide content and granin immunocytochemistry. *Appl Immunohistochem.* 1998;6:120-132.
12. Schmechel D, Marangos PJ, Brightman M. Neurone-specific enolase is a molecular marker for peripheral and central NE cells. *Nature.* 1978;276:834-836.
13. Haimoto H, Takahashi Y, Koshikawa T, et al. Immunohistochemical localization of gamma enolase in normal human tissues other than nervous and NE tissue. *Lab Invest.* 1985;52:257-263.
14. Schmechel DE. Gamma subunit of the glycolytic enzyme enolase: Nonspecific or neuron specific? *Lab Invest.* 1985;52:239-242.
15. Rode J, Dhillon AP, Doran JF, et al. PGP 9.5, a new marker for human NE tumors. *Histopathology.* 1985;9:147-158.
16. Li GL, Farooque M, Holtz A, Olsson Y. Expression of the ubiquitin carboxyl-terminal hydrolase PGP 9.5 in axons following spinal cord compression trauma. *APMIS.* 1997;105:384-390.
17. Wilson PO, Barber PC, Hamid QA, et al. The immunolocalization of protein gene product 9.5 using rabbit polyclonal and mouse monoclonal antibodies. *Br J Exp Pathol.* 1988;69:91-104.
18. Bordi C, Pilato FP, D'Adda T. Comparative study of several NE markers in pancreatic endocrine tumors. *Virchows Arch A Pathol Anat Histopathol.* 1988;413:387-398.
19. Tezel E, Hibi K, Nagasaka T, et al. PGP9.5 as a prognostic factor in pancreatic cancer. *Clin Cancer Res.* 2000;6:4764-4767.
20. Mendelsohn G. Histaminase localization in medullary thyroid carcinoma and small cell lung carcinoma. In: DeLellis RA, ed. *Diagnostic Immunohistochemistry.* New York: Masson; 1981:299-312.
21. Sasano H, Mason JI, Sasano N. Immunohistochemical analysis of cytochrome P450 17 alpha in human adrenocortical disorders. *Hum Pathol.* 1989;20:113-117.
22. Sasano H, Okamoto M, Sasano N. Immunohistochemical study of cytochrome P-450 11B hydroxylase in human adrenal cortex with mineralo- and glucocorticoid excess. *Virchows Arch A Pathol Anat Histopathol.* 1988;413:313-318.
23. Sasano H, Okamoto M, Mason JI, et al. Immunohistochemical studies of steroidogenic enzymes (aromatase, 17 alpha-hydroxylase and cholesterol side chain cleavage cytochrome P450) in sex cord stromal tumors of the ovary. *Hum Pathol.* 1989;20:452-457.
24. Lloyd RV, Wilson BS. Specific endocrine tissue marker defined by a monoclonal antibody. *Science.* 1983;222:628-630.
25. O'Connor DT, Burton D, Deftos LJ. Chromogranin A. Immunohistology reveals its universal occurrence in normal polypeptide hormone producing endocrine glands. *Life Sci.* 1983;33:1657-1663.
26. Wilson BS, Lloyd RV. Detection of chromogranin in NE cells with a monoclonal antibody. *Am J Pathol.* 1984;115:458-468.
27. Hagn C, Schmid KW, Fischer-Colbrie R, Winkler H. Chromogranin A, B, and C in human adrenal medulla and endocrine tissues. *Lab Invest.* 1986;55:405-411.
28. Huttner WB, Gerdes H-H, Rosa P. Chromogranins/secretogranins—widespread constituents of the secretory granule matrix in endocrine cells and neurons. In: Langley K, Gratzl M, eds. *Markers for Neural and Endocrine Cells: Molecular and Cell Biology.* Weinheim, Germany, VCH, 1991.
29. Portela-Gomes GM, Hacker GW, Weitgasser R. NE cell markers for pancreatic islets and tumors. *Appl Immunohistochem Mol Morphol.* 2004;12:183-192.
30. Fahrenkamp AG, Wibbeke C, Winde G. Immunohistochemical distribution of chromogranins A and B and secretogranin II in NE tumors of the gastrointestinal tract. *Virch Arch.* 1995;426:361-367.
31. Schmid KW, Kroll M, Hittmair A, et al. Chromogranin A and B in adenomas of the pituitary: An immunohistochemical study of 42 cases. *Am J Surg Pathol.* 1991;15:1072-1077.
32. Fischer-Colbrie R, Eder S, Lovisetti-Scamihorn P, et al. NE secretory protein-55: a novel marker for the constitutive secretory pathway. *Ann NY Acad Sci.* 2002;971:317-322.
33. Srivastava A, Padilla O, Fischer-Collbrie R, et al. NE secretory protein-55 (NESP-55) expression discriminates pancreatic endocrine tumors and pheochromocytomas from gastrointestinal and pulmonary carcinoids. *Am Surg J Pathol.* 2004;28:1371-1378.
34. Srivastava A, Hornick JL. Immunohistochemical staining for CDX2, PDX-1, NESP-55 and TTF-7 can help distinguish gastrointestinal carcinoid tumors from pancreatic endocrine and pulmonary carcinoid tumors. *Am J Surg Pathol.* 2008 (E.pub).
35. Gould VE, Lee I, Wiedenmann B, et al. Synaptophysin: A novel marker for neurons, certain NE cells and their neoplasms. *Hum Pathol.* 1986;17:979-983.
36. Komminoth P, Roth J, Schroder S, et al. Overlapping expression of immunohistochemical markers and synaptophysin mRNA in pheochromocytomas and adrenocortical carcinomas: Implications for the differential diagnosis of adrenal gland tumors. *Lab Invest.* 1995;72:424-431.
37. Portela-Gomes GM, Lukinius GM, Grimelius L. Synaptic vesicle protein 2: A new NE cell marker. *Am J Pathol.* 2000;157:1299-1309.
38. Bumming P Nilsson O, Ahlman H, et al. Gastrointestinal stromal tumors regularly express synaptic vesicle proteins: Evidence of a neuroendocrine phenotype. *Endocr Relat Cancer.* 2007;14:835-863.
39. Jakobsen AM, Anderson P, Saglik G, et al. Differential expression of vesicular monoamine transporter (VMAT) 1 and 2 in gastrointestinal endocrine tumors. *J Pathol.* 2001;195:463-472.
40. Gut A, Kiraly CE, Fukuda M, et al. Expression and localization of synaptotagmin isoforms in endocrine beta cells: their function in insulin exocytosis. *J Cell Sci.* 2001;114:1709-1716.
41. Adolfsen B, Saraswati S, Yoshihara M, Littleton JT. Synaptotagmins are trafficked to distinct subsellular domains including the post synaptic compartment. *J Cell Bol.* 2004;166:249-260.
42. Regazzi R, Wolheim CB, Lang J, et al. VAMP-2 and cellubrevin are expressed in pancreatic beta cells and are essential for Ca(2+) but not for GTP gamma S-induced insulin secretion. *EMBO J.* 1995;14:2723-2730.
43. Grabowski P, Schönfelder J, Ahnert-Hilger G, et al. Heterogeneous expression of NE marker proteins in human undifferentiated carcinoma of the colon and rectum. *Ann NY Acad Sci.* 2008;1014:270-274.
44. Arber DA, Weirs LM. CD57: A review. *Appl Immunohistochem.* 1995;3:137-152.
45. McGarry RC, Helfand SL, Quarles RH, Roder JC. Recognition of the myelin associated glycoprotein by the monoclonal antibody HNK-1. *Nature.* 1983;306:376-378.
46. Tischler AS, Mobtaker H, Mann K, et al. Anti-lymphocyte antibody Leu 7 (HNK-1) recognizes a constituent of NE granule matrix. *J Histochem Cytochem.* 1986;34:1213-1216.
47. Ghali VS, Jimenez EJS, Garcia RL. Distribution of Leu 7 antigen (HNK-1) in thyroid tumors: Its usefulness as a diagnostic marker for follicular and papillary carcinomas. *Hum Pathol.* 1992;23:21-25.
48. Langley K, Gratzl M. Neural cell adhesion molecule (NCAM) in neural and endocrine cells. In: Langley K, Gratzl M, eds. *Markers for Neural and Endocrine Cells: Molecular and Cell Biology. Diagnostic Applications.* Weinheim, Germany: VCH; 1991:133-177.
49. Shipley WR, Hammer RD, Lennington WJ, Macon WR. Paraffin immunohistochemical detection of CD56, a useful marker for neural cell adhesion molecule in normal and neoplastic fixed tissues. *Appl Immunohistochem.* 1997;5:87-93.
50. Jin L, Hemperly JJ, Lloyd RV. Expression of neural cell adhesion molecule in normal and neoplastic human NE tissues. *Am J Pathol.* 1991;138:961-969.
51. Komminoth P, Roth J, Saremaslani P, et al. Polysialic acid of the neural cell adhesion molecule in the human thyroid: A marker for medullary thyroid carcinoma and primary C-cell hyperplasia: An immunohistochemical study on 79 thyroid lesions. *Am J Surg Pathol.* 1994;18:399-411.
52. Komminoth P, Roth J, Lackie PM, et al. Polysialic acid of the neural cell adhesion molecule distinguishes small cell lung carcinoma from carcinoids. *Am J Pathol.* 1991;139:297-304.

53. Fuchs E, Weber K. Intermediate filaments: Structure, dynamics, function and disease. *Ann Rev Biochem*. 1994;63:345-382.
54. Hoefler H, Denk H, Lackinger E, et al. Immunocytochemical demonstration of intermediate filament cytoskeleton proteins in human endocrine tissues and (neuro-) endocrine tumors. *Virch Arch A Pathol Anat Histopathol*. 1986;409:609-626.
55. Wang NP, Zee S, Zarbo RJ, et al. Coordinate expression of cytokeratins 7 and 20 defines unique subsets of carcinomas. *Appl Immunohistochem*. 1995;3:99-107.
56. Trojanowski JQ, Lee VM, Schlaepfer WW. An immunohistochemical study of human central and peripheral nervous system tumors, using monoclonal antibodies against neurofilaments and glial filaments. *Hum Pathol*. 1984;15:248-257.
57. Perez MA, Saul SH, Trojanowski JQ. Neurofilament and chromogranin expression in normal and neoplastic NE cells of the human gastrointestinal tract and pancreas. *Cancer*. 1990;65: 1219-1227.
58. Kulig E, Lloyd RV. Transcription factors and endocrine disease. *Endocr Pathol*. 1996;1:245-250.
59. Reubi JC, Kappeler A, Waser B, et al. Immunohistochemical localization of somatostatin receptors sst2A in human tumors. *Am J Pathol*. 1998;153:233-245.
60. Erickson LA, Jin L, Wollen P, et al. Parathyroid hyperplasia, adenomas and carcinomas: differential expression of p27 Kip1 protein. *Am J Surg Pathol*. 1999;23:288-295.
61. LaRosa S, Sessa F, Capella C, et al. Prognostic criteria in nonfunctioning pancreatic endocrine tumors. *Virchows Arch*. 1996;429:323-333.
62. DeLellis RA. Proliferation markers in NE tumors: Useful or useless? A critical reappraisal. *Verh Dtsch Ges Pathol*. 1997;81: 53-61.
63. Vosse BA, Seelentag W, Bachmann A, et al. Background staining of visualization systems in immunohistochemistry: comparison of the avidin-biotin complex system and the EnVision + system. *Appl Immunohistochem Mol Morphol*. 2007;15:103-107.
64. Asa SL. *Atlas of Tumor Pathology: Tumors of the Pituitary Gland*. Washington, D.C.: Armed Forces Institute of Pathology; 1998.
65. Girod C, Trouillar J, Dubois MP. Immunocytochemical localization of S100 protein in stellate cells (folliculo-stellate cells) of the anterior lobe of the normal human pituitary. *Cell Tissue Res*. 1985;241:505-511.
66. Lloyd RV, Cano M, Rosa P, et al. Distribution of chromogranin A and secretogranin I (chromogranin B) in NE cells and tumors. *Am J Pathol*. 1988;130:296-304.
67. Hofler H, Walter GF, Denk H. Immunohistochemistry of folliculo-stellate cells in normal human adenohypophyses and in pituitary adenomas. *Acta Neuropathol (Berl)*. 1994;65:35-40.
68. Scheitauer BW, Kovacs K, Horvath E, et al. Pituitary carcinoma. In: DeLellis RA, Lloyd RV, Heitz P, Eng C, eds. *Tumours of the Endocrine Organs. WHO Classification of Tumours*. Lyon, France: IRC; 2004:36-39.
69. Thappar K, Kovacs K, Scheithauer BW, et al. Proliferative activity and invasiveness among pituitary adenomas and carcinomas: An analysis using the MIB-1 antibody. *Neurosurgery*. 1996;38:99-106.
70. Thappar K, Schaithauer BW, Kovacs K, et al. p53 expression in pituitary adenomas and carcinomas: Correlation with invasiveness and tumor growth fractions. *Neurosurgery*. 1996;38: 765-771.
71. Asa SL, Ezzat S. Genetics and proteomics of pituitary tumors. *Endocrine*. 2005;28(1):43-37.
72. Wierinckx A, Auger C, Devauchelle P, et al. A diagnostic marker set for invasion, proliferation and aggressiveness of prolactin pituitary tumors. *Endocrine-Related Cancer*. 2007;14:887-900.
73. Riss D, Jim L, Qian X, et al. Differential expression of galectin-3 in pituitary tumors. *Cancer Res*. 2003;63:2251-2255.
74. Asa SL. Practical pituitary pathology: What does the pathologist need to know? *Arch Pathol Lab Med*. 2008;132:1231-1240.
75. Burger PC, Scheithauer BW. *Atlas of Tumor Pathology: Tumors of the Central Nervous System. Series 4*. Washington, D.C: American Registry of Pathology in collaboration with Armed Forces Institute of Pathology; 2007.
76. Coca S, Vaquero J, Escandon J, et al. Immunohistochemical characterization of pineocytomas. *Clin Neuropathol*. 1992;11:298-303.
77. Hayashi K, Hoshida Y, Horie Y, et al. Immunohistochemical study on the distribution of α and β subunits of S100 protein in brain tumors. *Acta Neuropathol (Berl)*. 1991;81:657-663.
78. Korf HW, Klein DC, Zigler JS, et al. S-antigen-like immunoreactivity in a human pineocytoma. *Acta Neuropathol (Berl)*. 1986;69:165-167.
79. Perentes E, Rubinstein LJ, Herman MM, et al. S-antigen immunoreactivity in human pineal glands and pineal parenchymal tumors: A monoclonal antibody study. *Acta Neuropathol (Berl)*. 1986;71:224-227.
80. Arivazhagan A, Anandh B, Santash V, Chandramouli BA. Pineal parenchymal tumors-utility of immunohistochemical markers in prognostication. *Clin Neuropathol*. 2008;27:325-333.
81. Bocker W, Dralle H, Dorn G. Thyroglobulin: An immunohistochemical marker in thyroid disease. In: DeLellis RA, ed. *Diagnostic Immunohistochemistry*. New York: Masson; 1981:37-60.
82. Sambade C, Franssila K, Cameselle-Teijeiro J, et al. Hyalinizing trabecular adenoma: A misnomer for a peculiar tumor of the thyroid gland. *Endocr Pathol*. 1991;2:83-91.
83. Hirokawa M, Carney JA. Cell membrane and cytoplasmic staining for MIB-1 in hyalinizing trabecular adenoma of the thyroid. *Am J Surg Pathol*. 2000;24:575-578.
84. Leonardo E, Volante M, Barbareschi M, et al. Cell membrane reactivity of MIB-1 antibody to Ki-67 in human tumors: fact or artifact? *Appl Immunohistochem Mol Morphol*. 2007;15: 220-223.
85. Berge-Lefranc JL, Cartouzou G, DeMicco C, et al. Quantification of thyroglobulin messenger RNA by in-situ hybridization in differentiated thyroid cancers: Difference between well-differentiated and moderately differentiated histologic types. *Cancer*. 1985;56:345-350.
86. Keen CE, Szakacs S, Okon E, et al. CA125 and thyroglobulin staining in papillary carcinomas of thyroid and ovarian origin is not entirely specific for site of origin. *Histopathology*. 1999;34:113-117.
87. Carcangiu ML, Zampi G, Rosai J. Poorly differentiated ("insular") thyroid carcinoma: A reinterpretation of Langhans' "wuchernde Struma." *Am J Surg Pathol*. 1984;8:655-668.
88. Ordonez NG, El-Naggar AK, Hickey RC, Samaan NA. Anaplastic thyroid carcinoma: Immunocytochemical study of 32 cases. *Am J Clin Pathol*. 1991;96:15-24.
89. Carcangiu ML, Steeper T, Zampi G, Rosai J. Anaplastic thyroid cancer: A study of 70 cases. *Am J Clin Pathol*. 1985;83: 135-158.
90. Kawaoi A, Okano T, Nemoto N, et al. Simultaneous detection of thyroglobulin, (Tg) thyroxine (T4) and tri-iodothyronine (T3) in nontoxic thyroid tumors by the immunoperoxidase method. *Am J Pathol*. 1982;108:39-49.
91. Katoh R, Kawaoi A, Miyagi E, et al. Thyroid transcription factor 1 in normal, hyperplastic and neoplastic thyroid follicular thyroid cells examined by immunohistochemistry and non-radioactive *in situ* hybridization. *Mod Pathol*. 2000;13:570-576.
92. Lau SK, Luthringer DJ, Eisen RN. Thyroid transcription factor-1: A review. *Appl Immunohistochem Mol Morphol*. 2002;10:97-102.
93. Ordonez NG. Thyroid transcription factor 1 is a marker of lung and thyroid carcinomas. *Adv Anat Pathol*. 2000;7:123-127.
94. Kaufmann O, Dietel M. Thyroid transcription factor-1 is the superior immunohistochemical marker for pulmonary adenocarcinomas and large cell carcinomas compared to surfactant proteins A and B. *Histopathology*. 2000;36:8-16.
95. Byrd-Gloster AL, Khoor A, Glass LF, et al. Differential expression of thyroid transcription factor-1 in small cell lung carcinoma and Merkel cell tumor. *Hum Pathol*. 2000;31:58-62.
96. Agoff SN, Lamps LW, Philip AT, et al. Thyroid transcription factor-1 is expressed in extrapulmonary small cell carcinomas but not in other extrapulmonary NE tumors. *Mod Pathol*. 2000;13:238-242.
97. Nonaka D, Tang Y, Chiriboga L, Rivera M, and Ghossein R, et al. Diagnostic utility of thyroid transcription factors PAX8 and TTF2 (Fox E1) in thyroid epithelial neoplasms. *Mod Pathol*. 2008;21:192-200.
98. Henzen-Logmans SC, Mullink H, Ramaekers FC, et al. Expression of cytokeratins and vimentin in epithelial cells of normal and pathologic thyroid tissue. *Virchows Arch A Pathol Anat Histopathol*. 1987;410:347-354.

99. Miettinen M, Franssila K, Lehto V-P, et al. Expression of intermediate filament proteins in thyroid gland and thyroid tumors. *Lab Invest*. 1984;50:262-270.
100. Viale G, Dell'Orto P, Coggi G, Gambacorta M. Co-expression of cytokeratins and vimentin in normal and diseased thyroid glands: Lack of diagnostic utility of vimentin immunostaining. *Am J Surg Pathol*. 1989;13:1034-1040.
101. Schelfhout LJDM, van Muijen GN, Fleuren GJ. Expression of keratin 19 distinguishes papillary thyroid carcinoma from follicular carcinomas and follicular thyroid adenoma. *Am J Clin Pathol*. 1989;92:654-658.
102. Raphael SJ, McKeown-Eyssen G, Asa SL. High molecular weight cytokeratin and cytokeratin 19 in the diagnosis of thyroid tumors. *Mod Pathol*. 1994;7:295-300.
103. Fonseca E, Nesland JM, Hoie J, Sobrinho-Simoes M. Pattern of expression of intermediate cytokeratin filaments in the thyroid gland: An immunohistochemical study of simple and stratified epithelial-type cytokeratins. *Virchows Arch*. 1997;430:239-245.
104. Miettinen M, Kovatich AJ, Karkkainen P. Keratin subsets in papillary and follicular thyroid lesions: A paraffin section analysis with diagnostic implications. *Virchows Arch*. 1997;431:407-413.
105. Kragsterman B, Grimelius L, Wallin G, et al. Cytokeratin 19 expression in papillary thyroid carcinoma. *Appl Immunohistochem*. 1999;7:181-185.
106. Baloch ZW, Abraham S, Roberts S, LiVolsi VA. Differential expression of cytokeratins in follicular variant of papillary carcinoma: An immunohistochemical study and its diagnostic utility. *Hum Pathol*. 1999;30:1166-1171.
107. Fonseca E, Nesland J, Sobrinho-Simoes M. Expression of stratified epithelial cytokeratins in hyalinizing trabecular adenoma supports their relationship with papillary carcinoma of the thyroid. *Histopathology*. 1997;31:330-335.
108. Hirokawa M, Carney JA, Ohtsuki Y. Hyalinizing trabecular adenoma and papillary carcinoma of the thyroid express different cytokeratin patterns. *Am J Surg Pathol*. 2000;24:877-881.
109. Liberman E, Weidner N. Papillary and follicular neoplasms of the thyroid gland: Differential immunohistochemical staining with high molecular weight keratin and involucrin. *Appl Immunohistochem*. 2000;8:42-48.
110. Soares P, Cameselle-Teijeiro J, Sobrinho-Simoes M. Immunohistochemical detection of p53 in differentiated, poorly differentiated and undifferentiated carcinomas of the thyroid. *Histopathology*. 1994;24:205-210.
111. Holm R, Nesland JM. Retinoblastoma and p53 tumor suppressor gene protein expression in carcinomas of the thyroid gland. *J Pathol*. 1994;172:267-272.
112. Tallini G, Santoro M, Helie M, et al. RET/PTC oncogene activation defines a subset of papillary thyroid carcinomas lacking evidence of progression to poorly differentiated or undifferentiated tumor phenotypes. *Clin Cancer Res*. 1998;4:287-294.
113. Papotti M, Volante M, Guiliano A, et al. RET/PTC activation in hyalinizing trabecular tumors of the thyroid. *Am J Surg Pathol*. 2000;24:1615-1621.
114. Cheung CC, Boerner SL, MacMillan CM, et al. Hyalinizing trabecular tumor of the thyroid: A variant of papillary carcinoma proved by molecular genetics. *Am J Surg Pathol*. 2000;24:1622-1626.
115. LiVolsi VA. Hyalinizing trabecular tumor of the thyroid: Adenoma, carcinoma, or neoplasm of uncertain malignant potential? *Am J Surg Pathol*. 2000;24:1683-1684.
116. Kroll TG, Sarraf P, Pecciarini L, et al. PAX8-PPAR gamma 1 fusion oncogene in human thyroid carcinoma. *Science*. 2000;289:1357-1360.
117. Nikiforova MN, Biddinger PW, Candill CM, et al. PAX8-PPAR gamma rearrangement in thyroid tumors: RT-PCR and immunohistochemical analyzer. *Am J Surg Pathol*. 2002;26:1016-1023.
118. Marques AR, Espadinha C, Catarino AL, et al. Expression of PAX8-PPAR gamma/rearrangements in both follicular thyroid carcinoma and adenoma. *J Clin Endocrinol Metab*. 2002;87:3947-3952.
119. Cheung L, Messina M, Gill A, et al. Detection of the PAX8-PPAR gamma fusion oncogene in both follicular thyroid carcinomas and adenomas. *J Clin Endocrinol Metab*. 2003;88:354-357.
120. Sack MJ, Astengo-Osuna C, Lin BT, et al. HBME-1 immunostaining in thyroid fine needle aspirations: A useful marker in the diagnosis of carcinoma. *Mod Pathol*. 1997;10:668-674.
121. Miettinen M, Karkkainen P. Differential HBME-1 reactivity in benign vs. malignant thyroid tissue is helpful in the diagnosis of thyroid tumors. *[abstract] Mod Pathol*. 1996;5:50A.
122. Mase T, Funahashi H, Koshikawa T, et al. HBME-1 immunostaining in thyroid tumors especially in follicular neoplasms. *Endocr J*. 2003;50:173-177.
123. Casey MB, Lohse CM, Lloyd RV. Distinction between papillary thyroid hyperplasia and papillary thyroid carcinoma by immunohistochemical staining for cytokeratin 19, galectin-3 and HBME-1. *Endocr Pathol*. 2003;14:55-60.
124. Cheung CC, Ezzat S, Freeman JL, et al. Immunohistochemical diagnosis of papillary thyroid carcinoma. *Mod Pathol*. 2001;14:338-342.
125. Choi YL, Kim MK, Suh JW, et al. Immunoexpression of HBME-1, high molecular weight cytokeratin, cytokeratin 19, thyroid transcription factor-1 and E-cadherin in thyroid carcinoma. *J Korean Med Sci*. 2005;20:853-859.
126. Fischer S, Asa S. Application of immunohistochemistry to thyroid neoplasms. *Arch Pathol Lab Med*. 2008;132:359-372.
127. Xu XC, el-Naggar AK, Lotan R. Differential expression of galectin-1 and galectin-3 in thyroid tumors. Potential diagnostic implications. *Am J Pathol*. 1995;147:815-822.
128. Fernandez PL, Merino MJ, Gomez M, et al. Galectin-3 and laminin expression in neoplastic and non-neoplastic thyroid tissue. *J Pathol*. 1997;181:80-86.
129. Orlandi F, Saggiorato E, Pivano G, et al. Galectin-3 is a presurgical marker of human thyroid carcinoma. *Cancer Res*. 1998;58:3015-3020.
130. Herrmann ME, LiVolsi VA, Pasha TL, et al. Immunohistochemical expression of galectin 3 in benign and malignant lesions. *Arch Pathol Lab Med*. 2002;126:710-713.
131. Bartolazzi A, Gasbarri A, Papotti M, et al. Application of an immunodiagnostic method for improving pre-operative diagnosis of nodular thyroid lesions. *Lancet*. 2001;357:1644-1650.
132. Volante M, Bozzalla-Cassione F, DePompa R, et al. Galectin-3 and HBME-1 expression in oncocytic cell tumors of the thyroid. *Virchows Arch*. 2004;445:183-188.
133. Wiseman SM, Melck A, Masoudi H, et al. Molecular phenotype of thyroid tumors identifiers: A marker panel for differentiated thyroid cancer diagnosis. *Am Surg Oncol*. 2008;15:2811-2826.
134. Griffith OL, Chiu CG, Gown AM, et al. Biomarker panel diagnosis of thyroid cancer: A critical review. *Expert Rev Anticancer Ther*. 2008;8:1399-1413.
135. Prasad ML, Pellegata NS, Kloos RT, et al. CITED1 expression suggests papillary thyroid carcinoma in high throughput tissue microarray-based study. *Thyroid*. 2004;14:169-175.
136. Huang Y, Prasad M, Lemon WJ, et al. Gene expression in papillary thyroid carcinoma reveals highly consistent profiles. *Proc Nat'l Acad Sci USA*. 2001;98:15044-15049.
137. Prasad ML, Pellegata NS, Huang Y, et al. Galectin-3, fibronectin-1, CITED1, HBME-1 and cytokeratin-19 immunohistochemistry is useful for the differential diagnosis of thyroid tumors. *Mod Pathol*. 2005;18:48-57.
138. Sconamiglio T, Hyjek E, Kao J, et al. Diagnostic usefulness of HBME-1, galectin-3, CK19 and CITED1 and evaluation of their expression in encapsulated lesions with questionable features of papillary thyroid carcinoma. *Am J Clin Pathol*. 2006;126:700-708.
139. Scheumman GF, Hoang-Vu, Cetin Y, et al. Clinical significance of E-cadherin as a prognostic marker in thyroid carcinoma. *J Clin Endocrinol Metab*. 1995;80:2168-2172.
140. Garcia-Rostan G, Camp RL, Herreo A, et al. Beta catenin dysregulation in thyroid neoplasms: Down regulation, aberrant nuclear expression, and CTNNB1 exon 3 mutations are markers for aggressive tumor phenotypes and poor prognosis. *Am J Pathol*. 2001;158:987-996.
141. Wiseman SM, Griffith OL, Deen S, et al. Identification of molecular markers altered during transformation of differentiated into anaplastic thyroid carcinoma. *Arch Surg*. 2007;142:717-729.
142. Dasovic-Knezevic M, Bormer O, Holm R, et al. Carcinoembryonic antigen in medullary thyroid carcinoma: An immunohistochemical study applying six novel monoclonal antibodies. *Mod Pathol*. 1989;2:610-617.

143. Schroder S, Schwarz W, Rehpenning W, et al. Prognostic significance of Leu M1 immunostaining in papillary carcinomas of the thyroid gland. *Virchows Arch A Pathol Anat Histopathol.* 1987;411:435-439.
144. Loy TS, Darkow GV, Spollen LE, Diaz-Arias AA. Immunostaining for Leu 7 in the diagnosis of thyroid carcinoma. *Arch Pathol Lab Med.* 1994;118:172-174.
145. Ostrowski ML, Brown RW, Wheeler TM, et al. Leu 7 immunoreactivity in cytologic specimens of thyroid lesions with an emphasis on follicular neoplasms. *Diagn Cytopathol.* 1995;12:297-302.
146. Gatalica Z, Miettinen M. Distribution of carcinoma antigens CA19-9 and CA15-3: An immunohistochemical study of 400 tumors. *Appl Immunohistochem.* 1994;2:205-211.
147. Alves P, Soares P, Fonseca E, Sobrinho-Simoes M. Papillary thyroid carcinoma overexpresses fully and underglycosylated mucins together with native and sialylated simple mucin antigens and histo-blood group antigens. *Endocrine Pathol.* 1999;10:315-324.
148. Lee HM, Baek SK, Kwon SY, et al. Cyclooxygenase 1 and 2 expression in the human thyroid gland. *Eur Arch Otorhinolaryngol.* 2006;263:199-204.
149. Garcia-Gonzalez M, Abdulkader I, Boquete AV, et al. Cyclooxygenase 2 in normal hyperplastic and neoplastic follicular cells of the human thyroid gland. *Virchows Arch.* 2005;447:12-17.
150. Ito Y, Yoshida H, Nakano K, et al. Cyclooxygenase-2 expression in thyroid neoplasms. *Histopathol.* 2003;42:492-497.
151. Bur M, Shiraki W, Masood S. Estrogen and progesterone receptor detection in neoplastic and non-neoplastic thyroid tissue. *Mod Pathol.* 1993;6:469-472.
152. McLaren KM, Cossar DW. The immunohistochemical localization of S-100 in the diagnosis of papillary carcinoma of the thyroid. *Hum Pathol.* 1996;27:633-636.
153. Papotti M, Gugliotta P, Forte G, Bussolati G. Immunocytochemical identification of oxyphilic mitochondrion rich cells. *Appl Immunohistochem.* 1994;2:261-267.
154. Nylander K, Vojtesek B, Nenutil R, et al. Differential expression of p63 isoforms in normal tissues and neoplastic cells. *J Pathol.* 2002;198:417-427.
155. Hunt JL, LiVolsi VA, Barnes EL. p63 expression in sclerosing mucoepidermoid carcinomas with eosinophilia arising in the thyroid. *Mod Pathol.* 2004;17:526-529.
156. DeLellis RA, Wolfe HJ. The pathology of the human calcitonin C-cell. *Pathol Annu.* 1981;16:25-52.
157. Sikri KL, Varndell IM, Hamid QA, et al. Medullary carcinoma of the thyroid: An immunocytochemical and histochemical study of 25 cases using 8 separate markers. *Cancer.* 1985;56: 2481-2491.
158. Perry A, Molberg K, Albores-Saavedra J. Physiologic versus neoplastic C-cell hyperplasia of the thyroid: Separation of distinct histologic and biologic entities. *Cancer.* 1996;77:750-756.
159. Holm R, Sobrinho-Simoes M, Nesland JM, et al. Medullary carcinoma of the thyroid gland: An immunocytochemical study. *Ultrastruct Pathol.* 1985;8:25-41.
160. Uribe M, Fenoglio-Preiser CM, Grimes M, Feind C. Medullary carcinoma of the thyroid gland: Clinical, pathological and immunohistochemical features with a review of the literature. *Am J Surg Pathol.* 1985;9:577-594.
161. Zajac JD, Penschow J, Mason T, et al. Identification of calcitonin and calcitonin gene related peptide messenger RNA in medullary thyroid carcinoma by hybridization histochemistry. *J Clin Endocrinol Metab.* 1986;62:1037-1043.
162. Eusebi V, Damiani S, Riva C, et al. Calcitonin free oat cell carcinoma of the thyroid gland. *Virchows Arch A Pathol Anat Histopathol.* 1990;417:267-271.
163. Franc B, Rosenberg-Bourgin M, Caillou B, et al. Medullary thyroid carcinoma: Search for histological predictors of survival (109 proband case analysis). *Hum Pathol.* 1998;29:1078-1084.
164. Steenbergh PH, Hoppener JW, Zandberg J, et al. Calcitonin gene related peptide coding sequence is conserved in the human genome and is expressed in medullary thyroid carcinoma. *J Clin Endocrinol Metab.* 1984;59:358-360.
165. Scopsi L, Ferrari C, Pilotti S, et al. Immunocytochemical localization and identification of prosomatostatin gene products in medullary carcinoma of human thyroid gland. *Hum Pathol.* 1990;21:820-830.
166. Sunday ME, Wolfe HJ, Roos BA, et al. Gastrin releasing peptide gene expression in developing, hyperplastic and neoplastic thyroid C-cells. *Endocrinology.* 1988;122:1551-1558.
167. Heitz PU, von Herbay G, Kloppel G, et al. The expression of subunits of human chorionic gonadotropin (hCG) by nontrophoblastic, nonendocrine and endocrine tumors. *Am J Clin Pathol.* 1987;88:467-472.
168. DeLellis RA, Moore FM, Wolfe HJ. Thyroglobulin immunoreactivity in human medullary thyroid carcinoma. *Lab Invest.* 1983;48:20A.
169. Holm R, Sobrinho-Simoes M, Nesland JM, Johannessen JV. Concurrent production of calcitonin and thyroglobulin by the same neoplastic cells. *Ultrastruct Pathol.* 1986;10:241-248.
170. Ljungberg O, Bondeson L, Bondeson AG. Differentiated thyroid carcinoma, intermediate type: A new tumor entity with features of follicular and parafollicular cell carcinomas. *Hum Pathol.* 1984;15:218-228.
171. Volante M, Papotti M, Roth J, et al. Mixed medullary follicular thyroid carcinoma: Molecular evidence for a dual origin of tumor components. *Am J Pathol.* 1999;155:1499-1509.
172. Schmid KW, Fischer-Colbrie R, Hagn C, et al. Chromogranin A and B and secretogranin II in medullary carcinomas of the thyroid. *Am J Surg Pathol.* 1987;11:551-556.
173. Katsetos CD, Jami MM, Krishna L, et al. Novel immunohistochemical localization of 28,000 molecular-weight (Mr) calcium binding protein (calbindin-D28k) in enterochromaffin cells of the human appendix and neuroendocrine tumors (carcinoids and small-cell carcinomas) of the midgut and foregut. *Arch Pathol Lab Med.* 1994;118:633-639.
174. Viale G, Roncalli M, Grimelius L, et al. Prognostic value of bcl-2 immunoreactivity in medullary thyroid carcinoma. *Hum Pathol.* 1995;26:945-950.
175. DeLellis RA, Rule AH, Spiler I, et al. Calcitonin and carcinoembryonic antigen as tumor markers in medullary thyroid carcinoma. *Am J Clin Pathol.* 1978;70:587-594.
176. Schroder S, Kloppel G. Carcinoembryonic antigen and nonspecific cross reacting antigen in thyroid cancer: An immunocytochemical study using polyclonal and monoclonal antibodies. *Am J Surg Pathol.* 1987;11:100-108.
177. Mendelsohn G, Wills Jr SA, Baylin SB. Relationship of tissue carcinoembryonic antigen and calcitonin to tumor virulence in medullary thyroid carcinoma: An immunohistochemical study in early, localized and virulent disseminated stages of disease. *Cancer.* 1984;54:657-662.
178. Kimura N, Nakazato Y, Nagura H, Sasano N. Expression of intermediate filaments in NE tumors. *Arch Pathol Lab Med.* 1990;114:506-510.
179. Nikiforov YE. Thyroid carcinoma: Molecular pathways and therapeutic targets. *Mod Pathol.* 2008;21(Suppl 2):S37-S43.
180. Nikiforova MN, Nikiforov YE. Molecular genetics of thyroid cancer; implications for diagnostic treatment and prognosis. *Expert Rev Mol Diagn.* 2008;8:830-895.
181. DeLellis RA. Pathology and genetics of thyroid carcinoma. *J Surg Oncol.* 2006;94:662-669.
182. Ciampi R, Nikiforov YE. RET/PTC rearrangements and BRAF mutations in thyroid tumorigenesis. *Endocrinol.* 2007;148: 936-941.
183. Nikiforov Y. Genetic alterations involved in the transition from well to poorly differentiated and anaplastic carcinoma. *Endocr Pathol.* 2004;15:319-328.
184. Grieco M, Santoro M, Berlingieri MT, et al. PTC is a novel rearranged form of the ret proto-oncogene and is frequently detected *in vivo* in human thyroid papillary carcinomas. *Cell.* 1990;60:557-563.
185. Nikiforov YE, Rowland JM, Bove KE, et al. Distinct pattern of ret oncogene rearrangements in morphological variants of radiation induced and sporadic thyroid papillary carcinomas in children. *Cancer Res.* 1997;57:1690-1694.
186. Pierotti MA, Borgarzone I, Borello MG, et al. Cytogenetics and molecular genetics of carcinomas arising from thyroid epithelial follicular cells. *Genes Chromosomes Cancer.* 1996;16:1-14.
187. Kimura ET, Nikiforova MN, Zhu Z, et al. High prevalence of BRAP mutations in thyroid cancer. Genetic evidence for constitutive activation of the RET/PTC-RAS-BRAF signalling pathway in papillary thyroid carcinoma. *Cancer Res.* 2003;63: 1454-1457.

188. Soares P, Trovisco V, Rocha AS, et al. BRAF mutations and RET/PTC rearrangements all alternative events in the etiopathogenesis of PTC. *Oncogene*. 2003;22:4578-4580.
189. Nikiforova MN, Kimura ET, Gandhi M, et al. BRAF mutations in thyroid tumors are restricted to papillary carcinomas and anaplastic or poorly differentiated carcinomas arising from papillary carcinoma. *J Clin Endocrinol Metab*. 2003;88:5399-5404.
190. Zhu Z, Gandhi M, Nikiforova MN, et al. Molecular profile and clinical-pathological features of the follicular variant of papillary thyroid carcinoma. An unusually high prevalence of ras mutations. *Am J Clin Pathol*. 2003;120:71-77.
191. Esapa CT, Johnson SJ, Kendall-Taylor P, et al. Prevalence of Ras mutations in thyroid neoplasia. *Clin Endocrinol (Oxf)*. 1999;50:529-523.
192. Abu-Amero KK, Alzahrani AS, Zou M, Shi Y. High frequency of somatic mitochondrial DNA mutations in human thyroid carcinomas and complex 1 respiratory defect in thyroid cancer cell lines. *Oncogene*. 2005;24:1455-1460.
193. Botelho MV, Capela J, Soares P, et al. Somatic and germline mutation in GRIM-19, a dual function gene involved in mitochondrial metabolism and cell death, is linked to mitochondrion-rich (Hurthle cell) tumours of the thyroid. *Br J Cancer*. 2005;92:1817-1818.
194. Smallridge R, Marlow L, Copland J. Anaplastic thyroid cancer: Molecular pathogenesis and emerging therapies. *Endocr Relat Cancer*. 2008 (epub).
195. Eng C. RET proto-oncogene in the development of human cancer. *J Clin Oncol*. 1999;17:380-393.
196. Finley DJ, Arora N, Zhu B, et al. Molecular profiling distinguishes papillary carcinoma from benign thyroid nodules. *J Clin Endocrinol Metab*. 2004;89:3214-3223.
197. Giordano TJ, Kuick R, Thomas DG, et al. Molecular classification of papillary thyroid carcinoma: distinct BRAF, RAS, RET/PTC mutations-specific gene expression profiles discovered by DNA microarray analysis. *Oncogene*. 2005;24:6646-6656.
198. Frattini M, Ferrario C, Bressan P, et al. Alternative mutations of BRAF, RET and NTRK1 are associated with similar but distinct gene expression patterns in papillary thyroid cancer. *Oncogene*. 2004;23:7426-7440.
199. Ball DW. Medullary thyroid carcinoma: therapeutic targets and molecular markers. *Curr Opin Oncol*. 2007;19:18-23.
200. Miettinen M, Clark R, Lehto VP, et al. Intermediate filament proteins in parathyroid glands and parathyroid adenomas. *Arch Pathol Lab Med*. 1985;109:986-989.
201. Futrell JM, Roth SI, Su SP, et al. Immunocytochemical localization of parathyroid hormone in bovine parathyroid glands and human parathyroid adenomas. *Am J Pathol*. 1979;94:615-622.
202. Tomita T. Immunocytochemical staining patterns for parathyroid hormone and chromogranin in parathyroid hyperplasia, adenoma and carcinoma. *Endocr Pathol*. 1999;10:145-156.
203. Stork PJ, Herteaux C, Frazier R, et al. Expression and distribution of parathyroid hormone and parathyroid hormone messenger RNA in pathological conditions of the parathyroid gland. *Lab Invest*. 1992;61:169-174.
204. Weber CJ, Russell J, Chryssochoos JT, et al. Parathyroid hormone content distinguishes true normal parathyroids from parathyroids of patients with primary hyperparathyroidism. *World J Surg*. 1996;20:1010-1015.
205. Danks JA, Ebeling PR, Hayman J, et al. Parathyroid hormone related protein: Immunohistochemical localization in cancers and in normal skin. *J Bone Miner Res*. 1989;4:273-278.
206. Schmid KW, Morgan JM, Baumert M, et al. Calcitonin and calcitonin gene related peptide mRNA detection in a population of hyperplastic parathyroid cells, also expressing chromogranin B. *Lab Invest*. 1995;73:90-95.
207. Kahn A, Tischler AS, Patwardhan NA, DeLellis RA. Calcitonin immunoreactivity in neoplastic and hyperplastic parathyroid glands. *Endocr Pathol*. 2003;14:249-250.
208. Hellman P, Karlsson-Parra A, Klareskog L, et al. Expression and function of a CD4 like molecule in parathyroid tissue. *Surgery*. 1996;120:985-992.
209. McGregor DK, Khurana KK, Cao C, et al. Diagnosing primary and metastatic renal cell carcinoma: the use of the monoclonal antibody "Renal Cell Carcinoma Marker." *Am J Surg Pathol*. 2001;25:1485-1492.
210. Bakshi N, Kunju LP, Giordano T, Shah RB. Expression of renal carcinoma antigen in renal epithelial and non-renal tumors: Diagnostic implications. *Appl Immunohistochem Mol Morphol*. 2007;15:310-315.
211. Gokden N, Gokden M, Phan DC, McKenney JK. The utility of PAX-2 in distinguishing metastatic clear cell renal carcinoma from its morphologic mimics: an immunohistochemical study with renal cell carcinoma marker. *Am J Surg Pathol*. 2008;32:1462-1467.
212. Vasef MA, Brynes RK, Sturm M, et al. Expression of cyclin D1 in parathyroid carcinomas, adenomas and hyperplasias: A paraffin immunohistochemical study. *Mod Pathol*. 1999;12:412-416.
213. Abbona GC, Papotti M, Gasparri G, Bussolati G. Proliferative activity in parathyroid tumors as detected by Ki-67 immunostaining. *Hum Pathol*. 1995;26:135-138.
214. Vargas MP, Vargas HI, Kleiner DE, Merino MJ. The role of prognostic markers (MIB-1, RB, bcl-2) in the diagnosis of parathyroid tumors. *Mod Pathol*. 1997;10:12-17.
215. Cryns VL, Thor A, Xu H-J, et al. Loss of the retinoblastoma tumor suppressor gene in parathyroid carcinoma. *N Engl J Med*. 1994;330:757-761.
216. Farnebo F, Auer G, Farnebo LO, et al. Evaluation of retinoblastoma and Ki-67 immunostaining as diagnostic markers of benign and malignant parathyroid disease. *World J Surg*. 1999;23:68-74.
217. Kayath MJ, Martin LC, Vieira JG, et al. A comparative study of p53 immunoexpression in parathyroid hyperplasias secondary to uremia, primary hyperplasias, adenomas and carcinomas. *Eur J Endocrinol*. 1998;139:78-83.
218. Pearce SH, Trump D, Wooding C, et al. Loss of heterozygosity studies at the retinoblastoma and breast cancer susceptibility BRCA2 loci in pituitary, parathyroid, pancreatic and carcinoid tumors. *Clin Endocrinol (Oxf)*. 1996;45:195-200.
219. Cetani F, Pardi E, Viacava P, et al. A reappraisal of the Rb1 gene abnormalities in the diagnosis of parathyroid carcinoma. *Clin Endocrinol (Oxf)*. 2004;60:99-106.
220. Shattuck TM, Kim TS, Costa J, et al. Mutational analysis of RB and BRCA2 as candidate tumor suppressor genes in parathyroid carcinomas. *Clin Endocrinol (Oxf)*. 2003;59:180-189.
221. Carpten JD, Robbins CM, Villablanca A, et al. HRPT2 encoding parafibromin is mutated in hyperparathyroidism-jaw tumor syndrome. *Nat Genet*. 2002;32:676-680.
222. Teh BT, Sweet KM, Morrison CD. Hyperparathyroidism-jaw tumor syndrome. In: DeLellis RA, Lloyd RV, Heitz PN, Eng C (eds). *Pathology and Genetics of Tumours of Endocrine Organs (WHO Classification)*. Lyon, France: IARC Press; 2004:228-229.
223. Howell VM, Haven CJ, Kahnoski K, et al. HRPT2 mutations are associated with malignancy in sporadic parathyroid tumors. *J Med Genet*. 2003;40:657-663.
224. Shattuck TM, Valimaki S, Obara T, et al. Somatic and germline mutations of the HRPT2 gene in sporadic parathyroid carcinoma. *N Engl J Med*. 2003;349:1722-1729.
225. Tan MH, Morrison C, Wang P, et al. Loss of parafibromin immunoreactivity is a distinguishing feature of parathyroid carcinoma. *Clin Cancer Res*. 2004;10:6629-6637.
226. Juhlin C, Larsson C, Yakoleva T, et al. Loss of parafibromin expression in a subset of parathyroid adenomas. *Endocr Relat Cancer*. 2006;13:509-523.
227. Gill AJ, Clarkson A, Gimm O, et al. Loss of nuclear expression of parafibromin distinguishes parathyroid carcinomas and hyperparathyroidism-jaw tumor associated adenomas from sporadic parathyroid adenomas and hyperplasias. *Am J Surg Pathol*. 2006;30:1140-1149.
228. Cetani F, Ambrogini E, Viacava P, et al. Should parafibromin staining replace HRPT2 gene analysis as an additional tool for histologic diagnosis of parathyroid carcinoma? *Eur J Endocrinol*. 2007;156:547-554.
229. Juhlin CC, Villablanca A, Sandelin K, et al. Parafibromin immunoreactivity; its use as an additional diagnostic marker for parathyroid tumor classification. *Endocr Relat Cancer*. 2007;14:501-512.
230. Tominaga Y, Tsuzuki T, Matsuoka A, et al. Expression of parafibromin in distant metastatic parathyroid tumors in patients with advanced secondary hyperparathyroidism due to chronic kidney disease. *World J Surg*. 2008;32:815-821.

231. Mangray S, Kurek KC, Sabo E, DeLellis RA. Immunohistochemical expression of parafibromin is of limited value in distinguishing parathyroid carcinoma from adenoma. *Mod Pathol.* 2008;21:108A: (abstract).
232. Mangray S, DeLellis RA. Parafibromin as a tool for the diagnosis of parathyroid tumors (letter). *Adv Anat Pathol.* 2008;15:179.
233. Schroder S, Niendorf A, Achilles E, et al. Immunocytochemical differential diagnosis of adrenocortical neoplasms using the monoclonal antibody D11. *Virchows Arch A Pathol Anat Histopathol.* 1990;417:89-96.
234. Schroder S, Padberg BC, Achilles E, et al. Immunocytochemistry in adrenocortical tumors: A clinicopathological study of 72 neoplasms. *Virchows Arch A Pathol Anat Histopathol.* 1992;420:65-70.
235. Tartour E, Caillou B, Tenenbaum F, et al. Immunohistochemical study of adrenocortical carcinoma: Predictive value of the D11 monoclonal antibody. *Cancer.* 1993;72:3296-3303.
236. Sasano H, Shizawa S, Suzuki T, et al. Transcription factor adrenal 4 binding protein as a marker of adrenocortical malignancy. *Hum Pathol.* 1995;26:1154-1156.
237. Busam KJ, Iversen K, Coplan KA, et al. Immunoreactivity for A103, an antibody to melan-A (Mart-1) in adrenocortical and other steroid tumors. *Am J Surg Pathol.* 1998;22:57-63.
238. Renshaw AA, Granter SR. A comparison of A103 and inhibin reactivity in adrenal cortical tumors: Distinction from hepatocellular carcinoma and renal tumors. *Mod Pathol.* 1998;11:1160-1164.
239. Loy TS, Phillips RW, Linder CL. A103 immunostaining in the diagnosis of adrenal cortical tumors: An immunohistochemical study of 316 cases. *Arch Pathol Lab Med.* 2002;126:170-172.
240. Ghorab Z, Jorda M, Ganjei P, et al. Melan A (A103) is expressed in adrenocortical neoplasms but not in renal cell and hepatocellular carcinomas. *Appl Immunohistochem Mol Morphol.* 2003;11:330-333.
241. Shin SJ, Hoda RS, Ying L, DeLellis RA. Diagnostic utility of the monoclonal antibody A103 in fine-needle aspiration biopsies of the adrenal. *Am J Clin Pathol.* 2000;113:295-302.
242. Pelkey TJ, Frierson HF, Mills SE, Stoler MH. The α subunit of inhibin in adrenal cortical neoplasia. *Mod Pathol.* 1998;11:516-524.
243. Fetsch PA, Powers CN, Zakowski M, et al. Anti-alpha inhibin: Marker of choice for the consistent distinction between adrenocortical carcinoma (ACC) and renal cell carcinoma (RCC) in fine needle aspirations (FNA). *Cancer.* 1999;87:168-172.
244. McCluggage WG, Maxwell P, Patterson A, et al. Immunohistochemical staining of hepatocellular carcinoma with monoclonal antibody against inhibin. *Histopathology.* 1997;30:518-522.
245. Munro LM, Kennedy A, McNicol AM. The expression of inhibin/activin subunits in the human adrenal cortex and its tumors. *J Endocrinol.* 1999;161:341-347.
246. McCluggage WG, Maxwell P. Adenocarcinoma of various sites may exhibit immunoreactivity with anti-inhibin antibodies. *Histopathology.* 1999;35:216-220.
247. Brown FM, Gaffey TA, Wold LE, et al. Myxoid neoplasms of the adrenal cortex: a rare histologic variant. *Am J Surg Pathol.* 2000;24:396-410.
248. Arola J, Liu J, Heikkila P, et al. Expression of inhibin alpha in adrenocortical tumors reflects the hormonal status of the neoplasm. *J Endocrinol.* 2000;165:223-229.
249. Cho EY, Ahn GH. Immunoexpression of inhibin α-subunit in adrenal neoplasms. *Appl Immunohistochem Mol Morphol.* 2001;9:222-228.
250. Vargas MP, Vargas HI, Kleiner DE, Merino MJ. Adrenocortical neoplasms: Role of prognostic markers MIB-1, p53 and RB. *Am J Surg Pathol.* 1997;21:556-562.
251. Schmitt A, Saremaslani P, Schmid S, et al. IGF II and MIB-1 immunohistochemistry is helpful in the differentiation of benign from malignant adrenocortical tumors. *Histopathology.* 2006;49:298-307.
252. Miettinen M. NE differentiation in adrenocortical carcinoma: New immunohistochemical findings supported by electron microscopy. *Lab Invest.* 1992;66:169-174.
253. Chetty R, Pillay P, Jaichand V. Cytokeratin expression in adrenal phaeochromocytomas and extra-adrenal paragangliomas. *J Clin Pathol.* 1998;51:477-478.
254. Fogt F, Vortmeyer AO, Poremba C, et al. Bcl-2 expression in normal adrenal glands and in adrenal neoplasms. *Mod Pathol.* 1998;11:716-720.
255. Zhang PJ, Genega EM, Tomaszewski JE, et al. The role of calretinin, inhibin, melan-A, bcl-2, and c-kit in differentiating adrenal cortical and medullary tumors: an immunohistochemical study. *Mod Pathol.* 2003;16:591-597.
256. Jorda M, De Madeiros B, Nadji M. Calretinin and inhibin are useful in separating adrenocortical neoplasms from pheochromocytomas. *Appl Immunohistochem Mol Morphol.* 2002;10:67-70.
257. Miettinen M, Lehto V-P, Virtanen I. Immunofluorescence microscopic evaluation of the intermediate filament expression of the adrenal cortex and medulla and their tumors. *Am J Pathol.* 1985;118:360-366.
258. Gaffey MJ, Traweek ST, Mills SE, et al. Cytokeratin expression in adrenocortical neoplasia: An immunohistochemical and biochemical study with implications for the differential diagnosis of adrenocortical, hepatocellular and renal cell carcinoma. *Hum Pathol.* 1992;23:144-153.
259. Wick MR, Cherwitz DL, McGlennen RC, Dehner LP. Adrenocortical carcinoma: An immunohistochemical comparison with renal cell carcinoma. *Am J Pathol.* 1986;122:343-352.
260. Cote RJ, Cardon-Cardo C, Reuter VE, Rosen PP. Immunopathology of adrenal and renal cortical tumors: Coordinated change in antigen expression is associated with neoplastic conversion in the adrenal cortex. *Am J Pathol.* 1990;136:1077-1084.
261. Unger PD, Hoffman K, Thung SN, et al. HMB-45 reactivity in adrenal pheochromocytomas. *Arch Pathol Lab Med.* 1992;116:151-153.
262. Caya JG. HMB-45 reactivity in adrenal pheochromocytomas. *Arch Pathol Lab Med.* 1994;118:1169.
263. Soon PS, McDonald KL, Robinson BG, Sidhu SB. Molecular markers and the pathogenesis of adrenocortical cancer. *Oncologist.* 2008;13:548-561.
264. Velazquez-Fernandez D, Laurell C, Geli J, et al. Expression profiling of adrenocortical neoplasms suggests a molecular signature of malignancy. *Surgery.* 2005;138:1087-1094.
265. Giordano TJ, Thomas DG, Kuiche R, et al. Distinct transcriptional profiles of adrenocortical tumors uncovered by microarray analysis. *Am J Pathol.* 2003;162:521-531.
266. West AN, Neale GA, Pounds S, et al. Gene expression profiling of childhood adrenocortical tumors. *Cancer Res.* 2007;67:600-608.
267. Marx C, Bornstein SR, Wolkersdorfer GW, et al. Relevance of major histocompatibility complex class II expression as a hallmark for the cellular differentiation in the human adrenal cortex. *J Clin Endocrinol Metab.* 1997;82:2136-2140.
268. Kuruba R, Gallagher SF. Current management of adrenal tumors. *Curr Opin Oncol.* 2008;20:34-36.
269. Lloyd RV, Shapiro B, Sisson JC, et al. An immunohistochemical study of pheochromocytomas. *Arch Pathol Lab Med.* 1984;108:541-544.
270. Lloyd RV, Blaivas M, Wilson BS. Distribution of chromogranin and S100 protein in normal and abnormal adrenal medullary tissues. *Arch Pathol Lab Med.* 1985;109:633-635.
271. Verhofstad AAJ, Steinbusch HWM, Joosten JWJ, et al. Immunocytochemical localization of nonadrenaline, adrenaline and serotonin. In: Polak JM, Van Noordens S, eds. *Immunohistochemistry: Practical Applications in Pathology and Biology.* Bristol, England: Wright-PSG; 1983:143-168.
272. Trojanowski JQ, Lee VM. Expression of neurofilament antigens by normal and neoplastic human adrenal chromaffin cells. *N Engl J Med.* 1985;313:101-104.
273. Grignon DJ, Ro JY, MacKay B, et al. Paraganglioma of the urinary bladder: Immunohistochemical, ultrastructural and DNA flow cytometric studies. *Hum Pathol.* 1991;22:1162-1169.
274. Johnson TL, Zarbo RJ, Lloyd RV, Crissman JD. Paragangliomas of the head and neck: Immunohistochemical NE and intermediate filament typing. *Mod Pathol.* 1988;1:216-223.
275. Salim SA, Milroy C, Rode J, et al. Immunocytochemical characterization of NE tumors of the larynx. *Histopathology.* 1993;23:69-73.

276. Helman LJ, Cohen PS, Averbuch SD, et al. Neuropeptide Y expression distinguishes malignant from benign pheochromocytoma. *J Clin Oncol.* 1989;7:720-725.
277. Clarke MR, Weyant RJ, Watson CG, Carty SE. Prognostic markers in pheochromocytoma. *Hum Pathol.* 1998;29:522-526.
278. August C, August K, Schroeder S, et al. CGH and CD44/MIB-1 immunohistochemistry are helpful to distinguish metastasized sporadic pheochromocytomas. *Mod Pathol.* 2004;17:1119-1128.
279. Triche TJ, Askin F. Neuroblastoma and the differential diagnosis of small-, round-, blue-cell tumors. *Hum Pathol.* 1983;14:569-595.
280. Hachitanda Y, Tsuneyoshi M, Enjoji M. An ultrastructural and immunohistochemical evaluation of cytodifferentiation in neuroblastic tumors. *Mod Pathol.* 1989;2:13-19.
281. Pagani A, Forni M, Tonini GP, et al. Expression of members of the chromogranin family in primary neuroblastomas. *Diagn Mol Pathol.* 1992;1:16-24.
282. Carter RL, Al-Sams SZ, Corbett RP, et al. A comparative study of immunohistochemical staining for neuron-specific enolase, protein gene product 9.5 and s-100 in neuroblastoma, Ewing's sarcoma and other round cell tumors in children. *Histopathology.* 1990;16:461-467.
283. Wirnsberger GH, Becker H, Ziervogel K, et al. Diagnostic immunohistochemistry of neuroblastic tumors. *Am J Surg Pathol.* 1992;16:49-57.
284. Franquemont DW, Mills SE, Lack EE. Immunohistochemical detection of neuroblastomatous foci in composite adrenal pheochromocytoma-neuroblastoma. *Am J Clin Pathol.* 1994;102:163-170.
285. Argani P, Erlandson RA, Rosai J. Thymic neuroblastoma in adults: Report of three cases with special emphasis on its association with the syndrome of inappropriate secretion of antidiuretic hormone. *Am J Clin Pathol.* 1997;108:537-543.
286. Fellinger EJ, Garin-Chesa P, Triche TJ, et al. Immunohistochemical analysis of Ewing's sarcoma cell surface antigen p30/32 MIC2. *Am J Pathol.* 1991;39:317-325.
287. Stevenson AJ, Chatten J, Bertoni F, et al. CD99 (p30/32mic2) neuroectodermal/Ewing's sarcoma antigen as an immunohistochemical marker: Review of more than 600 tumors and the literature experience. *Appl Immunohistochem.* 1994;2:231-240.
288. Weidner N, Tjoe J. Immunohistochemical profile of monoclonal antibody 013: Antibody that recognizes glycoprotein p 30/32mic2 and is useful in diagnosing Ewing's sarcoma and peripheral neuroepithelioma. *Am J Surg Pathol.* 1994;18:486-494.
289. Scotlandi K, Serra M, Manara MC, et al. Immunostaining of the p30/32mic2 antigen and molecular detection of EWS rearrangements for the diagnosis of Ewing's sarcoma and peripheral neuroectodermal tumor. *Hum Pathol.* 1996;27:408-416.
290. Hess E, Cohen C, DeRose PB, et al. Nonspecificity of p30/32mic2 immunolocalization with the 013 monoclonal antibody in the diagnosis of Ewing's sarcoma: Application of an algorithmic immunohistochemical analysis. *Appl Immunohistochem.* 1997;5:94-103.
291. Pappo AS, Douglass ED, Meyer WH, et al. Use of HBA 71 and anti-B2-microglobulin to distinguish peripheral neuroepithelioma from neuroblastoma. *Hum Pathol.* 1993;24:880-885.
292. Miettinen M, Chatten J, Paetau A, et al. Monoclonal antibody NB84 in the differential diagnosis of neuroblastoma and other small round cell tumors. *Am J Surg Pathol.* 1998;22:327-332.
293. Folpe AL, Patterson K, Gown AM. Antineuroblastoma antibody NB-84 also identifies a significant subset of other small blue round cell tumors. *Appl Immunohistochem.* 1997;5:239-245.
294. Tischler AS. Pheochromocytoma and extra-adrenal paraganglioma: Update. *Arch Pathol Lab Med.* 2008;132:1272-1284.
295. Brouwers FM, Glasker S, Nave AF, et al. Proteomic profiling of von Hippel Lindau syndrome and multiple endocrine neoplasia type 2 pheochromocytomas reveal different expression of chromogranin B. *Endocr Relat Cancer.* 2007;14:463-471.
296. Brouwers FM, Elkahloun AG, Munson PJ, et al. Gene expression profiling of benign and malignant pheochromocytoma. *Ann NY Acad Sci.* 2006;1073:541-556.
297. Thouënnon E, Elkahloun A, Guillemot J, et al. Insights into the pathophysiology of pheochromocytoma malignancy. *J Clin Endocrinol Metab.* 2007;92:4865-4487.
298. Dayal Y. Endocrine cells of the gut and their neoplasms. In: Norris HT, ed. *Pathology of the Colon, Small Intestine and Anus.* New York: Churchill Livingstone; 1991:305-366.
299. Moll R, Franke WW. Cytoskeletal differences between human NE tumors: A cytoskeletal protein of molecular weight 46000 distinguishes cutaneous from pulmonary NE tumors. *Differentiation.* 1985;30:165-175.
300. Burke AP, Sobin LH, Federspiel BH, Shekitka KM. Appendiceal carcinoids: Correlation of histology and immunohistochemistry. *Mod Pathol.* 1989;2:630-637.
301. Miettinen M. Keratin 20: Immunohistochemical marker for gastrointestinal, urothelial, and Merkel cell carcinomas. *Mod Pathol.* 1995;8:384-388.
302. Al-Khafaji B, Noffsinger AE, Miller MA, et al. Immunohistologic analysis of gastrointestinal and pulmonary carcinoid tumors. *Hum Pathol.* 1998;29:992-999.
303. Kimura N, Pilichowska M, Okamoto H, et al. Immunohistochemical expression of chromogranins A and B, prohormone convertases 2 and 3, and amidating enzyme in carcinoid tumors and pancreatic endocrine tumors. *Mod Pathol.* 2000;13:140-146.
304. Thomas RM, Baybick JH, Elsayed AM, Sobin LH. Gastric carcinoids: An immunohistochemical and clinicopathologic study of 104 patients. *Cancer.* 1994;73:2053-2058.
305. Machlouf HR, Burke AP, Sobin LH. Carcinoid tumors of the ampulla of Vater: A comparison with duodenal carcinoid tumors. *Cancer.* 1999;85:1241-1249.
306. Sheibani K, Battifora H, Burke JS, Rappaport H. Leu-M1 antigen in human neoplasms: An immunohistologic study of 400 cases. *Am J Surg Pathol.* 1986;10:227-236.
307. Moskaluk CA, Zheng H, Powell SM, et al. CDX2 protein expression in normal and malignant human tissue: An immunohistochemical survey using tissue microarrrays. *Mod Pathol.* 2003;16:913-919.
308. Azumi N, Traweek ST, Battifora H. Prostatic acid phosphatase in carcinoid tumors: Immunohistochemical and immunoblot studies. *Am J Surg Pathol.* 1991;15:785-790.
309. Zikusoka MN, Kidd M, Eick G, et al. The molecular genetics of gastroenteropancreatic NE tumors. *Cancer.* 2005;104:2292-2309.
310. Fujimori M, Ikeda S, Shimizu Y, et al. Accumulation of beta-catenin gene in gastrointestinal carcinoid tumor. *Cancer Res.* 2001;61:6656-6659.
311. Su MC, Wang CC, Chen CC, et al. Nuclear translocation of beta-catenin and APC mutation in gastrointestinal carcinoid tumor. *Ann Surg Oncol.* 2006;13:1604-1609.
312. Shah IA, Schlageter M-O, Netto D. Immunoreactivity of neurofilament proteins in NE neoplasms. *Mod Pathol.* 1991;4:215-219.
313. Chejfec G, Falkmer S, Grimelius L, et al. Synaptophysin: A new marker for pancreatic NE tumors. *Am J Surg Pathol.* 1987;11:241-247.
314. Solcia E, Capella C, Kloppel G. *Atlas of Tumor Pathology: Tumors of the Pancreas.* Washington, DC: Armed Forces Institute of Pathology; 1997.
315. Heitz PU, Kasper M, Polak JM, Kloppel G. Pancreatic endocrine tumors: Immunocytochemical analysis of 125 tumors. *Hum Pathol.* 1982;13:263-271.
316. Perkins PL, McLeod MK, Jin L, et al. Analysis of gastrinomas by immunohistochemistry and in-situ hybridization histochemistry. *Diagn Mol Pathol.* 1992;1:155-164.
317. Le Bodic M-F, Heyman M-F, Lecomete M, et al. Immuno histochemical study of 100 pancreatic tumors in 28 patients with multiple endocrine neoplasia type I. *Am J Surg Pathol.* 1996;20:1378-1384.
318. Solcia E, Capella C, Riva C, et al. The morphology and NE profile of pancreatic epithelial VIPomas and extrapancreatic, VIP producing neurogenic tumors. *Ann NY Acad Sci.* 1988;527:508-517.
319. Heitz PU, Kasper M, Kloppel G, et al. Glycoprotein-hormone alpha-chain production by pancreatic endocrine tumors: A specific marker for malignancy: Immunocytochemical analysis of tumors of 155 patients. *Cancer.* 1983;51:277-282.

320. Graeme-Cook F, Nardi G, Compton CC. Immunocytochemical staining for human chorionic gonadotropin subunits does not predict malignancy in insulinomas. *Am J Clin Pathol.* 1990;93:273-276.
321. Viale G, Doglioni C, Gambacorta M, et al. Progesterone receptor immunoreactivity in pancreatic endocrine tumors: An immunocytochemical study of 156 NE tumors of the pancreas, gastrointestinal and respiratory tracts and skin. *Cancer.* 1992;70:2268-2277.
322. Pelosi G, Bresaola E, Bogina G, et al. Endocrine tumors of the pancreas: Ki-67 immunoreactivity on paraffin sections is an independent predictor for malignancy: A comparative study with proliferating-cell nuclear antigen and progesterone receptor protein immunostaining, mitotic index and other clinicopathological variables. *Hum Pathol.* 1996;27:1124-1134.
323. Heitz PU, Komminoth P, Perren A, et al. Pancreatic endocrine tumours: An introduction. In: DeLellis RA, Lloyd RV, Heitz PU, Eng C, eds. *Pathology and Genetics of Tumours of Endocrine Organs. WHO Classification of Tumours.* Lyon, France: IARC Press; 2004:177-182.
324. Deshpande V, Fernandez-del Castillo C, Muzikansky A, et al. Cytokeratin 19 is a powerful predictor of survival in pancreatic endocrine tumors. *Am J Surg Pathol.* 2004;28:1145-1153.
325. Goto A, Niki T, Terrado Y, et al. Prevalence of CD99 expression in pancreatic endocrine tumors (PETs). *Histopathology.* 2004;45:384-392.
326. Schmitt AM, Anlauf M, Rousson V, et al. WHO 2004 criteria and CK19 are reliable prognostic markers in pancreatic endocrine tumors. *Am J Surg Pathol.* 2007;31:1677-1682.
327. LaRosa S, Rigoli E, Uccella S, et al. Prognostic and biological significance of cytokeratin 19 in pancreatic endocrine tumors. *Histopathology.* 2007;50:597-606.
328. Shida T, Furuya M, Kishimoto T, et al. The expression of neuroD1 and MASH1 in the gastroenteropancreatic NE tumors. *Mod Pathol.* 2008;21:1363-1370.
329. Couvelard A, Hu J, Steers G, et al. Identification of potential therapeutic targets by gene expression profiling in pancreatic endocrine tumors. *Gastroenterology.* 2006;131:1597-1610.
330. Perren A, Anlauf M, Komminoth P. Molecular profiles of pancreatic endocrine tumors. *Virchows Arch.* 2007;451(Supp 1):S39-S46.
331. Gould VE, Linnoila RI, Memoli VA, Warren WH. NE components of the bronchopulmonary tract: Hyperplasias, dysplasias and neoplasias. *Lab Invest.* 1983;49:519-537.
332. Travis WD, Linnoila ID, Tsokos MG, et al. NE tumors of the lung with proposed criteria for large cell NE carcinoma: An ultrastructural, immunohistochemical and flow cytometric study of 35 cases. *Am J Surg Pathol.* 1991;15:529-553.
333. Blobel GA, Gould VE, Moll R, et al. Co-expression of NE markers and epithelial cytoskeletal proteins in bronchopulmonary NE neoplasms. *Lab Invest.* 1985;52:39-51.
334. Oliveira AM, Tazelaar HD, Myers JL, et al. Thyroid transcription factor-1 distinguishes metastatic pulmonary from well differentiated NE tumors of other sites. *Am J Surg Pathol.* 2001;25:815-819.
335. Du EZ, Goldstraw P, Zacharias J, et al. TTF-1 expression is specific for lung primary in typical and atypical carcinoids: TTF-1 positive carcinoids are predominantly in peripheral location. *Hum Pathol.* 2004;35:825-831.
336. Cai YC, Banner B, Glickman J, Odze RD. Cytokeratin 7 and 20 and thyroid transcription factor-1 can help distinguish pulmonary from gastrointestinal carcinoid and pancreatic endocrine tumors. *Hum Pathol.* 2001;32:1087-1093.
337. Jiang S-X, Kameya T, Shoji M, et al. Large cell NE carcinoma of the lung: A histological and immunohistochemical study of 22 cases. *Am J Surg Pathol.* 1998;22:526-537.
338. Xu H, Bourne PA, Spaulding BO, Wang HL. High-grade neuroendocrine carcinomas of the lung express K homology domain containing overexpressed in cancer by carcinoid tumors do not. *Human Pathol.* 2007;34:555-563.
339. LaPoint RJ, Bourne PA, Wang HL, Xu U. Coexpression of c-kit and bcl-2 in small cell carcinoma and large cell neuroendocrine carcinoma of the lung. *Appl Immunohistochem Mol Morph.* 2007;15:401-406.
340. Meyronet D, Massoma P, Thivolet F, et al. Extensive expression of a collapsin response mediation protein 5 (CRMP5) is a specific marker of high grade lung NE carcinoma. *Am J Surg Pathol.* 2008;32:1699-1708.
341. Gersell DJ, Mazoujian G, Mutch DG, Rudloff MA. Small cell undifferentiated carcinoma of the cervix: A clinicopathologic, ultrastructural and immunocytochemical study of 15 cases. *Am J Surg Pathol.* 1988;12:684-698.
342. Abeler VM, Holm R, Nesland JM, Kjorstad KE. Small cell carcinoma of the cervix: A clinicopathologic study of 26 patients. *Cancer.* 1994;73:672-677.
343. Gilks CB, Young RH, Gersell DJ, Clement PB. Large cell NE carcinoma of the uterine cervix: A clinicopathologic study of 12 cases. *Am J Surg Pathol.* 1997;21:905-914.
344. Chan JK, Suster S, Wenig B, et al. Cytokeratin 20 immunoreactivity distinguishes Merkel cell (primary cutaneous NE) carcinomas and salivary gland small cell carcinomas from small cell carcinomas of various sites. *Am J Surg Pathol.* 1997;21(2):226-234.
345. Ordonez NG. Value of thyroid transcription factor-1 immunostaining in distinguishing small cell lung carcinomas from other small cell carcinomas. *Am J Surg Pathol.* 2000;24:1217-1223.
346. Straughn JM, Richter HE, Conner MG, et al. Predictors of outcome in small cell carcinoma of the cervix—a case series. *Gynecol Oncol.* 2001;83:216-220.
347. Masumoto N, Fujii T, Ishikawa M, et al. p16 overexpression and human papillomavirus infection in small cell carcinoma of the uterine cervix. *Hum Pathol.* 2003;34:778-783.
348. Conner MG, Richter H, Moran CA, et al. Small cell carcinoma of the cervix: a clinicopathologic and immunohistochemical study of 23 cases. *Ann Diagn Pathol.* 2002;6:345-348.
349. Stoler MH, Mills SE, Gersell DJ, Walker AN, et al. Small cell NE carcinoma of the cervix: A human papillomavirus 18 associated cancer. *Am J Surg Pathol.* 1991;15:28-32.
350. Ishida GM, Kato N, Hayasaka T, et al. Small cell NE carcinomas of the uterine cervix: a histological, immunohistochemical, and molecular genetic study. *Int J Gynecol Pathol.* 2004;23:366-372.
351. Wang HL, Lu DW. Detection of human papillomavirus DNA and expression of p16, Rb, and p53 proteins in small cell carcinomas of the uterine cervix. *Am J Surg Pathol.* 2004;28:901-908.
352. Grayson W, Rhemtula HA, Taylor LF, et al. Detection of human papillomavirus in large cell NE carcinoma of the uterine cervix: A study of 12 cases. *J Clin Pathol.* 2002;55:108-114.
353. Matthews-Greer J, Dominguez-Malagon H, Herrera GA, et al. Human papillomavirus typing of rare cervical carcinomas. *Arch Pathol Lab Med.* 2004;128:553-556.
354. Wang K-L, Yang Y-C, Wang T-Y, et al. NE carcinoma of the uterine cervix: A clinicopathologic retrospective study of 31 cases with prognostic implications. *J Chemotherapy.* 2006;18:209-216.
355. Tangitgamol S, Ramirez PT, Sun CC, et al. Expression of HER-2/neu, epidermal growth factor receptor, vascular endothelial growth factor, cyclooxygenase-2, estrogen receptor, and progesterone receptor in small cell and large cell NE carcinoma of the cervix: A clinicopathologic and prognostic study. *Int J Gynecol Cancer.* 2005;15:646-656.
356. Zarka TA, Han AC, Edelson MI, et al. Expression of cadherins, p53 and bcl-2 in small cell carcinomas of the cervix: potential tumor suppressor role for N-cadherin. *Int J Gynecol Cancer.* 2003;13:240-243.
357. diSant'Agnese PA, de Mesy Jensen KL, Churukian CJ, et al. Human prostatic endocrine-paracrine (APUD) cells: Distributional analysis with a comparison of serotonin and neuron specific enolase immunoreactivity and silver stains. *Arch Pathol Lab Med.* 1985;109:607-612.
358. diSant'Agnese PA. NE differentiation in prostatic carcinoma: An update. *Prostate (Suppl).* 1998;8:74-79.
359. Schmid KW, Helpap B, Totsch M, et al. Immunohistochemical localization of chromogranins A and B and secretogranin II in normal, hyperplastic and neoplastic prostate. *Histopathology.* 1994;24:233-239.
360. Yuan TC, Veeraman S, Lin MF. NE-like prostate cancer cells: NE trans differentiation of prostate adenocarcinoma cells. *Endocr Relat Cancer.* 2007;14:531-547.

361. di Sant' Agnese PA. Divergent NE differentiation in prostatic carcinoma. *Sem Diagn Pathol.* 2000;17:4967-4161.
362. Ghannoum JE, DeLellis RA, Shin SJ. Primary carcinoid tumor of the prostate with concurrent adenocarcinoma: A case report. *Int J Surg Pathol.* 2004;12(2):167-170.
363. Azumi N, Shibuya H, Ishikura M. Primary prostatic carcinoid with intracytoplasmic prostatic acid phosphatase and prostate specific antigen. *Am J Surg Pathol.* 1984;8:545-550.
364. Goldstein NS. Immunophenotypic characterization of 225 prostate adenocarcinomas with intermediate or high Gleason scores. *Am J Clin Pathol.* 2002;117:471-477.
365. Kawai S, Hiroshima K, Tsukamoto Y, et al. Small cell carcinoma of the prostate expressing prostate-specific antigen and showing syndrome of inappropriate secretion of antidiuretic hormone: An autopsy case report. *Pathol Int.* 2003;53:892-896.
366. Azumi N, Shibuya H, Ishikura M. Primary prostatic carcinoid tumor with intracytoplasmic prostatic acid phosphatase and prostate-specific antigen. *Am J Surg Pathol.* 1984;8:545-550.
367. Bostwick DG, Dousa MK, Crawford BG, Wollan PC. NE differentiation in prostatic intraepithelial neoplasia and adenocarcinoma. *Am J Surg Pathol.* 1994;18:1240-1246.
368. Simon RA, diSant'Agnes PA, Huang L-S, et al. CD44 expression is a feature of prostatic small cell carcinoma and distinguishes it from its mimickers. *Hum Pathol.* 2009;40:252-258.
369. Sauer CG, Roemar A, Grobholz R. Genetic analysis of NE tumor cells in prostate carcinoma. *Prostate.* 2006;66:227-234.
370. Gould VE, Moll R, Moll I, et al. NE Merkel cells of the skin: Hyperplasias, dysplasias and neoplasms. *Lab Invest.* 1985;52: 334-353.
371. Leech SN, Kolar AJO, Barrett PD, et al. Merkel cell carcinoma can be distinguished from metastatic small cell carcinoma using antibodies to cytokeratin 20 and thyroid transcription factor 1. *J Clin Pathol.* 2001;54:727-729.
372. Cheuk W, Kwan MY, Suster S, et al. Immunostaining for thyroid transcription factor-1 and cytokeratin 20 aids the distinction of small cell carcinoma from Merkel cell carcinoma, but not pulmonary from extrapulmonary small cell carcinomas. *Arch Pathol Lab Med.* 2001;125:228-231.
373. Hanly AJ, Elgart GW, Jorda M, et al. Analysis of thyroid transcription factor-1 and cytokeratin 20 separates Merkel cell carcinoma from small cell carcinoma of lung. *J Cutan Pathol.* 2000;27:118-120.
374. Nicholson SA, McDermott MB, Swanson PE, Wick MR. CD99 and cytokeratin 20 in small cell and basaloid tumors of the skin. *Appl Immunohistochem Mol Morphol.* 2000;8:37-41.
375. Nagao T, Gaffey TA, Olsen KD, et al. Small cell carcinoma of the major salivary glands: Clinicopathologic study with emphasis on cytokeratin 20 immunoreactivity and clinical outcome. *Am J Surg Pathol.* 2004;28(6):762-770.
376. Jensen K, Kohler S, Rouse RV. Cytokeratin staining in Merkel cell carcinoma: An immunohistochemical study of cytokeratins 5/6, 7, 17, and 20. *Appl Immunohistochem Mol Morph.* 2000;8:310-315.
377. Drijkoningen M, de Wolf-Peeters C, van Limbergen E, Desmet V. Merkel cell tumor of the skin: An immunohistochemical study. *Hum Pathol.* 1986;17:301-307.
378. Liu Y, Mangini J, Saad R, et al. Diagnostic value of microtubule-associated protein-2 in Merkel cell carcinoma. 2003;11:326-329.
379. Sibley RK, Dahl D, Primary NE. (Merkel cell?) carcinoma of the skin. II: An immunohistochemical study of 21 cases. *Am J Surg Pathol.* 1985;9:109-116.
380. Dinh V, Feun L, Elgart G, et al. Merkel cell carcinomas. *Hematol Oncol Clin North Am.* 2007;21(3):527-544.
381. Brinkschmidt C, Stolze P, Fahrenkamp AG, et al. Immunohistochemical demonstration of chromogranin A, chromogranin B and secretoneunin in Merkel cell carcinoma of the skin: An immunohistochemical study suggesting two types of Merkel cell carcinoma. *Appl Immunohistochem.* 1995;3:37-44.
382. Sur M, AlArdati H, Ross C, Alowami S. TdT expression in Merkel cell carcinoma: Potential diagnostic pitfall with blastic hematological malignancies and expanded immunohistochemical analysis. *Mod Pathol.* 2007;20:1113-1120.
383. Buresh CT, Oliai BR. Reactivity with TdT in Merkel cell carcinoma: A potential diagnostic pitfall. *Am J Clin Pathol.* 2008;129:894-898.
384. Dong HY, Liu W, Cohen P, et al. B-cell activation protein encoded by the PAX-5 gene is commonly expressed in Merkel cell carcinoma and small cell carcinomas. *Am J Surg Pathol.* 2005;29:687-692.
385. Yang DT, Holden JA, Florell SR. CD117, CK20, TTF-1, and DNA topoisomerase II-α antigen expression in small cell tumors. *J Cutan Pathol.* 2004;31:254-261.
386. Su LD, Fullen DR, Lowe L, et al. CD117 (kit receptor) expression in Merkel cell carcinoma. *Am J Dermatopathol.* 2002;24:289-293.
387. Strong S, Shalders K, Carr R, et al. KIT receptor (CD117) expression in Merkel cell carcinoma. *Br J Dermatol.* 2004;150:384-385.
388. Han AC, Soler AP, Tang C-K, et al. Nuclear localization of E-cadherin expression in Merkel cell carcinoma. *Arch Pathol Lab Med.* 2000;124:1147-1151.
389. Tanaka Y, Sano T, Qian ZR, et al. Expression of adhesion molecules and cytokeratin 20 in merkel cell carcinomas. *Endocr Pathol.* 2004;15:117-129.
390. Ralston J, Chireboga L, Nonaka D. Mash1: A useful marker in differentiating pulmonary small cell carcinoma from Merkel cell carcinomas. *Mod Pathol.* 2009;21:1257-1362.
391. Pryor JG, Simon R, Bourne PA, et al. Merkel cell carcinoma expresses K homology domain-containing protein over expressed in cancer similar to other high grade neuroendocrine carcinomas. *Hum Pathol.* 2009;40:238-243.
392. Feng H, Shuda M, Chang Y, et al. Clonal integration of a polyomavirus in human Merkel cell carcinoma. *Science.* 2008;319:1096-1100.
393. Kassem A, Schöpflin A, Diaz C, et al. Frequent detection of Merkel cell polyomavirus in human Merkel cell carcinomas and identification of a unique deletion in the VP1gene. *Cancer Res.* 2008;68:5009-5013.
394. Kondapalli L, Soltani K, Lacouture ME. The promise of molecular targeted therapies: protein kinase inhibitors in the treatment of cutaneous malignancies. *J Am Acad Dermatol.* 2005;53:291-302.
395. Fenig E, Nordenberg J, Beery E, et al. Combined effect of aloe-emodin and chemotherapeutic agents on the proliferation of an adherent variant cell line of Merkel cell carcinomas. *Oncol Rep.* 2004;11:213-217.
396. Maluf HM, Koerner FC. Carcinomas of the breast with endocrine differentiation: A review. *Virchows Arch.* 1994;425:449-457.
397. Papotti M, Gherardi G, Eusebi V, et al. Primary oat cell (NE) carcinoma of the breast: Report of four cases. *Virchows Arch A Pathol Anat Histopathol.* 1992;420:103-108.
398. Adegbola T, Connolly CE, Mortimer G. Small cell neuroendocrine carcinoma of the breast: A report of 3 cases and review of the literature. *J Clin Pathol.* 2005;58:775-778.
399. Francois A, Chatikhine VA, Chevallier B, et al. NE primary small cell carcinoma of the breast: Report of a case and review of the literature. *Am J Clin Oncol.* 1995;18:133-138.
400. Sapino A, Righi L, Cassoni P, et al. Expression of the NE phenotype in carcinomas of the breast. *Semin Diagn Pathol.* 2000;17(2):127-137.
401. Viacava P, Castagna M, Bevilacqua G. Absence of NE cells in fetal and adult mammary gland: Are NE breast tumors real NE tumours? *Breast.* 1995;4:143-146.
402. Tavassoli F, Devilee P. *Tumours of the Breast and Female Genital Organs. WHO, Classification of Tumours.* Lyon, France: IARC Press; 2003.
403. Shin SJ, DeLellis RA, Ying BA, Rosen PP. Small cell carcinoma of the breast: A clinico-pathological and immunohistochemical study of 9 patients. *Am J Surg Pathol.* 2000;24:1231-1238.
404. Bergman S, Hoda SA, Geisinger KR, et al. E-cadherin-negative primary small cell carcinoma of the breast: Report of a case and review of the literature. *Am J Clin Pathol.* 2004;121:1170121.
405. Hoang MP, Maitra A, Gazdar AF, et al. Primary mammary small cell carcinoma: A molecular analysis of 2 cases. *Human Pathol.* 2001;32:753-757.
406. Yamasaki T, Shimazaki H, Aida S, et al. Case report: primary small cell (oat cell) carcinoma of the breast: Report of a case and review of the literature. *Pathol Int.* 2000;50:914-918.

407. Weigelt B, Horlings HM, Kreike B, et al. Refinement of breast cancer classification by molecular characterization of histological special types. *J Pathol*. 2008;216:141-150.
408. Perou CM, Sorlie T, Eisen MB, et al. Molecular portraits of human breast tumours. *Nature*. 2000;406:747-752.
409. Sorlie T, Perou CM, Tibshirani R, et al. Gene expression patterns of breast carcinomas distinguish tumor subclasses with clinical implications. *Proc Natl Acad Sci USA*. 2001;98:10869-10874.
410. Reis-Filho JS, Lakhani SR. Breast cancer special types: Why bother? *J Pathol*. 2008;Jul 31. [Epub ahead of print].
411. Klemm KM, Moran CA. Primary NE carcinoma of the thymus. *Semin Diagn Pathol*. 1999;16:32-41.
412. Moran CA, Suster S. Thymic NE carcinomas with combined features ranging from well-differentiated (carcinoid) to small cell carcinoma: A clinicopathologic and immunohistochemical study of 11 cases. *Am J Clin Pathol*. 2000;113:345-350.
413. De Montpreville VT, Macchiarini P, Dulmet E. Thymic NE carcinoma (carcinoid): A clinicopathologic study of fourteen cases. *J Thorac Cardiovasc Surg*. 1996;111:134-141.
414. Kaufmann O, Dietel M. Expression of thyroid transcription factor-1 in pulmonary and extrapulmonary small cell carcinomas and other NE carcinomas of various primary sites. *Histopathology*. 2000;36:415-420.
415. Moran CA, Suster S. NE carcinomas (carcinoid tumor) of the thymus. A clinicopathologic analysis of 80 cases. *Am J Clin Pathol*. 2000;114:100-110.
416. Hishima T, Fukayama M, Hayashi Y, et al. NE differentiation in thymic epithelial tumors with special reference to thymic carcinoma and atypical thymoma. *Hum Pathol*. 1998;29:330-338.
417. Goto K, Kodama T, Matsuno Y, et al. Clinicopathologic and DNA cytometric analysis of carcinoid tumors of the thymus. *Mod Pathol*. 2001;14:985-994.
418. Pan C-C, Jong Y-J, Chen Y-J. Comparative genomic hybridization analysis of thymic NE tumors. *Modern Pathol*. 2005;18:358-364.
419. Reiker RJ, Aulmann S, Penzel R, et al. Chromosomal imbalances in sporadic NE tumours of the thymus. *Cancer Letters*. 2004;223:169-174.

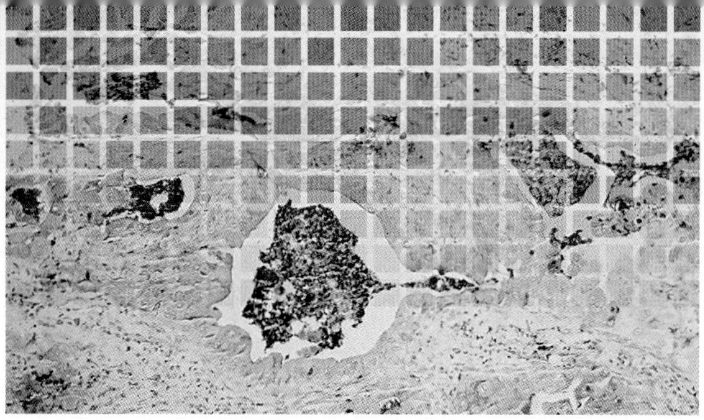

11

Immunohistology of the Mediastinum

Mark R. Wick

- Introduction 340
- Biology of Antigens and Antibodies 340
- Algorithmic Immunohistochemistry of Mediastinal Disease 340
- Immunohistologic Findings in Specific Diseases of the Mediastinum 341
- Prognostic Markers in Mediastinal Neoplasms 364

INTRODUCTION

The mediastinum is a relatively confined anatomic site, but it is capable of harboring a wide variety of non-neoplastic and neoplastic pathologic processes. These include proliferations of somatic epithelial, lymphoid, mesenchymal, and germ cell types. Surgical pathology of mediastinal disorders is all the more challenging because small biopsies (taken by either mediastinoscopy or closed needle biopsy) have become routine as the primary method of diagnosis.[1-6] Therefore, one is often faced with the need to perform numerous immunostains on such material in order to obtain a meaningful diagnosis in the absence of much morphologic detail. This chapter presents a synopsis of immunohistologic information as applied to this topic; however, it is not encyclopedic in regard to the scope of pathologic entities that may arise in the mediastinum or the panoply of immunoreactants assessed in them. This chapter will, however, emphasize practical differential diagnosis and the role that immunohistology plays in that process.

BIOLOGY OF ANTIGENS AND ANTIBODIES

Very few cellular proliferations of the mediastinum—neoplastic or otherwise—are unique to it. Therefore, the spectrum of immunoreactants that is of interest in this topographic region overlaps significantly with that considered in other chapters. Hence, this chapter will not recount the biochemical attributes of intermediate filament subtypes, the various membrane glycoproteins synthesized by epithelial and hematopoietic cells, or cytoplasmic differentiation-related proteins. Refer to specific chapters in this text for in-depth discussions of topics such as carcinomas, hematolymphoid lesions, specific mesenchymal proliferations, and so on. This chapter will, however, describe reactants that appear to be restricted to mediastinal disorders or are elaborated in a singular fashion in these diseases.

Thymic Hormones: Several hormonal proteins are apparently synthesized by epithelial cells of the thymus, and they are thought to have distant effects on the development or function of the immunologic system. Such moieties include thymopoietic, thymic humoral factor, thymosin, facteur thymique serique, thymic factor X, thymic plasma recirculating factor, thymotoxin, thymulin, and thymin.[7] Among them, only thymosin has been evaluated immunohistochemically in human neoplasms, primarily in thymomas, with reactivity being observed in >80% of cases.[8] Nevertheless, there have been no systematic studies of the differential diagnostic utility (or lack thereof) of thymic hormones, and their practical role in the surgical pathology laboratory is consequently unknown.

Keratin Subclasses: As in many other organs, keratin subsets have been analyzed in the normal thymus and in tumors deriving from it.[9,10] In particular, keratins 7, 13, and 18 appear to be expressed in this spectrum of tissues. Keratin 13 is restricted to epithelial cells of the thymic medulla but is shared by thymomas of all types. Keratins 7 and 18 likewise appear to be preferentially seen in neoplastic proliferations of this gland.

ALGORITHMIC IMMUNOHISTOCHEMISTRY OF MEDIASTINAL DISEASE

Perhaps in reaction to the overwhelming number of antibodies that one may now apply to diagnostic questions in surgical pathology, shotgun approaches to immunohistology have become worryingly common. Concerns over medicolegal liabilities also may prompt one to empty the reservoir of reagents in the evaluation of difficult cases. Nonetheless, published experience with well-characterized procedures and antibodies has made this temptation unnecessary. Indeed, a sufficient body of data on reagent specificity and sensitivity that one may codify by means of integration into algorithms is now available.

Adjunctive algorithmic diagnosis has several benefits. It provides reproducible strategies that can be used to resolve recurring problems in histopathology, gives one a prescribed sequence in which the results of predefined antibody-mediated stains may be interpreted, and compensates for the reality that no single reagent is likely to provide a definitive answer in any given case. The last of these points is important because it has been fashionable (but largely non-contextual and fatuous, in the author's opinion) to embrace the practice of "antibody bashing" with regard to the specificity of individual reagents.

Before immunohistochemical algorithms can be safely and effectively applied, one must heed the following caveats:

1. The user (pathologist) must control the processing of all tissues in his or her own laboratory under stringent conditions. When specimen fixation times or conditions vary wildly, antibody reactivity patterns will also vary.
2. The user (not the manufacturer or distributor) must personally determine the optimal dilutions of all antibody reagents. Simply following commercial recommendations is unwise; practical information can be found in published scientific papers on such reagents.
3. The user must accrue data on the spectra of reactivity for all antibodies, over a broad group of pathologic conditions or neoplasms, as processed and studied in his or her laboratory. Failing the feasibility of this approach, the user must adopt the exact method of fixation, processing, and staining that is used in published investigations containing the desired information.
4. Algorithms must be based on formal statistical analyses of specificity, sensitivity, and Bayesian predictive values, as applied to predefined differential diagnostic problems. This approach allows one to determine relative values for each determinant in well-characterized settings.
5. Relative statistical values must govern the sequence of interpretation of a group of immunostains and should move from most to least specific or from highest to lowest positive predictive value.
6. Distinct morphologic categories must be determined for application of the foregoing principles. For example, one can generically classify all morphologically indeterminate and undifferentiated neoplasms of the mediastinum into one of three major groups: small cell, large polygonal cell, and spindle cell/pleomorphic tumors.
7. Immunohistochemical data must be applied only in the context of thorough morphologic analysis and well-formulated differential diagnosis. Immunostains are merely diagnostic adjuncts, and they do not replace skill in the interpretation of slides stained with hematoxylin and eosin. A poor histodiagnostician would probably be a worse immunohistochemist! Hence, one must always ensure that clinical information, histologic differential diagnosis, and immunohistologic interpretations fit together in a sensible fashion.
8. Algorithms should be flexible. As new reagents are introduced and suitably characterized, they may be integrated into pre-existing schemes to replace or supplement older antibodies.

Working examples of practical algorithms used in the author's laboratory are presented in Chapter 12. The statistical data used to construct them were gathered over a period of several years using the following: specimens that were fixed routinely in 10% neutral-buffered formalin; primary antibody incubations at 4°C for 16 to 18 hours; the Elite avidin-biotin-peroxidase complex method of immunodetection (Vector Laboratories, Burlingame, Calif); and the antibody reagents listed in Table 11.1.

IMMUNOHISTOLOGIC FINDINGS IN SPECIFIC DISEASES OF THE MEDIASTINUM

Cystic Thymoma Versus Cystic Seminoma

In many respects, cystic thymomas are morphologically quite similar to thymic cysts.[11-13] However, more pertinently, they may also be confused with intrathymic seminomas, which manifest prominent cystic changes.[14,15] These lesions are usually separated from one another adequately by conventional microscopy, inasmuch as cystic seminoma typically displays a much greater degree of nuclear atypia than thymoma. However, in small biopsies this feature may be unclear. The periodic acid-Schiff stain is helpful in delineating the glycogen content that typifies seminomas, and it may be used to screen for the neoplastic cell aggregates in this particular setting. Similarly, immunostains for placental alkaline phosphatase (PLAP) and those with a broadly reactive mixture of monoclonal antibodies to keratin are helpful in this setting. With nuclear labeling, seminomas are uniformly positive for PLAP and podoplanin (with a cell-membranous pattern of reactivity) and for Oct-¾; <15% will label for keratin.[14-18] On the other hand, thymoma is universally keratin positive and lacks the other markers just cited.[19,20]

Differential Diagnosis of Other Thymoma Variants

The favored nosologic scheme for thymomas groups them into several discrete categories based on microscopic morphology: lymphocyte predominant (>66%

TABLE 11.1 Antibodies Used in the Algorithmic Immunohistochemical Analysis of Mediastinal Diseases

Antigen	Antibody (Clone)	Source	Dilution
Cytokeratins	AE1	Boehringer-Mannheim	1:100
	AE1/AE3	Boehringer-Mannheim	1:150
	CAM5.2	Becton-Dickinson	1:150
	MAK6	Triton BioSciences	1:40
CK20	ITKs2O.8	DAKO	1:40
Vimentin	V9	BioGenex	1:2000
Desmin	033	BioGenex	1:2000
Epithelial membrane antigen	E29	DAKO	1:400
Carcinoembryonic antigen	NG	Boehringer-Mannheim	1:4000
Epithelial antigen	BEREP4	DAKO	1:200
Calretinin	Polyclonal	Zymed	1:750
Neuron-specific enolase	Polyclonal	BioGenex	1:450
Chromogranin A	LK2H1O	Boehringer-Mannheim	1:4000
Synaptophysin	SY38	Boehringer-Mannheim	1:40
CD57	Leu7	Becton-Dickinson	1:20
S-100 protein	Polyclonal	DAKO	1:300
Antimelanoma	HMB-45	BioGenex	1:60
Tyrosinase	T311	Novocastra	1:20
MART-1	A103	BioGenex	1:25
Muscle-specific actin	HHF-35	BioGenex	1:400
Alpha-isoform actin	IA4	BioGenex	1:2
Myogenin	F5D	DAKO	1:10
Myo-D1	AntiMyoD1	DAKO	1:10
Placental alkaline phosphatase	Polyclonal	DAKO	1:800
Alpha fetoprotein	C3	BioGenex	1:40
CD31	JC/70A	DAKO	1:40
CD34	Myl 0	DAKO	1:800
CD45	PD7/26-2B111	DAKO	1:80
CD3	Polyclonal	DAKO	1:40
CD5	CD5/54/B4	Vector	1:4
	4C7	Vector	1:100
CD43	MT1	BioGenex	1:50
	DF-T1	DAKO	1:50
CD45RO	UCHL-1	DAKO	1:120
CD20	L26	DAKO	1:200
Membrane-bound B-cell antigen	MB2	BioGenex	1:80
CD74	LN2	BioGenex	1:8
CD15	LeuM1	Becton-Dickinson	1:150
CD30	BerH2	DAKO	1:40
Anti-Hodgkin disease	BLA.36	DAKO	1:200
Anti-large cell lymphoma	BNH9	DAKO	1:200
Lysozyme	Polyclonal	DAKO	1:400

TABLE 11.1 Antibodies Used in the Algorithmic Immunohistochemical Analysis of Mediastinal Diseases—cont'd

Antigen	Antibody (Clone)	Source	Dilution
Cathepsin B	Polyclonal	ICN Biomed	1:800
Myeloid/Histiocyte Antigen	MAC387	DAKO	1:800
CD68	KP1	DAKO	1:800
Myeloperoxidase	Polyclonal	DAKO	1:250
Ki-67	MIB-1	AMAC	1:200
PCNA	PC10	Novocastra	1:400
p53	D01	Oncogene Sci	1:160
	D07	DAKO	1:240
CD21	Clone 1F8	DAKO	1:100
CD23	Clone Tu1	NovoCastra	1:100
CD35	Clone BerMACDRC	DAKO	1:150
CD117	Clone A4502	DAKO	1:250
Oct-¾	Clone C10	Santa Cruz	1:300
Podoplanin	Clone NZ-1	AngioBio	1:200

NG, Not given by manufacturer.

lymphocytes), epithelial predominant (>66% epithelial cells), mixed lymphoepithelial (34% to 66% epithelial cells), and spindle cell (a subtype of epithelial-predominant thymoma featuring a nearly exclusive composition by fusiform tumor cells).[19,21-24] However, for this system to have clinical usefulness, thymoma must be defined as a cytologically bland epithelial neoplasm. This utility is not one of prognostication, but rather a cue to the consideration of dissimilar differential diagnostic categories that attend each of the four major histologic categories mentioned earlier. Salient diagnostic problems that are specific to these tumor subgroups are presented in the following paragraphs. Later in the discussion, we will consider the distinction between thymoma and primary thymic carcinoma (which may occasionally arise in transition *from* thymoma).

LYMPHOCYTE-PREDOMINANT THYMOMA VERSUS LYMPHOID HYPERPLASIA

In patients with myasthenia gravis, one must distinguish between true thymic hyperplasia[25] and thymoma in surgical specimens. In general, thymoma does not manifest the presence of internal lymphoid follicles, although the latter do occur rarely. In this circumstance, immunostaining for keratin reveals a finely arborized network of interconnecting epithelial cell processes between the lymphocytes in thymoma (Fig. 11.1), which is not seen in lymphoid hyperplasia.[20,21,26]

LYMPHOCYTE-PREDOMINANT THYMOMA VERSUS LYMPHOMA

The imitation of lymphoblastic lymphoma (LL) by selected lymphocyte-rich thymomas is enhanced by the peculiar features of infiltrating lymphocytes in some of the latter tumors; these may show convoluted nuclear contours, increased nucleocytoplasmic ratios, and brisk mitotic activity,[21] as typically seen in LL. Moreover, the immunophenotypes of the lymphocytes in thymomas and those of LL cells are remarkably comparable. Both populations are typically labeled for CD1a, CD2, CD3, CD5, CD43, CD99 (MIC-2),[27-29] and BCL-2,[29-31] as well as terminal deoxynucleotidyl transferase.[28,29,32-38] Consequently, immunohistochemical distinctions between these neoplasms must be made with extreme caution.

The most helpful immunostain in this differential diagnosis—and one that the author, through regrettable mistakes, has made routine—is an assessment of keratin reactivity. The elaborately interconnecting epithelial cells of lymphocyte-predominant thymoma (LPT), which are not seen in LL, are distinctive. This *pattern* is essential to differential diagnosis, because LL and other lymphomas of thymus may demonstrate entrapped nonneoplastic thymic epithelial cells that are visible (but widely separated and non-interconnecting) on keratin immunostains.[5,39] Another potential marker for thymic epithelium—p63 protein[40]—is not as useful in this particular contextual setting. That is true because LL may be p63-reactive as well.[41]

PREDOMINANTLY EPITHELIAL SPINDLE-CELL THYMOMA VERSUS FIBROUS HISTIOCYTOMA AND SOLITARY FIBROUS TUMOR/HEMANGIOPERICYTOMA

Predominantly epithelial thymomas (PET) that are constituted by spindle cells may be difficult to separate diagnostically from fibrous histiocytomas (FH) or solitary fibrous tumors/hemangiopericytomas (HPCs) by conventional histologic study.[21] Immunohistochemistry is a more discerning method toward that end, particularly

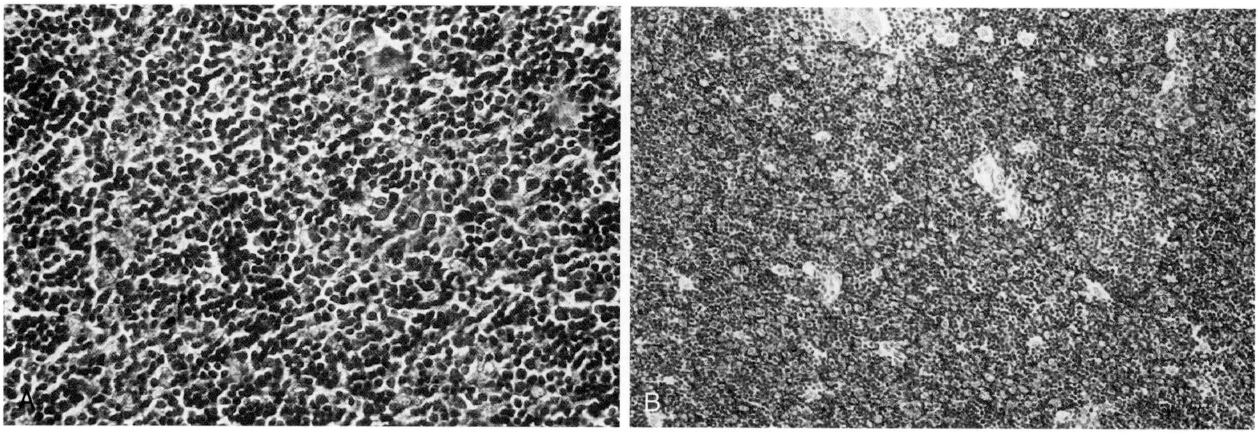

FIGURE 11.1 Keratin in lymphocyte-predominant thymoma **(A)**. Note the delicately interlocking pattern of reactivity **(B)**.

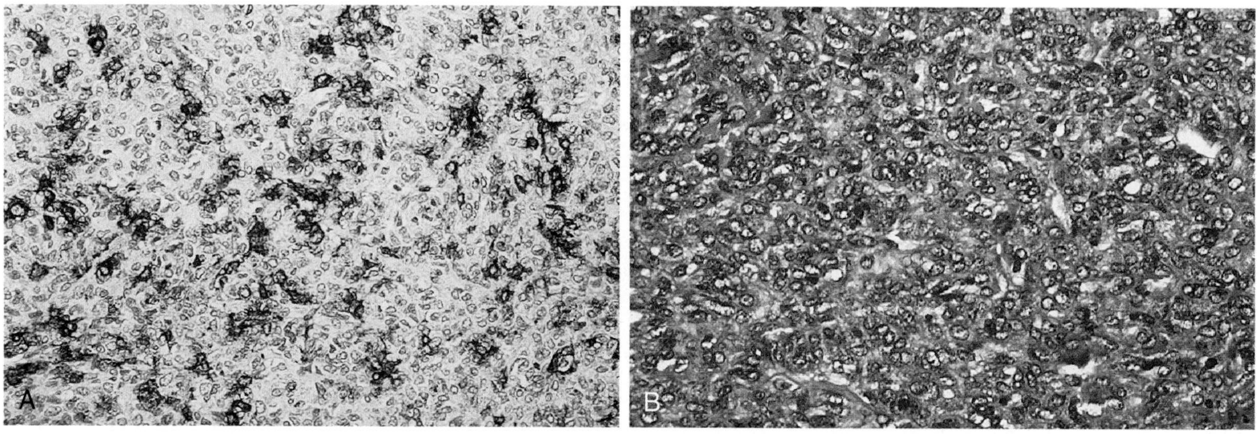

FIGURE 11.2 CD34 positivity **(A)** in true hemangiopericytoma **(B)** of the mediastinum.

when only small biopsy specimens are available for analysis. Pseudomesenchymal thymomas are universally positive for keratin and lack vimentin,[20] whereas FH and HPC show the opposite of that pattern.[42] In addition, HPC commonly demonstrates reactivity for CD34 (Fig. 11.2),[43] whereas the latter determinant is not expected in thymomas.

KEY DIAGNOSTIC POINTS

Thymus

- The elaborate keratin-positive meshwork of thymic epithelial cells is present in thymoma, but not in areas of thymic hyperplasia or lymphoma.
- Spindle cells of hemangiopericytoma, not thymoma, are CD34+.

Benign Peripheral Nerve Sheath Tumors and Ganglioneuromas

The overwhelming majority of neoplasms encountered in the posterior mediastinum are neurogenic in nature.[44-46] Therefore, they often show morphologic similarities to one another and consequently present diagnostic difficulties. Schwann-cell neoplasms (peripheral nerve sheath tumors; PNST) are usually subdivided into specific neurofibromas and neurilemmomas (schwannomas) because of their differing associations with von Recklinghausen disease and the risk of malignant transformation.[46-49] They also must be separated from ganglioneuromas.[45,50] All of these proliferations are reactive for vimentin and S-100 protein in a uniform manner. In fact, S-100 negativity should cast serious doubt on any of the three diagnoses under discussion. Fine and colleagues[51] have observed that calretinin is present in most schwannomas but is only present in a small number of neurofibromas, which makes this marker potentially useful in detailed diagnosis. A comparable statement can be made in reference to podoplanin.[52] Synaptophysin, a synaptic vesicle-related protein that is typical of neuronal and neuroendocrine lesions,[53] is a helpful determinant for the labeling of ganglion cells (which may be focal or widely scattered) in ganglioneuromas.

Fibrogenic and Myofibroblastic Proliferations

Four cytologically bland spindle-cell proliferations of the mediastinum may be mistaken for one another histologically; namely, solitary fibrous tumor (SFT),[54-56]

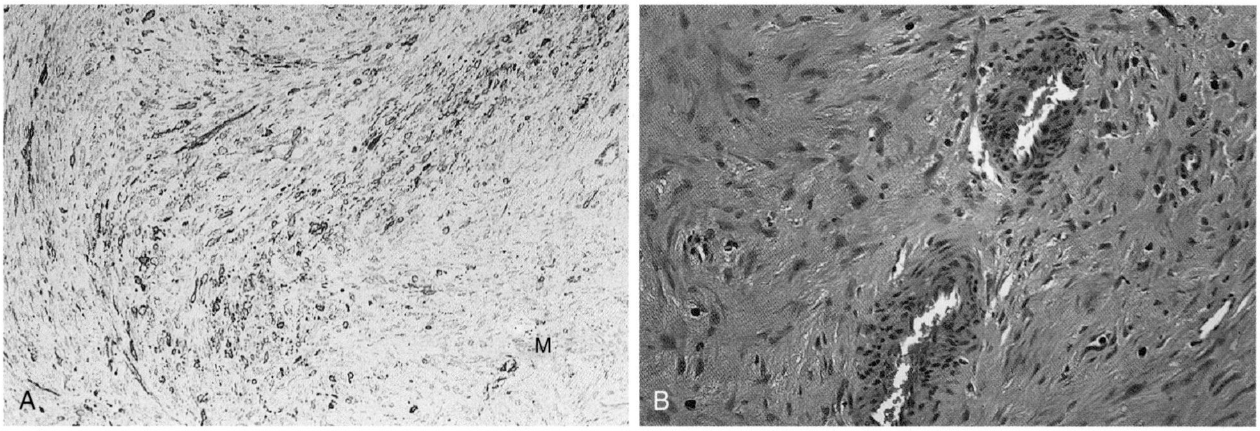

FIGURE 11.3 Muscle-specific actin (M) **(A)** is present in the proliferating cells of this mediastinal desmoid-type fibromatosis **(B)**.

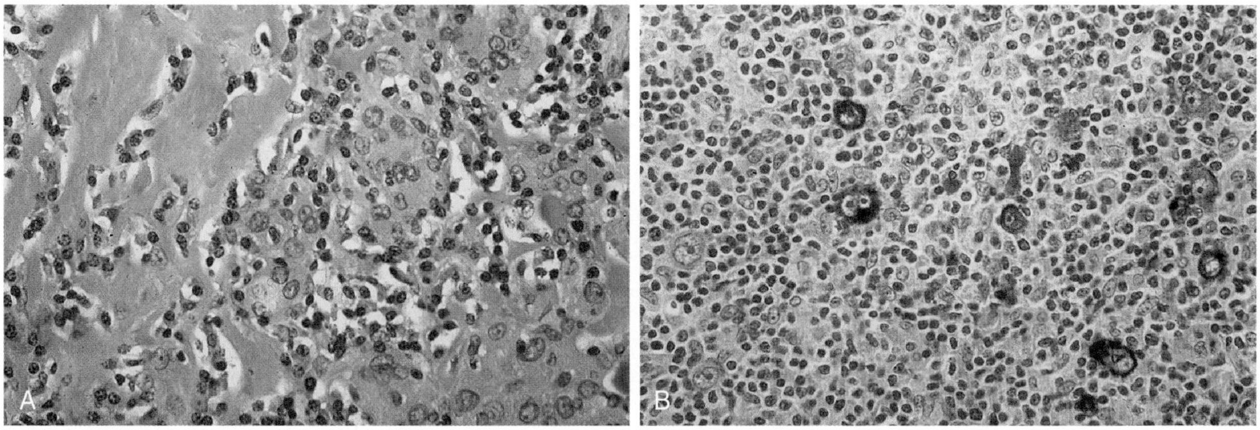

FIGURE 11.4 **(A)** This dense fibroinflammatory mass in the mediastinum has the appearance of a tumefactive fibroinflammatory lesion (fibrosing mediastinitis). However, biopsy of an adjacent lymph node **(B)** demonstrated classic Reed-Sternberg cells (labeled for CD30), which established a diagnosis of the total obliterative nodular sclerosing subtype of Hodgkin disease.

desmoid-type fibromatosis, sclerosing mediastinitis, and inflammatory myofibroblastic tumor (inflammatory pseudotumor).[56-60] The immunophenotype shows reactivity for vimentin and CD34, with a lack of keratin, epithelial membrane antigen, S-100 protein, desmin, and actin.

In contrast, fibromatoses and inflammatory myofibroblastic (pseudo-) tumors (IMTs) show a mixture of cells that label for vimentin and muscle-specific or alpha-isoform actin, with or without desmin (Fig. 11.3).[61-63] The distinction between the latter two lesions can usually be made on the basis of morphologic features alone; however, immunostains for anaplastic lymphoma kinase-1 (ALK-1) and nuclear beta-catenin (NBC) also may contribute. The first of these markers is seen in approximately 40% of IMTs, but not in fibromatoses. Conversely, NBC characterizes the great majority of desmoid-type fibromatosis cases.[64,65] Sclerosing mediastinitis (SM) is composed of spindle cells that are only reactive for vimentin. However, one must observe an important caution in reference to lesions thought to be SM. Selected malignant lymphomas (especially obliterative total sclerosis Hodgkin disease),[14,66] metastatic carcinomas, and desmoplastic mesotheliomas may engender a densely fibrotic response in the mediastinal soft tissue or lymph node groups. The actual tumor cells in such cases are consequently sparse and may be surprisingly bland cytologically. Accordingly, they may be overlooked and lead to diagnostic mistakes (Fig. 11.4).[67-69] Thus, stains for keratin, CD15, CD20, CD30, and CD45 should be routine in the assessment of putative cases of SM.

Malignant Small-Cell Mediastinal Neoplasms (Tables 11.2, 11.3; Figs. 11.5-11.8)

MEDIASTINAL SMALL-CELL NEUROENDOCRINE CARCINOMA (GRADE III NEUROENDOCRINE CARCINOMA, SMALL-CELL TYPE)

Nearly all small-cell neuroendocrine carcinomas (SCNCs) involving the mediastinum are metastatic,[70] usually from tumors of the lungs or esophagus. Immunophenotypically, SCNC commonly demonstrates perinuclear punctate labeling for keratin (Fig. 11.9),[20] which is a specific marker of neuroendocrine lineage in a small-cell neoplasm. Less frequently, it will show reactivity for one of several neuroendocrine markers such as chromogranin, synaptophysin, CD56, CD57, or specific neuropeptides.[71-76] There are currently no reliable discriminants to distinguish

TABLE 11.2	Immunoreactants Used in the Differential Diagnosis of Small Cell Indeterminate and Undifferentiated Neoplasms of the Mediastinum
Keratin (monoclonal mixture)	
Epithelial membrane antigen	
Vimentin	
Desmin	
Muscle-specific actin	
Myo-D1	
Myogenin	
Neuron-specific enolase	
Synaptophysin	
Chromogranin A	
CD15	
CD45	
CD99 (MIC-2 protein)	
Ber-EP4	
S-100 protein	
HMB-45	
MART-1	
Tyrosinase	
PNL2	
FLI-1	

between primary (thymic) and secondary mediastinal SCNCs; thyroid transcription factor-1 (TTF-1) is seen in 85% to 95% of pulmonary neuroendocrine tumors of this type,[77,78] but there are still no meaningful data on the expression of this marker in primary thymic endocrine tumors.

BASALOID SQUAMOUS CELL CARCINOMA OF THE MEDIASTINUM

Basaloid squamous cell carcinoma (BSCC) also may be either a primary thymic tumor[75,79,80] or a mediastinal metastasis from a primary neoplasm of the oropharynx, hypopharynx, larynx, esophagus, lungs, or anorectal region.[80] Keratin is universally present in BSCC with a diffuse cytoplasmic pattern of labeling, and reactivity for epithelial membrane antigen, keratin 5/6, and p63 may also be observed.[21,78,80,81] In the author's experience, neuroendocrine determinants have been consistently absent.

NEUROBLASTOMA OF THE MEDIASTINUM

Characteristically, neuroblastoma (NBL) is a disease of young children,[46,82] and it is usually located in the posterior mediastinum.[83,84] Nonetheless, rare examples of this tumor and its congeners in the anterior mediastinum have also been reported in adults.[85,86] The immunoprofile of NBL includes variable reactivity for vimentin and neurofilament protein; a substantial proportion of cases will lack both of these proteins.[87] Neural features are reflected by positivity for CD56, CD57, and synaptophysin (Fig. 11.10).[45,88] Neuroblastomas are universally devoid of markers of myogenous differentiation (desmin, actin, Myo-D1, myogenin), a hematolymphoid lineage (CD45), and epithelial character (keratin, epithelial membrane antigen).[57,85] NB84 is a monoclonal antibody that was raised specifically against NBL; although it is not specific for that neoplasm, this marker is seen in the great majority of neuroblastic tumors.[89]

MEDIASTINAL PRIMITIVE NEUROECTODERMAL TUMOR

The primitive neuroectodermal tumor (PNET) may rarely occur in the mediastinum, either in the anterior or in the posterior compartments.[90] The immunophenotype of PNET is similar to that of neuroblastoma, but the former of these lesions shows more uniform reactivity for vimentin and only occasionally is labeled for neurofilament protein.[42] Moreover, the CD99 (p30/32 [MIC-2]) and MB2 antigens and beta-2-microglobulin are consistently seen in PNET but not in NBL (Fig. 11.11).[91-94] Synaptophysin, CD56, and CD57 are detectable in many cases of PNET as well, and examples of this tumor with divergent differentiation will also demonstrate focal reactivity for keratin, desmin, and actin.[42,95] Such lesions also have been termed *desmoplastic small cell tumor of the peritoneum, rhabdomyosarcoma-like small cell tumors of soft tissue,* and *ectomesenchymomas,* among other designations. In some instances, it may be difficult to distinguish between a solid alveolar rhabdomyosarcoma (refer to the following section) that is MIC-2–positive and a PNET with divergent rhabdomyoblastic differentiation, especially if synaptophysin is absent. In such cases, one may have to rely on cytogenetic evaluations, seeking the characteristic t(2;13) or t(1;13) chromosomal translocations of alveolar rhabdomyosarcoma or the t(11;22) translocation of PNET. Another possible avenue of discrimination is represented by immunostaining for FLI-1, a nuclear transcription factor that is expressed in most PNETs. It has not been observed in histologically similar striated muscle sarcomas.[96]

RHABDOMYOSARCOMA OF THE MEDIASTINUM

Rhabdomyosarcoma (RMS) of the mediastinum is almost exclusively observed in children and adolescents[45,97,98] and may demonstrate embryonal or alveolar architectural features (see Chapter 17). Nearly all rhabdomyosarcomas express desmin (Fig. 11.12) and muscle-specific actin, together with vimentin. Myoglobin is observed only in large maturing rhabdomyoblasts and is therefore not a particularly useful marker of RMS in its purely small-cell form. Synaptophysin is lacking in RMS, but some cases will demonstrate labeling for CD56

TABLE 11.3 Percentages of Immunoreactivity for Selected Markers in Malignant Small Cell Tumors of the Mediastinum with Indeterminate or Undifferentiated Histologic Features

Tumor	KER	EMA	VIM	DES	MSA	MYO-D1	MYOGN	S-100	HMB-45	TYR	MART-1	NSE	SYN	CGA	BER-EP4	CD45	CD15	CD99
ES/PNET	10	0	87	1	3	3	3	10	0	0	0	91	74	0	70	0	0	81
RMS	0	0	91	93	97	91	92	7	0	0	0	37	0	0	0	0	0	20
LL/TAL*	0	0	23	0	0	0	0	10	0	0	0	11	0	0	0	90/78	85/52	10
SCMM	1	3	100	0	0	0	0	97	50	86	87	70	0	0	0	0	0	7
PNBL	0	0	56	0	0	0	0	37	0	0	0	99	65	71	0	0	0	0
MSCSCC	100	83	35	0	0	0	0	52	0	0	0	50	40	0	60	0	0	0
MSCADCA	100	99	12	0	0	0	0	5	0	0	0	44	15	0	92	0	69	0
SCNC	99	73	0	0	0	0	0	0	0	0	0	70	35	40	100	0	18	20
SCUS	0	0	100	0	0	0	0	0	0	0	0	10	0	0	0	0	0	0

*Unless otherwise indicated, the given percentage of reactivity applies to both tumor entities.

KER, keratin (mixture of monoclonal antibodies); EMA, epithelial membrane antigen; VIM, vimentin; DES, desmin; MSA, muscle-specific actin; MYOGN, myogenin; S-100, S-100 protein; TYR, tyrosinase; NSE, neuron-specific (gamma dimer) enolase; SYN, synaptophysin; CGA, chromogranin A; PNET, primitive neuroectodermal tumor; ES, Ewing's sarcoma; RMS, rhabdomyosarcoma; LL, lymphoblastic lymphoma; TAL, tumefactive acute myelogenous leukemia; SCMM, small cell malignant melanoma; PNBL, peripheral neuroblastoma; MSCSCC, metastatic small cell squamous cell carcinoma; MSCADCA, metastatic small cell adenocarcinoma; SCNC, small cell neuroendocrine carcinoma; SCUS, small cell undifferentiated sarcoma.

Data from Frisman D. Immunoquery (available at http://www.immunoquery.com) and the author's experience.

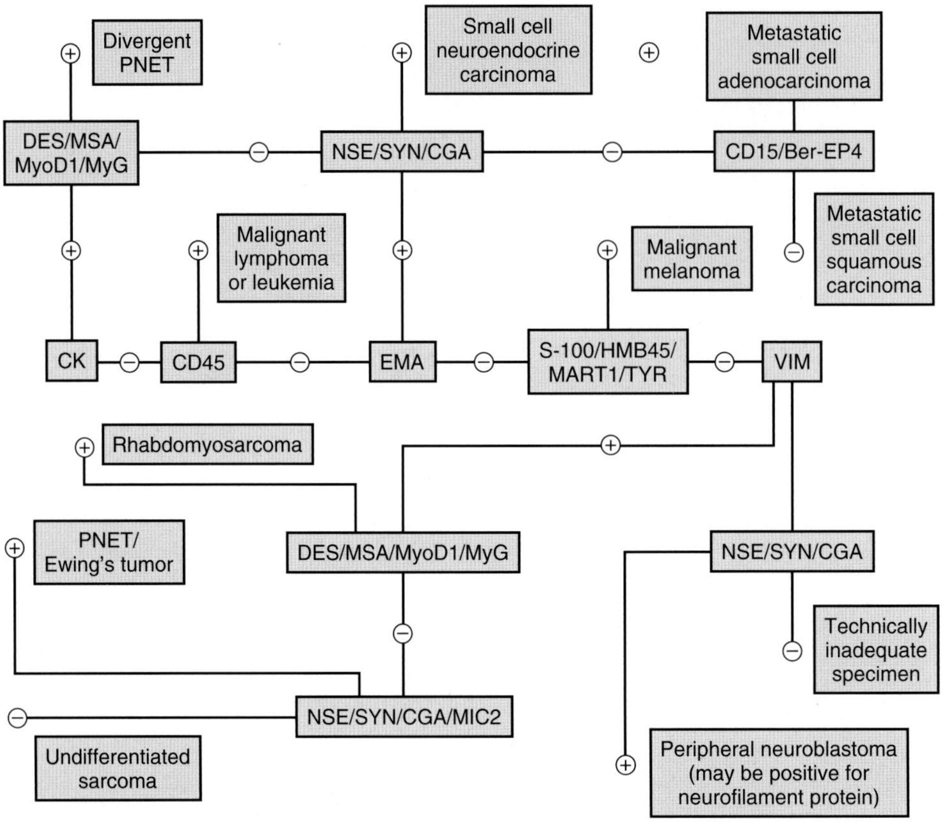

FIGURE 11.5 Algorithm for immunohistologic evaluation of malignant small-cell tumors of the mediastinum.

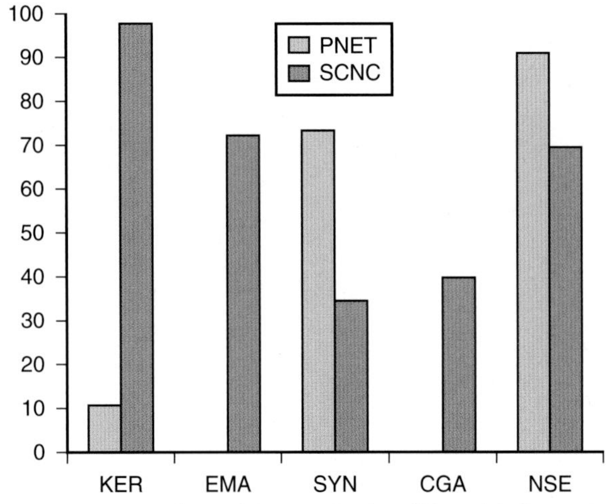

FIGURE 11.6 Markers of interest in the differential diagnosis of primitive neuroectodermal tumor (PNET) versus small-cell neuroendocrine carcinoma of the mediastinum (SCNC).

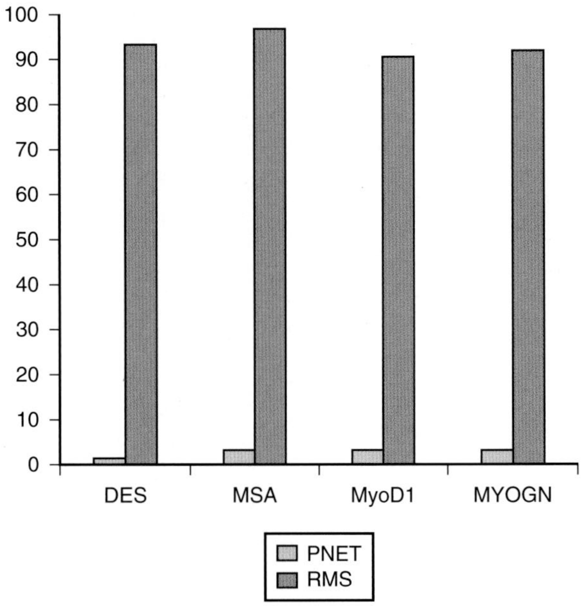

FIGURE 11.7 Markers of interest in the differential diagnosis of primitive neuroectodermal tumor (PNET) versus rhabdomyosarcoma of the mediastinum (RMS).

or CD57.[42,57,92,93,99] The specificity of desmin and actin for the diagnosis of RMS could be challenged because these determinants are also observed in smooth-muscle neoplasms. However, this argument seems superfluous to the author because a small-cell variant of leiomyosarcoma does not exist. In any event, nuclear proteins that are apparently restricted to striated muscle—namely, Myo-D1 and myogenin[99,100]—can be applied effectively to the differential diagnosis in question.

SMALL-CELL MALIGNANT LYMPHOMAS OF THE MEDIASTINUM

Several small-cell non-Hodgkin lymphomas (SCNHLs) may be observed in the mediastinum as primary lesions. These include lymphoblastic lymphoma (LL)[101-103]

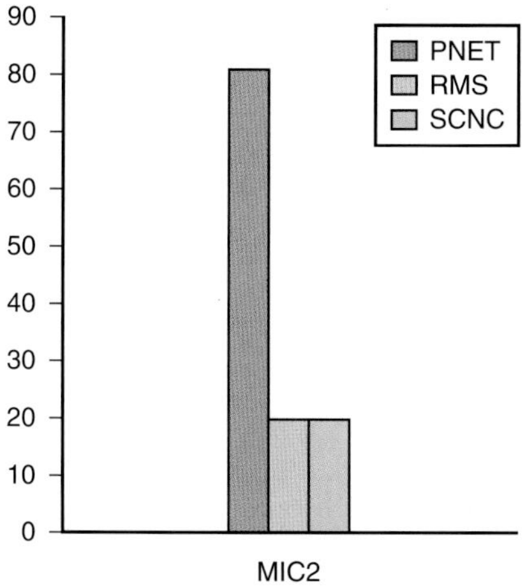

FIGURE 11.8 Relative rates of positivity for CD99 (MIC-2) in primitive neuroectodermal tumor (PNET) versus rhabdomyosarcoma (RMS) versus small-cell neuroendocrine carcinoma (SCNC) of the mediastinum.

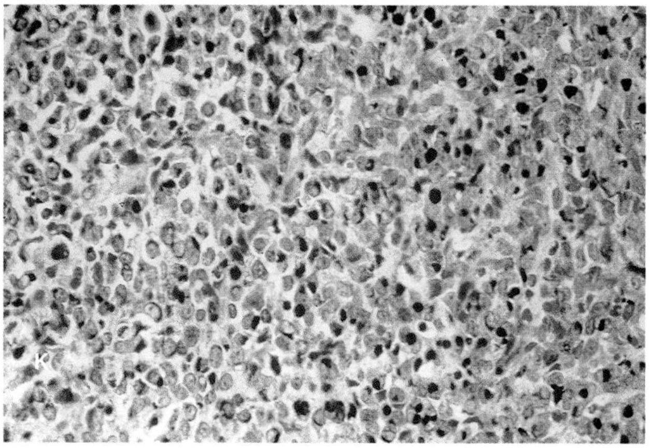

FIGURE 11.9 Characteristic perinuclear dots of immunoreactivity for keratin (K) are evident in this small-cell neuroendocrine carcinoma of the mediastinum.

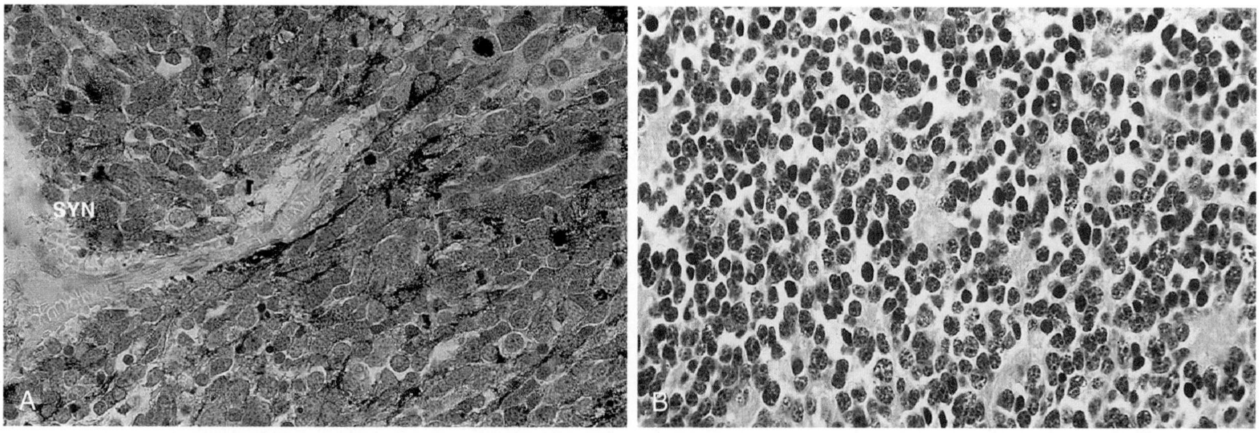

FIGURE 11.10 Diffuse reactivity for synaptophysin (SYN) **(A)** in mediastinal neuroblastoma **(B)**.

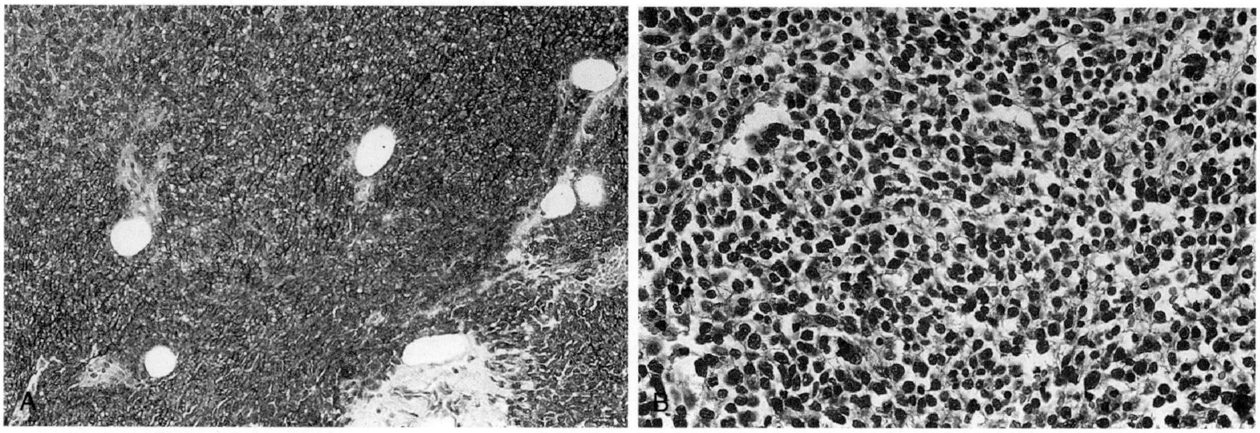

FIGURE 11.11 Labeling for CD99 (MIC-2) **(A)** in primitive neuroectodermal tumor of the mediastinum **(B)**.

(discussed earlier in the chapter), small noncleaved cell (Burkitt/non-Burkitt) lymphoma (SNCL),[104,105] and lymphomas of the mucosa-associated lymphoid tissue (MALTomas).[106-108]

Immunohistochemical analysis is helpful in diagnostically separating these tumor types. They usually express the CD45 (leukocyte common) antigen, although uncommon types of LL lack this marker. Lymphoblastic lymphoma also is commonly labeled with CD43 reagents (L60, Leu22, MT-1); CD99 antibodies such as HBA-71, O13, or 12E7; anti-CD10 (common acute lymphoblastic leukemia antigen); and antibodies to BCL-2 protein and TdT (Fig. 11.13).[29] SNCL expresses CD20, with or without BCL-2 protein.[29] Variants of the latter

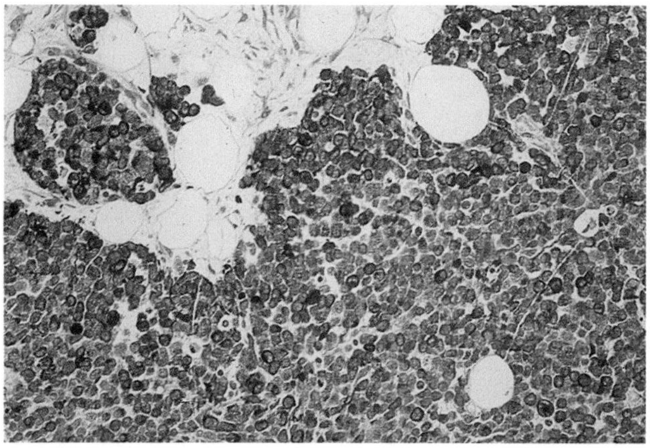

FIGURE 11.12 Immunoreactivity for desmin in rhabdomyosarcoma of the mediastinum.

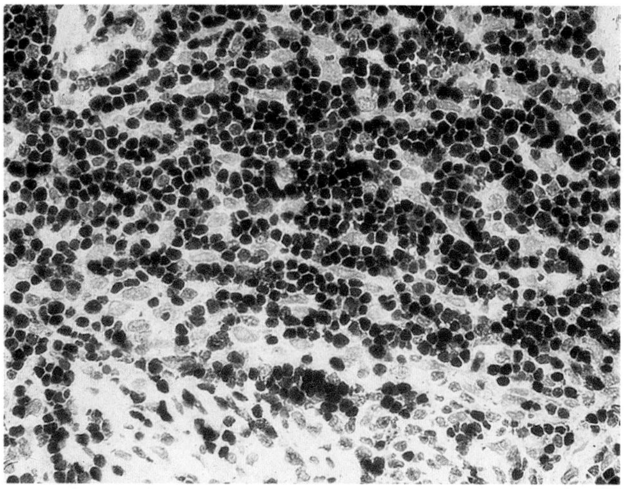

FIGURE 11.13 Nuclear labeling for terminal deoxynucleotidyl transferase in lymphoblastic lymphoma of the thymus.

tumor that harbor chromosomal translocations involving the *c-myc* gene also tend to show immunoreactivity for combinations of T-cell leukemia-1 antigen, CD38, and/or CD44.[107] In MALTomas (marginal-zone lymphomas), reactivity for CD20 and CD79a is evident, but CD10, CD43, CD99, BCL-2, and TdT are absent.[108-111] CD5 is variably present, but keratin, CD56, CD57, synaptophysin, desmin, actin, Myo-D1, and myogenin are not detectable in any of these three SCNHLs. Roughly 50% are positive for vimentin.[112]

OTHER SMALL-CELL MEDIASTINAL NEOPLASMS

In addition to the small-cell tumors presented in the foregoing sections, others of a metastatic nature also may involve the mediastinum. These include small-cell osteosarcoma and Ewing's sarcoma/primitive neuroectodermal tumor (PNET) of bone, as well as small-cell malignant melanoma. Except for the last of these possibilities, the primary lesion in such cases is typically obvious and there is no question of whether the intrathoracic neoplasm might have arisen there. Nonetheless, melanomas are certainly capable of producing distant metastasis in the absence of an obvious primary source.

TABLE 11.4 Immunoreactants Used in the Differential Diagnosis of Large Cell Indeterminate and Undifferentiated Neoplasms of the Mediastinum
Keratin (monoclonal mixture)
Vimentin
Synaptophysin
Chromogranin A
CD15
CD30
CD45
Placenta-like alkaline phosphatase
Carcinoembryonic antigen
Ber-EP4
Calretinin
S-100 protein
HMB-45
Tyrosinase
MART-1
PNL-2

Furthermore, they may assume the guise of a small-cell neoplasm, closely resembling SCNC.[113] Immunohistochemical characteristics of small-cell melanomas include uniform labeling for S-100 protein, tyrosinase, MART-1, and the PNL2 or HMB-45 antigens,[113-115] none of which is expected in other small-cell neoplasms of the mediastinum.

Large Polygonal-Cell Neoplasms of the Mediastinum (Tables 11.4, 11.5; Figs. 11.14-11.18)

PRIMARY THYMIC CARCINOMAS

Although primary thymic carcinoma (PTC) is an exciting diagnosis because of its rarity, most neoplasms thought to represent this entity will ultimately prove to represent metastases. Immunohistochemical analysis of PTCs reveals uniform labeling for keratin and p63,[116] and many cases also express epithelial membrane antigen (EMA). Carcinoembryonic antigen, secretory component, BG8, MOC-31, calretinin, HBME-1, Ber-EP4, and the TAG-72 antigen are variably seen as well, especially in tumors that show partial or uniform glandular differentiation.[111] However, vimentin, thrombomodulin, WT-1 protein, and TTF-1 are characteristically undetectable in polygonal-cell PTC variants.[20,112,116,117] The so-called *hepatoid variant* of PTC, which comprises sheets of large oncocytoid cells like those of metastatic hepatocellular carcinoma (MHCC), represents a potential pitfall in interpretation.[118] Indeed, hepatoid thymic carcinoma and MHCC share potential reactivity for Hep-PAR1, which is usually regarded as a hepatocytic marker.[119]

TABLE 11.5 Percentages of Immunoreactivity for Selected Markers in Malignant Large Polygonal Cell Tumors of the Mediastinum with Indeterminate or Undifferentiated Histologic Features

Tumor	KER	CEA	VIM	CALRET	PLAP	S-100	HMB-45	TYR	MART-1	SYN	CGA	BER-EP4	CD45	CD15	CD30
PTADCA	100	70	5	67	0	0	0	0	0	40	20	70	0	65	0
MADCA	100	75	12	10	10	10	0	0	0	3	5	90	0	70	0
PNEC	100	40	20	0	0	6	0	0	0	80	90	90	0	85	0
MNEC	100	62	20	0	0	10	0	0	0	80	75	90	0	20	0
LCL/TAL*	0	0/50	65	0	0	3	0	0	0	0	0	0	99/85	3/85	23/3
ALCL	0	0	100	0	0	10	0	0	0	0	0	0	90	13	99
SYNHD	0	0	50	0	0	0	0	0	0	0	0	0	6	90	90
MELAN	1	0	100	0	0	97	50	86	90	0	0	0	0	0	0
SEMIN	12	0	70	0	93	0	0	0	0	0	0	0	0	0	3
EMBCA	100	0	17	0	90	0	0	0	0	0	0	0	0	0	80
YST	100	0	50	0	50	0	0	0	0	0	0	0	0	0	20
EPSARCS[a]	V	0	100	V	0	V	0	0	0	0	0	V	0	0	0
PSCC	100	40	5	0	0	3	0	0	0	40	20	50	0	20	0
MSCC	100	50	30	33	10	10	0	0	0	20	3	50	0	20	0
LELCT	100	0	50	0	0	0	0	0	0	40	20	10	0	0	0
MESOTH	100	0	54	90	3	7	0	0	0	0	2	10	0	1	0
PARAGANG	2	0	40	0	0	40	0	0	0	100	100	0	0	0	0

*Unless otherwise indicated, the given percentage of reactivity applies to both tumor entities.

[a]Epithelioid synovial sarcoma is reactive for keratin in 100% of cases and Ber-EP4 in 90% of cases. Epithelioid malignant peripheral nerve sheath tumor is reactive for S-100 protein in 80% of cases.

V, variable, usually positive.

KER, keratin (mixture of monoclonal antibodies); CEA, carcinoembryonic antigen; VIM, vimentin; CALRET, calretinin; PLAP, placental alkaline phosphatase; S-100, S-100 protein; TYR, tyrosinase; SYN, synaptophysin; CGA, chromogranin A; PTADCA, primary thymic adenocarcinoma; MADCA, metastatic adenocarcinoma; PNEC, primary neuroendocrine carcinoma; MNEC, metastatic neuroendocrine carcinoma; LCL, large cell lymphoma; TAL, tumefactive acute myelogenous leukemia; ALCL, anaplastic large cell lymphoma; SYNHD, syncytial Hodgkin disease; MELAN, malignant melanoma; SEMIN, seminoma; EMBCA, embryonal carcinoma; YST, yolk sac tumor; EPSARCS, sarcomas with epithelioid features; PSCC, primary thymic squamous cell carcinoma; MSCC, metastatic squamous cell carcinoma; LELCT, lymphoepithelioma-like carcinoma of the thymus; MESOTH, mesothelioma; PARAGANG, malignant paraganglioma.

Data from Frisman D. Immunoquery (available at http://www.immunoquery.com) and the author's experience.

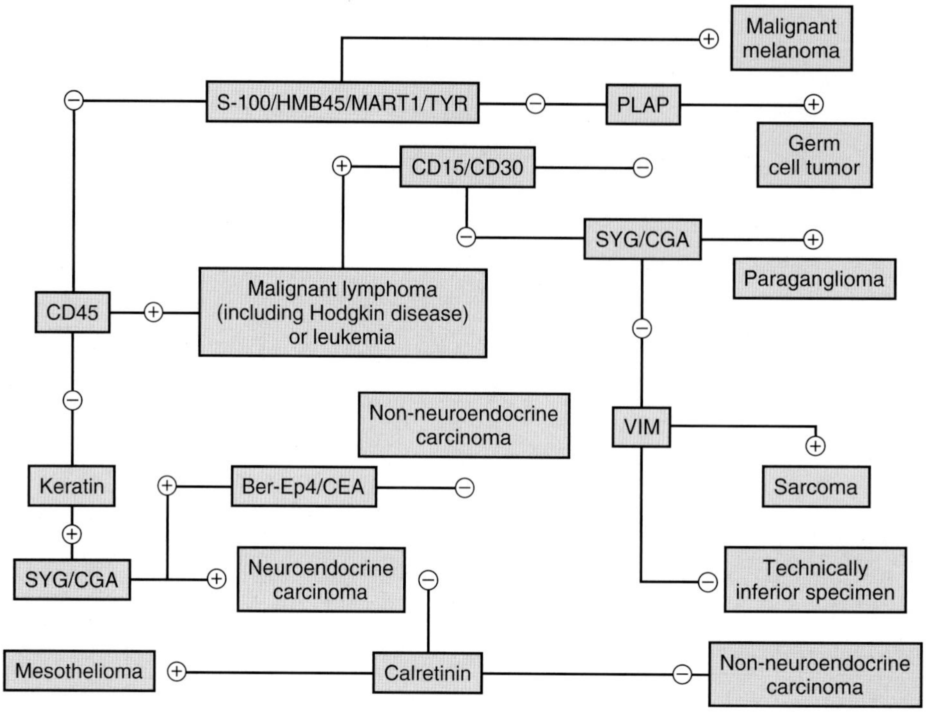

FIGURE 11.14 Algorithm for immunohistologic evaluation of malignant large polygonal cell tumors of the mediastinum.

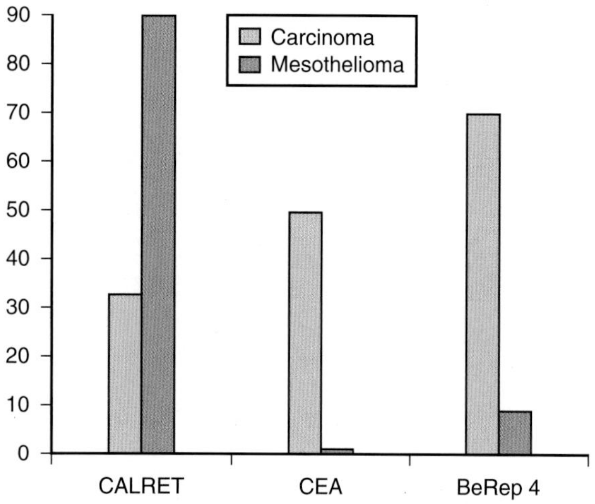

FIGURE 11.15 Markers of interest in the differential diagnosis of carcinoma versus mesothelioma.

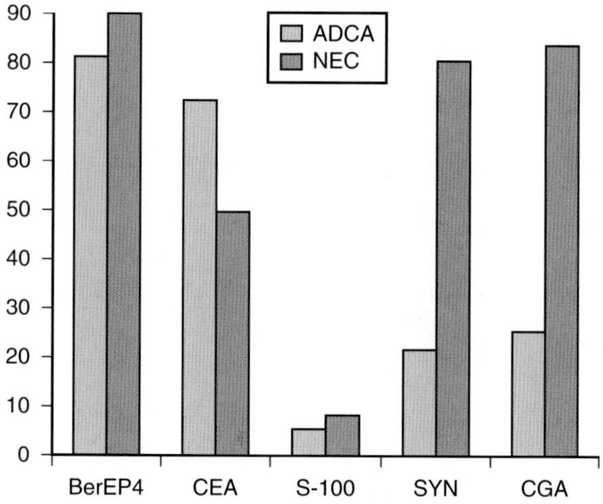

FIGURE 11.16 Markers of interest in the differential diagnosis between poorly differentiated adenocarcinoma (ADCA) and neuroendocrine carcinoma of the mediastinum (NEC).

Several reports have been made on the expression of CD5 by the epithelial cells of thymic carcinoma, but there are no reports on conventional thymoma available (Fig. 11.19).[112-114,120] This statement must be qualified in part, because *atypical* epithelial-predominant thymomas (i.e., those with evidence of cytologic atypia that is insufficient for an outright diagnosis of malignancy)[19,23,44] also show CD5 positivity in 40% of cases.[114] Saad and associates[117] also found that the majority of primary poorly differentiated lung carcinomas (the principal differential diagnostic alternative for PTC) also were CD5 reactive.

CD117 (c-*kit*) is a marker that is usually associated with seminoma in the context of mediastinal neoplasia. However, Nakagawa and colleagues[121] have shown that it is commonly present (80%) in PTC as well, often *together* with CD5. Comparisons with non-thymic tumors in their series indicated that all CD5+/CD117+ lesions were PTCs, whereas 13 of 16 that were CD5–/CD117– were metastatic carcinomas from the lung.

Some variability exists in the literature concerning mutant p53 protein as another potential discriminant between thymoma and thymic carcinoma.[122-124] In general, however, immunostains performed with the DO1 and DO3 antibodies against mutant p53 are much more likely to yield positive results in PTC than in conventional thymoma. Hence, this determinant could serve as an adjunct in making the diagnostic distinction between those two entities. Similar claims have been made for

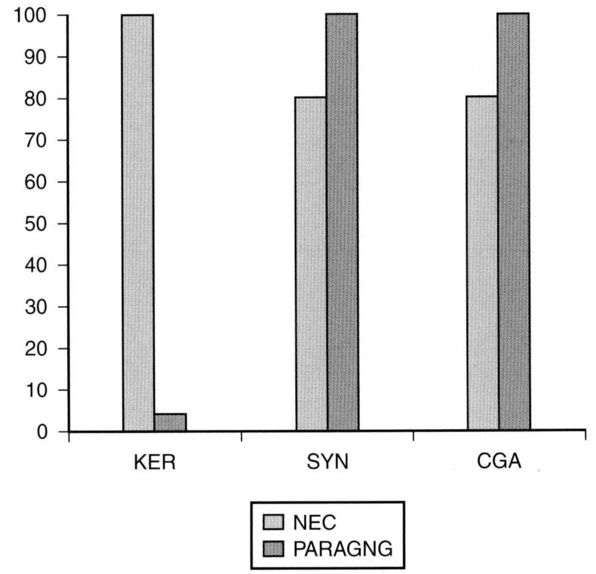

FIGURE 11.17 Relative reactivity patterns for neuroendocrine carcinoma (NEC) and malignant paraganglioma (PARAGNG) of the mediastinum.

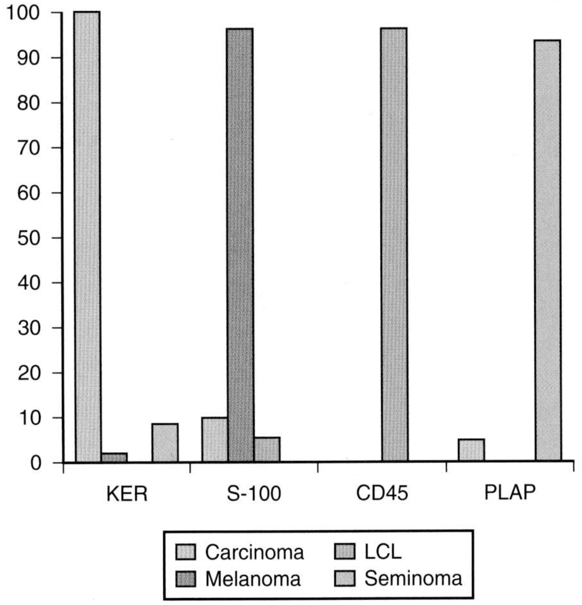

FIGURE 11.18 Markers of interest in the differential diagnosis of carcinoma versus metastatic melanoma versus large-cell non-Hodgkin lymphoma (LCL) versus seminoma of the mediastinum.

MCL-1 protein[125] and the *Fas* antigen,[126] but data on these reactants in thymic neoplasms are scarce. Other primary malignant tumors of the thymic region, such as germ cell tumors and lymphomas, are typically CD5-negative.[113,114,120] Future studies will be necessary to determine whether such observations withstand the test of time. On the other hand, it has been found in most cases that MIC-2–positive lymphocytes are lacking in both PTCs and metastatic carcinomas in the thymic region, which indicates that CD99 has no role in making the distinction between these neoplasms.[25]

Another facet of PTCs is their capacity for occult neuroendocrine differentiation. Even though no overt morphologic evidence of neuroendocrine features exists in such lesions, immunoreactivity may be observed for synaptophysin, chromogranin A, CD56, or CD57 (Fig. 11.20).[127] The biological significance of these findings is currently uncertain, but they are not sufficiently compelling to change the diagnostic classification of these tumors to that of outright neuroendocrine carcinoma.

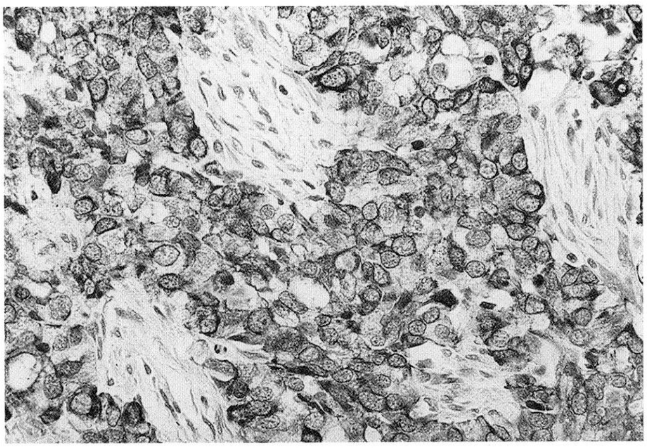

FIGURE 11.19 Diffuse immunoreactivity for CD5 in primary thymic carcinoma.

KEY DIAGNOSTIC POINTS

Primary Thymic Carcinoma

- Keratin and P63+; CD5 typically positive
- TTF-1 and WT-1 both negative

PARATHYROID CARCINOMA OF THE MEDIASTINUM

Parathyroid carcinoma (PAC) may be seen intrathymically or in the soft tissue of the anterosuperior mediastinum. It bears a considerable resemblance to thymic neuroendocrine carcinoma in some cases, and paraganglioma also enters into differential diagnosis.[128-130] The clinical diagnosis of malignant parathyroid lesions is typically straightforward because they are associated with striking levels of hypercalcemia. Nevertheless, nonsecretory PACs may require immunohistologic evaluation for definitive diagnosis. This can be accomplished by documenting the intracellular presence of parathyroid hormone, which is restricted to parathyroid lesions among contextual diagnostic possibilities (Fig. 11.21).[131] Otherwise, the immunophenotypes of PAC and other neuroendocrine carcinomas are largely superimposable.[130]

MALIGNANT MEDIASTINAL GERM CELL TUMORS

Pure or mixed mediastinal germ cell tumors with seminomatous, embryonal carcinomatous, endodermal sinus tumor, and choriocarcinomatous elements all have the potential to arise in the mediastinum or involve it metastatically.[15,16,132-136] Immunohistology is often indispensable for characterizing such neoplasms, especially

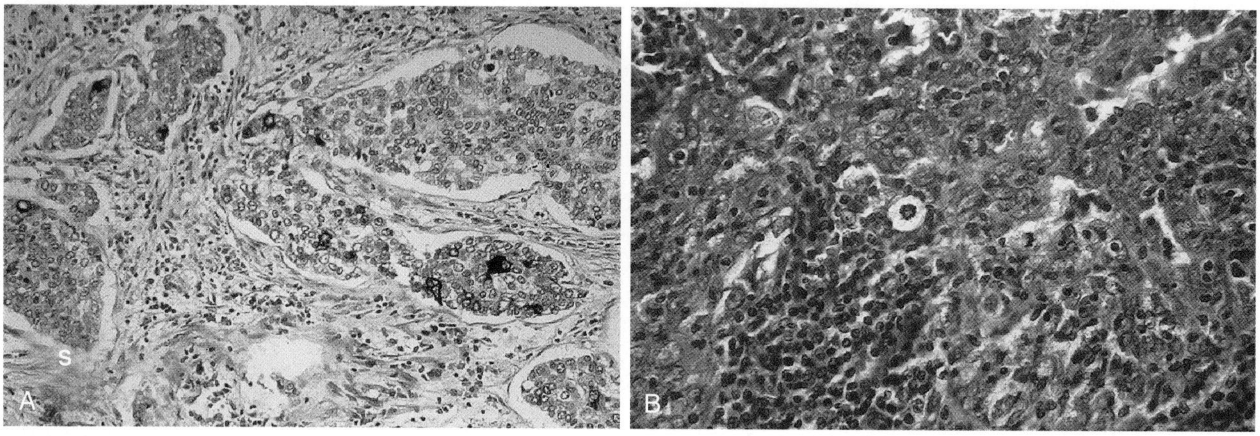

FIGURE 11.20 Occult labeling for synaptophysin (S) **(A)** in a primary thymic carcinoma that did not have neuroendocrine characteristics by conventional morphologic study **(B)**.

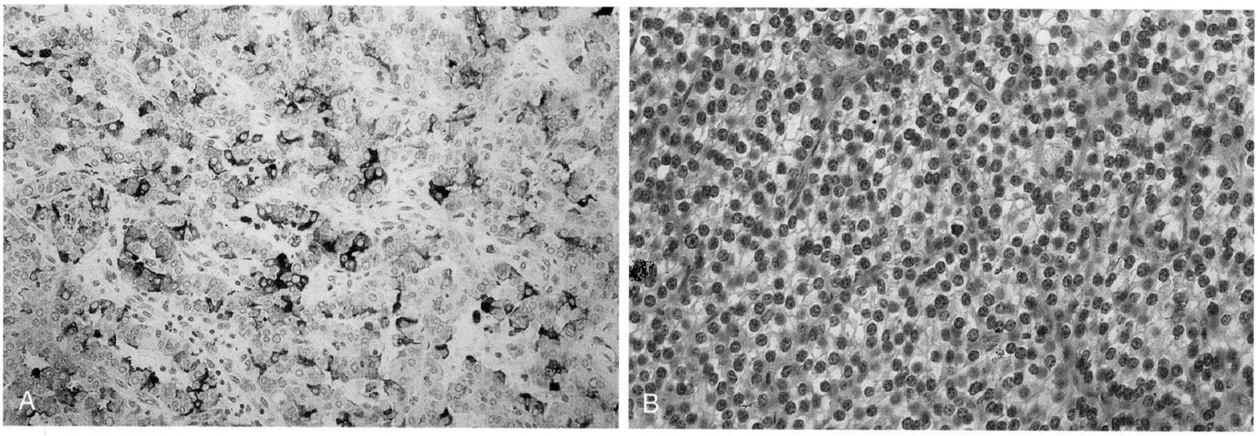

FIGURE 11.21 Immunoreactivity for parathyroid hormone **(A)** in primary mediastinal parathyroid carcinoma **(B)**.

in limited tissue samples. The typical phenotype of seminoma is that of a keratin- and EMA-negative tumor with uniform cell-membrane–based reactivity for CD117, podoplanin, Oct-¾, and PLAP (Fig. 11.22A-D).[16,137-141] Approximately 10% to 15% of such lesions, however, will indeed demonstrate limited labeling for keratin proteins.[16] Embryonal carcinomas and yolk sac carcinomas differ from the latter description in their acquisition of intense, diffuse keratin positivity and potential labeling for alpha fetoprotein (AFP).[16,135,142] In addition, embryonal carcinoma paradoxically manifests the presence of CD30 (Fig. 11.23),[143] which is typically conceptualized as a hematopoietic determinant. Choriocarcinoma is also globally keratin reactive, but it is further typified by the immunohistologic presence of EMA and beta–human chorionic gonadotropin.[16,144]

KEY DIAGNOSTIC POINTS

Mediastinal Germ Cell Tumors

- Seminoma is CD117+, PLAP+, keratin– (rarely focally +).
- Embryonal carcinoma is keratin+, CD30+; yolk sac tumor is keratin+, AFP+; choriocarcinoma is keratin+, EMA+.

MEDIASTINAL CARCINOID TUMOR (NEUROENDOCRINE CARCINOMA, GRADES I AND II)

Immunohistochemically, neuroendocrine carcinomas of the thymus show reproducible positivity for keratin, neuron-specific (gamma-dimeric) enolase, synaptophysin, CD56, CD57, and chromogranin.[20,145-149] Furthermore, even the lesions that have not produced a clinical endocrinopathy can show the presence of specific neuropeptides at an intracellular level.[150-152]

MEDIASTINAL PARAGANGLIOMAS

Intrathoracic paragangliomas (PGs) may arise in the anterior mediastinal compartment, in association with the aorticopulmonary root, or along the vertebral column.[148,153,154] Some of these lesions may demonstrate a prominently sclerotic stroma, which can obscure their true lineage.[155] Their neural nature is reflected by their lack of labeling for keratin and EMA. They instead express neurofilament protein, with or without vimentin, in likeness to NBL.[148] Stains for S-100 protein can be used to label sustentacular cells that surround cellular nests in PGs (Fig. 11.24),[156] and the tumor cells themselves often

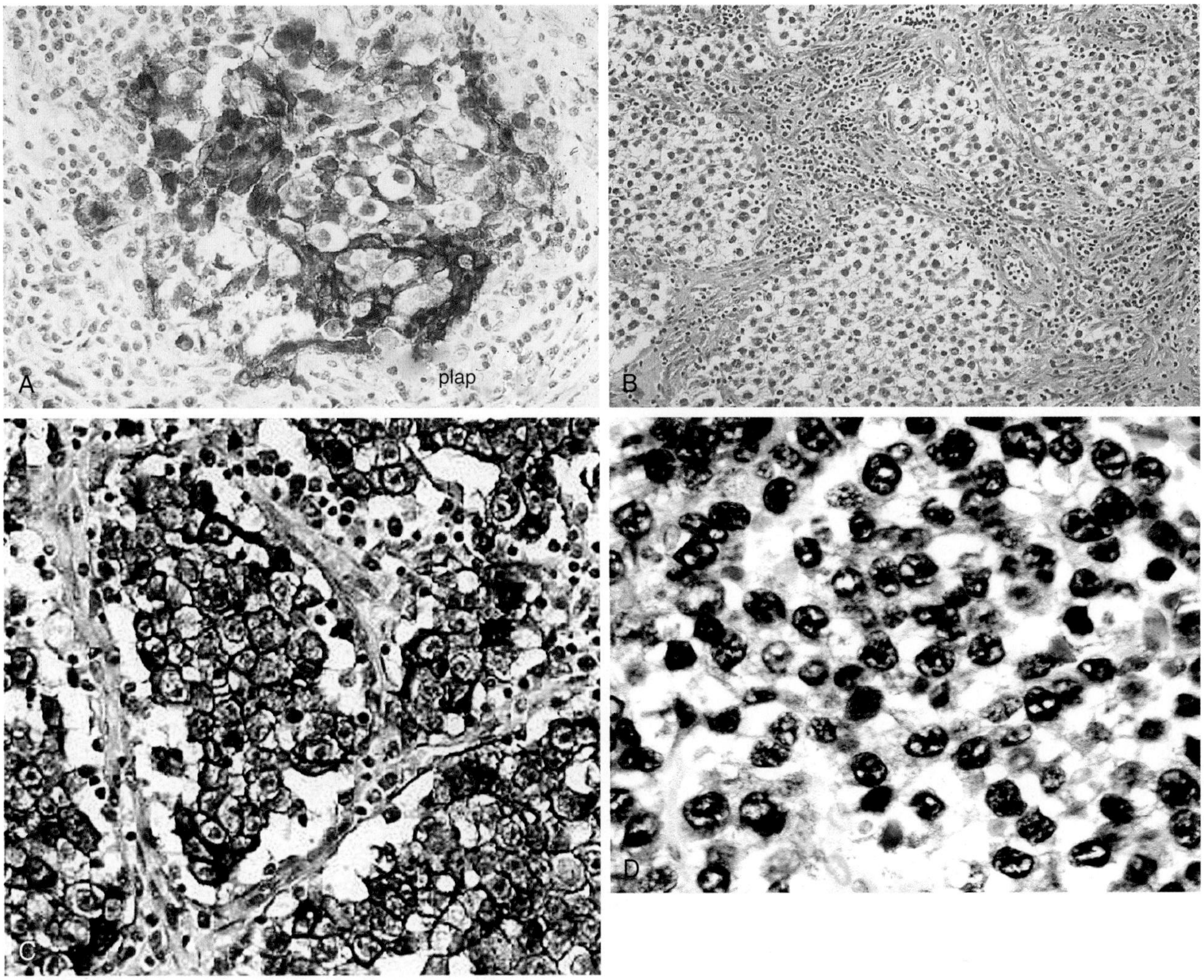

FIGURE 11.22 Membrane-based immunolabeling for placental alkaline phosphatase (PLAP) **(A)** in primary mediastinal seminoma **(B)**. Membrane-based immunostaining for podoplanin is typical of seminoma **(C)**. Nuclear staining for Oct-¾ in seminoma **(D)**.

contain one of the enkephalin peptides.[157] Labeling for chromogranin A is universal in these neoplasms.

MEDIASTINAL LARGE-CELL NON-HODGKIN LYMPHOMA (TABLE 11.6; FIG. 11.25)

After Hodgkin disease, large-cell non-Hodgkin lymphoma (LCNHL) is the most common primary malignancy of the mediastinum.[112] Immunohistology reveals crisp cell-membranous reactivity for CD45 in virtually all LCNHLs.[39,112,158-161] However, rare examples of Ki-1+ (CD30+) (large-cell anaplastic) lymphoma have been reported at this site,[162] some of which have been CD45 negative. Therefore, it is prudent to evaluate the possible presence of CD30 when assessing a possible LCNHL; in the context of simultaneous keratin negativity, this marker is specific for a diagnosis of lymphoma.[112] The belief that most mediastinal LCNHLs show B-cell differentiation is supported by their reactivity for CD20, PAX-5, and CD79a in most cases (Fig. 11.26),[160,161,163-165] including those with anaplastic features.[162] Only exceptional LCNHLs with T-cell or true histiocytic differentiation have been reported in the mediastinum.[112]

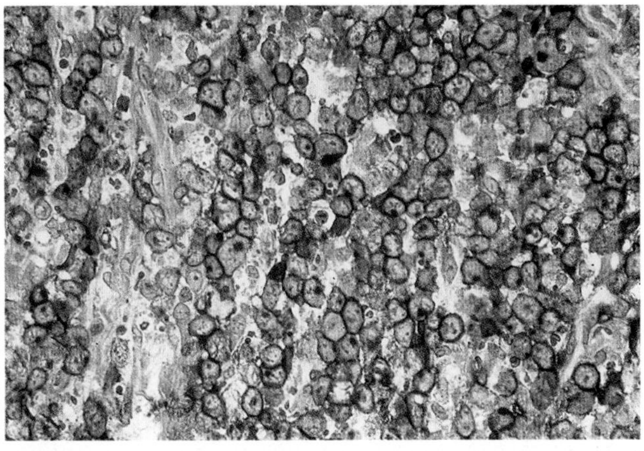

FIGURE 11.23 Diffuse positivity for CD30 in thymic embryonal carcinoma.

SYNCYTIAL MEDIASTINAL HODGKIN DISEASE

Hodgkin lymphoma (HL) is the most common cytologically malignant mediastinal neoplasm.[112] Although it is thought to arise in the thymus or perithymic lymph

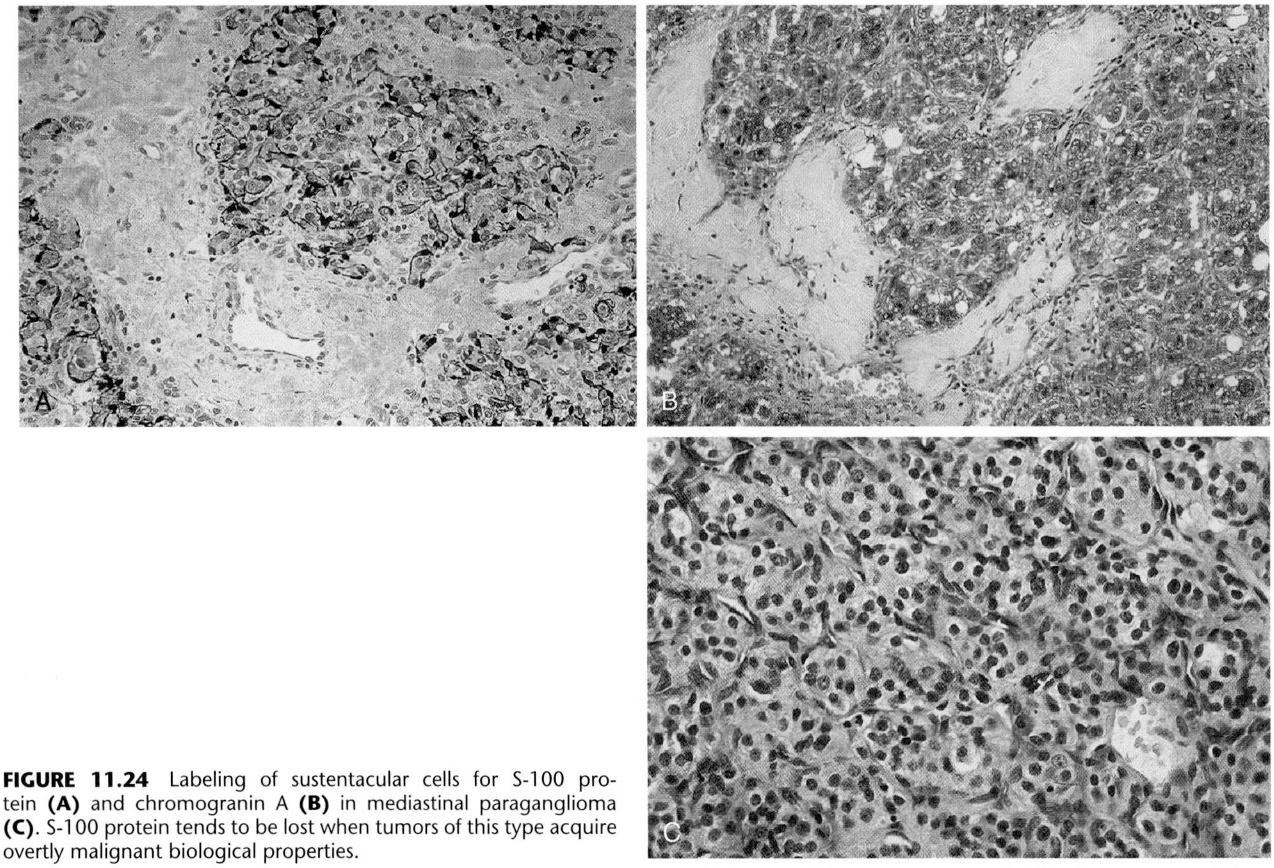

FIGURE 11.24 Labeling of sustentacular cells for S-100 protein **(A)** and chromogranin A **(B)** in mediastinal paraganglioma **(C)**. S-100 protein tends to be lost when tumors of this type acquire overtly malignant biological properties.

nodes in the thorax, this lesion also may involve other contiguous structures by direct extension.[166-168] Most examples of HL are recognizable without the need for immunohistology, but one of its variants, syncytial HL (in which mononuclear Reed-Sternberg cells are arranged in sheets) may closely simulate the appearance of a carcinoma or LCNHL.[169] The typical immunophenotype of the Reed-Sternberg cells in HL is CD45-negative; this is in contrast to its presence in almost all cases of LCNHL.[20,112] On the other hand, Reed-Sternberg cells in syncytial HL coexpress CD15 and CD30 (Fig. 11.27). CD15 is not seen in most LCNHLs, which enables one to make a distinction between these tumor types.[112] Nonetheless, there is a potential overlap between Hodgkin lymphoma and selected examples of CD30+ LCNHL. This makes cytogenetic studies (particularly for abnormalities at the 5q35 locus, which typify Ki-1+ large-cell lymphomas)[170,171] a wise inclusion in this context. In reference to its distinction from carcinomas in the mediastinum, syncytial HL uniformly lacks keratin,[20,112,169] unlike malignant epithelial neoplasms.

TABLE 11.6 Immunoreactants Used in the Differential Diagnosis of Hematopoietic Diseases of the Mediastinum

Keratin	CD45
HMB-45	CD45RO
MART-1	CD68
Tyrosinase	CD74
Placenta-like alkaline phosphatase	MB2
CD3	BLA.36
CD15	BNH9
CD20	Cathepsin-B
CD30	Lysozyme
CD43	Myeloperoxidase

OTHER MEDIASTINAL HEMATOPOIETIC TUMORS

Two other hematopoietic neoplasms that may present in the mediastinum are granulocytic sarcoma (extramedullary myelogenous leukemia; Fig. 11.28)[172,173] and extraosseous plasmacytoma.[174,175] Immunoreactivity for CD15, CD33, CD34, CD68, and myeloperoxidase is expected in granulocytic sarcoma but not in LCNHL.[176-178] Extraosseous plasmacytoma of the mediastinum (EPM) can potentially imitate the microscopic

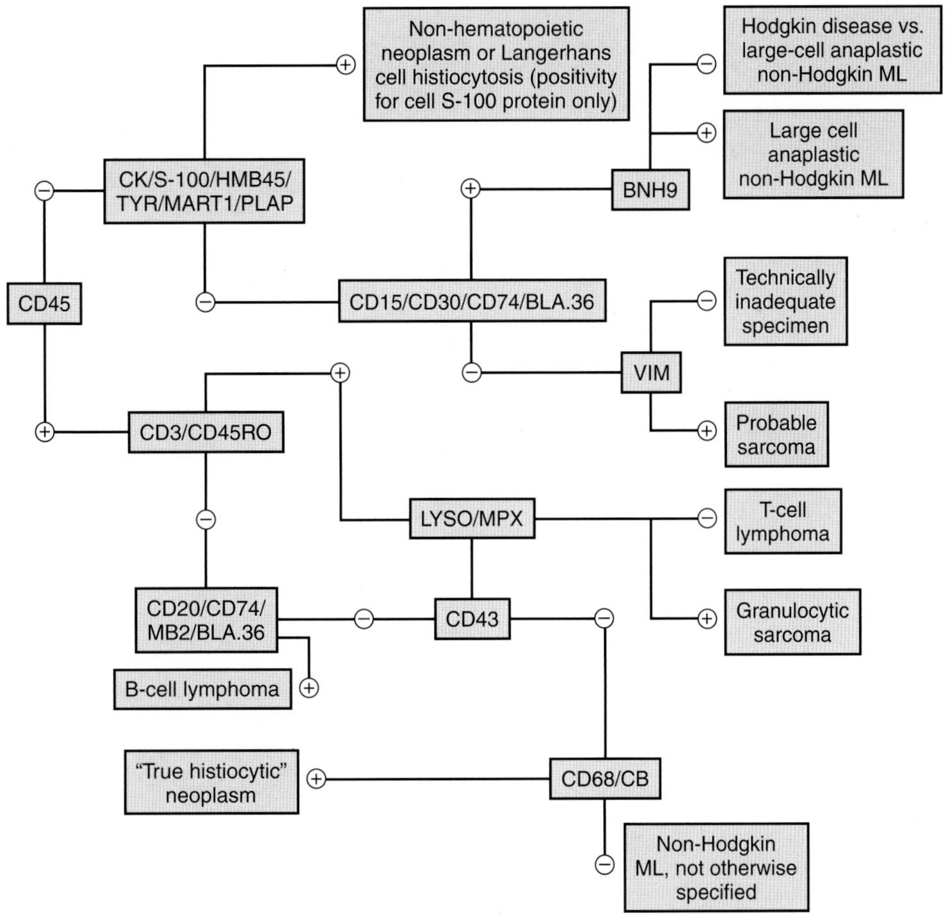

FIGURE 11.25 Algorithm for immunohistologic evaluation of hematopoietic neoplasms of the mediastinum.

appearance of neuroendocrine neoplasms, as well as that of large-cell lymphomas.[174,175] EPM is reactive for light-chain immunoglobulins (Fig. 11.29), CD38, and CD138 (syndecan-1),[179] but not for keratin, chromogranin A, or synaptophysin.[180] A special diagnostic trap attending this tumor is its potential to express an EMA-like substance;[181] this result may appear to support a mistaken interpretation of neuroendocrine neoplasia for the unwary.

Conversely, CD138 is not specific for plasmacellular proliferations. As shown by Kambham[182] and colleagues, it may be observed in a variety of mesenchymal and epithelial neoplasms as well.

MALIGNANT EPITHELIOID MESOTHELIOMA OF THE MEDIASTINUM

Although malignant mesotheliomas are usually regarded as tumors of the peripheral pleurae or the peritoneum, they also are seen in the mediastinum, where they likely originate from hilar reflections of the pleural surfaces. The immunophenotype of mesothelioma features keratin reactivity in all of its histologic variants, including the purely epithelioid form, and the same is potentially true of calretinin, WT-1, and podoplanin.[183-186] Vimentin coexpression also may be seen in roughly 50% of mesothelioma cases, and there is also heterogeneous (and not entirely specific) labeling for such determinants as HBME-1[187] and thrombomodulin.[188] Specialized markers of carcinomatous differentiation—including CEA, CD15, p63, TTF-1, blood group antigens (e.g., A, B, H, and Lewis), and the CA72-4 antigen (recognized by antibody B72.3)—are absent in mesotheliomas.[189-191]

METASTATIC MEDIASTINAL CARCINOMA AND MELANOMA

As stated earlier in this discussion, most non-hematopoietic malignancies of the mediastinum should be presumed metastatic until proven otherwise. Immunohistologic analysis is only variably productive in establishing a site of origin for secondary carcinomas in this location. If determinants are found that are unassociated with PTCs, such as TTF-1, thyroglobulin, prostate-specific antigen, S-100 protein, PLAP, CA 19-9 (an enteric carcinoma marker), or CA 125 (a serosal and Müllerian tract marker),[192] it is likely that the lesion is a metastasis. Conversely, the presence of coexpression of keratin 5/6, p63, and CD5 would, at least tentatively, appear to support a thymic origin for such a neoplasm.[120]

Mediastinal implants of an amelanotic malignant melanoma rarely represent the initial manifestation of

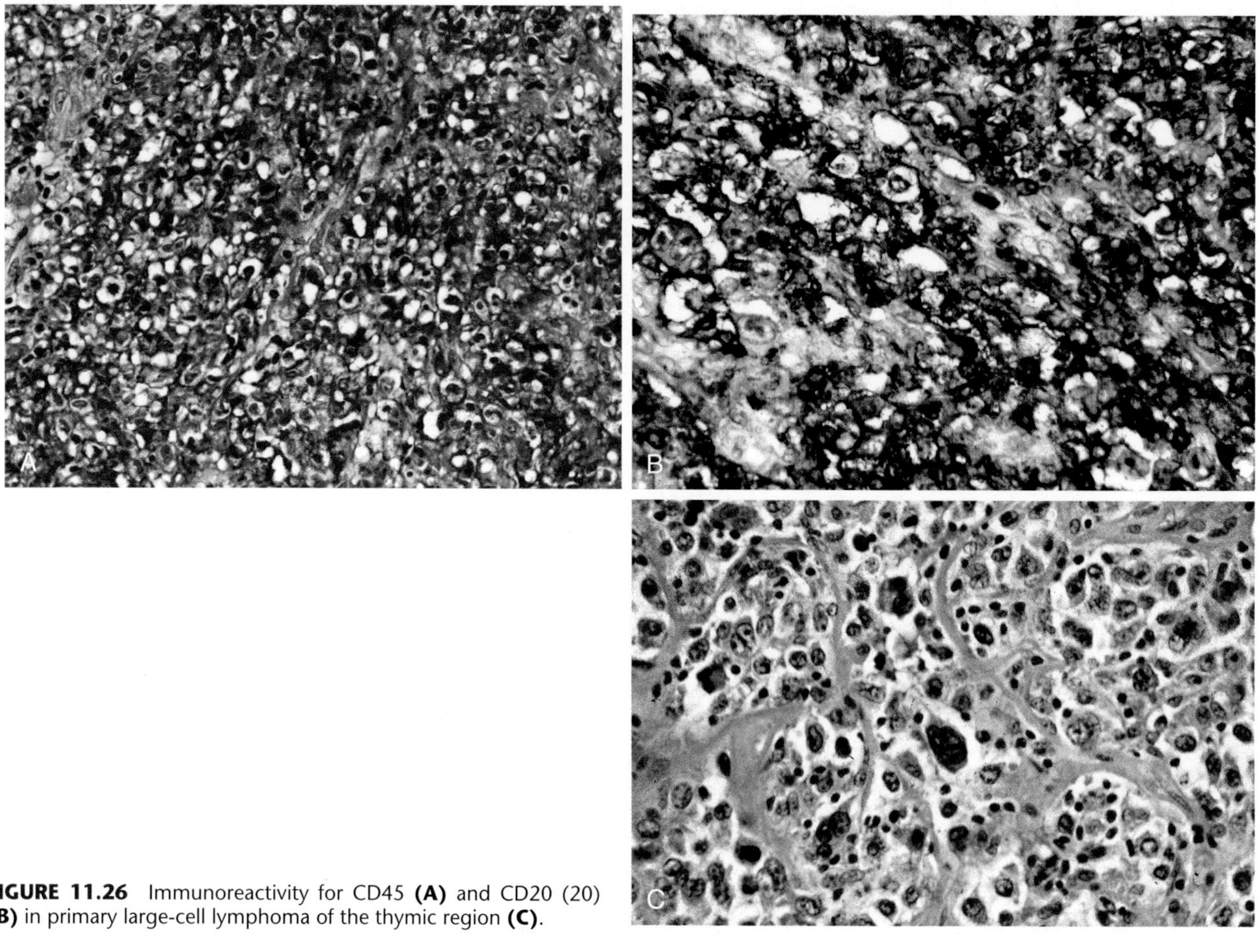

FIGURE 11.26 Immunoreactivity for CD45 **(A)** and CD20 (20) **(B)** in primary large-cell lymphoma of the thymic region **(C)**.

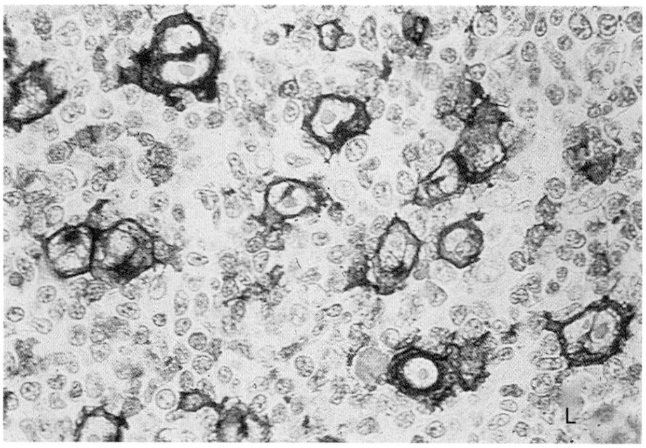

FIGURE 11.27 Typical cell-membranous and Golgi-zone labeling for CD15 in the Reed-Sternberg cells of mediastinal Hodgkin disease.

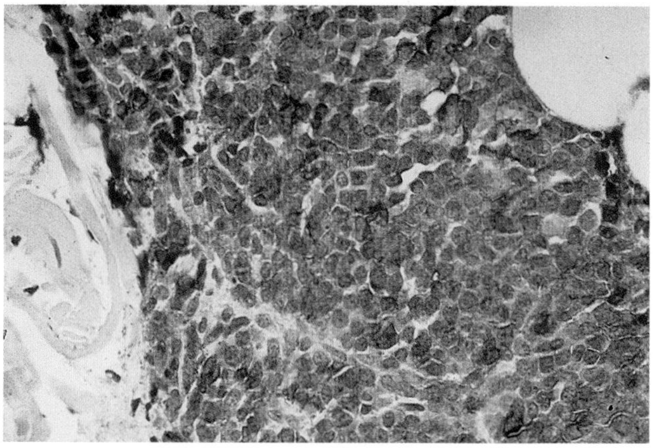

FIGURE 11.28 Diffuse cytoplasmic reactivity for myeloperoxidase in granulocytic sarcoma of the mediastinum.

this tumor[193] in the face of no detectable cutaneous or mucosal disease. In this scenario, the differential diagnosis would also include primary or metastatic somatic carcinomas, malignant germ cell tumors, and lymphomas. Immunohistochemical studies show that metastatic large-cell melanomas of the mediastinum are devoid of keratin, EMA, PLAP, CD15, CD30, and CD45. Instead, they react with antibodies to vimentin, S-100 protein, tyrosinase, MART-1, and PNL2.[114,192,194]

Mixed Small-Cell and Large-Cell Malignancies

MIXED LARGE-CELL AND SMALL-CELL NON-HODGKIN LYMPHOMA

There is still some controversy on the definition of mixed large- and small-cell non-Hodgkin lymphoma (MNHL), as it is distinguished from LCNHL. The author uses the rather arbitrary criterion that no more than 30% of large cells should be seen in mixed non-Hodgkin lymphomas.

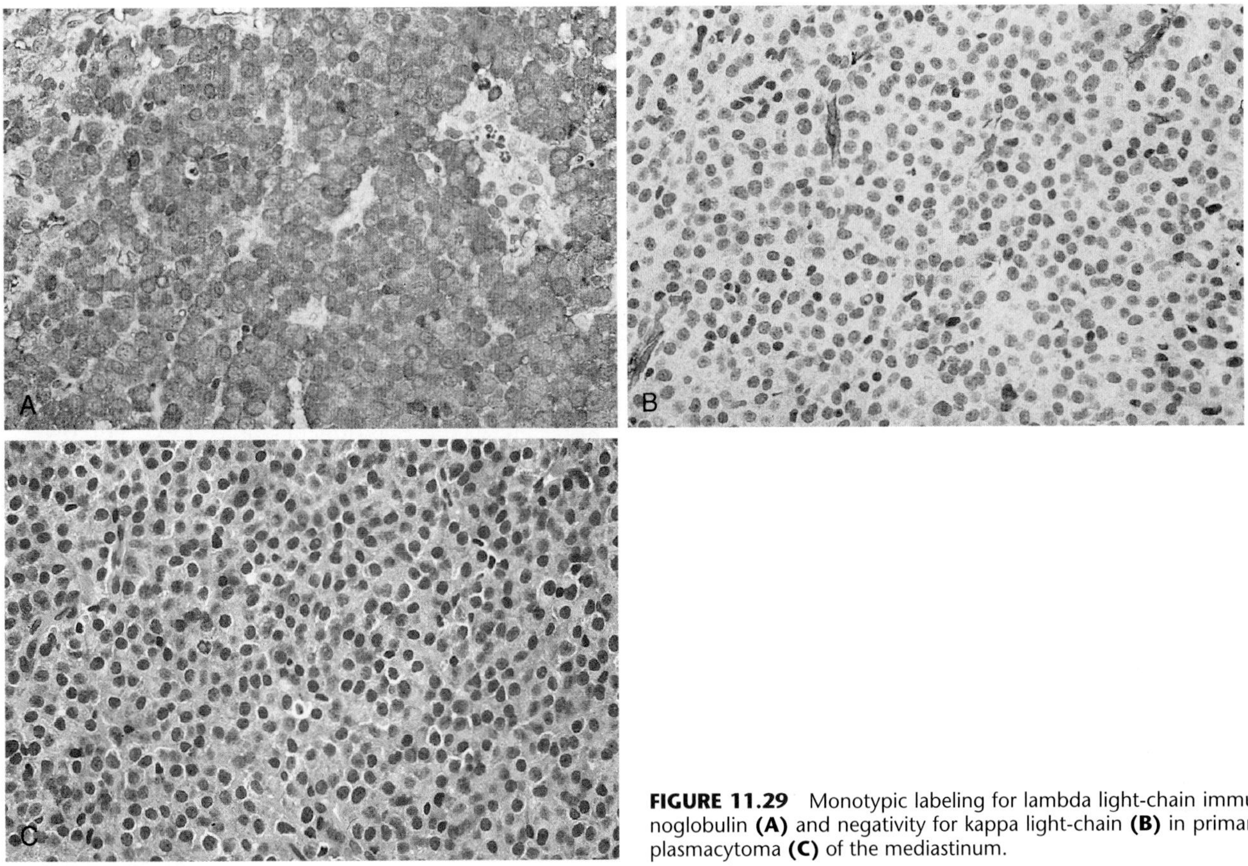

FIGURE 11.29 Monotypic labeling for lambda light-chain immunoglobulin **(A)** and negativity for kappa light-chain **(B)** in primary plasmacytoma **(C)** of the mediastinum.

The immunoprofile of MNHL separates it from other malignant mixed-cell neoplasms of the mediastinum. It includes reactivity for CD45 in all lesional cells, as well as positivity for CD20 in B-cell tumors or CD3, CD43, or CD45R0 in T-cell neoplasms.[195] Keratin is universally absent, but some p63 isoforms are variably expressed by non-Hodgkin lymphomas of various types.[196]

MIXED-CELLULARITY HODGKIN DISEASE

Mixed-cellularity Hodgkin disease is superficially similar histologically to MNHL; however, the former lesion fails to show labeling for CD45 in the large tumor cells (Reed-Sternberg cells). They also lack CD3, CD20, CD43, and CD45RO but express CD15 (with or without CD30, MUM-1, and PAX5), often with a distinctive Golgi zone and cell-membranous staining pattern.[112,169,197,198] EMA may be observed in some cases of mixed-cellularity Hodgkin disease, but keratin is consistently absent.[197]

LYMPHOEPITHELIOMA-LIKE CARCINOMA

Lymphoepithelioma-like carcinoma (LELC) of the thymus features an admixture of large epithelioid cells and small lymphocytes, in likeness to the image of classical nasopharyngeal carcinoma. All cases of LELC are immunoreactive for keratin (Fig. 11.30), p63, and EMA. Conversely, the large tumor cells are devoid of PLAP, CD3, CD15, CD20, CD30, CD43, CD45, and CD45R0.[20,76] As mentioned earlier, a proportion of LELCs also are reactive for CD5, CD117, or both.

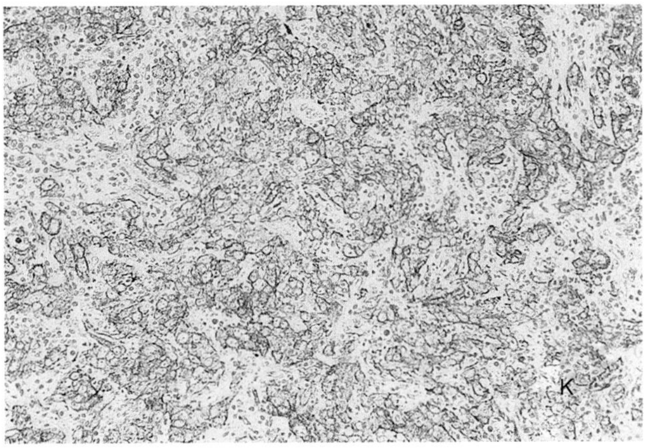

FIGURE 11.30 Delicately interlocking reactivity for keratin (K) in primary lymphoepithelioma-like carcinoma of the thymus.

Malignant Spindle Cell Mediastinal Tumors (Tables 11.7, 11.8; Figs. 11.31-11.33)

SARCOMATOID THYMIC CARCINOMA

Comparatively few examples of sarcomatoid thymic carcinoma (STC) have been reported.[69,199-201] Microscopically, this lesion is characterized by fascicles of fusiform and pleomorphic tumor cells, with little internal organization. Some cases, however, contain limited foci in which cohesive epithelioid cell nests are admixed with spindle-cell elements.[74] Biphasic STCs with carcinoidal elements have also been documented.[202] Snover and coworkers[74] reported an example of STC with focally well-defined rhabdomyogenic differentiation, complete with cytoplasmic cross-striations. Some observers may choose to label such lesions as carcinosarcomas,[203] but it is the author's opinion that they are basically epithelial in nature (i.e., metaplastic or sarcoma-like carcinomas).[204]

Immunohistochemically, the fusiform and pleomorphic cells of STCs express vimentin. Labeling for keratin and EMA is also seen, but it may be quite focal (Fig. 11.34).[21,204] This finding opens the door to the possibility that a small biopsy specimen could fail to demonstrate any epithelial markers because of sampling artifact.

TABLE 11.7 Immunoreactants Used in the Differential Diagnosis of Spindle Cell Indeterminate and Undifferentiated Neoplasms of the Mediastinum

Keratin (monoclonal mixture)
Epithelial membrane antigen
Calretinin
Vimentin
Desmin
Muscle-specific actin
Alpha fetoprotein
Synaptophysin
Chromogranin A
Podoplanin
CD21
CD23
CD35

Tumors that show divergent components, such as myogenic elements, may additionally exhibit immunoreactivity for desmin, actin, myoglobin, Myo-D1, or myogenin.[69,72] Obviously, these potential results underscore the difficulty in establishing a firm diagnosis of STC with limited tissue samples.

An especially troublesome differential diagnosis is the separation of primary mediastinal synovial sarcoma and PTC. This is because their clinical, electron microscopic, and immunophenotypic features are quite similar. The demonstration of t(X;18) chromosomal translocations in synovial sarcoma—by fluorescence *in situ* hybridization or traditional cytogenetic analyses—has now made this tumor consistently identifiable.[205] Mesothelioma also enters consideration in this context; notably, this tumor type shares possible reactivity for keratin and calretinin with sarcomatoid PTC and synovial sarcoma. However, only mesothelioma commonly expresses the WT-1 protein among these possibilities, and, unlike sarcomatoid PTC or synovial sarcoma, mesothelial tumors do not label for CD99.[206-209]

Another potential pitfall in the diagnosis of STC is the existence of thymomas, which incite the proliferation of an exuberant but reactive spindle-cell stroma.[210] This phenomenon produces a biphasic morphologic image and also yields a mutually exclusive immunophenotype in the two lesional components with respect to keratin and vimentin labeling. Hence, the superficial resemblance to carcinosarcoma is great, and attending to the cytologic blandness of the lesion will help avoid diagnostic errors.

SPINDLE CELL CARCINOID TUMOR OF THE THYMUS

The existence of a spindle cell variant of thymic carcinoid was first documented in 1976 by Levine and Rosai,[211] but it appears to be a very rare tumor subtype with only a limited number of additional examples having been identified.[212] For all practical purposes, the immunoprofile of this neoplastic variant is identical to that of polygonal-cell neuroendocrine

TABLE 11.8 Percentages of Immunoreactivity for Selected Markers in Malignant Small Cell Tumors of the Mediastinum with Indeterminate or Undifferentiated Histologic Features

Tumor	KER	EMA	VIM	CALRET	DES	MSA	AFP	SYN	CGA
MESOTH	100	3	86	100	20	90	0	0	0
SCYST	100	10	50	0	0	0	80	0	0
LMS	3	0	89	0	70	90	0	0	0
SPCCA	86	67	96	0	3	10	0	0	0
SYNSC	80	85	100	67	0	0	0	0	0
SPCNC	100	80	3	0	0	10	0	80	75
FS/MFH	1	1	100	0	0	0	0	0	0

KER, keratin (mixture of monoclonal antibodies); EMA, epithelial membrane antigen; VIM, vimentin; CALRET, calretinin; DES, desmin; MSA, muscle-specific actin; AFP, alpha fetoprotein; SYN, synaptophysin; CGA, chromogranin A; MESOTH, mesothelioma; SCYST, spindle cell yolk sac tumor; LMS, leiomyosarcoma; SPCCA, spindle cell carcinoma (either primary or metastatic); SYNSC, synovial sarcoma; SPCNC, spindle cell neuroendocrine carcinoma; FS, fibrosarcoma; MFH, malignant fibrous histiocytoma.

Data from Frisman D. Immunoquery (available at http://www.immunoquery.com) and the author's experience.

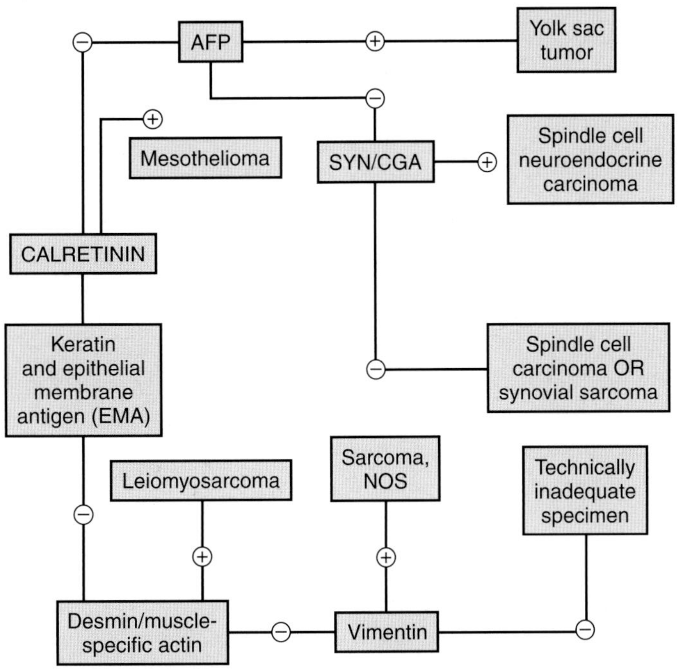

FIGURE 11.31 Algorithm for immunohistologic evaluation of malignant spindle-cell tumors of the mediastinum.

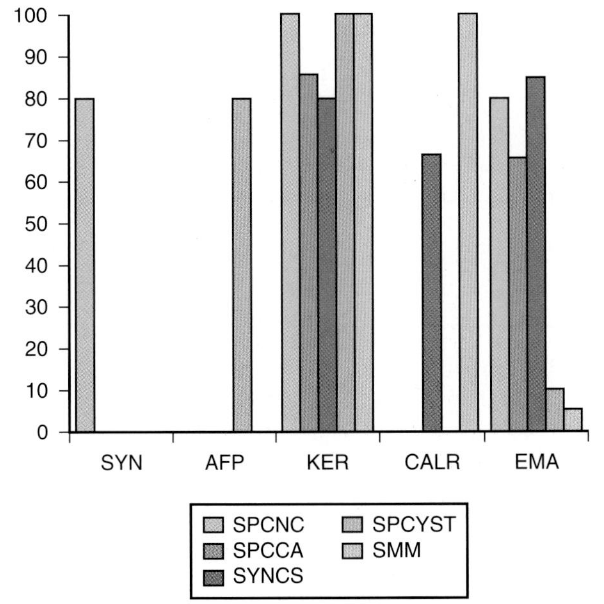

FIGURE 11.32 Markers of interest in the differential diagnosis of malignant epithelial spindle cell tumors of the mediastinum.

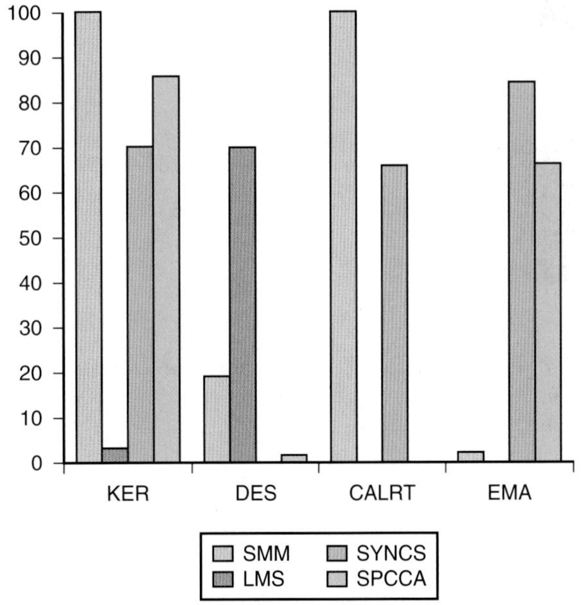

FIGURE 11.33 Pertinent markers in the differential diagnosis of leiomyosarcoma versus malignant epithelial spindle-cell tumors of the mediastinum.

carcinomas of the mediastinum, as discussed earlier in this section.

SARCOMATOID MEDIASTINAL MALIGNANT MESOTHELIOMA

Aside from its exclusive composition by fusiform and pleomorphic tumor cells, sarcomatoid mediastinal mesothelioma also is dissimilar from its epithelioid or biphasic counterparts in its ultrastructural and immunohistologic features. These closely approximate the specialized pathologic attributes of sarcomatoid carcinoma, as discussed earlier in this chapter. Mesothelial tumors differ from the latter entity in that mesotheliomas are reactive for WT-1, podoplanin, and calretinin, whereas carcinomas are not.[183,185,206]

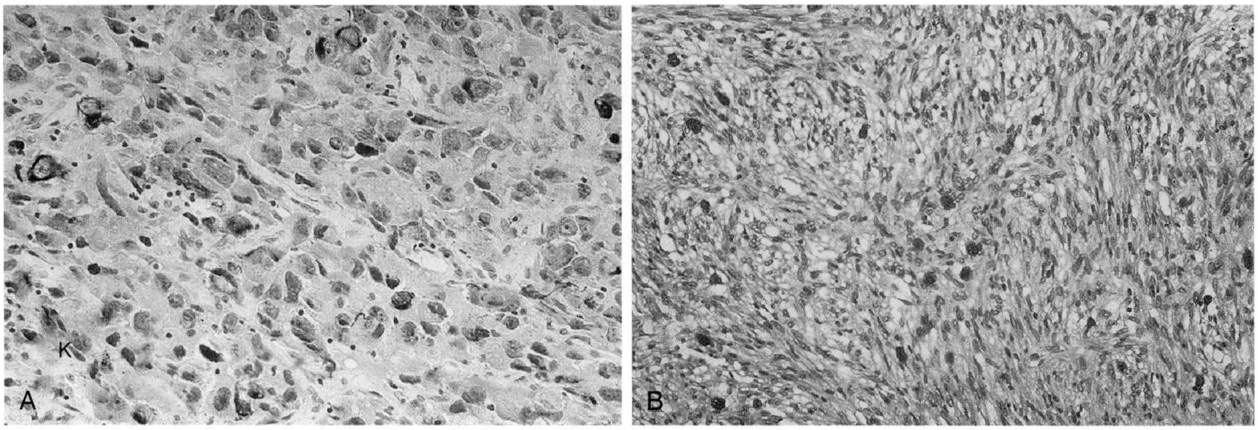

FIGURE 11.34 Focal immunolabeling for keratin (K) **(A)** in primary sarcomatoid carcinoma of the thymus **(B)**.

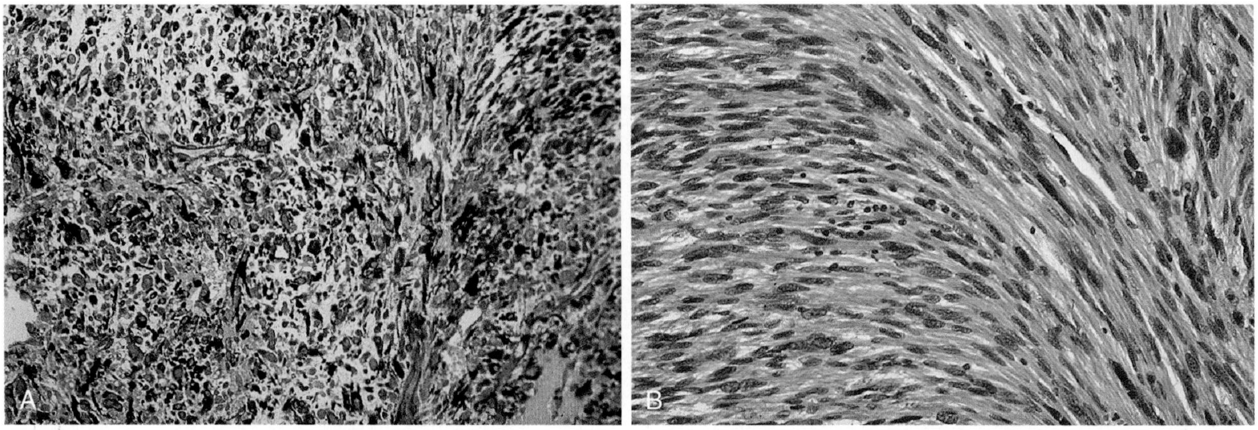

FIGURE 11.35 Immunoreactivity for desmin **(A)** in mediastinal leiomyosarcoma **(B)**.

SARCOMATOID THYMIC YOLK SAC TUMOR

A peculiar variant of primary mediastinal yolk sac tumor (MYST) has been documented by Moran and Suster.[213] Even though it features a predominance of spindle cells, and as such may be confused with the other neoplastic entities cited in this section, sarcomatoid MYST is identical immunohistologically to conventional endodermal sinus tumor (described in the previous paragraphs). Reactivity for keratin and AFP is expected in spindle-cell MYST. The second of these markers reproducibly excludes the diagnostic possibility of STC, which lacks AFP.[199-201,213]

MEDIASTINAL LEIOMYOSARCOMA

Moran and colleagues[214] have reported the existence of primary mediastinal leiomyosarcomas, which may be observed in either the anterior or posterior compartments. These spindle-cell malignancies are uniformly immunoreactive for desmin (Fig. 11.35), muscle-specific actin, alpha-isoform actin, caldesmon, and calponin[215]; vimentin also may be present. Conversely, EMA, keratin, Myo-D1, myoglobin, myogenin, and S-100 protein are absent in leiomyosarcomas.[42]

Mediastinal Solitary Fibrous Tumor

Solitary fibrous tumor (SFT) has been discussed in this chapter in connection with the immunohistologic differential diagnosis of thymoma variants. Occasionally, however, it may demonstrate significant cytologic atypia and produce confusion with respect to possible diagnoses of sarcomatoid carcinoma, synovial sarcoma, or mesothelioma (Fig. 11.36). In this particular context, SFT can be recognized by its concomitant immunoreactivity for CD34, CD99, or BCL-2 protein, in the absence of epithelial markers.[216] Synovial sarcoma also has the potential to label for the latter two of these determinants.[207] Another possible pitfall is associated with the ability of SFT to show podoplanin positivity, usually associated with mesotheliomas.[217]

Dendritic Cell Tumors/Sarcomas of The Mediastinum

Since the 1990s, neoplasms that show differentiation toward lymphoreticular dendritic cells have been increasingly recognized.[218,219] These may arise in the

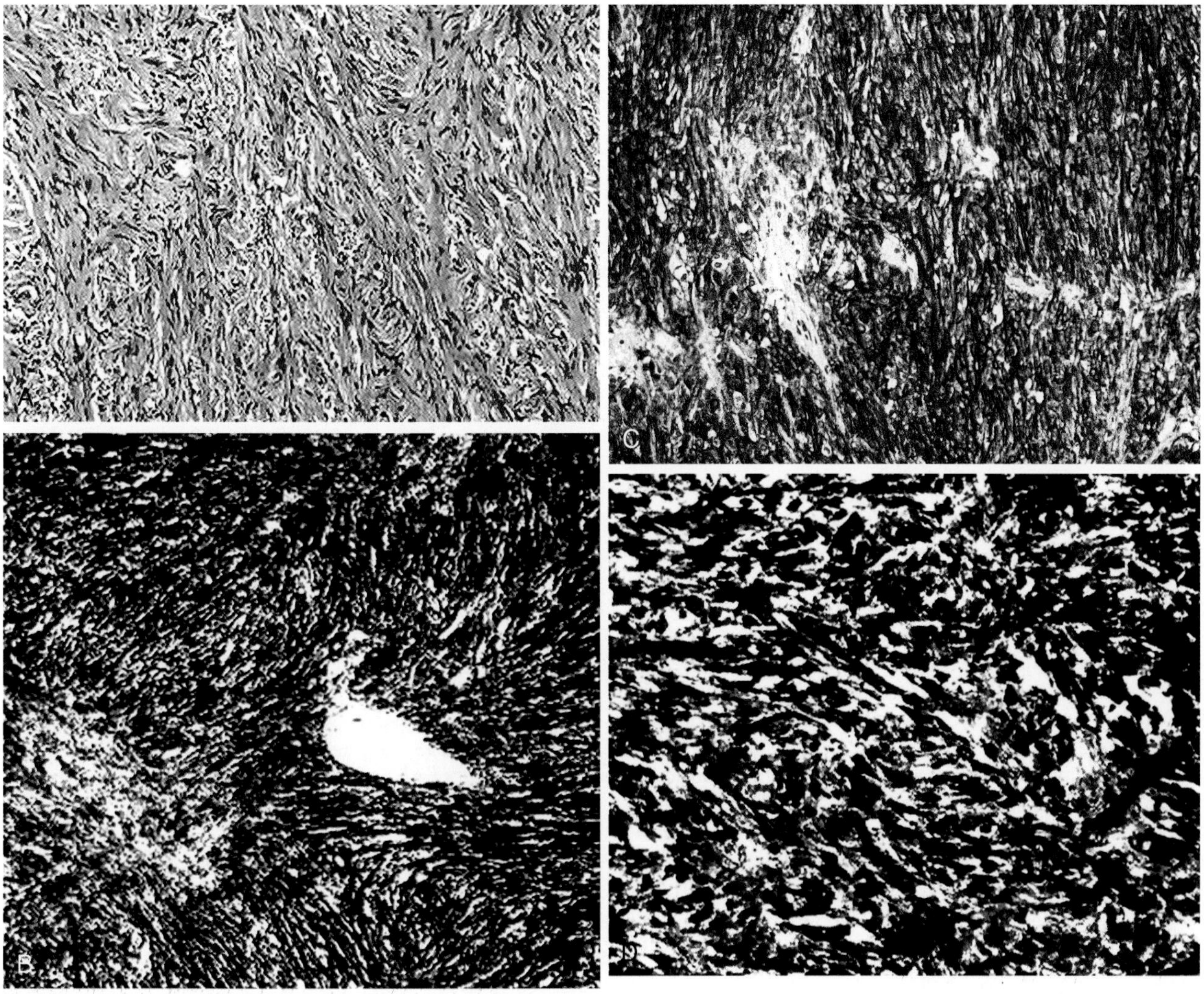

FIGURE 11.36 Solitary fibrous tumor **(A)** usually labels for CD34 **(B)**, and may also be reactive for CD99 **(C)** and BCL-2 protein **(D)**.

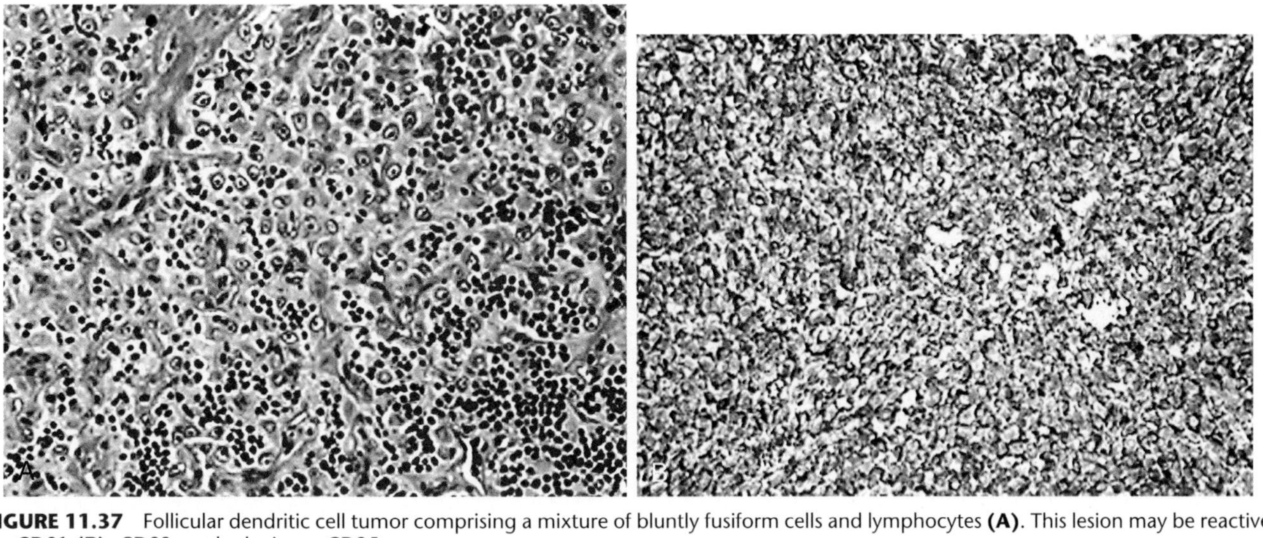

FIGURE 11.37 Follicular dendritic cell tumor comprising a mixture of bluntly fusiform cells and lymphocytes **(A)**. This lesion may be reactive for CD21 **(B)**, CD23, podoplanin, or CD35.

mediastinum, the lymph nodes, or the thymus and can be confused with spindle-cell thymomas. In the author's experience, CD99+ and TdT+ lymphocytes invested such a lesion in one case, causing a particularly strong resemblance to a thymic epithelial tumor (Fig. 11.37). Two main categories of mediastinal dendritic cell tumor/sarcoma (DCTS) are currently codified, namely, follicular and interdigitating DCTSs.[218]

In contrast to thymoma, dendritic cell tumors consistently lack keratin and p63. The constituent spindle cells are variably reactive for CD45; those in the follicular DCTS group label for combinations of CD21, CD23, CD35, CXCL13, and podoplanin, whereas interdigitating DCTS lacks these markers and is positive for S100 protein.[218-221]

PROGNOSTIC MARKERS IN MEDIASTINAL NEOPLASMS

Attempts at prognosticating the behavior of thymoma have involved immunohistologic semiquantitation of tumoral proliferative rates with anti-proliferating cell nuclear antigen (PCNA) and Ki-67[222,223] and detection of aberrant expression of BCL-2, *Fas*, or p53 gene products by immunostaining or blotting.[30,31,123,126] In general, these methods have not produced any consistently reproducible results. Comparable statements apply to the immunohistologic evaluation of E-cadherin expression.[224,225] Similarly, there are no uniformly effective molecular markers of prognosis for other mediastinal neoplasms. Thus, at the time of this writing, the author considers this aspect of contextual immunohistochemical analysis to be beyond the standard practice of surgical pathology.

SUMMARY

The application of immunohistology in the study of the incredibly complex mediastinum is challenging indeed. Most immunohistologic applications are performed on small biopsy materials, emphasizing the importance of proper tissue fixation and processing for optimal diagnostic, theranostic, and genomic investigations.

REFERENCES

1. Sterrett G, Whitaker D, Shilkin KB, et al. The fine needle aspiration cytology of mediastinal lesions. *Cancer*. 1983;51:127-135.
2. Gherardi G, Marveggio C, Placidi A. Neuroendocrine carcinoma of the thymus: Aspiration biopsy, immunocytochemistry, and clinicopathologic correlates. *Diagn Cytopathol*. 1995;35:158-164.
3. Heilo A. Tumors in the mediastinum: Ultrasound-guided histologic core-needle biopsy. *Radiology*. 1993;189:143-146.
4. Powers CN, Silverman JF, Geisinger KR, et al. Fine needle aspiration biopsy of the mediastinum: A multiinstitutional analysis. *Am J Clin Pathol*. 1996;105:168-173.
5. Yu GH, Salhany KE, Gokaslan ST, et al. Thymic epithelial cells as a diagnostic pitfall in the fine needle aspiration diagnosis of primary mediastinal lymphoma. *Diagn Cytopathol*. 1997;16:460-465.
6. Shin HJ, Katz RL. Thymic neoplasia as represented by fine needle aspiration biopsy of anterior mediastinal masses: A practical approach to the differential diagnosis. *Acta Cytol*. 1998;42:855-864.
7. Wick MR, Rosai J. The endocrine thymus. In: Kovacs K, Asa SL, eds. *Functional Endocrine Pathology*. 2nd ed. Oxford: Blackwell; 1998:869-894.
8. Hirokawa K, Utsuyama M, Moriizumi E, et al. Immunohistochemical studies in human thymomas: Localization of thymosin and various cell markers. *Virchows Arch B Cell Pathol*. 1988;55:371-380.
9. Fukai I, Masaoka A, Hashimoto T, et al. Cytokeratins in normal thymus and thymic epithelial tumors. *Cancer*. 1993;71:99-105.
10. Fukai I, Masaoka A, Hashimoto T, et al. Differential diagnosis of thymic carcinoma and lung carcinoma with the use of antibodies to cytokeratins. *J Thorac Cardiovasc Surg*. 1995;110:1670-1675.
11. Wick MR. Mediastinal cysts and intrathoracic thyroid tumors. *Semin Diagn Pathol*. 1990;7:285-294.
12. Sabiston D, Scott HW. Primary neoplasms and cysts of the mediastinum. *Ann Surg*. 1961;136:777-797.
13. LeRoux BT, Kallichurum S, Shama DM. Mediastinal cysts and tumors. *Curr Probl Surg*. 1984;21:1-77.
14. Suster S, Moran CA. Malignant thymic neoplasms that may mimic benign conditions. *Semin Diagn Pathol*. 1995;12:98-110.
15. Moran CA, Suster S. Mediastinal seminomas with prominent cystic changes: A clinicopathologic study of 10 cases. *Am J Surg Pathol*. 1995;25:1047-1053.
16. Niehans GA, Manivel JC, Copland GT, et al. Immunohistochemistry of germ cell and trophoblastic neoplasms. *Cancer*. 1988;62:1113-1123.
17. Yu H, Pinkus GS, Hornick JL. Diffuse membranous immunoreactivity for podoplanin (D2-40) distinguishes primary and metastatic seminomas from other germ cell tumors and metastatic neoplasms. *Am J Clin Pathol*. 2007;128:767-775.
18. Ulbright TM, Young RH. Seminoma with tubular, microcystic, and related patterns: A study of 28 cases of unusual morphologic variants that often cause confusion with yolk sac tumor. *Am J Surg Pathol*. 2005;29:500-505.
19. Suster S, Moran CA. Primary thymic epithelial neoplasms: Spectrum of differentiation and histological features. *Semin Diagn Pathol*. 1999;16:2-17.
20. Wick MR, Simpson RW, Niehans GA, et al. Anterior mediastinal tumors: A clinicopathologic study of 100 cases, with emphasis on immunohistochemical analysis. *Prog Surg Pathol*. 1990;11:79-119.
21. Wick MR, Rosai J. Epithelial tumors. In: Givel JC, ed. *Surgery of the Thymus*. Berlin: Springer-Verlag; 1990:79-107.
22. Walker AN, Mills SE, Fechner RE. Thymomas and thymic carcinomas. *Semin Diagn Pathol*. 1990;7:250-265.
23. Lewis JE, Wick MR, Scheithauer BW, et al. Thymoma: A clinicopathologic review. *Cancer*. 1987;60:2727-2743.
24. Rosai J, Sobin LH, Caillaud JM, et al. *WHO classification of thymic tumors*. Geneva: World Health Organization; 1999: 1-25.
25. Rice HE, Flake AW, Hori T, et al. Massive thymic hyperplasia: Characterization of a rare mediastinal mass. *J Pediatr Surg*. 1994;29:1561-1564.
26. Battifora H, Sun TT, Bahu RM, et al. The use of antikeratin antiserum as a diagnostic tool: Thymoma versus lymphoma. *Hum Pathol*. 1980;11:635-641.
27. Chan JKC, Tsang WY, Seneviratne S, et al. The MIC2 antibody O13: Practical application for the study of thymic epithelial tumors. *Am J Surg Pathol*. 1995;19:1115-1123.
28. Robertson PB, Neiman RS, Worapongpaiboon S, et al. O13 (CD99) positivity in hematologic proliferations correlates with TdT positivity. *Mod Pathol*. 1997;10:277-282.
29. Soslow RA, Bhargava V, Warnke RA. MIC2, TdT, bcl-2, and CD34 expression in paraffin-embedded high-grade lymphoma/acute lymphoblastic leukemia distinguishes between distinct clinicopathologic entities. *Hum Pathol*. 1997;28: 1158-1165.
30. Brocheriou I, Carnot F, Briere J. Immunohistochemical detection of bcl-2 protein in thymoma. *Histopathology*. 1995;27: 251-255.
31. Chen FF, Yan JJ, Jin YT, et al. Detection of bcl-2 and p53 in thymoma: expression of bcl-2 as a reliable marker of tumor aggressiveness. *Hum Pathol*. 1996;27:1089-1092.
32. Chan WC, Zaatari GS, Tabei S, et al. Thymoma: An immunohistochemical study. *Am J Clin Pathol*. 1984;82:160-166.

33. Knowles II DM . Lymphoid cell markers: Their distribution and usefulness in the immunopathologic analysis of lymphoid neoplasms. *Am J Surg Pathol.* 1985;9(Suppl):85-108.
34. Weiss LM, Bindl JM, Picozzi VJ, et al. Lymphoblastic lymphoma: An immunophenotypic study of 26 cases with comparison to T-cell acute lymphoblastic leukemia. *Blood.* 1986;67:474-478.
35. Picker LJ, Weiss LM, Medeiros LJ, et al. Immunophenotypic criteria for the diagnosis of non-Hodgkin's lymphoma. *Am J Pathol.* 1987;128:181-201.
36. Berrih-Aknin S, Safar D, Cohen-Kaminsky S. Analysis of lymphocyte phenotype in human thymomas. *Adv Exp Med Biol.* 1988;237:369-374.
37. Ito M, Taki T, Mihaye M, et al. Lymphocyte subsets in human thymoma studied with monoclonal antibodies. *Cancer.* 1988;61:284-287.
38. Perrone T, Frizzera G, Rosai J. Mediastinal diffuse large-cell lymphoma with sclerosis: A clinicopathologic study of 60 cases. *Am J Surg Pathol.* 1986;10:176-191.
39. Wick MR, Swanson PE, Manivel JC. Immunohistochemical analysis of soft tissue sarcomas: comparisons with electron microscopy. *Appl Pathol.* 1988;6:169-196.
40. Dotto J, Pelosi G, Rosai J. Expression of p63 in thymomas and normal thymus. *Am J Clin Pathol.* 2007;127:415-420.
41. Park CK, Oh YH. Expression of p63 in reactive hyperplasias and malignant lymphomas. *J Korean Med Sci.* 2005;20: 752-758.
42. Nappi O, Ritter JH, Pettinato G, et al. Hemangiopericytoma: Histopathological pattern or clinicopathologic entity? *Semin Diagn Pathol.* 1995;12:221-232.
43. Shimosato Y, Mukai K. Tumors of the mediastinum. In: Rosai J, ed. *Atlas of Tumor Pathology, Series 3, Fascicle* 21. Washington, DC: Armed Forces Institute of Pathology; 1997:33-273.
44. Swanson PE. Soft tissue neoplasms of the mediastinum. *Semin Diagn Pathol.* 1991;8:14-34.
45. Marchevsky AM. Mediastinal tumors of peripheral nervous system origin. *Semin Diagn Pathol.* 1999;16:65-78.
46. Chaves-Espinosa JI, Chaves-Fernandez JA, Hoyer OH, et al. Endothoracic neurogenic neoplasms: Analysis of 30 cases. *Rev Interamer Radiol.* 1980;5:49-54.
47. Gale AW, Jelihovsky T, Grant AF, et al. Neurogenic tumors of the mediastinum. *Ann Thorac Surg.* 1974;17:434-443.
48. Davidson KG, Walbaum PR, McCormack RJM. Intrathoracic neural tumors. *Thorax.* 1978;33:359-367.
49. Young DG. Thoracic neuroblastoma/ganglioneuroma. *J Pediatr Surg.* 1983;18:37-41.
50. Gould VE, Wiedenmann B, Lee I, et al. Synaptophysin expression in neuroendocrine neoplasms as determined by immunocytochemistry. *Am J Pathol.* 1987;126:243-257.
51. Fine SW, McClain SA, Li M. Immunohistochemical staining for calretinin is useful for differentiating schwannomas from neurofibromas. *Am J Clin Pathol.* 2004;122:552-559.
52. Jokinen CH, Dadras SS, Goldblum JR, et al. Diagnostic implications of podoplanin expression in peripheral nerve sheath neoplasms. *Am J Clin Pathol.* 2008;129:886-893.
53. Witkin GB, Rosai J. Solitary fibrous tumor of the mediastinum: A report of 14 cases. *Am J Surg Pathol.* 1989;13:547-557.
54. Balassiano M, Reichert N, Rosenman Y, et al. Localized fibrous mesothelioma of the mediastinum devoid of pleural connections. *Postgrad Med J.* 1989;65:788-790.
55. Hanau CA, Miettinen M. Solitary fibrous tumor: Histological and immunohistochemical spectrum of benign and malignant variants presenting at different sites. *Hum Pathol.* 1995;26:440-449.
56. Wick MR, Manivel JC, Swanson PE. Contributions of immunohistochemistry to the diagnosis of soft tissue tumors. *Prog Surg Pathol.* 1988;8:197-249.
57. England DM, Hochholzer L, McCarthy MJ. Localized benign and malignant fibrous tumors of the pleura: A clinicopathologic review of 223 cases. *Am J Surg Pathol.* 1989;13:640-658.
58. Swanson PE, Wick MR. Immunohistochemical diagnosis of soft tissue tumors. In: Colvin R, Bhan A, McCluskey R, eds. *Diagnostic Immunopathology.* 2nd ed. New York: Raven Press; 1995:599-632.
59. Dines DE, Payne WS, Bernatz PE, et al. Mediastinal granulomas and fibrosing mediastinitis. *Chest.* 1979;75:320-324.
60. Coffin CM, Watterson J, Priest JR, et al. Extrapulmonary inflammatory myofibroblastic tumor (inflammatory pseudotumor): A clinicopathologic and immunohistochemical study of 84 cases. *Am J Surg Pathol.* 1995;19:859-872.
61. Lukes RJ, Butler JJ, Hicks EB. Natural history of Hodgkin's disease as related to its pathologic picture. *Cancer.* 1966;19:317-344.
62. Matsubara O, Mark EJ, Ritter JH. Pseudoneoplastic lesions of the lungs, pleural surfaces, and mediastinum. In: Wick MR, Humphrey PA, Ritter JH, eds. *Pathology of Pseudoneoplastic Lesions.* Philadelphia: Lippincott-Raven; 1997:97-129.
63. Crotty TB, Colby TV, Gay PC, et al. Desmoplastic malignant mesothelioma masquerading as sclerosing mediastinitis: A diagnostic dilemma. *Hum Pathol.* 1992;23:79-82.
64. Cessna MH, Zhou H, Sanger WG, et al. Expression of ALK1 and p80 in inflammatory myofibroblastic tumor and its mesenchymal mimics: A study of 135 cases. *Mod Pathol.* 2002;15: 931-938.
65. Carlson JW, Fletcher CDM. Immunohistochemistry for beta-catenin in the differential diagnosis of spindle-cell lesions: Analysis of a series and review of the literature. *Histopathology.* 2007;51:509-514.
66. Ritter JH, Humphrey PA, Wick MR. Malignant neoplasms capable of simulating inflammatory (myofibroblastic) pseudotumors and tumefactive fibroinflammatory lesions: Pseudopseudotumors. *Semin Diagn Pathol.* 1998;15:111-132.
67. Rosai J, Levine GD, Weber WR, et al. Carcinoid tumors and oat cell carcinomas of the thymus. *Pathol Annu.* 1976;11:201-226.
68. Wick MR, Rosai J. Neuroendocrine neoplasms of the thymus. *Pathol Res Pract.* 1988;183:188-199.
69. Kuo TT, Chang JP, Lin FJ, et al. Thymic carcinomas: Histopathological varieties and immunohistochemical study. *Am J Surg Pathol.* 1990;14:24-34.
70. Truong LD, Mody DR, Cagle PT, et al. Thymic carcinoma: A clinicopathologic study of 13 cases. *Am J Surg Pathol.* 1990;14:151-166.
71. Shimizu J, Hayashi Y, Morita K, et al. Primary thymic carcinoma: A clinicopathological and immunohistochemical study. *J Surg Oncol.* 1994;56:159-164.
72. Suster S, Rosai J. Thymic carcinoma: A clinicopathologic study of 60 cases. *Cancer.* 1991;67:1025-1032.
73. Ritter JH, Wick MR. Primary carcinomas of the thymus gland. *Semin Diagn Pathol.* 1999;16:18-31.
74. Snover DC, Levine GD, Rosai J. Thymic carcinomas: Five distinctive histological variants. *Am J Surg Pathol.* 1982;6: 451-470.
75. Iezzoni JC, Nass LB. Thymic basaloid carcinoma: A case report and review of the literature. *Mod Pathol.* 1996;9:21-25.
76. DeLorimier AA, Bragg KU, Linden G. Neuroblastoma in childhood. *Am J Dis Child.* 1969;118:441-450.
77. Ordonez NG. Value of thyroid transcription factor-1 immunostaining in distinguishing small cell carcinomas from other small cell carcinomas. *Am J Surg Pathol.* 2000;24:1217-1223.
78. Kaufmann O, Fietze E, Mengs J, et al. Value of p63 and cytokeratin 5/6 as immunohistochemical markers for the differential diagnosis of poorly differentiated and undifferentiated carcinomas. *Am J Clin Pathol.* 2001;116:823-830.
79. Salter Jr JE, Gibson D, Ordonez NG, et al. Neuroblastoma of the anterior mediastinum in an 80 year old woman. *Ultrastruct Pathol.* 1995;19:305-310.
80. Hachitanda Y, Hata J. Stage IVS neuroblastoma: A clinical, histological, and biological analysis of 45 cases. *Hum Pathol.* 1996;27:1135-1138.
81. Jerome-Marson V, Mazieres J, Groussard O, et al. Expression of TTF-1 and cytokeratins in primary and secondary epithelial lung tumors: Correlation with histological type and grade. *Histopathology.* 2004;45:125-134.
82. Argani P, Erlandson RA, Rosai J. Thymic neuroblastoma in adults: Report of three cases with special emphasis on its association with the syndrome of inappropriate secretion of antidiuretic hormone. *Am J Clin Pathol.* 1997;108:537-543.
83. Asada Y, Marutsuka K, Mitsukawa T, et al. Ganglioneuroblastoma of the thymus: An adult case with the syndrome of inappropriate secretion of antidiuretic hormone. *Hum Pathol.* 1996;27:506-509.

84. Wirnsberger GH, Becker H, Ziervogel K, et al. Diagnostic immunohistochemistry of neuroblastic tumors. *Am J Surg Pathol.* 1992;16:49-57.
85. Dehner LP. Peripheral and central primitive neuroectodermal tumors: A nosologic concept seeking a consensus. *Arch Pathol Lab Med.* 1986;110:997-1005.
86. Fellinger EJ, Garin-Chesa P, Su SL, et al. Biochemical and genetic characterization of the HBA71 Ewing's sarcoma cell surface antigen. *Cancer Res.* 1991;51:336-340.
87. Dehner LP. Primitive neuroectodermal tumor and Ewing's sarcoma. *Am J Surg Pathol.* 1993;17:1-13.
88. Gluer S, Zense M, Radtke E, et al. Polysialylated neural cell adhesion molecule in childhood ganglioneuroma and neuroblastoma of different histological grade and clinical stage. *Langenbecks Arch Surg.* 1998;383:340-344.
89. Miettinen M, Chatten J, Paetau A, et al. Monoclonal antibody NB84 in the differential diagnosis of neuroblastoma and other small round cell tumors. *Am J Surg Pathol.* 1998;22:327-332.
90. Leong ASY, Wick MR, Swanson PE. *Immunohistology and electron microscopy of anaplastic and pleomorphic tumors.* Cambridge, UK: Cambridge Press; 1997:109-208.
91. Parham DM, Dias P, Kelly DR, et al. Desmin positivity in primitive neuroectodermal tumors of childhood. *Am J Surg Pathol.* 1992;16:483-492.
92. Pachter MR, Lattes R. Mesenchymal tumors of the mediastinum. I. Tumors of fibrous tissue, adipose tissue, smooth muscle, and striated muscle. *Cancer.* 1963;16:74-94.
93. Suster S, Moran CA, Koss MN. Rhabdomyosarcomas of the anterior mediastinum: Report of four cases unassociated with germ cell, teratomatous, or thymic carcinomatous components. *Hum Pathol.* 1994;25:349-356.
94. Tsokos M. The diagnosis and classification of childhood rhabdomyosarcoma. *Semin Diagn Pathol.* 1994;11:26-38.
95. Cui S, Hano H, Harada T, et al. Evaluation of new monoclonal anti-MyoD1 and anti-myogenin antibodies for the diagnosis of rhabdomyosarcoma. *Pathol Int.* 1999;49:62-68.
96. Rossi S, Orvieto E, Furlanetto A, et al. Utility of the immunohistochemical detection of FLI-1 expression in round cell and vascular neoplasms using a monoclonal antibody. *Mod Pathol.* 2004;17:547-552.
97. Nathwani BN, Kim H, Rappaport H. Malignant lymphoma, lymphoblastic. *Cancer.* 1976;38:964-983.
98. Nathwani BN, Diamond LW, Winberg CD, et al. Lymphoblastic lymphoma: A clinicopathologic study of 95 patients. *Cancer.* 1981;48:2347-2357.
99. Shikano T, Arioka H, Kobayashi R, et al. Acute lymphoblastic leukemia and non-Hodgkin's lymphoma with mediastinal mass—A study of 23 children; different disorders or different stages? *Leuk Lymphoma.* 1994;13:161-167.
100. Trump DL, Mann RB. Diffuse large cell and undifferentiated lymphomas with prominent mediastinal involvement: A poor prognostic subset of patients with non-Hodgkin's lymphoma. *Cancer.* 1982;50:277-282.
101. Majolino I, Marceno R, Magrin S, et al. Burkitt's cell leukemia with mediastinal mass and unusually good prognosis. *Haematologica.* 1983;68:287-288.
102. Isaacson PG, Chan JKC, Tang C, et al. Low-grade B-cell lymphoma of mucosa-associated lymphoid tissue arising in the thymus: A thymic lymphoma mimicking myoepithelial sialadenitis. *Am J Surg Pathol.* 1990;14:342-351.
103. Takagi N, Nakamura S, Yamamoto K, et al. Malignant lymphoma of mucosa-associated lymphoid tissue arising in the thymus of a patient with Sjögren's syndrome: A morphologic, phenotypic, and genotypic study. *Cancer.* 1992;69:1347-1355.
104. Ozdemirli M, Fanburg-Smith JC, Hartmann DP, et al. Precursor B-lymphoblastic lymphoma presenting as a solitary bone tumor and mimicking Ewing's sarcoma: A report of four cases and review of the literature. *Am J Surg Pathol.* 1998;22:795-804.
105. Zukerberg LR, Medeiros LJ, Ferry JA, et al. Diffuse low-grade B-cell lymphomas: Four clinically distinct subtypes defined by a combination of morphologic and immunophenotypic features. *Am J Clin Pathol.* 1993;100:373-385.
106. Banks PM, Isaacson PG. MALT lymphomas in 1997. *Am J Clin Pathol.* 1999;111(Suppl 1):S75-S83.
107. Rodig SJ, Vergilio JA, Shahsafaei A, et al. Characteristic expression patterns of TCL1, CD38, and CD44 identify aggressive lymphomas harboring a MYC translocation. *Am J Surg Pathol.* 2008;32:113-122.
108. Strickler JG, Kurtin PJ. Mediastinal lymphoma. *Semin Diagn Pathol.* 1991;8:2-13.
109. Nakhleh RE, Wick MR, Rocamora A, et al. Morphologic diversity in malignant melanomas. *Am J Clin Pathol.* 1990;93:731-740.
110. Fetsch PA, Marincola FM, Abati A. The new melanoma markers: MART-1 and Melan-A. *Am J Surg Pathol.* 1999;23:607-610.
111. Matsuno Y, Mukai K, Noguchi M, et al. Histochemical and immunohistochemical evidence of glandular differentiation in thymic carcinomas. *Acta Pathol Jpn.* 1989;39:433-438.
112. Kuo TT, Chan JKC. Thymic carcinoma arising in thymoma is associated with alterations in immunohistochemical profile. *Am J Surg Pathol.* 1998;22:1474-1481.
113. Berezowski K, Grimes MM, Gal A, et al. CD5 immunoreactivity of epithelial cells in thymic carcinoma and CASTLE using paraffin-embedded tissue. *Am J Clin Pathol.* 1996;106:483-486.
114. Hishima T, Fukayama M, Fujisawa M, et al. CD5 expression in thymic carcinoma. *Am J Pathol.* 1994;145:268-275.
115. Busam KJ, Kucukaol D, Sato E, et al. Immunohistochemical analysis of novel monoclonal antibody PNL2 and comparison with other melanocyte differentiation markers. *Am J Surg Pathol.* 2005;29:400-406.
116. Pan CC, Chen PC, Chou TY, et al. Expression of calretinin and other mesothelioma-related markers in thymic carcinoma and thymoma. *Hum Pathol.* 2003;34:1155-1162.
117. Saad RS, Landreneau RJ, Liu Y, et al. Utility of immunohistochemistry in separating thymic neoplasms from germ cell tumors and metastatic lung cancer involving the anterior mediastinum. *Appl Immunohistochem Molec Morphol.* 2003;11:107-112.
118. Franke A, Strobel P, Fackeldey V, et al. Hepatoid thymic carcinoma: Report of a case. *Am J Surg Pathol.* 2004;28:250-256.
119. Lugli A, Tornillo L, Mirlacher M, et al. Hepatocyte paraffin-1 expression in human normal and neoplastic tissues: Tissue microarray analysis on 3,940 tissue samples. *Am J Clin Pathol.* 2004;122:721-727.
120. Kornstein MJ, Rosai J. CD5 labeling of thymic carcinomas and other non-lymphoid neoplasms. *Am J Clin Pathol.* 1998;109:722-726.
121. Nakagawa K, Matsuno Y, Kunicoh H, et al. Immunohistochemical KIT (CD117) expression in thymic epithelial tumors. *Chest.* 2005;128:140-144.
122. Tateyama H, Eimoto T, Tada T, et al. p53 protein expression and p53 gene mutation in thymic epithelial tumors: An immunohistochemical and DNA sequencing study. *Am J Clin Pathol.* 1995;104:375-381.
123. Stefanaki K, Rontogianni D, Kouvidou CH, et al. Expression of p53, mdm2, p21/waf1, and bcl-2 proteins in thymomas. *Histopathology.* 1997;30:549-555.
124. Weirich G, Schneider P, Fellbaum C, et al. p53 alterations in thymic epithelial tumors. *Virchows Arch A.* 1997;431:17-23.
125. Chen FF, Yan JJ, Chang KC, et al. Immunohistochemical localization of Mcl-1 and bcl-2 proteins in thymic epithelial tumors. *Histopathology.* 1996;29:541-547.
126. Tateyama H, Eimoto T, Tada T, et al. Apoptosis, bcl-2 protein, and Fas antigen in thymic epithelial tumors. *Mod Pathol.* 1997;10:983-991.
127. Lauriola L, Erlandson RA, Rosai J. Neuroendocrine differentiation is a common feature of thymic carcinoma. *Am J Surg Pathol.* 1998;22:1059-1066.
128. Clark OH. Mediastinal parathyroid tumors. *Arch Surg.* 1988;123:1096-1100.
129. Nathaniels EK, Nathaniels AM, Wang CA. Mediastinal parathyroid tumors: A clinical and pathological study of 84 cases. *Ann Surg.* 1970;171:165-170.
130. Murphy MN, Glennon PG, Diocee MS, et al. Nonsecretory parathyroid carcinoma of the mediastinum. *Cancer.* 1986;58:2468-2476.

131. Ordonez NG, Ibanez ML, Samaan NA, et al. Immunoperoxidase study of uncommon parathyroid tumors. *Am J Surg Pathol.* 1983;7:535-542.
132. Dehner LP. Germ cell tumors of the mediastinum. *Semin Diagn Pathol.* 1990;7:266-284.
133. Wick MR, Ritter JH, Humphrey PA, et al. Clear cell neoplasms of the endocrine system and thymus. *Semin Diagn Pathol.* 1997;14:183-202.
134. Knapp RH, Hurt RD, Payne WS, et al. Malignant germ cell tumors of the mediastinum. *J Thorac Cardiovasc Surg.* 1985;89:82-89.
135. Truong LD, Harris L, Mattioli C, et al. Endodermal sinus tumor of the mediastinum: A report of seven cases and review of the literature. *Cancer.* 1986;58:730-739.
136. Weidner N. Germ cell tumors of the mediastinum. *Semin Diagn Pathol.* 1999;16:42-50.
137. Moran CA, Suster S, Przygodzki RM, et al. Primary germ cell tumors of the mediastinum: II. Mediastinal seminomas—a clinicopathologic and immunohistochemical study of120 cases. *Cancer.* 1997;80:691-698.
138. Przygodzki RM, Hubbs AE, Zhao F, et al. Primary mediastinal seminomas: Evidence of single and multiple KIT mutations. *Lab Invest.* 2002;82:1369-1375.
139. Sonne SB, Herlihy AS, Hoei-Hansen CE, et al. Identity of M2A (D2-40) antigen and gp36 (Aggrus, T1A-2, podoplanin) in human developing testis, testicular carcinoma in situ and germ-cell tumours. *Virchows Arch.* 2006;449:200-206.
140. Sung MT, Maciennan GT, Lopez-Beltran A, et al. Primary mediastinal seminoma: A comprehensive assessment integrated with histology, immunohistochemistry, and fluorescence in-situ hybridization for chromosome 12p abnormalities in 23 cases. *Am J Surg Pathol.* 2008;32:146-155.
141. Iczkowski KA, Butler SL, Shanks JH, et al. Trials of new germ cell immunohistochemical stains in 93 extragonadal and metastatic germ cell tumors. *Hum Pathol.* 2008;39:275-281.
142. Moran CA, Suster S. Hepatoid yolk sac tumors of the mediastinum: A clinicopathologic and immunohistologic study of four cases. *Am J Surg Pathol.* 1997;21:1210-1214.
143. Suster S, Moran CA, Dominguez-Malagon H, et al. Germ cell tumors of the mediastinum and testis: A comparative immunohistochemical study of 120 cases. *Hum Pathol.* 1998;29:737-742.
144. Moran CA, Suster S. Primary mediastinal choriocarcinomas: A clinicopathologic and immunohistochemical study of eight cases. *Am J Surg Pathol.* 1997;21:1007-1012.
145. Klemm KM, Moran CA. Primary neuroendocrine carcinomas of the thymus. *Semin Diagn Pathol.* 1999;16:32-41.
146. de Montpréville VT, Macchiarini P, Dulmet E. Thymic neuroendocrine carcinoma (carcinoid): A clinicopathologic study of fourteen cases. *J Thorac Cardiovasc Surg.* 1996;111:134-141.
147. Caceres W, Baldizon C, Sanchez J. Carcinoid tumor of the thymus: A unique neoplasm of the mediastinum. *Am J Clin Oncol.* 1998;21:82-83.
148. Wick MR, Rosai J. Neuroendocrine neoplasms of the mediastinum. *Semin Diagn Pathol.* 1991;8:35-51.
149. Moran CA, Suster S. Cystic well-differentiated neuroendocrine carcinoma (carcinoid tumor): A clinicopathologic and immunohistochemical study of two cases. *Am J Clin Pathol.* 2006;126:377-380.
150. Valli M, Fabris GA, Dewar A, et al. Atypical carcinoid tumor of the thymus: A study of eight cases. *Histopathology.* 1994;24:371-375.
151. Wick MR, Scheithauer BW. Thymic carcinoid: A histologic, immunohistochemical, and ultrastructural study of 12 cases. *Cancer.* 1984;53:475-484.
152. Herbst WM, Kumner W, Hofmann W, et al. Carcinoid tumors of the thymus: An immunohistochemical study. *Cancer.* 1987;60:2465-2470.
153. Odze R, Begin LR. Malignant paraganglioma of the posterior mediastinum. *Cancer.* 1990;65:564-569.
154. Olson JL, Salyer WR. Mediastinal paraganglioma (aortic body tumor): A report of four cases, and a review of the literature. *Cancer.* 1978;41:2405-2412.
155. Plaza JA, Wakely Jr PE, Moran C, et al. Sclerosing paraganglioma: Report of 19 cases of an unusual variant of neuroendocrine tumor that may be mistaken for an aggressive malignant neoplasm. *Am J Surg Pathol.* 2006;30:7-12.
156. Schroder HD, Johannsen L. Demonstration of S100 protein in sustentacular cells of phaeochromocytomas and paragangliomas. *Histopathology.* 1986;10:1023-1033.
157. DeLellis RA, Tischler AS, Lee AK, et al. Leu-enkephalin-like immunoreactivity in proliferative lesions of the human adrenal medulla and extra-adrenal paraganglia. *Am J Surg Pathol.* 1983;7:29-37.
158. Lamarre L, Jacobson JO, Aisenberg AC, et al. Primary large cell lymphoma of the mediastinum: A histologic and immunophenotypic study of 29 cases. *Am J Surg Pathol.* 1989;13:730-739.
159. Suster S. Primary large-cell lymphomas of the mediastinum. *Semin Diagn Pathol.* 1999;16:51-64.
160. Davis RE, Dorfman RF, Warnke RA. Primary large-cell lymphoma of the thymus: A diffuse B-cell neoplasm presenting as primary mediastinal lymphoma. *Hum Pathol.* 1990;21:1262-1268.
161. Al-Sharabati M, Chittal S, Duga-Neulat, et al. Primary anterior mediastinal B-cell lymphoma: A clinicopathologic and immunohistochemical study of 16 cases. *Cancer.* 1991;67:2579-2587.
162. Suster S, Moran CA. Pleomorphic large cell lymphomas of the mediastinum. *Am J Surg Pathol.* 1996;20:224-232.
163. Addis BJ, Isaacson PG. Large-cell lymphoma of the mediastinum: A B-cell tumor of probable thymic origin. *Histopathology.* 1986;10:379-390.
164. Torlakovic E, Torlakovic G, Nguyen PL, et al. The value of anti-PAX-5 immunostaining in routinely fixed and paraffin-embedded sections: A novel pan pre-B and B-cell marker. *Am J Surg Pathol.* 2002;26:1343-1350.
165. Martelli M, Ferreri AJ, Johnson P. Primary mediastinal large B-cell lymphoma. *Crit Rev Oncol Hematol.* 2008;68:256-263.
166. Fechner RE. Hodgkin's disease of the thymus. *Cancer.* 1969;23:16-23.
167. Katz A, Lattes R. Granulomatous thymoma or Hodgkin's disease of thymus? A clinical and histologic study and a re-evaluation. *Cancer.* 1969;23:1-15.
168. Lazzarino M, Orlandi E, Paulli M, et al. Treatment outcome and prognostic factors for primary mediastinal (thymic) B-cell lymphoma: A multicenter study of 106 patients. *J Clin Oncol.* 1997;15:1646-1653.
169. Strickler JG, Michie SA, Warnke RA, et al. The "syncytial variant" of nodular sclerosing Hodgkin's disease. *Am J Surg Pathol.* 1986;10:470-477.
170. Frizzera G. The distinction of Hodgkin's disease from anaplastic large cell lymphoma. *Semin Diagn Pathol.* 1992;9:291-296.
171. Menestrina F, Chilosi M, Scarpa A. Nodular lymphocyte predominant Hodgkin's disease and anaplastic large cell (CD30+) lymphoma: Distinct entities or nonspecific patterns? *Semin Diagn Pathol.* 1995;12:256-269.
172. Kubonishi I, Ohtsuki Y, Machida K, et al. Granulocytic sarcoma as a mediastinal mass. *Am J Clin Pathol.* 1984;83:730-734.
173. Chubachi A, Miura I, Takahashi N, et al. Acute myelogenous leukemia associated with a mediastinal tumor. *Leuk Lymphoma.* 1993;12:143-146.
174. Niwa K, Tanaka T, Mori H, et al. Extramedullary plasmacytoma of the mediastinum. *Jpn J Clin Oncol.* 1987;17:95-100.
175. Miyazaki T, Kohno S, Sakamoto A, et al. A rare case of extramedullary plasmacytoma in the mediastinum. *Intern Med.* 1992;31:1363-1365.
176. Meis JM, Butler JJ, Osborne BM, et al. Granulocytic sarcoma in nonleukemic patients. *Cancer.* 1986;58:2697-2709.
177. Quintanilla-Martinez L, Zukerberg LR, Ferry JA, et al. Extramedullary tumors of lymphoid or myeloid blasts: The role of immunohistology in diagnosis and classification. *Am J Clin Pathol.* 1995;104:431-443.
178. Goldstein NS, Ritter JH, Argenyi ZB, et al. Granulocytic sarcoma: Potential diagnostic clues from immunostaining patterns seen with anti-lymphoid antibodies. *Int J Surg Pathol.* 1995;2:199-206.
179. Aref S, Goda T, El-Sherbiny M. Syndecan-1 in multiple myeloma: Relationship to conventional prognostic factors. *Hematology.* 2003;8:221-228.
180. Tong AW, Lee JC, Stone MJ. Characterization of a monoclonal antibody having selective reactivity with normal and neoplastic plasma cells. *Blood.* 1987;69:238-245.
181. Petruch UR, Horny HP, Kaiserling E. Frequent expression of haematopoietic and non-haematopoietic antigens by neoplastic plasma cells: An immunohistochemical study using formalin-fixed, paraffin-embedded tissue. *Histopathology.* 1992;20:35-40.

182. Kambham N, Kong C, Longacre TA, et al. Utility of syndecan-1 (CD138) expression in the diagnosis of undifferentiated malignant neoplasms: A tissue microarray study of 1754 cases. *Appl Immunohistochem Mol Morphol.* 2005;13:304-310.
183. Ordonez NG. Role of immunohistochemistry in differentiating epithelial mesothelioma from adenocarcinoma: Review and update. *Am J Clin Pathol.* 1999;112:75-89.
184. Hinterberger M, Reineke T, Storz M, et al. D2-40 and calretinin: A tissue microarray analysis of 341 malignant mesotheliomas with emphasis on sarcomatoid differentiation. *Mod Pathol.* 2007;20:248-255.
185. Padgett DM, Cathro HP, Wick MR, et al. Podoplanin is a better immunohistochemical marker for sarcomatoid mesothelioma than calretinin. *Am J Surg Pathol.* 2008;32:123-127.
186. Marchevsky AM. Application of immunohistochemistry to the diagnosis of malignant mesothelioma. *Arch Pathol Lab Med.* 2008;132:397-401.
187. Kennedy AD, King G, Kerr KM. HBME-1 and antithrombomodulin in the differential diagnosis of malignant mesothelioma of pleura. *J Clin Pathol.* 1997;50:859-862.
188. Ordonez NG. Value of thrombomodulin immunostaining in the diagnosis of mesothelioma. *Histopathology.* 1997;31:25-30.
189. Wick MR, Loy T, Mills SE, et al. Malignant epithelioid pleural mesothelioma versus peripheral pulmonary adenocarcinoma: A histochemical, ultrastructural, and immunohistologic study of 103 cases. *Hum Pathol.* 1990;21:759-766.
190. Riera JR, Astengo-Osuna C, Longmate JA, et al. The immunohistochemical diagnostic panel for epithelial mesothelioma: A reevaluation after heat-induced epitope retrieval. *Am J Surg Pathol.* 1997;21:1409-1419.
191. Khoor A, Whitsett JA, Stahlman MT, et al. Utility of surfactant protein B precursor and thyroid transcription factor 1 in differentiating adenocarcinoma of the lung from malignant mesothelioma. *Hum Pathol.* 1999;30:695-700.
192. Wick MR. Immunohistochemistry in the diagnosis of "solid" malignant tumors. In: Jennette JC, ed. *Immunohistology in Diagnostic Pathology.* Boca Raton: CRC Press; 1989:161-191.
193. Feldman L, Kricun ME. Malignant melanoma presenting as a mediastinal mass. *JAMA.* 1979;241:396-397.
194. Kaufmann O, Koch S, Burghardt J, et al. Tyrosinase, melan-A, and KBA62 as markers for the immunohistochemical identification of metastatic amelanotic melanomas on paraffin sections. *Mod Pathol.* 1998;11:740-746.
195. Andrade RE, Wick MR, Frizzera G, et al. Immunophenotyping of hematopoietic malignancies in paraffin sections. *Hum Pathol.* 1988;19:394-402.
196. Nylander K, Vojtesek B, Nenutil R, et al. Differential expression of p63 isoforms in normal tissues and neoplastic cells. *J Pathol.* 2002;198:417-427.
197. Said JW. The immunohistochemistry of Hodgkin's disease. *Semin Diagn Pathol.* 1992;9:265-271.
198. Buettner M, Greiner A, Avramidou A, et al. Evidence of abortive plasma cell differentiation in Hodgkin and Reed-Sternberg cells of classical Hodgkin lymphoma. *Hematol Oncol.* 2005;23:127-132.
199. Suster S, Moran CA. Spindle cell thymic carcinoma: A clinicopathologic and immunohistochemical study of a distinctive variant of primary thymic epithelial neoplasm. *Am J Surg Pathol.* 1999;23:691-700.
200. Suster S, Moran CA. Thymic carcinoma: Spectrum of differentiation and histologic types. *Pathology (Australasian).* 1998;30:111-122.
201. Moran CA, Suster S. Primary thymic carcinomas. *Pathology (American).* 1996;4:141-153.
202. Kuo TT. Carcinoid tumor of the thymus with divergent sarcomatoid differentiation: Report of a case with histogenetic considerations. *Hum Pathol.* 1994;25:319-323.
203. Suarez-Vilela D, Salas-Valien JS, Gonzalez-Moran MA, et al. Thymic carcinosarcoma associated with a spindle cell thymoma: An immunohistochemical study. *Histopathology.* 1992;21:263-268.
204. Wick MR, Swanson PE. Carcinosarcomas—Current perspectives and a historical review of nosological concepts. *Semin Diagn Pathol.* 1993;10:118-127.
205. DeLeeuw B, Suijkerbuijk RF, Olde-Weghuis D, et al. Distinct Xp11.2 breakpoint regions in synovial sarcoma revealed by metaphase and interphase FISH: Relationship to histologic subtypes. *Cancer Genet Cytogenet.* 1994;73:89-94.
206. Miettinen M, Limon J, Niezabitowski A, et al. Calretinin and other mesothelioma markers in synovial sarcoma: Analysis of antigenic similarities and differences with malignant mesothelioma. *Am J Surg Pathol.* 2001;25:610-617.
207. Suster S, Moran CA. Primary synovial sarcomas of the mediastinum: A clinicopathologic, immunohistochemical, and ultrastructural study of 15 cases. *Am J Surg Pathol.* 2005;29:569-578.
208. Yoo SH, Han J, Kim TJ, Chung DH. Expression of CD99 in pleomorphic carcinomas of the lung. *J Korean Med Sci.* 2005;20:50-55.
209. Sun B, Sun Y, Wang J, et al. The diagnostic value of SYT-SSX detected by reverse transcriptase-polymerase chain reaction (RT-PCR) and fluorescence in-situ hybridization (FISH) for synovial sarcoma: A review and prospective study of 255 cases. *Cancer Sci.* 2008;99:1355-1361.
210. Suster S, Moran CA, Chan JKC. Thymoma with pseudosarcomatous stroma: Report of an unusual histologic variant of thymic epithelial neoplasm that may simulate carcinosarcoma. *Am J Surg Pathol.* 1997;21:1316-1323.
211. Levine GD, Rosai J. A spindle-cell variant of thymic carcinoid tumor: A clinical, histologic, and fine structural study with emphasis on its distinction from spindle-cell thymoma. *Arch Pathol Lab Med.* 1976;100:293-300.
212. Moran CA, Suster S. Spindle-cell neuroendocrine carcinomas of the thymus (spindle-cell thymic carcinoid): A clinicopathologic and immunohistochemical study of seven cases. *Mod Pathol.* 1999;12:587-591.
213. Moran CA, Suster S. Yolk sac tumors of the mediastinum with prominent spindle cell features: A clinicopathologic study of three cases. *Am J Surg Pathol.* 1997;21:1173-1177.
214. Moran CA, Suster S, Perino G, et al. Malignant smooth muscle tumors presenting as mediastinal soft tissue masses: A clinicopathologic study of 10 cases. *Cancer.* 1994;74:2251-2260.
215. Hisaoka M, Wei-Qi S, Jian W, et al. Specific but variable expression of H-caldesmon in leiomyosarcomas: An immunohistochemical reassessment of a new myogenic marker. *Appl Immunohistochem Molec Morphol.* 2001;9:302-308.
216. Gannon BR, O'Hara CD, Reid K, et al. Solitary fibrous tumor of the anterior mediastinum: A rare extrapleural neoplasm. *Tumori.* 2007;93:508-510.
217. Naito Y, Ishii G, Kawai O, et al. D2-40 positive solitary fibrous tumors of the pleura: Diagnostic pitfall of biopsy specimens. *Pathol Int.* 2007;57:618-621.
218. Kairouz S, Hashash J, Kabbara W, et al. Dendritic cell neoplasms: An overview. *Am J Hematol.* 2007;82:924-928.
219. Pileri SA, Grogan TM, Harris NL, et al. Tumours of histiocytes and accessory dendritic cells: An immunohistochemical approach to classification from the International Lymphoma Study Group based on 61 cases. *Histopathology.* 2002;41:1-29.
220. Xie Q, Chen L, Fu K, et al. Podoplanin (D2-40): A new immunohistochemical marker for reactive follicular dendritic cells and follicular dendritic cell sarcomas. *Int J Clin Exp Pathol.* 2008;1:276-284.
221. Vermi W, Lonardi S, Bosisio D, et al. Identification of CXCL13 as a new marker for follicular dendritic cell sarcoma. *J Pathol.* 2008;216:356-364.
222. Yang WI, Efird JT, Quintanilla-Martinez L, et al. Cell kinetic study of thymic epithelial tumors using PCNA (PC10) and Ki-67 (MIB-1) antibodies. *Hum Pathol.* 1996;27:70-76.
223. Pan CC, Ho DM, Chen WY, et al. Ki-67 labeling index correlates with stage and histology but not significantly with prognosis in thymoma. *Histopathology.* 1998;33:453-458.
224. Yang WI, Yang KM, Hong SW, et al. E-cadherin expression in thymomas. *Yonsei Med J.* 1998;39:37-44.
225. Pan CC, Ho DM, Chen WY, et al. Expression of E-cadherin and alpha- and beta-catenins in thymoma. *J Pathol.* 1998;184:207-211.

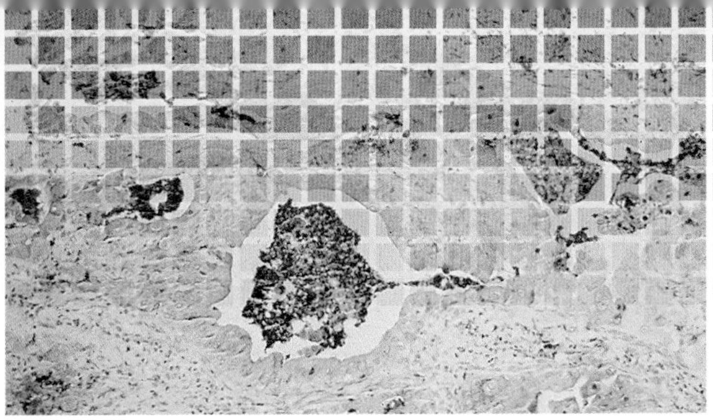

12

Immunohistology of Lung and Pleural Neoplasms

Samuel P. Hammar • Sanja Dacic

Introduction 369
Primary Lung Neoplasms 369
Primary Intrapulmonary Thymoma 397
Summary 452

INTRODUCTION

Immunohistochemistry is an effective, commonly used, adjuvant technique used to diagnose primary and metastatic neoplasms of the lung and pleura. Because of its relative ease of use and specificity, immunohistochemistry has largely replaced mucin histochemistry and electron microscopy in diagnosing pulmonary and pleural neoplasms. In some instances, electron microscopy is diagnostically superior to immunohistochemistry. In other cases, neither immunohistochemistry nor electron microscopy is specific for a given neoplasm. As described in this chapter, immunohistochemistry is now being used for therapeutic/prognostic reasons.

Since the time of the writing of the first edition of this book, significant new information has accumulated concerning the immunohistochemical features of lung and pleural neoplasms. As might be expected, specificities and sensitivities of some markers have changed; new and highly sensitive and specific markers have been developed; and markers thought to initially be restricted to certain neoplasms have been observed in neoplasms not thought to express such markers. Some antibodies are now being used to determine the degree of differentiation of a neoplasm and predictors of prognosis.[1-7]

For example, Pelosi and colleagues[6] evaluated fascin, an actin-bundling protein that induces cell membrane protrusions and increases the motility of normal and transformed epithelial cells for predicting lymph node metastases in typical and atypical carcinoids. The authors found that fascin immunoreactivity was closely correlated with occurrence of lymph node metastases in typical carcinoid and atypical carcinoid tumors. However, the authors found no correlation in high-grade neuroendocrine tumors of the lung. Fascin expression was also associated with an increased proliferative activity (Ki-67). Pelosi and associates[7] evaluated fascin immunoreactivity in stage I non–small cell lung cancer and concluded that fascin was up-regulated and that invasive and more aggressive non–small cell lung cancers were an independent, not a prognostic, predictor of unfavorable clinical course. The authors also suggested that targeting the fascin pathway could be used in a therapeutic sense.

Since the time of the writing of the second edition, the majority of immunohistochemical reports have dealt with diagnostic and therapeutic issues. We will discuss these issues later in this chapter.

An overview of immunohistochemistry titled *Immunohistochemistry: Then and Now* by Jaishree Jagirdar[8] is an excellent review of persons who have been involved in diagnostic immunohistochemistry from the beginning and those who are entering the discipline.

Most primary lung cancers can be diagnosed using histologic criteria alone, although immunohistochemical techniques are often employed to confirm or eliminate a pathologic diagnosis when lung neoplasms are poorly differentiated and clinical situations are complicated. In addition, many neoplasms of different primary origins are morphologically similar to primary lung and pleural neoplasms, and immunohistochemistry is an effective way to distinguish them from each other.

PRIMARY LUNG NEOPLASMS

A wide variety of primary neoplasms occur in the lung. Four major types make up 85% to 90% of primary lung neoplasms: adenocarcinoma, squamous cell carcinoma, small cell carcinoma, and large-cell undifferentiated carcinoma.[9] Adenocarcinoma is currently the most frequently diagnosed primary lung cancer in the United States[10,11] and usually occurs in a subpleural location, although occasionally is central or intrabronchial. Squamous cell carcinoma is the second most common primary lung cancer and occurs predominantly in a central distribution arising from mainstem and lobar bronchi.

Approximately 10% of primary pulmonary squamous cell carcinomas occur in the periphery of the lung. Small cell lung cancers occur in the central region of the lung arising from neuroendocrine cells in the mainstem bronchi and lobar bronchi, although up to 10% of small cell lung cancers occur in the periphery of the lung. Large cell undifferentiated carcinomas potentially may occur in any location in the lung and comprise approximately 8% to 10% of primary lung cancers.

Biology of Antigens and Antibodies

Several antibodies are useful in confirming or eliminating primary lung cancers. Those employed are dependent on the type of neoplasm suspected and the clinical situation encountered. A list of the antibodies commonly used in detecting, confirming, or eliminating primary lung carcinomas (excluding neuroendocrine carcinomas, which we will discussed later in the chapter) is shown in Table 12.1. A list of tumor-specific markers and their staining patterns are shown in Table 12.2.

ANTIBODIES USED TO DETECT NON-NEUROENDOCRINE LUNG NEOPLASMS

Keratins are a family of polypeptides that have been separated according to molecular weight and isoelectric point (acidic or basic). Twenty molecular species exist and have been catalogued by Moll and colleagues[12,13] CK7 is expressed in many pulmonary epithelial cells, although is found in a variety of other epithelial cells and in a variety of nonpulmonary carcinomas.[14] CK7 is the most commonly found molecular species of keratin in primary pulmonary adenocarcinoma. CK5 is found

TABLE 12.1 Antibodies Commonly Used to Evaluate Potential Lung Neoplasms*

Antibody Directed Against	Clone	Characteristics of Antigen	Immunogen	Manufacturer	Dilution	Type of Antigen Retrieval
Keratin	AE1/AE3	AE1—acidic subfamily 40,48,50, 56.5 kD AE3—basic subfamily 52, 56, 58, 59, 64, 65-67 kD	Human epidermal keratin	Dako	1:200	HIER
Keratin	5D3	CK8, CK18	Colorectal carcinoma cell line	BioGenex	1:100	HIER
Keratin	MAK6	CK8, CK14-CK16, CK18, CK19	Extracellular antigen from MCF-tissue culture and from human sole epidermis	Zymed	1:100	HIER
Keratin	35βH11	CK8—54 kD	Hep3B hepatocellular carcinoma line	Dako	1:50	HIER
Keratin	34βE12	Keratins—Moll numbers 1, 5, 10 and 14	Human stratum corneum keratin	Dako	1:100	HIER
CK5/6	D5/16B4	Intermediate filament CK5/CK6 and to slight degree CK4	Purified CK5	Biocare Medical	1:100	HIER
CK7	OV-TL 12/30	Moll CK7—54 kD	OTN 11 ovarian cell carcinoma line	Cell Marque	NA	HIER
CK20	Ks20.8	Moll CK20	Cytoskeletal protein from human duodenal mucosa	Cell Marque	NA	HIER
Vimentin	Vim 3B4	Intermediate filament—57 kD	Vimentin from bovine eye lens	Dako	1:100	HIER
Epithelial membrane antigen (EMA)	E29	Glycoprotein—250-400 kD	Delipidated extract of human milk fat	Ventana	NA	HIER
Human milk fat globule protein-2 (HMFG-2)	115D8	MAM-6 mucus glycoprotein > 400 kD	Purified human milk fat globule protein	BioGenex	1:25	HIER

TABLE 12.1 Antibodies Commonly Used to Evaluate Potential Lung Neoplasms—cont'd*

Polyclonal carcinoembryonic antigen (pCEA)	–	Antibody recognizes CEA and CEA-like proteins, including nonspecific cross-reacting substance and biliary glycoprotein	Human CEA isolated from metastatic colonic adenocarcinoma	Ventana	NA	HIER
CD15 (LeuM1)	C3D-1	3-fucosyl-N-acetyllactosamine	Purified neutrophils from normal human peripheral blood	Ventana	NA	HIER
Tumor-associated glycoprotein	B72.3	Glycoprotein in a variety of adenocarcinomas	Membrane-enriched fraction of metastatic breast carcinoma	Cell Marque	NA	HIER
Human epithelial antigen	VU-1D9	Glycoproteins of 34 and 49 kD on surface and in cytoplasm of all epithelial cells except squamous epithelium, hepatocytes, and parietal cells	MCF-7 cell line	Ventana	NA	HIER
Thyroid transcription factor-1 (TTF-1)	8G7G3/1	40-kD member of NKx2 family of homeodomain transcription factors	Mouse ascites	Cell Marque	NA	HIER
S-100 protein	–	S-100 protein A and B	S-100 protein isolated from cow brain	Dako	1:3,000	HIER
Surfactant apoprotein A (SP-A)	PE-10	Surfactant A	Surfactant apoproteins isolated from lung lavages of patients with alveolar proteinosis	Dako	1:100	HIER
CDX2	CDX2-88	Homeobox family of intestine-specific transcription factor regulates proliferation and differentiation of intestinal epithelial cells	Full length CDX2	BioGenex	NA	HIER
p63	4A4	Human p63 protein, a member of the p53 family	Mouse monoclonal antibody	Cell Marque	1:100	HIER
Fascin	55K-2	55-kD actin-bundling protein	Fascin purified from HeLa cells	Dako	1:1000	HIER

*Excludes neuroendocrine lung neoplasms.
HIER, heat-induced epitope retrieval.

predominantly in squamous cell carcinoma. When used diagnostically, CK7 is often used with CK20 and non-keratin antibodies in diagnosing and classifying glandular neoplasms. Most primary pulmonary carcinomas contain several molecular species of keratins, with the exception of small cell carcinoma, which typically contains low molecular weight keratins, including CK7.

Chu and colleagues[15] evaluated 435 epithelial neoplasms from various organs using immunohistochemistry with CK7 and CK20 antibodies. CK7 was seen in the majority of carcinoma cases, with the exception of carcinomas arising from the colon, prostate, kidney, and thymus; carcinoid tumors of the lung and gastrointestinal tract; and Merkel cell carcinomas of the skin. The majority of squamous cell carcinomas from various organs were CK7-negative, with the exception of cervical squamous cell carcinoma. CK20 was seen in almost all colorectal carcinomas and in Merkel cell carcinomas. CK20 expression was also observed in 62% of pancreatic carcinomas, 50% of gastric carcinomas,

TABLE 12.2 Tumor-Specific Markers and Their Staining Patterns

Marker	Tumor	Staining Pattern
Calretinin	Mesothelioma, sex cord–stromal, adrenocortical	Nuclear/cytoplasmic
CDX2	Colorectal/duodenal	Nuclear
D2-40	Mesothelioma, lymphatic endothelial cell marker	Membranous
ER/PR (estrogen receptor/progesterone receptor)	Breast, ovary, endometrium	Nuclear
GCDFP-15 (gross cystic disease fluid protein 15)	Breast	Cytoplasmic
HepPar-1 (hepatocyte paraffin)	Hepatocellular	Cytoplasmic
Inhibin	Sex cord–stromal, adrenocortical	Cytoplasmic
Mammaglobin	Breast	Cytoplasmic
Melan-A	Adrenocortical, melanoma	Cytoplasmic
Mesothelin	Mesothelioma	Cytoplasmic/membranous
PAP (prostate acid phosphatase)	Prostate	Cytoplasmic
PSA (prostate specific antigen)	Prostate	Cytoplasmic
RCC marker (renal cell carcinoma)	Renal	Membranous
Thyroglobulin	Thyroid	Cytoplasmic
TTF-1 (thyroid transcription factor-1)	Lung, thyroid	Nuclear
Uroplakin III	Urothelial	Membranous
Villin	Gastrointestinal (epithelia with brush border)	Apical
WT1	Ovarian serous, mesothelioma, Wilms' desmoplastic, small round cell	Nuclear

43% of cholangiocarcinomas, and 29% of transitional cell carcinomas. As shown in Table 12.3, CK7 expression was seen in 10 of 10 (100%) adenocarcinomas, 3 of 7 (43%) small cell lung carcinomas, 2 of 9 (22%) carcinoid tumors, and 0 of 15 (0%) squamous cell lung carcinomas. As shown in Table 12.4, CK20 expression was seen in 1 of 10 (10%) adenocarcinomas, 0 of 7 (0%) small cell lung carcinomas, 0 of 9 (0%) carcinoid tumors, and 0 of 15 (0%) squamous cell lung carcinomas. An update of CK7 and CK20 expression in various neoplasms is shown in Table 12.5.

Vimentin is a 58-kD intermediate filament found predominantly in mesenchymal cells. However, vimentin is expressed in most spindle cell carcinomas[16] and is reported by some to be expressed in a relatively high percentage of pulmonary adenocarcinomas.[17] Thyroid transcription factor-1 (TTF-1), a 38- to 40-kD transcription factor member of the NKx2 family of homeodomain transcription factors, is expressed in thyroid and pulmonary epithelial cells.[18,19] TTF-1 binds to and activates the promoters for Clara cell secretory protein and surfactant proteins A, B, and C.[20,21] As reported in the literature and as observed by this author (SPH), TTF-1 is expressed in the nuclei of 60% to 75% of pulmonary adenocarcinomas[22-25] and in most small cell lung cancers, atypical carcinoids, large cell neuroendocrine carcinomas, and approximately 35% of typical carcinoids.[26] Data concerning TTF-1 expression in various tumors are shown in Table 12.6.

Another member of the p53 family is p63, which is significant in the development of epithelial tissue and squamous cell carcinomas. p63 expression was evaluated in 408 cases of lung cancer by tissue microarray in two different laboratories by Au and associates.[27] Table 12.7 shows the results for p63 expression in lung carcinoma for both laboratories. As expected, the majority of squamous cell carcinomas expressed p63, as did a sizable number of large cell neuroendocrine carcinomas and small cell carcinomas. p63 expression was stated to be of prognostic significance in neuroendocrine carcinomas with high-grade tumors more likely to express p63 than low-grade tumors. From a practical point of view, this author uses p63 expression as a marker of squamous cell differentiation (Fig. 12.1).

Sheikh and coworkers[28] evaluated 33 cases of adenocarcinoma, 43 cases of benign lungs with fibrosis and metaplasia, 5 cases of atypical adenomatous hyperplasia, 5 cases of adenosquamous carcinoma, and 3 cases of squamous carcinomas for nuclear p63 expression by immunohistochemistry. The benign lung conditions included usual interstitial pneumonia, parenchymal scar, cryptogenic organizing pneumonia, and diffuse alveolar damage. In a normal lung, p63 was expressed in the reserve cells of large and small airways and occasional

TABLE 12.3 CK7 in Epithelial Neoplasms

Organ	Tumor Type	Total Cases	Positive Cases	% Positive
Lung	Adenocarcinoma	10	10	100
Ovary	Adenocarcinoma	24	24	100
Pancreas	Adenocarcinoma	13	12	92
Stomach	Adenocarcinoma	8	3	38
Colon	Adenocarcinoma	20	1	5
Prostate	Adenocarcinoma	18	0	0
Lung	Carcinoid tumor	9	2	22
Gastrointestinal tract	Carcinoid tumor	15	2	13
Kidney	Carcinoma	19	2	11
Liver	Cholangiocarcinoma	14	13	93
Adrenal	Cortical carcinoma	10	0	0
Breast	Ductal and lobular carcinoma	26	25	96
Uterus	Endometrial carcinoma	10	10	100
Soft tissue	Epithelioid sarcoma	12	0	0
Germ cell	Germ cell tumor	14	1	7
Liver	Hepatoma	11	1	9
Skin	Merkel cell tumor	9	0	0
Mesothelium	Mesothelioma, malignant	17	11	65
Lung, liver, small bowel	Neuroendocrine carcinoma	9	5	56
Lung	Small cell carcinoma	7	3	43
Cervix	Squamous cell carcinoma	15	13	87
Head and neck	Squamous cell carcinoma	30	8	27
Esophagus	Squamous cell carcinoma	14	3	21
Lung	Squamous cell carcinoma	15	0	0
Thymus	Thymoma	8	0	0
Bladder	Transitional cell carcinoma	24	21	88
Salivary gland	Tumors, all	9	9	100
Thyroid	Tumors, all	55	54	98

cells of distal lobular unit. In the fibrotic reactive processes, nuclear staining was observed in the basal cells of the airways and the bronchiolar and squamous metaplastic epithelium. p63 immunoreactivity was stated to be less uniformly expressed in acute lung injury. Strong reactivity was shown in 1 of 33 pulmonary adenocarcinomas and in most epithelial cells of 2 of 5 atypical adenomatous hyperplasias. Three pulmonary adenocarcinomas were stated to highlight only rare tumor cells. The authors concluded that their results highlighted the differential p63 expression across various bronchioloalveolar lesions and that p63 could be helpful in distinguishing reactive from neoplastic glandular proliferations in the lung.

A variety of epithelial cell markers (carcinoembryonic antigen [CEA], human milk fat globule protein-2 [HMFG-2], epithelial membrane antigen [EMA], LeuM1 [CD15], B72.3, BerEP4, and surfactant apoprotein) are expressed in primary lung carcinomas, predominantly pulmonary adenocarcinomas. Most are nonspecific and are frequently used in distinguishing epithelial mesothelioma from pulmonary and nonpulmonary adenocarcinoma (see the paragraphs that follow) and in evaluating metastatic adenocarcinoma of unknown primary origin (see Chapter 8).[29]

The immunohistogram of common non-neuroendocrine lung neoplasms is shown in Fig. 12.2. Additional immunohistochemical findings in lung neoplasms are listed in Table 12.8).[15,30-37] Table 12.9 shows an update on the differential expression of TTF-1, CK7, and CK20 in common primary and metastatic tumors of the lung.

Napsin-A (Nap-A) is an aspartic proteinase that is expressed in normal lung parenchymal type II pneumocytes, and in proximal and convoluted tubules of the kidney.[38] It is present in lysosomes of type II pneumocytes

TABLE 12.4 CK20 in Epithelial Neoplasms

Organ	Tumor Type	Total Cases	Positive Cases	% Positive
Colon	Adenocarcinoma	20	20	100
Pancreas	Adenocarcinoma	13	8	62
Stomach	Adenocarcinoma	8	4	50
Lung	Adenocarcinoma	10	1	10
Ovary	Adenocarcinoma	24	1	4
Prostate	Adenocarcinoma	18	0	0
Gastrointestinal tract	Carcinoid tumor	15	1	7
Lung	Carcinoid tumor	9	0	0
Kidney	Carcinoma	19	0	0
Liver	Cholangiocarcinoma	14	6	43
Adrenal	Cortical carcinoma	10	0	0
Uterus	Endometrial carcinoma	10	0	0
Soft tissue	Epithelioid sarcoma	12	0	0
Germ cell	Germ cell tumor	14	0	0
Liver	Hepatocellular carcinoma	11	1	9
Breast	Lobular and ductal carcinoma	26	0	0
Skin	Merkel cell tumor	9	7	78
Mesothelium	Mesothelioma, malignant	17	0	0
Lung, liver, small bowel	Neuroendocrine carcinoma	9	0	0
Lung	Small cell carcinoma	7	0	0
Head and neck	Squamous cell carcinoma	30	2	6
Cervix	Squamous cell carcinoma	15	0	0
Esophagus	Squamous cell carcinoma	14	0	0
Lung	Squamous cell carcinoma	15	0	0
Thymus	Thymoma	8	0	0
Bladder	Transitional cell carcinoma	24	7	29
Salivary gland	Tumors, all	9	0	0
Thyroid	Tumors, all	55	0	0

and alveolar macrophages, presumably secondary to phagocytosis, and to a lesser degree in pancreatic acini and ducts. Napsin is thought to be involved in the maturation of biologically active surfactant protein B peptide. Napsin-A is strongly expressed in the cytoplasm of up to 80% of primary lung adenocarcinomas studied using immunohistochemistry. Poorly differentiated cancers do not stain as well as well-differentiated cancers. Squamous cell carcinomas and small cell carcinomas of the lung are reported negative for Nap-A expression.[38]

Sainz and colleagues[39] studied the presence of Nap-A in 967 lung neoplasms. The authors[39] found that less than 5% of carcinomas of the bladder, pancreas, breast, liver, biliary tract, colon, ovary, uterus, lung squamous cell carcinoma, and lung small cell carcinoma were positive for Nap-A and that 74% of lung adenocarcinomas were positive for Nap-A versus 63% positive for TTF-1. Also, 11% of lung adenocarcinomas detected by Nap-A were missed by TTF-1 staining. The authors[39] concluded that Napsin A was a valuable marker for detecting lung adenocarcinomas versus other adenocarcinomas such as those from the breast, colon, biliary tract, pancreas, urinary bladder, and ovary. It was less useful in distinguishing primary pulmonary adenocarcinomas from thyroid carcinomas and renal carcinomas.

Neuroendocrine Lung Neoplasms

Small cell carcinoma (small cell lung cancer) is the most common neuroendocrine neoplasm of the lung.[40,41] The previously described subtypes (lymphocyte-like, intermediate-polygonal/fusiform) are currently lumped together as small cell lung cancer.[42] The entity referred to as *large cell–small cell carcinoma* has been eliminated.

TABLE 12.5 Carcinomatous Tumors

CK7+/CK20+	CK7+/CK20–		CK7-/CK20+	CK7–/CK20–	
Urothelial carcinoma uroplakin+ thrombomodulin+ p63+ CK5/6 (~1/2+)	*Breast carcinoma* ER/PR+ GCDFP+ mammaglobin+ CEA+	*Lung small cell carcinoma* (majority) TTF-1+ NE* markers+ p63– *Neuroendocrine markers, including synaptophysin, chromogranin, and CD56	*Colorectal adenocarcinoma* CDX2+ CEA+ MUC-2+ MUC5-AC–	*Prostate adenocarcinoma* PSA+ PAP+ CEA– uroplakin– thrombomodulin– p63– CK5/6–	*Nonseminoma GCTs** PLAP+ EMA– *Yolk sac tumor:* AFP+ *Embryonal CA:* OCT3/4+ CD30+ *Note: seminoma is keratin negative, OCT3/4 positive
Pancreatic adenocarcinoma (~2/3) CEA+ CA19-9+ MUC5-AC+ MUC-2– CDX2 (variable)	*Endometrial adenocarcinoma* vimentin+ ER/PR+ CEA–	*Mesothelioma* (~2/3) calretinin+ WT1+ CK5/6+ thrombomodulin+ D2-40+ mesothelin+ p63– CEA– MOC31– BerEP4– TTF-1–	*Merkel cell carcinoma* NE* markers+ *Neuroendocrine markers, including synaptophysin, chromogranin, and CD56	*Squamous cell carcinoma* p63+ CK5/6+ thrombomodulin+	*Mesothelioma* (~1/3)
Ovarian mucinous carcinoma MUC5-AC+ MUC-2– CDX2 (variable)	*Endocervical adenocarcinoma* CEA+ vimentin– ER/PR–	*Thyroid carcinoma* TTF-1+* thyroglobulin+* CEA–(except medullary CA) *Note: undifferentiated anaplastic thyroid carcinoma is often negative for TTF1 and thyroglobulin	*Gastric adenocarcinoma* (subset)	*Renal cell carcinoma* vimentin+ RCC marker+ CD10+ CEA–	*Lung small cell carcinoma* (minor subset)
Bladder adenocarcinoma thrombomodulin+ CDX2 (variable)	*Ovarian serous carcinoma* WT1+ ER/PR+ mesothelin+ CEA–	*Squamous cell carcinoma of cervix*		*Hepatocellular carcinoma* HepPar1+ pCEA+* CD10+* MOC31– CK19– *Note: characteristic canalicular pattern	*Gastric adenocarcinoma* (subset)
Gastric adenocarcinoma (subset)	*Lung adenocarcinoma* TTF-1+ CEA+ CK5/6- p63–	*Salivary gland tumor*		*Adrenocortical carcinoma* inhibin+ calretinin+ melanA+ vimentin+ CEA–	
Cholangiocarcinoma (minor subset)	*Cholangiocarcinoma* CEA+ CK19+	*Urothelial carcinoma* (subset)			
	MOC31+ CA19-9+ CDX2 (variable) HepPar1–	*Pancreatic and gastric adenocarcinoma* (subset)			

TABLE 12.6 Thyroid Transcription Factor-1 Expression In Tumors

Diagnosis	% Positive	Diagnosis	% Positive
Adenocarcinoma, bronchioloalveolar, mixed	91	Carcinoma, large cell, metastatic	63
		Carcinoma, large cell, neuroendocrine	46
Adenocarcinoma, bronchioloalveolar, mucinous	21	Carcinoma, large cell, not otherwise specified	20
Adenocarcinoma, bronchioloalveolar, nonmucinous	87	Carcinoma, oat cell, pulmonary	88
Adenocarcinoma, colorectal	2	Carcinoma, rhabdoid features, lung, nonrhabdoid component	56
Adenocarcinoma, colorectal, metastatic	4	Carcinoma, small cell, bladder	34
Adenocarcinoma, endometrial	6	Carcinoma, small cell, cervix	20
Adenocarcinoma, enteric differentiation, lung	70	Carcinoma, small cell, esophageal	34
		Carcinoma, small cell, gastrointestinal	17
Adenocarcinoma, lung and metastases	77	Carcinoma, small cell, metastatic to lung	50
Adenocarcinoma, mucinous, lung	73		
Adenocarcinoma, peritoneal, primary	8	Carcinoma, small cell, prostate	58
Adenocarcinoma, thyroid (note: anaplastic carcinomas of thyroid are less frequently positive)	100	Carcinoma, small cell, vaginal	34
		Carcinoma, squamous cell, lung	7
Alveolar adenoma	100	Carcinoma, undifferentiated type, metastatic	34
Carcinoid tumor, atypical, lung	100	Cystadenocarcinoma, ovarian	2
Carcinoid tumor, intestinal	2	Mesothelioma, all types	0
Carcinoid tumor, lung	57	Sarcoma, not otherwise specified	6
Carcinoid tumor, metastatic, lung primary	80	Sclerosing hemangioma of lung—cuboidal cells and polygonal cells	100
Carcinoid, atypical	26		
Carcinoid, not otherwise specified	24	Signet ring cell carcinoma, lung	85
Carcinoma, adenosquamous, lung	75	Synovial sarcoma	20

The World Health Organization (WHO) International Histologic Classification of Tumors defines small cell carcinoma as "a malignant epithelial tumor consisting of small cells with scant cytoplasm, ill-defined cell borders, finely granular nuclear chromatin, and absent or inconspicuous nucleoli. The cells are round, oval and spindle shaped, and nuclear molding is prominent. The mitotic count is high." A variant of small cell carcinoma is referred to as *combined small cell carcinoma* and is defined as "a small cell carcinoma combined with an additional component that consists of any of the histologic types of non–small cell carcinoma, usually adenocarcinoma, squamous cell carcinoma, or large cell carcinoma, but less commonly, spindle cell or giant cell carcinoma."

Other primary neuroendocrine neoplasms of the lung include typical carcinoid, atypical carcinoid, and large cell neuroendocrine carcinoma. The WHO definition of typical carcinoid is "a tumor with carcinoid morphology and less than 2 mitoses/10 high power field (2 mm^2) lacking necrosis and 0.5 cm or larger."

There has been significant confusion concerning the entity *atypical carcinoid,* and several different names applied to the entity. The designation *atypical carcinoid* was used by Arrigoni and associates[43] to describe a neuroendocrine lung neoplasm that differed from typical carcinoid. Atypical carcinoid has been referred to as *malignant carcinoid,*[44] *well-differentiated neuroendocrine carcinoma,*[45] *peripheral small cell carcinoma of lung resembling carcinoid tumor,*[46] and *Kulchitzky cell carcinoma II.*[47] The current *WHO International Histological Typing of Lung,* along with Travis and colleagues[48] describe atypical carcinoid as a tumor with neuroendocrine morphology with between 2 and 10 mitoses/10 high power fields (2 mm^2) and/or with foci of punctate necrosis, or both.

Additional reports have been published comparing typical and atypical pulmonary carcinoids.[49,50] A report by Thomas and colleagues[49] provides evidence that atypical pulmonary carcinoid tumors with regional lymph node metastasis have a high likelihood of developing recurrent disease if treated with surgical resection only and that patients have a significantly worse outcome than those who have typical carcinoids with thoracic lymph node involvement.

TABLE 12.7 p63 Expression in Lung Carcinoma

PhenoPath Laboratory Results					
Tumor Type	**Negative**	**Weak**	**Strong**	**Uninterpretable**	**% Positive**
Adenocarcinoma	56	14	10	13	30.0
Atypical carcinoid	18	4	4	5	30.8
Classic carcinoid	51	1	0	16	1.9
Large cell carcinoma	34	5	15	14	37.0
Large cell neuroendocrine carcinoma	4	3	1	3	50.0
Small cell carcinoma	3	5	5	1	76.9
Squamous cell carcinoma	3	1	93	26	96.9
GPEC Laboratory Results					
Tumor Type	**Negative**	**Weak**	**Strong**	**Uninterpretable**	**% Positive**
Adenocarcinoma	74	2	5	12	8.6
Atypical carcinoid	23	1	3	4	14.8
Classic carcinoid	57	0	1	10	1.7
Large cell carcinoma	42	3	10	13	23.6
Large cell neuroendocrine carcinoma	9	0	0	2	0
Small cell carcinoma	9	2	2	1	30.8
Squamous cell carcinoma	4	11	89	19	96.2

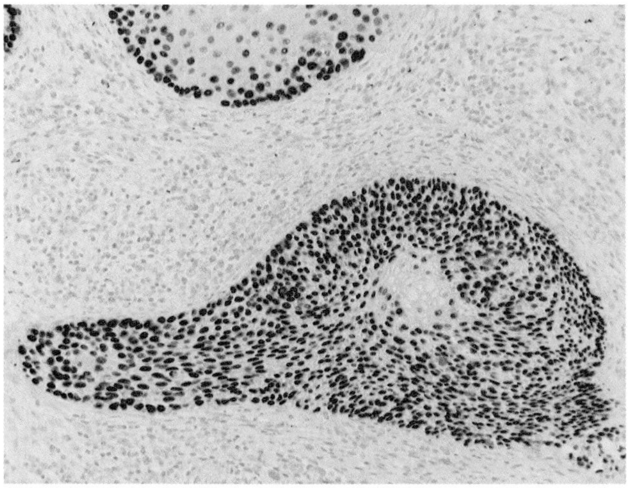

FIGURE 12.1 Nuclear p63 expression in a poorly differentiated squamous cell carcinoma of lung. X 100.

The existence of large cell neuroendocrine carcinoma of the lung was suggested by Gould and Chejfec[51] in 1978 and was further described by Hammond and Sause[52] in 1985, Neal and coworkers[53] in 1986, and Barbareschi and associates[54] in 1989. It is uncertain whether the neoplasms described by McDowell[55] in 1981 were large cell neuroendocrine carcinomas or non–small cell lung carcinomas showing neuroendocrine differentiation.

Travis and colleagues[56] reported on 35 neuroendocrine lung neoplasms in 1991, including 5 large cell neuroendocrine lung neoplasms. They included the following criteria for diagnosing a neoplasm as a large cell neuroendocrine carcinoma:

- A neuroendocrine appearance by light microscopy that included an organoid, trabecular, palisading, or rosette pattern
- Large cells with most cells greater than the nuclear diameter of three small resting lymphocytes
- A low nuclear to cytoplasmic ratio, polygonal-shaped cells, finely granular eosinophilic cytoplasm with an eosinophilic hue, coarse nuclear chromatin, and frequent nucleoli
- A mitotic rate greater than 10 mitoses per 10 high power fields
- Necrosis
- Neuroendocrine features by immunohistochemistry, electron microscopy, or both

The *WHO International Histological Classification of Tumors* describes a large cell neuroendocrine carcinoma as a "large cell carcinoma showing histologic features such as organoid, nesting, trabecular, rosette-like, and palisading patterns that suggest neuroendocrine differentiation in which the latter can be confirmed by immunohistochemistry or electron microscopy."

As published by this author in 1989,[57] there is a wide spectrum of differentiation for neuroendocrine lung neoplasms, and some do not fit into a well-defined category.

Additional data has been published on large cell neuroendocrine carcinoma.[58-64] These more recent articles continue to show that large cell neuroendocrine carcinoma of the lung is an aggressive neoplasm. The publication by Peng and colleagues[64] showed that the immunohistochemical features of large cell neuroendocrine

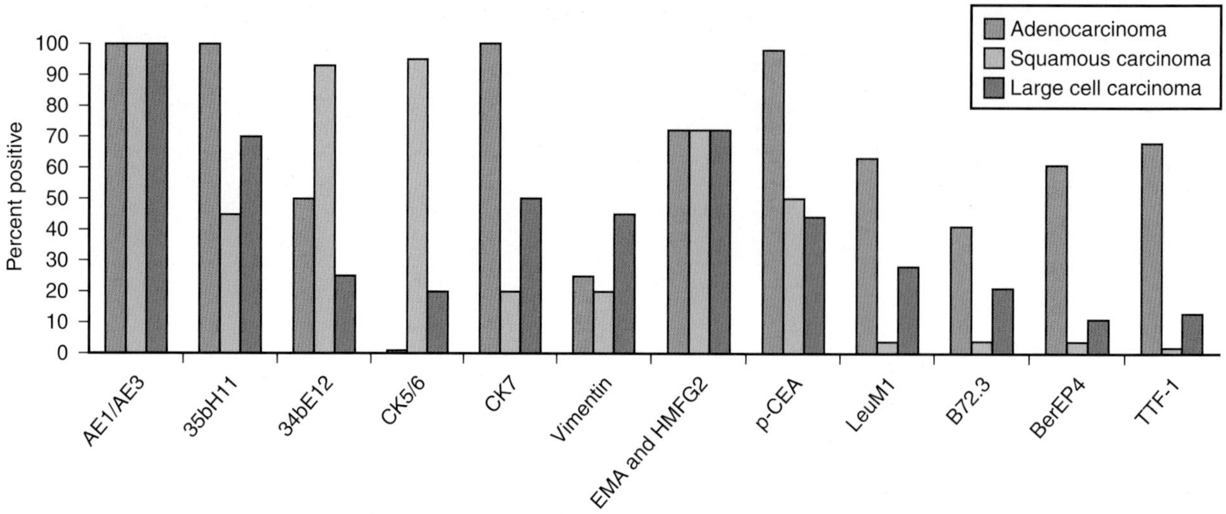

FIGURE 12.2 Immunohistogram of common primary pulmonary carcinomas, excluding small cell carcinoma.

carcinoma had a similar biological marker profile to small cell lung cancer and a different biological profile than large cell carcinoma with neuroendocrine features. However, there was a loss of heterozygosity at 3p in both large cell neuroendocrine carcinoma, large cell carcinoma with neuroendocrine features, and small cell lung cancer. The authors suggested that morphologic neuroendocrine differentiation might not be identical to biological neuroendocrine differentiation in large cell carcinomas of the lung.

ANTIBODIES USED TO DETECT NEUROENDOCRINE LUNG NEOPLASMS

Neuroendocrine cells occur in many organs and tissues in the body and are part of the diffuse neuroendocrine system, as described by Pearse[65] and the dispersed neuroendocrine system, described by Gould and DeLellis.[66] Not surprisingly, neuroendocrine cells and neoplasms formed by cells exhibiting neuroendocrine differentiation show similar immunohistochemical features. They contain a variety of biogenic amines, peptide hormones, and neurotransmitters that can be identified biochemically or immunohistochemically.[67] Immunohistochemical markers are useful in showing neuroendocrine differentiation by a neoplasm but are not usually specific. The antibodies commonly employed in demonstrating neuroendocrine differentiation are shown in Table 12.10.

Synaptophysin is a 38-kD glycoprotein component of pre-synaptic vesicles isolated from bovine neurons.[68,69] In this author's opinion, it is the most sensitive antibody for identifying neuroendocrine neoplasms. Synaptophysin has occasionally been observed in non-neuroendocrine, non–small cell lung carcinomas.

Chromogranins are a family of acidic proteins that contain high concentrations of glutamic acid located in the matrix of neuroendocrine granules in normal and neoplastic neuroendocrine cells.[70,71] In 1965 Chromogranin A was discovered in adrenal medullary cells by Banks and Helle.[72] Antibodies against chromogranin A are the most specific marker of normal and neoplastic neuroendocrine cells. Expression in a given neoplasm generally correlates with the number of cytoplasmic neuroendocrine granules visualized ultrastructurally.

Neuron-specific enolase (NSE) catalyzes the interconversion of 2-phosphoglycerate and phosphoenolpyruvate in the glycolytic pathway. Enolases are dimers composed of three subunits: alpha (α), beta (β) and gamma (γ). Neuron-specific enolase contains a high concentration of gamma enolase and is usually present in high concentrations in neurons and neuroendocrine cells. Unfortunately, neuron-specific enolase is not neuron or neuroendocrine cell specific. Neuron-specific enolase has been identified in a wide variety of non-neuron, non-neuroendocrine cells, including smooth muscle cells, myoepithelial cells, renal epithelial cells, plasma cells, and megakaryocytes.[73,74] Neuron-specific enolase is not uncommonly referred to as *non-specific enolase*. Despite its low specificity, it is a highly sensitive marker for neoplastic neuroendocrine cells.

Other neuroendocrine markers that are occasionally used to identify normal neuroendocrine lung cells and neoplastic neuroendocrine cells include neurofilaments,[75] neural cell adhesion molecules (N-CAM),[76,77] and Leu7.[78] The most frequent neuropeptides, neuroamines, and hormones found in neuroendocrine lung neoplasms are listed in Table 12.11. TTF-1 is found in a high percentage of small cell carcinomas, atypical carcinoids, and large cell neuroendocrine carcinomas, but in less than 50% of typical carcinoids.

Matsuki and colleagues[79] evaluated histidine decarboxylase, an enzyme of the amine precursor uptake and decarboxylation system known to be distributed in mast cells and enterochromaffin-like cells, with the hypothesis that this enzyme was a marker for neuroendocrine differentiation. The authors[79] found that the anti-histidine decarboxylase antibody stained most small cell lung cancers (18 of 23; sensitivity 0.78) and was rarely reactive with non-neuroendocrine lung tumors

TABLE 12.8 Expression of Keratins, TTF-1, and SP-A in Primary Pulmonary Neoplasms

Reference	Number of Cases Studied	Histologic Type of Lung Cancer	CK5	CK7	Cam5.2 CK8	CK20	TTF-1	SP-A
Chu P, et al. *Mod Pathol.* 2000;13: 962-972	10	Adenocarcinoma	Not done	10(100%)	Not done	1 (10%)	Not done	Not done
	15	Squamous cell carcinoma	Not done	0 (0%)	Not done	0 (0%)	Not done	Not done
	7	Small cell carcinoma	Not done	3 (43%)	Not done	0 (0%)	Not done	Not done
	9	Typical carcinoid	Not done	2 (22%)	Not done	0 (0%)	Not done	Not done
Amin, et al. *Am J Surg Pathol.* 2002;26: 358-364	15	Micropapillary adenocarcinoma	Not done	14 (93%)	Not done	2 (13%)	12 (80%)	Not done
Nakamura N, et al. *Mod Pathol.* 2002;15: 1058-1067	52	Adenocarcinoma	Not done	Not done	Not done	Not done	50 (96.2%)	38 (73.1%)
	19	Well differentiated	Not done	Not done	Not done	Not done	19 (100%)	17 (89.5%)
	29	Moderately differentiated	Not done	Not done	Not done	Not done	27 (93%)	18 (62%)
	4	Poorly differentiated	Not done	Not done	Not done	Not done	4 (100%)	2 (50%)
	26	Squamous cell carcinoma	Not done	Not done	Not done	Not done	0 (0%)	0 (0%)
	18	Small cell carcinoma	Not done	Not done	Not done	Not done	16 (88.9%)	0 (0%)
	8	Large cell undifferentiated	Not done	Not done	Not done	Not done	0 (0%)	0 (0%)
Lau SK, et al. *Mod Pathol.* 2002;15:538-542	67	Bronchioloalveolar:						
	48	Nonmucinous	Not done	46 (96%)	Not done	0 (0%)	36 (75%)	Not done
	12	Mucinous	Not done	10 (83%)	Not done	3 (25%)	0 (0%)	Not done
	7	Mixed	Not done	7 (100%)	Not done	0 (0%)	6 (86%)	Not done
Simsir A, et al. *Am J Clin Pathol.* 2004;121: 350-357	16	Bronchioloalveolar:						
	6	Mucinous	Not done	4 (67%)	Not done	4 (67%)	0 (0%)	Not done
	4	Nonmucinous	Not done	4 (100%)	Not done	0 (0%)	2 (50%)	Not done
	6	Mixed	Not done	6 (100%)	Not done	6 (100%) Focally +	5 (83%)	Not done
Johansson L. *Ann Diagn Pathol.* 2004;8:259-267	12	Squamous cell carcinoma	12 (100%)	3 (25%)	12 (100%)	0 (0%)	0 (0%)	Not done
	13	Small cell carcinoma	0 (0%)	13 (100%)	13 (100%)	0 (0%)	13 (100%)	Not done
	11	Adenocarcinoma	0 (0%)	11 (100%)	11 (100%)	0 (0%)	11 (100%)	Not done
	9	Large cell pleomorphic	0 (0%)	5 (55%)	9 (100%)	0 (0%)	5 (55%)	Not done

Continued

TABLE 12.8 Expression of Keratins, TTF-1, and SP-A in Primary Pulmonary Neoplasms—cont'd

Reference	Number of Cases Studied	Histologic Type of Lung Cancer	CK5	CK7	Cam5.2 CK8	CK20	TTF-1	SP-A
Yatabe Y, et al. *Am J Surg Pathol.* 2002;26:767-773	64	Adenocarcinoma	Not done	Not done	Not done	Not done	54 (84.4%)	41 (64.1%)
Chang Y, et al. *Lung Cancer.* 2004;44:149-157	99	Squamous carcinoma	Not done	Not done	Not done	Not done	4 (4%)	Not done
	176	Adenocarcinoma	Not done	Not done	Not done	Not done	169 (96%)	Not done
	12	Adenosquamous CA	Not done	Not done	Not done	Not done	12 (100%)	Not done
	0	Squamous cell carcinoma						
	36	Small cell carcinoma	Not done	Not done	Not done	Not done	19 (53%)	Not done
		Large cell undifferentiated	Not done	Not done	Not done	Not done	0 (0%)	Not done
	23	Pleomorphic						
	25	Lymphoepithelial-like						
	8	Typical carcinoid	Not done	Not done	Not done	Not done	0 (0%)	Not done
	3	Atypical carcinoid	Not done	Not done	Not done	Not done	0 (0%)	Not done
	44	Sclerosing hemangioendothelioma	Not done	Not done	Not done	Not done	39 (89%)	Not done
	1	Mesothelioma	Not done	Not done	Not done	Not done	0 (0%)	Not done
	1	Pseudomesothelioma	Not done	Not done	Not done	Not done	0 (0%)	Not done
	83	Metastatic* lung neoplasm	Not done	Not done	Not done	Not done	5	Not done
	125	Non-lung metastatic neoplasm	Not done	Not done	Not done	Not done	0 (0%)	Not done
Saad RS, et al. *Hum Pathol.* 2004;35:3-7	50	"Conventional" adenocarcinomas	Not done	Not done	Not done	Not done	30 (60%)	Not done
		Bronchioloalveolar:						
	32	Nonmucinous	Not done	Not done	Not done	Not done	20 (62.5%)	Not done
	18	Mucinous	Not done	Not done	Not done	Not done	4 (22.2%)	Not done

*Positive—all thyroid cancers.

TABLE 12.9 Differential Expression of TTF-1, CK7, and CK20 in Common Primary and Metastatic Lung Neoplasms

Diagnosis	TTF-1 %	CK7 %	CK20 %
TTF-1+CK7+CK20+ Bronchioloalveolar Carcinoma			
Adenocarcinoma, bronchioloalveolar, mixed	91	100	64
Adenocarcinoma, mucinous, lung	21	87	67
TTF-1+CK7+CK20– Tumors			
Adenocarcinoma, bronchioloalveolar, nonmucinous	87	99	4
Adenocarcinoma, enteric differentiation, lung	70	100	24
Adenocarcinoma, follicular, papillary thyroid	94	100	0
Adenocarcinoma, lung	77	97	9
Adenocarcinoma, lung, metastatic	77	98	9
Sclerosing hemangioma of lung	99	100	0
Signet ring cell carcinoma, lung	85	100	0
TTF-1–CK7+CK20+ Tumors			
Adenocarcinoma, ampullary	0	83	58
Adenocarcinoma, bronchioloalveolar, mucinous	21	98	83
Carcinoma, signet ring, stomach	0	69	35
Carcinoma, transitional cell, not otherwise specified	0	91	40
Cystadenocarcinoma, mucinous, ovarian, not otherwise specified	0	93	70
TTF-1+CK7–CK20– Tumors			
Carcinoma, oat cell, pulmonary	88	13	3
TTF-1–CK7+CK20–			
Adenocarcinoma, endometrial	6	95	5
Adenocarcinoma, gallbladder	0	94	28
Adenocarcinoma, gastric	1	70	45
Adenocarcinoma, metastatic	0	100	0
Adenocarcinoma, pancreas	0	94	43
Adenocarcinoma, peritoneal, primary	8	100	0
Carcinoma, breast	0	88	0
Carcinoma, breast, metastatic	0	88	2
Carcinoma, embryonal, not otherwise specified	0	79	0
Carcinoma, large cell, not otherwise specified	20	80	12
Carcinoma, signet ring, breast	0	100	4
Carcinoma, squamous cell, cervical	0	87	0
Cholangiocarcinoma	0	95	44
Cystadenocarcinoma, ovarian	2	97	16
Mesothelioma, malignant, localized	0	100	0
Mesothelioma, not otherwise specified	0	77	4
Mucoepidermoid carcinoma, lung	0	77	4
Neuroendocrine carcinoma, high grade, ampulla of Vater	0	88	38
Papillary cystadenocarcinoma, metastatic	0	100	0

TABLE 12.10 Antibodies Commonly Used to Identify Neuroendocrine Lung Neoplasms

Antibody Directed Against	Clone	Characteristics of Antigen	Immunogen	Manufacturer	Dilution	Type of Antigen Retrieval
Synaptophysin	–	38-kD membrane component of synaptic vesicles	Synthetic human synaptophysin coupled to ovalbumin	Dako	1:100	HIER
Chromogranin A	DAK-A3	439 amino acid protein encoded on chromosome 14 residing in neuroendocrine granules	C-terminal 20-kD fragment of chromogranin-A	Dako	1:100	HIER
Neuron-specific enolase	–	46-kD gamma-gamma isoenzyme of enolase	NSE isolated from human brain	Dako	1:400	HIER
Leu7 CD57	NK-1	110-kD human myeloid cell-associated surface glycoprotein	Antigen from human natural killer cells	BioGenex	1:20	HIER
Neural cell adhesion molecule (NCAM)	UJ13A	125-kD sialo glycoprotein	Sixteen-week-old fetal human brain homogenates	Dako	1:20	HIER
Thyroid transcription factor-1 (TTF-1)	8G7G3/1	40-kD member of NKx2 family of homeodomain transcription factors in lung and thyroid	Mouse ascites	Cell Marque	NA	HIER
CD117	–	145-kD band of transmembrane receptor	Rabbit	Dako	1:400	HIER
Ki-67	–	Ki-67 nuclear antigen in proliferating cells	Mouse monoclonal antibody	Ventana	NA	HIER

TABLE 12.11 Neuropeptides, Neuroamines, and Hormones Frequently Found in Neuroendocrine Lung Neoplasms

Adrenocorticotropic hormone (ACTH)
Arginine vasopressin
Bombesin
Calcitonin
Gastrin
Leu-enkephalin
Neurotensin
Serotonin
Somatostatin
Vasoactive intestinal polypeptide

(2 of 44; specificity 0.95). The authors ascertained that the reaction was similar to that obtained with CD56.[79] They noted that histidine decarboxylase was expressed in 6 of 12 large cell neuroendocrine carcinomas and 4 of 7 gastrointestinal small cell carcinomas. Matsuki and coworkers[79] concluded that histidine decarboxylase was useful for distinguishing small cell lung carcinoma from non-neuroendocrine lung carcinoma and for demonstrating neurendocrine differentiation.

The antibodies this author uses to evaluate lung neoplasms for neuroendocrine differentiation include low molecular weight keratin, high molecular weight keratin, synaptophysin, chromogranin A, TTF-1, and leukocyte common antigen. Carcinoembryonic antigen is occasionally expressed in neuroendocrine lung neoplasms,[80] and neuron-specific enolase is expressed in nearly all neuroendocrine lung neoplasms. In Figure 12.3, an immunohistogram shows characteristic immunohistochemical staining reactions in neuroendocrine lung neoplasms.

Small cell carcinomas make up about 20% to 25% of all primary lung cancers. They show immunostaining for low molecular weight keratins (CAM5.2, 35βH11), but not for high molecular weight keratins. Small cell carcinomas also show immunostaining for synaptophysin, neuron-specific enolase, and carcinoembryonic antigen (Fig. 12.4); variable staining for chromogranin A; and frequent nuclear immunostaining for thyroid TTF-1 (Fig. 12.5). The pattern of staining for low molecular weight keratin and chromogranin is usually punctate (Figs. 12.6 and 12.7). In our experience, many small cell lung cancers do not express chromogranin A, although

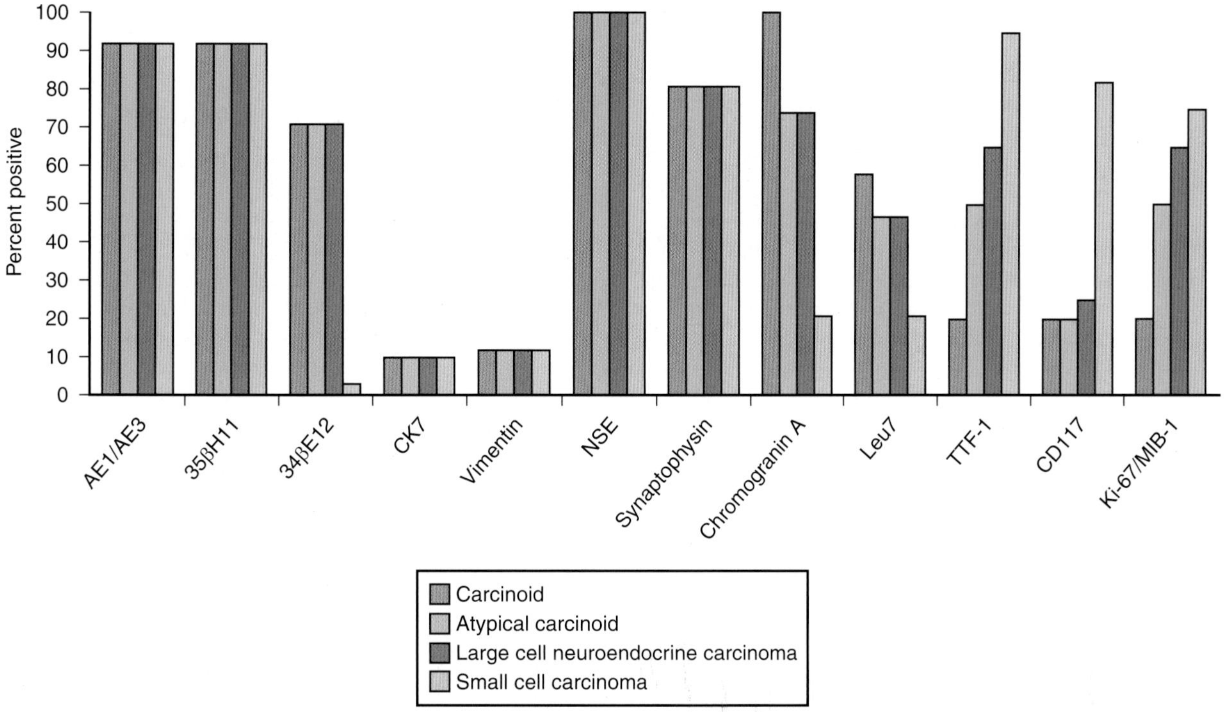

FIGURE 12.3 Immunohistogram of neuroendocrine lung carcinomas.

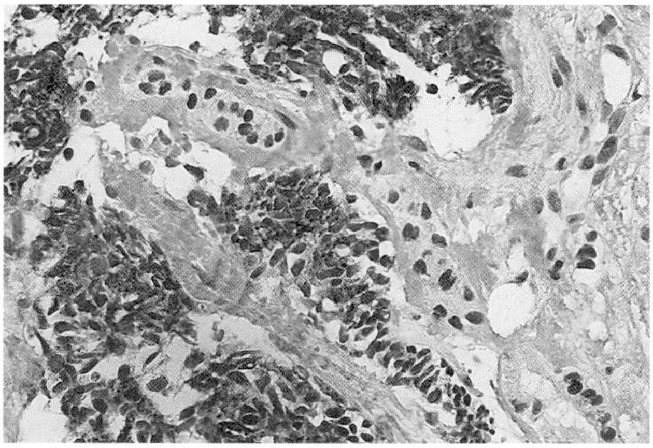

FIGURE 12.4 Many small cell lung carcinomas express carcinoembryonic antigen. X 200.

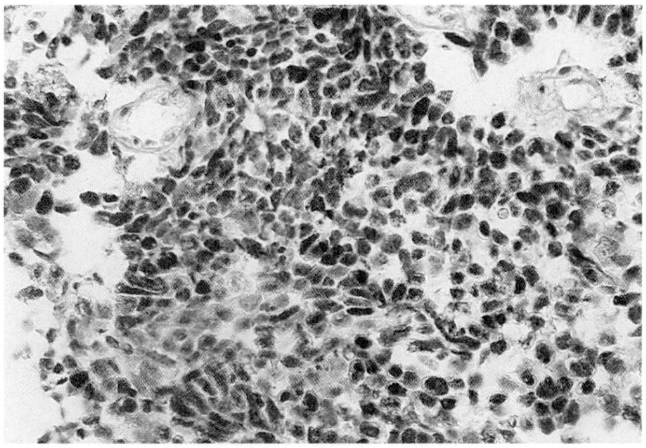

FIGURE 12.5 This small cell carcinoma of lung shows intense nuclear immunostaining for thyroid transcription factor-1. X 200.

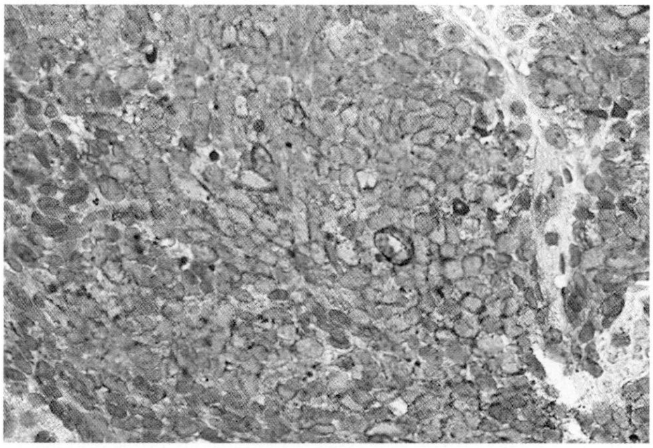

FIGURE 12.6 Most small cell carcinomas of lung show punctate immunostaining for low molecular weight keratin. X 400.

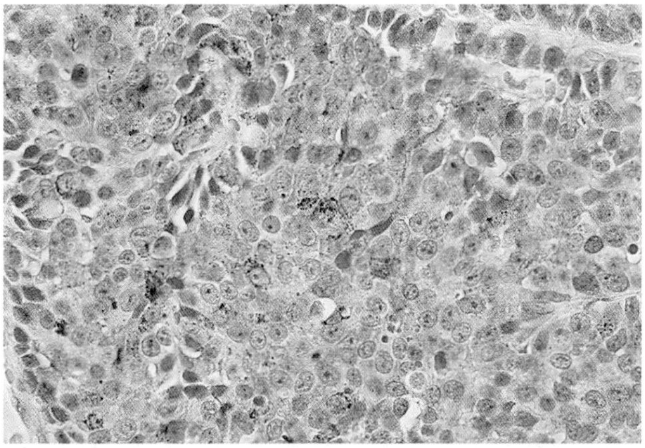

FIGURE 12.7 As shown in this photograph, the immunostaining pattern for chromogranin A in this small cell lung carcinoma is punctate. X 400.

expression is dependent upon how many neuroendocrine granules are in the cytoplasm of the neoplastic cells. When studied by electron microscopy, one can observe occasional small cell carcinomas whose tumor cells contain a moderate number of neuroendocrine granules (Fig. 12.8).

Typical carcinoids, atypical carcinoids, and large cell neuroendocrine carcinomas characteristically express low and high molecular weight keratins, synaptophysin, and chromogranin A. Atypical carcinoids and large cell neuroendocrine carcinomas frequently express TTF-1. Immunohistochemical tests can help identify these neoplasms as neuroendocrine, but they often cannot help separate specific neoplasms from one another. Chromogranin A shows the greatest staining intensity in typical carcinoids (Fig. 12.9), which correlates with their relatively frequent cytoplasmic neuroendocrine granules.

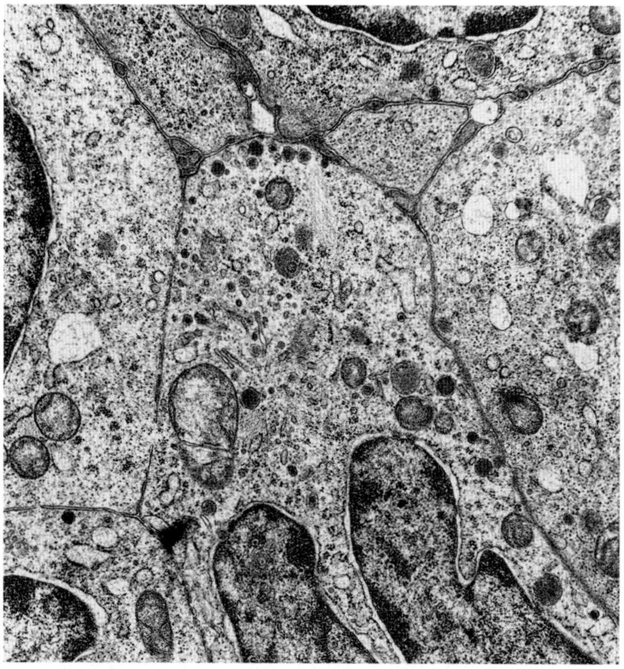

FIGURE 12.8 In this small cell carcinoma, the neoplastic cells contain a moderate number of cytoplasmic dense core neuroendocrine granules. X 16,000.

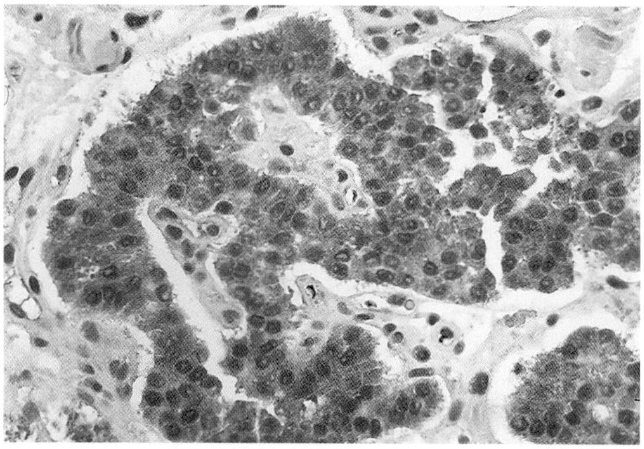

FIGURE 12.9 This typical carcinoid shows intense cytoplasmic immunostaining for chromogranin A. X 400.

Rare Primary Lung Neoplasms

Pathologists occasionally encounter a variety of rare primary lung neoplasms that may cause diagnostic confusion. None are frequent. Examples include sarcomatoid carcinoma (carcinosarcoma, spindle cell carcinoma), pulmonary blastoma, malignant hemangioendothelioma (intravascular bronchioloalveolar tumor [IVBAT], sarcoma, lymphoproliferative disorder—lymphoma, pulmonary Langerhans cell histiocytosis, Kaposi's sarcoma, clear cell neoplasm (sugar tumor, PEComa), rhabdoid tumor, sclerosing hemangioma, and inflammatory pseudotumor.[81]

SARCOMATOID CARCINOMA

Sarcomatoid carcinoma, also referred to as *carcinosarcoma, spindle cell carcinoma, blastoma,* and *teratocarcinoma*, are neoplasms of epithelial derivation that show variable differentiation. Sarcomatoid carcinoma has been reviewed conceptually by Wick and Swanson.[82] Several studies have evaluated sarcomatoid carcinoma by immunohistochemistry using keratin antibodies and/or electron microscopy. These studies concluded that the spindle cell component of the neoplasm was of epithelial derivation.[83-87] In most instances, the spindle cells coexpress keratin and vimentin (Figs. 12.10 and 12.11) or occasionally keratin and other intermediate filaments such as desmin or actin.

PLEOMORPHIC CARCINOMA

Pleomorphic carcinoma, as defined by Fishback and associates,[88] is a neoplasm that occurs predominantly in older patients and is composed predominantly of spindle cells and large pleomorphic giant cells. In 78 cases, the authors found foci of squamous differentiation in 8% of cases, large cell undifferentiated carcinoma in 25% of cases, and adenocarcinoma in 45% of cases. The remaining 22% of the neoplasms were composed of neoplastic

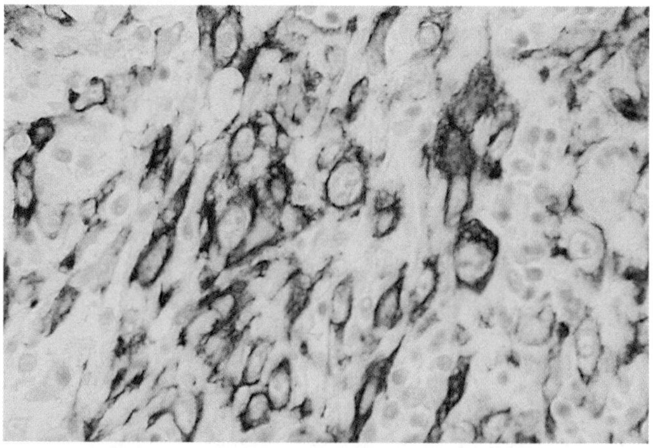

FIGURE 12.10 This region of sarcomatoid carcinoma shows immunostaining of the spindle cells for low molecular weight keratin. X 400.

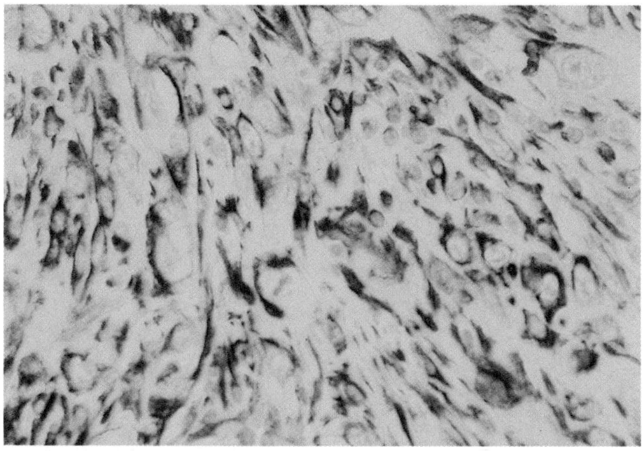

FIGURE 12.11 Same neoplasm shown in Figure 12.10. Neoplastic spindle cells show intense immunostaining for vimentin. X 400.

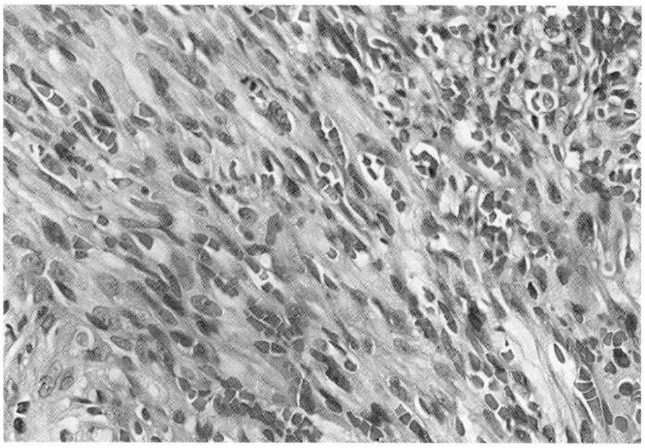

FIGURE 12.12 The neoplastic cells in Kaposi's sarcoma are spindle-shaped and are in a lymphatic distribution. X 400.

spindle cells and giant cells. The neoplastic spindle cells usually express only vimentin. The immunostaining pattern of the epithelial component of the neoplasm depends on what type of differentiation it shows.

Pelosi and colleagues[89] evaluated 31 cases of pleomorphic carcinomas of the lung that showed neoplastic epithelial cells and a spindle and/or giant cell component for cytokeratins, EMA, CEA, vimentin, S-100 protein, smooth muscle actin, desmin, cell cycle control and apoptosis (p53, p21Waf1, p27Kip1, FHIT), tumor growth (proliferative fraction assessed by Ki-67 antigen and microvascular density assessed by CD34 immunostaining), and tumor cell motility (fascin). The authors found that the epithelial component of these tumors was more immunoreactive for cytokeratins, EMA, CEA, cell cycle inhibitors, and tumor suppressor gene expression, whereas the sarcomatoid component (independent of tumor stage and size) was more immunoreactive for vimentin, fascin, and microvascular density. The authors suggested a model of tumorigenesis whereby the mesenchymal phenotype of the pleomorphic cells was likely induced by selective activation and segregation of several molecules involved in cell differentiation, cell cycle control, and tumor cell growth and motility.

PULMONARY BLASTOMA

Pulmonary blastomas are composed of an epithelial component (which forms glandular structures that often resemble endometrial glands or fetal glands) and a spindle cell component. The epithelial tumor cells occasionally form squamous morulae. As reported by Koss and colleagues[90] and Yousem and colleagues,[91] these neoplasms differentiate in divergent ways and occasionally show neuroendocrine differentiation. The epithelial cells form glands and immunostain for keratin, CEA, and EMA. The spindle cells express vimentin and, depending on the type of differentiation of the sarcomatoid component, desmin, actin, and S-100 protein. Those that contain neuroendocrine elements show markers of neuroendocrine cells. The epithelial component of pulmonary blastoma typically expresses beta-catenin.

PRIMARY SARCOMA

Primary sarcomas of the lung are rare, and a variety of them occur. The immunophenotype of the neoplastic cells that form such neoplasms is essentially identical to that of sarcomas that occur in soft tissue and other organs (see Chapter 4). Etienne-Mastroianni and associates[92] performed a clinicopathologic study of 12 cases of primary sarcomas of the lung. The histologic diagnosis of these 12 neoplasms was confirmed by detailed immunohistochemistry. There were 7 leiomyosarcomas, 2 monophasic synovial sarcomas, 1 peripheral nerve sheath tumor, 1 epithelioid sarcoma, and 1 malignant fibrous histiocytoma. Nine of the 12 patients had surgery; 3 pneumonectomies, and 6 lobectomies with further resection in 2 cases. Four patients received chemotherapy, and 2 patients had radiation therapy. Follow-up was available on all 12 patients. Survival ranged from 3 to 144 months, with a mean of 42 months. Long-term survival up to 3 years was observed in 5 patients. Overall 5-year survival rate was 38%. The authors concluded that primary sarcomas of the lung were rare and aggressive neoplasms, and that treatment and prognosis did not differ from that used for other soft tissue sarcomas.

KAPOSI'S SARCOMA

Kaposi's sarcoma is more common since the advent of acquired immunodeficiency syndrome (AIDS), and in most cases it is a metastatic neoplasm in the lung.[93-102] Kaposi's sarcoma follows lymphatic pathways in the lung and often involves lymph nodes. The neoplastic cells are spindle-shaped (Fig. 12.12) and immunostain for vimentin and endothelial cell markers such as CD31 (Fig. 12.13).

HEMANGIOENDOTHELIOMA

Malignant hemangioendothelioma, also referred to as *intravascular bronchioloalveolar tumor (IVBAT)*, usually occurs in relatively young women, is bilateral, and takes the form of multiple small nodules that fill alveolar spaces and undergo degeneration, necrosis, and

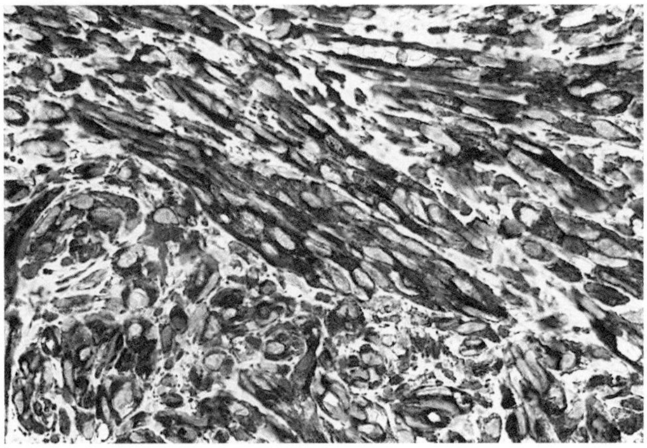

FIGURE 12.13 Kaposi's sarcoma tumor cells express vascular markers such as CD31. X 400.

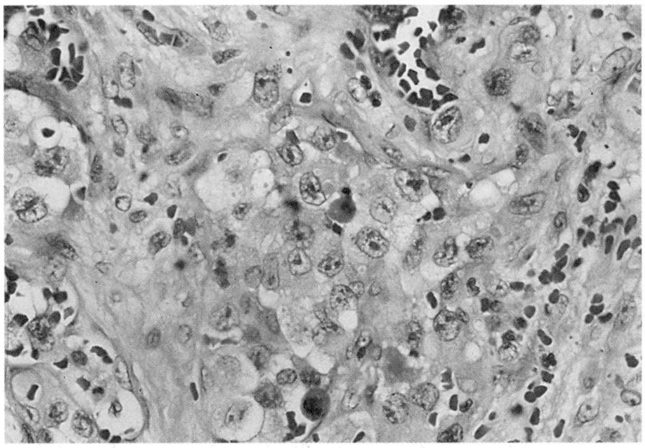

FIGURE 12.14 In this malignant epithelioid hemangioendothelioma, the neoplastic cells have an epithelial appearance and can be confused with carcinomas. X 400.

calcification.[81] This neoplasm was initially thought to be of alveolar cell origin. Histologically, the tumor cells are round or polygonal and have an epithelial appearance (Fig. 12.14). They characteristically express endothelial markers such as CD31, CD34, and factor VIII antigen, and they immunostain for vimentin. Rarely, epithelioid hemangioendotheliomas express keratin (Fig. 12.15). Ultrastructurally, the neoplastic cells often contain Weibel-Palade bodies, which are pathognomonic markers of endothelial cells (Fig. 12.16).

ANGIOSARCOMA

Primary angiocarcinomas are rare and can be de-differentiated without forming obvious vascular channels. The neoplastic cells usually show the same immunohistochemical profile as malignant hemangioendotheliomas. Adem and coworkers[103] reported on 7 patients with metastatic angiosarcoma that masqueraded as diffuse pulmonary hemorrhage. Of the 7 patients ranging in age between 31 and 73 years, 6 were men and 1 was a woman. Six patients presented with hemoptysis, and all had diffuse abnormalities on radiographic studies.

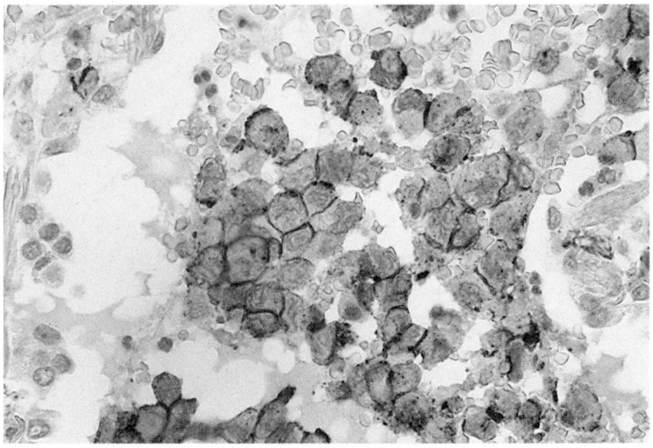

FIGURE 12.15 Occasional neoplastic epithelioid hemangioendothelioma cells show cytoplasmic immunostaining for keratin. X 400.

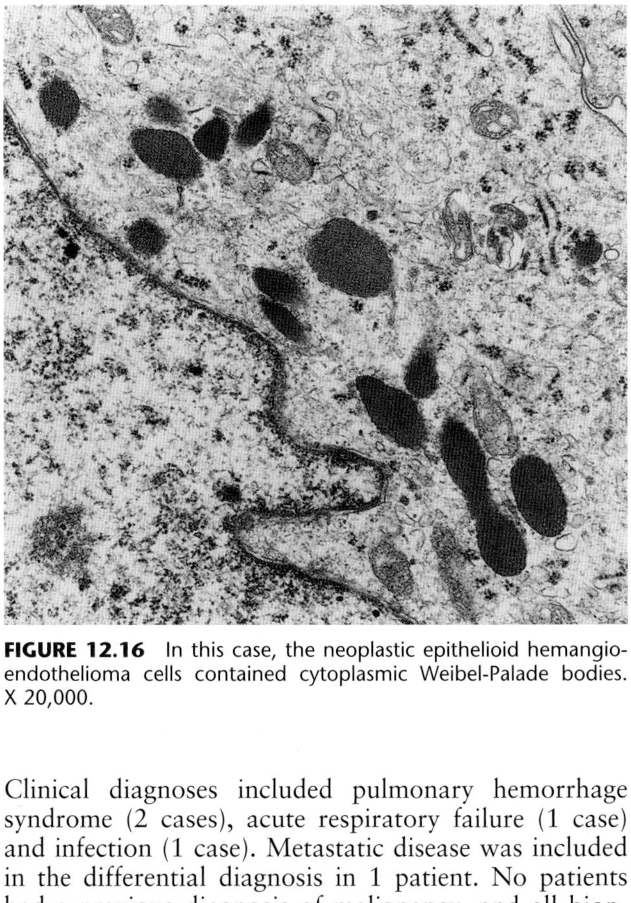

FIGURE 12.16 In this case, the neoplastic epithelioid hemangioendothelioma cells contained cytoplasmic Weibel-Palade bodies. X 20,000.

Clinical diagnoses included pulmonary hemorrhage syndrome (2 cases), acute respiratory failure (1 case) and infection (1 case). Metastatic disease was included in the differential diagnosis in 1 patient. No patients had a previous diagnosis of malignancy, and all biopsies showed hemorrhage associated with atypical epithelioid and spindle cells forming anastomosing vascular channels distributed along and within lymphatics and arteries. The neoplastic cells were stated to be immunoreactive for factor VIII–related protein and CD31. Three patients with complete follow-up died of their disease, and three patients underwent autopsy examination in which primary sites outside of the lung were identified. Two angiosarcomas arose in the heart, and one arose in the pelvic soft tissue. One patient likely had a primary site in the right atrium identified by cardiac ultrasound. The authors concluded that angiosarcoma should be

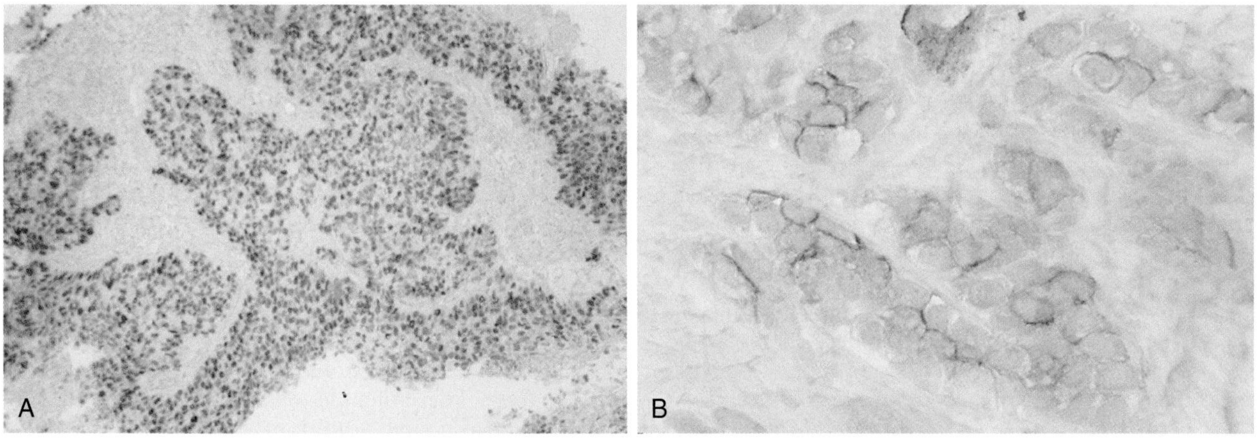

FIGURE 12.17 Angiosarcoma, lung—**(A)** H&E; **(B)** CD31 immunostain.

included in the differential diagnosis of diffuse hemorrhage, especially in young adults. The authors observed a similar case in which the cells had a much more epithelioid morphology and presented as multiple nodules in the lung, although no primary tumor was identified (Fig. 12.17).

Lymphoproliferative Disorders of the Lung

A variety of non-neoplastic and neoplastic lymphoproliferative disorders involve the lung (see Chapters 5 and 6). There has been a significant evolution with respect to classification of lymphoproliferative lung lesions as sophisticated molecular biology and genetic studies have become available. Conditions thought to be non-neoplastic several years ago have now been shown to be low-grade lymphomas.

BRONCHIAL-ASSOCIATED LYMPHOID TISSUE

Bronchial-associated lymphoid tissue (BALT) is inconspicuous or absent in most normal adult human lung tissue. There is debate as to whether bronchial-associated lymphoid tissue is seen in normal human adult lungs.[104] Exogenous or endogenous antigenic stimulation of a variety of types causes lymphoid tissue to appear in human lung tissue, and it usually occurs in a fairly distinct anatomic location (i.e., in association with bronchi and bronchioles). It is referred to as *bronchial associated lymphoid tissue (BALT)*. In non-smoking adults, lymphoid tissue is seldom seen in lung tissue and, when present, occurs as small aggregates usually found at bronchial divisions and adjacent to respiratory bronchioles. In smokers, there is a significant increase in BALT with occasional large lymphoid follicles, some of which have germinal centers.[105] As recently reviewed by Swigris and colleagues, BALT is part of a larger system referred to as *mucosal associated lymphoid tissue (MALT)*, is uncommonly seen in the normal adult lung, and is commonly seen in other mammals such as rats, rabbits, and sheep. The lymphoid tissue is usually poorly organized and consists of aggregates of lymphocytes around small bronchi and at bronchial divisions. Some lymphocytes reside in the bronchial epithelium between the epithelial cells. It is thought that lymphoid cells populate these areas by cell surface homing receptors such as integrins contacting specific intrapulmonary vascular adhesion molecules, such as those seen in post capillary vascular endothelial cells. Approximately 60% of BALT is composed of B cells, and the remaining percentage is composed of T cells. It is thought that BALT plays an essential role in the prevention of infection of inhaled microorganisms and is a site for lymphoid differentiation where lymphocytes come in contact with inhaled antigens to become antigen-specific memory or immune effector cells. When primed by an antigen, it is thought that these cells circulate throughout the BALT and remaining lung parenchyma and are ready to react to antigen exposure. Other cells such as dendritic macrophages (Langerhans cells) are involved in the immunologic response. The respiratory epithelium overlying the BALT usually contains relatively few goblet cells and ciliated cells. The BALT-associated epithelial cells are surfaced by microvilli. The epithelium is infiltrated by predominantly CD8-positive and occasionally CD4-positive lymphocytes. According to Swigris and associates,[106] BALT does not express the secretory component of IgA and differs from other mucosal-associated lymphoid tissue such as that seen in the GI tract. Bienenstock and colleagues[107,108] were first to provide information on the morphologic and functional characteristics of BALT.

The majority of non-neoplastic and neoplastic lymphoid infiltrates in the lung are related to BALT. In neoplasia, BALT proliferations can explain most neoplastic pulmonary lymphoid diseases. As stated earlier in the chapter, pathologists may encounter difficulty in distinguishing between neoplastic and non-neoplastic lymphoid lesions. In many instances, molecular biology techniques such as flow cytometry are necessary to prove malignancy.[109,110]

A variety of recognizable benign conditions of the lung are associated with lymphoid infiltrates that seem haphazardly oriented. These include usual interstitial pneumonia; desquamative interstitial pneumonia; collagen vascular associated lung disease; the cellular phase of non-specific interstitial pneumonia; hypersensitivity pneumonitis; the early phase of sarcoidosis; Wegener granulomatosis; Churg-Strauss granulomatosis; microscopic polyarteritis nodosa; and infiltrates associated with certain drugs such as sulfasalazine. Detailed information concerning most lymphoproliferative diseases of the lung is provided in references 111 to 116.

Most pulmonary lymphoid lesions represent hyperplasias of BALT and neoplastic lymphoproliferative disorders arising from BALT. Kradin and Mark[117] were the first to discard the terms *pseudolymphoma* and *lymphoid interstitial pneumonitis* and replace them with *nodular* and *diffuse hyperplasias of BALT*. As discussed in detail by Koss,[116] localized hyperplasias of BALT (also called *follicular bronchitis/bronchiolitis*) are due to a proliferation of BALT in the region of small bronchi and bronchioles. Lymphoid hyperplasias are seen in a number of clinical conditions including chronic infections, congenital immune deficiency syndromes, obstructive pneumonias, and collagen vascular diseases. Pathologically, they are characterized by collections of lymphoid nodules with or without germinal centers in a peribronchial/peribronchiolar distribution.

Nodular lymphoid hyperplasia BALT has replaced the term *pseudolymphoma* and is characterized by reactive lymphoid proliferation that characteristically shows numerous lymphoid follicles with large germinal centers usually occurring in middle-aged people, most of whom are asymptomatic. Approximately 10% to 15% of patients have a collagen vascular disease such as systemic lupus erythematosus or an immune disease of uncertain etiology, and they frequently exhibit polyclonal gammopathy. Polytypic plasma cells are common. Marker studies show a mixed population of CD4- and CD8-positive T cells. Most cases occur as solitary nodules and reoccur in up to 15% of surgically excised cases.

LYMPHOCYTIC INTERSTITIAL PNEUMONIA-PNEUMONITIS

Lymphocytic interstitial pneumonia-pneumonitis (LIP) is thought to be a diffuse hyperplasia of the bronchial-associated lymphoid tissue.[118] It is thought to be a response to a variety of stimuli, including a wide spectrum of autoimmune diseases; systemic immunodeficiency states; allogenic bone marrow transplantation; pulmonary alveolar microlithiasis; uncommon infections such as Legionella pneumonia, tuberculosis, mycoplasma and Chlamydia; dilantin use; and pulmonary alveolar proteinosis. Most patients are women between 40 and 70 years of age. They may present with a variety of symptoms such as fever, hemoptysis, arthralgias, weight loss, and pleuritic chest pain. Some have Sjogren syndrome or myasthenia gravis. Chest radiographs usually show a diffuse reticular or reticulonodular infiltrate with occasionally nodular lesions. Some patients have hypergammaglobulinemia, and about 10% of adult patients have hypogammoglobulinemia. If LIP patients have a monoclonal gammopathy, it is usually due to a coexistent lymphoma. A significant number of patients with LIP respond to steroids, although about 30% to 50% die within five years, frequently from infectious complications and some as a result of treatment. Some patients develop lymphoma and immunoblastic sarcomas.

NODULAR LYMPHOID INFILTRATES OF UNCERTAIN NATURE

Nodular lymphoid lesions of uncertain etiology exist in the lung. These include plasma cell granulomas, pulmonary hyalinizing granulomas, and benign lymphocytic angiitis and granulomatosis (BLAG). Plasma cell granuloma, also referred to as *myofibroblastic tumors* or *inflammatory pseudotumors,* occur predominantly in younger patients and have been observed in a wide variety of organs and tissues, including trachea, thyroid, heart, stomach, liver, pancreas, spleen, lymph nodes, kidney, retroperitoneum, mesentery, bladder, pelvic soft tissue, breast, spinal cord meninges, and orbit.[81] The term *granuloma* may be somewhat misleading unless one realizes this term has been used loosely to describe inflammatory tissue similar to that observed in Wegener granulomatosis and lymphomatoid granulomatosis. Histologically, an inflammatory infiltrate composed predominantly of plasma cells and a proliferation of myofibroblasts comprises these nodules. Some studies suggest plasma cell granulomas are neoplastic. Inflammatory pseudotumors are discussed in some detail in the following paragraphs.

Pulmonary hyalinizing granuloma occurs most frequently as single or occasionally multiple nodules. Some individuals are asymptomatic, and others have cough, shortness of breath, chest pain, or weight loss. The dominant histological finding is one of dense lamellar collagen bundles that are oriented parallel to one another and an associated lymphoid infiltrate frequently in a bronchial distribution.

Benign lymphocytic angiitis and granulomatosis was described in 1977 by Saldana and colleagues[119] and by Israel and associates.[120] This entity was described as being less common than Wegener granulomatosis and lymphomatoid granulomatosis. Most patients are middle-aged, and in most instances they have multiple nodular pulmonary lesions. Histologically, the nodules are composed of a dense lymphoid infiltrate with occasional giant cells, including multinucleated histiocytic giant cells (but without well-defined granuloma formation). Lymphoid infiltrates around arteries and veins are frequent, and lymphocytes invade vessel walls and occasionally produce occlusion of vascular lumina. Differential diagnoses include lymphocytic lymphoma and lymphomatoid granulomatosis when the lesions are multiple.

LYMPHOMAS OF THE LUNG

Few neoplasms have received as much emphasis on classification and subtyping as lymphoma. Histology/cytology, immunohistochemistry, flow cystometry, and other molecular biology techniques have been extensively employed for the classification of lymphoma. The proper handling and recommendations for classification and reporting of lymphoid neoplasms was published in 2002.[121] Immunohistochemical criteria for diagnosing such neoplasms was reported in detail in 2001.[122]

PULMONARY NON-HODGKIN LYMPHOMA

Most non-Hodgkin lymphomas that occur in the lung are low-grade B-cell lymphomas, and it is thought that they are derived from BALT. As mentioned earlier in the chapter, there can be considerable difficulty in differentiating a low-grade B-cell lymphoma from a non-neoplastic process. Routine immunohistochemical markers such as kappa and lambda light chains are of occasional value in separating neoplastic from non-neoplastic processes. Flow cyometric analysis and PCR should be employed to evaluate most cases. Low-grade B-cell lymphomas clinically are associated with a good prognosis.

T-cell lymphomas occur in the lung but are much less common than B-cell lymphomas.[123] Occasional primary lymphomas in the lung show prominent plasma cell differentiation.[124] The predominant criteria for diagnosing primary non-Hodgkin lymphoma of the lung are: 1) involvement of the lung or a lobar or mainstem bronchus, either unilaterally or bilaterally with or without mediastinal lymph node involvement; and 2) no evidence of extra-thoracic lymphoma at the time of diagnosis or for three months afterwards.[125] Patients with primary non-Hodgkin lymphoma of the lung are usually older than 60 years of age, and 50% of them are asymptomatic. Most patients have an abnormal chest radiograph. Symptomatic patients usually have B-symptoms consisting of fever, night sweats, and weight loss, and they occasionally experience dyspnea on exertion, cough, and chest pain. A significant number of patients with non-Hodgkin lymphoma of the lung have associated von Willebrand syndrome, erythema nodosum, or Sjogren syndrome.

Primary lymphomas of the lung comprise less than 1% of all primary pulmonary neoplasms. Small cell lymphomas comprise about 80 to 90% of all primary pulmonary lymphomas with marginal zone B-cell lymphoma representing over 90% of cases.

MARGINAL ZONE B-CELL LYMPHOMA OF MALT TYPE

Marginal zone B-cell lymphoma of MALT type (MZBCL/MALT) is a low-grade extranodal lymphoma composed of small B lymphoid cells with phenotypic features of marginal zone B lymphocytes. MZBCL/MALT occurs mostly in adult patients, although it may occur in children, particularly those infected with HIV. Although most MALT lymphomas are suspected to arise as a result of chronic antigenic stimulation such as that caused by *Helicobacter pylori* in cases of gastric MALT lymphoma, no specific etiologic agent has been found for MZBCL/MALTs in the lung. Most patients present with nonspecific pulmonary complaints and have a mass less than 5 cm in diameter or multiple masses. Hilar lymphadenopathy is almost always absent. A subset of patients may have a synchronous lymphoma of MALT type at another anatomic location in the body. The larger neoplasms are composed of small lymphocytes that show peripheral tracking along lymphatic pathways. Bronchial infiltration is often associated with the formation of lymphoepithelial lesions. Reactive germinal centers are frequently seen within the neoplasm adjacent to the bronchovascular structures or at the periphery. The neoplastic population replaces the expanded marginal zones of the germinal centers. Cytologically, the predominant cells are small lymphocytes that are usually round or may be lymphoplasmacytic. Some cells may have clear cytoplasm and may be referred to as *monocytoid cells.* Scattered plasma cells may be present. The lymphocytes of marginal zone lymphoma characteristically express pan B-cell markers such as CD20, PAX5, and CD79a (Table 12.12). They are typically negative for CD5, CD10, CD23, BCL6, and BCL1/cyclin D1. CD43 is expressed in up to 50% of lymphocytes, and nuclear expression of BCL10 may exist. Light chain restriction can be seen in plasma cells in about 25% of cases.

CHRONIC LYMPHOCYTIC LEUKEMIA–SMALL CELL LYMPHOCYTIC LYMPHOMA

Lung involvement in chronic lymphocytic leukemia–small cell lymphocytic lymphoma (CLL-SLL) usually occurs in patients with a long-standing history of CLL-SLL. In most cases, a biopsy is not necessary since the diagnosis can often be made on clinical grounds. Patients often present with progressive shortness of breath and cough and have interstitial infiltrates in chest radiographs. Some patients have endobronchial obstructions. Most patients are over 50, and the male-to-female ratio is usually 2:1. Histologically, the condition is characterized by a dense lymphoid infiltrate that follows bronchovascular bundles and/or is in a bronchiocentric distribution with a relative sparing of the remainder of the lung. The infiltrate is composed predominantly of a population of small, round lymphocytes with a mature chromatin pattern. Sometimes larger neoplastic cells are present, which would suggest a composite diffuse large B-cell lymphoma if there are larger cells present in sheets. The cells of CLL-SLL are B lymphocytes expressing B-cell marker CD20, PAX5 and CD79a (see Table 12.12). They often show coexpression of CD5, CD43, CD23, and BCL2. They are negative for CD10, BCL6, BCL1, and cyclin D1. Ki-67 is usually low (in the neighborhood of 10% to 20%). Molecular studies may show clonality of the immunoglobulin heavy or light chains. The cells frequently have abnormal karyotypes.

MANTLE CELL LYMPHOMA

The lung is an unusual site of involvement of mantle cell lymphoma, even in cases of advanced disease. The lymphoma is characterized by a monomorphic population of small- to intermediate-sized lymphoid cells with mild to marked irregular nuclei and relatively mature chromatin pattern without prominent nucleoli. There

TABLE 12.12 Immunohistochemical Features of Primary Lymphomas of Lung

	Antibody Directed Against													
Type of Lymphoma	CD20	PAX5	CD79a	CD43	CD5	CD10	CD23	CD15	CD30	Cyclin D1	BCL-2	BCL10	EBV	Monoclonal Light Chain
Marginal zone B-cell	+	+	+	S	N	N	N	N	N	N	N	S	N	S
Chronic lymphocytic leukemia/small cell lymphocytic lymphoma	+	+	+	S	S	N	N	N	N	+	S	N	N	S
Mantle cell lymphoma	+	+	+	S	S	N	N	N	N	S	S	N	N	S
Follicular lymphoma	+	+	+	N	N	S	N	N	N	N	S	N	N	S
Hodgkin lymphoma	S	S	S	N	N	N	N	S	S	N	S	N	S	N
Lymphomatoid granulomatosis	S	U	U	N	N	N	N	N	N	N	N	U	S	N
Intravascular lymphoma	+	+	+	R	S	U	N	N	N	N	S	U	U	U
Primary effusion lymphoma	N	N	N	S	N	N	N	N	S	U	U	U	S	N
Pyothorax-associated lymphoma	+	+	+	S	N	N	N	N	N	U	U	U	S	N

Reactivity:
+, almost always diffuse, strong positivity
S, sometimes positive
R, rare cells positive
N, almost always negative
U, uncertain

are occasional epithelioid macrophages associated with neoplastic lymphoid cells, but they do not aggregate into granulomas. There is a blastoid subtype in which about 10% of cases have a fine chromatin pattern resembling a lymphoblastic lymphoma. The neoplastic cells are similar to other small B-cell lymphomas in that they express pan B-cell marker CD20, PAX5, and CD79a (see Table 12.12). They also usually express CD5, CD43, BCL2, BCL1, and cyclin D1. They are negative for CD10, CD23, and BCL6. Ki-67 studies usually show reactivity in about 20% to 50% of the cells. A high percentage of these cases show a t(14;18) translocation involving the BCL2 gene.

FOLLICULAR LYMPHOMA

Follicular lymphoma involvement of the lung is rare and is usually a widespread process often clinically diagnosed as infection. The follicular pattern observed in a lymph node involved by follicular lymphoma is the same as that seen in the lung. The neoplastic lymphoid cells express pan B-cell markers CD20, PAX5, CD79a, BCL2, BCL6, and CD10. They show no immunostaining for CD5, CD43, and CD23. Molecular studies show clonality of immunoglobulin heavy and/or light chain genes, and approximately 90% of these cases show a t(14;18) translocation involving the BCL2 gene.

PRIMARY PULMONARY HODGKIN LYMPHOMA

Primary pulmonary Hodgkin lymphoma is uncommon and morphologically resembles Hodgkin lymphoma in lymph nodes. When Hodgkin lymphoma primarily involves the lung, it is usually misdiagnosed as an inflammatory process or as an organizing pneumonia. In 1990, Radin[126] reported on 61 cases of primary pulmonary Hodgkin lymphoma. In their series, there were 36 female patients and 25 male patients with an average of 42.5 years of age and a range of 12 to 82 years. The most common histologic type of Hodgkin lymphoma identified was nodular sclerosing; mixed cellular type was the second most frequent. The criteria used for diagnosing primary pulmonary Hodgkin lymphoma included documentation of pulmonary parenchymal involvement that primarily affected the lung with only minimal enlargement or no enlargement of hilar and mediastinal lymph nodes. The most frequent symptoms before diagnosis included cough, weight loss, chest pain, dyspnea, hemoptysis,

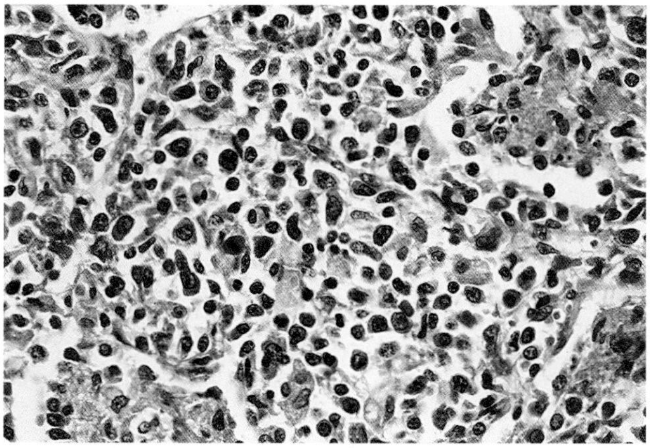

FIGURE 12.18 Lymphomatoid granulomatosis is composed of a variegated lymphoid infiltrate. X 100.

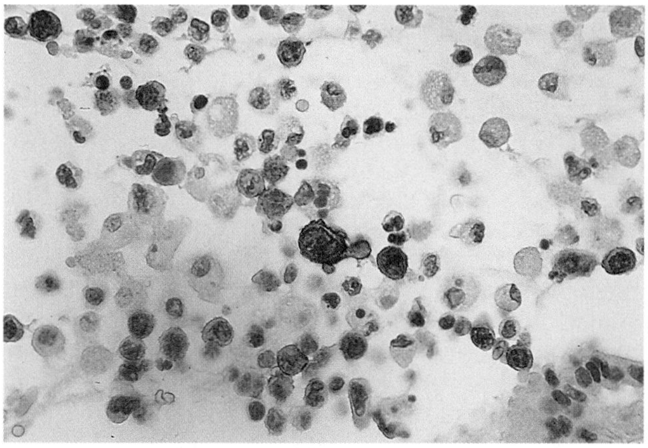

FIGURE 12.19 The large atypical cells in lymphomatoid granulomatosis express B-cell antigen CD20. X 400.

fatigue, rash, night sweats, and wheezing. Physical examination was often normal. Bronchoscopic evaluation in 35 of 61 patients was normal in 18 patients and abnormal in 16. Radiologic abnormalities were dominated by nodular-like masses in 45 of 61 patients and pneumonic infiltrates in 13 of 61 patients. To diagnose primary pulmonary Hodgkin lymphoma, one has to think of the diagnosis and identify the same histologic pattern seen in lymph nodes involved in Hodgkin lymphoma. Immunohistochemistry can facilitate the diagnosis in that Reed-Sternberg cells are frequently CD15- and CD30-positive and may occasionally express CD20 (see Table 12.12).

RARE PRIMARY LYMPHOMAS IN THE LUNG AND CHEST CAVITY

Several rare lymphomas exist in the lung. The most notable is lymphomatoid granulomatosis. Other rare lymphomas include intravascular lymphoma, primary effusion lymphoma, pyothorax-associated lymphoma, secondary lymphomas/leukemias, and Erdheim-Chester syndrome.

Lymphomatoid Granulomatosis

Lymphomatoid granulomatosis (LYG) was first reported by Liebow and coworkers.[127] This publication contains the best pathologic description of the entity. Forty patients were included in the study, and more than 50% presented with "B" symptoms frequently seen in patients with lymphoma. Over 50% of the patients died within one year of diagnosis. In 1979 Katzenstein and colleagues[128] reviewed information concerning the clinicopathologic features of lymphomatoid granulomatosis. They noted that patients who had adverse outcomes included those less than 25 years of age; patients with an increased white blood cell count, neurologic abnormalities, or hepatosplenomegaly; and those whose pulmonary infiltrates showed atypical lymphoid cells. Over the years, lymphomatoid granulomatosis evolved into a condition thought to represent an angiocentric lymphoma, specifically, an angiocentric T-cell lymphoma based on immunohistochemical studies. Guinee and colleagues[129] analyzed ten cases of lymphomatoid granulomatosis using immunohistochemistry and *in situ* hybridization for CD20 and Epstein-Barr virus, and by polymerase chain reaction for IGg heavy chain gene rearrangement. The authors found that in all cases, the majority of small and medium-sized lymphocytes were CD45RO-positive T lymphocytes. A much smaller population of large atypical cells were CD20-positive B cells, and in each case combined immunohistochemistry and *in situ* hybridization confirmed Epstein-Barr virus in the CD20-positive B cells. The authors concluded that the proliferating cell in lymphomatoid granulomatosis was a large B lymphocyte and was probably a manifestation of an Epstein-Barr virus–associated disease. Lymphomatoid granulomatosis continues to be somewhat of an enigma to clinicians and pathologists with respect to its exact nature and clinical course. Most patients who develop LYG have a rapidly downhill course and die, although some have responded rather dramatically with treatment by Cytoxan.[130] Pathologically, LYG is composed of distinct nodules composed of a variegated lymphoid infiltrate with large atypical lymphoid cells (Fig. 12.18). There is a tendency to infiltrate pulmonary veins and to cause necrosis. The large atypical cells in lymphomatoid granulomatosis express B-cell antigen CD20 as shown in Fig. 12.19.

Intravascular Lymphoma

Intravascular lymphomas are neoplasms of large B cells that occur in an extranodal distribution and are characterized by neoplastic cells in the lumens of small vessels, particularly capillaries. These have also been referred to as *angioendotheliosis proliferans*.[131-137] The intravascular growth pattern is thought to be secondary to a defect in homing receptors on the neoplastic cells. These studies suggest that neoplastic B cells lack adhesion molecules. Intravascular lymphomas commonly involve central nervous system and skin but can present as primary lymphomas in the lungs. They can be a challenging diagnosis unless considered as a possibility. Immunohistochemical studies are usually necessary to make the diagnosis.

Primary Effusion Lymphoma

This neoplasm of large B cells presents as a serous effusion with no detectable tumor masses elsewhere in the body.[138-141] Primary effusion lymphoma (PEL) is known to be associated with human herpesvirus 8 (Kaposi's sarcoma–associated herpesvirus [KSHV]) and most frequently occurs in the setting of AIDS. Patients typically present with pleural effusions in the absence of lymphadenopathy or organomegaly. Neoplastic cells are stated to mark for KSHV in all cases. The neoplastic cells are CD45-positive and are negative for B-cell markers. They are negative for surface immunoglobulin. They often express CD30, CD38, or CD138.

Pyothorax-Associated Lymphoma

Pyothorax-associated lymphoma (PAL) is a rare type of lymphoma that arises in patients with chronic pyothorax often decades after the initial pleural injury.[142-144] The disease was first described in Japan, and the largest series originated there. Clinical presentation includes effusion, chest pain, weight loss, and dyspnea. Men are more frequently affected than women. Patients typically do not have a history of HIV infection or immunosuppression. The cause of the pyothorax is usually tuberculosis. The postulated pathogenesis includes chronic antigenic stimulation analogous to MALT lymphomas of the stomach. Gross findings include a mass often 10 cm or greater associated with pleural fibrosis with direct invasion of adjacent structures. The neoplastic cells are large B lymphoblastic cells. Lymphoplasmacytic cells comprise a smaller number of cases. At autopsy, over 50% of the patients had disease limited to the intrathoracic region, and the remaining patients had extrathoracic extension. The neoplastic cells characteristically are CD45-, CD20-, and CD79a-positive. Some cells are CD138-positive, and most cells are CD3-negative.

SECONDARY LYMPHOMAS INVOLVING THE LUNG AND LEUKEMIC INFILTRATES

In all instances in which a lymphoma is identified in the lung, the patient should be evaluated with respect to whether there is a known lymphoma outside of the lung. If so, the lymphoma should be reviewed and compared morphologically to the lymphoma occurring in the lung. Sometimes transformation of lymphomas can make it difficult to determine if a lymphoma is primary within or metastatic to the lung. Chronic lymphocytic leukemia is the most common leukemia to infiltrate the lung and can be indistinguishable from primary or secondary small lymphocytic lymphomas. When Hodgkin lymphoma secondarily involves the lung, it usually infiltrates along bronchovascular structures with neoplastic cells oriented around blood vessels. While leukemic infiltrates in the lung are found histologically at autopsy in 25% to 64% of cases, they are relatively infrequently found during life. In patients with acute leukemia, non-lymphocytic–type leukemias more frequently infiltrate lung than acute lymphocytic leukemias.

Erdheim-Chester Disease

Erdheim-Chester disease is a rare, non-familial, histiocytic disorder identified by William Chester in 1930 that primarily affects middle-aged and older adults, predominantly involving long bones of the extremities. The etiology of the disease is unknown. According to a report by Allen and associates,[145] approximately 50% of patients have involvement of other tissues, including skin, retro-orbital and periorbital tissue, pituitary-hypothalamic axis, heart, kidney, retroperitoneum, breast, skeletal muscle, and sinonasal mucosa. About 20% have pulmonary involvement. This report lists 24 cases of Erdheim-Chester disease involving the lung. Pulmonary involvement is fairly characteristic and is in a subpleural interlobar septal/bronchovascular distribution. Erdheim-Chester disease is a primary neoplastic histiocytic disorder and the neoplastic cells show immunostaining for CD68 and XIIIa. S-100 protein has been identified in some cells, although studies to date have not identified Langerhans cell granules. These are generally treated as a histiocytic lymphoma.

Pulmonary Langerhans Cell Histiocytosis

A conceptual understanding of pulmonary Langerhans cell histiocytosis (PLCH; also called *histiocytosis X* or *eosinophilic granuloma*) is based on an understanding of normal Langerhans cells.[146] Langerhans cells were identified in 1869 by Paul Langerhans and compose about 3% to 8% of cells in the epidermis. They occur in a variety of organs, including epidermis, esophagus, anus/rectum, cervix, thymus, lymph nodes, and occasionally in normal lung. In the lung, they are usually associated with BALT and are frequently located between epithelial cells. In 1961 Michael Birbeck identified unusual cytoplasmic inclusions in Langerhans cells called *Birbeck granules* or *Langerhans cell granules*. Normal Langerhans cells are large dendritic cells that process antigen and present antigen to T lymphocytes.

Pulmonary Langerhans cell histiocytosis occurs almost exclusively in cigarette smokers and occurs more frequently in younger patients. The individual histiocytic cells are much smaller than normal Langerhans cells and do not show extensive dendritic processes. The histiocytic cells typically contain Langerhans cell granules and show immunostaining for S-100 protein (Fig. 12.20), CD1A, CD68, and CD31. The lesions first occur in a bronchial distribution and can progress from a cellular phase to a fibrotic phase. In some instances, the fibrotic phase is difficult to diagnose because the number of histiocytic cells is few. Patients with PLCH may be asymptomatic, or they may have relatively severe symptoms with an elevated sedimentation rate, fever, and weight loss. On chest radiograph, the nodules can occasionally be large enough to suggest metastatic cancer. In rare cases, the disease presents as a single nodule, although in most cases there are multiple nodules with sparing of the lower lobes. Cystic change occurs frequently, and the diagnosis usually is suspected by high resolution CT scans. Transbronchial biopsy

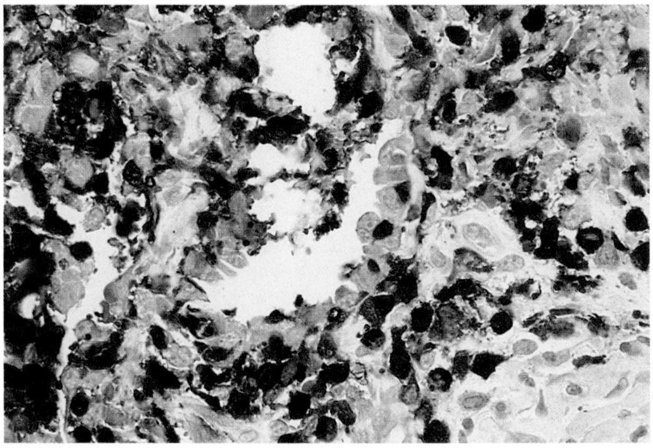

FIGURE 12.20 Langerhans cells show nuclear and cytoplasmic immunostaining for S-100 protein. X 400.

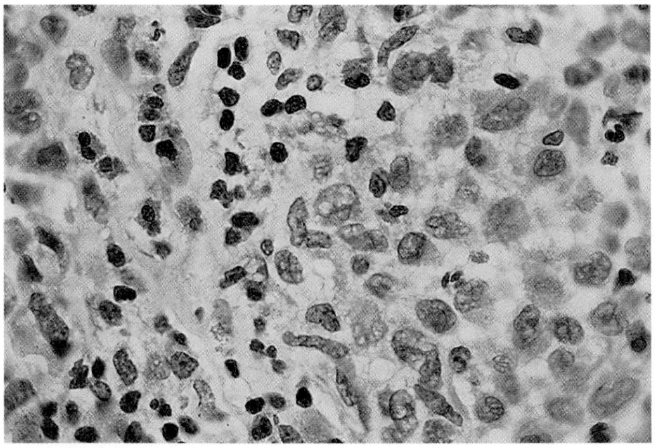

FIGURE 12.21 Portion of a nodule of pulmonary Langerhans cell granulomatosis. Langerhans cells are smaller than mature alveolar macrophages and have highly convoluted nuclei and a small amount of pale cytoplasm. Note the associated inflammatory cells. X 400.

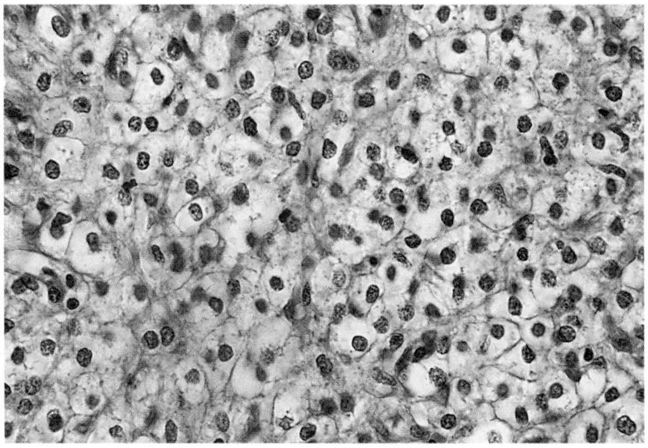

FIGURE 12.22 This clear cell tumor of lung is composed of relatively uniform cells. The clear cytoplasm is due to glycogen. X 400.

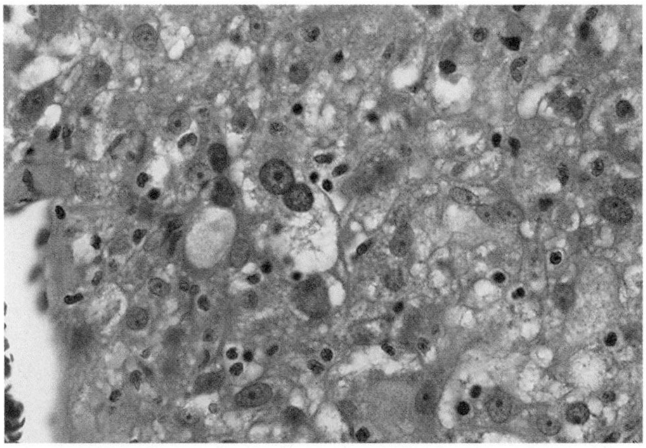

FIGURE 12.23 This clear cell tumor of lung is composed of significantly more pleomorphic cells than those shown in Figure 12.22. X 400.

specimens may be sufficient to diagnose the disease, but in most instances an open lung biopsy is necessary. The nodules of PLCH are composed of histiocytosis X cells admixed with varying numbers of lymphocytes, plasma cells, eosinophils, neutrophils, and cigarette smoker's macrophages. Histiocytosis X cells are smaller than mature alveolar macrophages and mature Langerhans cells, and they contain extensively convoluted nuclei (Fig. 12.21).

Clear Cell Neoplasm/Sugar Tumor/PEComa

Clear cell neoplasms of the lung occur as unencapsulated discrete nodules, are often referred to as *sugar tumors,* and are a member of the PEComa family of tumors.[147] PEComas include angiomyolipoma, lymphangioleiomyomatosis, clear cell tumor of the lung, clear cell myomelanocytic tumor of ligamentum teres/falciform ligament, and abdominopelvic sarcoma of perivascular epithelioid cells.[148] These tumors coexpress HMB-45 and muscle markers. Usually they are histologically composed of cells that are relatively uniform in size, shape, and nuclear appearance (Fig. 12.22), although they can be more pleomorphic (Fig. 12.23). The neoplastic cells characteristically contain large amounts of glycogen in their cytoplasm that ultrastructurally is membrane bound. The neoplastic cells show immunostaining for vimentin and frequently express HMB-45 (Fig. 12.24) and S-100 protein. In some cases, the neoplastic cells express neuron-specific enolase, Leu7, synaptophysin, and HMB-50. They are keratin-negative. They have recently been reported to express Myo-D1.[149] As described by Gaffey and colleagues,[150] some neoplastic cells contain melanosomes (Fig. 12.25), as demonstrated ultrastructurally.

Lymphangioleiomyomatosis

A rare, proliferative, but non-neoplastic pulmonary condition, lymphangioleiomyomatosis, is briefly mentioned because the proliferative cells in this condition express HMB-45.[151,152] This disease primarily affects women in the reproductive age and is characterized by proliferation of atypical smooth cells surrounding lymphatics and

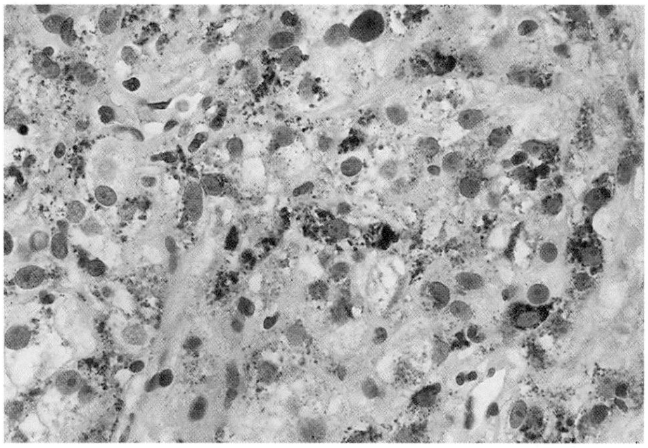

FIGURE 12.24 The neoplastic cells of this clear cell tumor express HMB-45. X 400.

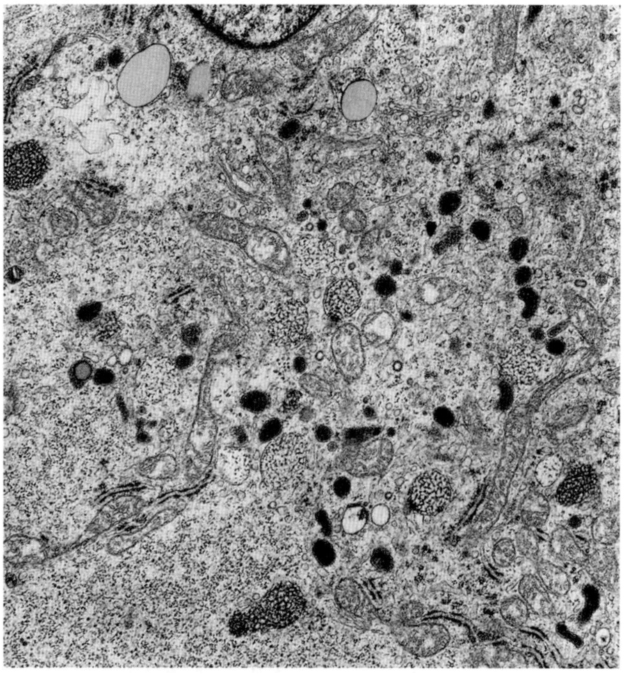

FIGURE 12.25 The neoplastic cells of this clear lung neoplasm contain melanosomes. X 16,000.

blood vessels with cystic space formation. These cells may express actin, vimentin, estrogen receptor protein, progesterone receptor protein, and HMB-45. Patients with lymphangioleiomyomatosis frequently have renal angiomyolipomas.

Sclerosing Hemangioma

Sclerosing hemangioma is one of the most extensively studied rare pulmonary neoplasms, and it usually occurs as a round-oval solitary subpleural mass,[153,154] the majority of which occur in relatively young women.[155] Most sclerosing hemangiomas are

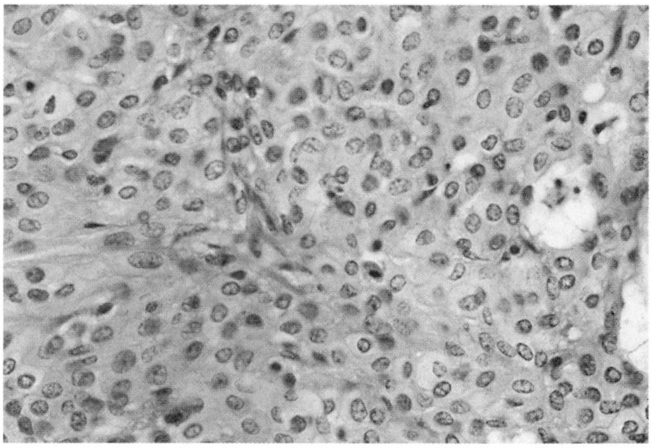

FIGURE 12.26 In the solid region of this sclerosing hemangioma, the majority of the neoplastic cells are round, oval, and occasionally slightly spindle-shaped. X 400.

TABLE 12.13 Reported Immunohistochemical Findings in Sclerosing Hemangiomas of Lung

Cells in Solid Regions of Tumor		Cells Lining Spaces in Tumor	
Positive Reactions	**Negative Reactions**	**Positive Reactions**	**Negative Reactions**
Vimentin	Keratin	Keratin	Vimentin
EMA	S-100 protein	Vimentin	S-100 protein
Keratin (rare)		EMA	Clara cell antigen
TTF-1		Surfactant apoprotein	CEA
			TTF-1

EMA, epithelial membrane antigen; CEA, carcinoembryonic antigen; TTF-1, thyroid transcription factor-1.

histologically variegated, showing cellular areas, various-sized spaces occasionally containing blood, sclerosis, and papillary structures. In the solid cellular regions, the neoplastic cells are round, oval, and slightly spindle-shaped (Fig. 12.26). The spaces are usually lined by cuboidal or columnar cells that appear morphologically as epithelial cells and are often different than adjacent tumor cells. Most sclerosing hemangiomas contain varying types and numbers of inflammatory cells, especially mast cells. Dail reviewed several immunohistochemical studies of sclerosing hemangiomas.[81] Positive and negative immunohistochemical reactions of the neoplastic cells in the solid areas are contrasted to positive and negative immunohistochemical reactions reported for the lining cells in Table 12.13. In a recent case evaluated by this author, the lining cells and tumor cells in solid areas showed intense immunostaining for epithelial membrane antigen (Fig. 12.27) and moderately intense cytoplasmic

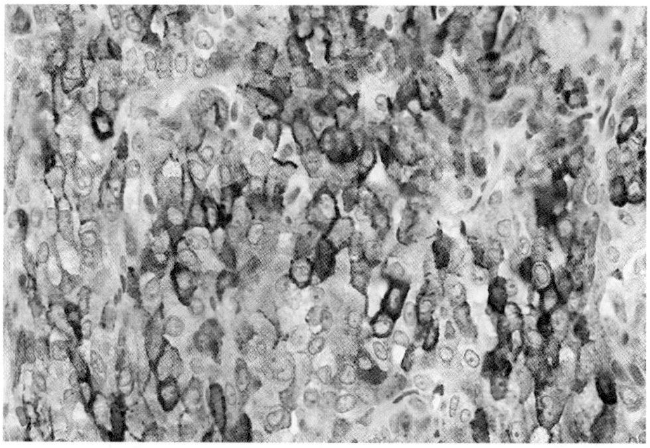

FIGURE 12.27 This sclerosing hemangioma is composed of cells that show relatively intense immunostaining for epithelial membrane antigen. X 400.

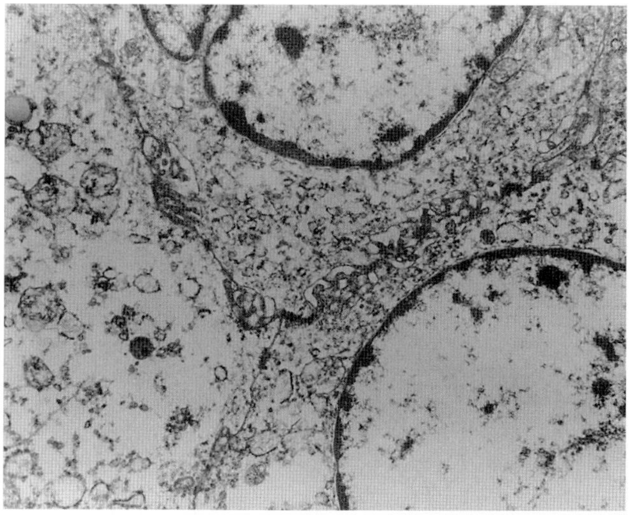

FIGURE 12.28 Ultrastructurally, the central cells of sclerosing hemangioma exhibit epithelioid features with short microvillus processes and small intercellular junctions. X 10,000.

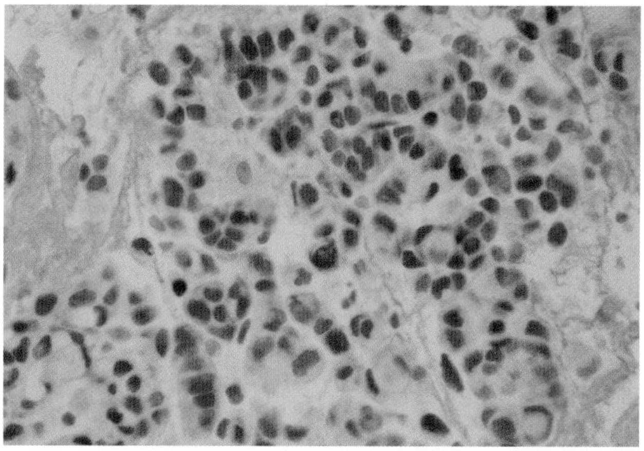

FIGURE 12.29 The neoplastic cells of sclerosing hemangiomas characteristically express TTF-1.

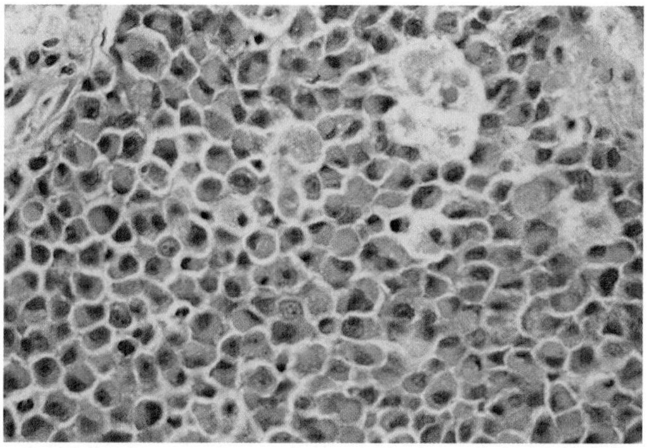

FIGURE 12.30 This primary rhabdoid tumor of lung is composed of large cells with large, globular eosinophilic inclusions. X 400.

immunostaining for vimentin. Occasional lining cells showed low intensity immunostaining for keratin. The lining cells and neoplastic cells in solid areas showed no immunostaining for actin, desmin, S-100 protein, HMB-45, CD31, and factor VIII antigen. Ultrastructurally, the neoplastic cells in solid areas had epithelioid features with short microvillus processes and small intercellular junctions (Fig. 12.28).

The neoplastic cells of sclerosing hemangiomas characteristically express TTF-1[156] (Fig. 12.29). An endobronchial variant has been described,[157] as have cases associated with lymph node metastases.[158]

Rhabdoid Tumor

Malignant rhabdoid tumors of the kidney were described in 1978 by Beckwith and Palmer[159] as highly malignant tumors of infants and children initially thought to represent a variant of Wilms' tumor. Similar neoplasms were described in extrarenal sites and in adults.[160-173] Those that resemble rhabdoid tumors in the kidney but occur in non-renal sites are frequently designated as *pseudorhabdoid tumors*. They have a diverse immunohistochemical phenotype,[160-173] although the majority of them express vimentin and many coexpress vimentin and keratin.

Six lung tumors with rhabdoid morphology were described by Cavazza and coworkers[174] in 1996. These neoplasms were composed predominantly of large, round cells with ovoid nuclei, large nucleoli, and large eosinophilic globular inclusions that compress the nucleus toward one side of the cell (Fig. 12.30). These six primary rhabdoid tumors of lung were evaluated immunohistochemically with 17 antibodies in 5 cases and 18 antibodies in one case. The rhabdoid component of the tumor immunostained for vimentin in all cases, with a high staining intensity in most cases. The cytoplasmic eosinophilic inclusions showed immunostaining for EMA and neuron-specific enolase in 5 of 6 cases, chromogranin and broad-spectrum keratin in 3 of 6 cases, CAM5.2 keratin in 2 of 6 cases, neurofilament in 2 of 6 cases, and Leu7 and gliofibrillary

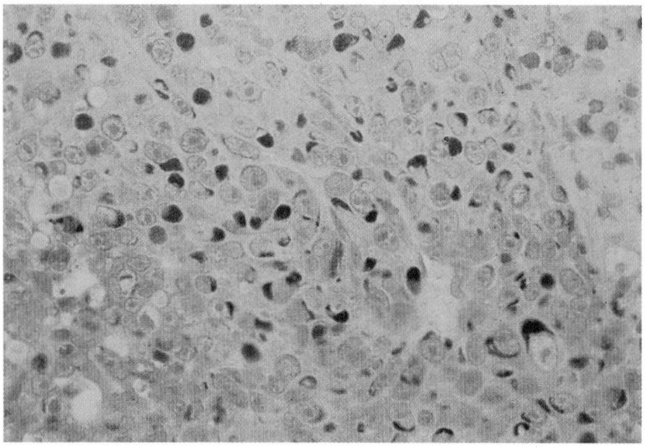

FIGURE 12.31 The globular inclusions in this primary rhabdoid tumor of lung show intense immunostaining for vimentin. X 200.

acidic protein in 1 of 6 cases. Synaptophysin was focally positive in 3 of 6 cases and CD34 in 1 of 6 cases but did not stain the globular inclusions. Diffuse granular cytoplasmic immunostaining for myoglobin was observed in 1 case. The neoplastic cells showed no immunostaining for factor VIII antigen, actin, desmin, S-100 protein, HMB-45, and light chain immunoglobulin (evaluated in 1 case). In this author's experience with 6 cases primary in the lung, 5 showed immunostaining for vimentin (Fig. 12.31) and 1 showed coexpression of vimentin and keratin. Miyagi and associates[175] described 3 cases of primary lung rhabdoid tumor, all associated with an adenocarcinoma. The authors concluded that the rhabdoid cells in these cases represented dedifferentiated components of an adenocarcinoma.

Inflammatory Pseudotumor

Inflammatory pseudotumor of lung, also referred to as *plasma cell granuloma of lung,* represent less than 1% of all lung tumors.[176] Most occur in patients less than 40 years of age, and 15% arise in persons 1 to 10 years of age.[177,178] They cause symptoms/signs of cough, chest pain, dyspnea, hemoptysis, clubbing, and fever. Radiographically, they are usually circumscribed but may be irregularly shaped. Macroscopically, they are yellowish white, well-circumscribed, and can infiltrate normal lung tissue, causing its destruction. Histologically they are composed of mature plasma cells, macrophages (including multinucleated histiocytic great cells), lymphocytes, mast cells, neutrophils, and spindle cells. The differential pathologic diagnoses usually include sclerosing hemangioma, malignant fibrous histiocytoma, malignant plasmacytoma, and reactive lymphoid proliferation. Immunohistochemically, the plasma cells show polyclonal expression of light chain immunoglobulin. The spindle cells usually stain as myofibroblasts expressing vimentin and actin, and the spindle cells express keratin in rare cases. These tumors can be invasive and resemble low-grade sarcomas.[179,180] It has been reported that expression of tumor suppressor gene product p53 is helpful in differentiating sarcoma from inflammatory pseudotumor,[181] although this marker has been controversial in differentiating other inflammatory conditions from neoplasms (e.g., fibrosing pleuritis versus desmoplastic mesotheliomas). Cytogenetic clonal changes have recently been reported in inflammatory pseudotumor of lung.[182] Yousem and colleagues[183] described the chromosomal abnormalities of inflammatory pseudotumors of lung and reported that 3 of 9 primary pulmonary inflammatory pseudotumors showed changes in the 2p23 and anaplastic lymphoma kinase (ALK) gene regions. The authors suggested that immunohistochemical detection of anaplastic lymphoma kinase (ALK) might be helpful in predicting the future biological behavior of inflammatory pseudotumors. Freeman and colleagues[184] suggested that ALK 1 expression can be useful in diagnosing inflammatory pseudotumors.

Desmoplastic Small Round Cell Tumor

Desmoplatic small round cell tumors occur primarily in the abdominal cavity.[185] The neoplasms characteristically show immunostaining for desmin (a dot-like pattern), WT1, keratin, neuron-specific enolase, CD99, and actin. They also show the EWS-WT1 gene fusion transcript. A desmoplastic, small, round cell tumor was reported primary in the lung by Syed and coworkers.[186] Ultrastructurally, this tumor showed intracytoplasmic whorls of intermediate filaments, presumably desmin. A desmoplastic, small, round cell tumor was also reported as a primary neoplasm in the pleura.[187]

Epithelial-Myoepithelial Neoplasm

Epithelial-myoepithelial neoplasms have been reported primary in the lung.[188-191] These neoplasms are composed of an inner epithelial cell layer that immunostains for keratin, CEA, and EMA, and an outer cell layer of myoepithelial cells that immunostain for S-100 protein and actin.

Granular Cell Tumor

Granular cell tumors are thought to be derived from Schwann cells and may occur as solitary pulmonary neoplasms.[192] The neoplastic cells typically express S-100 protein, neuron-specific enolase, vimentin, and actin.

Salivary Gland Neoplasm

Salivary gland-like neoplasms rarely occur in the lung. They show the same immunohistochemical profile as those that arise in salivary glands[193] and are thought to arise from minor salivary glands in the bronchial mucosa.

PRIMARY INTRAPULMONARY THYMOMA

Moran and associates[194] reported on 8 cases of primary intrapulmonary thymoma in which there was no evidence of mediastinal masses radiographically or at surgery. The masses varied from 0.5 to 10 cm in diameter. Five were located close to the hilum, and 3 were in a subpleural location. The masses were composed of mixtures of lymphocytes and epithelial cells that were separated by fibrous bands. The epithelial cells immunostained for keratins and epithelial membrane antigen.

Pulmonary Meningothelial Nodules

Minute pulmonary meningothelial-like nodules (MPMN), previously referred to as *minute chemodectoma-like bodies,* are most frequently found incidentally in the lung. They are composed of spindle-shaped cells and form nodules centered around small veins. Ionescu and colleagues[195] reported on 16 cases, yielding 33 separate MPMN and 10 cases of meningiomas. The cells forming MPMN showed immunostaining for vimentin in 96.6% of cases, EMA in 33.3% of cases and S-100 protein in 3% of cases. All cases were negative for cytokeratin and synaptophysin. They found that the MPMN lacked mutational damage, consistent with a reactive origin. In contrast, the four cases with multiple MPMNs (MPMomatosis) showed genotypic findings suggestive of transition between reactive and neoplastic transformation. The 10 meningiomas evaluated showed the highest frequency of loss of heterozygosity.

Mukhopadhyay and colleagues[196] evaluated 400 consecutive surgical lung biopsies of various types to further evaluate meningothelial-like nodules in surgical lung biopsies, lobectomies, and pediatric autopsies to clarify their incidence, distribution, and relation to age and underlying disease, and to shed potential light on their origin. Tissue sections were immunostained for progesterone receptor protein, CD56, EMA, TTF-1, CD99, CD34, CD31, and Ki-67. Meningothelial-like nodules were stated to have been roundly distributed in alveolar septa and were rarely present in scars. There was no relation to venules, although small vessels were common in the nodules. The vessels appeared to be entrapped. Immunostains were stated to have been positive for progesterone receptor in 14 of 14 cases, CD56 in 14 of 14 cases, and EMA in 10 of 10 cases; they were negative for TTF-1 in 0 of 4 cases, CD99 in 0 of 11cases, CD34 in 0 of 6 cases, and CD31 in 0 of 6 cases. Ki-67 was focally positive in 2 of 12 cases. The authors concluded that the incidence of meningothelial-like nodules in their study was higher than previously appreciated. The presence in nearly half of the extensively sampled lobectomy specimens suggested that they may be present in all lungs if sufficiently sampled. The absence of meningothelial-like nodules in patients less than 20 years of age suggests that they are not congenital rests. Staining for CD56 was novel but had been reported in meningotheliomas, thus supporting the concept that meningothelial-like nodules were of meningothelial origin. They suggested a more appropriate term for these would be *meningothelial nodules*. The lesions were stated to have no clinical significance.

Placental Transmogrification of Lung

Brief mention is made of placental transmogrification of the lung. It occurs in association with lipomatosis[197] and bullous emphysema[198] and is composed of placental villus-like structures in the lung parenchyma. The epithelium surfacing the placentoid structures shows immunostaining for TTF-1 in most cases. The stromal cells express vimentin and are non-reactive for TTF-1. Mast cells are common in the stromal tissue.

Variables and Pitfalls

Squamous cell carcinomas of lung show a variety of histologic forms and can be poorly differentiated. Small cell squamous carcinomas of lung can be confused with small cell neuroendocrine carcinomas. These two neoplasms are contrasted in Table 12.14. The main difference is that small cell squamous carcinomas do not express neuroendocrine markers, usually express high molecular weight keratin, and show no immunostaining for TTF-1, whereas small cell neuroendocrine carcinomas typically express neuroendocrine markers, do not show immunostaining for high molecular weight keratin, show punctate immunostaining for low molecular weight keratin, and express TTF-1 in a high percentage of cases. Small cell squamous carcinomas are usually positive for p63, whereas in our experience, small cell lung carcinoma is usually negative for p63 (although it has been reported in neuroendocrine lung neoplasms).

Squamous carcinomas frequently show spindle cell features. The neoplastic spindle squamous cells often coexpress keratin and vimentin. Some spindle cell squamous carcinomas express predominantly vimentin and relatively small amounts of keratin.

Basaloid carcinoma is a relatively rare lung neoplasm[199] that may be confused with neuroendocrine carcinoma. Basaloid carcinomas are composed predominantly of nests of relatively small undifferentiated cells with extensive necrosis and palisading of the peripheral cell layer (Fig. 12.32). They may show squamous and glandular differentiation, although the degree of this differentiation is usually poorly developed. The glandular component is often composed of small cells. Basaloid carcinoma can be confused with small cell carcinoma, atypical carcinoid and large cell neuroendocrine carcinoma. Basaloid carcinomas usually express low and high molecular weight keratins and do not express neuroendocrine markers.

Sturm and colleagues evaluated TTF-1 and 34βE12 (cytokeratins 1, 5, 10, and 14) expression in basaloid and large cell neuroendocrine carcinomas.[59] The authors did not observe TTF-1 expression in basaloid carcinomas, and they observed expression of high molecular weight keratin (34βE12) in only one large cell neuroendocrine carcinoma. Basaloid carcinoma is contrasted with small

TABLE 12.14 Immunohistochemical Features of Small Cell Squamous Carcinoma of Lung and Small Cell Neuroendocrine Carcinoma of Lung

	Antibody Directed Against								
Type of Neoplasm	Low molecular weight keratin	High molecular weight keratin	CK5/ CK6	CK7	CK20	Synaptophysin	Chromogranin A	Thyroid transcription factor-1	p63
Small cell squamous carcinoma	S	S	S	N	R	N	N	N	S
Small cell neuroendocrine carcinoma	+*	N	N	R	R	+	S†	+	S

*Pattern of staining is usually punctate using antibody 35βH11.
†Pattern of staining is usually punctate.
Reactivity:
+, almost always diffuse, strong positivity
S, sometimes postive
R, rare cells positive
N, almost always negative

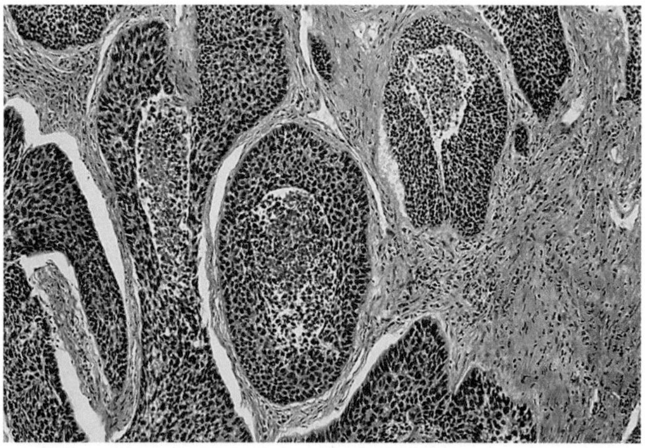

FIGURE 12.32 This basaloid carcinoma of lung is composed of undifferentiated, relatively small cells and often resembles primary pulmonary neuroendocrine carcinomas. X 200.

cell carcinoma, atypical carcinoid, and large cell neuroendocrine carcinoma in Table 12.15.

Kargi and associates[200] reported on the diagnostic value of TTF-1, CK5/6, and p63 in the classification of lung carcinomas. The authors evaluated bronchoscopic biopsies of 77 lung cancers in which the morphology of the tumor was stated to have been easily studied.[200] All cases were immunostained for p63, CK5/6, and TTF-1. The results of their study are shown in Table 12.16. Of the 39 squamous cell carcinomas, 32 were positive for p63, 31 were positive for CK5/6, 27 were positive for p63 and CK5/6, and 36 were positive for p63 or CK5/6. With respect to small cell lung cancers, 2 of 28 were positive for CK5/6, and 2 of 28 showed p63 or CK5/6 positivity. Of the 10 adenocarcinomas, 2 of 10 expressed CK5/6 positivity, and 2 of 20 expressed p63 or CK5/6 positivity. The authors concluded that to achieve as accurate as possible histologic typing of lung cancer, TTF-1 in combination with p63 and CK5/6 might be useful components of analyzing poorly differentiated lung carcinomas in biopsy tissues.

Pulmonary adenocarcinomas are currently the most common primary lung cancer,[10,11] and they show a wide range of differentiation. In most cases, pulmonary adenocarcinomas show more than one histologic pattern. Several mucinous forms of primary pulmonary adenocarcinomas exist, including a cystic mucinous form and signet ring adenocarcinoma. Histologically, it is often difficult to differentiate a primary mucinous pulmonary adenocarcinoma from a metastatic adenocarcinoma from the GI tract, such as colon. Ultrastructurally, it is usually impossible to differentiate these neoplasms with respect to their site of origin. The immunohistochemical profile of pulmonary adenocarcinoma is contrasted with metastatic colonic adenocarcinoma in Table 12.17. In general, primary pulmonary adenocarcinomas typically express CK7 and TTF-1 and do not express CK20. Metastatic colonic adenocarcinomas to lung typically express CK20 and CDX2 and show no expression of CK7 or TTF-1. As stated previously, TTF-1 is the most specific marker in differentiating primary pulmonary adenocarcinomas from adenocarcinomas of other sites. Approximately 60% to 75% of primary pulmonary adenocarcinomas express TTF-1. Caution is urged in that mucin-producing pulmonary adenocarcinomas can express CDX2, as we will discuss later in this chapter.

One must be aware of cytoplasmic TTF-1 immunoreactivity in other neoplasms. Bejarano and Mousavi[201] evaluated 361 neoplasms from 29 organ sites, including primary and metastatic neoplasms. Twenty-three (6.3%) tumors showed cytoplasmic staining for TTF-1. In 13 of these cases, the primary site of origin was established with certainty: 7 were lung carcinomas (3 primary lung adenocarcinomas, 1 primary large cell carcinoma, 1 metastatic small cell carcinoma to the liver, 1 metastatic adenocarcinoma to a neck lymph node, and 1 metastatic adenocarcinoma to thigh soft tissue); 3 colonic adenocarcinomas (2 metastatic to vertebrae and

TABLE 12.15 Immunohistochemical Features of Basaloid Carcinoma of Lung Compared with Small Cell Carcinoma, Atypical Carcinoid, and Large Cell Neuroendocrine Carcinoma of Lung

	Antibody Directed Against								
Type of Tumor	Low molecular weight keratin (35βH11)	High molecular weight keratin (34βE12)	CK5/6	CK7	CK20	Synaptophysin	Chromogranin A	Carcinoembryonic antigen	TTF-1
Basaloid carcinoma	S	S	S	S	R	N	N	S	R
Small cell carcinoma	+	N	N	R	N	+	S	S	+
Atypical carcinoid carcinoma	S	S	N	R	N	S	+	S	S
Large cell neuroendocrine carcinoma	S	R	R	R	N	S	+	S	S

TTF-1, Thyroid transcription factor-1.
Reactivity:
+, almost always diffuse, strong positivity
S, sometimes postive
R, rare cells positive
N, almost always negative

TABLE 12.16 Immunohistochemical Reactivities of Squamous Cell Carcinoma, Adenocarcinoma, and Small Cell Lung Carcinoma for CK5/6, TTF-1, and p63

Markers	SCC (n = 39) Positive (n)	AC (n = 10) Positive (n)	SCLC (n = 28) Positive (n)
CK5/6	31	2	2
TTF-1	0	4	28
p63	32	0	0

1 to lung); 1 metastatic breast ductal adenocarcinoma to femur; 1 metastatic laryngeal squamous cell carcinoma to liver; and 1 meningioma involving the orbit bone. The authors concluded that occasional cytoplasmic immunostaining for TTF-1 was observed in several different types of neoplasms but was a nonspecific finding and should be disregarded for diagnostic purposes.

With the passage of time, some immunohistochemical reactions become less specific. Lau and coworkers[32] evaluated TTF-1, CK7, and CK20 expression in 48 nonmucinous, 12 mucinous, and 7 mixed histology bronchioloalveolar carcinomas. The 12 mucinous bronchioloalveolar carcinomas were TTF-1-negative, and there was a trend toward absence of TTF-1 expression in the mucinous component of bronchioloalveolar carcinomas of mixed histology. Sixty-three of 67 (94%) bronchioloalveolar cell carcinomas were CK7-positive with no difference in expression of different subtypes. The 3 bronchioloalveolar carcinomas that were CK20-positive exhibited a mucinous morphology. These results indicated that mucinous bronchioloalveolar carcinomas were frequently TTF-1-negative and could express CK20.

Simsir and colleagues[33] evaluated 6 mucinous bronchioloalveolar cell carcinomas, 4 nonmucinous bronchioloalveolar carcinomas and 6 with focal mucinous differentiation. Four of six (67%) of the mucinous bronchioloalveolar carcinomas were CK7-positive, CK20-positive, and TTF-1-negative. All 4 nonmucinous bronchioloalveolar carcinomas were CK7-positive and CK20-negative. Two of 4 were TTF-1-positive. The 6 mixed bronchioloalveolar carcinomas were diffusely positive for CK7 and focally positive for CK20; 5 (83%) were TTF-1-positive. The authors concluded that mucinous and mixed bronchioloalveolar carcinomas had an immunophenotype that was different from conventional pulmonary adenocarcinoma.

CDX2 transcription factor is characteristically expressed in gastrointestinal adenocarcinomas.[202] Rossi and colleagues[203] evaluated 13 primary mucinous (colloid) carcinomas of the lung immunohistochemically. All 11 goblet cell–type mucinous carcinomas strongly immunostained for CDX2 and MUC2. Eight reacted with TTF-1, 6 with CK20, 9 with CK7, and 2 with MUC-5AC. The 2 signet ring mucinous carcinomas immunostained for TTF-1, CK7, and MUC-5AC but did not immunostain for CDX2 and CK20. The authors concluded that since goblet cell–type mucinous carcinomas strongly immunostained for CDX2, MUC2, and CK20, the differential diagnosis with metastatic colorectal carcinoma was challenging and required appropriate clinical correlation.

Mazziotta and associates[204] evaluated a number of types of adenocarcinomas for CDX2 expression, including 84 lung adenocarcinomas. Ten of 84 lung cancers showed areas of fairly strong immunoreactivity for

TABLE 12.17 Comparison of Immunohistochemical Features of Primary Mucinous Pulmonary Adenocarcinomas versus Metastatic Colonic Adenocarcinomas

	Antibody Directed Against						
Type of Neoplasm	CK5/6	CK7	CK20	Carcinoembryonic antigen	Surfactant apoprotein A	TTF-1	CDX2
Primary pulmonary mucinous tumors	R	S	S	+	S	S	R
Metastatic colonic mucin-producing adenocarcinoma	N	S	S	+	N	N	S

TTF-1, Thyroid transcription factor-1.
Reactivity:
+, almost always diffuse, strong positivity
S, sometimes postive
R, rare cells positive
N, almost always negative

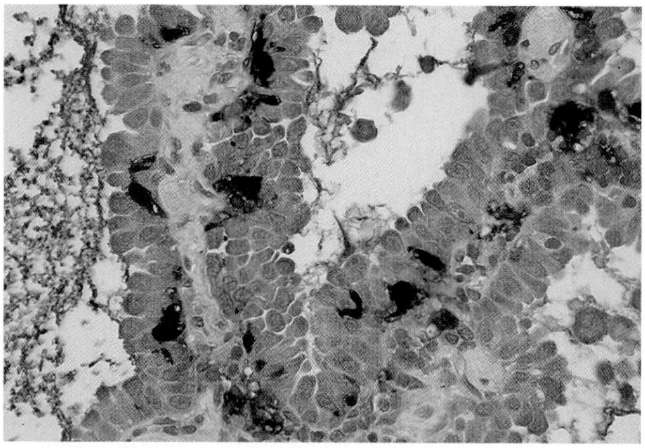

FIGURE 12.33 This nonmucinous bronchioloalveolar cell carcinoma shows numerous S-100 protein–positive dendritic cells admixed with the tumor cells. X 400.

CDX2. Seven of the lung cancers were adenocarcinomas, and 3 were large cell undifferentiated carcinomas. Three of 7 adenocarcinomas and 1 large cell carcinoma were positive for TTF-1 and CK7 and were negative for CK20. In 7 of 8 cases evaluated, gene expression of CDX2 was identified. The authors concluded that CDX2 was a relatively specific marker for tumors with intestinal differentiation with the caveat that CDX2 expression could be seen in some primary adenocarcinomas and large cell carcinomas of the lung and mucinous carcinomas of the ovary.

Some peripheral pulmonary adenocarcinomas with acinar and papillary patterns with abundant extracellular mucin may also express GCDFP-15 in addition to TTF-1. Striebel [205] and colleagues reviewed 211 adenocarcinomas and found that 5.2% expressed GCDFP-15, a specific marker used in breast pathology. Eighty-one percent of these cases also expressed TTF-1, but none expressed hormone receptors. One needs to exercise caution when hunting for breast metastasis in the lung because GCDFP-15 has a very high specificity for breast carcinoma.

A few primary pulmonary adenocarcinomas may show low intensity immunostaining for S-100 protein.[206] However, it is more common in primary pulmonary adenocarcinomas, especially non-mucinous bronchioloalveolar cell carcinomas, to show S-100 protein–positive dendritic cells admixed with the neoplastic cells[207] (Fig. 12.33). These S-100 protein–positive cells represent Langerhans cells (Fig. 12.34). Adenocarcinomas may secrete a factor that is chemotactic for the Langerhans cells.[208] Langerhans cells, however, can be seen in a wide variety of neoplasms and non-neoplastic pulmonary conditions.[209] Dorion and colleagues[210] studied the utility of S-100 protein in differentiating lung adenocarcinoma from papillary and follicular carcinoma of the thyroid. They found that pulmonary adenocarcinoma showed nuclear and cytoplasmic staining for S-100 protein in 31 of 39 cases, whereas all cases of papillary carcinoma of the thyroid and follicular carcinoma of the thyroid were negative for S-100 protein. The authors, however, did not mention that Langerhans cells are S-100 protein–positive and can frequently be seen in pulmonary adenocarcinomas and thus easily be misinterpreted as cancer cells.

Nonmucinous bronchioloalveolar cell carcinomas frequently show intranuclear inclusions that are PAS-diastase–positive[211-214] (Fig. 12.35). The intranuclear PAS-positive inclusions immunostain for the apoprotein portion of surfactant (Fig. 12.36). When examined ultrastructurally, these intranuclear inclusions consist of 45-nm–diameter tubules that attach to the inner nuclear membrane (Fig. 12.37).

Antibodies against surfactants are commercially available and have been evaluated in diagnosing pulmonary adenocarcinomas. Surfactant antibodies are not 100% specific for surfactant-producing pulmonary adenocarcinomas. Bejarano and coworkers[22] used immunohistochemical markers to distinguish between primary non–small cell lung carcinoma and metastatic breast carcinoma. They studied 57 primary non–small cell lung cancers, including 46 adenocarcinomas and 51 adenocarcinomas of the breast. They found surfactant protein A, surfactant protein B, and TTF-1 in 49%,

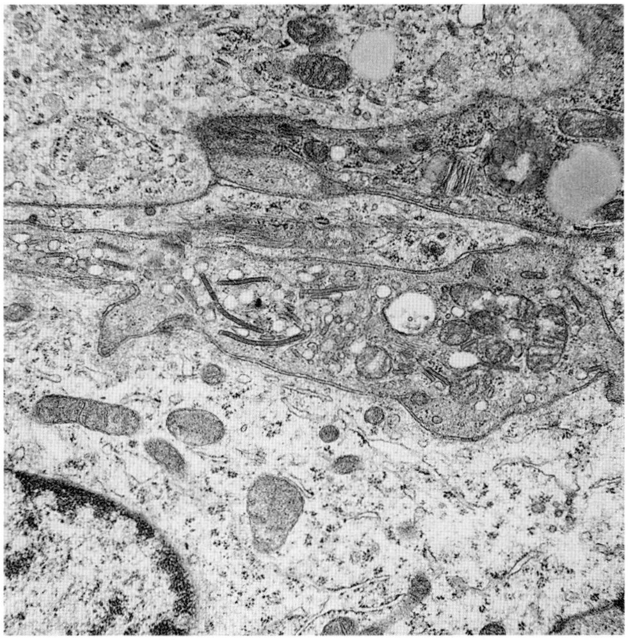

FIGURE 12.34 Ultrastructurally, the S-100 protein-positive cells represent Langerhans cells. Langerhans cells are antigen presenting–processing macrophages that contain peculiar cytoplasmic organelles referred to as *Langerhans cells granules* or *Birbeck granules.* X 20,000.

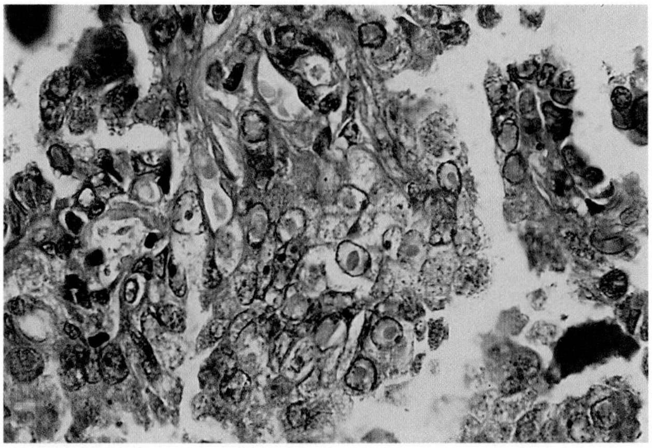

FIGURE 12.35 This nonmucinous bronchioloalveolar cell carcinoma shows intranuclear PAS-positive inclusions. X 400.

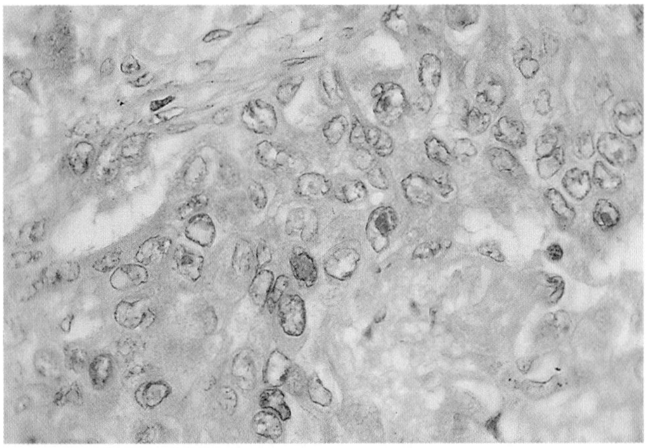

FIGURE 12.36 The intranuclear inclusions in nonmucinous bronchioloalveolar cell carcinomas immunostain for the apoprotein portion of surfactant A. X 400.

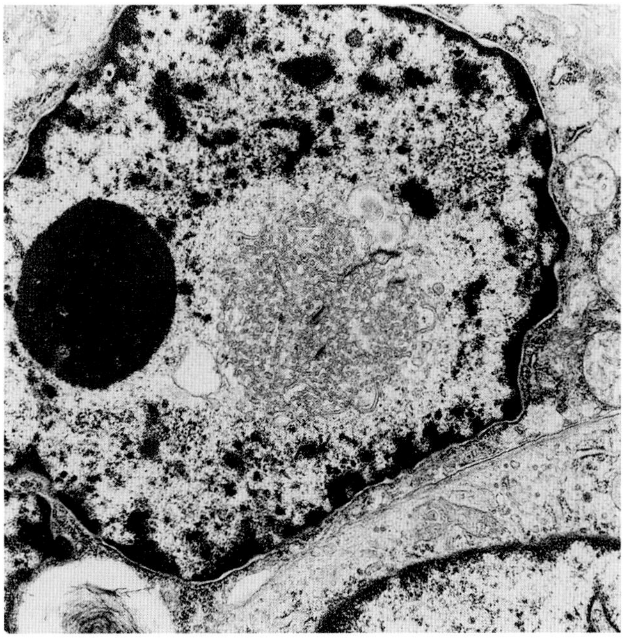

FIGURE 12.37 Ultrastructurally, the intranuclear inclusions are composed of 45-nm-diameter tubules that connect to the inner nuclear membrane. X 20,000.

53%, and 63% of non–small cell pulmonary carcinomas, respectively, and 54%, 63%, and 76% of primary pulmonary adenocarcinomas, respectively. Squamous cell lung carcinomas rarely stained with these antibodies. Fifty-one breast carcinomas showed no immunostaining for TTF-1 and surfactant B, although four breast cancers immunostained for surfactant A.

As shown in Table 12.8, recent studies of primary pulmonary adenocarcinomas have shown that those that express TTF-1 usually express surfactant protein-A (SP-A). This is not unexpected because TTF-1 is a transcription factor for surfactant in primary pulmonary adenocarcinomas.

Nonaka and Chiriboga[215] studied basal cell differentiation in 108 cases of stage 1 primary lung adenocarcinoma by immunohistochemistry using tissue microarrays with immunostains for p63, TTF-1, CK7, CK20, 34βE12 (high molecular weight keratin), CK14, CK17, SP-A, surfactant protein-C (SP-C), clara cell protein-16 (CC16), and CD208 (DC-LAMP). The results are given in their report. They concluded that p63-positive cells were common components in lung adenocarcinomas and that most showed a CK14-negative/CK17-positive immunophenotype, which corresponded to a basal cell (reserve cell) of the distal airway (type B basal cell). p63 and/or 34βE12-positive cells in lung carcinoma did not always indicate squamous cell differentiation, and the possibility of a tumor with a basal cell phenotype should be considered.

Tigrani and Weydert[216] studied inhibin-alpha expression in 48 primary pulmonary non–small cell carcinomas using immunohistochemistry. It was stated that inhibin was a glycoprotein hormone that was known to be expressed in carcinomas of adrenocortical and germ cell origins. Inhibin was occasionally identified in other tumor cells. The authors found inhibin-alpha expression in 9 of 48 cases. The extent of expression was limited to less than 25% of the tumors. The authors concluded that primary lung carcinoma was not excluded by a positive staining for inhibin-alpha. The extent of positive staining in lung carcinoma, however, appeared to be limited to the minority of cells in the given tumor.

Zhang and colleagues[217] studied inhibin-alpha expression in non–small cell carcinoma of the lung with a focus on adenocarcinomas. Their results suggested that a significant percentage of pulmonary adenocarcinomas showed inhibin-alpha expression. They stated that caution should therefore be taken when using inhibin-alpha as a key antibody to evaluate primary lung cancer. Their study was similar to the study by Tigrani and associates[216] The lung is the site of numerous metastatic neoplasms, and pathologists must be acutely aware of this.[218,219] Metastatic neoplasms to lung are more common than primary tumors. The problem with differentiating primary from metastatic lung neoplasms is compounded by their similar histologic appearances. Adenocarcinoma as a group is the most difficult neoplasm to differentiate primary from metastatic. Metastatic tumors to the lung must always be considered when making a diagnosis of primary lung cancer, even when considering solitary pulmonary nodules.

As discussed by these authors[21] and others,[220] antibodies against CK7 and CK20 are helpful in distinguishing primary from metastatic carcinoma, although they are not specific. Many GI tract cancers, a few renal cell carcinomas, gynecological neoplasms, and bladder neoplasms express CK7. TTF-1 is the most specific antibody in identifying pulmonary adenocarcinoma, but it is negative in 25% to 40% of cases of primary pulmonary adenocarcinomas. As discussed earlier in the chapter, there is variability, especially with mucin-producing pulmonary adenocarcinomas, mucinous bronchioloalveolar carcinomas, and the goblet-cell variant of primary mucinous carcinomas of the lung. Some primary pulmonary adenocarcinomas, especially those that are mucin-producing, may express CK20 and CDX2.

Carcinomas of breast frequently metastasize to pleura and lung, often many years after the initial diagnosis.[219] Ollayos and colleagues evaluated the sensitivity of estrogen receptor protein by immunohistochemistry in known cases of adenocarcinoma of colon, pancreas, and lung.[221] Forty-three colon adenocarcinomas and 18 pancreatic adenocarcinomas showed no nuclear immunostaining for estrogen receptor proteins, whereas 3 of 42 primary pulmonary adenocarcinomas immunostained for estrogen receptor protein.

Canver and coworkers[222] studied sex hormone receptor expression by immunohistochemistry in 64 non–small lung cancers. It was stated that specimens had been acetone-fixed. They found no immunostaining for sex hormone receptors in normal lung. However, 62 of 64 non–small cell lung carcinomas showed nuclear immunostaining for estrogen receptor protein. Immunostaining for progesterone receptor protein was not found in 50 cases (78%) and was weakly positive in 14 cases (22%). Bacchi and colleagues[223] reported expression of nuclear estrogen and progesterone receptor proteins in a few pulmonary carcinoids and small cell carcinomas. DiNunno and associates[224] evaluated 248 consecutive cases of stage I and II non–small cell lung cancers for estrogen and progesterone receptors using formalin-fixed paraffin-embedded tissue. No nuclear or cytoplasmic expression of estrogen and progesterone receptors was found. The authors concluded that finding estrogen and progesterone receptor in a lung carcinoma was supportive of a non-pulmonary metastatic carcinoma to the lung. In contrast, Dabbs and colleagues evaluated 45 resected primary pulmonary adenocarcinomas, of which 25 were nonmucinous bronchioloalveolar carcinomas and 20 were moderately differentiated adenocarcinomas not otherwise specified, for estrogen and progesterone receptors using monoclonal antibodies to two different clones (clone 6F11 and clone 1D5) on formalin-fixed paraffin-embedded tissue. [225] Nuclear estrogen receptor expression was seen in 56% of the nonmucinous bronchioloalveolar carcinomas and 80% of the primary pulmonary adenocarcinomas not otherwise specified with antibody clone 6F11. No estrogen receptor immunostaining was observed with antibody clone 1D5. No progesterone expression was detectable in any neoplasm. The authors concluded that further study is warranted to discern the nature of the 6F11 clone anti-estrogen antibody and that the clinical significance and ramifications of estrogen receptor in pulmonary adenocarcinomas remains unknown.

Selvaggi and associates[226] evaluated 130 primary lung carcinomas (60 squamous, 48 adenocarcinoma, and 22 large cell undifferentiated) for HER2/neu expression. Six of 60 squamous carcinomas, 6 of 48 adenocarcinomas, and 3 of 22 large cell undifferentiated carcinomas expressed HER2/neu. On multivariate analysis, HER2/neu expression and extent of tumor were an independent factor for disease-related survival. The median survival time (85 weeks versus 179 weeks) and overall survival rate were significantly lower in patients with greater than 5% HER2/neu-positive tumor cells.

This author has observed several cases of nuclear estrogen receptor protein by immunohistochemistry in pulmonary adenocarcinoma using heat epitope antigen retrieval. A few cases of small cell carcinoma showed nuclear estrogen and progesterone receptor protein expression.

The immunophenotype of large cell undifferentiated neoplasms of lung is unpredictable. Most large cell undifferentiated neoplasms are carcinomas and coexpress keratin and vimentin. Some express only vimentin. There are large cell neoplasms that look like carcinomas but, in fact, are not. Another area of potential confusion is related to observations that non-neuroendocrine, non–small cell carcinomas as determined by histologic appearances express neuroendocrine markers by immunohistochemistry. We will discuss this concept later in this chapter.

Lymphoepithelioma-like carcinoma, a subtype of primary large cell undifferentiated carcinoma, may occur as a primary lung cancer composed of large anaplastic cells and be confused with lymphomas and other neoplasms.[227] Most express low and high molecular weight keratin and show ultrastructural features of epithelial differentiation, including desmosomes and intracellular tonofilaments. Some express Epstein-Barr virus and BCL-2.[228] Giant cell carcinoma of lung is a subtype of large cell undifferentiated carcinoma composed of at least 40% of cells greater than 40 μm in diameter.[229] They usually coexpress keratin and vimentin. They must be differentiated from metastatic sarcomas and melanomas. Some show cytoplasmic immunostaining for CEA.

Some large cell anaplastic lymphomas have an epithelioid appearance and show immunostaining for keratin.[230] Most Ki-1 (CD30)-positive anaplastic lymphomas express epithelial membrane antigen.[231] Some large cell anaplastic lymphomas have ultrastructural features suggesting epithelial differentiation.[232] A list of large cell undifferentiated neoplasms and their immunophenotype is shown in Table 12.18.

Chu and coworkers[233] recently reported finding significant numbers of nonhematopoietic epithelioid neoplasms expressing T/NK cell antigens, although few were of diagnostic significance (Table 12.19).

As known by most surgical pathologists, malignant melanomas may show significant variability in differentiation. Nearly all show immunostaining for S-100 protein and vimentin. Approximately 50% immunostain for human melanoma black-45 (HMB-45) antigen. Most stain for pan melanoma antibody. Rare melanomas immunostain for keratin,[234] which can cause diagnostic confusion.

The mediastinum contains a variety of neoplasms, including those of germ cell origin. One can encounter difficulty when determining if a neoplasm is primary in the lung, is invading the mediastinum, or is primary in the mediastinum and invading lung. In addition, thymic carcinomas show significant variability in differentiation, including cases that show germ cell differentiation. This problem can be compounded because primary lung cancers have been reported to express germ cell markers. Yoshimoto and colleagues[235] reported a case of a poorly differentiated mucin-producing primary pulmonary neoplasm whose tumor cells showed immunostaining for CEA, alpha-fetoprotein, and human chorionic gonadotropin (hCG). Autopsy tissue showed these substances in different tumor cells, which the authors interpreted to suggest that the lung cancer consisted of at least three clones of cancer cells with different phenotypes. Kuida and associates[236] found hCG expression in 4 of 11 primary lung cancers. The application of TTF-1 would potentially help clarify some cases with respect to a primary mediastinal or pulmonary origin of the neoplasm.

Trophoblastic expression was evaluated for hCG and its derivatives, leutenizing hormone (LH, LHβ), follicle stimulating hormone (FSH, FSHβ), placental lactogen (PL), and growth hormone (GH-227) in 40 neuroendocrine lung neoplasms, 29 primary pulmonary adenocarcinomas, 20 squamous cell carcinomas, and 1 adenosquamous carcinoma.[237] Trophoblastic hormone immunoreactivity was found in 28 of 90 (31%) of all lung carcinomas but primarily in typical carcinoids.

Rare primary lung neoplasms resembling hepatocellular carcinoma, referred to as *hepatoid carcinomas,* may express high concentrations of alpha-fetoprotein and abnormal prothrombin.[238]

Pathologists and clinicians continue to extensively evaluate neuroendocrine neoplasms. Cooper and colleagues[239] evaluated 77 patients retrospectively who underwent surgical resection. Of the 77 neoplasms, 50 were typical carcinoids, 5 were atypical carcinoids, 9 were large cell neuroendocrine carcinomas, 4 were classified as mixed large cell–small cell neuroendocrine carcinomas, and 9 were small cell neuroendocrine carcinomas. Follow-up was obtained in 62 of 77 patients for an average of 38.1 months (range 2 to 132 months). Eight of 13 deaths were disease-related: 4 deaths in patients with large cell neuroendocrine carcinoma; 2 deaths in small cell carcinoma patients; 1 death in an atypical carcinoid patient; and 1 death in a patient with mixed small cell-large cell carcinoma. The mean disease-free intervals for patients with neuroendocrine neoplasms were: typical carcinoid, 41.3 months; atypical carcinoid, 20 months; large cell neuroendocrine carcinoma, 25 months; and small cell neuroendocrine carcinoma, 48 months. The authors acknowledged the limitations of the study and the controversial role of surgery in high-grade neuroendocrine carcinomas.

Lyda and Weiss[240] immunostained 142 primary lung carcinomas for B72.3, 34βE12 (CKs 1, 5, 10, 14), CK7, CK17, synaptophysin, and chromogranin to determine the utility of neuroendocrine markers and epithelial markers in diagnosing primary lung cancers. Eighty-four percent (37 of 44) of the large cell and small cell neuroendocrine carcinomas were chromogranin-positive; 64% (21 of 36 small cell carcinomas and 6 of 6 large cell neuroendocrine carcinomas) were synaptophysin-positive; 5% (2 of 43) were keratin 34βE12-positive; 9% (4 of 44) were CK7-positive; and 5% (2 of 37) small cell carcinomas and 50% (3 of 6) large cell neuroendocrine carcinomas were B72.3-positive. Among 98 non-neuroendocrine carcinomas, 5% (5 of 98) were chromogranin-positive; 3% (3 of 98) were synaptophysin-positive; 97% (95 of 98) were positive for 34βE12 or CK7; and 99% (97 of 98) were positive for either keratin 34βE12, CK7, or B72.3. An antibody panel consisting of CK7, 34βE12, chromogranin, and synaptophysin separated 132 of 141 (94%) tumors into distinct groups. As discussed, this author believes that there are better panels than proposed by Lyda and Weiss[240] to differentiate neuroendocrine from non-neuroendocrine primary lung neoplasms.

Sturm and coworkers[241] evaluated 227 neuroendocrine proliferations and tumors for TTF-1, a factor that regulates lung morphogenesis and differentiation. Immunostaining was detected in 47 of 55 (85.5%) small cell lung cancers; in 31 of 64 (49%) large cell carcinomas; and in 0 of 15 (0%) neuroendocrine hyperplasias, 23 tumorlets, 27 typical carcinoid, and 23 atypical carcinoids. In 19 of 20 (95%) combined small cell lung cancers and large cell neuroendocrine carcinomas, TTF-1 was expressed in the neuroendocrine and non-neuroendocrine components of the tumor. The authors concluded that their findings challenged the concept of a spectrum of neuroendocrine neoplasms and suggested that the findings lended credence to the alternative

TABLE 12.18 Immunohistochemical Features of Various Types of Large Cell Undifferentiated Neoplasms Involving Lung

	Antibody Directed Against														
Type of Neoplasm	AE1/AE3	Low molecular weight keratin	High molecular weight keratin	CK7	CK20	Vimentin	Epithelial membrane antigen	CEA	S-100 Protein	HMB-45	CD30	CD20	Neuron-specific enolase	SYN	CGA
Large cell undifferentiated carcinoma of lung	+	+	S	S	–	S	S	S	R	N	N	N	S	R	R
Giant cell carcinoma of lung	+	+	S	S	–	S	S	S	R	N	N	N	S	R	R
Lymphoepithelioma-like carcinoma of lung	S	S	S	S	–	S	S	S	R	N	N	N	R	R	R
Large cell neuroendocrine carcinoma	S	S	S	S	–	S	S	S	R	N	N	N	+	+	S
Malignant melanoma	R	R	R	R	–	+	R	R	S	S	R	N	S	R	R
Anaplastic lymphoma	R	R	R	N	N	S	S	R	R	N	S	S	R	N	N

CEA, carcinoembryonic antigen; SYN, synaptophysin; CGA, chromogranin A.
Reactivity:
+, almost always diffuse, strong positivity
S, sometimes postive
R, rare cells positive
N, almost always negative

TABLE 12.19 Frequencies of CD2, CD3, CD4, CD5, CD7, CD8, CD56, and CD138 Expression in 447 Nonhematopoietic Neoplasms with Epithelioid Features

		Number of Positive Cases							
Tumor Type	**Total**	**CD2**	**CD3**	**CD4**	**CD5**	**CD7**	**CD8**	**CD56**	**CD138**
Lung									
Lung adenocarcinoma	21	0	0	0	2	8	0	1	11
Small cell carcinoma	6	0	0	0	0	0	0	6	0
Gastrointestinal tract									
Colon	10	0	0	0	5	6	0	0	9
Pancreatic carcinoma	13	0	0	0	6	9	0	0	4
Gastric adenocarcinoma	15	0	0	0	0	3	0	0	2
Hepatocellular carcinoma	25	0	0	0	0	0	0	0	15
Cholangiocarcinoma	14	0	0	0	12	13	0	3	13
Genitourinary tract									
Prostate carcinoma	18	0	0	0	4	0	0	1	6
Renal cell carcinoma	19	0	0	0	1	0	0	2	12
Transitional cell carcinoma	24	0	0	0	5	9	0	0	22
Female reproductive system									
Breast (ductal and lobular)	26	0	0	0	7	3	0	1	18
Ovarian carcinoma	24	0	0	0	3	8	0	2	10
Endometrial adenocarcinoma	10	0	0	0	0	3	0	1	9
Skin									
Squamous cell carcinoma	25	0	0	0	0	2	0	0	25
Basal cell carcinoma	20	0	0	0	0	2	0	0	14
Thyroid tumors									
Follicular adenoma	24	0	0	0	0	0	0	17	10
Papillary carcinoma	9	0	0	0	0	0	0	9	2
Medullary carcinoma	17	0	0	0	0	0	0	15	2
Neuroendocrine tumors									
Adrenal cortical neoplasm	20*	0	0	0	2	1	0	18	7
Neuroendocrine carcinoma	9	0	0	0	0	0	0	9	3
Carcinoid tumor	10	0	0	0	0	0	0	9	2
Merkel cell carcinoma	9	0	0	0	0	0	0	9	2
Miscellaneous									
Thymoma	8	0	0	0	0	0	0	0	0
Germ cell tumor	14	0	0	0	0	0	0	0	0
Malignant melanoma	20	0	0	0	2	8	0	1	1
Salivary gland tumor	11	0	0	0	1	1	0	0	3
Malignant mesothelioma	16†	0	0	0	2	4	0	0	0
Epithelioid sarcoma	10	0	0	0	3	7	0	2	0
Total	447	0 (0.0)	0 (0.0)	0 (0.0)	55 (12.3%)	87 (19.5%)	0 (0.0)	106 (23.7%)	202 (45.2%)

*An additional 10 cases of adrenocortical carcinomas were studied for CD56 expression. Of 30 cases, 25 were CD56-positive.
†An additional 5 cases of malignant mesothelioma were studied for CD138 expression. Of 21 cases, 1 was CD138-positive.
Reproduced from: Chu PG, Arber DA, Weiss LM. Expression of T/NK-cell and plasma cell antigens in nonhematopoietic epithelioid neoplasms: An immunohistochemical study of 447 cases. *Am J Clin Pathol.* 2003;120:64-70.

hypothesis of a common derivation for small cell lung carcinomas and non–small cell lung carcinomas. It is this author's opinion that Sturm and colleagues'[241] conclusion is difficult to accept because there is abundant biochemical, histochemical, and ultrastructural evidence of the association between different neuroendocrine lung neoplasms. In addition, as discussed previously, others have found TTF-1 expression in typical carcinoids and atypical carcinoids.

Barbareschi and associates[242] evaluated CDX-2 expression in routine samples of 20 normal endocrine/neuroendocrine tissues and 299 samples of well-differentiated neuroendocrine tumors and high-grade neuroendocrine carcinomas from different sites. CDX-2 was expressed at high levels in 81% of intestinal neuroendocrine carcinomas. Somewhat unexpectedly, CDX-2 was seen in 39% of neuroendocrine carcinomas of other sites. Reactivity was stated to have frequently overlapped TTF-1 expression, suggesting deregulated expression of homeobox genes in neuroendocrine carcinomas. The authors concluded that these findings resulted in a limited diagnostic role for CDX-2 in neuroendocrine carcinomas because of its frequent expression in non-gastrointestinal tumors.

Lin and colleagues[243] studied the value of CDX-2 and TTF-1 expression in separating metastatic neuroendocrine neoplasms of unknown origin. The authors[243] studied 155 primary neuroendocrine tumors, including 60 pulmonary, 60 gastrointestinal, 30 pancreatic, and 5 neuroendocrine tumors from other sites. In addition, they evaluated 13 metastatic neuroendocrine tumors, including 11 gastrointestinal and 2 pulmonary. CDX-2 was stated to have been expressed in 28 of 60 (47%) gastrointestinal neuroendocrine tumors. Of those that expressed CDX-2, 11 of 11 (100%) were appendiceal neuroendocrine tumors, 12 of 14 (86%) were small intestinal, 3 of 4 (75%) were colonic, 2 of 11 (18%) were rectal, and 0 of 20 (0%) were gastric. TTF-1 was stated to have been expressed in 13 of 30 (43%) pulmonary carcinoid tumors and in 27 of 30 (90%) pulmonary small cell lung cancers. In contrast to the study by Barbareschi and colleagues,[242] Lin and coworkers[243] concluded that CDX-2 expression was highly specific in identifying neuroendocrine tumors of intestinal origin and that TTF-1 expression was helpful in identifying neuroendocrine tumors of pulmonary origin.

Proliferation marker Ki-67 (MIB-1 clone) has been used to determine low-grade versus high-grade neuroendocrine carcinomas as reported by Lin and associates.[244] The authors stated that when MIB-1 immunoreactivity was considered, all low-grade neuroendocrine neoplasms showed immunoreactivity in less than 25% of the neoplastic cells in contrast to high-grade neuroendocrine neoplasms that showed MIB-1 immunoreactivity in greater than 50% of the neoplastic cells.

This observation was further expanded upon by Pelosi and colleagues[245] who observed seven patients with typical or atypical carcinoid tumors that were overdiagnosed as small cell lung cancers in bronchial biopsy specimens. The authors studied bronchial biopsies from 9 consecutive small cell lung carcinoma patients, histologically and immunohistochemically (cytokeratins,

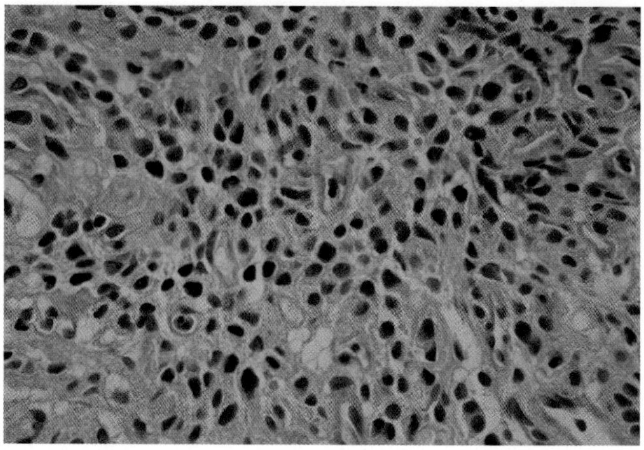

FIGURE 12.38 This transbronchial biopsy was initially diagnosed as a small cell lung cancer. X 400.

chromogranin A, synaptophysin, Ki-67/MIB-1, and TTF-1). The typical carcinoid tumors were centrally or peripherally located and composed of tumor cells with a granular or coarse nuclear chromatin pattern, intense chromogranin A and synaptophysin reactivity, and a low (<20%) Ki-67/MIB-1 labeling index. The carcinoid tumors' stroma contained thin-walled blood vessels. The small cell lung carcinomas were in a central location, had finely dispersed nuclear chromatin, and showed less intense immunostaining for chromogranin A and synaptophysin and a high (>50%) Ki-67/MIB-1 labeling index. The authors concluded that overdiagnosis of carcinoid tumors as small cell lung cancer in small, crushed bronchial biopsies remained a significant problem. They stated that careful evaluation of hematoxylin and eosin-stained sections was the most important tool in arriving at the correct diagnosis with evaluation of the tumor cell proliferation index by Ki-67/MIB-1 being the most useful ancillary technique for detection.

This author recently saw three such cases in which two neoplasms had initially been diagnosed as small cell carcinoma. All three patients were nonsmokers.

- The first patient was a 67-year-old man with a history of asbestos exposure and asbestosis who was initially diagnosed as small cell lung cancer. His tumor was in the right upper lobe and was surgically resected. The tumor was 3-cm in diameter, well-demarcated, and composed of uniform, round to slightly spindle-shaped cells with less than one mitoses per 50 high power fields and showing intense immunostaining for chromogranin A and synaptophysin and no immunostaining for TTF-1. The Ki-67 labeling index was less than 20%.
- The second patient was a 71-year-old woman whose transbronchial biopsy showed focal areas of crushed cells (Fig. 12.38) and was initially diagnosed as small cell lung cancer. On review, the neoplastic cells were round to slightly spindle shaped, had a uniform chromatin pattern, and showed no mitotic activity. The cytoplasm of the neoplastic cells showed intense immunostaining for chromogranin A and synaptophysin (Fig. 12.39) and no

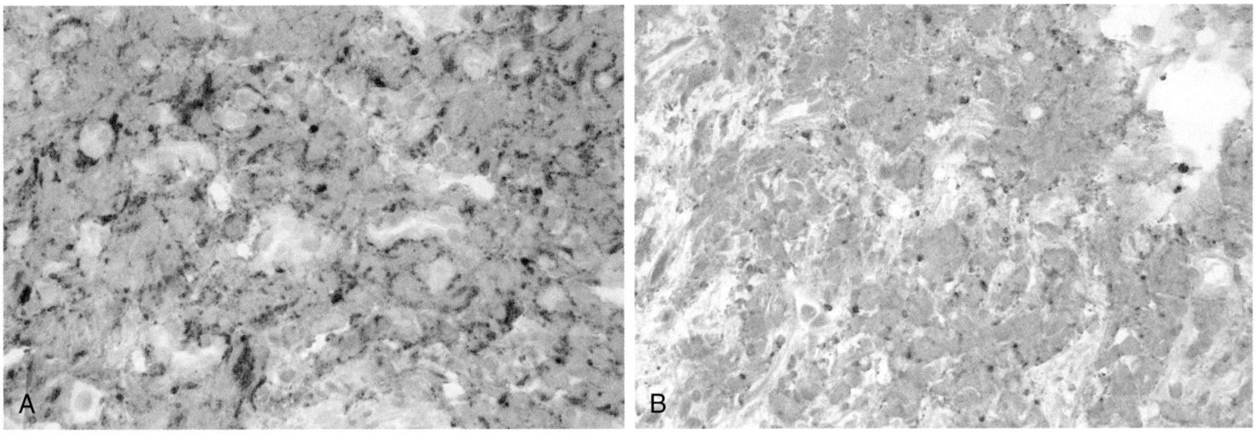

FIGURE 12.39 When evaluated by immunohistochemistry, the neoplastic cells showed intense immunostaining for synaptophysin **(A)** and chromogranin A **(B)**.

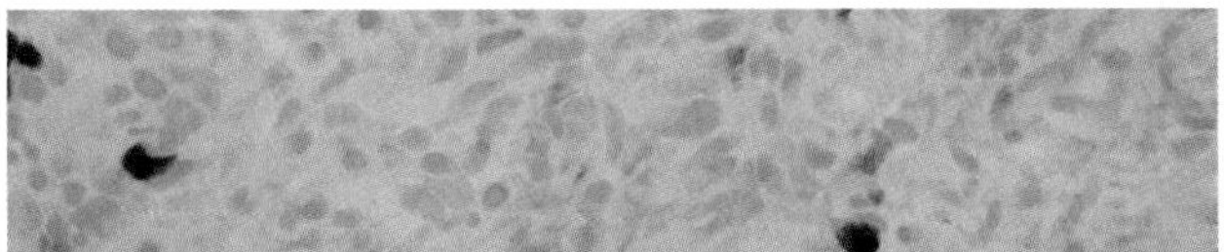

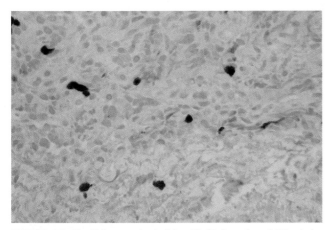

FIGURE 12.40 When evaluated for Ki-67, less than 20% of the neoplastic cells showed nuclear immunostaining.

immunostaining for TTF-1. The Ki-67 labeling index was less than 20% (Fig. 12.40).

- The third patient was a 70-year-old man whose transbronchial biopsy showed a uniform population of cells with focal crush artifact but no necrosis or mitotic activity. The neoplastic cells showed no immunostaining for TTF-1 but showed intense immunostaining for chromogranin A and synaptophysin. The Ki-67 labeling index was less than 20%.

Non–small cell primary lung neoplasms may show neuroendocrine differentiation. This can cause confusion if the neoplasm being evaluated is considered histologically to have features suggestive of a non-neuroendocrine tumor. Visscher and coworkers[246] evaluated 56 poorly differentiated non–small cell primary lung neoplasms with monoclonal antibodies directed against chromogranin A, synaptophysin, S-100 protein, keratin, vimentin, and neurofilament antigen. These neoplasms were stated to show no histologic features of neuroendocrine differentiation. Using frozen, unfixed tissue sections, 5 of 17 (29%) large cell undifferentiated carcinomas and 4 of 19 (21%) adenocarcinomas showed immunostaining for chromogranin A or synaptophysin. Diffuse intense immunostaining for synaptophysin was observed in two large cell undifferentiated carcinomas and one poorly differentiated adenocarcinoma. One of 20 (5%) poorly differentiated squamous carcinomas expressed synaptophysin. Of interest, 10 of 17 (58.8%) large cell undifferentiated carcinomas and 10 of 19 (52.6%) poorly differentiated adenocarcinomas expressed vimentin or neurofilament antigen. The authors concluded that immunohistologic evidence of neuroendocrine differentiation was observed in a significant number of large cell undifferentiated carcinomas and poorly differentiated adenocarcinomas and was accompanied by heterogeneous intermediate filament expression. This author has evaluated neurofilament expression in undifferentiated or poorly differentiated primary lung carcinomas, and over half of such neoplasms coexpressed keratin and vimentin, even if they did not show neuroendocrine differentiation by immunohistochemistry.

Linnoila and colleagues[247] evaluated 113 surgically resected primary lung neoplasms with antibodies against chromogranin A, Leu7, neuron-specific enolase, serotonin, bombesin, calcitonin, ACTH, vasopressin, neurotensin, CEA, keratin, vimentin, and neurofilament using formalin-fixed paraffin-embedded sections. They observed that the majority of typical carcinoids and small cell carcinomas expressed multiple neuroendocrine markers in a high percentage of tumor cells and that approximately 50% of non–small cell lung carcinomas contained subpopulations of tumor cells expressing neuroendocrine markers. They found occasional non–small cell lung carcinomas that showed immunostaining patterns indistinguishable from small cell carcinoma. They also found that neuroendocrine markers were expressed more frequently in large cell undifferentiated carcinomas and in adenocarcinomas than in squamous carcinomas.

Mooi and associates[248] evaluated 11 resected primary lung neoplasms classified as large cell carcinoma or squamous cell carcinoma but showing some microscopic resemblance to bronchial carcinoid and small cell carcinoma. All cases were neuron-specific enolase and protein gene product 9.5-positive, which the authors stated was indicative of neuroendocrine differentiation. Bombesin and chromogranin were positive in 2 cases each, and C-terminal peptide was expressed in 5 cases. In 6 of 7 cases evaluated by electron microscopy, dense core neuroendocrine granules were observed. Based on the published photographs of the neoplasms, one might argue that the neoplasms reported represented mixed neuroendocrine—non-neuroendocrine tumors.

Wick and colleagues[249] compared 12 large cell carcinomas of lung showing neuroendocrine differentiation with 15 large cell pulmonary neoplasms showing no neuroendocrine differentiation. From data presented, the large cell neoplasms showing neuroendocrine differentiation would have been classified by Travis and colleagues'[56] criteria as large cell neuroendocrine carcinomas and not as large cell undifferentiated carcinomas showing focal neuroendocrine differentiation. Of interest and potential importance, the large cell neoplasms with neuroendocrine differentiation had a significantly worse prognosis than those that did not show neuroendocrine differentiation. The authors suggested that immunohistochemistry and electron microscopy were necessary to diagnose such neoplasms and that they were probably underdiagnosed. Some medical oncologists suggest that all large cell carcinomas of lung be evaluated for neuroendocrine differentiation because of potential differences in chemotherapeutic treatment. This may or may not be appropriate based on a study discussed later in this chapter.

Loy and coworkers[250] evaluated 66 neoplasms that had been examined ultrastructurally and with a battery of neuroendocrine markers, including neuron-specific enolase, chromogranin A, Leu7, and synaptophysin, and with a non-neuroendocrine marker (B72.3). They studied 11 small cell carcinomas, 4 low-grade neuroendocrine carcinomas (? atypical carcinoids), 2 large cell carcinomas with neuroendocrine differentiation (? large cell neuroendocrine carcinomas), 26 adenocarcinomas, 10 squamous cell carcinomas, and 11 large cell undifferentiated carcinomas. Four of 10 squamous carcinomas, 3 of 26 adenocarcinomas, and 1 of 11 large cell undifferentiated carcinomas showed immunostaining for chromogranin A. Zero of 10 squamous carcinomas, 4 of 26 adenocarcinomas, and 0 of 11 large cell undifferentiated carcinomas showed immunostaining for Leu7. Six of 10 squamous carcinomas, 15 of 26 adenocarcinomas, and 7 of 11 large cell undifferentiated carcinomas showed immunostaining for neuron-specific enolase. Six of 10 squamous carcinomas, 16 of 26 adenocarcinomas, and 7 of 11 large cell undifferentiated carcinomas showed immunostaining for synaptophysin. Overall, 34 of 47 (79%) carcinomas without neuroendocrine features expressed at least one neuroendocrine immunohistochemical marker. Nineteen of 19 (100%) of neuroendocrine carcinomas expressed at least one neuroendocrine marker.

Xu and associates[251] used immunohistochemical analysis to study novel protein K homology domain containing protein overexpressed in cancer (KOC) in neuroendocrine lung cancers. KOC was stated to be a member of the insulin-like growth factor (IGF) messenger RNA-binding protein family and was expressed during embryogenesis and certain malignancies. The authors studied neuroendocrine lung neoplasms. Ten small cell lung cancers exhibited strong cytoplasmic staining—nine with diffuse positivity and one with focal positivity. Fourteen large cell neuroendocrine carcinomas expressed KOC; 9 of them exhibited strong and diffuse cytoplasmic staining, and 5 cases showed focal immunoreactivity. In contrast, no KOC was detected in 21 typical and atypical carcinoids, except for 1 atypical carcinoid with oncocytic features. The authors stated that although small cell lung cancers exhibited a strong and diffuse staining pattern more frequently than large cell neuroendocrine carcinomas, the difference did not reach statistical significance. The authors concluded that their findings of equivalent IGF-II expression in KOC-positive SCLC and LCNEC and KOC-negative carcinoid tumors suggested different regulatory mechanisms in the control of IGF-II expression in these tumors. This perhaps could be another way for pathologists to avoid the trap of misdiagnosing typical carcinoids as small cell lung cancers or atypical carcinoids.

Schleusener and colleagues[252] evaluated 107 patients with stage III A, stage III B and stage IV non–small cell lung carcinomas (62 adenocarcinomas, 22 squamous cell carcinomas, 18 large cell carcinomas, 5 adenosquamous carcinomas) immunohistochemically with antibodies against keratin, synaptophysin, Leu7, and chromogranin A. Keratin was used as a control and was positive in 99.1% of cases. Thirty-five percent of adenocarcinomas, 41% of squamous carcinomas, and 33% of large cell carcinomas expressed at least one neuroendocrine marker. Somewhat surprising was the finding of increased survival in patients whose tumors expressed one or more neuroendocrine markers. However, there was no correlation between neuroendocrine markers and response to chemotherapy.

The bottom line for pathologists is that lung neoplasms that are not classified by histologic criteria as being a neuroendocrine neoplasm may express neuroendocrine markers by immunohistochemistry. A summary of these studies showing the frequency of expression of chromogranin A, synaptophysin, neuron-specific enolase, and Leu7 is shown in Fig. 12.41.

Ralston and colleagues[253] evaluated MASH1 as a marker in differentiating small cell lung cancer from Merkel cell carcinoma. The authors pointed out that Merkel cell carcinoma is a rare aggressive neoplasm of the skin with a neuroendocrine phenotype and was regarded as the cutaneous counterpart of small cell carcinoma. The authors correctly pointed out that, morphologically, metastatic small cell carcinoma could be confused with Merkel cell carcinoma. The authors pointed out that achaete-scute complex-like 1 (ASCL1), also called *mammalian* or *human achaete-scute complex homolog-1 (MASH1, HASH1)*, was a basic helix-loop-helix transcription factor that was crucial for neuroendocrine cell differentiation. The authors stated that MASH1 had been reported to be expressed in some neuroendocrine neoplasms, including small cell lung cancer. The authors studied 30 cases

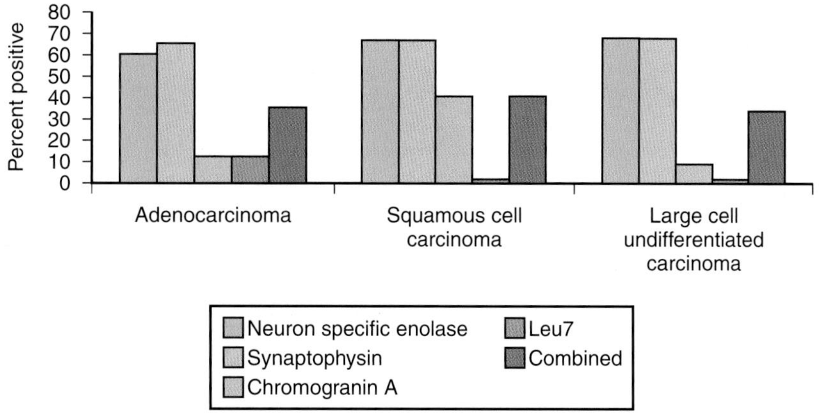

FIGURE 12.41 Summary of expression of neuroendocrine markers in histologically diagnosed non-neuroendocrine neoplasms. Neuroendocrine expression in non-neuroendocrine lung neoplasms is usually focal and is usually of low intensity.

of Merkel cell carcinoma and 59 cases of small cell lung cancer that were immunostained for MASH1 and TTF-1 antibodies. Of the 59 small cell lung carcinomas, 49 (83%) expressed MASH1 in a nuclear staining pattern, whereas out of 59 small cell lung carcinomas, 43 (73%) expressed TTF-1 in a nuclear staining pattern. MASH1 was stated to be completely negative in all 30 Merkel cell carcinomas, whereas TTF-1 expression was seen in 1 of 30 (3%) Merkel cell carcinomas. The authors concluded that MASH1 was a useful adjunct for differentiating small cell carcinoma of the lung from Merkel cell carcinoma.

KEY DIAGNOSTIC POINTS

Immunohistologic Pitfalls of Primary versus Metastatic Carcinoma in Lung

- CDX2 expression may be seen in primary mucinous "colloid" pulmonary carcinomas. They may also express CK20 and lack CK7 and TTF-1. Clinical correlation and imaging may be critically necessary in these situations.
- GCDFP-15 may be expressed in up to 5% of primary lung adenocarcinomas. These tumors often have abundant extracellular mucin, and they typically express TTF-1 and synaptophysin. Caution is in order in the hunt for metastatic breast carcinoma in this situation.
- Alpha inhibin may be seen in nearly 25% of primary lung carcinomas. Additional panel markers, especially keratins, will obviate this pitfall.
- Some clones of estrogen receptor may demonstrate positive immunostaining in primary lung adenocarcinoma. Estrogen receptor should not be used as a diagnostic application in this setting.

Theranostic Applications

More than 50 protein markers have been assessed by immunohistochemistry for their prognostic value in NSCLC patients.[254] To date, none is sufficiently robust for adoption in patient care. More recent studies conducted on tumor samples of patients involved in large phase III placebo controlled randomized adjuvant chemotherapy trials have revealed optimism about some IHC markers. The International Adjuvant Lung Trial (IALT) demonstrated that immunohistochemical assessment of ERCC1 (excision repair cross-complementation group 1) expression in non–small cell lung cancer before chemotherapy is an independent predictor of the effect of adjuvant chemotherapy.[255] ERCC1 is 1 of 16 genes that encode the proteins of the nucleotide excision repair complex. Patients with completely resected non–small cell lung cancer and ERCC1-negative tumors showed a substantial benefit from adjuvant cisplatin-based chemotherapy, compared with patients with ERCC1-positive tumors.[255,256]

The significance of EGFR protein expression in NSCLC in predicting response to tyrosine kinase inhibitors (TKI) remains contradictory and a standard method has not been adopted.[257-259] Recently reported results of comparative analysis of EGFR protein expression in NSCLC by immunohistochemistry using the Dako EGFR PharmDx kit (scoring percent of positive tumor cells) and Zymed monoclonal antibody clone 31G7 (combined scoring of percent of positive cells and intensity of staining) suggested that the Dako PharmDx kit and percentage of positive staining may provide more accurate prediction of gefitinib treatment on survival.[260] Recent studies suggest that EGFR immunopositivity may play a role as selection criteria for cetuximab-based therapy, but this needs to be further validated.

Several markers including HER2/neu, Ki-67, p53, and BCL-2 were suggested to be important as prognostic markers by meta-analysis.[254] Cyclin E, VEGF A, $p16^{INK4A}$, $p27^{kip1}$, and β-catenin are promising candidates but need further study in large randomized clinical trial samples using standardized assays and scoring systems.[254]

Beyond Immunohistochemistry: Anatomic Molecular Diagnostic Applications

A high likelihood of response to EGFR TKIs in lung adenocarcinoma patients correlates with somatic mutations in the exons 18-21 of the TK domain of the EGFR

TABLE 12.20 Methods for Detecting EGFR Mutations in Lung Cancer Specimens

Technique	Sensitivity (% Mutant DNA)	Mutations Identified	Comprehensive Detection of Deletions and Insertions
Direct sequencing	25	Known and new	Yes
PCR-SSCP	10	Known and new	Yes
TaqMan PCR	10	Known only	No
Loop-hybrid mobility shift assay	7.5	Known only	Yes
Cycleave PCR	5	Known only	Yes
PCR-RFLP and length analysis	5	Known only	Yes
MALDI-TOF MS-based genotyping	5	Known only	No
PNA-LNA PCR clamp	1	Known only	No
Scorpions ARMS	1	Known only	No
dHPLC	1	Known and new	Yes
Single-molecule sequencing	0.2	Known and new	Yes
Mutant-enriched PCR	0.2	Known only	No
SMAP	0.1	Known only	No

SSCP, single-strand conformation polymorphism; PNA-LNA, peptide nucleic acid-locked nucleic acid; MALDI-TOF MS, matrix-assisted laser desorption/ionization time-of-flight mass spectrometry; ARMS, amplified refractory mutation system; dHPLC, denaturing high performance liquid chromatography.

Modified from Pao W, Ladanyi M. Epidermal growth factor receptor mutation testing in lung cancer: Searching for the ideal method. [comment]. *Clin Cancer Res.* 2007:13:4954-4955.

gene.[261-263] The most common are in-frame deletions in exon 19 (45%), followed by a point mutation (CTG to CGG) in exon 21 at nucleotide 2573, which results in substitution of leucine by arginine at codon 858 (L858R) (41%). Other less common mutations that are associated with sensitivity to EGFR TKIs include G719 mutations in exon 18 and L861 mutations in exon 21. Exon 19 deletions are also associated with better survival independent of EGFR TKI treatment.[264] These data suggest that EGFR mutations in addition to predictive value have prognostic significance. Direct DNA sequencing is the most common method of mutational analysis, but other more sensitive methods summarized in Table 12.20 are also used in a clinical practice.[265] These assays can be performed on a fresh, frozen, and archival FFPE tissue, including surgical resection specimens or fine needle biopsies.[266,267] Resistance mutation D790M in exon 20 has been identified in up to 50% of patients who were initially sensitive to TKIs.[268] Resistance is also associated with MET oncogene amplification, which could be detected by FISH in only 3% of primary naïve lung adenocarcinomas and about 21% of EGFR TKI treated adenocarcinomas that developed resistance.[269,270]

KRAS mutations of codon 12 are negative predictors of lung adenocarcinoma response to EGFR TKI therapy and are an adverse prognostic factor.[271,272] HER2 (3%) and BRAF (1%) mutations are rarely identified in lung adenocarcinomas but are mutually exclusive with EGFR mutations.[273]

Development of new targeted therapies has resulted in clinical testing in lung adenocarcinomas beyond EGFR mutational status. Some clinical laboratories have put into practice a comprehensive mutational profile for lung adenocarcinomas (Fig. 12.42).

EGFR mutations are frequently associated with increased EGFR gene copy numbers. There is still ongoing discussion about most appropriate clinical testing for establishing EGFR status in lung adenocarcinoma, particularly gene copy number analysis (FISH or CISH).[274-278] The main issue with EGFR FISH is lack of standardized interpretation criteria. Conflicting results regarding prediction of tumor response to EGFR TKIs were demonstrated in multiple studies using University of Colorado scoring system for EGFR FISH (see Table 12.20).[274,276,277] Some studies also used qPCR. Increased EGFR copy number detected by FISH may be a predictor of a patient's response to cetuximab.[279]

Recent literature also explored chromogenic in-situ hybridization (CISH) as a method of choice for detection of EGFR copy number in FFPE tissue.[280] The results showed good correlation with FISH analysis, however chromosome 7 polysomy cannot be readily distinguished from EGFR amplification. The importance of distinguishing polysomy from gene amplification is still uncertain.

Several recent abstracts/articles have discussed theranostic applications in primary lung cancer. Barletta and coworkers[281] studied 125 consecutive patients with lung adenocarcinomas treated at the Brigham and Women's Hospital between 1997 and 1999. The authors found that TTF-1 protein expression identified by immunohistochemistry was highly correlated with TTF-1 gene amplification and was associated with a better overall survival in patients with high levels of TTF-1 expression. TTF-1 gene amplification was a predictor of poor

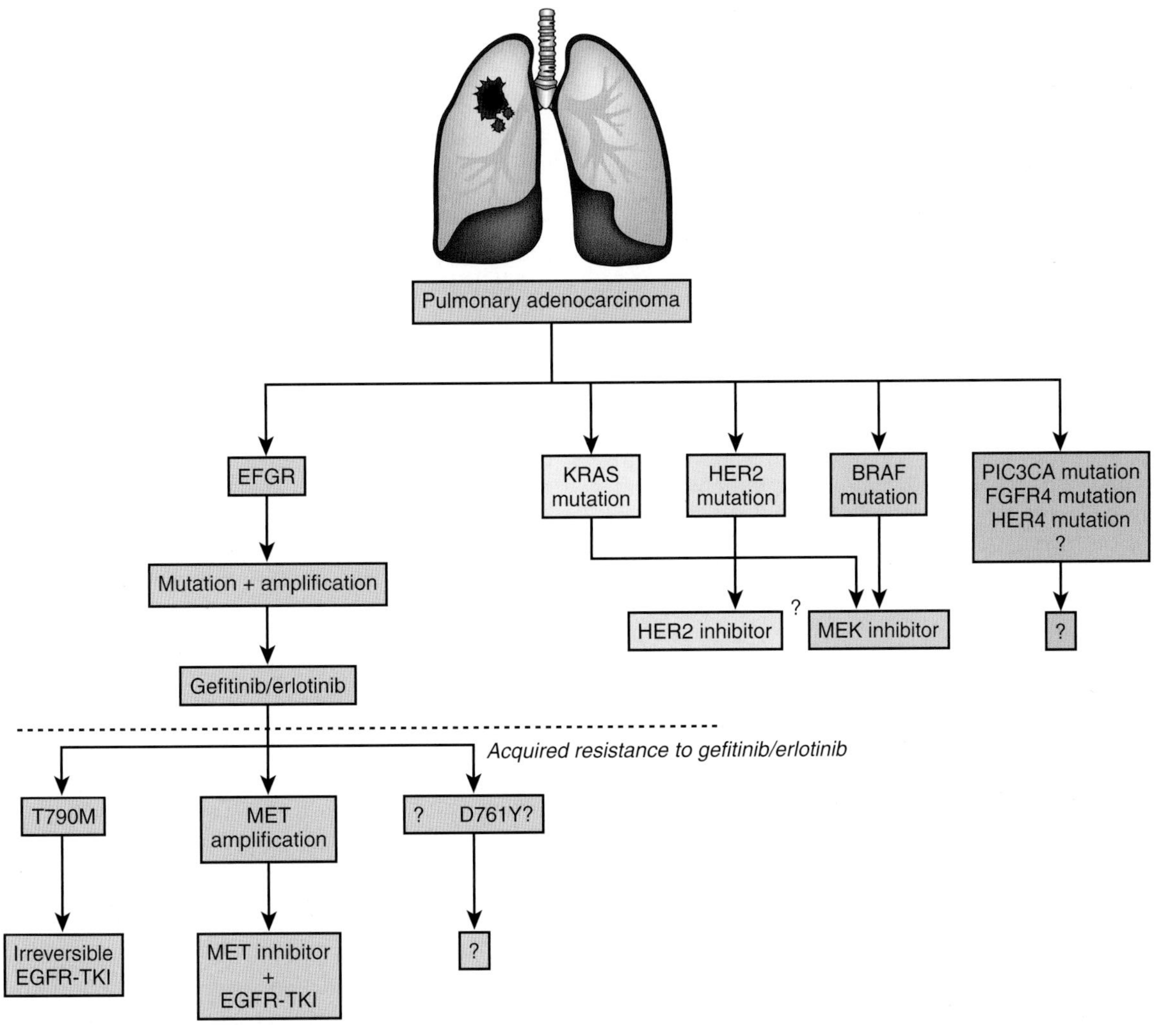

FIGURE 12.42 Comprehensive mutational profile for lung adenocarcinoma.

outcome. Their results indicated that TTF-1 expression by immunohistochemistry and TTF-1 gene amplification by FISH could be significant prognostic factors for patients with lung adenocarcinomas.

Beasley and associates[282] studied hypoxia-induced factor-1 alpha (HIF-1) in 187 adenocarcinomas, 90 squamous cell carcinomas, 70 non–small cell lung cancers not otherwise specified, 40 typical carcinoids, 5 atypical carcinoids, 11 large cell neuroendocrine carcinomas, and 39 small cell carcinomas. The authors found that HIF-1 was expressed in the majority of pulmonary neuroendocrine carcinomas regardless of grade and was seen more frequently in neuroendocrine carcinomas than in non–small cell lung carcinomas. The finding of HIF-1 in the majority of typical carcinoids suggested that HIF-1 was not necessarily an independent marker for an aggressive behavior in neuroendocrine carcinomas. In contrast, low-level expression of HIF-1 in adenocarcinomas/BAC carcinomas compared to non–small cell lung cancers was reflected the less aggressive behavior of adenocarcinoma/BAC adenocarcinomas. The authors stated that a high level of HIF-1 expression in neuroendocrine carcinomas could indicate a role for HIF-1 targeted therapy.

Beheshti and colleagues[283] studied TTF-1 positivity as a predictor of epidermal growth factor receptor mutation and treatment response in pulmonary adenocarcinomas. The authors found that strong/extensive TTF-1 staining was a statistically significant and sensitive predictor of EGFR mutation and response to tyrosine kinase inhibitor treatment. Weak/absent TTF-1 staining had a very high negative predictive value for treatment response. The authors concluded that in centers where EGFR analysis was not available, a pathologist's interpretation of weak/absent TTF-1 (score <2+) might help exclude patients from EGFR testing and/or tyrosine kinase inhibitor therapy.

Kundu and colleagues[284] evaluated alpha-methylacyl-coA-racemase (AMACR) in tissue microarrays made from 240 non–small cell lung cancers. The authors concluded that AMACR expression in poorly differentiated large cell carcinomas of the lung was statistically associated with a poor five-year survival in early stage patients with prior presumably curative resection. The authors suggested that AMACR expression may serve in stratifying these patients into a category of increased risk of death from their cancer despite resection. The authors stated that increased AMACR expression in lung cancers might serve as a target for molecular radiology and therapy.

Perner and colleagues[285] evaluated TTF-1 amplification with respect to TTF-1 overexpression in 198 lung adenocarcinomas using FISH. The authors found a significantly higher TTF-1 expression in adenocarcinomas with TTF-1 amplification as compared to adenocarcinomas without amplification. There was a trend toward patients with TTF-1 amplification having a worse outcome than patients without TTF-1 amplification. The authors concluded that TTF-1 expression might be a prognostic biomarker for lung adenocarcinomas.

Vohra and associates[286] studied IMP3 expression in 247 primary non–small cell lung cancers (187 adenocarcinomas, 90 squamous cell carcinomas) by immunohistochemistry. IMP3 is an oncofetal RNA-binding protein and member of the insulin growth factor family and has been proven useful as a biomarker of disease progression in renal cell carcinoma. The authors stated that IMP3 immunostaining was found in 98 (52.4%) adenocarcinomas and 69 (76.6%) squamous cell carcinomas. The authors concluded that IMP3 expression in greater than 30% of tumor cells showed a strong positive trend in predicting a better 5-year survival in early stage squamous cell carcinomas of the lung. The authors stated that this marker could be useful in stratifying squamous cell carcinomas in studies of new therapies and as a potential target for molecular therapies.

Cutz and colleagues[287] used immunohistochemistry to evaluate epidermal growth factor and downstream effectors such as extracellular signal-regulated kinase (ERK). The authors studied 44 patients who received curative chemoradiation therapy and found a radiographic response of 50.15±15% at 6 weeks post-therapy with an overall survival of 14.13±9.6 months. The authors observed a statistically significant negative correlation between membrane and cytoplasmic p-EGFR and overall survival. Cytoplasmic p-Erk levels correlated negatively with radiographic response. The authors concluded that their study suggested p-EGFR levels (and not total-EGFR levels as measured by IHC) served as an independent poor prognostic factor in a subset of patients. The authors found that IHC scores of cytoplasmic p-Erk appeared to predict poor radiographic response to curative chemoradiation therapy in locally advanced non–small cell lung cancers.

Li and coworkers[288] studied overexpression of NRF2 and p53 in pulmonary papillary adenocarcinomas by immunohistochemistry on tissue microarrays. The authors found that NRF2 and p53 were strongly expressed in papillary adenocarcinoma cancer cells and that NRF2 overexpression correlated with p53 expression and was independent of tumor size and stage. The authors concluded that NRF2 overexpression by virtually all cancer cells in papillary adenocarcinoma differed from results in other non–small cell lung cancers and could relate to poor prognosis and chemotherapeutic response. The authors stated that the regulation mechanism of NRF2 could involve several signaling pathways, and that further studies were needed to understand chemotherapeutic resistance in patients with this type of cancer.

Luu and colleagues[289] studied the prognostic value of aspartyl (asparaginyl) hydroxylase (AAH) in 375 lung carcinomas using tissue microarrays studied by immunohistochemistry. The authors concluded that among lung carcinomas, AAH expression was associated with a poor prognosis for bronchioloalveolar cell carcinoma and squamous cell carcinoma, and a strong trend for poor prognosis for large cell undifferentiated carcinoma.

Shahjahan and associates[290] studied ProEx C, a biomarker reagent containing antibodies to minichromosome maintenance protein 2 (MCM2) and topoisomerase II A (TOP2A) used to detect aberrant S-phase induction in cells. The authors studied 289 non–small cell lung cancers using immunohistochemistry and found ProEx C expression in more than two-thirds of the cancers and an association between strong expression and a longer 5-year survival in certain cellular subtypes. The findings suggested a role in tumor progression of these cancer cells and might be a potential basis for targeted therapy.

Sienko and colleagues[291] evaluated galectin-4 expression in 264 stage I and II non–small cell lung cancers by immunohistochemistry. Galectin-4 was stated to be a member of the galectin family of binding proteins (beta-galactosides) that play a major role in regulation of cell differentiation, cell proliferation, and apoptosis. The authors stated that their study showed an association between galectin-4 overexpression and a trend toward a worse prognosis in early stage non–small cell lung cancers. They stated that galectin-4 could prove to be a useful prognostic marker in non–small cell lung cancers and for therapeutic targets.

Song and colleagues[292] studied c-Met expression in pulmonary neuroendocrine tumors. The authors stated that c-Met was a tyrosine kinase receptor that played an important role in tumor growth, invasion, metastasis, and drug resistance. The authors studied 44 carcinoids, 35 small cell lung cancers, and 9 large cell neuroendocrine carcinomas by immunochemistry. c-Met expression was stated to have been frequently observed in all three categories of neuroendocrine lung tumors, supporting the potential use of c-Met as a therapeutic target in tumors, including small cell lung cancer and large cell neuroendocrine carcinoma.

Haque and coworkers[293] studied tissue micro-arrays constructed from 43 small cell lung cancers that were immunostained with E-cadherin and pan-cadherin. The authors stated that E-cadherin and pan-cadherin expression was seen in 40% of tumors, and that there was a significant inverse correlation between E-cadherin and pan-cadherin in the expression and presence of metastasis at diagnosis. Reduced or lack of E-cadherin expression and pan-cadherin in small cell lung cancers was associated with metastasis and, consequently, a higher stage and poorer prognosis. The authors suggested that the regulation of cadherin-mediated adhesion might be a potential therapeutic target for control of small cell lung cancer metastasis.

Homan and associates[294] studied down-regulation of GADD45a protein expression in non–small cell lung cancers. Decreased GADD45a expression was observed in 69 of 115 (60%) non–small cell lung cancers, including 66% of squamous cell carcinomas, 51% of adenocarcinomas, and 64% of bronchioloalveolar lung cancers (BACs). Down-regulation was noted in 100% of cases in which death occurred within one year of diagnosis and 78% within five years versus 40% of cases of death beyond five years. The authors concluded that GADD45a expression was significantly decreased in non–small cell lung cancers compared with adjacent non-neoplastic bronchial epithelium. Squamous cell carcinomas of higher stage and those with decreased survival showed a down-regulation of GADD45a protein expression. The authors stated that the results showed evidence for an association between altered GADD45a expression and tumorigenesis.

Malik and colleagues[295] studied RON, a member of MET proto-oncogene family of tyrosine kinase receptors in 175 cases of primary and metastatic lung cancer by immunohistochemistry. The authors found that RON was widely expressed and constitutively phosphorylated in all histotypes of lung cancer with a potential role as a novel therapeutic target. The authors found a positive correlation between RON/p-RON expression levels, higher tumor stage, and more regional spread of tumors, suggesting RON was likely involved with a more malignant state through its proliferative, motile, and morphologic effects. The authors stated that RON provided prognostic information and helped to identify patients who required adjuvant therapy for small cell lung cancer and more extensive resection for non–small cell lung cancer patients.

CD117 (c-*kit*) is a transmembrane tyrosine kinase receptor that has been immunolocalized in various neoplasms, the most notable of which is gastrointestinal stromal tumors where c-*kit* is felt to be a relatively specific and sensitive immunohistochemical marker of gastrointestinal stromal tumors. If a gastrointestinal stromal tumor expresses CD117, it is usually treated with Gleevec. CD117 has been evaluated in lung and pleural neoplasms.[296-299]

Lonardo and colleagues[296] evaluated c-*kit* expression in primary lung cancer and mesothelioma using two antibodies with and without heat-induced epitope retrieval. Positive reactivity was observed predominantly in small cell lung cancers and, infrequently, in other cancers. Using the Dako antibody, 7 of 33 mesotheliomas showed immunostaining. The authors concluded that c-*kit* expression in small cell lung cancer suggests that it plays an important role in the biology of this malignancy and could be targeted in subsets of patients for therapy using c-*kit* inhibitors.

In the report by Pelosi and colleagues,[297] membranous CD117 immunostaining was observed in 19 of 88 adenocarcinomas (22%) and 15 of 113 squamous cell carcinomas (13%). Cytoplasmic labeling was seen in 28 adenocarcinomas and 8 squamous cell carcinomas. In the tumors that showed membranous immunostaining for CD117, immunoreactivity was associated with a higher proliferative fraction and with features of more aggressive tumor behavior, including higher stage, size, and grade, as well as occurrence of clinical symptoms and other changes. Immunoreactive tumors exhibited increased levels of BCL-2, cyclin-E, HER2/neu, p27, and fascin. The authors concluded that CD117 immunoreactivity identified a peculiar subset of stage I adenocarcinomas and squamous cell carcinomas of lung that could have prognostic relevance in patients whose tumor expressed CD117. They also suggested that targeting the CD117 pathway could be a novel therapeutic strategy in treating a subset of primary lung cancers.

The study by Casali and associates[298] investigated c-*kit* protein overexpression in large cell neuroendocrine carcinomas because it had been observed in small cell lung cancers and was associated with a poor prognosis. They used a polyclonal c-*kit* antibody and evaluated 33 patients who had undergone radical resection. Overall, one-, three- and five-year survival rates were 79%, 58%, and 51%, respectively in tumors that expressed c-*kit*. The authors stated that survival analysis showed no difference for any clinicopathologic features except for CD117 immunostaining. One and 3-year survival rates were 91% and 82%, respectively, for CD117-negative large cell neuroendocrine carcinomas and 72% and 44%, respectively, for CD117-positive ones. The authors also stated that CD117 expression was associated with an elevated recurrence rate (60% versus 23% for CD117-positive and CD117-negative large cell neuroendocrine carcinomas, respectively). These authors concluded that c-*kit* protein was frequently expressed in large cell neuroendocrine carcinoma and represented a negative prognostic factor.

Butnor and colleagues[299] used a polyclonal c-*kit* antibody to evaluate 61 lung/pleural cancers, including 11 small cell carcinomas, 4 large cell neuroendocrine carcinomas, 22 squamous cell carcinomas, 23 adenocarcinomas, 11 pulmonary typical carcinoid tumors, 19 pleural malignant mesotheliomas, and 6 localized pleural fibrous tumors. Small cell lung cancers demonstrated c-*kit* staining in 82% of cases, nearly all of which demonstrated moderate to intense immunoreactivity. Immunostaining was observed in 25% of large cell neuroendocrine carcinomas, and focal staining was observed in 9% of squamous cell carcinomas and 17% of adenocarcinomas. Typical pulmonary carcinoid tumors showed no reactivity. Moderately intense immunostaining was noted in 50% of localized fibrous tumors of the lung, and malignant mesotheliomas were nonreactive for c-*kit* in 95% of cases. The authors concluded that the high frequency of c-*kit* immunostaining in small cell lung carcinoma could have important potential therapeutic implications.

Maddau and coworkers[300] used immunohistochemical detection to evaluate the expression of p53 and Ki-67 in non–small cell lung cancer. They found that overexpression of p53 was associated with a significantly worse patient outcome in stage I disease, whereas no excess risk was evident in stages II and III disease. The same pattern was observed with Ki-67 expression. The authors found that excess risk in stage I cases with p53 and Ki-67 overexpression was observed only in adenocarcinoma.

Kobayashi and colleagues[301] evaluated endogenous secretory receptor for advanced glycation end products in 182 non–small cell lung cancer surgical specimens. The authors found that endogenous secretory receptor for advanced glycation end-product expression in cytoplasm was reduced or absent in 137 of 182 (75%) carcinomas in contrast to normal lung tissue. mRNA expression was also suppressed in the cancer cells. The authors found that among patients with low expression of the cytoplasmic secretory receptor, the overall survival rate was significantly lower than that of patients with normal expression. The authors concluded that cytoplasmic endogenous secretory receptor for advanced glycation end-product expression had the potential to be a prognostic factor for predicting outcome of curative surgery in patients with non–small cell lung cancer.

Allen and colleagues[302] studied the expression of glutathione S-transferase p and glutathione synthase in 201 non–small cell lung cancers by immunohistochemistry with antibodies against GST-p and GSH2 using standard immunostaining techniques. Nuclear staining with GST-p in greater than 10% of cells was closely associated with decreased survival in stage I and II squamous cell carcinomas (n = 40). Cytoplasmic staining showed a similar trend that did not reach statistical significance. No significant correlation between GST-p staining and survival was determined for other histologic types of non–small cell lung cancer. Cytoplasmic GSH2 staining in greater than 80% of tumor cells was associated with a trend toward improved survival for stage I adenocarcinoma ($P = .08$) but did not show a relationship to survival for other histologic types. The authors concluded that GST-p expression predicted prognosis in stage I and II squamous cell lung cancer, and that GSH2 expression may indicate better survival in early stage adenocarcinoma of the lung. The authors also stated that manipulation of GST-p and GSH2 had the potential basis for treatment of some non–small cell lung cancers.

Lee and associates[303] studied the significance of extranodal expression of regional lymph nodes in surgically resected non–small cell lung cancer. The authors studied 199 non–small cell lung cancer patients who were found to have regional lymph node involvement after resection. Histologic examination included tumor cell type, grade of differentiation, vascular invasion, regional lymph node metastasis emphasizing the number and station of lymph node involvement, the presence or absence of extranodal extension, and the immunohistochemistry of p53 expression. The authors found that extranodal extension was significantly higher in women, in those with adenocarcinoma, in advanced stage disease, in tumors with vascular invasion, or with p53 overexpression. Multivariate analysis of survival, the presence or total number of lymph nodes with extranodal extension, tumor stage, and p53 expression were significant prognostic factors.

Fukuoka and colleagues[304] studied desmoglein 3, a desmosomal protein of the cadherin family, in primary non–small cell lung cancers and neuroendocrine tumors by immunohistochemical analysis. The authors found that negative immunohistochemical staining with desmoglein 3 was associated with a shorter survival for all lung cancer patients, regardless of histologic type (5-year survival of 20.9% versus 49.5%, $P < .001$). In patients with atypical carcinoid tumors that lacked desmoglein 3 expression, the 5-year survival rate was 0% compared with 36.8% for cases that showed desmoglein 3 expression. The authors concluded that desmoglein 3 status indicated a poor prognosis in lung cancers and portended a more aggressive behavior for atypical carcinoid tumors.

Aviel-Ronen and coworkers[305] studied glypican-3 expression in lung cancer at the protein and mRNA levels and correlated these findings with clinical, histological, and genomic characteristics such as RAS mutation status. They performed these studies using immunohistochemistry on tissue microarrays in 97 patients. The authors stated that glypican-3 immunostaining was negative in all normal lung tissues and positive in 23% of lung carcinoma samples. High protein and mRNA expression was associated with squamous histology. Among smokers, glypican-3 mRNA expression was reduced in adenocarcinoma patients and elevated in those with squamous cell carcinoma. Patients with tumors staining positively for glypican-3 smoked significantly more than patients with tumors staining negatively. No association was found between glypican-3 expression and patient outcome. The authors concluded that glypican-3 was overexpressed in cancerous versus normal lung tissue and that adenocarcinoma and squamous cell carcinoma had differential expression of glypican-3, with apredilection to squamous cell carcinoma patients who smoked. The authors also stated that glypican-3 expression in squamous cell carcinoma as an oncofetal protein could be a potential candidate marker for early detection of squamous cell lung cancer.

LaPoint and colleagues[306] evaluated coexpression of c-*kit* and BCL-2 in small cell carcinoma and large cell neuroendocrine carcinoma of the lung. C-*kit* is a proto-oncogene encoding a type III transmembrane tyrosine kinase receptor (CD117). C-*kit* is almost universally expressed in gastrointestinal stromal tumors and in chronic myelocytic leukemia, but it is rarely seen in other cancers, including small cell lung cancer and large cell neuroendocrine carcinoma. Immunohistochemical analysis was performed on 5μm formalin-fixed paraffin-embedded tissue sections that used antigen retrieval for antibodies against synaptophysin, CD56, and BCL-2, but no antigen retrieval for chromogranin or c-*kit*. Using a polyclonal antibody against c-*kit* and a monoclonal antibody against BCL-2, the authors found that 7 of 7 (100%) small cell lung cancers were positive for c-*kit* and BCL-2. For large cell neuroendocrine carcinomas, 7 of 14 (50%) immunostained for c-*kit*, and 9 of 14 (64%) expressed BCL-2. All cases of high-grade neuroendocrine carcinomas (small cell lung cancers and large cell neuroendocrine carcinomas) that expressed c-*kit* coexpressed BCL-2. In contrast, all typical and atypical carcinoids were negative for c-*kit*, and only 1 of 16 (6.3%) typical carcinoids and 1 of 6 (16.7%) atypical carcinoids stained positive for BCL-2. The authors stated there was progressive increase of c-*kit* and BCL-2 expression and coexpression from carcinoid tumors and atypical carcinoids to large cell neuroendocrine carcinomas and small cell lung cancers. They also stated that high-grade neuroendocrine carcinomas were more likely to coexpress c-*kit* and BCL-2 when compared with carcinoid tumors. The high expression and coexpression of these two molecules in high-grade neuroendocrine carcinomas suggested that they may be involved in the carcinogenic pathway and that therapeutic targeting for c-*kit* and BCL-2 molecules might be beneficial in the management of patients with high-grade neuroendocrine carcinomas. Another potential use of this information would be separating typical carcinoids and atypical carcinoids from small cell lung cancer and large cell neuroendocrine carcinomas in bronchial biopsy specimens.

Meyronet and associates[307] pointed out that high-grade neuroendocrine carcinomas show unfavorable outcome and should receive multimodal therapy. The authors pointed out that this type of neoplasm can be mistaken for a poorly differentiated non–small cell carcinoma or carcinoid. The authors stated that no immunohistochemical marker currently distinguishes between histologic lung subtypes. The authors pointed out that because the collapsin response mediator protein (CRMP) family was involved in an autoimmune disease associated with small cell lung carcinoma, they felt it was worthwhile to explore the relationship between CRMP5 expression and lung tumor behavior. The authors evaluated 123 neuroendocrine lung tumors and 41 randomly selected non-neuroendocrine tumors. CRMP5 expression in tumors, metastases, and healthy lung tissue was assessed using immunostaining methods. Strong and extensive CRMP5 expression was seen in 98.6% of high-grade neuroendocrine lung tumors, including small cell lung cancer and large cell neuroendocrine cancer, but not in pulmonary squamous cell carcinoma or pulmonary adenocarcinomas. In contrast, the majority of low-grade neuroendocrine lung tumors were negative for CRMP5 staining, although weak CRMP5 expression was seen in some, with two different staining patterns. The authors concluded that their findings suggested CRMP5 was a novel marker for routine pathologic evaluation of lung tumor surgical samples in distinguishing between highly aggressive neuroendocrine carcinoma and other lung cancers.

Yousem and colleagues[308] evaluated 220 adenocarcinomas of lung lacking KRAS and EGFR mutations and identified 10 adenocarcinomas with BRAF-V600E mutations. All BRAF-V600E mutations were heterozygous. There was a slight female predilection (6:4) in these elderly patients averaging 67 years if age who were found to have a greater than expected incidence of intralobar satellite nodules and N2 nodal involvement. The adenocarcinomas were described as being largely of mixed type with a high incidence of papillary (80%) and lepidic growth (50%). The authors concluded that adenocarcinomas with this clinicopathologic phenotype might be worthwhile investigating for BRAF-V600E mutations as more genetically oriented drug therapies emerge.

Pleural Neoplasms

Neoplasms of the pleura are relatively uncommon, and more metastatic tumors involve the pleura than primary tumors.[219,309] The differentiation of primary from metastatic pleural neoplasms is an area that has received extensive attention in the discipline of immunohistochemistry. In part, this has been due to an increased understanding of the biology of the serosal membranes and the pathology/pathobiology of mesotheliomas.

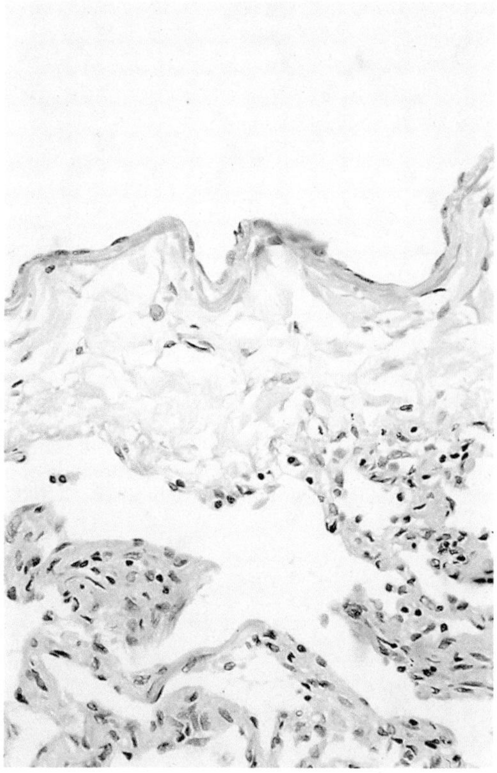

FIGURE 12.43 In the resting state, the normal pleura are composed of a slightly flattened layer of mesothelial cells with underlying spindle cells, collagen, and elastic tissue. X 200.

The celomic cavity develops relatively early in embryogenesis and gives rise to the pleural, peritoneal, and pericardial cavities by partitioning membranes that divide the celomic cavity.[310] Mesotheliomas arise from the serosal tissue of the body cavities. The biology and morphology of the normal pleura has been extensively studied. In the resting state, the pleura are composed of a layer of relatively flattened mesothelial cells that are separated from the underlying connective tissue components by a basement membrane (Fig. 12.43). The sub-basement membrane cells are spindle shaped and are associated with elastic tissue and collagen that is best seen in elastic tissue stained sections. Epithelial mesothelial cells and pleural spindle cells show a marked reaction to injury and increase in number and size (Fig. 12.44). The pleural spindle cells are interesting in that, by immunohistochemistry, they express keratin, vimentin, actin, and calretinin (Fig. 12.45), and ultrastructurally have the appearance of myofibroblasts (Fig. 12.46). In 1986, these authors[311] extensively studied the pleura and its reaction to injury and related the histologic, immunohistochemical, and ultrastructural features of mesotheliomas to the reactive pleural cells. Although doubted by some, there is evidence that epithelial mesothelial cells are derived from a proliferation of sub-basement membrane spindle cells that differentiate into epithelial-mesothelial cells. We named these cells *multipotential-subserosal cells.*

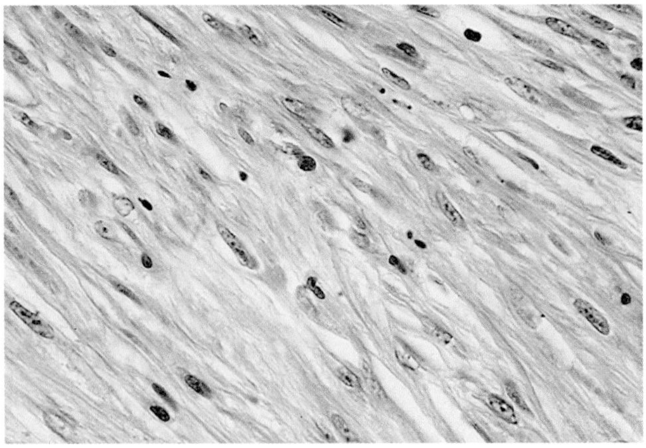

FIGURE 12.44 When injured, the pleura show hypertrophy and hyperplasia of lining mesothelial cells and a proliferation of underlying spindle cells that have features of myofibroblasts. X 400.

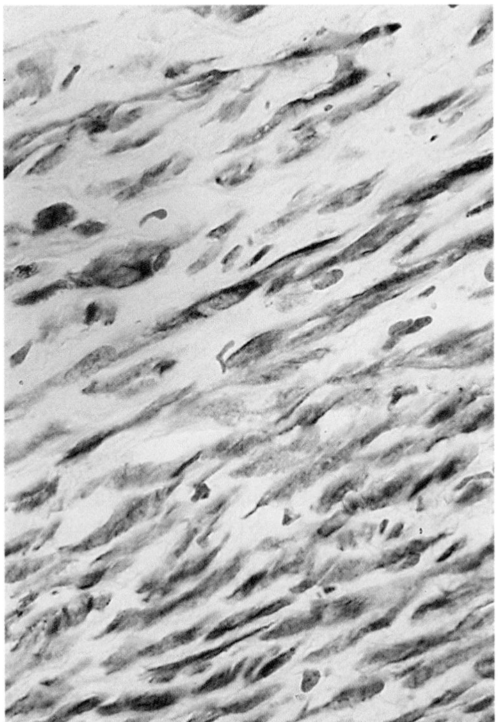

FIGURE 12.45 The proliferating myofibroblasts of the pleura immunostain keratin, vimentin, actin, and calretinin. This photograph shows immunostaining for calretinin. X 400.

Except for a cohort of insulators studied by Selikoff and colleagues,[312] pleural mesotheliomas account for approximately 90% of all mesotheliomas.

Pleural mesotheliomas show a wide range of histologic differentiation, although they can be divided into four major subtypes: 1) epithelial; 2) sarcomatoid [fibrous, sarcomatous]; 3) biphasic; and 4) desmoplastic [a variant of a sarcomatoid mesothelioma].

Immunohistochemistry is the predominant technique used for accurately diagnosing mesotheliomas and differentiating them from primary lung cancers

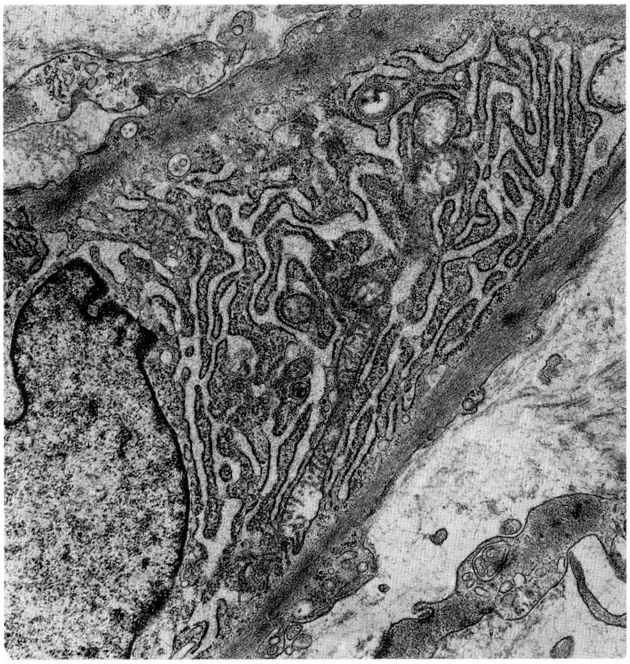

FIGURE 12.46 The proliferating spindle cells have ultrastructural features of myofibroblasts. X 40,000.

that invade the pleura and from primary lung cancers and neoplasms outside of the chest cavity that metastasize to pleura. The four major histologic types of pleural mesothelioma represent a marked oversimplification of what exists. For example, there are approximately 20 different epithelial subtypes (Table 12.21; Figs. 12.47A-W).

A well-differentiated papillary form of mesothelioma exists in the peritoneal cavity and pleural cavity that is important to recognize because unlike other mesotheliomas, it is usually clinically benign or has a low malignant potential.[313-315] In addition, serosal membranes are extremely reactive tissues and show a variety of changes when injured, which can be misinterpreted as malignant.[316] Immunohistochemistry may not be helpful diagnostically in differentiating atypical reactive pleural processes from malignant ones, but is often helpful in identifying cells in these processes as either epithelial mesothelial cells or pleural spindle cells.[317]

As discussed later in this chapter, immunohistochemical studies have been used to separate reactive mesothelial hyperplasias from epithelioid mesotheliomas.

A variety of antibodies have been used to understand and help diagnose mesotheliomas. They can be divided into three main categories: 1) antibodies that are relatively specific for mesothelial cells and mesotheliomas, which when positive serve as a positive marker for mesotheliomas; 2) antibodies that show no reaction for mesothelial cells or mesotheliomas and when negative serve as a negative marker for mesotheliomas; and 3) other antibodies that may react with mesothelial cells and mesotheliomas but are relatively nonspecific.

As stated, mesotheliomas show a variety of histologic patterns and exhibit a wide range of differentiation. The

TABLE 12.21	Epithelial Mesothelioma Subtypes
A	Adenoid cystic
B	Adenomatoid
C	Bakery roll
D	Clear cell
E	Deciduoid
F	Gaucher-like
G	Glandular/acinar
H	Glomeruloid
I	Histiocytoid/epithelioid
J	In association with excess amounts of hyaluronic acid or proteoglycan
K	In situ
L	Macrocystic
M	Microcystic
N	Mucin positive
O	Placentoid
P	Pleomorphic
Q	Poorly differentiated
R	Rhabdoid
S	Signet ring
T	Single file
U	Small cell
V	Tubulopapillary
W	Well-differentiated papillary

See Fig. 12.47 A-W.

selection of a panel of antibodies to evaluate a suspected mesothelioma varies depending on the type of differentiation the suspected mesothelioma shows.

The antibodies that are frequently used in diagnosing suspected mesotheliomas are listed and characterized in Table 12.22.

Positive Markers

Keratins are found in nearly 100% of mesotheliomas. Keratin antibodies are used primarily to identify neoplastic mesothelial cells, to determine invasion in suspected mesotheliomas, to diagnose sarcomatoid mesotheliomas, and to differentiate sarcomatoid mesothelioma from sarcoma, localized fibrous tumors of the pleura, and other neoplasms that are usually keratin-negative. Low and high molecular weight keratins are detectable in most mesotheliomas, especially low molecular weight cytokeratins (CAM5.2, 35βH11). We use AE1/AE3 keratin as a broad-spectrum keratin screening antibody. Cytokeratin expression in mesotheliomas have been reviewed by Henderson and coworkers[318] and Ordonez.[319] In 1985 Blobel and colleagues[320] reported that normal and neoplastic mesothelial cells express CK7, CK8, CK18, and CK19, which were cytokeratins typically seen in simple epithelial cells and in adenocarcinomas. They found some epithelial mesotheliomas contained CK4, CK14, CK16, and CK17. In a previous publication,[321] they reported that adenocarcinomas contained CK7, CK8, CK18, and CK19 and that squamous carcinomas showed a more complex cytokeratin pattern containing simple epithelial cytokeratins (CK7, CK8, CK18, and CK19) and stratified epithelium-type keratins, specifically CK5/6. In 1989 Moll and associates[322] used antibody AE14 to demonstrate CK5 reactivity in 12 of 13 epithelial and biphasic mesotheliomas but in 0 of 21 pulmonary adenocarcinomas. They concluded that CK5 was a helpful marker in distinguishing between pulmonary adenocarcinomas and epithelial-biphasic mesotheliomas. Unfortunately, the AE14 antibody did not work on formalin-fixed paraffin-embedded tissue. It wasn't until 1997 that Clover and colleagues[323] used commercial monoclonal antibody D5/16B4 (which reacted with CK5 and CK6 in formalin-fixed paraffin-embedded tissue) to obtain reactivity in 23 of 23 (100%) epithelial mesotheliomas. The authors observed reactivity in 5 of 27 (18.5%) pulmonary adenocarcinomas. In 4 of 5 (90%) pulmonary adenocarcinomas, the authors noted that reactivity was weak or equivocal. In one, it was described as being patchy. Ordonez,[319] using the same antibody as Clover and colleagues,[323] found positive staining in 40 of 40 (100%) epithelial mesotheliomas, 15 of 15 (100%) squamous carcinomas of lung, and 0 of 30 pulmonary adenocarcinomas. Focal or weak reactivity was noted in 14 of 93 (15.1%) nonpulmonary adenocarcinomas: specifically 10 of 30 (33.3%) ovarian adenocarcinomas, 2 of 10 (20%) endometrial adenocarcinomas, 1 of 18 (5.6%) breast carcinomas, 1 of 7 (14.3%) thyroid carcinomas, 0 of 10 renal carcinomas, 0 of 10 colonic adenocarcinomas, and 0 of 8 prostatic adenocarcinomas. Cytokeratin profiles of epithelial mesothelioma, pulmonary adenocarcinoma, and squamous cell carcinoma of lung are contrasted in Table 12.23.

Kahn and coworkers[324] reported a difference in the pattern of keratin distribution in benign and malignant mesothelial cells compared to adenocarcinomas. In mesothelial cells, the authors observed keratin filaments in a perinuclear or peripheral distribution, whereas in adenocarcinomas they saw an arborizing pattern. In a more extensive study, 10 adenocarcinomas, 10 typical carcinoids, and 4 mesotheliomas were evaluated for keratin intermediate filament distribution using three monoclonal and three polyclonal antibodies against keratin. [325] When the authors allowed the diaminobenzidine color reaction to proceed for less than two minutes, they observed a web-like pattern of reactivity in adenocarcinomas, a punctate crescentic pattern in carcinoids, and a perinuclear-staining pattern in mesotheliomas. While the perinuclear distribution of keratin intermediate filaments is common in epithelial mesotheliomas, it is not seen in all cases, and some pulmonary adenocarcinomas show a perinuclear distribution of keratin. Hence we do not use the distribution pattern of keratin diagnostically.

Although 100% of epithelial mesotheliomas express keratin, the percentage of sarcomatoid mesotheliomas reported in the literature to express keratin is variable.

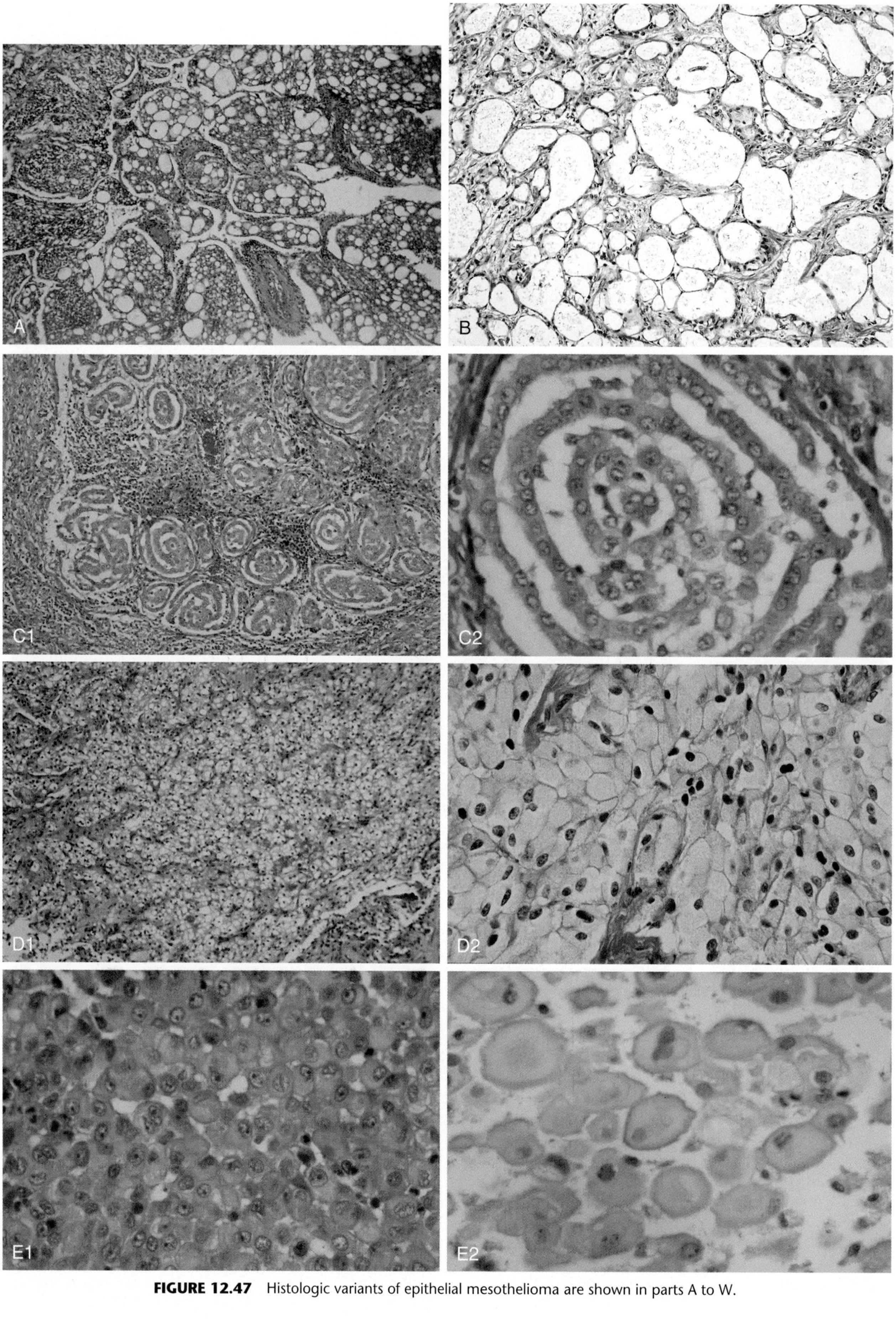

FIGURE 12.47 Histologic variants of epithelial mesothelioma are shown in parts A to W.

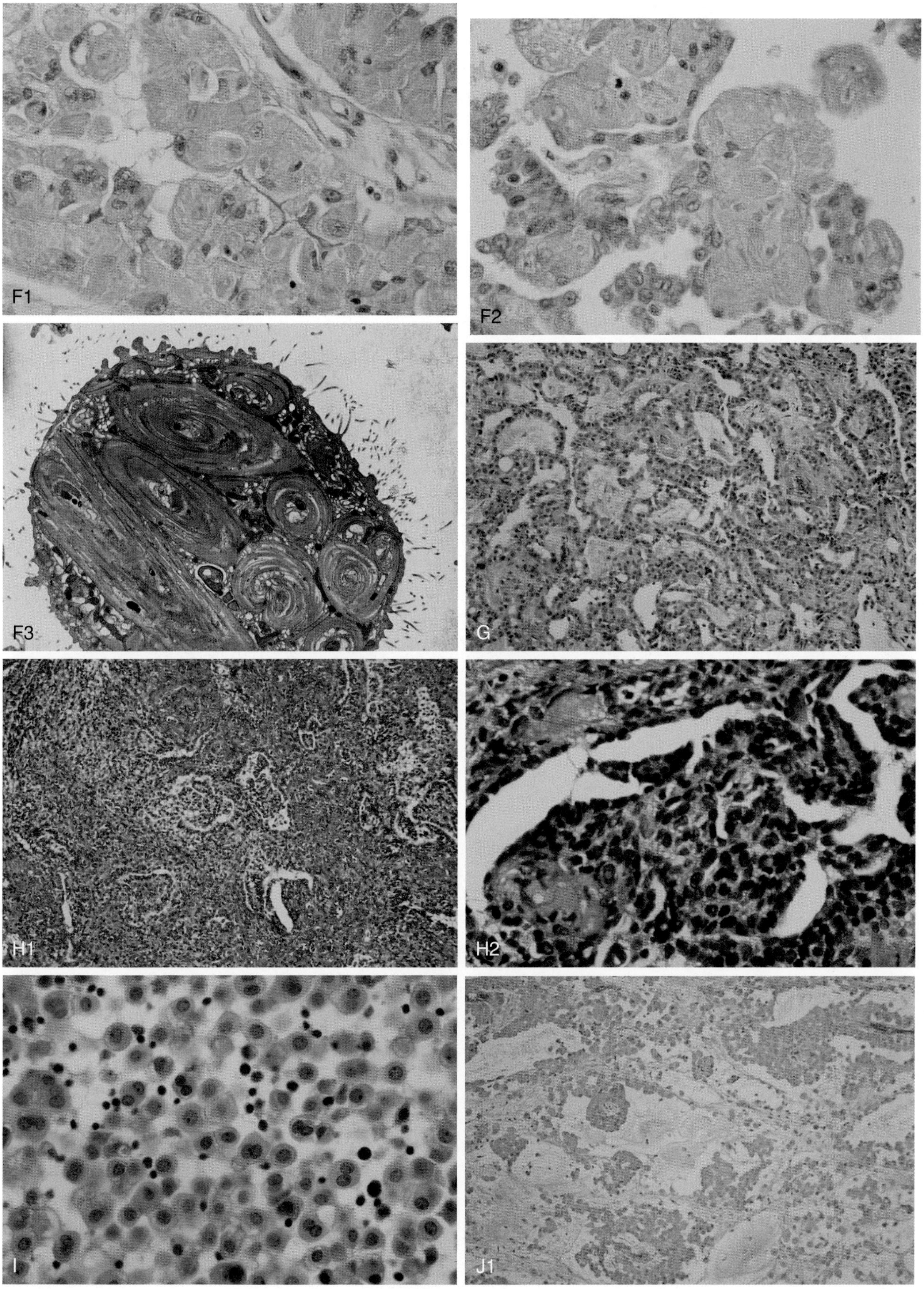

FIGURE 12.47, cont'd

Continued

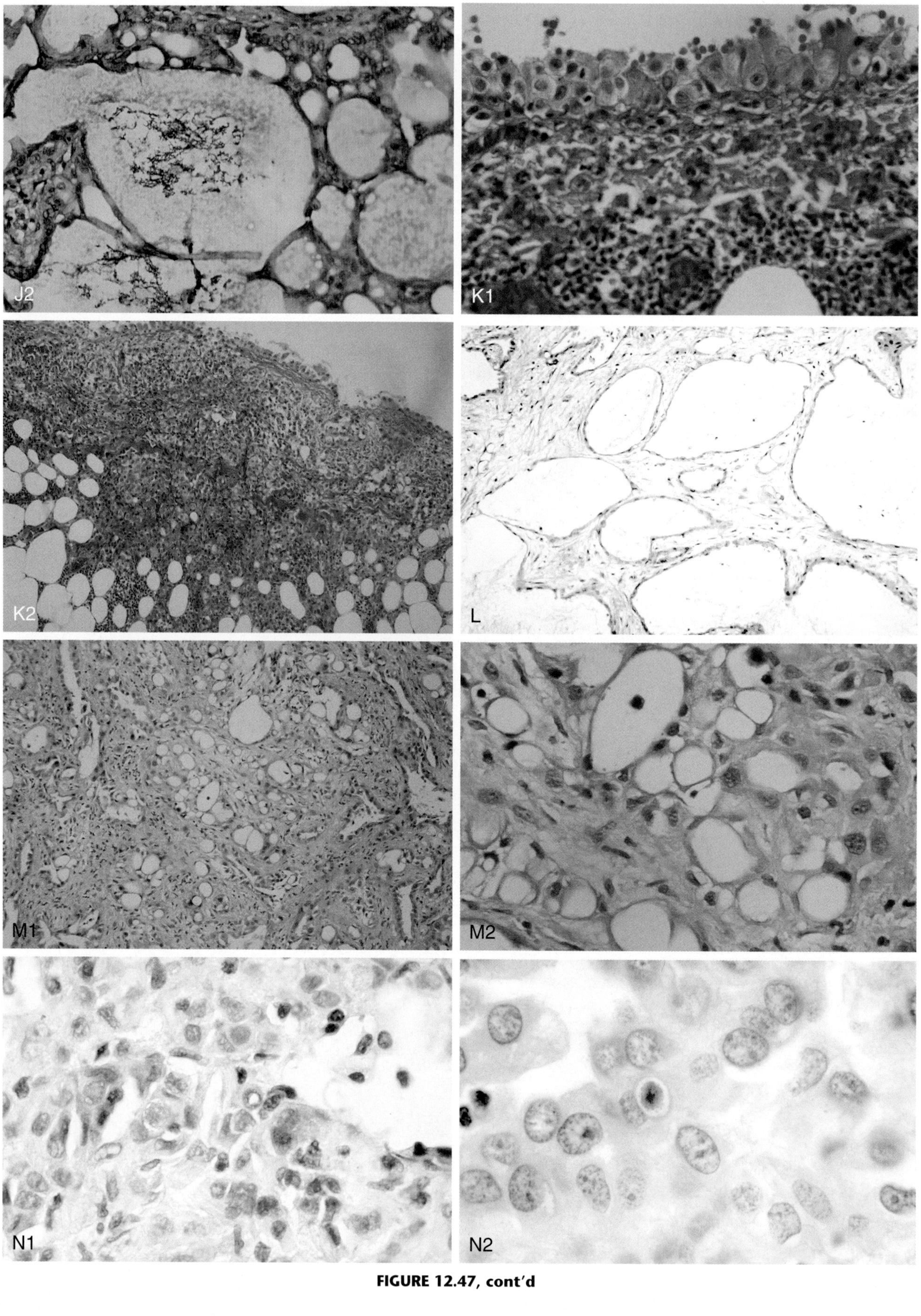

FIGURE 12.47, cont'd

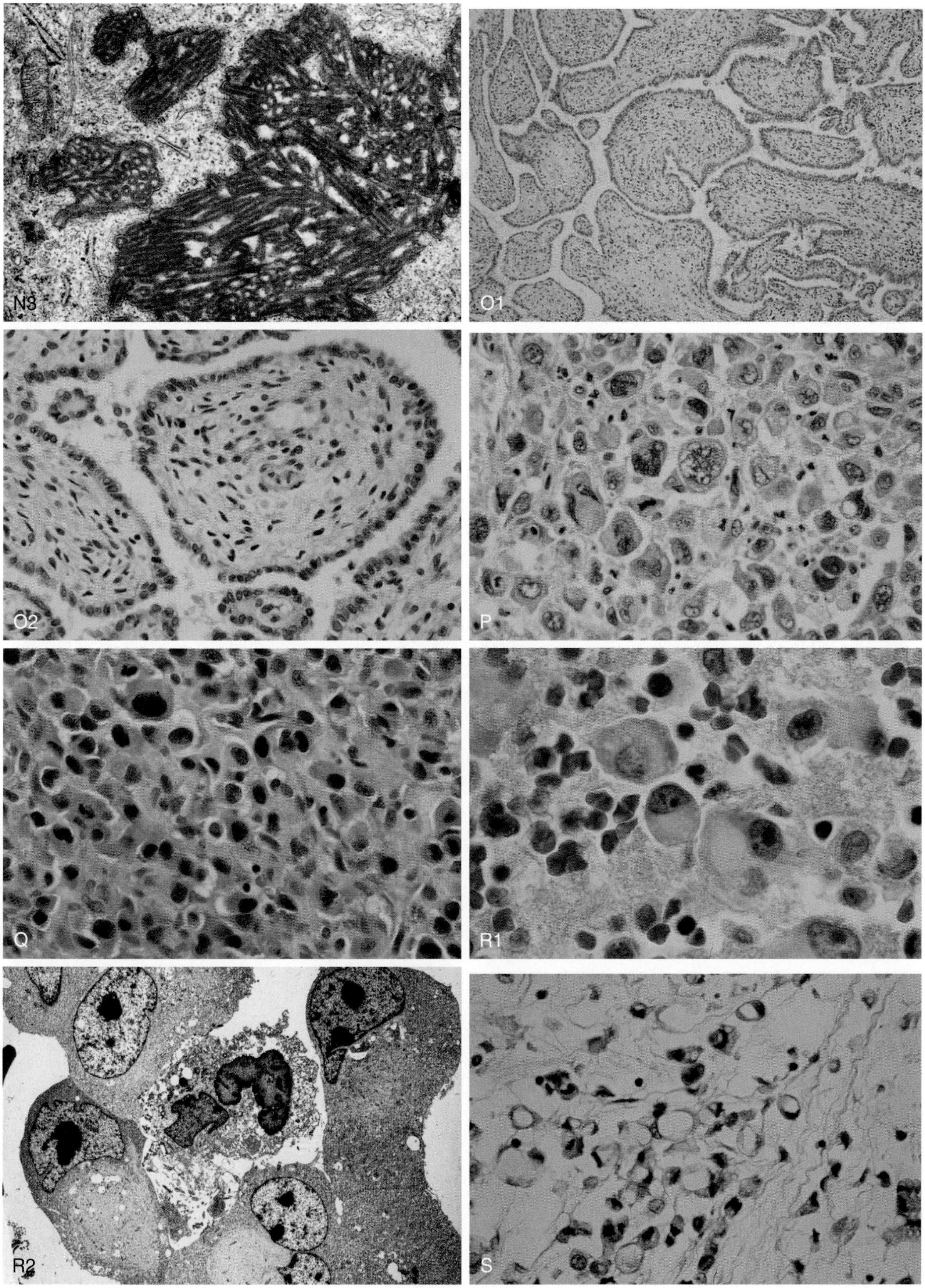

FIGURE 12.47, cont'd

Continued

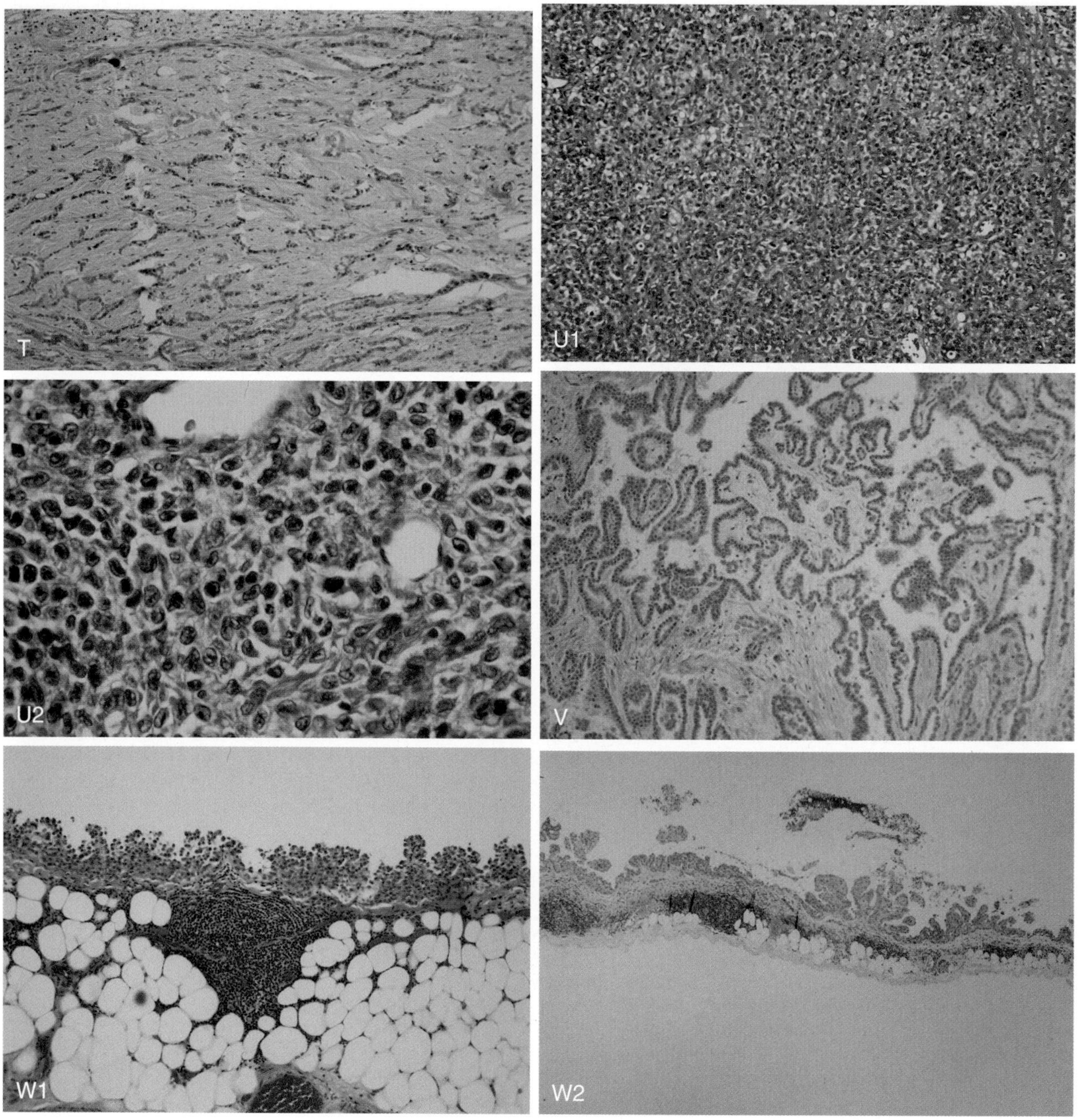

FIGURE 12.47, cont'd

Montag and colleagues[326] detected keratins in 16 of 16 (100%) sarcomatoid mesotheliomas. Their findings were identical to those of Battifora,[327] who observed keratins in 100% of over 20 sarcomatoid mesotheliomas examined. In contrast, some investigations have failed to detect keratin in over 40% of sarcomatoid mesotheliomas.[320,328-334] The U.S./Canadian Mesothelioma Panel recognizes cases of keratin-negative sarcomatoid mesothelioma. In our experience with large samples of well-fixed autopsy tissue, keratin expression in sarcomatoid mesotheliomas can be highly variable. Some regions of a sarcomatoid mesothelioma show intense immunostaining for keratin, and other regions of the same tumor show no keratin staining. This has been observed with broad-spectrum keratin antibodies (AE1/AE3) and with antibodies against low molecular weight keratin (35βH11, CAM5.2).

Lucas and colleagues[335] immunostained 20 mesotheliomas with sarcomatoid components (10 biphasic and 10 sarcomatoid) for pan cytokeratin, CK5/6, calretinin, WT1, thrombomodulin, and smooth muscle actin. They compared the immunophenotypic profile of these tumors with 24 high-grade sarcomas, 10 pulmonary sarcomatoid carcinomas, and 16 epithelioid mesotheliomas. The 10 pulmonary sarcomatoid carcinomas were also immunostained for TTF-1. Their results are shown in Table 12.24. They concluded that: 1) there was a decrease in epithelial and mesothelial epitopes in sarcomatoid mesothelioma; 2) there was a wide immunophenotypic overlap among sarcomatoid

TABLE 12.22 Antibodies Used to Confirm, Eliminate, or Classify Suspected Mesotheliomas

Antibody Directed Against	Clone	Characteristics of Antigens Recognized	Immunogen	Manufacturer	Dilution	Type of Antigen Retrieval
Keratin	AE1/AE3	Keratins—Moll numbers 1-5, 6, 8, 9, 10, 14-16, and 18	Human epidermal keratin	Dako	1:200	HIER
Keratin	MAK-6	Keratins—Moll numbers 8, 14-16, 18, and 19	Extracellular antigen from MCF-tissue culture and from human sole epidermis	Zymed	1:100	HIER
Keratin	5D3	Keratins—Moll numbers 8 and 18	Colorectal carcinoma cell line	BioGenex	1:100	HIER
Keratin	35βH11	Keratin—Moll number 8	Hep3B hepatocellular carcinoma cell line	Dako	1:50	HIER
Keratin	34βE12	Keratins—Moll numbers 1, 5, 10, and 14	Human stratum corneum keratin	Dako	1:100	HIER
CK5/CK6	D5/16B4	Keratins—Moll numbers 5, 6 (and 4—to a slight degree)	Purified cytokeratin 5	Biocare Medical	1:100	HIER
CK7	OV-TL 12/30	Keratin—Moll number 7	OTN 11 ovarian carcinoma cell line	Cell Marque	NA	HIER
CK20	Ks20.8	Keratin—Moll number 20	Villi of human duodenal mucosa	Cell Marque	NA	HIER
Vimentin	Vim3B4	Intermediate filament57-kD	Vimentin from bovine eye lens	Dako	1:100	HIER
Alpha actin	1A4	Alpha–smooth muscle isoform of actin	N-terminal decapeptide of human α smooth-muscle actin	Cell Marque	NA	HIER
Muscle-specific actin	HHF-35	42-kD protein in preparations of purified skeletal muscle actin and extracts of aorta, uterus, diaphragm, and heart	SDS extracted protein fraction of human myocardium	Cell Marque	NA	HIER
Desmin	NCL-DE-R-11	53-kD intermediate filament in muscle cells, recognizing 18-kD rod piece of molecule	Desmin purified from porcine stomach	Ventana	NA	HIER
Calretinin	–	29-kD calcium-binding protein	Human recombinant calretinin	Cell Marque	NA	HIER
Mesothelioma antigen	HBME-1	Antigen present in membrane of mesothelial cells	Suspension of human mesothelial cells from malignant epithelial mesothelioma	Dako	1:400	HIER
Thrombomodulin	1009	Transmembrane glycoprotein of 75-kD molecular weight containing 6 repeated domains homologous with epidermal growth factor	Recombinant thrombomodulin	Dako	1:50	HIER
Epithelial membrane antigen (EMA)	E29	250-400 kD glycoprotein of milk fat globule protein family	Delipidated extract of human milk fat	Ventana	NA	HIER
Human milk fat globule protein-2 (HMFG-2)	115D8	MAM-6 mucus glycoprotein of >400 kD in glycocalyx of epithelial cells	Purified human milk fat globule protein	BioGenex	1:25	HIER
N-Cadherin	389	Transmembrane glycoprotein involved in calcium-dependent cell adhesion	Intracellular domain of chicken N-cadherin	Zymed	1:100	HIER

Continued

TABLE 12.22 Antibodies Used to Confirm, Eliminate, or Classify Suspected Mesotheliomas—cont'd

Antibody Directed Against	Clone	Characteristics of Antigens Recognized	Immunogen	Manufacturer	Dilution	Type of Antigen Retrieval
Polyclonal carcinoembryonic antigen (CEA)	–	CEA and CEA-like proteins including nonspecific cross-reacting substance and biliary glycoprotein	Human CEA isolated from metastatic colonic adenocarcinoma	Ventana	NA	HIER
CD15 (LeuM1)	C3D-1	3-fucosyl-N-acetyl-lactosamine	Purified neutrophils from normal human peripheral blood	Ventana	NA	HIER
Tumor-associated glycoprotein	B72.3	Tumor-associated glycoprotein of a wide variety of human adenocarcinomas	Membrane-enriched fraction of metastatic breast carcinoma	Cell Marque	NA	HIER
Human epithelial antigen	VU-1D9	34- and 49-kD glycoproteins on the surface and in cytoplasm of most epithelial cells (except squamous epithelium, hepatocytes, and parietal cells)	MCF-7 cell line	Ventana	NA	HIER
Thyroglobulin	2H11+6E1	Thyroglobulin	Thyroglobulin from human thyroid glands	Cell Marque	NA	HIER
Thyroid transcription factor-1 (TTF-1)	8G7G3/1	40-kD member of NKx2 family of homeodomain transcription factors	Mouse ascites	Cell Marque	NA	HIER
Prostate specific antigen (PSA)	ER-PR8	330-kD prostate-specific antigen	Purified human prostate-specific antigen	Ventana	NA	HIER
Prostatic acid phosphatase (PAP)	PASE/4LJ	52-kD human prostatic acid phosphatase	Purified prostatic acid phosphatase from human seminal plasma	Ventana	NA	HIER
Human epithelial-related antigen	MOC-31	40-kD transmembrane glycoprotein present on most normal and malignant epithelial cells	Neuraminidase treated cells from small cell carcinoma cell line	Dako	1:50	HIER
Lewis Y antigen	BG8-F3	Difucosylated tetrasaccharide found on type 2 blood group oligosaccharide	SK-LU-3 lung cancer cell line	Signet	1:40	HIER
E-cadherin	4A2C7	Transmembrane glycoprotein in calcium-dependent cell adhesion	Recombinant protein of human E-cadherin	Ventana	NA	HIER
Gross cystic disease fluid protein-15 (BRST-2)	D6	Pathologic secretion of breast composed of several glycoproteins including 15-kD monomer protein	Gross cystic disease fluid protein-15	Signet	1:50	HIER
Estrogen receptor protein	1D5	66-kD protein member of nuclear hormone receptor that acts as a ligand-activated transcription factor	Human recombinant estrogen receptor protein	Ventana	NA	HIER
c-erbB-2 oncoprotein	–	190-kD protein product of c-erbB-2 proto-oncogene	Synthetic human c-erbB-2 oncoprotein peptide	Dako	1:500	HIER
Human leukocyte antigen CD45	Dako-LCA	Five or more high molecular weight glycoproteins on the surface of most human leukocytes	Human peripheral blood lymphocytes maintained in T-cell growth factor	Ventana	NA	HIER

CD20 Human B-lymphocyte antigen	L26	33-kD non-glycosylated membrane spanning protein	Human tonsil B lymphocyte	Ventana	NA	HIER
CD3 Human T-lymphocyte antigen	–	Intracytoplasmic portion of CD3 antigen	Synthetic human CD3 peptide	Ventana	NA	HIER
CD30 Ki-1 antigen	Ber-H2	120-kD transmembrane glycoprotein	Co cell line cells	Ventana	NA	HIER
Bcl-2 oncoprotein	124	25-kD integral protein localized in mitochondria that inhibits apoptosis	Synthetic peptide sequence amino acids 41-54 of bcl-2 protein	Ventana	NA	HIER
Neuron-specific enolase	–	Gamma subunit of enolase	Neuron-specific enolase isolated from human brain	Dako	1:400	HIER
Chromogranin A	DAK-A3	Member of secretogranin/chromogranin class of proteins in secretory granules of endocrine and neuron cells	C-terminal 20-kD fragment of chromogranin A	Ventana	NA	HIER
Synaptophysin	–	38-kD membrane component of neuron synaptic vesicles	Synthetic human synaptophysin peptide coupled to ovalbumin	Cell Marque	NA	HIER
S-100 protein	–	S-100 protein A and B	S-100 protein isolated from cow brain	Ventana	NA	HIER
Melanoma antigen	HMB-45	Neuraminidase-sensitive oligosaccharide side chain of glycoconjugate in immature melanosomes	Extract of pigmented melanoma metastases from lymph nodes	Dako	1:200	HIER
CD34	My10	105- to 120-kD single-chain transmembrane glycoprotein associated with human hematopoietic progenitor cells	CD34 antigen	Ventana	NA	HIER
CD31	JC/70A	100-kD glycoprotein in endothelial cells and 130 kD glycoprotein in platelets	Membrane preparation of spleen from patient with hairy cell leukemia	Cell Marque	NA	HIER
Factor VIII antigen	–	Human von Willebrand factor	von Willebrand factor isolated from human plasma	Cell Marque	NA	HIER
Mesothelin	5B2	Amino acids present in the mesothelin molecule	Mouse myeloma	Novocastra	NA	HIER
WT1	6F-H2	Suppressor gene on chromosome 11p13	Tissue culture supernatant of mouse antibodies	Cell Marque	NA	HIER
D2-40	D2-40	Oncofetal antigen M2A	Mouse ascites	Signet	NA	HIER
Surfactant apoprotein A (SP-A)	PE-10	Surfactant A	Surfactant apoproteins isolated from lung lavages of patients with alveolar proteinosis	Dako	1:100	HIER
CDX2	CDX2-88	Homeobox family of intestine-specific transcription factor regulates proliferation and differentiation of intestinal epithelial cells	Full length CDX2	BioGenex	NA	HIER
p63	4A4	Human p63 protein, a member of the p53 family	Mouse monoclonal antibody	Cell Marque	1:100	HIER

*HIER, heat-induced epitope retrieval.

TABLE 12.23 Cytokeratin Profiles of Epithelial Mesothelioma, Pulmonary Adenocarcinoma, and Squamous Cell Carcinoma of Lung

	Cytokeratin Moll Number, Molecular Weight, and Isoelectric pH																			
Type of Neoplasm	1 68 kD 7.8	2 65.5 kD 7.8	3 63 kD 7.5	4 59 kD 7.3	5 58 kD 7.4	6 56 kD 7.8	7 54 kD 6.0	8 52.5 kD 6.1	9 64 kD 5.4	10 56.5 kD 5.3	11 56 kD 5.3	12 55 kD 4.9	13 54 kD 5.1	14 50 kD 5.3	15 50 kD 4.9	16 48 kD 5.1	17 46 kD 5.1	18 45 kD 5.7	19 40 kD 5.2	20 46 kD 5.2
Primary pulmonary adeno-carcinoma	N	N	N	N	N	N	S	S	N	N	N	N	N	N	N	N	N	S	S	R
Epithelial mesothelioma	N	N	N	N	S	S	S	S	N	N	N	N	N	S	N	N	S	S	S	R
Primary pulmonary squamous cell carcinoma	N	N	N	S	S	S	R	S	N	N	N	N	N	S	S	S	S	S	S	R

Reactivity:
+, almost always diffuse, strong positivity
S, sometimes positive
R, rare cells positive
N, almost always negative

TABLE 12.24 Percentage of Immunohistochemically Positive Mesotheliomas and Sarcomas Based on Histological Type

	Pan-CK	CK5/6	Calretinin	WT1	Thrombomodulin	Smooth-Muscle Actin
Epithelioid mesothelioma	100	100	100	69	81	50
Biphasic mesothelioma with epithelioid component	100	40	90	60	90	20
Biphasic mesothelioma with sarcomatoid component	90	10	60	20	50	60
Sarcomatoid mesothelioma	70	0	70	10	70	60
Sarcoma	17	4	17	4	38	58
Sarcomatoid carcinoma	90	0	60	0	40	10

Pan-CK, pan cytokeratin; CK5/6, cytokeratin 5/6.
Reprinted from: Lucas DR, Pass HI, Madan SK, et al. Sarcomatoid mesothelioma and its histological mimics: A comparative immunohistochemical study. *Histopathology.* 2003;42:270-279.

mesothelioma, sarcoma, and sarcomatoid carcinoma; 3) cytokeratin and calretinin had the most value in differentiating sarcomatoid mesothelioma from sarcoma; 4) with the exception of smooth muscle actin, all other markers studied showed a similar distribution in sarcomatoid mesothelioma and sarcomatoid carcinoma, including frequent calretinin and thrombomodulin expression in both tumors; 5) since cytokeratin expression can be absent in sarcomatoid mesothelioma, the distinction between it and sarcoma is arbitrary; and 6) immunohistochemistry plays a more limited role in the differential diagnosis of sarcomatoid tumors versus epithelioid neoplasms, and the macroscopic distribution of the neoplasm correlates with microscopic and immunohistochemical findings.

Attanoos and associates[336] evaluated 31 sarcomatoid mesotheliomas and a spectrum of other spindle cell neoplasms with antibodies directed against cytokeratin, thrombomodulin, calretinin, and CK5/6. Twenty-four of 31 (77%) sarcomatoid mesotheliomas expressed cytokeratin, 9 of 31 (29%) expressed thrombomodulin, 12 of 31 (39%) expressed calretinin, and 9 of 31 (29%) expressed CK5/6. Two of 9 (22%) sarcomas not otherwise specified expressed broad-spectrum cytokeratin and thrombomodulin, and 1 of 9 (11%) expressed CK5/6. As might be expected, 100% of synovial sarcomas expressed broad-spectrum keratin but showed no immunostaining for thrombomodulin, calretinin, and CK5/6. Two of 3 (67%) angiosarcomas expressed thrombomodulin, which is not surprising since thrombomodulin stains normal endothelial cells. The authors concluded that a combination of a broad-spectrum cytokeratin with calretinin resulted in a high sensitivity (77% for AE1/AE3 keratin) and high specificity (100% for calretinin) for sarcomatoid mesothelioma. They stated that the mesothelial markers thrombomodulin and CK5/6 were not useful alone in diagnosing sarcomatoid mesothelioma. Their study also found that 3% of sarcomatoid mesotheliomas did not express broad-spectrum keratin, which would again support the notion that there are cytokeratin-negative sarcomatoid mesotheliomas.

We have not found the expression of broad-spectrum keratin (AE1/AE3 keratin) in sarcomas or the degree of calretinin expression in sarcomatoid mesotheliomas, sarcomas, or sarcomatoid carcinomas noted by Lucas and coworkers.[335] In our experience, broad-spectrum keratin is rarely found (<1% of cases) in sarcomas. Calretinin expression is found in a maximum of 20% of sarcomatoid mesotheliomas and is not seen in sarcomas or sarcomatoid carcinomas. Others have found similar immunoreactions (see the paragraphs that follow).

Vimentin is a 58-kD intermediate filament found predominantly in cells of mesenchymal derivation. Although initially touted in the late 1970s and early 1980s as being useful in separating carcinomas from sarcomas, vimentin is observed in normal epithelial cells and in a variety of carcinomas.[17,337-339] In our experience, vimentin is expressed in all sarcomatoid mesotheliomas—usually intensely—and in most poorly differentiated and transitional mesotheliomas. Churg[340] reported vimentin expression in 2 alcohol-fixed epithelial mesotheliomas, 1 of which was a tubulopapillary variant. Jasani and colleagues observed vimentin expression in 75% of 44 malignant mesotheliomas of all histologic types.[341] However, 46% of 24 of pulmonary adenocarcinomas also demonstrated vimentin by immunohistochemical analysis. Mullink and colleagues[342] found it more common for epithelial mesotheliomas than for pulmonary adenocarcinomas to coexpress keratin and vimentin. We observed that 30% to 45% of epithelial mesotheliomas coexpressed keratin and vimentin.

In our opinion, antibody against calretinin is the most specific and reproducible positive marker of epithelial mesothelioma. Calretinin is a calcium-binding protein similar to S-100 protein.[343,344] It has a molecular weight of 29-kD and is found in the central and peripheral nervous systems and in a wide spectrum of non-neural cells (including steroid-producing cells of ovaries and testes, fat cells, renal tubular epithelial cells, eccrine glands, thymic epithelial cells, and mesothelial cells). Gotzos[345] found calretinin immunostaining in 7 of 7 (100%) epithelial mesotheliomas and in the epithelial component of 15 of 15 (100%) biphasic mesotheliomas. They found no immunostaining in sarcomatoid components of biphasic mesotheliomas or in a single case of sarcomatoid mesothelioma. The four lung adenocarcinomas evaluated showed no immunostaining for calretinin. Doglioni and colleagues[346] found calretinin immunostaining in 44 of 44 (100%) epithelial mesotheliomas and focal staining in 28 of 294 (9.5%) adenocarcinomas of various origin. Doglioni and associates[346] found positive staining in 3 of 3 (100%) sarcomatoid

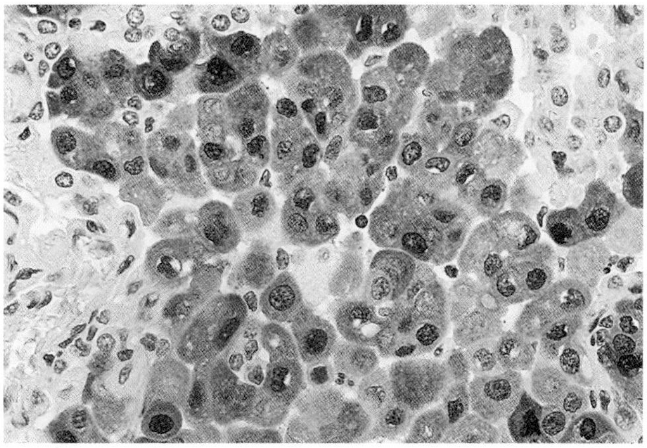

FIGURE 12.48 Most well and moderately well differentiated epithelial mesotheliomas and a few sarcomatoid mesotheliomas show cytoplasmic and nuclear immunostaining for calretinin. X 400.

mesotheliomas and in the sarcomatoid component of 5 biphasic mesotheliomas. Studying cells in serous fluids, Barberis and coworkers found immunostaining for calretinin in 8 of 8 (100%) epithelial mesotheliomas and low intensity immunostaining in 3 of 13 (23.1%) adenocarcinomas.[347] The authors did not state if the staining was cytoplasmic or nuclear. Leers and colleagues observed calretinin immunostaining in 20 of 20 (100%) epithelial mesotheliomas and weak immunostaining in 1 of 21 (4.8%) adenocarcinomas (with the location of staining not specified).[348]

Ordonez compared two commercially available calretinin antibodies.[349] Using a calretinin antibody obtained from Zymed Laboratories, the author found calretinin immunostaining in 8 of 38 (21.1%) epithelial mesotheliomas and focal, generally weak immunostaining in 14 of 155 (9%) adenocarcinomas of various types. In contrast, 28 of 38 (73.1%) epithelial mesotheliomas and 6 of 155 (3.8%) adenocarcinomas showed immunostaining for calretinin using a calretinin antibody from Chemicon International. In our experience using a calretinin antibody from Biocare, 198 of 210 (94%) epithelial mesotheliomas showed immunostaining for calretinin. As with S-100 protein, the immunostaining pattern for calretinin was cytoplasmic and nuclear (Fig. 12.48). Reactive multipotential subserosal spindle cells typically express calretinin in a cytoplasmic and nuclear distribution.

Additional studies have shown a high degree of specificity and sensitivity for calretinin in differentiating epithelial mesotheliomas from pulmonary adenocarcinomas and other epithelioid neoplasms.[350-353]

The use of the ME1 antibody was initially reported by O'Hara and colleagues in 1990.[354] ME1 is a monoclonal antibody generated from the mesothelial cell line SPC111 and reacted with normal mesothelial cells and malignant epithelial mesotheliomas. Their antibody was only useful on frozen section tissue and showed immunostaining of 40 of 40 (100%) epithelial mesotheliomas. Nineteen well and moderately differentiated primary pulmonary adenocarcinomas failed to stain with the ME1 antibody, but one poorly differentiated pulmonary adenocarcinoma showed intense immunostaining.

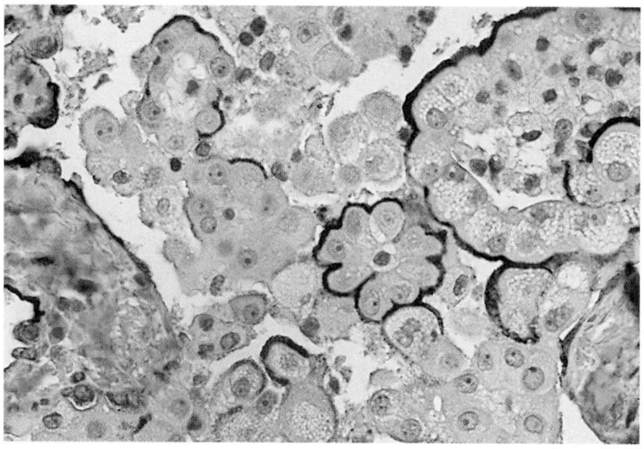

FIGURE 12.49 Most well to moderately well differentiated epithelial mesotheliomas show thick cell membrane immunostaining for HBME-1. X 400.

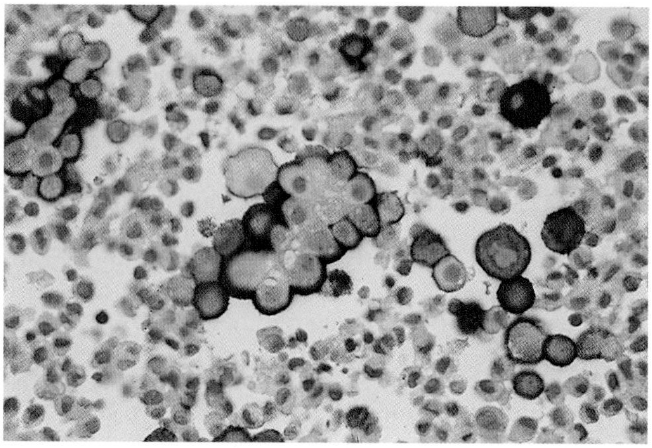

FIGURE 12.50 Most well to moderately well differentiated epithelial mesotheliomas show thick cell membrane staining for epithelial membrane antigen. X 400.

As reviewed by Sheibani and colleagues,[355] Battifora produced an ME1 monoclonal antibody designated HBME-1 that worked on paraffin-embedded formalin-fixed tissue. As reported by these authors, this antibody showed immunostaining of a relatively high percentage of epithelial mesotheliomas in a cell membrane distribution (Fig. 12.49). In our experience, the intensity of this reaction varies from one case to another. Dako's product specification sheet states that 17 of 19 (89.5) epithelial mesotheliomas showed immunostaining for HBME-1. The antibody also reacted with 19 of 50 (38%) adenocarcinomas. The specification sheet suggests using the antibody at a dilution of 1:100. However, in our experience, the antibody should be used at a much greater dilution, (1:7500 in this author's laboratory). As reported by Henderson and associates, they use HBME-1 antibody in a dilution between 1:5000 and 1:15,000.[318] They found that when lower dilutions (higher concentrations) were used, the cytoplasm of many mesotheliomas stained and a significant number of adenocarcinomas showed cytoplasmic immunostaining. These findings suggest that it is necessary to use HBME-1 at a higher dilution to effectively differentiate epithelial mesotheliomas from other neoplasms. Of interest, HBME-1 reacts with respiratory epithelium and occasionally shows cell membrane staining of primary pulmonary squamous cell carcinomas.

Epithelial membrane antigen (EMA) and human milk fat globule protein-2 (HMFG-2) are similar glycoproteins of high molecular weight (250 to 400-kD) and are known as human milk fat globule proteins. These glycoproteins are found in milk fat and in a variety of normal and neoplastic epithelial cells. Antibodies against EMA and HMFG-2 are of use in diagnosing epithelial mesotheliomas in that the majority of epithelial mesotheliomas show immunostaining in a cell membrane distribution (only anti-EMA is currently available). This is different from most adenocarcinomas and other carcinomas, which usually show cytoplasmic immunostaining. We detected epithelial membrane antigen in 50 of 64 (78.1%) epithelial mesotheliomas, 37 of 60 (61.7%) adenocarcinomas, and 8 of 19 (42%) squamous cell carcinomas.[356] Walz and Koch demonstrated EMA expression in 33 of 44 epithelial mesotheliomas.[357] Wick and coworkers found immunostaining in 43 of 51 (84%) epithelial mesotheliomas.[358] As stated, the antigen is concentrated in the cell membrane and produces a thick cell membrane reaction (Fig. 12.50) in most well-differentiated to moderately well differentiated epithelial mesotheliomas owing to the extensive microvillus surface of epithelial mesotheliomas. Henderson and colleagues demonstrated strong cell surface epithelial membrane antigen staining in epithelial mesotheliomas and found immunostaining in a surface distribution in some lymphoid cells.[359] In our experience, most reactive (benign) epithelial mesothelial cells show no immunostaining for EMA. We have found relatively intense EMA cell membrane staining in cases of nonmucinous bronchioloalveolar cell carcinomas and in pulmonary papillary adenocarcinomas.

Thrombomodulin is a plasma membrane–related glycoprotein that has anticoagulant activity. Thrombomodulin antigen is found in several cell types, including mesangial cells, synovial cells, mesothelial cells, endothelial cells, megakaryocytes, and some squamous epithelial cells. Fink and colleagues demonstrated immunostaining for thrombomodulin in 8 epithelial mesotheliomas and 2 mesothelial cell lines.[360] The cell lines were shown by *in situ* hybridization to possess messenger RNA for thrombomodulin. In contrast, 14 of 15 (93.3%) adenocarcinomas were negative for thrombomodulin, and 1 showed focal positivity. Collins and colleagues[361] found thrombomodulin expression in 31 of 31 (100%) epithelial mesotheliomas and 4 of 48 (8.3%) pulmonary adenocarcinomas. In contrast, Brown and coworkers observed only 60% of epithelial and biphasic mesotheliomas to express thrombomodulin, whereas 58% of pulmonary adenocarcinomas were positive.[362] Ascoli and colleagues identified thrombomodulin in 33 of 33 (100%) epithelial mesotheliomas, in reactive mesothelial cells in 35 effusions, and in 57 of 145 (39.3%) carcinomas in effusions.[363] They reported a different immunohistochemical pattern of staining in benign reactive mesothelial cells, malignant epithelial mesotheliomas, and carcinomas. In benign reactive mesothelial cells, thin linear staining was observed. Thick membrane staining was seen in malignant epithelial mesotheliomas, and cytoplasmic staining was observed in most cases of carcinoma.

Cadherins are a family of adhesion proteins that are important during morphogenesis for sorting cells into specialized tissues.[364,365] The cadherin family includes epithelial (E) cadherin, nerve (N) cadherin, retina (R) cadherin, osteoblast (OB) cadherin, and placental (P) cadherin. N-cadherin is a 135,000-kD protein found in nerve cells, developing muscle cells, and mesothelial cells.[366] Peralta-Soler and associates used 13A9 anti-N-cadherin monoclonal antibody on frozen sections and observed a strong immunoreactivity in 19 of 19 (100%) epithelial mesotheliomas and a focal weak reactivity in 3 of 16 (18.8%) pulmonary adenocarcinomas.[367] Using antigen retrieval methodology on paraffin-embedded tissue sections, Han and colleagues reported 12 of 13 (92.3%) epithelial mesotheliomas and 1 of 14 (7.1%) pulmonary adenocarcinomas to be positive for N-cadherin.[368]

Ordonez evaluated 31 epithelioid mesotheliomas and 29 pulmonary adenocarcinomas for E-cadherin and N-cadherin expression. They used the 5H9, HECD-1, and clone 36 anti–E-cadherin antibodies and the 3B9 and clone 32 anti–N-cadherin antibodies.[369] Sixty-eight percent, 52%, and 19% of the epithelial mesotheliomas reacted with anti–E-cadherin clone 36, clone HECD-1, and 5H9, respectively. Seventy-four percent and 71% of epithelial mesotheliomas reacted with anti–N-cadherin clone 3B9 and clone 32, respectively. Ninety-three percent, 90%, and 90% of pulmonary adenocarcinomas reacted with anti–E-cadherin clone 36, clone HECD-1, and clone 5H9, respectively. Forty-five percent and 34% of pulmonary adenocarcinomas reacted with anti–N-cadherin clone 32 and clone 3B9, respectively. Ordonez concluded that the 5H9 anti–E-cadherin antibody had some utility in discriminating between pleural epithelioid mesothelioma and pulmonary adenocarcinoma.

Wilms' tumor suppressor gene (WT1) resides on the 11p13 chromosome whose inactivation causes susceptibility to Wilms' tumor. This gene is found predominantly in tissues of mesodermal origin. Using frozen tissue sections, Amin and colleagues[370] observed nuclear immunostaining in 20 of 21 (95.2%) malignant mesotheliomas and in 0 of 26 nonmesothelioma tumors involving lung, including 20 primary non–small cell lung carcinomas. Kumar-Singh and coworkers used an antibody adaptable to formalin-fixed paraffin-embedded tissue and found positive staining of Wilms' tumor suppressor gene products in 39 of 42 (92.9%) mesotheliomas, 2 of 2 (100%) papillary carcinomas of ovary, and 1 of 1 (100%) renal cell carcinoma.[371] Twelve adenocarcinomas of lung, 4 squamous cell carcinomas of lung, 8 metastatic breast adenocarcinomas, and 3 metastatic adenocarcinomas of colon did not express Wilms' tumor suppressor gene products. This antibody is potentially useful in diagnosing mesotheliomas. Using molecular biology techniques, Walker and colleagues found WT1 transcripts in 23 of 26 (88.5%) mesothelioma cell lines and in 5 of 8 (62.5%) human malignant mesotheliomas, but not in non–small cell lung cancer cell lines or in a few other biopsy specimens.[372]

Mesothelin is a 40-kD glycoprotein of unknown function that is strongly expressed in mesothelial cells, ovarian serous cells, and pancreatic-bile duct cells. Using monoclonal antibody 5B2, Ordonez found it to immunostain normal mesothelial cells, mesotheliomas, nonmucinous ovarian carcinomas, and occasionally other neoplasms. Ordonez concluded that mesothelin staining could be used to diagnose mesotheliomas, although it was expressed in 14 of 14 ovarian carcinomas, 12 of 14 pancreatic ductal adenocarcinomas, 7 of 12 desmoplastic small round cell tumors, and 9 of 9 synovial sarcomas. Therefore, this antibody should be interpreted carefully.

D2-40, a clone of podoplanin, is a recently developed commercially available antibody directed against the M2A antigen, a 40,000-kD sialoglycoprotein associated with germ cells and lymphatic endothelium. Chu and colleagues evaluated 53 cases of mesothelioma, 28 cases of reactive pleural tissue, 30 cases of pulmonary adenocarcinoma, 35 cases of renal cell carcinoma, 26 cases of ovarian serous carcinoma, 16 cases of invasive breast carcinoma, 11 cases of prostatic adenocarcinoma, and 7 cases of urothelial carcinoma.[374] The authors found D2-40 expression in 51 of 53 (96%) mesotheliomas, 27 of 28 (96%) reactive pleural tissues, and 17 of 26 (65%) ovarian serous carcinomas. They did not find D2-40 in the other tumors examined. The authors also observed that the neoplastic cells immunostained in a cell membrane distribution.

h-Caldesmon is a cytoskeleton-associated protein present in smooth and non-smooth muscle cells. It combines with calmodulin, tropomyosin and actin, and is involved in the regulation of cellular contraction. Comin and associates used immunohistochemical analysis with an antibody for h-caldesmon (a specific marker for smooth muscle tumors) to examine 70 cases of epithelial mesothelioma and 70 cases of lung adenocarcinoma.[375] In addition, immunohistochemistry for muscle markers such as desmin, alpha–smooth-muscle actin, muscle-specific actin, myoglobin, myogenin, myosin, and Myo-D1 was performed on all mesothelioma cases. The authors found reactivity for h-caldesmon in 68 of 70 (97%) epithelial mesotheliomas, but in none of the adenocarcinoma cases. All mesotheliomas were stated to be negative for other muscle markers. The authors concluded that h-caldesmon was a highly sensitive and specific marker and suggested its inclusion in the immunohistochemical panel for the differential diagnosis of epithelioid mesothelioma versus pulmonary adenocarcinoma.[375]

Negative Markers

Of all the antibodies used as exclusionary for diagnosing epithelial mesothelioma, polyclonal-CEA has been used most frequently. Carcinoembryonic antigen (CEA) is a glycoprotein of approximately 200 kD that contains approximately 50% carbohydrate.[376-379] CEA is referred to as a family[380] and is coded by 29 genes, 18 of which are expressed (7 belong to the CEA subgroup, and 11 belong to the pregnancy-specific subgroup).

Often referred to as an oncofetal antigen, CEA is expressed in normal adult tissues and in a variety of epithelial neoplasms. The CEA subgroup includes biliary glycoprotein and nonspecific cross-reacting substance. The antibody we use is polyclonal, and the immunogen is CEA isolated from hepatic metastases of a colonic adenocarcinoma. The antibody reacts with nonspecific cross-reacting substance and biliary glycoprotein. Nonspecific cross-reacting substance is present in granulocytes and monocytes, and biliary glycoprotein is expressed by a large number of normal epithelial cells and by granulocytes, lymphocytes, and possibly endothelial cells. Therefore, it is likely that built-in positive control staining exists in most tissue sections for polyclonal CEA.

Polyclonal CEA shows no immunostaining in most epithelial mesotheliomas.[381-383] In contrast, it is found in a high percentage (85% to 100%) of pulmonary adenocarcinomas. Henderson and colleagues analyzed data from 21 separate reports evaluating 598 cases of diffuse malignant mesothelioma and found 58 cases (9.7%) reported to express CEA.[359] In the majority of cases where a positive reaction was observed, it was usually focal and weak. In the same analysis, 359 of 404 (88.9%) pulmonary adenocarcinomas expressed CEA. We have rarely observed CEA-positive staining in mesotheliomas. It occurred predominantly in epithelial mucin-positive mesotheliomas, which correlated with those producing large quantities of hyaluronic acid or proteoglycan. In our experience, polyclonal CEA is the best negative marker of mesothelioma.

LeuM1 is a monoclonal antibody against the membrane-related trisaccharide fucoysl-N-acetyllactosamine on myelomonocytic cells, where the epitope is also known as CD15 or X-hapten. LeuM1 is found in Reed-Sternberg cells in most cases of Hodgkin lymphoma. In 1985, Sheibani and Battifora[384] reported LeuM1 in a metastatic, poorly differentiated pulmonary adenocarcinoma. In 1986 Sheibani and colleagues[385] performed immunohistochemical analyses on 400 malignant neoplasms and found LeuM1 immunostaining in 105 of 179 (58.7%) adenocarcinomas and 0 of 18 epithelial mesotheliomas. Sheibani and coworkers subsequently studied 50 primary pulmonary adenocarcinomas and 28 pleural epithelial mesotheliomas, finding expression in 47 of 50 (94%) pulmonary adenocarcinomas and 0 of 28 epithelial mesotheliomas.[386] In another study, Sheibani and associates reported no immunostaining for LeuM1 in 127 cases of malignant mesothelioma.[387] Wick and colleagues identified LeuM1 in 52 of 52 (100%) pulmonary adenocarcinomas and 0 of 51 epithelial mesotheliomas.[260] In contrast, Otis and colleagues[388] observed LeuM1 immunostaining in only 50% of pulmonary adenocarcinomas and reported LeuM1 expression in epithelial mesotheliomas. Battifora and McCaughey observed focal LeuM1 expression in epithelial mesotheliomas.[313] This author has observed several LeuM1-positive epithelial mesotheliomas, and the staining is usually focal. In contrast to what has been reported in the literature and despite using heat-induced antigen retrieval, we have observed a positive reaction for LeuM1 (CD15) in only approximately 50% of primary pulmonary adenocarcinomas.

B72.3 is an antibody that recognizes a high molecular weight glycoprotein complex, tumor associated glycoprotein 72 (TAG-72), which is derived from a membrane- enriched fraction of human metastatic breast carcinoma. Szpak and colleagues[389] and Ordonez[390] reported immunostaining in 38 of 45 (84.4%) pulmonary adenocarcinomas in comparison with 1 of 38 (2.6%) epithelial mesotheliomas. Wick and associates reported that 43 of 52 (82.6%) pulmonary adenocarcinomas expressed B72.3, whereas all 51 epithelial mesotheliomas were negative.[358] In an evaluation of peritoneal mesotheliomas and serous papillary adenocarcinomas of the peritoneum, Bollinger and coworkers reported 43 of 46 (93.4%) serous papillary carcinomas positive for B72.3, whereas 8 epithelial mesotheliomas were negative.[391] Ordonez tabulated the reported literature and found 69 of 684 (10.1%) epithelial mesotheliomas to show immunostaining for B72.3 (0 to 48% of cases) and 578 of 607 (95.2%) adenocarcinomas to show positivity (47 to 100%).[319] When positive for B72.3, epithelial mesotheliomas usually show a small percentage of cells to be positive. However, Henderson and colleagues reported more extensive B72.3 expression in the cytoplasm of epithelial mesotheliomas and described one case of intracytoplasmic crescentic staining that correlated ultrastructurally with intracytoplasmic glycogen.[318]

Ber-EP4 is a monoclonal antibody that recognizes the protein moiety of two 34-kD and 39-kD glycopolypeptides on human epithelial cells. Latza and colleagues observed Ber-EP4reactivity in 142 of 144 (98.6%) adenocarcinomas from various sites and in 0 of 14 epithelial mesotheliomas.[392] Sheibani and associates observed Ber-EP4immunoreactivity in 1 of 115 (0.86%) epithelial mesotheliomas and 72 of 83 (86.7%) adenocarcinomas of various sites.[393] Eight of 25 breast carcinomas and 3 renal cell carcinomas studied were negative for BerEP4. Gaffey and colleagues found different results.[394] They reported 103 of 120 (83%) adenocarcinomas to be positive. Ten of 49 (20%) epithelial mesotheliomas were also reactive, as were 2 of 9 (22%) adenomatoid tumors. Gaffey and coworkers reported one epithelial mesothelioma diffusely positive.[394] Staining for Ber-EP4was usually in a cell membrane distribution. A possible explanation for the difference in these results is that Sheibani and colleagues used protease type 14 pre-digestion before Ber-EP4staining;[393] Gaffey and associates used 0.4% pepsin pre-digestion for 30 minutes before staining.[394] We currently use heat-induced epitope retrieval and observe approximately 20% of epithelial mesotheliomas to show predominantly low intensity cell membrane staining for BerEP4. Occasional epithelial mesotheliomas show intense cell membrane immunostaining. Ordonez reviewed published studies of Ber-EP4reactivity in epithelial mesotheliomas and adenocarcinomas of various types.[319] Seventy-six of 611 (12.4%) epithelial mesotheliomas (0 to 88%) and 940 of 1399 (67.2%) adenocarcinomas (35% to 100%) immunostained for BerEP4.

MOC31 is a monoclonal antibody that reacts with a 38-kD epithelial-associated transmembrane glycoprotein of small cell lung carcinoma known as epithelial glycoprotein-2.[395,396] DeLeij and colleagues reported MOC31 activity in all pulmonary carcinomas, including 28 of 28 (100%) adenocarcinomas.[397] Normal mesothelial cells and neoplastic epithelial mesothelial cells did not react with the antibody. In 1991 Delahaye and colleagues studied cytologic preparations of serous fluid and found positive MOC31 staining in 2 of 24 (8.3%) epithelial mesotheliomas and in 18 of 31 (58.1%) adenocarcinomas of various origins.[398] Ruitenbeek and coworkers found MOC31 reactivity in 62 of 63 (98.4%) adenocarcinomas and in 0 of 5 epithelial mesotheliomas.[396] Ordonez reported intense MOC31 reactivity in 37 of 40 (92.5%) pulmonary adenocarcinomas, 11 of 11 (100%) colon adenocarcinomas, 20 of 21 (95.2%) ovarian adenocarcinomas, 9 of 10 (90%) breast adenocarcinomas, and 5 of 13 (38.5%) kidney adenocarcinomas.[399] MOC31 reactivity was seen in 2 of 38 (5.3%) epithelial mesotheliomas, although the degree of staining was usually focal, involving less than 10% of cells. Ordonez reviewed published studies of MOC31 reactivity in epithelial mesotheliomas and various types of adenocarcinomas.[319] Immunostaining was found in 307 of 333 (92.2%) adenocarcinomas (58 to 100%) and 23 of 158 (14.6%) epithelial mesotheliomas (0 to 88%).

Monoclonal antibody BG8 reacts with SK-LU-3 lung cancer cells that recognize the Lewis Y blood group antigen. Jordon and colleagues reported reactivity in 18 of 18 (100%) pulmonary adenocarcinomas and in 7 of 30 (23.3%) epithelial mesotheliomas.[400] Reactivity in mesotheliomas was usually focal and limited to a few cells, whereas reactivity in pulmonary adenocarcinomas was usually strong and diffuse. Riera and colleagues[401] evaluated BG8 antibody and found expression in 114 of 123 (92.7%) pulmonary adenocarcinomas and 5 of 57 (8.8%) epithelial mesotheliomas. The staining in epithelial mesotheliomas was usually focal and weak.

E-cadherin is a 120-kD cell adhesion molecule expressed in epithelial cells.[364,402] Loss of E-cadherin expression is associated with a higher degree of invasiveness and an increase in malignant potential in several carcinomas, including lung cancers.[403] Peralta-Soler and associates reported intense immunostaining for E-cadherin (epithelial cadherin) in 16 of 16 (100%) pulmonary adenocarcinomas and 8 of 19 (42.1%) epithelial mesotheliomas, with the staining usually involving only a few cells.[367] Using formalin-fixed heat-induced epitope antigen retrieval, 13 of 14 (92.9%) pulmonary carcinomas were positive for E-cadherin and 0 of 13 epithelial mesotheliomas were reactive. Leers and colleagues reported positive reactivity in 20 of 21 (95.2%) adenocarcinomas of various origin and in 3 of 20 (15%) epithelial mesotheliomas.[348] Using the commercially available 5H9 anti-E-cadherin antibody on sections of formalin-fixed paraffin-embedded tissue, Ordonez found reactivity in 15 of 18 (83.3%) pulmonary adenocarcinomas and 0 of 17 epithelial mesotheliomas.[319] When Ordonez used anti–E-cadherin monoclonal antibody clone 36 (Transduction Laboratory, Lexington, Kentucky), strong reactivity was seen in 6 of 6 (100%) epithelial mesotheliomas. It would therefore appear that caution needs to be exercised using this antibody and that the 5H9 anti-E-cadherin antibody would be the appropriate one to use. As discussed earlier in the chapter, Ordonez concluded that only 5H9 clone anti-E-cadherin antibody had utility in differentiating epithelial mesothelioma from pulmonary adenocarcinoma.[369]

Blood group–related antigen expression has been used to evaluate epithelial mesotheliomas and pulmonary adenocarcinomas. Wick and coworkers found ABH iso-antigen expression in 35 of 52 (67.3%) adenocarcinomas and in 0 of 51 epithelial mesotheliomas.[358] Kawai and associates evaluated 20 epithelial, 3 biphasic, and 6 sarcomatoid mesotheliomas; 5 reactive mesothelial cell lesions; and 38 well-differentiated pulmonary adenocarcinomas using ABH blood group-related antigen (BGRA-g) antibody and *Helix pomotia* agglutinin (HPAgg).[404] The reactive mesothelial lesions and the mesotheliomas showed no expression for BGRA-g or HPAgg, irrespective of the blood group type. Positive staining for A, B, or H blood group–related antigen was seen in 40 of 48 (83%) adenocarcinomas in compatible blood group–type patients. A positive reaction for HPAgg was seen in 16 of 17 (94.1%) cases of blood type A and in all blood type AB patients. Positive staining for HPAgg was observed in 4 of 5 (80%) blood group type B patients and in 4 of 12 (33.3%) with blood group type O.

Riera and colleagues[401] used heat-induced epitope retrieval to study 268 paraffin-embedded, formalin-fixed tumors, including 57 epithelial mesotheliomas and 211 adenocarcinomas of various origin. After statistical analysis, they found that CEA, BerEP4, and BG8 were the best discriminators between adenocarcinoma and epithelial mesothelioma within the entire panel, and that the mesothelioma-associated antibodies HBME-1, calretinin, and thrombomodulin were less sensitive and less specific, but useful in only certain cases. They observed all adenocarcinomas and mesotheliomas to show intense immunohistochemical staining for keratin with no discernible difference in staining pattern between adenocarcinoma and mesothelioma. Forty-six of 57 (81.5%) mesotheliomas and 66 of 211 (31.2%) adenocarcinomas expressed vimentin. The authors stated that the intensity and distribution of vimentin staining was greater in mesotheliomas than in adenocarcinomas. CEA immunoreactivity was observed in 175 of 211 (82.9%) adenocarcinomas and in no mesotheliomas. Ovarian and breast adenocarcinomas showed 44.8% and 79.3% CEA-positive staining, respectively. Focal immunostaining for Ber-EP4was observed in 63.7% of adenocarcinomas and in no mesotheliomas. BG8 reactivity was observed in 88.6% of adenocarcinomas and 5 of 57 (8.7%) mesotheliomas, with the neoplastic cells in mesotheliomas staining only focally positivity and with less intensity. B72.3 immunostaining was observed in 170 of 211 (80.5%) adenocarcinomas and 2 of 57 (3.5%) mesotheliomas. In mesotheliomas, immunostaining for B72.3 was focal but intense. Granular cytoplasmic staining for LeuM1 was found in 159 of 211 (75.3%) adenocarcinomas and 104 of 123 (84.5%) pulmonary adenocarcinomas. Two of 57 (3.5%) mesotheliomas showed predominantly focal membrane staining for LeuM1. Diffuse, moderately intense cytoplasmic

TABLE 12.25 Sensitivity and Specificity of Immunohistochemical Tests Used to Evaluate Adenocarcinomas*

	1		2		3	
Scoring	Sensitivity	Specificity	Sensitivity	Specificity	Sensitivity	Specificity
CEA-I	83	100	79	100	75	100
CEA-D			75	100	64	100
BG8-I	89	91	82	91	50	96
BG8-D			75	100	42	100
BerEP4-I	64	100	64	100	39	100
BerEP4-D			55	100	29	100
B72.3-I	81	96	77	96	68	96
B72.3-D			50	98	19	98
LeuM1-I	75	96	71	96	55	96
LeuM1-D			55	100	33	100
HMFG-2-CI	85	72	64	79	19	89
HMFG-2-CD		72	73	77	40	89

*Heat-induced epitope retrieval (HIER) used when appropriate.
Values are percentages.
I, intensity of staining; D, distribution of staining.
Reproduced from Riera JR, Astengo-Osuna C, Longmate JA, et al. The immunohistochemical diagnostic panel for epithelial mesothelioma: A reevaluation after heat-induced epitope retrieval. *Am J Surg Pathol.* 1997;21:1409-1419.

TABLE 12.26 Sensitivity and Specificity of Immunohistochemical Tests Used to Evaluate Mesotheliomas*

	1		2		3	
Scoring	Sensitivity	Specificity	Sensitivity	Specificity	Sensitivity	Specificity
Calretinin-I	42	94	31	96	8	100
Calretinin-D	49	94	39	97	16	98
Thrombomodulin-I	49	94	46	95	35	97
Thrombomodulin-D	49	94	32	96	32	96
HBME-1-I†	79	61	74	72	53	91
HBME-2-D†	79	61	65	73	39	89

*HIER (heat-induced epitope retrieval) used when appropriate.
†Only membrane staining interpreted.
I, intensity of staining; D, distribution of staining.
Reproduced from Riera JR, Astengo-Osuna C, Longmate JA, et al. The immunohistochemical diagnostic panel for epithelial mesothelioma: A reevaluation after heat-induced epitope retrieval. *Am J Surg Pathol.* 1997;21:1409-1419.

staining was observed for Ber-EP4in 180 of 211 (85.3%) adenocarcinomas and 16 of 57 (28.1%) mesotheliomas. Most adenocarcinomas were stated to show cytoplasmic reactivity. In contrast, 33 of 57 (57.8%) epithelial mesotheliomas showed cell membrane staining usually without cytoplasmic staining. In several cases, a thick pattern of membrane staining was observed similar to that found with HBME-1.

Concerning mesothelial-related antigens, 28 of 57 (49.1%) epithelial mesotheliomas immunostained for thrombomodulin compared to 13 of 211 (6.1%) adenocarcinomas, of which 7 were pulmonary adenocarcinomas. HBME-1 immunoreactivity was observed in 45 of 57 (78.9%) epithelial mesotheliomas, usually in a circumferentially thick or moderately thick distribution, and in 83 of 211 (39.3%) adenocarcinomas, usually in a thin pattern restricted to the apical region. A thick membrane pattern was observed in 19 of 211 (9%) adenocarcinomas, usually in an apical distribution. Twenty-four of 57 (42.1%) epithelial mesotheliomas showed immunostaining for calretinin (cytoplasmic, finely granular, and diffuse in 22 cases and focal in 2 cases), whereas 13 of 211 (6.1%) adenocarcinomas showed weak or moderate staining.

The sensitivity and specificity of the adenocarcinoma and mesothelioma markers observed by Riera and colleagues[401] are shown in Tables 12.25 and 12.26, respectively.

The study by Riera and colleagues[401] provides a great deal of practical information. Of interest in their study was that the HBME-1 antibody was used in a dilution of 1:40, which is in contrast to what we use (1:7500) and what Henderson[318] uses (1:5000 to 1:15,000). We have found a much higher positive staining reaction for calretinin (approximately 95%) in epithelial mesothelioma than Riera and associates[401] did.

Miscellaneous Antibodies

Expression of p53 tumor suppressor gene products has been evaluated as a method of discriminating between mesothelioma and reactive mesothelial hyperplasia.[405,406] Ramael and coworkers[406] evaluated 40 cases of non-neoplastic reactive pleural mesothelial proliferative lesions and 36 epithelial mesotheliomas for p53 tumor suppressor gene product. Using DO-7 and CM-1 antibodies, nuclear immunolabeling for p53 was observed in 25% of mesotheliomas. No reactivity was observed using antibody PAb240. There was no significant difference in reactivity for the p53 tumor suppressor gene product between histologic subtypes of mesothelioma. Mayall and colleagues[405] evaluated p53 gene product expression using DO-7 and CM-1 antibodies in pepsin pre-digested tissue sections and found positive reactions in 10 of 16 (62.5%) epithelial mesotheliomas, 9 of 19 (47.4%) biphasic mesotheliomas, 2 of 12 (16.7%) sarcomatoid mesotheliomas, and in 0 of 20 reactive mesothelial cell proliferations. Mayall and colleagues[407] found no difference in p53 gene product expression in asbestos-induced mesotheliomas versus mesotheliomas that were not caused by asbestos, which suggests that asbestos is not the cause of p53 gene mutation.

Using formalin-fixed paraffin-embedded tissue sections, Hurlimann[408] reported immunohistochemical desmin expression in 9 of 16 (56.3%) mesotheliomas (8 epithelial and 1 biphasic). Staining was described as focal or was found only in rare tumor cells. Cases showed positive reactivity more frequently with heat-induced epitope retrieval. Four of 16 (25%) mesotheliomas (3 epithelial and 1 biphasic) expressed neuron-specific enolase, 5 of 16 (31.3%) immunostained for chromogranin (4 epithelial, 1 biphasic) and 5 of 16 (31.3%) mesotheliomas (all epithelial) were positive for S-100 protein. Only rare tumor cells expressed these neuroepithelial markers.

Azumi and associates used immunohistochemistry to study 33 mesotheliomas (32 pleural, 1 peritoneal, 18 epithelial, 10 biphasic, 4 sarcomatoid, 1 desmoplastic) and 37 adenocarcinomas for hyaluronate. Three of 37 (8.1%) adenocarcinomas and all mesotheliomas immunostained for hyaluronate.[409] The location of the staining reaction in the mesotheliomas was membranous in 30 cases, cytoplasmic in 21 cases, and membranous and cytoplasmic in 19 cases. The staining reaction in mesotheliomas was classified as moderate or greater in 27 of 33 (81.8%) cases. The authors concluded that the demonstration of hyaluronate should be considered an important adjunct to other immunohistochemical tests and electron microscopy in diagnosing epithelial mesotheliomas.

Hyaluronan detection in pleural fluid has been advocated as a method of diagnosing mesothelioma.[410] Among 13 patients with pleural fluid hyaluronan concentrations above 225 mg/L, no other diagnosis but mesothelioma was identified. The specificity for mesothelioma was 96%, with a cutoff level of 75 mg/L hyaluronan and 100% with a cutoff level of 225 mg/L hyaluronan.

Martensson and colleagues evaluated hyaluronan in pleural fluid from 19 male patients with mesothelioma.[411] Tumor volume was estimated on transilluminated CT scans with a digital planimeter. The authors found an elevated (7,100 mg/L) concentration of hyaluronan in the pleural fluid in 13 of 19 (68.4%) patients. They also found a positive correlation between the initial concentration of hyaluronan in the serum and the concentration of hyaluronan in the pleural fluid. Increasing concentration of circulating hyaluronan correlated positively with an increasing tumor volume in the hyaluronan-producing mesotheliomas, but not in the non-hyaluronan–producing mesotheliomas.

Thylen and coworkers evaluated the immunohistochemical differences between hyaluronan and non-hyaluronan–producing malignant mesothelioma and found a significantly higher reactivity to EMA, a higher reactivity to CAM5.2 keratin, and a lower reactivity to vimentin in the hyaluronan-producing epithelial mesotheliomas. [412] All tumors were stated to be negative for CEA. Our experience is different from that of Thylen and colleagues in that the mesotheliomas that produce excess amounts of hyaluronic acid and/or proteoglycans are more likely to be mucin-positive and to express the negative markers of epithelial mesothelioma, such as CEA, LeuM1, and B72.3.

CA-125 is a glycoprotein identified in the cell membrane in celomic epithelium during embryogenesis and in neoplasms of the female genital tract.[413-416] The antibody to detect CA-125 in histologic sections, OC-125 was initially thought to work only in frozen tissue sections but was adapted to work in formalin-fixed paraffin-embedded sections using enzymatic digestion[417] or heat-induced epitope retrieval. It soon became apparent that OC-125 reactivity was not restricted to the gynecologic tract. OC-125 reactivity was observed in breast neoplasms,[418] lung neoplasms,[419,420] and neoplasms of the pleura and peritoneal linings.[421,422] The authors stated that M-11, the second-generation antibody against CA 125, showed greater intensity staining than OC-125.[423] M-11 reactivity was demonstrated in mesothelial linings of spontaneous abortion specimens of 6 to 14 weeks gestation.[424] This author has observed several cases of usually low/moderate intensity cell membrane immunostaining of epithelial mesotheliomas for OC-125.

In rare instances, unusual substances have been demonstrated immunohistochemically in mesotheliomas. Okamoto and colleagues reported two neoplasms consistent with primary pleural mesotheliomas that contained anaplastic tumor giant cells that contained hCG, as demonstrated by immunohistochemistry.[425]

McAuley and colleagues evaluated a patient with malignant mesothelioma who had hypercalcemia and an elevated serum concentration of parathyroid-like hormone.[426] They evaluated 9 epithelial mesotheliomas

TABLE 12.27 Sensitivity and Specificity of Each Marker Using a Fixed 10% Positive Cutoff

	Sensitivity	Specificity	Specificity excluding ovarian tumors
For Diagnosing Mesothelioma			
Thrombomodulin	68%	92%	
CK5/6	95%	87%	
Vimentin	69%	84%	
Mesothelin	75%	71%	9%
WT1	78%	62%	81%
HBME-1	84%	48%	
Caldesmon	97%	45%	
For Diagnosing Adenocarcinoma			
Bg8	95%	98%	
CEA	63%	98%	
CD15 (LeuM1)	51%	97%	
BerEP4	74%	95%	
MOC-31	92%	87%	

for parathyroid-like peptide and found abundant immunopositive cells in 8 of 9 cases. They also observed parathyroid-like peptide immunoreactivity in normal and reactive epithelial mesothelial cells.

Tateyama and associates reported CD5 expression in thymic carcinoma and atypical thymoma and in 9 of 13 (69.2%) mesotheliomas (5 epithelial, 3 biphasic, 1 sarcomatoid).[427] All CD5-positive mesotheliomas showed intense intracytoplasmic staining. Eight of 13 (61.5%) pulmonary adenocarcinomas showed low to moderately intense, predominantly cell membrane staining for CD5. A significant number of mesotheliomas show immunostaining for various CD antigens such as CD30, CD56, and CD99.

Diagnostic Considerations

These authors use a battery of antibodies to evaluate mesothelial proliferative lesions, including reactive and neoplastic processes. Keratin antibodies, with the exception of CK5/6, are generally not used to differentiate an epithelial mesothelioma from another neoplasm or from a reactive process, but are used to identify the extent of a neoplastic or reactive mesothelial cell process. The antibodies we use to differentiate a well or moderately well differentiated epithelial mesothelioma from a pulmonary adenocarcinoma or nonpulmonary adenocarcinoma include AE1/AE3 cytokeratin, CK5/6, CK7, CK20, vimentin, EMA, HBME-1, calretinin, mesothelin, WT1, D2-40, caldesmon, CEA, LeuM1, B72.3, BerEP4, and TTF-1.

Yaziji and coworkers evaluated 133 neoplasms using immunohistochemistry, including 65 epithelial mesotheliomas, 22 lung adenocarcinomas, 27 ovarian serous carcinomas, 24 breast carcinomas, and 5 gastric carcinomas.[428] The diagnoses was made on clinical, histologic, ultrastructural, and/or immunohistochemical findings. Deparaffinized sections were immunostained with 13 antibodies to confirm antigenicity. These included calretinin, mesothelin, WT1, HBME-1, CK5/6, vimentin, epithelial glycoprotein (MOC31), epithelial glycoprotein (BerEP4), epithelial glycoprotein (Bg8), CEA, CD15, and pan cytokeratin (AE1/AE3 keratin). The sensitivity and specificity of each marker using a fixed 10% positive cutoff are listed in Table 12.27. Calretinin was found to have the best sensitivity for mesothelioma (95%) followed by HBME-1 (84%), WT1 (78%), CK5/6 (76%), mesothelin (75%), vimentin (69%), and thrombomodulin (68%). Thrombomodulin had the best specificity for mesothelioma (92%) followed by CK5/6 (89%), calretinin (87%), vimentin (84%), and HBME-1 (48%). When ovarian carcinomas were excluded from the analysis, the specificity of mesothelin and WT1 for the diagnosis of mesothelioma increased to 90% and 81%, respectively. The authors found that the sensitivity of the nonmesothelial antigens for adenocarcinoma was organ dependent, with Bg8 performing best in the breast cancer group (96%), and BerEP4, Bg8, and MOC-31 performing best in the lung cancer group (100%).[428] The specificity of the nonmesothelial antigens for adenocarcinoma was 98% for Bg8 and CEA, 97% for CD15, 95% for BerEP4, and 87% for MOC-31. A statistical analysis technique employing logic regression analysis identified a three-antibody immunohistochemical panel, including calretinin, Bg8, and MOC-31, which provided over 96% sensitivity and specificity for distinguishing epithelioid mesothelioma from adenocarcinoma.

Marchevsky recently reviewed the application of immunohistochemistry to the diagnosis of malignant mesothelioma. [429] Marchevsky stated that antibody panels that had been proposed for the distinction between malignant mesothelioma and other neoplasms included two or more epithelial markers used to exclude the diagnosis of carcinoma (e.g., monoclonal and polyclonal CEA, BerEP4, B72.3, CD15, MOC-31,

TABLE 12.28 Immunostains in Malignant Mesothelioma and Other Malignant Neoplasms

Antibody	Epithelial Mesothelioma	Sarcomatoid Mesothelioma	Adenocarcinoma	Squamous Cell Carcinoma	Renal Cell Carcinoma
Epithelial Markers					
pCEA	5%	0%	83%	7%	0%
mCEA	3%	–	81%	–	–
BerEP4	10%	0%	80%	40%	0-58%
B72.3	7%	0%	80%	87%	–
CD15 (LeuM1)	7%	0%	72%	30%	25%-100%
MOC-31	7%	0%	93%	97%	0%-75%
TTF-1	Negative	0%	Lung: 72% Other: Negative	Negative	–
Lewis-BG8	7%	0%	93%	80%	0%-33%
Mesothelial Markers					
CK5/6	83%	13%	14.9%	100%	5%
Calretinin	82%	88%	15%	40%	10%
HBME-1	85%	–	57%	–	–
Thrombomodulin	61%	13%	20%	–	0%-32%
WT1	77%	13%	4%	Negative	0%-4%
Mesothelin	100%	0%	–	27%	–
D2-40	86%-100%	0%	36% (weak)	–	–
Podoplanin	86%-93%	0%	–	15%	–

pCEA, polyclonal carcinoembryonic antigen; mCEA, monoclonal carcinoembryonic antigen; TTF-1, thyroid transcription factor-1.

TTF-1, and Bg8) and two or more mesothelial markers used to confirm the diagnosis (e.g., CK5/6, calretinin, HBME-1, WT1, mesothelin, thrombomodulin, and podoplanin [D2-40]). Marchevsky concluded that antibody panels provided excellent sensitivity and specificity between malignant epithelial mesothelioma and adenocarcinoma, but with a lower accuracy for the diagnosis of sarcomatoid malignant mesothelioma. Marchevsky summarized the data in Table 12.28. As noted, even the antibodies used to mark adenocarcinomas and those that were negative in malignant mesothelioma were positive in 5%, 3%, 10%, 7%, 7%, and 7% of cases for pCEA, mCEA, BerEP4, B72.3, CD15 (LeuM1), and MOC-31, respectively. TTF-1 was the only adenocarcinoma marker that was completely negative in every case of mesothelioma. With respect to mesothelioma, Marchevsky found that the mesothelial markers CK5/6, calretinin, HBME-1, thrombomodulin, WT1, mesothelin, and podoplanin were positive in 83%, 82%, 85%, 61%, 77%, 100%, and 86% to 93% of cases, respectively. Marchevsky used Bayesian statistics to analyze the review data published by King and colleagues and concluded that the best odds ratio for the differential diagnosis between epithelial mesothelioma and pulmonary adenocarcinoma can be achieved by using panels composed of only two antibodies—one mesothelial and one epithelial, such as WT1 and TTF-1, or two epithelial epitopes, such as MOC-31 and TTF-1.

The immunohistogram of a well to moderately well differentiated epithelial mesothelioma is shown in Fig. 12.51. A comparison of the immunohistochemical profile of well to moderately well differentiated epithelial mesothelioma and pulmonary adenocarcinoma is shown in Table 12.29.

According to the Guidelines for Pathologic Diagnosis of Malignant Mesothelioma: Consensus from the International Mesothelioma Interest Group, an immunohistochemical panel that can be useful for the evaluation of sarcomatoid tumors involving the pleura should include cytokeratins, calretinin, and D2-40.[430] As stated earlier in the chapter, multiple cytokeratin antibodies, including AE1/AE3 keratin, CAM5.2 keratin (CK18), and CK7 usually are expressed in sarcomatoid mesotheliomas. D2-40 and calretinin are the two positive markers that are most frequently expressed in sarcomatoid mesotheliomas in a variable percentage of cases.[374,431-433]

Marchevsky[429] evaluated sarcomatoid mesotheliomas and correctly pointed out that the diagnosis of sarcomatoid mesothelioma was particularly difficult as the sensitivity and specificity of mesothelial markers was considerably lower in these lesions than in malignant epithelial mesothelioma. Marchevsky correctly stated that immunostains for calretinin, thrombomodulin, and WT1 were positive in fewer than 20% of sarcomatoid mesotheliomas. Marchevsky stated that immunostaining for AE1/AE3 keratin was the most helpful in that it showed staining in almost all cases of sarcomatoid

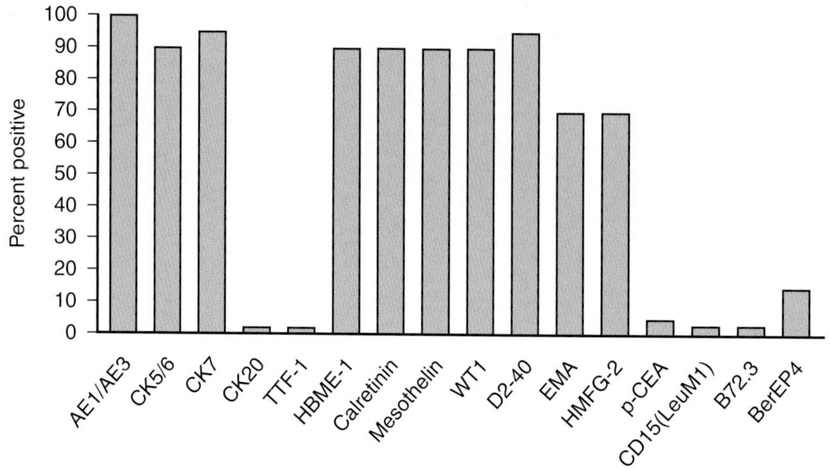

FIGURE 12.51 Immunohistogram of a well to moderately well differentiated epithelial mesothelioma.

mesothelioma. Marchevsky also pointed out that other types of sarcomatoid neoplasms involving the pleura, such as synovial sarcoma and sarcomatoid carcinoma, can show positive staining for AE1/AE3 keratin. Marchevsky also stated that podoplanin (D2-40) stained the epithelioid cells of a biphasic synovial sarcoma.

Most sarcomatoid mesotheliomas express keratin (usually low molecular weight keratin), vimentin, and frequently muscle-specific/alpha actin. In our experience, a relatively small percent (10% to 20%) of sarcomatoid mesotheliomas express calretinin, and most sarcomatoid mesotheliomas do not express cytokeratin 5/6. Most sarcomatoid mesotheliomas express CK7, often intensely. In our experience, sarcomatoid mesotheliomas (and tumors with which they may be confused) do not express the "negative" markers used to evaluate potential epithelial mesotheliomas, including CEA, LeuM1, B72.3, BerEP4, BG8, and TTF-1. Therefore, we would not include these antibodies in a "screen" of a malignant spindle cell proliferative lesion of the pleura.

With respect to sarcomatoid malignant mesothelioma and the diagnosis of sarcoma, Marchevsky correctly noted that the diagnosis of sarcomatoid mesothelioma was particularly difficult because the sensitivity and specificity of mesothelial markers was considerably lower in these lesions than in malignant epithelial mesothelioma.[429] Marchevsky correctly stated that immunostains for calretinin, thrombomodulin, and WT1 were positive in fewer than 20% of sarcomatoid mesotheliomas. Immunostaining for AE1/AE3 keratin was probably the most helpful because it showed staining in most if not all cases of sarcomatoid mesothelioma. Marchevsky also correctly pointed out that other types of sarcomatoid neoplasms, such as synovial sarcoma and sarcomatoid carcinoma, can show positive staining for AE1/AE3 keratin. Marchevsky also noted that podoplanin (D2-40) stained the epithelioid cells of a biphasic synovial sarcoma.

Klebe and associates reported 27 cases of malignant mesothelioma that had heterologous elements.[434] Of 27 cases, 16 (59%) were sarcomatoid, 10 (37%) were biphasic, and 1 was epithelioid. Eleven cases (40%) showed osteosarcomatous elements only; 19% showed areas of rhabdomyosarcoma only; 19% showed areas of chondrosarcomatous differentiation only; and 22% showed osteochondromatous elements. The authors stated that immunohistochemical labeling for cytokeratins was exhibited in the majority of cases. These tumors had a very poor prognosis with a median survival of only 6 months. The authors pointed out that lack of labeling for cytokeratins in a spindle cell/sarcomatoid tumor did not exclude the diagnosis of mesothelioma irrespective of the presence of heterologous elements. The authors suggested that if the anatomic distribution of the tumor conformed to that of a mesothelioma, a diagnosis of heterologous mesothelioma should be made in preference to a diagnosis of a primary pleural osteosarcoma or chondrosarcoma, regardless of cytokeratin positivity (as for conventional non-heterologous sarcomatoid mesothelioma).

Rare sarcomatoid mesotheliomas show heterologous differentiation composed of fat (Figs. 12.52 and 12.53).[435] The immunohistogram of a sarcomatoid mesothelioma is shown in Figure 12.54. The most important immunohistochemical finding in sarcomatoid mesothelioma is coexpression of keratin and vimentin.

As mesotheliomas become more poorly differentiated such as those we[311] refer to as *transitional*, they usually only express broad-spectrum keratin and vimentin.

Metastatic tumors to the pleura are more common than primary neoplasms. It is imperative that metastases be considered a possibility for any tumor involving the pleura that is being evaluated by immunohistochemistry. In this context, it is important to know clinical information concerning the patient, which may have an influence on the immunohistochemical tests performed. However, the pathologic diagnosis is based on objective findings and not on the clinical history.

Metastatic tumors of unknown primary origin are discussed in Chapter 8, and may involve the pleura. These and other authors have shown that the most cost-effective way of evaluating a suspected metastatic

TABLE 12.29 Comparison of Immunohistochemical Profiles of Well to Moderately Well Differentiated Epithelial Mesotheliomas and Well to Moderately Well Differentiated Pulmonary Adenocarcinomas

Type of Neoplasm	Antibody Directed Against									
	AE1/AE3	Low molecular weight keratin (35βH11)	High molecular weight keratin (34βE12)	CK5/6	CK7	CK20	Vimentin	HBME-1	Calretinin	Caldesmon
Well to moderately well differentiated epithelial mesothelioma	+	+	+	S	+	S	S	S*	S**	+
Well to moderately well differentiated pulmonary adenocarcinoma	+	+	S	R	+	S	S	R	R	N

Type of Neoplasm	Antibody Directed Against									
	Epithelial membrane antigen	Carcinoembryonic antigen	CD15 (LeuM1)	BerEP4	B72.3	Thyroid transcription factor-1	WT1	Mesothelin	D2-40	Human milk fat globule protein-2
Well to moderately well differentiated epithelial mesothelioma	S*	R	R	S	R	N	+	+	+	S*
Well to moderately well differentiated pulmonary adenocarcinoma	S†	+	S	S	S	S	N	N	N	S†

*Cell membrane distribution.
†Cytoplasmic distribution.
**Nuclear and cytoplasmic immunostaining.
Reactivity:
+, almost always diffuse, strong positivity
S, sometimes positive
R, rare cells positive
N, almost always negative

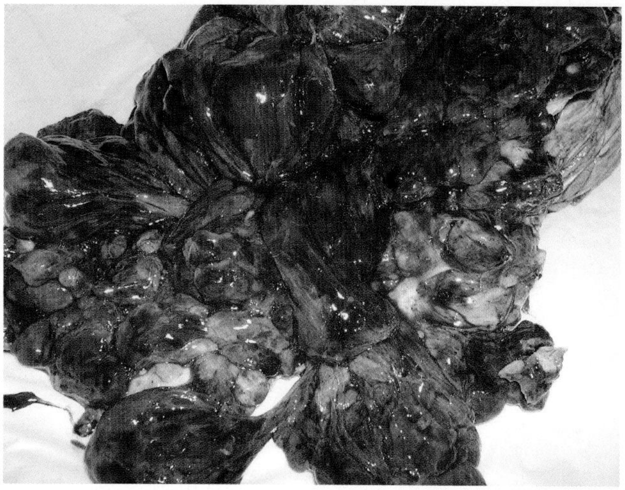

FIGURE 12.52 This neoplasm was in a diffuse pleural distribution and had the consistency of fat.

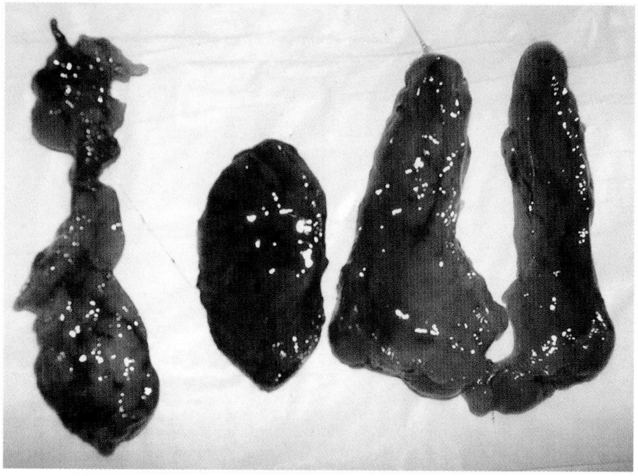

FIGURE 12.53 Portions of tumor having morphology consistent with fat.

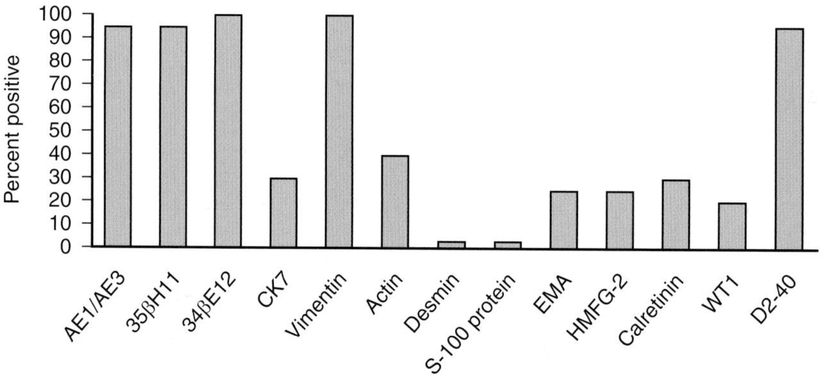

FIGURE 12.54 Immunohistogram of a sarcomatoid mesothelioma.

tumor of unknown primary origin is by pathologic techniques, including immunohistochemistry and electron microscopy.[436,437] The histologic appearance of the tumor dictates the antibody selection in such neoplasms. Pathologists should remember the variable histologic spectrum of mesotheliomas so that uncommon histologic types of mesothelioma are not misdiagnosed as metastatic neoplasms. In cases of suspected pleural mesothelioma, clinical information may be helpful by demonstrating radiographically that a tumor is encasing the lung and by providing evidence that a neoplasm is not identified in other organs or tissues.

Localized malignant mesotheliomas occur[438,439] and show the same histologic and immunohistochemical features of diffuse malignant mesotheliomas. However, mesotheliomas may be diffuse and beyond the resolution of current radiographic techniques (e.g., computed tomography and magnetic resonance imaging) and initially appear as localized.

Pleomorphic mesotheliomas exist[440] and are composed of pleomorphic epithelioid and sarcomatoid cells. Occasional multinucleated macrophage giant cells are associated with the tumor cells. Pleomorphic mesotheliomas need to be differentiated from pleomorphic carcinomas of the lung. In most instances, pleomorphic mesotheliomas express pan cytokeratin and vimentin, and in 10% to 20% of cases they express more specific markers such as calretinin, CK5/6, CK7, and rarely mesothelin and WT1.

A difficult area in mesothelioma pathology involves differentiating reactive mesothelial hyperplasia from mesothelioma. Table 12.30 contrasts the difference between mesothelial hyperplasia and mesothelioma. Table 12.31 compares the immunohistochemical features of reactive mesothelial hyperplasia versus epithelial mesothelioma. Several publications have evaluated the issue of reactive mesothelial hyperplasia versus mesothelioma.

Attanoos and colleagues used the avidin-biotin complex method to evaluate 60 cases of malignant pleural mesothelioma and 40 cases of reactive mesothelial hyperplasia with antibodies stained against desmin, epithelial membrane antigen (EMA), p53, BCL-2, P-glycoprotein, and platelet derived growth factor receptor (PDGF-R) beta chain.[441] The cohort of malignant pleural mesotheliomas were immunoreactive to desmin, EMA, and p53 in 6 of 60 (10%), 48 of 60 (80%), and 27 of 60 (45%), respectively. In contrast, the cohort of reactive mesothelial hyperplasia were immunoreactive to desmin, EMA and p53 in 34 of 40 (85%), 8 of 40 (20%), and 0 of 40 (0%), respectively. In a smaller cohort (n = 15) of malignant pleural mesotheliomas, BCL-2, P-glycoprotein, and PDGF-R beta were expressed in 0 of 15 (0%),

TABLE 12.30 Differentiating Reactive Mesothelial Hyperplasia from Mesothelioma

Characteristics	Reactive Mesothelial Hyperplasia	Mesothelioma
Stromal invasion	Absent (beware of entrapment and en face cuts)	Usually apparent (highlight with pan cytokeratin staining)
Cellularity	May be prominent but within the mesothelial space and not the stroma	Dense, including cells surrounded by stroma
Papillae	Simple; single cell layers	Complex; tubules, cellular stratification
Necrosis	Rare	Occasionally present
Inflammation	Common	Usually minimal
Growth	Uniform (highlighted with cytokeratin staining)	Disorganized; expansile nodules (highlighted on cytokeratin staining)
EMA, p53	Usually negative	Often positive
Desmin	Often positive	Often negative
Mitotic activity	Usually not useful	
Cytologic atypia	Usually not useful	

2 of 15 (13%), and 15 of 15 (100%), respectively. In a small cohort of reactive mesothelial hyperplasias (n = 15), BCL-2, P-glycoprotein, and PDGF-R beta were immunoreactive in 0 of 15 (0%), 0 of 15 (0%), and 6 of 15 (40%), respectively. The authors concluded that desmin and EMA appeared to be the most useful markers in distinguishing benign from malignant mesothelial cell proliferation. Desmin appeared to be preferentially expressed in reactive mesothelium, and EMA was preferentially expressed in neoplastic mesothelium. Immunohistochemical detection of mutated p53 oncoprotein appeared to be of less utility in this study on account of the low marker sensitivity for malignant mesothelioma. BCL-2, P-glycoprotein, and PDGF-R beta chain appeared to be of no use in distinguishing reactive from neoplastic mesothelium.

Wu and colleagues evaluated benign and malignant mesothelial tissue samples for the presence of X-link inhibitor of apoptosis protein (XIAP), a potent constituent of the inhibitor of apoptosis family of caspase inhibitors.[442] The authors studied 31 malignant mesotheliomas, 2 well-differentiated peritoneal mesotheliomas, 13 pleural mesothelial hyperplasias, and 9 benign mesothelial tissues from archival formalin-fixed paraffin-embedded surgical tissue blocks with citrate-based antigen retrieval. The authors found that all 9 normal mesothelial samples were negative for XIAP. Of the 13 mesothelial hyperplasias, 1 (8%) was weakly positive in fewer than 10% of cells, as was 1 of 2 well-differentiated papillary peritoneal mesotheliomas. Of the 31 malignant mesotheliomas, 25 (81%) expressed XIAP positivity. The authors concluded that XIAP immunostaining, when strong, allowed for distinction of malignant from benign and hyperplastic mesothelial cell populations and was a potential useful immunodiagnostic marker in small samples and morphologically controversial cases. The authors concluded that elevated XIAP expression could contribute to tumorigenesis in mesothelioma.

Kato and coworkers evaluated GLUT-1 expression in reactive and neoplastic mesothelioma.[443] The authors stated that to date no immunohistochemical marker allowed for unequivocal discrimination of reactive mesothelium from malignant pleural mesothelioma. The authors stated that a family of glucose transporter isoform (GLUT), of which GLUT-1 was a member, facilitated the entry of glucose into cells. GLUT-1 was largely undetectable by immunohistochemistry in normal epithelial tissues and benign tumors, but was also expressed in a variety of malignancies. The authors studied whether or not GLUT-1 appeared to be a potential marker of malignant transformations and stated that studies had shown GLUT-1 expression was useful for distinguishing benign from malignant lesions. The purpose of the study was to evaluate the diagnostic utility of GLUT-1 expression for the differential

TABLE 12.31 Comparison of Immunohistochemical Features of Reactive Mesothelial Hyperplasia and Epithelial Mesothelioma

Antibody	Mesothelial Hyperplasia	Epithelial Mesothelioma
Desmin	S	R
Epithelial membrane antigen	R	S
GLUT-1	N	+
XIAP	R	S
BCL-2	N	N
p-Glycoprotein	N	R
PDGF-R	S	+

Reactivity:
+, almost always diffuse, strong positivity
S, sometimes positive
R, rare cells positive
N, almost always negative

TABLE 12.32 Differentiating Fibrosing Pleuritis from Desmoplastic Mesothelioma

Characteristics	Fibrous Pleurisy	Desmoplastic Mesothelioma
Storiform pattern	Not prominent	Often prominent
Stromal invasion	Absent	Present (use pan cytokeratin to confirm)
Necrosis	If present, at surface and often associated with acute inflammation	Bland paucicellular collagenized tissue
Thickness	Uniform	Uneven with disorganized growth, expansile nodules, and abrupt changes in cellularity
Maturation	Hypercellularity at the surface and deep, decreased cellularity (so-called *zonation*)	Lack of maturation from the surface to depths of the process
Orientation	Perpendicularly oriented	Without paucity of vessels
Cellularity	Usually not useful	
Atypia (unless severe)	Usually not useful	
Mitotic activity (unless numerous atypical mitotic figures)	Usually not useful	

diagnosis between reactive mesothelium and malignant pleural mesotheliomas. The authors found immunohistochemical GLUT-1 expression in 40 of 40 (100%) of malignant pleural mesotheliomas and in all cases the expression was demonstrated by linear plasma membrane staining, sometimes with cytoplasmic staining in addition. GLUT-1 expression was also observed in 56 of 58 (96.5%) of lung carcinomas. No reactive mesothelium cases were stated to have expressed GLUT-1. The authors concluded that GLUT-1 was a sensitive and specific immunohistochemical marker enabling differential diagnosis of reactive mesothelioma from malignant pleural mesothelioma, although it was not useful in discriminating malignant pleural epithelial mesothelioma from lung carcinoma.

Acurio and colleagues evaluated immunohistochemical profiles of 85 mesothelial tissues, including 20 normal, 20 hyperplastic, and 45 malignant mesotheliomas, using desmin, epithelial membrane antigen, p53 protein, and GLUT-1.[444] The authors concluded that p53 failed to distinguish between benign and malignant mesothelial lesions. Desmin was stated to have identified benign mesothelium and distinguished it from malignant mesothelioma. They also stated that EMA and GLUT-1 had been positive in the majority of malignant mesotheliomas and negative or only weakly positive in benign mesothelial tissues. The authors stated that since some malignant lesions were negative for EMA and GLUT-1, diagnosis should not be based exclusively on immunoreactivity. Instead, desmin, EMA, and GLUT-1 could be used as part of an IHC profile and as adjuncts to histomorphology in the diagnosis of malignant mesothelioma.

Another area of difficulty in pleural pathology is differentiating between fibrosing pleuritis and desmoplastic mesothelioma. Immunohistochemistry is not particularly useful in differentiating fibrosing pleuritis from desmoplastic mesothelioma in that the spindle cells of both conditions characteristically express keratin and vimentin. A comparison for differentiating fibrosing pleuritis from desmoplastic mesothelioma is shown in Table 12.32.

Rare Primary Pleural Neoplasms

SOLITARY FIBROUS TUMORS OF THE PLEURA

Solitary localized fibrous tumors of the pleura are uncommon neoplasms that are thought to arise from subpleural connective tissue cells.[445-447] They occur as neoplasms in the subvisceral-subpleural zone of the lung and are either located within the pleural space attached to the pleura (usually visceral) by a small pedicle or in a subparietal pleural location. Such neoplasms may become extremely large and can be associated with unusual clinical situations such as hypoglycemia. Histologically, these neoplasms are composed of spindle cells with varying degrees of cellularity and various amounts of extracellular collagen. Identifying these neoplasms as malignant can be difficult, with malignant criteria including more than 4 mitoses/10 high-power fields, hemorrhage, necrosis, and invasion into lung and chest wall.[447] One hundred percent of localized fibrous tumors of the pleura express vimentin, and they are uniformly negative for keratin. About 75 to 80% express CD34,[448,449] and a slightly greater percentage express the anti-apoptosis substance BCL-2.[450] Rare localized fibrous tumors of the pleura express actin.[447]

Schirosi and associates performed a clinicopathologic, immunohistochemical, and molecular study of 88 cases of pleuropulmonary solitary fibrous tumors[451] confirming the prognostic value of the de Perrot staging system[452], p53 expression, c-*kit*, BRAF, PDGFR-alpha, PDGFR-beta, c-Met, and EGFR. The de Perrot staging system is shown in Table 12.33. The authors found that 52 cases (59%) had at least one clinicopathologic feature related to malignancy, whereas mortality and recurrences occurred in 10.2% and 18.2% of cases, respectively. The authors found that de Perrot staging and a high p53 expression were significantly related to conventional clinicopathologic prognostic features, as well as to overall survival and disease-free survival. With respect to multivariate analysis, high p53 expression and tumor necrosis were the only parameters associated with overall survival and disease-free survival (p = 0.017 and p = 0.012, respectively). The authors found that immunohistochemical expression was frequently detected for PDGFR-alpha (97.7%), PDGFR-beta (86.5%), and hepatocyte growth factor receptor (96.6%). Missense mutations were only identified in two cases, both involving PDGFR-beta (exons 18 and 20). The authors concluded that de Perrot stratification of solitary fibrous tumors was a reliable prognostic indicator and merited consideration in view of its suggestions for the management of these tumors in daily practice. p53 was stated to possibly represent a valid and easy to test prognostic factor significantly related to overall survival and disease-free interval. The authors stated that although mutations of the corresponding genes were rare events in solitary fibrous tumors, PDGFR-alpha, PDGFR-beta, and hepatocyte growth factor receptor tyrosine kinases should be further investigated given the availability of specific inhibitory molecules that might provide useful and novel therapeutic approaches for patients with solitary fibrous tumors.

Localized fibrous tumors of the pleura are contrasted to sarcomatoid mesotheliomas and sarcomas in Table 12.34.

TABLE 12.33 Staging System of Pleuropulmonary Solitary Fibrous Tumor

Stage 0	Tumor with peduncle Without features of malignancy at histology
Stage 1	Tumor with sessile or "inverted" appearance Without features of malignancy at histology
Stage 2	Tumor with peduncle With features of malignancy at histology
Stage 3	Tumor with sessile or "inverted" appearance With features of malignancy at histology
Stage 4	Multiple metastatic tumor

Modified from Schirosi L, Lantuejoul S, Cavazza A, et al. Pleuropulmonary solitary fibrous tumors: A clinicopathologic, immunohistochemical, and molecular study of 88 cases confirming the prognostic value of de Perrot staging system and p53 expression, and evaluating the role of c-kit, BRAF, PDGFRs (alpha/beta), c-met, and EGFR. *Am J Surg Pathol.* 2008;32:1627-1642.

PSEUDOMESOTHELIOMATOUS CARCINOMAS OF THE LUNG

Rare primary neoplasms of lung grow in a distribution characteristic of mesothelioma. Five such neoplasms were described by Babolini and Blasi in 1956.[453] In 1976, six examples were reported by Harwood and colleagues, who introduced the term *pseudomesotheliomatous carcinoma*.[454] In 1992, Koss and colleagues reported on 30 cases of pseudomesotheliomatous adenocarcinoma of lung, 15 of which were from a review of published literature and 15 from the files of the Armed Forces Institute of Pathology.[455] Hartman and Schutz reported on 72 cases and designated these neoplasms as *mesothelioma-like tumors of the pleura*.[456] In 1998 Koss and coworkers described 29 cases of pseudomesotheliomatous adenocarcinoma of lung.[457] These authors reported on 17 cases of pseudomesotheliomatous carcinoma of lung in abstract form,[458] and we are currently preparing a report on over 160 cases of pseudomesotheliomatous lung cancer, including rare varieties. In 2003, Attanoos and Gibbs reported an additional 53 cases of pseudomesotheliomatous carcinoma.[459]

These neoplasms macroscopically look almost identical to pleural mesothelioma (Fig. 12.55). As reported by Koss and colleagues[455,457] and in our experience,[458] the majority of pseudomesotheliomatous lung neoplasms are adenocarcinomas, and the most common histologic subtype is what we refer to as a *tubulodesmoplastic*

TABLE 12.34 Comparison of Immunohistochemical Features of Localized Fibrous Tumors of the Pleura, Sarcomatoid Mesothelioma, and Soft Tissue Sarcomas

	Antibody Directed Against									
Type of Neoplasm	AE1/AE3 keratin	Low molecular weight keratin	High molecular weight keratin	CK7	Vimentin	Actin	Desmin	S-100 protein	CD34	BCL-2
Sarcomatoid mesothelioma	S	S	S	S	+	S	R	R	R	R
Localized fibrous tumor of pleura	N	N	N	N	+	S	N	N	+	+
Soft tissue sarcoma	R	R	R	R	+	S*	S*	S*	R*	R*

*Positivity depends on type of soft tissue sarcoma.
Reactivity:
+, almost always diffuse, strong positivity
S, sometimes positive
R, rare cells positive
N, almost always negative

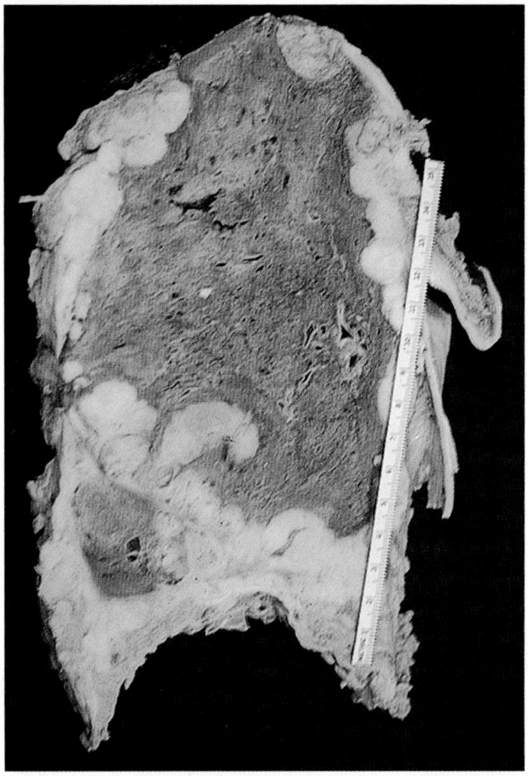

FIGURE 12.55 Macroscopically, pseudomesotheliomatous adenocarcinomas of lung look like diffuse malignant mesotheliomas.

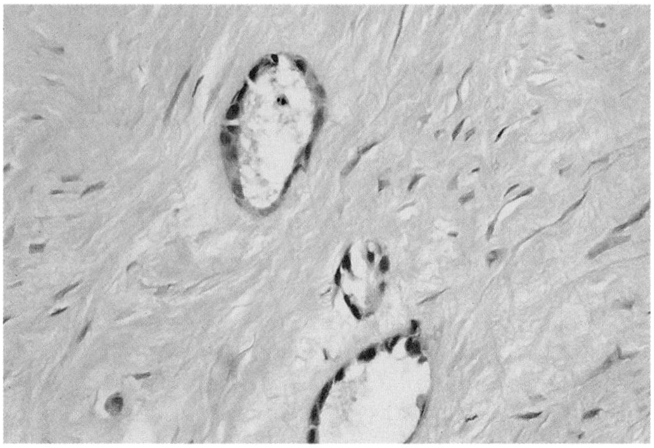

FIGURE 12.56 The most common histologic appearance of pseudomesotheliomatous adenocarcinoma is a tubulodesmoplastic pattern. X 400.

pseudomesotheliomatous adenocarcinoma (Fig. 12.56). Pseudomesotheliomatous pulmonary adenocarcinomas are usually mucin-positive and express the immunohistochemical markers of a pulmonary adenocarcinoma. Occasionally, these neoplasms show squamous and small cell neuroendocrine differentiation. Some are large cell undifferentiated carcinomas, and some may be poorly differentiated and difficult to differentiate from a poorly differentiated mesothelioma. The poorly differentiated pseudomesotheliomatous carcinomas usually coexpress keratin and vimentin and may not express specific carcinoma or mesothelioma markers, thus it is usually not possible to differentiate them from mesothelioma. Koss and associates reported two biphasic variants,[455,457] and we observed one.[458]

The immunohistochemical profile of a pseudomesotheliomatous adenocarcinoma of the lung is the same as for the typical primary pulmonary adenocarcinoma. As reported by these authors[458] and Koss and colleagues,[455,457] a significant percentage of these neoplasms occur in individuals who were exposed to asbestos and who have elevated concentrations of asbestos in their lung tissue.

PSEUDOMESOTHELIOMATOUS EPITHELIOID HEMANGIOENDOTHELIOMA

Rare neoplasms composed of endothelial cells resembling epithelial mesotheliomas are referred to as *pseudomesotheliomatous epithelioid hemangioendothelioma* or as *epithelioid hemangioendothelioma mimicking mesothelioma*.[460,461] this author contributed to a series by Lin and colleagues.[461] In this case, a 50-year-old male patient had a history of potential exposure to asbestos while working at a hardware store at age 20. He presented with a right pleural effusion and a tumor encasing the right lung. The initial biopsy was diagnosed by the treating pathologist as adenocarcinoma and by another pathologist as an epithelial mesothelioma. The case was referred to this author. The pattern of immunoreactivity was confusing in that the neoplastic cells expressed low molecular weight (35βH11) and high molecular weight (34βE12) keratins; vimentin; CD31; factor VIII antigen (Fig. 12.57); and CD34. Ultrastructurally, the neoplastic cells resembled endothelial cells and contained Weibel-Palade bodies in their cytoplasm (Fig. 12.58). Of note, keratin expression has been reported in normal endothelial cells and in vascular neoplasms.[462]

CALCIFYING FIBROUS PSEUDOTUMOR OF THE PLEURA

Calcifying fibrous pseudotumor of the pleura is a newly recognized fibrous soft tissue tumor of the pleura that occurs predominantly in younger patients and presents as a pleural mass radiographically.[463] Patients with this neoplasm usually present with chest pain and/or cough and vague chest discomfort. The tumor consists of circumscribed but unencapsulated masses of dense hyalinized collagenous tissue interspersed with a lymphoplasmacytic infiltrate and calcium deposits, many of which have the appearance of psammoma bodies. This author has seen four such lesions, and the spindle cells show immunostaining for vimentin and no immunostaining for keratin, alpha actin, desmin, S-100 protein, CD34, BCL-2, or CD117.

PRIMARY DESMOID TUMORS OF THE PLEURA

These tumors resemble desmoid tumors in other locations and show infiltration of adjacent fat and skeletal muscle by plump spindle cells.[464] Immunohistochemically,

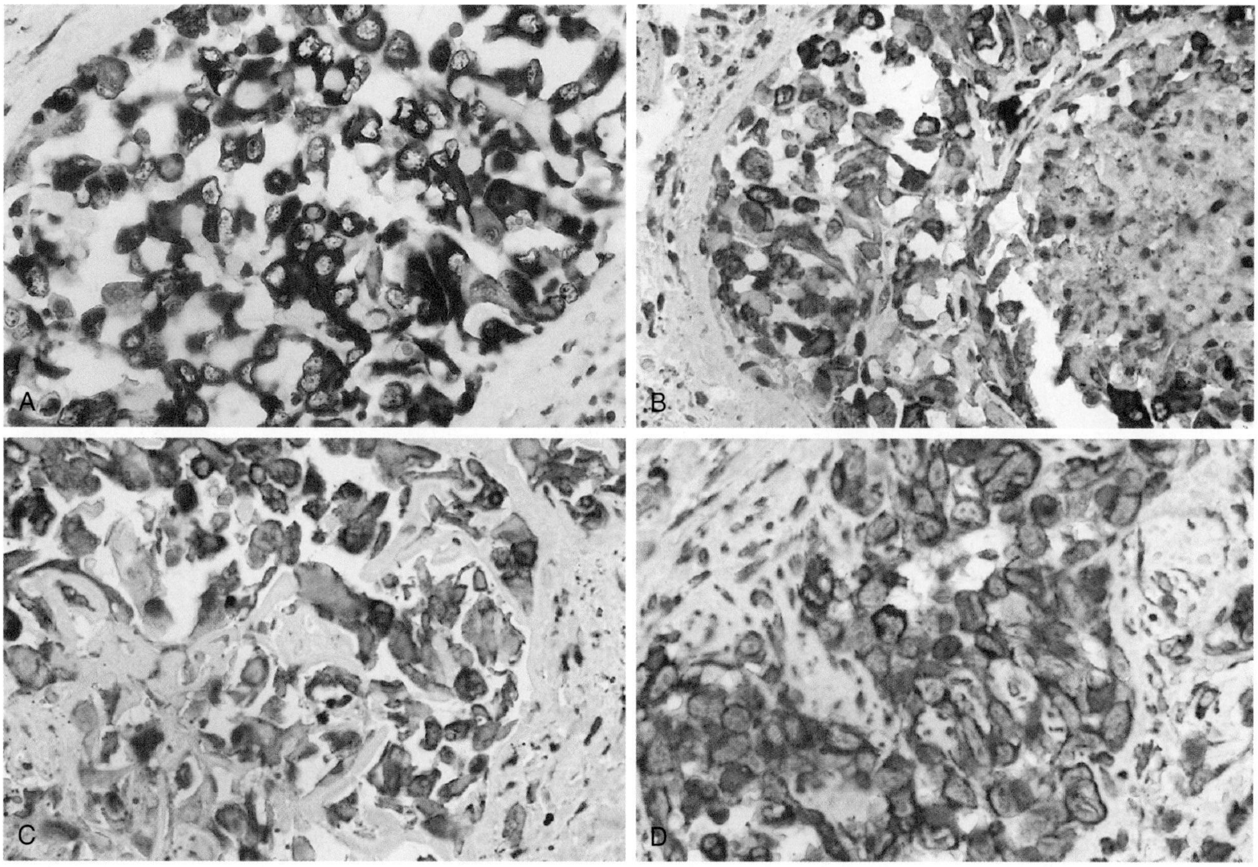

FIGURE 12.57 This pseudomesotheliomatous epithelioid hemangioendothelioma was initially diagnosed as an adenocarcinoma and then as an epithelial mesothelioma. In this case, the neoplastic cells expressed keratin and endothelial cell markers CD31, factor VIII antigen, and vimentin. X 400.

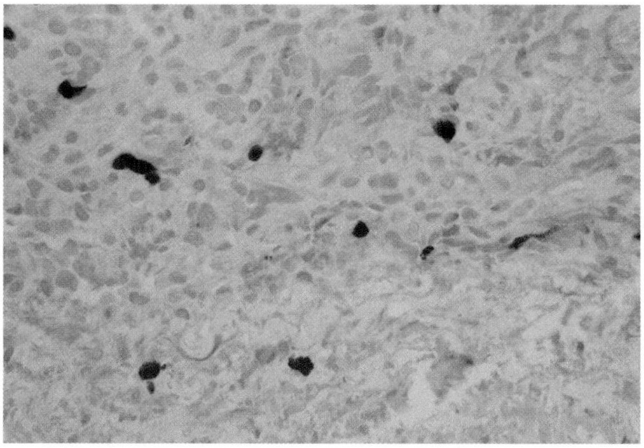

FIGURE 12.58 Ultrastructurally, this pseudomesotheliomatous epithelioid hemangioendothelioma contained Weibel-Palade bodies in many of the neoplastic cells. X 42,000.

the neoplastic spindle cells show immunostaining for vimentin, desmin, smooth muscle actin, and muscle-specific actin. They are negative for S-100 protein and keratin. Ultrastructurally, the neoplastic cells resemble myofibroblasts.

Andino and associates evaluated the expression of β-catenin and cyclin D1 in desmoid tumors and solitary fibrous tumors. They compared the utility of β-catenin and cyclin D1 for distinguishing between these entities with those of other more commonly used stains.[465] The authors studied formalin-fixed paraffin-embedded sections of 4 desmoid tumors (1 pulmonary, 1 pleural, and 2 pleural/chest wall), and 5 benign and 6 malignant solitary fibrous tumors of the pleura with β-catenin, cyclin D1, ALK1, CD34, vimentin, desmin, smooth muscle actin, muscle-specific actin, S-100 protein, and pan cytokeratin. The authors stated that staining intensity and the percentage of stained tumor cells were assessed semiquantitatively. The authors found diffuse moderate or strong nuclear staining for β-catenin in all desmoid tumors, 4 of 5 benign solitary fibrous tumors, and 2 of 6 malignant solitary fibrous tumors. All cases except 1 benign solitary fibrous tumor showed concurrent cytoplasmic staining. Nuclear and cytoplasmic cyclin D1 staining was observed in all groups. The best distinction between desmoid tumors and solitary fibrous tumors was provided by CD34 with none of the desmoid tumors staining and 8 of 11 solitary fibrous tumors expressing CD34. Muscle specific actin expression was observed in 4 desmoid tumors but none of the 11 solitary fibrous tumors. The authors concluded that alterations in the adenomatous polyposis coli/β-catenin pathway and cyclin D1 dysregulation may have contributed to the pathogenesis of pleuropulmonary desmoid tumors and solitary fibrous tumors. The authors stated that CD34 and smooth muscle actin stains were of particular usefulness in differentiating between desmoid tumors and solitary fibrous tumors.

PRIMARY PLEURAL THYMOMAS

Thymomas may occur in the pleura and can be confused with mesothelioma.[466-469] These neoplasms may be confused with a sarcomatoid mesothelioma with a heavy lymphoid infiltrate or with a lymphohistiocytoid mesothelioma. None of the cases presented by Moran and coworkers showed radiographic evidence of a mediastinal tumor, however 6 cases showed histologic features of a "mixed" (lymphocyte-epithelial) thymoma.[466] The neoplastic thymic epithelial cells express keratin and CD5.

SYNOVIAL SARCOMAS

Synovial sarcomas may occur as primary neoplasms in the pleura and can be confused histologically with biphasic and sarcomatoid mesotheliomas.[470-472] The neoplastic epithelial cells express keratin and show glandular differentiation. The cells forming the glandular structures frequently express CEA and Ber-EP4and are positive for neutral mucins, which are absent findings in most epithelial mesotheliomas. Ultrastructurally, the neoplastic epithelial cells in a synovial sarcoma are different than epithelial mesotheliomas, having short microvilli and showing glycocalyceal bodies.[474] Monophasic synovial sarcomas are difficult to differentiate from sarcomatoid mesotheliomas. Sarcomatoid synovial sarcoma tumor cells usually show BCL-2 expression and may express CD99. Colwell and colleagues and Yano and colleagues reported SYT and SYX fusion genes in synovial sarcomas that can be identified by fluorescence *in situ* hybridization.[472,473] A variety of other sarcomas can occur in the lung and pleura. These are beautifully described and illustrated by Litzky.[475]

PLEUROPULMONARY BLASTOMA

Pleuropulmonary blastomas are rare neoplasms that occur predominantly in infants and children and involve the lung and/or pleura.[476,477] Rare cases occur in adults.[478] The neoplasm is frequently cystic, with the cysts lined by benign metaplastic epithelium that can be ciliated. The malignant component is composed of differentiated and/or anaplastic sarcomatous elements, including fibrosarcoma, chondrosarcoma, embryonal rhabdomyosarcoma, and mixtures of these elements. The immunohistologic findings are dependent on what type of sarcomatous differentiation occurs.

LYMPHOMAS INVOLVING THE PLEURA

Relatively little information exists concerning pleura involvement of lymphoma. In 1992 Ceiloglu and associates reviewed involvement of the pleura by lymphomas.[479] In 2006 Vega and colleagues reported on pleural involvement by lymphoma.[480] The authors stated that pleural involvement was relatively common, although there were very few clinicopathologic studies concerning lymphomas involving the pleura.[480] The authors reviewed clinicopathologic features of 34 patients with lymphoma involving the pleura proven by biopsy and classified according to the WHO classification. Of the 34 cases, 22 were men and 12 were women with an average age of 62 years and a range of 22 to 88 years. Nine (26.5%) patients had pleural involvement as the only site of disease, whereas 22 (64.7%) had other sites of involvement, and 3 (8.8%) had inadequate staging data. The authors found that 18 (56.2%) of the 32 patients with adequate clinical data had a history of lymphoma, including 3 patients with pleural involvement as the only disease site. In 29 (85.3%) cases, a specific diagnosis according to the WHO classification can be made: 17 (58.6%) diffuse large B-cell lymphomas; 5 (17.2%) follicular lymphomas, including a case with areas of diffuse large B-cell lymphoma; 2 (6.9%) small lymphocytic lymphoma/chronic lymphocytic leukemias; 2 (6.9%) precursor T-cell lymphoblastic lymphoma/leukemias; and 1 (3.4%) each of mantle cell lymphoma, post-transplant lymphoproliferative disorder, and classical Hodgkin lymphoma. Five cases were B-cell lymphomas that could not be further classified. The authors stated that although any type of lymphoma can potentially involve the pleura, in their study diffuse large B-cell lymphoma was the most frequent type found followed by follicular lymphoma (approximately 60% and 20%, respectively). Obviously, immunohistochemistry is very important in classifying these lymphomas, as shown in Table 1 of the authors' report. As stated in the section on lung cancer, primary effusion lymphomas and pyogenic lymphomas occur.

Variabilities and Pitfalls

An important pitfall in accurately diagnosing mesothelioma is the failure of pathologists to recognize the many histologic patterns exhibited by epithelial and sarcomatoid mesotheliomas. Most immunohistochemical literature discussing mesothelioma concerns epithelial mesothelioma, specifically well differentiated and moderately well differentiated epithelial mesotheliomas. Most antibodies used to differentiate mesothelioma from adenocarcinoma include tumors that are well or moderately well differentiated. As mesotheliomas become more poorly differentiated, many relatively specific positive markers such as HBME-1, calretinin, and CK5/6 fail to stain. Poorly differentiated mesotheliomas characteristically express low molecular weight keratin, occasionally high molecular weight keratin, and vimentin. An absolute diagnosis of such mesotheliomas may be difficult, and the diagnosis may have to state that histologic and immunohistologic findings are consistent with a poorly differentiated mesothelioma. The clinical (diffuse pleural) distribution of a pleural neoplasm can help support the diagnosis of mesothelioma.

Several articles have been published discussing immunohistochemical tests used in distinguishing epithelial mesotheliomas from pulmonary adenocarcinomas and other carcinomas.[352,353,481-484] These have been extensively reviewed by Ordonez.[484-486] The most recent review by Ordonez evaluated 60 unequivocal epithelial mesotheliomas and 50 lung adenocarcinomas with a

TABLE 12.35 Antibodies Used to Distinguish Epithelial Mesothelioma from Pulmonary Adenocarcinoma and Other Carcinomas

Marker	Source	Type	Dilution	Antigen retrieval
B72.3	BioGenox (San Ramon, CA)	B72.3	1:300	No
Ber-EP4	Dako Corporation	MAb	1:30	Yes (enzymatic digestion)
BG-8 (Lewis Y)	Signet (Dedham, MA)	BG-8 MAb	1:50	Yes (citrate)
CA19-9	Dako Corporation	MAb	1:50	Yes (citrate)
Calretinin	Zymed (South San Francisco, CA)	PAb (rabbit)	1:20	Yes (citrate)
CD44S	Vector Laboratories (Burlingame, CA)	F10-44.2 MAb	1:75	Yes (citrate)
Carcinoembryonic antigen	NeoMarkers (Fremont, CA)	PAb (rabbit)	1:175	No
Cytokeratin 5/6	Boehringer-Mannheim (Indianapolis, IN)	D5/16B4 MAb	1:25	Yes (citrate)
E-cadherin	Zymed	HECD-1 MAb	1:20	Yes (citrate)
Epithelial membrane antigen	Dako Corporation	E29 MAb	1:20	Yes (citrate)
HBME-1	Dako Corporation	MAb	1:50	Yes (citrate)
Leu-M1 (CD15)	Becton-Dickinson (Mountain View, CA)	Leu-M1 (MAb)	1:40	Yes (Tris-EDTA)
Mesothelin	Novocastra (Newcastle-upon-Tyne, UK)	5B2 Mab	1:30	Yes (Tris-EDTA)
MOC-31	Dako Corporation	MAb	1:50	Yes (citrate)
N-cadherin	Zymed	3B9 MAb	1:20	Yes (Tris-EDTA)
Thrombomodulin	Dako Corporation	1005 MAb	1:50	Yes (citrate)
Thyroid transcription factor-1	Dako Corporation	BG7G3/1 MAb	1:25	Yes (citrate)
Vimentin	Dako Corporation	V9 MAb	1:500	Yes (citrate)
WT1	Dako Corporation (Carpinteria, CA)	6F-H2 MAb	1:40	Yes (Tris-EDTA)

large panel of antibodies (Table 12.35).[486] The results of his evaluation are shown in Table 12.36. The results of published immunohistochemical studies concerning the various immunohistochemical tests are listed in Tables 12.4 to 12.17 of the Ordonez article[484] and are summarized in Table 12.37. Based on their sensitivity and specificity, Ordonez concluded that calretinin, CK5/6, and WT1 were the best positive markers. Ordonez stated that calretinin and CK5/6 were more sensitive than WT1. Thrombomodulin was found to be less sensitive and less specific than calretinin, CK5/6, and WT1. Ordonez found that mesothelin was a highly sensitive marker for epithelial mesothelioma, although it was less specific. Ordonez stated that HBME-1, N-cadherin, and CD44S were not helpful. Ordonez found that CEA, MOC31, BerEP4, BG8, and B72.3 were the most specific and sensitive negative epithelial mesothelioma markers, and that TTF-1, LeuM1 (CD15), and CA19-9 were highly specific but less sensitive. Ordonez concluded that from a practical viewpoint, a panel of four markers (two positive and two negative) allowed for the distinction between epithelial mesothelioma and pulmonary adenocarcinoma.[486] Ordonez's recommendation was calretinin and CK5/6 (or WT1) for the positive markers, and CEA and MOC-31 (or B72.3, BerEP4, or BG8) for the negative markers.[486] Ordonez noted that with respect to positive markers, WT1 was absent in lung adenocarcinoma but was strongly expressed in serous ovarian carcinoma. Others have come to a slightly different selection of positive and negative markers.[487] Calretinin expression has been reported in a fairly diverse group of non-mesothelial neoplasms, but it is often identified only in the cytoplasm.[488-491] WT1 expression has also been identified in a variety of other neoplasms,[492-495] and nerve growth factor receptors TfkA and p75 have also been reported.[496] As reported by Henderson and coworkers, non-neoplastic reactive proliferative pleural lesions may very closely simulate mesothelioma.[316] This may be the most difficult area of diagnostic pleural pathology. As discussed earlier in the chapter, differentiating fibrosing pleuritis from desmoplastic mesothelioma, and epithelial mesothelioma from reactive mesothelial proliferations can be difficult.

Unusual/uncommon types of mesothelioma should be mentioned because they can cause diagnostic confusion. Mucin-positive epithelial mesotheliomas are not uncommon.[497] Between 1% and 5% of all moderately well to well differentiated epithelial mesotheliomas show mucicarmine and/or PAS-diastase staining (Fig. 12.59). Patterns of mucin staining have been extensively described by this author.[498] Mucin-positive epithelial mesotheliomas most frequently express immunohistochemical markers that are negative in most epithelial mesotheliomas and usually positive in pulmonary adenocarcinomas (CEA, LeuM1, B72.3, BerEP4). Mucin-positive epithelial mesotheliomas express calretinin and

TABLE 12.36 Immunohistochemical Results of Epithelial Mesotheliomas and Pulmonary Adenocarcinomas

	Epithelial Mesotheliomas Grade of reactivity						Pulmonary Adenocarcinomas Grade of reactivity					
Marker	(n = 60) + cases (%)	Trace	1+	2+	3+	4+	(n = 50) + cases (%)	Trace	1+	2+	3+	4+
B72.3 (TAG-72)	0 (0%)	0	0	0	0	0	42 (84%)	0	7	12	15	8
Ber-EP4	11 (18%)	2	9	0	0	0	50 (100%)	0	0	0	13	37
BG-8 (Lewis Y)	4 (7%)	2	2	0	0	0	48 (96%)	1	6	7	15	21
CA19-9	0 (0%)	0	0	0	0	0	24 (48%)	0	6	10	6	2
Calretinin	60 (100%)	0	0	0	15	45	4 (8%)	2	2	0	0	0
Carcinoembryonic antigen	0 (0%)	0	0	0	0	0	44 (88%)	0	3	8	17	16
CD44S	44 (73%)	5	7	4	11	17	24 (48%)	0	14	7	2	1
Cytokeratin 5/6	60 (100%)	2	3	7	16	32	1 (2%)	0	1	0	0	0
E-cadherin	24 (40%)	0	14	5	2	3	44 (88%)	0	9	8	20	7
Epithelial membrane antigen	56 (93%)	0	7	9	19	21	50 (100%)	0	3	12	10	25
HBME-1	51 (85%)	0	7	11	14	28	34 (68%)	0	4	5	9	16
LeuM1 (CD15)	0 (0%)	0	0	0	0	0	36 (72%)	0	4	9	13	7
Mesothelin	60 (100%)	0	11	4	17	28	19 (38%)	0	8	5	5	1
MOC-31	5 (8%)	2	3	0	0	0	50 (100%)	0	3	7	19	21
N-cadherin	44 (73%)	1	5	13	14	11	15 (30%)	2	4	3	6	0
Thrombomodulin	46 (77%)	0	10	16	16	3	7 (14%)	2	5	0	0	0
Thyroid transcription factor-1	0 (0%)	0	0	0	0	0	37 (74%)	0	4	10	15	8
Vimentin	33 (55%)	1	28	4	0	0	19 (38%)	1	16	2	0	0
WT1	56 (93%)	0	4	9	16	27	0 (0%)	0	0	0	0	0

HBME-1 and show cell membrane staining for EMA and HMFG-2. Ultrastructurally, mucin-positive epithelial mesotheliomas frequently contain crystalloid material (Fig. 12.60) in intracellular neolumens, in glandular spaces formed by neoplastic cells, or in the extracellular space. In our experience, this crystalloid material is unique to epithelial mesotheliomas.

Some mesotheliomas are composed of small cells and may be confused with small cell lung carcinoma.[498] Mayall and Gibbs reported on 13 cases of small cell mesothelioma that had areas of atypical epithelial mesothelioma and 7 cases in which 90% of the neoplastic cells were small cells.[498] Mayall and colleagues reported neuron-specific enolase staining in 46 of 48 (96%) mesotheliomas and Leu7 expression in 14 of 20 (70%) mesotheliomas.[499] Unlike that observed by Hurlimann, the mesotheliomas showed no expression of chromogranin A and bombesin.[408] Falconieri and associates reported on 4 cases of pseudomesotheliomatous small cell carcinoma of lung that could be confused with small cell mesothelioma.[500]

van Hengel reported on 2 cases of atypical carcinoid presenting as mesothelioma.[501] In both cases, the patients had been exposed to asbestos. This author recently saw a neoplasm composed of nodules of fleshy tumor involving the visceral and parietal pleura (Fig. 12.61). In this case, the tumor was composed of neoplastic cells that showed carcinoid-like features with the individual cells showing a very high mitotic rate (up to 10 per high-power field) and focal areas of necrosis (Fig. 12.62). These neoplastic cells showed immunostaining for synaptophysin, chromogranin-A, and TTF-1 (Figs. 12.63 to 12.65).

We believe that the best way to differentiate pseudomesotheliomatous small cell lung cancer from small cell mesothelioma is with TTF-1 (positive in 90% of small cell lung cancer; negative in mesothelioma), CEA (positive in approximately 30% to 50% of small cell lung cancer; negative in small cell mesothelioma), and synaptophysin (positive in 90% of small cell lung cancer; negative in most small cell mesotheliomas).

Lymphohistiocytoid mesothelioma is a rare form of sarcomatoid mesothelioma that was initially histologically diagnosed as a lymphoma.[502] Lymphohistiocytoid mesothelioma is composed of large, mostly round cells admixed with numerous inflammatory cells (Fig. 12.66). This neoplasm can be misdiagnosed as a large cell lymphocytic lymphoma. The neoplastic cells characteristically express low molecular weight keratin, high molecular

TABLE 12.37 Summary of Immunohistochemical Tests Referred to by Ordonez[484]

Antigen Tested For	Epithelial Mesothelioma				Primary Pulmonary Adenocarcinoma				Conclusion of Study				
	Number of Cases	Positive Cases	Range of % Positive Cases	Average % Positive Cases	Number of Cases	Positive Cases	Range of % Positive Cases	Average % Positive Cases	Useful	Not Useful	Sometimes Useful	Not Applicable	No Conclusion
B72.3	797	68	0-48	8.0	490	412	35-100	82.1	Not given				
BerEP4	1055	139	0-88	10.5	222	210	57-100	93.8	Not given				
BG8 (Lewis Y)	316	34	6-24	13.2	108	105	96-100	98	Not given				
Calretinin	805	648	50-100	86.2	238	74	0-70	9.5	16	8	2		
CD44S	495	336	47-100	72	159	100	15-57	54	Not given				
CEA	1392	68	0-45	5.0	1023	840	25-100	81.6	Not given				
CK5/6	309	286	64-100	90.1	183	16	0-19	6.2	Not given				
E-cadherin	224	101	0-100	51.9	123	116	84-100	96.2	3	6		1	1
HBME-1	613	516	57-100	86.2	249	175	55-100	71.7	5	9	1		
LeuM1 (CD15)	1423	173	0-33	5.0	693	521	44-100	84.6	Not given				
MOC-31	265	34	0-88	19.5	173	167	90-100	97.5	Not given				
Thrombo-modulin	637	501	30-100	51.4	430	109	5-77	21.9	Not given				
Vimentin	715	418	16-100	60.3	354	73	0-50	19.5	6	9	-	-	2
WT1	298	231	43-95	77.7	154	8	0-20	10	Not given				

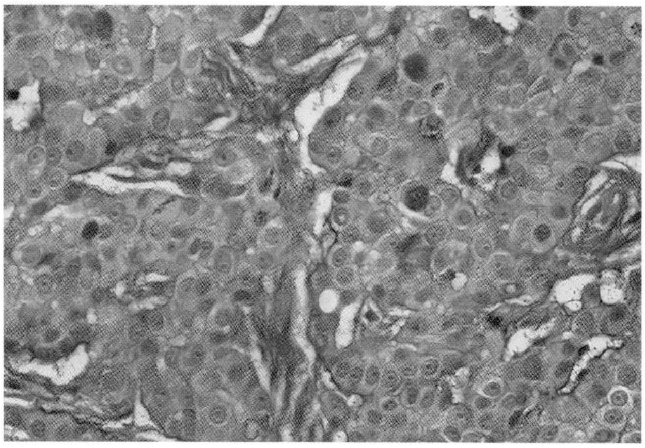

FIGURE 12.59 This mucin-positive epithelial mesothelioma shows intracellular mucicarmine staining. This reaction can result in an incorrect diagnosis of a mucin-producing adenocarcinoma. X 400.

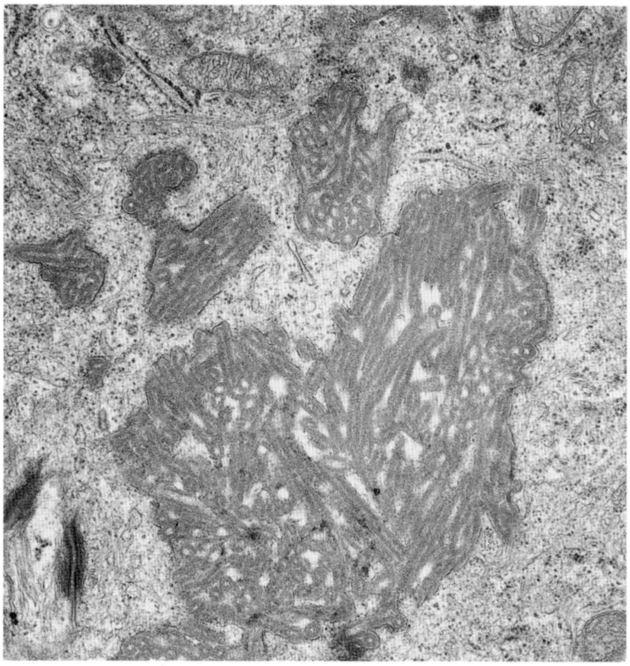

FIGURE 12.60 In this mucin-positive epithelial mesothelioma, crystalloid material is located in glandular spaces formed by the neoplastic cells and in intracellular neolumens. X 20,000.

weight keratin, and vimentin. Most lymphohistiocytoid mesotheliomas are negative for calretinin, HBME-1, and EMA. Ultrastructurally, the neoplastic cells show intercellular junctions and intracellular tonofilaments.

Well-differentiated papillary epithelial mesothelioma can cause diagnostic confusion, often because pathologists are not familiar with this neoplasm.[313-315,503] Most cases occur in the peritoneal cavity of young women (20 to 30 years of age), although some have been recently reported in the pleura.[315,504] Macroscopically, they present as multiple serosal surface nodules typically involving the omentum, mesentery, pelvic cavity, and the pleura. The nodules vary from a few millimeters to several centimeters in maximum dimension. Histologically, they show tubulopapillary differentiation and are composed of well-differentiated, relatively uniform cuboidal cells (Fig. 12.67). The immunohistochemical pattern is generally that of a typical well-differentiated epithelial mesothelioma, and most cases we have seen show cell membrane immunostaining for EMA and no immunostaining for desmin. These tumors differ from typical epithelial mesotheliomas in that they usually have a good prognosis and do not rapidly progress. However, some cases will progress, invade, and cause death.

Some epithelial mesotheliomas are composed of small cysts formed by uniform cuboidal mesothelial cells and associated numerous blood vessels (Fig. 12.68). This type of mesothelioma may be difficult to differentiate from a vascular neoplasm. The epithelial mesothelial cells may contain intracytoplasmic hemosiderin (Fig. 12.69). The immunophenotype of such neoplasms is identical to that of other epithelial mesotheliomas. The vascular proliferation may be related to an endothelial growth factor produced by neoplastic mesothelial cells.[505] Adenomatoid tumors are localized benign mesothelial proliferations that most frequently occur in the epididymus and cornua of the uterus.[516] Adenomatoid tumors have been identified in the adrenal gland[507] and pancreas.[508] These tumors are formed by uniform small cuboidal cells and can appear invasive. They express keratin and other markers of mesothelial cells and have the characteristic ultrastructural features of mesothelial cells. Adenomatoid tumors have also been reported in the pleura.[440] Hyperplastic mesothelial cells may be found in mediastinal lymph nodes and simulate metastatic epithelial mesothelioma or carcinoma.[509,510] These atypical mesothelial cells typically occur in nodal sinuses and are most prominent in the subcapsular sinuses. They may be confused with macrophages. In fact, Ordonez and colleagues reported on lesions composed of cells that were thought to represent reactive mesothelial cells, but were, in fact, macrophages.[511] The mesothelial cells express the usual positive epithelial mesothelial cell markers and are negative for the antigens that are characteristically negative in epithelial mesothelioma. One must be aware, however, that epithelial mesotheliomas may present as metastatic tumors of unknown primary origin in lymph nodes.[512] Well-differentiated epithelial mesotheliomas and well-differentiated papillary epithelial mesotheliomas need to be differentiated from primary papillary serous carcinomas of the serosa, nearly all of which occur in the peritoneal cavity of women.[391,513-521] One case was reported in a male patient,[528] and rare cases involve the pleural cavity.[318] Histologically, these neoplasms are well differentiated and exhibit a papillary morphology. Psammoma bodies are more commonly seen in primary papillary carcinomas than in papillary epithelial mesotheliomas, although psammoma bodies are seen in papillary mesotheliomas. Primary serosal papillary carcinomas are usually mucicarmine and PAS-diastase–negative. Using immunohistochemistry, the staining pattern can be similar to epithelial mesotheliomas, although Khoury and colleagues found serous papillary tumors to express one or more of the antigens CEA, LeuM1 (CD15), and TAG-72 (B72.3).[521] In 17 of 20 cases, 7 expressed monoclonal CEA, 6 expressed LeuM1, and 13 were positive for B72.3 when tissue sections were predigested with pepsin. Ultrastructurally, primary papillary serous carcinomas show occasional cilia

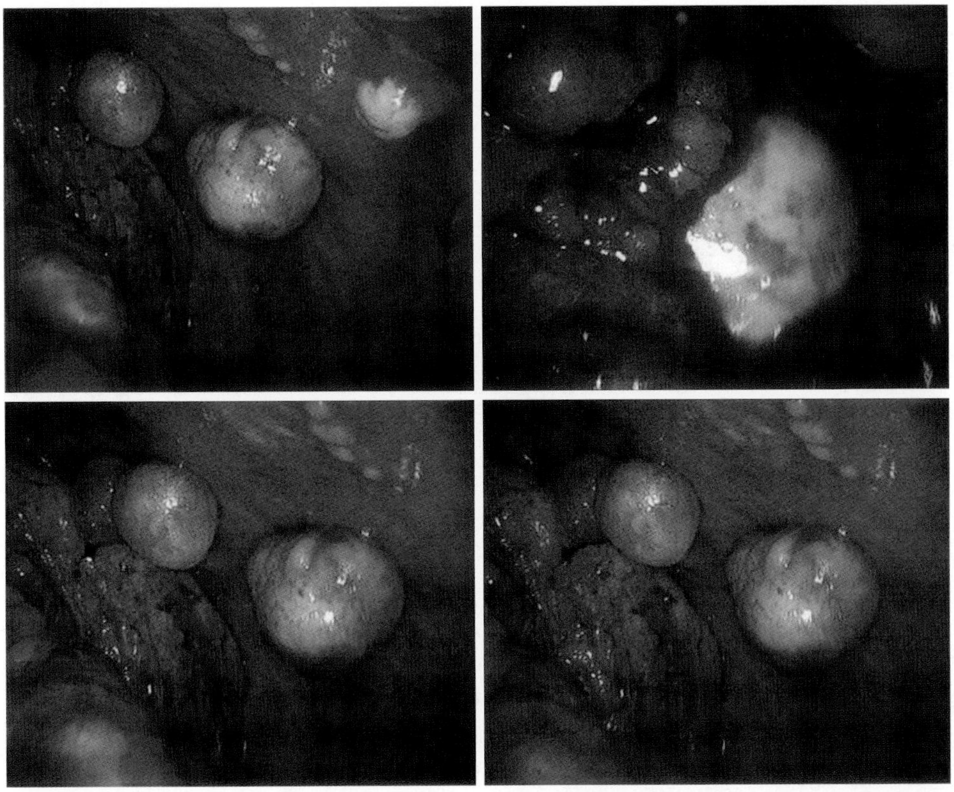

FIGURE 12.61 This neoplasm consists of fleshy nodules attached to the visceral and parietal pleura.

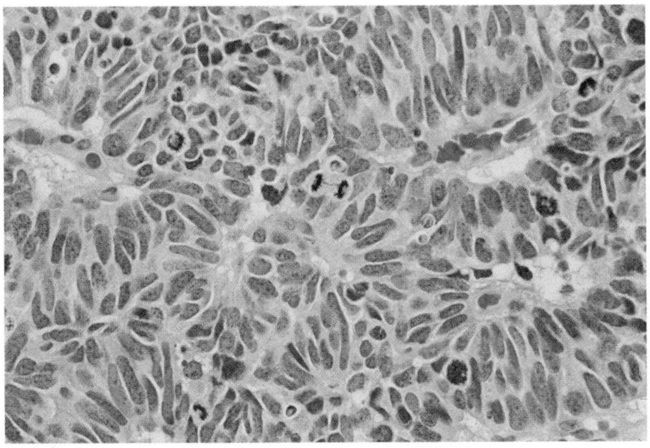

FIGURE 12.62 Histologically, the neoplasm had the features of an atypical carcinoid.

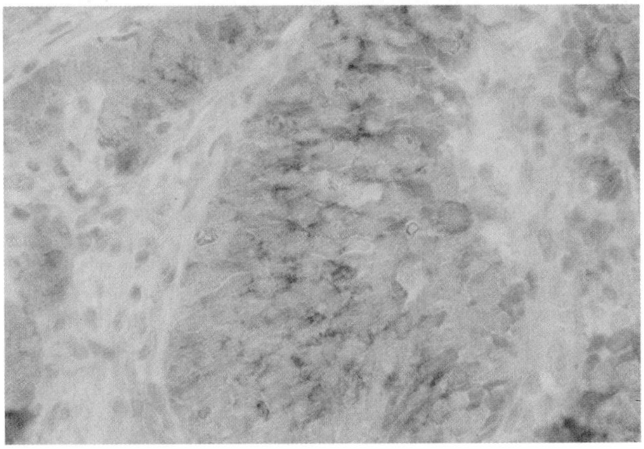

FIGURE 12.63 The neoplastic cells expressed synaptophysin.

and outpouchings of straight and relatively short microvilli that are covered by a fuzzy glycocalyx. Sometimes the microvilli are longer and are branched.

Sarcomatoid renal cell carcinomas can metastasize to the pleura in a macroscopic distribution identical to mesothelioma and very closely simulate a sarcomatoid mesothelioma.[522] This tumor is considered as a pseudomesotheliomatous carcinoma but not a primary pulmonary pseudomesotheliomatous carcinoma. The immunostaining pattern of such neoplasms can be identical to a sarcomatoid mesothelioma. The situation can be further complicated because sarcomatoid mesotheliomas can metastasize to the kidney. If an individual is known to have a sarcomatoid renal cell carcinoma and has a spindle cell neoplasm of the pleura, one must consider the possibility of a metastatic sarcomatoid renal cell carcinoma. If the tumor shows a clear cell and a sarcomatoid pattern, metastatic renal cell carcinoma is most likely, although mesotheliomas may show a clear cell pattern.[523]

Pathologists should be aware that renal cell carcinoma-associated markers such as erythropoietin and CD10 can be identified in diffuse malignant mesotheliomas and in metastatic renal cell carcinomas. Butnor and coworkers evaluated 100 diffuse malignant mesotheliomas and 20 metastatic renal cell carcinomas for erythropoietin immunoexpression.[524] These cases and an additional 45 diffuse malignant mesotheliomas were evaluated for CD10 and renal cell carcinoma marker RCCMA. The authors found that erythropoietin was expressed in 100% of diffuse malignant mesotheliomas and metastatic renal cell

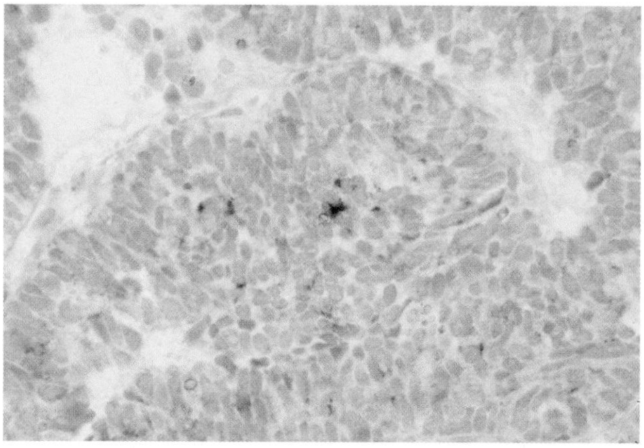

FIGURE 12.64 The neoplastic cells expressed chromogranin A.

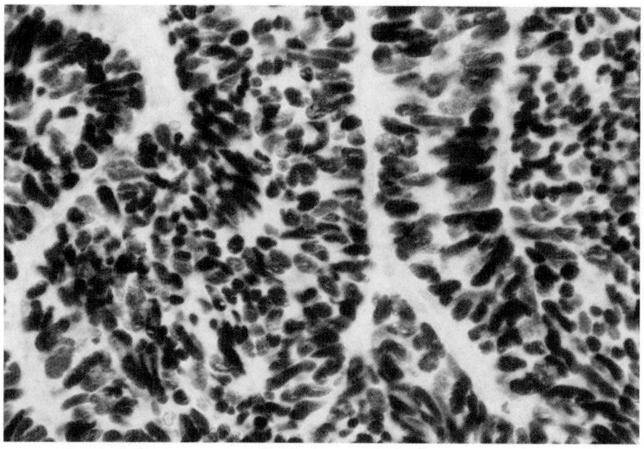

FIGURE 12.65 The nuclei of the neoplastic cells showed immunostaining for TTF-1.

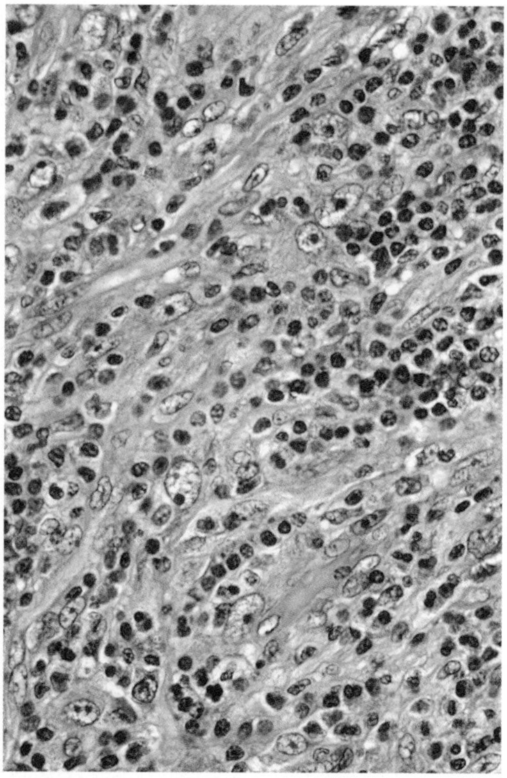

FIGURE 12.66 This mesothelioma is composed of large round cells admixed with numerous lymphoid cells. Histologically this tumor resembles a lymphoma.

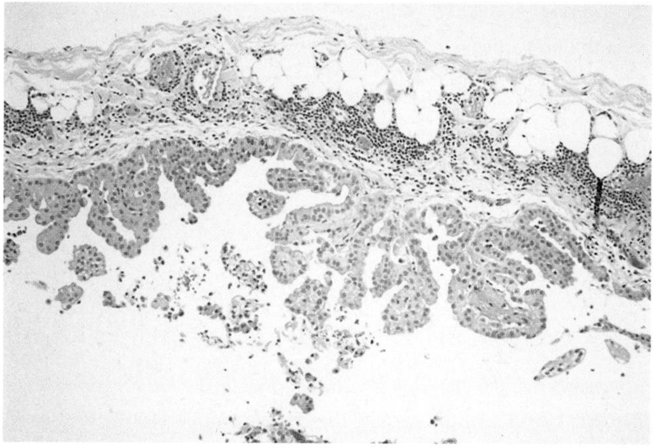

FIGURE 12.67 This well-differentiated papillary epithelial mesothelioma involving pleura shows papillary differentiation and is composed of relatively small, uniform cuboidal cells. This type of mesothelioma usually pursues a benign clinical course. X 200.

carcinomas. Staining for CD10 was observed in 54% of diffuse malignant mesotheliomas and 100% of metastatic renal cell carcinomas. Renal cell carcinoma marker stained 26% of diffuse malignant mesotheliomas and 55% of metastatic renal cell carcinomas. The authors concluded that given the overlap in the expression of renal cell carcinoma markers in metastatic renal cell carcinoma and diffuse malignant mesothelioma, these markers must be interpreted cautiously and should be used in conjunction with mesothelial-associated markers. The authors also concluded that differences in expression may potentially help distinguish metastatic renal cell carcinoma from diffuse malignant mesothelioma inasmuch as strong and diffuse expression of renal cell carcinoma marker and CD10 supported a diagnosis of metastatic renal cell carcinoma over diffuse malignant mesothelioma.

Molecular Biology and Theranostic Features in Diffuse Malignant Mesothelioma

One of the most common genetic alterations in mesothelioma is the homozygous deletion of the 9p21 locus within a cluster of genes that includes CDKN2A, CDKN2B, and MTAP.[525,526] Several cytogenetic and molecular studies have reported p16/CDKN2A deletions in up to 72% of primary mesotheliomas.[527,528] Recent studies demonstrated this alteration detected by FISH may be useful for differentiating benign from malignant mesothelial proliferations in surgical and cytology specimens.[529,530] Homozygous deletion of 9p21 is an adverse prognostic factor in malignant mesotheliomas.[526,531]

Allen and associates[532] constructed a tissue microarray of 19 cases of diffuse malignant mesothelioma that included 19 cases of diffuse malignant mesothelioma

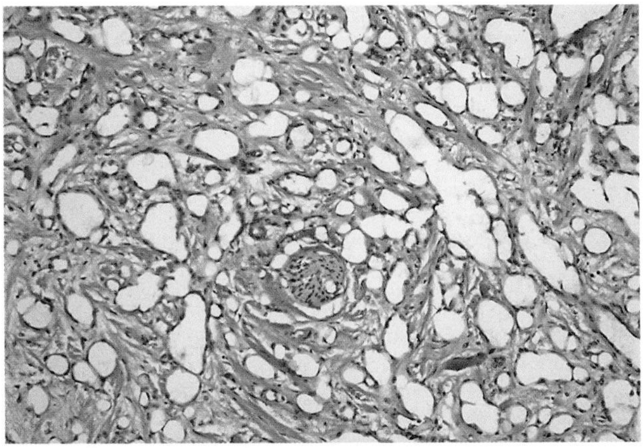

FIGURE 12.68 This epithelial mesothelioma is composed of small cysts associated with numerous blood vessels. X 200.

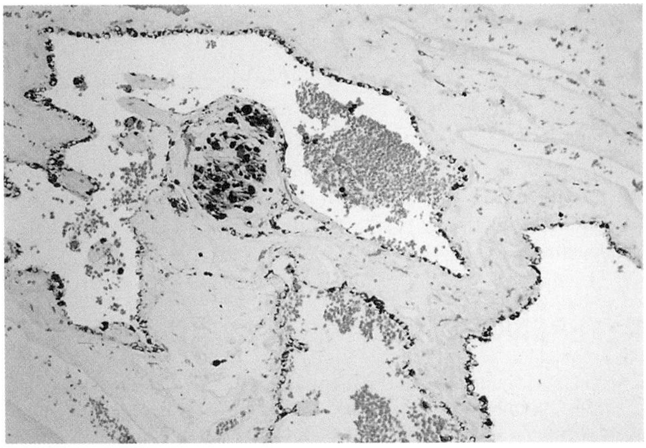

FIGURE 12.69 The neoplastic mesothelial cells showed abundant intracytoplasmic hemosiderin as demonstrated in this Prussian-Blue iron stained section. X 200.

with rare long survival (more than 3 years) and 21 cases that were typical of diffuse malignant mesothelioma with short survival. The authors found that osteopontin and HIF-1 were commonly over-expressed in diffuse malignant mesothelioma, including both diffuse malignant mesothelioma with long survival and diffuse malignant mesothelioma with short survival. The authors found that the lack of osteopontin and HIF-1 were observed only in the long survival diffuse malignant mesothelioma cases, which suggests that lack of osteopontin and HIF-1 expression may have had some role in prolonging survival.

Chung and colleagues studied dual-color FISH for p16 and chromosome 9 on paraffin-embedded sections in 56 biopsy or resected malignant mesothelioma cases (43 epithelioid, 1 sarcomatoid, 12 biphasic), 11 reactive mesothelial proliferations, and 8 equivocal biopsy cases for which a histopathologic distinction between benign and malignant was uncertain.[533] The authors found a high prevalence of p16 deletion in malignant mesothelioma, which was consistent with the findings by others. The authors stated they were first to document the use of FISH for p16 deletion in paraffin-embedded sections of malignant mesothelioma and stated that this test could help distinguish malignant mesothelioma in a difficult biopsy case with the exception of desmoplastic mesothelioma. The findings of p16 homozygous or hemizygous deletion by FISH added further support for a malignant diagnosis.

Xu and colleagues used immunohistochemistry to study KOC/IMP3 in 53 malignant pleural mesotheliomas and 12 reactive mesothelial hyperplasias. The authors stated that K homology domain contained proteins over-expressed in cancer (KOC), also known as IMP3 and L523S, and that they were members of the insulin-like growth factor family.[534] The authors found that KOC/IMP3 was strongly and diffusely expressed in a large proportion of malignant pleural mesotheliomas and only occasionally expressed in reactive mesothelial hyperplasias, which suggests that this marker can be used to distinguish malignant mesothelioma from benign mesothelial lesions. The authors stated that the high frequency of expression in sarcomatoid and biphasic malignant pleural mesotheliomas suggests that KOC expression may be associated with an aggressive biologic behavior.

Gardner and associates studied the expression of matrix metalloproteinase-7 (MMP-7) in 45 diffuse malignant mesotheliomas.[535] The authors used a tissue microarray that was immunohistochemically stained for MMP-7. The authors found positive staining for MMP-7 in 43 of 45 cases of malignant mesothelioma. Of these 43 positive cases, 36 (84%) exhibited strong staining, 2 (5%) exhibited moderate staining, and 5 (11%) exhibited weak staining. All positive cases stained diffusely with 50% to 100% of tumor cells staining for MMP-7. The staining pattern was cytoplasmic in 77%, nuclear in 2%, and nuclear and cytoplasmic in 21% of cases. The authors concluded that strong MMP-7 expression in their series indicated that MMP-7 was likely to play a role in the progression of malignant mesothelioma. The authors suggested that MMP-7 could be a target for chemotherapeutic intervention in malignant mesothelioma.

Moore and colleagues[536] studied topoisomerase II-alpha, minichromosome maintenance protein 2 (MCM2), and X-linked mammalian inhibitor of apoptosis protein (XIAP) expression in diffuse pleural malignant mesotheliomas using tissue microarrays immunostained for these substances. The authors found increased expression of ProExC and XIAP in a substantial percentage of diffuse pleural malignant mesothelioma with a higher positive rate in epithelioid versus sarcomatoid subtype. The authors stated that since these proteins were under investigation as targets for new cancer therapies, further studies needed to be done.

Westerhoff and associates used immunohistochemistry to study c-Met receptor tyrosine kinase (c-Met) in 24 malignant mesotheliomas (18 epithelioid, 3 sarcomatoid, and 3 biphasic).[537] The authors found that PKCβ2 (phosphorylated protein kinase) expression was an adverse prognostic factor in malignant mesothelioma. Westerhoff and colleagues also found that c-Met expression was an adverse prognostic factor and that p-Met expression correlated with the downstream target of VEGFR2/KDR p-PKCβ2. Their study suggested that dual targeting of c-Met and p-PKCβ2 could be an important therapeutic strategy for malignant mesothelioma.

SUMMARY

Immunohistochemistry is a valuable technique used to accurately diagnose primary and metastatic tumors of the lung and pleura. As with all adjuvant diagnostic pathologic techniques, the results of immunohistochemical tests must be correlated with histological, histochemical, and ultrastructural observations and with clinical observations.

REFERENCES

1. Han H, Landreneaux RJ, Santucci TS, et al. Prognostic value of immunohistochemical expression of p53, HER-2-neu and bcl-2 in stage I non-small cell lung cancer. *Hum Pathol.* 2002;33:105-110.
2. Minami K, Saito Y, Imamura H. Okamura. Prognostic significance of p53, Ki67, VEGF and GLUT-1 in resected stage I adenocarcinoma of the lung. *Lung Cancer.* 2002;38:51-57.
3. Nakanishi K, Kawai T, Kumaki F, et al. Survivin expression in atypical adenomatous hyperplasia of the lung. *Am J Clin Pathol.* 2003;120:712-719.
4. Yamaguchi NH, Lichetenfels AJ, Demarchi LMM, et al. Cox-2, MMP-9 and Noguchi classification provide additional prognostic information about adenocarcinomas of the lung: A study of 117 patients from Brazil. *Am J Clin Pathol.* 2004;121:78-86.
5. Saad RS, Liu Y, Han H, et al. Prognostic significance of HER2/neu, p53 and vascular endothelial growth factor expression in early stage conventional adenocarcinoma and bronchioloalveolar carcinoma of the lung. *Mod Pathol.* 2004;17:1234-1242.
6. Pelosi G, Pasini F, Fraggetta F, et al. Independent value of fascin immunoreactivity for predicting lymph node metastases in typical and atypical pulmonary carcinoids. *Lung Cancer.* 2003;42:203-213.
7. Pelosi G, Pastorini O, Pasini F, et al. Independent prognostic value of fascin immunoreactivity in stage I nonsmall cell lung cancer. *Br J Cancer.* 2003;88:537-547.
8. Jagirdar J. Immunohistochemistry: Then and Now. *Arch. Pathol Lab Med.* 2008;132:323-325.
9. Hammar SP. Common neoplasms. In: Dail DH, Hammar SP, eds. *Pulmonary Pathology.* 2nd ed. New York: Springer-Verlag; 1994:1487-1579.
10. Dodds L, Davis S, Polissar L. A population-based study of lung cancer incidence by histological type. *J Natl Cancer Inst.* 1986;76:21-29.
11. Thun MJ, Lally CA, Flannery JT, et al. Cigarette smoking and changes in the histopathology of lung cancer. *J Natl Cancer Inst.* 1997;89:1580-1586.
12. Moll R, Franke WW, Schiller DL, et al. The catalog of human cytokeratins: Patterns of expression in normal epithelia, tumors and cultured cells. *Cell.* 1982;31:11-24.
13. Moll R, Lowe A, Laufer J, et al. Cytokeratin 20 in human carcinomas. A new histodiagnostic marker detected by monoclonal antibodies. *Am J Surg Pathol.* 1992;140:427-447.
14. Ramaekers F, Huysmans A, Schaart G, et al. Tissue distribution of keratin 7 as monitored by a monoclonal antibody. *Exp Cell Research.* 1987;170:235-249.
15. Chu P, Wu E, Weiss LM. Cytokeratin 7 and cytokeratin 20 expression in epithelial neoplasms: A survey of 435 cases. *Mod Pathol.* 2000;13:962-972.
16. Hammar SP, Hallman KO. Unusual primary lung neoplasms: spindle cell and undifferentiated carcinomas expressing only vimentin. *Ultrastruct Pathol.* 1990;14:407-422.
17. Upton MP, Hirohashi S, Tome Y, et al. Expression of vimentin in surgically resected adenocarcinomas and large cell carcinomas of lung. *Am J Surg Pathol.* 1986;10:560-567.
18. Guazzi S, Price M, DeFelice M, et al. Thyroid nuclear factor-1 (TTF-1) contains a homeodomain and displays a novel DNA-binding specificity. *EMBO J.* 1990;9:3631-3639.
19. Lazzaro D, Price M, DeFelice M, et al. The transcription factor TTF-1 expressed at the onset of thyroid and lung morphogenesis and in the restricted regions of the foetal brain. *Development.* 1991;113:1093-1094.
20. Bohinski RJ, DiLauro R, Whitsett JA. The lung specific surfactant protein B promoter is a target for thyroid transcription factor-1 and hepatocyte nuclear factor 3, indicating common factors for organ-specific gene expression along the Foregut axis. *Mol Cell Biol.* 1994;14:5671-5678.
21. Bohinski RJ, Huffman JA, Whitsett JA, et al. Cis-active elements controlling lung cell-specific expression of human pulmonary surfactant B gene. *J Biol Chem.* 1993;268:11160-11166.
22. Bejarano PA, Baughman RP, Biddinger PW, et al. Surfactant proteins and thyroid transcription factor-1 in pulmonary and breast carcinomas. *Mod Pathol.* 1996;9:445-452.
23. Fabbro D, DiLoreto C, Stamerra O, et al. TTF-1 gene expression in human lung tumors. *Eur J Cancer.* 1996;32A:512-573.
24. DiLoreto C, DiLauro V, Puglisi F, et al. Immunohistochemical expression of tissue specific transcription factor-1 in lung carcinoma. *J Clin Pathol.* 1997;50:30-32.
25. Holzinger A, Dingle S, Bejarano PA, et al. Monoclonal antibody to thyroid transcription factor-1: Production, characterization and usefulness in tumor diagnosis. *Hybridoma.* 1996;15:49-53.
26. Folpe AL, Gown AM, Lamps LW, et al. Thyroid transcription factor-1: Immunohistochemical evaluation in pulmonary neuroendocrine tumors. *Mod Pathol.* 1999;12:5-8.
27. Au NHC, Gown AM, Cheang M, et al. p63 expression in lung carcinomas: A tissue microarray study of 408 cases. *Appl Immunohistochem Mol Morphol.* 2004;12:240-247.
28. Sheikh HA, Fuhrer K, Cieply K, et al. p63 expression in assessment of bronchioloalveolar proliferations of the lung. *Mod Pathol.* 2004;17:1134-1140.
29. Hammar SP. Metastatic adenocarcinoma of unknown primary origin. *Hum Pathol.* 1998;29:1393-1402.
30. Amin MB, Tamboli P, Merchant SH. Micropapillary component in lung adenocarcinoma: A distinctive histologic feature with possible prognostic significance. *Am J Surg Pathol.* 2002;26:358-364.
31. Nakamura N, Miyagi E, Murata S, et al. Expression of thyroid transcription factor-1 in normal and neoplastic lung tissues. *Mod Pathol.* 2002;15:1058-1067.
32. Lau SK, Desrochers MJ, Luthringer DJ. Expression of thyroid transcription factor-1, cytokeratin 7 and cytokeratin 20 in bronchioloalveolar carcinomas: an immunohistochemical evaluation of 67 cases. *Mod Pathol.* 2002;15:538-542.
33. Simsir A, Wei XJ, Yee H, et al. Differential expression of cytokeratins 7 and 20 and thyroid transcription factor-1 in bronchioloalveolar carcinoma: an immunohistochemical study in fine needle aspiration biopsy specimens. *Am J Clin Pathol.* 2004;121:350-357.
34. Johansson L. Histopathologic classification of lung cancer: relevance of cytokeratin and TTF-1 immunophenotyping. *Ann Diagn Pathol.* 2004;8:259-267.
35. Yatabe Y, Mitsudomi T, Takahashi T. TTF-1 expression in pulmonary adenocarcinomas. *Am J Surg Pathol.* 2002;26:767-773.
36. Chang Y, Lee Y, Lia W, et al. The utility and limitation of thyroid transcription factor-1 protein in primary and metastatic pulmonary neoplasms. *Lung Cancer.* 2004;44:149-157.
37. Saad RS, Liu YL, Han H, et al. Prognostic significance of thyroid transcription factor-1 expression in both early-stage conventional adenocarcinoma and bronchioloalveolar carcinoma of the lung. *Hum Pathol.* 2004;35:3-7.
38. Jagirdar J. Application of immunohistochemistry to the diagnosis of primary and metastatic carcinoma to the lung. *Arch Pathol Lab Med.* 2008;132:384-396.
39. Sainz IM, Fukuoka J, Cagle PT, et al. A new marker for lung adenocarcinoma is complementary and more sensitive than TTF-1 (thyroid transcription factor-1): Evaluation of 967 cases by tissue microarray. *Mod Pathol.* 2008;21:349A.
40. Yesner R. Small cell tumors of the lung. *Am J Surg Pathol.* 1983;7:775-785.
41. Carter D. Small-cell carcinoma of the lung. *Am J Surg Pathol.* 1983;7:787-795.
42. Yesner R. Classification of lung cancer histology. *N Engl J Med.* 1985;312:652-653.
43. Arrigoni MG, Woolner LB, Berantz PE. Atypical carcinoid tumors of the lung. *J Thorac Cardiovasc Surg.* 1972;64:413-421.
44. Leschke H. Über nur regionär bösartige und über krebsig entartete Bronchusadenome bzw. *Carcinoide. Virch Arch [Pathol Anat].* 1956;328:635-657.

45. Warren WH, Memoli VA, Gould VE. Immunohistochemical and ultrastructural analysis of bronchopulmonary neuroendocrine neoplasms: II. Well-differentiated neuroendocrine carcinomas. *Ultrastruct Pathol.* 1984;7:185-199.
46. Mark EJ, Ramirerz JF. Peripheral small-cell carcinoma of the lung resembling carcinoid tumor: A clinical and pathologic study of 14 cases. *Arch Pathol Lab Med.* 1985;109:263-269.
47. Paladugu RR, Benfield JR, Pak HY, et al. Bronchopulmonary Kulchitzky cell carcinomas. *Cancer.* 1985;55:1303-1311.
48. Travis WD, Colby TV, Corrin B, et al. *Histological Typing of Lung and Pleural Tumors.* New York: Springer-Verlag; 1999.
49. Thomas CF, Tazelaar HD, Jett JR. Typical and atypical pulmonary carcinoids: Outcome in patients presenting with regional lymph node involvement. *Chest.* 2001;119:1143-1150.
50. Slodkowska J, Langfort R, Rudzinski P, et al. Typical and atypical pulmonary carcinoids—Pathologic and clinical analysis of 77 cases. *Pneumonol Alergol Pol.* 1998;66:297-303.
51. Gould VE, Chejfec G. Ultrastructural and biochemical analysis of pulmonary "undifferentiated" carcinomas. *Hum Pathol.* 1978;9:377-384.
52. Hammond ME, Sause WT. Large cell neuroendocrine tumors of the lung: Clinical significance and histological definition. *Cancer.* 1985;56:1624-1629.
53. Neal MH, Kosinki R, Cohen P, et al. Atypical endocrine tumors of the lung: A histologic, ultrastructural and clinical study of 19 cases. *Hum Pathol.* 1986;17:1264-1277.
54. Barbareschi M, Mariscotti C, Barberis M, et al. Large cell neuroendocrine of the lung. *Tumor.* 1989;75:583-588.
55. McDowell EM, Wilson TS, Trump BF. Atypical endocrine tumors of the lung. *Arch Pathol Lab Med.* 1981;105:20-28.
56. Travis WD, Linnoila I, Tsokos MG, et al. Neuroendocrine tumors of the lung with proposed criteria for large cell neuroendocrine carcinoma: An ultrastructural, immunohistochemical and flow cytometric study of 35 cases. *Am J Surg Pathol.* 1991;15:529-533.
57. Hammar S, Bockus D, Remington F, Cooper L. The unusual spectrum of neuroendocrine lung neoplasms. *Ultra Pathol.* 1989;13:515-560.
58. Jiang SX, Kameya T, Shoji M, et al. Large cell neuroendocrine carcinoma of the lung: a histologic and immunohistochemical study of 22 cases. *Am J Surg Pathol.* 1998;22:526-537.
59. Sturm N, Lantuejoul S, Laverriere MH, et al. Thyroid transcription factor-1 and cytokeratins 1, 5, 10, 14 (34βE12) expression in basaloid and large cell neuroendocrine carcinomas of the lung. *Hum Pathol.* 2001;32:918-925.
60. Jung KJ, Lee KS, Han J, et al. Large cell neuroendocrine carcinoma of the lung: Clinical, CT and pathologic findings in 11 patients. *J Thorac Imaging.* 2001;16:156-162.
61. Mazieres J, Daste G, Molinier L, et al. Large cell neuroendocrine carcinoma of the lung: pathological study and clinical outcome of 18 resected cases. *Lung Cancer.* 2002;37:287-292.
62. Paci M, Cavazza A, Annessi V, et al. Large cell neuroendocrine carcinoma of the lung: A 10 year clinicopathologic retrospective study. *Ann Thorac Surg.* 2004;77:1163-1167.
63. Doddoli C, Barlesi F, Chetaille B, et al. Large cell neuroendocrine carcinoma of the lung: An aggressive disease potentially treatable with surgery. *Ann Thorac Surg.* 2004;77:1168-1172.
64. Peng WX, Sano T, Oyama T, et al. Large cell neuroendocrine carcinoma of the lung: A comparison with large cell carcinoma with neuroendocrine morphology and small cell carcinoma. *Lung Cancer.* 2005;47:225-233.
65. Pearse AGE. The diffuse neuroendocrine system: An extension of the APUD concept. In: Taylor S, ed. *Endocrinology.* London: Heinemann; 1972:145-222.
66. Gould VE, DeLellis RA. The neuroendocrine cell system: Its tumors, hyperplasias and dysplasias. In: Silverberg SG, ed. *Principles and practice of surgical pathology.* New York: John Wiley; 1983:1488-1501.
67. Hammar SP, Gould VE. Neuroendocrine neoplasms. In: Azar HA, ed. *Pathology of Human Neoplasms: An Atlas of Diagnostic Electron Microscopy and Immunohistochemistry.* New York: Raven Press; 1988:333-404.
68. Jahn B, Schibler W, Ouimet C, et al. A 38,000 dalton membrane protein (p38) present in synaptic vesicles. *Proc Natl Acad Sci USA.* 1985;82:4137-4141.
69. Wiedenmann B, Franke WW. Identification and localization of synaptophysin, an integral membrane glycoprotein of Mr 38,000 characteristic of presynaptic vesicles. *Cell.* 1985;41:1017-1028.
70. Carmichael SW, Winkler H. The adrenal chromaffin cell. *Sci Am.* 1985;253:40-49.
71. O'Connor DT, Frigon RP. Chromogranin A, the major catecholamine storage vesicle protein. *J Biol Chem.* 1984;259:3237-3247.
72. Banks P, Helle K. The release of protein from the stimulated adrenal medulla. *Biochem J.* 1965;97:40C-41C.
73. Haimoto H, Takahashi V, Koshikawa T, et al. Immunohistochemical localization of gamma-enolase in normal human tissues other than nervous and neuroendocrine tissues. *Lab Invest.* 1985;52:257-263.
74. Pahlman S, Esscher T, Nilsson K. Expression of gamma-subunit of enolase, neuron-specific enolase in human non-neuroendocrine tumors and derived cell lines. *Lab Invest.* 1986;54:554-560.
75. Leoncini P, DeMarco EB, Bognoli M, et al. Expression of phosphorylated and non-phosphorylated neurofilament subunits and cytokeratins in neuroendocrine lung tumors. *Pathol Res Pract.* 1989;185:848-855.
76. Komminoth P, Roth J, Lackie PM, et al. Polysialic acid of the neural cell adhesion molecule distinguishes small cell carcinoma from carcinoids. *Am J Pathol.* 1991;139:297-304.
77. Kibbelaar RE, Moolenaar CEC, Michalides RJAM, et al. Expression of the embryonal neural cell adhesion molecule N-CAM in lung carcinoma: Diagnostic usefulness of monoclonal antibody 735 for the distinction between small cell lung cancer and non–small cell lung cancer. *J Pathol.* 1989;159:23-28.
78. Bunn P, Linnoila I, Minna J, et al. Small-cell lung cancer, endocrine cells of the fetal bronchus and other neuroendocrine cells express Leu-7 antigenic determinant present on natural killer cells. *Blood.* 1985;65:764-768.
79. Matsuki Y, Tanimoto A, Hamada T, et al. Histidine decarboxylase expression as a new sensitive and specific marker for small cell lung carcinoma. *Mod Pathol.* 2003;16:72-78.
80. Gibbs AR, Whimster WF. Tumors of the lung and pleura. In: Fletcher CDM, ed. *Diagnostic Histopathology of Tumors.* Edinburg: Churchill Livingstone; 1995:127-150.
81. Dail DH. Uncommon neoplasms. In: Dail DH, Hammar SP, eds. *Pulmonary Pathology.* 2nd ed. New York: Springer-Verlag; 1994:1279-1461.
82. Wick MR, Swanson PE. Carcinosarcomas: current perspective and a historical review of nosologic concepts. *Semin Diag Pathol.* 1993;10:118-127.
83. Addis BJ, Corrin B. Pulmonary blastoma, carcinosarcoma and spindle cell carcinoma: An immunohistochemical study of keratin intermediate filaments. *J Pathol.* 1985;147:291-301.
84. Zarbo RJ, Crissman JD, Venkat H, et al. Spindle cell carcinoma of the upper aerodigestive tract mucosa: An immunohistologic and ultrastructural study of 18 biphasic tumors and comparison with seven monophasic spindle cell tumors. *Am J Surg Pathol.* 1986;10:741-753.
85. Humphrey PA, Scroggs MW, Roggli VL, et al. Pulmonary carcinomas with a sarcomatoid element: An immunohistochemical and ultrastructural analysis. *Hum Pathol.* 1988;19:155-165.
86. Colby TV, Bilbao JE, Battifora H, et al. Primary osteosarcoma of the lung: A re-appraisal following immunohistologic study. *Arch Pathol Lab Med.* 1989;113:1147-1150.
87. Nappi O, Glasner SD, Swanson PE, et al. Biphasic and monophasic sarcomatoid carcinomas of the lung: A re-appraisal of "carcinosarcomas" and "spindle cell carcinomas." *Am J Clin Pathol.* 1994;102:331-340.
88. Fishback NF, Travis WD, Moran CA, et al. Pleomorphic (spindle/giant cell) carcinoma of the lung. *Cancer.* 1994;73:2936-2945.
89. Pelosi G, Fraggetta F, Nappi O, et al. Pleomorphic carcinomas of the lung show a selective distribution of gene products involved in cell differentiation, cell cycle control, tumor growth and tumor cell motility: A clinicopathologic and immunohistochemical study of 31 cases. *Am J Surg Pathol.* 2003;27:1203-1215.
90. Koss MN, Hochholzer L, O'Leary T. Pulmonary blastomas. *Cancer.* 1983;73:265-294.
91. Yousem SA, Wick MR, Randhawa P, et al. Pulmonary blastoma: An immunohistochemical analysis and comparison with fetal lung in its pseudoglandular stage. *Am J Clin Pathol.* 1990;93:167-175.

92. Etienne-Mastroianni B, Falchero L, Chalabreysse L, et al. Primary sarcomas of the lung: A clinicopathologic study of 12 cases. *Lung Cancer*. 2002;38:283-290.
93. Ognibene FP, Steis RG, Macher AM, et al. Kaposi's sarcoma causing pulmonary infiltrates and respiratory failure in the acquired immunodeficiency syndrome. *Ann Intern Med*. 1985;102:471-475.
94. Garay SM, Belenko M, Fazzini E, et al. Pulmonary manifestations of Kaposi's sarcoma. *Chest*. 1987;91:39-43.
95. White DA, Matthay RA. Noninfectious pulmonary complications of infection with the human immunodeficiency virus. *Am Rev Respir Dis*. 1989;140:1763-1787.
96. McLoud TC, Naidich DP. Thoracic disease in the immunocompromised patient. *Radiol Clin North Am*. 1992;30:525-554.
97. Ognibene FP, Shelhamer JH. Kaposi's sarcoma. *Clin Chest Med*. 1988;9:459-465.
98. Heitzman ER. Pulmonary neoplastic lymphoproliferative disease in AIDS: A review. *Radiology*. 1990;177:347-351.
99. Purdy LJ, Colby TV, Yousem SA, et al. Pulmonary Kaposi's sarcoma. Premortem histologic diagnosis. *Am J Surg Pathol*. 1986;10:301-311.
100. Hymes KB, Cheung T, Greene JB, et al. Kaposi's sarcoma in homosexual men: A report of eight cases. *Lancet*. 1981;2:598-600.
101. Kaposi's sarcoma and pneumocystis pneumonia in homosexual men—New York City and California. *MMWR*. 1981;30:305-308.
102. Gottlieb GJ, Ackerman AB. Kaposi's sarcoma: An extensively disseminated form in young homosexual men. *Hum Pathol*. 1982;13:882-892.
103. Adem C, Aubry MC, Tazelaar HD, et al. Metastatic angiosarcoma masquerading as diffuse pulmonary hemorrhage: Clinicopathologic analysis of 7 new patients. *Arch Pathol Lab Med*. 2001;125:1562-1565.
104. Tschernig T, Pabst R. Bronchus-associated lymphoid tissue (BALT) is not present in the normal adult lung but in different disease. *Pathobiology*. 2000;68:1-8.
105. Richmond I, Pritchard GE, Ashcroft T, et al. Bronchus associated lymphoid tissue (BALT) in human lungs: Its distribution in smokers and nonsmokers. *Thorax*. 1993;48:1130-1134.
106. Swigris JJ, Berry GJ, Raffin TA, et al. Lymphoid interstitial pneumonia. A narrative review. *Chest*. 2002;122:2150–1064.
107. Bienenstock J, Johnston N, Perey DYE. Bronchial lymphoid tissue. I. Morphologic characteristics. *Lab Invest*. 1973;28:686-692.
108. Bienenstock J, Johnston N, Perey DYE. Bronchial lymphoid tissue II. Functional characteristics. *Lab Invest*. 1973;28:693-698.
109. Pisani RJ, Witzit TE, Li CY, et al. Confirmation of lymphomatous pulmonary involvement by immunophenotypic and gene rearrangement analysis of broncho-alveolar lavage fluid. *Mayo Clin Proc*. 1990;65:651-656.
110. Kuroso K, Yumo T, Rom WN, et al. Oligoclonal T cell expansions in pulmonary lymphoproliferative disorders: Demonstration of the frequent occurrence of oligoclonal T cells in human Immunodeficiency virus-related lymphoid interstitial pneumonia. *Am J Respir Crit Care Med*. 2002;165:254-259.
111. Colby TV. Lymphoproliferative diseases. In: Dail DH, Hammar SP, Colby TV, eds. *Pulmonary Pathology Tumors*. New York: Springer Verlag; 1995:343-368.
112. Lymphoproliferative Disorders and Leukemia. In: Fraser RS, Pare PD, Muller NL, Colmann, eds. *Diagnosis of Diseases of the Chest*. 4th ed. Philadelphia: Saunders; 1999:1269-1330.
113. Jaffe ES, Harris NL, Stein H, et al. *Genetics of tumours of hematopoietic and lymphoid tissues*. Lyon: IARC Press; 2001.
114. Nicholson AG. Lymphoproliferative lung disease. In: Corrin B, ed. *Pathology of Lung Tumors.*. New York: Churchill Livingstone; 1997:213-223.
115. Yousem SA. Lung tumors in the immunocompromised host. In: Corrin B, ed. New York: Churchill Livingstone; 1997:189-212.
116. Koss MN. Pulmonary lymphoid disorders. *Sem Diag Pathol*. 1995:158-171.
117. Kradin RL, Mark EG. Benign lymphoid disorders of the lung with a theory regarding their development. *Human Pathol*. 1983;14:857-867.
118. Colby TV. Lymphoproliferative diseases. In: Dail DH, Hammar SP, eds. 2nd ed. New York: Springer-Verlag; 1994:1097-1122.
119. Saldana MJ, Patchfsky AS, Israel HL, et al. Pulmonary angiitis and granulomatosis. The relationship between histologic features, organ involvement and response to treatment. *Hum Pathol*. 1977;8:391-409.
120. Israel HL, Patchfsky AS, Saldana MJ. Wegener's granulomatosis, lymphomatoid granulomatosis, and benign lymphocytic angiitis and granulomatosis of lung. Recognition and treatment. *Ann Intern Med*. 1977;87:691-699.
121. Jaffe ES, Banks PM, Natwhani B, et al. Recommendations for reporting of lymphoid neoplasms: A report from the association of directors of anatomic and surgical pathology. The ad hoc committee of reporting of lymphoid neoplasms. *Hum Pathol*. 2002;33:1064-1068.
122. His ED, Yegaptan S. Lymphoma Immunophenotyping: A new era in paraffin-sectioned immunohistochemistry. *Advances in Anatomic Pathology*. 2001;8:218-239.
123. Rosenow C, Wilson WR, Cockerill FR. Pulmonary disease in the immunocompromised host. *Mayo Clin Proc*. 1985;60:473-487.
124. Lin Y, Rodriguez GD, Turner JF, et al. Plasmablastic lymphoma of the lung: Report of a unique case and review of the literature. *Arch Pathol and Laboratory Medicine*. 2001;125:282-285.
125. L'Hoste RJ, Filippa DA, Lieberman PH, et al. Primary pulmonary lymphomas: A clinicopathologic analysis of 36 cases. *Cancer*. 1984;54:1397-1406.
126. Radin AI. Primary pulmonary Hodgkin's disease. *Cancer*. 1990;65:550-563.
127. Liebow AA, Carrington CB, Friedman PJ. Lymphomatoid granulomatosis. *Hum Pathol*. 1972;3:457-558.
128. Katzenstein AL, Carrington CB, Liebow AA. Lymphomatoid granulomatosis: A clinicopathologic study of 152 cases. *Cancer*. 1979;43:360-373.
129. Guinee D, Kingma D, Fishback N, et al. Pulmonary lesions with features of lymphomatoid granulomatosis/angiocentric immunoproliferative lesion (LYT/AIL); evidence for Epstein-Barr virus within B lymphocytes. 1994;USCAP Abstract #881.
130. Fauci AS, Haynes BF, Costa J, et al. Lymphomatoid granulomatosis: Prospective, clinical and therapeutic experience over 10 years. *N Engl J Med*. 1982;306:68-74.
131. Demirer T, Dail DH, Aboulafia DM. Four varied cases of intravascular lymphomatosis and a literature review. *Cancer*. 1994;73:1738-1745.
132. Tan TB, Spaander PJ, Blaisse M, et al. Angiotropic large cell lymphoma presenting as interstitial lung disease. *Thorax*. 1988;43:578-579.
133. Snyder LS, Harmon KR, Estensen RD. Intravascular lymphomatosis (malignant angioendotheliomatosis) presenting as pulmonary hypertension. *Chest*. 1989;96:1199-1200.
134. Yousem SA, Colby TB. Intravascular lymphomatosis presenting in the lung. *Cancer*. 1990;65:349-353.
135. Pellicone JT, Goldstein HB. Pulmonary malignant angioendotheliomatosis: Presentation with fever and syndrome of inappropriate anti-diuretic hormone. *Chest*. 1990;98:1292-1294.
136. Takamura K, Nasuhara Y, Mishina T, et al. Intravascular lymphomatosis diagnosed by transbronchial lung biopsy. *Eur Respir J*. 1997;10:955-957.
137. Walls JG, Hong YG, Cox JE, et al. Pulmonary intravascular lymphomatosis: Presentation with dyspnea and air trapping. *Chest*. 1999;115:1207-1210.
138. Ansari MQ, Dawson DB, Nador R, et al. Primary body cavity-based AIDS-related lymphomas. *Am J Clin Pathol*. 1996;105:221-229.
139. Banks PM, Warnke RA. Primary effusion lymphoma. In: *WHO Classification of Tumors of Hematopoietic and Lymphoid Tissues*. Lyon: IARC Press; 2001:179-180.
140. Banks PM, Harris NL, Warnke RA. Primary effusion lymphoma. In: Travis WD, Brambilla E, eds. *WHO Classification of Tumors of the Lung, Pleura and Mediastinum*. Lyon: IARC Press; 2004.
141. Cesarman E, Chang Y, Moore PS, et al. Kaposi's sarcoma-associated herpes virus-like DNA sequencing in age-related body cavity lymphoma. *N Engl J Med*. 1995;332:1186-1191.
142. Aozasa K, Ohsaw AM, Kanno H. Pyothorax-associated lymphoma: A distinctive type of lymphoma strongly associated with Epstein-Barr virus. *Adv in Anat Pathol*. 1997;4:58-63.

143. Gaulard P, Harris NL. Pyothorax-associated lymphoma. In: Travis WD, Brambilla E, eds. *WHO Classification of Tumors of the Lung, Pleura and Mediastinum*. Lyon: IARC Press; 2004.
144. Ibuka T, Fukayama M, Hayashi Y, et al. Pyothorax-associated pleural lymphoma. *Cancer*. 1994;73:738-744.
145. Allen TC, Barrios-Chevez P, Shetlar DJ, et al. Pulmonary and opthalmic involvement with Erdheim-Chester disease; a case report and review of the literature. *Arch Pathol Lab Med*. 2004;128:1428-1431.
146. Hammar SP. Pulmonary histiocytosis-X (Langerhans cell granulomatosis). In: Dail DH, Hammar SP, eds. *Pulmonary Pathology*. 2nd ed: New York: Springer-Verlag; 1994:567-596.
147. Carter D, Patchefsky AS, Mountain CF. Clear cell lesions. In: Carter D, Patchefsky AS, eds. *Tumors and Tumor-like Lesions of the Lung*. Philadelphia: WB Saunders; 1998:271-274.
148. Bonetti F, Pea M, Martigoni G, et al. Clear cell ("sugar tumor") of the lung is a lesion strictly related to angiomyolipoma—the concept of a family of lesions characterized by the presence of the perivascular epithelioid cells (PEC). *Pathology*. 1994;26:230-236.
149. Panizo-Santos A, Sola I, de Alava E, et al. Angiomyolipoma and PEComa are immunoreactive for MyoD1 in cell cytoplasmic staining pattern. *Appl Immunohistochem Mol Morphol*. 2003;11:156-160.
150. Gaffey M, Mills S, Zarbo R, et al. Clear cell tumor of the lung: Immunohistochemical and ultrastructural evidence of melanogenesis. *Am J Surg Pathol*. 1991;15:644-653.
151. Sullivan EJ. Lymphangioleiomyomatosis: A review. *Chest*. 1998;114:1689-1703.
152. Johnson S. Lymphangioleiomyomatosis: Clinical features, management and basic mechanism. *Thorax*. 1999;54:254-264.
153. Liebow AA, Hubbell DS. Sclerosing hemangioma (histiocytoma, xanthoma) of the lung. *Cancer*. 1956;9:53-75.
154. Sogio K, Yokoyama H, Kanedo S, et al. Sclerosing hemangioma of the lung: radiographic and pathologic study. *Ann Thorac Surg*. 1992;53:295-300.
155. Katzenstein A-LA, Gmelich JT, Carrington CB. Sclerosing hemangioma of the lung: A clinicopathologic study of 51 cases. *Am J Surg Pathol*. 1982;4:343-356.
156. Devouassoux-Shisheboran M, Hayashi T, Linnoila RI, et al. A clinicopathologic study of 100 cases of pulmonary sclerosing hemangioma with immunohistochemical studies: TTF-1 is expressed in both round and surface cells, suggesting an origin from primitive respiratory epithelium. *Am J Surg Pathol*. 2000;24:906-916.
157. Devouassoux-Shisheboran M, de la Fouchardiere A, Thivolet-Bejui F, et al. Endobronchial variant of sclerosing hemangioma of the lung: Histological and cytological features on endobronchial material. *Mod Pathol*. 2004;17:252-257.
158. Miyagawa-Hayashino A, Tazelaar HD, Langel DJ, et al. Pulmonary sclerosing hemangioma with lymph node metastases: Report of 4 cases. *Arch Pathol Lab Med*. 2003;127:321-325.
159. Beckwith JB, Palmer NF. Histopathology and prognosis of Wilms' tumor: Results from the first national Wilms' tumor study. *Cancer*. 1978;55:2850-2853.
160. Small EJ, Gordon GJ, Dahms BB. Malignant rhabdoid tumor of the heart in an infant. *Cancer*. 1985;55:2850-2853.
161. Balaton AJ, Vaury P, Videgrain M. Paravertebral malignant rhabdoid tumor in an adult: A case report of immunocytochemical study. *Pathol Res Pract*. 1987;182:713-718.
162. Harris M, Eyden BP, Joglekar VM. Rhabdoid tumour of the bladder: A histological, ultrastructural and immunohistochemical study. *Histopathology*. 1987;11:1083-1089.
163. Biggs PJ, Garren PD, Posers JM, et al. Malignant rhabdoid tumor of the central nervous system. *Hum Pathol*. 1987;18:332-337.
164. Dervan PA, Cahalane SF, Kneafsey P, et al. Malignant rhabdoid tumor of soft tissue: An ultrastructural and immunohistological study of a pelvic tumour. *Histopathol*. 1987;11:183-190.
165. Parham DM, Peiper S, Robicheaux G, et al. Malignant rhabdoid tumor of the liver: Evidence for epithelial differentiation. *Arch Pathol Lab Med*. 1988;112:61-64.
166. Jakate SM, Mardsen HB, Ingram L. Primary rhabdoid tumour of the brain. *Virch Arch [A]*. 1988;412:393-397.
167. Uchida H, Yokoyama S, Nakayama I, et al. An autopsy case of malignant rhabdoid tumor arising from soft parts in the left inguinal region. *Acta Pathol Jpn*. 1988;38:1087-1096.
168. Patron M, Palacious J, Rodriguez-Peralto JL, et al. Malignant rhabdoid tumor of the tongue: A case report with immunohistochemical and ultrastructural findings. *Oral Surg Oral Med Oral Path*. 1988;65:67-70.
169. Carter RL, McCarthy KP, al-Sam SZ, et al. Malignant rhabdoid tumour of the bladder with immunohistochemical and ultrastructural evidence suggesting histiocytic origin. *Histopathology*. 1989;14:179-190.
170. Jsujimura T, Wasa A, Kawano K, et al. A case of malignant rhabdoid tumor arising from soft parts of the prepubic region. *Acta Pathol Jpn*. 1989;37:677-682.
171. Cho KR, Rosenshein NB, Epstein JI. Malignant rhabdoid tumor of the kidney and soft tissues: evidence for a diverse morphological and immunocytochemical phenotype. *Arch Pathol Lab Med*. 1989;113:115-120.
172. Tsokos M, Kouraklis G, Chandra RS, et al. Malignant rhabdoid tumor of the kidney and soft tissues: Evidence for a diverse morphological and immunocytochemical phenotype. *Arch Pathol Lab Med*. 1989;113:115-120.
173. Molenaar WM, DeJong B, Dam-Meiring A, et al. Epithelioid sarcoma or malignant rhabdoid tumor of soft tissue. Epithelioid immunophenotype and rhabdoid karyotype. *Hum Pathol*. 1989;20:347-351.
174. Cavazza A, Colby TV, Tsokos M, et al. Lung tumors with a rhabdoid phenotype. *Am J Clin Pathol*. 1996;105:182-188.
175. Miyagi J, Tsuhako K, Kinjo T, et al. Rhabdoid tumor of the lung is a dedifferentiated phenotype of pulmonary adenocarcinoma. *Histopathology*. 2000;37:37-44.
176. Bahadori H, Liebow AA. Plasma cell granuloma of the lung. *Cancer*. 1973;31:191-208.
177. Lane JD, Krohn S, Kolozzi W, et al. Plasma cell granuloma of the lung. *Dis Chest*. 1955;27:216-221.
178. Berardi RS, Lee SS, Chen HP, et al. Inflammatory pseudotumors of the lung. *Surg Gynecol Obstet*. 1983;156:89-96.
179. Tang TT, Segura AD, Oechler HW, et al. Inflammatory myofibrohistiocytic proliferation simulating sarcoma in children. *Cancer*. 1990;65:1626-1634.
180. Tan-Liu NS, Matsubara MD, Grillo HC, et al. Invasive fibrous tumor of the tracheobronchial tree: Clinical and pathological study of seven cases. *Hum Pathol*. 1989;20:180-184.
181. Ledet SC, Brown RW, Cagle PT. p53 immunostaining of the differentiation of inflammatory pseudotumor from sarcoma involving the lung. *Mod Pathol*. 1995;8:282-286.
182. Snyder CS, Dell-Aquila M, Haghighi P, et al. Clonal changes in inflammatory pseudotumor of the lung. *Cancer*. 1995;76:1545-1549.
183. Yousem SA, Shaw H, Cieply K. Involvement of 2p23 pulmonary inflammatory pseudotumors. *Hum Pathol*. 2001;32:428-433.
184. Freeman A, Geddes N, Munson P, et al. Anaplastic lymphoma kinase (ALK 1) staining and molecular analysis in inflammatory myofibroblastic tumors of the bladder: A preliminary clinicopathologic study of nine cases and review of the literature. *Mod Pathol*. 2004;17:765-771.
185. Lae ME, Roche PC, Jin L, et al. Desmoplastic small round cell tumor: A clinicopathologic, immunohistochemical and molecular study of 32 tumors. *Am J Surg Pathol*. 2002;26:823-835.
186. Syed S, Hague AK, Hawkins HK, et al. Desmoplastic small round cell tumor of the lung. *Arch Pathol Lab Med*. 2002;126:1226-1228.
187. Ostoros G, Orosz Z, Kovacs G, et al. Desmoplastic small round cell tumor of the pleura: A case report with unusual follow-up. *Lung Cancer*. 2002;36:333-336.
188. Tsuji N, Tateishi R, Ishigoro S, et al. Adenomyoepithelioma of the lung. *Am J Surg Pathol*. 1995;19:956-962.
189. Veeramechaneni R, Gulic J, Halldorsson AO, et al. Benign myoepithelioma of the lung: A case report and review of the literature. *Arch Pathol Lab Med*. 2001;125:1494-1496.
190. Pelosi G, Fraggetta F, Maffini F, et al. Pulmonary epithelial-myoepithelial tumor of unproven malignant potential: Report of a case and review of the literature. *Mod Pathol*. 2001;14:521-526.
191. Ro K, Srivastava A, Tischer AS. Bronchial epithelial-myoepithelial carcinoma. *Arch Pathol Lab Med*. 2004;128:92-94.
192. Dearers M, Guinee D, Koss MN, et al. Granular cell tumors of the lung: Clinicopathologic study of 20 cases. *Am J Surg Pathol*. 1995;19:627-635.

193. de Araujo VC, de Sousa SOM, Carvalho YR, et al. Application of immunohistochemistry to the diagnosis of salivary gland tumors. *Appl Immunohist Mol Morphol.* 2000;8:195-202.
194. Moran CA, Suster S, Fishback NF, et al. Primary intrapulmonary thymoma: A clinicopathologic and immunohistochemical study of eight cases. *Am J Surg Pathol.* 1995;19:304-312.
195. Ionescu DN, Sasatomi E, Aldeeb D, et al. Pulmonary meningothelial-like nodules: A genotypic comparison with meningiomas. *Am J Surg Pathol.* 2004;28:207-214.
196. Mukhopadhyay S, El-Zammar OA, Katzenstein A- LA. Pulmonary meningothelial-like nodules: New insights into a common but poorly understood entity. *Mod Pathol.* 2008;21:348A.
197. Hochholzer L, Moran CA, Koss MN. Pulmonary lipomatosis: A variant of placental transmogrification. *Mod Pathol.* 1997;10:846-849.
198. Fidler ME, Koomen M, Sebek B, et al. Placental transmogrification of the lung, a histologic variant of giant bullous emphysema. *Am J Surg Pathol.* 1995;19:563-570.
199. Brambilla E. Basaloid carcinoma of the lung. In: Corrin B, ed. *Pathology of Lung Tumors.* New York: Churchill Livingstone; 1997:71-82.
200. Kargi A, Gurel D, Tuna B. The diagnostic value of TTF-1, CK5/6, and p63 immunostaining in classification of lung carcinomas. *Appl Immunohistochem Mol Morphol.* 2007;15:415-420.
201. Bejarano PA, Mousavi F. Incidence and significance of cytoplasmic thyroid transcription factor-1 immunoreactivity. *Arch Pathol Lab Med.* 2003;127:193-195.
202. Kaimaktchiev V, Terracciano L, Tornillo L, et al. The homeobox intestinal differentiation factor CDX2 is selectively expressed in gastrointestinal carcinomas. *Mod Pathol.* 2004;17:1392-1399.
203. Rossi G, Murer B, Cavazza A, et al. Primary mucinous (so-called colloid) carcinomas of the lung: A clinicopathologic and immunohistochemical study with special reference to CDX2 homeobox gene and MUC2 expression. *Am J Surg Pathol.* 2004;28:442-452.
204. Mazziotta RM, Borczuk AC, Powell CA, et al. CDX2 immunostaining as a gastrointestinal marker: Expression in lung carcinomas is a potential pitfall. *Appl Immunohistochem Mol Morphol.* 2005;13:55-60.
205. Striebel JM, Dacic S, Yousem SA. Gross Cystic Disease Fluid Protein (GCDFP-15): expression in primary lung adenocarcinoma. *Am J Surg Pathol.* 2008;32:426-432.
206. Herrera GA, Turbat-Herrera EA, Lott RL. S100 protein expression by primary and metastatic adenocarcinoma. *Am J Clin Pathol.* 1988;89:168-176.
207. Hammar SP, Bockus D, Remington F, et al. Langerhans cells and serum precipitating antibodies against fungal antigens in bronchioloalveolar cell carcinomas: Possible association with eosinophilic granuloma. *Ultrastruct Pathol.* 1980;1:19-37.
208. Colasante A, Castrilli G, Aiello FB, et al. Role of cytokines in the distribution of dendritic cells/Langerhans cell lineage in human primary carcinomas of the lung. *Hum Pathol.* 1995;26:866-872.
209. Hammar SP, Bockus D, Remington F, et al. The widespread distribution of Langerhans cells in pathologic tissues: An ultrastructural and immunohistochemical study. *Hum Pathol.* 1986;17:894-905.
210. Dorion P, Shi J, Zhang K, et al. Utility of S100 protein in differentiating adenocarcinoma of the lung from papillary carcinoma and follicular carcinoma of the thyroid. *Modern Pathol.* 2008;21:340.
211. Torikata C, Ishiwata K. Intranuclear tubular structures observed in the cells of alveolar cell carcinomas of the lung. *Cancer.* 1977;40:1194-1201.
212. Singh G, Katyal SL, Torikata C. Carcinoma of type II pneumocytes: Immunodiagnosis of a subtype of bronchioloalveolar carcinoma. *Am J Pathol.* 1981;102:195-208.
213. Singh G, Katyal SL, Torikata C. Carcinoma of type II pneumocytes: PAS staining as a screening test for nuclear inclusions of surfactant-specific apoprotein. *Cancer.* 1982;50:946-948.
214. Ghadially FN, Harawi S, Khan W. Diagnostic ultrastructural markers in alveolar cell carcinoma. *J Submicrosc Cytol.* 1985;17:269-278.
215. Nonaka D, Chiriboga L. Basal cell differentiation in lung adenocarcinoma. *Mod Pathol.* 2008;21:348A.
216. Tigrani DY, Weydert JA. Expression of inhibin-alpha in primary pulmonary non-small cell carcinomas by immunohistochemistry. *Mod Pathol.* 2008;21:352A.
217. Zhang K, Shi J, Lin F. Expression of inhibin-alpha in non-small cell carcinoma of the lung with a focus on adenocarcinoma: A diagnostic pitfall in the evaluation of metastatic pulmonary carcinoma. *Modern Pathol.* 2008;21:353A.
218. Abrams HJ, Spiro R, Goldstein N. Metastases in carcinoma, analysis of 1000 autopsied cases. *Cancer.* 1950;3:74-85.
219. Dail DH. Metastases to and from the lung. In: Dail DH, Hammar SP, Colby TV, eds. *Pulmonary Tumors.* New York: Springer-Verlag; 1995:369-403.
220. Wang NP, Zee S, Zarbo RJ, et al. Coordinate expression of cytokeratins 7 and 20 defines unique subsets of carcinomas. *Appl Immunohist.* 1995;3:99-107.
221. Ollayos CW, Riordan P, Rushin JM. Estrogen receptor detection in paraffin section of adenocarcinoma of colon, pancreas and lung. *Arch Pathol Lab Med.* 1994;118:630-632.
222. Canver CC, Memoli VA, Vanderveer PL, et al. Sex hormones in non-small cell lung cancer in human beings. *J Thorac Cardiovasc Surg.* 1994;108:153-157.
223. Bacchi CE, Garcia RL, Gown AM. Immunolocalization of estrogen and progesterone receptors in neuroendocrine tumors of lung, skin, gastrointestinal and female genital tracts. *Appl Immunohist.* 1997;5:17-22.
224. DiNunno LD, Larsson LG, Rinehart JJ, et al. Estrogen and progesterone receptors in non-small cell lung cancer in 248 consecutive patients who underwent surgical resection. *Arch Pathol Lab Med.* 2000;124:1467-1470.
225. Dabbs DJ, Landreneau RJ, Liu Y, et al. Detection of estrogen receptor by immunohistochemistry in pulmonary adenocarcinoma. *Ann Thorac Surg.* 2002;73:403-406.
226. Selvaggi G, Scagliotti GV, Torri V, et al. HER-2/neu overexpression in patients with radically resected nonsmall cell lung carcinoma: Impact on long-term survival. *Cancer.* 2002;94:2669-2674.
227. Butler AE, Colby TV, Weiss L, et al. Lymphoepithelioma-like carcinoma of lung. *Am J Surg Pathol.* 1989;13:632-639.
228. Chen F, Yan J, Lai W, et al. Epstein-Barr virus-associated non-small cell lung carcinoma: Undifferentiated "lymphoepithelioma-like" carcinomas as a distinct entity with better prognosis. *Cancer.* 1998;82:2334-2342.
229. Ginsberg SS, Buzaid AC, Stern H, et al. Giant cell carcinoma of the lung. *Cancer.* 1992;70:606-610.
230. Gustmann C, Altmannsberger M, Osborn M, et al. Cytokeratin expression and vimentin content in large cell anaplastic lymphoma and other non-Hodgkin's lymphoma. *Am J Pathol.* 1991;38:1413-1422.
231. Delsol G, AlSaati T, Gatter KC, et al. Coexpression of epithelial membrane antigen (EMA), Ki-1 and interleukin-2 receptor by anaplastic large cell lymphomas. Diagnostic value in so-called malignant histiocytosis. *Am J Pathol.* 1988;130:59-70.
232. Osborne BM, Mockay B, Butler JJ, et al. Large cell lymphoma with microvillus-like projections: An ultrastructural study. *Am J Clin Pathol.* 1983;79:433-450.
233. Chu PG, Arber DA, Weiss LM. Expression of T/NK-cell and plasma cell antigens in nonhematopoietic epithelioid neoplasms: An immunohistochemical study of 447 cases. *Am J Clin Pathol.* 2003;120:64-70.
234. Bishop PW, Menasce LP, Yates AJ, et al. An immunophenotypic survey of malignant melanomas. *Histopathology.* 1993;23:159-166.
235. Yoshimoto T, Higashino K, Hada T, et al. A primary lung carcinoma producing alpha-fetoprotein, carcinoembryonic antigen and human chorionic gonadotropin. *Cancer.* 1987;60:2744-2750.
236. Kuida CA, Braunstein GD, Shintaku P, et al. Human chorionic gonadotropin expression in lung, breast and renal carcinomas. *Arch Pathol Lab Med.* 1988;112:282-285.
237. Dirnhofer S, Freund M, Rogatsch H, et al. Selective expression of trophoblastic hormones by lung carcinoma: Neuroendocrine tumors produce human chorionic gonadotropin alpha-subunit (hCGα). *Hum Pathol.* 2000;31:966-972.

238. Nasu M, Soma T, Fukushima H, et al. Hepatoid carcinoma of the lung with production of alpha fetoprotein and abnormal prothrombin: An autopsy case report. *Mod Pathol.* 1997;10:1054-1058.
239. Cooper WA, Thourani VH, Gal AA, et al. The surgical spectrum of pulmonary neuroendocrine neoplasms. *Chest.* 2001;119: 14-18.
240. Lyda MH, Weiss LM. Immunoreactivity for epithelial and neuroendocrine antibodies are useful in the differential diagnosis of lung carcinomas. *Hum Pathol.* 2000;31:980-987.
241. Sturm N, Rossi G, Lantuejoul S, et al. Expression of thyroid transcription factor-1 in the spectrum of neuroendocrine cell lung proliferations with special interest in carcinoids. *Hum Pathol.* 2002;33:175-182.
242. Barbareschi M, Roldo C, Zamboni G, et al. CDX-2 homeobox gene product expression in neuroendocrine tumors: Its role as a marker of intestinal neuroendocrine tumors. *Am J Surg Pathol.* 2004;28:1169-1176.
243. Lin X, Saad RS, Luckasevic TM, et al. Diagnostic value of CDX-2 and TTF-1 expressions in separating metastatic neuroendocrine neoplasms of unknown origin. *Appl Immunohistochem Mol Morphol.* 2007;15:407-414.
244. Lin O, Olgac S, Green I, et al. Immunohistochemical staining of cytologic smears with MIB-1 helps distinguish low-grade from high-grade neuroendocrine neoplasms. *Am J Clin Pathol.* 2003;120:209-216.
245. Pelosi G, Rodriguez J, Viale G, et al. Typical and atypical pulmonary carcinoid tumor overdiagnosed as small cell carcinoma on biopsy specimens: A major pitfall in the management of lung cancer patients. *Am J Surg Pathol.* 2005;29:179-187.
246. Visscher DW, Zarbo RJ, Trojanowski JQ, et al. Neuroendocrine differentiation in poorly-differentiated lung carcinomas: A light microscopic and immunohistochemical study. *Mod Pathol.* 1990;3:508-512.
247. Linnoila RI, Mulshine JL, Steinberg SM, et al. Neuroendocrine differentiation in endocrine and nonendocrine lung carcinomas. *Am J Clin Pathol.* 1988;90:641-652.
248. Mooi WJ, Dewar A, Springall D, et al. Non-small cell lung carcinomas with neuroendocrine features: A light microscopic, immunohistochemical and ultrastructural study of 11 cases. *Histopathology.* 1988;13:329-337.
249. Wick MR, Berg LC, Hertz MI. Large cell carcinoma of the lung with neuroendocrine differentiation: A comparison with large cell "undifferentiated" pulmonary tumors. *Am J Clin Pathol.* 1992;97:796-805.
250. Loy TS, Darkow GVD, Quesenberry JT. Immunostaining in the diagnosis of pulmonary neuroendocrine carcinomas: An immunohistochemical study with ultrastructural correlations. *Am J Surg Pathol.* 1995;19:173-182.
251. Xu H, Bourne PA, Spaulding BO, et al. High-grade neuroendocrine carcinomas of the lung express K homology domain containing protein overexpressed in cancer but carcinoid tumors do not. *Hum Pathol.* 2007;38:555-563.
252. Schleusener JT, Tazelaar HD, Jung S, et al. Neuroendocrine differentiation is an independent prognostic factor in chemotherapy-treated non-small cell lung carcinoma. *Cancer.* 1996;77:1284-1291.
253. Ralston J, Chiriboga L, Nonaka D. MASH1: A useful marker in differentiating pulmonary small cell carcinoma from Merkel cell carcinoma. *Mod Pathol.* 2008;21:1357-1362.
254. Zhu CQ, Shih W, Ling CH, et al. Immunohistochemical markers of prognosis in non-small cell lung cancer: A review and proposal for a multiphase approach to marker evaluation. *J Clin Pathol.* 2006;59:790-800.
255. Olaussen KA, Dunant A, Fouret P, et al. DNA repair by ERCC1 in non-small-cell lung cancer and cisplatin-based adjuvant chemotherapy.[see comment]. *N Engl J Med.* 2006;355:983-991.
256. Simon G, Sharma A, Li X, et al. Feasibility and efficacy of molecular analysis-directed individualized therapy in advanced non-small-cell lung cancer. *J Clin Oncol.* 2007;25: 2741-2746.
257. Clark GM, Zborowski DM, Culbertson JL, et al. Clinical utility of epidermal growth factor receptor expression for selecting patients with advanced non-small cell lung cancer for treatment with erlotinib. *J Thorac Oncol.* 2006;1:837-846.
258. Jeon YK, Sung S-W, Chung J-H, et al. Clinicopathologic features and prognostic implications of epidermal growth factor receptor (EGFR) gene copy number and protein expression in non-small cell lung cancer. *Lung Cancer.* 2006;54:387-398.
259. Tsao M-S, Sakurada A, Cutz J-C, et al. Erlotinib in lung cancer—molecular and clinical predictors of outcome. [see comment][erratum appears in *N Engl J Med.* 2006:355(16):1746]. *N Engl J Med.* 2005;353:133–144.
260. Hirsch FR, Dziadziuszko R, Thatcher N, et al. Epidermal growth factor receptor immunohistochemistry: Comparison of antibodies and cutoff points to predict benefit from gefitinib in a phase 3 placebo-controlled study in advanced nonsmall-cell lung cancer. *Cancer.* 2008;112:1114-1121.
261. Lynch TJ, Bell DW, Sordella R, et al. Activating mutations in the epidermal growth factor receptor underlying responsiveness of non-small-cell lung cancer to gefitinib.[see comment]. *N Engl J Med.* 2004;350:2129-2139.
262. Paez JG, Janne PA, Lee JC, et al. EGFR mutations in lung cancer: Correlation with clinical response to gefitinib therapy.[see comment]. *Science.* 2004;304:1497-1500.
263. Pao W, Miller V, Zakowski M, et al. EGF receptor gene mutations are common in lung cancers from "never smokers" and are associated with sensitivity of tumors to gefitinib and erlotinib. *Proc Natl Acad Sci U S A.* 2004;101:13306-13311.
264. Jackman DM, Yeap BY, Sequist LV, et al. Exon 19 deletion mutations of epidermal growth factor receptor are associated with prolonged survival in non-small cell lung cancer patients treated with gefitinib or erlotinib. *Clin Cancer Res.* 2006;12:3908-3914.
265. Pao W, Ladanyi M. Epidermal growth factor receptor mutation testing in lung cancer: Searching for the ideal method. [comment]. *Clin Cancer Res.* 2007;13:4954-4955.
266. Sequist LV, Joshi VA, Janne PA, et al. Epidermal growth factor receptor mutation testing in the care of lung cancer patients. *Clin Cancer Res.* 2006;12:4403s-4408s.
267. Shih JY, Gow CH, Yu CJ, et al. Epidermal growth factor receptor mutations in needle biopsy/aspiration samples predict response to gefitinib therapy and survival of patients with advanced nonsmall cell lung cancer. [see comment]. *Int J Cancer.* 2006;118:963-969.
268. Shih JY, Gow CH, Yang PC. EGFR mutation conferring primary resistance to gefitinib in non-small-cell lung cancer. *N Engl J Med.* 2005;353:207-208.
269. Bean J, Brennan C, Shih JY, et al. MET amplification occurs with or without T790M mutations in EGFR mutant lung tumors with acquired resistance to gefitinib or erlotinib. *Proc Natl Acad Sci U S A.* 2007;104:20932-20937.
270. Engelman JA, Zejnullahu K, Mitsudomi T, et al. MET amplification leads to gefitinib resistance in lung cancer by activating ERBB3 signaling. *Science.* 2007;316:1039-1043.
271. Ahrendt SA, Decker PA, Alawi EA, et al. Cigarette smoking is strongly associated with mutation of the K-ras gene in patients with primary adenocarcinoma of the lung. *Cancer.* 2001;92:1525-1530.
272. Eberhard DA, Johnson BE, Amler LC, et al. Mutations in the epidermal growth factor receptor and in KRAS are predictive and prognostic indicators in patients with non-small-cell lung cancer treated with chemotherapy alone and in combination with erlotinib.[see comment]. *J Clin Oncol.* 2005;23:5900-5909.
273. Shigematsu H, Gazdar AF. Somatic mutations of epidermal growth factor receptor signaling pathway in lung cancers. *Int J Cancer.* 2006;118:257-262.
274. Cappuzzo F, Hirsch FR, Rossi E, et al. Epidermal growth factor receptor gene and protein and gefitinib sensitivity in non-small-cell lung cancer.[see comment][comment]. *J Natl Cancer Inst.* 2005;97:643-655.
275. Daniele L, Macri L, Schena M, et al. Predicting gefitinib responsiveness in lung cancer by fluorescence in situ hybridization/chromogenic in situ hybridization analysis of EGFR and HER2 in biopsy and cytology specimens. *Mol Cancer Ther.* 2007;6:1223-1229.
276. Gallegos Ruiz MI, Floor K, Vos W, et al. Epidermal growth factor receptor (EGFR) gene copy number detection in non-small-cell lung cancer; a comparison of fluorescence in situ hybridization and chromogenic in situ hybridization. *Histopathology.* 2007;51:631-637.

277. Hirsch FR, Varella-Garcia M, McCoy J, et al. Increased epidermal growth factor receptor gene copy number detected by fluorescence in situ hybridization associates with increased sensitivity to gefitinib in patients with bronchioloalveolar carcinoma subtypes: A Southwest Oncology Group Study. [see comment]. *J Clin Oncol.* 2005;23:6838-6845.
278. Johnson BE, Janne PA. Selecting patients for epidermal growth factor receptor inhibitor treatment: A FISH story or a tale of mutations?[see comment][comment]. *J Clin Oncol.* 2005;23:6813-6816.
279. Hirsch FR, Herbst RS, Olsen C, et al. Increased EGFR gene copy number detected by fluorescent in situ hybridization predicts outcome in non-small-cell lung cancer patients treated with cetuximab and chemotherapy. *J Clin Oncol.* 2008;26:3351-3357.
280. Sholl LM, John Iafrate A, Chou YP, et al. Validation of chromogenic in situ hybridization for detection of EGFR copy number amplification in nonsmall cell lung carcinoma. *Mod Pathol.* 2007;20:1028-1035.
281. Barletta JA, Weir BA, Perner S, Johnson L, Rubin MA, et al. Clinical significance of TTF-1 protein expression and TTF-1 gene amplification in lung adenocarcinomas. *Mod Pathol.* 2008;21:335A.
282. Beasley MB, Castro CY, Garza L, et al. Expression of HIF-1 alpha in pulmonary non-small cell carcinomas and neuroendocrine carcinomas—a tissue microarray analysis of 442 cases. *Mod Pathol.* 2008;21:336A.
283. Beheshti J, Sabo E, Janne PA, et al. TTF-1 positivity is a sensitive predictor of EGFR mutation and treatment response in pulmonary adenocarcinomas, by pathologist interpretation and by image analysis. *Mod Pathol.* 2008;21:336A.
284. Kundu UR, Li W, Tan D, et al. Alpha-methylacyl-co-a-racemase (AMACR) expression is a biomarker of poor prognosis in stage 1 and 2 large cell carcinomas of the lung. *Mod Pathol.* 2008;21:345A.
285. Perner S, Demichelis F, Johnson L, et al. TTF1 amplification defines TTF1 overexpression in lung adenocarcinomas. *Mod Pathol.* 2008;21:349A.
286. Vohra P, Cagle PT, Allen TC, et al. Tissue microarray study of RNA-binding protein IMP3 in primary non-small cell lung cancers: Prediction of survival in early stage squamous cell carcinomas. *Mod Pathol.* 2008;21:352A.
287. Cutz J-C, Tsakaridis TS, Wright J, et al. Immunohistochemistry for phosphorylated EGF receptor predicts survival and phosphorylated ERK predicts tumor response to chemo-radiotherapy in unresectable, locally advanced non-small cell lung cancer patients. *Mod Pathol.* 2008;21:339A.
288. Li QK, Tully E, Askin FB, et al. Overexpression of NRF2 is correlated with elevated p53 levels in pulmonary papillary adenocarcinoma by tissue microarray analysis. *Mod Pathol.* 2008;21:345A.
289. Luu M, Sabo E, Resnick M, et al. Prognostic value of aspartyl (asparaginyl) hydroxylase (AAH) in lung carcinomas: Correlation with survival. *Mod Pathol.* 2008;21:346A.
290. Shahjahan M, Zhai QJ, Allen TC, et al. ProEx C expression in non-small cell lung cancers (NSCLC) is associated with longer patient survival. *Mod Pathol.* 2008;21:350A.
291. Sienko AE, Allen TC, Barrios R, et al. Expression of galectin-4 in non-small cell lung carcinoma (NSCLC) and correlation with survival. *Mod Pathol.* 2008;21:351A.
292. Song J, Tretiakova MS, Salgia R, et al. c-Met expression in pulmonary neuroendocrine tumors. *Mod Pathol.* 2008;21:351A-352A.
293. Haque AK, Singhal N, Allen T, et al. Lack of E-cadherin and Pan-cadherin immunoexpression is associated with metastasis in small cell lung cancer. *Mod Pathol.* 2008;21:342A.
294. Homan SM, Sheehan CE, Ross JS, et al. Downregulation of GADD45a protein expression is associated with advanced tumor stage and decreased survival in squamous cell carcinoma of the lung. *Mod Pathol.* 2008;21:343A.
295. Malik A, Krishnaswamy S, Gong C, et al. RON overexpression and activation in primary and metastatic lung carcinoma. *Mod Pathol.* 2008;21:346A.
296. Lonardo F, Pass HI, Lucas DR. Immunohistochemistry frequently detects c-Kit expression in pulmonary small cell carcinoma and may help select clinical subsets for a novel form of chemotherapy. *Appl Immunohist Mol Morphol.* 2003;11:51-55.
297. Pelosi G, Barisella M, Pasini F, et al. CD117 immunoreactivity in stage I adenocarcinoma and squamous carcinoma of the lung: Relevance to prognosis in a subset of adenocarcinoma patients. *Mod Pathol.* 2004;17:711-721.
298. Casali C, Stefani A, Rossi G, et al. The prognostic role of c-Kit protein expression in resected large cell neuroendocrine carcinoma of the lung. *Ann Thorac Surg.* 2004;77:252-253.
299. Butnor KJ, Burchette JL, Sporn TA, et al. The spectrum of Kit (CD117) immunoreactivity in lung and pleural tumors: A study of 96 cases using a single-source antibody with a review of the literature. *Arch Pathol Lab Med.* 2004;128:538-543.
300. Maddau C, Confortini M, Bisanzi S, et al. Prognostic significance of p53 and Ki-67 antigen expression in surgically treated non-small cell lung cancer: Immunocytochemical detection with imprint cytology. *Am J Clin Pathol.* 2006;125:425-431.
301. Kobayashi S, Kubo H, Suzuki T, et al. Endogenous secretory receptor for advanced glycation end products in non-small cell lung carcinoma. *Am J Respir Crit Care Med.* 2007;175:184-189.
302. Allen TC, Granville LA, Cagle PT, et al. Expression of glutathione S-transferase p and glutathione synthase correlates with survival in early stage non-small cell carcinomas of the lung. *Hum Pathol.* 2007;38:220-227.
303. Lee Y-C, Wu C-T, Kuo S-W, et al. Significance of extranodal extension of regional lymph nodes in surgically resected non-small cell lung cancer. *Chest.* 2007;131:993-999.
304. Fukuoka J, Dracheva T, Shih JH, et al. Desmoglein 3 as a prognostic factor in lung cancer. *Hum Pathol.* 2007;38:276-283.
305. Aviel-Ronen S, Lau SK, Pintilie M, et al. Glypican-3 is overexpressed in lung squamous cell carcinoma, but not in adenocarcinoma. *Mod Pathol.* 2008;21:817-825.
306. LaPoint RJA, Bourne PA, Wang HL, et al. Coexpression of c-kit and bcl-2 in small cell carcinoma and large cell neuroendocrine carcinoma of the lung. *Appl Immunohistochem Mol Morphol.* 2007;15:401-406.
307. Meyronet D, Massoma P, Thivolet F, et al. Extensive expression of collapsing response mediator protein 5 (CRMP5) is a specific marker of high-grade neuroendocrine carcinoma. *Am J Surg Pathol.* 2008;32:1699-1708.
308. Yousem SA, Nikiforova M, Nikiforov Y. The histopathology of BRAF-V600E-mutated lung adenocarcinoma. *Am J Surg Pathol.* 2008;32:1317-1321.
309. Hammar SP. Pleural diseases. In: Dail DH, Hammar SP, Colby TV, eds. *Pulmonary Pathology Tumors.* New York: Springer-Verlag; 1995:405-530.
310. Davies J. *Human Developmental Anatomy.* New York: Roland Press; 1963:51-52.
311. Bolen JW, Hammar SP, McNutt MA. Reactive and neoplastic serosal tissue: A light-microscopic, ultrastructural and immunocytochemical study. *Am J Surg Pathol.* 1986;10:34-47.
312. Selikoff IJ, Seidman H. Asbestos-associated deaths among insulation workers in the United States and Canada, 1967-1987. *Ann NY Acad Sci.* 1991;643:1-14.
313. Battifora H, McCaughey WTE. *Tumors of the serosal membranes.* Washington DC: Armed Forces Institute of Pathology; 1995:17-88.
314. Butnor KJ, Sporn TA, Hammar SP, et al. Well-differentiated papillary mesothelioma. *Am J Surg Pathol.* 2001;25:1304-1309.
315. Galateau-Salle F, Vignaud J, Burke L, et al. Well-differentiated papillary mesothelioma of the pleura: A series of 24 cases. *Am J Surg Pathol.* 2004;28:534-540.
316. Henderson DW, Shilkin KB, Whitaker D. Reactive mesothelial hyperplasia vs. mesothelioma, including mesothelioma in situ: A brief review. *Am J Clin Pathol.* 1998;110:397-404.
317. US-Canadian Mesothelioma Reference Panel, Churg A, Colby TV, Cagle P, Corson J, Gibbs AR, Gilks B, Grimes M, Hammar S, Roggli V, Travis WD. The separation of benign and malignant mesothelial proliferations. *Am J Surg Pathol.* 2000;24:1183-1200.
318. Henderson DW, Comin CE, Hammar SP, et al. Malignant mesothelioma of the pleura: Current surgical pathology. In: Corrin B, ed. *Pathology of Lung Tumors.* New York: Churchill Livingstone; 1997:241-280.
319. Ordonez NG. The immunohistochemical diagnosis of epithelial mesothelioma. *Hum Pathol.* 1999;30:313-323.

320. Blobel GA, Moll R, Franke WW, et al. The intermediate filament cytoskeleton of malignant mesothelioma and its diagnostic significance. *Am J Pathol.* 1985;121:235-247.
321. Blobel GA, Moll R, Franke WW, et al. Cytokeratins in normal lung and lung carcinomas. I. Adenocarcinomas, squamous cell carcinomas and cultured cell lines. *Virchows Arch Cell Pathol.* 1984;45:407-429.
322. Moll R, Dhovailly D, Sun TT. Expression of keratin 5 as a distinctive feature of epithelial and biphasic mesotheliomas: An immunohistochemical study using monoclonal antibody AE14. *Virchows Archiv B Cell Pathol.* 1989;58:129-145.
323. Clover J, Oates J, Edwards C. Anti-cytokeratin 5/6: A positive marker for epithelial mesothelioma. *Histopathology.* 1997;31:140-143.
324. Kahn HJ, Thorner PS, Yeager H, et al. Immunohistochemical localization of pre-keratin filaments in benign and malignant cells in effusions: Comparison with intermediate filament distribution by electron microscopy. *Am J Pathol.* 1982;109:206-214.
325. Kahn HJ, Thorner PS, Yeger H, et al. Distinct keratin patterns demonstrated by immunoperoxidase staining of adenocarcinomas, carcinoids and mesotheliomas using polyclonal and monoclonal keratin antibodies. *Am J Clin Pathol.* 1986;86:566-574.
326. Montag AG, Pinkus GS, Corson JM. Keratin protein reactivity immunoreactivity of sarcomatoid and mixed types of diffuse malignant mesotheliomas: An immunoperoxidase study of 30 cases. *Hum Pathol.* 1988;19:336-342.
327. Battifora H. The pleura. In: Sternberg SS, ed. *Diagnostic Surgical Pathology*, Volume I. New York: Raven Press; 1989:829-855.
328. Roggli VL, Kolbeck J, Sanfilippo F, et al. Pathology of human mesothelioma: Etiologic and diagnostic considerations. *Pathol Annu.* 1987;22(pt 2):91-131.
329. Al-Izzi M, Thurlow NP, Corrin B. Pleural mesothelioma of connective tissue type, localized fibrous tumour of the pleura and reactive submesothelial hyperplasia: An immunohistochemical comparison. *J Pathol.* 1989;157:41-44.
330. Mayall FG, Goddard H, Gibbs AR. Intermediate filament expression in mesotheliomas: leiomyoid mesotheliomas are not uncommon. *Histopathol.* 1992;21:453-457.
331. Yousem SA, Hochholzer L. Malignant mesotheliomas with osseous and cartilaginous differentiation. *Arch Pathol Lab Invest.* 1987;111:62-66.
332. Wirth PR, Legler J, Wright GL. Immunohistochemical evaluation of seven monoclonal antibodies for differentiation of pleural mesothelioma from lung adenocarcinoma. *Cancer.* 1991;67:655-662.
333. Carter D, Otis CN. Three types of spindle cell tumors of pleura: Fibroma, sarcoma and sarcomatoid mesothelioma. *Am J Surg Pathol.* 1988;12:747-753.
334. Azumi N, Battifora H, Carlson G, et al. Sarcomatous (spindle-cell) mesothelioma of pleura: Immunohistochemical study. *Lab Invest.* 1989;60:4A.
335. Lucas DR, Pass HI, Madan SK, et al. Sarcomatoid mesothelioma and its histological mimics: A comparative immunohistochemical study. *Histopathology.* 2003;42:270-279.
336. Attanoos RL, Dojcinov SD, Webb R, Gibbs AR. Anti-mesothelial markers in sarcomatoid mesothelioma and other spindle cell neoplasms. *Histopathology.* 2000;37:224-231.
337. McNutt MA, Bolen JW, Gown AM, et al. Coexpression of intermediate filaments in human epithelial neoplasms. *Ultrastruct Pathol.* 1985;9:31-43.
338. Azumi N, Battifora H. The distribution of vimentin and keratin in epithelial and non-epithelial neoplasms. A comprehensive study on formalin and alcohol-fixed tumors. *Am J Clin Pathol.* 1987;88:286-296.
339. Raymond WA, Leong ASY. Vimentin—a new prognostic marker in breast carcinoma. *J Pathol.* 1989;158:107-114.
340. Churg A. Immunohistochemical staining for vimentin and keratin in malignant mesothelioma. *Am J Surg Pathol.* 1985;9:360-365.
341. Jasani B, Edwards RE, Thomas ND, et al. The use of vimentin antibodies in the diagnosis of malignant mesothelioma. *Virch Arch A Pathol Anat.* 1985;406:441-448.
342. Mullink H, Henzen-Logmans SC, Alons-van Kordelaan JJM, et al. Simultaneous immunoenzyme staining of vimentin and cytokeratins with monoclonal antibodies as an aid in the differential diagnosis of malignant mesothelioma from pulmonary adenocarcinoma. *Virch Arch B Pathol Anat.* 1986;42:55-65.
343. Andersen C, Blumcke I, Celio MR. Calcium-binding proteins: Selective markers of nerve cells. *Cell Tissue Res.* 1993;271:181-208.
344. Schwaller B, Buchwald P, Blucke I, et al. Characterization of a polyclonal antiserum against the purified human recombinant calcium binding protein calretinin. *Cell Calcium.* 1993;14:639-648.
345. Gotzos V, Schwaller B, Hertzel N, et al. Expression of the calcium binding protein calretinin in Wi Dr cells and its correlation to their cell cycle. *Exp Cell Res.* 1992;202:292-302.
346. Doglioni C, Dei Tos AP, Laurino L, et al. Calretinin: A novel immunocytochemical marker for mesothelioma. *Am J Surg Pathol.* 1996;20:1037-1046.
347. Barberis MCP, Faleri M, Veronese S, et al. Calretinin: A selective marker of normal and neoplastic mesothelial cells in serous effusions. *Acta Cytol.* 1997;41:1757-1761.
348. Leers MPG, Aarts MMJ, Theunissen PHMH. E-cadherin and calretinin: A useful combination of immunochemical markers for differentiation between mesothelioma and metastatic adenocarcinoma. *Histopathol.* 1998;32:209-216.
349. Ordonez NG. Value of calretinin immunostaining in differentiating epithelial mesothelioma from lung adenocarcinoma. *Mod Pathol.* 1998;10:929-933.
350. Chenard-Neu MP, Kabou A, Mechine A, et al. Immunohistochemistry in the differential diagnosis of mesothelioma and adenocarcinoma: evaluation of 5 new and 6 traditional antibodies. *Ann Pathol.* 1998;18:460-465.
351. Cury PM, Butcher DN, Fisher C, et al. Value of mesothelium-associated antibodies thrombomodulin, cytokeratin 5/6, calretinin and CD44H in distinguishing epithelioid mesothelioma from adenocarcinoma metastatic to the pleura. *Mod Pathol.* 2000;13:107-112.
352. Oates J, Edwards C. HBME-1, MOC-31, WT1 and calretinin: An assessment of recently described markers for mesothelioma and adenocarcinoma. *Histopathol.* 2000;36:341-347.
353. Chieng DC, Yee H, Schaefer D, et al. Calretinin staining pattern aids in the differentiation of mesothelioma from adenocarcinoma in serous effusions. *Cancer.* 2000;25:194-200.
354. O'Hara CJ, Corson JM, Pinkus GS, et al. ME1: A monoclonal antibody that distinguishes epithelial-type mesothelioma from pulmonary adenocarcinoma and extra-pulmonary malignancies. *Am J Pathol.* 1990;136:421-428.
355. Sheibani K, Esteban JM, Bailey A, et al. Immunopathologic and molecular studies as an aid to the diagnosis of malignant mesothelioma. *Hum Pathol.* 1992;23:107-116.
356. Hammar SP, Bolen JW, Bockus D, et al. Ultrastructural and immunohistochemical features of common lung tumors: An overview. *Ultrastruct Pathol.* 1985;9:283-318.
357. Walz R, Koch HK. Malignant pleural mesotheliomas: Some aspects of epidemiology, differential diagnosis and prognosis. Histological and immunohistochemical evaluation and follow-up of mesotheliomas diagnosed from 1964 to January 1985. *Pathol Res Pract.* 1990;186:124-134.
358. Wick MR, Loy T, Mills SE, et al. Malignant epithelioid pleural mesothelioma versus peripheral pulmonary adenocarcinoma: A histochemical, ultrastructural and immunohistologic study of 103 cases. *Hum Pathol.* 1990;21:759-766.
359. Henderson DW, Shilkin KB, Whitaker D, et al. The pathology of mesothelioma, including immunohistology and ultrastructure. In: Henderson DW, Shilkin KB, Langlois SL, Whitaker D, eds. *Malignant Mesothelioma.* New York: Hemisphere; 1992: 69-139.
360. Fink L, Collins CL, Schaefer R, et al. Thrombomodulin expression can be used to differentiate between mesotheliomas and adenocarcinomas. *Lab Invest.* 1992;66:113A.
361. Collins CL, Ordonez NG, Schaefer R, et al. Thrombomodulin expression and pulmonary adenocarcinoma. *Am J Pathol.* 1992;141:827-833.
362. Brown RW, Clark GM, Tandon AK, et al. Multiple-marker immunohistochemical phenotypes distinguishing malignant pleural mesothelioma from pulmonary adenocarcinoma. *Hum Pathol.* 1993;24:347-354.
363. Ascoli V, Scalzo CC, Taccogna S, et al. The diagnostic value of thrombomodulin immunolocalization in serous effusions. *Arch Pathol Lab Med.* 1995;119:1136-1140.

364. Geiger B, Ayalon O. Cadherins. *Annu Rev Cell Biol.* 1992;8: 307-332.
365. Takeichi M. Cadherin cell adhesion receptors as a morphogenetic regulator. *Science.* 1991;251:1451-1455.
366. Hatta K, Takagi S, Fujisawa H, et al. Spatial and temporal expression pattern of N-cadherin cell adhesion molecules correlated with morphogenetic processes of chicken embryos. *Dev Biol.* 1987;120:215-227.
367. Peralta-Soler A, Knudsen KA, Jaurand MC, et al. The differential expression of N-cadherin, E-cadherin distinguished pleural mesotheliomas from lung adenocarcinomas. *Hum Pathol.* 1995;26:1363-1369.
368. Han AC, Peralta-Soler A, Knudsen KA, et al. Differential expression of N-cadherin in pleural mesotheliomas and E-cadherin in lung adenocarcinomas in formalin-fixed, paraffin-embedded tissues. *Hum Pathol.* 1997;28:641-645.
369. Ordonez NG. Value of E-cadherin and N-cadherin immunostaining in the diagnosis of mesothelioma. *Hum Pathol.* 2003;34:749-755.
370. Amin KM, Litzky LA, Smythe WR, et al. Wilms' tumor 1 susceptibility (WT1) gene products are selectively expressed in malignant mesothelioma. *Am J Pathol.* 1995;146:344-356.
371. Kumar-Singh S, Segers K, Rodeck O, et al. WT1 mutation in malignant mesothelioma and WT1 immunoreactivity in relation to p53 growth factor expression, cell-type transition and prognosis. *J Pathol.* 1997;181:67-74.
372. Walker C, Rutlen F, Yuan X, et al. Wilms' tumor suppressor gene expression in rat and human mesothelioma. *Cancer Res.* 1994;54:1301-1306.
373. Ordonez NG. Application of mesothelin immunostaining in tumor diagnosis. *Am J Surg Pathol.* 2003;27:1418-1428.
374. Chu AY, Litzky LA, Pasha TL, et al. Utility of D2-40, a novel mesothelial marker, in the diagnosis of malignant mesothelioma. *Mod Pathol.* 2005;18:105-110.
375. Comin CE, Dini S, Novelli L, et al. h-Caldesmon, a useful positive marker in the diagnosis of pleural malignant mesothelioma, epithelioid type. *Am J Surg Pathol.* 2006;30:463-469.
376. Shivley JE, Beatty JD. CEA-related antigens: Molecular biology and clinical significance. *CRC Crit Rev Oncol Hematol.* 1985;2:355-399.
377. Thompson J, Grunert F, Zimmermann W. Carcinoembryonic antigen gene family: Molecular biology and clinical perspectives. *J Clin Labor Anal.* 1991;5:344-366.
378. Hammarstrom S, Khan WN, Teglund S, et al. The carcinoembryonic antigen family. In: Van Regenmortel MHV, ed. *Structure of Antigens.* Boca Raton: CRC Press; 1993:341-376.
379. Hammarstrom S, Olsen A, Teglund S, et al. The nature and expression of the human CEA family. In: Stanners C, ed. *Cell Adhesion and Clinical Perspectives..* Amsterdam: Harwood Academic Publishers; 1997:1-30.
380. Hammarstrom S. The carcinoembryonic antigen (CEA) family: Structures, suggested functions and expression in normal and malignant tissues. *Cancer Biol.* 1999;9:67-81.
381. Wang N-S, Huang S-N, Gold P. Absence of carcinoembryonic antigen-like material in mesothelioma: An immunohistochemical differentiation from other lung cancers. *Cancer.* 1979;44:437-943.
382. Whitaker D, Shilkin KB. Carcinoembryonic antigen in the tissue diagnosis of malignant mesothelioma. *Lancet.* 1981;1:1369-1370.
383. Whitaker D, Sterret GF, Shilkin KB. Detection of tissue CEA-like substance as an aid in the differential diagnosis of malignant mesothelioma. *Pathology.* 1982;14:255-258.
384. Sheibani K, Battifora H. Leu-M1 positivity is not specific for Hodgkin's disease. *Am J Clin Pathol.* 1985;84:682.
385. Sheibani K, Battifora H, Burke JS, et al. Leu-M1 in human neoplasms: An immunohistologic study of 400 cases. *Am J Surg Pathol.* 1986;10:227-236.
386. Sheibani K, Battifora H, Burke J. Antigenic phenotype of malignant mesotheliomas and pulmonary adenocarcinomas: An immunohistologic analysis demonstrating the value of Leu-M1 antigen. *Am J Pathol.* 1986;123:212-219.
387. Sheibani K, Azumi N, Battifora H. Further evidence demonstrating the value of LeuM1 antigen in differential diagnosis of malignant mesothelioma and adenocarcinoma: An immunohistologic evaluation of 395 cases. *Lab Invest.* 1988;58:84A.
388. Otis CN, Carter O, Cole S, et al. Immunohistochemical evaluation of pleural mesothelioma and pulmonary adenocarcinoma. *Am J Surg Pathol.* 1987;11:445-456.
389. Szpak CA, Johnston WW, Roggli V, et al. The diagnostic distinction between malignant mesothelioma and adenocarcinoma of the lung as defined by a monoclonal antibody (B72.3). *Am J Pathol.* 1986;122:252-260.
390. Ordonez NG. The immunohistochemical diagnosis of mesothelioma: Differentiation of mesothelioma and lung adenocarcinoma. *Am J Surg Pathol.* 1989;13:276-291.
391. Bollinger DJ, Wick MR, Dehner LP, et al. Peritoneal malignant mesothelioma versus serous papillary adenocarcinoma: A histochemical and immunohistochemical comparison. *Am J Surg Pathol.* 1989;13:659-670.
392. Latza V, Niedobitek G, Schwarting R, et al. Ber-EP4: New monoclonal antibody which distinguishes epithelia from mesothelia. *J Clin Pathol.* 1990;43:213-219.
393. Sheibani K, Shin SS, Kezirian J, et al. Ber-EP4 antibody as a discriminant in the differential diagnosis of malignant mesothelioma versus adenocarcinoma. *Am J Surg Pathol.* 1991;15:779-784.
394. Gaffey MJ, Mills SE, Swanson PE, et al. Immunoreactivity for Ber-EP4 in adenocarcinomas, adenomatoid tumors and malignant mesotheliomas. *Am J Surg Pathol.* 1992;16:593-599.
395. Souhami RL, Beverly PCL, Bobrow LG. Antigens of small cell lung cancer. First International Workshop. *Lancet.* 1987;2:325-326.
396. Riutenbeek T, Gouw ASH, Poppema S. Immunocytology of body cavity fluids: MOC-31, a monoclonal antibody discriminating between mesothelial and epithelial cells. *Arch Pathol Lab Med.* 1994;118:265-269.
397. DeLeij L, Broers J, Ramaekers F, et al. Monoclonal antibodies in clinical and experimental pathology of lung cancer. In: Roiter DJ, Fleuren GJ, Warner SO, eds. *Applications of Monoclonal Antibodies in Tumor Pathology.* Dordrecht: Martinus Nijhoff; 1987:191-210.
398. Delahaye M, Hoogsteden HC, van der Kwast TH. Immunocytochemistry of malignant mesothelioma: OV632 as a marker of malignant mesothelioma. *J Pathol.* 1991;165:137-143.
399. Ordonez NG. Value of MOC-31 monoclonal antibody in differentiating epithelial pleural mesothelioma from lung adenocarcinoma. *Hum Pathol.* 1998;29:166-169.
400. Jordon D, Jagirdar J, Kaneko M. Blood group antigens Lewis x and Lewis y in the diagnostic discrimination of malignant mesothelioma versus adenocarcinoma. *Am J Pathol.* 1989;135:931-937.
401. Riera JR, Astengo-Osuna C, Longmate JA, et al. The immunohistochemical diagnostic panel for epithelial mesothelioma. A reevaluation after heat-induced epitope retrieval. *Am J Surg Pathol.* 1997;21:1409-1419.
402. Kinsella AR, Green B, Lepts GC, et al. The role of cell-cell adhesion molecule E-cadherin in large bowel tumour cell invasion and metastasis. *Br J Cancer.* 1993;67:904-909.
403. Williams CL, Hayes VY, Hummel AM, et al. Regulation of E-cadherin mediated adhesion by muscarinic acetylcholine receptor in small cell lung carcinoma. *J Cell Biol.* 1993;121:643-654.
404. Kawai T, Suzuki M, Torikata C, et al. Expression of blood group-related antigens and Helix pomatia agglutinin in malignant pleural mesothelioma and pulmonary adenocarcinoma. *Hum Pathol.* 1991;22:118-124.
405. Mayall FG, Goddard H, Gibbs AR. p53 immunostaining in the distinction between benign and malignant mesothelial proliferations using formalin-fixed paraffin sections. *J Pathol.* 1992;168:377-381.
406. Ramael M, Lemmens G, Eerdekens C, et al. Immunoreactivity for p53 protein in malignant mesothelioma and non-neoplastic mesothelium. *J Pathol.* 1992;168:371-375.
407. Mayall FG, Goddard H, Gibbs AR. The frequency of p53 immunostaining in asbestos-associated mesotheliomas. *Histopathology.* 1993;22:383-386.
408. Hurlimann J. Desmin and neural marker expression in mesothelial cells and mesotheliomas. *Hum Pathol.* 1994;25:753-757.
409. Azumi N, Underhill CB, Kagan E, et al. A novel biotinylated probe specific for hyaluronate. *Am J Surg Pathol.* 1992;16:116-121.
410. Thylen A, Wallin J, Martensson G. Hyaluronan in serum as an indicator of progressive disease in hyaluronan-producing malignant mesothelioma. *Cancer.* 1999;86:2000-2005.

411. Martensson G, Thylen A, Lindquist U, et al. The sensitivity of hyaluronan analysis of pleural fluid from patients with malignant mesothelioma and a comparison of different methods. *Cancer*. 1994;73:1406-1410.
412. Thylen A, Levin-Jacobsen AM, Hjerpe A, et al. Immunohistochemical differences between hyaluronan and non-hyaluronan-producing malignant mesothelioma. *Eur Respir J*. 1997;10: 404-408.
413. Kabawat SE, Bast RC, Bhan AK, et al. Immunopathologic characterization of a monoclonal antibody that recognizes common surface antigens of human ovarian tumors of serous, endometrioid and clear cell types. *Am J Clin Pathol*. 1983;79:98-104.
414. Kabawat SE, Bast RC, Bhan AK, et al. Tissue distribution of celomic epithelium related antigen recognized by monoclonal antibody OC-125. *Int J Gynecol Pathol*. 1983;2:275-285.
415. Dabbs DJ, Geisinger KR. Selective application of immunohistochemistry in gynecological neoplasms. *Pathol Annu*. 1993;28(pt 1):329-353.
416. Bast RC, Freeney M, Lazarus H, et al. Reactivity of a monoclonal antibody with human ovarian carcinoma. *J Clin Invest*. 1981;68:1331-1337.
417. Koelma IA, Nap M, Rodenburg CJ, et al. The value of tumor marker CA-125 in surgical pathology. *Histopathology*. 1987;11:287-294.
418. Nanbu Y, Fujii S, Konishi I, et al. Immunohistochemical localization of CA-130 in fetal tissue and in normal and neoplastic tissues of the female genital tract. *Asia Oceania J Obstet Gynecol*. 1990;16:379-387.
419. Tamura S, Yamaguchi K, Terada M, et al. Immunohistochemical analysis of CA19-9, SLX and CA-125 in adenoidcystic carcinoma of trachea and bronchus. *Nippon Kyobu Shikkan Gakkai Zasshi*. 1992;3:407-411.
420. Zhou J, Iwasa Y, Konishi I, et al. Papillary serous carcinoma of the peritoneum in women: A clinicopathologic and immunohistochemical study. *Cancer*. 1995;76:429-436.
421. Nouwen EJ, Pollet DE, Eerdekens MW, et al. Immunohistochemical localization of placental alkaline phosphatase, carcinoembryonic antigen and cancer antigen 125 in normal and neoplastic human lung. *Cancer Res*. 1986;46:866-876.
422. Bateman AC, al-Talib RK, Newman T, et al. Immunohistochemical phenotype of malignant mesothelioma: Predictive value of CA-125 and HBME-1 expression. *Histopathology*. 1997;30:49-56.
423. Nap M. Immunohistochemistry of CA-125: Unusual expression in normal tissues, distribution in the human fetus and questions around its application in diagnostic pathology. *Int J Biol Markers*. 1998;13:210-215.
424. O'Brien TJ, Raymond LM, Bannon GA, et al. New monoclonal antibodies identify the glycoprotein carrying the CA-125 epitope. *Am J Obst Gynecol*. 1991;61:1857-1864.
425. Okamoto H, Matsuno Y, Noguchi M, et al. Malignant pleural mesothelioma producing chorionic gonadotropin: Report of two cases. *Am J Surg Pathol*. 1992;16:969-974.
426. McAuley P, Asa SL, Chiv B, et al. Parathyroid hormone-like peptide in normal and neoplastic mesothelial cells. *Cancer*. 1990;66:1975-1979.
427. Tateyama H, Eimoto T, Tada T, et al. Immunoreactivity of a new CD5 antibody with normal epithelium and malignant tumors including thymic carcinoma. *Am J Clin Pathol*. 1999;111:235-240.
428. Yaziji H, Battifora H, Barry TS, et al. Evaluation of 12 antibodies for distinguishing epithelioid mesothelioma from adenocarcinoma: Identification of a three-body immunohistochemical panel with maximal sensitivity and specificity. *Mod Pathol*. 2006;19:514-523.
429. Marchevsky AM. Application of immunohistochemistry to the diagnosis of malignant mesothelioma. *Arch Pathol Lab Med*. 2008;132:397-401.
430. Husain AN, Colby TV, Ordonez NG, et al. Guidelines for pathologic diagnosis of malignant mesothelioma: A consensus statement from the International Mesothelioma Interest Group. *Arch Pathol Lab Med* [in press].
431. Chirieac L, Pinkus G, Pinkus J. Sarcomatoid malignant mesothelioma: Immunohistochemical characteristics of 24 cases. *Mod Pathol*. 2006;19:305A:Abstract 1422.
432. Ordonez NG. D2-40 and podoplanin are highly specific and sensitive immunohistochemical markers of epithelioid malignant mesothelioma. *Hum Pathol*. 2005;36:372-380.
433. Hinterberger M, Reineke T, Storz M, et al. D2-40 and calretinin: A tissue microarray analysis of 341 malignant mesotheliomas with emphasis on sarcomatoid differentiation. *Mod Pathol*. 2007;20:248-255.
434. Klebe S, Mahar A, Henderson DW, et al. Malignant mesothelioma with heterologous elements: Clinicopathological correlation of 27 cases and literature review. *Mod Pathol*. 2008;21:1084-1094.
435. Krishna J, Haqqani MT. Liposarcomatous differentiation in diffuse pleural mesothelioma. *Thorax*. 1993;48:409-410.
436. Hammar SP, Bockus D, Remington F. Metastatic tumors of unknown origin: An ultrastructural analysis of 265 cases. *Ultrastruct Pathol*. 1987;11:209-250.
437. Gaber AO, Rice P, Eaton C, et al. Metastatic malignant disease of unknown origin. *Am J Surg Pathol*. 1983;145:493-497.
438. Crotty TB, Myers JL, Katzenstein AL, et al. Localized malignant mesothelioma: A clinicopathologic and flow cytometric study. *Am J Surg Pathol*. 1994;18:357-363.
439. Allen TC, Cagle PT, Churg AM, et al. Localized malignant mesothelioma. *Am J Surg Pathol*. 2005;29:866-873.
440. Hammar SP, Henderson DW, Klebe S, et al. Neoplasms of the pleura. In: Tomashefski JF, ed. *Dail and Hammar's Pulmonary Pathology*. 3rd ed. New York: Springer; 2008:558-734.
441. Attanoos RL, Griffin A, Gibbs AR, et al. The use of immunohistochemistry in distinguishing reactive from neoplastic mesothelium: A novel use for desmin and comparative evaluation with epithelial membrane antigen, p53, platelet-derived growth factor-receptor, P-glycoprotein and Bcl-2. *Histopathology*. 2003;43:231-238.
442. Wu M, Sun Y, Li G, et al. Immunohistochemical detection of XIAP in mesothelium and mesothelial lesions. *Am J Clin Pathol*. 2007;128:783-787.
443. Kato Y, Tsuta K, Ski K, et al. Immunohistochemical detection of GLUT-1 can discriminate between reactive mesothelium and malignant mesothelioma. *Mod Pathol*. 2007;20:215-220.
444. Acurio A, Arif Q, Gattuso P, et al. Value of immunohistochemical markers in differentiating benign from malignant mesothelial lesions. *Mod Pathol*. 2008;21:334A.
445. Briselli M, Mark EJ, Dickersin GR. Solitary fibrous tumors of the pleura: Eight new cases and review of 360 cases in the literature. *Cancer*. 1981;47:2678-2689.
446. Doucet J, Dardick I, Srigley JR, et al. Localized fibrous tumour of serosal surfaces. *Virch Arch Pathol Anat*. 1986;409:349-363.
447. England DM, Hochholzer L, McCarthy MJ. Localized benign and malignant fibrous tumors of the pleura. A clinicopathologic review of 223 cases. *Am J Surg Pathol*. 1989;13:640-658.
448. van de Rijn M, Lombard CM, Rouse RV. Expression of CD34 by solitary fibrous tumors of the pleura, mediastinum and lung. *Am J Surg Pathol*. 1994;18:814-820.
449. Flint A, Weiss SW. CD-34 and keratin expression distinguishes solitary fibrous tumor (fibrous mesothelioma) of pleura from desmoplastic mesothelioma. *Hum Pathol*. 1995;26:428-431.
450. Hasegawa T, Matsuno Y, Shimoda T, et al. Frequent expression of bcl-2 protein in solitary fibrous tumors. *Jpn J Clin Oncol*. 1998;28:86-91.
451. Schirosi L, Lantuejoul S, Cavazza A, et al. Pleuro-pulmonary solitary fibrous tumors: A clinicopathologic, immunohistochemical, and molecular study of 88 cases confirming the prognostic value of de Perrot staging system and p53 expression, and evaluating the role of c-kit, BRAF, PDGFRs (alpha/beta), c-met, and EGFR. *Am J Surg Pathol*. 2008;32:1627-1642.
452. de Perrot M, Fischer S, Bründler MA, et al. Solitary fibrous tumors of the pleura. *Ann Thorac Surg*. 2002;74:285-293.
453. Babolini G, Blasi A. The pleural form of primary cancer of the lung. *Dis of Chest*. 1956;29:314-323.
454. Harwood TR, Gracey DR, Yokoo H. Pseudomesotheliomatous carcinoma of the lung. *Am J Clin Pathol*. 1976;65:159-167.
455. Koss M, Travis W, Moran C, et al. Pseudomesotheliomatous adenocarcinoma: A reappraisal. *Semin Diag Pathol*. 1992;9:117-123.
456. Hartman C-A, Schutze H. Mesothelioma-like tumors of the pleura: A review of 72 cases. *Cancer Res Clin Oncol*. 1994;120:331-347.

457. Koss MN, Fleming M, Przygodzki RM, et al. Adenocarcinoma simulating mesothelioma: A clinicopathologic and immunohistochemical study of 29 cases. *Ann Diagn Pathol.* 1998;2:93-102.
458. Robb JA, Hammar SP, Yokoo H. Pseudomesotheliomatous carcinoma of lung. *Lab Invest.* 1993;68:134A.
459. Attanoos RL, Gibbs AR. "Pseudomesotheliomatous" carcinomas of the pleura: A 10-year analysis of cases from the Environmental Lung Disease Research Group. *Cardiff Histopathol.* 2003;43:444-452.
460. Battifora H. Epithelioid hemangioendothelioma imitating mesothelioma. *Appl Immunohistochem.* 1993;1:220-221.
461. Lin BT-Y, Colby T, Gown AM, et al. Malignant vascular tumors of the serous membranes mimicking mesothelioma: A report of 14 cases. *Am J Surg Pathol.* 1996;20:1431-1439.
462. Gray MH, Rosenberg AE, Dickersin GR, et al. Cytokeratin expression in epithelioid vascular neoplasms. *Hum Pathol.* 1990;21:212-217.
463. Pinkard NB, Wilson RW, Lawless N, et al. Calcifying fibrous pseudotumor of pleura: A report of three cases of a newly described entity involving the pleura. *Am J Clin Pathol.* 1996;105:189-194.
464. Wilson RW, Galateau-Salle F, Moran CA. Desmoid tumors of the pleura: A clinicopathologic mimic of localized fibrous tumor. *Mod Pathol.* 1999;12:9-14.
465. Andino L, Cagle PT, Murer B, et al. Pleuropulmonary desmoids tumors: Immunohistochemical comparison with solitary fibrous tumors and assessment of β-catenin and cyclin D1 expression. *Arch Pathol Lab Med.* 2006;130:1503-1509.
466. Moran CA, Travis WD, Rosada-de-Christenson M, et al. Thymomas presenting as pleural tumors: Report of eight cases. *Am J Surg Pathol.* 1992;16:138-144.
467. Payne Jr CB, Morningstar WA, Chester EH. Thymoma of the pleura masquerading as diffuse mesothelioma. *Am Rev Respir Dis.* 1966;94:441-446.
468. Honma K, Shimada K. Metastasizing ectopic thymoma arising in the right thoracic cavity and mimicking diffuse pleural mesothelioma: An autopsy study of a case with review of the literature. *Wien Klin Wschr.* 1986;98:14-20.
469. Shih D, Wang J, Tseng H, et al. Primary pleural thymoma. *Arch Pathol Lab Med.* 1997;121:79-82.
470. Gaertner E, Zeren H, Fleming MV, et al. Biphasic synovial sarcomas arising in the pleural cavity: A clinicopathologic study of five cases. *Am J Surg Pathol.* 1996;20:36-45.
471. Nicholson AG, Goldstraw P, Fischer C. Synovial sarcoma of the pleura and its differentiation from other primary pleural tumors: A clinicopathological and immunohistochemical review of three cases. *Histopathol.* 1998;33:508-513.
472. Colwell AS, D'Cunha J, Vargas SO, et al. Synovial sarcoma of the pleura: A clinical and pathologic study of three cases. *J Thorac Cardiovasc Surg.* 2002;124:828-832.
473. Yano M, Toyooka S, Tsukuda K, et al. SYT-SSX fusion genes in synovial sarcoma of the thorax. *Lung Cancer.* 2004;44:391-397.
474. Ordonez NG, Mahfouz SM, Mackay B. Synovial sarcoma: An immunohistochemical and ultrastructural study. *Hum Pathol.* 1990;21:733-749.
475. Litzky LA. Pulmonary sarcomatous tumors. *Arch Pathol Lab Med.* 2008;132:1104-1117.
476. Hachitanda Y, Aoyama C, Sato JK, et al. Pleuropulmonary blastoma in childhood. A tumor of divergent differentiation. *Am J Surg Pathol.* 1993;17:382-391.
477. Priest JR, McDermott MB, Bhatia S, et al. Pleuropulmonary blastoma: A clinicopathologic study of 50 cases. *Cancer.* 1997;80:147-161.
478. Hill DA, Sadeghi S, Schultz MZ, et al. Pleuropulmonary blastoma in an adult: An initial case report. *Cancer.* 1999;85:2368-2374.
479. Celikoglu F, Teirstein AS, Krellenstein DJ, et al. Pleural effusion in non-Hodgkin's lymphoma. *Chest.* 1992;101:1357-1360.
480. Vega F, Padula A, Valbuena JR, et al. Lymphomas involving the pleura: A clinicopathologic study of 34 cases diagnosed by pleural biopsy. *Arch Pathol Lab Med.* 2006;130:1497-1502.
481. Fetsch PA, Abati A, Hijazi YM. Utility of the antibodies CA-19-9, HBME-1 and thrombomodulin in the diagnosis of malignant mesothelioma and adenocarcinoma in cytology. *Cancer.* 1998;84:101-108.
482. Khoor A, Whitsett JA, Stahlman MT, et al. Utility of surfactant protein B precursor and thyroid transcription factor-1 in differentiating adenocarcinoma of the lung from malignant mesothelioma. *Hum Pathol.* 1999;30:695-700.
483. Curry PM, Butcher DN, Fisher C, et al. Value of the mesothelium associated antibodies thrombomodulin, cytokeratin 5/6, calretinin and CD44H in distinguishing epithelioid pleural mesothelioma from adenocarcinoma metastatic to the pleura. *Mod Pathol.* 2000;13:107-112.
484. Ordonez NG. Role of immunohistochemistry in differentiating epithelial mesothelioma from adenocarcinoma: Review and update. *Am J Clin Pathol.* 1999;112:75-89.
485. Ordonez NG. Immunohistochemical diagnosis of epithelioid mesotheliomas: A critical review of old markers, new markers. *Hum Pathol.* 2002;33:953-967.
486. Ordonez NG. The immunohistochemical diagnosis of mesothelioma: A comparative study of epithelioid mesothelioma and lung adenocarcinoma. *Am J Surg Pathol.* 2003;27:1031-1051.
487. Comin CE, Novelli L, Boddi V, et al. Calretinin, thrombomodulin, CEA and CD15: A useful combination of immunohistochemical markers for differentiating pleural epithelial mesothelioma from peripheral pulmonary adenocarcinoma. *Hum Pathol.* 2001;32:529-536.
488. Zhang PJ, Genega EM, Tomaszewski JE, et al. The role of calretinin, inhibin, melan-A, BCL-2 and C-kit in differentiating adrenal cortical and medullary tumors: An immunohistochemical study. *Mod Pathol.* 2003;16:591-597.
489. Laskin WB, Miettinen M. Epithelioid sarcoma: New insights based on an extended immunohistochemical analysis. *Arch Pathol Lab Med.* 2003;127:1161-1168.
490. Pan C, Chen DC, Choo T, et al. Expression of calretinin and other mesothelioma-related markers in thymic carcinoma and thymoma. *Hum Pathol.* 2003;34:1155-1162.
491. Fine SW, McClain SA, Li M. Immunohistochemical staining for calretinin is useful for differentiating schwannomas from neurofibromas. *Am J Clin Pathol.* 2004;122:552-559.
492. Bergmann L, Maurer U, Weidmann E. Wilms tumor gene expression in acute myeloid leukemias. *Leuk Lymphoma.* 1997;25:435-443.
493. Sugiyama H. Wilms tumor gene (WT1) as a new marker for the detection of minimal residual disease in leukemia. *Leuk Lymphoma.* 1998;30:55-61.
494. Hwang H, Quenneville L, Yaziji H, et al. Wilms tumor gene product: Sensitive and contextually specific marker of serous carcinoma of ovarian surface epithelial origin. *Appl Immunohistochem Mol Morphol.* 2004;12:122-126.
495. Carpentieri DF, Nichols K, Chou PM, et al. The expression of WT-1 in the differentiation of rhabdomyosarcoma from other pediatric small round blue cell tumors. *Mod Pathol.* 2002;15:1080-1086.
496. Davidson B, Reich R, Lazarovici P, et al. Expression of the nerve growth factor receptor TrkA and p75 in malignant mesothelioma. *Lung Cancer.* 2004;44:159-165.
497. Hammar SP, Bockus DE, Remington FL, et al. Mucin-positive epithelial mesotheliomas: A histochemical, immunohistochemical and ultrastructural comparison with mucin-producing pulmonary adenocarcinomas. *Ultra Pathol.* 1996;20:293-325.
498. Mayall FG, Gibbs AR. The histology and immunohistochemistry of small cell mesothelioma. *Histopathology.* 1992;20:47-51.
499. Mayall FG, Jasani B, Gibbs AR. Immunohistochemical positivity for neuron specific enolase and Leu 7 in malignant mesotheliomas. *J Pathol.* 1992;165:325-328.
500. Falconieri G, Zanconati F, Bussani R, et al. Small cell carcinoma of lung simulating mesothelioma. *Pathol Res Pract.* 1995;191:1147-1151.
501. van Hengel P, van Geffen F, Kazzaz BA, et al. Atypical carcinoid presenting as mesothelioma. *Neth J Med.* 2001;58:185-190.
502. Henderson DW, Atwood HD, Constance TJ, et al. Lymphohistiocytoid mesothelioma: A rare lymphomatoid variant of predominantly sarcomatoid mesothelioma. *Ultrastruct Pathol.* 1988;12:367-384.
503. Daya D, McCaughey WTE. Well-differentiated papillary mesothelioma of the peritoneum: A clinicopathologic study of 22 cases. *Cancer.* 1990;65:292-296.

504. Yesner R, Hurwitz A. Localized pleural mesothelioma of epithelial type. *J Thorac Surg*. 1953;26:325-329.
505. Thickett DR, Armstrong L, Millar AB. Vascular endothelial growth factor (VEGF) in inflammatory and malignant pleural effusions. *Thorax*. 1999;54:707-710.
506. Golden A, Ash J. Adenomatoid tumors of genital tract. *Am J Pathol*. 1990;14:63-80.
507. Isotalo PA, Keeney GL, Sebo TJ, et al. Adenomatoid tumor of the adrenal gland: A clinicopathologic study of five cases and review of the literature. *Am J Surg Pathol*. 2003;27:969-977.
508. Overstreet K, Wixum C, Shabaik A, et al. Adenomatoid tumor of the pancreas: A case report with comparison of histology and aspiration cytology. *Mod Pathol*. 2003;16:613-617.
509. Argani P, Rosai J. Hyperplastic mesothelial cells in lymph nodes. Report of six cases of a benign process that simulate metastatic involvement by mesothelioma or carcinoma. *Am J Surg Pathol*. 1998;29:339-346.
510. Brooks JSJ, LiVolsi VA, Pietra GG. Mesothelial cell inclusions in mediastinal lymph nodes mimicking metastatic carcinoma. *Am J Clin Pathol*. 1990;93:741-748.
511. Ordonez NG, Ro JY, Ayal AG. Lesions described as nodular mesothelial hyperplasia are primarily composed of histiocytes. *Am J Surg Pathol*. 1998;22:285-292.
512. Sussman J, Rosai J. Lymph node metastasis as the initial manifestation of malignant mesothelioma: Report of six cases. *Am J Surg Pathol*. 1990;14:819-828.
513. Kannerstein M, Churg J, McCaughey WTE, et al. Papillary tumors of the peritoneum in women: Mesothelioma or papillary carcinoma. *Am J Obstet Gynecol*. 1977;127:306-314.
514. Foyle A, Al-Jabi M, McCaughey WTE. Papillary peritoneal tumors in women. *Am J Surg Pathol*. 1981;5:241-249.
515. Mills SE, Andersen WA, Fechner RE, et al. Serous surface papillary carcinomas: A clinicopathologic study of 10 cases and comparison with stage III-IV ovarian serous carcinoma. *Am J Surg Pathol*. 1988;12:827-834.
516. Raju U, Fine G, Greenwald KA, et al. Primary papillary serous neoplasia of the peritoneum: A clinicopathologic and ultrastructural study of eight cases. *Hum Pathol*. 1989;20:426-436.
517. Bell DA, Scully RE. Benign and borderline serious lesions of the peritoneum in women. *Pathol Annu*. 1989;24(pt 2):1-21.
518. Rutledge ML, Silva EG, McLemore D, et al. Serous surface carcinoma of the ovary and peritoneum: A flow cytometric study. *Pathol Annu*. 1989;24(pt 2):227-235.
519. Bell DA, Scully RE. Serous borderline tumors of the peritoneum. *Am J Surg Pathol*. 1990;14:230-239.
520. Truong LD, Maccato ML, Awalt H, et al. Serous surface carcinoma of the peritoneum: A clinicopathologic study of 22 cases. *Hum Pathol*. 1990;21:99-110.
520. Shah IA, Jayram L, Gani OS, et al. Papillary serous carcinoma of the peritoneum in a man. *Cancer*. 1998;82:860-866.
521. Biscotti CV, Hart WR. Peritoneal serous micropapillomatosis of low malignant potential (serous borderline tumors of the peritoneum): A clinicopathologic study of 17 cases. *Am J Surg Pathol*. 1992;16:467-475.
521a. Khoury N, Raju R, Crissman JD, et al. A comparative immunohistochemical study of peritoneal and ovarian tumors, and mesotheliomas. *Hum Pathol*. 1990;21:811-819.
522. Taylor DR, Page W, Huges D, et al. Metastatic renal cell carcinoma mimicking pleural mesothelioma. *Thorax*. 1987;42:901-902.
523. Ordonez NG, Myhre M, Mackay B. Clear cell mesothelioma. *Ultrastruct Pathol*. 1996;20:331-336.
524. Butnor KJ, Nicholson AG, Allred DC, et al. Expression of renal cell carcinoma-associated markers erythropoietin, CD10, and renal cell carcinoma marker in diffuse malignant mesothelioma and metastatic renal cell carcinoma. *Arch Pathol Lab Med*. 2006;130:823-827.
525. Illei PB, Rusch VW, Zakowski MF, et al. Homozygous deletion of CDKN2A and codeletion of the methylthioadenosine phosphorylase gene in the majority of pleural mesotheliomas. *Clinical Cancer Research*. 2003;9:2108-2113.
526. Lopez-Rios F, Chuai S, Flores R, et al. Global gene expression profiling of pleural mesotheliomas: Overexpression of aurora kinases and P16/CDKN2A deletion as prognostic factors and critical evaluation of microarray-based prognostic prediction. *Cancer Research*. 2006;66:2970-2979.
527. Prins JB, Williamson KA, Kamp MM, et al. The gene for the cyclin-dependent-kinase-4 inhibitor, CDKN2A, is preferentially deleted in malignant mesothelioma. *Int J Cancer*. 1998;75:649-653.
528. Xio S, Li D, Vijg J, et al. Codeletion of p15 and p16 in primary malignant mesothelioma. *Oncogene*. 1995;11:511-515.
529. Chiosea S, Krasinskas A, Cagle PT, et al. Diagnostic importance of 9p21 homozygous deletion in malignant mesotheliomas. *Mod Pathol*. 2008;21:742-747.
530. Illei PB, Ladanyi M, Rusch VW, et al. The use of CDKN2A deletion as a diagnostic marker for malignant mesothelioma in body cavity effusions. *Cancer*. 2003;99:51-56.
531. Dacic S, Kothmaier H, Land S, et al. Prognostic significance of P16/CDKN2Alossinpleuralmalignantmesotheliomas.VirchowsArchives (in press).
532. Allen TC, Popper HH, Kothmaier H, et al. Osteopontin (OPN) and HIF-1 expression in diffuse malignant mesothelioma (DMM) with long-term (>3 year) survival (LS) versus short-term survival (SS). *Mod Pathol*. 2008;21:335A.
533. Chung CT-S, Santos GC, Hwang DM, et al. p16/CDKN2A deletion as a diagnostic marker to distinguish benign from malignant mesothelial proliferations. *Mod Pathol*. 2008;21:338A.
534. Xu H, Simon R, Bourne PA, et al. Immunohistochemical analysis of KOC/IMP3 in malignant pleural mesothelioma. *Mod Pathol*. 2008;21:353A.
535. Gardner JM, Allen TC, Jagirdar J, et al. Expression of matrix metalloproteinase-7 (MMP-7) in 45 diffuse malignant mesotheliomas (MM): Potential target for therapy. *Mod Pathol*. 2008;21:342A.
536. Moore BH, Cagle PT, Allen TC, et al. Topoisomerasae II-alpha, minichromosome maintenance protein 2 (MCM2), and X-linked mammalian inhibitor of apoptosis protein (XIAP) expression in pleural diffuse malignant mesothelioma (PDMM): Possible role for chemotherapeutic intervention. *Mod Pathol*. 2008;21:347A.
537. Westerhoff M, Faoro L, Loganathan S, et al. Immunohistochemical (IHC) expression of c-Met receptor tyrosine kinase (c-Met) has prognostic significance and its activation is related to phosphorylated protein kinase Cβ (p-PKC β) in malignant mesothelioma (MM). *Mod Pathol*. 2008;21:353A.

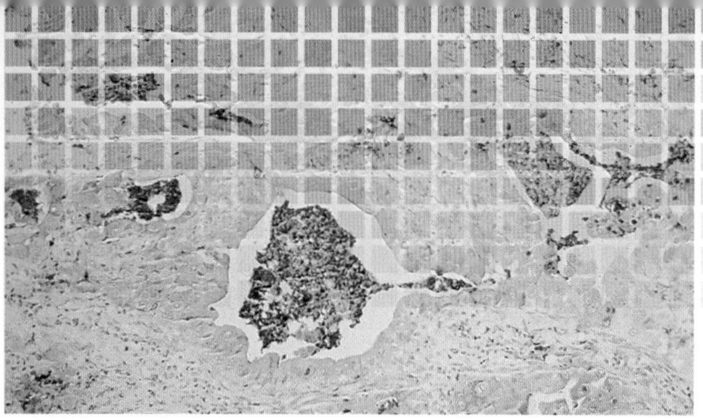

13

Immunohistology of Skin Tumors

Mark R. Wick • Paul E. Swanson • James W. Patterson

- Introduction 464
- Epithelial Tumors of the Skin 464
- Cutaneous Lymphohematopoietic Disorders 472
- Mesenchymal Tumors of the Skin 479
- Special Topics in Cutaneous Immunohistochemistry 489

INTRODUCTION

The skin is a complex microenvironment. The normal structures of the epidermis, dermis, and cutaneous adnexae are morphologically and functionally complicated, and the histologic entities that occur in this tissue compartment are numerous as well. Cutaneous lesions may also be a part of systemic proliferations or have exact morphologic counterparts in other sites. Principal examples of such disorders are lymphoreticular diseases and mesenchymal tumors. Because the diagnostic and immunohistochemical issues pertaining to those conditions are covered in detail elsewhere in this text, comments on them are relatively limited in scope, mainly centering on lesions that are peculiar to the skin. Finally, it should be understood that this chapter primarily focuses on those antigenic profiles that can be obtained with routinely processed, formalin-fixed tissues and commercially available reagents.

EPITHELIAL TUMORS OF THE SKIN

Because of the many forms of differentiated epidermal and adnexal epithelia in the skin, the nosologic categorization of corresponding cutaneous tumors is potentially confusing. From a pragmatic viewpoint, however, the diagnostic applications of immunohistochemistry require that only five basic patterns of epithelial differentiation be recognized: epidermal, sweat glandular, sebaceous, pilar, and endocrine.

Epidermal Tumors

Tumors with differentiation toward epidermal cells are the most common epithelial neoplasms of the skin. The most important of these are squamous cell carcinoma (SCC) and basal cell carcinoma (BCC).

SCC is a tumor that is usually composed of relatively uniform keratinizing polygonal cells, and as such, it poses few diagnostic challenges. However, several microscopic subtypes of SCC have been described, each of which may occasionally mimic both glandular and mesenchymal neoplasms in skin. These include adenoid (acantholytic), pleomorphic, small-cell, and spindle-cell forms.[1-3] Because of the latter variants, an understanding of the immunohistologic attributes of squamous carcinoma is important to the differential diagnosis of cutaneous tumors in general. Fortunately, all forms of SCC show similar antigenic profiles, with minor exceptions.

SCC contains an abundance of cytokeratin intermediate filament proteins that range from 40 to 68 kD in molecular weight.[4-8] The cells of those neoplasms that are well differentiated synthesize high-molecular-weight cytokeratin (CK); in contrast, more poorly differentiated tumors express low-molecular-weight keratin peptides. The concomitant expression of both cytokeratins and vimentin characterizes spindle-cell, pleomorphic, and some acantholytic squamous carcinomas (Fig. 13.1).[3,9]

Sarcomatoid carcinomas may sometimes express keratin focally, and the best approach to their recognition is to employ a broadly reactive mixture of monoclonal antikeratins as a screening reagent. Keratin 5/6 could be included as a specific target therein because it is squamous-cell selective.

Another epithelial determinant displayed in SCC is epithelial membrane antigen (EMA). Although variable amounts of this glycoprotein are encountered in most examples of SCC,[10] the authors have observed that diffuse EMA reactivity is usually only a feature of poorly differentiated tumors (Broders grades 3 and 4).

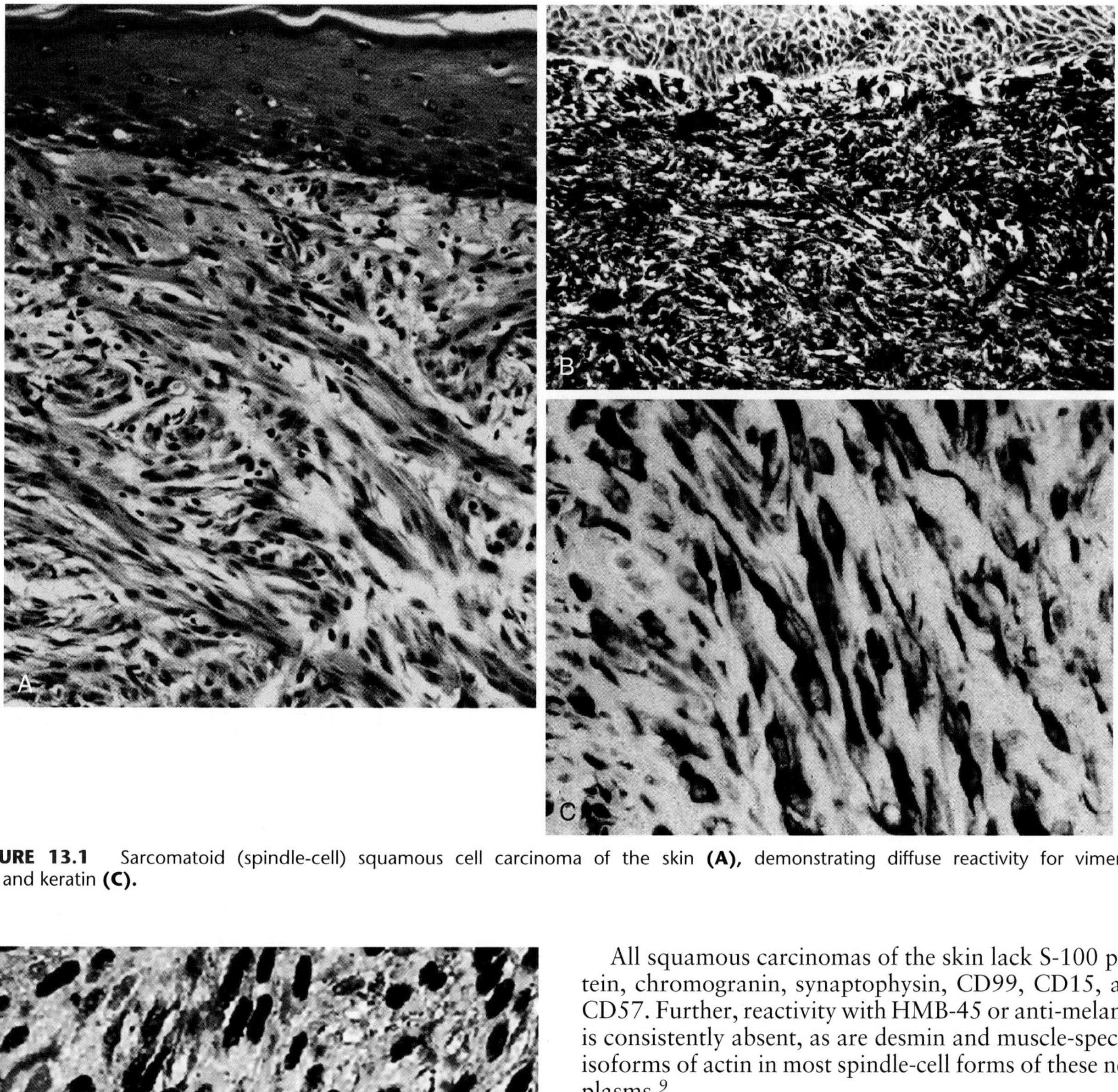

FIGURE 13.1 Sarcomatoid (spindle-cell) squamous cell carcinoma of the skin **(A)**, demonstrating diffuse reactivity for vimentin **(B)** and keratin **(C)**.

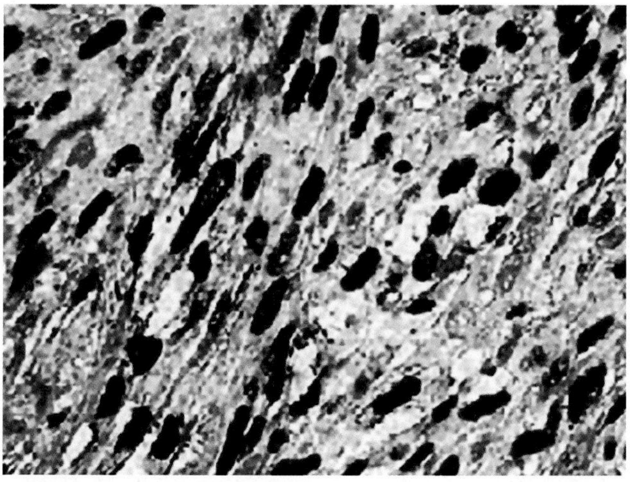

FIGURE 13.2 Positivity for p63 protein in poorly differentiated squamous cell carcinoma of the skin.

Carcinoembryonic antigen (CEA) staining has been described in SCC,[11] but in our experience, such reactivity is generally lacking. p63 Protein is a nuclear determinant that is seen in squamous, basal cell, and appendageal malignancies in the skin (Fig. 13.2). It is a member of the p53 family, which includes the p53, p63, and p73 polypeptides.[5,6]

All squamous carcinomas of the skin lack S-100 protein, chromogranin, synaptophysin, CD99, CD15, and CD57. Further, reactivity with HMB-45 or anti-melan-A is consistently absent, as are desmin and muscle-specific isoforms of actin in most spindle-cell forms of these neoplasms.[9]

Unfortunately, there are no well-characterized proteins that exclusively define epidermal differentiation. Substances associated with epidermal keratinization such as filaggrin and involucrin[12-16] are preferentially expressed in SCC, and, as such, have sometimes been touted as markers of malignancy among keratinocytic proliferations. Such claims, however, have generally proven to be unfounded, and the authors contend that no well-characterized marker has reliably separated benign cutaneous (or extracutaneous) neoplasms from histologically similar malignant tumors. This point has particular relevance to filaggrins and involucrin because both have been detected in keratoacanthomas and a variety of benign keratinocytic proliferations.[14,17] Although they may help to distinguish SCC from BCC, those markers cannot separate SCC from adnexal tumors of the skin,[13,18] particularly those of the pilar apparatus. Hence although these determinants may enhance our understanding of neoplastic keratinocytes, they have proven less useful as diagnostic aids.

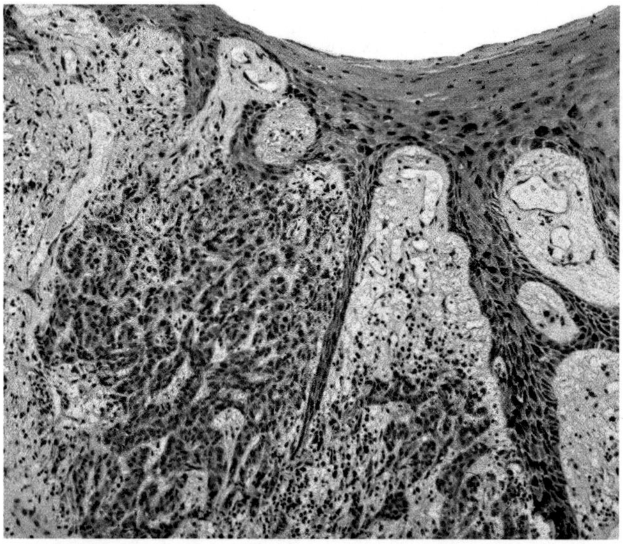

FIGURE 13.3 Nonreactivity for epithelial membrane antigen (EMA) in basal cell carcinoma. The overlying epidermis demonstrates facultative expression of EMA.

BCC, like SCC, has several distinctive variants, all of which invoke dissimilar differential diagnoses. Among the better-recognized subtypes of BCC are the morpheaform, adenoid, clear cell, keratotic, and metatypical (squamoid) forms.[19]

In general, BCC lacks complex patterns of antigenic expression. Like SCC, this tumor displays reactivity for cytokeratin (CK) polypeptides; however, these intermediate filaments are typically less than 50 kilodaltons (kD) in molecular weight.[4,20] In contrast to SCC, EMA is not observed in any variant of pure BCC (Fig. 13.3).[10,21,22]

Rare examples of BCC display reactivity with HMB45. Similarly, a few lesions exhibit staining for endocrine-associated peptides including CD56, synaptophysin, and chromogranin A (CG).[23-26] It should be noted, however, that most analyses do not demonstrate reactivity for those markers. The apparent ability of BCC to express such specialized determinants, as well as alpha-isoform actin,[26] has been used to support the premise that the cells of that lesion recapitulate the properties of epidermal "stem" cells. Nevertheless, the absence of vimentin, CEA, S-100 protein, CD57, and CD15[27] suggests that there may be flaws in the "stem cell hypothesis" as applied to BCC. BCC with additional patterns of differentiation such as "eccrine epithelioma,"[28] "apocrine epithelioma,"[29] and "basosebaceous epithelioma"[19] may indeed show positivity for EMA, CEA, or CD15 in histologically divergent areas.

Another useful glycoproteinaceous marker that is present in most BCCs is recognized by the antibody BerEP4, directed at two epitopes (34 kD and 39 kD) on human epithelial cells (Fig. 13.4).[30] In the skin, BerEP4 labels not only BCCs but also the cells of Paget disease, Merkel cell carcinoma, and other selected appendageal neoplasms. It is probably most useful in separating metatypical (squamoid) BCC from basaloid SCC, which is BerEP4 negative.[31] Conversely, squamous tumors bind to the L-Fucose-specific lectin, *Ulex europaeus* I, which lacks affinity for BCC.[32,33] The distinction between basaloid SCC and BCC is diagnostically crucial in certain anatomic locations such as the anal and perianal skin.

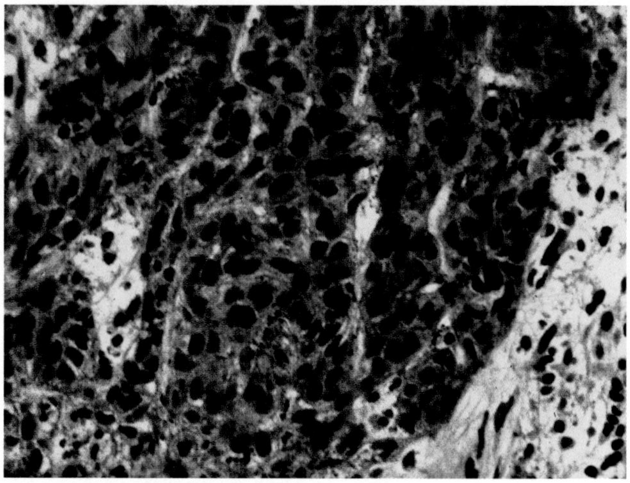

FIGURE 13.4 Diffuse immunoreactivity for the BerEP4 antigen in basal cell carcinoma.

KEY DIAGNOSTIC POINTS

Epithelial Tumors

- Adenoid (acantholytic), pleomorphic, small cell and spindle cell forms are variants of squamous cell carcinoma (SCC).
- SCC is decorated with AE1/AE3, K903, and CK5/6.
- Poorly differentiated SCC is decorated with CAM5.2, AE1/AE3.
- SCC is EMA+, P63+, BerEp4–.
- BCC is EMA–, BerEP4+.

Sudoriferous Tumors

The eccrine and apocrine glandular adnexae comprise the sudoriferous structures of skin. The neoplasms of these structures are histologically diverse[34] but share certain immunohistologic features. All of these tumors demonstrate CK reactivity and the potential for expression of CEA, tumor-associated glycoprotein-72 (TAG-72; also known as CA72.4) (Fig. 13.5), EMA, CD15, and p63.[35-40] The last three of these substances are seen in varying proportions in both sweat gland adenomas and carcinomas. EMA is more often observed in malignant sudoriferous neoplasms than in benign ones; indeed, certain benign lesions of the eccrine sweat gland including spiradenoma and cylindroma typically lack this determinant. In contrast, CEA and CD15 may be detected in roughly 70% to 80% of all eccrine and apocrine[21,35,41,42] regardless of their biologic potentials; CA72.4 appears to show a predilection for apocrine lesions and is usually not seen in eccrine tumors.[43,44] This profile proves useful in the separation of sudoriferous neoplasms from other cutaneous glandular and epidermal neoplasms. It has also been instrumental in

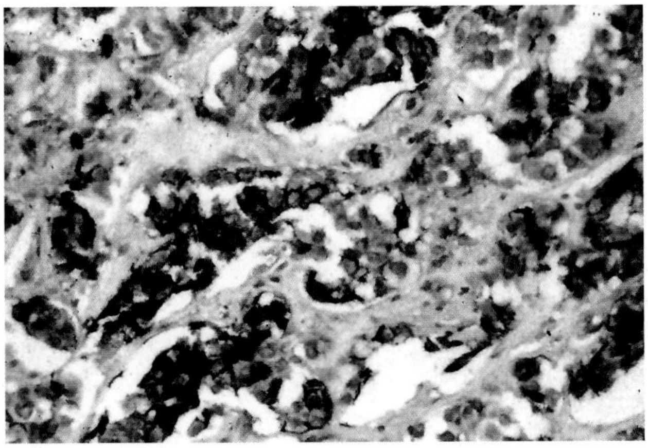

FIGURE 13.5 Positivity for CA72.4 (recognized by antibody B72.3) in sweat gland carcinoma.

verifying the presence of sweat glandular differentiation in occasional examples of lymphoepithelioma-like carcinoma of the skin, a poorly differentiated tumor showing histologic similarities to nasopharyngeal "lymphoepithelioma."[45]

Immunophenotypic differences between eccrine and apocrine neoplasms may occasionally be exploited to diagnostic advantage. For instance, eccrine carcinomas express S-100 protein in almost 50% of cases, whereas apocrine carcinomas including invasive extramammary Paget disease (EPD) are generally negative for that marker.[46] Conversely, gross cystic disease fluid protein[16] (GCDFP-15) is selectively expressed by apocrine cells and neoplasms (Fig. 13.6),[35,47] along with CA72.4. Together with CK7, CD23, and BerEP4, those markers represent discriminants that can separate EPD from superficial spreading malignant melanoma and Pagetoid Bowen disease (intraepidermal squamous carcinoma) diagnostically because they are present only in the first of those three tumors.[48-51] Keratin 20 also may be observed in cases of perineal or perianal EPD that are associated with regional visceral carcinomas (e.g., of the rectum or endocervix).[52-54] In contrast, Bowen disease is singular among them in its expression of high-molecular-weight keratin (as is typical of other SCCs),[55] and, only melanoma reacts with HMB-45, MART-1, and antibodies to S-100 protein among this group of lesions (see Chapter 7).[46]

Alpha-methylacyl coenzyme A racemase-reactivity has also been observed in EPD.[56] However, that enzyme is potentially present in SCC and melanoma as well[57] and therefore has lesser diagnostic value compared with the aforementioned determinants.

GCDFP-15 is not absolutely specific for apocrine cells; several eccrine carcinomas studied in the authors' laboratories have also been reactive for that marker.[35]

However, the selectivity of this determinant has proven useful in the evaluation of some benign sudoriferous lesions. For example, although sporadic GCDFP-15 staining in encountered in a minority of eccrine sweat gland adenomas, it is consistently displayed in tumors with known apocrine differentiation.[47] The apparent exception has been that of benign mixed tumor

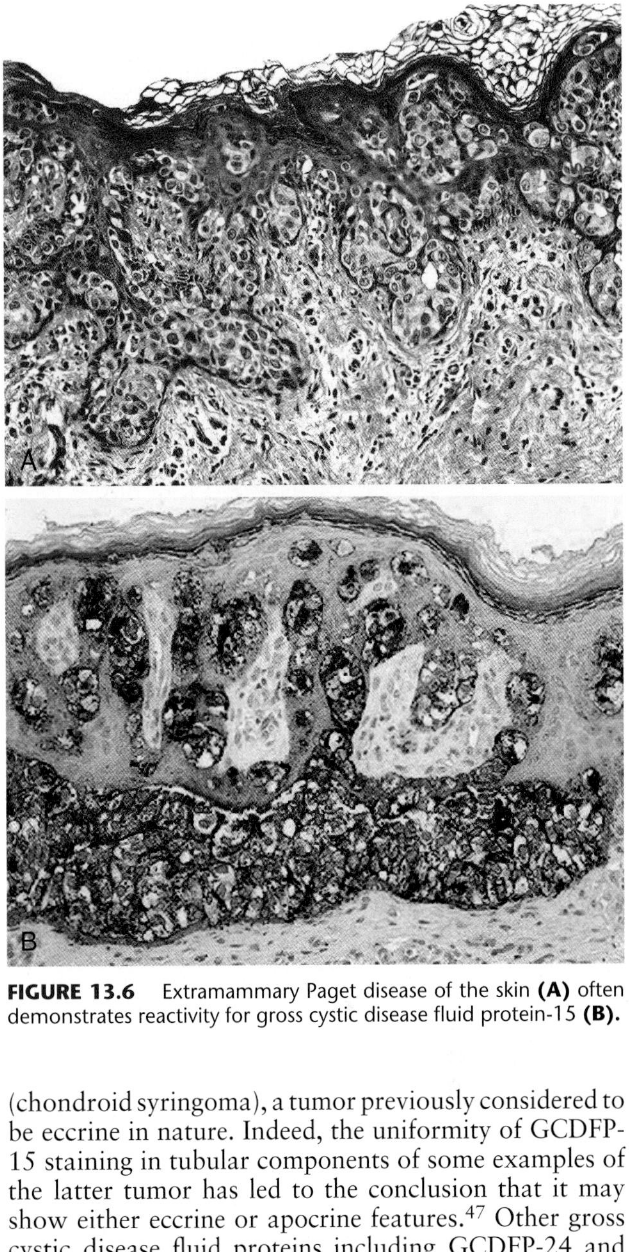

FIGURE 13.6 Extramammary Paget disease of the skin **(A)** often demonstrates reactivity for gross cystic disease fluid protein-15 **(B).**

(chondroid syringoma), a tumor previously considered to be eccrine in nature. Indeed, the uniformity of GCDFP-15 staining in tubular components of some examples of the latter tumor has led to the conclusion that it may show either eccrine or apocrine features.[47] Other gross cystic disease fluid proteins including GCDFP-24 and zinc-alpha-2-glycoprotein are less selective markers in this context.[58]

Some papers have described the selective expression of specific cytokeratin peptides and other cellular determinants in eccrine tumors. Antibodies to these substances including "EKH5," "EKH6," and "IKH-4"[59,60] may indeed show a preference for eccrine tumors, but the lack of systematic study of cutaneous and extracutaneous neoplasms for similar reactivity leaves the issue of their specificity an open one.

One difficult problem centering on the diagnosis of sweat gland carcinoma is its distinction from metastatic adenocarcinoma in the skin (Fig. 13.7).[61] The best way of achieving that goal is still by paying attention to the clinical history. Primary adnexal tumors are typically solitary and slowly growing (present for at least 6 months), whereas metastases are multiple and rapidly evolving. However, data from some studies suggest that p63 reactivity may be helpful in this context as well.[36,37]

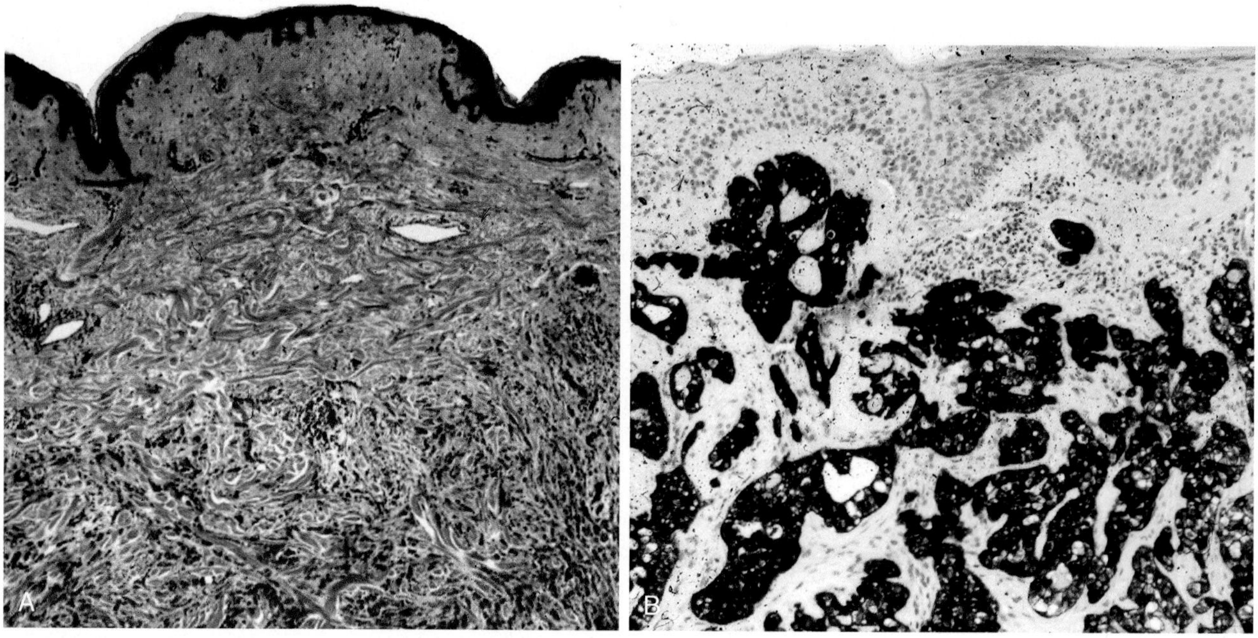

FIGURE 13.7 Metastatic adenocarcinoma in the skin **(A)**, showing diffuse positivity for carcinoembryonic antigen **(B)**. Many determinants such as that one are shared by primary and secondary cutaneous glandular malignancies.

It has been observed in the majority of sweat gland carcinomas but has generally not been seen commonly in metastatic adenocarcinomas. Nevertheless, Kanitakis and Chouvet reported p63-reactivity in 11% of cutaneous metastatic epithelial tumors.[38] Additional markers that may contribute to the separation of primary and secondary carcinomas in the skin are represented by CK 5/6 and podoplanin.[36,39,40] Like p63, they are principally seen in primary cutaneous appendage tumors.

KEY DIAGNOSTIC POINTS

Sudoriferous Tumors

- Express CK, CEA, CA72.4, CD15, and p63
- Epithelial membrane antigen more common in malignant neoplasms
- Eccrine carcinomas S-100+, apocrine S-100–, GCDFP-15+
- Paget disease: CK7+, GCDFP-15+, BerEP4+, CA72.4+
- Malignant melanoma: negative for Paget disease markers, HMB-45+, melan-A+, S-100+
- Bowen disease: AE1/AE3 and K903+, negative for Paget disease and melanoma markers

Sebaceous Tumors

Although it is a glandular adnexal structure, the sebaceous gland is topographically and ontogenetically related to the hair sheath. Hence antigenic similarities between the isthmus of the outer hair sheath and germinative basaloid cells of the sebaceous gland are not unexpected. Similarly, the occasional admixture of basosebaceous and hair sheath elements (as in superficial epithelioma with sebaceous differentiation and "sebaceoma") is understandable. The common expression of both high- and low-molecular-weight species of cytokeratin in pilar and sebaceous neoplasms, but not most eccrine or apocrine tumors, also points to similar patterns of cellular differentiation.[51] In addition, the architectural features of sebaceous neoplasms bear more resemblance to those of pilar neoplasms than to sudoriferous tumors. It follows from these observations that many antigens associated with sweat gland tumors (including S-100 protein, CA72.4, GCDFP-15, and CEA) are absent in sebaceous neoplasms.

Reactivity for EMA and related substances is often obtained in sebaceous tumors,[62] and these substances are typically displayed in a unique manner in these neoplasms. In both benign and malignant sebaceous proliferations, a characteristic microvesicular or "bubbly" cytoplasmic profile of the mature sebocyte is often maintained (Fig. 13.8). EMA staining in such neoplasms is comparable to that seen in non-neoplastic sebaceous epithelium, in that cytoplasmic lipid vesicles are rimmed by EMA reactivity. Even in poorly differentiated sebaceous carcinomas, EMA stains may highlight otherwise inapparent cytoplasmic multivacuolization.[63]

Other diagnostically relevant determinants shared by sebaceous and sweat gland neoplasms are CD15 and BerEP4.[30,42] However, an antibody panel directed at EMA, S-100 protein, and CEA will allow for separation between those tumors in most instances. To date, specific markers of sebaceous differentiation have not been characterized.[62] Some studies have reported selective labeling of sebaceous cells and their neoplasms for nuclear androgen receptor protein (ARP), but with somewhat contradictory results. Bayer-Garner and colleagues[64] found that all sebaceous tumors were ARP reactive, whereas Shikata and colleagues[65] suggested that sebaceous carcinomas lacked ARP. Incidentally,

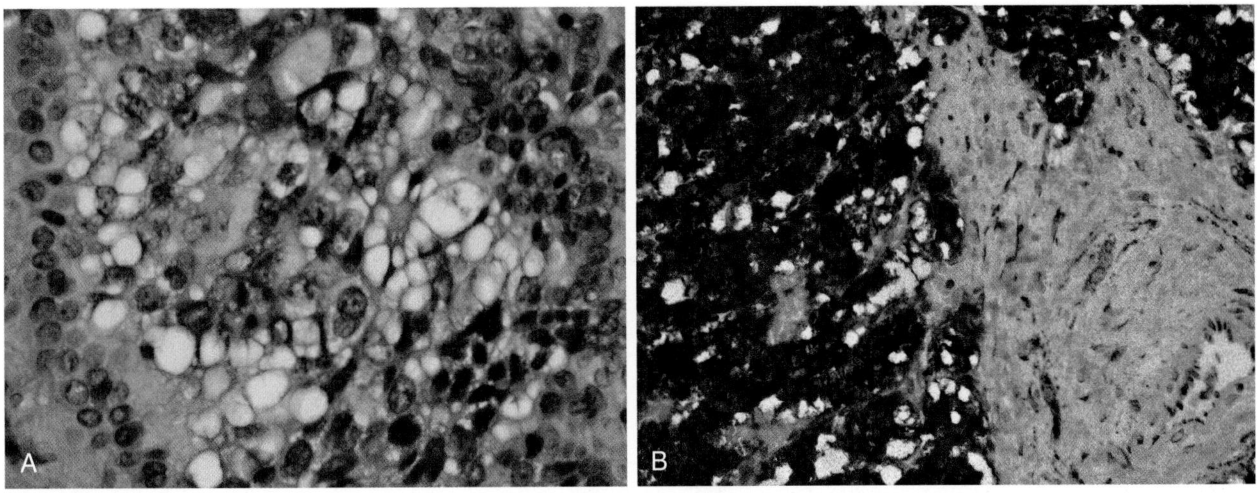

FIGURE 13.8 Sebaceous carcinoma **(A)** usually demonstrates diffuse reactivity for epithelial membrane antigen **(B)**, often with a "bubbly" cytoplasmic pattern of staining.

the authors of the first of those two publications also reported that poorly differentiated sebaceous carcinomas failed to show "bubbly" EMA reactivity, as described earlier. Other publications have suggested that reactivity for immunoglobulin A, lipase, milk fat globule–associated (ovarian carcinoma–associated) sebaceous antigen OV-2, and the OKM5 (CD36) antigen may be selective for sebaceous lesions.[62] However, the presence of those markers in extracutaneous lesions has not been assessed systematically to date.

The pathologic distinction between primary sebaceous carcinoma and metastatic renal cell carcinoma (RCC; an important differential diagnostic alternative with a clear-cell appearance) is similar to that made earlier in reference to sweat gland carcinomas. Slow evolution of a solitary skin tumor favors a primary lesion. In addition, immunostaining for podoplanin is effective in this context; that determinant is consistently present in sebaceous tumors,[40] whereas it is absent in RCC.[66] CD10 is potentially seen in both lesional categories.[67,68]

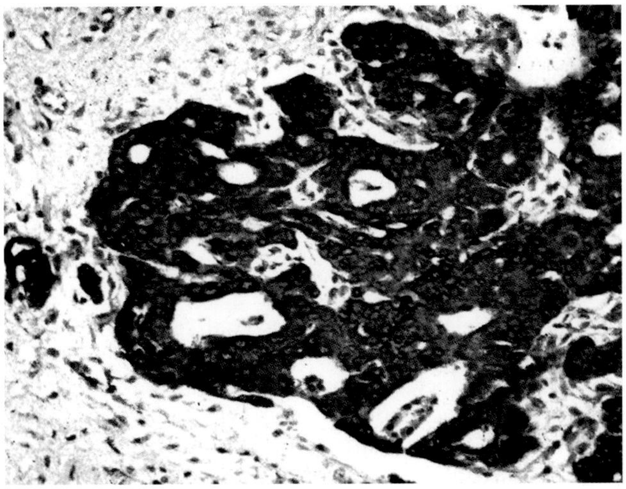

FIGURE 13.9 Positivity for bcl-2 protein in basal cell carcinoma.

KEY DIAGNOSTIC POINTS

Sebaceous Tumors

- Absent expression of S-100, CA72.4, GCDFP-15, CEA compared with sweat gland tumors, which are positive for these markers
- Sebaceous and sweat gland tumors CD15+ and BerEP4+
- EMA characteristic "bubbly" cytoplasmic decoration

Pilar Tumors

The multiplicity of diagnoses assigned to benign pilar tumors[69] reflects the protean morphologic manifestations of trichogenic differentiation. Unfortunately, most commercially available antibodies fail to select among those various patterns including lesions with features of the germinal matrix, cortex, inner hair sheath, outer hair sheath, and infundibulum. Indeed, the antigenic profiles of all benign pilar tumors are generally similar. They generally contain BerEP4 antigen, p63, and cytokeratin polypeptides over 50 kD in molecular weight,[4,5,70] but except for occasional proliferating pilar tumors, trichogenic neoplasms are EMA negative.[70] CEA, S-100, CD15, CA72.4, the HMB-45 antigen, and GCDFP-15 are also not detected in these tumors. As such, the immunophenotype of pilar adenomas is generally similar to that of BCC.

The last statement has several diagnostic corollaries. First, much of the literature on "classic" trichoepithelioma (CTE) still contends that it is conceptually distinct from BCC. Accordingly, some studies have been devoted to the analysis of immunohistochemical markers with which the two tumor types putatively can be separated from one another. For example, it has been suggested that bcl-2 protein staining (Fig. 13.9) of the epithelial cells and CD34 labeling of peritumoral stromal cells are diagnostic of BCC and CTE, respectively, in this narrow context.[71,72] Moreover, Lum and Binder[73] found that

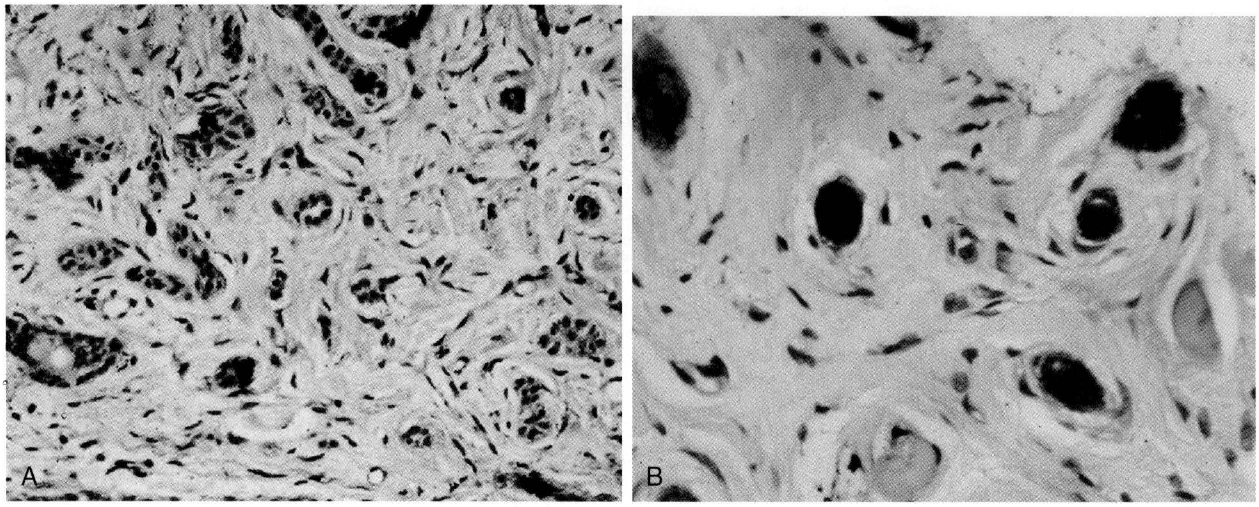

FIGURE 13.10 Reactivity for chromogranin A **(A)** and keratin 20 **(B)** is apparent in scattered cell nests in desmoplastic trichoepithelioma. Those determinants are typically absent in sclerosing basal cell carcinoma, which is the principal differential diagnostic consideration.

a Ki-67 index of greater than 25% and p21 protein expression were also discriminatory, with both favoring a diagnosis of BCC. The experience of the authors and others[74] with this subject has led to more nihilistic conclusions. In short, the authors do not believe that BCC and CTE can be distinguished reliably from one another immunohistochemically because CTE is probably a highly differentiated form of BCC. Increasing numbers of case reports on the "transformation" of CTE into BCC[75-79] and demonstration of a shared cytogenetic aberration (deletion of chromosomal segment 9q22.3) in CTE and BCC[80] provide support for that conclusion.

A more productive comparison can be made between desmoplastic trichoepithelioma (DTE) and infiltrative BCC (IBCC), which share histologic similarities in small biopsy specimens. The epithelial cells in DTE more often show EMA positivity and divergent neuroendocrine differentiation (with multifocal reactivity for CD56, chromogranin A, and keratin 20) than those in IBCC (Fig. 13.10)[81,82]; conversely, peritumoral stromal cells are reactive for stromelysin-3 (a proteolytic enzyme) in IBCC but not DTE.[83]

Selected evaluations of pilar and surface epidermal neoplasms by various authors have identified patterns of keratin expression that characterize predefined groups of follicular lesions.[84,85] The most intriguing finding from these investigations is that "hard keratins" recognized by the antibodies AE12 and AE13 are selectively expressed in cells exhibiting matrical differentiation. Pilomatricoma, as the prototypical matrical neoplasm, is diffusely reactive with AE13, whereas diminutive or abortive hair follicles represent the only reactive population in trichofolliculoma. Tumors with trichilemmal patterns of differentiation such as proliferating pilar tumor and tricholemmoma are AE13 negative but may instead be labeled with AE14 (Fig. 13.11). The latter reagent is a monoclonal antibody that recognizes both a cortical sulfur-containing moiety and a low-molecular-weight cytokeratin.[85] The latter substance is typically expressed by most adnexal epithelia and epidermal basal cells,

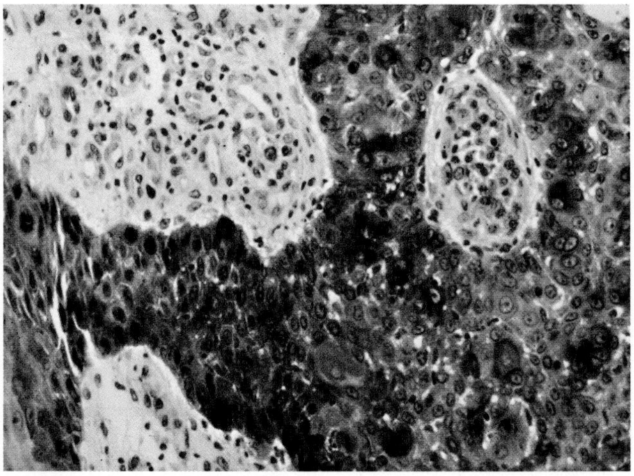

FIGURE 13.11 Immunoreactivity for "pilar-type" keratin in low-grade malignant proliferating pilar tumor, as recognized with antibody AE14.

and, as such, it is not as useful a marker as AE13. Interestingly, occasional small keratotic cysts in desmoplastic trichoepithelioma are AE13 positive, whereas examples of "classic" trichoepithelioma are uniformly negative with that antibody. Consistent AE13 staining is also seen in the small keratin cysts of microcystic adnexal carcinoma, indicating partial pilar differentiation in that tumor (Fig. 13.12).[86]

The expression of keratin proteins labeled by the antibodies HKN5, HKN6, and HKN7[84] and anti–human hair keratin (HHK) antibodies[87] may also reflect specialized patterns of pilar differentiation. Substances recognized by HKN6/7 are found only in cuticular, cortical, and inner hair sheath cells, whereas HKN5 also labels a cellular component of the outer hair sheath. Pilomatricomas typically express the HKN6/7 and HHK antigens; the latter is also present in malignant pilomatricoma.[87] In contrast, most other pilar tumors, BCCs, and other epidermal proliferations do not contain these substances. The expression of HKN5 is shared by pilar

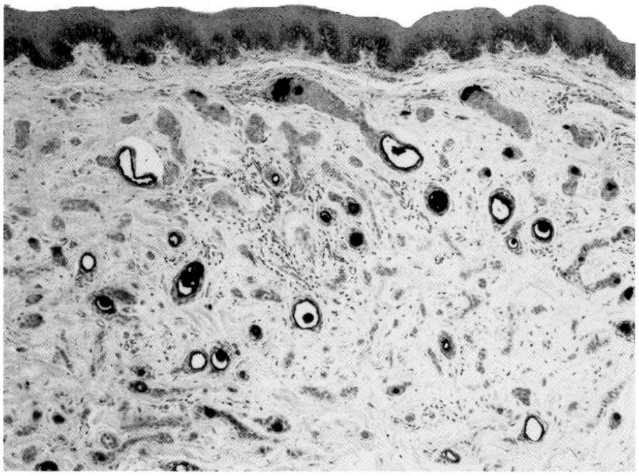

FIGURE 13.12 Multifocal positivity is seen with antibody AE13 in microcystic adnexal carcinoma of the skin. That reagent recognizes a keratin subtype that is related to the hair bulb.

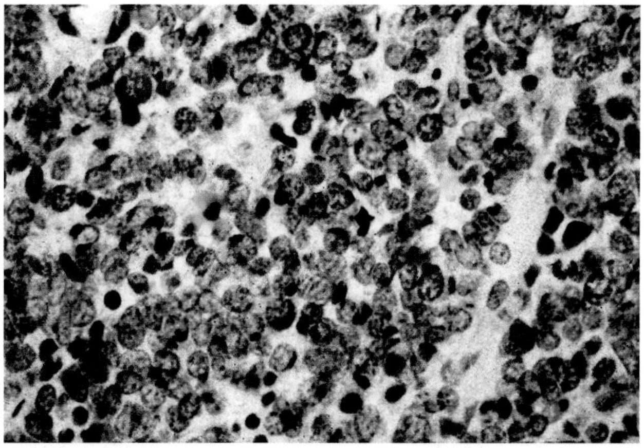

FIGURE 13.13 Perinuclear "globules" of keratin reactivity in Merkel cell carcinoma. That staining pattern simultaneously identifies the tumor as epithelial and neuroendocrine.

tumors and BCCs but is not seen in seborrheic keratoses. The detection of HKN5, 6, and 7 in some examples of the "Borst-Jadassohn" (clonal) type of intraepidermal carcinoma suggests that those lesions may have pilar characteristics.[84]

With malignant transformation, the immunophenotypes of pilar neoplasms become somewhat more complex. Pilar carcinomas (squamous carcinoma-like neoplasms arising in proliferating pilar tumors ["high-grade malignant proliferating pilar tumors"])[88] often display EMA, and trichilemmal carcinoma (a tumor with architectural and cytologic similarities to tricholemmoma) has the potential to manifest both CEA and S-100 protein, although such reactivity is generally focal.[89] No other commonly studied markers, with the exception of selected cytokeratins and p63, are shared by pilar and sudoriferous neoplasms.

KEY DIAGNOSTIC POINTS

Pilar Tumors

- Pilar adenoma immunoprofile is similar to basal cell carcinoma (BCC) of skin: epithelial membrane antigen (EMA), carcinoembryonic antigen, S100, CD15, and CA72.4 are negative.
- Desmoplastic trichoepithelioma versus infiltrative BCC: EMA, CD15, chromogranin, CK20; these markers are largely negative in invasive BCC.
- IBCC stromal cells are stromelysin-3+.

Endocrine Tumors

Primary cutaneous neuroendocrine carcinoma (PCNC) was originally described with the designation of "trabecular carcinoma of the skin" but is now best known as "Merkel cell carcinoma." After 30 years, it remains an object of biochemical and immunohistochemical interest. Some authors have postulated that PCNC displays neurotactile differentiation, emulating "Merkel" cells of the normal skin and oral mucosa.[90] Other studies have failed to substantiate or negate this hypothesis definitively. Non-neoplastic Merkel cells are reactive for cytokeratin 20, CG, MOC-31, neurofilament protein, CD56, met-enkephalin, vasoactive intestinal polypeptide (VIP), and blood group antigen Pr(h) but in general appear to lack the ability to synthesize other endocrine determinants consistently.[91-96] Reactivity for pankeratin, keratin 20, neurofilament protein, CD15, CD56, CD57, EMA, MOC-31 antigen, BerEP4 antigen, chromogranin A, calcitonin, somatostatin, adrenocorticotropic hormone, VIP, pancreatic polypeptide, and substance P is typically encountered in most (but not all) PCNCs.[97-101]

It has also been suggested that PCNC is closely related to sweat gland carcinomas.[102] However, despite having studied more than 200 cases of Merkel cell carcinoma, the authors have never observed any reactivity in that lesion for CEA, S-100 protein, CA72.4, or GCDFP15, as seen in sudoriferous tumors.

Because of its capacity for diffuse or medullary patterns of growth, and its uniform, occasionally dyshesive small-cell constituency, PCNC is potentially mistaken for lymphoma cutis. That problem is readily resolved by immunohistochemical analyses. Whereas lymphoma is reactive for CD45, PCNC is not. Moreover, keratin filaments in Merkel cell carcinomas are often clustered in the perinuclear cytoplasm, yielding a characteristic "dot" of chromogenic precipitate (Fig. 13.13).[103] Such an image is simultaneously diagnostic of epithelial and neuroendocrine differentiation in a small-cell cutaneous neoplasm, even if such markers as chromogranin, synaptophysin, and CD56 are absent in the tumor. Keratin assumes particular importance in making the distinction between PCNC and lymphoma because both of those tumor types share the potential for expression of PAX-5 and terminal deoxynucleotidyl transferase.[104-106]

Histologic features cannot reliably distinguish PCNC from metastatic small cell neuroendocrine carcinoma

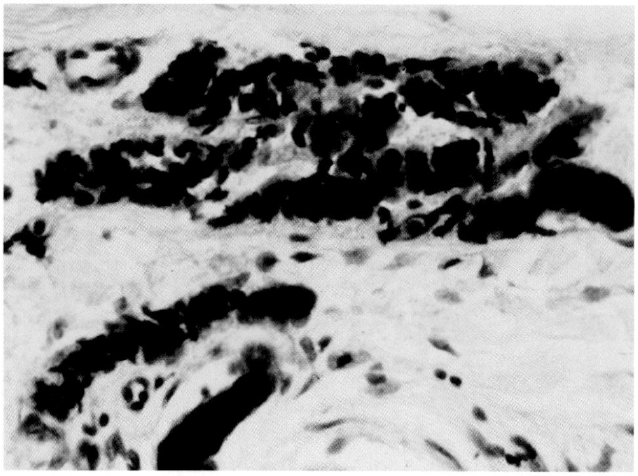

FIGURE 13.14 Diffuse nuclear positivity for thyroid transcription factor-1, in metastatic small-cell neuroendocrine carcinoma arising in the lung and involving the skin. That marker is consistently lacking in Merkel cell carcinoma.

originating in the lungs or other visceral sites. Nonetheless, a battery of antibodies to CEA, keratin 20, neurofilament protein (NFP), and thyroid transcription factor-1 is useful in this context. Bronchogenic small cell neuroendocrine carcinoma typically shows reactivity for CEA or TTF-1 (Fig. 13.14), or both, but it lacks keratin 20 and NFP.[107-109] Conversely, keratin 20 and NFP are often selectively expressed by PCNC and are generally absent in extracutaneous neuroendocrine carcinomas.[101] Despite such findings, thorough clinical evaluations including detailed imaging studies of the thorax are still advisable in most cases before metastasis is excluded diagnostically.

A second differential diagnostic consideration in cases of deeply seated PCNC is that of primary Ewing sarcoma/primitive neuroectodermal tumor (ES/PNET) of the subcutis.[110-115] Although both of those tumor types share possible reactivity for CD56, CD57, FLI-1, synaptophysin, and CD99 (Fig. 13.15A), pankeratin reactivity is unusual in PNET and positivity for keratin 20 and EMA has not been described in that lesion.[112,113,115-118] Conversely, most examples of PNET can be labeled for vimentin, but PCNC consistently lacks that filament protein.

PCNC may also be mistaken morphologically for BCC in selected instances.[119] The potential for endocrine differentiation in the latter tumor has already been mentioned, but it is never as global as that seen in PCNC. Moreover, CK20 and EMA are not seen in BCC, as they are in Merkel cell carcinoma, and the perinuclear keratin reactivity pattern of PCNC is absent in BCC.

Zembowicz and colleagues[120] have described another primary cutaneous carcinoma with histologic features that are entirely dissimilar from PCNC; namely, "endocrine mucin-producing sweat gland carcinoma." That lesion histologically resembled mucinous carcinoma of the skin and was immunoreactive for estrogen and progesterone receptor proteins in addition to endocrine markers.

Expected immunoreactivity patterns in various cutaneous epithelial tumors are shown in Figure 13.15B.

KEY DIAGNOSTIC POINTS

Endocrine Tumors

- Primary cutaneous neuroendocrine carcinoma (PCNC) positive for CK20 (dot-pattern), neurofilament, CD15, CD56, CD57, chromogranin, and various neuroendocrine hormones
- Pulmonary small-cell carcinoma metastatic in skin is CEA+, TTF-1+, CK20−; PCNC shows converse profile
- Cutaneous Ewing's sarcoma/PNET: CK is focal if positive, vimentin+, CK20−, and EMA−

CUTANEOUS LYMPHOHEMATOPOIETIC DISORDERS

Given the histologic diversity of T-cell and B-cell lymphoid and histiocytic proliferations of skin, complete consideration of each of those conditions is well beyond the scope of this chapter; indeed, detailed information on the immunohistology of hematopoietic lesions in general is provided in Chapters 5 and 6. Histopathologic criteria for the separation of benign and malignant lymphoreticular processes, although not without limitations, are certainly applicable to lesions of skin. Nonetheless, definitive determinations of cell lineage in several of these disorders are often difficult or impossible if only their morphologic and clinical attributes are considered. This discussion emphasizes selected aspects of immunophenotyping that have special relevance to hematologic lesions of the skin.

Lymphoma and Leukemia in the Skin

An effective arsenal of antibodies to various lymphoid antigens is applicable to skin biopsies that are felt to show hematopoietic lesions.[121-136] Virtually all examples of lymphoma and leukemia cutis are reactive for CD45 in paraffin sections,[137] allowing for the exclusion of histologically similar nonhematologic cellular proliferations. In addition, several lineage-selective reagents may be employed including CD3, CD4, CD5, CD7, CD8, CD43, and CD45RO as effective T-cell markers; CD20, 4KB5 CD45R, CD79a, PAX-5, CD179, and cyclin-D1 as B-cell markers; CD68, MAC387, factor XIIIa, and cathepsin B as histiocyte/monocyte markers; and CD30 and ALK-1 as selective markers in primary and secondary anaplastic large cell lymphomas (ALCLs) (Fig. 13.16).[121-136,138] Hodgkin's lymphoma of the skin is vanishingly rare,[139] and therefore it is not considered here, except to say that ALCL appears to be separable from that entity because of its common reactivity for CD99; Hodgkin lymphoma lacks the latter marker.[140-142]

Among the other markers listed earlier, most are closely restricted to their respective lymphoid lineages. However, CD43 may be seen in selected B-cell lesions, T-cell infiltrates, and myeloid proliferations.[143] The last

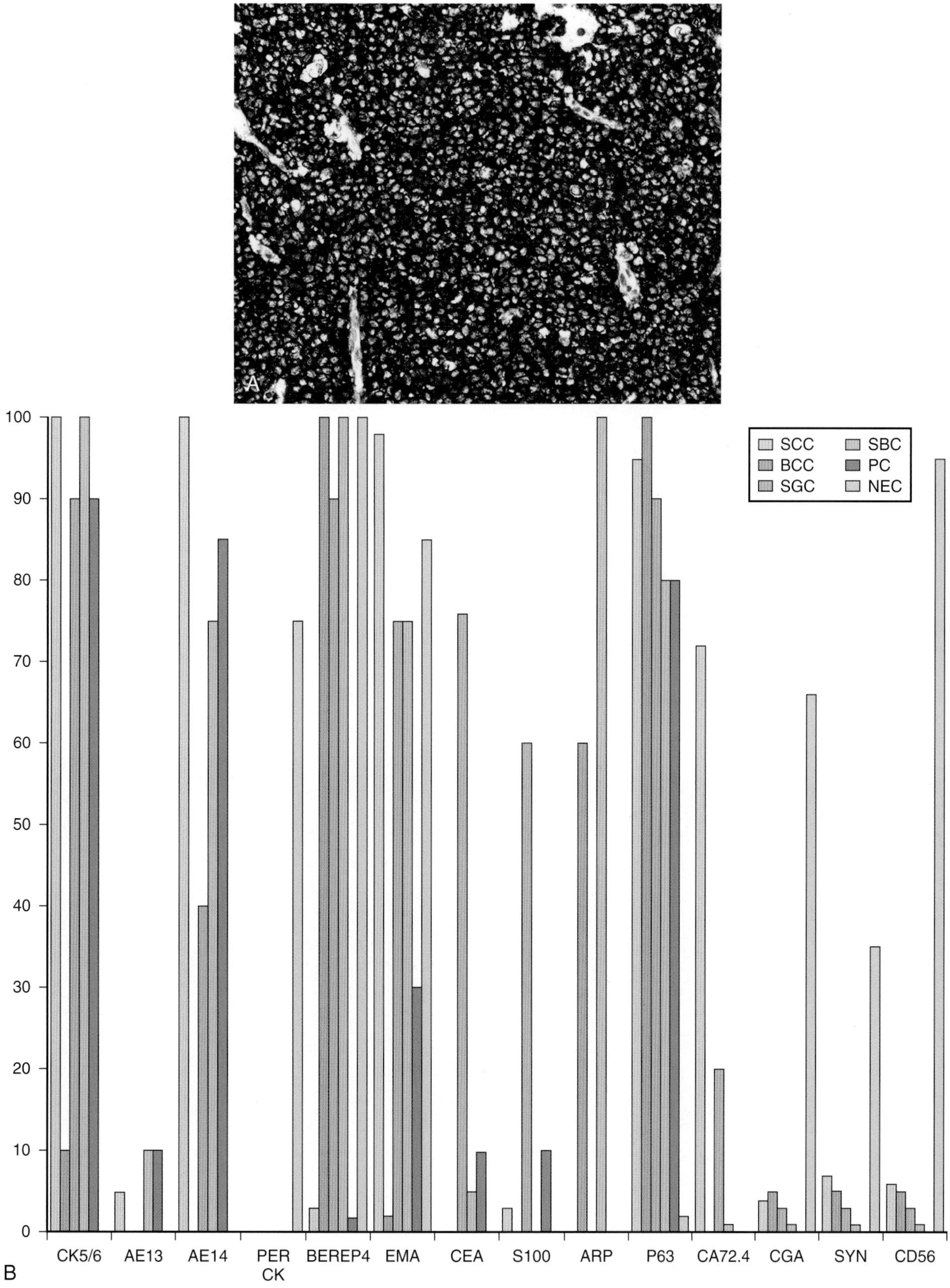

FIGURE 13.15 Immunoreactivity for CD99 in primitive neuroectodermal tumor of the subcutis **(A).** That determinant may also be seen in Merkel cell carcinoma. **B,** Expected immunoreactivity patterns in various carcinoma morphotypes in the skin. SCC, squamous cell carcinoma; BCC, basal cell carcinoma; SGC, sweat gland carcinoma; SBC, sebaceous carcinoma; PC, pilar carcinomas; NEC, neuroendocrine carcinoma; CK 5/6, keratin 5/6; AE13, AE14, pilar-related keratins; PER CK, perinuclear globular reactivity for keratin; EMA, epithelial membrane antigen; CEA, carcinoembryonic antigen; S100, S-100 protein; ARP, androgen receptor protein; CA72.4, TAG-72, tumor-associated glycoprotein-72; CGA, chromogranin A; SYN, synaptophysin.

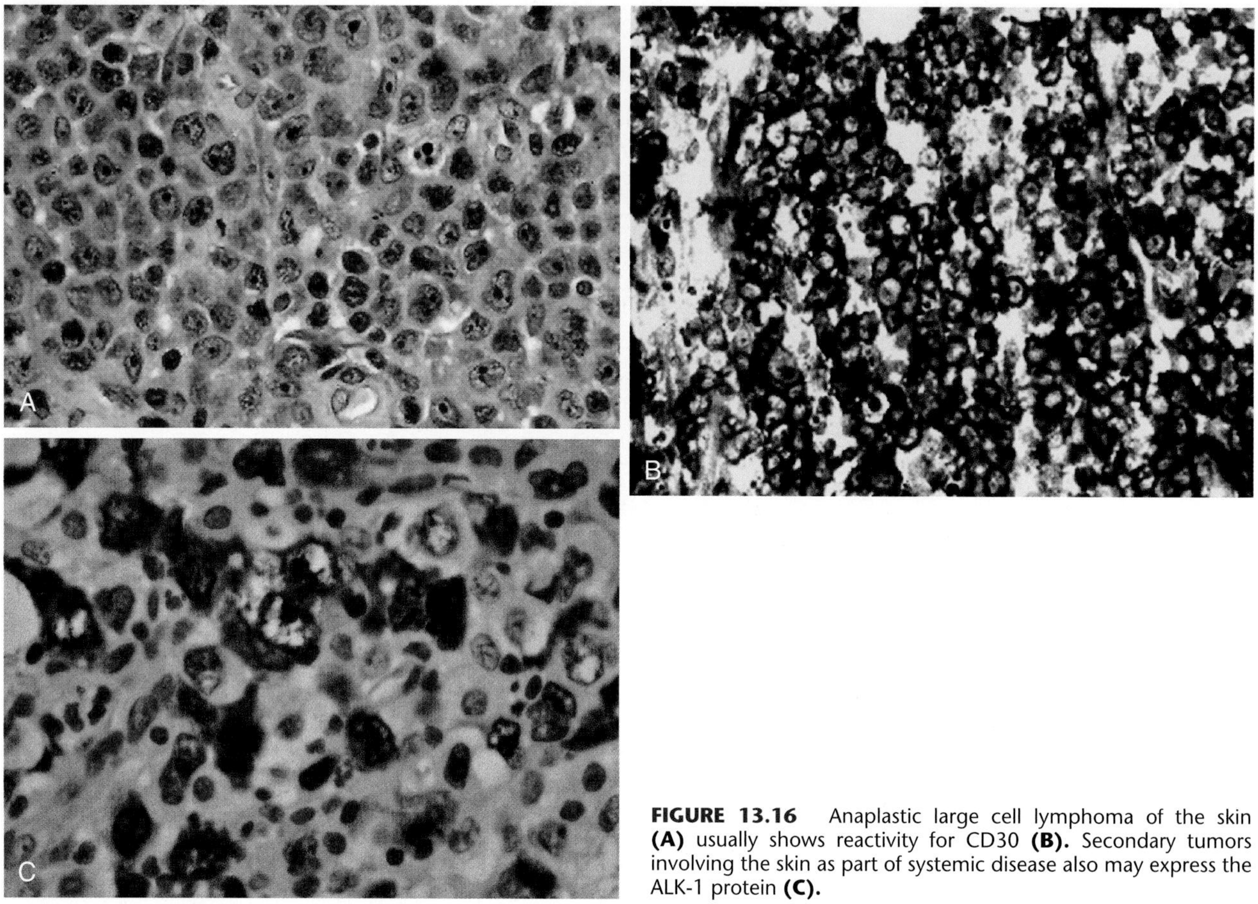

FIGURE 13.16 Anaplastic large cell lymphoma of the skin **(A)** usually shows reactivity for CD30 **(B).** Secondary tumors involving the skin as part of systemic disease also may express the ALK-1 protein **(C).**

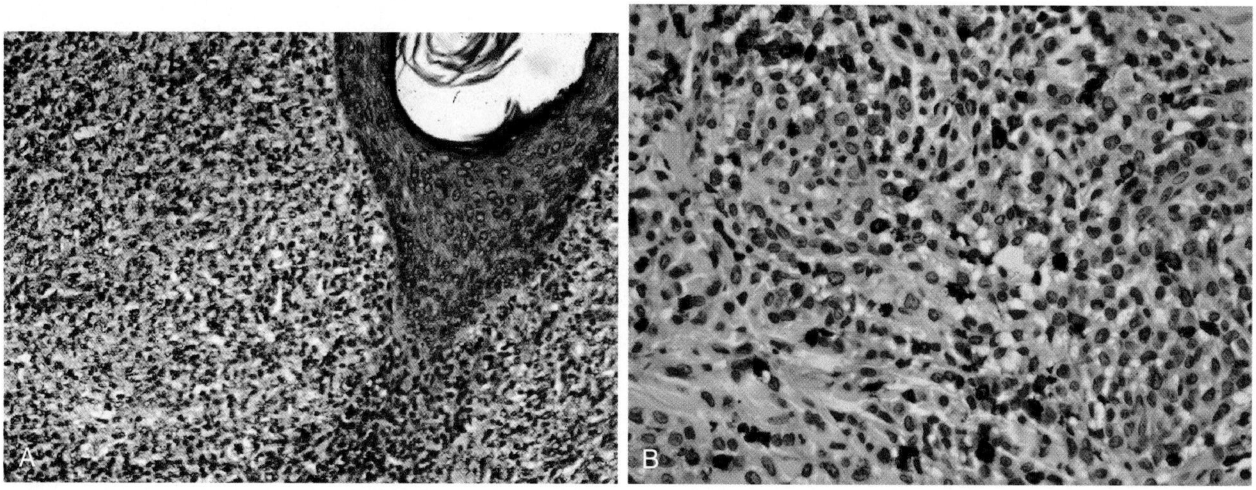

FIGURE 13.17 Extramedullary myeloid tumor of the skin (myeloid leukemia cutis; granulocytic sarcoma) **(A),** showing multifocal reactivity for myeloperoxidase **(B).**

of those is noteworthy; cutaneous myelomonocytic infiltrates are typically CD43 positive, but they are often only weakly reactive for CD45.[144] A possible diagnosis of myeloid leukemia cutis (extramedullary myeloid tumor; granulocytic sarcoma) for a "CD43-only" lesion can then be pursued by evaluating additional granulocyte- and monocyte-related markers such as myeloperoxidase, CD117, and cathepsin-B (Fig. 13.17).[130,131,136] In young children, lymphoblastic leukemia/lymphoma may also present with a CD43-only phenotype in the skin. That proliferation can be further assessed using stains for CD10, CD99, PAX-5, terminal deoxynucleotidyl transferase (Fig. 13.18), and CD179.[127,145,146] Positivity for the latter determinants would support the diagnosis of a lymphoblastic infiltrate.

One important limitation of immunophenotypic analysis of paraffin sections is that, for the most part, the markers listed earlier do not delineate differences

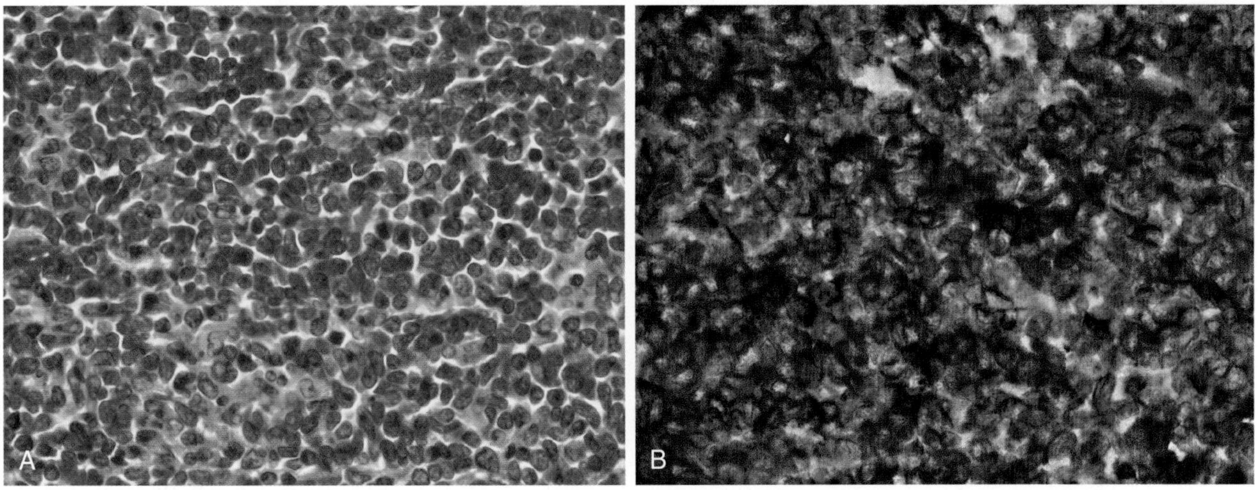

FIGURE 13.18 Lymphoblastic lymphoma in the skin **(A)**, demonstrating diffuse labeling for CD10 **(B)**.

between benign cellular infiltrates and malignant lymphoreticular proliferations. That separation is most satisfactorily demonstrated by genotypic analysis using Southern blotting or polymerase chain reaction–based technologies.[147,148] This problem is made even more vexing by the recent recognition that "cutaneous lymphoid hyperplasia" and lymphoma cutis probably comprise a continuum rather than mutually exclusive entities.[149,150] Hence it may not always be possible to distinguish between those disorders, even with the use of "molecular" methods.

With that having been said, however, the presence of functionally and immunophenotypically mature lymphoid follicles and a mixed inflammatory infiltrate often distinguishes benign cutaneous B-cell infiltrates from most B-cell lymphomas. Many cutaneous B-cell malignancies also show monotypic cell-surface or cytoplasmic immunoglobulin kappa or lambda light chains.[133] Commercially available anti-kappa and anti-lambda reagents work poorly in fixed tissue but may be adequately sensitive and specific in frozen sections and cell suspensions. The demonstration of lymphoid monotypism by *in situ* hybridization is definitely preferable methodologically in paraffin sections.[151] Genotypic evidence of clonal heavy- or light-chain immunoglobulin gene rearrangements in cutaneous B-cell lymphomas is also confirmatory.[148,152]

Immunophenotypic markers of monoclonal T-cell proliferations have not been identified. However, subtle alterations in broadly active T-cell selective ("pan-T-cell") determinants may be helpful in selected cases. Cutaneous T-cell lymphomas (CTCL) characteristically express "aberrant" phenotypes, represented either by the relative absence of the pan-T-cell markers CD3, CD5, CD43, and CD7 (especially the last of those) or by the concordant expression or loss of both CD4 and CD8 (Fig. 13.19).[153,154] Those results are not expected in most mature reactive (benign) T-cell populations.[122,155,156] Unfortunately, some examples of CTCL fail to exhibit aberrant phenotypes, limiting the value of these attributes in the separation of such lymphomas from T-cell-rich dermatitides,[122,155] and, conversely, benign infiltrates may occasionally show abnormal antigenic profiles.[154] More definitive evidence of T-cell neoplasia may be obtained from genotypic analyses, confirming the presence of clonal rearrangement of T-cell receptor genes.[147,157]

Certain aberrant B-cell phenotypes may also have diagnostic value. The most important example is the coexpression of CD5 or CD43 with CD20 in B-cell infiltrates.[122,158] Those constellations correlate well with light-chain immunoglobulin monotypism.

In the following material, only selected diagnostic settings are considered in which hematopoietic infiltrates in the skin may be the source of particular confusion. Further discussion of the immunohistology of other cutaneous neoplasms in this general category is available elsewhere.[159-161]

Special Pseudoneoplastic Lymphoid Lesions of the Skin

EPIDERMOTROPIC INFILTRATES RESEMBLING MYCOSIS FUNGOIDES

Selected drug-induced pseudolymphomatous infiltrates, chronic lichenoid and spongiotic dermatitides, and actinic reticuloid are the principal conditions that have the capacity to mimic mycosis fungoides (MF) histologically.[155,162-164] This is so because they may feature the presence of grouped lymphocytes in the epidermis, as well as the dermal interstitium, and such cells commonly demonstrate at least a modest degree of "activation" and nuclear atypia. Nearly universally, these elements are also T cells, as are the proliferating cells of MF.[163,165]

If it is available, frozen tissue can be studied immunohistologically to assess the presence or absence of an aberrant T-cell phenotype. The latter is said to be defined by the loss of one or more "pan-T-cell" determinants (CD2, 3, 5, and 7), as mentioned earlier, or by the coexpression of antigens that are usually mutually exclusive (e.g., both CD4 and CD8 in the same cell population).[122,166] CD7 is the pan-T-cell antigen cluster

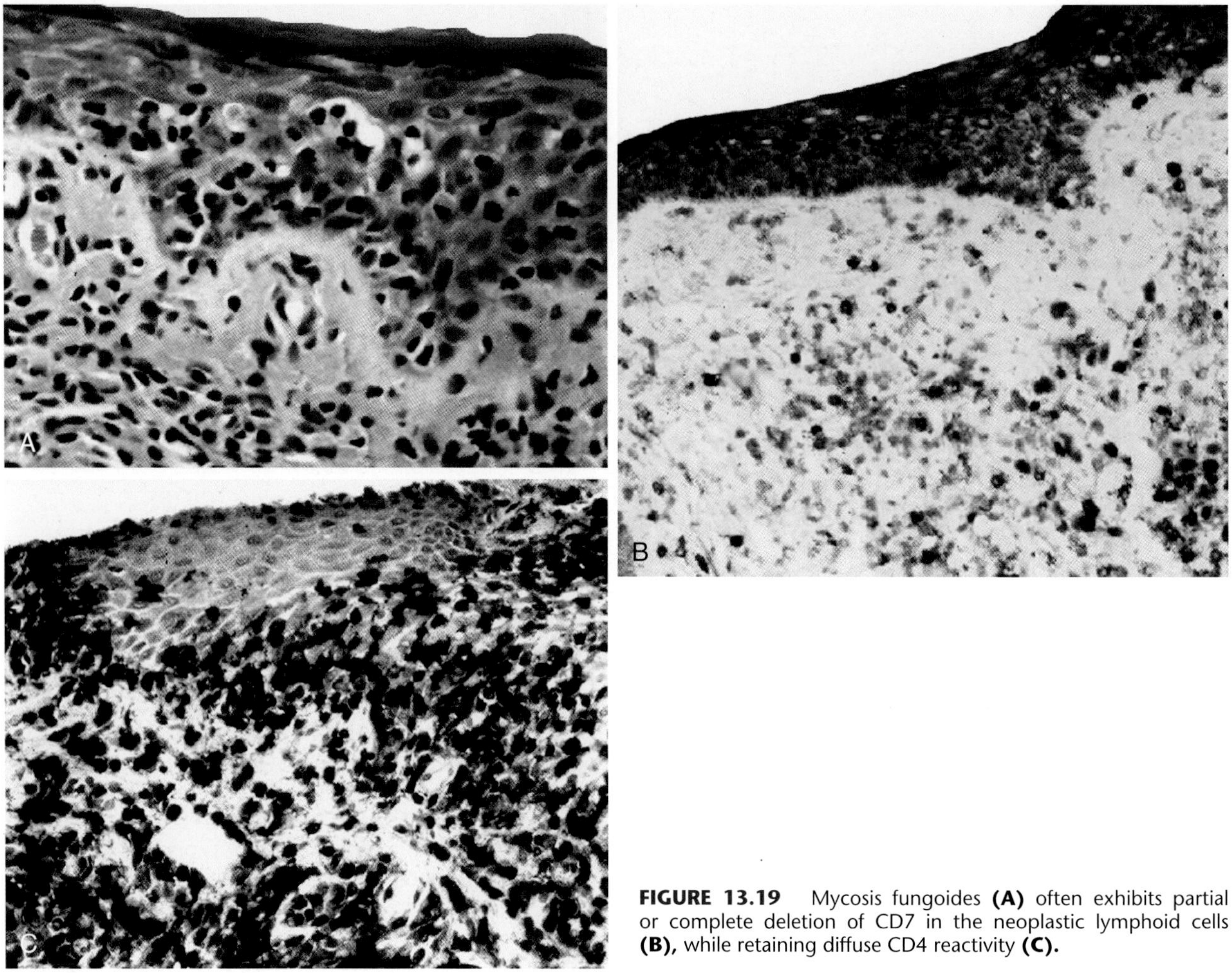

FIGURE 13.19 Mycosis fungoides **(A)** often exhibits partial or complete deletion of CD7 in the neoplastic lymphoid cells **(B)**, while retaining diffuse CD4 reactivity **(C)**.

that is most often lost in MF, which is characteristically a proliferation of CD4+ cells.[122,153] Nonetheless, this is not a universal finding in cutaneous T-cell lymphoma and it has been reported in benign inflammatory conditions as well.[154] On the other hand, actinic reticuloid and most other chronic dermatitides usually do retain pan-T-cell markers. Drug-induced pseudo-MF may have an immunophenotype like that of chronic spongiotic dermatitis, or it may simulate the profile of MF perfectly.[122,163] If the latter fact is disheartening, it is made more so by the knowledge that even genotyping studies may show T-cell receptor gene rearrangements in drug-related pseudolymphomas that are like those observed in MF.[167] In the final analysis, withdrawal of all medications—within feasible boundaries—and continued clinical surveillance over time may be the only means whereby pseudo-MF and true cutaneous T-cell lymphoma (CTCL) can be distinguished from one another in selected cases.

Paraffin sections are also acceptable substrates for the immunohistologic separation of benign and malignant T-cell infiltrates of the skin. As alluded to earlier, the authors have found that CD4-predominant intraepidermal lymphoid infiltrates, which also show concurrent negativity for CD3, CD5, CD7, CD43, or CD45RO, are more often seen in MF than in benign T-cell infiltrates of the skin.

Deep Lymphoid Infiltrates Simulating Small Cell or Mixed B-Cell Lymphomas

Generally speaking, "bulky" deep lymphoid infiltrates of the dermis and subcutis raise the specter of a B-cell lymphoma, rather than one of CTCL or peripheral T-cell lymphoma.[168] Some of the former conditions are relatively easy to recognize as benign disorders because they are composed principally of T lymphocytes or show a roughly equal admixture of B and T cells. Such lesions include Jessner's infiltrates, active cutaneous lupus erythematosus, and inflammatory cutaneous "pseudotumors."[122] However, other infiltrates such as lymphadenoma benigna cutis, lymphocytoma cutis, and follicular variants of cutaneous lymphoid hyperplasia (CLH) do, in fact, contain a large number of B lymphocytes and can cause substantial diagnostic difficulty.[122,161,169-171]

Frozen section studies or *in situ* hybridization analyses are helpful if they show restriction of lambda or kappa light-chain immunoglobulin expression by the

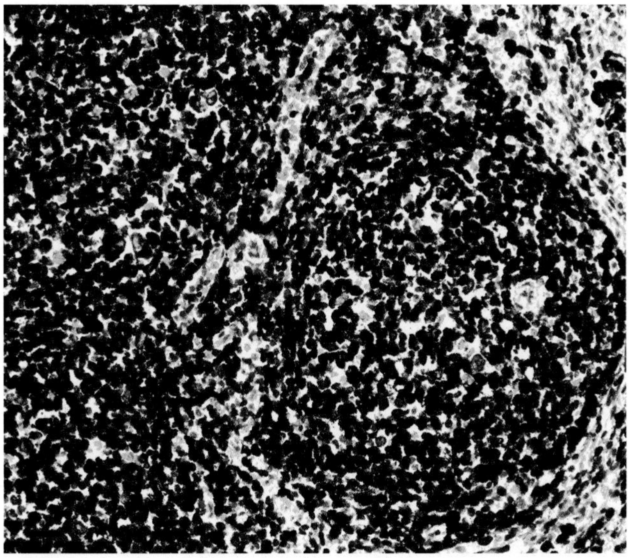

FIGURE 13.20 Labeling for bcl-2 protein is seen only inconsistently in primary follicular lymphomas of the skin and is principally represented in low-grade tumors.

constituent B cells.[172] By convention, this profile must demonstrate a ratio of at least 10:1 when one light chain is compared with the other.

Other determinants may also be used successfully in separating B-cell lymphomas from variants of CLH in paraffin sections. B-cell lymphoma is the likely diagnosis when CD20 and CD43 are coexpressed by the same population of lymphocytes, when more than 75% of the infiltrate are marked as B cells, and when more than 30% of the cells are positive for proliferating cell nuclear antigen or Ki-67.[158] These results parallel those that were obtained by Ngan and colleagues[173] in an analysis of extracutaneous lymphoid lesions.

The utility of another marker—the bcl-2 protein (BCLP)—has been analyzed in several studies of cutaneous lymphoid infiltrates. That moiety is an inhibitor of apoptosis, and it is overexpressed in malignant lymphoid cells that demonstrate a t(14;18) chromosomal translocation.[174] The latter is most characteristically seen in follicular lymphomas (Fig. 13.20). However, it would appear that BCLP unexpectedly has limited differential diagnostic usefulness in the narrower context of cutaneous lymphoproliferations. Many examples of CLH, CTCL, and various B-cell lymphomas of the skin are BCLP positive, and one must restrict attention only to overtly follicular proliferations in order to realize any benefit from this marker. Follicular CLH is BCLP negative, but follicular lymphoma in the skin also shows inconsistent positivity for that marker.[175-181]

Cutaneous Large Cell Lymphoproliferations Simulating Large B-Cell Lymphoma

Occasional examples of follicular CLH may contain such a strikingly large number of reactive immunoblasts that they mimic the microscopic appearance of a nodular B-cell lymphoma of the large-cell type.[168] Similarly, Kikuchi disease—a rare benign lymphoproliferative disorder that is much more often seen in Asia than in the United States—also comprises large atypical lymphoid elements that may cause confusion with a malignant process.[182-185]

In the first of these scenarios, that of florid follicular CLH, particular benefit is realized from routinely applying a broad panel of immunostains. These demonstrate a large number of B cells among the large-cell population, but they also show the presence of normal follicular mantles, interfollicular zones rich in T cells, and accentuation of Ki-67 reactivity in the central aspects of the follicular aggregates. In other words, the results mirror those seen in lymph nodal hyperplasia. It should also be remembered with caution that CD30—a marker associated with certain large-cell lymphomas[186]—is also potentially seen in *benign* immunoblastic proliferations in the skin and elsewhere.[187,188] Hence the presence of this determinant should never be used as sole support for a diagnosis of lymphoid malignancy.

Kikuchi disease (KD) features the presence of large, atypical mononuclear cells in the dermis, admixed with neutrophils and zones of necrosis; as such, it is a potential imitator of a subtype of ALCL.[182-185] However, KD is apparently a true histiocytic proliferation; it is correspondingly labeled by the monoclonal antibody MAC-387 and those in the CD68 group (e.g., KP-1), but not by CD20 or pan-T-cell reagents.[189] Inasmuch as examples of cutaneous "malignant histiocytosis" have essentially vanished in the wake of nosologic reclassification,[186] the latter findings constitute strong evidence for the presence of a benign disorder.

Langerhans Cell Histiocytosis ("Histiocytosis X")

Langerhans cell histiocytosis (LCH), like other prototypical hematopoietic infiltrates of the skin, is often readily diagnosed when all of its expected clinicopathologic features are present.[190] LCH is typically a disorder of children and often presents as a multifocal macular or papular eruption represented by vaguely defined or nodular histologic infiltrates of histiocytoid cells with characteristically folded or grooved nuclei. Patients with LCH often have prior or concurrent disease in extracutaneous sites, but LCH may occasionally present as a solitary skin lesion. Adults may develop limited cutaneous LCH as well in exceptional cases.[191-193] In each of these circumstances, the clinical and morphological differential diagnosis may include lymphoma cutis, malignant melanoma, and poorly differentiated epithelial and mesenchymal lesions.

Regardless of its mode of presentation in the skin, LCH has a consistent immunophenotype. Like nonneoplastic intraepidermal Langerhans histiocytes, the constituent cells of LCH are usually reactive for S-100 protein, fascin, CD1a, langerin, and CD31 (Fig. 13.21).[194-198] This phenotype is readily seen in paraffin sections and serves as supportive evidence of LCH if other determinants such as CD21 and melan-A are

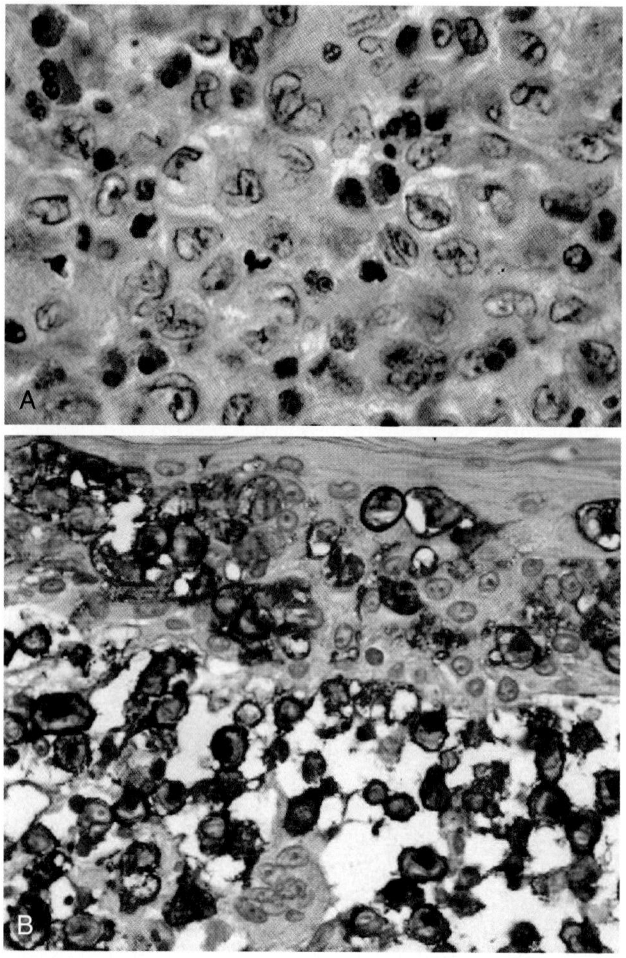

FIGURE 13.21 Langerhans cell histiocytosis of the skin ("histiocytosis X") **(A)**, showing positivity for CD1a **(B)**.

absent.[194,199] S-100 protein reactivity is otherwise limited to a few examples of non-LCH histiocytic infiltrates including reticulum-cell proliferations and extranodal cutaneous infiltrates of sinus histiocytosis with massive lymphadenopathy (Rosai-Dorfman disease).[200,201] Additional evidence of Langerhans cell differentiation may be gained from the ultrastructural demonstration of Birbeck granules in the lesional cells, but those inclusions are not seen in all examples of LCH.[200]

Diagnostic difficulties are uncommonly posed by other cutaneous histiocytoses that affect children, among them the so-called "congenital self-healing reticulohistiocytosis" (CSHR)[202,203] and "benign cephalic histocytosis."[204-206] The former of those conditions is unequivocally a proliferation of Langerhans cells and shares all immunophenotypic and ultrastructural attributes with LCH.[202] In fact, CSHR is generally regarded as a localized form of LCH. Benign cephalic histiocytosis (BCH) also demonstrates S-100 protein-positive histiocytes, but it shares few other clinical or morphologic attributes with LCH. The infiltrates of BCH are generally more well circumscribed and limited to the superficial dermis. They also lack the nuclear features of Langerhans cells, as well as CD1a reactivity and the synthesis of Birbeck granules.[206]

KEY DIAGNOSTIC POINTS

Pseudoneoplastic Lymphoid Proliferations

- CD4+ intraepidermal lymphocytes that are negative for CD3, CD5, CD7, CD43, or CD45R0 are more likely to be seen in mycosis fungoides than benign conditions.
- B-cell lymphoma is more likely when there is coexpression of CD20 and CD43, when greater than 75% of lymphocytes are B cells, and if Ki-67 is greater than 30% of cells.
- Cells in Kikuchi disease are true histiocytes: negative for B- and T-cell markers, positive for CD68 and MAC387.
- Langerhans histiocytosis cells express S-100, fascin, CD1a, and CD31.

Cutaneous "Pseudopseudolymphomas"

Among all lymphohematopoietic lesions of the skin, those that present as recurrent eruptions may be the source of considerable diagnostic difficulty. Two of them, namely, so-called "regressing atypical histiocytosis"/cutaneous ALCL and lymphomatoid papulosis, historically were considered to be benign cutaneous proliferations ("pseudolymphomas"), but careful clinical evaluation and immunophenotypic analyses have demonstrated that they have the pathologic features of malignant diseases. As such, these two entities might be labeled as "pseudopseudolymphomas."

In 1982 Flynn and colleagues[207] described a distinctive lesion of the skin that was composed of large, anaplastic, pleomorphic lymphoid cells that effaced the dermis and subcutis. Despite the appearance of this infiltrate, affected patients initially followed a favorable clinical course; the cutaneous lesions regressed spontaneously, and there were relatively long periods of apparent remission. The disease was given the name "regressing atypical histiocytosis" (RAH) to emphasize its indolent nature. Unfortunately, the original patients with RAH, as well as many others who were reported subsequently, eventually developed aggressive cutaneous and extracutaneous lymphoproliferations with the immunophenotypic characteristics of "Ki-1" (CD30+) ALCL.[208-211]

Immunohistochemically, the cells of RAH/ALCL are usually reactive for CD3, CD5, CD45, CD30, CD43, CD45RO, and CD99 in paraffin sections (Fig. 13.22).[141,208,211-216] This phenotype supports the interpretation of most of these lesions (≈80%) as T-cell neoplasms. The remaining cases demonstrate "null-cell" differentiation. Primary ALCLs in the skin are typically negative for the ALK-1 protein, whereas systemic ALCLs that *involve* the skin are ALK-1 reactive.

In contrast to RAH/ALCL, lymphomatoid papulosis (LYP) follows a more consistently indolent course, and, as such, it is still not uniformly accepted as a malignant disease.[217-219] LYP may arise in virtually any cutaneous or mucocutaneous surface, although axial sites are most common. The typical lesions are small papules that may undergo central hemorrhage and necrosis before healing

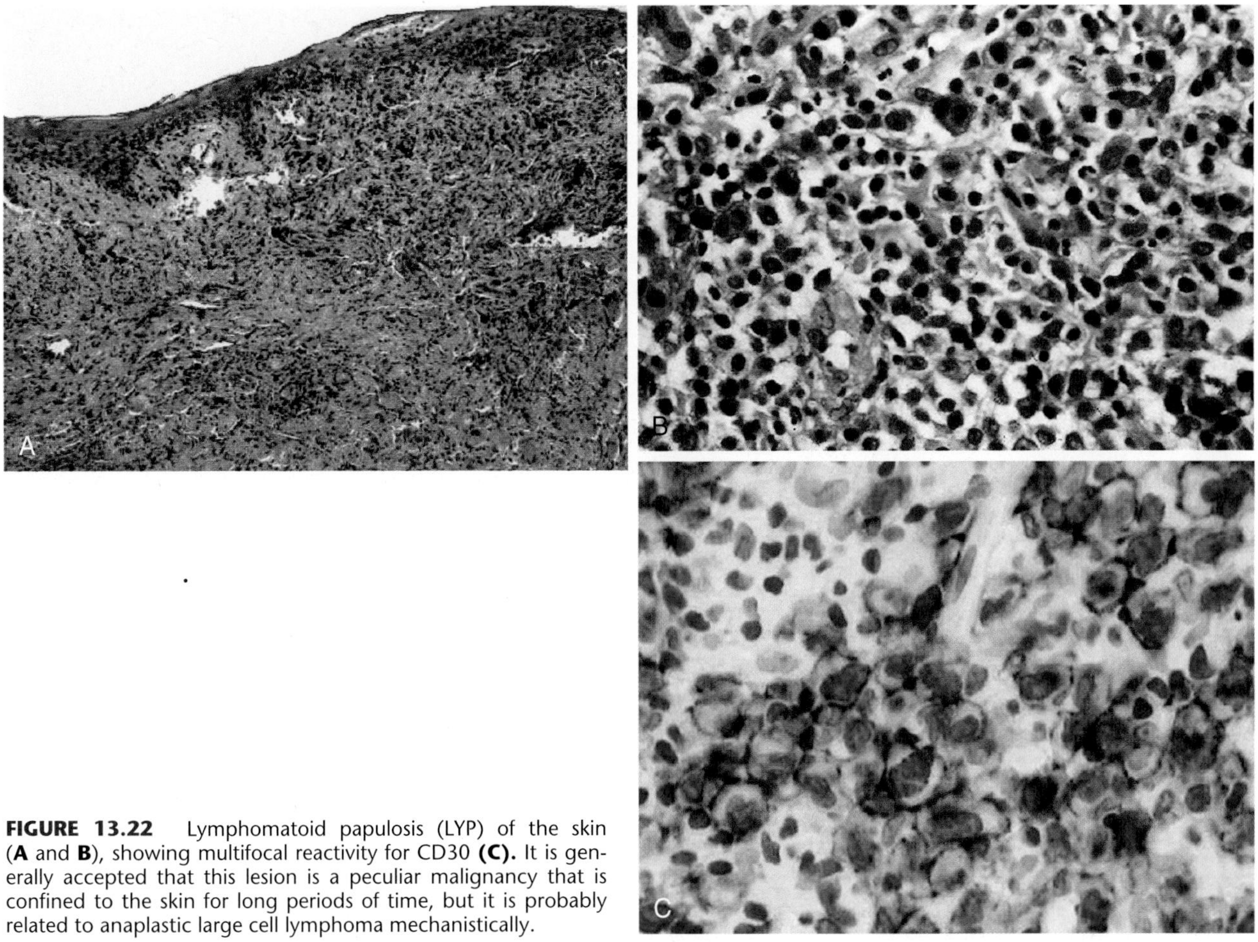

FIGURE 13.22 Lymphomatoid papulosis (LYP) of the skin (**A** and **B**), showing multifocal reactivity for CD30 **(C)**. It is generally accepted that this lesion is a peculiar malignancy that is confined to the skin for long periods of time, but it is probably related to anaplastic large cell lymphoma mechanistically.

spontaneously. Some may persist indefinitely, and local or distant recurrences are common.[220]

Histologically, LYP is a superficial and deep perivascular and interstitial infiltrate, often with a wedge-shaped configuration, which may have a lichenoid component in the superficial dermis. The overlying epidermis is often spongiotic and parakeratotic. The infiltrate of LYP is mixed, and constituent lymphocytes are usually smaller than those seen in ALCL. However, a minority of tumor cells in LYP have highly atypical cytologic features; in some cases, they may be multinucleated and contain pathologic mitotic figures. The latter are more prevalent in active lesions, whereas resolving or healing lesions contain fewer atypical elements.[212,215,216] Less commonly, the large cells in LYP may form tumoral nodules or sheets; in such cases, despite the presence of clinical features of LYP, a diagnosis of outright ALCL is more tempting.

LYP is considered by most observers to be a peculiar T-cell lymphoma that is "contained" within the skin by an effective immunologic host response.[212,218,221] Immunophenotypic analyses of LYP support this view because in most instances an aberrant phenotype that is comparable to that of ALCL is detected.[215,222,223] CD4 positivity is common in both of those conditions. Clonal T-cell receptor gene rearrangements in LYP further solidify the conclusion that it is inherently a malignancy[157,221] because they are uncommon in benign reactive T-cell infiltrates. Eventually, approximately 10% to 20% of patients with LYP will eventually develop a systemic lymphoma.[215,224,225]

MESENCHYMAL TUMORS OF THE SKIN

Patterns of mesenchymal differentiation in cutaneous neoplasms are no less diverse than those encountered in deeper soft tissues. Fibroblastic or myofibroblastic, "fibrohistiocytic," muscular, neural, epithelial, and vascular lesions may be seen as primary tumors in the dermis and subcutis. As is also true in deep soft tissues, the histologic evaluation of those neoplasms may fail to provide an unequivocal diagnosis. Hence immunophenotyping has proven to be valuable in this context. The diagnostic separation of various spindle-cell, polygonal-cell, epithelioid-cell, and small-cell lesions of the skin is assisted in many settings by immunohistochemical analysis.

Fibroblastic/Myofibroblastic Neoplasms

In general, tumors showing pure fibroblastic or myofibroblastic differentiation are uncommon. Only three cutaneous neoplastic proliferations fall into that

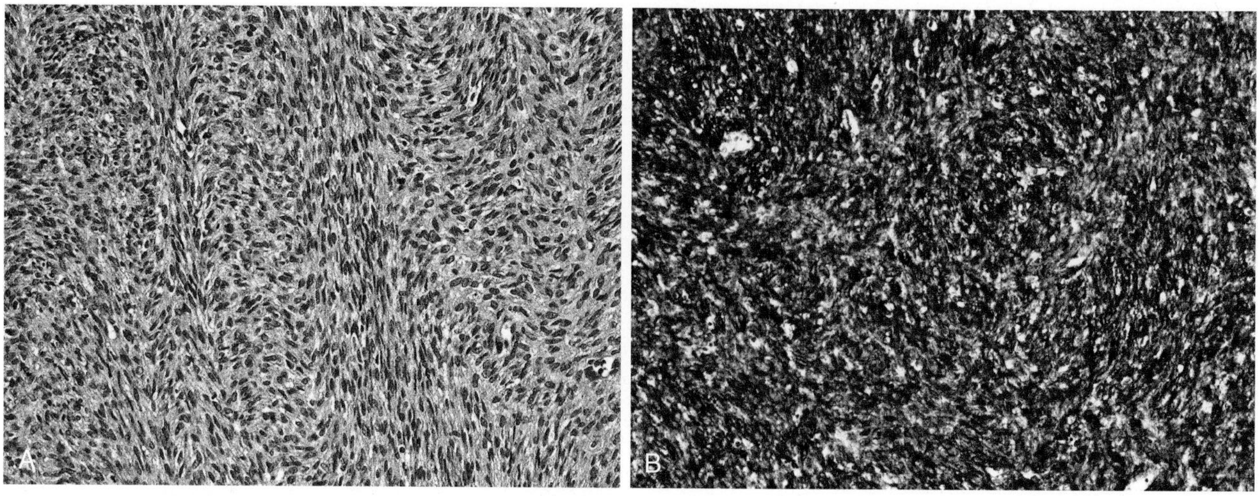

FIGURE 13.23 Fibrosarcoma of the dermis and subcutis **(A)**, showing diffuse vimentin positivity **(B)**.

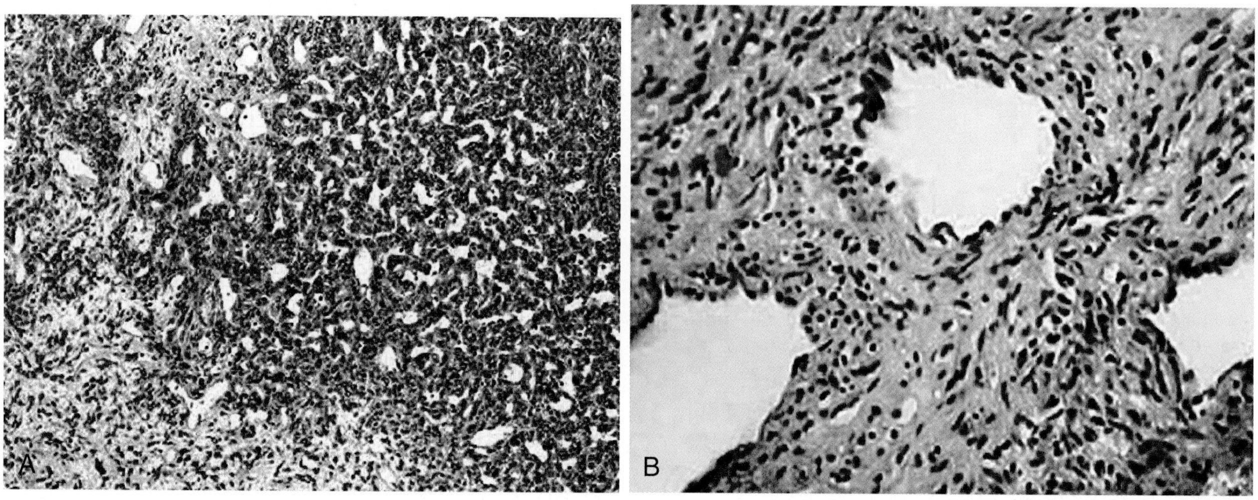

FIGURE 13.24 "Hemangiopericytoma" of the dermis and subcutis **(A)** is currently regarded as a form of myofibromatosis and is therefore expected to demonstrate reactivity for actins **(B)**.

category—recurrent digital fibroma/digital fibromatosis,[226-229] cutaneous fibrosarcoma,[230,231] and congenital superficial "hemangiopericytoma."[232,233] The first of those tumors typically occurs on the hands of children; in many instances, it is multifocal. Ultrastructural analysis has shown that digital fibroma (DF) is composed of myofibroblasts [226]; accordingly, it exhibits uniform reactivity for vimentin and muscle-specific isoforms of actin.

In the experience of the authors, desmin may be detected as well, although others have disagreed on that point.[234] The ultrastructural and biochemical attributes of myofibroblastic contractile elements are essentially identical to those of smooth muscle cells. Notably, the peculiar intracytoplasmic inclusions that are present in DF correspond to aggregates of immunoreactive actin filaments.[227-229]

Fibrosarcoma of the skin has been reported in association with burn scars, surgical scars, smallpox vaccinations, and other injection sites.[231] This exceedingly uncommon neoplasm is composed exclusively of fibroblastic elements and stains only for vimentin, to the exclusion of the other specialized mesenchymal determinants that are associated with nonfibroblastic differentiation (Fig. 13.23). A more common source of fibrosarcoma (FS) in the skin is the "dedifferentiation" (clonal transformation) of dermatofibrosarcoma protuberans (DFSP), as discussed later.

Congenital hemangiopericytoma—so-named because of the peculiar "staghorn" vascular pattern that characterizes this tumor in young children—is a lesion that shares clinical and histologic features with the myofibromatoses of childhood and with solitary acquired myofibroma of adults.[235-237] Unlike true hemangiopericytomas, which lack muscle-specific actin, "congenital hemangiopericytomas" are usually diffusely reactive for that marker (Fig. 13.24).[237]

"Fibrohistiocytic" Neoplasms

The concept that such tumors as atypical fibroxanthoma (AFX), malignant fibrous histiocytoma (MFH), and DFSP display "fibrohistiocytic" cellular features is more of a historical concept than a currently accepted tenet. Although

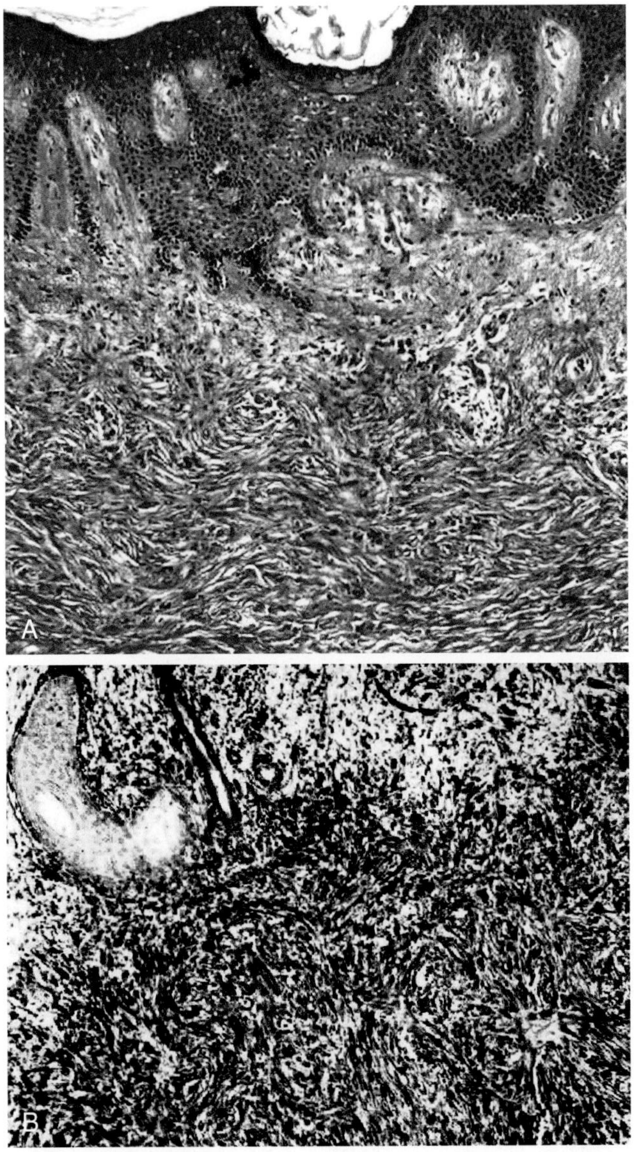

FIGURE 13.25 Dermatofibroma **(A)** usually shows diffuse positivity for factor XIIIa **(B)**.

there is some disagreement on this point,[238] only a small minority of these lesions express specialized hematopoietic determinants. The latter include CD14, CD16, CD18, CD36, CD43, and CD68, all of which have been associated with bone marrow–derived monocytes and histocytes.[238,239] The presence of HLA-DR in MFH has been substantiated in some reports as well,[238] but analyses of other soft tissue malignancies also have shown the presence of that class II histocompatibility antigen.[240,241]

Similarly, cellular proteases such as alpha-l-anti-chymotrypsin and cathepsin-B (CB) are regularly present not only in AFX, MFH, and DFSP[242] but also in many other spindle-cell tumors of the skin.[199,239] MAC387, an antibody to a cytoplasmic determinant (the L1 antigen) that is characteristic of functionally mature monocytes and macrophages, also frequently is observed in multinucleated, and, less commonly, fusiform elements in MFH, AFX, and DFSP. However, MAC387 likewise may be observed in virtually every other type of malignant cutaneous neoplasm.[243] Finally, immunoreactivity for factor XIIIa, a coagulation factor expressed by fibroblasts and "dermal dendrocytes," is seen in dermatofibromas (Fig. 13.25), AFX, and MFH, but it is also encountered in other sarcomas, granular cell tumors, and neurofibromas.[244-248]

As one would expect, MFH, AFX, and DFSP demonstrate diffuse reactivity for vimentin.[249] Muscle-specific actins and caldesmon have also been detected in some of these neoplasms, particularly in AFX.[250,251] CD34 positivity separates DFSP—which is virtually always diffusely reactive for that marker (Fig. 13.26)—from most other spindle-cell neoplasms of the dermis and subcutis, with the exception of selected peripheral nerve sheath tumors, acral fibromyxoma, and spindle cell lipoma.[252-258] Incidentally, it should also be noted that giant-cell fibroblastoma, giant-cell angiofibroma, and cutaneous solitary fibrous tumor are entities which are closely related to DFSP biologically, and they share its immunophenotypic properties.[259-268] CD34 staining is not necessary to make the diagnosis of DFSP in most instances, and it has its greatest value in small biopsies where the architecture of the lesion is not well represented. Moreover, it should be recognized that dermatofibromas sometimes show peripheral-lesional "leading-edge" positivity for CD34 as well (Fig. 13.27), with the central aspect of the lesion being negative; that finding should not dissuade one from making a benign interpretation. Another peculiarity of DFSP is the focal presence of myoid differentiation in some instances, with regional positivity for actins and desmin.[269-273] That property is shared by selected examples of dermatofibroma as well.

As mentioned earlier, fibrosarcoma *ex* DFSP is a special variant of dermatofibrosarcoma. Two immunoprofiles may be observed in this "composite" tumor: It may be diffusely reactive for CD34 throughout, or the fibrosarcomatous component may lack that marker, producing biphasic immunoreactivity.[270-277]

Another subtype of DFSP in which CD34 labeling is diagnostically beneficial is its "atrophic" form. In that lesion the prototypically bulky and protuberant nodular histologic image of DFSP is lacking, and one sees an "alternating stair-step" pattern of spindle-cell proliferation in the subcutis (Fig. 13.28).[278] Diffuse CD34 reactivity in such tumors helps one to avoid mistaking them for benign lesions.

It is likely that "MFH" is not a unified entity in the skin or elsewhere, but instead represents a histologic pattern that is a common final pathway of differentiation for several modes of mesenchymal neoplasia. That concept was first espoused by Brooks.[279] Thus an MFH-like pattern may be seen in conjunction with other mesenchymal images in the same tumor mass, as a consequence of clonal evolution. An unqualified diagnosis of MFH can be made immunohistologically only if one is dealing with a pleomorphic malignant tumor that is vimentin reactive and lacks epithelial, myogenous, neural, and endothelial markers. At present, there are no "proactive" determinants that define this neoplasm.

The authors regard AFX as a special superficial variant of MFH, and therefore comments applying to the

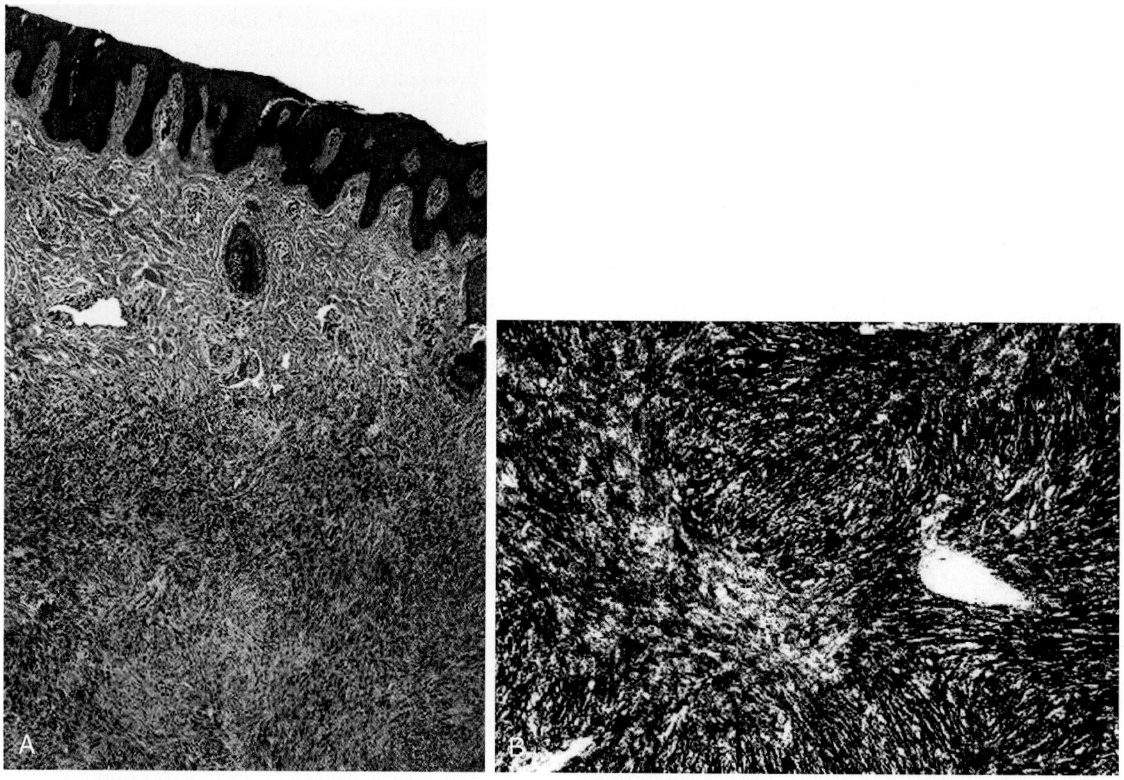

FIGURE 13.26 Dermatofibrosarcoma protuberans **(A)** typically shows global reactivity for CD34 **(B)**.

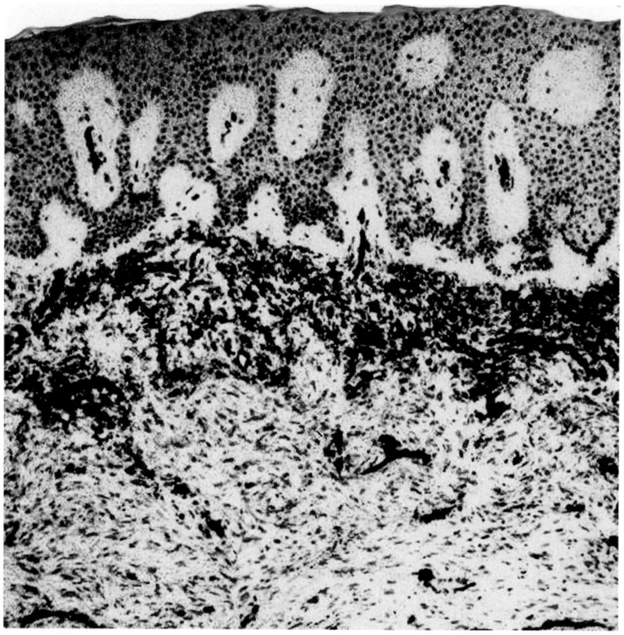

FIGURE 13.27 If dermatofibromas express CD34, as shown here, it is restricted to the "leading edge" of the tumor, in contrast to the expected pattern in dermatofibrosarcoma.

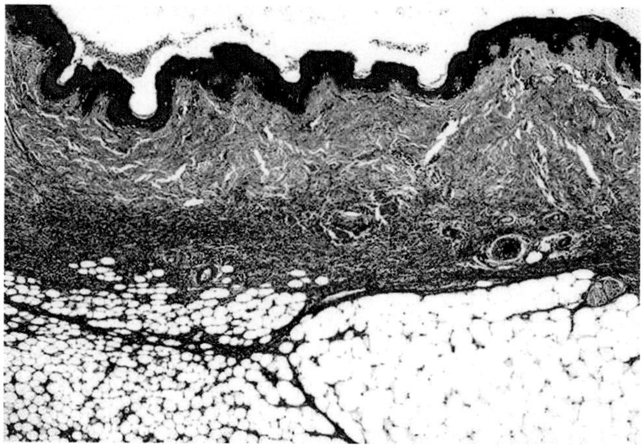

FIGURE 13.28 "Atrophic" dermatofibrosarcoma shows irregular growth into the subcutis and can be difficult to recognize diagnostically. CD34 immunolabeling is a valuable diagnostic adjunct.

latter lesion are also apropos of atypical fibroxanthoma. CD99 has been touted by some authors as a helpful marker of AFX,[280] but the authors' experience with it has not corroborated that contention. Many cases of AFX studied in the authors' laboratory have been CD99 negative; conversely, the authors and others have also observed CD99 reactivity in DFSP, solitary fibrous tumor, and even spindle-cell melanoma.[281] CD10 is associated with similar comments. Despite the fact that AFX usually expresses that marker, more than 50% of sarcomatoid squamous carcinomas and some sarcomatoid melanomas do so as well.[282-285]

Dermatofibromas and their variants (e.g., nodular histiocytoma, xanthogranuloma, transitional histiocytoma, nodular subepidermal fibroma, aneurysmal cutaneous fibrous histiocytoma, palisading fibrous histiocytoma, epithelioid reticulohistiocytoma) all share reactivity for vimentin, factor XIIIa, CD10, CD68,

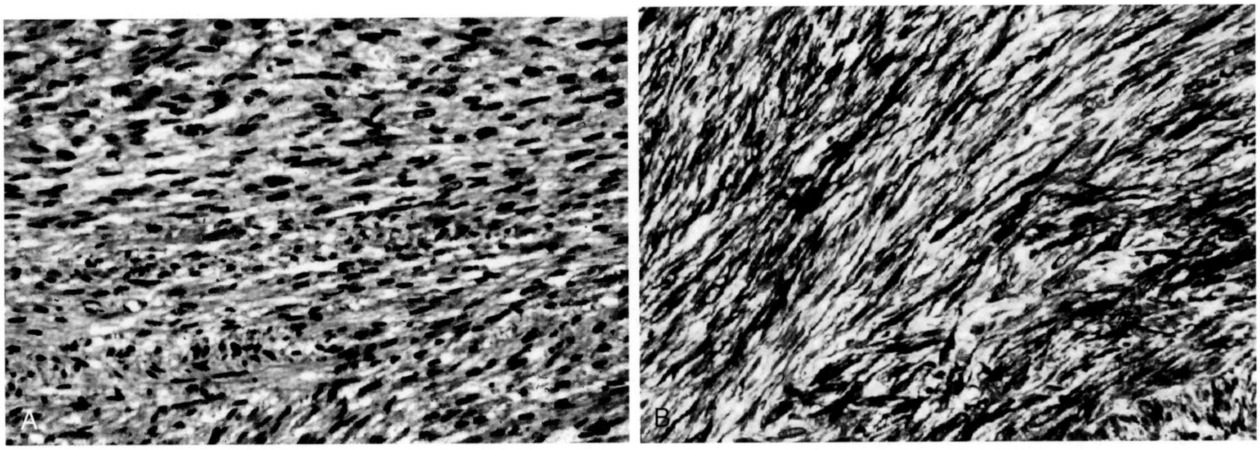

FIGURE 13.29 Leiomyosarcoma of the subcutis **(A)**, showing diffuse labeling for desmin **(B)**.

CD163, and stromelysin-3.[286-289] However, the morphologic attributes of these lesions are typically distinctive enough that immunohistochemical studies are not necessary for their recognition except in small biopsy samples.

KEY DIAGNOSTIC POINTS

Fibrohistiocytic Tumors

- DFSP is diffusely CD34+, factor XIIIa–; dermatofibroma is CD34–, factor XIIIa+; leading edge of dermatofibromas may be CD34+.
- MFH and AFX have no specific immunoprofile.

Tumors with "Pure" or Partial Smooth Muscle Differentiation

As is true of extracutaneous leiomyomas and leiomyosarcomas, those in the skin are diffusely labeled by antibodies to vimentin, desmin, caldesmon, and muscle-related actins (Fig. 13.29).[290-295] Nonetheless, one must recognize that the latter immunoprofile is not specific; myofibroblastic proliferations including cellular scars, post-traumatic spindle-cell nodules, and nodular fasciitis also exhibit a comparable "myogenic" immunophenotype. Therefore the integration of immunophenotypes together with morphologic findings is paramount diagnostically in this specific setting.

Some immunohistologic peculiarities exist in reference to smooth muscle tumors of the skin. Roughly 30% of dermal leiomyomas and leiomyosarcomas are S-100 protein reactive, and a similar proportion of subcuticular tumors are labeled for CD57.[290] It has been speculated that those findings reflect pilar-smooth muscular and vascular-smooth muscular differentiation, respectively. They have practical importance as well because of shared patterns of reactivity with peripheral nerve sheath tumors of the skin. Fortunately, few of the latter lesions are expected to exhibit positivity for myogenic markers, as seen in smooth muscle tumors.

Another contentious issue concerns the "aberrant" expression of keratin and EMA in smooth muscle tumors. Although some authors have reported a high incidence of that phenomenon in general, with no particular reference to specific soft tissue sites,[296] the authors' experience indicates that cutaneous leiomyomas and leiomyosarcomas only rarely show the presence of epithelial markers.

Glomus tumors, glomangiomas, myopericytomas, and glomangiosarcomas are also related to tumors of smooth muscle, in that they show features of specialized perivascular smooth muscle (pericytic) differentiation.[297-301] However, they differ from other myogenous tumors in that desmin positivity is usually absent. It has been suggested in the past that glomangiocellular tumors should be classified as vascular neoplasms; however, they lack specific endothelial markers and, therefore, the authors believe that assertion to be incorrect. Nevertheless, reactivity for CD34 may be seen occasionally in glomus tumors.[302]

Still other cutaneous lesions with partial myogenous differentiation are represented by so-called "PEComas" (tumors of perivascular epithelioid cells), also known as "myomelanocytomas." Although such neoplasms have been reported in the skin only relatively recently,[303] they are analogous in every way to PEComas in the lung, kidney, and soft tissue.[304] A histologic composition by epithelioid and fusiform cells with variably granular or clear cytoplasm is typical (Fig. 13.30). The term "myomelanocytoma" is preferred for these tumors by the authors because of its descriptive nature, reflecting immunoreactivity for HMB-45, tyrosinase, MART-1, or PNL2, together with muscle-specific actin or desmin.[304]

Nerve Sheath Tumors

The most common cutaneous nerve sheath tumors are neurofibromas; often, such tumors are multiple and occur in the setting of von Recklinghausen's neurofibromatosis. Neurilemmomas (schwannomas), granular cell tumors, perineuriomas, and neurothekeomas are represented in the skin as well.[305] In contrast, *malignant* cutaneous peripheral nerve sheath tumors are rare.[230,306-308]

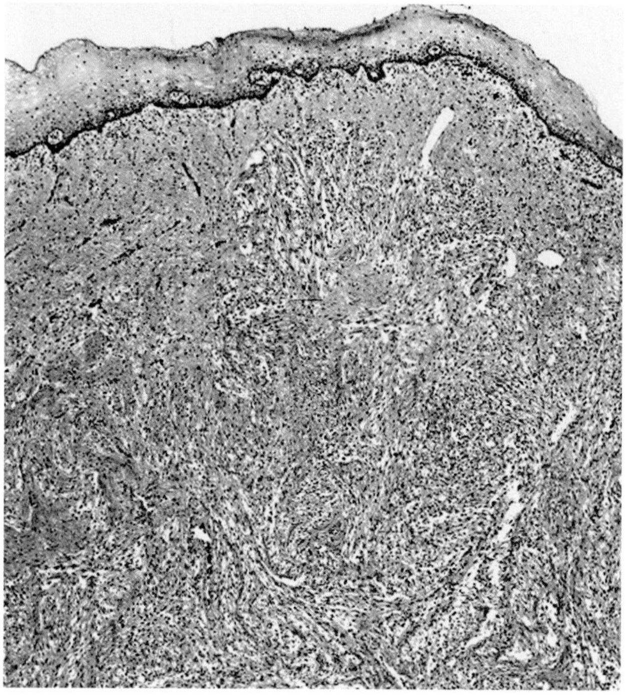

FIGURE 13.30 Myomelanocytoma of the skin.

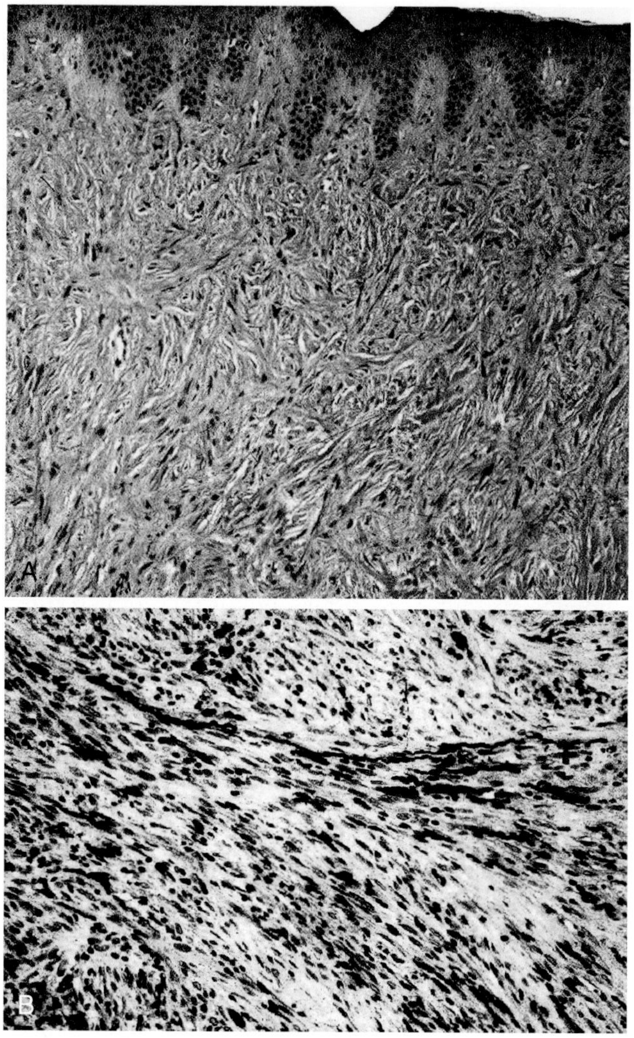

FIGURE 13.31 Malignant peripheral nerve sheath tumor of the dermis in a patient with neurofibromatosis **(A).** The tumor shows multifocal staining for S-100 protein **(B).**

Most arise primarily in the dermis or subcutaneous tissues, but secondary involvement of the skin by more deeply seated lesions may also occur.

The immunophenotypic attributes that typify most peripheral nerve sheath tumors (PNSTs) include staining for vimentin, along with S-100 protein, CD56, or CD57 (Fig. 13.31).[306,309-311]

Detection of the latter three markers, alone or in combination, provides for the reliable identification of PNSTs if all myogenous and epithelial determinants are concurrently absent. In particular, neurilemmoma essentially always shows diffuse and intense reactivity for S-100 protein, but neurofibromas are more heterogeneous immunohistologically.[310] Other determinants also have been detected in selected PNSTs including glial fibrillary acidic protein, neuron-specific enolase, and nerve growth factor receptor.[310,312]

It is commonly accepted that most granular cell tumors (GCTs) of the skin show Schwann cell differentiation,[313] but some examples of leiomyoma, leiomyosarcoma, BCC, and angiosarcoma also may demonstrate a granular-cell appearance.[314,315] Accordingly, most (80%) but not all granular-cell tumors are reactive for S-100 protein,[316] CD56, or CD57. GCT also shares with neurofibroma (but not neurilemmoma) the expression of factor XIIIa,[244] and it is also potentially reactive for protein gene product 9.5, calretinin, and inhibin (Fig. 13.32).[317] Malignant GCTs of the skin are exceedingly rare, but, like their benign counterparts, most exhibit nerve sheath differentiation.

Perineuriomas are distinctive PNSTs that are uncommon in the skin.[318-332] They are heterogeneous morphologically; some demonstrate a constituency of bland spindle cells that form vaguely concentric profiles in partially myxoid stroma, whereas others may resemble dermatofibroma, solitary fibrous tumor, or storiform collagenoma.[328] Additional variants show a reticular or plexiform architecture.[329] The hallmark of these lesions is their lack of markers that are usually associated with Schwann cells, as discussed earlier, an absence of keratin, and consistent positivity for EMA (Fig. 13.33).[324,330] That profile parallels the immunophenotype of non-neoplastic perineurial fibroblasts. Differential diagnosis from cutaneous meningothelial proliferations, which share a closely similar immunoprofile, relies largely on morphologic and ultrastructural evaluation.[323] Folpe and colleagues[333] have also cited the use of claudin-1 (a tight junction-associated protein) in the identification of perineurial cell tumors.

Neurothekeomas (NTKs) are distinctive and probably heterogeneous neoplasms that are only seen in the skin, in the authors' opinion. They have been subdivided nosologically into three groups: "conventional" NTK, "dermal nerve sheath myxoma," and "cellular NTK."[305,334] The first of those categories shows variable reactivity for schwannian and neuroectodermal markers,[327,334,335] the second group typically labels for vimentin and S-100

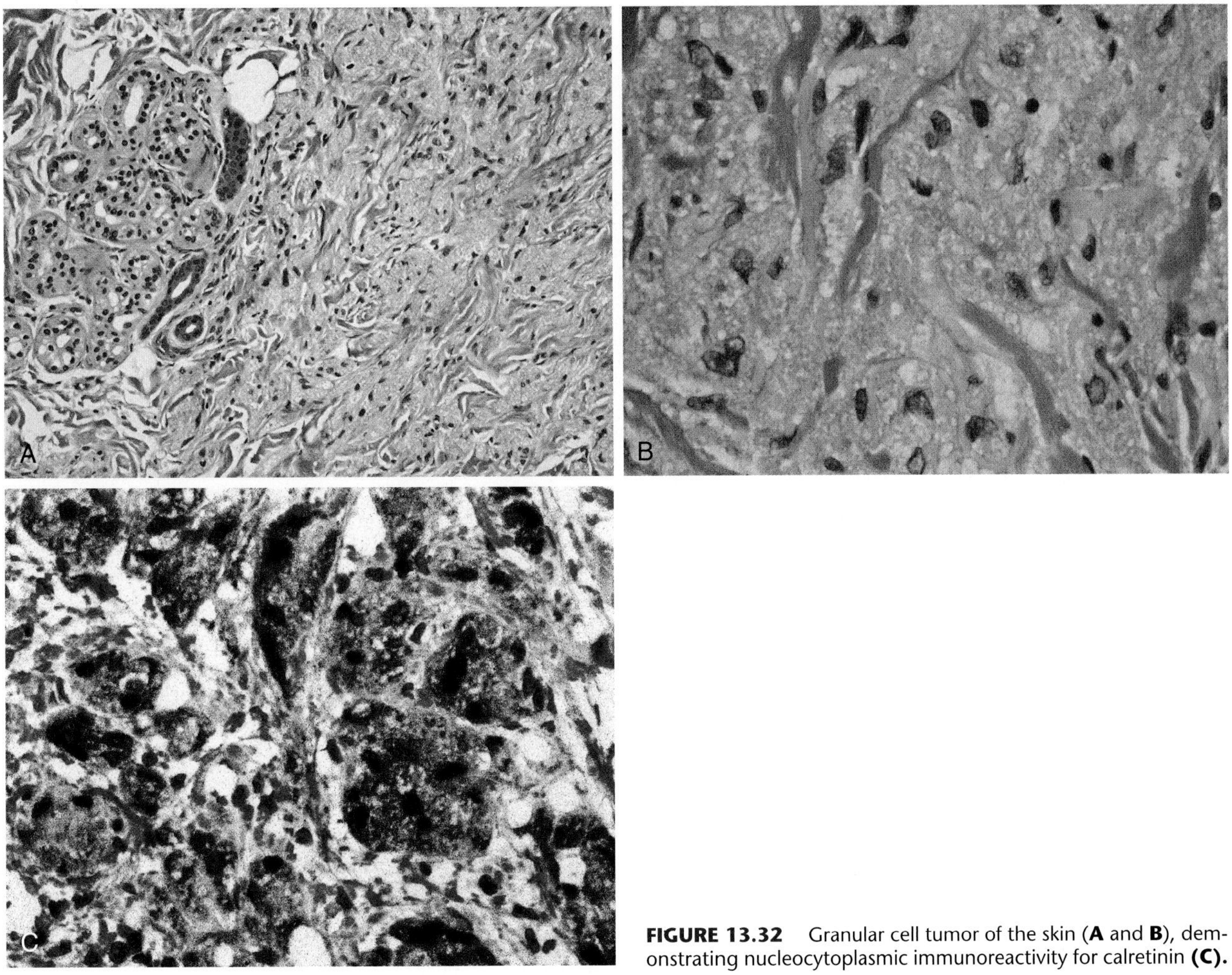

FIGURE 13.32 Granular cell tumor of the skin (**A** and **B**), demonstrating nucleocytoplasmic immunoreactivity for calretinin **(C)**.

protein (Fig. 13.34),[336] and the third shows myogenous or "histiocytic" features (with actin or CD68 reactivity) rather than neural characteristics.[37-340]

KEY DIAGNOSTIC POINTS

Peripheral Nerve Sheath Tumors

- S-100 distribution dependent on pattern
- Typically CD56+, CD57+
- Granular cell tumors and neurofibromas: factor XIIIa+, calretinin+, inhibin+
- Perineuriomas EMA+, negative for other markers

Vascular Neoplasms

Perhaps because of the wide spectrum of morphologic images associated with vascular tumors of the skin, a great deal of attention has been paid to their immunohistochemical characterization.[341] At this point, several potential markers of endothelial differentiation are available for clinical use, but most of them need to be employed with several other reagents to allow for a final diagnostic conclusion. That is true because neoplastic endothelial cells have the potential to express some proteins that are not seen in nontumoral blood vessels, and which are also shared with nonvascular neoplasms. The latter statement principally applies to malignant tumors, but some hemangiomas also may exhibit unexpected immunophenotypes in selected instances. In the interest of brevity, the many individual cutaneous vascular tumor entities that are now recognized[342] are not considered here. Instead, they are discussed as a group, with special comments on selected lesions.

The determinants that are generically associated with endothelial differentiation include factor VIII-related antigen (von Willebrand factor [vWF]); CD31, CD34, CD141 (thrombomodulin), FLI-1, vascular endothelial growth factor receptor-3 (VEGFR3), podoplanin (PPN), and fucose-rich cell membrane binding sites for *Ulex europaeus* I lectin (UEL) (Fig. 13.35).[343-351] Of those, the last four have sufficient sensitivity to recommend their use in diagnostic work, but vWF does not. Another issue that is of conceptual interest to some people is whether endothelial lesions show *vascular*-endothelial or *lymphatic*-endothelial differentiation.[350] The authors consider that topic to be peripheral to practical dermatopathology and it is not addressed further.

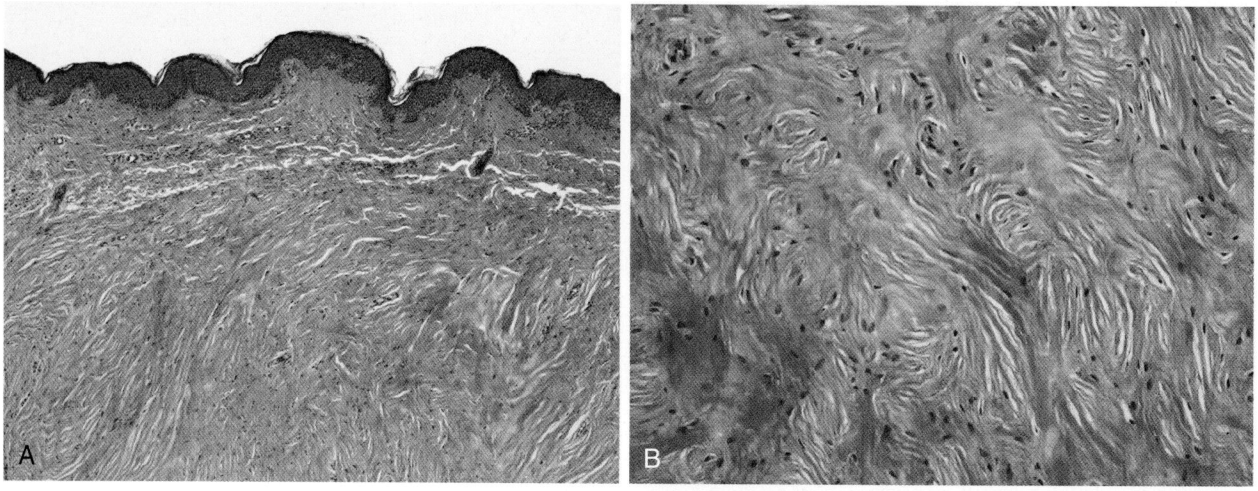

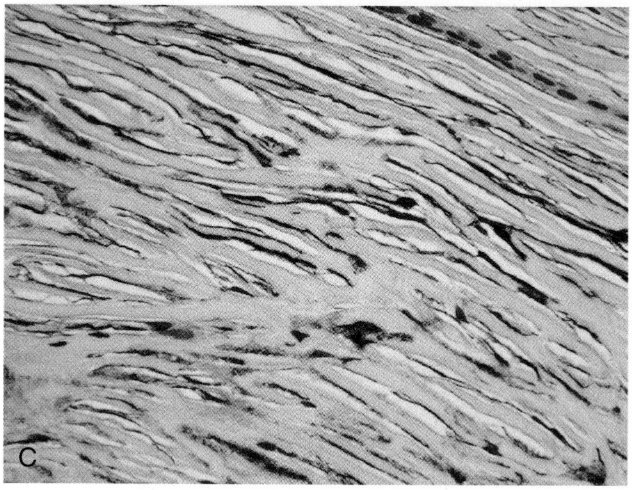

FIGURE 13.33 Cutaneous perineurioma (**A** and **B**), showing diffuse positivity for epithelial membrane antigen **(C)**.

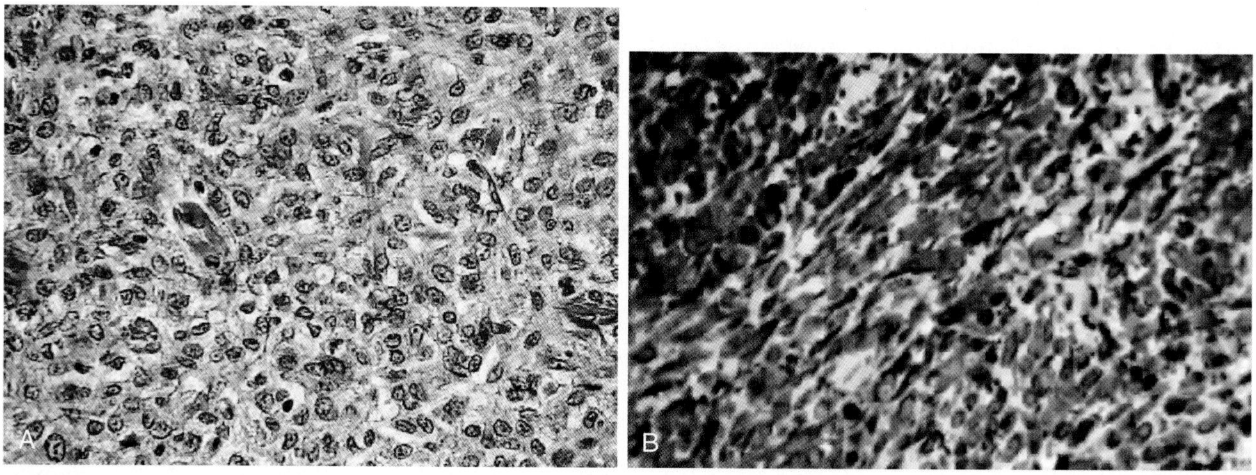

FIGURE 13.34 "Cellular neurothekeoma" **(A)** shows a "histiocytic" phenotype in this case, with diffuse labeling of the tumor cells for CD68 **(B)** and an absence of other specialized determinants.

The usual approach to characterization of a vascular tumor is to employ a battery of endothelial-selective markers together with several reagents directed at epithelial and muscle-related determinants. That is because selected endothelial tumors may histologically simulate carcinomas or sarcomas with myogenic differentiation (and vice versa). Moreover, epithelioid vascular neoplasms have a recognized capacity for "aberrant" keratin synthesis[352,353]; thus it is essential that other potential indicators of epithelial differentiation—such as EMA, p63, E-cadherin, and desmoplakin—should be evaluated along with CD31, CD34, CD141, FLI-1,

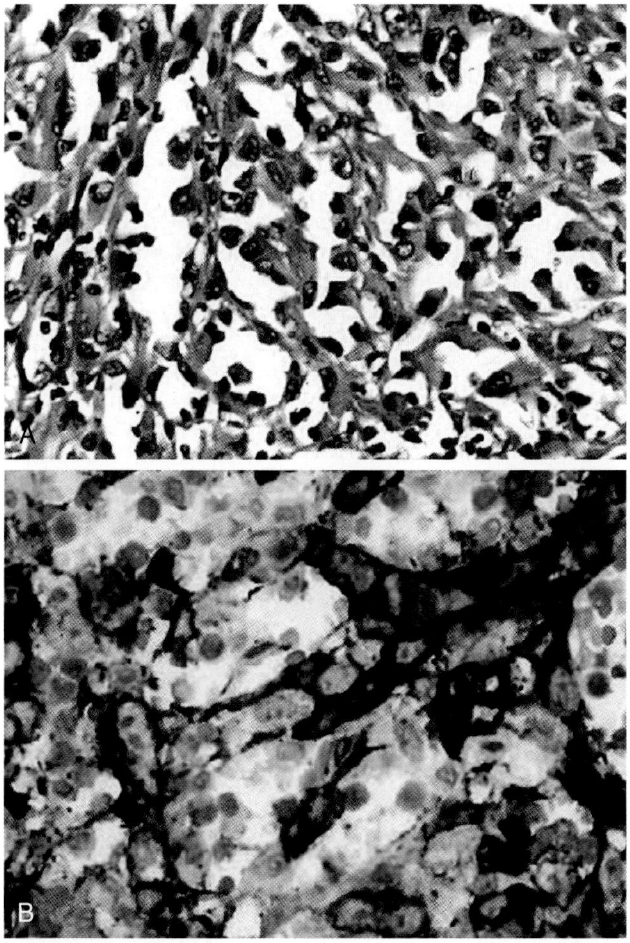

FIGURE 13.35 Cutaneous angiosarcoma **(A)**, showing immunoreactivity for CD31 **(B)**.

VEGFR2, PPN, or UEL binding before making a final interpretation.

Until recently, immunohistology had little if any role in the diagnosis of Kaposi's sarcoma (KS), one of the most common vascular malignancies. That was true because in its "patch" stage, KS is easily recognizable on morphologic grounds alone, whereas in its spindle-cell or "nodular" stage, the tumor cells in KS tend to lose endothelial-related markers. However, several studies have now shown that an antibody to human herpesvirus 8–latent nuclear antigen-1 (HH8LNA) is highly selective for KS regardless of its morphologic iterations (Fig. 13.36). The majority of KS cases (80% in our experience) are labeled for that marker, whereas none of its morphologic simulators shows HH8LNA reactivity.[354-356]

Lesions classified as "hemangioendotheliomas," generally conceptualized as "borderline" endothelial tumors, have increased in number in recent years.[357-360] These have immunophenotypes that parallel those of other vascular neoplasms, with one notable exception. Billings and colleagues have described a peculiar tumor in this group that closely simulates the image of epithelioid sarcoma (EPS, see next section) on conventional microscopy.[361] It has accordingly been named "epithelioid sarcoma-like hemangioendothelioma" (Fig. 13.37) (ESLH). Indeed, that entity shares immunoreactivity for keratin and vimentin with true EPS, but ESLH paradoxically lacks CD34 (which is seen in EPS[362] and most other hemangioendotheliomas) and additionally labels for CD31 and FLI-1.

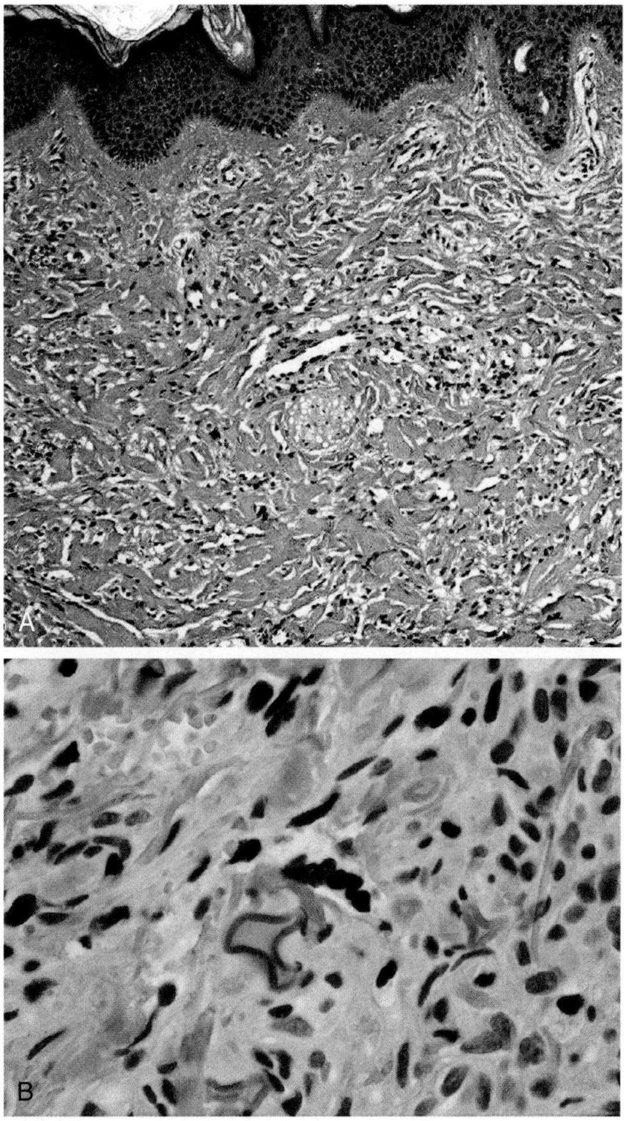

FIGURE 13.36 Kaposi sarcoma of the skin **(A)** demonstrates nuclear positivity for human herpesvirus 8–latent nuclear antigen-1 **(B)**.

KEY DIAGNOSTIC POINTS

Vascular Neoplasms

- Best panel includes CD31, CD141, CD34, and FLI-1 or Ulex.
- Epithelioid angiosarcomas often show expression of keratin with both AE1/AE3 and CAM5.2, emphasizing the need to use the vascular panel to avoid diagnostic pitfall.
- Antibody HH8LNA (herpesvirus latent nuclear antigen) is highly sensitive and specific for Kaposi's sarcoma.
- ESLH is positive for CD31 and FLI-1 but negative for CD34, whereas epithelioid sarcoma is CD34+.

Epithelioid Sarcoma

EPS is a polygonal-cell neoplasm of the dermis and subcutis that may assume varied microscopic appearances.[363] These may easily result in its confusion with other lesions.

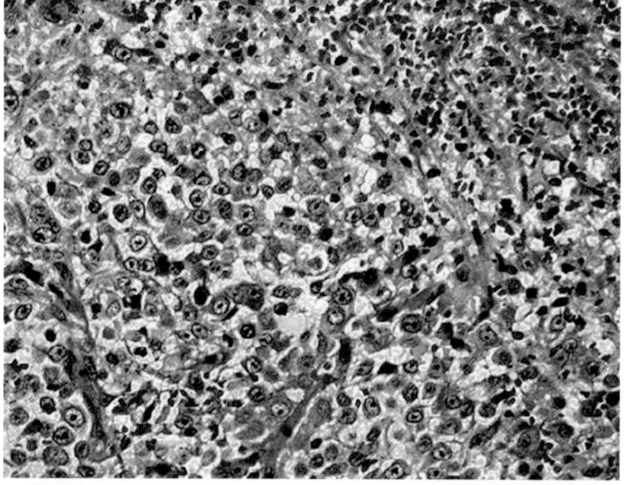

FIGURE 13.37 Epithelioid sarcoma-like hemangioendothelioma of the subcutis. This tumor is unusual among endothelial lesions in that it is reproducibly keratin positive, but it lacks CD34. CD31 staining is also typical.

When it manifests a predominantly solid pattern of growth, EPS may be mistaken for metastatic carcinoma or malignant melanoma; alternatively, a granulomatoid pattern of growth, with palisading of neoplastic cells around areas of necrosis, can impart a similarity to necrobiotic granulomas (e.g., rheumatoid nodule, deep granuloma annulare). Pseudoangiomatous areas in EPS may likewise make the histologic separation of that tumor from hemangioendotheliomas a challenge.[361,363-365]

Among epithelioid mesenchymal tumors of the superficial soft tissues, only EPS is *consistently* immunoreactive for keratin (Fig. 13.38)[363,366-369]; this attribute is shared by some monophasic synovial sarcomas, but the latter lesions are more typically situated in the deeper soft tissues. Keratin reactivity in epithelioid vascular neoplasms[370] has also been considered in the previous section. The potential immunophenotypic overlap between EPS and metastatic carcinoma is accentuated by the presence of EMA in 70% to 80% of EPS cases and CA-125 in some examples.[363-365,371,372] Virtually all examples of EPS demonstrate CD34 positivity as well,[362] however, and that marker is rare in carcinoma. In contrast, Lin and colleagues[373] and Laskin and Miettinen[369] have shown that reactivity for keratin 5/6 and p63 protein is consistent in SCC, but it is lacking in most examples of EPS. A similar pattern pertains to E-cadherin reactivity.[369,374] The separation of EPS from

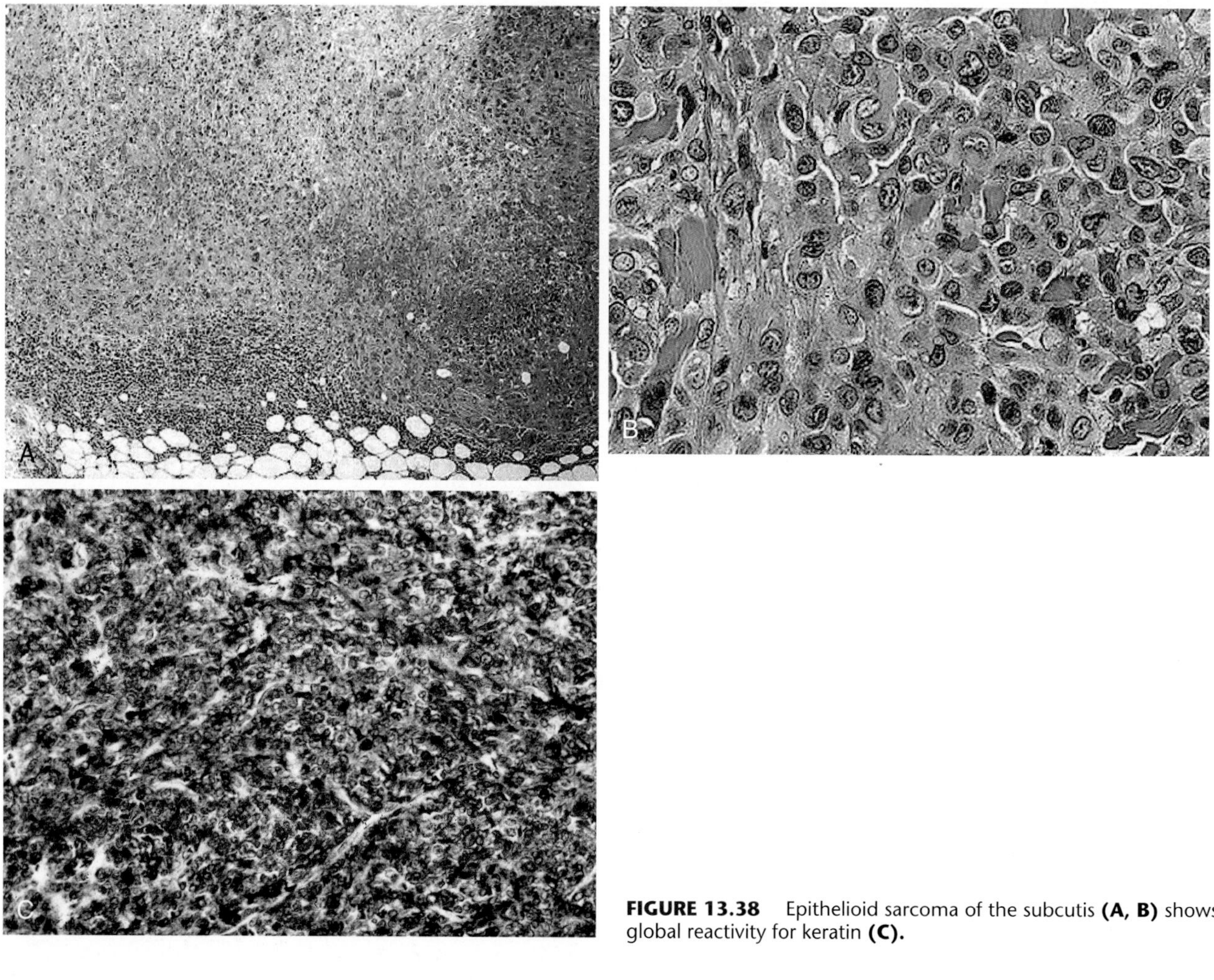

FIGURE 13.38 Epithelioid sarcoma of the subcutis **(A, B)** shows global reactivity for keratin **(C)**.

melanoma or clear cell sarcoma (melanoma of soft parts) is more straightforward because fewer than 15% of EPS cases are S-100 protein reactive and none of them manifests labeling for HMB-45, tyrosinase, or MART-1, as seen in melanocytic lesions.[363]

As mentioned earlier, the distinction between EPS and ESLH principally relies on a demonstration of specific endothelial markers in the latter of those neoplasms. CD31 and FLI-1 are the most discriminatory.[361] In fact, the same rule applies to the diagnostic separation between all vascular tumors and EPS.

SMALL ROUND CELL MESENCHYMAL TUMORS

Small cell neoplasms of the skin and subcutis may include Merkel cell carcinoma, small cell squamous carcinoma, small cell eccrine carcinoma, small cell melanoma, peripheral neuroectodermal tumor/ extraskeletal Ewing's sarcoma (PNET/ES), lymphoma, or rhabdomyosarcoma (RMS) (Fig. 13.39).[117,375] Mesenchymal tumors in that group constitute a small minority. RMS consistently expresses desmin, myogenin, and muscle-specific actin, in the absence of keratin, whereas PNET/ES uniformly exhibits CD99 reactivity and may be labeled for CD56, CD57, and synaptophysin, as well as focally for keratin.[112-117] Neither of those tumor groups is reactive for EMA, CD45, S-100 protein, CEA, or HMB-45.

SPECIAL TOPICS IN CUTANEOUS IMMUNOHISTOCHEMISTRY

Estrogen and Progesterone Receptor Proteins

Selected hormone receptor proteins were originally targeted as diagnostic discriminants between eccrine carcinomas and histologically similar metastases of mammary carcinoma.[376] However, that expectation was not realized. Several analyses have shown that estrogen receptor protein (ERP) is common in selected benign apocrine neoplasms (especially hidradenoma papilliferum), as well as eccrine carcinomas (Fig. 13.40).[377-380] Progesterone receptor proteins (PRPs) may also be present in some eccrine carcinomas.[380,381] The relationship of these observations to prognosis or treatment/response of the immunoreactive lesions is unclear because systematic therapeutic trials of hormonal antagonists have not been attempted for sweat gland carcinomas as yet. Interestingly, examples of apocrine adenocarcinoma or extramammary Paget disease typically *fail* to stain for ERP or PRP.[376,377]

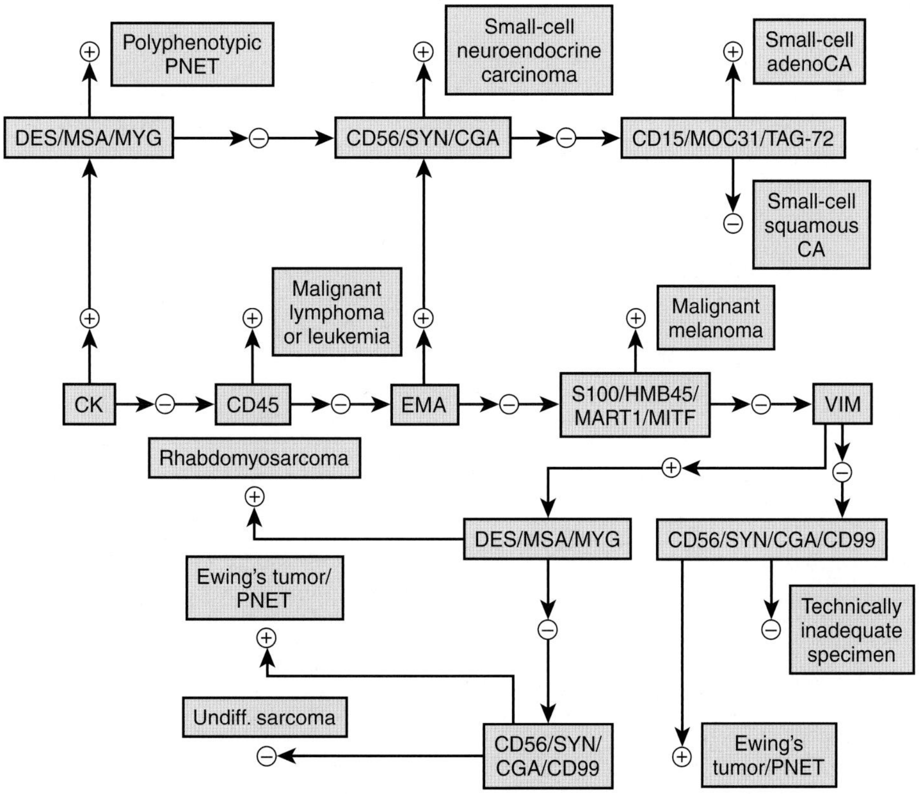

FIGURE 13.39 Algorithm showing the sequence of immunohistologic interpretation associated with diagnosis of small-cell undifferentiated tumors of the skin and subcutis (CK, cytokeratin; DES, desmin; MSA, muscle-specific actin; MYG, myogenin; SYN, synaptophysin; CGA, chromogranin A; TAG-72, tumor-associated glycoprotein-72 [CA72.4]; EMA, epithelial membrane antigen; MITF, microophthalmia transcription factor; PNET, primitive neuroectodermal tumor; AdenoCA, adenocarcinoma; CA, carcinoma; Undiff., undifferentiated).

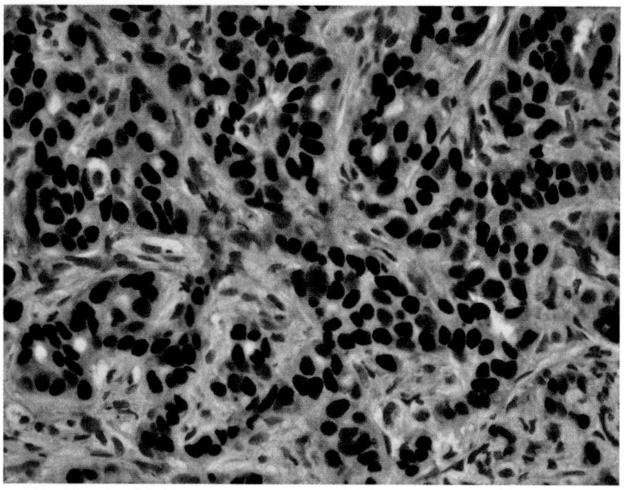

FIGURE 13.40 Positivity for estrogen receptor protein in primary eccrine carcinoma of the skin.

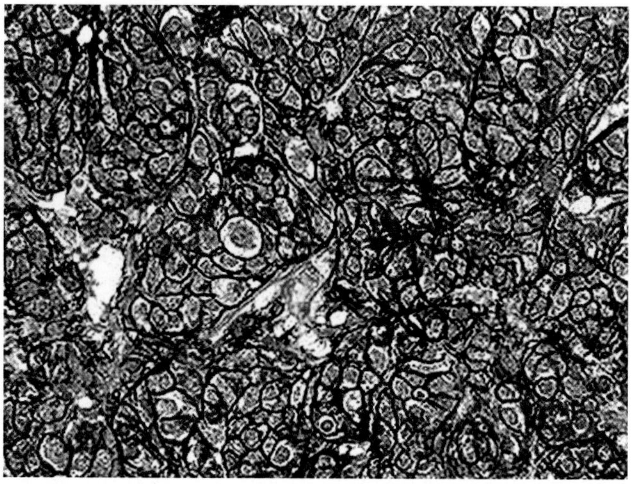

FIGURE 13.41 Diffuse reactivity for epidermal growth factor receptor in poorly differentiated squamous cell carcinoma of the skin.

Oncogenes and Other Possibly Prognostic Markers

The role of oncogene expression in the initiation and modulation of neoplastic growth in the skin has considerable interest, but it is an area that has yet to yield an abundance of practical information. Two oncogenes that have been studied in detail in the skin are epidermal growth factor receptor (EGFR) and the *c-erbB-2* (neu) oncogene. The latter is a 185 kD transmembrane glycoprotein with tyrosine kinase activity that is functionally and structurally related to the 175 kD EGFR gene product. Although its precise role in cell differentiation and proliferation is uncertain, it appears to function as a true growth factor receptor when expressed in its physiologic state. In normally differentiated and developing cells, native forms of both EGFR and *c-erbB-2* are expressed, but each may be altered or overexpressed in certain epithelial neoplasms.

Not surprisingly, EGFR expression is characteristic of SCC (Fig. 13.41),[383,384] but there is little evidence that the presence or amount of the native receptor molecule or truncated forms of it is related to either the grade or clinical behavior of SCC. EGFR has also been detected in BCC, but fewer than 50% of such lesions are immunoreactive.[383,384] EGFR may also be encountered in benign keratinocytic proliferations including acrochordons and seborrheic keratoses, as well as adnexal carcinomas of the skin.[380,385] The receptor is increased in density in the latter lesions in pregnant women, patients who are taking exogenous estrogenic or progestational hormones, and those who have the dysplastic nevus syndrome.[385]

Although *c-erbB-2* is overexpressed in some aggressive breast carcinomas, that molecule does not seem to reproducibly predict unfavorable behavior in malignant sudoriferous neoplasms. In our analysis of eccrine carcinoma, 27% exhibited *c-erbB-2*-immunoreactivity; all of those tumors were of low or moderate grade, and none metastasized or recurred (Swanson PE, Wick MR; unpublished observations). In contrast, Hasebe and colleagues[386] did report a relationship between *c-erbB-2* expression and prognosis in sweat gland carcinomas. Extramammary Paget disease also may stain for *c-erbB-2*.[387]

CD44 is a cell-surface protein involved in cell-to-cell and cell-to-matrix adhesion and lymphocyte-homing activity. It is expressed in epidermal keratinocytes, hair follicles, and sebaceous and eccrine cells.[388,389] Aberrant CD44 expression has been reported in a variety of tumors, and expression of CD44 has been correlated with more aggressive behavior. For example, BCCs do not exhibit immunolabeling for CD44, in contrast to squamous cell carcinomas and metastatic adenocarcinomas, in which almost 100% of cells are labeled.[390] CD44 expression by Merkel cell carcinoma also may correlate with metastatic risk.[391]

It is clear that we do not yet know how, or to what extent, many single oncogenes initiate or modulate the intracellular cascade of events that results in uncontrolled cellular growth. Although some oncogene products can immortalize cells or maintain a transformed phenotype of cells in culture, the ultimate importance of many of these effects *in vitro* is not yet understood. There may well be validity to claims that overexpression of various oncopeptides may relate to the aggressiveness of cutaneous tumors, but it seems unlikely that any one of them will have sufficient importance to serve as an independent predictor of behavior. Modeling of future studies to correlate oncogene expression with histopathologic or clinical data should rely on analyses of *several* oncogene products in concert, in a manner analogous to the immunophenotypic panels that aid the diagnostic pathologist.

REFERENCES

1. Lohmann CM, Solomon AR. Clinicopathologic variants of cutaneous squamous cell carcinoma. *Adv Anat Pathol.* 2001;8:27-36.
2. Petter G, Haustein UF. Histologic subtyping and malignancy: assessment of cutaneous squamous cell carcinoma. *Dermatol Surg.* 2000;26:521-530.

3. Nappi O, Pettinato G, Wick MR. Adenoid (acantholytic) squamous cell carcinoma of the skin. *J Cutan Pathol.* 1989;16:114-121.
4. van Muijen GNP, Ruiter DJ, Ponec M, et al. Monoclonal antibodies with different specificities against cytokeratins: an immunohistochemical study of normal tissues and tumors. *Am J Pathol.* 1984;114:9-17.
5. Reis-Filho JS, Simpson PT, Martins A, et al. Distribution of p63, cytokeratins 5/6 and cytokeratin 14 in 51 normal and 400 neoplastic human tissue samples using TARP-4 multi-tumor tissue microarray. *Virchows Arch.* 2003;443:122-132.
6. Dotto JE, Glusac EJ. p63 is a useful marker for cutaneous spindle-cell squamous cell carcinoma. *J Cutan Pathol.* 2006;33:413-417.
7. Suo Z, Holm R, Nesland JM. Squamous cell carcinomas: an immunohistochemical study of cytokeratins and involucrin in primary and metastatic tumors. *Histopathology.* 1993;23:45-54.
8. Sigel JE, Skacel M, Bergfeld WF, et al. The utility of cytokeratin 5/6 in the recognition of cutaneous spindle cell squamous cell carcinoma. *J Cutan Pathol.* 2001;28:520-524.
9. Wick MR, Fitzgibbon JF, Swanson PE. Cutaneous sarcomas and sarcomatoid neoplasms of the skin. *Semin Diagn Pathol.* 1993;10:148-158.
10. Pinkus GS, Kurtin PJ. Epithelial membrane antigen: a diagnostic discriminant in surgical pathology. *Hum Pathol.* 1985;16:929-940.
11. Egawa K, Honda Y, Ono T, et al. Immunohistochemical demonstration of carcinoembryonic antigen and related antigens in various cutaneous keratinous neoplasms and verruca vulgaris. *Br J Dermatol.* 1998;139:178-185.
12. Dale BA, Gown AM, Fleckman P, et al. Characterization of two monoclonal antibodies to human epidermal keratohyaline: reactivity with filaggrin and related proteins. *J Invest Dermatol.* 1987;88:306-313.
13. Hashimoto T, Inamato N, Nakamura K, et al. Involucrin expression in skin appendage tumors. *Br J Dermatol.* 1987;117:325-332.
14. Klein-Szanto AJP, Barr RJ, Reiners JJ, et al. Filaggrin distribution in keratoacanthomas and squamous cell carcinomas. *Arch Pathol Lab Med.* 1984;108:888-890.
15. Said JW, Sassoon AF, Shintaku JP, et al. Involucrin in squamous and basal cell carcinomas of the skin: an immunohistochemical study. *J Invest Dermatol.* 1984;82:449-452.
16. Smoller BR, Kwan TH, Said JW. Keratoacanthoma and squamous cell carcinoma of the skin: immunohistochemical localization of involucrin and keratin proteins. *J Am Acad Dermatol.* 1986;14:225-236.
17. Murphy CF, Flynn RC, Rice RH, et al. Involucrin expression in normal and neoplastic human skin: a marker for keratinocyte differentiation. *J Invest Dermatol.* 1984;82:453-457.
18. Kanitakis J, Zambruno G, Viae J, et al. Involucrin expression in adnexal skin tumors: an immunohistochemical study. *Virchows Archiv.* 1986;408:527-540.
19. Strutton GM. Pathological variants of basal cell carcinoma. *Australas J Dermatol.* 1997;38(Suppl 1):S31-S35.
20. Shimizu N, Ito M, Tazawa T, et al. Immunohistochemical study of keratin expression in certain cutaneous epithelial neoplasms. Basal cell carcinoma, pilomatricoma, and seborrheic keratosis. *Am J Dermatopathol.* 1989;11:534-540.
21. Heyderman E, Graham RM, Chapman DV, et al. Epithelial markers in primary skin cancer: an immunoperoxidase study of the distribution of epithelial membrane antigen (EMA) and carcinoembryonic antigen (CEA) in 65 primary skin carcinomas. *Histopathology.* 1984;8:423-434.
22. Wick MR, Swanson PE. Primary adenoid cystic carcinoma of the skin: a clinical, histologic, and immunohistochemical comparison with adenoid cystic carcinoma of salivary glands, and adenoid basal cell carcinoma. *Am J Dermatopathol.* 1986;8:2-13.
23. George E, Swanson PE, Wick MR. Neuroendocrine differentiation in basal cell carcinoma: an immunohistochemical study. *Am J Dermatopathol.* 1989;11:131-135.
24. Foschini MP, Eusebi V. Divergent differentiation in endocrine and nonendocrine tumors of the skin. *Semin Diagn Pathol.* 2000;17:162-168.
25. Collina G, Macri L, Eusebi V. Endocrine differentiation in basocellular carcinoma. *Pathologica.* 2001;93:208-212.
26. Tsukamoto H, Hayashibe K, Mishima Y, et al. The altered expression of alpha-smooth muscle actin in basal cell epithelioma and its surrounding stroma, with special reference to proliferating cell nuclear antigen expression and adenoid differentiation. *Br J Dermatol.* 1994;130:189-194.
27. Grando SA, Schofield OM, Skubitz AP, et al. Nodular basal cell carcinoma in vivo vs. in vitro. Establishment of pure cell cultures, cytomorphologic characteristics, ultrastructure, immunophenotype, biosynthetic activities, and generation of antisera. *Arch Dermatol.* 1996;132:1185-1193.
28. Sanchez NP, Winkelmann RK. Basal cell tumor with eccrine differentiation (eccrine epithelioma). *J Am Acad Dermatol.* 1982;6:514-518.
29. Sakamoto F, Ito M, Sato S, et al. Basal cell tumor with apocrine differentiation: apocrine epithelioma. *J Am Acad Dermatol.* 1985;13:355-363.
30. Jimenez FJ, Burchette Jr JL, Grichnik JM, et al. Ber-EP4 immunoreactivity in normal skin and cutaneous neoplasms. *Mod Pathol.* 1995;8:854-858.
31. Swanson PE, Fitzpatrick MM, Ritter JH, et al. Immunohistologic differential diagnosis of basal cell carcinoma, squamous cell carcinoma, and trichoepithelioma in small cutaneous biopsy specimens. *J Cutan Pathol.* 1998;25:153-159.
32. Ko T, Muramatsu T, Shirai T. Distribution of lectin UEA-I in trichilemmal carcinoma, squamous cell carcinoma, and other epithelial tumors of the skin. *J Dermatol.* 1996;23:389-393.
33. Heng MC, Fallon-Friendlander S, Bennett R. Expression of Ulex europaeus agglutinin I lectin-binding sites in squamous cell carcinomas and their absence in basal cell carcinomas. Indicator of tumor type and differentiation. *Am J Dermatopathol.* 1992;14:216-219.
34. Urso C, Bondi R, Paglierani M, et al. Carcinomas of sweat glands: report of 60 cases. *Arch Pathol Lab Med.* 2001;125:498-505.
35. Swanson PE, Cherwitz DL, Neumann MP, et al. Eccrine sweat gland carcinoma: a histologic and immunohistochemical study of 32 cases. *J Cutan Pathol.* 1987;14:65-86.
36. Qureshi HS, Ormsby AH, Lee MW, et al. The diagnostic utility of p63, CK5/6, CK7, and CK20 in distinguishing primary cutaneous adnexal neoplasms from metastatic carcinomas. *J Cutan Pathol.* 2004;31:145-152.
37. Ivan D, Hareez-Diwan A, Prieto VG. Expression of p63 in primary cutaneous adnexal neoplasms and adenocarcinoma metastatic to the skin. *Mod Pathol.* 2005;18:137-142.
38. Kanitakis J, Chouvet B. Expression of p63 in cutaneous metastases. *Am J Clin Pathol.* 2007;128:753-758.
39. Plumb SJ, Argenyi ZB, Stone MS, DeYoung BR. Cytokeratin 5/6 immunostaining in cutaneous adnexal neoplasms and metastatic adenocarcinoma. *Am J Dermatopathol.* 2004;26:447-451.
40. Liang H, Wu H, Giorgadze TA, et al. Podoplanin is a highly sensitive and specific marker to distinguish primary skin adnexal carcinomas from adenocarcinomas metastatic to skin. *Am J Surg Pathol.* 2007;31:304-310.
41. Metze D, Grunert F, Neumaier M, et al. Neoplasms with sweat gland differentiation express various glycoproteins of the carcinoembryonic antigen (CEA) family. *J Cutan Pathol.* 1996;23:1-11.
42. Ansai S, Koseki S, Hozumi Y, et al. An immunohistochemical study of lysozyme, CD15 (Leu-M1), and gross cystic disease fluid protein-15 in various skin tumors: assessment of the specificity and sensitivity of markers of apocrine differentiation. *Am J Dermatopathol.* 1995;17:249-255.
43. Tsubura A, Senzaki H, Sasaki M, et al. Immunohistochemical demonstrated of breast-derived and/or carci-noma-associated glycoproteins in normal skin appendages and their tumors. *J Cutan Pathol.* 1992;19:73-79.
44. Santos-Juanes J, Bernaldo-de Quiros JF, Galache-Osuna C, et al. Apocrine carcinoma, adenopathies, and raised TAG72 serum tumor marker. *Dermatol Surg.* 2004;30:566-569.
45. Wick MR, Swanson PE, LeBoit PE, et al. Lymphoepithe-lioma-like carcinoma of the skin with adnexal differentiation. *J Cutan Pathol.* 1991;18:93-102.

46. Ramachandra S, Gillette CE, Millis RR. A comparative immunohistochemical study of mammary and extramammary Paget's disease and superficial spreading melanoma, with particular emphasis on melanocytic markers. *Virchows Arch*. 1996;429: 371-376.
47. Mazoujian G, Margolis R. Immunohistochemistry of gross cystic disease fluid protein (GCDFP-15) in 65 benign sweat gland tumors of the skin. *Am J Dermatopathol*. 1988;10:28-35.
48. Battles OE, Page DL, Johnson JE. Cytokeratins, CEA, and mucin histochemistry in the diagnosis and characterization of extramammary Paget's disease. *Am J Clin Pathol*. 1997;108: 6-12.
49. Hitchcock A, Topham S, Bell J, et al. Routine diagnosis of mammary and extramammary Paget's disease: a modern approach. *Am J Surg Pathol*. 1992;16:58-61.
50. Mazoujian G, Pinkus GS, Haagensen Jr DE. Extramammary Paget's disease—evidence for an apocrine origin: an immunoperoxidase study of gross cystic disease fluid protein-15, carcinoembryonic antigen, and cytokeratin proteins. *Am J Surg Pathol*. 1984;8:43-50.
51. Carvalho J, Fullen D, Lowe L, et al. The expression of CD23 in cutaneous non-lymphoid neoplasms. *J Cutan Pathol*. 2007;34:693-698.
52. Nowak MA, Guerriere-Kovach P, Pathan A, et al. Perianal Paget's disease: distinguishing primary and secondary lesions using immunohistochemical studies including gross cystic disease fluid protein-15 and cytokeratin 20 expression. *Arch Pathol Lab Med*. 1998;122:1077-1081.
53. Ohnishi T, Watanabe S. The use of cytokeratins 7 and 20 in the diagnosis of primary and secondary extramammary Paget's disease. *Br J Dermatol*. 2000;142:243-247.
54. Haga R, Suzuki H. Rectal carcinoma associated with pagetoid phenomenon. *Eur J Dermatol*. 2003;13:93-94.
55. Raju RR, Goldblum JR, Hart WR. Pagetoid squamous cell carcinoma in situ (Pagetoid Bowen's disease) of the external genitalia. *Int J Gynecol Pathol*. 2003;22:127-135.
56. Mayes DC, Patterson JW, Ramnani DM, Mills SE. Alpha-methylacyl coenzyme A racemase is immunoreactive in extramammary Paget disease. *Am J Clin Pathol*. 2007;127:567-571.
57. Nasser A, Amin MB, Sexton DG, Cohen C. Utility of alpha-methylacyl coenzyme A racemase (p504S antibody) as a diagnostic immunohistochemical marker for cancer. *Appl Immunohistochem Mol Morphol*. 2005;13:252-255.
58. Mazoujian G. Immunohistochemistry of GCDFP-24 and zinc-alpha-2-glycoprotein in benign sweat gland tumors. *Am J Dermatopathol*. 1990;12:452-457.
59. Hashimoto K, Eto H, Matsumoto M, et al. Antikeratin antibodies: production, specificity, and applications. *J Cutan Pathol*. 1983;10:529-539.
60. Ishihara M, Mehregan OR, Hashimoto K, et al. Staining of eccrine and apocrine neoplasms and metastatic adenocarcinoma with IKH-4, a monoclonal antibody specific for the eccrine gland. *J Cutan Pathol*. 1998;25:100-105.
61. Ormsby AH, Snow JL, Su WPD, et al. Diagnostic immunohistochemistry of cutaneous metastatic breast carcinoma: a statistical analysis of the utility of gross cystic disease fluid-protein-15 and estrogen receptor protein. *J Am Acad Dermatol*. 1995;32:711-716.
62. Latham JA, Redferm CP, Thody AJ, et al. Immunohistochemical markers of human sebaceous gland differentiation. *J Histochem Cytochem*. 1989;37:729-734.
63. Swanson PE. Monoclonal antibodies to human milk fat globule proteins. In: Wick MR, Siegal GP, eds. *Monoclonal Antibodies in Diagnostic Immunohistochemistry*. New York: Marcel Dekker; 1988:227-283.
64. Bayer-Garner IB, Givens V, Smoller BR. Immunohistochemical staining for androgen receptors: a sensitive marker of sebaceous differentiation. *Am J Dermatopathol*. 1999;21:426-431.
65. Shikata N, Kurokawa I, Andachi H, et al. Expression of androgen receptors in skin appendage tumors: an immunohistochemical study. *J Cutan Pathol*. 1995;22:149-153.
66. Browning L, Bailey D, Parker A. D2-40 is a sensitive and specific marker in differentiating primary adrenal cortical tumors from both metastatic clear cell renal cell carcinoma and pheochromocytoma. *J Clin Pathol*. 2008;61:293-296.
67. Perna AG, Smith MJ, Krishnan B, Reed JA. CD10 is expressed in cutaneous clear cell lesions of different histogenesis. *J Cutan Pathol*. 2005;32:248-251.
68. Bahrami S, Malone JC, Lear S, Martin AW. CD10 expression in cutaneous adnexal neoplasms and a potential role for differentiating cutaneous metastatic renal cell carcinoma. *Arch Pathol Lab Med*. 2006;130:1315-1319.
69. Headington JT. Tumors of the hair follicle: a review. *Am J Pathol*. 1976;85:480-505.
70. Manivel JC, Wick MR, Mukai K. Pilomatrix carcinoma: an immunohistochemical comparison with benign pilomatrixoma and other benign cutaneous lesions of pilar origin. *J Cutan Pathol*. 1986;13:22-29.
71. Basarab TG, Orchard R, Russell-Jones R. The use of immunostaining for bcl-2 and CD34 and the lectin peanut agglutinin in differentiating between basal cell carcinoma and trichoepithelioma. *Am J Dermatopathol*. 1998;20:448-452.
72. Kirchmann TT, Prieto VG, Smoller BR. CD34 staining pattern distinguishes basal cell carcinoma from trichoepithelioma. *Arch Dermatol*. 1994;21:332-336.
73. Lum CA, Binder SW. Proliferative characterization of basal cell carcinoma and trichoepithelioma in small biopsy specimens. *J Cutan Pathol*. 2004;31:550-554.
74. Poniecka AW, Alexis JB. An immunohistochemical study of basal cell carcinoma and trichoepithelioma. *Am J Dermatopathol*. 1999;21:332-336.
75. Hunt SJ, Abell E. Malignant hair matrix tumor ("malignant trichoepithelioma") arising in the setting of multiple hereditary trichoepithelioma. *Am J Dermatopathol*. 1991;13:275-281.
76. Johnson SC, Bennett RG. Occurrence of basal cell carcinoma among multiple trichoepitheliomas. *J Am Acad Dermatol*. 1993;28:322-326.
77. Wallace ML, Smoller BR. Trichoepithelioma with an adjacent basal cell carcinoma: transformation or collision?. *J Am Acad Dermatol*. 1997;37:343-345.
78. Yamamoto N, Gonda K. Multiple trichoepitheliomas with basal cell carcinoma. *Ann Plast Surg*. 1999;43:221-222.
79. Martinez CA, Priolli DG, Piovesan H, et al. Nonsolitary giant perianal trichoepithelioma with malignant transformation into basal cell carcinoma: report of a case and review of the literature. *Dis Colon Rectum*. 2004;47:773-777.
80. Harada H, Hashimoto K, Toi Y, et al. Basal cell carcinoma occurring in multiple familial trichoepithelioma: detection of loss of heterozygosity in chromosome 9q. *Arch Dermatol*. 1997;133:666-667.
81. Hartschuh W, Schulz T. Merkel cells are integral constituents of desmoplastic trichoepithelioma: an immunohistochemical and electron microscopic study. *J Cutan Pathol*. 1995;22:413-421.
82. Abesamis-Cubillan E, El-Shabrawi-Caelen L, LeBoit PE. Merkel cells and sclerosing epithelial neoplasms. *Am J Dermatopathol*. 2000;22:311-315.
83. Thewes M, Worret WI, Engst R, et al. Stromelysin-3: a potent marker for histopathologic differentiation between desmoplastic trichoepithelioma and morphealike basal cell carcinoma. *Am J Dermatopathol*. 1998;20:140-142.
84. Ito M, Tazawa T, Shimuzu N. Cell differentiation in human anagen hair and hair follicles studied with anti-hair keratin monoclonal antibodies. *J Invest Dermatol*. 1986;86:563-569.
85. Lynch MH, O'Guin M, Hardy C, et al. Acidic and basic hair/nail (hard) keratins: their colocalization in upper cortical and cuticle cells of the human hair follicle and their relationship to soft keratins. *J Cell Biol*. 1986;103:2593-2606.
86. Wick MR, Cooper PH, Swanson PE, et al. Microcystic adnexal carcinoma: an immunohistochemical comparison with other cutaneous appendage tumors. *Arch Dermatol*. 1990;126:189-194.
87. Tateyama H, Eimoto T, Tada T, et al. Malignant pilomatrixoma: an immunohistochemical study with antihair keratin antibody. *Cancer*. 1992;69:127-132.
88. Amaral ALMP, Nascimento A, Goellner JR. Proliferating pilar (trichilemmal) cyst: report of two cases, one with carcinomatous transformation, and one with distant metastases. *Arch Pathol Lab Med*. 1984;108:808-810.
89. Swanson PE, Marrogi AJ, Williams DJ, et al. Tricholemmal carcinoma: clinicopathologic study of 10 cases. *J Cutan Pathol*. 1992;19:100-109.

90. Dreno B, Mousset S, Stalder JF, et al. A study of intermediate filaments (cytokeratin, vimentin, neurofilament) in two cases of Merkel cell tumor. *J Cutan Pathol.* 1985;12:37-45.
91. Hartschuh W, Reinecke M, Weihe E, et al. VIP-immuno-reactivity in the skin of various mammals: immunohistochemical, radioimmunological, and experimental evidence for a dual localization in cutaneous nerves and Merkel cells. *Peptides.* 1984;5:239-245.
92. Chen-Chew SB, Leung PY. Species variability in the expression of met- and leu-enkephalin-like immunoreactivity in mammalian Merkel cell dense-core granules: a light and electron microscopic immunohistochemical study. *Cell Tissue Res.* 1992;269: 347-351.
93. Narisawa Y, Hashimoto K, Kohda H. Immunohistochemical demonstration of the expression of neurofilament proteins in Merkel cells. *Acta Derm Venereol.* 1994;74:441-443.
94. Gallego R, Garcia-Caballero T, Fraga M, et al. Neural cell adhesion molecule immunoreactivity in Merkel cells and Merkel cell tumors. *Virchows Arch.* 1995;426:317-321.
95. Fantini F, Johansson O. Neurochemical markers in human cutaneous Merkel cells: an immunohistochemical investigation. *Exp Dermatol.* 1995;4:365-371.
96. Kanitakis J, Bourchany D, Faure M, et al. Merkel cells in hyperplastic and neoplastic lesions of the skin: an immunohistochemical study using an antibody to keratin 20. *Dermatology.* 1998;196:208-212.
97. Jensen K, Kohler S, Rouse RV. Cytokeratin staining in Merkel cell carcinoma: an immunohistochemical study of cytokeratins 5/6, 7, 17, and 20. *Appl Immunohistochem Mol Morphol.* 2000;8:310-315.
98. Kurokawa M, Nabeshima K, Akiyama Y, et al. CD56: a useful marker for diagnosing Merkel cell carcinoma. *J Dermatol Sci.* 2003;31:219-224.
99. Garcia-Caballero T, Pintos E, Gallego R, et al. MOC-31/ Ep-CAM immunoreactivity in Merkel cells and Merkel cell carcinomas. *Histopathology.* 2003;43:480-484.
100. Mott RT, Smoller BR, Morgan MB. Merkel cell carcinoma: a clinicopathologic study with prognostic implications. *J Cutan Pathol.* 2004;31:217-223.
101. Bickle K, Glass LF, Messina JL, et al. Merkel cell carcinoma: a clinical, histopathologic, and immunohistochemical review. *Semin Cutan Med Surg.* 2004;23:46-53.
102. Heenan PJ, Cole JM, Spagnolo DV. Primary cutaneous neuroendocrine carcinoma (Merkel cell tumor): an adnexal epithelial neoplasm. *Am J Dermatopathol.* 1990;12:7-16.
103. Battifora H, Silva EG. The use of antikeratin antibodies in the immunohistochemical distinction between neuroendocrine (Merkel cell) carcinoma of the skin, lymphoma, and oat cell carcinoma. *Cancer.* 1986;58:1040-1046.
104. Buresh CJ, Oliai BR, Miller RT. Reactivity with TdT in Merkel cell carcinoma: a potential diagnostic pitfall. *Am J Clin Pathol.* 2008;129:894-898.
105. Mhawech-Fauceglia P, Saxena R, Zhang S, et al. PAX-5 immunoexpression in various types of benign and malignant tumors: a high-throughput tissue microarray analysis. *J Clin Pathol.* 2007;60:709-714.
106. Dong HY, Liu W, Cohen P, et al. B-cell specific activation protein encoded by the PAX-5 gene is commonly expressed in Merkel cell carcinoma and small cell carcinomas. *Am J Surg Pathol.* 2005;29:687-692.
107. Lau SK, Luthringer DJ, Eisen RN. Thyroid transcription factor-1: a review. *Appl Immunohistochem Mol Morphol.* 2002;10:97-102.
108. Leech SN, Kolar AJ, Barrett PD, et al. Merkel cell carcinoma can be distinguished from metastatic small cell carcinoma using antibodies to cytokeratin 20 and thyroid transcription factor-1. *J Clin Pathol.* 2001;54:727-729.
109. Bobos M, Hytiroglou P, Kostopoulos I, et al. Immunohistochemical distinction betweem Merkel cell carcinoma and small cell carcinoma of the lung. *Am J Dermatopathol.* 2006;28:99-104.
110. Jacinto CM, Grant-Kels JM, Knibbs DR, et al. Malignant primitive neuroectodermal tumor presenting as a scalp nodule. *Am J Dermatopathol.* 1991;13:63-70.
111. Patterson JW, Maygarden SJ. Extraskeletal Ewing's sarcoma with cutaneous involvement. *J Cutan Pathol.* 1986;13:46-58.
112. Banerjee SS, Agbamu DA, Eyden BP, et al. Clinicopathological characteristics of peripheral primitive neuroectodermal tumor of skin and subcutaneous tissue. *Histopathology.* 1997;31:355-366.
113. Hasegawa SL, Davison JM, Rutten A, et al. Primary cutaneous Ewing's sarcoma: immunophenotypic and molecular cytogenetic evaluation of five cases. *Am J Surg Pathol.* 1998;22:310-318.
114. Chao TK, Chang YL, Sheen TS. Extraskeletal Ewing's sarcoma of the scalp. *J Laryngol Otol.* 2000;114:73-75.
115. Taylor GB, Chan YF. Subcutaneous primitive neuroectodermal tumor in the abdominal wall of a child: long-term survival after local excision. *Pathology.* 2000;32:294-298.
116. Nicholson SA, McDermott MB, Swanson PE, et al. CD99 and cytokeratin-20 in small-cell and basaloid tumors of the skin. *Appl Immunohistochem Mol Morphol.* 2000;8:37-41.
117. Devoe K, Weidner N. Immunohistochemistry of small round-cell tumors. *Semin Diagn Pathol.* 2000;17:216-224.
118. Rossi S, Orvieto E, Furlanetto A, et al. Utility of the immunohistochemical detection of FLI-1 expression in round-cell and vascular neoplasms using a monoclonal antibody. *Mod Pathol.* 2004;17:547-552.
119. Ball NJ, Tanhuanco-Kho G. Merkel cell carcinoma frequently shows histologic features of basal cell carcinoma: a study of 30 cases. *J Cutan Pathol.* 2007;34:612-619.
120. Zembowicz A, Carcia CF, Tannous ZS, et al. Endocrine mucin-producing sweat gland carcinoma: twelve new cases suggest that it is a precursor of some invasive mucinous carcinomas. *Am J Surg Pathol.* 2005;29:1330-1339.
121. Faure P, Chittal S, Gorguet B, et al. Immunohistochemical profile of cutaneous B-cell lymphoma on cryostat and paraffin sections. *Am J Dermatopathol.* 1990;12:122-133.
122. Ralfkiaer E. Immunohistological markers for the diagnosis of cutaneous lymphomas. *Semin Diagn Pathol.* 1991;8:62-72.
123. Rest EB, Horn TD. Immunophenotypic analysis of benign and malignant cutaneous lymphoid infiltrates. *Clin Dermatol.* 1991;9:261-272.
124. Hsi ED, Yegappan S. Lymphoma immunophenotyping: a new era in paraffin section immunohistochemistry. *Adv Anat Pathol.* 2001;8:218-239.
125. Chen CC, Raikow RB, Sonmez-Alpan E, et al. Classification of small B-cell lymphoid neoplasms using a paraffin section immunohistochemical panel. *Appl Immunohistochem Mol Morphol.* 2000;8:1-11.
126. Baldassano MF, Bailey EM, Ferry JA, et al. Cutaneous lymphoid hyperplasia and cutaneous marginal zone lymphoma: comparison of morphologic and immunophenotypic features. *Am J Surg Pathol.* 1999;23:88-96.
127. Schmitt IM, Manente L, DiMatteo A, et al. Lymphoblastic lymphoma of the pre-B phenotype with cutaneous presentation. *Dermatology.* 1997;195:289-292.
128. Dorfman DM, Kraus M, Perez-Atayde AR, et al. CD99 (p30/32-MIC2) immunoreactivity in the diagnosis of leukemia cutis. *Mod Pathol.* 1997;10:283-288.
129. deBoer CJ, van Krieken JH, Schuuring E, et al. Bcl-1/cyclin-D1 in malignant lymphoma. *Ann Oncol.* 1997;8(Suppl 2):109-117.
130. Quintanilla-Martinez L, Zukerberg LR, Ferry JA, et al. Extramedullary tumors of lymphoid or myeloid blasts: the role of immunohistology in diagnosis and classification. *Am J Clin Pathol.* 1995;104:431-443.
131. Audouin J, Comperat E, LeTourneau A, et al. Myeloid sarcoma: clinical and morphologic criteria useful for diagnosis. *Int J Surg Pathol.* 2003;11:271-282.
132. Segal GH, Stoler MH, Fishleder AJ, et al. Reliable and cost-effective paraffin section immunohistology of lymphoproliferative disorders. *Am J Surg Pathol.* 1991;15:1034-1041.
133. Cerroni L, Smolle J, Soyer HP, et al. Immunophenotyping of cutaneous lymphoid infiltrates in frozen and paraffin-embedded tissue sections: a comparative study. *J Am Acad Dermatol.* 1990;22:405-413.
134. Fartasch M, Goerdt S, Hornstein OP. Possibilities and limits of paraffin-embedded cell markers in diagnosis of primary cutaneous histiocytosis. *Hautarzt.* 1995;46:144-153.

135. Nemes Z, Thomazy V. Diagnostic significance of histiocyte-related markers in malignant histiocytosis and true histiocytic lymphoma. *Cancer*. 1988;62:1970-1980.
136. Andrade RE, Wick MR, Frizzera G, et al. Immunophenotyping of hematopoietic malignancies in paraffin sections. *Hum Pathol*. 1988;19:394-402.
137. Kurtin PJ, Pinkus GS. Leukocyte common antigen—a diagnostic discriminant between hematopoietic and non-hematopoietic neoplasms in paraffin sections using monoclonal antibodies: correlation with immunologic studies and ultrastructural localization. *Hum Pathol*. 1985;16:353-365.
138. Falini B, Mason DY. Proteins encoded by genes involved in chromosomal alterations in lymphoma and leukemia: clinical value of their detection by immunocytochemistry. *Blood*. 2002;99:409-426.
139. Cerroni L, Beham-Schmid C, Kerl H. Cutaneous Hodgkin's disease: an immunohistochemical analysis. *J Cutan Pathol*. 1995;22:229-235.
140. Shiran MS, Tan GC, Savariah AR, et al. Small cell variant of anaplastic large cell lymphoma with positive immunoreactivity for CD99. *Med J Malaysia*. 2008;63:150-151.
141. Sung CO, Ko YH, Park S, et al. Immunoreactivity for CD99 in non-Hodgkin's lymphoma: unexpected frequent expression in ALK-positive anaplastic large cell lymphoma. *J Korean Med Sci*. 2005;20:952-956.
142. Lee IS, Kim SH, Song HG, Park SH. The molecular basis for the generation of Hodgkin and Reed-Sternberg cells in Hodgkin's lymphoma. *Int J Hematol*. 2003;77:330-335.
143. Segal GH, Stoler MH, Tubbs RR. The "CD43 only" phenotype. An aberrant, nonspecific immunophenotype requiring comprehensive analysis for lineage resolution. *Am J Clin Pathol*. 1992;97:861-865.
144. Goldstein NS, Ritter JH, Argenyi ZB, et al. Granulocytic sarcoma: potential diagnostic clues from immunostaining patterns seen with "anti-lymphoid" antibodies. *Int J Surg Pathol*. 1995;2:199-206.
145. Kiyokawa N, Sekino T, Matsui T, et al. Diagnostic importance of CD179a/b as markers of precursor B-cell lymphoblastic lymphoma. *Mod Pathol*. 2004;17:423-429.
146. Torlakovic E, Torlakovic G, Nguyen PL, et al. The value of anti-pax-5 immunostaining in routinely fixed and paraffin-embedded sections: a novel pan pre-B and B-cell marker. *Am J Surg Pathol*. 2002;26:1343-1350.
147. Fucich LF, Freeman SF, Boh EE, et al. Atypical cutaneous lymphoid infiltrates and a role for quantitative immunohistochemistry and gene rearrangement studies. *Int J Dermatol*. 1999;38:749-756.
148. Yang B, Tubbs RR, Finn W, et al. Clinicopathologic reassessment of primary cutaneous B-cell lymphomas with immunophenotypic and molecular genetic characterization. *Am J Surg Pathol*. 2000;24:694-702.
149. Nihal M, Mikkola D, Horvath N, et al. Cutaneous lymphoid hyperplasia: a lymphoproliferative continuum with lymphomatous potential. *Hum Pathol*. 2003;34:617-622.
150. Gilliam AC, Wood GS. Cutaneous lymphoid hyperplasias. *Semin Cutan Med Surg*. 2000;19:133-141.
151. Magro CM, Crowson AN, Porcu P, et al. Automated kappa and lambda light chain mRNA expression for the assessment of B-cell clonality in cutaneous B-cell infiltrates: its utility and diagnostic application. *J Cutan Pathol*. 2003;30:504-511.
152. Leinweber B, Colli C, Chott A, et al. Differential diagnosis of cutaneous infiltrates of B lymphocytes with follicular growth pattern. *Am J Dermatopathol*. 2004;26:4-13.
153. Alaibac M, Pigozzi B, Belloni-Fortina A, et al. CD7 expression in reactive and malignant human skin T-lymphocytes. *Anticancer Res*. 2003;23:2707-2710.
154. Murphy M, Fullen D, Carlson JA. Low CD7 expression in benign and malignant cutaneous lymphocytic infiltrates: experience with an antibody reactive with paraffin-embedded tissue. *Am J Dermatopathol*. 2002;24:6-16.
155. Rijlaarsdam U, Willemze R. Cutaneous pseudo-T-cell lymphomas. *Semin Diagn Pathol*. 1991;8:102-108.
156. Smolle J, Tome R, Soyer HP, et al. Immunohistochemical classification of cutaneous pseudolymphomas: delineation of distinct patterns. *J Cutan Pathol*. 1990;17:149-159.
157. Griesser H, Feller AC, Sterry W. T-cell receptor and immunoglobulin gene rearrangements in cutaneous T-cell-rich pseudolymphomas. *J Invest Dermatol*. 1990;95:292-295.
158. Ritter JH, Adesokan PN, Fitzgibbon JF, et al. Paraffin section immunohistochemistry as an adjunct to morphologic analysis in the diagnosis of cutaneous lymphoid infiltrates. *J Cutan Pathol*. 1994;21:481-493.
159. Van Vloten WA. *Cutaneous Lymphoma*. Basel, Switzerland: S. Karger; 1989.
160. Giannotti B, Pimpinelli N. Modern diagnosis of cutaneous lymphoma. *Recent Results Cancer Res*. 2002;160:303-306.
161. Cerroni L, Goteri G. Differential diagnosis between cutaneous lymphoma and pseudolymphoma. *Anal Quant Cytol Histol*. 2003;25:191-198.
162. Toonstra J. Actinic reticuloid. *Semin Diagn Pathol*. 1991;8:109-116.
163. Magro CM, Crowson AN, Kovatich AJ, et al. Drug-induced reversible lymphoid dyscrasia: a clonal lymphomatoid dermatitis of memory and activated T cells. *Hum Pathol*. 2003;34:119-129.
164. Burg G, Dummer R, Haeffner A, et al. From inflammation to neoplasia: mycosis fungoides evolves from reactive inflammatory conditions (lymphoid infiltrates) transforming into neoplastic plaques and tumors. *Arch Dermatol*. 2001;137:949-952.
165. LeBoit PE. Variants of mycosis fungoides and related cutaneous T-cell lymphomas. *Semin Diagn Pathol*. 1991;8:73-81.
166. Wood GS, Abel EA, Hoppe RT, et al. Leu-8 and Leu-9 antigen phenotypes: immunological criteria for the distinction of mycosis fungoides from cutaneous inflammation. *J Am Acad Dermatol*. 1986;14:1006-1013.
167. Bignon YJ, Souteyrand P. Genotyping of cutaneous T-cell lymphomas and pseudolymphomas. *Curr Prob Dermatol*. 1990;19:114-123.
168. Ceballos KM, Gascoyne RD, Martinka M, et al. Heavy multinodular cutaneous lymphoid infiltrates: clinicopathologic features and B-cell clonality. *J Cutan Pathol*. 2002;29:159-167.
169. Kerl H, Smolle J. Classification of cutaneous pseudolymphomas. *Curr Prob Dermatol*. 1989;19:167-176.
170. Hurt MA, Santa Cruz DJ. Cutaneous inflammatory pseudotumors. *Am J Surg Pathol*. 1990;14:764-772.
171. Toyota N, Matsuo S, Iizuka H. Immunohistochemical differential diagnosis between lymphocytoma cutis and malignant lymphoma in paraffin-embedded sections. *J Dermatol*. 1991;18:586-591.
172. Picker LJ, Weiss LM, Medeiros LJ, et al. Immunophenotypic criteria for the diagnosis of non-Hodgkin's lymphoma. *Am J Pathol*. 1987;128:181-201.
173. Ngan BY, Picker LJ, Medeiros LJ, et al. Immunophenotypic diagnosis of non-Hodgkin's lymphoma in paraffin sections: coexpression of L60 (Leu-22) and L26 antigens correlates with malignant histologic findings. *Am J Clin Pathol*. 1989;91:579-583.
174. Utz GL, Swerdlow SH. Distinction of follicular hyperplasia from follicular lymphoma in B5-fixed tissues: comparison of MT2 and bcl-2 antibodies. *Hum Pathol*. 1993;24:1155-1158.
175. Triscott JA, Ritter JH, Swanson PE, et al. Immunoreactivity for bcl-2 protein in cutaneous lymphomas and lymphoid hyperplasias. *J Cutan Pathol*. 1995;22:2-10.
176. Mirza I, Macpherson N, Paproski S, et al. Primary cutaneous follicular lymphoma: an assessment of clinical, histopathologic, immunophenotypic, and molecular features. *J Clin Oncol*. 2002;20:647-655.
177. Goodlad JR, Krajewski AS, Batstone PJ, et al. Primary cutaneous follicular lymphoma: a clinicopathologic and molecular study of 16 cases in support of a distinct entity. *Am J Surg Pathol*. 2002;26:733-741.
178. Lawnicki LC, Weisenburger DD, Aoun P, et al. The t(14;18) and bcl-2 expression are present in a subset of primary cutaneous follicular lymphoma: association with lower grade. *Am J Clin Pathol*. 2002;118:765-772.
179. Kim BK, Surti U, Pandya AG, et al. Primary and secondary cutaneous diffuse large B-cell lymphomas: a multiparameter analysis of 25 cases including fluorescence in-situ hybridization for t(14;18) translocation. *Am J Surg Pathol*. 2003;27:356-364.

180. Hoefnagel JJ, Vermeer MH, Jansen PM, et al. Bcl-2, Bcl-6 and CD10 expression in cutaneous B-cell lymphoma: further support for a follicle centre cell origin and differential diagnostic significance. *Br J Dermatol.* 2003;149:1183-1191.
181. Vergier B, Belaud-Rotureau MA, Benassy MN, et al. Neoplastic cells do not carry bcl-2-JH rearrangements detected in a subset of primary cutaneous follicle center B-cell lymphomas. *Am J Surg Pathol.* 2004;28:748-755.
182. Kuo TT. Cutaneous manifestations of Kikuchi's histiocytic necrotizing lymphadenitis. *Am J Surg Pathol.* 1990;14:872-879.
183. Spies J, Foucar K, Thompson CT, et al. The histopathology of cutaneous lesions of Kikuchi's disease (necrotizing lymphadenitis): a report of five cases. *Am J Surg Pathol.* 1999;23:1040-1047.
184. Lee CS, Lim HW. Cutaneous diseases in Asians. *Dermatol Clin.* 2003;21:669-677.
185. Yen HR, Lin PY, Chuang WY, et al. Skin manifestations of Kikuchi-Fujimoto disease: case report and review. *Eur J Pediatr.* 2004;163:210-213.
186. Kaudewitz P, Burg G. Lymphomatoid papulosis and Ki-1 (CD30)-positive cutaneous large cell lymphomas. *Semin Diagn Pathol.* 1991;8:117-124.
187. Stein H, Mason DY, Gerdes J, et al. The expression of the Hodgkin's disease-associated antigen Ki-1 in reactive and neoplastic tissue. *Blood.* 1985;66:848-858.
188. Cepeda LT, Pieretti M, Chapman SF, et al. CD30-positive atypical lymphoid cells in common non-neoplastic cutaneous infiltrates rich in neutrophils and eosinophils. *Am J Surg Pathol.* 2003;27:912-918.
189. Kuo TT. Kikuchi's disease (histiocytic necrotizing lymphadenitis): a clinicopathologic study of 79 cases with an analysis of histologic subtypes, immunohistology, and DNA ploidy. *Am J Surg Pathol.* 1995;19:798-809.
190. Ruzicka T, Evers J. Clinical course and therapy of Langerhans cell histiocytosis in children and adults. *Hautarzt.* 2003;54:148-155.
191. Singh A, Prieto VG, Czelusta A, et al. Adult Langerhans cell histiocytosis limited to the skin. *Dermatology.* 2003;207:157-161.
192. Aoki M, Aoki R, Akimoto M, et al. Primary cutaneous Langerhans cell histiocytosis in an adult. *Am J Dermatopathol.* 1998;20:281-284.
193. Stefanato CM, Andersen WK, Calonje E, et al. Langerhans cell histiocytosis in the elderly: a report of three cases. *J Am Acad Dermatol.* 1998;39:375-378.
194. Rowden G, Connelly EM, Winkelmann RK. Cutaneous histiocytosis X: the presence of S100 protein and its use in diagnosis. *Arch Dermatol.* 1983;119:553-559.
195. Emile JF, Wechsler J, Brousse N, et al. Langerhans cell histiocytosis: definitive diagnosis with the use of monoclonal antibody O10 on routinely paraffin-embedded samples. *Am J Surg Pathol.* 1995;19:636-641.
196. Pinkus GS, Lones MA, Matsumura F, et al. Langerhans cell histiocytosis: immunohistochemical expression of fascin, a dendritic cell marker. *Am J Clin Pathol.* 2002;118:335-343.
197. Slone SP, Fleming DR, Buchino JJ. Sinus histiocytosis with massive lymphadenopathy and Langerhans cell histiocytosis express the cellular adhesion molecule CD31. *Arch Pathol Lab Med.* 2003;127:341-344.
198. Lau SK, Chu PG, Weiss LM. Immunohistochemical expression of Langerin in Langerhans cell histiocytosis and non-Langerhans cell histiocytic disorders. *Am J Surg Pathol.* 2008;32:615-619.
199. Weiss LM, Grogan TM, Muller-Hermelink HK, et al. *Follicular dendritic cell sarcoma/tumor. Tumors of Haematopoeitic and Lymphoid Tissues.* Washington, DC: WHO/IARC Press; 2001, 286-288.
200. Favara BE, Feller AC, Pauli M, et al. Contemporary classification of histiocytic disorders: the WHO Committee on Histiocytic/Reticulum Cell Proliferations. Reclassification Working Group of the Histiocyte Society. *Med Pediatr Oncol.* 1997;29:157-166.
201. Shamoto M, Hosokawa S, Shinzato M, et al. Comparison of Langerhans cells and interdigitating reticulum cells. *Adv Exp Med Biol.* 1993;329:311-314.
202. Davaris DXG, Ling FCK, Prentice RSA. Congenital self-healing histiocytosis: report of two cases with histochemical and ultrastructural studies. *Am J Dermatopathol.* 1991;13:481-487.
203. Kapila PK, Grant-Kels JM, Allred C, et al. Congenital spontaneously regressing histiocytosis: case report and review of the literature. *Pediatr Dermatol.* 1985;2:312-317.
204. Gianotti R, Alessi E, Caputo R. Benign cephalic histiocytosis: a distinct entity or a part of a wide spectrum of histiocytic proliferative disorders of children? A histopathological study. *Am J Dermatopathol.* 1993;15:315-319.
205. Pena-Penabad C, Unamuno P, Garcia-Silva J, et al. Benign cephalic histiocytosis: case report and literature review. *Pediatr Dermatol.* 1994;11:164-167.
206. Jih DM, Salcedo SL, Jaworsky C. Benign cephalic histiocytosis: a case report and review. *J Am Acad Dermatol.* 2002;47:908-913.
207. Flynn KJ, Dehner LP, Gajl-Peczalska KJ, et al. Regressing atypical histiocytosis: a cutaneous proliferation of atypical neoplastic histiocytes with unexpectedly indolent biological behavior. *Cancer.* 1982;49:959-970.
208. Headington JT, Roth MS, Schnitzer B. Regressing atypical histiocytosis: a review and critical appraisal. *Semin Diagn Pathol.* 1987;4:28-37.
209. Headington JT, Roth MS, Ginsburg D, et al. T-cell receptor gene rearrangement in regressing atypical histiocytosis. *Arch Dermatol.* 1987;123:1183-1187.
210. Motley RJ, Jasani B, Ford AM, et al. Regressing atypical histiocytosis, a regressing cutaneous phase of Ki-1-positive anaplastic large cell lymphoma: immunocytochemical, nucleic acid, and cytogenetic studies of a new case in view of current opinion. *Cancer.* 1992;70:476-483.
211. Turner ML, Gilmour HM, McLaren KM, et al. Regressing atypical histiocytosis: report of two cases with progression to high-grade T-cell non-Hodgkin's lymphoma. *Hematol Pathol.* 1993;7:33-47.
212. Drews R, Samel A, Kadin ME. Lymphomatoid papulosis and anaplastic large cell lymphomas of the skin. *Semin Cutan Med Surg.* 2000;19:109-117.
213. Stein H, Foss HD, Durkop H, et al. CD30+ anaplastic large cell lymphoma: a review of its histopathologic, genetic, and clinical features. *Blood.* 2000;96:3681-3695.
214. Kadin ME, Carpenter C. Systemic and primary cutaneous anaplastic large cell lymphoma. *Semin Hematol.* 2003;40:244-256.
215. Liu HL, Hoppe RT, Kohler S, et al. CD30+ cutaneous lymphoproliferative disorders: the Stanford experience in lymphomatoid papulosis and primary cutaneous anaplastic large cell lymphoma. *J Am Acad Dermatol.* 2003;49:1049-1058.
216. Willemze R, Meijer CJ. Primary cutaneous CD30-positive lymphoproliferative disorders. *Hematol Oncol Clin North Am.* 2003;17:1319-1332.
217. Cerio R, Black MM. Regressing atypical histiocytosis and lymphomatoid papulosis: variants of the same disorder? *Br J Dermatol.* 1990;123:515-521.
218. Yashiro N, Kitajima J, Kobayashi H, et al. Primary anaplastic large-cell lymphoma of the skin: a case report suggesting that regressing atypical histiocytosis and lymphomatoid papulosis are subsets. *J Am Acad Dermatol.* 1994;30:358-363.
219. Camisa C, Helm TN, Sexton C, et al. Ki-1-positive anaplastic large-cell lymphoma can mimic benign dermatoses. *J Am Acad Dermatol.* 1993;29:696-700.
220. Brown JR, Skarin AT. Clinical mimics of lymphoma. *Oncologist.* 2004;9:406-416.
221. Steinhoff M, Hummel M, Anagnostopoulos I, et al. Single-cell analysis of CD30+ cells in lymphomatoid papulosis demonstrates a common clonal T-cell origin. *Blood.* 2002;15:578-584.
222. Banerjee SS, Heald J, Harris M. Twelve cases of Ki-1-posi-tive anaplastic large cell lymphoma of skin. *J Clin Pathol.* 1991;44:119-125.
223. Beljaards RC, Meijer CJ, Scheffer E. Prognostic significance of CD30 (Ki-1/Ber-H2) expression in primary cutaneous large-cell lymphoma of T-cell origin: a clinicopathologic and immunohistochemical study of 20 patients. *Am J Pathol.* 1989;135:1169-1178.
224. Kadin ME, Levi E, Kempf W. Progression of lymphomatoid papulosis to systemic lymphoma is associated with escape from growth inhibition by transforming growth factor-beta and CD30 ligand. *Ann NY Acad Sci..* 2001;94:59-68.

225. ten Berge RL, Oudejans JJ, Ossenkoppele GJ, et al. ALK-negative systemic anaplastic large-cell lymphoma: differential diagnostic and prognostic aspects—a review. *J Pathol.* 2003;200:4-15.
226. Bhawan J, Bacchetta C, Joris I, et al. A myofibroblastic tumor: infantile digital fibroma (recurrent digital fibrous tumor of childhood). *Am J Pathol.* 1979;94:9-28.
227. Blusje LG, Bastiaens M, Chang A, et al. Infantile-type digital fibromatosis tumor in an adult. *Br J Dermatol.* 2000;143:1107-1108.
228. Kanwar AJ, Kaur S, Thami GP, et al. Congenital infantile digital fibromatosis. *Pediatr Dermatol.* 2002;19:370-371.
229. Kang SK, Chang SE, Choi JH, et al. A case of congenital infantile digital fibromatosis. *Pediatr Dermatol.* 2002;19:462-463.
230. Guillen DR, Cockerell CJ. Cutaneous and subcutaneous sarcomas. *Clin Dermatol.* 2001;19:262-268.
231. Diaz-Cascajo C, Borghi S, Weyers W, et al. Fibroblastic/myofibroblastic sarcomas of the skin: a report of five cases. *J Cutan Pathol.* 2003;30:128-134.
232. Hayes MM, Dietrich BE, Uys CJ. Congenital hemangiopericytomas of skin. *Am J Dermatopathol.* 1986;8:148-153.
233. Ferreira CM, Maceira JM, Coelho JM. Congenital hemangiopericytoma of the skin. *Int J Dermatol.* 1997;36:521-523.
234. Schurch W, Seemayer TA, Lagace R, et al. The intermediate filament cytoskeleton of myofibroblasts: an immunofluorescence and ultrastructural study. *Virchows Archiv.* 1984;403:323-336.
235. Coffin CM, Neilson KA, Ingels S, et al. Congenital generalized myofibromatosis: a disseminated angiocentric myofibromatosis. *Pediatr Pathol Lab Med.* 1995;15:571-587.
236. Beham A, Badve S, Suster S, et al. Solitary myofibroma in adults: clinicopathological analysis of a series. *Histopathology.* 1993;22:335-341.
237. Mentzel T, Calonje E, Nascimento AG, et al. Infantile hemangiopericytoma versus infantile myofibromatosis: study of a series suggesting a continuous spectrum of infantile myofibroblastic lesions. *Am J Surg Pathol.* 1994;18:922-930.
238. Strauchen JA, Dimitriu-Bona A. Malignant fibrous histiocytoma: expression of monocyte/macrophage differentiation antigens detected with monoclonal antibodies. *Am J Pathol.* 1986;124:303-309.
239. Mechterscheimer G. Towards the phenotyping of soft tissue tumors by cell surface markers. *Virchows Arch.* 1991;419:7-28.
240. Mechterscheimer G, Staudter M, Majdie O. Expression of HLA-A, B, C, beta-microglobulin, HLA-DR, -DP, -DQ, and HLA-D-associated invariant chain in soft tissue tumors. *Int J Cancer.* 1990;46:813-823.
241. Swanson PE, Wick MR. HLA-DR (Ia-like) reactivity in tumors of bone and soft tissue: an immunohistochemical comparison of monoclonal antibodies LN3 and LK803 in routinely processed specimens. *Mod Pathol.* 1990;3:113-119.
242. Crocker J, Burnett D, Jones EL. Immunohistochemical demonstration of cathepsin B in the macrophages of benign and malignant lymphoid tissues. *J Pathol.* 1984;142:87-94.
243. Loftus B, Loh LC, Curran B, et al. MAC387: its non-specificity as a tumor marker or marker of histiocytes. *Histopathology.* 1991;17:251-255.
244. Cerio R, Spaull J, Oliver GF, et al. A study of factor XIIIa and MAC387 immunolabeling in normal and pathological skin. *Am J Dermatopathol.* 1990;12:221-233.
245. Gray MH, Smoller BR, McNutt NS, et al. Neurofibromas and neurotized nevi are immunohistochemically distinct neoplasms. *Am J Dermatopathol.* 1990;12:234-241.
246. Nemes Z, Thomazy V. Factor XIIIa and the classic histiocytic markers in malignant fibrous histiocytoma: a comparative immunohistochemical study. *Hum Pathol.* 1988;19:822-829.
247. Silverman JS, Tamsen A. High-grade malignant fibrous histiocytomas have bimodal cycling populations of factor XIIIa+ dendrophages and dedifferentiated mesenchcymal cells possibly derived from CD34+ fibroblasts. *Cell Vis.* 1998;5:73-76.
248. Nikkels AF, Arrese-Estrada J, Pierard-Franchimont C, et al. CD68 and factor XIIIa expressions in granular-cell tumor of the skin. *Dermatology.* 1993;186:106-108.
249. Hirose T, Kudo E, Hasegawa T, et al. Expression of intermediate filaments in malignant fibrous histiocytomas. *Hum Pathol.* 1989;20:871-877.
250. Longacre TA, Smoller BR, Rouse RV. Atypical fibroxanthoma: multiple immunohistologic profiles. *Am J Surg Pathol.* 1993;17:1199-1209.
251. Hasegawa T, Hasegawa F, Hirose T, et al. Expression of smooth muscle markers in so-called malignant fibrous histiocytomas. *J Clin Pathol.* 2003;56:666-671.
252. Abenoza P, Lillemoe T. CD34 and factor XIIIa in the differential diagnosis of dermatofibroma and dermatofibrosarcoma protuberans. *Am J Dermatopathol.* 1993;15:429-434.
253. Altman DA, Nickoloff BJ, Fivenson DP. Differential expression of factor XIIIa and CD34 in cutaneous mesenchymal tumors. *J Cutan Pathol.* 1993;20:154-158.
254. Goldblum JR, Tuthill RJ. CD34 and factor XIIIa—immunoreactivity in dermatofibrosarcoma protuberans and dermatofibroma. *Am J Dermatopathol.* 1997;19:147-153.
255. Wick MR, Ritter JH, Lind AC, et al. The pathological distinction between "deep penetrating" dermatofibroma and dermatofibrosarcoma protuberans. *Semin Cutan Med Surg.* 1999;18:91-98.
256. Weiss SW, Nickoloff BJ. CD34 is expressed by a distinctive cell population in peripheral nerve, nerve sheath tumors, and related lesions. *Am J Surg Pathol.* 1993;17:1039-1045.
257. Suster S, Fisher C. Immunoreactivity for the human hematopoietic progenitor cell antigen (CD34) in lipomatous tumors. *Am J Surg Pathol.* 1997;21:195-200.
258. Fetsch JF, Laskin WB, Miettinen M. Superficial acral fibromyxoma: a clinicopathologic and immunohistochemical analysis of 37 cases of a distinctive soft tissue tumor with a predilection for the fingers and toes. *Hum Pathol.* 2001;32:704-714.
259. Cowper SE, Kilpatrick T, Proper S, et al. Solitary fibrous tumor of the skin. *Am J Dermatopathol.* 1999;21:213-219.
260. Ramdial PK, Madaree A. Aggressive CD34-positive fibrous scalp lesion of childhood: extrapulmonary solitary fibrous tumor. *Pediatr Devel Pathol.* 2001;4:267-275.
261. Hardisson D, Cuevas-Santos J, Contreras F. Solitary fibrous tumor of the skin. *J Am Acad Dermatol.* 2002;46(Suppl 2):S37-S40.
262. Goldblum JR. Giant cell fibroblastoma: a report of three cases with histologic and immunohistochemical evidence of a relationship to dermatofibrosarcoma protuberans. *Arch Pathol Lab Med.* 1996;120:1052-1055.
263. Terrier-Lacombe MJ, Guillou L, Maire G, et al. Dermatofibrosarcoma protuberans, giant cell fibroblastoma, and hybrid lesions in children: a clinicopathologic comparative analysis of 28 cases with molecular data—a study from the French Federation of Cancer Centers Sarcoma Group. *Am J Surg Pathol.* 2003;27:27-39.
264. Silverman JS, Tamsen A. A cutaneous case of giant cell angiofibroma occurring with dermatofibrosarcoma protuberans and showing bimodal CD34+ fibroblastic and factor XIIIa+ histiocytic immunophenotype. *J Cutan Pathol.* 1998;25:265-270.
265. Sandberg AA, Bridge JA. Update on the cytogenetics and molecular genetics of bone and soft tissue tumors: dermatofibrosarcoma protuberans and giant cell fibroblastoma. *Cancer Genet Cytogenet.* 2003;140:1-12.
266. Billings SD, Folpe AL. Cutaneous and subcutaneous fibrohistiocytic tumors of intermediate malignancy: an update. *Am J Dermatopathol.* 2004;26:141-155.
267. Mori T, Misago N, Yamamoto O, et al. Expression of nestin in dermatofibrosarcoma protuberans in comparison to dermatofibroma. *J Dermatol.* 2008;35:419-425.
268. Erdag G, Qureshi HS, Patterson JW, Wick MR. Solitary fibrous tumors of the skin: a clinicopathologic study of 10 cases and review of the literature. *J Cutan Pathol.* 2007;34:844-850.
269. Zelger B. It's a dermatofibroma: CD34 is irrelevant! *Am J Dermatopathol.* 2002;24:453-454.
270. O'Connell JX, Trotter MJ. Fibrosarcomatous dermatofibrosarcoma protuberans with myofibroblastic differentiation: a histologically distinctive variant. *Mod Pathol.* 1996;9:273-278.
271. Diaz-Cascajo C. Myoid differentiation in dermatofibrosarcoma protuberans and its fibrosarcomatous variant. *J Cutan Pathol.* 1997;24:197-198.
272. Zamecnik M. Myoid cells in the fibrosarcomatous variant of dermatofibrosarcoma protuberans. *Histopathology.* 2000;36:186.

273. Morimitsu Y, Hisaoka M, Okamoto S, et al. Dermatofibrosarcoma protuberans and its fibrosarcomatous variant with areas of myoid differentiation: a report of three cases. *Histopathology*. 1998;32:547-551.
274. Diaz-Cascajo C, Weyers W, Borrego L, et al. Dermatofibrosarcoma protuberans with fibrosarcomatous areas: a clinicopathologic and immunohistochemical study of four cases. *Am J Dermatopathol*. 1997;19:562-567.
275. Mentzel T, Beham A, Katenkamp D, et al. Fibrosarcomatous (high-grade) dermatofibrosarcoma protuberans: clinicopathologic and immunohistochemical study of a series of 41 cases with emphasis on prognostic significance. *Am J Surg Pathol*. 1998;22:576-587.
276. Sigel JE, Bergfeld WF, Goldblum JR. A morphologic study of dermatofibrosarcoma protuberans: expansion of a histologic profile. *J Cutan Pathol*. 2000;27:159-163.
277. Diedhiou A, Larsimont D, Vandeweyer E, et al. Fibrosarcomatous variant of dermatofibrosarcoma protuberans: clinicopathologic analysis of 4 cases. *Ann Pathol*. 2001;21:164-167.
278. Davis DA, Sanchez RL. Atrophic and plaque-like dermatofibrosarcoma protuberans. *Am J Dermatopathol*. 1998;20:498-501.
279. Brooks JJ. The significance of double phenotypic patterns and markers in human sarcomas: a new model of mesenchymal differentiation. *Am J Pathol*. 1986;125:113-123.
280. Monteagudo C, Calduch L, Navarro S, et al. CD9 immunoreactivity in atypical fibroxanthoma: a common feature of diagnostic value. *Am J Clin Pathol*. 2002;117:126-131.
281. Diwan AH, Skelton III HG, Horenstein MG, et al. Dermatofibrosarcoma protuberans and giant cell fibroblastoma exhibit CD99 positivity. *J Cutan Pathol*. 2008;35:647-650.
282. De Feraudy S, Mar N, McCalmont TH. Evaluation of CD10 and procollagen I expression in atypical fibroxanthoma and dermatofibroma. *Am J Surg Pathol*. 2008;32:1111-1122.
283. Hall JM, Saenger JS, Fadare O. Diagnostic utility of p63 and CD10 in distinguishing cutaneous spindle cell/sarcomatoid squamous cell carcinoma and atypical fibroxanthoma. *Int J Clin Exp Pathol*. 2008;1:524-530.
284. Kanitakis J, Bourchany D, Claudy A. Expression of the CD10 antigen (neutral endopeptidase) by mesenchymal tumors of the skin. *Anticancer Res*. 2000;20:3539-3544.
285. Hultgren TL, DiMaio DJ. Immunohistochemical staining of CD10 in atypical fibroxanthomas. *J Cutan Pathol*. 2007;34:415-419.
286. Prieto VG, Reed JA, Shea CR. Immunohistochemistry of dermatofibromas and benign fibrous histiocytomas. *J Cutan Pathol*. 1995;22:336-341.
287. Sachdev R, Sundram U. Expression of CD163 in dermatofibroma, cellular fibrous histiocytoma, and dermatofibrosarcoma protuberans: comparison with CD68, CD34, and factor XIIIa. *J Cutan Pathol*. 2006;33:353-360.
288. Kim HJ, Lee JY, Kim SH, et al. Stromelysin-3 expression in the differential diagnosis of dermatofibroma and dermatofibrosarcoma protuberans: comparison with factor XIIIa and CD34. *Br J Dermatol*. 2007;157:319-324.
289. Miettinen M, Fetsch JF. Reticulohistiocytoma (solitary epithelioid histiocytoma): a clinicopathologic and immunohistochemical study of 44 cases. *Am J Surg Pathol*. 2006;30:521-528.
290. Swanson PE, Stanley MW, Scheithauer BW, et al. Primary cutaneous leiomyosarcoma: a histologic and immunohistochemical study of nine cases, with ultrastructural correlation. *J Cutan Pathol*. 1988;15:129-141.
291. Spencer JM, Amonette RA. Tumors with smooth muscle differentiation. *Dermatol Surg*. 1996;22:761-768.
292. Watanabe K, Kusakabe T, Hoshi N, et al. H-caldesmon in leiomyosarcoma and tumors with smooth muscle cell-like differentiation: its specific expression in the smooth muscle cell tumor. *Hum Pathol*. 1999;30:392-396.
293. Schadendorf D, Haas N, Ostmeier H, et al. Primary leiomyosarcoma of the skin: a histological and immunohistochemical analysis. *Acta Derm Venereol*. 1993;73:143-145.
294. Jensen ML, Jensen OM, Michalski W, et al. Intradermal and subcutaneous leiomyosarcoma: a clinicopathological and immunohistochemical study of 41 cases. *J Cutan Pathol*. 1996;23:458-463.
295. Altinok G, Dogan AL, Aydin SO, et al. Primary leiomyosarcomas of the skin. *Scand J Plast Reconstr Surg Hand Surg*. 2002;36:56-59.
296. Iwata J, Fletcher CDM. Immunohistochemical detection of cytokeratin and epithelial membrane antigen in leiomyosarcoma: a systematic study of 100 cases. *Pathol Int*. 2000;50:7-14.
297. Dervan PA, Tobbia IN, Casey M, et al. Glomus tumors: an immunohistochemical profile of 11 cases. *Histopathology*. 1989;14:483-491.
298. Kaye VN, Dehner LP. Cutaneous glomus tumor: a comparative immunohistochemical study with pseudoangiomatous intradermal melanocytic nevi. *Am J Dermatopathol*. 1991;13:2-6.
299. Haupt HM, Stern JB, Berlin SJ. Immunohistochemistry in the differential diagnosis of nodular hidradenoma and glomus tumor. *Am J Dermatopathol*. 1992;14:310-314.
300. Park JH, Oh SH, Yang MH, et al. Glomangiosarcoma of the hand: a case report and review of the literature. *J Dermatol*. 2003;30:827-833.
301. Mentzel T, Dei Tos AP, Sapi Z, Kutzner H. Myopericytoma of skin and soft tissues: clinicopathological and immunohistochemical study of 54 cases. *Am J Surg Pathol*. 2006;30:104-113.
302. Mentzel T, Hugel H, Kutzner H. CD34-positive glomus tumor: clinicopathologic and immunohistochemical analysis of six cases with myxoid stromal changes. *J Cutan Pathol*. 2002;29:421-425.
303. Mentzel T, Reisshauer S, Rutten A, et al. Cutaneous clear cell myomelanocytic tumor: a new member of the growing family of perivascular epithelioid cell tumors (PEComas). Clinicopathological and immunohistochemical analysis of seven cases. *Histopathology*. 2005;46:498-504.
304. Hornick JL, Fletcher CDM. PEComa: what do we know so far? *Histopathology*. 2006;48:75-82.
305. Requena L, Sangueza OP. Benign neoplasms with neural differentiation: a review. *Am J Dermatopathol*. 1995;17:75-96.
306. George E, Swanson PE, Wick MR. Malignant peripheral nerve sheath tumors of the skin. *Am J Dermatopathol*. 1989;11:213-221.
307. Demir Y, Tokyol C. Superficial malignant schwannoma of the scalp. *Dermatol Surg*. 2003;29:879-881.
308. Leroy K, Dumas V, Martin-Garcia N, et al. Malignant peripheral nerve sheath tumors associated with neurofibromatosis type 1: a clinicopathologic and molecular study of 17 patients. *Arch Dermatol*. 2001;137:908-913.
309. Wick MR, Swanson PE, Scheithauer BW, et al. Malignant peripheral nerve sheath tumor: an immunohistochemical study of 62 cases. *Am J Clin Pathol*. 1987;87:425-433.
310. Swanson PE, Scheithauer BW, Wick MR. Peripheral nerve sheath neoplasms: clinicopathologic and immunochemical observations. *Pathol Ann*. 1995;30(Pt.2):1-82.
311. Miettinen M, Cupo W. Neural cell adhesion molecule distribution in soft tissue tumors. *Hum Pathol*. 1993;24:62-66.
312. Gray MH, Rosenberg AE, Dickersin GR, et al. Glial fibrillary acidic protein and keratin expression by benign and malignant peripheral nerve sheath tumors. *Hum Pathol*. 1989;20:1089-1096.
313. Stefansson K, Wollman RL. S100 protein in granular cell tumors (granular cell myoblastomas). *Cancer*. 1982;49:1834-1838.
314. LeBoit PE, Barr RJ, Burall S, et al. Primitive polypoid granular cell tumor and other cutaneous granular cell neoplasms of apparent non-neural origin. *Am J Surg Pathol*. 1991;15:48-58.
315. Hitchcock MG, Hurt MA. Santa Cruz DJ. Cutaneous granular cell angiosarcoma. *J Cutan Pathol*. 1994;21:256-262.
316. Le BH, Boyer PJ, Lewis JE, et al. Granular cell tumor: immunohistochemical assessment of inhibin-alpha, protein gene product 9.5, S100 protein, CD68, and Ki-67 proliferative index with clinical correlation. *Arch Pathol Lab Med*. 2004;128:771-775.
317. Fine SW, Li M. Expression of calretinin and the alpha-subunit of inhibin in granular cell tumors. *Am J Clin Pathol*. 2003;119:259-264.
318. Skelton HG, Williams J, Smith KJ. The clinical and histologic spectrum of cutaneous fibrous perineuriomas. *Am J Dermatopathol*. 2001;23:190-196.
319. Baran R, Perrin C. Subungual perineurioma: a peculiar location. *Br J Dermatol*. 2002;146:125-128.

320. Zamecnik M, Koys F, Gomoleak P. Atypical cellular perineurioma. *Histopathology*. 2002;40:296-299.
321. Baran R, Perrin C. Perineurioma: a tendon-sheath-fibroma-like variant in a distal subungual location. *Acta Derm Venereol*. 2003;83:60-61.
322. Mentzel T. Cutaneous perineurioma: clinical and histological findings and differential diagnosis. *Pathologe*. 2003;24:207-213.
323. Hewan-Lowe K, Furlong B, Mackay B. Perineurial cell differentiation in benign tumors and tumor-like proliferations of peripheral nerves. *Ultrastruct Pathol*. 1993;17:263-270.
324. Mentzel T, Dei Tos AP, Fletcher CDM. Perineurioma (storiform perineurial fibroma): clinicopathological analysis of four cases. *Histopathology*. 1994;25:261-267.
325. Giannini C, Scheithauer BW, Jenkins RB, et al. Soft tissue perineurioma: evidence for an abnormality of chromosome 22, criteria for diagnosis, and review of the literature. *Am J Surg Pathol*. 1997;21:164-173.
326. Fetsch JF, Miettinen M. Sclerosing perineurioma: a clinicopathologic study of 19 cases of a distinctive soft tissue lesion with a predilection for the fingers and palms of young adults. *Am J Surg Pathol*. 1997;21:1433-1442.
327. Hirose T, Scheithauer BW, Sano T. Perineurial malignant peripheral nerve sheath tumor (MPNST): a clinicopathologic, immunohistochemical, and ultrastructural study of seven cases. *Am J Surg Pathol*. 1998;22:1368-1378.
328. Hornick JL, Fletcher CD. Soft tissue perineurioma: clinicopathologic analysis of 81 cases including those with atypical histologic features. *Am J Surg Pathol*. 2005;29:845-858.
329. Mentzel T, Kutzner H. Reticular and plexiform perineurioma: clinicopathological and immunohistochemical analysis of two cases and review of perineurial neoplasms of skin and soft tissue. *Virchows Arch*. 2005;447:677-682.
330. Zelger B, Weinlich G, Zelger B. Perineurioma: a frequently unrecognized entity with emphasis on a plexiform variant. *Adv Clin Pathol*. 2000;4:25-33.
331. Burgues O, Monteagudo C, Noguera R, et al. Cutaneous sclerosing Pacinian-like perineurioma. *Histopathology*. 2001;39:498-502.
332. Rosenberg AS, Langee CL, Stevens GL, et al. Malignant peripheral nerve sheath tumor with perineurial differentiation: "malignant perineurioma. *J Cutan Pathol*. 2002;29:362-367.
333. Folpe AL, Billings SD, McKenney JK, et al. Expression of claudin-1, a recently described tight junction-associated protein, distinguishes soft tissue perineurioma from potential mimics. *Am J Surg Pathol*. 2002;26:1620-1626.
334. Laskin WB, Fetsch JF, Miettinen M. The "neurothekeoma:" immuohistochemical analysis distinguishes the true nerve sheath myxoma from its mimics. *Hum Pathol*. 2000;31:1230-1241.
335. Page RN, King R, Mihm Jr MC, et al. Microophthalmia transcription factor and NKI/C3 expression in cellular neurothekeoma. *Mod Pathol*. 2004;17:230-234.
336. Fullen DR, Lowe L, Su LD. Antibody to S100 A6 protein is a sensitive immunohistochemical marker for neurothekeoma. *J Cutan Pathol*. 2003;30:118-122.
337. Misago N, Satoh T, Narisawa Y. Cellular neurothekeoma with histiocytic differentiation. *J Cutan Pathol*. 2004;31:568-572.
338. Calonje E, Wilson-Jones E, Smith NP, et al. Cellular neurothekeoma: an epithelioid variant of pilar leiomyoma? Morphological and immunohistochemical analysis of a series. *Histopathology*. 1992;20:397-404.
339. Fetsch JF, Laskin WB, Miettinen M. Nerve sheath myxoma: a clinicopathologic and immunohistochemical analysis of 57 morphologically distinctive, S100 protein- and GFAP-positive, myxoid peripheral nerve sheath tumors with a predilection for the extremities and a high local recurrence rate. *Am J Surg Pathol*. 2005;29:1615-1624.
340. Hornick JL, Fletcher CD. Cellular neurothekeoma: detailed characteristics in a series of 133 cases. *Am J Surg Pathol*. 2007;31:329-340.
341. Swanson PE, Wick MR. Immunohistochemical evaluation of vascular neoplasms. *Clin Dermatol*. 1991;9:243-253.
342. Requena L, Sangueza OP. Cutaneous vascular proliferations: Part III: Malignant neoplasms, other cutaneous neoplasms with a significant vascular component, and disorders erroneously considered as vascular neoplasms. *J Am Acad Dermatol*. 1998;38:143-175.
343. Miettinen M, Holthofer H, Lehto VP, et al. Ulex europaeus I lectin as a marker for tumors derived from endothelial cells. *Am J Clin Pathol*. 1983;79:32-36.
344. Leader M, Collins M, Patel J, et al. Staining for factor VIII-related antigen and Ulex europaeus agglutinin I (UEA-I) in 230 tumors. An assessment of their specificity for angiosarcoma and Kaposi's sarcoma. *Histopathology*. 1986;10:1153-1162.
345. Ramani P, Bradley NJ, Fletcher CDM. QBEND/10, a new monoclonal antibody to endothelium: assessment of its diagnostic utility in paraffin sections. *Histopathology*. 1990;17:237-242.
346. Suster S, Wong TY. On the discriminatory value of anti-HPCA-1 (CD34) in the differential diagnosis of benign and malignant cutaneous vascular proliferations. *Am J Dermatopathol*. 1994;16:355-363.
347. DeYoung BR, Swanson PE, Argenyi ZB, et al. CD31 immunoreactivity in mesenchymal neoplasms of the skin and subcutis: report of 145 cases and review of putative immunohistological markers of endothelial differentiation. *J Cutan Pathol*. 1995;22:215-222.
348. Appleton MA, Attanoos RL, Jasani B. Thrombomodulin as a marker of vascular and lymphatic tumors. *Histopathology*. 1996;29:153-157.
349. Breiteneder-Geleff S, Soleiman A, Kowalski H, et al. Angiosarcomas express mixed endothelial phenotypes of blood and lymphatic capillaries: podoplanin as a specific marker for lymphatic endothelium. *Am J Pathol*. 2999;154:385-394.
350. Folpe AL, Veikkola T, Valtola R, Weiss SW. Vascular endothelial growth factor receptor-3 (VEGFR3): a marker of vascular tumors with presumed lymphatic differentiation, including Kaposi's sarcoma, Kaposiform and Dabska-type hemangioendotheliomas, and a subset of angiosarcomas. *Mod Pathol*. 2000;13:180-185.
351. Folpe AL, Chand EM, Goldblum JR, et al. Expression of FLI-1, a nuclear transcription factor, distinguishes vascular neoplasms from potential mimics. *Am J Surg Pathol*. 2001;25:1061-1066.
352. Gray MH, Rosenberg AE, Dickersin GR, et al. Cytokeratin expression in epithelioid vascular neoplasms. *Hum Pathol*. 1990;21:212-217.
353. Traweek ST, Liu J, Battifora H. Keratin gene expression in non-epithelial tissues: detection with polymerase chain reaction. *Am J Pathol*. 1993;142:1111-1118.
354. Robin YM, Guillou L, Michels JJ, et al. Human herpesvirus8 immunostaining: a sensitive and specific method for diagnosing Kaposi's sarcoma in paraffin-embedded sections. *Am J Clin Pathol*. 2004;121:330-334.
355. Cheuk W, Wong KO, Wong CS, et al. Immunostaining for human herpesvirus 8 latent nuclear antigen-1 helps distinguish Kaposi's sarcoma from its mimickers. *Am J Clin Pathol*. 2004;121:335-342.
356. Patel RM, Goldblum JR, His ED. Immunohistochemical detection of human herpes virus-8 latent nuclear antigen-1 is useful in the diagnosis of Kaposi's sarcoma. *Mod Pathol*. 2004;17:456-460.
357. O'Hara CD, Nascimento AG. Endothelial lesions of soft tissues: a review of reactive and neoplastic entities with emphasis on low-grade malignant (borderline) vascular tumors. *Adv Anat Pathol*. 2003;10:69-87.
358. Fletcher CDM, Beham A, Schmid C. Spindle-cell hemangioendothelioma: a clinicopathological and immunohistochemical study indicative of a non-neoplastic lesion. *Histopathology*. 1991;18:291-301.
359. Mentzel T, Beham A, Calonje E, et al. Epithelioid hemangioendothelioma of skin and soft tissues: clinicopathologic and immunohistochemical study of 30 cases. *Am J Surg Pathol*. 1997;21:363-374.
360. Mentzel T, Mazzoleni G, Dei Tos AP, et al. Kaposiform hemangioendothelioma in adults: clinicopathologic and immunohistochemical analysis of three cases. *Am J Clin Pathol*. 1997;108:450-455.
361. Billings SD, Folpe AL, Weiss SW. Epithelioid sarcoma-like hemangioendothelioma. *Am J Surg Pathol*. 2003;27:48-57.
362. Arber DA, Kandalaft PL, Mehta P, et al. Vimentin-negative epithelioid sarcoma. The value of an immunohistochemical panel that includes CD34. *Am J Surg Pathol*. 1993;17:302-307.

363. Manivel JC, Wick MR, Dehner LP, et al. Epithelioid sarcoma: an immunohistochemical study. *Am J Clin Pathol.* 1987;87: 319-326.
364. Wick MR, Manivel JC. Epithelioid sarcoma and isolated necrobiotic granuloma: a comparative immunohistochemical study. *J Cutan Pathol.* 1986;13:253-260.
365. Wick MR, Manivel JC. Epithelioid sarcoma and epithelioid hemangioendothelioma: an immunohistochemical and lectin-histochemical comparison. *Virchows Arch.* 1987;410:309-316.
366. Chase DR, Enzinger FM, Weiss SW, et al. Keratin in epithelioid sarcoma: an immunohistochemical study. *Am J Surg Pathol.* 1984;8:435-441.
367. Wakely Jr P. Epithelioid/granular soft tissue lesions: correlation of cytopathology and histopathology. *Ann Diagn Pathol.* 2000;4:316-328.
368. Humble SD, Prieto VG, Horenstein MG. Cytokeratin 7 and 20 expression in epithelioid sarcoma. *J Cutan Pathol.* 2003;30:242-246.
369. Laskin WB, Miettinen M. Epithelioid sarcoma: new insights based on an extended immunohistochemical analysis. *Arch Pathol Lab Med.* 2003;127:1161-1168.
370. Miettinen M, Fetsch JF. Distribution of keratins in normal endothelial cells and a spectrum of vascular tumors: implications in tumor diagnosis. *Hum Pathol.* 2000;31:1062-1067.
371. Lee HI, Kang KH, Cho YM, et al. Proximal-type epithelioid sarcoma with elevated CA-125: report of a case with CA-125 immunoreactivity. *Arch Pathol Lab Med.* 2006;130:871-874.
372. Kato H, Hatori M, Kokubun S, et al. CA-125 expression in epithelioid sarcoma. *Jpn J Clin Oncol.* 2004;34:149-154.
373. Lin L, Skacel M, Sigel JE, et al. Epithelioid sarcoma: an immunohistochemical analysis evaluating the utility of cytokeratin 5/6 in distinguishing superficial epithelioid sarcoma from spindled squamous cell carcinoma. *J Cutan Pathol.* 2003;30:114-117.
374. Laskin WB, Miettinen M. Epithelial-type and neural-type cadherin expression in malignant noncarcinomatous neoplasms with epithelioid features that involve the soft tissues. *Arch Pathol Lab Med.* 2002;126:425-431.
375. Peydro-Olaya A, Llombart-Bosch A, Carda-Batalla C, et al. Electron microscopy and other ancillary techniques in the diagnosis of small round-cell tumors. *Semin Diagn Pathol.* 2003;20:25-45.
376. Lloveras B, Googe PB, Goldberg DE, et al. Estrogen receptors in skin appendage tumors and extramammary Paget's disease. *Mod Pathol.* 1991;4:487-490.
377. Swanson PE, Mazoujian G, Mills SE, et al. Immunoreactivity for estrogen receptor protein in sweat gland tumors. *Am J Surg Pathol.* 1991;15:835-841.
378. Wallace ML, Longacre TA, Smoller BR. Estrogen and progesterone receptors and anti-gross cystic disease fluid protein-15 (BRST-2) fail to distinguish metastatic breast carcinoma from eccrine neoplasms. *Mod Pathol.* 1995;8:897-901.
379. Wick MR, Ockner DM, Mills SE, et al. Homologous carcinomas of the breasts, skin, and salivary glands: a histologic and immunohistochemical comparison of ductal mammary carcinoma, ductal sweat gland carcinoma, and salivary duct carcinoma. *Am J Clin Pathol.* 1998;109:75-84.
380. Busam KJ, Tan LK, Granter SR, et al. Epidermal growth factor, estrogen, and progesterone receptor expression in primary sweat gland carcinomas and primary and metastatic mammary carcinomas. *Mod Pathol.* 1999;12:786-793.
381. Voytek TM, Ricci Jr A, Cartun RW. Estrogen and progesterone receptors in primary eccrine carcinoma. *Mod Pathol.* 1991;4:582-585.
382. Baujnedcht T, Gross G, Hagedorn M. Epidermal growth factor receptors in different skin tumors. *Dermatologica.* 1985;171:16-20.
383. Nazini MN, Dykes RI, Marks R. Epidermal growth factor receptors in human epidermal tumors. *Br J Dermatol.* 1990;123:153-161.
384. Springer EA, Robinson JK. Patterns of epidermal growth factor receptors in basal cell carcinomas and squamous cell carcinomas. *J Dermatol Surg Oncol.* 1991;17:20-24.
385. Ellis DL, Nanney LB, King Jr LE. Increased epidermal growth factor receptors in seborrheic keratoses and acrochordons of patients with the dysplastic nevus syndrome. *J Am Acad Dermatol.* 1990;23:1070-1077.
386. Hasebe T, Mukai K, Yamaguchi N, et al. Prognostic value of immunohistochemical staining for proliferating cell nuclear antigen, p53, and c-erbB-2 in sebaceous gland carcinoma and sweat gland carcinomas: comparison with histopathological parameters. *Mod Pathol.* 1994;7:37-43.
387. Wolber RA, Dupuis BA, Wick MR. Expression of c-erbB-2 oncoprotein in mammary and extramammary Paget's disease. *Am J Clin Pathol.* 1991;96:243-247.
388. Seelentag WK, Gunthert U, Saremaslani P, et al. CD44 standard and variant isoform expression in normal human skin appendages and epidermis. *Histochem Cell Biol..* 1996;106:283-289.
389. Hale LP, Patel DD, Clark RE, et al. Distribution of CD44 variant isoforms in human skin: differential expression in components of benign and malignant epithelia. *J Cutan Pathol.* 1995;22:536-545.
390. Prieto VG, Reed JA, McNutt NS, et al. Differential expression of CD44 in malignant cutaneous epithelial neoplasms. *Am J Dermatopathol.* 1995;17:447-451.
391. Penneys NS, Shapiro S. CD44 expression in Merkel cell carcinoma may correlate with risk of metastasis. *J Cutan Pathol.* 1994;21:22-26.

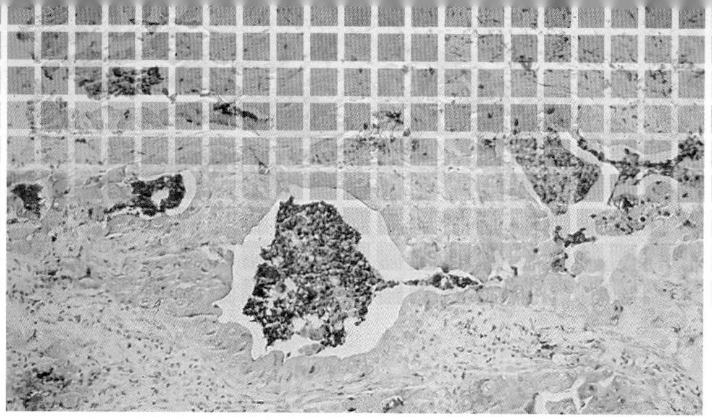

14

Immunohistology of the Gastrointestinal Tract

Alyssa M. Krasinskas • Jeffrey D. Goldsmith

- Introduction 500
- Biology of Antigens: General and Tissue Specific 500
- Diagnostic Immunohistochemistry 501
- Genomic Applications 528
- Theranostic Applications 528
- Beyond Immunohistochemistry: Anatomic Molecular Diagnostic Applications 529

INTRODUCTION

This chapter divides the discussion of immunohistochemistry (IHC) of the luminal gastrointestinal tract into three sections: (1) epithelial pathology, (2) neuroendocrine lesions, and (3) spindle cell lesions. We have attempted to compile the innumerable immunohistochemical studies that have been applied to these organs into a cogent, useful, and relevant text.

BIOLOGY OF ANTIGENS: GENERAL AND TISSUE SPECIFIC

This section includes a brief discussion of antigens/epitopes that are often used in gastrointestinal pathology. See Table 14.1 for representative assay conditions for these antibodies. Note that the conditions listed in this table are meant to be guides. All new antibodies must be thoroughly validated by the laboratory performing the test.

GENERAL CYTOKERATINS For the purposes of diagnostic IHC, carcinomas that stain with low- and high-molecular-weight cytokeratins include esophageal and gastric carcinomas. Carcinomas that stain predominantly with low-molecular-weight cytokeratin antibodies include colorectal adenocarcinomas, carcinoids, and high-grade neuroendocrine carcinomas.[1] Carcinomas that stain with predominantly high-molecular-weight cytokeratin antibodies include esophageal and anal squamous cell carcinomas (SCCs).

BETA-CATENIN This protein is an 88 kD member of the catenin family of proteins that are important constituents of the cytoskeleton. Beta-catenin is also important in gene expression and is a member of the Wnt signaling cascade. In certain conditions, when the normal degradation of B-catenin is disrupted, this protein accumulates in the cytoplasm and abnormally translocates to the nucleus where it can disrupt normal gene expression.[2, 3]

CYTOKERATIN 7 Keratin 7 is an intermediate filament expressed predominantly by ductal epithelial cells of the pancreaticobiliary tract, renal collecting ducts, and proximal gastrointestinal tract. Expression of CK7 keratin is limited to subtypes of adenocarcinomas and squamous carcinomas arising within noncornified mucosa.

CYTOKERATIN 20 In the small intestine, CK20 stains only the highly differentiated small bowel villous enterocytes (cytokeratin 18 stains the more immature basilar, proliferative zone cells). In the colon, CK20 stains only the surface epithelial cell layer. CK20 staining is more extensive and stronger in small bowel neoplasms than colonic carcinomas.[4]

CDX2 CDX2 is a homeobox gene that is an integral component of intestinal cell proliferation and differentiation.[5] It appears to function as a tumor suppressor gene in colorectal and some pancreaticobiliary and gastric adenocarcinomas.[6]

CHROMOGRANIN A This protein is an acidic soluble glycoprotein located within neurosecretory granules.[7,8] Chromogranin A undergoes post-translational modification which varies between gastrointestinal sites and their associated neoplasms.[9] Chromogranin is more specific, but less sensitive than synaptophysin.[8] Most non-neoplastic neuroendocrine lesions and low-grade neuroendocrine neoplasms diffusely and strongly stain with chromogranin, and this is proportional to the number of intracytoplasmic neurosecretory granules. However, some carcinoids stain weakly with chromogranin, which may

TABLE 14.1 Assay Conditions for Representative Antibodies

Antibody	Clone	Dilution	Retrieval
Beta-catenin	17C2	1:200	pH 6.1
c-kit (CD117)	104D2	1:200	pH 9.0
CDX2	CDX2-88	1:50	pH 6.1
Chromogranin A	DAK-A3	1:800	pH 9.0
Cytokeratin 7	OV-TL 12/30	1:400	Proteinase K
Cytokeratin 20	Ks20.8	1:25	Proteinase K
COX2	SP-21	1:100	pH 8.5
MLH1	CM220C	1:10	Proprietary solution
MOC31	MOC-31	1:25	Proteinase K
MSH2	FE11	1:25	Proprietary solution
MSH6	70834	1:100	pH 9.0
MUC1	Ma95	1:100	pH 8.5
MUC2	Ccp58	1:25	pH 8.5
MUC5AC	CLH2	1:100	pH 8.5
MUC6	CLH5	1:25	pH 8.5
p53	DO-7	1:25	pH 9.0
p63	4A4	1:50	pH 9.0
PMS2	A16-4	1:10	pH 9.0
Synaptophysin	Sv38	1:100	pH 6.1
Villin	CWWB1	1:100	Citrate, pH 6.0

reflect differences in the type of amines contained within the tumor cell cytoplasm.

COX 2 This enzyme is the rate-limiting enzyme in the production of various prostaglandins from arachidonic acid.[10] It is expressed in a variety of neoplasms, including colorectal,[11,12] gastric,[13] and pancreatic carcinomas.[14,15]

C-KIT (CD117) The antibody against this protein stains the transmembrane and cytoplasmic KIT protein which is a type 3 tyrosine kinase receptor. This antibody is useful for identifying gastrointestinal stromal tumors (GISTs).

DNA MISMATCH REPAIR PROTEINS (MLH1, MSH2, MSH6, PMS2) These antibodies are directed at protein components of the mismatch repair complex. These proteins function as heterodimers; MLH1 associates with PMS2 while MSH2 associates with MSH6. As such, these pairs of proteins can show loss of expression in concert. Decreased or absent staining is indicative of quantitative protein deficiencies or mutated protein.[17]

MOC31 MOC31 is one of the myriad of monoclonal antibodies against the epithelial adhesion molecule, Ep-CAM.[18,19] MOC-31 is expressed in a host of benign epithelia and is expressed in many carcinomas including those derived from the colon, stomach, breast, pancreas, ovary, and bile ducts.[20,21]

MUCS Mucin core polypeptides are the backbone molecule of gastrointestinal tract mucin and are responsible for the mucus-gel layer, which covers the mucosa.[22] MUC1 is normally expressed by enterocytes and intestinal goblet cells, MUC2 is normally secreted by intestinal goblet cells, MUC5AC is expressed by gastric foveolar mucus cells and neoplastic goblet cells, and MUC6 is secreted by gastric antral and fundic gland cells.

NESP-55 NESP-55 is a recently described member of the granin family of proteins that are localized to dense core secretory granules present in various endocrine cells.[23,24] It is highly expressed in the adrenal medulla, pituitary gland, and brain.[25]

P53 Normal p53 protein has an extremely short half-life and is found in small quantities inside cells. As such, p53 cannot be detected in normal cells using immunohistochemistry. The p53 protein from abnormal p53 genes has a longer half-life than normal p53 protein, builds up inside cells, and can be detected with anti-p53 antibodies. In theory, p53 overexpression, as a surrogate marker for p53 gene mutations, is an immunohistochemical test for neoplasia (dysplasia). However, this is not the case in practice because correlation between staining and gene abnormalities is not precise.[26]

P63 This molecule is a member of the p53 family of proteins; it exists as multiple protein variants, which are a result of alternative transcript splicing events. The relative concentrations of these protein variants affect the expression and functionality of wild-type p63 and p53 proteins.[27] The p63 protein is expressed in a nuclear pattern in various myoepithelia and is present in the basal layer of squamous epithelium.[28,29]

SYNAPTOPHYSIN This protein is a membrane glycoprotein found in calcium channels of cells. Its expression is independent of chromogranin A.[8]

VILLIN Villin is a brush border, microfilament-associated, actin-binding protein related to rootlet formation. Staining in colorectal adenocarcinomas is diffusely cytoplasmic with brush border accentuation.[30-33]

DIAGNOSTIC IMMUNOHISTOCHEMISTRY

Epithelial Lesions of the Gastrointestinal Tract

ESOPHAGUS

Barrett Esophagus and the Gastric Cardia

Barrett esophagus (BE) is defined as intestinal metaplasia in association with endoscopically recognized columnar metaplasia of the gastroesophageal junction. This

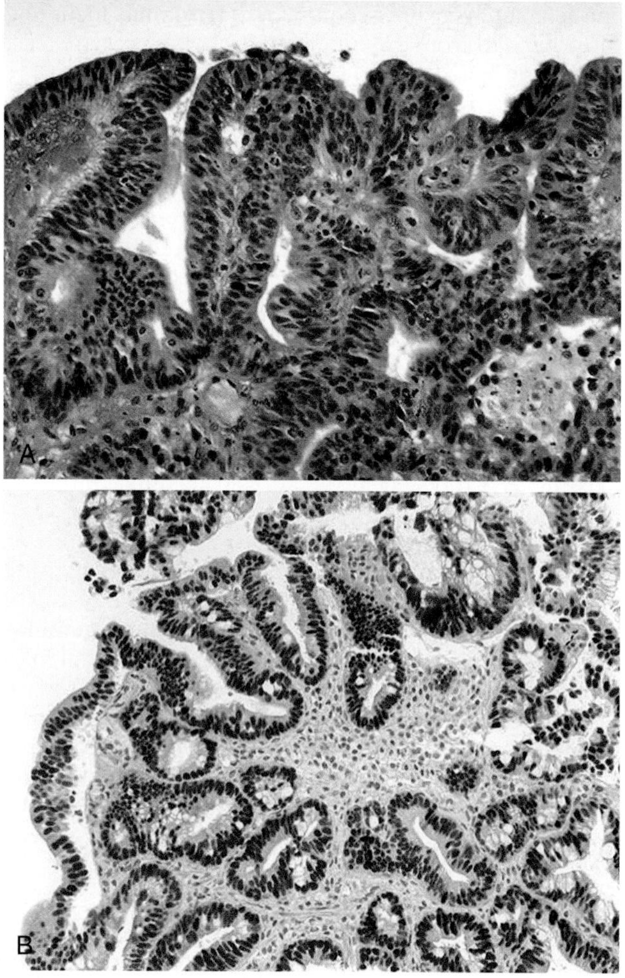

FIGURE 14.1 **A,** High-grade dysplasia in Barrett esophagus typically shows strong and diffuse nuclear staining with p53 **(B)**. However, there can be substantial overlap of the patterns of p53 reactivity in epithelial cells that are reactive and those that show low-grade dysplasia.

finding is distinct from intestinal metaplasia of the gastric cardia.[34] IHC has been used to distinguish these two mucosae with variable success.[35-43] Published in 2003, a consensus conference on the morphology of BE stated that immunohistochemical stains, including cytokeratins 7 and 20, MUCs, or CDX2 were not essential for the diagnosis.[44] Thus, the use of immunohistochemistry to diagnose BE or distinguish BE from gastric cardia mucosa with intestinal metaplasia is currently investigational, and should not be used in routine clinical practice.

DYSPLASIA IN BARRETT ESOPHAGUS Numerous molecular alterations associated with the development of neoplasia within BE have been described.[45-51] Many of these genetic alterations were used as the foundation for IHC to assist in the morphologic diagnosis and grading of dysplasia;[45,48,49] Of these altered proteins, p53 is the only antibody with any established utility in the diagnosis of dysplasia. p53 immunoreactivity in BE is weak and focal over a morphologic spectrum of cases including reactive, indeterminate for dysplasia, and low-grade dysplasia. Cells of high-grade epithelial dysplasia usually show strong and diffuse nuclear staining (Fig. 14.1).[52] As a result, some authors have suggested that p53 nuclear reactivity can be used as an adjunct to the histologic evaluation of dysplasia in BE.[53] The clinical utility of p53 is limited, however, because there is substantial overlap of the patterns of p53 reactivity in epithelia that are negative for dysplasia, those that show reactive changes, and epithelia with low-grade dysplasia.[26,54,55] p53 appears to be most useful in biopsies that are distorted by crush artifact, tangential sectioning, ulceration, or fragmentation for helping to distinguish between BE with reactive cytologic features and high-grade epithelial dysplasia. However, one should not use p53 staining as a sole criterion to establish the diagnosis of dysplasia in BE.

KEY DIAGNOSTIC POINTS

Barrett Esophagus

- IHC is not reliable for distinguishing Barrett esophagus from intestinal metaplasia of the gastric cardia.
- p53 can help distinguish high-grade dysplasia from nondysplastic columnar mucosa if the result is extensively and strongly positive; however, p53 expression must be combined with histologic features to make a diagnosis of dysplasia.

Esophageal Adenocarcinoma

Esophageal adenocarcinomas typically express cytokeratins AE1/AE3, Cam 5.2, CK19, and CK7; a minority of cases express CK20. CDX2 expression is variable; while many tumors may show focal positivity, a significant minority are completely negative and only a few are uniformly positive.[56] Villin expression is more uniform, present in approximately 75% of tumors.[56] Most studies have found that esophageal adenocarcinomas are immunophenotypically identical to adenocarcinomas of the gastric cardia (see below).[57-60] Some[50,61,62] but not all[36] studies suggest that esophageal and gastric cardia adenocarcinomas have different CK7/CK20 staining patterns based on statistical comparison of a large number of cases. However, the overlap in staining patterns between the two groups in these studies is substantial, resulting in a limited use of CK7/CK20 staining to differentiate esophageal adenocarcinomas from proximal gastric adenocarcinomas.

KEY DIAGNOSTIC POINTS

Esophageal Adenocarcinoma

Esophageal adenocarcinoma is immunophenotypically similar to proximal gastric adenocarcinoma. There is currently no reliable immunohistochemical panel to distinguish these two entities.

Esophageal Squamous Cell Carcinoma

SCCs generally stain strongly with medium- and high-molecular-weight cytokeratins; expression of low molecular weight keratins is typically weak (Fig. 14.2).

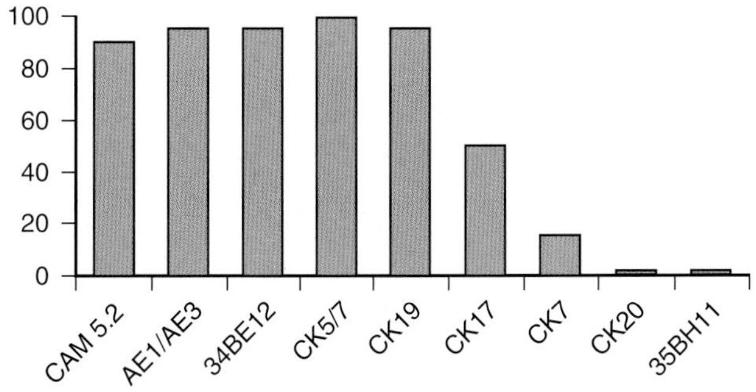

FIGURE 14.2 Cytokeratin reactivity in esophageal squamous cell carcinoma.

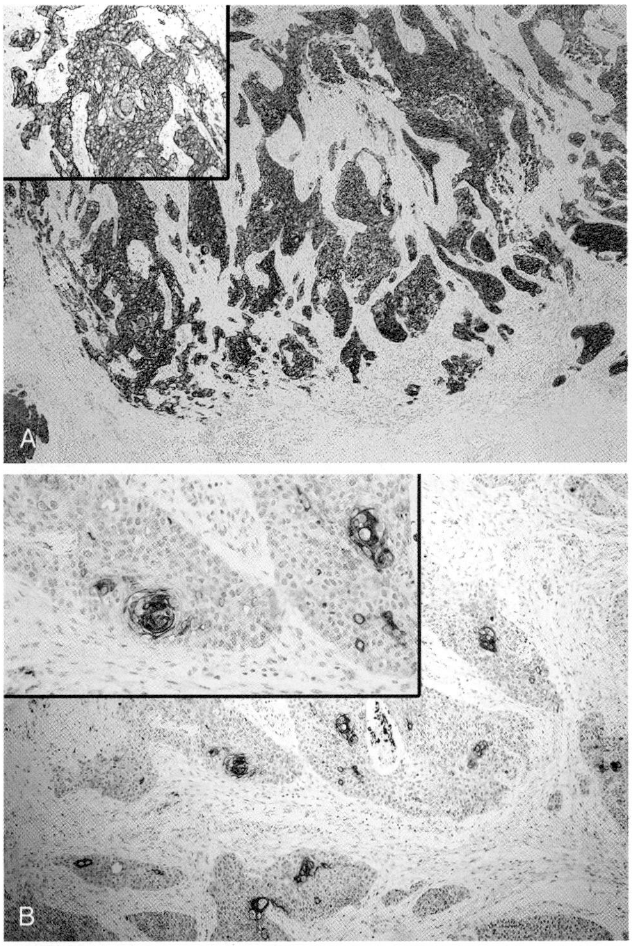

FIGURE 14.3 **A,** Esophageal squamous cell carcinoma stains diffusely and strongly with cytokeratin 34βE12. *Inset:* Central keratin whirl is clearly outlined against surrounding strongly staining tumor cells. **B,** In contrast, cytokeratin 5/6 staining is predominantly confined to the central keratinized cell whirls. *Inset:* Rare, isolated tumor cells also stain strongly.

Accordingly, most SCCs stain diffusely and strongly with cytokeratin antibodies CAM5.2, AE1/AE3, 34bE12, CK5/6, CK14, and CK19.[63-71] Cytokeratin 34bE12 usually produces stronger and more diffuse staining than CK5/6 (Fig. 14.3).

The intensity of cytokeratin 19 expression increases with higher tumor grade. Approximately 70% of low-grade SCCs stain with CK19 in less than half of the neoplastic cells, whereas almost all high-grade neoplasms are diffusely and strongly reactive.[66] Squamous carcinoma *in situ* is also positive for CK19, whereas benign squamous mucosa is negative (Fig. 14.4). Other diagnostically useful antibodies that are typically strongly positive are p63, which stains in a nuclear pattern,[72] thrombomodulin, epithelial membrane antigen, and selected monoclonal CEAs.[73,74]

Nonreactive antibodies include CK7, CK20, CK 35bH11, Ber-EP4, TTF-1, and WT1.[70,71,75,76] Although CK7 is included in this group, approximately 15% to 30% of SCCs have occasional and scattered clusters of cells that are CK7 positive.[66,67] However, if one defines a positive result as expression in more than 50% of tumor cells, esophageal SCCs are considered CK7/CK20 negative.

Primary pulmonary SCC can occasionally be distinguished from esophageal SCC with TTF-1. Although both neoplasms are usually nonreactive, occasional pulmonary squamous cell carcinomas may show extensive and strong nuclear TTF-1 staining, whereas esophageal SCCs are consistently negative for TTF-1.[77]

It is occasionally important to distinguish between poorly differentiated SCC and poorly differentiated adenocarcinoma. Cytokeratins 7, 20, and 5/6 are useful in this context.[67] SCCs including poorly differentiated nonkeratinizing neoplasms are CK7–, CK20–, and CK5/6+, whereas adenocarcinomas of the esophagus, stomach, and lung are typically CK7+, CK20+, and CK5/6–.

Distinction between SCC and thymic carcinoma is also occasionally required. CD5 can be diffusely and strongly positive in primary thymic carcinoma and nonreactive in esophageal SCCs. Importantly, selective CD5 reactivity of thymic carcinomas is highly dependent on the pH of the antigen retrieval solution and the antibody clone. Some CD5 antibodies diffusely and strongly stain both thymic carcinomas and esophageal squamous carcinomas.[78,79]

Mesothelioma can occasionally be morphologically and clinically similar to poorly differentiated, nonkeratinizing, primary esophageal SCC. Both neoplasms are immunoreactive with calretinin and CK5/6, leaving WT1 as the single positive diagnostic marker for mesothelioma.[80]

KEY DIAGNOSTIC POINTS

Esophageal Squamous Cell Carcinoma

- Squamous cell carcinomas stain strongly and diffusely with CAM5.2, AE1/3, CK5/6, and p63.
- Cytokeratin 7, cytokeratin 20, and CEA are either negative or focally positive in poorly differentiated squamous cell carcinomas, whereas these antibodies are strongly positive in poorly differentiated adenocarcinomas.
- CD5, if performed correctly, can be used to distinguish thymic carcinoma from esophageal squamous cell carcinoma.

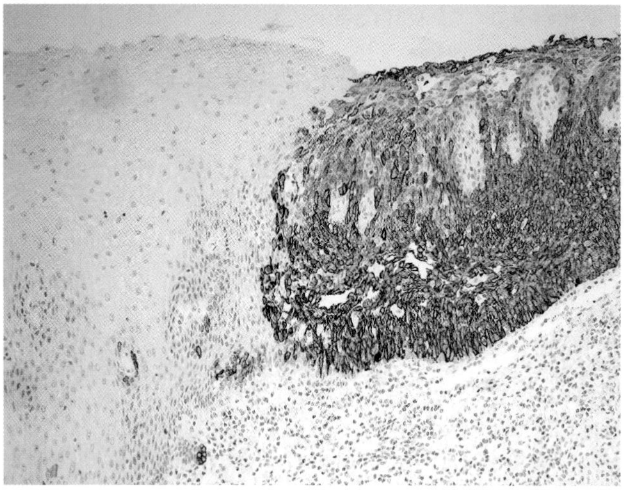

FIGURE 14.4 CK19 strongly stains the squamous cell carcinoma *in situ* on the right, whereas the benign epithelium on the left is nonreactive.

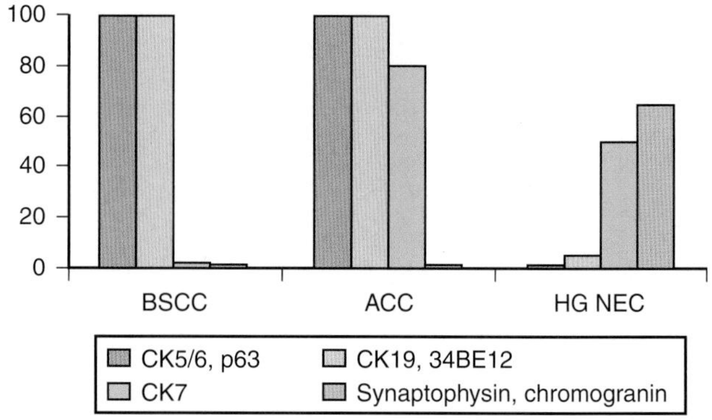

FIGURE 14.5 Differential staining patterns of basaloid-patterned esophageal carcinomas. ACC, adenoid cystic carcinoma; BSCC, basaloid squamous cell carcinoma; HG NEC, high-grade neuroendocrine carcinoma.

Squamous Cell Carcinoma Variants

BASALOID SQUAMOUS CELL CARCINOMA Basaloid squamous cell carcinoma (SCC) is a morphologic and genetic variant of poorly differentiated squamous cell carcinoma.[81] Mixed basaloid/classic squamous cell carcinomas or mixed basaloid squamous cell carcinoma/adenocarcinoma neoplasms may be seen. Bcl-2 has been reported to immunostain basaloid squamous cell carcinomas, while it is nonreactive in poorly differentiated, conventional squamous carcinomas.[82] CK5/6, CK monoclonal-OSCAR, CK13, CK14, CK19, AE1/3 and p63 typically are diffusely and strongly reactive in basaloid squamous cell carcinomas, whereas cytokeratins CAM5.2, and 35bH11 are often negative or weakly immunoreactive.[83-89] Typically, the central cells within each nest are strongly cytokeratin 5/6 and p63 positive. Moreover, the pseudopalisading, single cell layer at the periphery of carcinoma nests typically shows myoepithelial differentiation, including reactivity with CK19, S-100, and smooth muscle actin.[85] Similar to some high-grade breast carcinomas, immunohistochemical features of myoepithelial cell differentiation can be diffuse.[90]

ADENOID CYSTIC CARCINOMA Most reported esophageal adenoid cystic carcinomas are basaloid SCCs; true adenoid cystic carcinomas of the esophagus are extremely rare.[85] Esophageal salivary gland–type adenoid cystic carcinomas stain diffusely and strongly with CAM5.2 and AE1/AE3. 34bE12 and CEA stain the ductal-type cells, whereas S-100, actin, and vimentin stain the basaloid-type cells.[85-87]

Basaloid SCCs with a solid growth pattern, basaloid SCCs with a cribriform growth pattern that mimics adenoid cystic carcinoma, salivary gland-type adenoid cystic carcinomas, and high-grade neuroendocrine carcinomas are often morphologically similar and may be difficult to separate, especially in small biopsy fragments. Immunohistochemistry is useful in this context (Fig. 14.5). CK5/6, CK7, 34bE12, CK19, p63, CEA, chromogranin, and synaptophysin are useful for distinguishing among these three entities.[63,86] Cytokeratin 7 is often the single positive marker in high-grade neuroendocrine carcinoma. Care should be given to avoid misinterpreting the nonspecific synaptophysin staining of necrotic debris found in basaloid SCCs as true cytoplasmic granular immunoreactivity.

KEY DIAGNOSTIC POINTS

Squamous Cell Carcinoma Variants

- Central areas or nests of basaloid squamous cell carcinoma are CK5/6 and p63 positive, whereas the peripheral rim of palisading cells may be CK19 positive.
- Most adenoid cystic-like carcinomas are basaloid squamous cell carcinomas. True adenoid cystic carcinomas of the esophagus are extremely rare.
- High-grade (small cell) neuroendocrine carcinoma is diffusely synaptophysin and CK7 positive.

Esophageal Carcinomas with Spindle Cell or Mesenchymal Differentiation

Esophageal carcinomas can rarely show spindle cell or mesenchymal differentiation; however, the spindle cell component is often associated with recognizable epithelial differentiation. Not surprisingly, this mesenchymal differentiation shows decreased cytokeratin expression. The cytokeratin clones OSCAR and CK5/6 produce the strongest and most diffuse immunoreactivity. CK OSCAR is the preferred antibody for distinguishing neoplastic spindle cells from reactive myofibroblasts; CAM5.2, 35bH11, and AE1/AE3 are usually nonreactive.[91-94] Among these three antibodies, AE1/AE3 produces the strongest and most diffuse staining.[95] Neoplastic spindle cells can stain with actin antibodies; however, desmin is usually negative, providing the immunohistochemical distinction from leiomyosarcoma. True spindle cell rhabdomyosarcomatous differentiation can also occur, in which the cells stain with pan-muscle actin, desmin, and other markers of rhabdomyoblastic differentiation.[91,96]

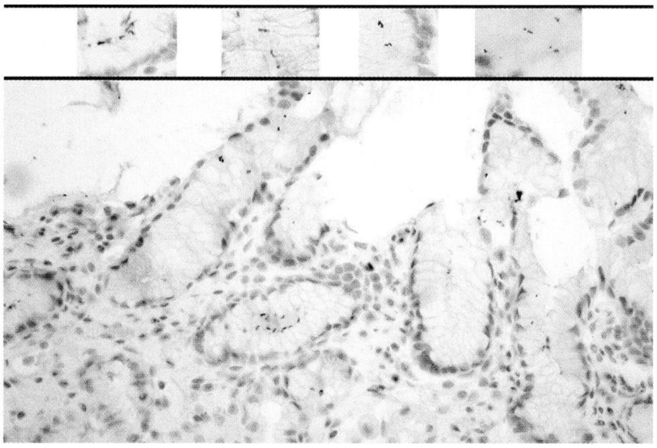

FIGURE 14.6 Gastric antral mucosa with numerous *Helicobacter pylori.* Many of the microorganisms are insinuated between the cell membranes of adjacent columnar mucus cells. The inset images across the top of the figure demonstrate the broad range of bacterial shapes including coccoid, spiral, bacilliform, and barbell.

STOMACH

Non-neoplastic Conditions

LYMPHOCYTIC GASTRITIS Lymphocytic gastritis is usually a manifestation of celiac disease and, occasionally, of *Helicobacter pylori* infection. In celiac disease patients the density of surface intraepithelial lymphocytes (IELs) is usually lower than that seen in the duodenum. Gastric IELs are T lymphocytes that stain with CD45RO, CD3, CD7, CD8, and TIA-1[97,98]

HELICOBACTER PYLORI Proton pump inhibitor and *H. pylori* eradication medications decrease the density of *H. pylori* organisms and alter their shape from spiral to coccoid.[99-101] Coccoid-shaped *H. pylori* can be difficult to distinguish from small mucin globules or extracellular debris on modified Giemsa or other histochemical stains. Immunohistochemistry is a more reliable and sensitive method for detecting *H. pylori,* especially when the organisms are few in number or when coccoid in shape (Fig. 14.6).[100-105] Additionally, most *H. pylori* antibodies cross-react with *Helicobacter heilmannii,* which can occasionally be useful when the morphology of these organisms does not unequivocally allow for their identification on routine stains.[106]

ATROPHIC GASTRITIS, AUTOIMMUNE TYPE Immunohistochemistry can be a useful adjunct in the diagnosis of autoimmune gastritis. Most cases of autoimmune gastritis show hyperplasia of the enterochromaffin-like (ECL) cell compartment secondary to hypergastrinemia. This phenomenon can be highlighted using synaptophysin and/or chromogranin immunohistochemistry. Normal mucosa shows occasional synaptophysin and/or chromogranin positive cells within the epithelial compartment. In autoimmune gastritis, intraepithelial linear arrays and/or extraepithelial nodules of synaptophysin/chromogranin positive ECL cells may be seen (Fig. 14.7).[107-109]

In addition to the detection of ECL hyperplasia, immunohistochemistry for gastrin can be helpful in separating atrophic "antralized" oxyntic mucosa with complete loss of both parietal and chief cells from true antral mucosa. In fully developed autoimmune gastritis, these two types of mucosa can be difficult to separate on routine histology. Gastrin-staining cells are present in the antrum and are absent in atrophic ("antralized") mucosa.[109-111] Of note, when assessing gastric biopsies for the presence of body-predominant atrophic gastritis, these three stains (synaptophysin, chromogranin, and gastrin) must be assessed in areas free of intestinal metaplasia because the intestinal metaplasia contains its own neuroendocrine cells that may be gastrin positive (see Fig. 14.7).

FUNDIC GLAND POLYPS Fundic gland polyps occur as sporadic lesions and may be associated with long-term proton pump inhibitor therapy. Additionally, fundic gland polyps may arise in association with familial adenomatous polyposis (FAP) and Zollinger-Ellison syndromes. Morphologic distinctions between the sporadic and syndromic polyps can be subtle. Cytokeratin 7 has been reported to stain sporadic polyps and Zollinger-Ellison syndrome-associated polyps, whereas beta-catenin expression has been described in sporadic polyps but not in FAP-associated polyps.[112-115] However, IHC is not routinely used to evaluate fundic gland polyps.

KEY DIAGNOSTIC POINTS

Non-neoplastic Stomach

- T-cell markers can be used to highlight intraepithelial lymphocytes (IELs) in suspected cases of lymphocytic gastritis associated with celiac disease or *Helicopter pylori* infection.
- IHC staining for *H. pylori* is useful when treatment-associated changes reduce the number of organisms or alter their normal appearance.
- In cases of suspected autoimmune gastritis, gastrin immunohistochemistry can be used to distinguish antral from atrophic body or fundic mucosa; synaptophysin and chromogranin immunohistochemistry is useful in the detection of enterochromaffin-like cell hyperplasia, a characteristic feature of autoimmune gastritis.

Gastric Adenocarcinoma

Although it is important for pathologists to characterize gastric adenocarcinomas into one of the two main morphologic subtypes, either intestinal-type or diffuse (signet ring cell)–type,[116] the immunohistochemical staining pattern of these two subtypes is similar. As a result, both types are discussed together in this section. Gastric adenocarcinomas stain with various cytokeratins (Fig. 14.8). The reactivity of several other antibodies is listed in Table 14.2. Some of these antibodies are now discussed in more detail.

CYTOKERATINS Gastric adenocarcinomas are diffusely and strongly positive for AE1/AE3 and 35BH11.[70] Cytokeratin CAM5.2 produces diffuse strong staining in

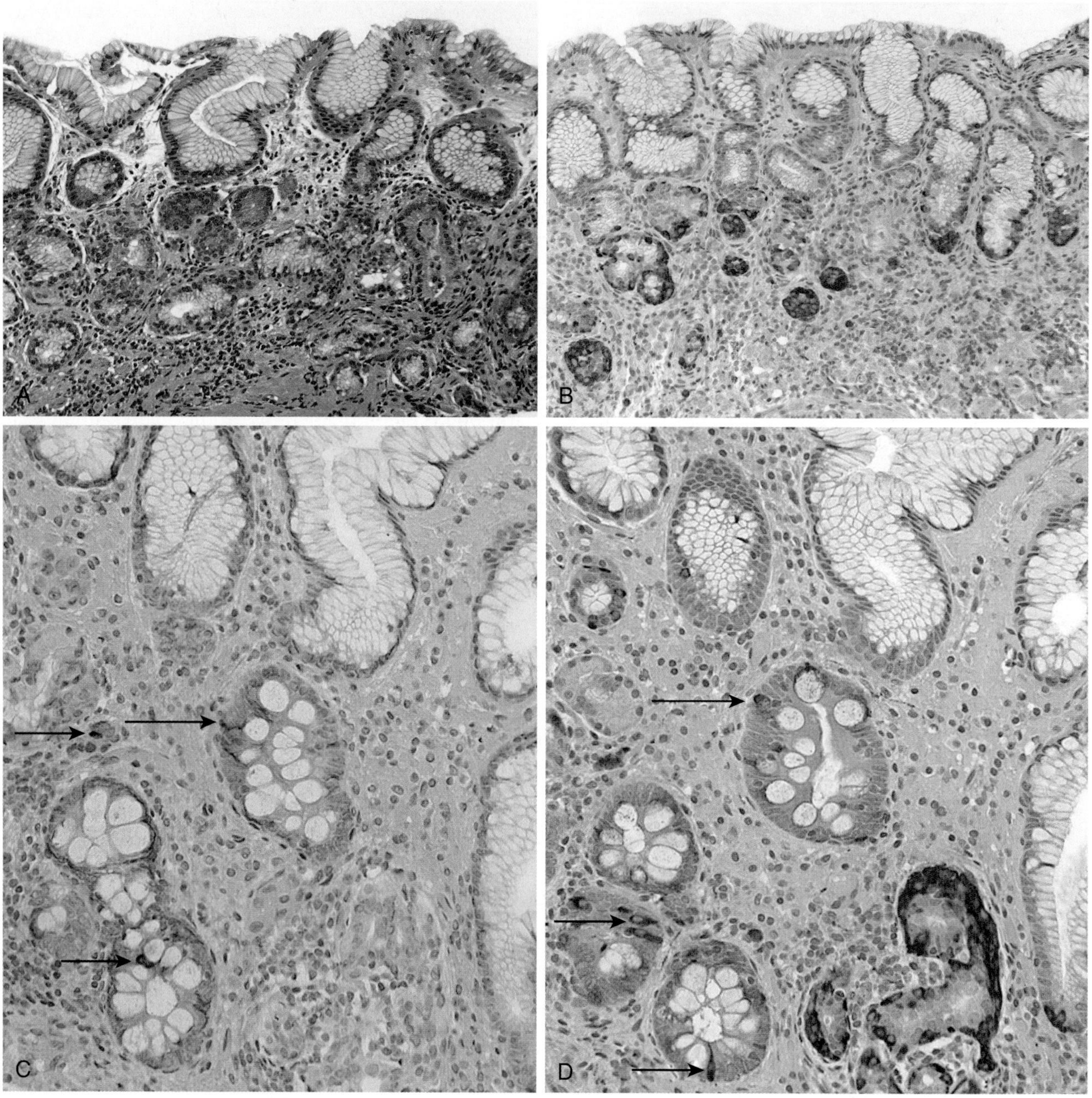

FIGURE 14.7 Autoimmune gastritis. **A,** This biopsy from the gastric body lacks oxyntic glands, and instead, the mucosa has the appearance of antral mucosa. However, this is not true antral mucosa; there are no G cells present on the gastrin immunostain (not shown). **B,** Synaptophysin highlights ECL cell hyperplasia within this atrophic body mucosa. Both linear (more than five positive cells in a line) and nodular (small round clusters) forms of ECL cell hyperplasia are present in this image. When interpreting immunostains in cases of possible autoimmune gastritis, it is important to ignore areas of intestinal metaplasia because metaplastic G cells or EC cells can often be present within the intestinal-type epithelium and they can stain with **(C)** gastrin *(arrows)* and **(D)** synaptophysin (*arrows;* true ECL cell hyperplasia is also present in the lower right of the figure).

approximately two thirds of these neoplasms and weak to moderate, patchy staining in the other third.[117] Cytokeratins 18 and 19 are diffusely and strongly positive.[50,118-121]

CYTOKERATIN 7 CK7 expression is an important marker of committed gastric epithelial cells and gastric adenocarcinoma. Approximately 50% of gastric adenocarcinomas are strongly positive in a diffuse or patchy distribution; 30% have rare clusters of strongly reactive cells, and 20% are weakly positive or negative (Fig. 14.9).[118-120,122-125]

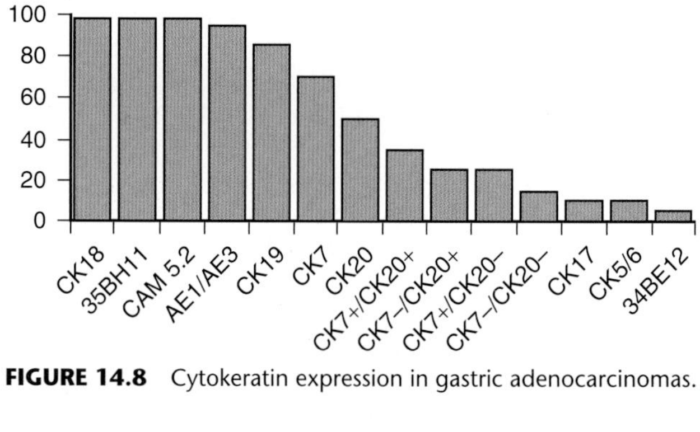

FIGURE 14.8 Cytokeratin expression in gastric adenocarcinomas.

TABLE 14.2 Expression of Various Antibodies (Excluding Cytokeratins) in Gastric Adenocarcinomas

Antibody	Reactivity	Comments	References
AMACR (p504s)	+	More commonly expressed in intestinal-type and high-grade dysplasia	Lee,* Huang†
B72.3	+		117, 169
BerEP4	+		117
CA-125	S	Single cells or small foci	118, 175
CA19-9	+		232
Calretinin	N		Doglioni‡
CD99	S	Staining confined to intestinal-type neoplasms	Jung§
CDX2	S	Heterogeneous and variable staining in 20% to 90% of cases	56, 133-135
CEA	+	Monoclonal antibody is more discriminatory	60, 117
DAS-1	S		138
EMA	+		220
GCDFP-15	N	Rare (<1%) signet ring cells can be positive	126, 171
HepPar1	S	High-grade and signet-ring cells can be focally positive	155, 156
Inhibin-alpha	N		McCluggage¶
MUC1	R		135, 137
MUC2	S	Up to 50% cases can be positive	134-138
MUC4	S		137, 139
MUC5AC	+	38-70% cases can be positive	134-138
MUC6	S		120, 134-138
p63	R	Patchy staining in high grade and squamoid carcinomas	65
S-100	S	About 20% neoplasms can have focal positivity	Herrera¶¶
TTF-1	N		77, 247
Villin	S		56, 136
Vimentin	R	Positive in spindle cell (sarcomatoid) carcinomas	152, 154, 303

N, negative; R, rarely positive; S, sometimes; +, positive.

*Lee WA. Alpha-methylacyl-CoA-racemase expression in adenocarcinoma, dysplasia and non-neoplastic epithelium of the stomach. *Oncology*. 2006;71:246-250.

†Huang W, Zhao J, Li L, et al. a-Methylacyl coenzyme A racemase is highly expressed in the intestinal-type adenocarcinoma and high-grade dysplasia lesions of the stomach. *Histol Histopathol*. 2008;23:1315-1320.

‡Doglioni C, Dei Tos AP, Laurino L, et al. A novel immunocytochemical marker for mesothelioma. *Am J Surg Pathol*. 1996;20:1037-1046.

§Jung KC, Park WS, Bae YM, et al. Immunoreactivity of CD99 in stomach cancer. *J Korean Med Sci*. 2002;17:483-489.

¶McCluggage WC, Maxwell P. Adenocarcinomas of various sites may exhibit immunoreactivity with anti-inhibin antibodies. *Histopathology*. 1999:216-220.

¶¶Herrera GA, Turbat-Herrera EA, Lott RL. S-100 protein expression by primary and metastatic adenocarcinomas. *Am J Clin Pathol*. 1988;89:168-176.

CYTOKERATIN 20 Approximately 40% of gastric adenocarcinomas are strongly positive in a patchy or diffuse distribution, 20% are weakly positive in a patchy distribution, and 40% are negative (Fig. 14.10).[118,119,124-127]

CYTOKERATINS 7 AND 20 COORDINATE STAINING Gastric adenocarcinoma is extremely heterogeneous in its CK7/CK20 coordinate staining patterns. The search for a predominant pattern has been complicated by the use of different cut-off points at which staining is considered positive. The percentage of positively staining cells in the literature ranges from 1% to 25%. Given these findings, there is no predominant pattern of coordinate CK7/20 staining; a significant minority of gastric adenocarcinomas stain with each of the four possible CK7/CK20 patterns. Approximately 35% of gastric adenocarcinomas are CK7+/CK20+, 25% are CK7−/CK20+, 25% are CK7+/CK20−, and 15% are CK7−/CK20−.[1,118,119,124,128-132] These percentages vary by up to 30% depending on the cut-off point used in the study.

CDX2 AND VILLIN Several studies examined CDX2 expression in gastric adenocarcinomas. CDX2 appears to be variably expressed (percent positivity ranges from 20% to 90%), but even when present, CDX2 expression tends to be heterogeneous as compared with strong

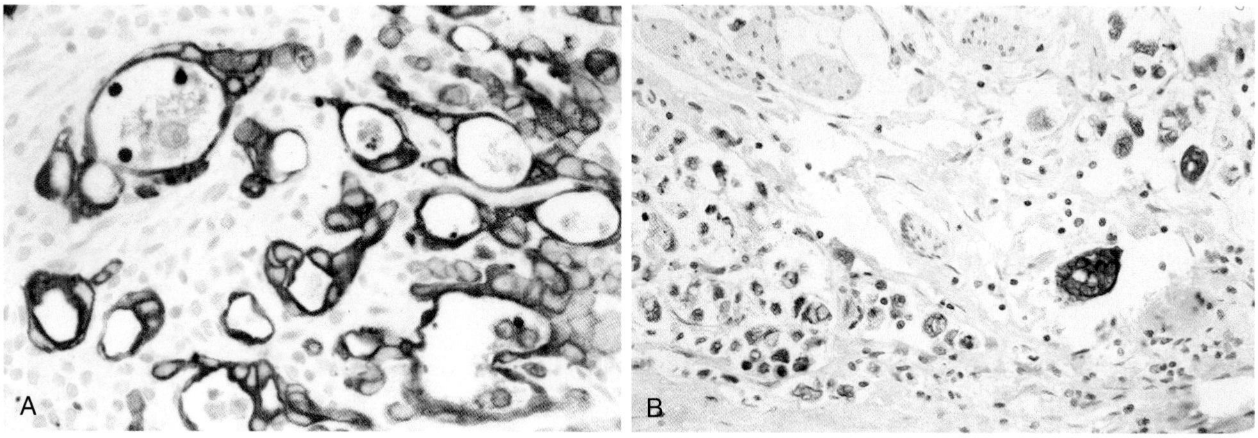

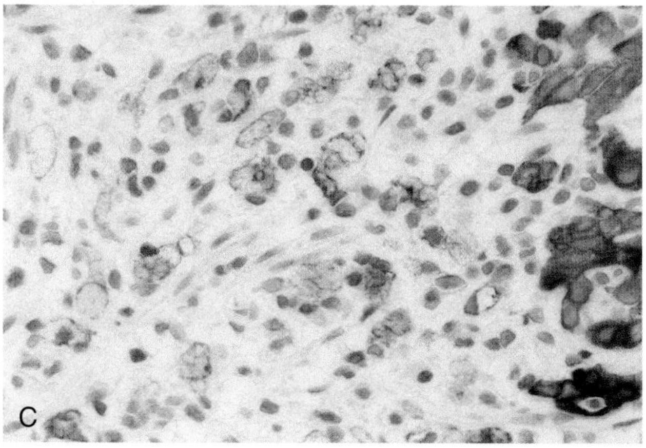

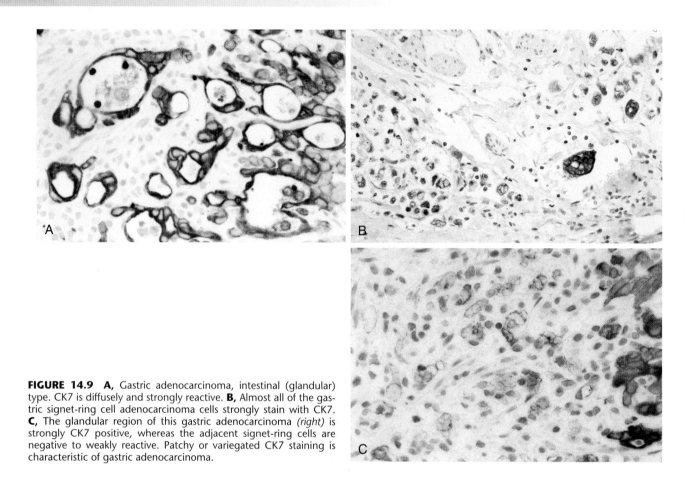

FIGURE 14.9 **A,** Gastric adenocarcinoma, intestinal (glandular) type. CK7 is diffusely and strongly reactive. **B,** Almost all of the gastric signet-ring cell adenocarcinoma cells strongly stain with CK7. **C,** The glandular region of this gastric adenocarcinoma *(right)* is strongly CK7 positive, whereas the adjacent signet-ring cells are negative to weakly reactive. Patchy or variegated CK7 staining is characteristic of gastric adenocarcinoma.

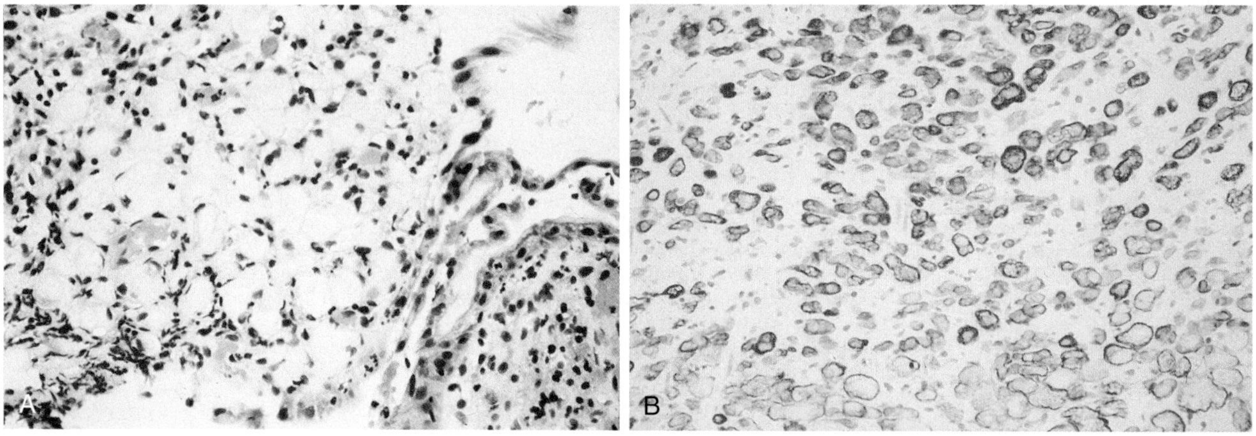

FIGURE 14.10 **A,** Gastric signet-ring cells are relatively inconspicuous within the lamina propria. **B,** CK20 reveals the numerous neoplastic signet-ring cells, which were not easily seen on hematoxylin and eosin stain.

and diffuse staining with true intestinal adenocarcinomas.[56,133-135] Villin also has variable expression and may be slightly more reliable than CDX2.[136]

APOMUCINS Overall, the various mucin stains may not be as helpful as one would like. The gastric mucin MUC5AC is positive, but only in 38% to 70% of cases.[134-138] MUC6, another gastric mucin, is only positive in 30% to 40% of cases.[120,134-138] MUC2 is positive in up to 50% of cases; MUC4 has inconsistent results in the literature, staining from 57% to 100% of cases; and MUC1 stains only a minority of cases.[137,139]

ESTROGEN RECEPTOR (ER) AND PROGESTERONE RECEPTOR (PR) The issue of estrogen receptor (ER) positivity in gastric adenocarcinomas has been debated for many years. Faint ER staining of gastric adenocarcinomas was initially interpreted to be a false-positive reaction. Nuclear staining was later deemed a true positive, with the lack of staining considered to be a false-negative result. The immunohistochemical detection of low-level ER expression is dependent on the antibody clone and IHC procedure, but in most studies, gastric adenocarcinomas are negative for ER.[135,138,140-144] Well-differentiated adenocarcinomas are reactive more often than poorly undifferentiated neoplasms.[145] Gastric adenocarcinomas are also generally negative for progesterone receptor (PR), but a few studies have reported infrequent staining with PR.[126,138,141,146] Although typically negative, focal or diffuse weak staining with ER or PR does not exclude a gastric primary.

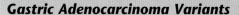

KEY DIAGNOSTIC POINTS

Gastric Adenocarcinoma

- Many cytokeratins stain gastric adenocarcinoma diffusely and strongly.
- Gastric adenocarcinoma is immunophenotypically similar to esophageal adenocarcinoma; there is currently no reliable immunohistochemical panel to distinguish these two entities.
- The CK7/CK20 coordinate staining pattern is not useful in distinguishing gastric adenocarcinoma from other adenocarcinomas.
- Weak estrogen receptor or progesterone receptor staining in a metastatic adenocarcinoma does not rule out a primary gastric carcinoma.

Gastric Adenocarcinoma Variants

LYMPHOEPITHELIAL-LIKE CARCINOMA Gastric lymphoepithelial-like carcinomas are undifferentiated (medullary-type) carcinomas with a lymphocyte-rich stroma. These tumors are often associated with either Epstein-Barr virus (see later) or a high-level level of microsatellite instability (MSI, Fig. 14.11). MSI characterizes a group of carcinomas that develop as a result of deficiencies of the DNA mismatch repair complex. Microsatellite unstable adenocarcinomas can be syndromic (e.g., hereditary nonpolyposis colorectal cancer; HNPCC) or sporadic. Antibodies against MLH1, MSH2, MSH6, and PMS2, proteins of the DNA mismatch repair complex, can detect MSI by their lack of staining in tumor cell nuclei. Syndromic patients can show a loss of any of these antibodies, most commonly MSH2. Almost all MSI-high (MSI-H) gastric adenocarcinomas are sporadic and show loss of MLH1 protein.[147,148] Authors who have classified gastric adenocarcinomas according to cell type have found that tumors with a foveolar phenotype are often microsatellite unstable, whereas carcinomas with an intestinal phenotype are usually microsatellite stable. Intestinal-type carcinomas harbor deletions of tumor suppressor genes that can be demonstrated by staining with p53.[149,150]

SPINDLE CELL DIFFERENTIATION (SARCOMATOID CARCINOMA) Similar to the colon and esophagus, spindle cell differentiation has been described in gastric carcinomas. These neoplasms usually stain with vimentin and EMA and variably with cytokeratin.[151-154] See "Esophagus" earlier for additional discussion.

YOLK-SAC, HEPATOID, AND CHORIOCARCINOMATOUS DIFFERENTIATION

So-called yolk-sac, clear-cell, or hepatoid differentiation is frequent in gastric carcinomas. Although areas of yolk-sac and/or hepatoid differentiation in an otherwise typical adenocarcinoma are common, pure tumors are rare. The morphology of these areas histologically resembles yolk-sac or hepatocellular carcinoma. Single cells or small clusters of cells strongly stain with alpha fetoprotein (AFP) in areas with yolk sac differentiation. Additionally, tumors with hepatoid differentiation may stain with HepPar1 in its typical, granular staining pattern.[155-158] Focal immunoreactivity with HepPar1 and/or AFP can also be seen in otherwise typical intestinal-type and signet-ring cell adenocarcinomas.[117,159,160] Thus AFP or HepPar1 staining alone is not sufficient for the diagnosis of yolk-sac or hepatoid differentiation. Additionally, yolk-sac or hepatoid differentiation has no prognostic significance.

Choriocarcinoma-like differentiation may also be present in otherwise usual-type adenocarcinomas. These foci usually stain with beta-human chorionic gonadotropin (β-hCG) and placental alkaline phosphatase. β-hCG staining of usual-type intestinal or signet-ring adenocarcinomas is common: approximately 33% stain strongly with polyclonal β-hCG and 60% are immunoreactive with the monoclonal antibody.[161-163]

GASTRIC ADENOCARCINOMA WITH NEUROENDOCRINE DIFFERENTIATION

Typical gastric adenocarcinomas of either the intestinal or signet-ring cell type may stain with chromogranin and synaptophysin without histologic evidence of neuroendocrine differentiation.[8,164,165] Staining with either antibody can be extensive in this setting and can be increased by using more sensitive methodologies.[166] Staining with chromogranin or synaptophysin is so common that it could be considered within the normal immunophenotype of gastric adenocarcinoma. Gastric tumors without morphologic features of neuroendocrine differentiation that stain with synaptophysin or chromogranin should not be considered neuroendocrine carcinomas, but rather adenocarcinomas that express neuroendocrine markers.

KEY DIAGNOSTIC POINTS

Gastric Adenocarcinoma Variants

- Lymphoepithelial-like gastric carcinomas have a unique morphologic pattern and most show either loss of MLH1 or expression of EBV by *in situ* hybridization.
- Other morphologic variants of gastric carcinomas have been described including spindle cell, yolk-sac, hepatoid, and choriocarcinoma variants. These variants have a corresponding IHC staining pattern that helps to confirm the morphologic impression.
- Some antibodies that stain morphologic variants such as AFP, HepPar1, and β-hCG can also stain the cells of morphologically typical adenocarcinomas. Immunostaining alone should not be used as evidence of variant differentiation without morphologic correlation.
- Chromogranin and synaptophysin can also be positive in typical adenocarcinomas. Thus, staining with neuroendocrine markers is not sufficient evidence for the diagnosis of neuroendocrine carcinoma.

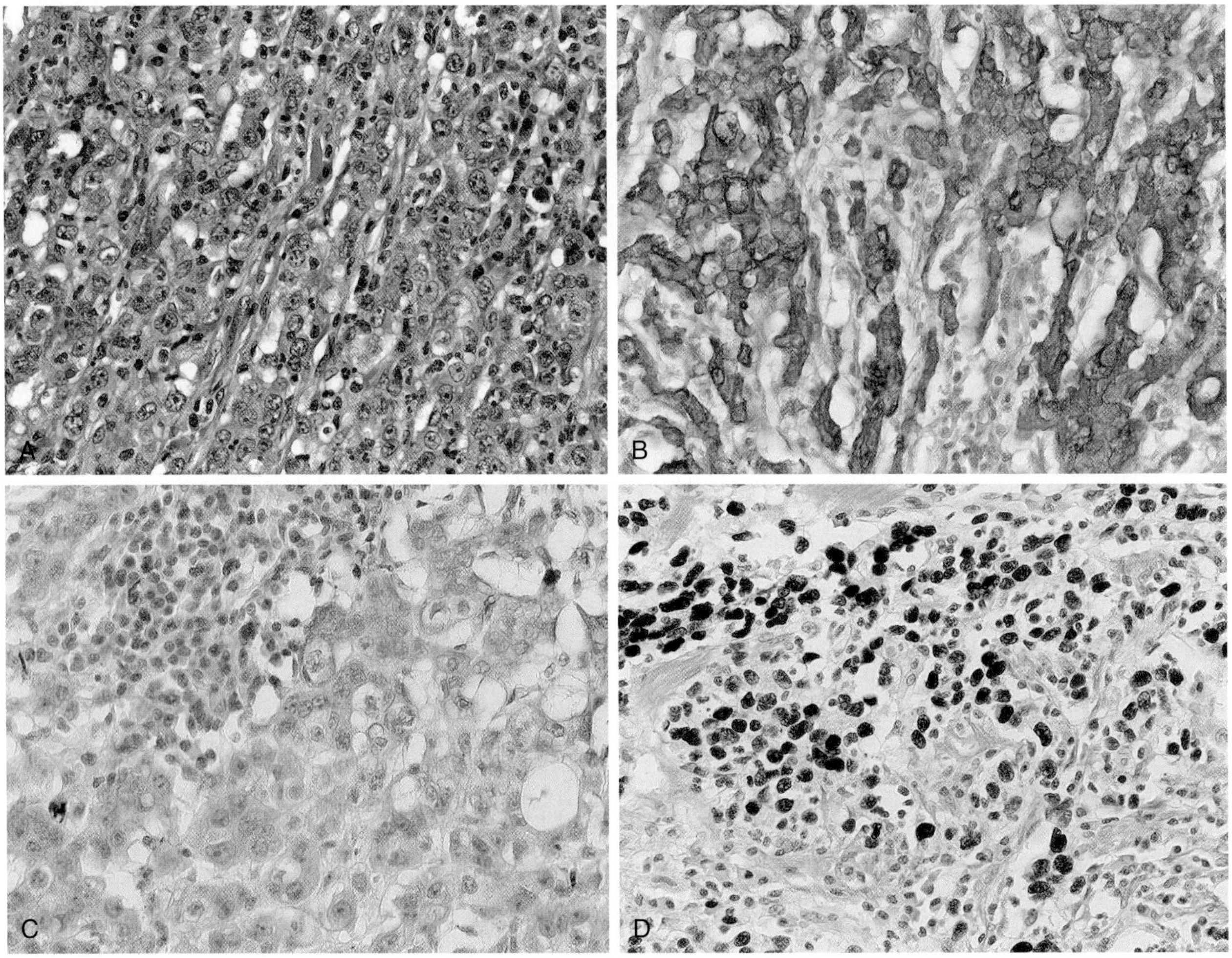

FIGURE 14.11 Lymphoepithelioma-like gastric carcinoma. **A,** The large neoplastic cells have prominent nucleoli and blend in with the background inflammatory cells. **B,** An AE1/AE3 cytokeratin stain highlights the carcinoma cells. **C,** In this neoplasm, MLH-1 is lost in the tumor cell nuclei as compared with the intact (positive) staining of lymphocyte and stromal cell nuclei. **D,** In this example, the tumor cell nuclei are positive for Epstein-Barr virus mRNA (*in situ* hybridization) and the inflammatory and stromal cells are negative.

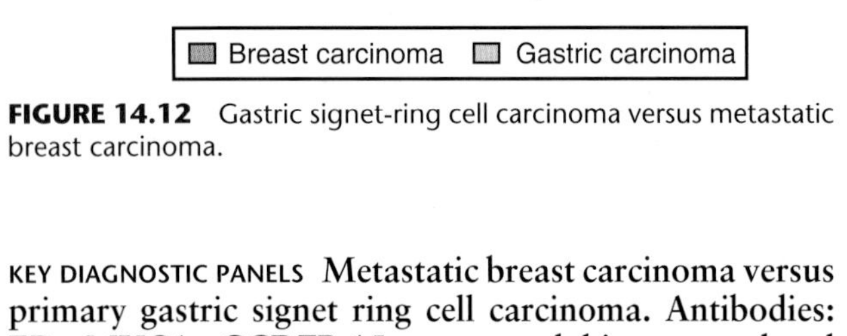

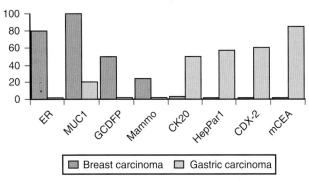

FIGURE 14.12 Gastric signet-ring cell carcinoma versus metastatic breast carcinoma.

KEY DIAGNOSTIC PANELS **Metastatic breast carcinoma versus primary gastric signet ring cell carcinoma. Antibodies: ER, MUC1, GCDFP-15, mammaglobin, monoclonal CEA, CDX2/villin, CK20, and HepPar1** (Fig. 14.12). Gastric signet ring cell carcinoma and metastatic lobular breast carcinoma can be morphologically similar; IHC can be useful in this differential diagnosis. GCDFP-15 and mammaglobin are positive in approximately 50% and 75% of breast carcinomas, respectively[167]; these markers are negative in gastric carcinomas.[126,168-172] Although several authors have reported ER positivity in gastric carcinoma, almost all recent studies have reported uniformly negative staining (see earlier discussion for additional information). The majority of lobular/signet ring cell carcinomas of breast show positive ER staining in most of the cells.[135,138,168] Expression of markers of intestinal differentiation such as villin and CDX2 are supportive of a gastric primary, whereas breast ductal carcinomas are villin and CDX2 negative.[30,32,56,133,144,173,174] Gastric signet ring cell carcinomas are often CK20 positive, compared with 2% of gastric carcinomas.[137,138,144] Monoclonal CEA is diffusely positive in gastric adenocarcinoma and is negative in breast carcinoma. Other CEA antibodies share epitopes and can be positive in both neoplasms.

Pancreaticobiliary versus gastric adenocarcinoma. Antibodies: CK17, CA 125. There is substantial immunophenotypic overlap between pancreaticobiliary and gastric adenocarcinomas. CK17 is expressed in up to 88% of pancreaticobiliary cancers but is only positive

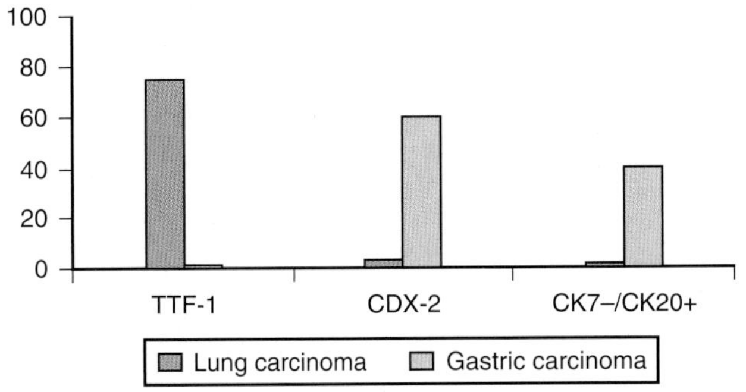

FIGURE 14.13 Gastric signet-ring cell carcinoma versus lung adenocarcinoma.

in 28% of gastric cancers.[174a] CA-125 is often present in less than 10% of cells in gastric carcinoma; a tumor with more than 50% cells staining would support a pancreaticobiliary adenocarcinoma.[175] Cytokeratins 7 and 20 do not play a role in the differential diagnosis because the staining patterns are similar in both tumors.[132]

Lung versus gastric adenocarcinoma. Antibodies: CK7, CK20, TTF-1, surfactant-A, CDX2 (Fig. 14.13). Primary pulmonary signet ring cell carcinomas can be morphologically identical to gastric signet ring cell adenocarcinoma.[176] Cytokeratins 7 and 20 are only useful in differentiating between these entities when a neoplasm expresses the CK7–/CK20+ pattern. This pattern is seen in approximately 40% of gastric adenocarcinomas compared with 0% of primary lung adenocarcinomas with signet ring differentiation.[122,124,125,127,132,170,176-179] Thyroid transcription factor-1 (TTF-1) and surfactant-A are positive in the majority of pulmonary adenocarcinomas and are negative in gastric adenocarcinomas.[176,177,180,181] Approximately 60% of gastric adenocarcinomas are CDX2 positive, whereas lung adenocarcinomas, except the colloid variant, are CDX2 negative.[56,174,182,183]

SMALL INTESTINE

Celiac Disease

Celiac disease is one of the diseases that show increased numbers of intraepithelial lymphocytes (IELs) as a key histologic feature. In celiac disease, most IELs are activated T cells including both alpha/beta and delta/gamma type T cells. The dominant IEL T-cell immunophenotype in celiac disease is CD3+/CD8+.[184] In general, staining for CD3 is not indicated for routine evaluation of duodenal biopsies for celiac disease. However, when the numbers of IELs are equivocally increased or if a section is difficult to evaluate for technical reasons, CD3 immunohistochemistry might be helpful.

Adenocarcinoma of the Small Intestine

Small intestinal adenocarcinomas stain diffusely and strongly with CKs 18 and 19.[120] In contrast to normal small intestinal epithelium, nonampullary small intestinal adenocarcinomas tend to develop CK7 expression and lose CK20 expression.[120,185] Approximately two thirds of small intestinal adenocarcinomas coexpress both CK7 and CK20, and the remaining 33% are CK7+/CK20–; no tumors were CK7–/CK20+ or CK7–/CK20–.[185] They also stain with villin and CDX2 in 60% to 70% of cases, a slightly lower rate than colorectal adenocarcinomas (Fig. 14.14).[56,186] Approximately 50% stain with MUC1 or MUC2, and 38% stain with MUC5A.[120,186] Alpha-methylacyl coenzyme A racemase (AMACR) is rarely expressed in small intestinal adenocarcinomas, but it stains 62% of colorectal adenocarcinomas.[187] The presence of CK7 staining and lack of AMACR staining can help differentiate small intestinal from colorectal adenocarcinomas. Similar to colon cancers, a minority of small bowel adenocarcinomas arise via the MSI pathway, but, immunohistochemically, the vast majority of cases show loss of nuclear staining of the mismatch repair protein MLH1 and preserved (intact) staining with MSH2.[188,189] Adenocarcinomas arising in the ampulla of Vater are discussed in Chapter 15.

KEY DIAGNOSTIC POINTS

Small Intestinal Adenocarcinomas

- The majority (66%) of nonampullary small bowel adenocarcinomas are CK7+/CK20+, which differs from colorectal adenocarcinomas, which tend to be CK7–/CK20+.
- Fewer small intestinal adenocarcinomas (60% to 70%) express CDX2 and villin, compared with colorectal adenocarcinomas.
- CK7 and AMACR can help differentiate small intestinal adenocarcinomas (CK7+/AMACR–) from colorectal adenocarcinomas (CK7–/AMACR+).

APPENDIX, COLON, AND RECTUM

Appendix

Some appendiceal epithelial neoplasms are similar to their colonic counterparts, whereas others are unique to the appendix. Similar to the colon, typical hyperplastic polyps and classic colonic-type adenomas do exist, but they are rare. Lesions with serrated, mucinous, or villous features with or without definite epithelial dysplasia are more common. An obvious assumption is that sessile serrated adenomas of the type seen in the right colon also occur in the appendix. This may be so, but the evidence to support this assumption is lacking at this time. Some propose the use of the term "low-grade appendiceal mucinous neoplasm" to encompass sessile villous adenomas, cystadenomas, and serrated mucinous lesions, especially when associated with intraluminal mucin accumulation that may spread into the peritoneal cavity and cause the clinically recognized entity pseudomyxoma peritonei. These low-grade appendiceal mucinous neoplasms, as well as low-grade mucinous adenocarcinomas, have some different immunohistochemical staining characteristics compared with colorectal mucinous adenocarcinomas (Fig. 14.15).[120,190-195] In addition to expressing CK20, about one third of mucinous lesions of the appendix coexpress CK7, with approximately 25% to 75% of cells staining (Figs. 14.16 to 14.18). The proportion of CK7-positive cells in this group of lesions is substantially greater than the pattern of rare cells

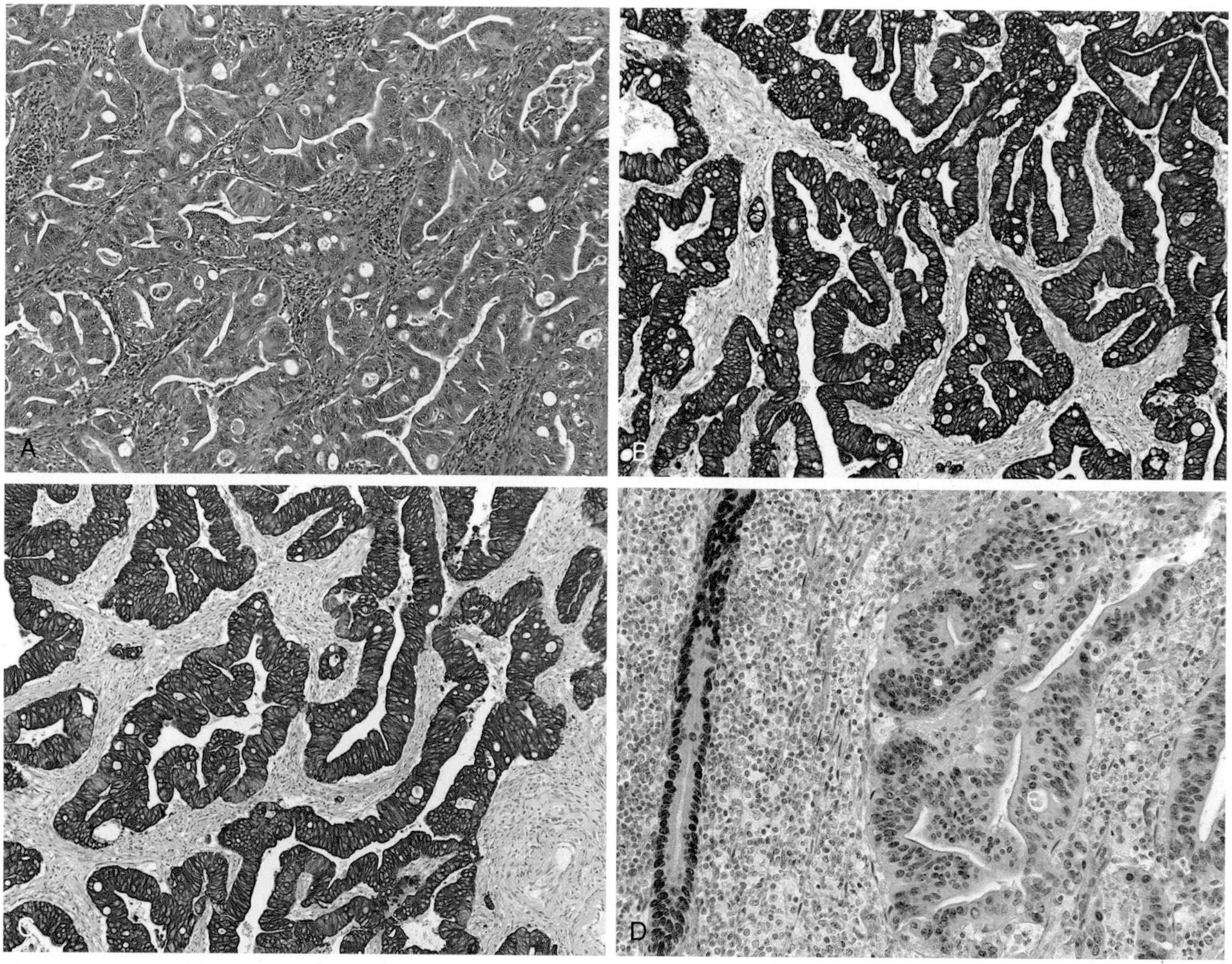

FIGURE 14.14 Small intestinal adenocarcinoma (**A,** H&E stain). This is an example of a small intestinal adenocarcinoma that strongly expresses CK7 **(B)**, CK20 **(C)**, and CDX2 **(D)**.

and occasional cluster of positive cells that is typical of colorectal adenocarcinomas. More than 80% of appendiceal mucinous adenocarcinomas are MUC5A positive, which is similar to the proportions stained in gastric, pancreatic, ovarian primary mucinous tumors (see Fig. 14.15). In contrast, only up to 33% of colorectal mucinous adenocarcinomas are MUC5A positive.[192] Similar to colorectal mucinous adenocarcinomas, appendiceal mucinous tumors diffusely and strongly stain with cytokeratins 8, 13, 18, 19, 20, MUC2, CDX2, and DPC4.[120,192,196,197] Nonmucinous, intestinal-type adenocarcinomas of the appendix are rare and are immunophenotypically similar to colonic adenocarcinomas.

The immunohistochemical distinction of primary and metastatic mucinous adenocarcinomas can be problematic, especially when they involve the ovary.[198,199] There can be overlap of the CK7/CK20 immunohistochemical profile of appendiceal and ovarian tumors.[188,193] An antibody panel of CK7, CK20, CDX2, MUC2, and MUC5A yields the most informative results (Fig. 14.15). Lack of CK7 and diffuse, strong CK20 staining is supportive of a colorectal adenocarcinoma, whereas diffuse CK7 staining and nonreactive CK20 is supportive of a primary ovarian neoplasm. Even in cases where focal or patchy staining of CK7 or CK20 is noted, the pattern of staining can be helpful. Ovarian tumors tend to show diffuse CK7 and patchy CK20 staining, whereas colorectal and appendiceal tumors tend to show patchy CK7 and diffuse CK20 staining.[192] Strong and diffuse nuclear CDX2 staining is supportive of a primary colorectal or appendiceal mucinous adenocarcinoma; CDX2 reactivity in ovarian and pancreatic mucinous neoplasms is characteristically less intense and extensive.[56,174,197,200]

KEY DIAGNOSTIC POINTS

Mucinous Appendiceal Neoplasms

- Appendiceal mucinous neoplasms can be distinguished from colonic mucinous adenocarcinomas by their comparatively greater CK7 staining and MUC5A reactivity, whereas colonic neoplasms tend to be nonreactive.
- An antibody panel of CK7, CK20, CDX2, MUC2, and MUC5A can aid in the distinction between primary and metastatic mucinous adenocarcinomas.

Hirschsprung Disease

The diagnosis of Hirschsprung disease relies on the histopathologic assessment of rectal biopsies. Acetylcholinesterase histochemistry can be used to highlight

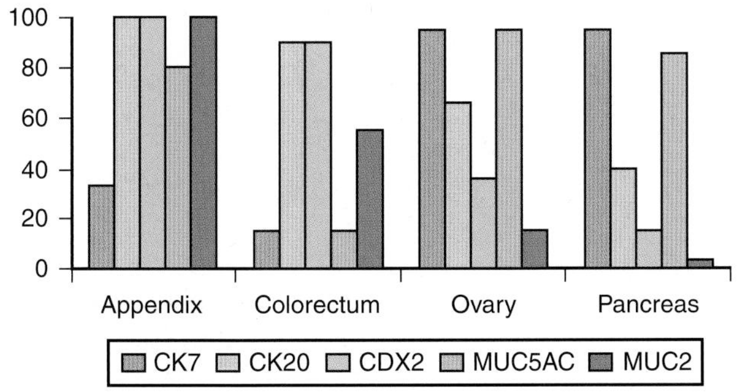

FIGURE 14.15 Immunophenotypes of mucinous adenocarcinomas.

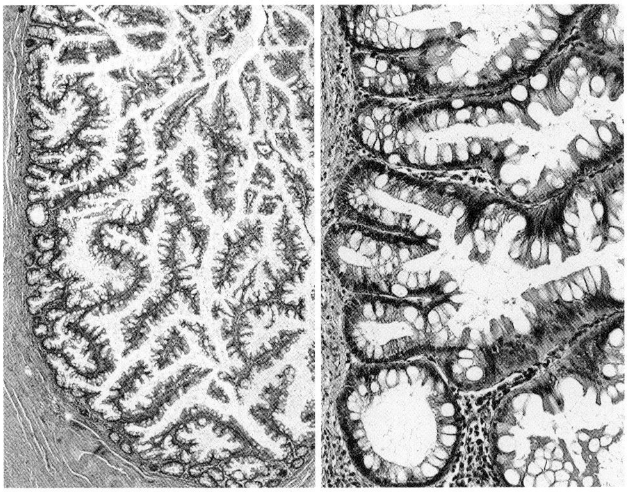

FIGURE 14.16 Appendiceal mucinous neoplasm, low-grade, noninvasive. At higher magnification, the neoplastic cells are morphologically similar to those comprising so-called ovarian-primary mucinous borderline neoplasms.

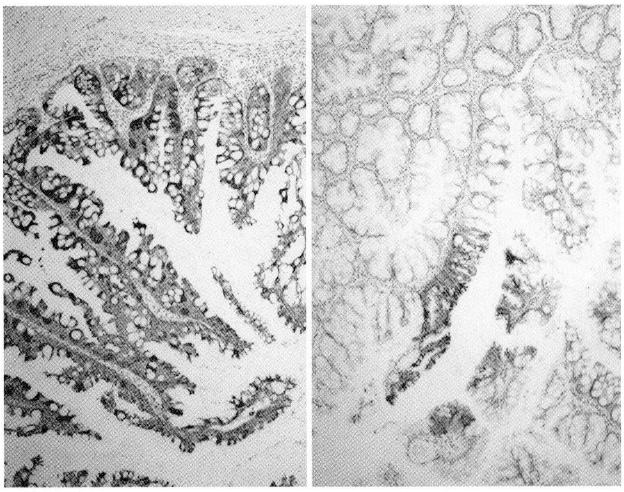

FIGURE 14.17 Most appendiceal-primary mucinous neoplasms are CK20 positive *(left)* and either negative or focally reactive with CK7 *(right)*.

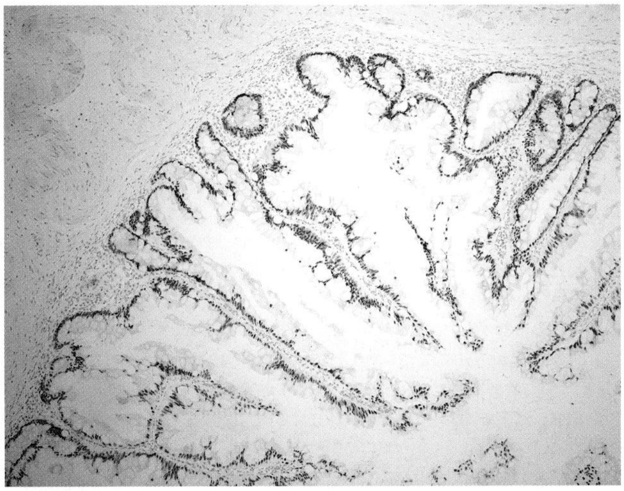

FIGURE 14.18 CDX2 is typically strongly reactive in the cell nuclei of appendiceal mucinous neoplasms.

increased nerve fibers, but this method requires special tissue handling. Routine immunohistochemistry can also aid in the diagnosis. Neuron-specific enolase, cathepsin D, bcl-2, and calretinin, which normally stain ganglion cells, can be used to identify ganglion cells or the lack thereof.[201-203] S-100 and NSE can be used to highlight hypertrophic nerve fibers within an aganglionic segment.[204] In addition to staining ganglion cells, calretinin stains normal nerve fibers. The presence of calretinin-positive nerve fibers in the muscularis mucosae and superficial submucosa correlates strongly with the presence of ganglion cells and may be superior to acetylcholinesterase histochemistry.[201]

Colonic Polyps

There was not much need to determine protein expression in colorectal polyps until the sessile serrated adenoma (SSA) was described as a new entity. Although SSAs share similar morphologic features to hyperplastic polyps (HPs), these polyps appear to arise via distinct genetic pathways and they have different risks of progression to malignancy. Because our understanding of both SSAs and HPs is still evolving, the following summary of the immunophenotypic features of these polyps is a review of the current literature and is also likely to evolve over a short period of time.

In one study, compared with typical (e.g., tubular or tubulovillous) adenomas, HPs, SSAs, and traditional serrated adenomas overexpressed MUC5AC, trefoil factor 1 (TFF1), and PDX1. These lesions also showed preserved staining with MUC2 and had decreased expression of TFF3. CDX2 was downregulated in HPs and SSAs.[205] SSA-associated cancers may arise via the MSI pathway, a theory that is supported by the finding of loss of MLH1 and PMS2 immunoexpression in areas of dysplasia and cancer but not in adjacent SSA or normal mucosa.[206] COX2 is expressed in adenomas (typical adenomas and traditional serrated adenomas) but not in SSAs or HPs.[207]

A few markers show promise in being able to distinguish SSAs from HPs, but these markers need to be verified with additional studies. One study found that SSAs express MUC6 in the deep glands, whereas left-sided

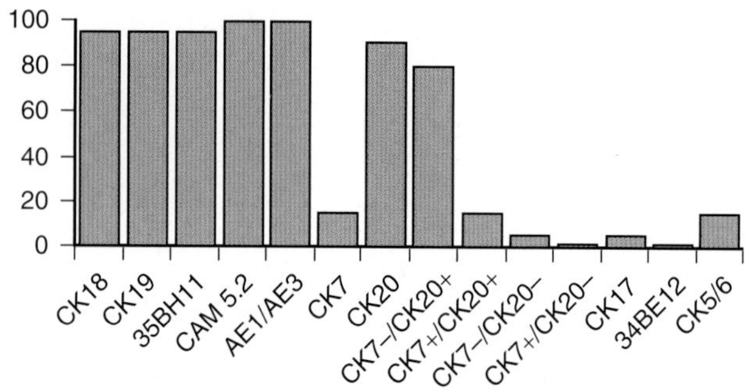

FIGURE 14.19 Cytokeratin expression in colorectal adenocarcinoma.

hyperplastic polyps do not.[208] Another study found distinct patterns of CK7, CK20, and ki-67 staining, which may help distinguish SSAs from HPs.[209]

Dysplasia in Inflammatory Bowel Disease

Patients with long-standing inflammatory bowel disease are at an increased risk for developing dysplasia and colorectal carcinoma. Surveillance colonoscopy with mucosal biopsies is currently the best and most widely used method to detect dysplasia and cancer in patients with IBD. However, for the pathologist, the assessment of dysplasia, especially in inflamed mucosa, can be challenging. IHC for p53 and ki-67 can help confirm a histologic impression of dysplasia. Both p53 and ki-67 tend to be overexpressed in areas of dysplasia compared with reactive and nonneoplastic epithelium.[210-215] Similar to the assessment of dysplasia in Barrett esophagus, there can be overlap of the patterns of p53 and ki-67 expression in reactive or inflamed epithelium. Surface involvement above the basal third of the crypts by these antibodies and strong p53 positivity supports the presence of dysplasia.[210,214,215] Increased AMACR expression also appears to be emerging as a useful marker of dysplasia and cancer in IBD.[213,216,217]

Colorectal Adenocarcinoma

Colorectal adenocarcinomas arise through different genetic pathways and should no longer be considered one disease. The majority of colorectal cancers arise via the chromosomal instability pathway with dysfunction of the APC/β-catenin/WNT signaling pathway. However, a subset of colorectal cancers arises via the MSI pathway, owing to either a germline mutation (Lynch syndrome) or epigenetic gene silencing secondary to hypermethylation. Because all older studies on colorectal cancer viewed this cancer as one disease, the majority of this section describes the immunophenotype of colon cancer in general. But evidence is now emerging that the tumors arising through these two main pathways have different immunophenotypic features. These differences are highlighted at the end of this section.

Colorectal cancer cells contain mostly low-molecular-weight cytokeratins, predominantly cytokeratins 8, 18, 19, and 20 (Fig. 14.19). They also stain with a broad molecular-weight spectrum of antibodies including AE1/AE3 and CAM5.2.[120,218-220]

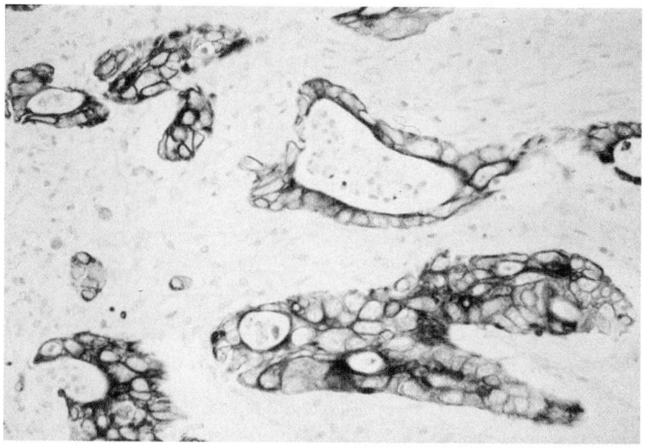

FIGURE 14.20 The most common pattern of CK20 staining in colorectal adenocarcinomas.

CYTOKERATINS 7 AND 20 Most (80% to 100%) adenocarcinomas are diffusely and strongly positive for CK20, but some tumors will show no or only focal positivity (Fig. 14.20).[120,127,218,221-223] Decreased CK20 staining occurs in microsatellite unstable adenocarcinomas (see later). In general, colorectal adenocarcinomas infrequently express CK7. Up to about 13% of cases can express CK7 and this frequency is independent of site (primary versus metastatic) and mucinous subtype.[120,124,125,129,130,131,221,223,224] On the basis of these staining patterns, colorectal adenocarcinoma is the major neoplasm that can be diffusely and strongly CK20 positive and completely CK7 negative.

CDX2 CDX2 is a marker of intestinal differentiation and stains the nuclei of about 90% of colorectal adenocarcinomas, but the range of tumor positivity in the literature is variable, from 72% to 100%.[56,174,225-227] Similar to CK7, fewer poorly differentiated and mucinous colorectal adenocarinomas are positive for CDX2,[133] which may be related to MSI (see later). In addition, CDX2 is not specific for colorectal adenocarcinomas. Staining can be seen in adenocarcinomas of pancreaticobiliary, gastric, small bowel, lung, ovarian (mucinous and endometrioid) and bladder origin, especially if they show intestinal differentiation.[226-229]

VILLIN Villin stains the brush border of the intestines and is thus commonly positive in colorectal adenocarcinomas. The staining pattern is diffusely cytoplasmic with brush border accentuation and is seen in approximately 92% of cases (Fig. 14.21); however, villin expression is not as specific as CDX2.[30,31,33,56,227] It also stains other intestinal-type tumors such as lung and bladder adenocarcinomas.[30,33,227]

OTHER ANTIBODIES Several other antibodies are typically positive in colorectal adenocarcinoma—such as MOC31, monoclonal CEA, and COX2—and these are shown in Table 14.3.[20,169,221,230,231] CA19-9 is positive

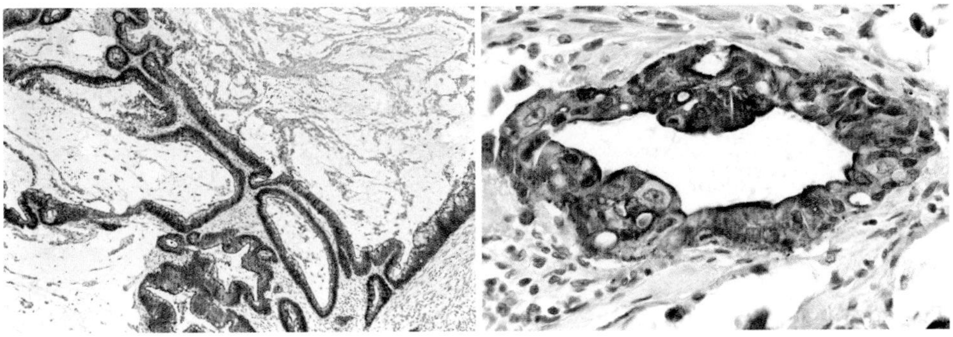

FIGURE 14.21 High and low magnifications of a mucinous colorectal adenocarcinoma stained with villin showing diffuse homogeneous cytoplasmic immunoreactivity with a microvillous luminal, membranous microvillous brush border accentuation. Although noncolonic adenocarcinomas can stain with villin, the microvillous brush border pattern is characteristic of colorectal adenocarcinomas.

TABLE 14.3 Expression of Various Antibodies (Excluding Cytokeratins) in Colorectal Adenocarcinomas

Antibody	Reactivity	Comments	References
BerEP4	+		117
CA125	R	Positive tumors usually show focal staining	118, 175
CA19-9	S		169, 224, 232
Calretinin	R		Doglioni*
CDX2	+		56, 225-227, 296
COX2	+		231
ER & PR	N		141, 144, 259
GCDFP	N		126, 169, 170
mCEA	+		60, 144, 169, 221, 231
MOC31	+		20, 230
MUC1	S		120
MUC2	+		120, 144
MUC5AC	R		120, 144
S-100	R	Positive tumors usually show focal staining	Herrera†
Synaptophysin & chromogranin	R	Focal positivity can be seen in colonic adenocarcinomas without neuroendocrine features	8, 165, 308
TTF-1	N		144
Villin	+		30, 31, 33, 56, 227

N, negative; R, rarely positive; S, sometimes; +, positive.
*Doglioni C, Dei Tos AP, Laurino L, et al. A novel immunocytochemical marker for mesothelioma. *Am J Surg Pathol.* 1996;20:1037-1046.
†Herrera GA, Turbat-Herrera EA, Lott RL. S-100 protein expression by primary and metastatic adenocarcinomas. *Am J Clin Pathol.* 1988;89:168-176.

in colorectal adenocarcinoma.[224,232] Other antibodies such as CK5/6, MUC5AC, and CA125 are typically negative (see Table 14.3).[63,144,169,175]

COLORECTAL ADENOCARCINOMA WITH MICROSATELLITE INSTABILITY

Approximately 15% to 20% of colorectal adenocarcinomas arise from deficiencies in mismatch repair complex function, resulting in MSI.[233,234] Four main proteins, MLH1, MSH2, MSH6, and PMS2, comprise the mismatch repair complex. Carcinomas arising via the MSI pathway tend to have characteristic pathologic features including right-sided location, age younger than 50, tumor-infiltrating lymphocytes, a lack of "dirty necrosis," the presence of a Crohn-like reaction, mucinous differentiation, medullary features, and/or well differentiation.[233] In nonhereditary, sporadic adenocarcinomas, hypermethylation of the *MLH1* mismatch repair promoter gene leads to deficiencies in MLH1 protein expression, resulting in loss of nuclear protein expression in the tumor cells. In hereditary adenocarcinomas (Lynch syndrome), germline mutations most commonly involve the *MSH2* gene but can also involve the *MLH1, MSH6,* and *PMS2* genes, resulting in loss of nuclear staining of the particular protein (Figs. 14.22 and 14.23).[234,235] Antibodies to MLH1, MSH2, MSH6, and PMS2 proteins can be used to screen for MSI-H neoplasms.[234,236,237] Another screening method is the use of molecular testing to detect MSI[238]; this is discussed further in the section "Beyond Immunohistochemistry." Such screening methods can identify patients who should have additional genetic testing and counseling. The results of the mismatch repair proteins need to

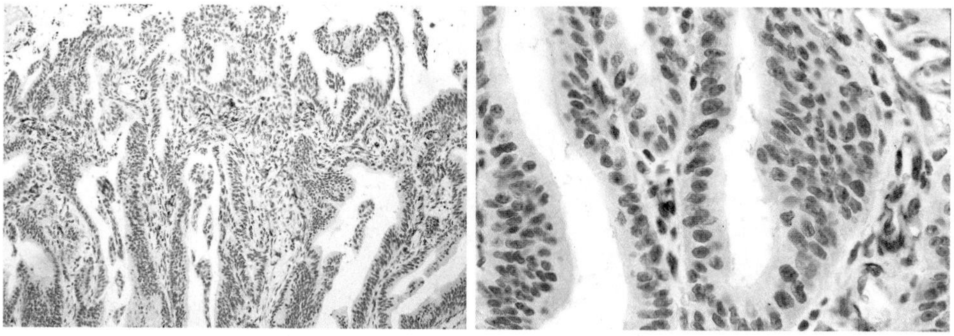

FIGURE 14.22 High and low magnification of an invasive cecal adenocarcinoma from a 46-year-old patient with hereditary nonpolyposis colon cancer syndrome (Lynch syndrome). Neoplastic cell nuclei are completely devoid of MLH2 immunoreactivity, whereas cell nuclei of the surrounding stromal cells stain strongly. Only the complete absence of nuclear staining should be interpreted as a marker of a mismatch repair enzyme defect.

be interpreted with caution. These antibodies can have substantial run-to-run variation in staining. Therefore complete absence of nuclear staining with an adequate internal control is required for a "positive" result. Compared with typical glandular adenocarcinomas, signet ring cell and mucinous adenocarcinomas are more often MSI-H and will have absent nuclear immunoreactivity with one of the mismatch repair proteins.

MSI-H adenocarcinomas can aberrantly express CDX2 and CK20. CK20 can be negative in up to 32% of MSI-H colon cancers,[240,241] while CDX2 has been reported to be negative in 22% of MSI-H tumors.[241] Interestingly, reduced or absent CDX2 expression increases dramatically, to over 85% of cases, when medullary-type MSI-H tumors are analyzed.[239] As mentioned earlier, CK7 can be expressed in a minority of colon cancers, and this includes both MSI-H and microsatellite stable tumors.[241] To avoid potential erroneous diagnoses, especially when assessing small biopsy specimens and metastases of unknown origin, it is important to be aware that some cases of colorectal cancer can aberrantly express CK20, CDX2, and/or CK7. Assessment of MSI can be helpful in such challenging cases.

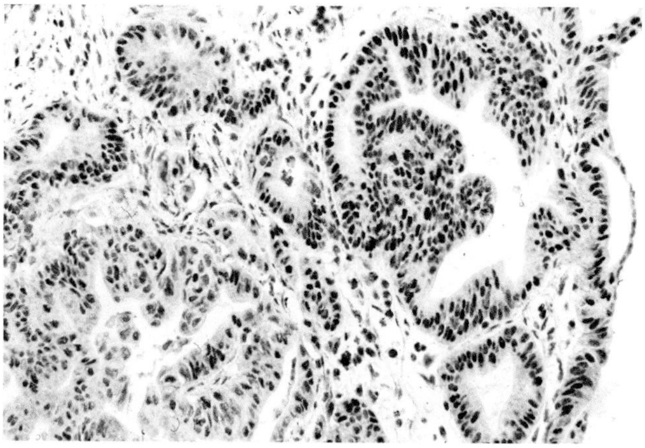

FIGURE 14.23 Characteristic intact nuclear staining with MLH1 in a patient with a microsatellite stable cancer. This pattern of staining would be present for all four mismatch repair protein antibodies (MLH1, MSH2, MSH6, and PMS2).

KEY DIAGNOSTIC POINTS

Colorectal Carcinomas

- Colorectal adenocarcinomas are typically positive for CK20, CDX2, and villin and negative for CK7.
- Stains for the mismatch repair proteins MLH1, MSH2, MSH6, and PMS2 can be used to screen for MSI-high neoplasms.
- MSI-H colonic adenocarcinomas can show decreased or absent CDX2 and/or CK20 staining.

Adenocarcinoma Variants and Subtypes

SIGNET RING CELL ADENOCARCINOMA In general, colonic signet ring cell adenocarcinomas show similar CK7, CK20, and CDX2 staining patterns compared with glandular colon adenocarcinomas.[118,135] However, a higher percentage of signet ring cell carcinomas are positive for MUC2 (100%) and MUC5AC (89%) and a lesser percentage are positive for E-cadherin (56%).[135] As noted earlier, microsatellite unstable cancers with signet ring cell morphology may show atypical expression of CK7, CK20, and CDX2.

CLEAR CELL ADENOCARCINOMA Most clear cell adenocarcinomas are immunophenotypically identical to usual-type colorectal adenocarcinomas.[242] Rare cases of primary colonic, clear cell carcinoma stain with alpha fetoprotein.

UNDIFFERENTIATED NEOPLASMS AND CARCINOMAS WITH RHABDOID DIFFERENTIATION These neoplasms are immunohistochemically similar to poorly differentiated carcinomas with spindle cell differentiation.[243] The two most common gastrointestinal locations for rhabdoid carcinomas are the colon and stomach.[244] This variant most often occurs as a component within typical adenocarcinoma.

Key Diagnostic Panels

COLON VERSUS LUNG ADENOCARCINOMA **Antibodies: CK7, CK20, CDX2 and TTF-1** (Fig. 14.24). Diffuse CK20 staining is strongly supportive of a colorectal adenocarcinoma, whereas diffuse, strong CK7 staining is strongly supportive of a lung adenocarcinoma.[69] Focal staining with either antibody should be considered noncontributory because it can be seen in either lung or colorectal adenocarcinomas.[69,127,178,245] TTF-1 (as well as surfactant-A) stains almost all low-grade nonmucinous

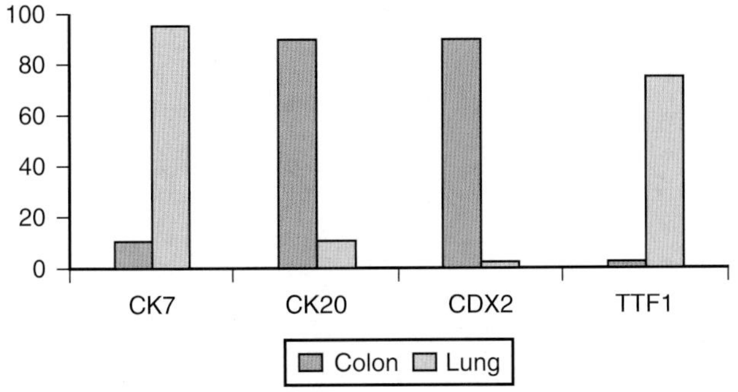

FIGURE 14.24 Colorectal adenocarcinoma versus lung adenocarcinoma.

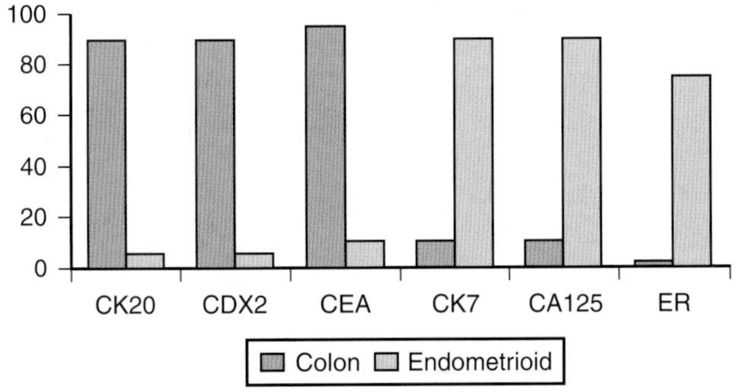

FIGURE 14.25 Colorectal adenocarcinoma versus müllerian endometrioid adenocarcinoma.

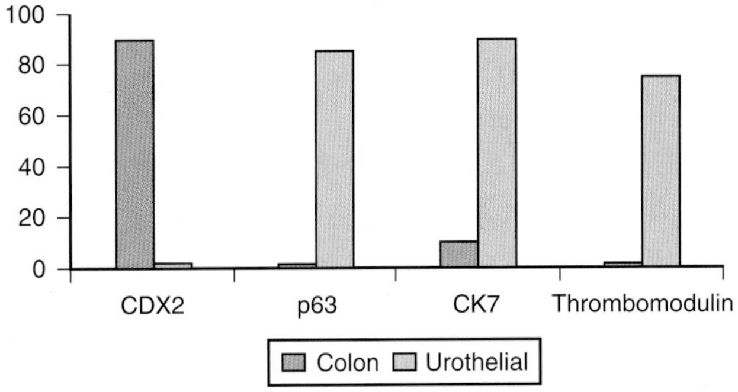

FIGURE 14.26 Colorectal adenocarcinoma versus urothelial carcinoma.

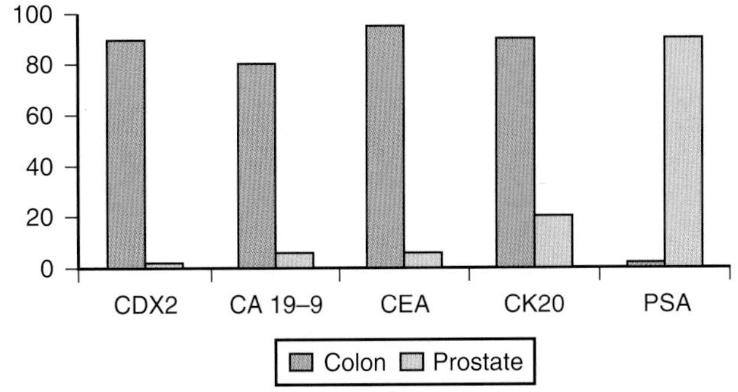

FIGURE 14.27 Colorectal adenocarcinoma versus prostatic adenocarcinoma.

pulmonary adenocarcinomas, compared with 0% of colon adenocarcinomas.[180,246-252] Colorectal adenocarcinomas are CDX2 positive, whereas nonmucinous pulmonary adenocarcinomas are CDX2 negative.[56,174] Primary pulmonary mucinous bronchioloalveolar and goblet cell adenocarcinomas are immunophenotypically different from usual-type pulmonary adenocarcinoma.[32,253,254] This subset of adenocarcinomas can stain with CDX2 and CK20, simulating metastatic colorectal adenocarcinoma.[255,256] Importantly, the intensity and extent of CDX2 staining in pulmonary mucinous adenocarcinomas is moderate and focal, unlike the diffuse, strong immunoreactivity seen in colorectal adenocarcinomas.

Colon versus müllerian endometrioid adenocarcinoma. Antibodies: CK7, CK20, CEA, CDX2, ER (Fig. 14.25). CK7 is a useful initial antibody because it is positive in greater than 95% of endometrioid adenocarcinomas and minimally reactive in colorectal adenocarcinomas. Conversely, CK20 is nonreactive in endometrioid adenocarcinomas and positive in colorectal adenocarcinomas.[124,127,128,218,221,245,257,258] An antibody panel that also includes monoclonal CEA (note, not polyclonal),[117,169,221,224] CDX2,[56,174] CA-125,[169,175,224,258] and ER[144,259] can aid in the distinction between these two lesions.

Colon adenocarcinoma versus urothelial carcinoma. Antibodies: CK7, CDX2, p63, and thrombomodulin (Fig. 14.26). In this differential diagnosis, CDX2 is currently the only antibody that definitively allows for the positive identification of colorectal adenocarcinoma because it has been consistently negative in transitional cell carcinomas. Diffuse, strong CK7 and thrombomodulin staining are characteristic of many transitional cell carcinomas, and either is useful for supporting a transitional cell carcinoma diagnosis if positive.[260] Many poorly differentiated transitional cell carcinomas undergo squamous differentiation that stain with CK5/6, 34bE12, and p63. Extensive staining with p63 in particular is supportive of a urothelial adenocarcinoma.[261,262] The lack of staining should be interpreted as a noncontributory finding rather than supportive of a primary colonic neoplasm.

Colon adenocarcinoma versus prostate adenocarcinoma. Antibodies: CDX2, CA 19-9, CEA, CK20, and PSA (Fig. 14.27). CDX2 and CA 19-9 stain colorectal adenocarcinomas and are nonreactive in prostate adenocarcinomas. CK20 and CEA support a diagnosis of colorectal adenocarcinoma only when they are diffusely and strongly reactive; both can focally stain high-grade prostatic adenocarcinomas. PSA is positive in prostatic adenocarcinoma and nonreactive in colorectal adenocarcinomas. Similar to other antibodies, the lack of staining with PSA should not be used to support the diagnosis of nonprostatic adenocarcinoma; many high-grade prostatic adenocarcinomas are PSA negative.[127,232,245,263-265]

ANUS

Squamous Cell Carcinoma

There is an increasing incidence of anal SCC in the United States, and these tumors share some similarities with their uterine cervical counterparts including association with high-risk human papilloma virus (HPV) infection.[266] Similar to other sites such as the head, neck,

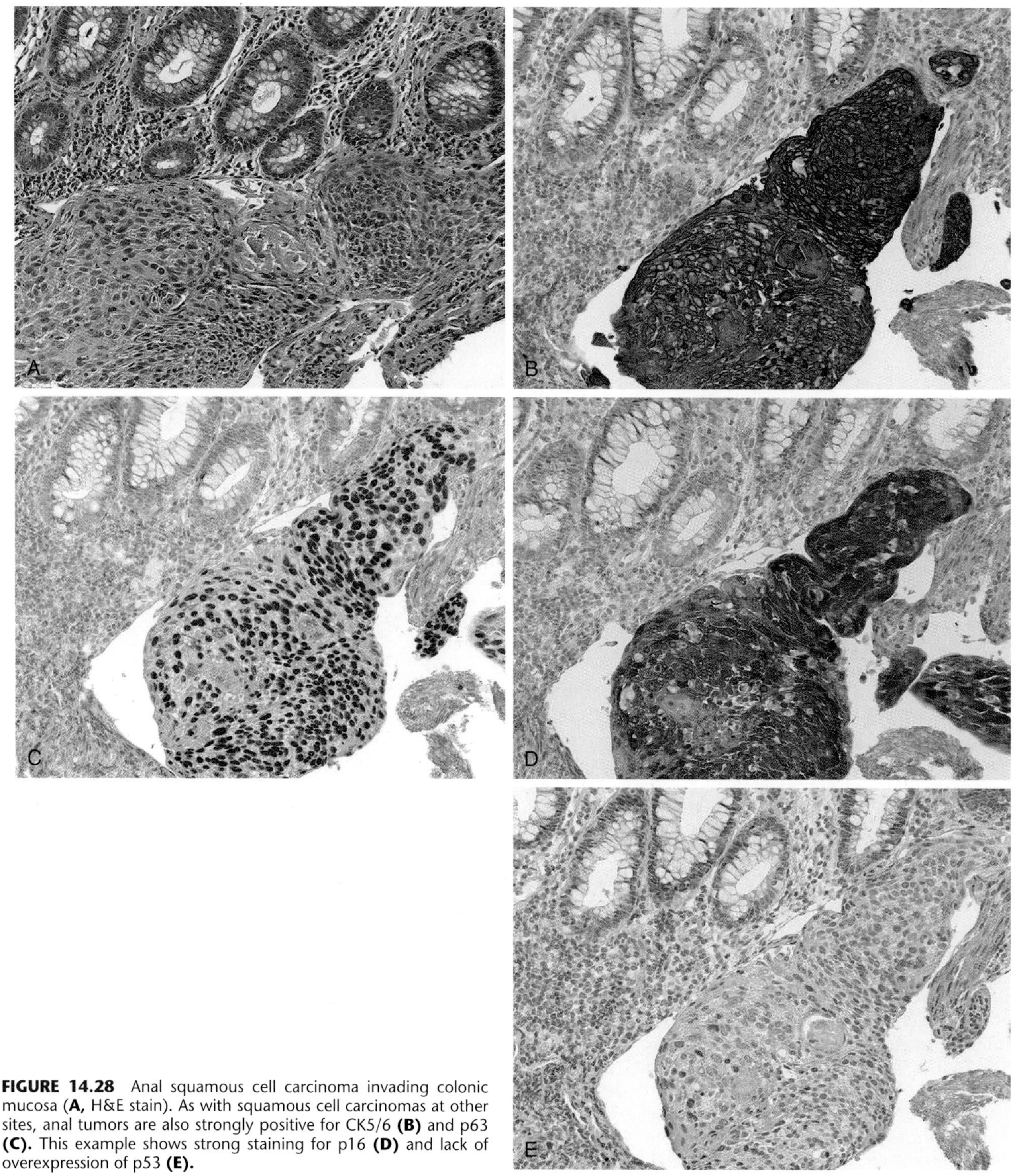

FIGURE 14.28 Anal squamous cell carcinoma invading colonic mucosa (**A,** H&E stain). As with squamous cell carcinomas at other sites, anal tumors are also strongly positive for CK5/6 **(B)** and p63 **(C).** This example shows strong staining for p16 **(D)** and lack of overexpression of p53 **(E).**

lung, and uterine cervix, CK5/6 and p63 are expressed in anal SCCs (Fig. 14.28A to C).[65,267] CK7 is usually negative, unless the carcinoma is a basaloid SCC with an adenoid cystic pattern.[268] Emerging evidence indicates two different histopathologic types of squamous cell *in situ* lesions/invasive carcinomas of the anus.[269] A bowenoid morphology of AIN or invasive cancer is associated with positive p16 staining and lack of p53 staining (Fig. 14.28D to E), whereas a "differentiated" morphology that maintains squamous maturation is associated with positive p53 staining and lack of p16 staining.

Anal Gland Adenocarcinoma

Anal gland adenocarcinoma is typically composed of small glands with scant mucin production. It invades the anorectal wall, has no identifiable intraluminal component, and has no association with a fistula.[270] Anal gland adenocarcinoma is diffusely positive for CK7 and negative for CK20, CDX2, p63, and CK5/6.[270,271]

Anal Paget Disease

The intraepidermal adenocarcinoma cells of anal Paget disease stain diffusely with AE1/AE3, CAM5.2, and CK7.[272-274] Cytokeratin 7 is useful because it diffusely stains the neoplastic cells while the surrounding normal squamous epithelium is nonreactive. GCDFP-15 is also expressed in cases of primary anal Paget disease. When associated with an underlying rectal or urothelial adenocarcinoma, the pagetoid cells tend to coexpress CK20 and lack GCDFP-15 expression.[275-277] MUC5AC and MUC1 stain most cases of anal Paget disease, whereas MUC2 is positive in cases with associated colorectal adenocarcinoma.[278,279] CEA and Ber-EP4 are also expressed in the tumor cells.[274-278]

KEY DIAGNOSTIC POINTS

Anal Malignancies

- Anal squamous cell carcinomas express CK5/6 and p63.
- Anal gland adenocarcinomas are CK7+/CK20− and negative for CDX2, p63, and CK5/6.
- Paget cells in primary anal disease are CK7+/CK20−/GCDFP+, whereas Paget cells associated with an underlying malignancy tend to be CK7+/CK20+/GCDFP-/MUC2+.

Neuroendocrine Lesions of the Gastrointestinal Tract

Neuroendocrine tumors (NETs) arise from different types of neuroendocrine cells that are present throughout the gastrointestinal (GI) tract. At least 15 distinct neuroendocrine cell types have been described. The biology and behavior of GI NETs is quite variable and is associated, in part, on the cell and site of origin. Because of these regional differences, GI NETs can be divided into foregut (stomach, duodenum, upper jejunum, and pancreas); midgut (lower jejunum, ileum, appendix, and cecum); and hindgut (colon and rectum) tumors.[280] Because even very small "benign-appearing" NETs can metastasize, all NETs of the GI tract should be considered potentially malignant. The older term for these tumors is *carcinoid tumor,* but this term is no longer commonly used and has been replaced by *well-differentiated NET.* In this chapter the term NET represents a well-differentiated neuroendocrine tumor; all poorly differentiated, high-grade neuroendocrine carcinomas are noted as such.

The general immunophenotype of GI NETs is similar to neuroendocrine tumors elsewhere in the body. They are positive for low-weight cytokeratins (Cam5.2) and often, but not always, high-molecular-weight cytokeratins (AE1/3). CK20 is positive in up to 25% of GI NETs and CK7 is positive in only 11% of cases.[281] The most commonly used antibodies to detect neuroendocrine differentiation are synaptophysin and chromogranin A. Other useful positively staining antibodies include CD56 (NCAM), CD57 (Leu7), and NSE. NESP-55, a member of the chromogranin family, is a promising marker of pancreatic neuroendocrine tumors, but it is typically negative in GI NETs.[282] Some grading schemes including the World Health Organization use Ki-67 to categorize GI NETs.[283] NETs at each specific site in the GI tract are now discussed including additional site-specific immunohistochemical stains that can be used.

NEUROENDOCRINE TUMORS OF THE ESOPHAGUS

Most esophageal neuroendocrine lesions are high-grade, poorly differentiated neuroendocrine carcinomas that are often large cell (rather than small cell) type and may have a component of adenocarcinoma.[284] Well-differentiated NETs, often presenting as small polypoid lesions in association with Barrett esophagus, also exist and may be found incidentally.[285,286] Primary high-grade small cell neuroendocrine carcinomas are rare and present mainly as a component of an SCC.[287-289]

Immunophenotypically, NETs stain diffusely and strongly with synaptophysin and chromogranin, whereas high-grade, large cell carcinomas may only be positive for synaptophysin.[286] Small cell carcinomas that arise in association with SCC may express CEA,[289] and up to one half of esophageal small cell carcinomas may be immunoreactive with TTF-1.[290,291]

KEY DIAGNOSTIC POINTS

Esophageal Neuroendocrine Tumors

- Synaptophysin and chromogranin are the immunohistochemistry mainstays of diagnosis.
- Cytokeratin CAM5.2 is preferred over other cytokeratins.

NEUROENDOCRINE TUMORS OF THE STOMACH

Three types of gastric neuroendocrine tumors exist: those that are physiologic and arise in the setting of autoimmune gastritis (type I), those that arise in association with multiple endocrine neoplasia type I (MEN1) or Zollinger-Ellison syndrome (type II), and those that are sporadic (type III). It is important to distinguish type I from type III NETs because type I tumors have nearly no metastatic risk, whereas type III tumors are much more aggressive.[286] Poorly differentiated neuroendocrine carcinomas are rare but could be considered the fourth type of gastric NET; some poorly differentiated tumors may arise as a component of gastric adenocarcinoma.

The cell of origin for type I, type II, and the vast majority of type III NETs are the enterochromaffin-like (ECL) cells that reside within oxyntic mucosa. These cells stain strongly for synaptophysin and chromogranin and will stain for the marker VMAT2 (vesicular monoamine transporter 2), which recognizes these histamine-producing cells.[286,292] Synaptophysin and chromogranin will also detect ECL-cell hyperplasia in the setting of autoimmune gastritis (Fig. 14.7). The rare poorly differentiated carcinomas are positive for synaptophysin but may be negative for chromogranin. In general, gastric

KEY DIAGNOSTIC POINTS

Gastric Neuroendocrine Tumors

- Synaptophysin and chromogranin A stain the ECL cells that give rise to the majority of gastric NETs.
- Synaptophysin and chromogranin A also highlight the proliferation of ECL cells in the oxyntic (fundic/body) mucosa in hypergastrinemia, hypochlorhydria, and Zollinger-Ellison syndrome.
- The positive staining for AE1/AE3 and CAM5.2 that is seen in gastric carcinoids can help distinguish them from secondary involvement of the gastrointestinal tract by other neuroendocrine tumors such as pheochromocytoma and retroperitoneal paraganglioma.

carcinoids are positive for AE1/AE3 and CAM5.2, approximately 10% are positive for CK7, and they are negative for CDX2 and CK20.[225,281,293]

NEUROENDOCRINE TUMORS OF THE SMALL BOWEL

NETs of the small bowel have different etiologies and prognosis, depending on the site, and are thus typically divided into two groups by location: duodenal/proximal jejunal NETs and distal jejunal/ileal NETs. Both groups of neoplasms are usually well-differentiated and stain with synaptophysin and chromogranin. They tend to be CK7 and TTF-1 negative and approximately 20% are CK20 positive.[281,294]

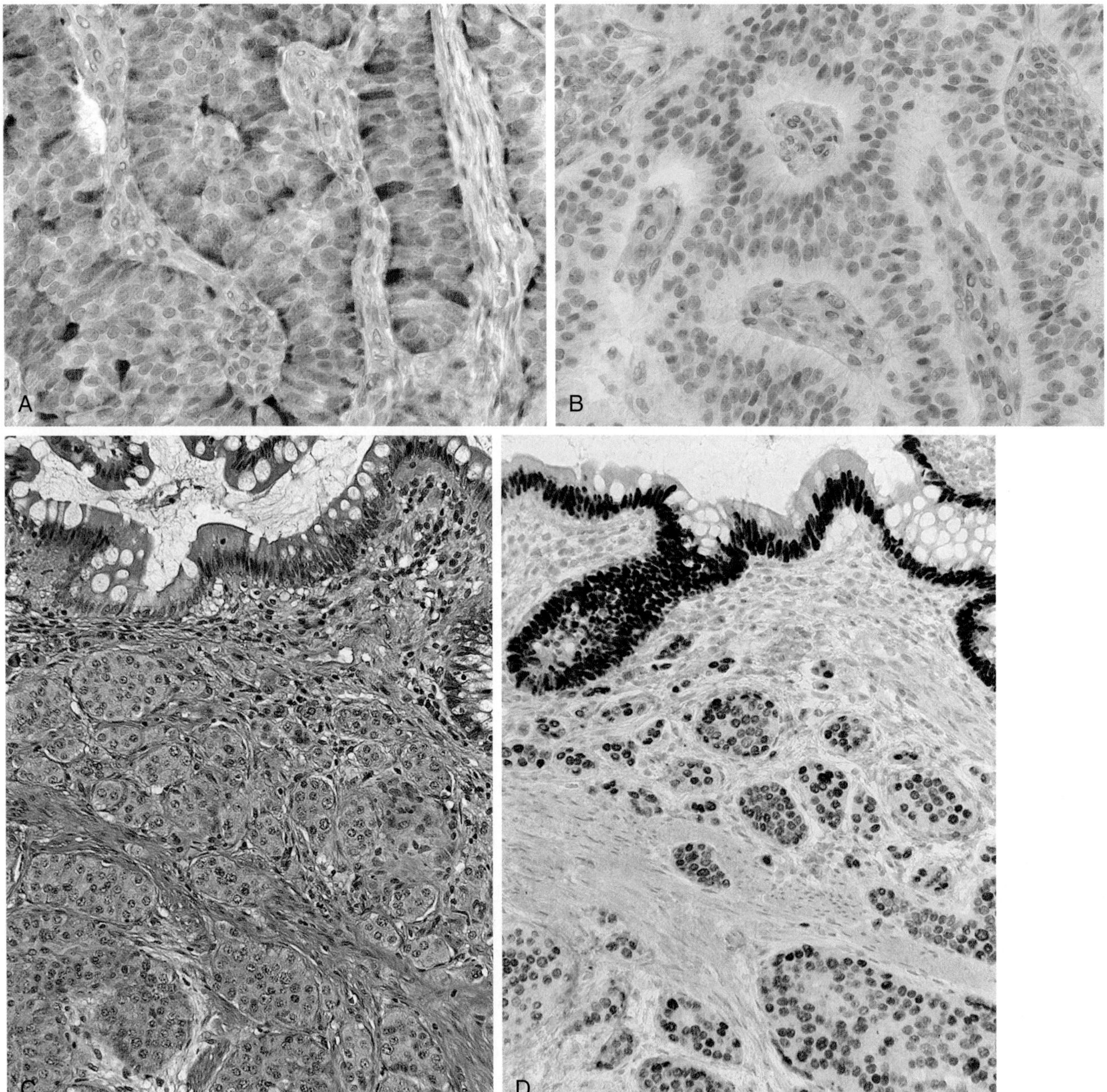

FIGURE 14.29 Gastrointestinal well-differentiated neuroendocrine tumors. Duodenal NETs are usually positive for gastrin **(A)** and lack staining for CDX2 **(B)**. Terminal ileal NETs (**C,** H&E stain) are positive for CDX2 **(D)**, whereas rectal NETs (**E,** H&E stain) are negative for CDX2 **(F)**.

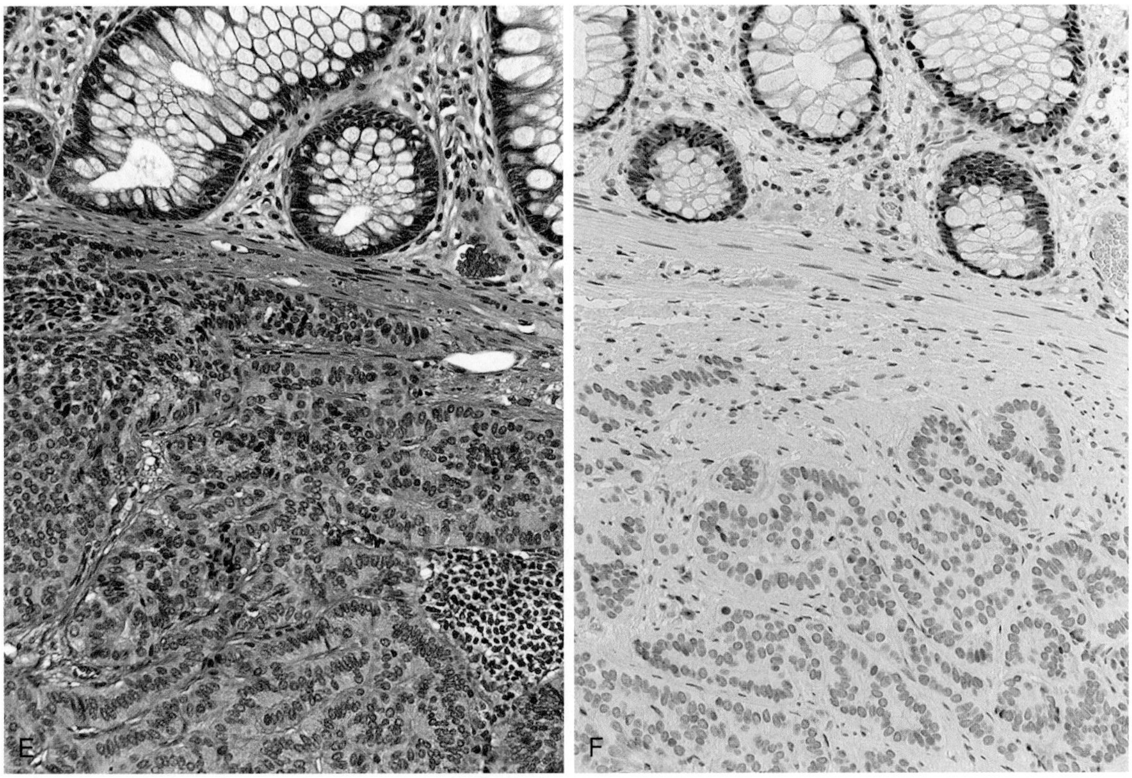

FIGURE 14.29, cont'd

Most duodenal NETs are gastrin positive (gastrinomas), and a subset are functionally active and result in the Zollinger-Ellison syndrome (Fig. 14.29). The most common site of gastrinomas is the duodenal bulb. Approximately 20% of duodenal NETs produce (and stain for) somatostatin. About one half of these tumors lack chromogranin A positivity but do stain with synaptophysin. Somatostatin-producing tumors tend to arise near the papilla of Vater. Duodenal NETs are positive for the pancreatic-duodenal homeobox 1 transcription factor PDX-1[295] and tend to be negative (or weakly staining) for CDX2 (see Fig. 14.29).[295,296]

Gangliocytic paragangliomas are a rare form of NET. They tend to arise in the second portion of the duodenum. Cytokeratins (CAM5.2), synaptophysin, and chromogranin will stain the nests of epithelial/endocrine cells, S-100 will stain the neurally derived spindle cells and the ganglion cells, and neurofilament would also stain the ganglion cells, if needed. Poorly differentiated NETs do exist and tend to involve the papilla of Vater.

Most NETs of the distal small bowel occur in the terminal ileum and arise from serotonin-producing enterochromaffin (EC) cells. Because CDX2 is positive in EC cells, nearly all terminal ileal NET express CDX2 (see Fig. 14.29).[296-298] These distal small bowel NETs are negative for PDX-1.[295] Even at small sizes (1 to 2 cm), these are aggressive tumors, often presenting with lymph node and hepatic metastases. When these tumors metastasize to the liver, patients can develop a carcinoid syndrome.

KEY DIAGNOSTIC POINTS

Small Bowel Neuroendocrine Tumors

- Proximal small bowel neuroendocrine tumors (those arising in the duodenum and proximal jejunum) tend to behave less aggressively and have different immunophenotypes than distal small bowel tumors (those that arise in the terminal ileum).
- Duodenal tumors often produce gastrin, are positive for PDX-1, and are negative for CDX-2; somatostatin-producing tumors are often found at the papilla of Vater.
- Terminal ileal NETs are positive for CDX-2 and about two thirds are positive for CEA; they are negative for PDX-1.

NEUROENDOCRINE TUMORS OF THE APPENDIX

Well-differentiated NETs of the appendix tend to arise in the tip. These are usually small (<1 cm), found incidentally, and have little to no chance of metastasizing. Occasionally, well-differentiated NETs can occur toward the base of the appendix and grow to a larger size; these tumors should be considered potentially malignant, as is the case with most other NETs of the GI tract. Similar to ileal NETs, appendiceal NETs typically arise from EC cells and, as such, are positive for CDX2.[295-297] These well-differentiated NET tend to be negative for both CK7 and CK20,[299] but they often have S-100-positive sustentacular cells around the cell nests.[299-301]

Appendiceal goblet cell carcinoids have a mixed phenotype, showing both neuroendocrine and glandular differentiation. Although these tumors stain for the

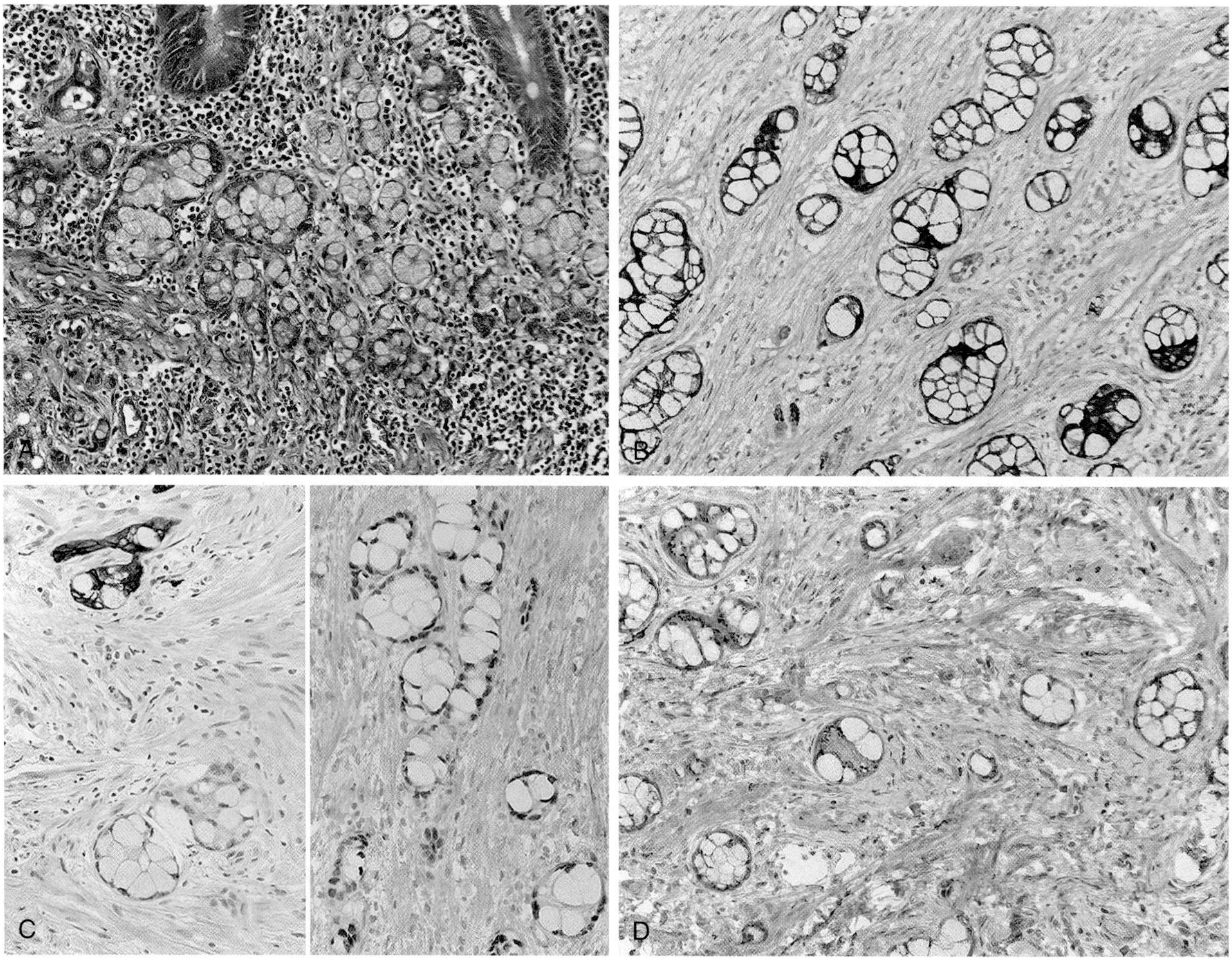

FIGURE 14.30 Appendiceal goblet cell carcinoid. **A,** Neoplastic goblet-shaped cells are present beneath two normal appendiceal crypts (H&E stain). **B,** Goblet cell carcinoids are typically positive for CK20. **C,** *Left:* CK7 staining can be variable (note scattered cells that are positive for CK7 and a separate cluster of tumor cells that are completely negative); *right:* CDX2 is positive. **D,** Staining with synaptophysin (shown) and chromogranin (not shown) can be variably positive.

neuroendocrine markers synaptophysin and chromogranin, the pattern is more focal, with only 5% to 25% of the cells staining, as compared with the more diffuse staining of well-differentiated NETs.[302] Most goblet cell carcinoid tumors are positive for CK20 and up to 70% are positive for CK7 (Fig. 14.30).[299] They show preserved staining with B-catenin and E-cadherin, are positive for MUC2, and are negative for MUC1 and p53.[302] Although typical appendiceal NETs are generally negative for CEA, goblet cell carcinoid tumors are positive.[300] When the goblet cell carcinoid tumors are associated with a poorly differentiated adenocarcinoma component, the poorly differentiated cells stain for p53 and MUC1 and lose MUC2 staining.[302]

KEY DIAGNOSTIC POINTS

Appendiceal Neuroendocrine Tumors

- Typical well-differentiated appendiceal neuroendocrine tumors (carcinoid tumors) are CDX-2+/CK7−/CK20−.
- Goblet cell carcinoids differ from typical appendiceal NETs, showing positive staining for CK7, CK20, MUC2 and CEA, as well as only focal staining with synaptophysin and chromogranin A.
- Both goblet cell and typical appendiceal carcinoids stain with E-cadherin and beta-catenin, unlike the more aggressive colorectal signet-ring cell carcinomas.

NEUROENDOCRINE TUMORS OF THE COLON AND RECTUM

Most well-differentiated NETs of the colorectum occur in the rectum. Rectal (hindgut) NETs are positive for synaptophysin and prostatic acid phosphatase and are usually negative for chromogranin.[303-306] Unlike adenocarcinomas of the prostate, hindgut carcinoids do not stain with prostatic-specific antigen or P504s.[264] CEA weakly stains approximately 25% of these tumors and glucagon is positive in about 10%.[304] CDX2 is negative or shows only weak staining in a small percentage of cells (see Fig. 14.29).[295-297] NETs can occur in the colon, and when they do, they tend to be right sided. The right-sided tumors are midgut tumors that have similar immunophenotypic profiles as ileal NETs.

KEY DIAGNOSTIC POINTS

Colorectal Neuroendocrine Tumors

- Hindgut (rectal) neuroendocrine tumors (NETs) are positive for synaptophysin and prostatic acid phosphatase and typically lack staining for chromogranin and CDX2.
- Cecal and other right-sided NETs have a similar immunophenotypic profile to other midgut NETs such as ileal NETs.

KEY DIAGNOSTIC PANEL FOR METASTATIC WELL-DIFFERENTIATED NETS OF UNKNOWN PRIMARY

An immunohistochemical panel using CDX-2, PDX-1, NESP-55, and TTF-1 can be used to distinguish gastrointestinal well-differentiated NETs from pancreatic endocrine and pulmonary carcinoid tumors (Fig. 14.31).[295]

HIGH-GRADE (POORLY DIFFERENTIATED) NEUROENDOCRINE CARCINOMAS

High-grade neuroendocrine carcinomas of the GI tract are rare. Those that arise in the esophagus are described above under "neuroendocrine tumors of the esophagus," since most neuroendocrine tumors of the esophagus are high grade.

Primary high grade neuroendocrine carcinomas of the stomach are positive for synaptophysin and may be focally positive for chromogranin. High grade neuroendocrine carcinomas of the stomach can also present in conjunction with and as a component of typical gastric adenocarcinoma. The morphologic features of a neuroendocrine carcinoma, often small cell type, need to be present, in contrast to usual-type gastric adenocarcinomas with immunohistochemical features of neuroendocrine differentiation discussed earlier. It is best to require synaptophysin and/or chromogranin immunoreactivity in such a neoplasm to avoid confusing crushed, usual-type adenocarcinoma cells with true neuroendocrine differentiation. These neuroendocrine neoplasms are CK20 and CK5/6 negative and they rarely stain with TTF-1.[63,291,307]

High-grade, poorly differentiated neuroendocrine carcinomas of the duodenum occur primarily in the region of the papilla of Vater and are covered in detail in Chapter 15.

High-grade neuroendocrine carcinomas in the colon and rectum most commonly occur as a component of poorly differentiated adenocarcinomas; more than 50% of the tumor should show neuroendocrine differentiation in order to be called a neuroendocrine carcinoma.[308] Both small cell and non–small cell types exist, and both tend to stain with low-molecular-weight cytokeratin (CAM5.2) in a perinuclear dot pattern, as well as with synaptophysin, chromogranin, and/or NSE (Fig. 14.32).[308,309] CD117 stains a substantial minority of high-grade neuroendocrine carcinomas; however, immunoreactivity has not been linked to c-*kit* juxtamembrane (exon 11) mutations.[310,311]

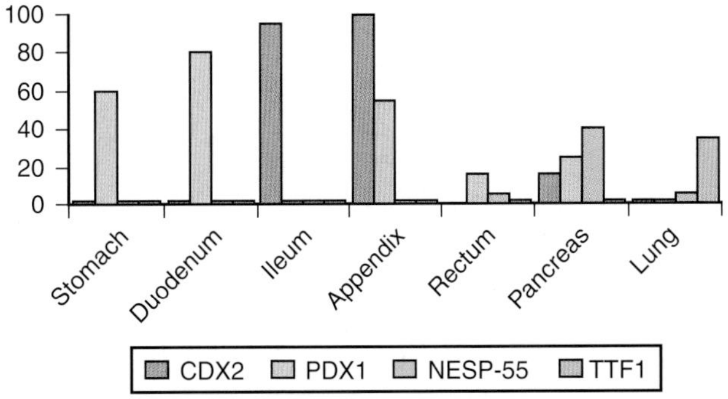

FIGURE 14.31 Well-differentiated NETs. *(Adapted from Srivastava A, Hornick JL. Immunohistochemical staining for CDX-2, PDX-1, NESP-55, and TTF-1 can help distinguish gastrointestinal carcinoid tumors from pancreatic endocrine and pulmonary carcinoid tumors. Am J Surg Pathol. 2009; 33:626-632.)*

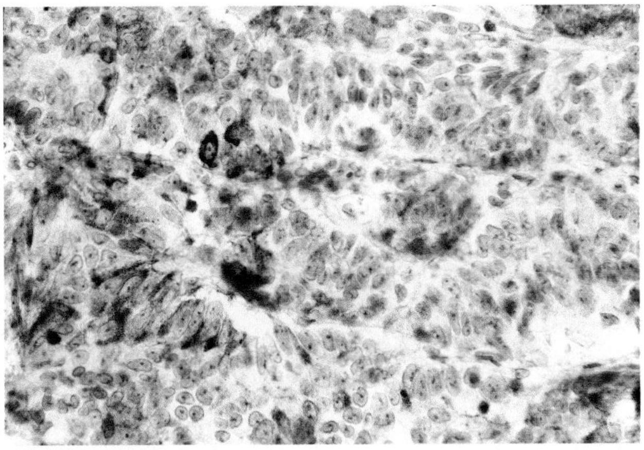

FIGURE 14.32 High-grade colonic neuroendocrine carcinoma with focal, moderate synaptophysin reactivity.

KEY DIAGNOSTIC POINTS

High-Grade (Poorly Differentiated) Neuroendocrine Carcinomas

- High-grade (poorly differentiated) small cell and non–small cell neuroendocrine carcinomas can occur throughout the gastrointestinal tract but are rare.
- In the stomach, they can occur as a primary neoplasm or in conjunction with an adenocarcinoma; in the colon, they tend to occur in association with an adenocarcinoma.
- By definition, they need to have morphologic features of a neuroendocrine carcinoma and stain with neuroendocrine markers such as synaptophysin or chromogranin.

Mesenchymal Lesions of the Gastrointestinal Tract

MESENCHYMAL LESIONS PRESENTING AS MURAL MASSES

Gastrointestinal Stromal Tumor (GIST)

CD117 AND C-*KIT* GENE The classification and diagnosis of GISTs radically changed with the recognition of the c-*kit* proto-oncogene mutation as the key molecular event

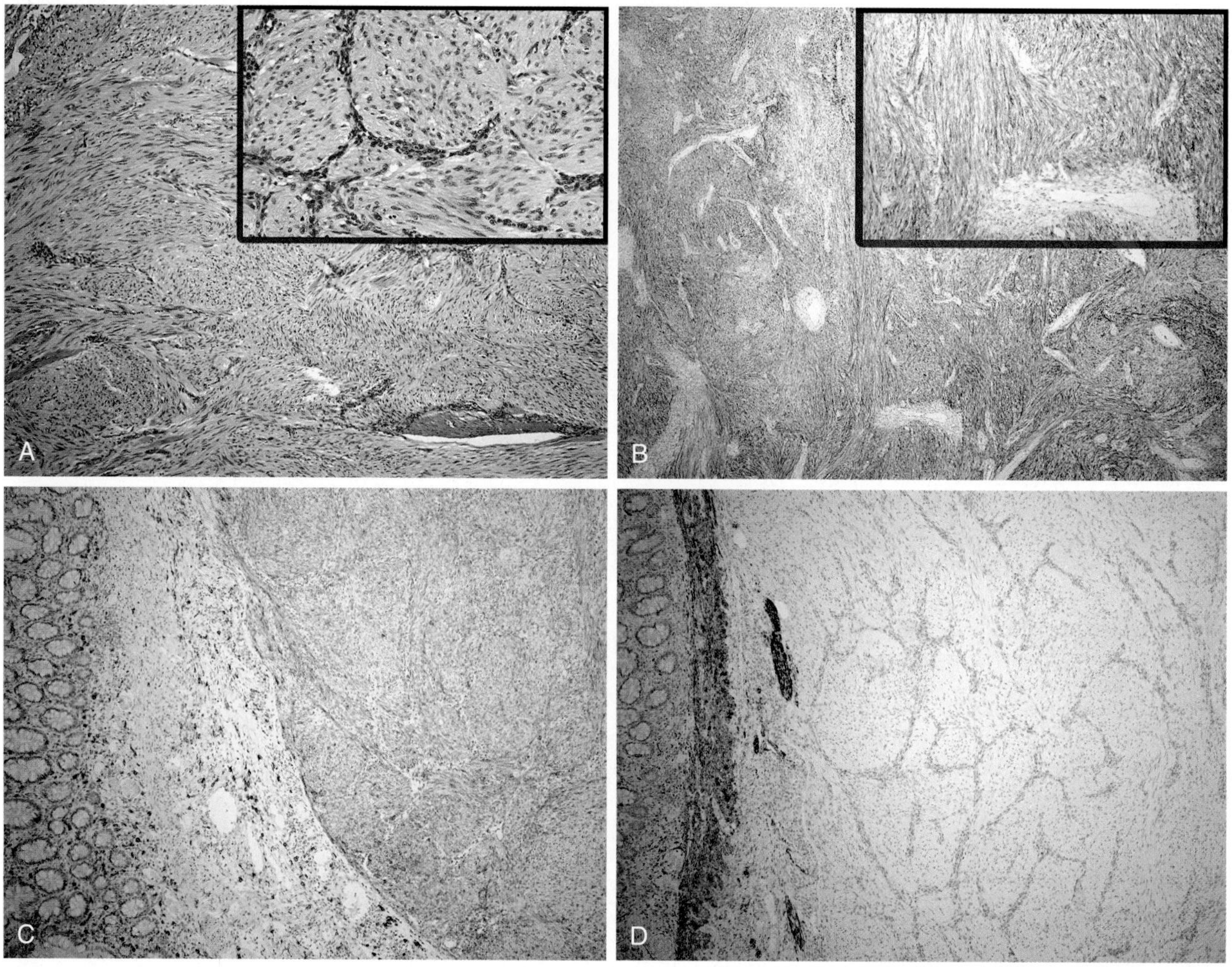

FIGURE 14.33 Gastric gastrointestinal stromal tumor. **A,** H&E stain. **B,** The neoplastic cells stain strongly and diffusely with CD117. *Inset:* The perivascular connective tissue stroma is negative. **C,** Mast cells also stain strongly for CD117 and provide a positive internal control. **D,** Most (90%) GISTs are negative for desmin, whereas the fibers of the muscularis mucosae are strongly positive.

in gastric GISTs. In excess of 85% of GISTs, c-*kit* or platelet-derived growth factor alpha (PDGFR-A) mutations are detected.[312-318] The c-*kit* mutation, most often in exon 11, results in constitutive activation of the Kit receptor, which is thought to promote proliferation and/or decrease apoptosis. The KIT protein can be immunohistochemically detected with antibodies to c-*kit,* which has been assigned to the 117 cluster designation (CD) antigen group. c-*kit* activating mutations and CD117 staining have been identified in neoplasms previously classified as leiomyomas, leiomyosarcomas, gastric autonomic nerve tumors, and some schwannomas, resulting in unification and substantial simplification of this group of neoplasms.[319-322] CD117 also stains interstitial cells of Cajal, which are involved in the regulation of gut motility, leading to the suggestion that GISTs are derived from this cell type.[323,324] Although c-*kit* gene mutations almost always result in CD117 immunoreactivity, CD117-positive lesions do not invariably indicate a c-*kit* mutation. For example, approximately 25% of neurofibromatosis type I patients develop GISTs that stain with CD117 and CD34 but lack c-*kit* gene mutations. Instead, these lesions have the typical *NF1* (17q11.2) gene mutations that are found in NF1-associated neurofibromas.[320]

CD117 STAINING IN GISTS CD117 stains approximately 95% of GISTs. CD117 immunoreactivity in GISTs is typically strongly and uniformly positive in a cytoplasmic pattern (Fig. 14-33), although a membranous pattern of staining can be seen. Additionally, approximately 50% of GISTs can show a dotlike pattern of expression; these tumors are more likely to be extraintestinal in location and may show an epithelioid pattern of growth.[325] The absence of CD117 staining in GISTs occurs in approximately 5% of cases and is strongly associated with a mutated platelet-derived growth receptor-alpha (PDGFR-A) gene.[326,327] These CD117-negative GISTs typically have an epithelioid morphology and occur in the omentum or peritoneum.[320,328-330] Markers for PDGFR-A[331,332] and DOG1[16,333] have been shown to have good sensitivity and specificity for c-kit–negative GISTs. However, because their performance has not been adequately studied to date, these antibodies should be used with caution.

CD117 IN NONGIST LESIONS CD117 immunoreactivity is not restricted to GISTs and has been reported in a number of other neoplasms including melanoma, renal cell carcinoma, and seminoma.[334-336] Sarcomas that have been reported to stain with c-kit include angiosarcoma, clear cell sarcoma, Ewing sarcoma/primitive neuroectodermal tumor, neuroblastoma, and Kaposi sarcoma.[337-339] In some series, intra-abdominal desmoid-type fibromatosis was reported to stain with c-kit in up to 75% of cases; typically this pattern of expression was noted to be weak and granular.[325,340] More recently, however, it has been shown that the use of optimal primary antibody dilution and a lack of antigen retrieval step resulted in only minimal cytoplasmic staining in 5% of intraabdominal desmoid tumors.[337,341,342]

OTHER ANTIBODIES GISTs have variable degrees of neural or smooth muscle differentiation.[320,324,343-360] CD34 strongly and diffusely stains approximately 70% of GISTs; the percentage of CD34-positive tumors varies by location with 47% of small intestinal GISTs, 96% of rectal GISTs, and 100% of esophageal GISTs showing CD34 expression.[325,350,361] In GISTs with neural differentiation, fewer cells stain positive for CD34 and the intensity of staining is lower compared with GISTs with smooth muscle differentiation. CD34 is not specific for GISTs; other CD34-positive neoplasms include solitary fibrous tumors, inflammatory fibroid polyps, and dedifferentiated liposarcoma. CD99 is also diffusely and strongly positive in most GISTs. Muscle-specific actin (HHF-35) and smooth muscle actins stain strongly in 10% to 47% of cases. Like CD34, the likelihood of actin expression in GISTs varies by location; up to 47% of small intestinal and 10% to 13% of rectal tumors are positive for actin.[350,362] Up to 10% of GISTs stain with desmin. Desmin-positive GISTs are more likely to show an epithelioid morphology compared with the typical spindle-cell pattern of growth.[342,362-364] Additionally, other markers of smooth muscle differentiation such as h-caldesmon commonly stain GISTs.[365] Cytoplasmic and nuclear expression of S-100 is restricted to 5% to 10% of GISTs.[350,362,363,366] Typically those GISTs that are S-100 positive are present in the small intestine.[350] Cytokeratins, most commonly CAM5.2 and 35bH11, stain GISTs in a patchy pattern, which occasionally can be of strong intensity. Cytokeratin AE1/AE3 is usually less intense and stains rare individual cells and small clusters of cells. Signet-ring GISTs are negative with cytokeratin antibodies. Synaptophysin can be strongly and diffusely positive in gastric GISTs, but chromogranin is nonreactive.

KEY DIAGNOSTIC POINTS

Gastrointestinal Stromal Tumors

- CD117 is typically expressed when mutation of the *c-kit* gene results in elevated KIT protein, a sensitive marker for GIST.
- CD117 may be negative in GISTs, owing to either limited tumor sampling or rarely (~5%) a unique subset of CD117-negative GISTs that typically show an epithelioid morphology and are more likely to harbor a PDGFR-A mutation.
- Although CD117 is the mainstay of IHC for diagnosis of GISTs, these tumors may also stain for other antigens including CD34, CD99, HHF-35, smooth muscle actins, S-100, and low-molecular-weight cytokeratins.

Other Mesenchymal Lesions Presenting as Mural Masses

SCHWANNOMA Schwannomas of the gastrointestinal tract are uncommon neoplasms that share morphologic features with GISTs.[351,354,367,368] Schwannomas are uniformly diffusely and strongly positive in both a nuclear and cytoplasmic pattern for S-100. Other positive markers in schwannomas include CD57 (Leu7) and GFAP. They do not stain with CD117, CD34, or smooth muscle actin.

GRANULAR CELL TUMOR Granular cell tumors of the GI tract typically present as mucosal or submucosal masses and are most common within the esophagus. These tumors have an immunophenotype identical to granular cell tumors of other sites. S-100 protein, CD57, and vimentin are usually strongly and diffusely reactive. The pattern of desmin staining in granular cell tumors can be useful in distinguishing these neoplasms from smooth muscle tumors with granular cytoplasmic change. Desmin is usually negative or weakly positive in rare cells in granular cell tumors, but strongly and diffusely positive in leiomyomas. Cytokeratin, epithelial membrane antigen, and monoclonal CEA are negative.[369,370]

DESMOID-TYPE FIBROMATOSIS Desmoid-type fibromatoses are rarely CD117 positive (see earlier).[371] In difficult cases, nuclear staining for beta-catenin can be useful in separating desmoid-type fibromatoses from other tumors because beta-catenin shows nuclear expression in approximately 75% of desmoid tumors (Fig. 14.34).[371-374] Of note, many tumors in the differential diagnosis of desmoid-type fibromatosis may show cytoplasmic staining for beta-catenin. Thus only a nuclear pattern of staining should be considered a significant finding. CD34 can stain lesional cells weakly and in a patchy distribution, and it is typically less intense than CD34 staining seen in solitary fibrous tumors. Most desmoid tumors are reactive with smooth muscle actin and desmin.[350]

SOLITARY FIBROUS TUMOR AND PSEUDOTUMOR Solitary fibrous tumors infrequently arise in the upper abdomen and mesentery.[350,375-377] They are positive with CD34, CD99, and smooth muscle actin but do not stain with CD117.[350,368,378] Also, approximately 25% of solitary fibrous tumors stain with beta-catenin in a nuclear pattern.[373] Nodular fibrous pseudotumors are rare lesions in this location. They share strong CD117 reactivity with GISTs; however, they are morphologically distinct from GISTs.

SMOOTH MUSCLE NEOPLASMS The distal third of the esophagus is a common site for leiomyomas; these neoplasms stain diffusely and strongly with desmin and actins; leiomyomas are negative for CD34 and CD117.[348,352] Most smooth muscle neoplasms arising as mural lesions outside of the esophagus are classified as leiomyosarcomas. These tumors stain with smooth muscle actin (SMA) in 63% to 100% of cases[151,325,379,380] and desmin in 33% to 100% of cases.[325,381-383] The degree of desmin and

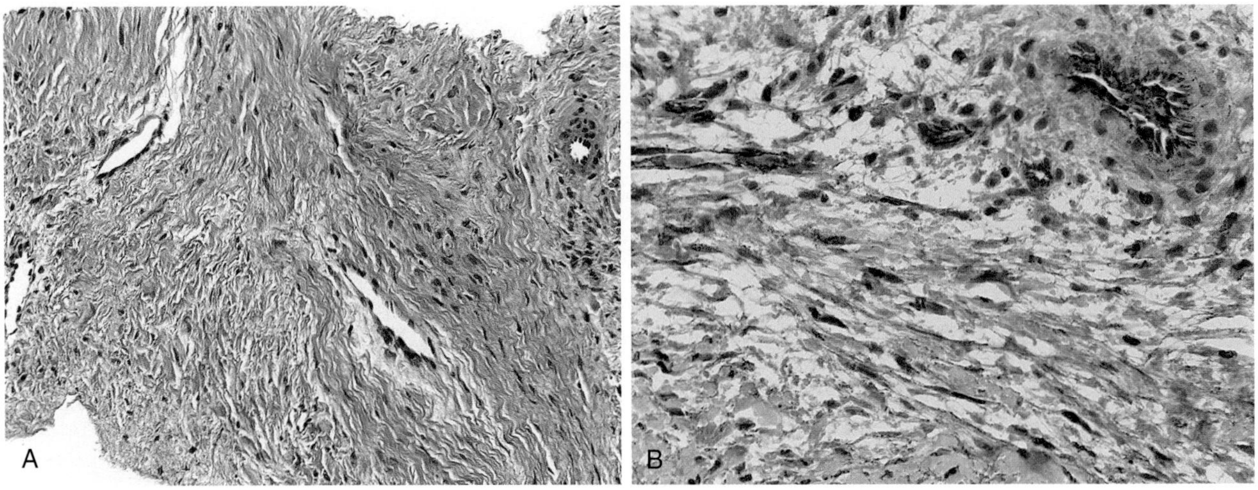

FIGURE 14.34 Desmoid-type fibromatosis (**A,** H&E stain). **B,** The nuclei are positive for beta-catenin.

SMA expression decreases with increased grade of the tumor. Leiomyosarcomas are negative for c-kit, CD34, beta-catenin, and S-100 protein.

MELANOMA The small intestine is a common metastatic site of cutaneous melanomas; primary melanomas arise rarely in the gastrointestinal tract and are most common in the anorectum and esophagus. Their immunophenotype is identical to their cutaneous counterparts; they stain with vimentin, S-100, HMB-45, melan-A, and tyrosinase (Fig. 14.35).[384-386] As noted earlier, c-kit may be positive in a subset of melanomas.

Differential Diagnoses

The immunohistochemical differential diagnosis of a mesenchymal neoplasm in the upper abdomen includes GIST, schwannoma, solitary fibrous tumor, desmoid-type fibromatosis, and leiomyosarcoma.[350,387] These lesions can share many morphologic features, especially in small-needle core biopsy specimens. The antibodies CD117, CD34, S-100, GFAP, CD99, beta-catenin, and desmin provide a useful diagnostic antibody panel (Fig. 14.36).

KEY DIAGNOSTIC POINTS

Mural Mesenchymal Lesions

- IHC aids in separating many of the lesions that may show morphologic overlap with GIST including schwannoma, desmoid-type fibromatosis, solitary fibrous tumor, and leiomyosarcoma.
- A panel of antibodies including CD117, CD34, S100, GFAP, CD99, beta-catenin, and desmin is useful in the diagnosis of these mesenchymal lesions.

MESENCHYMAL LESIONS PRESENTING AS POLYPOID LESIONS

Spindle cell lesions uncommonly manifest as endoscopically biopsied or resected polyps of the luminal GI tract. The differential diagnosis of these lesions includes neural lesions such as neurofibroma, ganglioneuroma, and perineurioma; fibroblastic lesions that include inflammatory fibroid polyp; and so-called "benign fibroblastic polyps" and leiomyomas of the muscularis mucosae. Importantly, in the evaluation of these lesions, a GIST presenting as a polypoid lesion should always be kept in the differential diagnosis; as such, c-kit immunohistochemistry should be always ordered on these lesions.

Neural Lesions

Neural lesions are common polypoid, spindle-cell lesions of the GI tract and are most often present in the colon. These lesions typically show a spindled cell morphology with interdigitation of the neoplastic cells between colonic crypts; in the case of ganglioneuroma, intermixed ganglion-type cells are seen (Fig. 14.37). Both neurofibroma and ganglioneuroma stain with S-100 protein, and the ganglion cells stain with neurofilament protein and synaptophysin.[388-390] Of note, both neurofibromas and ganglioneuromas are associated with neurofibromatosis, type I.[320,391-393] Although most ganglioneuromas are solitary, there is an additional association with multiple endocrine neoplasia, type IIb, and various polyposis syndromes.[393]

Perineurioma of the GI tract is a relatively recently described entity that rarely presents as a polypoid lesion. These lesions are composed of a bland spindle cell proliferation with delicate cytoplasmic protrusions that emanate from either side of an elongated nucleus. Like neurofibroma, this lesion grows around and entraps adjacent intestinal crypts. Analogous to perineuriomas of the soft tissues, intestinal perineuriomas almost uniformly stain with epithelial membrane antigen (EMA); a subset of these lesions expresses claudin-1. These lesions are negative for smooth muscle markers, S-100 protein, and c-*kit*.

Fibroblastic Lesions

Inflammatory fibroid polyp is a lesion that most commonly presents in the gastric antrum and the distal small intestine.[394] This lesion is composed of bland spindle

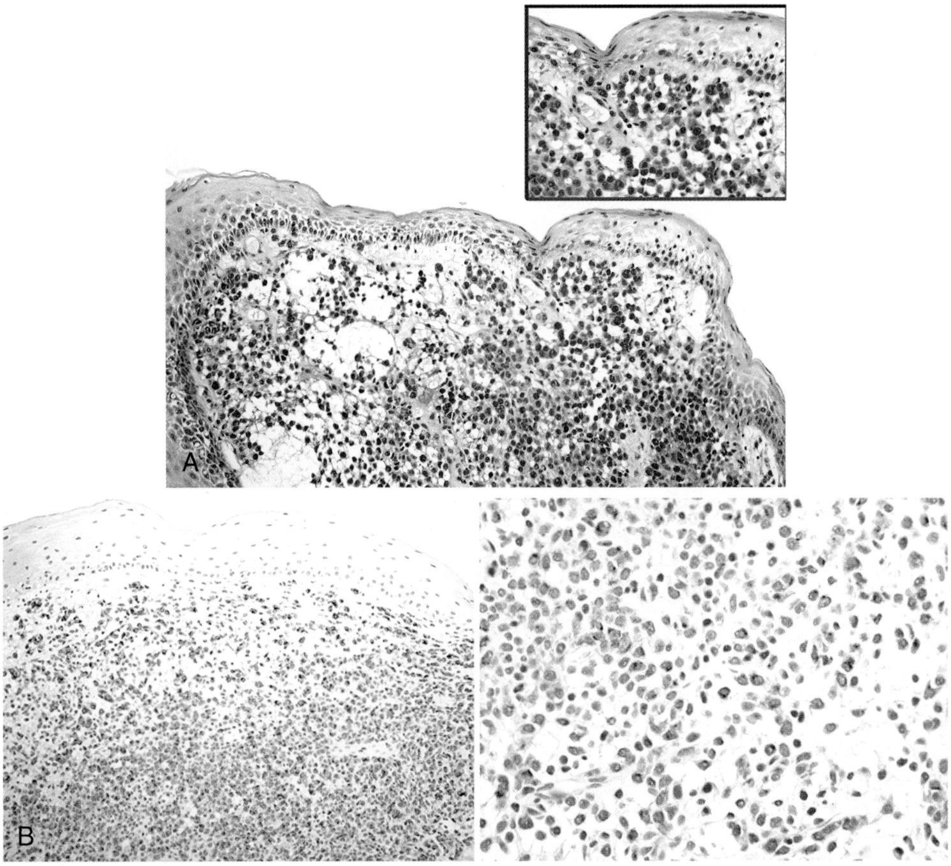

FIGURE 14.35 **A,** Esophageal melanoma. Subjacent to a normal squamous mucosa, undifferentiated, dyshesive neoplastic cells expand the submucosa. **B,** Esophageal melanoma. Tyrosinase diffusely stains the neoplastic cells with moderate intensity. Many cells have a perinuclear dot, Golgi-zone accentuation in addition to homogeneous cytoplasmic staining.

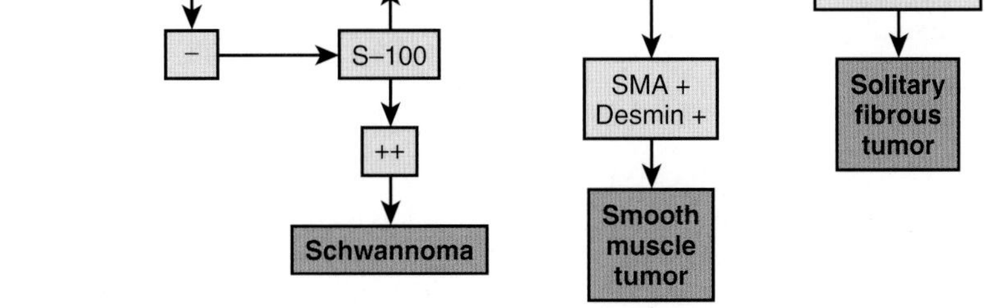

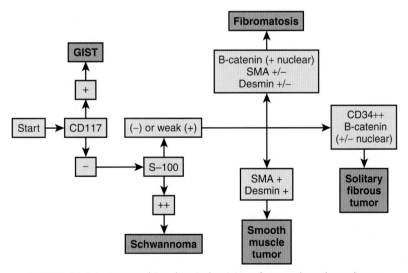

FIGURE 14.36 Immunohistochemical staining of mesenchymal neoplasms.

cells set in a vascularized and hyalinized stroma with abundant inflammatory cells, which contain a large number of eosinophils. These tumors are thought to be derived from fibroblasts or dendritic cells. As such, these tumors stain with CD34; fascin; CD35; calponin; and, less likely, smooth muscle actin.[395,396] Expression of c-*kit* in these tumors has been reported but is rare.[397]

Benign fibroblastic polyp is another recently described entity in the colon and is histologically similar to perineurioma.[398-401] However, unlike perineurioma, these lesions do not stain with EMA and do not show evidence of smooth muscle or neural differentiation. Benign fibroblastic polyps do express vimentin and may express smooth muscle actin and CD34.

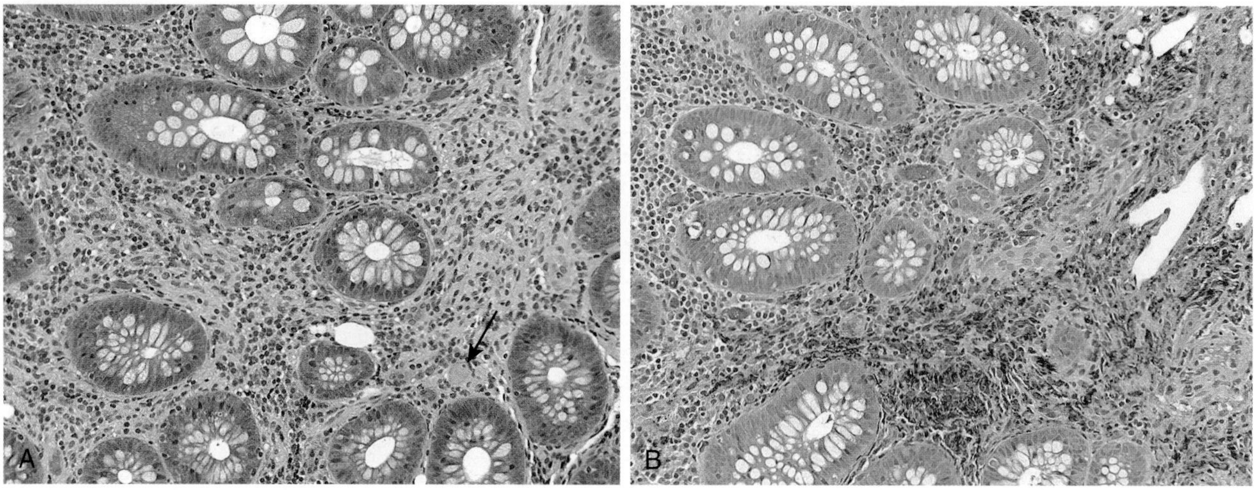

FIGURE 14.37 Mucosal ganglioneuroma. **A,** H&E stain showing spindled stroma and one ganglion cell *(arrow)*; eosinophils are prominent in this example. **B,** S-100 (red chromogen) strongly stains the stromal spindle cells, which wrap around negatively staining colonic crypts. The ganglion cells stain for neurofilament and synaptophysin (not shown).

Smooth Muscle Lesions

Leiomyoma of the muscularis mucosae is the most common mucosal-based mesenchymal lesion of the GI tract that may present as a polypoid mass.[402,403] These tumors often arise in the colon; leiomyomas are also likely to occur within the wall of the esophagus.[382] Unlike many of the previously mentioned lesions, this tumor displaces the colonic crypts and does not grow between crypts. As with leiomyomas elsewhere, these lesions stain strongly with smooth muscle actin and desmin and are negative for c-*kit*.

GENOMIC APPLICATIONS

Epithelial Lesions

COLORECTAL ADENOCARCINOMA Most colorectal adenocarcinomas arise through mutations of the β-catenin or APC genes or other genes in the Wnt signaling pathway. Dysfunction of this pathway can lead to translocation of β-catenin protein into the nucleus, where it can act as a transcriptional activator of other genes such as c-myc and cyclin D1. Nuclear β catenin expression was highly associated with progression of colorectal tissue from normal epithelial tissue, polyps, and adenomas to carcinomas.[404,405]

A subset of colorectal cancers arises via the MSI pathway owing to mutations or alterations in specific mismatch repair proteins. This pathway is discussed further later.

Neuroendocrine Lesions

About 5% to 10% of GI neuroendocrine tumors are associated with a hereditary disease. The inherited syndromes and their associated genes include multiple endocrine neoplasia type I (*MEN1* gene), neurofibromatosis type 1 (*NF1* gene), von Hippel-Lindau disease (*VHL* gene), and the tuberous sclerosis complex (*TSC1* or *TSC2* gene).[406]

Mesenchymal Lesions

GASTROINTESTINAL STROMAL TUMORS As noted earlier, the classification of spindle cell lesions of the gastrointestinal tract was immeasurably aided by the discovery of activating mutations in the KIT gene in approximately 80% of cases. Additionally, 5% to 7% of cases show a mutated *PDGFR-A* gene and the remaining 15% of cases show a lack of mutated KIT and PDGFR-A proteins.[326,407,408] A vast majority of these tumors show expression of the KIT protein using immunohistochemistry.

DESMOID-TYPE FIBROMATOSIS Up to 60% of desmoid-type fibromatoses harbor mutations in the beta-catenin gene, and an additional 10% of these tumors show mutations in the APC gene.[409-414] Mutations in either of these two genes result in abnormal accumulation of the beta-catenin protein in the nucleus.[411,415] This abnormal accumulation can be detected by immunohistochemistry, as noted earlier, and has utility in the diagnosis of desmoid-type fibromatosis.

THERANOSTIC APPLICATIONS

Epithelial Lesions

REFRACTORY CELIAC DISEASE Recently, immunohistochemistry has been shown to have utility in the evaluation of patients with refractory celiac disease. These patients continue to suffer from symptoms despite adherence to a gluten-free diet and are more likely to develop further complications such as ulcerative jejunoileitis and enteropathy-associated T-cell lymphoma. The group of patients with refractory sprue and loss of CD8 expression in more than 50% of the CD3-positive intraepithelial lymphocytes are more likely to develop enteropathy-associated T-cell lymphoma.[416] These patients with an abnormal T-cell phenotype are more likely to receive more aggressive immunosuppressive therapy.

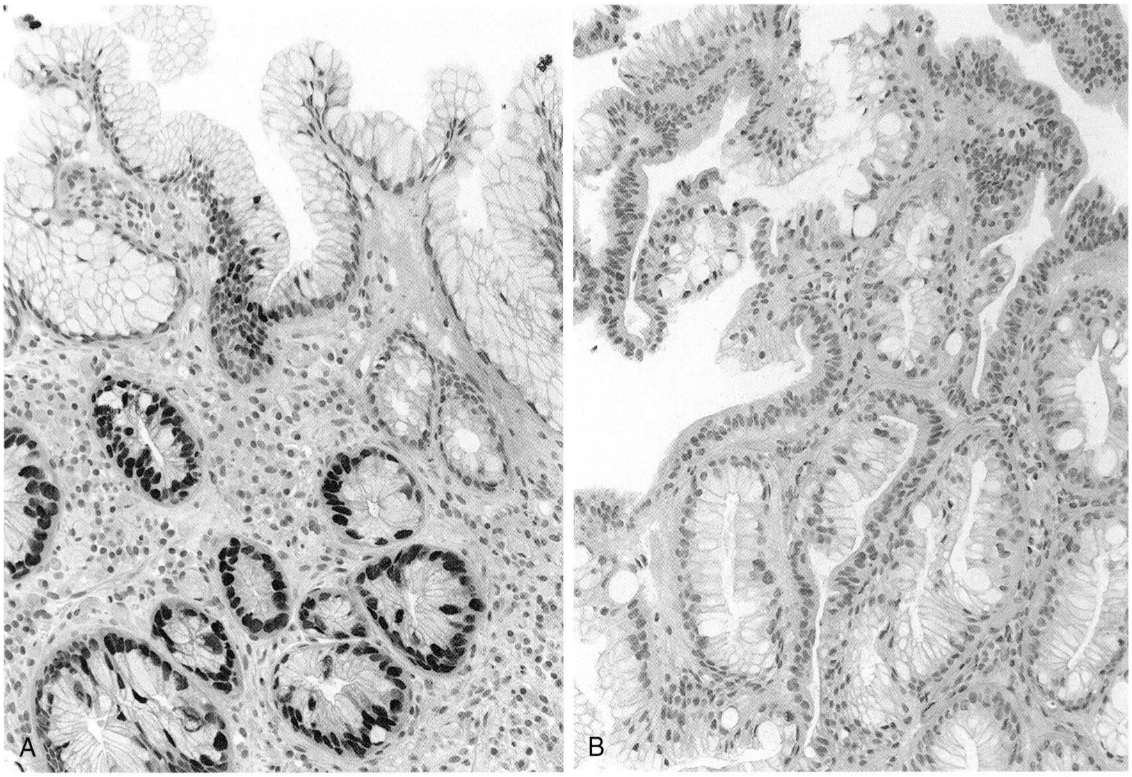

FIGURE 14.38 **A,** Low-grade dysplasia in Barrett esophagus showing overexpression of p53, compared with **B,** low-grade dysplasia without p53 expression.

BARRETT ESOPHAGUS Currently, high-grade dysplasia remains the most reliable predictor of progression to adenocarcinoma in Barrett esophagus. However, it would be more helpful to be able to predict progression in earlier lesions. One study found that p53 protein overexpression in low-grade dysplasia, as assessed by IHC, is predictive of progression (Fig. 14.38).[417] Of the 21% of cases of low-grade dysplasia that overexpressed p53 in their study, 60% progressed to high-grade dysplasia or carcinoma on follow-up biopsies, 25% had persistent low-grade dysplasia, and 13% "regressed." Although the results of this study are promising, they have not yet been incorporated into routine clinical use.

GASTRIC ADENOCARCINOMA Nuclear regulatory and cell cycle molecule E-cadherin, p16, and CDX2 have been studied as markers of poor prognosis.[418,419] Interest in Rb, cyclin D1, p53, and Ki-67 (MIB-1) are useful adjunctive tests for distinguishing between intestinal metaplasia and well-differentiated adenocarcinoma. Combinations of MUC1, MUC5A, and MUC5B staining, reflecting so-called intestinal or gastric type differentiation, appear to be prognostically significant.[420-423] MUC antibodies do not appear useful in distinguishing between adenocarcinomas of different sites.[120,424]

COLORECTAL ADENOCARCINOMA EGFR is a tyrosine kinase receptor. Humanized monoclonal antibody chemotherapy to EGFR blocks its functional activation. Immunohistochemical documentation of EGFR reactivity within colorectal cancers was once necessary to initiate anti-EGFR therapy. Currently, the initiation of therapy relies on documentation of a normal (wild-type) KRAS gene because tumors with KRAS mutations do not respond to anti-EGFR therapy (see later).

MSI-H/mismatch repair protein–deficient colorectal cancers, evaluated by either MSI testing or IHC, may have a better survival in subsets of colon cancer patients.[425] This effect may be related to the CpG island methylator phenotype (widespread promoter methylation).[426] MSI-H tumors may also respond differently to 5-fluorouracil-based chemotherapy.[427]

Mesenchymal Lesions

In the appropriate histologic context, documentation of either KIT protein expression by immunohistochemistry or a mutation in the KIT/PDGFRA genes is among the criteria for a diagnosis of GIST. The primary modality of medical treatment of these tumors is administration of the KIT/PDGFRA inhibitors imatinib mesylate and sunitinib malate. Thus expression of KIT using immunohistochemistry is an important predictive marker in mesenchymal tumors of the gastrointestinal tract.

BEYOND IMMUNOHISTOCHEMISTRY: ANATOMIC MOLECULAR DIAGNOSTIC APPLICATIONS

Epithelial Lesions

EPSTEIN-BARR VIRUS–ASSOCIATED GASTRIC CARCINOMAS Approximately 4% of gastric carcinomas are associated with EBV infection (Fig. 14.11D).[428,429] These tumors have a typical, lymphocyte-rich stroma that is a clue to the proper diagnosis.[147] These tumors show EBV-encoded RNA by *in situ* hybridization[430,431] and have a better prognosis compared with typical gastric adenocarcinoma.[147,432-434]

BARRETT ESOPHAGUS As mentioned earlier, histomorphology is the best tool to predict behavior in Barrett esophagus. There are promising biomarkers on the horizon using various techniques, but they need to be validated. Two techniques that have been used to stratify risk in Barrett esophagus are DNA content analysis (by flow cytometry) and loss of heterozygosity (LOH) (by PCR). In one study, patients with no DNA content abnormalities at baseline biopsy had 0% incidence of adenocarcinoma at 5 years, whereas patients with aneuploidy or increased tetraploidy (4N) at baseline biopsy had a 28% incidence of adenocarcinoma at 5 years.[435] In another study, of patients with baseline 17p LOH (p53 locus), 37% (20/54) progressed to adenocarcinoma and in patients with no loss at 17p, 3% (6/202) progressed to adenocarcinoma.[436]

COLORECTAL ADENOCARCINOMA As mentioned earlier, a subset of colorectal cancers arises via the MSI pathway. Molecular testing for MSI using a panel of microsatellite markers can detect microsatellite unstable (MSI-H) tumors.[238] Most MSI-H colorectal cancers are sporadic and arise from epigenetic gene silencing (hypermethylation) of one of the mismatch repair protein genes, most commonly *MLH1*. A minority of MSI-H colorectal cancers are inherited (hereditary nonpolyposis colorectal cancer) and arise from germline mutations of one of the mismatch repair protein genes *MLH1, MSH2, MSH6,* or *PMS2*. Patients with Lynch syndrome have HNPCC and, after additional testing, a confirmed mismatch repair gene germline mutation. The most common gene to be mutated in Lynch syndrome is MSH2.[234] As mentioned earlier, defects in the various mismatch repair proteins can be detected by immunohistochemistry. Zhang and Shia discuss the utility of MSI testing and immunohistochemistry, respectively, for screening colorectal cancer patients at risk for hereditary nonpolyposis colorectal cancer (Lynch) syndrome.[237,238]

***KRAS* MUTATIONAL ANALYSIS** Cetuximab is a monoclonal antibody that binds EGFR and competitively inhibits ligand binding. In the past, cetuximab was approved for irinotecan-resistant metastatic colorectal cancers that expressed EGFR by IHC. However, only a minority of these patients respond to anti-EGFR therapy.[437] More recently, it was discovered that tumors with KRAS gene mutations were resistant to cetuximab and had an overall poorer survival.[438,439] Hence KRAS mutational analysis, performed on either the primary or metastatic tumor, is becoming a routine test for patients with metastatic colorectal cancers, and cetuximab is given to those with no evidence of *KRAS* mutations (KRAS wild-type status).

Mesenchymal Lesions

KIT MUTATION STATUS AND CHEMOTHERAPY SUSCEPTIBILITY Imatinib mesylate and sunitinib malate chemotherapy inhibits the tyrosine kinase activity of the KIT and PDGFR-A proteins. This drug has proven itself to be a potent inhibitor of GIST growth in most patients.[440] However, the efficacy of these agents does vary with the particular KIT or PDGFR-A mutation. For example, GISTs with exon 11 KIT mutations are more sensitive to tyrosine kinase inhibitors than those tumors with either wild-type KIT or exon 9 mutated GISTs.[407,441,442] As a result of this information, many centers perform KIT and/or PDGFR-A mutation analysis to determine potential chemotherapeutic sensitivity.

SUMMARY

Immunohistochemistry is a powerful tool in the lumenal GI tract, providing essential theranostic and genomic applications in addition to crucial diagnostic applications.

REFERENCES

1. Gown AM. Immunohistochemical determination of primary sites of carcinomas. *J Histotechnology*. 1999;22:209-215.
2. Bracke ME, Van Roy FM, Mareel MM. The E-cadherin/catenin complex in invasion and metastasis. *Curr Top Microbiol Immunol*. 1996;213(Pt 1):123-161.
3. Willert K, Nusse R. Beta-catenin: a key mediator of Wnt signaling. *Curr Opin Genet Dev*. 1998;8:95-102.
4. Zhou Q, Toivola DM, Feng N, et al. Keratin 20 helps maintain intermediate filament organization in intestinal epithelia. *Mol Biol Cell*. 2003;14:2959-2971.
5. Hinoi T, Lucas PC, Kuick R, et al. CDX2 regulates liver intestine-cadherin expression in normal and malignant colon epithelium and intestinal metaplasia. *Gastroenterology*. 2002;123:1565-1577.
6. Bonhomme C, Duluc I, Martin E, et al. The Cdx2 homeobox gene has a tumour suppressor function in the distal colon in addition to a homeotic role during gut development. *Gut*. 2003;52:1465-1471.
7. Capella C, Heitz PU, Hofler H, et al. Revised classification of neuroendocrine tumours of the lung, pancreas and gut. *Virchows Arch*. 1995;425:547-560.
8. Mertz H, Vyberg M, Paulsen SM. Immunohistochemical detection of neuroendocrine markers in tumors of the lungs and gastrointestinal tract. *Appl Immunohistochem*. 1998;6:175-180.
9. Portela-Gomes GM, Stridsberg M. Chromogranin A in the human gastrointestinal tract: an immunocytochemical study with region-specific antibodies. *J Histochem Cytochem*. 2002;50:1487-1492.
10. Hla T, Neilson K. Human cyclooxygenase-2 cDNA. *Proc Natl Acad Sci U S A*. 1992;89:7384-7388.
11. Sano H, Kawahito Y, Wilder RL, et al. Expression of cyclo-oxygenase-1 and -2 in human colorectal cancer. *Cancer Res*. 1995;55:3785-3789.
12. Sheehan KM, Sheahan K, O'Donoghue DP, et al. The relationship between cyclooxygenase-2 expression and colorectal cancer. *JAMA*. 1999;282:1254-1257.
13. Lim HY, Joo HJ, Choi JH, et al. Increased expression of cyclo-oxygenase-2 protein in human gastric carcinoma. *Clin Cancer Res*. 2000;6:519-525.
14. Okami J, Yamamoto H, Fujiwara Y, et al. Overexpression of cyclooxygenase-2 in carcinoma of the pancreas. *Clin Cancer Res*. 1999;5:2018-2024.
15. Tucker ON, Dannenberg AJ, Yang EK, et al. Cyclooxygenase-2 expression is up-regulated in human pancreatic cancer. *Cancer Res*. 1999;59:987-990.

16. Espinosa I, Lee CH, Kim MK, et al. A novel monoclonal antibody against DOG1 is a sensitive and specific marker for gastrointestinal stromal tumors. *Am J Surg Pathol.* 2008;32:210-218.
17. Chiaravalli AM, Furlan D, Facco C, et al. Immunohistochemical pattern of hMSH2/hMLH1 in familial and sporadic colorectal, gastric, endometrial and ovarian carcinomas with instability in microsatellite sequences. *Virchows Arch.* 2001;438:39-48.
18. Myklebust AT, Beiske K, Pharo A, et al. Selection of anti-SCLC antibodies for diagnosis of bone marrow metastasis. *Br J Cancer.* 1991(Suppl)14:49-53.
19. Winter MJ, Nagtegaal ID, van Krieken JH, Litvinov SV. The epithelial cell adhesion molecule (Ep-CAM) as a morphoregulatory molecule is a tool in surgical pathology. *Am J Pathol.* 2003;163:2139-2148.
20. Morrison C, Marsh Jr W , Frankel WL. A comparison of CD10 to pCEA, MOC-31, and hepatocyte for the distinction of malignant tumors in the liver. *Mod Pathol.* 2002;15:1279-1287.
21. Niemann TH, Hughes JH, De Young BR. MOC-31 aids in the differentiation of metastatic adenocarcinoma from hepatocellular carcinoma. *Cancer.* 1999;87:295-298.
22. Van Klinken BJ, Dekker J, Buller HA, et al. Biosynthesis of mucins (MUC2-6) along the longitudinal axis of the human gastrointestinal tract. *Am J Physiol.* 1997;273:G296-G302.
23. Ischia R, Lovisetti-Scamihorn P, Hogue-Angeletti R, et al. Molecular cloning and characterization of NESP55, a novel chromogranin-like precursor of a peptide with 5-HT1B receptor antagonist activity. *J Biol Chem.* 1997;272:11657-11662.
24. Leitner B, Lovisetti-Scamihorn P, Heilmann J, et al. Subcellular localization of chromogranins, calcium channels, amine carriers, and proteins of the exocytotic machinery in bovine splenic nerve. *J Neurochem.* 1999;72:1110-1116.
25. Lovisetti-Scamihorn P, Fischer-Colbrie R, Leitner B, et al. Relative amounts and molecular forms of NESP55 in various bovine tissues. *Brain Res.* 1999;829:99-106.
26. Ireland AP, Clark GW, DeMeester TR. Barrett's esophagus. The significance of p53 in clinical practice. *Ann Surg.* 1997;225:17-30.
27. Yang A, Kaghad M, Wang Y, et al. p63, a p53 homolog at 3q27-29, encodes multiple products with transactivating, death-inducing, and dominant-negative activities. *Mol Cell.* 1998;2:305-316.
28. Marin MC, Kaelin Jr WG. p63 and p73: old members of a new family. *Biochim Biophys Acta.* 2000;1470:M93-M100.
29. Daniely Y, Liao G, Dixon D, et al. Critical role of p63 in the development of a normal esophageal and tracheobronchial epithelium. *Am J Physiol Cell Physiol.* 2004;287:C171-C181.
30. Bacchi CE, Gown AM. Distribution and pattern of expression of villin, a gastrointestinal-associated cytoskeletal protein, in human carcinomas: a study employing paraffin-embedded tissue. *Lab Invest.* 1991;64:418-424.
31. Nishizuka S, Chen ST, Gwadry FG, et al. Diagnostic markers that distinguish colon and ovarian adenocarcinomas: identification by genomic, proteomic, and tissue array profiling. *Cancer Res.* 2003;63:5243-5250.
32. Savera AT, Torres FX, Lindin MD, et al. Primary versus metastatic pulmonary adenocarcinoma: an immunohistochemical study using villin and cytokeratins 7 and 20. *Appl Immunohistochem.* 1996;4:86-94.
33. Tan J, Sidhu G, Greco MA, et al. Villin, cytokeratin 7, and cytokeratin 20 expression in pulmonary adenocarcinoma with ultrastructural evidence of microvilli with rootlets. *Hum Pathol.* 1998;29:390-396.
34. Odze RD. Update on the diagnosis and treatment of Barrett esophagus and related neoplastic precursor lesions. *Arch Pathol Lab Med.* 2008;132:1577-1585.
35. Kilgore SP, Ormsby AH, Gramlich TL, et al. The gastric cardia: fact or fiction? *Am J Gastroenterol.* 2000;95:921-924.
36. Flucke U, Steinborn E, Dries V, et al. Immunoreactivity of cytokeratins (CK7, CK20) and mucin peptide core antigens (MUC1, MUC2, MUC5AC) in adenocarcinomas, normal and metaplastic tissues of the distal oesophagus, oesophago-gastric junction and proximal stomach. *Histopathology.* 2003;43:127-134.
37. Glickman JN, Wang H, Das KM, et al. Phenotype of Barrett's esophagus and intestinal metaplasia of the distal esophagus and gastroesophageal junction: an immunohistochemical study of cytokeratins 7 and 20, Das-1 and 45 MI. *Am J Surg Pathol.* 2001;25:87-94.
38. Jovanovic I, Tzardi M, Mouzas IA, et al. Changing pattern of cytokeratin 7 and 20 expression from normal epithelium to intestinal metaplasia of the gastric mucosa and gastroesophageal junction. *Histol Histopathol.* 2002;17:445-454.
39. Kurtkaya-Yapicier O, Gencosmanoglu R, Avsar E, et al. The utility of cytokeratins 7 and 20 (CK7/20) immunohistochemistry in the distinction of short-segment Barrett esophagus from gastric intestinal metaplasia: is it reliable? *BMC Clin Pathol.* 2003;3:5.
40. Latchford A, Eksteen B, Jankowski J. The continuing tale of cytokeratins in Barrett's mucosa: as you like it. *Gut.* 2001;49:746-747.
41. Mohammed IA, Streutker CJ, Riddell RH. Utilization of cytokeratins 7 and 20 does not differentiate between Barrett's esophagus and gastric cardiac intestinal metaplasia. *Mod Pathol.* 2002;15:611-616.
42. Odze R. Cytokeratin 7/20 immunostaining: Barrett's oesophagus or gastric intestinal metaplasia? *Lancet.* 2002;359:1711-1713.
43. Ormsby AH, Goldblum JR, Rice TW, et al. Cytokeratin subsets can reliably distinguish Barrett's esophagus from intestinal metaplasia of the stomach. *Hum Pathol.* 1999;30:288-294.
44. Faller G, Borchard F, Ell C, et al. Histopathological diagnosis of Barrett's mucosa and associated neoplasias: results of a consensus conference of the Working Group for Gastroenterological Pathology of the German Society for Pathology on 22 September 2001 in Erlangen. *Virchows Arch.* 2003;443:597-601.
45. Chatelain D, Flejou JF. High-grade dysplasia and superficial adenocarcinoma in Barrett's esophagus: histological mapping and expression of p53, p21 and Bcl-2 oncoproteins. *Virchows Arch.* 2003;442:18-24.
46. Copelli SB, Mazzeo C, Gimenez A, et al. Molecular analysis of p53 tumor-suppressor gene and microsatellites in preneoplastic and neoplastic lesions of the colon and esophagus. *Oncol Rep.* 2001;8:923-929.
47. Croft J, Parry EM, Jenkins GJ, et al. Analysis of the premalignant stages of Barrett's oesophagus through to adenocarcinoma by comparative genomic hybridization. *Eur J Gastroenterol Hepatol.* 2002;14:1179-1186.
48. Raouf AA, Evoy DA, Carton E, et al. Loss of Bcl-2 expression in Barrett's dysplasia and adenocarcinoma is associated with tumor progression and worse survival but not with response to neoadjuvant chemoradiation. *Dis Esophagus.* 2003;16:17-23.
49. Reid BJ, Blount PL, Rabinovitch PS. Biomarkers in Barrett's esophagus. *Gastrointest Endosc Clin N Am.* 2003;13:369-397.
50. Taniere P, Borghi-Scoazec G, Saurin JC, et al. Cytokeratin expression in adenocarcinomas of the esophagogastric junction: a comparative study of adenocarcinomas of the distal esophagus and of the proximal stomach. *Am J Surg Pathol.* 2002;26:1213-1221.
51. Weiss MM, Kuipers EJ, Hermsen MA, et al. Barrett's adenocarcinomas resemble adenocarcinomas of the gastric cardia in terms of chromosomal copy number changes, but relate to squamous cell carcinomas of the distal oesophagus with respect to the presence of high-level amplifications. *J Pathol.* 2003;199:157-165.
52. Symmans PJ, Linehan JM, Brito MJ, Filipe MI. p53 expression in Barrett's oesophagus, dysplasia, and adenocarcinoma using antibody DO-7. *J Pathol.* 1994;173:221-226.
53. Cawley HM, Meltzer SJ, De Benedetti VM, et al. Anti-p53 antibodies in patients with Barrett's esophagus or esophageal carcinoma can predate cancer diagnosis. *Gastroenterology.* 1998;115:19-27.
54. Ramel S, Reid BJ, Sanchez CA, et al. Evaluation of p53 protein expression in Barrett's esophagus by two-parameter flow cytometry. *Gastroenterology.* 1992;102:1220-1228.
55. Levine DS. Barrett's oesophagus and p53. *Lancet.* 1994;344:212-213.
56. Werling RW, Yaziji H, Bacchi CE, Gown AM. CDX2, a highly sensitive and specific marker of adenocarcinomas of intestinal origin: an immunohistochemical survey of 476 primary and metastatic carcinomas. *Am J Surg Pathol.* 2003;27:303-310.
57. Deamant FD, Pombo MT, Battifora H. Estrogen receptor immunohistochemistry as a predictor of site of origin in metastatic breast cancer. *Appl Immunohistochem.* 1993;1:188-192.
58. Driessen A, Nafteux P, Lerut T, et al. Identical cytokeratin expression pattern CK7+/CK20- in esophageal and cardiac cancer: etiopathological and clinical implications. *Mod Pathol.* 2004;17:49-55.

59. Gulmann C, Counihan I, Grace A, et al. Cytokeratin 7/20 and mucin expression patterns in oesophageal, cardia and distal gastric adenocarcinomas. *Histopathology*. 2003;43:453-461.
60. Sheahan K, O'Brien MJ, Burke B, et al. Differential reactivities of carcinoembryonic antigen (CEA) and CEA-related monoclonal and polyclonal antibodies in common epithelial malignancies. *Am J Clin Pathol*. 1990;94:157-164.
61. Ormsby AH, Goldblum JR, Rice TW, et al. The utility of cytokeratin subsets in distinguishing Barrett's-related oesophageal adenocarcinoma from gastric adenocarcinoma. *Histopathology*. 2001;38:307-311.
62. Shen B, Ormsby AH, Shen C, et al. Cytokeratin expression patterns in noncardia, intestinal metaplasia-associated gastric adenocarcinoma: implication for the evaluation of intestinal metaplasia and tumors at the esophagogastric junction. *Cancer*. 2002;94:820-831.
63. Chu PG, Weiss LM. Expression of cytokeratin 5/6 in epithelial neoplasms: an immunohistochemical study of 509 cases. *Mod Pathol*. 2002;15:6-10.
64. Clover J, Oates J, Edwards C. Anti-cytokeratin 5/6: a positive marker for epithelioid mesothelioma. *Histopathology*. 1997;31:140-143.
65. Kaufmann O, Fietze E, Mengs J, Dietel M. Value of p63 and cytokeratin 5/6 as immunohistochemical markers for the differential diagnosis of poorly differentiated and undifferentiated carcinomas. *Am J Clin Pathol*. 2001;116:823-830.
66. Lam KY, Loke SL, Shen XC, Ma LT. Cytokeratin expression in non-neoplastic oesophageal epithelium and squamous cell carcinoma of the oesophagus. *Virchows Arch*. 1995;426:345-349.
67. Moll R. Cytokeratins as markers of differentiation in the diagnosis of epithelial tumors. *Subcell Biochem*. 1998;31:205-262.
68. Ordonez NG. Value of cytokeratin 5/6 immunostaining in distinguishing epithelial mesothelioma of the pleura from lung adenocarcinoma. *Am J Surg Pathol*. 1998;22:1215-1221.
69. Scarpatetti M, Tsybrovsky O, Popper HH. Cytokeratin typing as an aid in the differential diagnosis of primary versus metastatic lung carcinomas, and comparison with normal lung. *Virchows Arch*. 2002;440:70-76.
70. Shah KD, Tabibzadeh SS, Gerber MA. Comparison of cytokeratin expression in primary and metastatic carcinomas. Diagnostic application in surgical pathology. *Am J Clin Pathol*. 1987;87:708-715.
71. Suo Z, Holm R, Nesland JM. Squamous cell carcinomas. An immunohistochemical study of cytokeratins and involucrin in primary and metastatic tumours. *Histopathology*. 1993;23:45-54.
72. Di Como CJ, Urist MJ, Babayan I, et al. p63 expression profiles in human normal and tumor tissues. *Clin Cancer Res*. 2002;8:494-501.
73. Ikeda Y, Kuwano H, Ikebe M, et al. Immunohistochemical detection of CEA, CA19-9, and DF3 in esophageal carcinoma limited to the submucosal layer. *J Surg Oncol*. 1994;56:7-12.
74. Lager DJ, Callaghan EJ, Worth SF, et al. Cellular localization of thrombomodulin in human epithelium and squamous malignancies. *Am J Pathol*. 1995;146:933-943.
75. Moll R, Lowe A, Laufer J, Franke WW. Cytokeratin 20 in human carcinomas. A new histodiagnostic marker detected by monoclonal antibodies. *Am J Pathol*. 1992;140:427-447.
76. Rossen K, Thomsen HK. Ber-EP4 immunoreactivity depends on the germ layer origin and maturity of the squamous epithelium. *Histopathology*. 2001;39:386-389.
77. Lau SK, Luthringer DJ, Eisen RN. Thyroid Transcription Factor—1: A review. *Appl Immunohistochem Mol Morphol*. 2002;10:97-102.
78. Kornstein MJ, Rosai J. CD5 labeling of thymic carcinomas and other nonlymphoid neoplasms. *Am J Clin Pathol*. 1998;109:722-726.
79. Tateyama H, Eimoto T, Tada T, et al. Immunoreactivity of a new CD5 antibody with normal epithelium and malignant tumors including thymic carcinoma. *Am J Clin Pathol*. 1999;111:235-240.
80. Ordonez NG. Value of calretinin immunostaining in differentiating epithelial mesothelioma from lung adenocarcinoma. *Mod Pathol*. 1998;11:929-933.
81. Owonikoko T, Loberg C, Gabbert HE, Sarbia M. Comparative analysis of basaloid and typical squamous cell carcinoma of the oesophagus: a molecular biological and immunohistochemical study. *J Pathol*. 2001;193:155-161.
82. Sarbia M, Bittinger F, Porschen R, et al. bcl-2 expression and prognosis in squamous-cell carcinomas of the esophagus. *Int J Cancer*. 1996;69:324-328.
83. Banks ER, Frierson HF Jr, Mills SE, et al. Basaloid squamous cell carcinoma of the head and neck. A clinicopathologic and immunohistochemical study of 40 cases. *Am J Surg Pathol*. 1992;16:939-946.
84. Luna MA, el Naggar A, Parichatikanond P, et al. Basaloid squamous carcinoma of the upper aerodigestive tract. Clinicopathologic and DNA flow cytometric analysis. *Cancer*. 1990;66:537-542.
85. Tsang WY, Chan JK, Lee KC, et al. Basaloid-squamous carcinoma of the upper aerodigestive tract and so-called adenoid cystic carcinoma of the oesophagus: the same tumour type? *Histopathology*. 1991;19:35-46.
86. Tsubochi H, Suzuki T, Suzuki S, et al. Immunohistochemical study of basaloid squamous cell carcinoma, adenoid cystic and mucoepidermoid carcinoma in the upper aerodigestive tract. *Anticancer Res*. 2000;20:1205-1211.
87. Li TJ, Zhang YX, Wen J, et al. Basaloid squamous cell carcinoma of the esophagus with or without adenoid cystic features. *Arch Pathol Lab Med*. 2004;128:1124-1130.
88. Abe K, Sasano H, Itakura Y, et al. Basaloid-squamous carcinoma of the esophagus. A clinicopathologic, DNA ploidy, and immunohistochemical study of seven cases. *Am J Surg Pathol*. 1996;20:453-461.
89. Kawahara K, Makimoto K, Maekawa T, et al. An immunohistochemical examination of basaloid squamous cell carcinoma of the esophagus: report of a case. *Surg Today*. 2001;31:655-659.
90. Popnikolov NK, Ayala AG, Graves K, Gatalica Z. Benign myoepithelial tumors of the breast have immunophenotypic characteristics similar to metaplastic matrix-producing and spindle cell carcinomas. *Am J Clin Pathol*. 2003;120:161-167.
91. Guarino M, Reale D, Micoli G, Forloni B. Carcinosarcoma of the oesophagus with rhabdomyoblastic differentiation. *Histopathology*. 1993;22:493-498.
92. Lauwers GY, Grant LD, Scott GV, et al. Spindle cell squamous carcinoma of the esophagus: analysis of ploidy and tumor proliferative activity in a series of 13 cases. *Hum Pathol*. 1998;29:863-868.
93. Ooi A, Kawahara E, Okada Y, et al. Carcinosarcoma of the esophagus. An immunohistochemical and electron microscopic study. *Acta Pathol Jpn*. 1986;36:151-159.
94. Rosty D, Prevot S, Tiret E. Adenocarcinosarcoma in Barrett's esophagus: Report of a case. *Int J Surg Pathol*. 1996;4:43.
95. Iezzoni JC, Mills SE. Sarcomatoid carcinomas (carcinosarcomas) of the gastrointestinal tract: a review. *Semin Diagn Pathol*. 1993;10:176-187.
96. Amatya VJ, Takeshima Y, Kaneko M, Inai K. Esophageal carcinosarcoma with basaloid squamous carcinoma and rhabdomyosarcoma components with TP53 mutation. *Pathol Int*. 2004;54:803-809.
97. Drut R, Drut RM. Lymphocytic gastritis in pediatric celiac disease—immunohistochemical study of the intraepithelial lymphocytic component. *Med Sci Monit*. 2004;10:CR38-CR42.
98. Alsaigh N, Odze R, Goldman H, et al. Gastric and esophageal intraepithelial lymphocytes in pediatric celiac disease. *Am J Surg Pathol*. 1996;20:865-870.
99. Andersen LP, Dorland A, Karacan H, et al. Possible clinical importance of the transformation of Helicobacter pylori into coccoid forms. *Scand J Gastroenterol*. 2000;35:897-903.
100. Cao J, Li ZQ, Borch K, Petersson F, Mardh S. Detection of spiral and coccoid forms of Helicobacter pylori using a murine monoclonal antibody. *Clin Chim Acta*. 1997;267:183-196.
101. Goldstein NS. Chronic inactive gastritis and coccoid Helicobacter pylori in patients treated for gastroesophageal reflux disease or with *H pylori* eradication therapy. *Am J Clin Pathol*. 2002;118:719-726.
102. Ashton-Key M, Diss TC, Isaacson PG. Detection of Helicobacter pylori in gastric biopsy and resection specimens. *J Clin Pathol*. 1996;49:107-111.
103. Jonkers D, Houben G, de Bruine A, et al. Prevalence of gastric metaplasia in the duodenal bulb and distribution of Helicobacter pylori in the gastric mucosa. A clinical and histopathological study in 96 consecutive patients. *Ital J Gastroenterol Hepatol*. 1998;30:481-483.

104. Rotimi O, Cairns A, Gray S, et al. Histological identification of Helicobacter pylori: comparison of staining methods. *J Clin Pathol.* 2000;53:756-759.
105. van der Wouden EJ, Thijs JC, van Zwet AA, et al. Reliability of biopsy-based diagnostic tests for Helicobacter pylori after treatment aimed at its eradication. *Eur J Gastroenterol Hepatol.* 1999;11:1255-1258.
106. Singhal AV, Sepulveda AR. *Helicobacter heilmannii* gastritis: a case study with review of literature. *Am J Surg Pathol.* 2005;29:1537-1539.
107. Bordi C, Annibale B, Azzoni C, et al. Endocrine cell growths in atrophic body gastritis. Critical evaluation of a histological classification. *J Pathol.* 1997;182:339-346.
108. Solcia E, Rindi G, Fiocca R, et al. Distinct patterns of chronic gastritis associated with carcinoid and cancer and their role in tumorigenesis. *Yale J Biol Med* 1992;65:793-804; discussion 827-829.
109. Torbenson M, Abraham SC, Boitnott J, et al. Autoimmune gastritis: distinct histological and immunohistochemical findings before complete loss of oxyntic glands. *Mod Pathol.* 2002;15:102-109.
110. Stolte M, Baumann K, Bethke B, et al. Active autoimmune gastritis without total atrophy of the glands. *Z Gastroenterol.* 1992;30:729-735.
111. Ohchi T, Misumi A, Akagi M. A study on the distribution of G-cells in human gastric mucosa. *Gastroenterol Jpn.* 1984;19:41-52.
112. Burt RW. Gastric fundic gland polyps. *Gastroenterology.* 2003;125:1462-1469.
113. Declich P, Isimbaldi G, Sironi M, et al. Sporadic fundic gland polyps: an immunohistochemical study of their antigenic profile. *Pathol Res Pract.* 1996;192:808-815.
114. Sekine S, Shibata T, Yamauchi Y, et al. Beta-catenin mutations in sporadic fundic gland polyps. *Virchows Arch.* 2002;440:381-386.
115. Hassan A, Yerian LM, Kuan SF, et al. Immunohistochemical evaluation of adenomatous polyposis coli, beta-catenin, c-Myc, cyclin D1, p53, and retinoblastoma protein expression in syndromic and sporadic fundic gland polyps. *Hum Pathol.* 2004;35:328-334.
116. Lauren P. The two histological main types of gastric carcinoma: diffuse and so-called intestinal-type carcinoma. an attempt at a histo-clinical classification. *Acta Pathol Microbiol Scand.* 1965;64:31-49.
117. Ma CK, Zarbo RJ, Frierson Jr HF, Lee MW. Comparative immunohistochemical study of primary and metastatic carcinomas of the liver. *Am J Clin Pathol.* 1993;99:551-557.
118. Goldstein NS, Long A, Kuan SF, Hart J. Colon signet ring cell adenocarcinoma: immunohistochemical characterization and comparison with gastric and typical colon adenocarcinomas. *Appl Immunohistochem Mol Morphol.* 2000;8:183-188.
119. Kim MA, Lee HS, Yang HK, Kim WH. Cytokeratin expression profile in gastric carcinomas. *Hum Pathol.* 2004;35:576-581.
120. Lee MJ, Lee HS, Kim WH, et al. Expression of mucins and cytokeratins in primary carcinomas of the digestive system. *Mod Pathol.* 2003;16:403-410.
121. McKinley M, Listrom MB, Fenoglio-Preiser C. Cytokeratin 19: a potential marker of colonic differentiation. *Surg Pathol.* 1990;3:107-113.
122. Baars JH, De Ruijter JL, Smedts F, et al. The applicability of a keratin 7 monoclonal antibody in routinely Papanicolaou-stained cytologic specimens for the differential diagnosis of carcinomas. *Am J Clin Pathol.* 1994;101:257-261.
123. Ramaekers F, van Niekerk C, Poels L, et al. Use of monoclonal antibodies to keratin 7 in the differential diagnosis of adenocarcinomas. *Am J Pathol.* 1990;136:641-655.
124. Tot T. Adenocarcinomas metastatic to the liver: the value of cytokeratins 20 and 7 in the search for unknown primary tumors. *Cancer.* 1999;85:171-177.
125. Wauters CC, Smedts F, Gerrits LG, et al. Keratins 7 and 20 as diagnostic markers of carcinomas metastatic to the ovary. *Hum Pathol.* 1995;26:852-855.
126. Kaufmann O, Deidesheimer T, Muehlenberg M, et al. Immunohistochemical differentiation of metastatic breast carcinomas from metastatic adenocarcinomas of other common primary sites. *Histopathology.* 1996;29:233-240.
127. Miettinen M. Keratin 20: immunohistochemical marker for gastrointestinal, urothelial, and Merkel cell carcinomas. *Mod Pathol.* 1995;8:384-388.
128. Cathro HP, Stoler MH. Expression of cytokeratins 7 and 20 in ovarian neoplasia. *Am J Clin Pathol.* 2002;117:944-951.
129. Chu P, Wu E, Weiss LM. Cytokeratin 7 and cytokeratin 20 expression in epithelial neoplasms: a survey of 435 cases. *Mod Pathol.* 2000;13:962-972.
130. Kende AI, Carr NJ, Sobin LH. Expression of cytokeratins 7 and 20 in carcinomas of the gastrointestinal tract. *Histopathology.* 2003;42:137-140.
131. Park SY, Kim HS, Hong EK, Kim WH. Expression of cytokeratins 7 and 20 in primary carcinomas of the stomach and colorectum and their value in the differential diagnosis of metastatic carcinomas to the ovary. *Hum Pathol.* 2002;33:1078-1085.
132. Wang NP, Zee S, Zarbo RJ. Coordinate expression of cytokeratins 7 and 20 defines unique subsets of carcinomas. *Appl Immunohistochem.* 1995;3:99-107.
133. Kaimaktchiev V, Terracciano L, Tornillo L, et al. The homeobox intestinal differentiation factor CDX2 is selectively expressed in gastrointestinal adenocarcinomas. *Mod Pathol.* 2004;17:1392-1399.
134. Liu Q, Teh M, Ito K, et al. CDX2 expression is progressively decreased in human gastric intestinal metaplasia, dysplasia and cancer. *Mod Pathol.* 2007;20:1286-1297.
135. Chu PG, Weiss LM. Immunohistochemical characterization of signet-ring cell carcinomas of the stomach, breast, and colon. *Am J Clin Pathol.* 2004;121:884-892.
136. Tian MM, Zhao AL, Li ZW, Li JY. Phenotypic classification of gastric signet ring cell carcinoma and its relationship with clinicopathologic parameters and prognosis. *World J Gastroenterol.* 2007;13:3189-3198.
137. Nguyen MD, Plasil B, Wen P, Frankel WL. Mucin profiles in signet-ring cell carcinoma. *Arch Pathol Lab Med.* 2006;130: 799-804.
138. O'Connell FP, Wang HH, Odze RD. Utility of immunohistochemistry in distinguishing primary adenocarcinomas from metastatic breast carcinomas in the gastrointestinal tract. *Arch Pathol Lab Med.* 2005;129:338-347.
139. Llinares K, Escande F, Aubert S, et al. Diagnostic value of MUC4 immunostaining in distinguishing epithelial mesothelioma and lung adenocarcinoma. *Mod Pathol.* 2004;17:150-157.
140. Cameron BL, Butler JA, Rutgers J, et al. Immunohistochemical determination of the estrogen receptor content of gastrointestinal adenocarcinomas. *Am Surg.* 1992;58:758-760.
141. Nash JW, Morrison C, Frankel WL. The utility of estrogen receptor and progesterone receptor immunohistochemistry in the distinction of metastatic breast carcinoma from other tumors in the liver. *Arch Pathol Lab Med.* 2003;127:1591-1595.
142. Vang R, Gown AM, Barry TS, et al. Immunohistochemistry for estrogen and progesterone receptors in the distinction of primary and metastatic mucinous tumors in the ovary: an analysis of 124 cases. *Mod Pathol.* 2006;19:97-105.
143. Lee BH, Hecht JL, Pinkus JL, Pinkus GS. WT1, estrogen receptor, and progesterone receptor as markers for breast or ovarian primary sites in metastatic adenocarcinoma to body fluids. *Am J Clin Pathol.* 2002;117:745-750.
144. Park SY, Kim BH, Kim JH, et al. Panels of immunohistochemical markers help determine primary sites of metastatic adenocarcinoma. *Arch Pathol Lab Med.* 2007;131:1561-1567.
145. Theodoropoulos GE, Lazaris AC, Panoussopoulos D, et al. Significance of estrogen receptors and cathepsin D tissue detection in gastric adenocarcinoma. *J Surg Oncol.* 1995;58:176-183.
146. van Velthuysen ML, Taal BG, van der Hoeven JJ, Peterse JL. Expression of oestrogen receptor and loss of E-cadherin are diagnostic for gastric metastasis of breast carcinoma. *Histopathology.* 2005;46:153-157.
147. Grogg KL, Lohse CM, Pankratz VS, et al. Lymphocyte-rich gastric cancer: associations with Epstein-Barr virus, microsatellite instability, histology, and survival. *Mod Pathol.* 2003;16:641-651.
148. Jung HY, Jung KC, Shim YH, et al. Methylation of the hMLH1 promoter in multiple gastric carcinomas with microsatellite instability. *Pathol Int.* 2001;51:445-451.

149. Endoh Y, Tamura G, Ajioka Y, et al. Frequent hypermethylation of the hMLH1 gene promoter in differentiated-type tumors of the stomach with the gastric foveolar phenotype. *Am J Pathol.* 2000;157:717-722.
150. Ohmura K, Tamura G, Endoh Y, et al. Microsatellite alterations in differentiated-type adenocarcinomas and precancerous lesions of the stomach with special reference to cellular phenotype. *Hum Pathol.* 2000;31:1031-1035.
151. Azumi N, Ben-Ezra J, Battifora H. Immunophenotypic diagnosis of leiomyosarcomas and rhabdomyosarcomas with monoclonal antibodies to muscle-specific actin and desmin in formalin-fixed tissue. *Mod Pathol.* 1988;1:469-474.
152. Ueyama T, Nagai E, Yao T, Tsuneyoshi M. Vimentin-positive gastric carcinomas with rhabdoid features. A clinicopathologic and immunohistochemical study. *Am J Surg Pathol.* 1993;17:813-819.
153. Nakayama Y, Murayama H, Iwasaki H, et al. Gastric carcinosarcoma (sarcomatoid carcinoma) with rhabdomyoblastic and osteoblastic differentiation. *Pathol Int.* 1997;47:557-563.
154. Randjelovic T, Filipovic B, Babic D, et al. Carcinosarcoma of the stomach: a case report and review of the literature. *World J Gastroenterol.* 2007;13:5533-5536.
155. Maitra A, Murakata LA, Albores-Saavedra J. Immunoreactivity for hepatocyte paraffin 1 antibody in hepatoid adenocarcinomas of the gastrointestinal tract. *Am J Clin Pathol.* 2001;115:689-694.
156. Plaza JA, Vitellas K, Frankel WL. Hepatoid adenocarcinoma of the stomach. *Ann Diagn Pathol.* 2004;8:137-141.
157. Roberts CC, Colby TV, Batts KP. Carcinoma of the stomach with hepatocyte differentiation (hepatoid adenocarcinoma). *Mayo Clin Proc.* 1997;72:1154-1160.
158. Terracciano LM, Glatz K, Mhawech P, et al. Hepatoid adenocarcinoma with liver metastasis mimicking hepatocellular carcinoma: an immunohistochemical and molecular study of eight cases. *Am J Surg Pathol.* 2003;27:1302-1312.
159. Villari D, Caruso R, Grosso M, et al. Hep Par 1 in gastric and bowel carcinomas: an immunohistochemical study. *Pathology.* 2002;34:423-426.
160. Kumashiro Y, Yao T, Aishima S, et al. Hepatoid adenocarcinoma of the stomach: histogenesis and progression in association with intestinal phenotype. *Hum Pathol.* 2007;38:857-863.
161. Jan YJ, Chen JT, Ho WL, et al. Primary coexistent adenocarcinoma and choriocarcinoma of the stomach. A case report and review of the literature. *J Clin Gastroenterol.* 1997;25:550-554.
162. Saigo PE, Brigati DJ, Sternberg SS, et al. Primary gastric choriocarcinoma. An immunohistological study. *Am J Surg Pathol.* 1981;5:333-342.
163. Hirano Y, Hara T, Nozawa H, et al. Combined choriocarcinoma, neuroendocrine cell carcinoma and tubular adenocarcinoma in the stomach. *World J Gastroenterol.* 2008;14:3269-3272.
164. Blumenfeld W, Chandhoke DK, Sagerman P, Turi GK. Neuroendocrine differentiation in gastric adenocarcinomas. An immunohistochemical study. *Arch Pathol Lab Med.* 1996;120:478-481.
165. Park JG, Choe GY, Helman LJ, et al. Chromogranin-A expression in gastric and colon cancer tissues. *Int J Cancer.* 1992;51:189-194.
166. Qvigstad G, Sandvik AK, Brenna E, et al. Detection of chromogranin A in human gastric adenocarcinomas using a sensitive immunohistochemical technique. *Histochem J.* 2000;32:551-556.
167. Bhargava R, Beriwal S, Dabbs DJ. Mammaglobin vs GCDFP-15: an immunohistologic validation survey for sensitivity and specificity. *Am J Clin Pathol.* 2007;127:103-113.
168. Battifora H. Metastatic breast carcinoma to the stomach simulating linitis plastica. *Appl Immunohistochem.* 1994;2:225-228.
169. Brown RW, Campagna LB, Dunn JK, Cagle PT. Immunohistochemical identification of tumor markers in metastatic adenocarcinoma. A diagnostic adjunct in the determination of primary site. *Am J Clin Pathol.* 1997;107:12-19.
170. Perry A, Parisi JE, Kurtin PJ. Metastatic adenocarcinoma to the brain: an immunohistochemical approach. *Hum Pathol.* 1997;28:938-943.
171. Raju U, Ma CK, Shaw A. Signet ring variant of lobular carcinoma of the breast: a clinicopathologic and immunohistochemical study. *Mod Pathol.* 1993;6:516-520.
172. Sentani K, Oue N, Tashiro T, et al. Immunohistochemical staining of Reg IV and claudin-18 is useful in the diagnosis of gastrointestinal signet ring cell carcinoma. *Am J Surg Pathol.* 2008;32:1182-1189.
173. Drier JK, Swanson PE, Cherwitz DL, Wick MR. S100 protein immunoreactivity in poorly differentiated carcinomas. Immunohistochemical comparison with malignant melanoma. *Arch Pathol Lab Med.* 1987;111:447-452.
174. Barbareschi M, Murer B, Colby TV, et al. CDX-2 homeobox gene expression is a reliable marker of colorectal adenocarcinoma metastases to the lungs. *Am J Surg Pathol.* 2003;27:141-149.
174a. Sarbia M, Fritze F, Geddert H, et al. Differentiation between pancreaticobiliary and upper gastrointestinal adenocarcinomas: Is analysis of cytokeratin 17 expression helpful? *Am J Clin Pathol.* 2007;128:255-259.
175. Loy TS, Quesenberry JT, Sharp SC. Distribution of CA 125 in adenocarcinomas. An immunohistochemical study of 481 cases. *Am J Clin Pathol.* 1992;98:175-179.
176. Merchant SH, Amin MB, Tamboli P, et al. Primary signet-ring cell carcinoma of lung: immunohistochemical study and comparison with non-pulmonary signet-ring cell carcinomas. *Am J Surg Pathol.* 2001;25:1515-1519.
177. Harlamert HA, Mira J, Bejarano PA, et al. Thyroid transcription factor-1 and cytokeratins 7 and 20 in pulmonary and breast carcinoma. *Acta Cytol.* 1998;42:1382-1388.
178. Loy TS, Calaluce RD. Utility of cytokeratin immunostaining in separating pulmonary adenocarcinomas from colonic adenocarcinomas. *Am J Clin Pathol.* 1994;102:764-767.
179. Moch H, Oberholzer M, Dalquen P, et al. Diagnostic tools for differentiating between pleural mesothelioma and lung adenocarcinoma in paraffin embedded tissue. Part I: Immunohistochemical findings. *Virchows Arch A Pathol Anat Histopathol.* 1993;423:19-27.
180. Bejarano PA, Baughman RP, Biddinger PW, et al. Surfactant proteins and thyroid transcription factor-1 in pulmonary and breast carcinomas. *Mod Pathol.* 1996;9:445-452.
181. Di Loreto C, Puglisi F, Di Lauro V, et al. TTF-1 protein expression in pleural malignant mesotheliomas and adenocarcinomas of the lung. *Cancer Lett.* 1998;124:73-78.
182. Rossi G, Marchioni A, Romagnani E, et al. Primary lung cancer presenting with gastrointestinal tract involvement: clinicopathologic and immunohistochemical features in a series of 18 consecutive cases. *J Thorac Oncol.* 2007;2:115-120.
183. Jagirdar J. Application of immunohistochemistry to the diagnosis of primary and metastatic carcinoma to the lung. *Arch Pathol Lab Med.* 2008;132:384-396.
184. Ferguson A, Arranz E, O'Mahony S. Clinical and pathological spectrum of coeliac disease—active, silent, latent, potential. *Gut.* 1993;34:150-151.
185. Chen ZM, Wang HL. Alteration of cytokeratin 7 and cytokeratin 20 expression profile is uniquely associated with tumorigenesis of primary adenocarcinoma of the small intestine. *Am J Surg Pathol.* 2004;28:1352-1359.
186. Zhang MQ, Lin F, Hui P, et al. Expression of mucins, SIMA, villin, and CDX2 in small-intestinal adenocarcinoma. *Am J Clin Pathol.* 2007;128:808-816.
187. Chen ZM, Ritter JH, Wang HL. Differential expression of alpha-methylacyl coenzyme A racemase in adenocarcinomas of the small and large intestines. *Am J Surg Pathol.* 2005;29:890-896.
188. Planck M, Ericson K, Piotrowska Z, et al. Microsatellite instability and expression of MLH1 and MSH2 in carcinomas of the small intestine. *Cancer.* 2003;97:1551-1557.
189. Svrcek M, Jourdan F, Sebbagh N, et al. Immunohistochemical analysis of adenocarcinoma of the small intestine: a tissue microarray study. *J Clin Pathol.* 2003;56:898-903.
190. Guerrieri C, Franlund B, Boeryd B. Expression of cytokeratin 7 in simultaneous mucinous tumors of the ovary and appendix. *Mod Pathol.* 1995;8:573-576.
191. Guerrieri C, Franlund B, Fristedt S, et al. Mucinous tumors of the vermiform appendix and ovary, and pseudomyxoma peritonei: histogenetic implications of cytokeratin 7 expression. *Hum Pathol.* 1997;28:1039-1045.
192. Ji H, Isacson C, Seidman JD, et al. Cytokeratins 7 and 20, Dpc4, and MUC5AC in the distinction of metastatic mucinous carcinomas in the ovary from primary ovarian mucinous tumors: Dpc4 assists in identifying metastatic pancreatic carcinomas. *Int J Gynecol Pathol.* 2002;21:391-400.

193. Ronnett BM, Kurman RJ, Shmookler BM, et al. The morphologic spectrum of ovarian metastases of appendiceal adenocarcinomas: a clinicopathologic and immunohistochemical analysis of tumors often misinterpreted as primary ovarian tumors or metastatic tumors from other gastrointestinal sites. *Am J Surg Pathol.* 1997;21:1144-1155.
194. Ronnett BM, Shmookler BM, Diener-West M, et al. Immunohistochemical evidence supporting the appendiceal origin of pseudomyxoma peritonei in women. *Int J Gynecol Pathol.* 1997;16:1-9.
195. Seidman JD, Elsayed AM, Sobin LH, Tavassoli FA. Association of mucinous tumors of the ovary and appendix. A clinicopathologic study of 25 cases. *Am J Surg Pathol.* 1993;17:22-34.
196. O'Connell JT, Hacker CM, Barsky SH. MUC2 is a molecular marker for pseudomyxoma peritonei. *Mod Pathol.* 2002;15:958-972.
197. Tornillo L, Moch H, Diener PA, et al. CDX-2 immunostaining in primary and secondary ovarian carcinomas. *J Clin Pathol.* 2004;57:641-643.
198. Lee KR, Young RH. The distinction between primary and metastatic mucinous carcinomas of the ovary: gross and histologic findings in 50 cases. *Am J Surg Pathol.* 2003;27:281-292.
199. Seidman JD, Kurman RJ, Ronnett BM. Primary and metastatic mucinous adenocarcinomas in the ovaries: incidence in routine practice with a new approach to improve intraoperative diagnosis. *Am J Surg Pathol.* 2003;27:985-993.
200. Fraggetta F, Pelosi G, Cafici A, et al. CDX2 immunoreactivity in primary and metastatic ovarian mucinous tumours. *Virchows Arch.* 2003;443:782-786.
201. Kapur RP, Reed RC, Finn L, et al. Calretinin immunohistochemistry versus acetylcholinesterase histochemistry in the evaluation of suction rectal biopsies for Hirschsprung disease. *Pediatr Dev Pathol.* 2008:1.
202. MacKenzie JM, Dixon MF. An immunohistochemical study of the enteric neural plexi in Hirschsprung's disease. *Histopathology.* 1987;11:1055-1066.
203. Wester T, Olsson Y, Olsen L. Expression of bcl-2 in enteric neurons in normal human bowel and Hirschsprung disease. *Arch Pathol Lab Med.* 1999;123:1264-1268.
204. Monforte-Munoz H, Gonzalez-Gomez I, Rowland JM, Landing BH. Increased submucosal nerve trunk caliber in aganglionosis: a "positive" and objective finding in suction biopsies and segmental resections in Hirschsprung's disease. *Arch Pathol Lab Med.* 1998;122:721-725.
205. Mochizuka A, Uehara T, Nakamura T, et al. Hyperplastic polyps and sessile serrated 'adenomas' of the colon and rectum display gastric pyloric differentiation. *Histochem Cell Biol.* 2007;128:445-455.
206. Sheridan TB, Fenton H, Lewin MR, et al. Sessile serrated adenomas with low- and high-grade dysplasia and early carcinomas: an immunohistochemical study of serrated lesions "caught in the act." *Am J Clin Pathol.* 2006;126:564-571.
207. Kawasaki T, Nosho K, Ohnishi M, et al. Cyclooxygenase-2 overexpression is common in serrated and non-serrated colorectal adenoma, but uncommon in hyperplastic polyp and sessile serrated polyp/adenoma. *BMC Cancer.* 2008;8:33.
208. Owens SR, Chiosea SI, Kuan SF. Selective expression of gastric mucin MUC6 in colonic sessile serrated adenoma but not in hyperplastic polyp aids in morphological diagnosis of serrated polyps. *Mod Pathol.* 2008;21:660-669.
209. Torlakovic EE, Gomez JD, Driman DK, et al. Sessile serrated adenoma (SSA) vs. traditional serrated adenoma (TSA). *Am J Surg Pathol.* 2008;32:21-29.
210. Wong NA, Mayer NJ, MacKell S, et al. Immunohistochemical assessment of Ki67 and p53 expression assists the diagnosis and grading of ulcerative colitis-related dysplasia. *Histopathology.* 2000;37:108-114.
211. Harpaz N, Peck AL, Yin J, et al. p53 protein expression in ulcerative colitis-associated colorectal dysplasia and carcinoma. *Hum Pathol.* 1994;25:1069-1074.
212. Bruwer M, Schmid KW, Senninger N, Schurmann G. Immunohistochemical expression of P53 and oncogenes in ulcerative colitis-associated colorectal carcinoma. *World J Surg.* 2002;26:390-396.
213. Marx A, Wandrey T, Simon P, et al. Combined alpha-methylacyl coenzyme A racemase/p53 analysis to identify dysplasia in inflammatory bowel disease. *Hum Pathol.* 2009; 40:166-173.
214. Andersen SN, Rognum TO, Bakka A, Clausen OP. Ki-67: a useful marker for the evaluation of dysplasia in ulcerative colitis. *Mol Pathol.* 1998;51:327-332.
215. Sjoqvist U, Ost A, Lofberg R. Increased expression of proliferative Ki-67 nuclear antigen is correlated with dysplastic colorectal epithelium in ulcerative colitis. *Int J Colorectal Dis.* 1999;14:107-113.
216. Dorer R, Odze RD. AMACR immunostaining is useful in detecting dysplastic epithelium in Barrett's esophagus, ulcerative colitis, and Crohn's disease. *Am J Surg Pathol.* 2006;30:871-877.
217. Strater J, Wiesmuller C, Perner S, et al. Alpha-methylacyl-CoA racemase (AMACR) immunohistochemistry in Barrett's and colorectal mucosa: only significant overexpression favours a diagnosis of intraepithelial neoplasia. *Histopathology.* 2008;52:399-402.
218. Maeda T, Kajiyama K, Adachi E, et al. The expression of cytokeratins 7, 19, and 20 in primary and metastatic carcinomas of the liver. *Mod Pathol.* 1996;9:901-909.
219. O'Hara BJ, Paetau A, Miettinen M. Keratin subsets and monoclonal antibody HBME-1 in chordoma: immunohistochemical differential diagnosis between tumors simulating chordoma. *Hum Pathol.* 1998;29:119-126.
220. Thomas P, Battifora H. Keratins versus epithelial membrane antigen in tumor diagnosis: an immunohistochemical comparison of five monoclonal antibodies. *Hum Pathol.* 1987;18:728-734.
221. Berezowski K, Stastny JF, Kornstein MJ. Cytokeratins 7 and 20 and carcinoembryonic antigen in ovarian and colonic carcinoma. *Mod Pathol.* 1996;9:426-429.
222. Tot T. Cytokeratins 20 and 7 as biomarkers: usefulness in discriminating primary from metastatic adenocarcinoma. *Eur J Cancer.* 2002;38:758-763.
223. Vang R, Gown AM, Barry TS, et al. Cytokeratins 7 and 20 in primary and secondary mucinous tumors of the ovary: analysis of coordinate immunohistochemical expression profiles and staining distribution in 179 cases. *Am J Surg Pathol.* 2006;30:1130-1139.
224. Lagendijk JH, Mullink H, Van Diest PJ, et al. Tracing the origin of adenocarcinomas with unknown primary using immunohistochemistry: differential diagnosis between colonic and ovarian carcinomas as primary sites. *Hum Pathol.* 1998;29:491-497.
225. Moskaluk CA, Zhang H, Powell SM, et al. Cdx2 protein expression in normal and malignant human tissues: an immunohistochemical survey using tissue microarrays. *Mod Pathol.* 2003;16:913-919.
226. De Lott LB, Morrison C, Suster S, et al. CDX2 is a useful marker of intestinal-type differentiation: a tissue microarray-based study of 629 tumors from various sites. *Arch Pathol Lab Med.* 2005;129:1100-1105.
227. Suh N, Yang XJ, Tretiakova MS, et al. Value of CDX2, villin, and alpha-methylacyl coenzyme A racemase immunostains in the distinction between primary adenocarcinoma of the bladder and secondary colorectal adenocarcinoma. *Mod Pathol.* 2005;18:1217-1222.
228. Vang R, Gown AM, Wu LS, et al. Immunohistochemical expression of CDX2 in primary ovarian mucinous tumors and metastatic mucinous carcinomas involving the ovary: comparison with CK20 and correlation with coordinate expression of CK7. *Mod Pathol.* 2006;19:1421-1428.
229. Inamura K, Satoh Y, Okumura S, et al. Pulmonary adenocarcinomas with enteric differentiation: histologic and immunohistochemical characteristics compared with metastatic colorectal cancers and usual pulmonary adenocarcinomas. *Am J Surg Pathol.* 2005;29:660-665.
230. Proca DM, Niemann TH, Porcell AI, DeYoung BR. MOC31 immunoreactivity in primary and metastatic carcinoma of the liver. Report of findings and review of other utilized markers. *Appl Immunohistochem Mol Morphol.* 2000;8:120-125.
231. Wendum D, Svrcek M, Rigau V, et al. COX-2, inflammatory secreted PLA2, and cytoplasmic PLA2 protein expression in small bowel adenocarcinomas compared with colorectal adenocarcinomas. *Mod Pathol.* 2003;16:130-136.

232. Loy TS, Sharp SC, Andershock CJ, Craig SB. Distribution of CA 19-9 in adenocarcinomas and transitional cell carcinomas. An immunohistochemical study of 527 cases. *Am J Clin Pathol.* 1993;99:726-728.
233. Greenson JK, Huang SC, Herron C, et al. Pathologic predictors of microsatellite instability in colorectal cancer. *Am J Surg Pathol.* 2009;33:126-133.
234. Hampel H, Frankel WL, Martin E, et al. Feasibility of screening for lynch syndrome among patients with colorectal cancer. *J Clin Oncol.* 2008;26:5783-5788.
235. Wright CL, Stewart ID. Histopathology and mismatch repair status of 458 consecutive colorectal carcinomas. *Am J Surg Pathol.* 2003;27:1393-1406.
236. Jover R, Paya A, Alenda C, et al. Defective mismatch-repair colorectal cancer: clinicopathologic characteristics and usefulness of immunohistochemical analysis for diagnosis. *Am J Clin Pathol.* 2004;122:389-394.
237. Shia J. Immunohistochemistry versus microsatellite instability testing for screening colorectal cancer patients at risk for hereditary nonpolyposis colorectal cancer syndrome. Part I. The utility of immunohistochemistry. *J Mol Diagn.* 2008;10:293-300.
238. Zhang L. Immunohistochemistry versus microsatellite instability testing for screening colorectal cancer patients at risk for hereditary nonpolyposis colorectal cancer syndrome. Part II. The utility of microsatellite instability testing. *J Mol Diagn.* 2008;10:301-307.
239. Hinoi T, Tani M, Lucas PC, et al. Loss of CDX2 expression and microsatellite instability are prominent features of large cell minimally differentiated carcinomas of the colon. *Am J Pathol.* 2001;159:2239-2248.
240. McGregor DK, Wu TT, Rashid A, et al. Reduced expression of cytokeratin 20 in colorectal carcinomas with high levels of microsatellite instability. *Am J Surg Pathol.* 2004;28:712-718.
241. Lugli A, Tzankov A, Zlobec I, et al. Differential diagnostic and functional role of the multi-marker phenotype CDX2/CK20/CK7 in colorectal cancer stratified by mismatch repair status. *Mod Pathol.* 2008;21:1403-1412.
242. Jewell LD, Barr JR, McCaughey WT, et al. Clear-cell epithelial neoplasms of the large intestine. *Arch Pathol Lab Med.* 1988;112:197-199.
243. Yang AH, Chen WY, Chiang H. Malignant rhabdoid tumour of colon. *Histopathology.* 1994;24:89-91.
244. Amrikachi M, Ro JY, Ordonez NG, Ayala AG. Adenocarcinomas of the gastrointestinal tract with prominent rhabdoid features. *Ann Diagn Pathol.* 2002;6:357-363.
245. Wang NP, Zee S, Zarbo RJ, et al. Coordinate expression of cytokeratins 7 and 20 defines unique subsets of carcinomas. *Appl Immunohistochem.* 1995;3:99-107.
246. Chang YL, Lee YC, Liao WY, Wu CT. The utility and limitation of thyroid transcription factor-1 protein in primary and metastatic pulmonary neoplasms. *Lung Cancer.* 2004;44:149-157.
247. Kaufmann O, Dietel M. Thyroid transcription factor-1 is the superior immunohistochemical marker for pulmonary adenocarcinomas and large cell carcinomas compared to surfactant proteins A and B. *Histopathology.* 2000;36:8-16.
248. Moldvay J, Jackel M, Bogos K, et al. The role of TTF-1 in differentiating primary and metastatic lung adenocarcinomas. *Pathol Oncol Res.* 2004;10:85-88.
249. Nicholson AG, McCormick CJ, Shimosato Y, et al. The value of PE-10, a monoclonal antibody against pulmonary surfactant, in distinguishing primary and metastatic lung tumours. *Histopathology.* 1995;27:57-60.
250. Reis-Filho JS, Carrilho C, Valenti C, et al. Is TTF1 a good immunohistochemical marker to distinguish primary from metastatic lung adenocarcinomas? *Pathol Res Pract.* 2000;196:835-840.
251. Srodon M, Westra WH. Immunohistochemical staining for thyroid transcription factor-1: a helpful aid in discerning primary site of tumor origin in patients with brain metastases. *Hum Pathol.* 2002;33:642-645.
252. Zamecnik J, Kodet R. Value of thyroid transcription factor-1 and surfactant apoprotein A in the differential diagnosis of pulmonary carcinomas: a study of 109 cases. *Virchows Arch.* 2002;440:353-361.
253. Goldstein NS, Thomas M. Mucinous and nonmucinous bronchioloalveolar adenocarcinomas have distinct staining patterns with thyroid transcription factor and cytokeratin 20 antibodies. *Am J Clin Pathol.* 2001;116:319-325.
254. Shah RN, Badve S, Papreddy K, et al. Expression of cytokeratin 20 in mucinous bronchioloalveolar carcinoma. *Hum Pathol.* 2002;33:915-920.
255. Saad RS, Cho P, Silverman JF, Liu Y. Usefulness of Cdx2 in separating mucinous bronchioloalveolar adenocarcinoma of the lung from metastatic mucinous colorectal adenocarcinoma. *Am J Clin Pathol.* 2004;122:421-427.
256. Yatabe Y, Koga T, Mitsudomi T, Takahashi T. CK20 expression, CDX2 expression, K-ras mutation, and goblet cell morphology in a subset of lung adenocarcinomas. *J Pathol.* 2004;203:645-652.
257. Loy TS, Calaluce RD, Keeney GL. Cytokeratin immunostaining in differentiating primary ovarian carcinoma from metastatic colonic adenocarcinoma. *Mod Pathol.* 1996;9:1040-1044.
258. Young RH, Hart WR. Metastatic intestinal carcinomas simulating primary ovarian clear cell carcinoma and secretory endometrioid carcinoma: a clinicopathologic and immunohistochemical study of five cases. *Am J Surg Pathol.* 1998;22:805-815.
259. Slattery ML, Samowitz WS, Holden JA. Estrogen and progesterone receptors in colon tumors. *Am J Clin Pathol.* 2000;113:364-368.
260. Ordonez NG. Value of thrombomodulin immunostaining in the diagnosis of mesothelioma. *Histopathology.* 1997;31:25-30.
261. Tamboli P, Mohsin SK, Hailemariam S, Amin MB. Colonic adenocarcinoma metastatic to the urinary tract versus primary tumors of the urinary tract with glandular differentiation: a report of 7 cases and investigation using a limited immunohistochemical panel. *Arch Pathol Lab Med.* 2002;126:1057-1063.
262. Wang HL, Lu DW, Yerian LM, et al. Immunohistochemical distinction between primary adenocarcinoma of the bladder and secondary colorectal adenocarcinoma. *Am J Surg Pathol.* 2001;25:1380-1387.
263. Goldstein NS. Immunophenotypic characterization of 225 prostate adenocarcinomas with intermediate or high Gleason scores. *Am J Clin Pathol.* 2002;117:471-477.
264. Jiang Z, Fanger GR, Woda BA, et al. Expression of alpha-methylacyl-CoA racemase (P504s) in various malignant neoplasms and normal tissues: a study of 761 cases. *Hum Pathol.* 2003;34:792-796.
265. Torbenson M, Dhir R, Nangia A, et al. Prostatic carcinoma with signet ring cells: a clinicopathologic and immunohistochemical analysis of 12 cases, with review of the literature. *Mod Pathol.* 1998;11:552-559.
266. Longacre TA, Kong CS, Welton ML. Diagnostic problems in anal pathology. *Adv Anat Pathol.* 2008;15:263-278.
267. Owens SR, Greenson JK. Immunohistochemical staining for p63 is useful in the diagnosis of anal squamous cell carcinomas. *Am J Surg Pathol.* 2007;31:285-290.
268. Chetty R, Serra S, Hsieh E. Basaloid squamous carcinoma of the anal canal with an adenoid cystic pattern: histologic and immunohistochemical reappraisal of an unusual variant. *Am J Surg Pathol.* 2005;29:1668-1672.
269. Roma AA, Goldblum JR, Fazio V, Yang B. Expression of 14-3-3sigma, p16 and p53 proteins in anal squamous intraepithelial neoplasm and squamous cell carcinoma. *Int J Clin Exp Pathol.* 2008;1:419-425.
270. Hobbs CM, Lowry MA, Owen D, Sobin LH. Anal gland carcinoma. *Cancer.* 2001;92:2045-2049.
271. Lisovsky M, Patel K, Cymes K, et al. Immunophenotypic characterization of anal gland carcinoma: loss of p63 and cytokeratin 5/6. *Arch Pathol Lab Med.* 2007;131:1304-1311.
272. Battles OE, Page DL, Johnson JE. Cytokeratins, CEA, and mucin histochemistry in the diagnosis and characterization of extramammary Paget's disease. *Am J Clin Pathol.* 1997;108:6-12.
273. Helm KF, Goellner JR, Peters MS. Immunohistochemical stains in extramammary Paget's disease. *Am J Dermatopathol.* 1992;14:402-407.
274. Smith KJ, Tuur S, Corvette D, et al. Cytokeratin 7 staining in mammary and extramammary Paget's disease. *Mod Pathol.* 1997;10:1069-1074.

275. Nowak MA, Guerriere-Kovach P, Pathan A, et al. Perianal Paget's disease: distinguishing primary and secondary lesions using immunohistochemical studies including gross cystic disease fluid protein-15 and cytokeratin 20 expression. *Arch Pathol Lab Med.* 1998;122:1077-1081.
276. Ohnishi T, Watanabe S. The use of cytokeratins 7 and 20 in the diagnosis of primary and secondary extramammary Paget's disease. *Br J Dermatol.* 2000;142:243-247.
277. Ramalingam P, Hart WR, Goldblum JR. Cytokeratin subset immunostaining in rectal adenocarcinoma and normal anal glands. *Arch Pathol Lab Med.* 2001;125:1074-1077.
278. Kondo Y, Kashima K, Daa T, et al. The ectopic expression of gastric mucin in extramammary and mammary Paget's disease. *Am J Surg Pathol.* 2002;26:617-623.
279. Kuan SF, Montag AG, Hart J, et al. Differential expression of mucin genes in mammary and extramammary Paget's disease. *Am J Surg Pathol.* 2001;25:1469-1477.
280. Williams ED, Sandler M. The classification of carcinoid tumours. *Lancet.* 1963;1:238-239.
281. Cai YC, Banner B, Glickman J, Odze RD. Cytokeratin 7 and 20 and thyroid transcription factor 1 can help distinguish pulmonary from gastrointestinal carcinoid and pancreatic endocrine tumors. *Hum Pathol.* 2001;32:1087-1093.
282. Srivastava A, Padilla O, Fischer-Colbrie R, et al. Neuroendocrine secretory protein-55 (NESP-55) expression discriminates pancreatic endocrine tumors and pheochromocytomas from gastrointestinal and pulmonary carcinoids. *Am J Surg Pathol.* 2004;28:1371-1378.
283. Solcia E, Kloppel G, Sobin LH. *World Health Organization International Histological Classification of Tumours: Histological Typing of Endocrine Tumours.* 2nd ed. Berlin: Springer; 2000.
284. Capella C, Solcia E, Sobin LH, Arnold R. Endocrine tumours of the oesophagus. In: Hamilton SR, Aaltonen LA, eds. *Pathology and genetics, tumours of the digestive system: WHO classification of tumours.* Lyon, France: IARC; 2000: 26-27.
285. Hoang MP, Hobbs CM, Sobin LH, Albores-Saavedra J. Carcinoid tumor of the esophagus: a clinicopathologic study of four cases. *Am J Surg Pathol.* 2002;26:517-522.
286. Kloppel G, Rindi G, Anlauf M, et al. Site-specific biology and pathology of gastroenteropancreatic neuroendocrine tumors. *Virchows Arch.* 2007;451(Suppl 1):S9-27.
287. Osugi H, Takemura M, Morimura K, et al. Clinicopathologic and immunohistochemical features of surgically resected small cell carcinoma of the esophagus. *Oncol Rep.* 2002;9:1245-1249.
288. Takubo K, Nakamura K, Sawabe M, et al. Primary undifferentiated small cell carcinoma of the esophagus. *Hum Pathol.* 1999;30:216-221.
289. Yamamoto J, Ohshima K, Ikeda S, et al. Primary esophageal small cell carcinoma with concomitant invasive squamous cell carcinoma or carcinoma in situ. *Hum Pathol.* 2003;34:1108-1115.
290. Cheuk W, Chan JK. Thyroid transcription factor-1 is of limited value in practical distinction between pulmonary and extrapulmonary small cell carcinomas. *Am J Surg Pathol.* 2001;25:545-546.
291. Cheuk W, Kwan MY, Suster S, Chan JK. Immunostaining for thyroid transcription factor 1 and cytokeratin 20 aids the distinction of small cell carcinoma from Merkel cell carcinoma, but not pulmonary from extrapulmonary small cell carcinomas. *Arch Pathol Lab Med.* 2001;125:228-231.
292. Rindi G, Paolotti D, Fiocca R, et al. Vesicular monoamine transporter 2 as a marker of gastric enterochromaffin-like cell tumors. *Virchows Arch.* 2000;436:217-223.
293. Saqi A, Alexis D, Remotti F, Bhagat G. Usefulness of CDX2 and TTF-1 in differentiating gastrointestinal from pulmonary carcinoids. *Am J Clin Pathol.* 2005;123:394-404.
294. Oliveira AM, Tazelaar HD, Myers JL, et al. Thyroid transcription factor-1 distinguishes metastatic pulmonary from well-differentiated neuroendocrine tumors of other sites. *Am J Surg Pathol.* 2001;25:815-819.
295. Srivastava A, Hornick JL. Immunohistochemical staining for CDX-2, PDX-1, NESP-55, and TTF-1 can help distinguish gastrointestinal carcinoid tumors from pancreatic endocrine and pulmonary carcinoid tumors. *Am J Surg Pathol.* 2009; 33:626-632.
296. Barbareschi M, Roldo C, Zamboni G, et al. CDX-2 homeobox gene product expression in neuroendocrine tumors: its role as a marker of intestinal neuroendocrine tumors. *Am J Surg Pathol.* 2004;28:1169-1176.
297. Jaffee IM, Rahmani M, Singhal MG, Younes M. Expression of the intestinal transcription factor CDX2 in carcinoid tumors is a marker of midgut origin. *Arch Pathol Lab Med.* 2006;130:1522-1526.
298. La Rosa S, Rigoli E, Uccella S, et al. CDX2 as a marker of intestinal EC-cells and related well-differentiated endocrine tumors. *Virchows Arch.* 2004;445:248-254.
299. Alsaad KO, Serra S, Schmitt A, et al. Cytokeratins 7 and 20 immunoexpression profile in goblet cell and classical carcinoids of appendix. *Endocr Pathol.* 2007;18:16-22.
300. Burke AP, Sobin LH, Federspiel BH, Shekitka KM. Appendiceal carcinoids: correlation of histology and immunohistochemistry. *Mod Pathol.* 1989;2:630-637.
301. Moyana TN, Satkunam N. A comparative immunohistochemical study of jejunoileal and appendiceal carcinoids. Implications for histogenesis and pathogenesis. *Cancer.* 1992;70:1081-1088.
302. Tang LH, Shia J, Soslow RA, et al. Pathologic classification and clinical behavior of the spectrum of goblet cell carcinoid tumors of the appendix. *Am J Surg Pathol.* 2008;32:1429-1443.
303. Azumi N, Battifora H. The distribution of vimentin and keratin in epithelial and nonepithelial neoplasms. A comprehensive immunohistochemical study on formalin- and alcohol-fixed tumors. *Am J Clin Pathol.* 1987;88:286-296.
304. Federspiel BH, Burke AP, Sobin LH, Shekitka KM. Rectal and colonic carcinoids. A clinicopathologic study of 84 cases. *Cancer.* 1990;65:135-140.
305. Fahrenkamp AG, Wibbeke C, Winde G, et al. Immunohistochemical distribution of chromogranins A and B and secretogranin II in neuroendocrine tumours of the gastrointestinal tract. *Virchows Arch.* 1995;426:361-367.
306. Nash SV, Said JW. Gastroenteropancreatic neuroendocrine tumors. A histochemical and immunohistochemical study of epithelial (keratin proteins, carcinoembryonic antigen) and neuroendocrine (neuron-specific enolase, bombesin and chromogranin) markers in foregut, midgut, and hindgut tumors. *Am J Clin Pathol.* 1986;86:415-422.
307. Kaufmann O, Dietel M. Expression of thyroid transcription factor-1 in pulmonary and extrapulmonary small cell carcinomas and other neuroendocrine carcinomas of various primary sites. *Histopathology.* 2000;36:415-420.
308. Bernick PE, Klimstra DS, Shia J, et al. Neuroendocrine carcinomas of the colon and rectum. *Dis Colon Rectum.* 2004;47:163-169.
309. Sarsfield P, Anthony PP. Small cell undifferentiated ('neuroendocrine') carcinoma of the colon. *Histopathology.* 1990;16:357-363.
310. Akintola-Ogunremi O, Pfeifer JD, Tan BR, et al. Analysis of protein expression and gene mutation of c-kit in colorectal neuroendocrine carcinomas. *Am J Surg Pathol.* 2003;27:1551-1558.
311. Ishikubo T, Akagi K, Kurosumi M, et al. Immunohistochemical and mutational analysis of c-kit in gastrointestinal neuroendocrine cell carcinoma. *Jpn J Clin Oncol.* 2006;36:494-498.
312. Allander SV, Nupponen NN, Ringner M, et al. Gastrointestinal stromal tumors with KIT mutations exhibit a remarkably homogeneous gene expression profile. *Cancer Res.* 2001;61:8624-8628.
313. Bernet L, Zuniga A, Cano R. Characterization of GIST/GIPACT tumors by inmunohistochemistry and exon 11 analysis of c-kit by PCR. *Rev Esp Enferm Dig.* 2003;95:688-691:683-687.
314. Kitamura Y, Hirota S, Nishida T. Molecular pathology of c-kit proto-oncogene and development of gastrointestinal stromal tumors. *Ann Chir Gynaecol.* 1998;87:282-286.
315. Miettinen M, Lasota J. Gastrointestinal stromal tumors (GISTs): definition, occurrence, pathology, differential diagnosis and molecular genetics. *Pol J Pathol.* 2003;54:3-24.
316. Rubin BP, Singer S, Tsao C, et al. KIT activation is a ubiquitous feature of gastrointestinal stromal tumors. *Cancer Res.* 2001;61:8118-8121.
317. Taniguchi M, Nishida T, Hirota S, et al. Effect of c-kit mutation on prognosis of gastrointestinal stromal tumors. *Cancer Res.* 1999;59:4297-4300.
318. Miettinen M, Lasota J. Gastrointestinal stromal tumors: review on morphology, molecular pathology, prognosis, and differential diagnosis. *Arch Pathol Lab Med.* 2006;130:1466-1478.

319. Antonioli DA. Gastrointestinal autonomic nerve tumors. Expanding the spectrum of gastrointestinal stromal tumors. *Arch Pathol Lab Med.* 1989;113:831-833.
320. Fuller CE, Williams GT. Gastrointestinal manifestations of type 1 neurofibromatosis (von Recklinghausen's disease). *Histopathology.* 1991;19:1-11.
321. Lee JR, Joshi V, Griffin Jr JW, et al. Gastrointestinal autonomic nerve tumor: immunohistochemical and molecular identity with gastrointestinal stromal tumor. *Am J Surg Pathol.* 2001;25:979-987.
322. Miettinen M, El-Rifai W, L HLS, Lasota J. Evaluation of malignancy and prognosis of gastrointestinal stromal tumors: a review. *Hum Pathol.* 2002;33:478-483.
323. Chan JK. Mesenchymal tumors of the gastrointestinal tract: a paradise for acronyms (STUMP, GIST, GANT, and now GIPACT), implication of c-kit in genesis, and yet another of the many emerging roles of the interstitial cell of Cajal in the pathogenesis of gastrointestinal diseases? *Adv Anat Pathol.* 1999;6:19-40.
324. Sircar K, Hewlett BR, Huizinga JD, et al. Interstitial cells of Cajal as precursors of gastrointestinal stromal tumors. *Am J Surg Pathol.* 1999;23:377-389.
325. Yamaguchi U, Hasegawa T, Masuda T, et al. Differential diagnosis of gastrointestinal stromal tumor and other spindle cell tumors in the gastrointestinal tract based on immunohistochemical analysis. *Virchows Arch.* 2004;445:142-150.
326. Corless CL, Schroeder A, Griffith D, et al. PDGFRA mutations in gastrointestinal stromal tumors: frequency, spectrum and in vitro sensitivity to imatinib. *J Clin Oncol.* 2005;23:5357-5364.
327. Lasota J, Dansonka-Mieszkowska A, Sobin LH, Miettinen M. A great majority of GISTs with PDGFRA mutations represent gastric tumors of low or no malignant potential. *Lab Invest.* 2004;84:874-883.
328. Duensing A, Heinrich MC, Fletcher CD, Fletcher JA. Biology of gastrointestinal stromal tumors: KIT mutations and beyond. *Cancer Invest.* 2004;22:106-116.
329. Duensing A, Medeiros F, McConarty B, et al. Mechanisms of oncogenic KIT signal transduction in primary gastrointestinal stromal tumors (GISTs). *Oncogene.* 2004;23:3999-4006.
330. Hornick JL, Fletcher CD. The significance of KIT (CD117) in gastrointestinal stromal tumors. *Int J Surg Pathol.* 2004;12:93-97.
331. Miselli F, Millefanti C, Conca E, et al. PDGFRA immunostaining can help in the diagnosis of gastrointestinal stromal tumors. *Am J Surg Pathol.* 2008;32:738-743.
332. Rossi G, Valli R, Bertolini F, et al. PDGFR expression in differential diagnosis between KIT-negative gastrointestinal stromal tumours and other primary soft-tissue tumours of the gastrointestinal tract. *Histopathology.* 2005;46:522-531.
333. West RB, Corless CL, Chen X, et al. The novel marker, DOG1, is expressed ubiquitously in gastrointestinal stromal tumors irrespective of KIT or PDGFRA mutation status. *Am J Pathol.* 2004;165:107-113.
334. Guler ML, Daniels JA, Abraham SC, Montgomery EA. Expression of melanoma antigens in epithelioid gastrointestinal stromal tumors: a potential diagnostic pitfall. *Arch Pathol Lab Med.* 2008;132:1302-1306.
335. Memeo L, Jhang J, Assaad AM, et al. Immunohistochemical analysis for cytokeratin 7, KIT, and PAX2: value in the differential diagnosis of chromophobe cell carcinoma. *Am J Clin Pathol.* 2007;127:225-229.
336. Nikolaou M, Valavanis C, Aravantinos G, et al. Kit expression in male germ cell tumors. *Anticancer Res.* 2007;27:1685-1688.
337. Hornick JL, Fletcher CD. Immunohistochemical staining for KIT (CD117) in soft tissue sarcomas is very limited in distribution. *Am J Clin Pathol.* 2002;117:188-193.
338. Miettinen M, Lasota J. KIT (CD117): a review on expression in normal and neoplastic tissues, and mutations and their clinicopathologic correlation. *Appl Immunohistochem Mol Morphol.* 2005;13:205-220.
339. Parfitt JR, Rodriguez-Justo M, Feakins R, Novelli MR. Gastrointestinal Kaposi's sarcoma: CD117 expression and the potential for misdiagnosis as gastrointestinal stromal tumour. *Histopathology.* 2008;52:816-823.
340. Yantiss RK, Spiro IJ, Compton CC, Rosenberg AE. Gastrointestinal stromal tumor versus intra-abdominal fibromatosis of the bowel wall: a clinically important differential diagnosis. *Am J Surg Pathol.* 2000;24:947-957.
341. Lucas DR, al-Abbadi M, Tabaczka P, et al. c-Kit expression in desmoid fibromatosis. Comparative immunohistochemical evaluation of two commercial antibodies. *Am J Clin Pathol.* 2003;119:339-345.
342. Miettinen M. Are desmoid tumors kit positive? *Am J Surg Pathol.* 2001;25:549-550.
343. Brown DC, Theaker JM, Banks PM, Gatter KC, Mason DY. Cytokeratin expression in smooth muscle and smooth muscle tumours. *Histopathology.* 1987;11:477-486.
344. Dhimes P, Lopez-Carreira M, Ortega-Serrano MP, et al. Gastrointestinal autonomic nerve tumours and their separation from other gastrointestinal stromal tumours: an ultrastructural and immunohistochemical study of seven cases. *Virchows Arch.* 1995;426:27-35.
345. Franquemont DW, Frierson Jr HF. Muscle differentiation and clinicopathologic features of gastrointestinal stromal tumors. *Am J Surg Pathol.* 1992;16:947-954.
346. Greenson JK. Gastrointestinal stromal tumors and other mesenchymal lesions of the gut. *Mod Pathol.* 2003;16:366-375.
347. Herrera GA, Cerezo L, Jones JE, et al. Gastrointestinal autonomic nerve tumors. 'Plexosarcomas'. *Arch Pathol Lab Med.* 1989;113:846-853.
348. Miettinen M. Gastrointestinal stromal tumors. An immunohistochemical study of cellular differentiation. *Am J Clin Pathol.* 1988;89:601-610.
349. Miettinen M, Monihan JM, Sarlomo-Rikala M, et al. Gastrointestinal stromal tumors/smooth muscle tumors (GISTs) primary in the omentum and mesentery: clinicopathologic and immunohistochemical study of 26 cases. *Am J Surg Pathol.* 1999;23:1109-1118.
350. Miettinen M, Sobin LH, Sarlomo-Rikala M. Immunohistochemical spectrum of GISTs at different sites and their differential diagnosis with a reference to CD117 (KIT). *Mod Pathol.* 2000;13:1134-1142.
351. Miettinen M, Virolainen M, Maarit Sarlomo R. Gastrointestinal stromal tumors—value of CD34 antigen in their identification and separation from true leiomyomas and schwannomas. *Am J Surg Pathol.* 1995;19:207-216.
352. Saul SH, Rast ML, Brooks JJ. The immunohistochemistry of gastrointestinal stromal tumors. Evidence supporting an origin from smooth muscle. *Am J Surg Pathol.* 1987;11:464-473.
353. Shek TW, Luk IS, Loong F, Ip P, Ma L. Inflammatory cell-rich gastrointestinal autonomic nerve tumor. An expansion of its histologic spectrum. *Am J Surg Pathol.* 1996;20:325-331.
354. Suster S. Gastrointestinal stromal tumors. *Semin Diagn Pathol.* 1996;13:297-313.
355. Suster S, Fletcher CD. Gastrointestinal stromal tumors with prominent signet-ring cell features. *Mod Pathol.* 1996;9:609-613.
356. Tazawa K, Tsukada K, Makuuchi H, Tsutsumi Y. An immunohistochemical and clinicopathological study of gastrointestinal stromal tumors. *Pathol Int.* 1999;49:786-798.
357. Tworek JA, Goldblum JR, Weiss SW, et al. Stromal tumors of the anorectum: a clinicopathologic study of 22 cases. *Am J Surg Pathol.* 1999;23:946-954.
358. Tworek JA, Goldblum JR, Weiss SW, et al. Stromal tumors of the abdominal colon: a clinicopathologic study of 20 cases. *Am J Surg Pathol.* 1999;23:937-945.
359. Wong NA, Young R, Malcomson RD, et al. Prognostic indicators for gastrointestinal stromal tumours: a clinicopathological and immunohistochemical study of 108 resected cases of the stomach. *Histopathology.* 2003;43:118-126.
360. Yao T, Aoyagi K, Hizawa K. Gastric epithelioid tumor (leiomyoma) with granular changes. *Int J Surg Pathol.* 1996;4:37-42.
361. Natkunam Y, Rouse RV, Zhu S, et al. Immunoblot analysis of CD34 expression in histologically diverse neoplasms. *Am J Pathol.* 2000;156:21-27.
362. Miettinen M, Furlong M, Sarlomo-Rikala M, et al. Gastrointestinal stromal tumors, intramural leiomyomas, and leiomyosarcomas in the rectum and anus: a clinicopathologic, immunohistochemical, and molecular genetic study of 144 cases. *Am J Surg Pathol.* 2001;25:1121-1133.

363. Miettinen M, Lasota J. Gastrointestinal stromal tumors—definition, clinical, histological, immunohistochemical, and molecular genetic features and differential diagnosis. *Virchows Arch.* 2001;438:1-12.
364. Zhu X, Zhang XQ, Li BM, et al. Esophageal mesenchymal tumors: endoscopy, pathology and immunohistochemistry. *World J Gastroenterol.* 2007;13:768-773.
365. Miettinen MM, Sarlomo-Rikala M, Kovatich AJ, Lasota J. Calponin and h-caldesmon in soft tissue tumors: consistent h-caldesmon immunoreactivity in gastrointestinal stromal tumors indicates traits of smooth muscle differentiation. *Mod Pathol.* 1999;12:756-762.
366. Fletcher CD, Berman JJ, Corless C, et al. Diagnosis of gastrointestinal stromal tumors: A consensus approach. *Hum Pathol.* 2002;33:459-465.
367. Prevot S, Bienvenu L, Vaillant JC, de Saint-Maur PP. Benign schwannoma of the digestive tract: a clinicopathologic and immunohistochemical study of five cases, including a case of esophageal tumor. *Am J Surg Pathol.* 1999;23:431-436.
368. Sarlomo-Rikala M, Kovatich AJ, Barusevicius A, Miettinen M. CD117: a sensitive marker for gastrointestinal stromal tumors that is more specific than CD34. *Mod Pathol.* 1998;11:728-734.
369. Fanburg-Smith JC, Meis-Kindblom JM, Fante R, Kindblom LG. Malignant granular cell tumor of soft tissue: diagnostic criteria and clinicopathologic correlation. *Am J Surg Pathol.* 1998;22:779-794.
370. Goldblum JR, Rice TW, Zuccaro G, Richter JE. Granular cell tumors of the esophagus: a clinical and pathologic study of 13 cases. *Ann Thorac Surg.* 1996;62:860-865.
371. Montgomery E, Torbenson MS, Kaushal M, et al. Beta-catenin immunohistochemistry separates mesenteric fibromatosis from gastrointestinal stromal tumor and sclerosing mesenteritis. *Am J Surg Pathol.* 2002;26:1296-1301.
372. Bhattacharya B, Dilworth HP, Iacobuzio-Donahue C, et al. Nuclear beta-catenin expression distinguishes deep fibromatosis from other benign and malignant fibroblastic and myofibroblastic lesions. *Am J Surg Pathol.* 2005;29:653-659.
373. Carlson JW, Fletcher CD. Immunohistochemistry for beta-catenin in the differential diagnosis of spindle cell lesions: analysis of a series and review of the literature. *Histopathology.* 2007;51:509-514.
374. Ng TL, Gown AM, Barry TS, et al. Nuclear beta-catenin in mesenchymal tumors. *Mod Pathol.* 2005;18:68-74.
375. Fukunaga M, Naganuma H, Nikaido T, et al. Extrapleural solitary fibrous tumor: a report of seven cases. *Mod Pathol.* 1997;10:443-450.
376. Fukunaga M, Naganuma H, Ushigome S, et al. Malignant solitary fibrous tumour of the peritoneum. *Histopathology.* 1996;28:463-466.
377. Young RH, Clement PB, McCaughey WT. Solitary fibrous tumors ('fibrous mesotheliomas') of the peritoneum. A report of three cases and a review of the literature. *Arch Pathol Lab Med.* 1990;114:493-495.
378. Shidham VB, Chivukula M, Gupta D, et al. Immunohistochemical comparison of gastrointestinal stromal tumor and solitary fibrous tumor. *Arch Pathol Lab Med.* 2002;126:1189-1192.
379. Perez-Montiel MD, Plaza JA, Dominguez-Malagon H, Suster S. Differential expression of smooth muscle myosin, smooth muscle actin, h-caldesmon, and calponin in the diagnosis of myofibroblastic and smooth muscle lesions of skin and soft tissue. *Am J Dermatopathol.* 2006;28:105-111.
380. Rangdaeng S, Truong LD. Comparative immunohistochemical staining for desmin and muscle-specific actin. A study of 576 cases. *Am J Clin Pathol.* 1991;96:32-45.
381. Miettinen M, Kopczynski J, Makhlouf HR, et al. Gastrointestinal stromal tumors, intramural leiomyomas, and leiomyosarcomas in the duodenum: a clinicopathologic, immunohistochemical, and molecular genetic study of 167 cases. *Am J Surg Pathol.* 2003;27:625-641.
382. Miettinen M, Sarlomo-Rikala M, Sobin LH, Lasota J. Esophageal stromal tumors: a clinicopathologic, immunohistochemical, and molecular genetic study of 17 cases and comparison with esophageal leiomyomas and leiomyosarcomas. *Am J Surg Pathol.* 2000;24:211-222.
383. Miettinen M, Sarlomo-Rikala M, Sobin LH, Lasota J. Gastrointestinal stromal tumors and leiomyosarcomas in the colon: a clinicopathologic, immunohistochemical, and molecular genetic study of 44 cases. *Am J Surg Pathol.* 2000;24:1339-1352.
384. Chute DJ, Cousar JB, Mills SE. Anorectal malignant melanoma: morphologic and immunohistochemical features. *Am J Clin Pathol.* 2006;126:93-100.
385. Fetsch PA, Marincola FM, Filie A, et al. Melanoma-associated antigen recognized by T cells (MART-1): the advent of a preferred immunocytochemical antibody for the diagnosis of metastatic malignant melanoma with fine-needle aspiration. *Cancer.* 1999;87:37-42.
386. Lohmann CM, Hwu WJ, Iversen K, et al. Primary malignant melanoma of the oesophagus: a clinical and pathological study with emphasis on the immunophenotype of the tumours for melanocyte differentiation markers and cancer/testis antigens. *Melanoma Res.* 2003;13:595-601.
387. Graadt van Roggen JF, van Velthuysen ML, Hogendoorn PC. The histopathological differential diagnosis of gastrointestinal stromal tumours. *J Clin Pathol.* 2001;54:96-102.
388. Gould VE, Wiedenmann B, Lee I, et al. Synaptophysin expression in neuroendocrine neoplasms as determined by immunocytochemistry. *Am J Pathol.* 1987;126:243-257.
389. Marchevsky AM. Mediastinal tumors of peripheral nervous system origin. *Semin Diagn Pathol.* 1999;16:65-78.
390. Witkin GB, Rosai J. Solitary fibrous tumor of the mediastinum. A report of 14 cases. *Am J Surg Pathol.* 1989;13:547-557.
391. Davis GB, Berk RN. Intestinal neurofibromas in von Recklinghausen's disease. *Am J Gastroenterol.* 1973;60:410-414.
392. Hochberg FH, Dasilva AB, Galdabini J, Richardson Jr EP. Gastrointestinal involvement in von Recklinghausen's neurofibromatosis. *Neurology.* 1974;24:1144-1151.
393. Shekitka KM, Sobin LH. Ganglioneuromas of the gastrointestinal tract. Relation to Von Recklinghausen disease and other multiple tumor syndromes. *Am J Surg Pathol.* 1994;18:250-257.
394. Appelman HD. Mesenchymal tumors of the gastrointestinal tract. In: Ming SC, Goldman H, eds. *Pathology of the Gastrointestinal Tract.* 2nd ed. Baltimore: Williams and Wilkins; 1998:361-398.
395. Pantanowitz L, Antonioli DA, Pinkus GS, et al. Inflammatory fibroid polyps of the gastrointestinal tract: evidence for a dendritic cell origin. *Am J Surg Pathol.* 2004;28:107-114.
396. Hasegawa T, Yang P, Kagawa N, et al. CD34 expression by inflammatory fibroid polyps of the stomach. *Mod Pathol.* 1997;10:451-456.
397. Makhlouf HR, Sobin LH. Inflammatory myofibroblastic tumors (inflammatory pseudotumors) of the gastrointestinal tract: how closely are they related to inflammatory fibroid polyps? *Hum Pathol.* 2002;33:307-315.
398. Hornick JL, Fletcher CD. Intestinal perineuriomas: clinicopathologic definition of a new anatomic subset in a series of 10 cases. *Am J Surg Pathol.* 2005;29:859-865.
399. Groisman GM, Polak-Charcon S. Fibroblastic polyp of the colon and colonic perineurioma: 2 names for a single entity? *Am J Surg Pathol.* 2008;32:1088-1094.
400. Groisman GM, Amar M, Meir A. Expression of the intestinal marker Cdx2 in the columnar-lined esophagus with and without intestinal (Barrett's) metaplasia. *Mod Pathol.* 2004;17:1282-1288.
401. Kalof AN, Pritt B, Cooper K, et al. Benign fibroblastic polyp of the colorectum. *J Clin Gastroenterol.* 2005;39:778-781.
402. Miettinen M, Sarlomo-Rikala M, Sobin LH. Mesenchymal tumors of muscularis mucosae of colon and rectum are benign leiomyomas that should be separated from gastrointestinal stromal tumors—a clinicopathologic and immunohistochemical study of eighty-eight cases. *Mod Pathol.* 2001;14:950-956.
403. Moyana TN, Friesen R, Tan LK. Colorectal smooth-muscle tumors. A pathobiologic study with immunohistochemistry and histomorphometry. *Arch Pathol Lab Med.* 1991;115:1016-1021.
404. Chen RH, Ding WV, McCormick F. Wnt signaling to beta-catenin involves two interactive components. Glycogen synthase kinase-3beta inhibition and activation of protein kinase C. *J Biol Chem..* 2000;275:17894-17899.

405. He TC, Sparks AB, Rago C, et al. Identification of c-MYC as a target of the APC pathway. *Science*. 1998;281:1509-1512.
406. Anlauf M, Garbrecht N, Bauersfeld J, et al. Hereditary neuroendocrine tumors of the gastroenteropancreatic system. *Virchows Arch*. 2007;451(Suppl 1):S29-S38.
407. Debiec-Rychter M, Sciot R, Le Cesne A, et al. KIT mutations and dose selection for imatinib in patients with advanced gastrointestinal stromal tumours. *Eur J Cancer*. 2006;42:1093-1103.
408. Heinrich MC, Corless CL, Duensing A, et al. PDGFRA activating mutations in gastrointestinal stromal tumors. *Science*. 2003;299:708-710.
409. Alman BA, Li C, Pajerski ME, et al. Increased beta-catenin protein and somatic APC mutations in sporadic aggressive fibromatoses (desmoid tumors). *Am J Pathol*. 1997;151:329-334.
410. Miyoshi Y, Iwao K, Nawa G, et al. Frequent mutations in the beta-catenin gene in desmoid tumors from patients without familial adenomatous polyposis. *Oncol Res*. 1998;10:591-594.
411. Munemitsu S, Albert I, Souza B, et al. Regulation of intracellular beta-catenin levels by the adenomatous polyposis coli (APC) tumor-suppressor protein. *Proc Natl Acad Sci U S A*. 1995;92:3046-3050.
412. Saito T, Oda Y, Tanaka K, et al. beta-catenin nuclear expression correlates with cyclin D1 overexpression in sporadic desmoid tumours. *J Pathol*. 2001;195:222-228.
413. Tejpar S, Li C, Yu C, et al. Tcf-3 expression and beta-catenin mediated transcriptional activation in aggressive fibromatosis (desmoid tumour). *Br J Cancer*. 2001;85:98-101.
414. Tejpar S, Nollet F, Li C, et al. Predominance of beta-catenin mutations and beta-catenin dysregulation in sporadic aggressive fibromatosis (desmoid tumor). *Oncogene*. 1999;18:6615-6620.
415. Rubinfeld B, Albert I, Porfiri E, et al. Binding of GSK3beta to the APC-beta-catenin complex and regulation of complex assembly. *Science*. 1996;272:1023-1026.
416. Cellier C, Delabesse E, Helmer C, et al. Refractory sprue, coeliac disease, and enteropathy-associated T-cell lymphoma. French Coeliac Disease Study Group. *Lancet*. 2000;356:203-208.
417. Weston AP, Banerjee SK, Sharma P, et al. p53 protein overexpression in low grade dysplasia (LGD) in Barrett's esophagus: immunohistochemical marker predictive of progression. *Am J Gastroenterol*. 2001;96:1355-1362.
418. Chen HC, Chu RY, Hsu PN, et al. Loss of E-cadherin expression correlates with poor differentiation and invasion into adjacent organs in gastric adenocarcinomas. *Cancer Lett*. 2003;201:97-106.
419. Mizoshita T, Tsukamoto T, Nakanishi H, et al. Expression of Cdx2 and the phenotype of advanced gastric cancers: relationship with prognosis. *J Cancer Res Clin Oncol*. 2003;129:727-734.
420. Lee HS, Lee HK, Kim HS, et al. MUC1, MUC2, MUC5AC, and MUC6 expressions in gastric carcinomas: their roles as prognostic indicators. *Cancer*. 2001;92:1427-1434.
421. Wang JY, Chang CT, Hsieh JS, et al. Role of MUC1 and MUC5AC expressions as prognostic indicators in gastric carcinomas. *J Surg Oncol*. 2003;83:253-260.
422. Gurbuz Y, Kahlke V, Kloppel G. How do gastric carcinoma classification systems relate to mucin expression patterns? An immunohistochemical analysis in a series of advanced gastric carcinomas. *Virchows Arch*. 2002;440:505-511.
423. Pinto-de-Sousa J, David L, Reis CA, et al. Mucins MUC1, MUC2, MUC5AC and MUC6 expression in the evaluation of differentiation and clinico-biological behaviour of gastric carcinoma. *Virchows Arch*. 2002;440:304-310.
424. Wang RQ, Fang DC. Alterations of MUC1 and MUC3 expression in gastric carcinoma: relevance to patient clinicopathological features. *J Clin Pathol*. 2003;56:378-384.
425. Samowitz WS, Curtin K, Ma KN, et al. Microsatellite instability in sporadic colon cancer is associated with an improved prognosis at the population level. *Cancer Epidemiol Biomarkers Prev*. 2001;10:917-923.
426. Ogino S, Nosho K, Kirkner GJ, et al. CpG island methylator phenotype, microsatellite instability, BRAF mutation and clinical outcome in colon cancer. *Gut*. 2009;58:90-96.
427. Carethers JM, Smith EJ, Behling CA, et al. Use of 5-fluorouracil and survival in patients with microsatellite-unstable colorectal cancer. *Gastroenterology*. 2004;126:394-401.
428. Corvalan A, Koriyama C, Akiba S, et al. Epstein-Barr virus in gastric carcinoma is associated with location in the cardia and with a diffuse histology: a study in one area of Chile. *Int J Cancer*. 2001;94:527-530.
429. Horiuchi K, Mishima K, Ohsawa M, Aozasa K. Carcinoma of stomach and breast with lymphoid stroma: localisation of Epstein-Barr virus. *J Clin Pathol*. 1994;47:538-540.
430. Selves J, Bibeau F, Brousset P, et al. Epstein-Barr virus latent and replicative gene expression in gastric carcinoma. *Histopathology*. 1996;28:121-127.
431. Tokunaga M, Land CE, Uemura Y, et al. Epstein-Barr virus in gastric carcinoma. *Am J Pathol*. 1993;143:1250-1254.
432. Kijima Y, Ishigami S, Hokita S, et al. The comparison of the prognosis between Epstein-Barr virus (EBV)-positive gastric carcinomas and EBV-negative ones. *Cancer Lett*. 2003;200:33-40.
433. Nakamura S, Ueki T, Yao T, et al. Epstein-Barr virus in gastric carcinoma with lymphoid stroma. Special reference to its detection by the polymerase chain reaction and in situ hybridization in 99 tumors, including a morphologic analysis. *Cancer*. 1994;73:2239-2249.
434. van Beek J, zur Hausen A, Klein Kranenbarg E, et al. EBV-positive gastric adenocarcinomas: a distinct clinicopathologic entity with a low frequency of lymph node involvement. *J Clin Oncol*. 2004;22:664-670.
435. Reid BJ, Levine DS, Longton G, et al. Predictors of progression to cancer in Barrett's esophagus: baseline histology and flow cytometry identify low- and high-risk patient subsets. *Am J Gastroenterol*. 2000;95:1669-1676.
436. Reid BJ, Prevo LJ, Galipeau PC, et al. Predictors of progression in Barrett's esophagus II: baseline 17p (p53) loss of heterozygosity identifies a patient subset at increased risk for neoplastic progression. *Am J Gastroenterol*. 2001;96:2839-2848.
437. Cunningham D, Humblet Y, Siena S, et al. Cetuximab monotherapy and cetuximab plus irinotecan in irinotecan-refractory metastatic colorectal cancer. *N Engl J Med*. 2004;351:337-345.
438. De Roock W, Piessevaux H, De Schutter J, et al. KRAS wild-type state predicts survival and is associated to early radiological response in metastatic colorectal cancer treated with cetuximab. *Ann Oncol*. 2008;19:508-515.
439. Lievre A, Bachet JB, Boige V, et al. KRAS mutations as an independent prognostic factor in patients with advanced colorectal cancer treated with cetuximab. *J Clin Oncol*. 2008;26:374-379.
440. Singer S, Rubin BP, Lux ML, et al. Prognostic value of KIT mutation type, mitotic activity, and histologic subtype in gastrointestinal stromal tumors. *J Clin Oncol*. 2002;20:3898-3905.
441. Debiec-Rychter M, Dumez H, Judson I, et al. Use of c-KIT/PDGFRA mutational analysis to predict the clinical response to imatinib in patients with advanced gastrointestinal stromal tumours entered on phase I and II studies of the EORTC Soft Tissue and Bone Sarcoma Group. *Eur J Cancer*. 2004;40:689-695.
442. Heinrich MC, Corless CL, Demetri GD, et al. Kinase mutations and imatinib response in patients with metastatic gastrointestinal stromal tumor. *J Clin Oncol*. 2003;21:4342-4349.

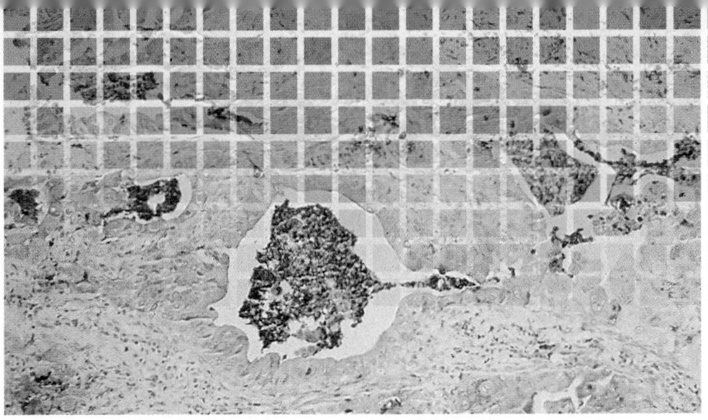

15

Immunohistology of the Pancreas, Biliary Tract, and Liver

Olca Basturk • Alton B. Farris III • N. Volkan Adsay

Pancreas 541
Extrahepatic Biliary Tract (Gallbladder and Extrahepatic Bile Ducts) 559
Ampulla 563
Liver 565
Summary 576

PANCREAS

The pancreas is one of the most versatile organs in the types of neoplasia it generates. This is partly because it is almost unique in harboring two functionally entirely distinct components, exocrine and endocrine, in an otherwise intimate mixture, and tumors arising from these two components have vastly different pathologic and biologic characteristics. Therefore pancreatic neoplasms are classified on the basis of their cellular lineage (i.e., which component of the organ they recapitulate: acinar, ductal, endocrine, or others); however, cross differentiation also does occur. For example, acinar carcinomas often contain numerous endocrine cells or a separate endocrine component. Additionally, the pancreas is one of a few organs, along with liver and kidney, that has an organ-specific "blastic" tumor of its own, pancreatoblastoma, which is characterized by differentiation along all components of this organ. Thus immunohistochemistry (IHC) plays a crucial role in delineating the differentiation of neoplasms that arise in this organ and is an invaluable adjunct in the often-challenging differential diagnosis. It has been an important tool in unraveling the mechanisms of tumorigenesis as well.

In this chapter the cellular lineage markers and the application of IHC in the diagnosis and management of specific tumor types are reviewed.

Here, the authors feel obliged to make a cautionary statement. It is the strong bias of these authors that IHC is an extremely powerful tool, but only if it is used cautiously and in combination with morphology. It is the authors' opinion (and experience) that there is no magic IHC marker that makes the diagnosis by itself. Exceptions always occur, and unfortunately, they tend to merge when IHC is necessary the most. This should not come as a surprise. Basic morphology and IHC are two different facets of the same phenotypic process in pathologic conditions. Where one is "unusual" or outside of the general realm, the other tends to be so as well.[1-3]

Biology of the Antigens and Antibodies

EPITHELIAL MARKERS

As expected, so-called "pan-epithelial" markers such as CAM 5.2, CK8, and CK18 are expressed in the pancreatic acini and ducts, as well as in the extrahepatic and peri-ampullary ducts[4]; however, certain subsets show differential expression patterns. Acinar cells generally do not label with AE1/AE3 or CK7 (Fig. 15.1) and CK19, whereas ductal cells are strongly positive for these markers. Both acini and ducts are typically negative for CK20, which is positive in the intestinal mucosa adjacent to ampulla. In general, expression of CKs, even the wide-spectrum CKs (CAM 5.2, AE1/AE3, CK8, and CK18), is typically less, if not absent, in islet cells compared with other elements.

GLANDULAR AND DUCTAL MARKERS

Mucin-Related Glycoproteins and Oncoproteins

In the pancreas and ampulla, the glandular/ductal system is characterized and distinguished by mucin production. With the exception of centroacinar cells/intercalated ducts in the pancreas and the serous cystadenomas that presumably recapitulate this earliest component of the ductal system, virtually all glandular elements

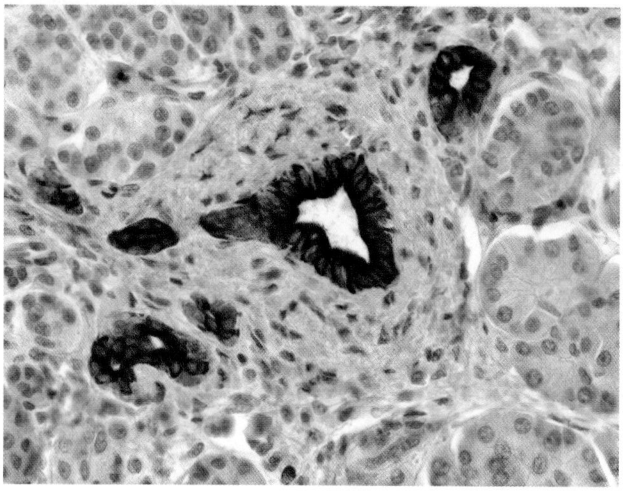

FIGURE 15.1 Pancreatic ductal cells are strongly positive for CK7, whereas acinar cells generally do not label with this marker.

and their neoplasms exhibit some degree and type of mucin formation. Among the mucin-related glycoproteins and oncoproteins that are commonly expressed in the glandular/ductal neoplasms of this region, the most widely are MUCs, CA19-9, carcinoembryonic antigen (CEA), B72.3 (TAG-72), and ductal-of-pancreas-2 (DUPAN-2).[5-10] Most of these are well described elsewhere in this book. The ones more pertinent to pancreas are discussed next.

MUCINS Mucins are high-molecular-weight glycoproteins, which are produced by various epithelial cells. They are categorized into membrane-associated mucins (MUC1, MUC3 MUC4, MUC12, MUC16, and MUC17), gel-forming mucins (MUC2, MUC5AC, MUC5B, and MUC6), and soluble mucin (MUC7).[11,12]

MUC1, *pan-epithelial membrane mucin* or the *"mammary-type" mucin,* is constitutively expressed in the cell apices of the centroacinar cells, intercalated ducts, intralobular ducts, and focally in the interlobular ducts, but not in the main pancreatic ducts, acini, or islets. It is thought to have an inhibitory role in cell-cell and cell-stroma interactions and in cytotoxic immunity.[13] MUC1 also appears to function as a signal transducer, closely interacting with the epidermal growth factor receptor (EGFR) family and participating in the progression of carcinogenesis.[13] It is expressed in almost all examples of *pancreatobiliary type* adenocarcinomas (invasive ductal adenocarcinomas of the pancreas, cholangiocarcinomas of the bile duct, and a subset of ampullary adenocarcinomas that presumably arise from peri-ampullary ductules). The expression is predominantly confined to the luminal membrane in the duct-forming areas, whereas it is also intracytoplasmic in the poorly differentiated areas. Therefore MUC1 is considered a marker of aggressiveness.[14,15]

MUC2, also known as *"intestinal-type" secretory mucin, "goblet-type" mucin,* or *gel-forming mucin,* is not constitutively expressed in the pancreas or ampullary ductules with the exception of the scattered goblet cells, where it functions as a protective barrier. It is a product of the MUC2 gene, which is known to have tumor suppressor properties, and as such considered to be responsible for the more indolent behavior of the tumors.[14,15] Carcinomas with prominent intestinal differentiation, namely villous/intestinal type pancreatic intraductal papillary mucinous neoplasms (IPMNs), colloid carcinomas that often arise in association with IPMNs, and intestinal type adenocarcinomas arising from the ampulla/duodenum, all typically show diffuse expression of MUC2 and CDX2. CDX2 is a transcription factor responsible for intestinal programming and is also an important upstream regulator of MUC2. Although diffuse expression of MUC2 is mostly confined to tumors with intestinal differentiation, CDX2 can be expressed to some degree in pancreatobiliary type tumors as well.

Like MUC1, MUC4 is a membrane-associated mucin; however, it is not expressed in normal pancreatic tissue. It is less well studied, but preliminary evidence suggests that, like MUC1, MUC4 may be a marker of ductal adenocarcinoma and a sign of aggressiveness.[16]

"Gastric-type" mucins, especially those marking gastric surface-epithelial (foveolar) mucin such as MUC5AC, are fairly ubiquitous in the gastrointestinal tract including the ampulla, wherever there are gastric-like glands, as well as the tumors arising from these sites, presumably due to the close embryologic foregut association with pancreatobiliary tissue. Normal pancreatic ducts, however, do not express this marker.[12] The expression of MUC6, *gastric pyloric glandular mucin* or *pyloric-type mucin,* is somewhat more restricted. In addition to decorating Brunner's glands, intercalated ducts of the pancreas, and the pyloric-like glands that occur in the walls of some preinvasive neoplasia such as IPMNs and mucinous cystic neoplasms (MCNs), MUC6 is also expressed extensively in some subsets of intraductal neoplasia that show oncocytic phenotype (intraductal oncocytic papillary neoplasms)[17] or those with nondescript morphology ("intraductal tubular carcinomas").[18]

ACINAR (ENZYMATIC) MARKERS

It has long been known that trypsin, one of the best-characterized serine proteinases, is produced as a zymogen (trypsinogen) in the acinar cells of the pancreas. It is secreted into the duodenum, activated into the mature form of trypsin by enterokinase, and functions as an essential food-digestive enzyme. It also catalyzes the cleavage of the other pancreatic proenzymes (e.g., chymotrypsinogen, prophospholipase, procarboxypeptidase, proelastase) to their active forms.[4,19] To date, four trypsin (or trypsinogen) genes—trypsin 1, 2, 3, and 4—have been characterized in humans and three of them—trypsins 1, 2, and 3—have been demonstrated as the zymogens in human pancreatic juice. Immunohistochemical methods demonstrate trypsin 1 in acinar cells along with pancreatic enzymes such as chymotrypsin, lipase, amylase, and elastase. Ductal and endocrine cells are negative for these enzymes. More importantly, although studies have shown that trypsins or trypsin-like enzymes are produced by other human cancer cells such as stomach, ovary, lung, and colon, immunohistochemical identification of pancreatic enzyme production is helpful in confirming the diagnosis of pancreatic acinar cell carcinoma (ACC).[19] Although this requires confirmation, it has been reported that the tumor-derived trypsin is likely to contribute to tumor invasion and metastasis by degrading extracellular matrix proteins and by activating the latent forms of matrix metalloproteinases (MMPs).[19]

ENDOCRINE MARKERS

The immunohistochemical demonstration of the specific endocrine cell peptides allows the classification of the pancreatic endocrine neoplasms (PENs). However, it is not always possible to demonstrate these in PENs. Therefore it is of diagnostic importance to use broad-spectrum endocrine cell markers for the general identification of the endocrine nature of islet cells and PENs. These protein markers, localized in the secretory granules in the cytosol or in the cellular membrane, are present in most (rarely in all) normal and neoplastic endocrine cells. The markers most commonly used in routine histopathology have been the secretory granule proteins chromogranin and synaptophysin and the cytosolic enzyme neuron-specific enolase (NSE).[20] Of these, chromogranin is the most specific but its sensitivity is about 80% to 90% (Fig. 15.2).

Chromogranins are a family of glycoproteins consisting of types A, B, and C. Among these, chromogranin A in particular has attracted great interest. Different chromogranin A antibodies are commercially available, and the staining results with these antibodies may vary. Also, the intensity of chromogranin varies with the amount of neurosecretory granules in the cytoplasm, which tend to be more abundant in the perivascular zones in normal islets.[20]

Synaptophysin, also called *protein p38,* is a glycoprotein initially found in small vesicle membranes of neurons and of chromaffin cells in the adrenal medulla. It has been routinely used as a broad-spectrum marker in normal and neoplastic neuroendocrine cells including those of the pancreas; however, strong synaptophysin immunoreactivity has been well-documented in tumors without any endocrine differentiation including solid-pseudopapillary neoplasm (SPN) of the pancreas, which is one of the most important differential diagnoses of endocrine neoplasia in this organ.[20]

NSE is a cytosolic isoenzyme of the glycolytic enzyme enolase, which catalyzes the conversion of 2-phosphoglycerate to phosphoenolpyruvate. It has been considered a marker for neuroendocrine cells and tumors including PENs. Its staining intensity is unrelated to the content of secretory granules and their peptide storage. Therefore NSE can immunostain even degranulated tumor cells. It may also be demonstrated in some non-neuroendocrine tumors. Thus the use of NSE as an endocrine marker requires careful evaluation, and it is important not to rely on NSE staining results alone but always to use them in combination with other markers of endocrine differentiation.[20]

Cell membrane–associated proteins such as neuronal cell adhesion molecule (NCAM, CD56) and leu-7 (CD57) have raised interest as neuroendocrine cell markers, but they lack specificity because they are also expressed in non-neuroendocrine cells and tumors.[20]

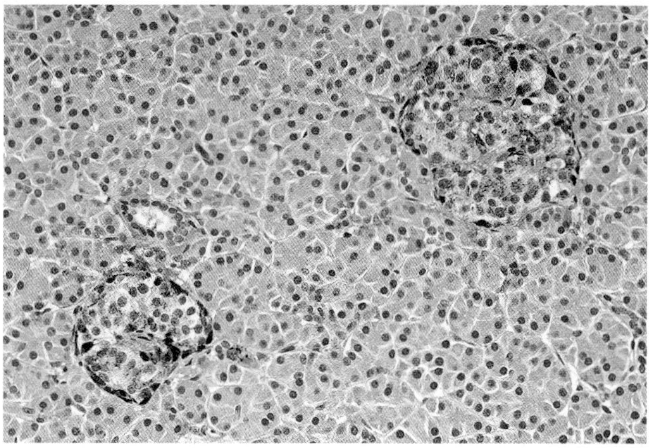

FIGURE 15.2 Immunohistochemistry for chromogranin shows strong positive staining in islets of Langerhans, more prominent in the peripheral cells. Ducts and acini are negative.

The authors' own experience and analysis of the literature also indicate a high incidence of "unexpected" or "unexplained" positivity reported with various antibodies in the islets.[21] For most of the antibodies, the staining pattern is faint and does not show any preferential staining pattern of the islet hormones, suggesting that it is a cross-reaction with a cytosolic component.[21]

ADHESION MOLECULES AND OTHER MARKERS

E-Cadherin

Cadherins are transmembrane glycoproteins that are prime mediators of cell-cell adhesion via calcium-dependent interactions. Different members of the family are found in different locations (e.g., E-cadherin is found in epithelial tissue, N-cadherin is found in muscle and adult neural tissues, P-cadherin is found in the placenta).[22]

E-cadherin plays a key role in the maintenance of epithelial integrity and polarity function.[23,24] Normal E-cadherin immunoexpression is localized to the cell membrane with a crisp staining pattern. Decrease in membrane staining compared with normal or complete absence of staining (with the antibody raised against the extracellular domain of E-cadherin) and/or nuclear staining (with the antibody recognizing the cytoplasmic domain of E-cadherin), as seen in a myriad of invasive cancers including solid-pseudopapillary neoplasms (SPNs) of the pancreas, is regarded as abnormal.[23,25] Therefore E-cadherin staining is of diagnostic use in the immunohistochemical workup of SPNs[23] because all cases will show either absence of membrane staining or nuclear positivity depending on the antibody that is employed.[24] The exact mechanism by which E-cadherin enters the nucleus is not known, but it is considered that it is closely related to several partner molecules such as β-catenin.[23] The cytoplasmic domain of E-cadherin interacts with the catenin molecules that mediate its binding to the actin cytoskeleton.[24] Cytoplasmic dotlike

TABLE 15.1 Immunohistogram of Pancreatic Ductal Adenocarcinoma with Selected Antibodies

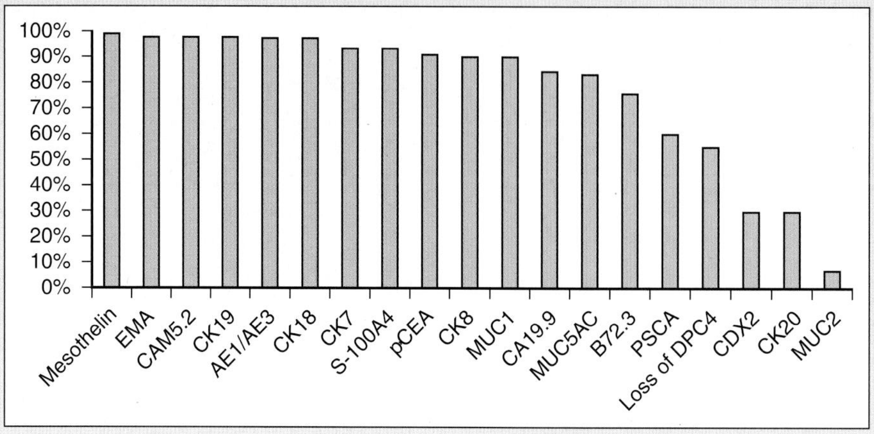

staining has also been described with the antibody to full-length E-cadherin.[23]

β-Catenin

β-catenin plays a key role in the Wnt signaling pathway as a transcriptional activator. Its normal immunoexpression shows distinct membrane decoration of the pancreatic acini and the ducts. Activating mutations in β-catenin gene *(CTNNB1)* result in (1) dysregulation and redistribution of β-catenin protein leading to characteristic strong cytoplasmic and nuclear immunoreactivity, which is seen in 100% of SPNs and in 50% to 80% of pancreatoblastomas, usually in the squamoid corpuscles and (2) overexpression of its target gene, cyclin D1, which is variably reported in 74% to 100% of SPNs[24] and in most pancreatoblastomas.

Exocrine Neoplasms

DUCTAL ADENOCARCINOMA

Ductal adenocarcinoma (DA) is the most common tumor of the pancreas (>85% of pancreatic tumors).[26] It often forms a solid mass, which can be closely mimicked by pancreatitis, and therefore most of the cases require FNA or core biopsy for diagnosis. Unfortunately, the tumor is usually scirrhous. It has abundant stromal component and low tumor cell yield, which makes the diagnosis of DA one of the most challenging in surgical pathology. Moreover, DA also has an insidious growth pattern. Along with ovarian cancer, it is the most common cause of "intra-abdominal carcinomatosis" and is one of the most common sources of carcinomas of unknown primary. Therefore it is important to know its immunolabeling pattern.[3] The immunohistogram in Table 15.1 is a summary for ductal adenocarcinomas.

Ductal adenocarcinomas express CKs and EMA. The keratins expressed consistently are CK7, CK8, CK18, CK19 (as normal ductal cells), CK13,[9,27-31] and in a lesser percentage CK4, CK10, CK17, and CK20.[9,27-50] Although CK7 is expressed relatively diffusely and strongly in the vast majority of the cases (Fig. 15.3A), CK20 expression is less common, detected

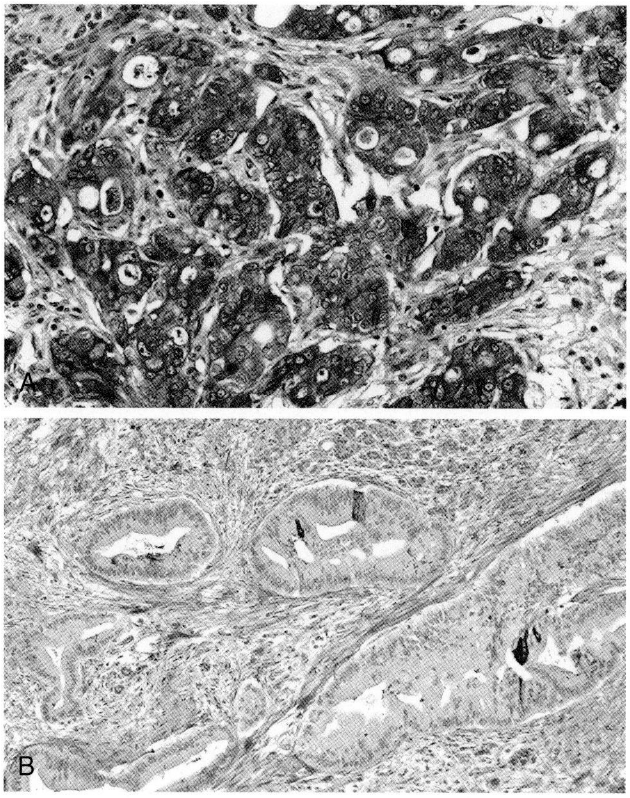

FIGURE 15.3 CK7 is expressed diffusely and strongly in the vast majority of ductal adenocarcinoma cases **(A)**; however, CK20 expression is less common and is usually focal **(B)**.

in about one third of the cases and is usually focal (Fig 15.3B).[31,34,35,37,39,42-44,48,51,52] This pattern of immunolabeling can be diagnostically useful because most acinar and endocrine neoplasms of the pancreas do not express CK7 and most colorectal cancers express CK20 but not CK7.[4] Areas of squamous differentiation in DA are also appropriately CK5/6 and p63 positive (Fig. 15.4).[45,53,54]

Ductal adenocarcinomas express several mucin-related glycoproteins including MUC1 (Fig. 15.5), which is reported to be associated with a poorer prognosis,[55-58]

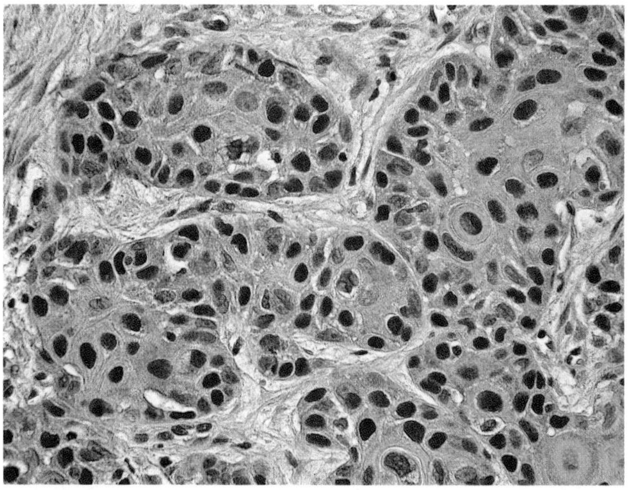

FIGURE 15.4 Among invasive carcinomas of the pancreas, p63 expression is detected only in areas with squamous differentiation.

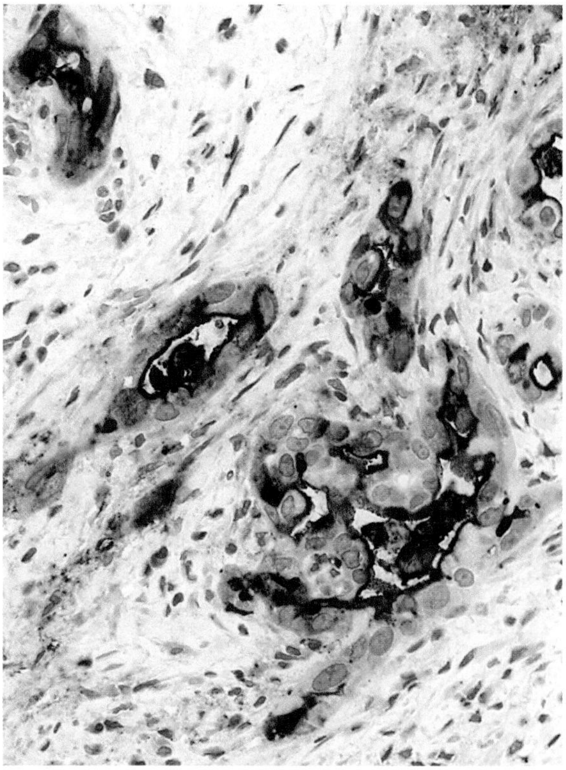

FIGURE 15.5 MUC1 is expressed in all *pancreatobiliary-type* adenocarcinomas (invasive ductal adenocarcinoma of the pancreas is shown here). The expression is predominantly confined to the luminal membrane in the duct-forming areas, whereas it is also intracytoplasmic in the poorly differentiated areas.

MUC3, MUC4, MUC5AC, and in a lesser percentage MUC6[36,55,56,59-65] but not MUC2. MUC2 is virtually nonexistent in DAs unless there is focal mucinous differentiation or there are metaplastic goblet cells. The intestinal differentiation marker CDX2 is also positive in only about 30% of DAs and its labeling is typically fainter and variegated compared with colonic adenocarcinomas.[66-69]

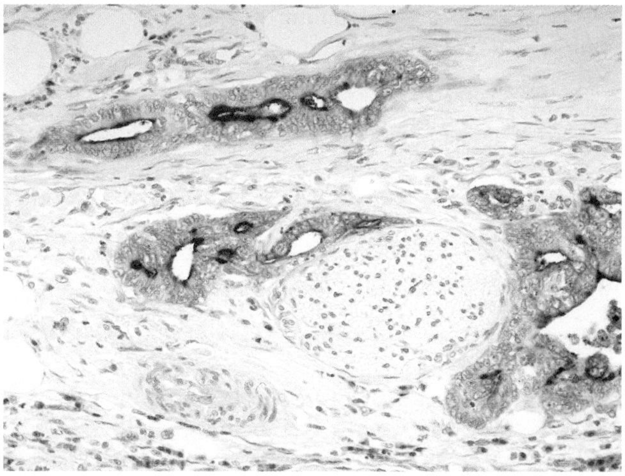

FIGURE 15.6 Carcinoembryonic antigen labeling in ductal adenocarcinoma, with areas of well-defined tubule formation showing more luminal surface labeling. Non-neoplastic glands are often negative or only focally positive for this marker. However, it should be kept in mind that overlaps occur.

Oncoproteins that are widely expressed in DAs include CA19-9, CEA, B72.3 (TAG-72), ductal-of-pancreas-2 (DUPAN-2), and CA125.[5-10,70-74] The expression of CEA (Fig. 15.6), B72.3, and CA125 may be useful in distinguishing DA or PanIN-3 from reactive glands because non-neoplastic glands are often negative or only focally positive for these markers.[5-10] However, caution needs to be exercised because overlaps are too common. Moreover, even the lower-grade PanINs (PanIN-1A) can express these markers. Recently another glycoprotein, CEACAM1 (a member of the CEA family), was reported to be positive in DA and not in normal pancreas or chronic pancreatitis, so serum levels of CEACAM1 might serve as a useful indicator for the presence of pancreatic cancer.[75]

DAs are typically negative for pancreatic enzymes such as trypsin, chymotrypsin, and lipase[70,76] unless there is a mixed acinar component, which is uncommon. They also fail to label with endocrine markers; however, in 30% of DAs there are scattered, possibly non-neoplastic, endocrine cells in close association with the neoplastic cells, which can be highlighted with immunostains for chromogranin A, synaptophysin, and NSE.[23-26,77-79] The latter two markers can occasionally show more diffuse expression, which should not be regarded as evidence of "neuroendocrine differentiation" if the tumor is an otherwise conventional adenocarcinoma.

The desmoplastic stroma associated with DAs expresses a variety of inflammatory and stromal markers. The inflammatory cells are mostly T cells (CD3 positive).[80] Scattered B cells (CD20 positive) and macrophages (MAC387 and KP1 positive) are also usually present.[80] The spindle cells express alpha-smooth muscle actin, smooth muscle myosin heavy chain, and collagen IV, markers of myofibroblastic differentiation.[81] They are also reported to be positive for heat shock protein 47 and fibronectin, as well as for proteins associated with tissue remolding such as urokinase-type plasminogen activator, the matrix metalloproteinases, and the tissue inhibitors of metalloproteinases.[82-85]

Genomic Applications of Immunohistochemistry

It has been recognized that DA, like other malignant processes, is a genetic disease produced by progressive mutations in cancer-related genes.

TUMOR SUPPRESSOR GENES Numerous studies have shown that inactivation of *TP53* gene occurs in 50% to 80% of cases.[86-96] As is well known, however, immunolabeling for the p53 protein is not entirely specific for a *TP53* gene mutation.[4]

DPC4 (Deleted in Pancreatic Carcinoma locus 4) or *SMAD4* (Mothers Against Decapentaplegic homolog 4) gene is inactivated in approximately 55% of the DAs but practically never in benign conditions.[87,97-100] Immunohistochemical labeling for the *SMAD4/DPC4* gene product has been shown to mirror *SMAD4/DPC4* gene status.[99] Therefore the immunohistochemical absence of its protein product in the ductal epithelium of a biopsy specimen is strongly suggestive of carcinoma,[92,101] as long as the in-built controls are labeling properly. Also, inactivation of *DPC4* gene is relatively uncommon in nonpancreatobiliary carcinomas. Thus loss of DPC4 may also serve as a marker of a pancreatic DA in small fine-needle aspirate samples and in metastatic sites.[97,102] This is particularly useful in the ovary in distinguishing metastatic pancreatic adenocarcinoma from primary ovarian tumors.

P16/CDKN2A is inactivated in approximately 95% of DAs (75% to 80% genetic inactivation plus 15% silencing by hypermethylation)[87-90,93,103-105]; however, because of the fact that a small minority of benign ductal epithelial cells also labels for its protein product (p16), loss of p16 is not as strongly suggestive of carcinoma.[91-93,106]

ONCOGENES The oncogene most frequently activated in pancreatic cancer is the *KRAS* oncogene,[107] which is discussed below, but a number of other oncogenes can be activated in DA including *HER2/neu* (overexpressed in ≈ 70% of the cases)[108-111] and *AKT2* (amplified in 10% to 20% of cases).[112,113]

NOVEL TUMOR MARKERS Gene expression analyses of DA have identified a large number of genes that are differentially overexpressed in DA compared with normal pancreatic tissue.[114-117] Among them, mesothelin is expressed in close to 100% of DAs,[62,118-120] sea urchin fascin in 95%,[83,120] a number of S-100 protein subtypes in 93%,[121-123] 14-3-3 sigma in 90%,[115] and prostate stem cell antigen (PSCA) in 60%.[124] The concurrent use of KOC and S-100A4 protein has been found in some studies to improve the diagnostic sensitivity of biliary brushings cytology and demonstrates similar specificity as cytology alone in the diagnosis of pancreatobiliary malignancy.[125] In addition, secreted or membranous proteins expressed in pancreatic cancer such as mesothelin or PSCA, which are shed into pancreatic secretions or blood, are under scrutiny as potential future markers for primary or recurrent disease.[126]

Beyond Immunohistochemistry: Anatomic Molecular Diagnostic Applications

DNA ploidy analyses have yielded aneuploid patterns in about half of the tumors, the incidence being higher with the poorly differentiated forms.[127-130] Also cytogenetic analyses of large series have revealed recurrent patterns of alterations in specific chromosomes[131-133] such as the most frequent whole chromosomal gains being chromosomes 20 and 7 and the most frequent whole chromosomal loss being chromosome 18.[131,132]

A number of studies have identified that *STK11/LKB1* Peutz-Jeghers gene, a tumor suppressor gene, is inactivated in a minority (5%) of DAs.[134-139] This is clinically important because patients with the Peutz-Jeghers syndrome have a greater than 130-fold increased risk of developing pancreatic cancer.[140] *STK11/LKB1* Peutz-Jeghers gene is also commonly altered in intraductal papillary mucinous neoplasms (see later).

Among all human cancers, DAs have the highest frequency of *KRAS* alterations, the oncogene being constitutively activated in approximately 90% of DAs.[87-90,107,136-139,141-145] However, it is important to point out that *KRAS* mutations are seen even in earliest forms of neoplastic transformation (namely PanIN-1A); they are a common incidental finding in pancreas, as well as in patients with chronic pancreatitis lacking invasive carcinoma[90,97]; thus they are by no means specific for "cancer." Other oncogenes that are found to be activated in pancreatic cancer include *AIB1, BRAF, c-MYC,* and *c-MYB*.[112,113,146-149]

Microsatellite instability (MSI) is a rare event in DAs and such cancers appear to have a distinct morphology called "medullary[150-153] (see later) and improved survival rate relative to those with conventional DAs.[150-153] The *MLH1* gene is often inactivated in MSI-high pancreatic carcinomas (characterized with loss of expression of hMLH1 at immunohistochemical level) by either mutation or hypermethylation.[150,152]

KEY DIAGNOSTIC POINTS

Ductal Adenocarcinoma

- Ductal adenocarcinomas (DAs) are consistently positive for CK7 diffusely and strongly, whereas CK20 is often either very focal or absent.
- Several mucin-related glycoproteins (MUC-1, MUC3, MUC4, and MUC5AC) and oncoproteins (CA19-9, CEA, B72.3, DUPAN-2, and CA125) are also typically positive in DAs to varying degrees. None of these is entirely specific for this tumor type.
- Scattered, possibly non-neoplastic endocrine cells in DAs can be demonstrated with immunostains for chromogranin A, synaptophysin, and NSE.
- Loss of DPC4 staining in the pancreatic ductal epithelium is suggestive of carcinoma provided that this loss is confirmed by the presence of in-built controls. DPC4 may also prove to be a helpful marker for differentiating pancreatic adenocarcinoma from other carcinomas in small fine-needle aspirate samples and in metastatic sites.

KEY DIFFERENTIAL DIAGNOSIS

Ductal Adenocarcinoma

Benign, noninvasive ducts versus ductal adenocarcinoma (DA):

- Strong cytoplasmic expression of MUC1 and CEA, which is often coupled with antigen leakage into stroma, is highly indicative of carcinoma (more common in high-grade areas).
- p53 and Ki-67 are significantly more abundant in carcinoma than in normal epithelium, although overlaps are common and should be used cautiously.
- Loss of DPC4 (SMAD4) is also a finding strongly in favor of adenocarcinoma, provided that in-built controls are working properly.
- Mesothelin, fascin, S-100, and PSCA are significantly more commonly expressed in carcinoma than in benign epithelium.[62]

Nonductal tumors versus DA:

- Colon versus DA: DA is consistently positive for CK7 diffusely and strongly. Approximately one third of DAs express CK20 and CDX2, but the expression is usually focal and weak. Colon carcinomas are negative for CK7 and they almost always express CK20 and CDX2. Additionally, although DA is MUC1+/MUC5AC+/MUC2−, colon carcinoma is more commonly MUC1−/MUC5AC−/MUC2+.
- Lung versus DA: TTF-1 and surfactant apoprotein A (PE-10) are usually positive in lung adenocarcinomas and are negative in DAs. In contrast, antibodies that can be focally positive in DAs such as CK20, CDX2, and CA125 are negative in lung carcinomas.
- Müllerian (gyn tract) versus DA: A panel composed of WT1, MUC5AC, and CK20 is advisable in distinguishing ovarian serous carcinomas from DAs in omental or peritoneal biopsies, which often proves to be a challenging differential diagnosis. WT1−/MUC5AC+ phenotype would point toward DA, whereas WT1+/MUC5AC− is highly in favor of ovarian primary. If present, CK20 and, less reliably, CDX2 would also be more compatible with a diagnosis of DA.[154] In one study, extensive CK17 reactivity has also been found to be supportive of a DA when the differential diagnosis includes ovarian serous and mucinous neoplasms.[37]

OTHER DUCTAL CARCINOMAS

Undifferentiated Carcinoma

In some DAs the hallmarks of ductal differentiation may be lacking. Such cases are classified as "undifferentiated carcinoma."[155] In some, epithelial-to-mesenchymal transition can be so complete that the tumor may resemble sarcomas (i.e., sarcomatoid carcinoma)[155] and only after adjunct studies such as immunohistochemistry can the ductal nature of the tumor be elucidated.[155]

Immunohistochemically, CKs are expressed in the well-formed epithelial component; however, the sarcomatoid component might be negative or focal/weak positive, hindering the differential diagnosis with sarcomas.[28,156,157] It should be kept in mind that sarcomas are exceedingly uncommon in the pancreas, and any sarcomatoid neoplasm ought to be regarded as suspect carcinoma rather than sarcoma. The keratin with the most diffuse and strongest staining has been reported to be the monoclonal so-called "pan-cytokeratins" (AE1/AE3 or OSCAR)[158]; however, these are also the keratins that are more prone to be expressed in true sarcomas. CAM 5.2, CK7, CK8, CK18, and CK19 are also positive in a variegated and less intense pattern.[28,156,157] As is typical of most undifferentiated carcinomas, the neoplastic cells diffusely and strongly stain with vimentin.[28,157,159,160] They may also express MUC1, CA19-9, CEA, and DUPAN-2.[156,161] EMA and B72.3 are negative in the majority of cases.[157] Immunolabeling for chromogranin, synaptophysin, and NSE is also negative.[4,162] In undifferentiated carcinomas with heterologous stromal elements, there may be immunoreactivity consistent with the line of mesenchymal differentiation (e.g., myoglobin or myogenin in striated muscle, S-100 protein in chondroid elements).[4]

Recently, it has been demonstrated that noncohesive pancreatic cancers including undifferentiated pancreatic carcinomas are characterized by the loss of E-cadherin protein expression, which might explain the poor cohesion of many undifferentiated carcinomas.[163]

Undifferentiated Carcinoma with Osteoclast-like Giant Cells

Osteoclast-like giant cells are not uncommon in sarcomatoid carcinomas, sarcomatoid mesotheliomas, and even some sarcomatoid melanomas.[164] In undifferentiated carcinoma with osteoclast-like giant cells of the pancreas, these cells are strikingly abundant, forming a sea of giant cells that may, in some cases, obscure the epithelial component of the tumor.[164] Recent studies confirmed that the osteoclast-like giant cells are in fact reactive in nature and that the malignant cells are actually the smaller, atypical mononuclear cells in the background.[164]

Immunohistochemically, the atypical mononuclear cells in the background, which are the true malignant cells representing the sarcomatoid carcinoma cells, almost always express vimentin, whereas only a minority expresses CKs (CAM 5.2, AE1/AE3 [Fig. 15.7A], or CK7); EMA; and CEA.[28,160,161,165-170] In some cases, all of the epithelial markers are negative. The osteoclast-like giant cells are positive for vimentin, leukocyte common antigen (LCA, CD45), histiocytic markers (CD68, KP1 [Fig. 15.7B]), and alpha-1-antichymotrypsin, whereas they are nonreactive for CKs, EMA, or CEA.[28,160,161,166-171] However, "tumor cannibalism" (i.e., presence of malignant cells in the benign giant cells) is fairly common in this entity and ought to be considered in evaluating these markers.

These neoplasms often have *TP53* gene mutations, and immunolabeling for the p53 protein has been shown to label the pleomorphic mononuclear cells but not the osteoclast-like giant cells.[140] Additionally, genetic analyses have demonstrated that the atypical mononuclear cells harbor *KRAS* mutations in about 90% of these neoplasms.[28,161,167,169,172,173] By contrast, the osteoclast-like giant cells do not harbor *KRAS* mutations.[169,170]

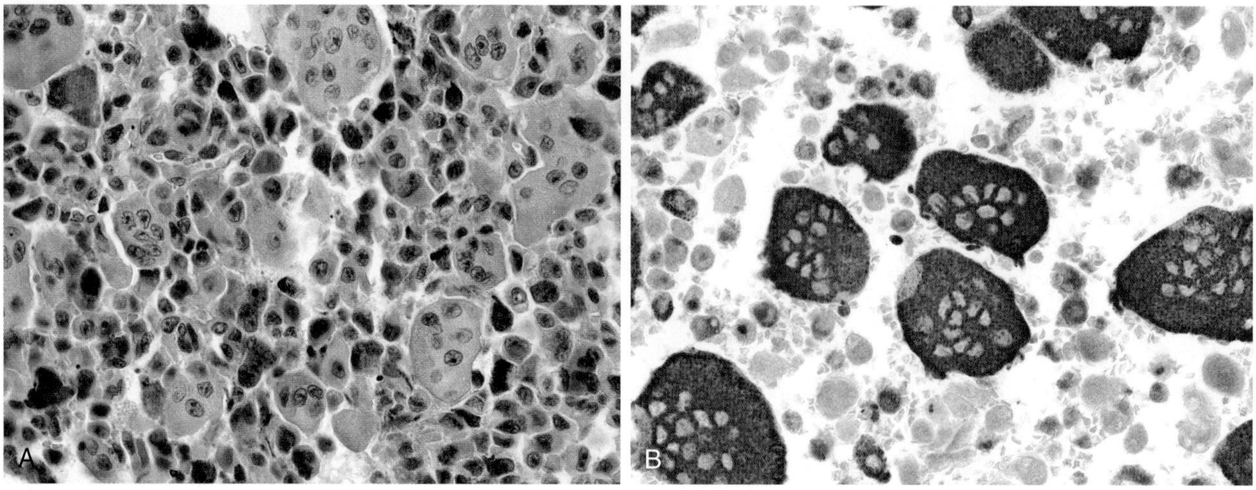

FIGURE 15.7 In undifferentiated carcinoma with osteoclast-like giant cells of the pancreas, the osteoclast-like giant cells are negative for AE1/AE3 **(A)** and positive for CD68 **(B)**.

Medullary Carcinoma

As in other organs (such as breast and tubular gastrointestinal [GI] tract), medullary carcinoma in the pancreas is defined as syncytial growth of poorly differentiated epithelioid tumor cells, often accompanied by dense lymphoplasmacytic inflammatory infiltrate.[150-153] Desmoplastic reaction is minimal.[150-153] The tumors may arise sporadically or in patients with the hereditary nonpolyposis colorectal cancer (HNPCC) syndrome.[153] Current experience is too limited to determine their biologic behavior and prognosis; however, in one study, the patients were found to have an improved survival rate relative to those with DAs.[150] Immunohistochemically, the epithelioid cells are labeled by antibodies to cytokeratins (CK),[150-153] whereas trypsin, chymotrypsin, lipase, chromogranin, and synaptophysin are usually negative. CD3 antibody highlights the presence of numerous intratumoral T lymphocytes.[152] Rare examples also contain Epstein-Barr virus RNA.[152]

Medullary carcinomas of the pancreas, like their colorectal counterparts, often show microsatellite instability, which is usually caused by somatic hypermethylation of the *MLH1* promoter in sporadic cases[174] and by an inherited mutation in MLH1 or MSH2 HNPCC syndrome.[153] Immunolabeling for MLH1 and MSH2 reveals loss of expression of one of these DNA mismatch repair proteins in many cases.

Adenosquamous Carcinoma

In the pancreas, squamous cells can be encountered in injured ductal epithelium as a result of a metaplastic process. The same metaplastic phenomenon also seems to take place focally in some examples of DA. When this finding is prominent (>25% of the tumor is the cut-off the authors use), the tumor is classified as adenosquamous carcinoma, and if it is exclusively squamous, then squamous cell carcinoma.[175] Most of the tumors express CKs (CAM 5.2, AE1/AE3, CK5/6, CK7, CK8, CK13, CK18, CK19, and CK20), EMA, CA19-9, CEA, and B72.3.[175,176] Typically, CK5/6, CK13, and p63 (see Fig. 15.4) are limited to the areas of squamous differentiation, whereas CK7, CK20, CA19-9, CEA, and B72.3 often label the glandular elements.[175,177,178]

The majority of the cases show nuclear p53 staining and loss of DPC4 protein similar to the molecular signature found in DA.[179] *KRAS* mutations are seen in the majority of cases.[175,180]

Colloid Carcinoma

Colloid carcinomas are characterized with well-delineated pools of stromal extracellular mucin containing scanty, floating carcinoma cells in clusters, strips, or as individual cells. By definition, mucin/epithelium ratio is typically high. Colloid carcinomas appear to have a distinctly better clinical course than other invasive carcinomas of ductal origin.[181,182] Five-year survival of resected cases is 55% as opposed to 10% in DAs.[181,182] The indolent behavior has been attributed to a combination of two factors: (1) There is inverse polarization of cells, which show secretory activity toward the "stroma-facing" surface of the cells, instead of the luminal surface, and (2) the mucin produced is a specific gel-forming mucin (MUC2) that acts as a containing factor, preventing the spread of the cells.[181,182]

Immunohistochemically, in addition to the conventional epithelial and ductal markers such as CKs, CEA, CA19-9, and B72.3, colloid carcinoma is unique among invasive carcinomas of the pancreas by expression of intestinal differentiation markers, MUC2, and CDX2 (Figs. 15.8 and 15.9, respectively).[182] Also, in contrast with DAs, they are negative for MUC1. Furthermore, the pattern of accentuated CEA labeling in the stroma-facing surface of the cells (Fig. 15.10) is specific to colloid carcinomas and is seldom seen in other invasive carcinomas of the pancreas.

As opposed to DAs, the expression of DPC4 is intact in almost all cases[183] and only one third harbors *KRAS* oncogene mutations.[182]

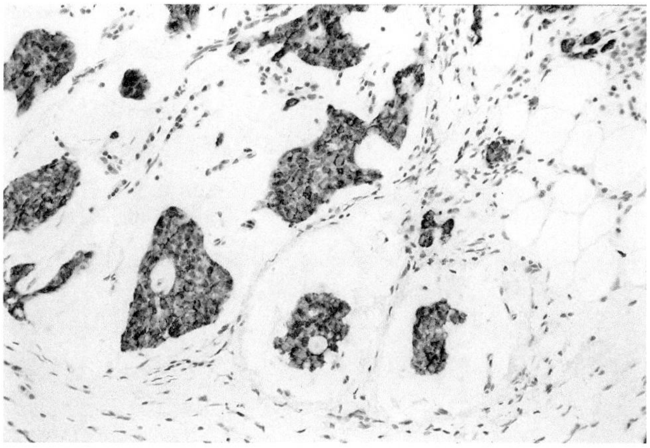

FIGURE 15.8 Strong and often diffuse intracytoplasmic MUC2 labeling is specific for colloid carcinoma.

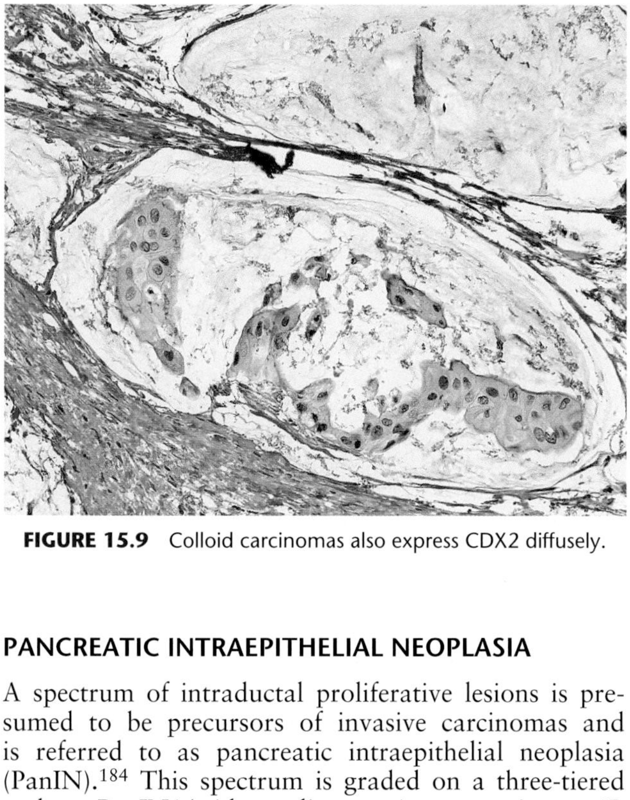

FIGURE 15.9 Colloid carcinomas also express CDX2 diffusely.

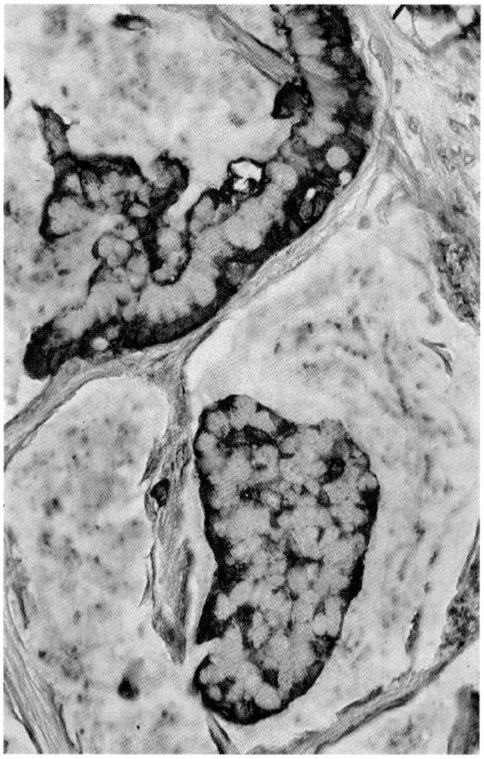

FIGURE 15.10 In contrast to MUC2, intracytoplasmic CEA labeling is much weaker in colloid carcinoma; however, there is strong CEA labeling in the stroma-facing surface of the cells.

PANCREATIC INTRAEPITHELIAL NEOPLASIA

A spectrum of intraductal proliferative lesions is presumed to be precursors of invasive carcinomas and is referred to as pancreatic intraepithelial neoplasia (PanIN).[184] This spectrum is graded on a three-tiered scale as PanIN1A (the earliest step), progressing to 1B and 2, and finally to PanIN3, which is considered carcinoma *in situ* (CIS). Lower-grade PanINs are relatively frequent incidental findings.[3] As a rule of thumb, it is considered that nearly 50% of adults older than the age of 50 have foci of PanIN1 in their pancreas. However, higher-grade PanINs, particularly PanIN3 (carcinoma *in situ*), are seldom encountered in isolation without a concomitant invasive adenocarcinoma.[2]

The immunohistochemical labeling pattern of PanINs parallels that of DA. None of the lesions express MUC2,[185] but most express MUC1, MUC4, MUC5AC, and MUC6.[55,185] In the multistep progression of DA, MUC1 expression within normal intralobular and interlobular ducts appears to be decreased in the low-grade PanINs and subsequently re-expressed in the advanced PanINs, increasing to 85% of PanIN3.[185] Unlike the case with MUC1, MUC5AC is expressed relatively uniformly throughout all grades of PanIN.[185] Increasing Ki-67 labeling indices has been shown with increasing grades of "dysplasia" in PanINs.[186]

Most of the molecular abnormalities identified within DAs have also been detected within PanIN. Among these, *p16* inactivation seems to be an "early" event. Its frequency increases with increasing grades of dysplasia (in 30% of PanIN1A lesions vs. in 85% of PanIN3 lesions), and it precedes both *p53* mutation and *DPC4* inactivation.[93,185] On the basis of nuclear cyclin D1 expression seen in one third of PanIN2 lesions, cyclin D1 abnormalities would best be classified as an "intermediate" event, also preceding *p53* mutation and *DPC4* inactivation.[185] *p53* mutation, as assessed by nuclear overexpression of p53 protein (>25% nuclei), is a "late" event in the progression model of DA, occurring only in PanIN3 (57% of the lesions). Similar to the case of the *p53* gene, inactivation of the *DPC4* gene appears to be a "late" event, seen only in PanIN3 (28% of the lesions).[187]

Comparative molecular/genetic analysis of microdissected normal and neoplastic ducts combined by immunohistochemistry has disclosed the upregulation of a cluster of extrapancreatic foregut markers (pepsinogen C, MUC6, KLF4, and TFF1) and various gastric epithelial markers (Sox-2, gastrin, HoxA5, and others) in PanINs, whereas the intestinal markers (CDX1 and CDX2) are rarely expressed, if at all, in either PanIN lesions

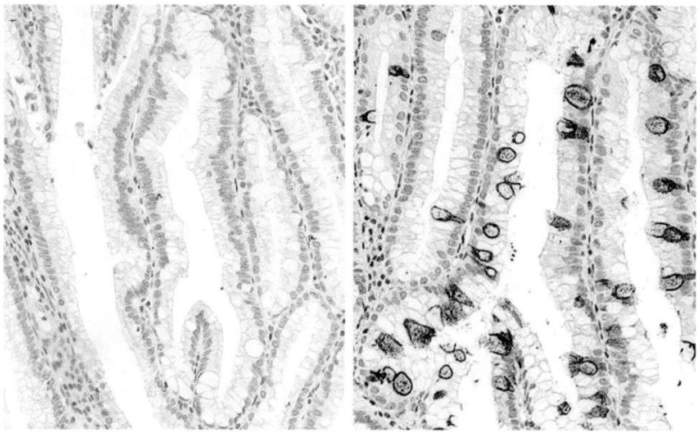

FIGURE 15.11 Intraductal papillary mucinous neoplasm with gastric/foveolar type papillae is usually negative for MUC1 *(left)*. MUC2 expression is only focal, marking goblet cells *(right)*.

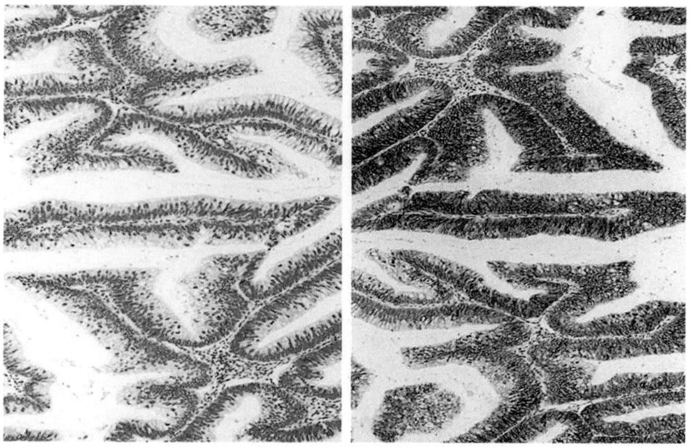

FIGURE 15.12 Most intestinal-type intraductal papillary mucinous neoplasm papillae are negative for MUC1 *(left)*. MUC2 expression is diffuse and strong *(right)*.

or invasive pancreatic cancer. These data suggest that PanIN development may involve Hedgehog-mediated conversion to a gastric epithelial differentiation program.[188]

INTRADUCTAL PAPILLARY MUCINOUS NEOPLASM

Intraductal papillary mucinous neoplasms (IPMNs) are characterized by intraductal proliferation of neoplastic mucinous cells, which usually form papillae and lead to cystic dilation of the pancreatic ducts, forming clinically and macroscopically detectable masses.[189] Microscopically, papillae with three distinct morphologic patterns can be seen: (1) pattern reminiscent of gastric foveolar epithelium or resembling PanIN1A with scattered goblet cells (gastric/foveolar), (2) pattern closely resembling colonic villous adenomas (villous/intestinal), (3) pattern characterized with more complex papillae lined by cuboidal cells (pancreatobiliary).[189] There is also a spectrum of cytoarchitectural atypia (IPMN with low-grade dysplasia, IPMN with moderate [borderline] dysplasia, and IPMN with high-grade dysplasia)[4,162] and approximately 30% of resected IPMNs have an associated invasive carcinoma. Gastric/foveolar and villous/intestinal-types IPMNs are usually associated with colloid carcinoma, and pancreatobiliary type is associated with tubular type invasion with all the morphologic features of DA.[189] Ki-67 and proliferating cell nuclear antigen (PCNA) labeling demonstrates a progressive increase in cell proliferation from normal duct epithelium, to IPMN with low-grade dysplasia to IPMN with moderate dysplasia and IPMN with high-grade dysplasia.[190,191] Also immunostaining of p53 protein is seen only in IPMNs with moderate and high-grade dysplasia and in DAs.[192]

MUC expression profile of IPMNs has been instrumental in delineating the differentiation and lineage of these neoplasms and in recognizing its subsets that are clinically significant[55,61,193-195]:

1. *Gastric/foveolar type papillae* appear to be full recapitulation of gastric mucosa, with more papillary areas expressing MUC5AC and only small glandular elements at the base labeling with MUC6. They are usually negative or only focally positive for MUC1 (Fig. 15.11) and CDX2. Scattered goblet cells can be highlighted by MUC2 (Fig. 15.11).[55,61,189,194,196]
2. *Villous/intestinal type papillae* do, in fact, show molecular characteristics of intestinal differentiation as evidenced by diffuse MUC2 (Fig. 15.12) and CDX2 expression but not MUC1 (Fig. 15.12).[55,61,189,194,196] Invasive carcinoma associated with villous/intestinal type, which is typically colloid carcinoma, also expresses MUC2 and CDX2 but not MUC1. In addition, villous/intestinal-type papillae are positive for MUC5AC and negative for MUC6.[55,61,182,189]
3. *Pancreatobiliary type papillae* typically do not express MUC2 and CDX2 but may instead express MUC1 (a "marker" of aggressive phenotype in the pancreas), as well as MUC5AC, and to a lesser degree, MUC6.[17,61] The invasive component also expresses MUC1 but not MUC2.[61] In general, IPMNs are reported to show weaker labeling for MUC4 (70%), MUC3 (60%), and MUC5B (35%)[194] and are almost always negative for MUC7.[4] IHC for IPMN is summarized in Table 15.2's immunohistogram.

As expected, virtually all IPMNs express CKs. They are positive for CAM 5.2, AE1/AE3, CKs 7, 8, 18, 19, and variably for CK20.[191,197,198] Some IPMNs, especially villous/intestinal type, also express CA19-9 and CEA.[198-200] In the villous/intestinal type, the degree of CEA expression increases with the degree of dysplasia.[201] Twenty percent of IPMNs label for DUPAN-2.[197,198,202] Scattered endocrine cells that are positive with chromogranin and synaptophysin are seen in most tumors but account for less than 5% of the tumor cells.[108,203] Cyclooxygenase-2 is also expressed in 60% to 80% of IPMNs.[204]

KRAS oncogene mutations have been reported in 30% to 60% of IPMNs.[90,192,197,205-216] The frequency of *TP53*[90,190,207,209,211,212,217-223] and *p16/CDKN2A* tumor suppressor gene mutations varies greatly between reported series.[90,209,217,223] However, in contrast to DAs, the protein product of the *SMAD4/DPC4* tumor suppressor gene is retained in virtually all cases

TABLE 15.2 Immunohistogram of Intraductal Papillary Mucinous Neoplasm with Selected Antibodies

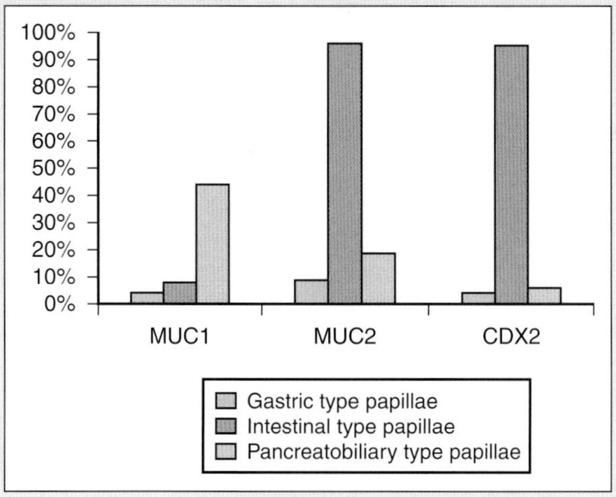

including the invasive carcinomas, suggesting a substantial difference in the pathogenesis of these two neoplasms.[61,90,183,205,209,217] Recently, human cripto-1 protein, which is thought to have a role in tumor progression, was reported to be expressed more abundantly in pancreatobiliary type than in other types.[224]

INTRADUCTAL ONCOCYTIC PAPILLARY NEOPLASM

Many authors regard intraductal oncocytic papillary neoplasm (IOPN) as a special subtype of IPMN,[225] although recent molecular findings suggest that it may be a distinct tumor type[226] but very similar to IPMN in several aspects. Distinctive morphologic features of IOPNs include (1) exuberant, complexly branching papillae in a relatively clean background; (2) oncocytic cells caused by an abundance of mitochondria; and (3) intraepithelial lumina, which are round, punched-out spaces within the epithelium. These intraepithelial lumina often contain mucin. Scattered goblet cells may be identified.[225]

Immunohistochemically, IOPNs usually label for MUC1[61,194,226] and MUC6,[17] whereas MUC2 and MUC5AC are largely restricted to goblet cells.[61,194,226] CDX2 is rarely expressed.[226] All cases are positive for B72.3, and some show focal, luminal staining for CEA. DPC4 is typically retained.[226] CA19-9 and DUPAN-2 are rarely positive.[225] IOPNs also label strongly with antibodies against mitochondrial antigens such as 111.3.[225,226] Interestingly, there is consistent immunolabeling with hepatocyte paraffin-1 (Hep Par-1) antibodies; however, *in situ* hybridization for albumin, a more specific test for hepatocellular differentiation, is consistently negative.[4]

Most interestingly, IOPNs, typically lack *KRAS2* mutations[205,226] in stark contrast with any other tumor types in the pancreas characterized by ductal-mucinous differentiation including greater than 90% of invasive ductal carcinomas and almost half of IPMNs.

MUCINOUS CYSTIC NEOPLASM

Mucinous cystic neoplasms (MCNs) are seen typically in perimenopausal women (95% of the patients are women; mean age, 50 years) and present as a thick-walled cyst, often multilocular, in the tail of the pancreas. Microscopically the cysts are lined by mucin-producing epithelium. A distinctive ovarian-like stroma is invariably present in the septa of the cysts.[227,228] Just as in IPMNs, MCNs also exhibit characteristics of an adenoma-carcinoma sequence (MCNs with low-grade dysplasia, MCNs with moderate [borderline] dysplasia, and MCNs with high-grade dysplasia or carcinoma *in situ*).[4,162,227,228] Invasive carcinoma can be seen in association with MCN in less than one fifth of MCNs. Invasive carcinoma is almost exclusively of tubular type with all the morphologic features of DA.[229,230] On occasion, sarcomatoid neoplasms arise in MCNs. It is debated whether these are sarcomatoid carcinomas originating from the epithelial component or sarcomatous transformation of the ovarian-type stroma.

The epithelial cells express immunoreactivity with CKs (CK7, 8, 18, and 19),[42,52,197,231] as well as with EMA, CA19-9, CEA, DUPAN-2, and CA125.[5,73,197,199,231-236] MUC1 is typically not expressed in noninvasive lesions of MCNs but is a marker of invasion observed in greater than 90% of cases with invasion, detected in both the *in situ* and invasive components.[233,237] MUC2 and CDX2 positivity can be seen, especially in the interspersed goblet cells; however, in contrast with villous/intestinal type IPMNs, the papillary dysplastic nodules are typically negative or only focal for these markers.[233,237] The lesions invariably express MUC5AC, which is also commonly expressed in DAs.[42,233] Although the papillary components of MCN are mostly MUC6 negative, the foveolar-like epithelium in nonpapillary areas is typically positive for MUC6.[17] Chromogranin- or synaptophysin-positive scattered endocrine cells are frequently noted within the epithelium.[203,232,235,238,239]

The ovarian-like stroma is immunoreactive for vimentin, smooth muscle actin, muscle-specific actin, desmin, h-caldesmon, bcl-2, and CD99, usually in a patchy distribution.[229,232,240-245] Progesterone receptors are also expressed fairly consistently (Fig. 15.13) and, in subtle cases, may help establish the diagnosis by highlighting the presence of this pathognomonic finding. Estrogen receptors are often negative by the current antibodies available; however, it is suspected that this lack of detection is related to the receptor subunit specificities of these antibodies. If present, the luteinized cells label with antibodies to tyrosine hydroxylase, α-inhibin, and calretinin, which have been shown to recognize ovarian hilar cells and testicular Leydig cells.[242,246]

By molecular/genetic analysis, *KRAS* mutations appear early and increase in frequency proportional to the degree of dysplasia.[218,247-249] p53 overexpression appears to occur relatively late in *in situ* and invasive mucinous cystadenocarcinomas.[218,247-249] Approximately half of the associated invasive carcinomas also show loss of DPC4 expression, which is not surprising because most of these carcinomas are conventional DAs.[183,232,233,241,250]

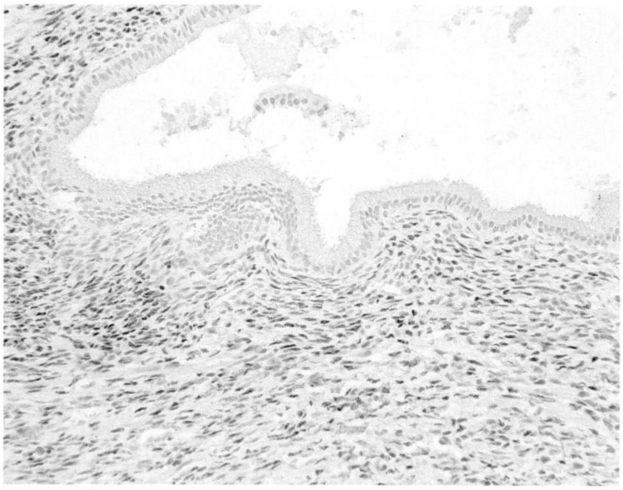

FIGURE 15.13 Progesterone receptors are expressed in the ovarian-like stroma cells and may be used to confirm the diagnosis in equivocal cases of mucinous cystic neoplasms.

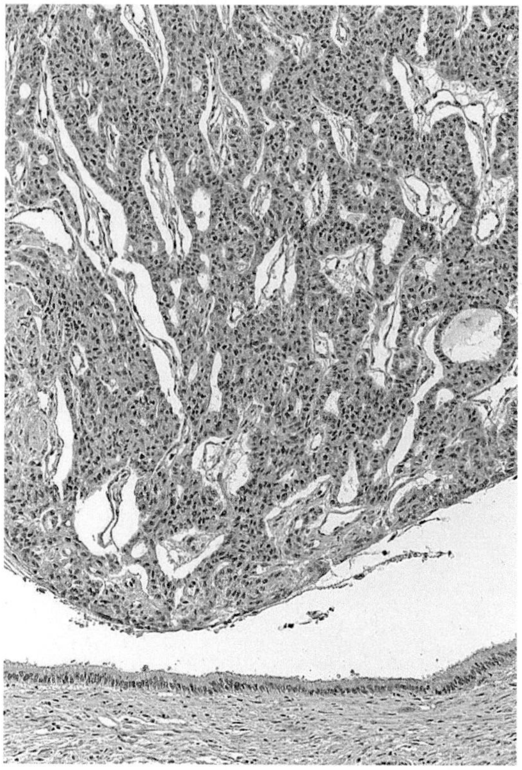

FIGURE 15.14 Intact DPC4 expression in the nuclei of the intraductal tubular carcinoma cells.

KEY DIAGNOSTIC POINTS

Mucinous Cystic Neoplasm

- Mucinous cystic neoplasms (MCNs) are mucinous/ductal type neoplasia and thus the epithelial cells are positive for CKs, as well as for EMA, CA19-9, and CEA.
- All MCNs express MUC5AC, but MUC1 is seen primarily in cases with an invasive component.
- Progesterone receptors are expressed in the ovarian-like stroma cells and may be used to confirm the diagnosis in equivocal cases of MCNs.
- The ovarian-like stroma cells also label with antibodies to smooth muscle actin, muscle-specific actin, desmin, h-caldesmon, and also variably for alpha-inhibin and calretinin.

INTRADUCTAL TUBULAR CARCINOMA

Intraductal tubular carcinoma is a recently described entity, the clinicopathologic characteristics of which have yet to be fully characterized.[18,251,252] It resembles IPMN by its intraductal nature and mimics acinar cell carcinoma (ACC) by its frequent acinar pattern. Approximately one third of the lesions have foci of invasion ranging from microscopic to larger foci.[18]

Immunohistochemically, intraductal tubular carcinomas are positive for AE1/AE3 (100%), CK7 (85%), and CK19 (85%), but not for CK20 and CDX2.[194,253-255] Most express CA19.9 (95%).[18] Focal linear immunoreactivity for CEA (40%) has been reported along the apical cytoplasm. The lesions also express MUC1 (90%) and MUC6 (60%), whereas MUC2 is negative,[194,253-256] placing them closer to the pancreatobiliary type IPMNs. However, MUC4 and MUC5AC are negative. The lesions almost always (>90%) show intact DPC4 labeling (Fig. 15.14).[18] Lack of acinar differentiation as demonstrated by negativity of trypsin and other acinar markers is essential in the differential diagnosis of intraductal tubular carcinomas from acinar cell carcinomas because the morphologic distinction of these two tumor types is often challenging.

SEROUS CYSTADENOMA

Serous cystadenoma (SCA) is the only nonmucinous example of ductal neoplasia in the pancreas and, unlike other ductal tumors, has virtually no tendency for malignant transformation.[257] It is also known to have a well-established association with von Hippel-Lindau (vHL) syndrome.[4,162]

The tumor cells have a clear cytoplasm because of the abundant intracytoplasmic glycogen and label with CAM 5.2, AE1/AE3, CK7, CK8, CK18, and CK19 but usually not with CK20.[257-263] A third of the cases are also positive for EMA.[258,260,261,264] Even though CA19-9 and B72.3 expression[261,265] is reported, immunolabeling for mucin markers is generally lacking with the exception of MUC6. CEA is uniformly negative, as are insulin, glucagon, somatostatin, vasoactive intestinal polypeptide, and vimentin.[260] Chromogranin- or synaptophysin-positive scattered endocrine cells are commonly detected.[5,231,258,259,261,265-267] Molecules implicated in clear cell tumorigenesis (glucose uptake and transporter-1 "GLUT-1" [Fig. 15.15], hypoxia-inducible factor-1a "HIF-1α," and carbonic anhydrase IX) are also consistently expressed.[268] As in other vHL-related clear cell tumors, there is a prominent capillary network immediately adjacent to the epithelium confirming that the clear cell-angiogenesis association is also valid for this tumor type.[268] This rich capillary

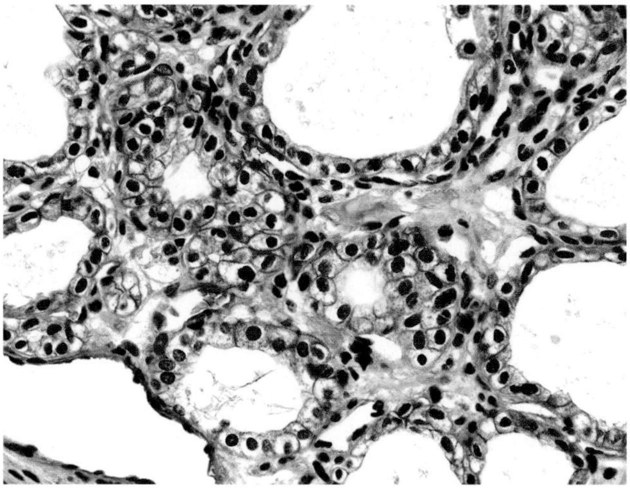

FIGURE 15.15 GLUT-1 expression in serous cystadenoma is detected predominantly in the cell membranes, but also in the cytoplasm.

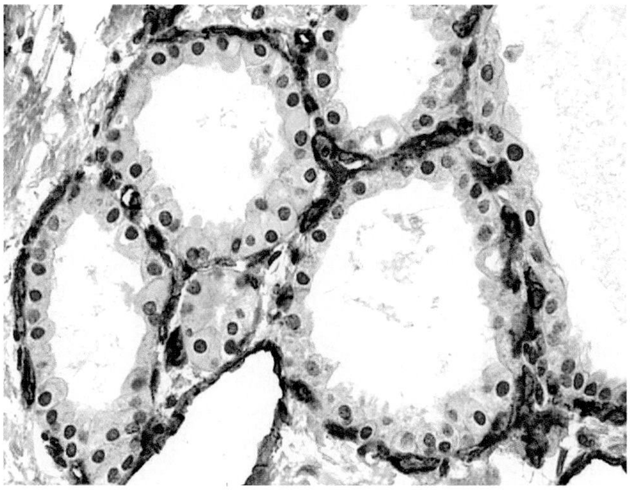

FIGURE 15.16 The remarkable intensity of capillary network immediately adjacent to the epithelium, highlighted by CD31, in serous cystadenoma.

network, which can be highlighted by CD31 stain (Fig. 15.16) may be helpful for surgical pathologists, especially as needle biopsies are becoming the norm for initial workup of the patients.[268] This finding may also be helpful in frozen sections where clear cell cytology is typically not evident owing to the preservation of glycogen.[268]

By molecular/genetic analysis, *vHL* gene (chromosome 3p) allelic deletions are detected in SCAs from patients with vHL, providing further evidence of their neoplastic nature and integral association with vHL syndrome.[269-271] Alterations of vHL gene may also be detected in sporadic cases.[249,269] Frequent (in 50% of patients) loss of heterozygosity has also been reported on chromosome 10q.[271] In contrast to DAs, activating mutations in the *KRAS* oncogene and inactivation of the *TP53* tumor suppressor gene have not been reported in SCAs.[218,249,265,270-272]

KEY DIAGNOSTIC POINTS

Serous Cystadenoma (SCA)

- SCA is virtually the only ductal tumor that does not show the pancreatic ductal differentiation markers (mucins, mucin-related oncoproteins, and KRAS mutation).
- Instead, it commonly expresses the markers of centroacinar-cell/intercalated duct system such as MUC6, as well as markers of clear cell tumorigenesis such as GLUT-1, HIF-1α, and carbonic anhydrase IX.
- Epithelial differentiation markers (CKs and EMA) are always positive.
- The rich capillary network, which can be highlighted by CD31 stain, may be helpful, especially in needle biopsies and frozen sections.

KEY DIFFERENTIAL DIAGNOSIS

Serous Cystadenoma (SCA)

- **Clear cell variant of pancreatic endocrine neoplasm versus serous cystadenoma:** Diffuse immunoreactivity for chromogranin and synaptophysin is highly in favor of an endocrine origin.
- **PEComa (sugar tumor) versus SCA:** HMB-45 and SMA are positive in PEComa, whereas the absence of such reactivity and immunolabeling for CKs and EMA is typical for SCA.

ACINAR CELL CARCINOMA

Acinar cell carcinomas (ACCs) are rare and fairly aggressive tumors, although prognostically not as dismal as DAs.[3] They can be seen in any age group but are more common in elderly patients. They are typically solid, cellular, stroma-poor tumors characterized by sheets of relatively uniform cells. Variable amounts of endocrine elements in forms of scattered individual cells, large zones, and hybrid foci or even as separate well-established nodules are commonly present in most cases if searched carefully. If the endocrine component is larger than 25% of the tumor, by convention the case is classified as "mixed."

ACC cells are also almost always positive for CAM 5.2, AE1/AE3, CK8, and CK18,[273,274] whereas CK7, CK19, and CK20 are generally negative. EMA is expressed in about half of the tumors.[273] Glycoproteins, characteristic of ductal differentiation (MUC1, MUC5AC, CEA, CA19-9, DUPAN-2, B72.3, and CA125), are either negative or only focally positive. Immunohistochemical identification of pancreatic enzyme production is helpful in confirming the diagnosis.[70,76,275-278] Both trypsin (Fig. 15.17) and chymotrypsin are detectable in more than 95% of cases, although some studies have shown less sensitivity for chymotrypsin.[275] Lipase is less commonly identified, in approximately 70% to 85% of cases. Other enzymes that are reportedly positive in ACC are alpha-1-antitrypsin, alpha-1-antichymotrypsin, phospholipase A2, and pancreatic secretory trypsin inhibitor. In daily practice the most useful antibody applied is trypsin.

The endocrine component shows immunoreactivity for chromogranin or synaptophysin[76,275,279,280] and, rarely, peptide hormones such as glucagon or somatostatin are expressed. In some cases of ACC, even the most typical acinar areas may show positivity with endocrine markers. Markers typically present in solid-pseudopapillary neoplasms (vimentin, CD56, and progesterone receptors) are negative.

Only rare cases exhibit abnormal nuclear accumulation of the p53 protein,[76,281-283] and DPC4 is retained.[90,284]

By molecular/genetic analysis, ACCs rarely, if at all, show *KRAS* mutations[76,90,281,283,285,286] in stark contrast with ductal cancers. Recent work has identified a high frequency of allelic loss on chromosomes 4q, 11p, and 16q.[284,287,288] In addition, 25% of ACCs have mutations in the *APC/β-catenin* pathway, a pattern similar to that of pancreatoblastoma.[76,283,284,287]

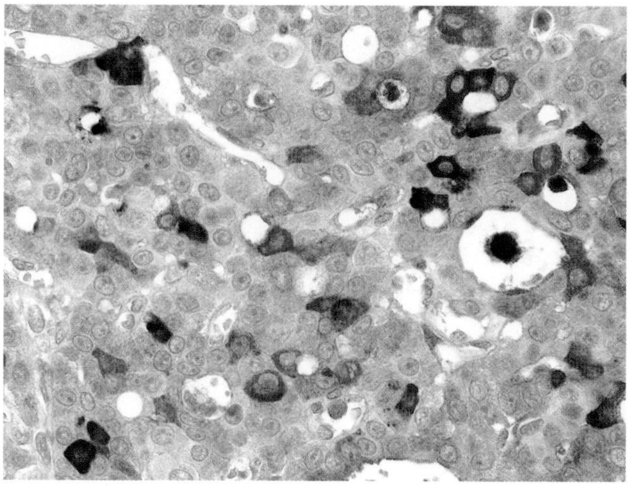

FIGURE 15.17 Immunohistochemical stains for acinar enzymes, in particular trypsin as shown here, are detectable in more than 95% of acinar cell carcinomas.

KEY DIAGNOSTIC POINTS

Acinar Cell Carcinoma (ACC)

- Immunohistochemical stains for acinar enzymes, particularly trypsin but also chymotrypsin, and lipases serve as highly specific markers of acinar differentiation.
- Pancreatic ductal differentiation markers (mucins and mucin-related oncoproteins) are either negative or only focally positive.
- Endocrine component is very commonly present and shows immunoreactivity for chromogranin or synaptophysin as well as other neuroendocrine markers.

KEY DIFFERENTIAL DIAGNOSIS

Acinar Cell Carcinoma (ACC)

- **Solid-pseudopapillary neoplasm (SPN) versus ACC:** SPN typically expresses a nonspecific acinar marker, α_1-antityripsin, similar to ACC; however, it also consistently expresses vimentin, CD56, β-catenin, CD10, and progesterone receptors. Furthermore, in SPN, in contrast with ACC, more specific acinar markers (trypsin, chymotrypsin, and lipases) are not expressed and epithelial markers are usually either focal or weak.
- **Pancreatic endocrine neoplasm versus ACC:** Scattered endocrine cells or a focal endocrine component are common in ACC; however, diffuse and strong reactivity for the endocrine markers (chromogranin and synaptophysin) throughout the tumor is characteristic of PENs. Additionally, PENs do not show immunoreactivity for acinar markers.

PANCREATOBLASTOMA

Pancreatoblastoma is a rare pancreatic tumor showing differentiation toward all three lineages in the pancreas (acinar, ductal, and endocrine) in variable amounts.[3] It is the most common pancreatic neoplasm of childhood, although one third of reported cases were in adults. Microscopically, the tumors show large, solid, nesting, and acinar growth patterns and have characteristic squamoid corpuscles that occasionally have optically clear nuclei rich in biotin.[289]

Many cases show labeling for markers of acinar, ductal, and endocrine differentiation in the respective areas, although acinar differentiation is the most common and the predominant pattern in the majority of the cases.[289] The acinar component labels with antibodies to CAM 5.2, AE1/AE3, CKs 7, 8, 18, and 19. Positivity for trypsin and chymotrypsin is found in nearly every case; lipase is less common.[70,290-295] The ductal elements, present in 50% to 65% of cases, express glycoprotein markers such as CEA, B72.3, and DUPAN-2.[70,291,292,296,297] Finally, endocrine markers chromogranin and synaptophysin are positive in two thirds of cases in a highly variable proportion of the cells.[70,296,297] Staining for islet peptides (insulin, glucagon, or somatostatin) is generally not found.[292] Immunohistochemical positivity for AFP has been detectable in cases with elevations in the serum levels of AFP.[292,298]

Morular formations that are referred as "squamoid corpuscles" are characteristic and entity-defining features of pancreatoblastoma, present in nearly every case. Immunohistochemical evaluation of the squamoid corpuscles has failed to define a reproducible line of differentiation for this component.[292] In fact, both by morphology and immunophenotype, they show more striking similarities to morules seen in tumors like endometrial carcinoma, pulmonary endodermal tumor, and cribriform-morular variant of papillary thyroid carcinoma, all of which are associated with β-catenin alteration just like squamoid corpuscles of pancreatoblastomas. In fact, the abnormal nuclear immunolabeling pattern for β-catenin is most prominent in squamoid corpuscles than other cell types that occur in pancreatoblastomas (Fig. 15.18). Squamoid corpuscles are also positive for EMA, which accentuates their similarities with meningothelial whorls. CEA can be focally

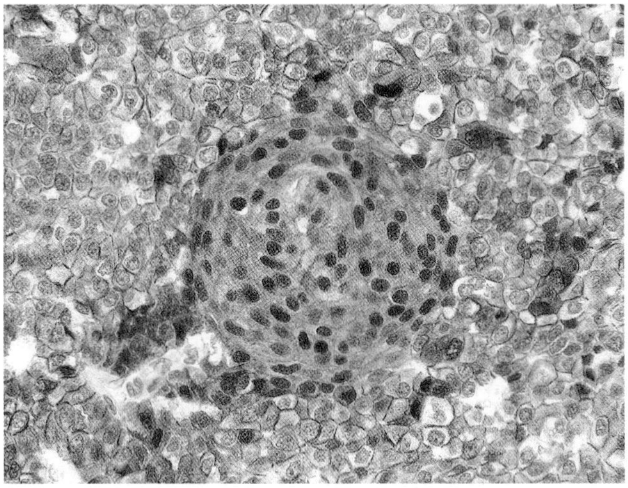

FIGURE 15.18 An abnormal cytoplasmic and nuclear immunolabeling pattern for the product of the β-catenin gene *(CTNNB1)* is seen in most pancreatoblastomas, predominantly in the squamoid corpuscles. Other areas usually display normal membranous immunolabeling.

positive[292] and so can CK8, CK18, and CK19, but not CK7.[293]

Genomic Applications of Immunohistochemistry

The distribution pattern of the β-catenin immunolabeling is characteristic for pancreatoblastomas. The acinar/ductular elements show mostly membranous (normal) expression of β-catenin, whereas the squamous corpuscles display diffuse nuclear/cytoplasmic (abnormal) expression (see Fig. 15.18) and overlapping cyclin D1 overexpression (>5% of tumor cells positive).[299,300]

Beyond Immunohistochemistry: Anatomic Molecular Diagnostic Applications

The most common genetic alteration identified to date is LOH of the highly imprinted region of chromosome 11p near the *WT2* gene locus.[301] Additionally, alterations in the adenomatous polyposis coli (APC)/β-*catenin* pathway have been reported in 50% to 80% of pancreatoblastomas.[299] Most often, these involve the β-catenin gene *(CTNNB1)*.[299,300] Unlike DAs, *TP53 and KRAS* mutations have not been detected.[284,299,301,302]

KEY DIAGNOSTIC POINTS

Pancreatoblastoma

- Most pancreatoblastomas show at least some labeling for acinar enzymatic markers (trypsin, chymotrypsin, and lipases).
- Endocrine and ductal markers are also often positive, but to a lesser degree, and positivity may be more focal.
- An abnormal nuclear and cytoplasmic immunolabeling pattern for the product of the β-catenin gene *(CTNNB1)* and overexpression of its target gene cyclin D1 is seen in most cases, usually in the squamoid corpuscles.

SOLID-PSEUDOPAPILLARY NEOPLASM

Solid-pseudopapillary neoplasm (SPN) is a peculiar tumor of indeterminate lineage. Although they have been described in all age groups, the mean age is 30. They are seen almost exclusively in females; however, they can also occur in males on occasion. Histomorphologically, SPNs typically show diffuse cellular proliferation of relatively bland cells admixed with variable degree of stroma. The preferential dyscohesiveness of the cells away from the microvasculature, presumably related to the alterations in cell adhesion molecules (β-catenin and E-cadherin), leads to the highly distinctive arrangement of cells that is referred as "pseudopapillary," although it is not present in all cases.[189] Eosinophilic globules composed of α_1-antitrypsin might also be seen. SPNs are low-grade malignancies that are curable with complete removal in 85% of the cases. No reliable criteria recognize the remaining 15% that will spread to the peritoneum or liver, but typically even these patients experience a protracted clinical course.

Despite intensive study, the line of differentiation of these neoplasms remains uncertain.[70,303-305] Both acinar and ductal markers, discussed previously, are consistently negative in SPN.[70,306,307] The tumors are also consistently negative for chromogranin. In only 5% of SPNs, there is focal chromogranin expression. The literature reflects conflicting data on this issue, but all experts now agree that if a tumor shows substantial chromogranin expression, it is not an SPN.[70,306,308,309] Peptide hormones are also usually negative or at most focally positive.[70,303-305,310,311] SPNs also fail to show any convincing neurosecretory granules by electron microscopy, which further corroborates that these are nonendocrine neoplasms. However, these tumors commonly react with some of the so-called neuroendocrine markers, synaptophysin, NSE, and neural cell adhesion molecule (NCAM or CD56).[70,303-306,309,311-321]

Even epithelial nature of SPN is dubious, although it has been referred to as "carcinoma" in the past. Cytokeratins (CAM 5.2, AE1/AE3) and other epithelial markers are typically either negative or only very focal in rare cases. Ultrastructural evidence of epithelial differentiation is also lacking. However, the neoplastic cells express vimentin and α_1-antitrypsin diffusely and strongly.[70,303-306,309,311-321] Another marker consistently expressed in SPN is CD10; however, this marker should be used cautiously in the differential diagnosis because DAs and PENs can also stain for CD10 (also known as common acute lymphocytic leukemia antigen, CALLA).[24,322] Progesterone receptors are also expressed in SPNs, regardless of whether it is in women or men.[314,317,323,324] Recently, C-kit (CD117)[325] and FLI-1[326] expressions have been reported in a portion of SPNs. SPNs usually do not stain with S-100,[70] calretinin,[327] or AFP.[306] IHC is summarized by immunohistogram in Table 15.3.

Genomic Applications of Immunohistochemistry

Greater than 90% of SPNs have mutations in exon 3 of the β-catenin gene *(CTNNB1)*.[2,67,68] In those cases not showing exon 3 mutations that would account

TABLE 15.3 Immunohistogram of Solid-Pseudopapillary Neoplasm with Selected Antibodies

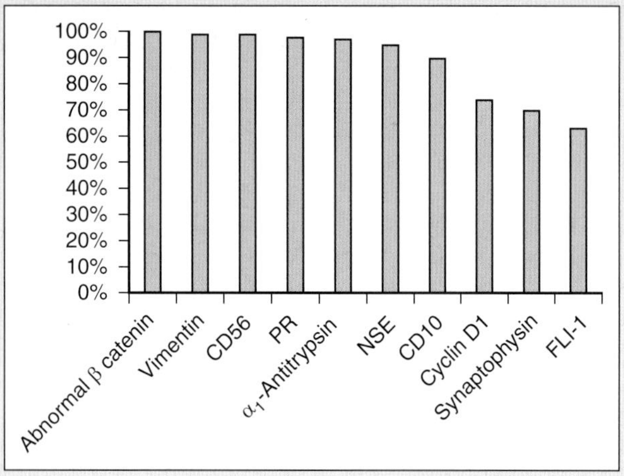

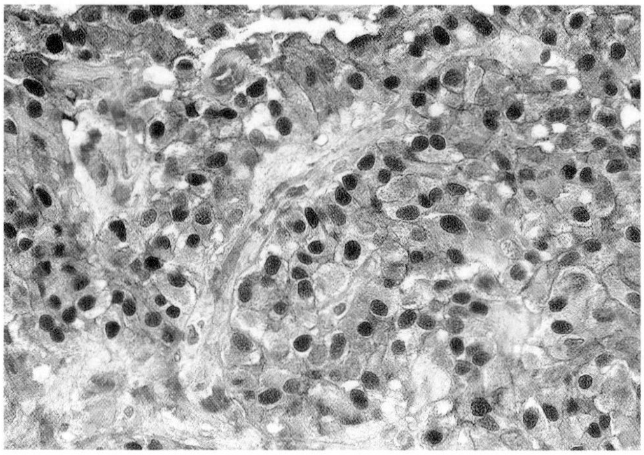

FIGURE 15.19 Solid-pseudopapillary neoplasm with diffuse cytoplasmic and nuclear β-catenin labeling.

for the remaining 10% of cases, it is likely that mutations are present in other exons.[24] Therefore 100% of SPNs show an abnormal cytoplasmic/nuclear pattern of labeling with antibodies to the β-catenin protein (Fig. 15.19).[314,318,326,328] This suggests a β-catenin gene *(CTNNB1)* mutation activating the Wnt-signaling pathway, which results in overexpression of cyclin D1 in the pathogenesis of these tumors.[90,218,247,315,318,319,329] In fact, in more than two thirds of the cases, a concomitant cyclin D1 expression is also seen.[318,319] In addition, through a mechanism that is not yet clear, the disruption of β-catenin interferes with E-cadherin and, as a result, using an E-cadherin antibody to the extracellular domain of the molecule illustrates complete membrane staining loss, whereas the antibody directed to the cytoplasmic fragment produces distinct nuclear staining of the tumor cells in virtually all cases.[23,326,330] This loss of E-cadherin may be responsible for the distinctive dyscohesiveness of the cells that creates the characteristic (and entity/name-defining) pseudopapillary appearance. Thus the most common genetic alterations in SPNs, β-catenin gene mutations, both help explain the poor cohesion of the neoplastic cells and provide a useful diagnostic tool-immunolabeling for β-catenin protein.[24,140]

The expression of CD56, progesterone receptor, and FLI-1, all located on chromosome 11q, has also been interpreted as evidence that chromosome 11q might be involved in a translocation or mutation that leads to the expression of some or all of these three proteins in SPNs.[326,331]

Beyond Immunohistochemistry: Anatomic Molecular Diagnostic Applications

In contrast to DAs, alterations in the *KRAS, p16/CDKN2A, TP53,* and *SMAD4/DPC4* genes have not been reported in SPNs. Besides, SPNs almost always exhibit β-catenin gene *(CTNNB1)* mutations.[218,247,313,315,318,328]

KEY DIAGNOSTIC POINTS

Solid-Pseudopapillary Neoplasm (SPN)

- Abnormal cytoplasmic/nuclear expression of β-catenin, as well as loss of membrane staining and/or abnormal nuclear staining for E-cadherin, combined with CD10 and progesterone receptor positivity, can be used to confirm the diagnosis of SPN even in small biopsy specimens.
- Diffuse and consistent immunoreactivity for vimentin and α_1-antitrypsin is also helpful.
- Nonspecific endocrine markers synaptophysin, CD56, and NSE are consistently positive in SPNs; however, the most specific endocrine marker, chromogranin, is consistently negative in SPNs.
- Cytokeratins (CAM 5.2, AE1/AE3) are usually negative or very focal and/or weak.

KEY DIFFERENTIAL DIAGNOSIS

Solid-Pseudopapillary Neoplasm (SPN)

SPN versus pancreatic endocrine neoplasia (PEN):

- Cytoplasmic/nuclear expression of β-catenin is consistent in SPN but uncommon in PENs. In contrast, most PENs show diffuse strong labeling for chromogranin and keratins, whereas virtually all SPNs are negative for these markers.
- Strong positivity of vimentin and progesterone receptors is also more common in SPNs than PENs.
- Synaptophysin, NSE, and CD56 are expressed consistently in both tumors and thus cannot be used in this differential diagnosis.

SPN versus ACC versus pancreatoblastoma:

- Expression of acinar enzymes, trypsin and chymotrypsin, coupled with diffuse keratin positivity, are diagnostic of ACCs and also present in pancreatoblastomas.
- Nuclear β-catenin expression and positivity of α_1-antitrypsin and antichymotrypsin (not to be confused with trypsin and chymotrypsin) are common to all three tumors and cannot be used in this differential.

Endocrine Neoplasms

Focal endocrine differentiation, especially in the form of scattered cells, is quite common in pancreatic neoplasia of ductal and acinar nature and is of no known biologic significance. However, if a tumor is predominantly composed of cells with endocrine lineage, it is classified as "endocrine."[3]

PANCREATIC ENDOCRINE NEOPLASMS

Pancreatic endocrine neoplasms (PENs) are the majority of the endocrine neoplasms in the pancreas.[332] Most PENs are sporadic. However, these tumors also constitute one of the major components of the multiple endocrine neoplasia I (MEN1) syndrome or may arise in patients with vHL syndrome. Those that are associated with increased serum levels of hormones and lead to corresponding symptoms are referred to as "functional" and are named according to which hormone they secrete (e.g., insulinoma—42% of all functional variants, gastrinoma—24%, glucagonoma—14%, VIPoma—10%, somatostatinoma—6%). Interestingly, the amount of hormone detected immunohistochemically in the tumor cells does not necessarily correlate with the functionality status.[289] Thus usage of hormone panel routinely in the diagnosis of PEN is a debated issue. Suffice it to say that serologic analysis or symptoms and signs of the tumor override the immunohistochemical findings in this regard. The tumor cells mimic the islet cells by forming nests, trabecules, and gyriform patterns and show the typical endocrine cytologic features including round monotonous nuclei, salt and pepper chromatin, and moderate amount of cytoplasm.[4,162]

Almost all PENs label for at least one of the endocrine differentiation markers such as chromogranin, synaptophysin, NSE, neural cell adhesion molecule (NCAM or CD56), and leu-7 (CD57).[333-349] Among these, chromogranin, the most specific endocrine marker, is detected in 85% to 95% of PENs. Synaptophysin is more consistently and diffusely expressed than chromogranin, but unfortunately it is less specific. For example, SPN, the main tumor in the differential diagnosis, is commonly positive for synaptophysin, as well as NSE and CD56.

Studies have shown that, in addition to the conventional peptide hormones of pancreatic islets (insulin, glucagon, somatostatin, and pancreatic polypeptide),[350,351] these tumors can also secrete (and express) ectopic peptides, in particular gastrin[350-352] and VIP (vasoactive intestinal peptide),[350-352] but on occasion also ACTH (adrenal corticotropic hormone),[353] antidiuretic hormone (ADH), MSH (melanocyte-stimulating hormone), calcitonin, neurotensin, secretoneurin,[267,354-356] PTH (parathyroid hormone-like peptide),[357] growth hormone and growth hormone releasing factor,[358-360] secretogranin II,[338] inhibin/activin,[361] prohormone convertases 2 and 3,[362] metallothionein,[363] and somatostatin receptors.[364] The pattern of labeling for these hormones varies widely.[350,365,366] It is common to demonstrate the production of more than one hormone in a single PEN. However, only occasionally does a true PEN produce detectable serotonin.[367] Therefore for practical purposes, a serotonin-producing tumor should be regarded as a carcinoid, and if it is in the pancreas, the possibility of metastasis from the GI tract or elsewhere ought to be ruled out.

TABLE 15.4 Immunohistogram of Pancreatic Endocrine Neoplasm with Selected Antibodies

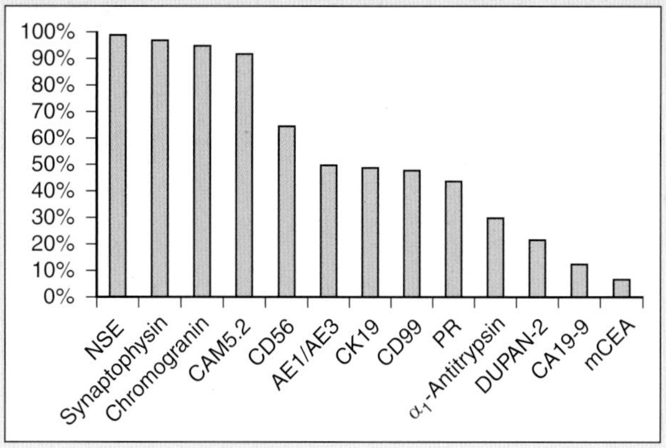

Most PENs also stain with CAM 5.2, CK8, and CK18 and approximately half with AE1/AE3. In general, the degree of keratin expression is weaker than it is in acinar and ductal tissue.[368-370] CK7 and CK20 are usually either negative or stain rare cells.[48,345,371,372] Scattered cells that are positive for acinar differentiation markers such as trypsin or chymotrypsin are commonly seen PENs.[373-375] If greater than 25% of the neoplastic cells in a predominantly endocrine neoplasm express markers of acinar differentiation, the neoplasm is classified as a "mixed acinar-endocrine carcinoma" by convention.[376] Limited experience suggests that these are more aggressive neoplasms, behaving like acinar carcinomas. PENs may also show labeling for glycoprotein markers of ductal differentiation. This may be encountered even in PENs with classical morphology and is not sufficient evidence for a diagnosis of "mixed ductal-endocrine carcinoma" unless a morphologically separate component of ductal adenocarcinoma is recognized.[4] Focal expression of DUPAN-2 or CA 19-9 is found in almost a quarter of conventional PENs.[373,374,377] CEA is much less commonly expressed. Some oncocytic PENs also label with hepatocyte paraffin-1 (Hep Par-1), which may be important in the differential diagnosis because these oncocytic PENs do resemble hepatocellular carcinomas.[378] Normal islet cells express progesterone receptors and CD99, but only some PENs retain expression of these markers.[373,379,380] The immunohistogram in Table 15.4 summarizes pancreatic endocrine neoplasms.

PENs are low- to intermediate-grade malignancies, but it is somewhat difficult to predict which examples are more prone for recurrence and metastasis. In the WHO classification, a constellation of clinical and microscopic findings (metastasis, extrapancreatic spread, size, mitotic activity, vascular/perineural/capsular invasion and Ki-67 [MIB-1] labeling index) is used to classify these tumors into prognostic categories as "tumor with

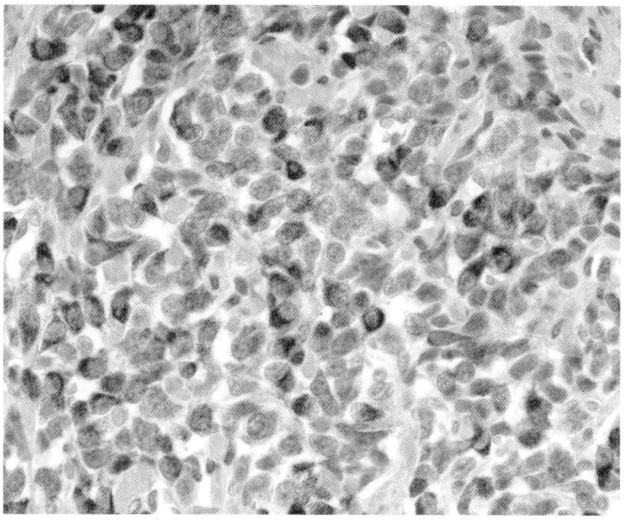

FIGURE 15.20 CK19 staining in pancreatic endocrine neoplasms is considered, by some authors, to be an independent predictor of aggressive behavior.

benign behavior," "tumor with uncertain behavior" and "carcinoma." A Ki-67 labeling index of more than 2% of the cells is considered an independent criterion to place the tumor into "uncertain behavior" rather than "benign behavior" category. Recently, it has been proposed to classify PENs on the basis of the Ki-67 labeling index of less than 2% as grade 1, 2% to 20% as grade 2, and greater than 20% as grade 3. If Ki-67 labeling index is high (>40%), the case ought to be reevaluated for the possibility of a different type of cancer or a poorly differentiated neuroendocrine carcinoma. Recently, several studies from various institutions have also shown that CK19 staining (Fig. 15.20) may serve as another reliable, independent predictor of aggressive behavior.[368,369] This has not yet been incorporated into the classification schemes, but many experts perform this stain routinely and report it in a comment. Functionality status has also been traditionally used as a prognostic parameter. It has been well documented that most insulinomas behave in a benign fashion and most glucagonomas exhibit a malignant course. However, it is now widely accepted that this association is through the stage of the tumor: Most insulinomas manifest early with symptoms and signs (Whipple triad: symptoms of hypoglycemia, low serum glucose, and relief of symptoms with glucose administration) before they achieve a size of 2 cm, whereas many glucagonomas are large and metastatic at presentation.

Other markers are under intense scrutiny as predictors of outcome in PENs. Chetty and colleagues[23,25] recently reported that aberrations of β-catenin (decrease in membranous staining compared with normal and/or abnormal cytoplasmic/nuclear staining) and E-cadherin expressions (decrease in membranous staining compared with normal and/or abnormal nuclear staining) occur in greater than 50% of PETs. They also showed that PENs with aberrant β-catenin and E-cadherin expressions tend to be larger than those with normal staining patterns and most of the cases with lymph node and liver involvement show concordant β-catenin and E-cadherin abnormal immunoexpression.[23,25,369] Whether or not these markers may be of use in identification of PENs with a potential for spread and hence poor outcome has yet to be fully characterized.

Beyond Immunohistochemistry: Anatomic Molecular Diagnostic Applications

Cytogenetic and molecular genetic studies have identified many chromosomal alterations in PENs (chromosomal losses are more common than gains).[381-383] Furthermore, a dominantly inherited defect in the *MEN1* gene has been described in patients with the MEN1 syndrome. Spontaneous *MEN1* gene abnormalities also occur in about 20% of sporadic PENs,[90,384-392] although a greater proportion show chromosomal losses in the same genetic region (11q13). It is believed that many of these PENs arise from the mutation in one locus of *MEN1*, followed by LOH. PENs arising in patients with the vHL syndrome also usually show biallelic inactivation of the *vHL* gene.[393] The *vHL* gene is normal in sporadic PENs.[90]

In contrast to DAs, *KRAS*, *TP53*, and *SMAD4/DPC4* are not mutated in most PENs with the exception of *p16/CDKN2A* abnormalities.[90,281,386,394-396]

KEY DIAGNOSTIC POINTS

Pancreatic Endocrine Neoplasms (PENs)

- Almost all PENs label for at least one of the endocrine differentiation markers such as chromogranin, synaptophysin, NSE, neural cell adhesion molecule (CD56), and leu-7 (CD57).
- They can express any of the pancreatic hormones, as well as ectopic peptides. In some cases, there is more than one hormone expressed. If an IHC "hormone panel" is to be used, the six hormones cover the vast majority of the cases: insulin, glucagon, somatostatin, PP, gastrin, and VIP; however, hormone IHC in the tumor does not necessarily correlate with the "functionality" status in all cases. Discrepancies do occur, and therefore serology and symptomatology are more reliable in classification of "functionality" status.
- For practical purposes, a serotonin-producing tumor should be regarded as a carcinoid, and if it is in the pancreas, the possibility of metastasis from the gastrointestinal tract or elsewhere should be ruled out.
- If greater than 25% of the neoplastic cells in a predominantly endocrine neoplasm express markers of acinar differentiation such as trypsin or chymotrypsin, the neoplasm should be classified as a "mixed acinar-endocrine carcinoma."
- Ki-67 labeling index is an important part of grading and classification of PENs.
- CK19 immunolabeling is also widely accepted to have prognostic significance.
- Normal islet cells are prone to bind antibodies nonspecifically,[21] and conceivably, the same problem may also exist for neoplastic endocrine cells. Therefore caution should be exercised before classifying islets (and PENs) as positive for any marker that is not verified by Western blot or other confirmatory methods.

KEY DIFFERENTIAL DIAGNOSIS

Pancreatic Endocrine Neoplasms (PENS)

- **Primary pancreas versus primary gastrointestinal tract versus primary lung neuroendocrine neoplasms:** Well-differentiated neuroendocrine (carcinoid) tumors of pulmonary and gastrointestinal origin show some morphologic similarities to PENs. Thus predicting the site of origin in a metastatic site may require aid from immunohistochemistry. The following facts have been reported[397,398]:
  - Nuclear expression of pancreatic duodenal homeobox-1 (PDX-1) and neuroendocrine secretory protein-55 (a new addition to the chromogranin family, NESP-55), especially if coupled with negative CDX-2 and TTF-1, would favor pancreatic origin.
  - Positivity of CDX-2 in the absence of PDX-1, NESP-55, and TTF-1 is highly in favor of a carcinoid of gastrointestinal primary.
  - TTF-1 positivity is compatible with pulmonary origin; however, it is not necessarily present in all lung neuroendocrine neoplasms.
  - Distinguishing full-blown PENs from reactive megaislets (up to several millimeters) can be accomplished by hormone stains showing a more clonal distribution in PENs with one or two peptides, whereas non-neoplastic islets often show more regional distribution of several hormones, similar to normal islets.

POORLY DIFFERENTIATED NEUROENDOCRINE CARCINOMA

These highly aggressive and rapidly fatal tumors constitute less than 1% of all pancreatic endocrine neoplasms. They are so uncommon that some authors believe a poorly differentiated neuroendocrine carcinoma occurring in the pancreas is most likely a metastasis from an occult primary in the lung. However, there are proven cases of primary in this region.[4,399-401] Many are in fact of ampullary origin, and few are pancreatic.[4,399-401] Some are akin to small cell carcinomas as defined in the lung, but more commonly they resemble large cell neuroendocrine carcinomas such as those common in the lung or elsewhere in the GI tract.[162]

Although defined by morphology and not reliant on the immunophenotype, immunohistochemical labeling commonly reveals positivity for chromogranin and synaptophysin even in the most poorly differentiated neuroendocrine carcinomas of the pancreas. It may, however, be very focal (especially for chromogranin).[4] CD56 and CD57 are frequently strongly positive in a membranous pattern.[402,403] In some studies, in contrast to DAs and well-differentiated PENs, poorly differentiated endocrine carcinomas were found to express the cell adhesion molecule L1 (CD171).[404,405] Parallel to the degree of mitotic activity and necrosis, the Ki-67 labeling index also tends to be high in these tumors.

Primitive neuroectodermal tumor (PNET), a tumor that shares some cytologic features with small cell carcinoma but occurs in younger patients, stains immunohistochemically for CD99[406] and FLI-1.

EXTRAHEPATIC BILIARY TRACT (GALLBLADDER AND EXTRAHEPATIC BILE DUCTS)

Epithelial Neoplasms

ADENOMA AND PAPILLOMA

Most adenomas of the extrahepatic biliary tract (EHBT) occur in the gallbladder and are usually detected incidentally.[407] In contrast, those in the extrahepatic bile ducts (EHBDs) present with signs and symptoms of obstruction. They can be multifocal, especially those with a papillary architecture. On the basis of the growth pattern, they have been classified traditionally as *tubular, papillary,* or *tubulopapillary,*[408-410] although the relevance of this classification independent of the degree of dysplasia is debatable.[2]

Another subclassification is based on the cytoarchitectural resemblance to different parts of the GI tract: *Pyloric gland–type adenomas* demonstrate glands that are virtually indistinguishable from pyloric glands of the stomach or Brunner glands of the duodenum. *Intestinal-type adenomas* are classified as such owing to their striking histologic resemblance to colonic adenomas.[408-411] *Biliary-type adenomas* are quite rare and less well characterized. Those papillary lesions that have more cuboidal-shaped cells than intestinal-type adenomas may also be included into this category.[408-410]

Another recently proposed classification system, which pertains mainly to adenoma in the EHBDs, divides them into two categories on the basis of the predominant cytologic features: "columnar-cell" and "cuboidal-cell" types.[412] This is analogous to the *villous/intestinal* and *pancreatobiliary* subsets of pancreatic IPMNs, respectively.[196]

The immunophenotype of adenomas corresponds to their particular lineage of cellular differentiation.[2] Most adenomas are CK7 positive and some express mucin-related glycoproteins and oncoproteins such as MUC1 and CEA, which are typically confined to the apical membrane of the cells. MUC5AC is expressed in about 30% of cases.[413] MUC2 expression parallels the degree of columnar-cell change and *intestinal* differentiation, whereas MUC6 is characteristically positive in the cuboidal-cell pattern and in cases with *pyloric* or *biliary* differentiation.[412] *Pyloric gland–type adenomas* are reported to be consistently positive for MUC6, as well as other pyloric gland markers such as M-GGMC-1.[413] Neuroendocrine markers such as chromogranin and synaptophysin highlight scattered endocrine cells, which also often show expression of serotonin and, on occasion, other hormones. Estrogen receptors have been detected in more than 50% of adenomas.[414]

As in other organs, there is a spectrum of carcinomatous transformation that can occur in exophytic biliary neoplasms. Although adenomas, especially pyloric gland adenomas, are typically negative for p53, carcinomas arising from these lesions may acquire p53 expression. Ki-67 labeling index increases with the degree of dysplasia. Unfortunately, there are no established thresholds to assign the dysplasia into specific grades on the basis of immunohistochemistry alone. Furthermore, areas of regenerative atypia associated with ulceration also commonly express these markers at a higher level. The pattern and intensity of some membrane-bound glycoproteins such as MUC1 and CEA also change during carcinomatous transformation. Often, frank CIS or invasive carcinoma arising from these preinvasive lesions displays more intense and intracytoplasmic labeling with these antibodies, as opposed to luminal-membranous labeling in lesser lesions.

Beyond Immunohistochemistry: Anatomic Molecular Diagnostic Applications

Molecular alterations of gallbladder adenomas are fairly different than those observed in the conventional dysplasia-carcinoma sequence. Mutations of the *p53* gene are virtually nonexistent in gallbladder adenomas and only rarely detected in EHBD tumors.[415] In contrast, *p53* abnormalities are quite common in flat dysplasia and invasive carcinoma.[416] Similarly, mutation of the *KRAS* oncogene is detected in only 25% of gallbladder adenomas.[415] In contrast, mutations of the β-*catenin* gene, which are uncommon in invasive biliary carcinomas, have been detected in 60% of adenomas,[417] mostly the *pyloric gland type,* and less commonly the *papillary* or *intestinal types*.[417]

MUCINOUS CYSTADENOMA

This adenoma represents the biliary counterpart of pancreatic mucinous cystic neoplasm (see "Pancreas" earlier for details).[418]

DYSPLASIA

Dysplasia is reported in 40% to 60% of the patients with invasive adenocarcinoma in EHBT; however, the incidence of dysplasia outside the setting of invasive adenocarcinoma is difficult to determine. It is also clear that the frequency varies significantly between different populations and risk groups and parallels that of adenocarcinoma.[419,420] For example, incidence of gallbladder dysplasia is high in regions with a high incidence of carcinoma, and incidence of bile duct dysplasia is higher in cases of primary sclerosing cholangitis or anomalous union of pancreatobiliary ducts or choledochal cysts.[2]

Microscopically, dysplasia is characterized by the disorderly intraepithelial proliferation of atypical columnar, cuboidal, or elongated biliary-type cells. However, biliary epithelium has tremendous capacity to develop marked cytologic atypia secondary to injury that may, at times, be impossible to distinguish from a true neoplastic process.[2]

If used cautiously, immunohistochemistry can be employed as an adjunct in the differential diagnosis of reactive versus dysplastic lesions. Nuclear p53 expression is present in more than 30% of all dysplasia in the EHBT (Fig. 15.21) and the incidence and the degree of expression is significantly higher in high-grade lesions,[421] whereas p53 is relatively uncommon in non-neoplastic epithelium. On the other hand, it can be present in areas

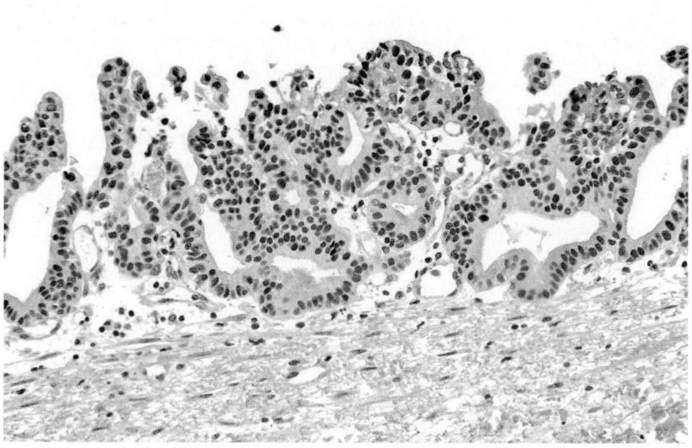

FIGURE 15.21 Immunohistochemical overexpression of p53 protein by dysplastic cells in gallbladder.

of marked regenerative changes as well, which limits its value as a sole diagnostic marker. Similarly, although Ki-67 labeling index is often substantially greater in dysplastic lesions and increases in quantity with increasing degrees of dysplasia, it can also be marked in areas of regenerative change.

INVASIVE ADENOCARCINOMA

Carcinomas of the gallbladder and extrahepatic bile ducts are rare.[2,422] They occur in elderly patients, seen predominantly in the seventh to eighth decades of life,[410] although those associated with primary sclerosing cholangitis tend to occur in younger patients. Most occur in the gallbladder, followed by the upper third of the EHBDs (above the cystic duct junction). There are well-established risk factors such as gallstones[423] for gallbladder cancer and parasitic infections[424] for EHBD carcinomas. The most common growth pattern is a scirrhous, gray-white, firm mass due to the prominence of desmoplasia.[410] Calculi are present in more than 80% of gallbladder cancers.[1,2]

EHBT carcinomas are similar, both morphologically and immunophenotypically, to other foregut carcinomas, namely pancreatic and gastro-esophageal cancers. Their similarity to pancreatic ductal carcinoma is such that they are often classified together as "pancreatobiliary-type" adenocarcinoma.[1] Mucin, in particular sialomucin,[425] nonsulfated, or neutral types, is demonstrable by histochemical or immunohistochemical stains in almost all cases and may be abundant.[1]

Immunohistochemically, CK7 is nearly always positive. CK20 may also be positive in some cases, which contrasts with intrahepatic cholangiocarcinomas that tend to be negative for CK20. Many surface-glycoproteins such as MUC1 and CEA (Fig. 15.22), normally limited to the apical membrane of the benign cells, are commonly detected in the cytoplasm of the adenocarcinoma cells.[1] For these markers, there appears to be a progressive increase in the level of expression from preinvasive to invasive and to poorly differentiated carcinomas, with dense intracytoplasmic expression detected mostly in advanced carcinomas. The tumors

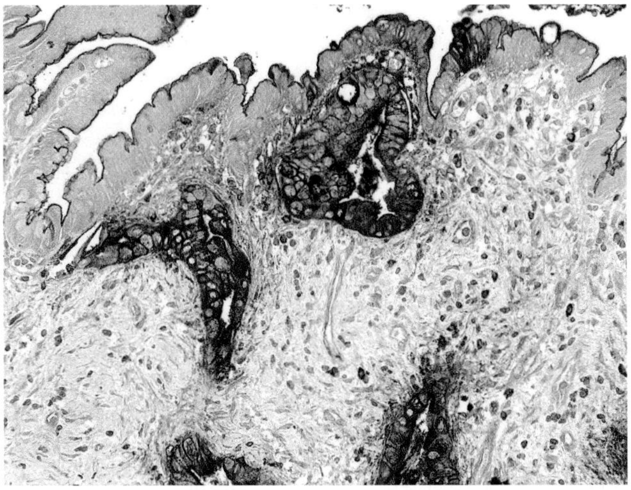

FIGURE 15.22 Carcinoembryonic antigen, which is generally limited to the apical membrane of the benign cells (surface), often shows intracytoplasmic staining in invasive carcinoma cells.

also usually express MUC5AC, CA19-9, B72.3, epidermal growth factor receptor, and pepsinogen I and II.[2,410,426] Estrogen receptors are only detectable in a small percentage of the cases.[414] Scattered endocrine cells, positive for chromogranin and synaptophysin stains, may also be found.[410]

Genomic Applications of Immunohistochemistry

In approximately 65% of the cases, there is positive immunoreactivity for the protein product of the *TP53* gene.[416,427] Some studies have shown this to be fairly specific for carcinoma, as opposed to non-neoplastic changes associated with primary sclerosing cholangitis[415]; however, it should be used cautiously because of significant overlap. Loss of DPC4, present in approximately half of pancreatic DAs, is almost as common in distal common bile duct carcinomas. However, DPC4 is retained in most proximal EHBD carcinomas.[428]

Beyond Immunohistochemistry: Anatomic Molecular Diagnostic Applications

Deletion of *p16* gene is observed in half of the gallbladder cancers[421,429,430] and is reported to be associated with a poor prognosis.[431,432] Although the frequency of KRAS mutations has differed widely in different studies, most investigators have found these mutations to be significantly higher in EHBD carcinomas than in gallbladder carcinomas.[427,433-437] Amplification of *HER2/neu* gene amplification is detected in half of the tumors as well.[438] Overexpression of *HER* family receptors including EGFR and c-met has also been reported.[439] Loss of pRB expression is rare in non–small cell gallbladder carcinoma but is common in small cell carcinoma of the gallbladder.[429] High-throughput microarrays have shown aberrant expression of several epithelial antigens such as mesothelin, prostate stem cell antigen, fascin, 14-3-3s, and topoisomerase II, as well as many peritumoral stromal proteins.[62] These have not yet been fully tested as diagnostic or prognostic markers.

KEY DIAGNOSTIC POINTS

Invasive Adenocarcinoma

Benign, noninvasive epithelium versus invasive carcinoma: Gallbladder adenocarcinomas may be deceptively bland appearing and, as such, may be difficult to distinguish from Aschoff-Rokitansky sinuses or Luschka's ducts. Although p53 and Ki-67 are significantly more common in neoplastic epithelium, overlaps are unfortunately too common for them to have a conclusive role in this distinction. Similarly, dense cytoplasmic expression of MUC1 and CEA is more characteristic of invasive adenocarcinomas. Unfortunately, this feature is not as evident in the more problematic well-differentiated carcinomas, in which the expression is more typically luminal membranous.

OTHER INVASIVE CARCINOMAS OF EXTRAHEPATIC BILIARY TRACT

Intestinal-type adenocarcinoma with all the features of conventional colonic adenocarcinomas is uncommon in the gallbladder; however, ordinary gallbladder adenocarcinomas, on occasion, may exhibit foci of columnar cells and pseudostratification and thus resemble intestinal carcinomas. Further complicating the issue, intestinal markers such as MUC2 and CDX2 may show some positivity in these tumors[1] and may be taken as further evidence of intestinal differentiation; however, it should be kept in mind that many classical foregut carcinomas also express these markers. It is advisable not to classify such cases as intestinal-type adenocarcinoma unless they exhibit all the characteristic morphologic features of colonic adenocarcinomas.[2]

Pure *mucinous (colloid) carcinomas* as seen in the breast, skin, or pancreas[182] are practically nonexistent in the gallbladder; however, mucinous carcinomas as described in the colon, in which the mucinous pattern constitute 50% to 90% of the tumor do occur.[440]

Hepatoid carcinomas showing many characteristics of hepatoid differentiation including positivity for hepatocyte-1 antigen (Hep Par-1), alpha feto-protein,[441] and a canalicular pattern with polyclonal CEA or CD10 may be seen, although uncommonly. However, unlike true hepatocellular carcinomas, they also express CK19 and CK20, which are more characteristic of biliary differentiation.[442,443]

Squamous differentiation is not uncommon in EHBT carcinomas, especially in the gallbladder. Most are focal and not reported. If the squamous areas constitute greater than 25% of the tumor, then the term *"adenosquamous"* is employed. By convention, even a small glandular component qualifies the tumor as adenosquamous, not squamous. The term *squamous cell carcinoma* is reserved for those rare "pure" examples, in which glandular elements cannot be documented by extensive sampling. The areas of squamous differentiation are typically positive for CK5/6, CK13, and nuclear p63, whereas glandular areas show CEA and B72.3 positivity.[2] In some studies, squamous/adenosquamous carcinomas of the gallbladder are reported to be associated with a better prognosis,[444,445] unlike those

branching architecture, and relatively smooth contours. Adenosquamous and squamous carcinomas of this region are rare. Similarly, sarcomatoid carcinomas are exceedingly uncommon.[1,410] The immunoprofile of these tumors is similar to their counterparts in the EHBT and pancreas as discussed in detail earlier.

GENOMIC APPLICATIONS OF IMMUNOHISTOCHEMISTRY

Mutations of *p53* have been detected in the majority of ampullary carcinomas with corresponding accumulation of the abnormal product as detected immunohistochemically.[461,462] EGFR is overexpressed in 50% to 65% of invasive ampullary carcinomas. Pancreatobiliary-type adenocarcinomas are more likely to overexpress EGFR than are intestinal-type tumors. Related growth factors c-erbB-2 and c-erbB-3 are also overexpressed in ampullary carcinoma.[410]

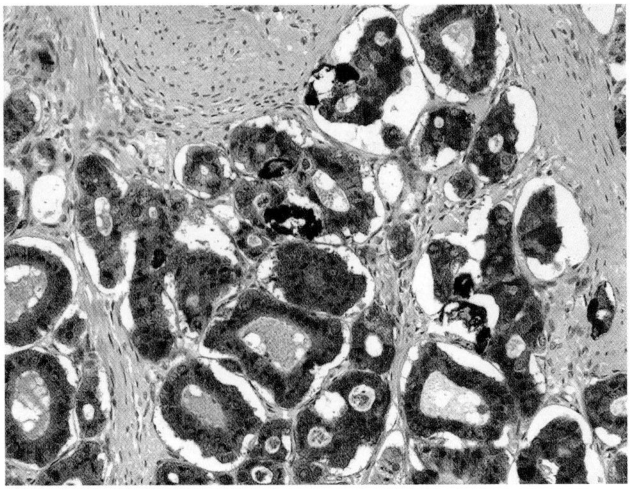

FIGURE 15.25 Diffuse and strong chromogranin positivity in ampullary somatostatinoma (glandular psammomatous carcinoid).

BEYOND IMMUNOHISTOCHEMISTRY: ANATOMIC MOLECULAR DIAGNOSTIC APPLICATIONS

Ampullary adenocarcinomas are less likely to show loss of *DPC4* gene expression[463] and *KRAS* gene mutations than pancreatic DAs,[464] probably corresponding to the incidences of these mutations in intestinal versus pancreatobiliary-type adenocarcinomas. Although rare, poorly differentiated ampullary carcinomas with morphologic features resembling medullary carcinomas of the large bowel have been reported to demonstrate microsatellite instability.[459]

KEY DIAGNOSTIC POINTS

Adenocarcinoma

- Most pancreatobiliary-type ampullary adenocarcinomas are CDX2−/MUC1+/MUC5AC+/MUC2−, and conversely, many intestinal-type ampullary adenocarcinomas are CDX2+/MUC1−/MUC5AC−/"MUC2+."
- CK7 is often strongly positive and CK20 more focal in pancreatobiliary-type ampullary adenocarcinomas, whereas intestinal-type ampullary adenocarcinomas tend to have more CK20 and less CK7.

Endocrine Neoplasms

A spectrum of endocrine differentiation may be seen in the ampullary region, which occurs in 3% of ampullary tumors.[410]

Most are *carcinoids*. Although the general characteristics of these are not too different from carcinoids elsewhere, there are some peculiarities worth mentioning. The majority of the "functioning" somatostatinomas occur in the ampulla. Moreover, whether functional or not, somatostatin-positive tumors of this region, in addition to the classical features of low-grade neuroendocrine neoplasms, also display tubule formation, focal intraluminal mucin, and psammomatous calcifications and may be associated with neurofibromatosis. This phenomenon is fairly specific to the ampulla.[465] All express diffuse and strong chromogranin (Fig. 15.25), synaptophysin, and somatostatin; however, they are not associated with the stigmata of somatostatin secretion, and therefore the term *glandular psammomatous carcinoid* of the ampulla is preferable to somatostatinomas. Other peptides may also be found. Even though lymph node metastasis is seen at presentation in more than 50% of the cases, surrogate signs of aggressiveness (high Ki-67 index and CK19 positivity) are not seen. Ki-67 index is typically low (<5%). Common S-100 expression is intriguing, especially considering the association with neurofibromatosis. Gland formation, intraluminal—but not intracytoplasmic—mucin, and infiltrative appearance may be mistaken as adenocarcinoma in small biopsies. Moreover, many cases show focal CA19-9 and CEA positivity.[465]

The ampulla is also included in the "gastrinoma triangle": Endocrine tumors associated with Zollinger-Ellison syndrome and multiple endocrine neoplasia-1 (MEN-1) are often localized in this region[410] and may be microscopic, and thus difficult to identify preoperatively and grossly.

High-grade neuroendocrine carcinomas may also be seen in the ampulla.[1,2] Although these account for an exceedingly small percentage of malignancies in the gastrointestinal tract, they appear to occur at a relatively higher proportion in the ampulla. Whether this is related to the abundance of endocrine cells seen also in the adenomas of this region is not known. Both small and large cell variants are recognized.[1]

Most high-grade neuroendocrine carcinomas are of the "small cell" type, similar to pulmonary small cell carcinoma. They tend to have a diffuse growth pattern. The tumor cells have minimal cytoplasm, indistinct cell borders, and polygonal nuclei having finely stippled chromatin and indistinct nucleoli. Some cases have more "large cell" phenotype with a more nested pattern and a moderate amount of cytoplasm. The nuclei are round and vesicular with often prominent nucleoli. High-grade neuroendocrine carcinomas are identified by brisk mitosis and easily identifiable necrosis. Cytokeratin and endocrine markers including chromogranin, synaptophysin, and NSE are often positive but may be focal and weak. As with their counterparts in other organs, these tumors are mostly defined by morphologic characteristics rather than detectability of neuroendocrine markers. CEA may be positive. Typically, Ki-67 labeling index is high, displaying positivity in the majority of the cells.[410] Loss of retinoblastoma protein is reported in 60% of high-grade neuroendocrine carcinomas but not in nonendocrine carcinomas. In contrast, loss of p27 is common in nonendocrine carcinomas but not in high-grade neuroendocrine carcinomas.[466]

KEY DIFFERENTIAL DIAGNOSIS

Endocrine Neoplasms of the Ampulla

- **High-grade neuroendocrine carcinoma versus carcinoid:** In general, there is more diffuse positivity for general neuroendocrine markers in carcinoid tumors. By definition,[467] proliferation markers such as Ki-67 are expressed significantly more commonly in high-grade carcinomas versus carcinoids.
- **High-grade neuroendocrine carcinoma versus lymphoma:** Immunohistochemical positivity for keratin and negative staining for lymphoid markers help exclude lymphoma.
- **High-grade neuroendocrine carcinoma versus poorly differentiated nonendocrine cancer:** By immunohistochemistry, the high-grade neuroendocrine carcinomas are positive for cytokeratins (AE1/AE3, CAM5.2, CK7, and in a lesser percentage CK20), similar to the pattern found in poorly differentiated nonendocrine carcinomas. However, if present, immunohistochemical expression of neuroendocrine markers is helpful in this regard. Also, loss of retinoblastoma protein expression, a characteristic finding in pulmonary small cell carcinomas, is present in almost half of ampullary high-grade neuroendocrine carcinomas. In contrast, p27 expression is lost in poorly differentiated nonendocrine carcinomas and retained in most high-grade neuroendocrine carcinomas.[466]

Duodenal Gangliocytic Paraganglioma

Duodenal gangliocytic paraganglioma is a lesion that is fairly specific to this area. It is a peculiar tumor of unknown origin that exhibits a mixture of (1) epithelioid (paraganglioma-like or carcinoid-like) elements, which are positive for keratins and neuroendocrine markers, chromogranin, synaptophysin, and NSE; (2) ganglion-like cells; and (3) spindle cells of nerve sheath,[10] which are negative for keratins, but express S100 instead. Specific peptides may also be found, especially pancreatic polypeptide and somatostanin.[410] The latter may be important in the differential from somatostatinomas because short of the ganglion-like and nerve sheath components, duodenal gangliocytic paragangliomas may be difficult to distinguish from glandular carcinoids (somatostatinomas) of this region.

LIVER

A wide variety of non-neoplastic (also referred to as "medical") and neoplastic diseases may affect the liver. Proper diagnosis of these entities is important because effective therapeutic options are becoming increasingly available including medical therapy for non-neoplastic diseases and resection for neoplastic diseases. In addition, liver transplantation has become an important modality for many chronic conditions. Immunohistochemistry (IHC) has an important role in the diagnosis of liver diseases. As discussed later, IHC can be useful in identifying hepatic infections, evaluating transplant biopsies, and classifying hepatic tumors. IHC has also been instrumental in elucidating the pathogenesis of many disorders of the liver.

Normal Hepatic Parenchyma

HEPATOCYTES

Embryonal hepatocytes contain cytokeratins (CK) 8, 18, and 19; however, mature ones contain only CK8 and 18, with CK19 being negative by the tenth week of gestation. CAM5.2 stains hepatocytes in the periportal zones and adjacent to venules. CK7, 19, and 20 are negative, as is epithelial membrane antigen (EMA) and vimentin. Although often not detectable in normal hepatocytes, α-fetoprotein can be positive in cirrhotic nodules.[46,468-474] Hepatocytes have significant amounts of biotin, which may lead to positive staining with standard immunohistochemical techniques if the endogenous biotin activity is not blocked, which is a major potential problem of "false positivity."[475-477] Hep Par-1 (human hepatocyte paraffin-1) stains hepatocytes in a diffuse granular cytoplasmic pattern without canalicular accentuation.[478-480] Thyroid transcription factor also stains the cytoplasm of hepatocytes in a coarsely granular pattern but does not stain the nuclei.[480] Bile canaliculi can be highlighted by a variety of antibodies against luminal-membranous glycoproteins such as polyclonal CEA and CD10.[473,481]

Bile Ducts

Intrahepatic bile ducts and peribiliary glands stain for cytokeratins 7, 8, 18, 19, 34βH11, 34βH12, and AE1/AE3.[468-470,479,482] CK20, CA19-9, and CEA are generally negative.[46,483]

Vasculature

The expression of many endothelial markers including CD34, factor VIII, CD31, or *Ulex europaeus* lectin is fairly weak in normal vasculature, whereas it can become quite prominent in pathologic conditions such as chronic liver disease and hepatocellular carcinoma.[473,484-486]

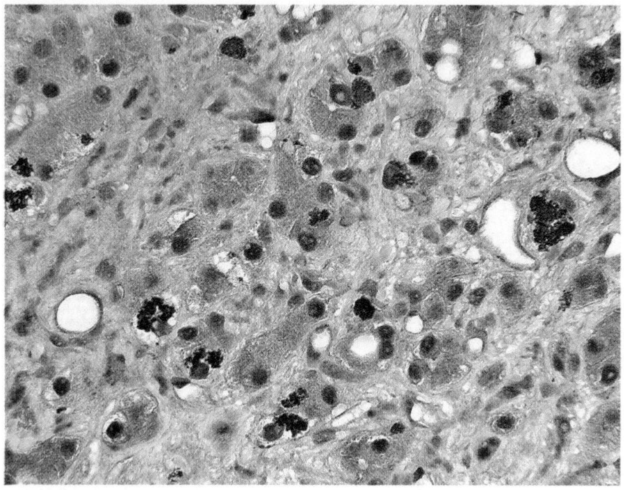

FIGURE 15.26 Ubiquitin immunohistochemistry demonstrating Mallory hyalines.

Interstitium

The interstitial matrix of the liver is composed of collagens, glycoproteins, proteoglycans, and glycosaminoglycans. Alterations in the extracellular matrix of the liver play an important role in fibrosis and the stromal milieu of both neoplastic and non-neoplastic processes. Type I collagen is the main collagen of portal tracts and in fibrotic liver and appears as thick, deep blue fibers on trichrome stains. Newly formed collagen is often composed of collagen type III and appears as fine, light blue fibers. Hepatic stellate cells have an important role in mediation of hepatic interstitial fibrosis and remodeling.[487-500] In some studies, they have been shown to have features of neural/neuroectodermal differentiation and stain with antibodies to synaptophysin, glial fibrillary acidic protein (GFAP), and neural cell adhesion molecule (N-CAM).[473,501-503] Activated stellate cells often acquire myofibroblastic features and show expression of vimentin, desmin, and smooth muscle actin.[473,504]

Medical Liver Diseases

STEATOHEPATITIS AND MALLORY'S BODIES

First described in alcoholic patients by Frank B. Mallory in 1911, Mallory hyalines/bodies also appear in other chronic liver diseases.[505] Sometimes they can be difficult to distinguish on biopsies, and ancillary immunohistochemistry with keratins CK18, 34βE12, and CAM5.2, as well as antibodies to ubiquitin (Fig. 15.26), may help by highlighting them. They are also occasionally positive for CK7 and CK19.[473,506,507]

VIRAL INFECTIONS

Viral infections may lead to hepatitis, which may become chronic, eventually leading to cirrhosis. In these infections, there is usually some degree of inflammatory mononuclear infiltrate in portal tracts, interface hepatitis, and lobular inflammation; however, since the inflammation is variable and does not always parallel the infectious activity, immunohistochemistry may need to be employed in highlighting infected hepatocytes. In chronic hepatitis B (HBV), infected ground-glass hepatocytes can be appreciated and confirmed by cytoplasmic staining for the hepatitis B surface antigen (HBsAg). Membranous staining for HBsAg is often indicative of active viral replication (Fig. 15.27A). Detection of HBsAg usually denotes chronic hepatitis because it is usually not detected in acute hepatitis. Hepatitis B core antigen (HBcAg) reactivity, on the other hand, which is usually appreciated in the nucleus (Fig. 15.27B) rather than in the cytoplasm, is used to measure the degree of viral replication. Patients who are immunocompromised or have received HBV through vertical transmission have both membranous HBsAg and nuclear HBcAg staining without a great deal of inflammation.[508-512] Hepatitis B immunohistochemistry may be particularly useful in identification of recurrent HBV after transplant for chronic HBV infection.[513] Delta virus, or hepatitis D, can also be detected immunohistochemically with cytoplasmic and nuclear staining.[509,514,515] It has been difficult to develop immunohistochemical antibodies that accurately detect hepatitis C virus (HCV) that can be applied on routine clinical specimens.[509,516-521] *In situ* hybridization techniques to detect hepatitis B, C, and D have been developed and have shown some utility.[522,523] Epstein-Barr virus (EBV) infection can be detected both immunohistochemically and through *in situ* hybridization. This is of particular use in EBV-driven posttransplant lymphoproliferative disorders (PTLDs) and in lymphoepithelioma-like hepatocellular and cholangiocarcinomas, which are associated with EBV.[509,524-527] Cytomegalovirus (CMV) is another important infection that can involve the liver and be detected with CMV immunohistochemical stains[509,528,529] and *in situ* hybridization.[522] Other infections of the liver that can be detected immunohistochemically include herpes simplex virus, herpes zoster virus, adenovirus, mycobacteria, and amoebiasis.[509,530]

CIRRHOSIS

Cirrhotic nodules may acquire some staining for α-fetoprotein (AFP); however, macroregenerative nodules are typically negative[474,531] for this marker. In cirrhotic regenerative nodules, peripheral hepatocytes may show ductular transformation and express both cytokeratin 7 and 19.[506,532-534] It is speculated that this is evidence of a stem-cell phenotype,[535-538] and the focal expression of AFP is also interpreted to provide further evidence for this.[474,539] Endothelial cells at the periphery of cirrhotic nodules adjacent to fibrous septa also have an altered phenotype, expressing CD31 and CD34, a feature that may be seen in other conditions including nodular regenerative hyperplasia.[473,484-486]

PRIMARY BILIARY CIRRHOSIS AND SCLEROSING CHOLANGITIS

Cytokeratin immunohistochemistry directed toward biliary epithelium can be useful in highlighting bile ductular proliferations that occur in a variety of conditions

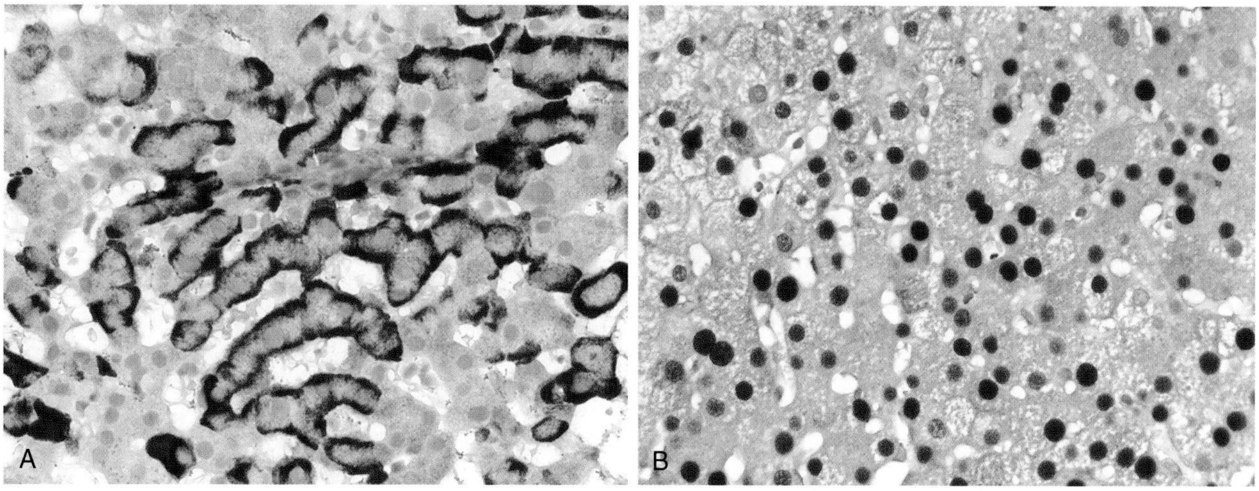

FIGURE 15.27 **A,** Hepatitis B surface antigen (HBsAg) immunohistochemistry showing both cytoplasmic and membranous positivity. **B,** Hepatitis B core antigen (HBcAg) immunohistochemistry showing nuclear positivity.

including primary biliary cirrhosis (PBC) and primary sclerosing cholangitis (PSC), regardless of the mechanism, whether it is a result of "ductular metaplasia" of limiting plate hepatocytes or primary proliferation of native ducts.[533,534] The utility of cytokeratin 7 in this context has been demonstrated.[540,541] Immunohistochemistry for endothelial markers such as CD31, CD34, factor VIII-related antigen, *Ulex europaeus,* and other lectins may also reveal differences in the microvasculature of the portal tracts in primary sclerosing cholangitis and primary biliary cirrhosis with the overall commonality to both disorders being a loss of capillary microvasculature. In PBC, vessels are often obliterated by granulomatous inflammation, whereas in PSC, the vessels are displaced by collagen deposits.[542-544] Recently, investigators have demonstrated that immunostaining of plasma cells with antibodies for IgM and IgG may be useful in the distinction between PBC and autoimmune hepatitis (AIH) with most of the plasma cells staining for IgM in PBC and most of the plasma cells staining for IgG in AIH. This parallels an increase in serum IgG that can be seen in AIH and increase in serum IgM that can be seen in PBC. However, it must be noted that IgG positive plasma cells can be seen in the liver in a number of disorders.[545]

IGG4-RELATED CHOLANGITIS

Recently lesions containing large numbers of immunoglobulin G4 (IgG4)-bearing plasma cells have been identified in a number of organs. Much interest has focused on the ones in the pancreas[546]; however, lesions of the intrahepatic and extrahepatic bile ducts may also contain large numbers of IgG4-bearing plasma cells. They are referred to by a number of descriptive names, notably IgG4-associated cholangitis (IAC), and may be confused with other lesions, particularly primary sclerosing cholangitis or autoimmune hepatitis. The lesions usually also contain prominent fibrous tissue in a stellate pattern with admixed inflammatory cells including lymphocytes and eosinophils. Obliterative phlebitis may be observed. The lesions may be quite florid with pseudotumor formation. Immunohistochemistry for IgG4 may be useful in properly categorizing these lesions.[546-552] The numeric threshold of IgG4-positive plasma cells required to place a lesion into this category has yet to be established. In the pancreas, this number has been advocated as a minimum of 10 per high-power field, with some authors requiring 20 or even 30.[553-558]

FOCAL NODULAR HYPERPLASIA

Focal nodular hyperplasia (FNH) is considered to be a hyperplastic reactive proliferation of hepatocytes due to localized abnormalities in blood flow. Classically, FNH has a central scar with radiating septa and hyperplastic hepatocyte nodules but is devoid of bile ducts. The diagnosis of FNH can be aided by CD34 immunohistochemistry, which highlights sinusoidal endothelial cells in the vicinity of fibrous septa in a linear pattern.[559,560] Hepatocytes at the periphery of cirrhotic-like nodules of FNH may stain with cytokeratins 7 and 19, and the cytokeratin 7 cells may be continuous with fibrous septa.[468,534]

Metabolic Disorders

Alpha-1-antitrypsin (α_1-AT) deficiency disease is associated with PAS-positive, diastase-resistant globules in the hepatocytes (Fig.15.28A). Immunohistochemical staining for α_1-AT may be useful in verifying the nature of these granules (Fig. 15.28B). In addition, early in α_1-AT deficiency, these globules may not be as visible and immunohistochemistry may be useful in highlighting α_1-AT (Fig. 15.28B). The α_1-AT stain may be positive as early as 19 weeks' gestation.[561-563]

Afibrinogenemia and hypofibrinogenemia (type I fibrinogen deficiencies) are rare congenital disorders in which plasma fibrinogen levels are low or immeasurable. Some cases of hypofibrinogenemia may actually be present as a "fibrinogen storage disease" in which

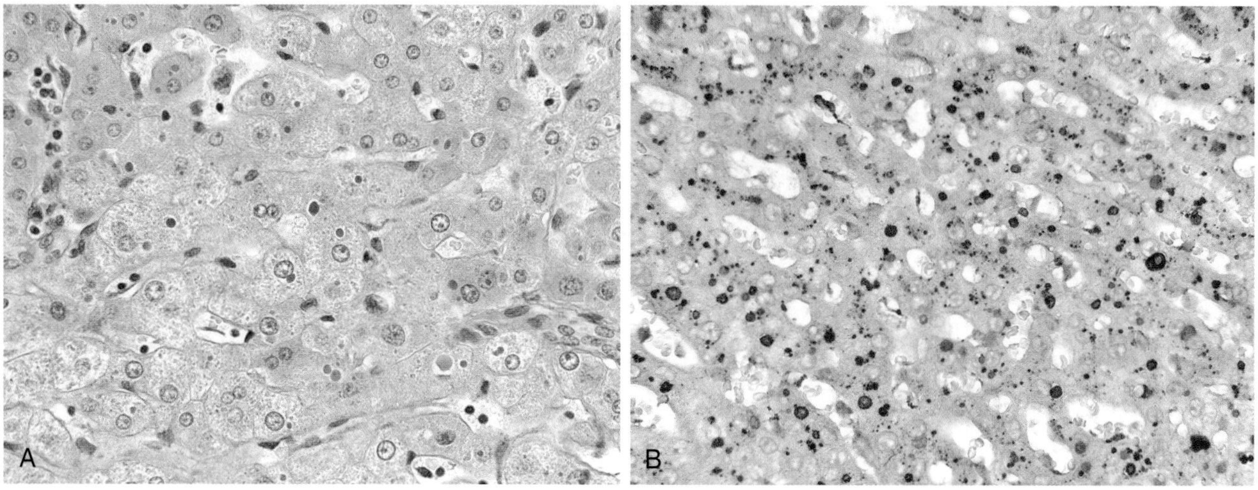

FIGURE 15.28 **A,** PAS/D stain showing prominent intracytoplasmic diastase-resistant globules. **B,** α_1-antitrypsin immunohistochemistry confirming that the globules contain α_1-antitrypsin.

fibrinogen is present in large quantities in hepatocytes, appreciable on routine stains as eosinophilic globules in hepatocytes, some of which have a dark core and some of which are vacuolated. Fibrinogen antibodies may be useful in determining that the intrahepatocytic material is fibrinogen.[563,564]

Liver Transplantation

Immunohistochemistry has two important applications in the evaluation of transplant biopsies: (1) identification of infectious agents and (2) determination of the mechanism (and thus etiology) of the immune injury. Immunohistochemistry for various organisms, particularly viral organisms, may be crucial in the interpretation of liver transplant biopsies. This may be particularly important for the identification of recurrent hepatitis B or C, as previously discussed.[565] Diagnosing liver allograft rejection, particularly antibody-mediated (humoral) rejection, can unfortunately be problematic. Immunohistochemistry for C4d, a marker frequently used in the interpretation of renal allograft biopsies, has been investigated in liver allografts, with mixed results.[566-581] Antibody-mediated rejection in the liver does appear to occur, as evidenced by antibody-mediated rejection of ABO incompatible livers. Deposition of C4d has been demonstrated in liver allografts and associated with decreased survival.[566] However, studies have pointed out different patterns of deposition of C4d in the liver including the following: stromal,[566] portal,[575,580] sinusoidal,[572,574,580] and hepatocytic pattern.[573,574]

Even though the sinusoidal and portal capillary endothelium patterns (Figs. 15.29A and 29B) seem to be most promising,[571,572,574] it is unclear which of these patterns actually has prognostic significance.[566]

This field, though yet imperfect, is in a rapid evolution, and there is no question that IHC will have an increasing role in the diagnosis of immune injury in the transplant setting in the future.

Neoplastic Liver Diseases

HEPATOCELLULAR NEOPLASMS

Hepatic Adenoma

Hepatic adenomas are benign tumors usually seen in women in their childbearing years. Long-term oral contraceptive steroid usage is a common risk factor. Grossly, the lesions are usually well demarcated and are yellow or tan, sometimes containing fibrosis, hemorrhage, or necrosis.[582] Microscopically, they are composed of plates of cells resembling normal hepatocytes separated by sinusoids. Immunohistochemically, estrogen and progesterone receptors are present in 75% of the lesions.[583] They might also express β-catenin.[584-586] This has also been observed in hepatocellular carcinomas associated with hepatitis C virus infection[582,587]; however, most hepatocellular carcinomas express glypican-3 and hepatic adenomas are negative for glypican-3.[588,589] Additionally, hepatocellular carcinomas typically show "complete" CD34 staining pattern (most sinusoidal spaces are CD34 positive throughout the lesion) and hepatic adenomas usually show "incomplete" staining (portal and periportal sinusoids are CD34 positive).[588]

Hepatoblastoma

Hepatoblastoma, the most common primary hepatic tumor in children, is a malignant tumor with embryonal features and divergent differentiation including striated muscle, fibrous tissue, and material resembling osteoid. Approximately one third of the cases have pure fetal epithelial differentiation resembling developing hepatocytes. The keratins expressed are generally of low-molecular-weight type (CK8 and 18, but sometimes also 19 and 7). Most tumor cells are also positive for EMA, vimentin, pCEA, Hep Par-1 and α-fetoprotein.[590,591]

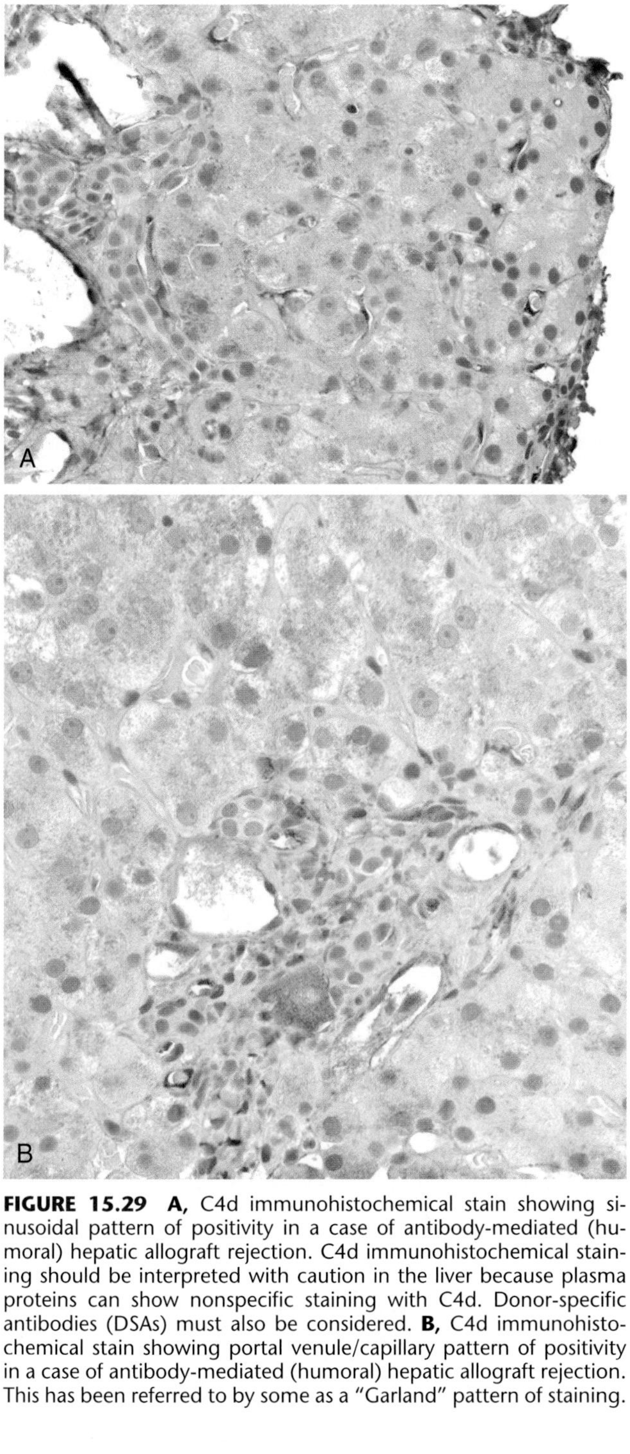

FIGURE 15.29 **A,** C4d immunohistochemical stain showing sinusoidal pattern of positivity in a case of antibody-mediated (humoral) hepatic allograft rejection. C4d immunohistochemical staining should be interpreted with caution in the liver because plasma proteins can show nonspecific staining with C4d. Donor-specific antibodies (DSAs) must also be considered. **B,** C4d immunohistochemical stain showing portal venule/capillary pattern of positivity in a case of antibody-mediated (humoral) hepatic allograft rejection. This has been referred to by some as a "Garland" pattern of staining.

Kupffer cells and endothelial cells lining sinusoids can be marked for UEA-1 and anti-CD34 in a pattern similar to HCC, more diffuse than normal liver.[591-593]

Hepatocellular Carcinoma

Hepatocellular carcinoma (HCC) is the single most common histologic type of epithelial primary liver tumor. Architecturally, HCC may have a number of different patterns, the most common being a trabecular or plate-like pattern. Other patterns include acinar, pseudoglandular, scirrhous, clear cell, spindle cell, and pleomorphic.[582]

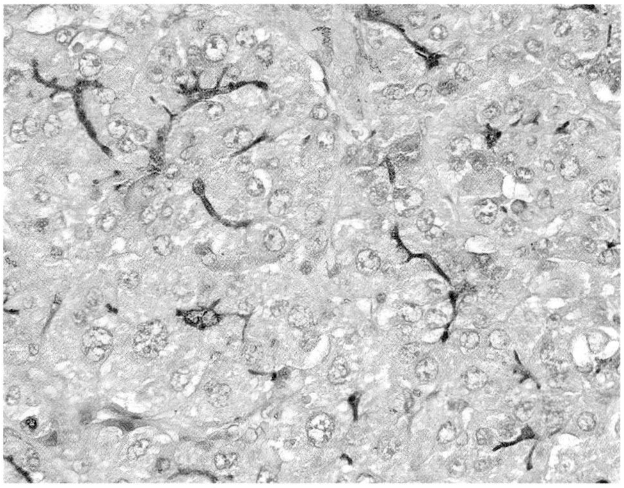

FIGURE 15.30 Polyclonal carcinoembryonic antigen positivity in hepatocellular carcinoma. Note the canalicular staining pattern.

CYTOKERATINS HCC reacts with antibodies directed against a variety of cytokeratins (CKs), particularly low-molecular-weight cytokeratins (CK8, CK18). Thus most HCCs stain with CAM 5.2 and 35βH11. They are usually negative for CK7, CK19, and CK20 or show patchy staining. AE1/AE3 is also typically patchy, but poorly differentiated HCCs often show clusters of positive cells.[41,46,594-599]

CARCINOEMBRYONIC ANTIGEN A canalicular staining pattern for polyclonal carcinoembryonic antigen (pCEA) is seen in 60% to 90% of HCCs[531,600] (Fig. 15.30) and is useful in discriminating hepatocellular tumors from other malignancies.[531,586] However, it should be remembered that abortive lumina formation in poorly differentiated adenocarcinomas can mimic canalicular pattern.

Hepatocellular carcinomas are nonreactive with monoclonal CEA, an important factor in the differential diagnosis with cholangiocarcinomas and metastatic carcinoma.[601]

HEP PAR-1 Hep Par-1 is an antigen reflecting hepatocytic differentiation (Fig. 15.31) and yields a diffuse cytoplasmic granular staining pattern in normal and neoplastic hepatocytes including approximately 80% to 90% of HCC cases. Therefore it is not useful for distinction of benign versus malignant hepatocellular lesions.[599] Hep Par-1 stains conventional adult HCC, as well as fibrolamellar and clear cell variants but not sclerosing HCC. Some investigators have reported decreased staining with more poorly differentiated HCC; however, this distinction is not completely clear. It should also be kept in mind that Hep Par-1 is not entirely specific for HCCs. It can be found in a variety of tumors, in particular those with oncocytoid morphology (abundant acidophilic, granular cytoplasm) including intraductal and cystic oncocytic neoplasia. Furthermore, rare carcinomas from the gastrointestinal tract and pancreas with hepatoid morphology (tumor cells with eosinophilic, granular cytoplasm) are positive for Hep Par-1.[472,479,531,586,599,602,603]

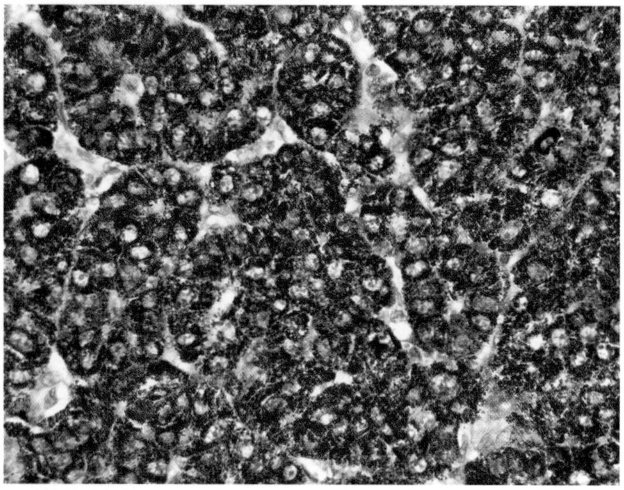

FIGURE 15.31 Hepatocellular carcinoma with positive Hep Par-1 immunohistochemistry.

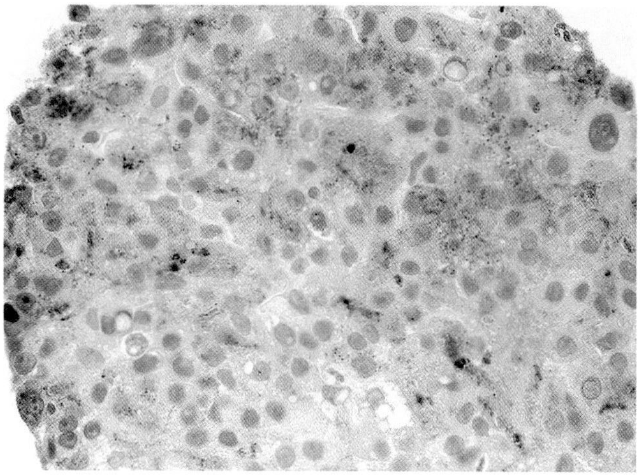

FIGURE 15.32 Hepatocellular carcinoma with focal glypican-3 staining.

GLYPICAN-3 Glypican-3 is a placenta and hepatic heparan sulfate proteoglycan, normally expressed in fetal liver but not in adult liver. Recently, much interest has been focused on its utility in the diagnosis of HCC. Because it is often negative in normal liver and adenomas,[588,589] it can be useful in distinguishing benign versus malignant hepatocellular lesions.[599] However, caution should be exercised in using glypican-3 in biopsy specimens because cirrhotic nodules can show positivity.[588,589,604]

Many studies have shown that glypican-3 is more sensitive than Hep Par-1 for HCC (Fig.15.32), particularly for poorly differentiated HCC,[589] and can be useful in the identification of poorly differentiated HCC. It is also used in the differential diagnosis of HCC versus cholangiocarcinoma (positive in 60% to 90% of HCCs and usually negative in cholangiocarcinomas).[588,589,599,604-608]

CD34 CD34, in conjunction with glypican-3, may be of some use in distinguishing HCC from its benign mimickers. Virtually all sinusoidal spaces in HCCs tend to have a "complete" staining pattern (most sinusoidal spaces are CD34 positive throughout the lesion), which is quite uncommon in benign lesions, with the exception of few hepatic adenomas and focal nodular hyperplasia.[588] If used selectively, this CD34 staining pattern may also be helpful in the distinction of HCC from adenocarcinomas. However, the sensitivity is low (20% to 40%) and because better antibodies are available, CD34 is not routinely used in this differential.[599]

ALBUMIN Albumin is a major serum transport protein synthesized by hepatocytes.[602] *In situ* hybridization (ISH) for the messenger RNA (mRNA) that encodes albumin shows positivity in non-neoplastic hepatocytes, as well as in hepatic adenomas, hepatoblastomas, and HCCs. Unfortunately, immunohistochemistry is not amenable to the detection of albumin because albumin is abundant in the serum, leading to nonspecific tissue staining. Up to 96% of HCC can show positivity with ISH, although staining can be diffuse, patchy, or focal.[592,602,609-613] One caveat is that other tumors including clear cell carcinoma of the ovary[614] and hepatoid carcinomas (e.g., hepatoid gastric and bladder carcinomas) are also positive.[609,615-618] Combination of albumin *in situ* hybridization and Hep Par 1 can yield 100% sensitivity for diagnosis of HCC.[613]

ALPHA-FETOPROTEIN α-Fetoprotein (AFP), an oncofetal glycoprotein, is frequently elevated in the serum of patients with HCC. Although high levels of serum AFP levels are fairly specific for HCC, some increase can also be seen in hepatitis and cirrhosis.[531,602,613,619] Its immunohistochemical expression in a tumor is specific for hepatocellular differentiation, but staining tends to be patchy and sensitivity is fairly low, 30% to 50%.[599] Moreover, serum increases and immunohistochemical staining of the tumor can be seen in cases of primary and metastatic hepatoid adenocarcinomas and yolk sac tumors as well.[620-622] Therefore AFP is a less useful option for diagnosis.[599,623]

MISCELLANEOUS MARKERS OF USE IN HEPATOCELLULAR CARCINOMA Thyroid transcription factor-1 (TTF-1), which is normally expressed in the nuclei of epithelial cells of thyroid and lung and in tumors that arise from them, shows cytoplasmic positivity in HCC (Fig. 15.33). Immunoreactivity varies with the antigen retrieval technique and the antibody clone used.[480,624,625] The significance of this cytoplasmic labeling and, in fact, whether it is "real" staining, is yet to be determined, but it can be of some value in identifying and differentiating HCC from some other carcinomas in select cases.

Epithelial membrane antigen (EMA) can be positive in 20% to 40% of HCC. There is some indication that higher-grade neoplasms have increased staining.[29,626-629]

CD10 (common acute lymphoblastic leukemia antigen, CALLA) can show a canalicular staining pattern similar to that of polyclonal-CEA in approximately half of HCCs.[531,600]

MOC-31 is a cell surface glycoprotein typically used as a marker of adenocarcinoma. Only a minority of HCC cases show labeling, often as weak staining, and studies show positivity in 0% to 20% of tumors.[602,630-632]

α_1-Antitrypsin (α_1-AT) can be positive in HCC with some studies indicating a high proportion (up to 86%) of HCC cases showing positivity.[633] However, this marker often shows some nonspecific labeling, which significantly limits its usability.

Factor VIII (FVIII) related antigen (von Willebrand Factor) positivity can be seen in sinusoidal endothelium in nearly all HCC cases, whereas the staining can be focal and even interpreted as being absent in normal livers. Some authors advocate the use of FVIII in conjunction with CD34.[486,634-638] Other studies have investigated similar patterns of the vascular endothelium in HCC with markers such as CD31, *Ulex europaeus* lectin, and ABH blood group antigens.[485,637,638] Unfortunately, these markers have not been found to be as reliable as CD34 in this regard.

Factor XIIIa (FXIIIa), a blood coagulation proenzyme, can be positive in histiocytes/macrophages and benign hepatocytes, as well as in HCC. Some have suggested that FXIII can be useful in differentiating HCC from cholangiocarcinoma, but other studies have indicated that FXIIIa is noncontributory in this differential diagnosis.[479,531,532,633]

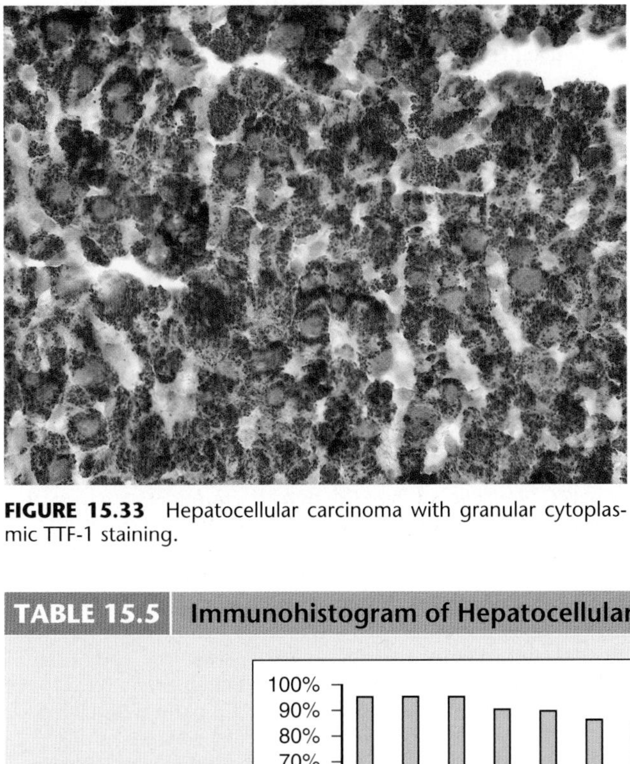

FIGURE 15.33 Hepatocellular carcinoma with granular cytoplasmic TTF-1 staining.

HCC may also react with antibodies directed against erythropoietin, C-reactive protein (CRP), acidic isoferritin, thioredoxin (RX), alkaline phosphatase, inhibin, α_1-antichymotripsin, and villin.[586,602] These markers are not widely used in routine practice.

Table 15.5 is an immunohistogram of selected antibodies for hepatocellular carcinoma.

Molecular and Genomic Applications of Immunohistochemistry

Immunohistochemical staining with various markers has been useful in elucidating potential explanations for the molecular pathogenesis of HCC. Nuclear accumulation of β-catenin, a component of the wingless/Wnt pathway, has been observed by immunohistochemistry in HCC. This correlated with mutations in the β-catenin gene, which were detected in 26% to 41% of HCCs,[582,587] particularly those associated with hepatitis C virus infections.[587] In addition, phosphoinositol 3-kinase/mammalian target of rapamycin (mTOR) pathway has been investigated in HCC using a number of methods including immunostaining. Investigators have also demonstrated the presence of microsatellite instability in HCC by both genetic molecular analysis and immunohistochemistry for the microsatellite markers (MLH1, MSH2, MSH6, and PMS2).[639-641]

Molecular insights into the pathogenesis of HCC may eventually guide therapy. Using everolimus (a rapamycin analog) to block mTOR signaling decelerated HCC tumor growth *in vitro* and in a xenograft model and increased survival.[642,643] Studies have shown that antibodies to molecules such as p53,[644-646] Ki-67,[644] and platelet-derived growth factor[647] may be useful in predicting prognosis in HCC.[644-647] In one study, platelet-derived growth factor receptor alpha (PDGFR-α) was found to be overexpressed in the endothelium of hepatocellular carcinoma with a high metastatic potential. In this study, STI571 (Gleevec, or imatinib mesylate) inhibited tumor growth, apparently through antiangiogenesis

TABLE 15.5 Immunohistogram of Hepatocellular Carcinoma with Selected Antibodies

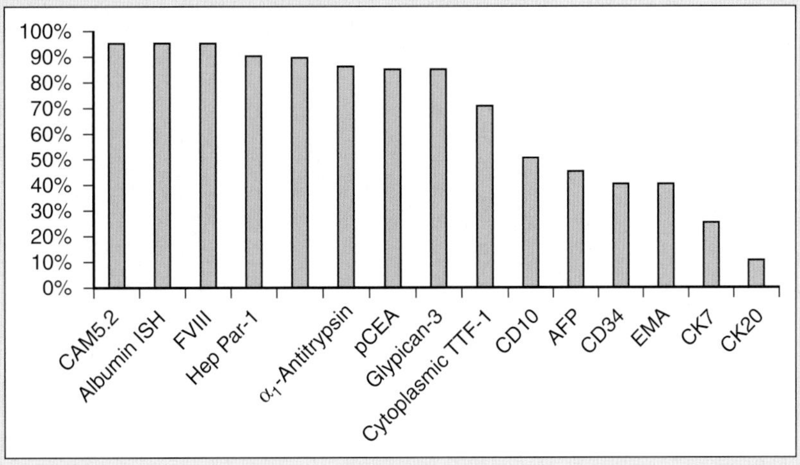

via inactivation of PDGFR-α, suggesting that PDGFR-α may serve as a biomarker for predicting metastasis and as a therapeutic target.[647] Much of this information, however, has not yet been fully verified and translated into daily practice.

Hepatocellular Carcinoma Variants

FIBROLAMELLAR HCC Fibrolamellar HCC is a distinct variant of HCC that occurs most often in noncirrhotic individuals from adolescence to young adulthood. It is characterized by sheets or trabeculae of neoplastic cells separated by collagen bundles in a lamellar configuration.[582] Tumor cells have granular eosinophilic (oncocytoid) cytoplasm and are large and polygonal. Fibrolamellar HCC has immunophenotypic similarities to the usual type of HCC[648]; however, unlike usual HCC, it may show strong CK7 expression.[649] Fibrolamellar HCC may sometimes stain with synaptophysin and on occasion focally even with chromogranin,[599,650,651] which complicates the differential diagnosis from neuroendocrine tumors. Increased expression of epidermal growth factor receptor (EGFR) may also be seen in fibrolamellar carcinoma, suggesting that treatment with EGFR antagonists may be considered in the future.[642,652,653]

SPINDLE CELL HCC High-grade/poorly differentiated HCC may have a spindle cell morphology.[582] Poorly differentiated HCC may be frankly sarcomatous with some cases having heterologous differentiation such as chondrosarcomatous.[654] Sarcomatous component often loses its epithelial differentiation and becomes negative for the conventional epithelial markers. In addition, they show the appropriate lineage markers reflecting their differentiation at histomorphologic level. For example, areas with chondrosarcomatous differentiation stain with S-100 and vimentin. However, some cells of the sarcomatous component also retain keratin in some cases.[654] Spindle cell carcinomas may also have osteoclast-like giant cells, in which case the osteoclast-like giant cells express histiocytic differentiation markers.[655]

CLEAR CELL HCC Clear cell HCC may be difficult to distinguish from other clear cell tumors such as adrenal cortical carcinoma and renal cell carcinoma using routine histology.[586] Renal cell carcinoma usually shows reactivity with vimentin, whereas only high-grade hepatocellular carcinoma or hepatocellular carcinoma with spindled morphology shows reactivity with vimentin.[586] Adrenal cortical carcinoma stains with Melan-A and inhibin, and hepatocellular carcinoma is usually negative with antibodies to these molecules. Furthermore, adrenal cortical carcinoma is negative for CAM 5.2.[586,656] Neuroendocrine carcinoma can sometimes have clear cell morphology. Neuroendocrine carcinomas are usually positive for synaptophysin and chromogranin, whereas HCC is usually negative for these markers.[586]

MEDULLARY (LYMPHOEPITHELIOMA-LIKE) CARCINOMA Carcinoma with a medullary (lymphoepithelioma-like) morphology has been reported in the liver. These cases consist of poorly differentiated carcinoma (Hep Par-1 positive) admixed with abundant lymphoid stroma. The presence of Epstein-Barr virus has been demonstrated by *in situ* hybridization.[525,527]

BILIARY-TYPE DIFFERENTIATION IN HCC Some hepatocellular carcinomas may express markers that are otherwise considered specific for biliary-duct differentiation and do not stain hepatocellular carcinomas. The expression of these markers, by itself, is not considered enough by most authors to qualify the tumor as "combined HCC and cholangiocarcinoma." Some authors refer to it as "biliary-type differentiation." HCC with "biliary-type differentiation" stains with monoclonal CEA, CK 7, CK 19, and AE1/AE3.[7,657,658]

KEY DIAGNOSTIC POINTS

Hepatocellular Carcinoma (HCC)

- HCC is positive for certain cytokeratins, particularly low-molecular-weight cytokeratins (CK8, CK18).
- The markers Hep Par-1 and glypican-3 are useful for the diagnosis of HCC.
- Polyclonal carcinoembryonic antigen (pCEA) and CD10 usually show canalicular staining in HCC, but this may be difficult to distinguish from abortive glandular areas in poorly differentiated cholangiocarcinomas.
- CD34 may help in highlighting the distinctive, "complete" sinusoidal vasculature of HCC.
- *In situ* hybridization for albumin may also be useful in HCC.

KEY DIFFERENTIAL DIAGNOSIS

Hepatocellular Carcinoma (HCC)

- **HCC versus benign hepatic tissue:** In the past, routine histology and histochemical stains were the mainstay in the distinction between benign hepatic tissue and HCC. Reticulin outlines the normal sinusoidal architecture in benign hepatic tissue and highlights thickened hepatocytic plates and abnormal nodules in HCC.[602] Currently, dealing with this differential diagnosis is also aided by immunohistochemistry. Recently, glypican-3 has gained attention for its utility in this regard because antibodies directed against it stain mainly neoplastic liver and only rarely cirrhotic liver.[482,588,589,602] In benign livers, CD34 shows a more selective ("incomplete") pattern highlighting the portal and periportal sinusoids, whereas in HCC, it labels the sinusoids throughout the lesion, showing a more widely spread ("complete") pattern.[588,602] Molecular studies that have been advocated to be of use include telomerase activity, comparative genomic hybridization, and measurement of proliferation status through counting of argyrophilic nucleolar organizer regions (AgNORs) with special silver staining,[602] although these have not found their way to routine practice.
- **HCC versus cholangiocarcinomas:** Cholangiocarcinoma is positive for both CK7 and CK19, whereas HCC is usually (though not always) negative for these antibodies. Hep Par-1, a marker commonly used to identify HCC, is not typically expressed in cholangiocarcinomas.[479,599]

- **HCC versus other adenocarcinomas:** In the differential diagnosis of HCC from other adenocarcinomas, generic adenocarcinoma markers such as MOC-31 B72.3, mCEA (cytoplasmic or diffuse noncanalicular positivity), CA19-9, MUC1, CK7, and CK20, which tend to be much more commonly positive in adenocarcinomas than in HCC, can be combined with the HCC markers. Depending on the clinico-morphologic differential diagnosis, more specific adenocarcinoma antibodies such as combination of mammoglobulin, breast-2, ER, PR, and HER2/neu for breast, or PSA for prostate (although metastasis to liver from prostate is exceedingly uncommon, it can occur) or others can be employed.[586,599,602]
- **HCC versus metastatic neuroendocrine tumors:** This is one differential in which immunohistochemistry can be of utmost importance. Numerous cytologic and architectural similarities exist between HCC and metastatic well-differentiated neuroendocrine neoplasia (carcinoids and pancreatic endocrine neoplasia): They are both cellular, stroma-poor tumors that have a delicate sinusoidal vasculature and relatively monotonous cells with fair amount of cytoplasm and round nuclei. A panel of "neuroendocrine markers" (chromogranin, synaptophysin, and CD56) combined with "hepatocytic" markers (Hep Par-1 and polyclonal-CEA, and FISH for albumin) can be helpful.
- **HCC and melanomas:** Melanomas can metastasize to liver. Because they can morphologically mimic HCC by showing monotonous cells with abundant cytoplasm, round nuclei, and prominent nucleoli, immunohistochemistry (e.g., keratins and melanoma markers including S-100, HMB45, Mart-1) is often crucial in this differential diagnosis.

BILE DUCT LESIONS

Bile Duct Hamartoma and Bile Duct Adenoma

Benign biliary ductular proliferations are seen in a variety of conditions associated with hepatic injury and subsequent metaplastic changes. Bile duct hamartomas (von Meyenburg complexes) are small collections of bile ductules displaying dilated ductules with contour irregularities, single layer of bland, cuboidal epithelium, and intraluminal bile.

Bile duct adenomas, on the other hand, are well circumscribed, firm, tan-white nodules resembling metastatic carcinoma. Nearly 85% are solitary. Microscopically, they contain numerous small tubular structures with small lumina, an important finding in differentiating from hamartomas. Lining epithelium lacks nuclear pleomorphism and hyperchromasia. Immunophenotype is that of peribiliary glands: There is reactivity for CK19, CEA and EMA. KRAS mutations have been reported in small percentage of the lesions.[659]

These benign biliary proliferations can be difficult to distinguish from well-differentiated carcinomas of *pancreatobiliary type* (cholangiocarcinomas or ductal adenocarcinomas). CD56 often shows labeling in these benign proliferations (except von Meyenburg complexes) but is lacking in adenocarcinomas (Fig. 15.36). Similarly, expression of p53, Ki-67, and B72.3 is significantly more common in malignant than in benign, but unfortunately overlaps are common and therefore, these ought to be used cautiously.

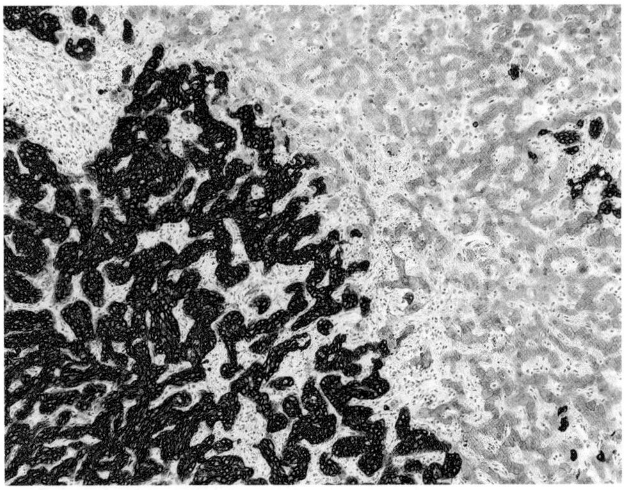

FIGURE 15.34 AE1/AE3 staining in cholangiocarcinoma. Note the interface of the tumor with normal liver.

Cholangiocarcinoma

Cholangiocarcinoma is a malignant tumor composed of cells recapitulating the biliary ductal cells, described as being intrahepatic (or peripheral) when arising in the liver or hilar when arising from the right or left hepatic ducts near their junction. It is a member of the generic category of "pancreatobiliary-type" adenocarcinomas, histologically similar, if not identical, to gallbladder carcinomas and pancreatic ductal adenocarcinomas. Many characteristics of these carcinomas are already discussed in detail in earlier sections. Cholangiocarcinoma typically shows malignant glands in a tubular configuration embedded in a fibrous stroma. There may be areas of adenosquamous, mucinous, and signet ring cell carcinoma. Variants include clear cell, mucinous, pleomorphic, and spindle cell types.[660] The lesions usually react with CK7, CK19, CAM5.2, AE1/AE3 (Fig. 15.34), CEA (both monoclonal and polyclonal in a noncanalicular pattern), and MOC-31. Cholangiocarcinoma is more likely to react with CK7 than other pancreatobiliary carcinomas and less likely to react with CK20, CK17, and p53.[586] CK19 is expressed in 85% to 100% of cholangiocarcinomas, whereas most HCCs either are negative or show patchy staining.[599] MOC-31 is consistently (80% to 100%) expressed in cholangiocarcinoma.[599] Ber-EP4 stains in a similar pattern to MOC-31.[632] Although not always included in diagnostic panels of cholangiocarcinoma, CA19-9 can be positive in up to 85% to 100% of cholangiocarcinomas (Fig. 15.35).[627,661-663] Mucins (e.g., MUC4, MUC5AC, MUC5B, MUC6) may be useful in classifying cholangiocarcinomas and predicting prognosis. A gastric mucin phenotype has been found in some studies to be associated with a worse prognosis.[457,586,664,665] α_1-Antitrypsin is typically negative with reports indicating that 0% to 10% of tumors stain.[633]

Cholangiocarcinoma may stain with parathyroid hormone-related peptide.[545,602] Table 15.6 summarizes select antibodies for cholangiocarcinoma.

KEY DIAGNOSTIC POINTS

Cholangiocarcinoma

- Cholangiocarcinoma is commonly positive for certain subtypes of cytokeratins (notably CK7 and CK19).
- Cholangiocarcinoma is positive for both monoclonal and polyclonal CEA in a noncanalicular pattern.
- Cholangiocarcinoma is also positive for various conventional "markers of adenocarcinoma" (e.g., MOC-31, Ber-EP4).

KEY DIFFERENTIAL DIAGNOSIS

Cholangiocarcinoma

Cholangiocarcinoma versus benign biliary ductular proliferations:

- If von Meyenburg complexes are excluded, CD56 can be used to differentiate benign biliary ductular proliferations from neoplastic proliferations. Reactive proliferating bile ductules are CD56 positive, whereas most cholangiocarcinomas are CD56 negative (Fig. 15.36).[666] However, exceptions do exist including cholangiocarcinomas with clear cell differentiation that are CD56 positive.[667]
- p53, Ki-67, and B72.3 can be employed but should be used cautiously because overlaps are common.
- **Cholangiocarcinoma versus HCC:** The distinction of cholangiocarcinoma from HCC can be aided by cytokeratin staining because cholangiocarcinoma shows staining for cytokeratins such as CK7 and CK19, whereas HCC is usually negative. Cholangiocarcinoma is usually negative for TTF-1, whereas HCC is often positive (cytoplasmic, not nuclear as it normally is in the lung or thyroid). Claudins, which are positive in cholangiocarcinoma and typically negative in HCC, have also been proposed as useful in the distinction of cholangiocarcinoma from HCC.[586,625,668,669]
- **Cholangiocarcinoma versus metastatic lesions:** Cholangiocarcinoma can be difficult to differentiate from adenocarcinomas metastatic from other sites, particularly gastrointestinal primaries (e.g., stomach, gallbladder, extrahepatic biliary tree, pancreas) using immunohistochemistry because cholangiocarcinoma shows an overlapping staining pattern with carcinomas of many sites.[599,602] Cholangiocarcinoma may react with CA125, making distinction from müllerian carcinomas difficult. However, cholangiocarcinoma does not usually react with estrogen receptor.[586,670]

Cholangiocarcinoma Variants

SPINDLE CELL (SARCOMATOID) CHOLANGIOCARCINOMA Spindle cell (sarcomatoid) cholangiocarcinoma usually occurs as a component of a more conventional or poorly differentiated cholangiocarcinoma. The spindled cell areas may be negative or stain only focally for cytokeratins.[671-674] Cases with a variety of sarcomatous differentiation have been reported including chondrosarcomatous elements[675] and rhabdoid.[75,676] Cells of the sarcomatous elements stain in a typical pattern for those sarcomas.[671,673,674] Rhabdoid elements are typically positive for vimentin,[674,676] which is typically true of other spindled/sarcomatous elements.[673] CEA positivity may be seen.[672,673] AFP is usually negative.[671,672]

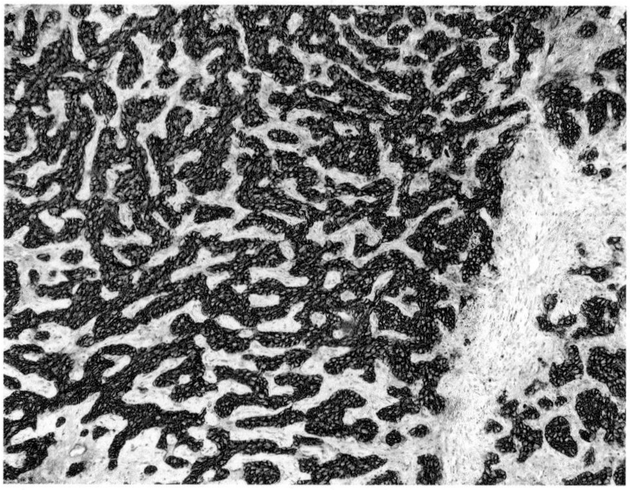

FIGURE 15.35 CA 19-9 positivity in cholangiocarcinoma.

TABLE 15.6 Immunohistogram of Cholangiocarcinoma with Selected Antibodies

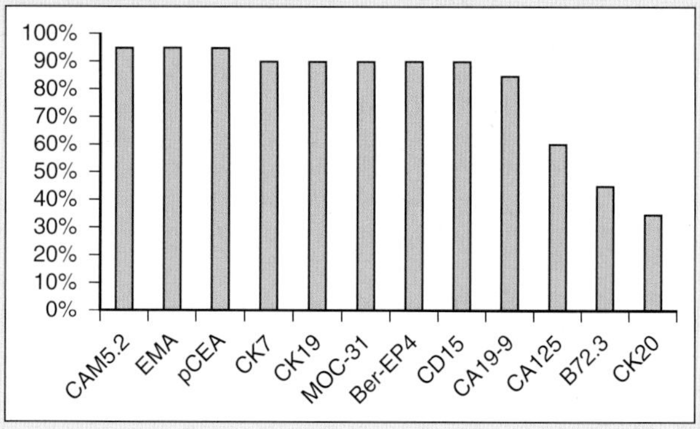

Mixed Hepatocellular and Cholangiocarcinoma

Existence of tumors that have both HCC and cholangiocarcinoma components has been well established in the literature. The proper classification and terminology of these tumors, however, which can exhibit a spectrum of cross differentiation, has been somewhat problematic. Although some cases have clearly distinct and easily identifiable HCC and cholangiocarcinoma components (with all the characteristic morphologic and immunophenotypical features of the respective tumors), in many, there are subtle transdifferentiation and a spectrum of hybrid phenotypes. The interpretation of this spectrum has also been variable among authors. Some employ the term "cholangiocellular carcinoma" for those that morphologically consist of biliary adenocarcinomas that have the immunohistochemical staining pattern of HCC.[677] In general, studies have shown that their molecular signature is closer to cholangiocarcinoma, suggesting they

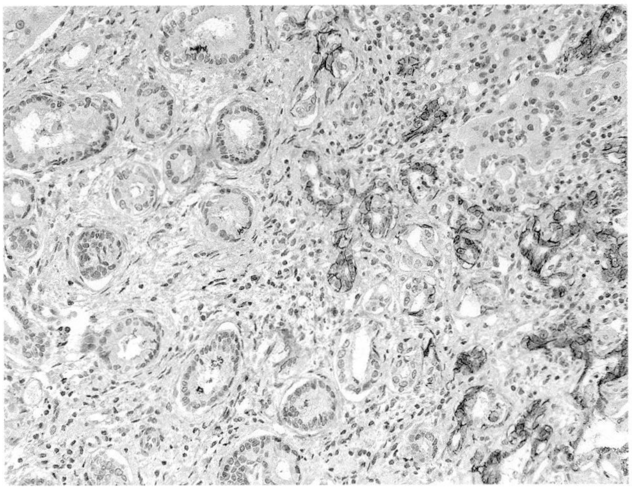

FIGURE 15.36 CD56 can be useful in distinguishing benign biliary ductular proliferations from neoplastic proliferations. Cholangiocarcinomas *(left)* are more commonly negative for CD56, whereas benign bile ductules *(right)* are positive.

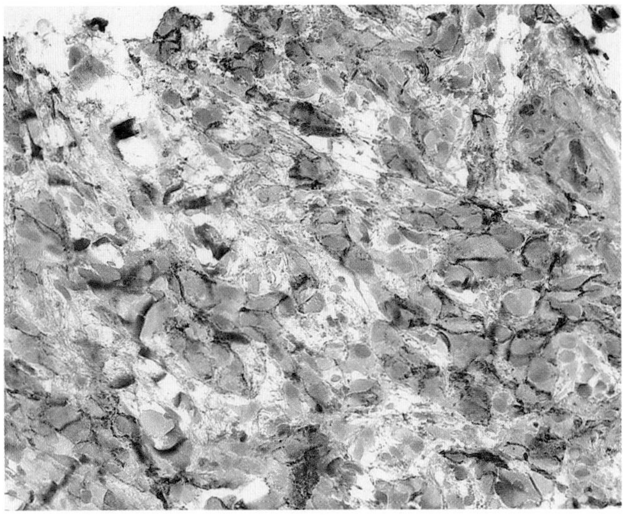

FIGURE 15.37 Endothelial markers (CD31 is shown here) are commonly expressed in epithelioid hemangioendothelioma and are extremely helpful in the differential diagnosis between adenocarcinomas and HCC.

may arise from cholangiocarcinoma. It should be kept in mind that some antibodies can produce seemingly discrepant results. For example, Hep Par-1 may stain some cholangiocarcinomas.[479,586,665,678-681] Overall, the cholangiocarcinoma component is usually more aggressive and appears to dictate the prognosis.

Biliary Cystadenoma and Cystadenocarcinoma

Biliary cystadenomas and cystadenocarcinomas have an immunohistochemical profile similar to pancreatobiliary cystadenomas and cystadenocarcinomas.[418,610,682-685] The epithelium typically shows staining for CK7, CK20, AE1/AE3, CEA, CA 19-9, and CA125.[418] Ovarian-type stroma may be present and may show staining for progesterone receptors.[686,687]

POORLY DIFFERENTIATED AND UNDIFFERENTIATED CARCINOMAS

Carcinosarcoma of the liver can occur, although it is rare.[675,688,689] In a series from China in which all of the patients were hepatitis B surface antigen positive, conventional hepatocellular carcinoma merged with areas of rhabdomyosarcoma, "malignant fibrous histiocytoma," and fibrosarcoma; and immunohistochemistry supported the diagnosis of carcinosarcoma.[689]

NEUROENDOCRINE NEOPLASMS

The overwhelming majority of neuroendocrine neoplasms occurring in the liver are metastatic. Well to moderately differentiated neuroendocrine neoplasms (e.g., carcinoids, pancreatic endocrine neoplasms, medullary thyroid carcinomas) may mimic primary hepatocellular processes, and thus immunohistochemistry with antibodies for chromogranin, synaptophysin, and CD56 can be extremely helpful, as discussed earlier. They may also be positive for MOC-31 but not for Hep Par-1. In contrast, HCC may occasionally show focal neuroendocrine differentiation and may stain for CD56,[690,691] synaptophysin, and chromogranin.[599,692] In particular, the fibrolamellar variant of HCC is often synaptophysin positive; however, HCCs are also positive for Hep Par-1.[599]

Metastatic high-grade neuroendocrine carcinomas ought to be differentiated from other high-grade malignancies, metastatic or primary. Wide-spectrum keratins are typically positive and helpful in confirming the epithelial nature of the tumor. Neuroendocrine markers (synaptophysin, chromogranin and CD56) can be fairly focal and thus ought to be evaluated carefully in high power. It should be remembered that these tumors are defined by morphologic features, and lack of neuroendocrine markers does not rule out this diagnosis by any means. If the differential diagnosis is with the lesser grade (well-moderately differentiated) endocrine lesions, Ki-67 labeling index, which is usually greater than 20% of the cells, can be helpful.

OTHER NEOPLASMS

Hemangioma is the most common primary hepatic tumor, usually an incidental finding at autopsy. Microscopically, most lesions are of cavernous type (see other chapters for details).

Epithelioid hemangioendothelioma of liver is often multifocal with involvement of both right and left liver lobes. Although it is generally regarded as a low-grade malignant neoplasm, in some cases it follows an aggressive clinical course. Nevertheless, the overall 5-year survival is estimated to be 50%, starkly different than that of cholangiocarcinoma for which it is often mistaken. Furthermore, transplant can be an effective treatment of this tumor type.[693] Histologically, subtle examples are typically dismissed as a non-neoplastic fibrosing disorder. More prominent and vessel-forming examples are misdiagnosed as metastatic adenocarcinoma or cholangiocarcinoma. Immunohistochemically, cytokeratins are often positive, further accentuating the challenge in distinguishing these lesions from glandular-epithelial lesions. Endothelial markers, CD34, CD31 (Fig. 15.37), and/or factor VIII, are commonly expressed and can be extremely helpful.[619,694] Less than 50% react with smooth muscle actin[586] as well.

Angiomyolipoma is a benign tumor thought to arise from perivascular epithelioid cells (also known as *PEC cells*) and consist of variable combinations of blood vessels, adipose tissue, and smooth muscle. Blood vessels may have thick walls and may be hyalinized. Extramedullary hematopoiesis may be present. The lesions are strongly positive for HMB-45 and Melan-A,[694,695] as well as ER, and weakly positive for actin and desmin.[696]

Embryonal (undifferentiated) sarcoma of the liver, also known as *mesenchymal sarcoma* or *malignant mesenchymoma,* occurs predominantly in children. Grossly, it is usually a large solitary and well-circumscribed mass measuring up to 30 cm in diameter, with degenerative changes including necrosis, hemorrhage, and cystic degeneration. Microscopically, the lesions are composed of highly atypical spindle to stellate cells and giant cells embedded in myxoid stroma. PAS-positive and diastase-resistant, large eosinophilic hyaline globules within the cytoplasm of tumor cells and in the stroma are characteristic. Scattered entrapped ducts are seen in most cases. Data regarding the immunophenotype of this rare tumor type are conflicting. Generally, they are considered to be positive for vimentin, smooth muscle actin, desmin, and keratin[697-699] but not myoglobin.[700]

SUMMARY

The array of medical and neoplastic diseases of the pancreas, extrahepatic and intrahepatic biliary tree, and liver are vast. Morphologic impressions remain the bedrock for proper interpretation of IHC and other specialized molecular anatomic tissue testing.

ACKNOWLEDGMENTS

The authors express their gratitude to Dr. Ipek Coban, Dr. Nevra Dursun, and Ms. Rhonda Everett for their assistance in preparing this chapter.

REFERENCES

1. Adsay NV. Gallbladder, Extrahepatic Biliary Tree and Ampulla. In: Mills SE, ed. Sternberg's Diagnostic Surgical Pathology. 5th ed. Philadelphia: Lippincott Williams & Wilkins; 2009.
2. Adsay NV, Klimstra DS. Benign and Malignant Tumors of the Gallbladder and Extrahepatic Biliary Tract. In: Odze RD, Goldblum JR, eds. *Surgical Pathology of the GI tract, Liver, Biliary Tract, and Pancreas.* Philadelphia: Elsevier; 2009: 845-875.
3. Klimstra DS, Adsay NV. Tumors of the Pancreas and Ampulla of Vater. In: Odze RD, Goldblum JR, eds. *Surgical Pathology of the GI tract, Liver, Biliary Tract, and Pancreas.* Philadelphia: Elsevier; 2009:909-960.
4. Hruban RH, Pitman MB, Klimstra DS. *Tumors of the Pancreas.* 4th ed. Washington, DC: ARP Press; 2007.
5. Batge B, Bosslet K, Sedlacek HH, et al. Monoclonal antibodies against CEA-related components discriminate between pancreatic duct type carcinomas and nonneoplastic duct lesions as well as nonduct type neoplasias. *Virchows Arch A Pathol Anat Histopathol.* 1986;408:361-374.
6. Klimstra DS, Hameed MR, Marrero AM, et al. Ductal Proliferative Lesions Associated with Infiltrating Ductal Adenocarcinoma of the Pancreas. *Int J Pancreatol.* 1994;16:224-225.
7. Ma CK, Zarbo RJ, Frierson Jr HF, Lee MW. Comparative immunohistochemical study of primary and metastatic carcinomas of the liver. *Am J Clin Pathol.* 1993;99:551-557.
8. Yamaguchi K, Enjoji M. Carcinoma of the pancreas: a clinicopathologic study of 96 cases with immunohistochemical observations. *Jpn J Clin Oncol.* 1989;19:14-22.
9. Luttges J, Vogel I, Menke M, et al. Clear cell carcinoma of the pancreas: an adenocarcinoma with ductal phenotype. *Histopathology.* 1998;32:444-448.
10. Yamaguchi K, Enjoji M, Tsuneyoshi M. Pancreatoduodenal carcinoma: a clinicopathologic study of 304 patients and immunohistochemical observation for CEA and CA19-9. *J Surg Oncol.* 1991;47:148-154.
11. Moniaux N, Escande F, Porchet N, et al. Structural organization and classification of the human mucin genes. *Front Biosci.* 2001;6:D1192-D1206.
12. Nagata K, Horinouchi M, Saitou M, et al. Mucin expression profile in pancreatic cancer and the precursor lesions. *J Hepatobiliary Pancreat Surg.* 2007;14:243-254.
13. Levi E, Klimstra DS, Andea A, et al. MUC1 and MUC2 in pancreatic neoplasia. *J Clin Pathol.* 2004;57:456-462.
14. Yonezawa S, Goto M, Yamada N, et al. Expression profiles of MUC1, MUC2, and MUC4 mucins in human neoplasms and their relationship with biological behavior. *Proteomics.* 2008;8:3329-3341.
15. Yonezawa S, Nakamura A, Horinouchi M, Sato E. The expression of several types of mucin is related to the biological behavior of pancreatic neoplasms. *J Hepatobiliary Pancreat Surg.* 2002;9:328-341.
16. Saitou M, Goto M, Horinouchi M, et al. MUC4 expression is a novel prognostic factor in patients with invasive ductal carcinoma of the pancreas. *J Clin Pathol.* 2005;58:845-852.
17. Khayyata S, Basturk O, Klimstra DS, et al. MUC6 Expression Distinguishes Oncocytic and Pancreatobiliary Type from Intestinal Type Papillae in Pancreatic Neoplasia: Delineation of a Pyloropancreatic Pathway. *Mod Pathol.* 2006;19:275A.
18. Klimstra DS, Adsay NV, Dhall D, et al. Intraductal tubular carcinoma of the pancreas: Clinicopathologic and immunohistochemical analysis of 18 cases. *Mod Pathol.* 2007;20:285A.
19. Koshikawa N, Hasegawa S, Nagashima Y, et al. Expression of trypsin by epithelial cells of various tissues, leukocytes, and neurons in human and mouse. *Am J Pathol.* 1998;153:937-944.
20. Portela-Gomes GM, Hacker GW, Weitgasser R. Neuroendocrine cell markers for pancreatic islets and tumors. *Appl Immunohistochem Mol Morphol.* 2004;12:183-192.
21. Nalbantoglu I, Basturk O, Thirabanjasak D, et al. Islets, the king of antigens? Non-specific reactivity of (especially the) islets is a common pitfall in immunohistochemical evaluation of the pancreas. *Mod Pathol.* 2007;20:288A.
22. Pignatelli M, Vessey CJ. Adhesion molecules: novel molecular tools in tumor pathology. *Hum Pathol.* 1994;25:849-856.
23. Chetty R, Serra S. Nuclear E-cadherin immunoexpression: from biology to potential applications in diagnostic pathology. *Adv Anat Pathol.* 2008;15:234-240.
24. Serra S, Chetty R. Revision 2: an immunohistochemical approach and evaluation of solid pseudopapillary tumour of the pancreas. *J Clin Pathol.* 2008;61:1153-1159.
25. Chetty R, Serra S, Asa SL. Loss of membrane localization and aberrant nuclear E-cadherin expression correlates with invasion in pancreatic endocrine tumors. *Am J Surg Pathol.* 2008;32: 413-419.
26. Evans DB, Abruzzese JL, Rich TA. Cancer of the pancreas. In: Devita VT, Hellman S, Rosenberg SA, eds. *Cancer: Principles and practice of oncology.* 6th ed. Philadelphia: Lippincott-Raven; 2001:1126-1161.
27. Moll R. Cytokeratins as markers of differentiation in the diagnosis of epithelial tumors. *Subcell Biochem.* 1998;31:205-262.
28. Hoorens A, Prenzel K, Lemoine NR, Kloppel G. Undifferentiated carcinoma of the pancreas: analysis of intermediate filament profile and Ki-ras mutations provides evidence of a ductal origin. *J Pathol.* 1998;185:53-60.
29. Thomas P, Battifora H. Keratins versus epithelial membrane antigen in tumor diagnosis: an immunohistochemical comparison of five monoclonal antibodies. *Hum Pathol.* 1987;18: 728-734.

30. Shimonishi T, Miyazaki K, Nakanuma Y. Cytokeratin profile relates to histological subtypes and intrahepatic location of intrahepatic cholangiocarcinoma and primary sites of metastatic adenocarcinoma of liver. *Histopathology*. 2000;37:55-63.
31. Alexander J, Krishnamurthy S, Kovacs D, Dayal Y. Cytokeratin profile of extrahepatic pancreatobiliary epithelia and their carcinomas. *Appl Immunohistochem Mol Morphol*. 1997;5:216-222.
32. Real FX, Vila MR, Skoudy A, et al. Intermediate filaments as differentiation markers of exocrine pancreas. II. Expression of cytokeratins of complex and stratified epithelia in normal pancreas and in pancreas cancer. *Int J Cancer*. 1993;54: 720-727.
33. Vlasoff DM, Baschinsky DY, Frankel WL. Cytokeratin 5/6 immunostaining in hepatobiliary and pancreatic neoplasms. *Appl Immunohistochem Mol Morphol*. 2002;10:147-151.
34. Duval JV, Savas L, Banner BF. Expression of cytokeratins 7 and 20 in carcinomas of the extrahepatic biliary tract, pancreas, and gallbladder. *Arch Pathol Lab Med*. 2000;124:1196-1200.
35. Goldstein NS, Bassi D. Cytokeratins 7, 17, and 20 reactivity in pancreatic and ampulla of vater adenocarcinomas. Percentage of positivity and distribution is affected by the cut-point threshold. *Am J Clin Pathol*. 2001;115:695-702.
36. Lee MJ, Lee HS, Kim WH, et al. Expression of mucins and cytokeratins in primary carcinomas of the digestive system. *Mod Pathol*. 2003;16:403-410.
37. Goldstein NS, Bassi D, Uzieblo A. WT1 is an integral component of an antibody panel to distinguish pancreaticobiliary and some ovarian epithelial neoplasms. *Am J Clin Pathol*. 2001;116: 246-252.
38. Ramaekers F, van Niekerk C, Poels L, et al. Use of monoclonal antibodies to keratin 7 in the differential diagnosis of adenocarcinomas. *Am J Pathol*. 1990;136:641-655.
39. Tot T. Adenocarcinomas metastatic to the liver: the value of cytokeratins 20 and 7 in the search for unknown primary tumors. *Cancer*. 1999;85:171-177.
40. Baars JH, De Ruijter JL, Smedts F, et al. The applicability of a keratin 7 monoclonal antibody in routinely Papanicolaou-stained cytologic specimens for the differential diagnosis of carcinomas. *Am J Clin Pathol*. 1994;101:257-261.
41. Chu P, Wu E, Weiss LM. Cytokeratin 7 and cytokeratin 20 expression in epithelial neoplasms: a survey of 435 cases. *Mod Pathol*. 2000;13:962-972.
42. Ji H, Isacson C, Seidman JD, et al. Cytokeratins 7 and 20, Dpc4, and MUC5AC in the distinction of metastatic mucinous carcinomas in the ovary from primary ovarian mucinous tumors: Dpc4 assists in identifying metastatic pancreatic carcinomas. *Int J Gynecol Pathol*. 2002;21:391-400.
43. Tot T. Cytokeratins 20 and 7 as biomarkers: usefulness in discriminating primary from metastatic adenocarcinoma. *Eur J Cancer*. 2002;38:758-763.
44. Rullier A, Le Bail B, Fawaz R, et al. Cytokeratin 7 and 20 expression in cholangiocarcinomas varies along the biliary tract but still differs from that in colorectal carcinoma metastasis. *Am J Surg Pathol*. 2000;24:870-876.
45. Tot T. The value of cytokeratins 20 and 7 in discriminating metastatic adenocarcinomas from pleural mesotheliomas. *Cancer*. 2001;92:2727-2732.
46. Moll R, Lowe A, Laufer J, Franke WW. Cytokeratin 20 in human carcinomas. A new histodiagnostic marker detected by monoclonal antibodies. *Am J Pathol*. 1992;140:427-447.
47. Kaufmann O, Deidesheimer T, Muehlenberg M, et al. Immunohistochemical differentiation of metastatic breast carcinomas from metastatic adenocarcinomas of other common primary sites. *Histopathology*. 1996;29:233-240.
48. Miettinen M. Keratin 20: immunohistochemical marker for gastrointestinal, urothelial, and Merkel cell carcinomas. *Mod Pathol*. 1995;8:384-388.
49. Wauters CC, Smedts F, Gerrits LG, et al. Keratins 7 and 20 as diagnostic markers of carcinomas metastatic to the ovary. *Hum Pathol*. 1995;26:852-855.
50. Schussler MH, Skoudy A, Ramaekers F, Real FX. Intermediate filaments as differentiation markers of normal pancreas and pancreas cancer. *Am J Pathol*. 1992;140:559-568.
51. Chen J, Baithun SI. Morphological study of 391 cases of exocrine pancreatic tumours with special reference to the classification of exocrine pancreatic carcinoma. *J Pathol*. 1985;146:17-29.
52. Cathro HP, Stoler MH. Expression of cytokeratins 7 and 20 in ovarian neoplasia. *Am J Clin Pathol*. 2002;117:944-951.
53. Chu PG, Weiss LM. Expression of cytokeratin 5/6 in epithelial neoplasms: an immunohistochemical study of 509 cases. *Mod Pathol*. 2002;15:6-10.
54. Di Como CJ, Urist MJ, Babayan I, et al. p63 expression profiles in human normal and tumor tissues. *Clin Cancer Res*. 2002;8:494-501.
55. Adsay NV, Merati K, Andea A, et al. The dichotomy in the preinvasive neoplasia to invasive carcinoma sequence in the pancreas: differential expression of MUC1 and MUC2 supports the existence of two separate pathways of carcinogenesis. *Mod Pathol*. 2002;15:1087-1095.
56. Monges GM, Mathoulin-Portier MP, Acres RB, et al. Differential MUC 1 expression in normal and neoplastic human pancreatic tissue. An immunohistochemical study of 60 samples. *Am J Clin Pathol*. 1999;112:635-640.
57. Swartz MJ, Batra SK, Varshney GC, et al. MUC4 expression increases progressively in pancreatic intraepithelial neoplasia. *Am J Clin Pathol*. 2002;117:791-796.
58. Masaki Y, Oka M, Ogura Y, et al. Sialylated MUC1 mucin expression in normal pancreas, benign pancreatic lesions, and pancreatic ductal adenocarcinoma. *Hepatogastroenterology*. 1999;46:2240-2245.
59. Andrianifahanana M, Moniaux N, Schmied BM, et al. Mucin (MUC) gene expression in human pancreatic adenocarcinoma and chronic pancreatitis: a potential role of MUC4 as a tumor marker of diagnostic significance. *Clin Cancer Res*. 2001;7:4033-4040.
60. Kim GE, Bae HI, Park HU, et al. Aberrant expression of MUC5AC and MUC6 gastric mucins and sialyl Tn antigen in intraepithelial neoplasms of the pancreas. *Gastroenterology*. 2002;123:1052-1060.
61. Luttges J, Zamboni G, Longnecker D, Kloppel G. The immunohistochemical mucin expression pattern distinguishes different types of intraductal papillary mucinous neoplasms of the pancreas and determines their relationship to mucinous noncystic carcinoma and ductal adenocarcinoma. *Am J Surg Pathol*. 2001;25:942-948.
62. Swierczynski SL, Maitra A, Abraham SC, et al. Analysis of novel tumor markers in pancreatic and biliary carcinomas using tissue microarrays. *Hum Pathol*. 2004;35:357-366.
63. Terada T, Ohta T, Sasaki M, et al. Expression of MUC apomucins in normal pancreas and pancreatic tumours. *J Pathol*. 1996;180:160-165.
64. Yonezawa S, Sueyoshi K, Nomoto M, et al. MUC2 gene expression is found in noninvasive tumors but not in invasive tumors of the pancreas and liver: its close relationship with prognosis of the patients. *Hum Pathol*. 1997;28:344-352.
65. Zhang H, Maitra A, Tabaczka P, et al. Differential MUC1, MUC2 and MUC5AC expression in colorectal, ampullary and pancreatobiliary carcinomas: Potential biologic and diagnostic implications (abstract). *Mod Pathol*. 2003;16:180A.
66. Werling RW, Yaziji H, Bacchi CE, Gown AM. CDX2, a highly sensitive and specific marker of adenocarcinomas of intestinal origin: an immunohistochemical survey of 476 primary and metastatic carcinomas. *Am J Surg Pathol*. 2003;27:303-310.
67. Moskaluk CA, Zhang H, Powell SM, et al. Cdx2 protein expression in normal and malignant human tissues: an immunohistochemical survey using tissue microarrays. *Mod Pathol*. 2003;16:913-919.
68. Barbareschi M, Murer B, Colby TV, et al. CDX-2 homeobox gene expression is a reliable marker of colorectal adenocarcinoma metastases to the lungs. *Am J Surg Pathol*. 2003;27:141-149.
69. Li MK, Folpe AL. CDX-2, a new marker for adenocarcinoma of gastrointestinal origin. *Adv Anat Pathol*. 2004;11:101-105.
70. Morohoshi T, Kanda M, Horie A, et al. Immunocytochemical markers of uncommon pancreatic tumors. Acinar cell carcinoma, pancreatoblastoma, and solid cystic (papillary-cystic) tumor. *Cancer*. 1987;59:739-747.

71. Ichihara T, Nagura H, Nakao A, et al. Immunohistochemical localization of CA 19-9 and CEA in pancreatic carcinoma and associated diseases. *Cancer*. 1988;61:324-333.
72. Osako M, Yonezawa S, Siddiki B, et al. Immunohistochemical study of mucin carbohydrates and core proteins in human pancreatic tumors. *Cancer*. 1993;71:2191-2199.
73. Sessa F, Bonato M, Frigerio B, et al. Ductal cancers of the pancreas frequently express markers of gastrointestinal epithelial cells. *Gastroenterology*. 1990;98:1655-1665.
74. Takeda S, Nakao A, Ichihara T, et al. Serum concentration and immunohistochemical localization of SPan-1 antigen in pancreatic cancer. A comparison with CA19-9 antigen. *Hepatogastroenterology*. 1991;38:143-148.
75. Simeone DM, Ji B, Banerjee M, et al. CEACAM1, a novel serum biomarker for pancreatic cancer. *Pancreas*. 2007;34:436-443.
76. Hoorens A, Lemoine NR, McLellan E, et al. Pancreatic acinar cell carcinoma. An analysis of cell lineage markers, p53 expression, and Ki-ras mutation. *Am J Pathol*. 1993;143:685-698.
77. Kamisawa T, Fukayama M, Tabata I, et al. Neuroendocrine differentiation in pancreatic duct carcinoma special emphasis on duct-endocrine cell carcinoma of the pancreas. *Pathol Res Pract*. 1996;192:901-908.
78. Pour PM, Permert J, Mogaki M, et al. Endocrine aspects of exocrine cancer of the pancreas. Their patterns and suggested biologic significance. *Am J Clin Pathol*. 1993;100:223-230.
79. Bommer G, Friedl U, Heitz PU, Kloppel G. Pancreatic PP cell distribution and hyperplasia. Immunocytochemical morphology in the normal human pancreas, in chronic pancreatitis and pancreatic carcinoma. *Virchows Arch A Pathol Anat Histol*. 1980;387:319-331.
80. Ademmer K, Ebert M, Muller-Ostermeyer F, et al. Effector T lymphocyte subsets in human pancreatic cancer: detection of CD8+CD18+ cells and CD8+CD103+ cells by multi-epitope imaging. *Clin Exp Immunol*. 1998;112:21-26.
81. Yen TW, Aardal NP, Bronner MP, et al. Myofibroblasts are responsible for the desmoplastic reaction surrounding human pancreatic carcinomas. *Surgery*. 2002;131:129-134.
82. Koshiba T, Hosotani R, Wada M, et al. Involvement of matrix metalloproteinase-2 activity in invasion and metastasis of pancreatic carcinoma. *Cancer*. 1998;82:642-650.
83. Maitra A, Iacobuzio-Donahue C, Rahman A, et al. Immunohistochemical validation of a novel epithelial and a novel stromal marker of pancreatic ductal adenocarcinoma identified by global expression microarrays: sea urchin fascin homolog and heat shock protein 47. *Am J Clin Pathol*. 2002;118:52-59.
84. Yamamoto H, Itoh F, Iku S, et al. Expression of matrix metalloproteinases and tissue inhibitors of metalloproteinases in human pancreatic adenocarcinomas: clinicopathologic and prognostic significance of matrilysin expression. *J Clin Oncol*. 2001;19:1118-1127.
85. Zhou W, Sokoll LJ, Bruzek DJ, et al. Identifying markers for pancreatic cancer by gene expression analysis. *Cancer Epidemiol Biomarkers Prev*. 1998;7:109-112.
86. Furukawa T, Horii A. Molecular pathology of pancreatic cancer: in quest of tumor suppressor genes. *Pancreas*. 2004;28:253-256.
87. Hruban RH, Iacobuzio-Donahue C, Wilentz RE, et al. Molecular pathology of pancreatic cancer. *Cancer J*. 2001;7:251-258.
88. Rozenblum E, Schutte M, Goggins M, et al. Tumor-suppressive pathways in pancreatic carcinoma. *Cancer Res*. 1997;57:1731-1734.
89. Moore PS, Sipos B, Orlandini S, et al. Genetic profile of 22 pancreatic carcinoma cell lines. Analysis of K-ras, p53, p16 and DPC4/Smad4. *Virchows Arch*. 2001;439:798-802.
90. Moore PS, Orlandini S, Zamboni G, et al. Pancreatic tumours: molecular pathways implicated in ductal cancer are involved in ampullary but not in exocrine nonductal or endocrine tumorigenesis. *Br J Cancer*. 2001;84:253-262.
91. DiGiuseppe JA, Hruban RH, Goodman SN, et al. Overexpression of p53 protein in adenocarcinoma of the pancreas. *Am J Clin Pathol*. 1994;101:684-688.
92. van Heek T, Rader AE, Offerhaus GJ, et al. K-ras, p53, and DPC4 (MAD4) alterations in fine-needle aspirates of the pancreas: a molecular panel correlates with and supplements cytologic diagnosis. *Am J Clin Pathol*. 2002;117:755-765.
93. Wilentz RE, Geradts J, Maynard R, et al. Inactivation of the p16 (INK4A) tumor-suppressor gene in pancreatic duct lesions: loss of intranuclear expression. *Cancer Res*. 1998;58:4740-4744.
94. Boschman CR, Stryker S, Reddy JK, Rao MS. Expression of p53 protein in precursor lesions and adenocarcinoma of human pancreas. *Am J Pathol*. 1994;145:1291-1295.
95. Li Y, Bhuiyan M, Vaitkevicius VK, Sarkar FH. Molecular analysis of the p53 gene in pancreatic adenocarcinoma. *Diagn Mol Pathol*. 1998;7:4-9.
96. Redston MS, Caldas C, Seymour AB, et al. p53 mutations in pancreatic carcinoma and evidence of common involvement of homocopolymer tracts in DNA microdeletions. *Cancer Res*. 1994;54:3025-3033.
97. Schutte M. DPC4/SMAD4 gene alterations in human cancer, and their functional implications. *Ann Oncol*. 1999;10(Suppl 4):56-59.
98. Hahn SA, Schutte M, Hoque AT, et al. DPC4, a candidate tumor suppressor gene at human chromosome 18q21.1. *Science*. 1996;271:350-353.
99. Wilentz RE, Su GH, Dai JL, et al. Immunohistochemical labeling for dpc4 mirrors genetic status in pancreatic adenocarcinomas: a new marker of DPC4 inactivation. *Am J Pathol*. 2000;156:37-43.
100. Iacobuzio-Donahue CA, Song J, Parmiagiani G, et al. Missense mutations of MADH4: characterization of the mutational hot spot and functional consequences in human tumors. *Clin Cancer Res*. 2004;10:1597-1604.
101. Tascilar M, Offerhaus GJ, Altink R, et al. Immunohistochemical labeling for the Dpc4 gene product is a specific marker for adenocarcinoma in biopsy specimens of the pancreas and bile duct. *Am J Clin Pathol*. 2001;116:831-837.
102. Ali S, Cohen C, Little JV, et al. The utility of SMAD4 as a diagnostic immunohistochemical marker for pancreatic adenocarcinoma, and its expression in other solid tumors. *Diagn Cytopathol*. 2007;35:644-648.
103. Bartsch D, Shevlin DW, Callery MP, et al. Reduced survival in patients with ductal pancreatic adenocarcinoma associated with CDKN2 mutation. *J Natl Cancer Inst*. 1996;88:680-682.
104. Schutte M, Hruban RH, Geradts J, et al. Abrogation of the Rb/p16 tumor-suppressive pathway in virtually all pancreatic carcinomas. *Cancer Res*. 1997;57:3126-3130.
105. Caldas C, Hahn SA, da Costa LT, et al. Frequent somatic mutations and homozygous deletions of the p16 (MTS1) gene in pancreatic adenocarcinoma. *Nat Genet*. 1994;8:27-32.
106. Geradts J, Hruban RH, Schutte M, et al. Immunohistochemical p16INK4a analysis of archival tumors with deletion, hypermethylation, or mutation of the CDKN2/MTS1 gene. A comparison of four commercial antibodies. *Appl Immunohistochem Mol Morphol*. 2000;8:71-79.
107. Almoguera C, Shibata D, Forrester K, et al. Most human carcinomas of the exocrine pancreas contain mutant c-K-ras genes. *Cell*. 1988;53:549-554.
108. Satoh K, Sasano H, Shimosegawa T, et al. An immunohistochemical study of the c-erbB-2 oncogene product in intraductal mucin-hypersecreting neoplasms and in ductal cell carcinomas of the pancreas. *Cancer*. 1993;72:51-56.
109. Day JD, Digiuseppe JA, Yeo C, et al. Immunohistochemical evaluation of HER-2/neu expression in pancreatic adenocarcinoma and pancreatic intraepithelial neoplasms. *Hum Pathol*. 1996;27:119-124.
110. Yamanaka Y, Friess H, Kobrin MS, et al. Overexpression of HER2/neu oncogene in human pancreatic carcinoma. *Hum Pathol*. 1993;24:1127-1134.
111. Dancer J, Takei H, Ro JY, Lowery-Nordberg M. Coexpression of EGFR and HER-2 in pancreatic ductal adenocarcinoma: a comparative study using immunohistochemistry correlated with gene amplification by fluorescent in situ hybridization. *Oncol Rep*. 2007;18:151-155.
112. Cheng JQ, Ruggeri B, Klein WM, et al. Amplification of AKT2 in human pancreatic cells and inhibition of AKT2 expression and tumorigenicity by antisense RNA. *Proc Natl Acad Sci U S A*. 1996;93:3636-3641.
113. Ruggeri BA, Huang L, Wood M, et al. Amplification and overexpression of the AKT2 oncogene in a subset of human pancreatic ductal adenocarcinomas. *Mol Carcinog*. 1998;21:81-86.

114. Iacobuzio-Donahue CA, Maitra A, Shen-Ong GL, et al. Discovery of novel tumor markers of pancreatic cancer using global gene expression technology. *Am J Pathol.* 2002;160:1239-1249.
115. Iacobuzio-Donahue CA, Ryu B, Hruban RH, Kern SE. Exploring the host desmoplastic response to pancreatic carcinoma: gene expression of stromal and neoplastic cells at the site of primary invasion. *Am J Pathol.* 2002;160:91-99.
116. Ryu B, Jones J, Hollingsworth MA, et al. Invasion-specific genes in malignancy: serial analysis of gene expression comparisons of primary and passaged cancers. *Cancer Res.* 2001;61:1833-1838.
117. Ryu B, Jones J, Blades NJ, et al. Relationships and differentially expressed genes among pancreatic cancers examined by large-scale serial analysis of gene expression. *Cancer Res.* 2002;62:819-826.
118. Argani P, Iacobuzio-Donahue C, Ryu B, et al. Mesothelin is overexpressed in the vast majority of ductal adenocarcinomas of the pancreas: identification of a new pancreatic cancer marker by serial analysis of gene expression (SAGE). *Clin Cancer Res.* 2001;7:3862-3868.
119. Armengol G, Knuutila S, Lluis F, et al. DNA copy number changes and evaluation of MYC, IGF1R, and FES amplification in xenografts of pancreatic adenocarcinoma. *Cancer Genet Cytogenet.* 2000;116:133-141.
120. Nichols LS, Ashfaq R, Iacobuzio-Donahue CA. Claudin 4 protein expression in primary and metastatic pancreatic cancer: support for use as a therapeutic target. *Am J Clin Pathol.* 2004;121:226-230.
121. Crnogorac-Jurcevic T, Missiaglia E, Blaveri E, et al. Molecular alterations in pancreatic carcinoma: expression profiling shows that dysregulated expression of S100 genes is highly prevalent. *J Pathol.* 2003;201:63-74.
122. Rosty C, Ueki T, Argani P, et al. Overexpression of S100A4 in pancreatic ductal adenocarcinomas is associated with poor differentiation and DNA hypomethylation. *Am J Pathol.* 2002;160:45-50.
123. Vimalachandran D, Greenhalf W, Thompson C, et al. High nuclear S100A6 (Calcyclin) is significantly associated with poor survival in pancreatic cancer patients. *Cancer Res.* 2005;65:3218-3225.
124. Argani P, Rosty C, Reiter RE, et al. Discovery of new markers of cancer through serial analysis of gene expression: prostate stem cell antigen is overexpressed in pancreatic adenocarcinoma. *Cancer Res.* 2001;61:4320-4324.
125. Ligato S, Zhao H, Mandich D, Cartun RW. KOC (K homology domain containing protein overexpressed in cancer) and S100A4-protein immunoreactivity improves the diagnostic sensitivity of biliary brushing cytology for diagnosing pancreaticobiliary malignancies. *Diagn Cytopathol.* 2008;36:561-567.
126. Iacobuzio-Donahue CA, Hruban RH. Gene expression in neoplasms of the pancreas: applications to diagnostic pathology. *Adv Anat Pathol.* 2003;10:125-134.
127. Porschen R, Remy U, Bevers G, et al. Prognostic significance of DNA ploidy in adenocarcinoma of the pancreas. A flow cytometric study of paraffin-embedded specimens. *Cancer.* 1993;71:3846-3850.
128. Yoshimura T, Manabe T, Imamura T, et al. Flow cytometric analysis of nuclear DNA content of duct cell carcinoma of the pancreas. *Cancer.* 1992;70:1069-1074.
129. Allison DC, Piantadosi S, Hruban RH, et al. DNA content and other factors associated with ten-year survival after resection of pancreatic carcinoma. *J Surg Oncol.* 1998;67:151-159.
130. Borg A, Sandberg T, Nilsson K, et al. High frequency of multiple melanomas and breast and pancreas carcinomas in CDKN2A mutation-positive melanoma families. *J Natl Cancer Inst.* 2000;92:1260-1266.
131. Griffin CA, Hruban RH, Long PP, et al. Chromosome abnormalities in pancreatic adenocarcinoma. *Genes Chromosomes Cancer.* 1994;9:93-100.
132. Griffin CA, Hruban RH, Morsberger LA, et al. Consistent chromosome abnormalities in adenocarcinoma of the pancreas. *Cancer Res.* 1995;55:2394-2399.
133. Johansson B, Bardi G, Pandis N, et al. Karyotypic pattern of pancreatic adenocarcinomas correlates with survival and tumour grade. *Int J Cancer.* 1994;58:8-13.
134. Coppola D, Lu L, Fruehauf JP, et al. Analysis of p53, p21WAF1, and TGF-beta1 in human ductal adenocarcinoma of the pancreas: TGF-beta1 protein expression predicts longer survival. *Am J Clin Pathol.* 1998;110:16-23.
135. van der Heijden MS, Yeo CJ, Hruban RH, Kern SE. Fanconi anemia gene mutations in young-onset pancreatic cancer. *Cancer Res.* 2003;63:2585-2588.
136. Su GH, Hruban RH, Bansal RK, et al. Germline and somatic mutations of the STK11/LKB1 Peutz-Jeghers gene in pancreatic and biliary cancers. *Am J Pathol.* 1999;154:1835-1840.
137. Su GH, Bansal R, Murphy KM, et al. ACVR1B (ALK4, activin receptor type 1B) gene mutations in pancreatic carcinoma. *Proc Natl Acad Sci U S A.* 2001;98:3254-3257.
138. Su GH, Hilgers W, Shekher MC, et al. Alterations in pancreatic, biliary, and breast carcinomas support MKK4 as a genetically targeted tumor suppressor gene. *Cancer Res.* 1998;58:2339-2342.
139. Goggins M, Shekher M, Turnacioglu K, et al. Genetic alterations of the transforming growth factor beta receptor genes in pancreatic and biliary adenocarcinomas. *Cancer Res.* 1998;58:5329-5332.
140. Shi C, Daniels JA, Hruban RH. Molecular characterization of pancreatic neoplasms. *Adv Anat Pathol.* 2008;15:185-195.
141. Hruban RH, Adsay NV. Molecular Classification of Neoplasms of the Pancreas (in press) Human Pathology. 2009.
142. Hruban RH, van Mansfeld AD, Offerhaus GJ, et al. K-ras oncogene activation in adenocarcinoma of the human pancreas. A study of 82 carcinomas using a combination of mutant-enriched polymerase chain reaction analysis and allele-specific oligonucleotide hybridization. *Am J Pathol.* 1993;143:545-554.
143. Luttges J, Diederichs A, Menke MA, et al. Ductal lesions in patients with chronic pancreatitis show K-ras mutations in a frequency similar to that in the normal pancreas and lack nuclear immunoreactivity for p53. *Cancer.* 2000;88:2495-2504.
144. Terhune PG, Phifer DM, Tosteson TD, Longnecker DS. K-ras mutation in focal proliferative lesions of human pancreas. *Cancer Epidemiol Biomarkers Prev.* 1998;7:515-521.
145. Moskaluk CA, Hruban RH, Kern SE. p16 and K-ras gene mutations in the intraductal precursors of human pancreatic adenocarcinoma. *Cancer Res.* 1997;57:2140-2143.
146. Aguirre AJ, Brennan C, Bailey G, et al. High-resolution characterization of the pancreatic adenocarcinoma genome. *Proc Natl Acad Sci U S A.* 2004;101:9067-9072.
147. Calhoun ES, Jones JB, Ashfaq R, et al. BRAF and FBXW7 (CDC4, FBW7, AGO, SEL10) mutations in distinct subsets of pancreatic cancer: potential therapeutic targets. *Am J Pathol.* 2003;163:1255-1260.
148. Miwa W, Yasuda J, Murakami Y, et al. Isolation of DNA sequences amplified at chromosome 19q13.1-q13.2 including the AKT2 locus in human pancreatic cancer. *Biochem Biophys Res Commun.* 1996;225:968-974.
149. Wallrapp C, Muller-Pillasch F, Solinas-Toldo S, et al. Characterization of a high copy number amplification at 6q24 in pancreatic cancer identifies c-myb as a candidate oncogene. *Cancer Res.* 1997;57:3135-3139.
150. Goggins M, Offerhaus GJ, Hilgers W, et al. Pancreatic adenocarcinomas with DNA replication errors (RER+) are associated with wild-type K-ras and characteristic histopathology. Poor differentiation, a syncytial growth pattern, and pushing borders suggest RER+. *Am J Pathol.* 1998;152:1501-1507.
151. Montgomery E, Wilentz RE, Argani P, et al. Analysis of anaphase figures in routine histologic sections distinguishes chromosomally unstable from chromosomally stable malignancies. *Cancer Biol Ther.* 2003;2:248-252.
152. Wilentz RE, Goggins M, Redston M, et al. Genetic, immunohistochemical, and clinical features of medullary carcinoma of the pancreas: a newly described and characterized entity. *Am J Pathol.* 2000;156:1641-1651.
153. Yamamoto H, Itoh F, Nakamura H, et al. Genetic and clinical features of human pancreatic ductal adenocarcinomas with widespread microsatellite instability. *Cancer Res.* 2001;61:3139-3144.
154. Ali-Fehmi R, Basturk O, Cheng JD, et al. Immunohistochemistry as a helpful adjunct in the differential diagnosis of intraabdominal carcinomatosis originating from the pancreas versus ovary. *Mod Pathol.* 2005;18:273A.

155. Alguacil-Garcia A, Weiland LH. The histologic spectrum, prognosis, and histogenesis of the sarcomatoid carcinoma of the pancreas. *Cancer*. 1977;39:1181-1189.
156. Paal E, Thompson LD, Frommelt RA, et al. A clinicopathologic and immunohistochemical study of 35 anaplastic carcinomas of the pancreas with a review of the literature. *Ann Diagn Pathol*. 2001;5:129-140.
157. Motoo Y, Kawashima A, Watanabe H, et al. Undifferentiated (anaplastic) carcinoma of the pancreas showing sarcomatous change and neoplastic cyst formation. *Int J Pancreatol*. 1997;21:243-248.
158. Goldstein NS, Bosler DS. Immunohistochemistry of the Gastrointestinal Tract, Pancreas, Bile Ducts, Gall Bladder and Liver. In: Dabbs D, ed. *Diagnostic Immunohistchemistry*. 2nd ed. Philadephia: Elsevier; 2006:442-508.
159. Nishihara K, Katsumoto F, Kurokawa Y, et al. Anaplastic carcinoma showing rhabdoid features combined with mucinous cystadenocarcinoma of the pancreas. *Arch Pathol Lab Med*. 1997;121:1104-1107.
160. Gatteschi B, Saccomanno S, Bartoli FG, et al. Mixed pleomorphic-osteoclast-like tumor of the pancreas. Light microscopical, immunohistochemical, and molecular biological studies. *Int J Pancreatol*. 1995;18:169-175.
161. Deckard-Janatpour K, Kragel S, Teplitz RL, et al. Tumors of the pancreas with osteoclast-like and pleomorphic giant cells: an immunohistochemical and ploidy study. *Arch Pathol Lab Med*. 1998;122:266-272.
162. Klimstra DS, Adsay NV. Benign and malignant tumors of the pancreas. In: Odze RD, Goldblum JR, Crawford JM, eds. *Surgical pathology of the GI tract, liver, biliary tract and pancreas*. Philadelphia: Saunders; 2004:699-731.
163. Winter JM, Ting AH, Vilardell F, et al. Absence of E-cadherin expression distinguishes noncohesive from cohesive pancreatic cancer. *Clin Cancer Res*. 2008;14:412-418.
164. Dhall D, Klimstra DS. The cellular composition of osteoclastlike giant cell-containing tumors of the pancreatobiliary tree. *Am J Surg Pathol*. 2008;32:335-337; author response 337.
165. Berendt RC, Shnitka TK, Wiens E, et al. The osteoclast-type giant cell tumor of the pancreas. *Arch Pathol Lab Med*. 1987;111:43-48.
166. Dizon MA, Multhaupt HA, Paskin DL, Warhol MJ. Osteoclastic giant cell tumor of the pancreas: an immunohistochemical study. *Arch Pathol Lab Med*. 1996;120:306-309.
167. Lukas Z, Dvorak K, Kroupova I, et al. Immunohistochemical and genetic analysis of osteoclastic giant cell tumor of the pancreas. *Pancreas*. 2006;32:325-329.
168. Molberg KH, Heffess C, Delgado R, et al. Undifferentiated carcinoma with osteoclast-like giant cells of the pancreas and periampullary region. *Cancer*. 1998;82:1279-1287.
169. Sakai Y, Kupelioglu AA, Yanagisawa A, et al. Origin of giant cells in osteoclast-like giant cell tumors of the pancreas. *Hum Pathol*. 2000;31:1223-1229.
170. Westra WH, Sturm P, Drillenburg P, et al. K-ras oncogene mutations in osteoclast-like giant cell tumors of the pancreas and liver: genetic evidence to support origin from the duct epithelium. *Am J Surg Pathol*. 1998;22:1247-1254.
171. Shiozawa M, Imada T, Ishiwa N, et al. Osteoclast-like giant cell tumor of the pancreas. *Int J Clin Oncol*. 2002;7:376-380.
172. Gocke CD, Dabbs DJ, Benko FA, Silverman JF. KRAS oncogene mutations suggest a common histogenetic origin for pleomorphic giant cell tumor of the pancreas, osteoclastoma of the pancreas, and pancreatic duct adenocarcinoma. *Hum Pathol*. 1997;28:80-83.
173. Imai Y, Morishita S, Ikeda Y, et al. Immunohistochemical and molecular analysis of giant cell carcinoma of the pancreas: a report of three cases. *Pancreas*. 1999;18:308-315.
174. Ueki T, Toyota M, Sohn T, et al. Hypermethylation of multiple genes in pancreatic adenocarcinoma. *Cancer Res*. 2000;60:1835-1839.
175. Kardon DE, Thompson LD, Przygodzki RM, Heffess CS. Adenosquamous carcinoma of the pancreas: a clinicopathologic series of 25 cases. *Mod Pathol*. 2001;14:443-451.
176. Ylagan LR, Scholes J, Demopoulos R. Cd44: a marker of squamous differentiation in adenosquamous neoplasms. *Arch Pathol Lab Med*. 2000;124:212-215.
177. Adsay NV, Hasteh F, Sarkar F, et al. Squamous cell and adenosquamous carcinomas of the pancreas: a clinicopathologic analysis of 11 cases. *Mod Pathol*. 2000;13:179a.
178. Basturk O, Khanani F, Sarkar F, et al. DeltaNp63 expression in pancreas and pancreatic neoplasia. *Mod Pathol*. 2005;18:1193-1198.
179. Witkiewicz AK, Brody JB, Constantino CL, et al. Adenosquamous carcinoma of the pancreas harbors KRAS2, DPC4 and TP53 molecular alterations similar to pancreatic ductal adenocarcinoma. *Mod Pathol*. 2009;22:325A.
180. Madura JA, Jarman BT, Doherty MG, et al. Adenosquamous carcinoma of the pancreas. *Arch Surg*. 1999;134:599-603.
181. Adsay NV, Merati K, Nassar H, et al. Pathogenesis of colloid (pure mucinous) carcinoma of exocrine organs: Coupling of gel-forming mucin (MUC2) production with altered cell polarity and abnormal cell-stroma interaction may be the key factor in the morphogenesis and indolent behavior of colloid carcinoma in the breast and pancreas. *Am J Surg Pathol*. 2003;27:571-578.
182. Adsay NV, Pierson C, Sarkar F, et al. Colloid (mucinous noncystic) carcinoma of the pancreas. *Am J Surg Pathol*. 2001;25:26-42.
183. Iacobuzio-Donahue CA, Klimstra DS, Adsay NV, et al. Dpc-4 protein is expressed in virtually all human intraductal papillary mucinous neoplasms of the pancreas: comparison with conventional ductal adenocarcinomas. *Am J Pathol*. 2000;157:755-761.
184. Hruban RH, Takaori K, Klimstra DS, et al. An illustrated consensus on the classification of pancreatic intraepithelial neoplasia and intraductal papillary mucinous neoplasms. *Am J Surg Pathol*. 2004;28:977-987.
185. Maitra A, Adsay NV, Argani P, et al. Multicomponent analysis of the pancreatic adenocarcinoma progression model using a pancreatic intraepithelial neoplasia tissue microarray. *Mod Pathol*. 2003;16:902-912.
186. Klein WM, Hruban RH, Klein-Szanto AJ, Wilentz RE. Direct correlation between proliferative activity and dysplasia in pancreatic intraepithelial neoplasia (PanIN): additional evidence for a recently proposed model of progression. *Mod Pathol*. 2002;15:441-447.
187. Adsay NV, Basturk O, Cheng JD, Andea AA. Ductal neoplasia of the pancreas: nosologic, clinicopathologic, and biologic aspects. *Semin Radiat Oncol*. 2005;15:254-264.
188. Prasad NB, Biankin AV, Fukushima N, et al. Gene expression profiles in pancreatic intraepithelial neoplasia reflect the effects of Hedgehog signaling on pancreatic ductal epithelial cells. *Cancer Res*. 2005;65:1619-1626.
189. Basturk O, Coban I, Adsay NV. Cystic Neoplasms of the Pancreas. *Arch Pathol Lab Med*. 2009; in press.
190. Mukawa K, Kawa S, Aoki Y, et al. Reduced expression of p53 and cyclin A in intraductal mucin-hypersecreting neoplasm of the pancreas compared with usual pancreatic ductal adenocarcinoma. *Am J Gastroenterol*. 1999;94:2263-2267.
191. Terada T, Ohta T, Kitamura Y, et al. Cell proliferative activity in intraductal papillary-mucinous neoplasms and invasive ductal adenocarcinomas of the pancreas: an immunohistochemical study. *Arch Pathol Lab Med*. 1998;122:42-46.
192. Tomaszewska R, Okon K, Nowak K, Stachura J. HER-2/Neu expression as a progression marker in pancreatic intraepithelial neoplasia. *Pol J Pathol*. 1998;49:83-92.
193. Nakamura A, Horinouchi M, Goto M, et al. New classification of pancreatic intraductal papillary-mucinous tumour by mucin expression: its relationship with potential for malignancy. *J Pathol*. 2002;197:201-210.
194. Terris B, Dubois S, Buisine MP, et al. Mucin gene expression in intraductal papillary-mucinous pancreatic tumours and related lesions. *J Pathol*. 2002;197:632-637.
195. Fukushima N, Sato N, Sahin F, et al. Aberrant methylation of suppressor of cytokine signalling-1 (SOCS-1) gene in pancreatic ductal neoplasms. *Br J Cancer*. 2003;89:338-343.
196. Adsay NV, Merati K, Basturk O, et al. Pathologically and biologically distinct types of epithelium in intraductal papillary mucinous neoplasms: delineation of an "intestinal" pathway of carcinogenesis in the pancreas. *Am J Surg Pathol*. 2004;28:839-848.

197. Paal E, Thompson LD, Przygodzki RM, et al. A clinicopathologic and immunohistochemical study of 22 intraductal papillary mucinous neoplasms of the pancreas, with a review of the literature. *Mod Pathol.* 1999;12:518-528.
198. Terada T, Ohta T, Nakanuma Y. Expression of oncogene products, anti-oncogene products and oncofetal antigens in intraductal papillary-mucinous neoplasm of the pancreas. *Histopathology.* 1996;29:355-361.
199. Nagai E, Ueki T, Chijiiwa K, et al. Intraductal papillary mucinous neoplasms of the pancreas associated with so-called "mucinous ductal ectasia." Histochemical and immunohistochemical analysis of 29 cases. *Am J Surg Pathol.* 1995;19:576-589.
200. Nagasaka T, Nakashima N. Problems in histological diagnosis of intraductal papillary-mucinous tumor (IPMT). *Hepatogastroenterology.* 2001;48:972-976.
201. Adsay NV, Pierson C, Sarkar F, et al. Comparative Immunohistochemical Analysis of Oncoprotein Expression in Various Components of IPMNs. *Pancreatology.* 2000;28:103A.
202. Tobi M, Hatfield J, Adsay V, et al. Prognostic Significance of the Labeling of Adnab-9 in Pancreatic Intraductal Papillary Mucinous Neoplasms. *Int J Gastrointest Cancer.* 2001;29:141-150.
203. Terada T, Ohta T, Kitamura Y, et al. Endocrine cells in intraductal papillary-mucinous neoplasms of the pancreas. A histochemical and immunohistochemical study. *Virchows Arch.* 1997;431:31-36.
204. Niijima M, Yamaguchi T, Ishihara T, et al. Immunohistochemical analysis and in situ hybridization of cyclooxygenase-2 expression in intraductal papillary-mucinous tumors of the pancreas. *Cancer.* 2002;94:1565-1573.
205. Patel SA, Adams R, Goldstein M, Moskaluk CA. Genetic analysis of invasive carcinoma arising in intraductal oncocytic papillary neoplasm of the pancreas. *Am J Surg Pathol.* 2002;26:1071-1077.
206. Fujii H, Inagaki M, Kasai S, et al. Genetic progression and heterogeneity in intraductal papillary-mucinous neoplasms of the pancreas. *Am J Pathol.* 1997;151:1447-1454.
207. Hoshi T, Imai M, Ogawa K. Frequent K-ras mutations and absence of p53 mutations in mucin-producing tumors of the pancreas. *J Surg Oncol.* 1994;55:84-91.
208. Izawa T, Obara T, Tanno S, et al. Clonality and field cancerization in intraductal papillary-mucinous tumors of the pancreas. *Cancer.* 2001;92:1807-1817.
209. Nakata B, Yashiro M, Nishioka N, et al. Very low incidence of microsatellite instability in intraductal papillary-mucinous neoplasm of the pancreas. *Int J Cancer.* 2002;102:655-659.
210. Satoh K, Sawai T, Shimosegawa T, et al. The point mutation of c-Ki-ras at codon 12 in carcinoma of the pancreatic head region and in intraductal mucin-hypersecreting neoplasm of the pancreas. *Int J Pancreatol.* 1993;14:135-143.
211. Satoh K, Shimosegawa T, Moriizumi S, et al. K-ras mutation and p53 protein accumulation in intraductal mucin-hypersecreting neoplasms of the pancreas. *Pancreas.* 1996;12:362-368.
212. Sessa F, Solcia E, Capella C, et al. Intraductal papillary-mucinous tumours represent a distinct group of pancreatic neoplasms: an investigation of tumour cell differentiation and K-ras, p53 and c-erbB-2 abnormalities in 26 patients. *Virchows Arch.* 1994;425:357-367.
213. Tada M, Omata M, Ohto M. Ras gene mutations in intraductal papillary neoplasms of the pancreas. Analysis in five cases. *Cancer.* 1991;67:634-637.
214. Yamaguchi K, Chijiiwa K, Noshiro H, et al. Ki-ras codon 12 point mutation and p53 mutation in pancreatic diseases. *Hepatogastroenterology.* 1999;46:2575-2581.
215. Yanagisawa A, Kato Y, Ohtake K, et al. c-Ki-ras point mutations in ductectatic-type mucinous cystic neoplasms of the pancreas. *Jpn J Cancer Res.* 1991;82:1057-1060.
216. Yoshizawa K, Nagai H, Sakurai S, et al. Clonality and K-ras mutation analyses of epithelia in intraductal papillary mucinous tumor and mucinous cystic tumor of the pancreas. *Virchows Arch.* 2002;441:437-443.
217. Biankin AV, Biankin SA, Kench JG, et al. Aberrant p16(INK4A) and DPC4/Smad4 expression in intraductal papillary mucinous tumours of the pancreas is associated with invasive ductal adenocarcinoma. *Gut.* 2002;50:861-868.
218. Flejou JF, Boulange B, Bernades P, et al. p53 protein expression and DNA ploidy in cystic tumors of the pancreas. *Pancreas.* 1996;13:247-252.
219. Islam HK, Fujioka Y, Tomidokoro T, et al. Immunohistochemical analysis of expression of molecular biologic factors in intraductal papillary-mucinous tumors of pancreas—diagnostic and biologic significance. *Hepatogastroenterology.* 1999;46:2599-2605.
220. Islam HK, Fujioka Y, Tomidokoro T, et al. Immunohistochemical study of genetic alterations in intraductal and invasive ductal tumors of the pancreas. *Hepatogastroenterology.* 2001;48:879-883.
221. Kawahira H, Kobayashi S, Kaneko K, et al. p53 protein expression in intraductal papillary mucinous tumors (IPMT) of the pancreas as an indicator of tumor malignancy. *Hepatogastroenterology.* 2000;47:973-977.
222. Kitagawa Y, Unger TA, Taylor S, et al. Mucus is a predictor of better prognosis and survival in patients with intraductal papillary mucinous tumor of the pancreas. *J Gastrointest Surg.* 2003;7:12-18; discussion 18-19.
223. Sasaki S, Yamamoto H, Kaneto H, et al. Differential roles of alterations of p53, p16, and SMAD4 expression in the progression of intraductal papillary-mucinous tumors of the pancreas. *Oncol Rep.* 2003;10:21-25.
224. Hong SP, Lee EK, Park JY, et al. Cripto-1 overexpression is involved in the tumorigenesis of gastric-type and pancreatobiliary-type intraductal papillary mucinous neoplasms of the pancreas. *Oncol Rep.* 2009;21:19-24.
225. Adsay NV, Adair CF, Heffess CS, Klimstra DS. Intraductal oncocytic papillary neoplasms of the pancreas. *Am J Surg Pathol.* 1996;20:980-994.
226. Chung SM, Hruban RH, Iacobuzio-Donahue CA, et al. Analysis of molecular alterations and differentiation pathways in intraductal oncocytic papillary neoplasm of the pancreas. *Mod Pathol.* 2005;18:277A.
227. Kloppel G, Luttges J. WHO-classification 2000: exocrine pancreatic tumors. *Verh Dtsch Ges Pathol.* 2001;85:219-228.
228. Kloppel G, Kosmahl M. Cystic lesions and neoplasms of the pancreas. The features are becoming clearer. *Pancreatology.* 2001;1:648-655.
229. Fukushima N, Mukai K. 'Ovarian-type' stroma of pancreatic mucinous cystic tumor expresses smooth muscle phenotype. *Pathol Int.* 1997;47:806-808.
230. Sarr MG, Carpenter HA, Prabhakar LP, et al. Clinical and pathologic correlation of 84 mucinous cystic neoplasms of the pancreas: can one reliably differentiate benign from malignant (or premalignant) neoplasms? *Ann Surg.* 2000;231:205-212.
231. Yamaguchi K, Enjoji M. Cystic neoplasms of the pancreas. *Gastroenterology.* 1987;92:1934-1943.
232. Thompson LD, Becker RC, Przygodzki RM, et al. Mucinous cystic neoplasm (mucinous cystadenocarcinoma of low-grade malignant potential) of the pancreas: a clinicopathologic study of 130 cases. *Am J Surg Pathol.* 1999;23:1-16.
233. Luttges J, Feyerabend B, Buchelt T, et al. The mucin profile of noninvasive and invasive mucinous cystic neoplasms of the pancreas. *Am J Surg Pathol.* 2002;26:466-471.
234. Ohta T, Nagakawa T, Fukushima W, et al. Immunohistochemical study of carcinoembryonic antigen in mucinous cystic neoplasm of the pancreas. *Eur Surg Res.* 1992;24:37-44.
235. van den Berg W, Tascilar M, Offerhaus GJ, et al. Pancreatic mucinous cystic neoplasms with sarcomatous stroma: molecular evidence for monoclonal origin with subsequent divergence of the epithelial and sarcomatous components. *Mod Pathol.* 2000;13:86-91.
236. Yu HC, Shetty J. Mucinous cystic neoplasm of the pancreas with high carcinoembryonic antigen. *Arch Pathol Lab Med.* 1985;109:375-377.
237. Khalifeh I, Basturk O, Zamboni G, et al. Villous-intestinal differentiation and progression to colloid carcinoma, characteristic of a major subset of IPMNs, are not features of mucinous cystic neoplasms. *Mod Pathol.* 2005;18:281A.
238. Albores-Saavedra J, Nadji M, Henson DE, et al. Entero-endocrine cell differentiation in carcinomas of the gallbladder and mucinous cystadenocarcinomas of the pancreas. *Pathol Res Pract.* 1988;183:169-175.

239. Albores-Saavedra J, Angeles-Angeles A, Nadji M, et al. Mucinous cystadenocarcinoma of the pancreas. Morphologic and immunocytochemical observations. *Am J Surg Pathol.* 1987;11:11-20.
240. Khalifeh I, Qureshi F, Jacques S, et al. The nature of "ovarian-like" mesenchyme of pancreatic and hepatic mucinous cystic neoplasms: A recapitulation of the periductal fetal mesenchme?. *Mod Pathol.* 2004;17:304A.
241. Wilentz RE, Albores-Saavedra J, Hruban RH. Mucinous cystic neoplasms of the pancreas. *Semin Diagn Pathol.* 2000;17:31-42.
242. Zamboni G, Scarpa A, Bogina G, et al. Mucinous cystic tumors of the pancreas: clinicopathological featurês, prognosis, and relationship to other mucinous cystic tumors. *Am J Surg Pathol.* 1999;23:410-422.
243. Izumo A, Yamaguchi K, Eguchi T, et al. Mucinous cystic tumor of the pancreas: immunohistochemical assessment of "ovarian-type stroma. *Oncol Rep.* 2003;10:515-525.
244. Weihing RR, Shintaku IP, Geller SA, Petrovic LM. Hepatobiliary and pancreatic mucinous cystadenocarcinomas with mesenchymal stroma: analysis of estrogen receptors/progesterone receptors and expression of tumor-associated antigens. *Mod Pathol.* 1997;10:372-379.
245. Ridder GJ, Maschek H, Klempnauer J. Favourable prognosis of cystadeno- over adenocarcinoma of the pancreas after curative resection. *Eur J Surg Oncol.* 1996;22:232-236.
246. Zheng W, Sung CJ, Hanna I, et al. Alpha and beta subunits of inhibin/activin as sex cord-stromal differentiation markers. *Int J Gynecol Pathol.* 1997;16:263-271.
247. Bartsch D, Bastian D, Barth P, et al. K-ras oncogene mutations indicate malignancy in cystic tumors of the pancreas. *Ann Surg.* 1998;228:79-86.
248. Jimenez RE, Warshaw AL, Z'Graggen K, et al. Sequential accumulation of K-ras mutations and p53 overexpression in the progression of pancreatic mucinous cystic neoplasms to malignancy. *Ann Surg.* 1999;230:501-509; discussion 509-511.
249. Kim SG, Wu TT, Lee JH, et al. Comparison of epigenetic and genetic alterations in mucinous cystic neoplasm and serous microcystic adenoma of pancreas. *Mod Pathol.* 2003;16:1086-1094.
250. Iacobuzio-Donahue CA, Wilentz RE, Argani P, et al. Dpc4 protein in mucinous cystic neoplasms of the pancreas: frequent loss of expression in invasive carcinomas suggests a role in genetic progression. *Am J Surg Pathol.* 2000;24:1544-1548.
251. Tajiri T, Tate G, Inagaki T, et al. Intraductal tubular neoplasms of the pancreas: histogenesis and differentiation. *Pancreas.* 2005;30:115-121.
252. Tajiri T, Tate G, Kunimura T, et al. Histologic and immunohistochemical comparison of intraductal tubular carcinoma, intraductal papillary-mucinous carcinoma, and ductal adenocarcinoma of the pancreas. *Pancreas.* 2004;29:116-122.
253. Albores-Saavedra J, Sheahan K, O'Riain C, Shukla D. Intraductal tubular adenoma, pyloric type, of the pancreas: additional observations on a new type of pancreatic neoplasm. *Am J Surg Pathol.* 2004;28:233-238.
254. Bakotic BW, Robinson MJ, Sturm PD, et al. Pyloric gland adenoma of the main pancreatic duct. *Am J Surg Pathol.* 1999;23:227-231.
255. Kato N, Akiyama S, Motoyama T. Pyloric gland-type tubular adenoma superimposed on intraductal papillary mucinous tumor of the pancreas. Pyloric gland adenoma of the pancreas. *Virchows Arch.* 2002;440:205-208.
256. Nakayama Y, Inoue H, Hamada Y, et al. Intraductal tubular adenoma of the pancreas, pyloric gland type: a clinicopathologic and immunohistochemical study of 6 cases. *Am J Surg Pathol.* 2005;29:607-616.
257. Compton CC. Serous cystic tumors of the pancreas. *Semin Diagn Pathol.* 2000;17:43-55.
258. Alpert LC, Truong LD, Bossart MI, Spjut HJ. Microcystic adenoma (serous cystadenoma) of the pancreas. A study of 14 cases with immunohistochemical and electron-microscopic correlation. *Am J Surg Pathol.* 1988;12:251-263.
259. Egawa N, Maillet B, Schroder S, et al. Serous oligocystic and ill-demarcated adenoma of the pancreas: a variant of serous cystic adenoma. *Virchows Arch.* 1994;424:13-17.
260. Kosmahl M, Wagner J, Peters K, et al. Serous cystic neoplasms of the pancreas: an immunohistochemical analysis revealing alpha-inhibin, neuron-specific enolase, and MUC6 as new markers. *Am J Surg Pathol.* 2004;28:339-346.
261. Shorten SD, Hart WR, Petras RE. Microcystic adenomas (serous cystadenomas) of pancreas. A clinicopathologic investigation of eight cases with immunohistochemical and ultrastructural studies. *Am J Surg Pathol.* 1986;10:365-372.
262. Sperti C, Pasquali C, Perasole A, et al. Macrocystic serous cystadenoma of the pancreas: clinicopathologic features in seven cases. *Int J Pancreatol.* 2000;28:1-7.
263. Yasuhara Y, Sakaida N, Uemura Y, et al. Serous microcystic adenoma (glycogen-rich cystadenoma) of the pancreas: study of 11 cases showing clinicopathological and immunohistochemical correlations. *Pathol Int.* 2002;52:307-312.
264. Perez-Ordonez B, Naseem A, Lieberman PH, Klimstra DS. Solid serous adenoma of the pancreas. The solid variant of serous cystadenoma? *Am J Surg Pathol.* 1996;20:1401-1405.
265. Ishikawa T, Nakao A, Nomoto S, et al. Immunohistochemical and molecular biological studies of serous cystadenoma of the pancreas. *Pancreas.* 1998;16:40-44.
266. Helpap B, Vogel J. Immunohistochemical studies on cystic pancreatic neoplasms. *Pathol Res Pract.* 1988;184:39-45.
267. Solcia E, Capella C, Kloppel G. *Tumors of the Pancreas.* 3rd ed. Washington, DC: American Registry of Pathology; 1997.
268. Thirabanjasak D, Basturk O, Altinel D, et al. Is serous cystadenoma of pancreas a model of clear cell associated angiogenesis and tumorigenesis? *Pancreatology.* 2008;9:182-188.
269. Mohr VH, Vortmeyer AO, Zhuang Z, et al. Histopathology and molecular genetics of multiple cysts and microcystic (serous) adenomas of the pancreas in von Hippel-Lindau patients. *Am J Pathol.* 2000;157:1615-1621.
270. Vortmeyer AO, Lubensky IA, Fogt F, et al. Allelic deletion and mutation of the von Hippel-Lindau (VHL) tumor suppressor gene in pancreatic microcystic adenomas. *Am J Pathol.* 1997;151:951-956.
271. Moore PS, Zamboni G, Brighenti A, et al. Molecular characterization of pancreatic serous microcystic adenomas: evidence for a tumor suppressor gene on chromosome 10q. *Am J Pathol.* 2001;158:317-321.
272. Santos LD, Chow C, Henderson CJ, et al. Serous oligocystic adenoma of the pancreas: a clinicopathological and immunohistochemical study of three cases with ultrastructural findings. *Pathology.* 2002;34:148-156.
273. Ordonez NG. Pancreatic acinar cell carcinoma. *Adv Anat Pathol.* 2001;8:144-159.
274. Hartman GG, Ni H, Pickleman J. Acinar cell carcinoma of the pancreas. *Arch Pathol Lab Med.* 2001;125:1127-1128.
275. Klimstra DS, Heffess CS, Oertel JE, Rosai J. Acinar cell carcinoma of the pancreas. A clinicopathologic study of 28 cases. *Am J Surg Pathol.* 1992;16:815-837.
276. Skacel M, Ormsby AH, Petras RE, et al. Immunohistochemistry in the differential diagnosis of acinar and endocrine pancreatic neoplasms. *Appl Immunohistochem Mol Morphol.* 2000;8:203-209.
277. Kuerer H, Shim H, Pertsemlidis D, Unger P. Functioning pancreatic acinar cell carcinoma: immunohistochemical and ultrastructural analyses. *Am J Clin Oncol.* 1997;20:101-107.
278. Ishihara A, Sanda T, Takanari H, et al. Elastase-1-secreting acinar cell carcinoma of the pancreas. A cytologic, electron microscopic and histochemical study. *Acta Cytol.* 1989;33:157-163.
279. Ohike N, Kosmahl M, Kloppel G. Mixed acinar-endocrine carcinoma of the pancreas. A clinicopathological study and comparison with acinar-cell carcinoma. *Virchows Arch.* 2004;445:231-235.
280. Basturk O, Zamboni G, Klimstra DS, et al. Intraductal and papillary variants of acinar cell carcinomas: a new addition to the challenging differential diagnosis of intraductal neoplasms. *Am J Surg Pathol.* 2007;31:363-370.
281. Pellegata NS, Sessa F, Renault B, et al. K-ras and p53 gene mutations in pancreatic cancer: ductal and nonductal tumors progress through different genetic lesions. *Cancer Res.* 1994;54:1556-1560.
282. Terhune PG, Heffess CS, Longnecker DS. Only wild-type c-Ki-ras codons 12, 13, and 61 in human pancreatic acinar cell carcinomas. *Mol Carcinog.* 1994;10:110-114.

283. Terhune PG, Memoli VA, Longnecker DS. Evaluation of p53 mutation in pancreatic acinar cell carcinomas of humans and transgenic mice. *Pancreas*. 1998;16:6-12.
284. Abraham SC, Wu TT, Hruban RH, et al. Genetic and immunohistochemical analysis of pancreatic acinar cell carcinoma: frequent allelic loss on chromosome 11p and alterations in the APC/beta-catenin pathway. *Am J Pathol*. 2002;160:953-962.
285. Longnecker DS. Molecular pathology of invasive carcinoma. *Ann N Y Acad Sci*. 1999;880:74-82.
286. Moore PS, Beghelli S, Zamboni G, Scarpa A. Genetic abnormalities in pancreatic cancer. *Mol Cancer*. 2003;2:7.
287. Rigaud G, Moore PS, Zamboni G, et al. Allelotype of pancreatic acinar cell carcinoma. *Int J Cancer*. 2000;88:772-777.
288. Taruscio D, Paradisi S, Zamboni G, et al. Pancreatic acinar carcinoma shows a distinct pattern of chromosomal imbalances by comparative genomic hybridization. *Genes Chromosomes Cancer*. 2000;28:294-299.
289. Klimstra DS. Nonductal neoplasms of the pancreas. *Mod Pathol*. 2007;20(Suppl 1):S94-112.
290. Henke AC, Kelley CM, Jensen CS, Timmerman TG. Fine-needle aspiration cytology of pancreatoblastoma. *Diagn Cytopathol*. 2001;25:118-121.
291. Kawamoto K, Matsuo T, Jubashi T, et al. Primary pancreatic carcinoma in childhood. Pancreatoblastoma. *Acta Pathol Jpn*. 1985;35:137-143.
292. Klimstra DS, Wenig BM, Adair CF, Heffess CS. Pancreatoblastoma: A clinicopathologic study and review of the literature. *Am J Surg Pathol*. 1995;19:1371-1389.
293. Nishimata S, Kato K, Tanaka M, et al. Expression pattern of keratin subclasses in pancreatoblastoma with special emphasis on squamoid corpuscles. *Pathol Int*. 2005;55:297-302.
294. Silverman JF, Holbrook CT, Pories WJ, et al. Fine needle aspiration cytology of pancreatoblastoma with immunocytochemical and ultrastructural studies. *Acta Cytol*. 1990;34:632-640.
295. Ohaki Y, Misugi K, Fukuda J, et al. Immunohistochemical study of pancreatoblastoma. *Acta Pathol Jpn*. 1987;37:1581-1590.
296. Cooper JE, Lake BD. Use of enzyme histochemistry in the diagnosis of pancreatoblastoma. *Histopathology*. 1989;15:407-414.
297. He L, Li P, Liu S, et al. [A clinicopathological study of pancreatoblastoma]. *Zhonghua Bing Li Xue Za Zhi*. 1999;28:337-339.
298. Iseki M, Suzuki T, Koizumi Y, et al. Alpha-fetoprotein-producing pancreatoblastoma. A case report. *Cancer*. 1986;57:1833-1835.
299. Abraham SC, Wu TT, Klimstra DS, et al. Distinctive molecular genetic alterations in sporadic and familial adenomatous polyposis-associated pancreatoblastomas: frequent alterations in the APC/beta-catenin pathway and chromosome 11p. *Am J Pathol*. 2001;159:1619-1627.
300. Tanaka Y, Kato K, Notohara K, et al. Significance of aberrant (cytoplasmic/nuclear) expression of beta-catenin in pancreatoblastoma. *J Pathol*. 2003;199:185-190.
301. Kerr NJ, Chun YH, Yun K, et al. Pancreatoblastoma is associated with chromosome 11p loss of heterozygosity and IGF2 overexpression. *Med Pediatr Oncol*. 2002;39:52-54.
302. Wiley J, Posekany K, Riley R, et al. Cytogenetic and flow cytometric analysis of a pancreatoblastoma. *Cancer Genet Cytogenet*. 1995;79:115-118.
303. Balercia G, Zamboni G, Bogina G, Mariuzzi GM. Solid-cystic tumor of the pancreas. An extensive ultrastructural study of fourteen cases. *J Submicrosc Cytol Pathol*. 1995;27:331-340.
304. Martin RC, Klimstra DS, Brennan MF, Conlon KC. Solid-pseudopapillary tumor of the pancreas: a surgical enigma? *Ann Surg Oncol*. 2002;9:35-40.
305. Miettinen M, Partanen S, Fraki O, Kivilaakso E. Papillary cystic tumor of the pancreas. An analysis of cellular differentiation by electron microscopy and immunohistochemistry. *Am J Surg Pathol*. 1987;11:855-865.
306. Yamaguchi K, Miyagahara T, Tsuneyoshi M, et al. Papillary cystic tumor of the pancreas: an immunohistochemical and ultrastructural study of 14 patients. *Jpn J Clin Oncol*. 1989;19:102-111.
307. Wunsch LP, Flemming P, Werner U, et al. Diagnosis and treatment of papillary cystic tumor of the pancreas in children. *Eur J Pediatr Surg*. 1997;7:45-47.
308. von Herbay A, Sieg B, Otto HF. Solid-cystic tumour of the pancreas. An endocrine neoplasm? *Virchows Arch A Pathol Anat Histopathol*. 1990;416:535-538.
309. Pettinato G, Manivel JC, Ravetto C, et al. Papillary cystic tumor of the pancreas. A clinicopathologic study of 20 cases with cytologic, immunohistochemical, ultrastructural, and flow cytometric observations, and a review of the literature. *Am J Clin Pathol*. 1992;98:478-488.
310. Lieber MR, Lack EE, Roberts Jr JR, et al. Solid and papillary epithelial neoplasm of the pancreas. An ultrastructural and immunocytochemical study of six cases. *Am J Surg Pathol*. 1987;11:85-93.
311. Stommer P, Kraus J, Stolte M, Giedl J. Solid and cystic pancreatic tumors. Clinical, histochemical, and electron microscopic features in ten cases. *Cancer*. 1991;67:1635-1641.
312. Yoon DY, Hines OJ, Bilchik AJ, et al. Solid and papillary epithelial neoplasms of the pancreas: aggressive resection for cure. *Am Surg*. 2001;67:1195-1199.
313. Lam KY, Lo CY, Fan ST. Pancreatic solid-cystic-papillary tumor: clinicopathologic features in eight patients from Hong Kong and review of the literature. *World J Surg*. 1999;23:1045-1050.
314. Kosmahl M, Seada LS, Janig U, et al. Solid-pseudopapillary tumor of the pancreas: its origin revisited. *Virchows Arch*. 2000;436:473-480.
315. Lee WY, Tzeng CC, Chen RM, et al. Papillary cystic tumors of the pancreas: assessment of malignant potential by analysis of progesterone receptor, flow cytometry, and ras oncogene mutation. *Anticancer Res*. 1997;17:2587-2591.
316. Notohara K, Hamazaki S, Tsukayama C, et al. Solid-pseudopapillary tumor of the pancreas: immunohistochemical localization of neuroendocrine markers and CD10. *Am J Surg Pathol*. 2000;24:1361-1371.
317. Zamboni G, Bonetti F, Scarpa A, et al. Expression of progesterone receptors in solid-cystic tumour of the pancreas: a clinicopathological and immunohistochemical study of ten cases. *Virchows Arch A Pathol Anat Histopathol*. 1993;423:425-431.
318. Abraham SC, Klimstra DS, Wilentz RE, et al. Solid-pseudopapillary tumors of the pancreas are genetically distinct from pancreatic ductal adenocarcinomas and almost always harbor beta-catenin mutations. *Am J Pathol*. 2002;160:1361-1369.
319. Muller-Hocker J, Zietz CH, Sendelhofert A. Deregulated expression of cell cycle-associated proteins in solid pseudopapillary tumor of the pancreas. *Mod Pathol*. 2001;14:47-53.
320. Chott A, Kloppel G, Buxbaum P, Heitz PU. Neuron specific enolase demonstration in the diagnosis of a solid-cystic (papillary cystic) tumour of the pancreas. *Virchows Arch A Pathol Anat Histopathol*. 1987;410:397-402.
321. Kloppel G, Maurer R, Hofmann E, et al. Solid-cystic (papillary-cystic) tumours within and outside the pancreas in men: report of two patients. *Virchows Arch A Pathol Anat Histopathol*. 1991;418:179-183.
322. Kim MJ, Jang SJ, Yu E. Loss of E-cadherin and cytoplasmic-nuclear expression of beta-catenin are the most useful immunoprofiles in the diagnosis of solid-pseudopapillary neoplasm of the pancreas. *Hum Pathol*. 2008;39:251-258.
323. Tien YW, Ser KH, Hu RH, et al. Solid pseudopapillary neoplasms of the pancreas: is there a pathologic basis for the observed gender differences in incidence? *Surgery*. 2005;137:591-596.
324. Nishihara K, Tsuneyoshi M, Ohshima A, Yamaguchi K. Papillary cystic tumor of the pancreas. Is it a hormone-dependent neoplasm? *Pathol Res Pract*. 1993;189:521-526.
325. Cao D, Antonescu C, Wong G, et al. Positive immunohistochemical staining of KIT in solid-pseudopapillary neoplasms of the pancreas is not associated with KIT/PDGFRA mutations. *Mod Pathol*. 2006;19:1157-1163.
326. Tiemann K, Heitling U, Kosmahl M, Kloppel G. Solid pseudopapillary neoplasms of the pancreas show an interruption of the Wnt-signaling pathway and express gene products of 11q. *Mod Pathol*. 2007;20:955-960.
327. Doglioni C, Tos AP, Laurino L, et al. Calretinin: a novel immunocytochemical marker for mesothelioma. *Am J Surg Pathol*. 1996;20:1037-1046.

328. Tanaka Y, Kato K, Notohara K, et al. Frequent beta-catenin mutation and cytoplasmic/nuclear accumulation in pancreatic solid-pseudopapillary neoplasm. *Cancer Res.* 2001;61:8401-8404.
329. Yamaue H, Tanimura H, Shono Y, et al. Solid and cystic tumor of the pancreas: clinicopathologic and genetic studies of four cases. *Int J Pancreatol.* 2000;27:69-76.
330. Chetty R, Serra S. Membrane loss and aberrant nuclear localization of E-cadherin are consistent features of solid pseudopapillary tumour of the pancreas. An immunohistochemical study using two antibodies recognizing different domains of the E-cadherin molecule. *Histopathology.* 2008;52:325-330.
331. Tiemann K, Kosmahl M, Ohlendorf J, et al. Solid pseudopapillary neoplasms of the pancreas are associated with FLI-1 expression, but not with EWS/FLI-1 translocation. *Mod Pathol.* 2006;19:1409-1413.
332. Heitz PU, Komminoth P, Perren A. Pancreatic endocrine tumors: Introduction. In: Delellis RA, Lloyd RV, Heitz PU, Eng C, eds. *WHO Classification of Tumors. Pathology and Genetics of Tumours od Endocrine Organs.* Lyon, France: IARC Press; 2004:177-182.
333. Lloyd RV, Mervak T, Schmidt K, et al. Immunohistochemical detection of chromogranin and neuron-specific enolase in pancreatic endocrine neoplasms. *Am J Surg Pathol.* 1984;8:607-614.
334. Thomas RM, Baybick JH, Elsayed AM, Sobin LH. Gastric carcinoids. An immunohistochemical and clinicopathologic study of 104 patients. *Cancer.* 1994;73:2053-2058.
335. Al-Khafaji B, Noffsinger AE, Miller MA, et al. Immunohistologic analysis of gastrointestinal and pulmonary carcinoid tumors. *Hum Pathol.* 1998;29:992-999.
336. Bordi C. Gastric carcinoids: an immunohistochemical and clinicopathologic study of 104 patients. *Cancer.* 1995;75:129-130.
337. Bordi C, Yu JY, Baggi MT, et al. Gastric carcinoids and their precursor lesions. A histologic and immunohistochemical study of 23 cases. *Cancer.* 1991;67:663-672.
338. Le Gall F, Vallet VS, Thomas D, et al. Immunohistochemical study of secretogranin II in 62 neuroendocrine tumours of the digestive tract and of the pancreas in comparison with other granins. *Pathol Res Pract.* 1997;193:179-185.
339. Burke AP, Federspiel BH, Sobin LH, et al. Carcinoids of the duodenum. A histologic and immunohistochemical study of 65 tumors. *Am J Surg Pathol.* 1989;13:828-837.
340. Makhlouf HR, Burke AP, Sobin LH. Carcinoid tumors of the ampulla of Vater: a comparison with duodenal carcinoid tumors. *Cancer.* 1999;85:1241-1249.
341. Lam KY, Lo CY. Pancreatic endocrine tumour: a 22-year clinico-pathological experience with morphological, immunohistochemical observation and a review of the literature. *Eur J Surg Oncol.* 1997;23:36-42.
342. Azzoni C, Doglioni C, Viale G, et al. Involvement of BCL-2 oncoprotein in the development of enterochromaffin-like cell gastric carcinoids. *Am J Surg Pathol.* 1996;20:433-441.
343. Hayashi H, Nakagawa M, Kitagawa S, et al. Immunohistochemical analysis of gastrointestinal carcinoids. *Gastroenterol Jpn.* 1993;28:483-490.
344. Rindi G, Ubiali A, Villanacci V. The phenotype of gut endocrine tumours. *Dig Liver Dis.* 2004;36(Suppl 1):S26-30.
345. Erickson LA, Lloyd RV. Practical markers used in the diagnosis of endocrine tumors. *Adv Anat Pathol.* 2004;11:175-189.
346. Chetty R, Asa SL. Pancreatic endocrine tumors: an update. *Adv Anat Pathol.* 2004;11:202-210.
347. Bostwick DG, Null WE, Holmes D, et al. Expression of opioid peptides in tumors. *N Engl J Med.* 1987;317:1439-1443.
348. Chejfec G, Falkmer S, Grimelius L, et al. Synaptophysin. A new marker for pancreatic neuroendocrine tumors. *Am J Surg Pathol.* 1987;11:241-247.
349. Simpson S, Vinik AI, Marangos PJ, Lloyd RV. Immunohistochemical localization of neuron-specific enolase in gastroenteropancreatic neuroendocrine tumors. Correlation with tissue and serum levels of neuron-specific enolase. *Cancer.* 1984;54:1364-1369.
350. Heitz PU, Kasper M, Polak JM, Kloppel G. Pancreatic endocrine tumors. *Hum Pathol.* 1982;13:263-271.
351. Mukai K. Functional pathology of pancreatic islets: immunocytochemical exploration. *Pathol Annu.* 1983;18(Pt 2):87-107.
352. Mukai K, Grotting JC, Greider MH, Rosai J. Retrospective study of 77 pancreatic endocrine tumors using the immunoperoxidase method. *Am J Surg Pathol.* 1982;6:387-399.
353. Clark ES, Carney JA. Pancreatic islet cell tumor associated with Cushing's syndrome. *Am J Surg Pathol.* 1984;8:917-924.
354. Schmid KW, Brink M, Freytag G, et al. Expression of chromogranin A and B and secretoneurin immunoreactivity in neoplastic and nonneoplastic pancreatic alpha cells. *Virchows Arch.* 1994;425:127-132.
355. Delis S, Bakoyiannis A, Giannakou N, et al. Asymptomatic calcitonin-secreting tumor of the pancreas. A case report. *JOP.* 2006;7:70-73.
356. Osamura RY, Oberg K, Perren A. Pancreatic endocrine tumours: ACTH and other ectopic hormone producing tumours. In: Delellis RA, Lloyd RV, Heitz PU, Eng C, eds. *WHO Classification of Tumours. Pathology and Genetics of Tumours of Endocrine Organs.* Lyon, France: IARC Press; 2004:199-200.
357. Miraliakbari BA, Asa SL, Boudreau SF. Parathyroid hormone-like peptide in pancreatic endocrine carcinoma and adenocarcinoma associated with hypercalcemia. *Hum Pathol.* 1992;23:884-887.
358. Berger G, Trouillas J, Bloch B, et al. Multihormonal carcinoid tumor of the pancreas. Secreting growth hormone-releasing factor as a cause of acromegaly. *Cancer.* 1984;54:2097-2108.
359. Bostwick DG, Quan R, Hoffman AR, et al. Growth-hormone-releasing factor immunoreactivity in human endocrine tumors. *Am J Pathol.* 1984;117:167-170.
360. Dayal Y, Lin HD, Tallberg K, et al. Immunocytochemical demonstration of growth hormone-releasing factor in gastrointestinal and pancreatic endocrine tumors. *Am J Clin Pathol.* 1986;85:13-20.
361. La Rosa S, Uccella S, Billo P, et al. Immunohistochemical localization of alpha- and betaA-subunits of inhibin/activin in human normal endocrine cells and related tumors of the digestive system. *Virchows Arch.* 1999;434:29-36.
362. Kimura N, Pilichowska M, Okamoto H, et al. Immunohistochemical expression of chromogranins A and B, prohormone convertases 2 and 3, and amidating enzyme in carcinoid tumors and pancreatic endocrine tumors. *Mod Pathol.* 2000;13:140-146.
363. Tomita T. Metallothionein in pancreatic endocrine neoplasms. *Mod Pathol.* 2000;13:389-395.
364. Papotti M, Bongiovanni M, Volante M, et al. Expression of somatostatin receptor types 1-5 in 81 cases of gastrointestinal and pancreatic endocrine tumors. A correlative immunohistochemical and reverse-transcriptase polymerase chain reaction analysis. *Virchows Arch.* 2002;440:461-475.
365. Larsson LI, Grimelius L, Hakanson R, et al. Mixed endocrine pancreatic tumors producing several peptide hormones. *Am J Pathol.* 1975;79:271-284.
366. Liu TH, Tseng HC, Zhu Y, et al. Insulinoma. An immunocytochemical and morphologic analysis of 95 cases. *Cancer.* 1985;56:1420-1429.
367. Osamura RY, Oberg K, Speel EJ, et al. Pancreatic endocrine tumours: serotonin-secreting tumour. In: Delellis RA, Lloyd RV, Heitz PU, Eng C, eds. *WHO Classification of Tumours. Pathology and Genetics of Tumours of Endocrine Organs.* Lyon, France: IARC Press; 2004:198.
368. Deshpande V, Fernandez-del Castillo C, Muzikansky A, et al. Cytokeratin 19 is a powerful predictor of survival in pancreatic endocrine tumors. *Am J Surg Pathol.* 2004;28:1145-1153.
369. Schmitt AM, Anlauf M, Rousson V, et al. WHO 2004 criteria and CK19 are reliable prognostic markers in pancreatic endocrine tumors. *Am J Surg Pathol.* 2007;31:1677-1682.
370. Ali A, Serra S, Asa SL, Chetty R. The predictive value of CK19 and CD99 in pancreatic endocrine tumors. *Am J Surg Pathol.* 2006;30:1588-1594.
371. Cai YC, Banner B, Glickman J, Odze RD. Cytokeratin 7 and 20 and thyroid transcription factor 1 can help distinguish pulmonary from gastrointestinal carcinoid and pancreatic endocrine tumors. *Hum Pathol.* 2001;32:1087-1093.
372. d'Amore ES, Manivel JC, Pettinato G, et al. Intestinal ganglioneuromatosis: mucosal and transmural types. A clinicopathologic and immunohistochemical study of six cases. *Hum Pathol.* 1991;22:276-286.

373. Hochwald SN, Zee S, Conlon KC, et al. Prognostic factors in pancreatic endocrine neoplasms: an analysis of 136 cases with a proposal for low-grade and intermediate-grade groups. *J Clin Oncol.* 2002;20:2633-2642.
374. Kamisawa T, Tu Y, Egawa N, et al. Ductal and acinar differentiation in pancreatic endocrine tumors. *Dig Dis Sci.* 2002;47:2254-2261.
375. Yantiss RK, Chang HK, Farraye FA, et al. Prevalence and prognostic significance of acinar cell differentiation in pancreatic endocrine tumors. *Am J Surg Pathol.* 2002;26:893-901.
376. Klimstra DS, Rosai J, Heffess CS. Mixed acinar-endocrine carcinomas of the pancreas. *Am J Surg Pathol.* 1994;18:765-778.
377. Arihiro K, Inai K. Malignant islet cell tumor of the pancreas with multiple hormone production and expression of CEA and CA19-9. Report of an autopsy case. *Acta Pathol Jpn.* 1991;41:150-157.
378. Hussain S, Arwini A, Chetty R, Klimstra DS. Oncocytic pancreatic endocrine neoplasms: a clinicopathologic and immnunohistochemical analysis of 21 cases. *Mod Pathol.* 2005;18:279A.
379. Goto A, Niki T, Terado Y, et al. Prevalence of CD99 protein expression in pancreatic endocrine tumours (PETs). *Histopathology.* 2004;45:384-392.
380. Viale G, Doglioni C, Gambacorta M, et al. Progesterone receptor immunoreactivity in pancreatic endocrine tumors. An immunocytochemical study of 156 neuroendocrine tumors of the pancreas, gastrointestinal and respiratory tracts, and skin. *Cancer.* 1992;70:2268-2277.
381. Speel EJ, Richter J, Moch H, et al. Genetic differences in endocrine pancreatic tumor subtypes detected by comparative genomic hybridization. *Am J Pathol.* 1999;155:1787-1794.
382. Stumpf E, Aalto Y, Hoog A, et al. Chromosomal alterations in human pancreatic endocrine tumors. *Genes Chromosomes Cancer.* 2000;29:83-87.
383. Zhao J, Moch H, Scheidweiler AF, et al. Genomic imbalances in the progression of endocrine pancreatic tumors. *Genes Chromosomes Cancer.* 2001;32:364-372.
384. Asteria C, Anagni M, Fugazzola L, et al. MEN1 gene mutations are a rare event in patients with sporadic neuroendocrine tumors. *Eur J Intern Med.* 2002;13:319-323.
385. Cupisti K, Hoppner W, Dotzenrath C, et al. Lack of MEN1 gene mutations in 27 sporadic insulinomas. *Eur J Clin Invest.* 2000;30:325-329.
386. Gortz B, Roth J, Krahenmann A, et al. Mutations and allelic deletions of the MEN1 gene are associated with a subset of sporadic endocrine pancreatic and neuroendocrine tumors and not restricted to foregut neoplasms. *Am J Pathol.* 1999;154:429-436.
387. Hessman O, Lindberg D, Einarsson A, et al. Genetic alterations on 3p, 11q13, and 18q in nonfamilial and MEN 1-associated pancreatic endocrine tumors. *Genes Chromosomes Cancer.* 1999;26:258-264.
388. Komminoth P. Review: multiple endocrine neoplasia type 1, sporadic neuroendocrine tumors, and MENIN. *Diagn Mol Pathol.* 1999;8:107-112.
389. Moore PS, Missiaglia E, Antonello D, et al. Role of disease-causing genes in sporadic pancreatic endocrine tumors: MEN1 and VHL. *Genes Chromosomes Cancer.* 2001;32:177-181.
390. Shan L, Nakamura Y, Nakamura M, et al. Somatic mutations of multiple endocrine neoplasia type 1 gene in the sporadic endocrine tumors. *Lab Invest.* 1998;78:471-475.
391. Wang EH, Ebrahimi SA, Wu AY, et al. Mutation of the MENIN gene in sporadic pancreatic endocrine tumors. *Cancer Res.* 1998;58:4417-4420.
392. Zhuang Z, Vortmeyer AO, Pack S, et al. Somatic mutations of the MEN1 tumor suppressor gene in sporadic gastrinomas and insulinomas. *Cancer Res.* 1997;57:4682-4686.
393. Lubensky IA, Pack S, Ault D, et al. Multiple neuroendocrine tumors of the pancreas in von Hippel-Lindau disease patients: histopathological and molecular genetic analysis. *Am J Pathol.* 1998;153:223-231.
394. Goebel SU, Iwamoto M, Raffeld M, et al. Her-2/neu expression and gene amplification in gastrinomas: correlations with tumor biology, growth, and aggressiveness. *Cancer Res.* 2002;62:3702-3710.
395. Chung DC, Smith AP, Louis DN, et al. A novel pancreatic endocrine tumor suppressor gene locus on chromosome 3p with clinical prognostic implications. *J Clin Invest.* 1997;100:404-410.
396. Scarpa A, Orlandini S, Moore PS, et al. Dpc4 is expressed in virtually all primary and metastatic pancreatic endocrine carcinomas. *Virchows Arch.* 2002;440:155-159.
397. Srivastava A, Hornick JL. Immunohistochemical staining for CDX-2, PDX-1, NESP-55, and TTF-1 can help distinguish gastrointestinal carcinoid tumors from pancreatic endocrine and pulmonary carcinoid tumors. *Am J Surg Pathol.* 2009; 33: 626-632.
398. Srivastava A, Padilla O, Fischer-Colbrie R, et al. Neuroendocrine secretory protein-55 (NESP-55) expression discriminates pancreatic endocrine tumors and pheochromocytomas from gastrointestinal and pulmonary carcinoids. *Am J Surg Pathol.* 2004;28:1371-1378.
399. Sellner F, Sobhian B, De Santis M, et al. Well or poorly differentiated nonfunctioning neuroendocrine carcinoma of the pancreas: a single institution experience with 17 cases. *Eur J Surg Oncol.* 2008;34:191-195.
400. Nilsson O, Van Cutsem E, Delle Fave G, et al. Poorly differentiated carcinomas of the foregut (gastric, duodenal and pancreatic). *Neuroendocrinology.* 2006;84:212-215.
401. Stukavec J, Jirasek T, Mandys V, et al. Poorly differentiated endocrine carcinoma and intraductal papillary-mucinous neoplasm of the pancreas: description of an unusual case. *Pathol Res Pract.* 2007;203:879-884.
402. Kaufmann O, Georgi T, Dietel M. Utility of 123C3 monoclonal antibody against CD56 (NCAM) for the diagnosis of small cell carcinomas on paraffin sections. *Hum Pathol.* 1997;28:1373-1378.
403. Capella C, Heitz PU, Hofler H, et al. Revised classification of neuroendocrine tumours of the lung, pancreas and gut. *Virchows Arch.* 1995;425:547-560.
404. Kaifi JT, Heidtmann S, Schurr PG, et al. Absence of L1 in pancreatic masses distinguishes adenocarcinomas from poorly differentiated neuroendocrine carcinomas. *Anticancer Res.* 2006;26:1167-1170.
405. Kaifi JT, Zinnkann U, Yekebas EF, et al. L1 is a potential marker for poorly-differentiated pancreatic neuroendocrine carcinoma. *World J Gastroenterol.* 2006;12:94-98.
406. Movahedi-Lankarani S, Hruban RH, Westra WH, Klimstra DS. Primitive neuroectodermal tumors of the pancreas: a report of seven cases of a rare neoplasm. *Am J Surg Pathol.* 2002;26:1040-1047.
407. O'Hara BJ, McCue PA, Miettinen M. Bile duct adenomas with endocrine component. Immunohistochemical study and comparison with conventional bile duct adenomas. *Am J Surg Pathol.* 1992;16:21-25.
408. Albores-Saavedra J, Vardaman CJ, Vuitch F. Non-neoplastic polypoid lesions and adenomas of the gallbladder. *Pathol Annu.* 1993;28(Pt 1):145-177.
409. Christensen AH, Ishak KG. Benign tumors and pseudotumors of the gallbladder. Report of 180 cases. *Arch Pathol.* 1970;90:423-432.
410. Albores-Saavedra J, Henson DE, Klimstra DS. *Tumors of the gallbladder, extrahepatic bile ducts and ampulla of Vater.* 3rd ed. Washington D.C: American Registry of Pathology; 2000.
411. Nakatani Y, Masudo K, Nozawa A, et al. Biotin-rich, optically clear nuclei express estrogen receptor-beta: tumors with morules may develop under the influence of estrogen and aberrant beta-catenin expression. *Hum Pathol.* 2004;35:869-874.
412. Shibahara H, Tamada S, Goto M, et al. Pathologic features of mucin-producing bile duct tumors: two histopathologic categories as counterparts of pancreatic intraductal papillary-mucinous neoplasms. *Am J Surg Pathol.* 2004;28: 327-338.
413. Nagata S, Ajioka Y, Nishikura K, et al. Co-expression of gastric and biliary phenotype in pyloric-gland type adenoma of the gallbladder: immunohistochemical analysis of mucin profile and CD10. *Oncol Rep.* 2007;17:721-729.
414. Yamamoto M, Nakajo S, Tahara E. Immunohistochemical analysis of estrogen receptors in human gallbladder. *Acta Pathol Jpn.* 1990;40:14-21.

415. Wistuba II , Miquel JF, Gazdar AF, Albores-Saavedra J. Gallbladder adenomas have molecular abnormalities different from those present in gallbladder carcinomas. *Hum Pathol.* 1999;30:21-25.
416. Tian Y, Ding RY, Zhi YH, et al. Analysis of p53 and vascular endothelial growth factor expression in human gallbladder carcinoma for the determination of tumor vascularity. *World J Gastroenterol.* 2006;12:415-419.
417. Chang HJ, Jee CD, Kim WH. Mutation and altered expression of beta-catenin during gallbladder carcinogenesis. *Am J Surg Pathol.* 2002;26:758-766.
418. Devaney K, Goodman ZD, Ishak KG. Hepatobiliary cystadenoma and cystadenocarcinoma. A light microscopic and immunohistochemical study of 70 patients. *Am J Surg Pathol.* 1994;18:1078-1091.
419. Ojeda VJ, Shilkin KB, Walters MN. Premalignant epithelial lesions of the gall bladder: a prospective study of 120 cholecystectomy specimens. *Pathology.* 1985;17:451-454.
420. Chan KW. Review of 253 cases of significant pathology in 7,910 cholecystectomies in Hong Kong. *Pathology.* 1988;20:20-23.
421. Wistuba II , Albores-Saavedra J. Genetic abnormalities involved in the pathogenesis of gallbladder carcinoma. *J Hepatobiliary Pancreat Surg.* 1999;6:237-244.
422. Stolzenberg-Solomon R, Fraumeni JF, Wideroff L. New Malignancies Following Cancer of the Digestive Tract, Excluding Colorectal Cancer (Chapter 4) New Malignancies Among Cancer Survivors: SEER. *Cancer Registries.* 2000:1973-2000.
423. Roa I, Ibacache G, Roa J, et al. Gallstones and gallbladder cancer-volume and weight of gallstones are associated with gallbladder cancer: a case-control study. *J Surg Oncol.* 2006;93:624-628.
424. Kumar S. Infection as a risk factor for gallbladder cancer. *J Surg Oncol.* 2006;93:633-639.
425. Esterly JR, Spicer SS. Mucin histochemistry of human gallbladder: changes in adenocarcinoma cystic fibrosis, and cholecystitis. *J Natl Cancer Inst.* 1968;40:1-10.
426. Lack EE. *Pathology of the pancreas, gallbladder, extrahepatic biliary tract and ampullary region.* New York: Oxford University Press; 2003.
427. Rashid A, Ueki T, Gao YT, et al. K-ras mutation, p53 overexpression, and microsatellite instability in biliary tract cancers: a population-based study in China. *Clin Cancer Res.* 2002;8:3156-3163.
428. Argani P, Shaukat A, Kaushal M, et al. Differing rates of loss of DPC4 expression and of p53 overexpression among carcinomas of the proximal and distal bile ducts. *Cancer.* 2001;91:1332-1341.
429. Parwani AV, Geradts J, Caspers E, et al. Immunohistochemical and genetic analysis of non-small cell and small cell gallbladder carcinoma and their precursor lesions. *Mod Pathol.* 2003;16:299-308.
430. Kim YT, Kim J, Jang YH, et al. Genetic alterations in gallbladder adenoma, dysplasia and carcinoma. *Cancer Lett.* 2001;169:59-68.
431. Shi YZ, Hui AM, Li X, et al. Overexpression of retinoblastoma protein predicts decreased survival and correlates with loss of p16INK4 protein in gallbladder carcinomas. *Clin Cancer Res.* 2000;6:4096-4100.
432. Quan ZW, Wu K, Wang J, et al. Association of p53, p16, and vascular endothelial growth factor protein expressions with the prognosis and metastasis of gallbladder cancer. *J Am Coll Surg.* 2001;193:380-383.
433. Rashid A. Cellular and molecular biology of biliary tract cancers. *Surg Oncol Clin N Am.* 2002;11:995-1009.
434. Masuhara S, Kasuya K, Aoki T, et al. Relation between K-ras codon 12 mutation and p53 protein overexpression in gallbladder cancer and biliary ductal epithelia in patients with pancreaticobiliary maljunction. *Pancreat Surg.* 2000;7:198-205.
435. Imai M, Hoshi T, Ogawa K. K-ras codon 12 mutations in biliary tract tumors detected by polymerase chain reaction denaturing gradient gel electrophoresis. *Cancer.* 1994;73:2727-2733.
436. Roa JC, Roa I, de Aretxabala X, et al. [K-ras gene mutation in gallbladder carcinoma]. *Rev Med Chil.* 2004;132:955-960.
437. Ajiki T, Fujimori T, Onoyama H, et al. K-ras gene mutation in gall bladder carcinomas and dysplasia. *Gut.* 1996;38:426-429.
438. Kim YW, Huh SH, Park YK, et al. Expression of the c-erb-B2 and p53 protein in gallbladder carcinomas. *Oncol Rep.* 2001;8:1127-1132.
439. Jan YY, Yeh TS, Yeh JN, et al. Expression of epidermal growth factor receptor, apomucins, matrix metalloproteinases, and p53 in rat and human cholangiocarcinoma: appraisal of an animal model of cholangiocarcinoma. *Ann Surg.* 2004;240:89-94.
440. Albores-Saavedra J, Molberg K, Henson DE. Unusual malignant epithelial tumors of the gallbladder. *Semin Diagn Pathol.* 1996;13:326-338.
441. Watanabe M, Hori Y, Nojima T, et al. Alpha-fetoprotein-producing carcinoma of the gallbladder. *Dig Dis Sci.* 1993;38:561-564.
442. Gakiopoulou H, Givalos N, Liapis G, et al. Hepatoid adenocarcinoma of the gallbladder. *Dig Dis Sci.* 2007;52:3358-3362.
443. Terracciano LM, Glatz K, Mhawech P, et al. Hepatoid adenocarcinoma with liver metastasis mimicking hepatocellular carcinoma: an immunohistochemical and molecular study of eight cases. *Am J Surg Pathol.* 2003;27:1302-1312.
444. Kim KW, Kim SH, Kim MA, et al. Adenosquamous carcinoma of the extrahepatic bile duct: clinicopathologic and radiologic features. *Abdom Imaging.* 2008.
445. Oohashi Y, Shirai Y, Wakai T, et al. Adenosquamous carcinoma of the gallbladder warrants resection only if curative resection is feasible. *Cancer.* 2002;94:3000-3005.
446. Chan S, Currie J, Malik AI, Mahomed AA. Paediatric cholecystectomy: shifting goalposts in the laparoscopic era. *Surg Endosc.* 2008;22:1392-1395.
447. Nishihara K, Tsuneyoshi M. Undifferentiated spindle cell carcinoma of the gallbladder: a clinicopathologic, immunohistochemical, and flow cytometric study of 11 cases. *Hum Pathol.* 1993;24:1298-1305.
448. Modlin IM, Sandor A. An analysis of 8305 cases of carcinoid tumors. *Cancer.* 1997;79:813-829.
449. Barron-Rodriguez LP, Manivel JC, Mendez-Sanchez N, Jessurun J. Carcinoid tumor of the common bile duct: evidence for its origin in metaplastic endocrine cells. *Am J Gastroenterol.* 1991;86:1073-1076.
450. Anjaneyulu V, Shankar-Swarnalatha G, Rao SC. Carcinoid tumor of the gall bladder. *Ann Diagn Pathol.* 2007;11:113-116.
451. Jun SR, Lee JM, Han JK, Choi BI. High-grade neuroendocrine carcinomas of the gallbladder and bile duct: report of four cases with pathological correlation. *J Comput Assist Tomogr.* 2006;30:604-609.
452. Papotti M, Cassoni P, Sapino A, et al. Large cell neuroendocrine carcinoma of the gallbladder: report of two cases. *Am J Surg Pathol.* 2000;24:1424-1428.
453. Kimura W, Futakawa N, Yamagata S, et al. Different clinicopathologic findings in two histologic types of carcinoma of papilla of Vater. *Jpn J Cancer Res.* 1994;85:161-166.
454. Fathallah L, Vyas P, Klimstra D, et al. MUC1 and MUC2 expression in carcinomas of ampullary region and their diagnostic and clinical significance. *Mod Pathol.* 2002;15:284A.
455. Chu PG, Schwarz RE, Lau SK, et al. Immunohistochemical staining in the diagnosis of pancreatobiliary and ampulla of Vater adenocarcinoma: application of CDX2, CK17, MUC1, and MUC2. *Am J Surg Pathol.* 2005;29:359-367.
456. Hansel DE, Maitra A, Lin JW, et al. Expression of the caudal-type homeodomain transcription factors CDX 1/2 and outcome in carcinomas of the ampulla of Vater. *J Clin Oncol.* 2005;23:1811-1818.
457. Paulsen FP, Varoga D, Paulsen AR, et al. Prognostic value of mucins in the classification of ampullary carcinomas. *Hum Pathol.* 2006;37:160-167.
458. Zhou H, Schaefer N, Wolff M, Fischer HP. Carcinoma of the ampulla of Vater: comparative histologic/immunohistochemical classification and follow-up. *Am J Surg Pathol.* 2004;28:875-882.
459. Sessa F, Furlan D, Zampatti C, et al. Prognostic factors for ampullary adenocarcinomas: tumor stage, tumor histology, tumor location, immunohistochemistry and microsatellite instability. *Virch Arch.* 2007;451:649-657.
460. Kamisawa T, Fukayama M, Koike M, et al. Carcinoma of the ampulla of Vater: expression of cancer-associated antigens inversely correlated with prognosis. *Am J Gastroenterol.* 1988;83:1118-1123.

461. Scarpa A, Capelli P, Zamboni G, et al. Neoplasia of the ampulla of Vater. Ki-ras and p53 mutations. *Am J Pathol.* 1993;142:1163-1172.
462. Takashima M, Ueki T, Nagai E, et al. Carcinoma of the ampulla of Vater associated with or without adenoma: a clinicopathologic analysis of 198 cases with reference to p53 and Ki-67 immunohistochemical expressions. *Mod Pathol.* 2000;13:1300-1307.
463. McCarthy DM, Hruban RH, Argani P, et al. Role of the DPC4 tumor suppressor gene in adenocarcinoma of the ampulla of Vater: analysis of 140 cases. *Mod Pathol.* 2003;16:272-278.
464. Howe JR, Klimstra DS, Cordon-Cardo C, et al. K-ras mutation in adenomas and carcinomas of the ampulla of vater. *Clin Cancer Res.* 1997;3:129-133.
465. Thirabanjasak D, Tang L, Klimstra DS, et al. Glandular carcinoids of the ampulla with psammoma bodies (so-called ampullary somatostatinomas): analysis of 12 cases of an underrecognized entity. *Modern Pathology.* 2008;20:623A.
466. Nassar H, Albores-Saavedra J, Klimstra DS. High-grade neuroendocrine carcinoma of the ampulla of vater: a clinicopathologic and immunohistochemical analysis of 14 cases. *Am J Surg Pathol.* 2005;29:588-594.
467. Rindi G, Kloppel G, Alhman H, et al. TNM staging of foregut (neuro)endocrine tumors: a consensus proposal including a grading system. *Virchows Arch.* 2006;449:395-401.
468. Van Eyken P, Sciot R, Desmet VJ. Immunocytochemistry of cytokeratins in primary human liver tumors. *APMIS.* 1991;23(Suppl):77-85.
469. Fischer HP, Altmannsberger M, Weber K, Osborn M. Keratin polypeptides in malignant epithelial liver tumors. Differential diagnostic and histogenetic aspects. *Am J Pathol.* 1987;127:530-537.
470. van Eyken P, Sciot R, van Damme B, et al. Keratin immunohistochemistry in normal human liver. Cytokeratin pattern of hepatocytes, bile ducts and acinar gradient. *Virch Arch A Pathol Anat Histopathol.* 1987;412:63-72.
471. Moll R, Franke WW, Schiller DL, et al. The catalog of human cytokeratins: patterns of expression in normal epithelia, tumors and cultured cells. *Cell.* 1982;31:11-24.
472. Zatloukal K, Stumptner C, Fuchsbichler A, et al. The keratin cytoskeleton in liver diseases. The diagnostic value of hepatocyte paraffin antibody 1 in differentiating hepatocellular neoplasms from nonhepatic tumors: a review. *J Pathol.* 2004;204:367-376.
473. Suriawinata AA, Thung SN. Liver. In: Mills SE, ed. *Histology for Pathologists.* 3rd ed. Philadelphia: Lippincott Williams & Wilkins; 2007:685-703.
474. Theise ND, Fiel IM, Hytiroglou P, et al. Macroregenerative nodules in cirrhosis are not associated with elevated serum or stainable tissue alpha-fetoprotein. *Liver.* 1995;15:30-34.
475. Dodson A, Campbell F. Biotin inclusions: a potential pitfall in immunohistochemistry avoided. *Histopathology.* 1999;34:178-179.
476. Iezzoni JC, Mills SE, Pelkey TJ, Stoler MH. Inhibin is not an immunohistochemical marker for hepatocellular carcinoma. An example of the potential pitfall in diagnostic immunohistochemistry caused by endogenous biotin. *Am J Clin Pathol.* 1999;111:229-234.
477. Bussolati G, Gugliotta P, Volante M, et al. Retrieved endogenous biotin: a novel marker and a potential pitfall in diagnostic immunohistochemistry. *Histopathology.* 1997;31:400-407.
478. Wennerberg AE, Nalesnik MA, Coleman WB. Hepatocyte paraffin 1: a monoclonal antibody that reacts with hepatocytes and can be used for differential diagnosis of hepatic tumors. *Am J Pathol.* 1993;143:1050-1054.
479. Leong AS, Sormunen RT, Tsui WM, et al. Hep Par 1 and selected antibodies in the immunohistological distinction of hepatocellular carcinoma from cholangiocarcinoma, combined tumours and metastatic carcinoma. *Histopathology.* 1998;33:318-324.
480. Wieczorek TJ, Pinkus JL, Glickman JN, Pinkus GS. Comparison of thyroid transcription factor-1 and hepatocyte antigen immunohistochemical analysis in the differential diagnosis of hepatocellular carcinoma, metastatic adenocarcinoma, renal cell carcinoma, and adrenal cortical carcinoma. *Am J Clin Pathol.* 2002;118:911-921.
481. Borscheri N, Roessner A, Rocken C. Canalicular immunostaining of neprilysin (CD10) as a diagnostic marker for hepatocellular carcinomas. *Am J Surg Pathol.* 2001;25:1297-1303.
482. Lai YS, Thung SN, Gerber MA, et al. Expression of cytokeratins in normal and diseased livers and in primary liver carcinomas. *Arch Pathol Lab Med.* 1989;113:134-138.
483. Nakajima T, Kondo Y. Well-differentiated cholangiocarcinoma: diagnostic significance of morphologic and immunohistochemical parameters. *Am J Surg Pathol.* 1989;13:569-573.
484. Terayama N, Terada T, Nakanuma Y. An immunohistochemical study of tumour vessels in metastatic liver cancers and the surrounding liver tissue. *Histopathology.* 1996;29:37-43.
485. Haratake J, Scheuer PJ. An immunohistochemical and ultrastructural study of the sinusoids of hepatocellular carcinoma. *Cancer.* 1990;65:1985-1993.
486. Ruck P, Xiao JC, Kaiserling E. Immunoreactivity of sinusoids in hepatocellular carcinoma. An immunohistochemical study using lectin UEA-1 and antibodies against endothelial markers, including CD34. *Arch Pathol Lab Med.* 1995;119:173-178.
487. Afdhal NH, Nunes D. Evaluation of liver fibrosis: a concise review. *Am J Gastroenterol.* 2004;99:1160-1174.
488. James J, Lygidakis NJ, van Eyken P, et al. Application of keratin immunocytochemistry and sirius red staining in evaluating intrahepatic changes with acute extrahepatic cholestasis due to hepatic duct carcinoma. *Hepatogastroenterology.* 1989;36:151-155.
489. Manning DS, Afdhal NH. Diagnosis and quantitation of fibrosis. *Gastroenterology.* 2008;134:1670-1681.
490. Desmet VJ. Histopathology of chronic cholestasis and adult ductopenic syndrome. *Clin Liver Dis.* 1998;2:249-264, viii.
491. Halfon P, Cacoub P. [Viral quantitation of hepatitis C virus: present and future]. *Rev Med Interne.* 2000;21:174-181.
492. Mardini H, Record C. Detection assessment and monitoring of hepatic fibrosis: biochemistry or biopsy? *Ann Clin Biochem.* 2005;42:441-447.
493. Lockwood DS, Yeadon TM, Clouston AD, et al. Tumor progression in hepatocellular carcinoma: relationship with tumor stroma and parenchymal disease. *J Gastroenterol Hepatol.* 2003;18:666-672.
494. Gulubova M. Immunohistochemical localization of collagen type III and type IV, laminin, tenascin and alpha-smooth muscle actin (alphaSMA) in the human liver in peliosis. *Pathol Res Pract.* 2002;198:803-812.
495. Torimura T, Ueno T, Inuzuka S, et al. The extracellular matrix in hepatocellular carcinoma shows different localization patterns depending on the differentiation and the histological pattern of tumors: immunohistochemical analysis. *J Hepatol.* 1994;21:37-46.
496. Schuppan D. Structure of the extracellular matrix in normal and fibrotic liver: collagens and glycoproteins. *Semin Liver Dis.* 1990;10:1-10.
497. Schuppan D, Ruehl M, Somasundaram R, Hahn EG. Matrix as a modulator of hepatic fibrogenesis. *Semin Liver Dis.* 2001;21:351-372.
498. Schuppan D, Porov Y. Hepatic fibrosis: from bench to bedside. *J Gastroenterol Hepatol.* 2002;17(Suppl 3):S300-305.
499. Bataller R, Brenner DA. Liver fibrosis. *J Clin Invest.* 2005;115:209-218.
500. Friedman SL. Mechanisms of hepatic fibrogenesis. *Gastroenterology.* 2008;134:1655-1669.
501. Knittel T, Aurisch S, Neubauer K, et al. Cell-type-specific expression of neural cell adhesion molecule (N-CAM) in Ito cells of rat liver. Up-regulation during in vitro activation and in hepatic tissue repair. *Am J Pathol.* 1996;149:449-462.
502. Neubauer K, Knittel T, Aurisch S, et al. Glial fibrillary acidic protein—a cell type specific marker for Ito cells in vivo and in vitro. *J Hepatol.* 1996;24:719-730.
503. Cassiman D, van Pelt J, De Vos R, et al. Synaptophysin: A novel marker for human and rat hepatic stellate cells. *Am J Pathol.* 1999;155:1831-1839.
504. Ogawa K, Suzuki J, Mukai H, Mori M. Sequential changes of extracellular matrix and proliferation of Ito cells with enhanced expression of desmin and actin in focal hepatic injury. *Am J Pathol.* 1986;125:611-619.

505. Zatloukal K, French SW, Stumptner C, et al. From Mallory to Mallory-Denk bodies: what, how and why? *Exp Cell Res.* 2007;313:2033-2049.
506. Van Eyken P, Sciot R, Desmet VJ. A cytokeratin immunohistochemical study of alcoholic liver disease: evidence that hepatocytes can express 'bile duct-type' cytokeratins. *Histopathology.* 1988;13:605-617.
507. Hazan R, Denk H, Franke WW, et al. Change of cytokeratin organization during development of Mallory bodies as revealed by a monoclonal antibody. *Lab Invest.* 1986;54:543-553.
508. Callea F. Immunohistochemical techniques for the demonstration of viral antigens in liver tissue. *Ric Clin Lab.* 1988;18:223-231.
509. Roskams T. The role of immunohistochemistry in diagnosis. *Clin Liver Dis.* 2002;6:571-589:x.
510. Booth JC, Goldin RD, Brown JL, et al. Fibrosing cholestatic hepatitis in a renal transplant recipient associated with the hepatitis B virus precore mutant. *J Hepatol.* 1995;22:500-503.
511. Chen CH, Chen PJ, Chu JS, et al. Fibrosing cholestatic hepatitis in a hepatitis B surface antigen carrier after renal transplantation. *Gastroenterology.* 1994;107:1514-1518.
512. Fang JW, Wright TL, Lau JY. Fibrosing cholestatic hepatitis in patient with HIV and hepatitis B. *Lancet.* 1993;342:1175.
513. Davies SE, Portmann BC, O'Grady JG, et al. Hepatic histological findings after transplantation for chronic hepatitis B virus infection, including a unique pattern of fibrosing cholestatic hepatitis. *Hepatology.* 1991;13:150-157.
514. Fischer HP, Willsch E, Bierhoff E, Pfeifer U. Histopathologic findings in chronic hepatitis C. *J Hepatol.* 1996;24:35-42.
515. Kasprzak A, Biczysko W, Adamek A, Zabel M. Morphological lesions detected by light and electron microscopies in chronic type B hepatitis. *Pol J Pathol.* 2002;53:103-115.
516. Sansonno D, Iacobelli AR, Cornacchiulo V, et al. Immunohistochemical detection of hepatitis C virus-related proteins in liver tissue. *Clin Exp Rheumatol.* 1995;13(Suppl 13):S29-32.
517. Lau JY, Krawczynski K, Negro F, Gonzalez-Peralta RP. In situ detection of hepatitis C virus—a critical appraisal. *J Hepatol.* 1996;24:43-51.
518. Scheuer PJ, Krawczynski K, Dhillon AP. Histopathology and detection of hepatitis C virus in liver. *Springer Semin Immunopathol.* 1997;19:27-45.
519. Gowans EJ. Distribution of markers of hepatitis C virus infection throughout the body. *Semin Liver Dis.* 2000;20:85-102.
520. Brody RI, Eng S, Melamed J, et al. Immunohistochemical detection of hepatitis C antigen by monoclonal antibody TORDJI-22 compared with PCR viral detection. *Am J Clin Pathol.* 1998;110:32-37.
521. Uchida T, Shikata T, Tanaka E, Kiyosawa K. Immunoperoxidase staining of hepatitis C virus in formalin-fixed, paraffin-embedded needle liver biopsies. *Virchows Arch.* 1994;424:465-469.
522. Negro F, Pacchioni D, Mondardini A, et al. In situ hybridization in viral hepatitis. *Liver.* 1992;12:217-226.
523. Negro F, Papotti M, Taraglio S, et al. Relationship between hepatocyte proliferation and hepatitis delta virus replication in neoplastic and non-neoplastic liver tissues. *J Viral Hepat.* 1997;4:93-98.
524. Raymond E, Tricottet V, Samuel D, et al. Epstein-Barr virus-related localized hepatic lymphoproliferative disorders after liver transplantation. *Cancer.* 1995;76:1344-1351.
525. Chen CJ, Jeng LB, Huang SF. Lymphoepithelioma-like hepatocellular carcinoma. *Chang Gung Med J.* 2007;30:172-177.
526. Chen TC, Ng KF, Kuo T. Intrahepatic cholangiocarcinoma with lymphoepithelioma-like component. *Mod Pathol.* 2001;14:527-532.
527. Vortmeyer AO, Kingma DW, Fenton RG, et al. Hepatobiliary lymphoepithelioma-like carcinoma associated with Epstein-Barr virus. *Am J Clin Pathol.* 1998;109:90-95.
528. Vanstapel MJ, Desmet VJ. Cytomegalovirus hepatitis: a histological and immunohistochemical study. *Appl Pathol.* 1983;1:41-49.
529. Lautenschlager I, Halme L, Hockerstedt K, et al. Cytomegalovirus infection of the liver transplant: virological, histological, immunological, and clinical observations. *Transpl Infect Dis.* 2006;8:21-30.
530. Humphrey DM, Weiner MH. Mycobacterial antigen detection by immunohistochemistry in pulmonary tuberculosis. *Hum Pathol.* 1987;18:701-708.
531. Lau SK, Prakash S, Geller SA, Alsabeh R. Comparative immunohistochemical profile of hepatocellular carcinoma, cholangiocarcinoma, and metastatic adenocarcinoma. *Human pathology.* 2002;33:1175-1181.
532. Hurlimann J, Gardiol D. Immunohistochemistry in the differential diagnosis of liver carcinomas. *Am J Surg Pathol.* 1991;15:280-288.
533. Van Eyken P, Sciot R, Desmet VJ. A cytokeratin immunohistochemical study of cholestatic liver disease: evidence that hepatocytes can express 'bile duct-type' cytokeratins. *Histopathology.* 1989;15:125-135.
534. van Eyken P, Sciot R, Callea F, Desmet VJ. A cytokeratin-immunohistochemical study of focal nodular hyperplasia of the liver: further evidence that ductular metaplasia of hepatocytes contributes to ductular "proliferation." *Liver.* 1989;9:372-377.
535. Sell S, Leffert HL. Liver cancer stem cells. *J Clin Oncol.* 2008;26:2800-2805.
536. Kamiya A, Gonzalez FJ, Nakauchi H. Identification and differentiation of hepatic stem cells during liver development. *Front Biosci.* 2006;11:1302-1310.
537. Gerber MA, Thung SN. Liver stem cells and development. *Lab Invest.* 1993;68:253-254.
538. Sell S. Is there a liver stem cell? *Cancer Res.* 1990;50:3811-3815.
539. Goldstein NS, Blue DE, Hankin R, et al. Serum alpha-fetoprotein levels in patients with chronic hepatitis C. Relationships with serum alanine aminotransferase values, histologic activity index, and hepatocyte MIB-1 scores. *Am J Clin Pathol.* 1999;111:811-816.
540. Cabibi D, Licata A, Barresi E, et al. Expression of cytokeratin 7 and 20 in pathological conditions of the bile tract. *Pathol Res Pract.* 2003;199:65-70.
541. Nakanuma Y, Ohta G. Immunohistochemical study on bile ductular proliferation in various hepatobiliary diseases. *Liver.* 1986;6:205-211.
542. Washington K, Clavien PA, Killenberg P. Peribiliary vascular plexus in primary sclerosing cholangitis and primary biliary cirrhosis. *Hum Pathol.* 1997;28:791-795.
543. Vertemati M, Minola E, Goffredi M, et al. Computerized morphometry of the cirrhotic liver: comparative analysis in primary biliary cirrhosis, alcoholic cirrhosis, and posthepatitic cirrhosis. *Microsc Res Tech.* 2004;65:113-121.
544. Kobayashi S, Nakanuma Y, Matsui O. Intrahepatic peribiliary vascular plexus in various hepatobiliary diseases: a histological survey. *Hum Pathol.* 1994;25:940-946.
545. Daniels JA, Torbenson M, Anders RA, Boitnott JK. Immunostaining of plasma cells in primary biliary cirrhosis. *Am J Clin Pathol.* 2009;131:243-249.
546. Deshpande V, Mino-Kenudson M, Brugge W, Lauwers GY. Autoimmune pancreatitis: more than just a pancreatic disease? A contemporary review of its pathology. *Arch Pathol Lab Med.* 2005;129:1148-1154.
547. Umemura T, Zen Y, Hamano H, et al. Immunoglobin G4-hepatopathy: association of immunoglobin G4-bearing plasma cells in liver with autoimmune pancreatitis. *Hepatology.* 2007;46:463-471.
548. Umemura T, Zen Y, Hamano H, et al. IgG4 associated autoimmune hepatitis: a differential diagnosis for classical autoimmune hepatitis. *Gut.* 2007;56:1471-1472.
549. Zen Y, Fujii T, Sato Y, et al. Pathological classification of hepatic inflammatory pseudotumor with respect to IgG4-related disease. *Mod Pathol.* 2007;20:884-894.
550. Zen Y, Fujii T, Harada K, et al. Th2 and regulatory immune reactions are increased in immunoglobin G4-related sclerosing pancreatitis and cholangitis. *Hepatology.* 2007;45:1538-1546.
551. Lefkowitch JH. Hepatobiliary pathology. *Current opinion in gastroenterology.* 2008;24:269-277.
552. Bjornsson E, Chari ST, Smyrk TC, Lindor K. Immunoglobulin G4 associated cholangitis: description of an emerging clinical entity based on review of the literature. *Hepatology.* 2007;45:1547-1554.

553. Park DH, Kim MHD, Chari ST. Recent advances in autoimmune pancreatitis. *Gut*. 2009.
554. Chari ST. Diagnosis of autoimmune pancreatitis using its five cardinal features: introducing the Mayo Clinic's HISORt criteria. *J Gastroenterol*. 2007;42(Suppl 18):39-41.
555. Kwon S, Kim MH, Choi EK. The diagnostic criteria for autoimmune chronic pancreatitis: it is time to make a consensus. *Pancreas*. 2007;34:279-286.
556. Kojima M, Sipos B, Klapper W, et al. Autoimmune pancreatitis: frequency, IgG4 expression, and clonality of T and B cells. *Am J Surg Pathol*. 2007;31:521-528.
557. Deshpande V, Chicano S, Finkelberg D, et al. Autoimmune pancreatitis: a systemic immune complex mediated disease. *Am J Surg Pathol*. 2006;30:1537-1545.
558. Zhang L, Notohara K, Levy MJ, et al. IgG4-positive plasma cell infiltration in the diagnosis of autoimmune pancreatitis. *Mod Pathol*. 2007;20:23-28.
559. Makhlouf HR, Abdul-Al HM, Goodman ZD. Diagnosis of focal nodular hyperplasia of the liver by needle biopsy. *Hum Pathol*. 2005;36:1210-1216.
560. Nguyen BN, Flejou JF, Terris B, et al. Focal nodular hyperplasia of the liver: a comprehensive pathologic study of 305 lesions and recognition of new histologic forms. *Am J Surg Pathol*. 1999;23:1441-1454.
561. Malone M, Mieli-Vergani G, Mowat AP, Portmann B. The fetal liver in PiZZ alpha-1-antitrypsin deficiency: a report of five cases. *Pediatr Pathol*. 1989;9:623-631.
562. Fairbanks KD, Tavill AS. Liver disease in alpha 1-antitrypsin deficiency: a review. *Am J Gastroenterol*. 2008;103:2136-2141:quiz 2142.
563. Portmann BC, Thompson RJ, Roberts EA, Paterson AC. Genetic and metabolic liver disease. In: Burt AD, Portmann BC, Ferrell LD, eds. *MacSween's Pathology of the Liver*. 5th ed. Philadelphia: Churchill Livingstone Elsevier; 2007:199-326.
564. Medicina D, Fabbretti G, Brennan SO, et al. Genetic and immunological characterization of fibrinogen inclusion bodies in patients with hepatic fibrinogen storage and liver disease. *Ann N Y Acad Sci*. 2001;936:522-525.
565. Demetris AJ, Adeyi O, Bellamy CO, et al. Liver biopsy interpretation for causes of late liver allograft dysfunction. *Hepatology*. 2006;44:489-501.
566. Haga H, Egawa H, Fujimoto Y, et al. Acute humoral rejection and C4d immunostaining in ABO blood type-incompatible liver transplantation. *Liver Transpl*. 2006;12:457-464.
567. Colvin RB. C4d in liver allografts: a sign of antibody-mediated rejection? *Am J Transplant*. 2006;6:447-448.
568. Schmeding M, Dankof A, Krenn V, et al. C4d in acute rejection after liver transplantation—a valuable tool in differential diagnosis to hepatitis C recurrence. *Am J Transplant*. 2006;6:523-530.
569. Bu X, Zheng Z, Yu Y, Zeng L, Jiang Y. Significance of C4d deposition in the diagnosis of rejection after liver transplantation. *Transplant Proc*. 2006;38:1418-1421.
570. Lorho R, Turlin B, Aqodad N, et al. C4d: a marker for hepatic transplant rejection. *Transplant Proc*. 2006;38:2333-2334.
571. Watson R, Kozlowski T, Nickeleit V, et al. Isolated donor specific alloantibody-mediated rejection after ABO compatible liver transplantation. *Am J Transplant*. 2006;6:3022-3029.
572. Troxell ML, Higgins JP, Kambham N. Evaluation of C4d staining in liver and small intestine allografts. *Arch Pathol Lab Med*. 2006;130:1489-1496.
573. Jain A, Ryan C, Mohanka R, et al. Characterization of CD4, CD8, CD56 positive lymphocytes and C4d deposits to distinguish acute cellular rejection from recurrent hepatitis C in post-liver transplant biopsies. *Clin Transplant*. 2006;20:624-633.
574. Bellamy CO, Herriot MM, Harrison DJ, Bathgate AJ. C4d immunopositivity is uncommon in ABO-compatible liver allografts, but correlates partially with lymphocytotoxic antibody status. *Histopathology*. 2007;50:739-749.
575. Sakashita H, Haga H, Ashihara E, et al. Significance of C4d staining in ABO-identical/compatible liver transplantation. *Mod Pathol*. 2007;20:676-684.
576. Ponticelli C. Renal transplantation 2004: where do we stand today? *Nephrol Dial Transplant*. 2004;19:2937-2947.
577. Krukemeyer MG, Moeller J, Morawietz L, et al. Description of B lymphocytes and plasma cells, complement, and chemokines/receptors in acute liver allograft rejection. *Transplantation*. 2004;78:65-70.
578. Terasaki PI. Humoral theory of transplantation. *Am J Transplant*. 2003;3:665-673.
579. Dankof A, Schmeding M, Morawietz L, et al. Portal capillary C4d deposits and increased infiltration by macrophages indicate humorally mediated mechanisms in acute cellular liver allograft rejection. *Virchows Arch*. 2005;447:87-93.
580. Sawada T, Shimizu A, Kubota K, et al. Lobular damage caused by cellular and humoral immunity in liver allograft rejection. *Clin Transplant*. 2005;19:110-114.
581. Michaels PJ, Fishbein MC, Colvin RB. Humoral rejection of human organ transplants. *Springer Semin Immunopathol*. 2003;25:119-140.
582. Hirohashi S, Ishak KG, Kojiro M, et al. Hepatocellular carcinoma. In: Hamilton SR, Aaltonen LA, eds. *Tumours of the Digestive System*. Lyon, France: International Agency for Research on Cancer (IARC); 2000:159-172.
583. Torbenson M, Lee JH, Choti M, et al. Hepatic adenomas: analysis of sex steroid receptor status and the Wnt signaling pathway. *Mod Pathol*. 2002;15:189-196.
584. Zucman-Rossi J, Jeannot E, Nhieu JT, et al. Genotype-phenotype correlation in hepatocellular adenoma: new classification and relationship with HCC. *Hepatology*. 2006;43:515-524.
585. Bioulac-Sage P, Balabaud C, Bedossa P, et al. Pathological diagnosis of liver cell adenoma and focal nodular hyperplasia: Bordeaux update. *J Hepatol*. 2007;46:521-527.
586. Geller SA, Dhall D, Alsabeh R. Application of immunohistochemistry to liver and gastrointestinal neoplasms: liver, stomach, colon, and pancreas. *Archives of Pathology & Laboratory Medicine*. 2008;132:490-499.
587. Huang H, Fujii H, Sankila A, et al. Beta-catenin mutations are frequent in human hepatocellular carcinomas associated with hepatitis C virus infection. *Am J Pathol*. 1999;155:1795-1801.
588. Coston WM, Loera S, Lau SK, et al. Distinction of hepatocellular carcinoma from benign hepatic mimickers using Glypican-3 and CD34 immunohistochemistry. *Am J Surg Pathol*. 2008;32:433-444.
589. Shafizadeh N, Ferrell LD, Kakar S. Utility and limitations of glypican-3 expression for the diagnosis of hepatocellular carcinoma at both ends of the differentiation spectrum. *Mod Pathol*. 2008;21:1011-1018.
590. Fasano M, Theise ND, Nalesnik M, et al. Immunohistochemical evaluation of hepatoblastomas with use of the hepatocyte-specific marker, hepatocyte paraffin 1, and the polyclonal anti-carcinoembryonic antigen. *Mod Pathol*. 1998;11:934-938.
591. Stocker JT, Schmidt D. Hepatoblastoma. In: Hamilton SR, Aaltonen LA, eds. *Tumours of the Digestive System*. Lyon, France: International Agency for Research on Cancer (IARC); 2000: 184-189.
592. Ruck P, Xiao JC, Pietsch T, et al. Hepatic stem-like cells in hepatoblastoma: expression of cytokeratin 7, albumin and oval cell associated antigens detected by OV-1 and OV-6. *Histopathology*. 1997;31:324-329.
593. Ruck P, Xiao JC, Kaiserling E. Immunoreactivity of sinusoids in hepatoblastoma: an immunohistochemical study using lectin UEA-1 and antibodies against endothelium-associated antigens, including CD34. *Histopathology*. 1995;26:451-455.
594. Moll R, Divo M, Langbein L. The human keratins: biology and pathology. *Histochem Cell Biol*. 2008;129:705-733.
595. Strnad P, Stumptner C, Zatloukal K, Denk H. Intermediate filament cytoskeleton of the liver in health and disease. *Histochem Cell Biol*. 2008;129:735-749.
596. Chu PG, Weiss LM. Keratin expression in human tissues and neoplasms. *Histopathology*. 2002;40:403-439.
597. Durnez A, Verslype C, Nevens F, et al. The clinicopathological and prognostic relevance of cytokeratin 7 and 19 expression in hepatocellular carcinoma. A possible progenitor cell origin. *Histopathology*. 2006;49:138-151.
598. Maeda T, Kajiyama K, Adachi E, et al. The expression of cytokeratins 7, 19, and 20 in primary and metastatic carcinomas of the liver. *Mod Pathol*. 1996;9:901-909.

599. Kakar S, Gown AM, Goodman ZD, Ferrell LD. Best practices in diagnostic immunohistochemistry: hepatocellular carcinoma versus metastatic neoplasms. *Arch Pathol Lab Med.* 2007;131:1648-1654.
600. Morrison C, Marsh Jr W, Frankel WL. A comparison of CD10 to pCEA, MOC-31, and hepatocyte for the distinction of malignant tumors in the liver. *Mod Pathol.* 2002;15:1279-1287.
601. Goodman ZD, Ishak KG, Langloss JM, et al. Combined hepatocellular-cholangiocarcinoma. A histologic and immunohistochemical study. *Cancer.* 1985;55:124-135.
602. Varma V, Cohen C. Immunohistochemical and molecular markers in the diagnosis of hepatocellular carcinoma. *Adv Anat Pathol.* 2004;11:239-249.
603. Wang L, Vuolo M, Suhrland MJ, Schlesinger K. HepPar1, MOC-31, pCEA, mCEA and CD10 for distinguishing hepatocellular carcinoma vs. metastatic adenocarcinoma in liver fine needle aspirates. *Acta Cytol.* 2006;50:257-262.
604. Libbrecht L, Severi T, Cassiman D, et al. Glypican-3 expression distinguishes small hepatocellular carcinomas from cirrhosis, dysplastic nodules, and focal nodular hyperplasia-like nodules. *Am J Surg Pathol.* 2006;30:1405-1411.
605. Llovet JM, Chen Y, Wurmbach E, et al. A molecular signature to discriminate dysplastic nodules from early hepatocellular carcinoma in HCV cirrhosis. *Gastroenterology.* 2006;131:1758-1767.
606. Wang XY, Degos F, Dubois S, et al. Glypican-3 expression in hepatocellular tumors: diagnostic value for preneoplastic lesions and hepatocellular carcinomas. *Hum Pathol.* 2006;37:1435-1441.
607. Yamauchi N, Watanabe A, Hishinuma M, et al. The glypican 3 oncofetal protein is a promising diagnostic marker for hepatocellular carcinoma. *Mod Pathol.* 2005;18:1591-1598.
608. Sakamoto M, Mori T, Masugi Y, et al. Candidate molecular markers for histological diagnosis of early hepatocellular carcinoma. *Intervirology.* 2008;51(Suppl 1):42-45.
609. Krishna M, Lloyd RV, Batts KP. Detection of albumin messenger RNA in hepatic and extrahepatic neoplasms. A marker of hepatocellular differentiation. *Am J Surg Pathol.* 1997;21:147-152.
610. D'Errico A, Deleonardi G, Fiorentino M, et al. Diagnostic implications of albumin messenger RNA detection and cytokeratin pattern in benign hepatic lesions and biliary cystadenocarcinoma. *Diagn Mol Pathol.* 1998;7:289-294.
611. Papotti M, Pacchioni D, Negro F, et al. Albumin gene expression in liver tumors: diagnostic interest in fine needle aspiration biopsies. *Mod Pathol.* 1994;7:271-275.
612. Papotti M, Sambataro D, Marchesa P, Negro F. A combined hepatocellular/cholangiocellular carcinoma with sarcomatoid features. *Liver.* 1997;17:47-52.
613. Kakar S, Muir T, Murphy LM, et al. Immunoreactivity of Hep Par 1 in hepatic and extrahepatic tumors and its correlation with albumin in situ hybridization in hepatocellular carcinoma. *Am J Clin Pathol.* 2003;119:361-366.
614. Oliveira AM, Erickson LA, Burgart LJ, Lloyd RV. Differentiation of primary and metastatic clear cell tumors in the liver by in situ hybridization for albumin messenger RNA. *Am J Surg Pathol.* 2000;24:177-182.
615. Supriatna Y, Kishimoto T, Uno T, et al. Evidence for hepatocellular differentiation in alpha-fetoprotein-negative gastric adenocarcinoma with hepatoid morphology: a study with in situ hybridisation for albumin mRNA. *Pathology.* 2005;37:211-215.
616. Lopez-Beltran A, Luque RJ, Quintero A, et al. Hepatoid adenocarcinoma of the urinary bladder. *Virch Arch.* 2003;442:381-387.
617. Tanigawa H, Kida Y, Kuwao S, et al. Hepatoid adenocarcinoma in Barrett's esophagus associated with achalasia: first case report. *Pathol Int.* 2002;52:141-146.
618. Roberts CC, Colby TV, Batts KP. Carcinoma of the stomach with hepatocyte differentiation (hepatoid adenocarcinoma). *Mayo Clin Proc.* 1997;72:1154-1160.
619. Minervini MI, Demetris AJ, Lee RG, et al. Utilization of hepatocyte-specific antibody in the immunocytochemical evaluation of liver tumors. *Mod Pathol.* 1997;10:686-692.
620. Lazaro J, Rubio D, Repolles M, Capote L. Hepatoid carcinoma of the ovary and management. *Acta Obstet Gynecol Scand.* 2007;86:498-499.
621. Hameed O, Xu H, Saddeghi S, Maluf H. Hepatoid carcinoma of the pancreas: a case report and literature review of a heterogeneous group of tumors. *Am J Surg Pathol.* 2007;31:146-152.
622. Yigit S, Uyaroglu MA, Kus Z, et al. Hepatoid carcinoma of the ovary: immunohistochemical finding of one case and literature review. *Int J Gynecol Cancer.* 2006;16:1439-1441.
623. Goodman ZD. Neoplasms of the liver. *Mod Pathol.* 2007;20(Suppl 1):S49-60.
624. Pan CC, Chen PC, Tsay SH, Chiang H. Cytoplasmic immunoreactivity for thyroid transcription factor-1 in hepatocellular carcinoma: a comparative immunohistochemical analysis of four commercial antibodies using a tissue array technique. *Am J Clin Pathol.* 2004;121:343-349.
625. Lei JY, Bourne PA, diSant'Agnese PA, Huang J. Cytoplasmic staining of TTF-1 in the differential diagnosis of hepatocellular carcinoma vs cholangiocarcinoma and metastatic carcinoma of the liver. *Am J Clin Pathol.* 2006;125:519-525.
626. Gaffey MJ, Traweek ST, Mills SE, et al. Cytokeratin expression in adrenocortical neoplasia: an immunohistochemical and biochemical study with implications for the differential diagnosis of adrenocortical, hepatocellular, and renal cell carcinoma. *Hum Pathol.* 1992;23:144-153.
627. Tsuji M, Kashihara T, Terada N, Mori H. An immunohistochemical study of hepatic atypical adenomatous hyperplasia, hepatocellular carcinoma, and cholangiocarcinoma with alpha-fetoprotein, carcinoembryonic antigen, CA19-9, epithelial membrane antigen, and cytokeratins 18 and 19. *Pathol Int.* 1999;49:310-317.
628. Pinkus GS, Kurtin PJ. Epithelial membrane antigen—a diagnostic discriminant in surgical pathology: immunohistochemical profile in epithelial, mesenchymal, and hematopoietic neoplasms using paraffin sections and monoclonal antibodies. *Hum Pathol.* 1985;16:929-940.
629. Christensen WN, Boitnott JK, Kuhajda FP. Immunoperoxidase staining as a diagnostic aid for hepatocellular carcinoma. *Mod Pathol.* 1989;2:8-12.
630. Proca DM, Niemann TH, Porcell AI, DeYoung BR. MOC31 immunoreactivity in primary and metastatic carcinoma of the liver. Report of findings and review of other utilized markers. *Appl Immunohistochem Mol Morphol.* 2000;8:120-125.
631. Niemann TH, Hughes JH, De Young BR. MOC-31 aids in the differentiation of metastatic adenocarcinoma from hepatocellular carcinoma. *Cancer.* 1999;87:295-298.
632. Porcell AI, De Young BR, Proca DM, Frankel WL. Immunohistochemical analysis of hepatocellular and adenocarcinoma in the liver: MOC31 compares favorably with other putative markers. *Mod Pathol.* 2000;13:773-778.
633. Fucich LF, Cheles MK, Thung SN, et al. Primary vs metastatic hepatic carcinoma. An immunohistochemical study of 34 cases. *Arch Pathol Lab Med.* 1994;118:927-930.
634. Gottschalk-Sabag S, Ron N, Glick T. Use of CD34 and factor VIII to diagnose hepatocellular carcinoma on fine needle aspirates. *Acta Cytol.* 1998;42:691-696.
635. Tanigawa N, Lu C, Mitsui T, Miura S. Quantitation of sinusoid-like vessels in hepatocellular carcinoma: its clinical and prognostic significance. *Hepatology.* 1997;26:1216-1223.
636. Terada T, Nakanuma Y. Expression of ABH blood group antigens, receptors of Ulex europaeus agglutinin I, and factor VIII-related antigen on sinusoidal endothelial cells in adenomatous hyperplasia in human cirrhotic livers. *Hum Pathol.* 1991;22:486-493.
637. Terada T, Nakanuma Y. Expression of ABH blood group antigens, Ulex europaeus agglutinin I, and type IV collagen in the sinusoids of hepatocellular carcinoma. *Arch Pathol Lab Med.* 1991;115:50-55.
638. Dhillon AP, Colombari R, Savage K, Scheuer PJ. An immunohistochemical study of the blood vessels within primary hepatocellular tumours. *Liver.* 1992;12:311-318.

639. Togni R, Bagla N, Muiesan P, et al. Microsatellite instability in hepatocellular carcinoma in non-cirrhotic liver in patients older than 60 years. *Hepatol Res*. 2009;39:266-273.
640. Chiappini F, Gross-Goupil M, Saffroy R, et al. Microsatellite instability mutator phenotype in hepatocellular carcinoma in non-alcoholic and non-virally infected normal livers. *Carcinogenesis*. 2004;25:541-547.
641. Wang L, Bani-Hani A, Montoya DP, et al. hMLH1 and hMSH2 expression in human hepatocellular carcinoma. *Int J Oncol*. 2001;19:567-570.
642. Llovet JM, Bruix J. Molecular targeted therapies in hepatocellular carcinoma. *Hepatology*. 2008;48:1312-1327.
643. Villanueva A, Chiang DY, Newell P, et al. Pivotal role of mTOR signaling in hepatocellular carcinoma. *Gastroenterology*. 2008;135:1972-1983, 1983 e1971–e1911.
644. Guzman G, Alagiozian-Angelova V, Layden-Almer JE, et al. p53, Ki-67, and serum alpha feto-protein as predictors of hepatocellular carcinoma recurrence in liver transplant patients. *Mod Pathol*. 2005;18:1498-1503.
645. Jing Z, Nan KJ, Hu ML. Cell proliferation, apoptosis and the related regulators p27, p53 expression in hepatocellular carcinoma. *World J Gastroenterol*. 2005;11:1910-1916.
646. Sugo H, Takamori S, Kojima K, et al. The significance of p53 mutations as an indicator of the biological behavior of recurrent hepatocellular carcinomas. *Surg Today*. 1999;29:849-855.
647. Zhang T, Sun HC, Xu Y, et al. Overexpression of platelet-derived growth factor receptor alpha in endothelial cells of hepatocellular carcinoma associated with high metastatic potential. *Clin Cancer Res Official J Am Assoc Cancer Res*. 2005;11:8557-8563.
648. Berman MA, Burnham JA, Sheahan DG. Fibrolamellar carcinoma of the liver: an immunohistochemical study of nineteen cases and a review of the literature. *Hum Pathol*. 1988;19:784-794.
649. Van Eyken P, Sciot R, Brock P, Casteels-Van Daele M, et al. Abundant expression of cytokeratin 7 in fibrolamellar carcinoma of the liver. *Histopathology*. 1990;17:101-107.
650. Gornicka B, Ziarkiewicz-Wroblewska B, Wroblewski T, et al. Carcinoma, a fibrolamellar variant—immunohistochemical analysis of 4 cases. *Hepatogastroenterology*. 2005;52:519-523.
651. Garcia de Davila MT, Gonzalez-Crussi F, Mangkornkanok M. Fibrolamellar carcinoma of the liver in a child: ultrastructural and immunohistologic aspects. *Pediatr Pathol*. 1987;7:319-331.
652. Buckley AF, Burgart LJ, Kakar S. Epidermal growth factor receptor expression and gene copy number in fibrolamellar hepatocellular carcinoma. *Hum Pathol*. 2006;37:410-414.
653. Thomas MB, Chadha R, Glover K, et al. Phase 2 study of erlotinib in patients with unresectable hepatocellular carcinoma. *Cancer*. 2007;110:1059-1067.
654. Ikebe T, Wakasa K, Sasaki M, et al. Hepatocellular carcinoma with chondrosarcomatous variation: case report with immunohistochemical findings, and review of the literature. *J Hepatobiliary Pancreat Surg*. 1998;5:217-220.
655. Sasaki A, Yokoyama S, Nakayama I, et al. Sarcomatoid hepatocellular carcinoma with osteoclast-like giant cells: case report and immunohistochemical observations. *Pathol Int*. 1997;47:318-324.
656. Pan CC, Chen PC, Tsay SH, Ho DM. Differential immunoprofiles of hepatocellular carcinoma, renal cell carcinoma, and adrenocortical carcinoma: a systemic immunohistochemical survey using tissue array technique. *Appl Immunohistochem Mol Morphol*. 2005;13:347-352.
657. Van Eyken P, Sciot R, Paterson A, et al. Cytokeratin expression in hepatocellular carcinoma: an immunohistochemical study. *Hum Pathol*. 1988;19:562-568.
658. Wu PC, Fang JW, Lau VK, et al. Classification of hepatocellular carcinoma according to hepatocellular and biliary differentiation markers. Clinical and biological implications. *Am J Pathol*. 1996;149:1167-1175.
659. Hruban RH, Sturm PD, Slebos RJ, et al. Can K-ras codon 12 mutations be used to distinguish benign bile duct proliferations from metastases in the liver? A molecular analysis of 101 liver lesions from 93 patients. *Am J Pathol*. 1997;151:943-949.
660. Nakanuma Y, Sripa B, Vatanasapt V, et al. Intrahepatic cholangiocarcinoma. In: Hamilton SR, Aaltonen LA, eds. *Tumours of the Digestive System*. Lyon: International Agency for Research on Cancer (IARC), 2000:173-180.
661. Haglund C, Lindgren J, Roberts PJ, Nordling S. Difference in tissue expression of tumour markers CA 19-9 and CA 50 in hepatocellular carcinoma and cholangiocarcinoma. *Br J Cancer*. 1991;63:386-389.
662. Ohshio G, Ogawa K, Kudo H, et al. Immunohistochemical studies on the localization of cancer associated antigens DU-PAN-2 and CA19-9 in carcinomas of the digestive tract. *J Gastroenterol Hepatol*. 1990;5:25-31.
663. Loy TS, Sharp SC, Andershock CJ, Craig SB. Distribution of CA 19-9 in adenocarcinomas and transitional cell carcinomas. An immunohistochemical study of 527 cases. *Am J Clin Pathol*. 1993;99:726-728.
664. Aishima S, Kuroda Y, Nishihara Y, et al. Gastric mucin phenotype defines tumour progression and prognosis of intrahepatic cholangiocarcinoma: gastric foveolar type is associated with aggressive tumour behaviour. *Histopathology*. 2006;49:35-44.
665. Cazals-Hatem D, Rebouissou S, Bioulac-Sage P, et al. Clinical and molecular analysis of combined hepatocellular-cholangiocarcinomas. *J Hepatol*. 2004;41:292-298.
666. Gutgemann I, Haas S, Berg JP, Zhou H, Buttner R, Fischer HP. CD56 expression aids in the differential diagnosis of cholangiocarcinomas and benign cholangiocellular lesions. *Virchows Arch*. 2006;448:407-411.
667. Kozaka K, Sasaki M, Fujii T, et al. A subgroup of intrahepatic cholangiocarcinoma with an infiltrating replacement growth pattern and a resemblance to reactive proliferating bile ductules: 'bile ductular carcinoma'. *Histopathology*. 2007;51:390-400.
668. Stroescu C, Herlea V, Dragnea A, Popescu I. The diagnostic value of cytokeratins and carcinoembryonic antigen immunostaining in differentiating hepatocellular carcinomas from intrahepatic cholangiocarcinomas. *J Gastrointest Liver Dis*. 2006;15:9-14.
669. Lodi C, Szabo E, Holczbauer A, et al. Claudin-4 differentiates biliary tract cancers from hepatocellular carcinomas. *Mod Pathol*. 2006;19:460-469.
670. Loy TS, Quesenberry JT, Sharp SC. Distribution of CA 125 in adenocarcinomas. An immunohistochemical study of 481 cases. *Am J Clin Pathol*. 1992;98:175-179.
671. Nakajima T, Tajima Y, Sugano I, et al. Intrahepatic cholangiocarcinoma with sarcomatous change. Clinicopathologic and immunohistochemical evaluation of seven cases. *Cancer*. 1993;72:1872-1877.
672. Imazu H, Ochiai M, Funabiki T. Intrahepatic sarcomatous cholangiocarcinoma. *J Gastroenterol*. 1995;30:677-682.
673. Sumiyoshi S, Kikuyama M, Matsubayashi Y, et al. Carcinosarcoma of the liver with mesenchymal differentiation. *World J Gastroenterol*. 2007;13:809-812.
674. Honda M, Enjoji M, Sakai H, et al. Case report: intrahepatic cholangiocarcinoma with rhabdoid transformation. *J Gastroenterol Hepatol*. 1996;11:771-774.
675. Nomura K, Aizawa S, Ushigome S. Carcinosarcoma of the liver. *Arch Pathol Lab Med*. 2000;124:888-890.
676. Lim BJ, Kim KS, Lim JS, et al. Rhabdoid cholangiocarcinoma: a variant of cholangiocarcinoma with aggressive behavior. *Yonsei Med J*. 2004;45:543-546.
677. Kanamoto M, Yoshizumi T, Ikegami T, et al. Cholangiolocellular carcinoma containing hepatocellular carcinoma and cholangiocellular carcinoma, extremely rare tumor of the liver:a case report. *J Med Invest*. 2008;55:161-165.
678. Wakasa T, Wakasa K, Shutou T, et al. A histopathological study on combined hepatocellular and cholangiocarcinoma: cholangiocarcinoma component is originated from hepatocellular carcinoma. *Hepatogastroenterology*. 2007;54:508-513.
679. Taguchi J, Nakashima O, Tanaka M, et al. A clinicopathological study on combined hepatocellular and cholangiocarcinoma. *J Gastroenterol Hepatol*. 1996;11:758-764.
680. Tickoo SK, Zee SY, Obiekwe S, et al. Combined hepatocellular-cholangiocarcinoma: a histopathologic, immunohistochemical, and in situ hybridization study. *Am J Surg Pathol*. 2002;26:989-997.
681. Jarnagin WR, Weber S, Tickoo SK, et al. Combined hepatocellular and cholangiocarcinoma: demographic, clinical, and prognostic factors. *Cancer*. 2002;94:2040-2046.
682. Siren J, Karkkainen P, Luukkonen P, et al. A case report of biliary cystadenoma and cystadenocarcinoma. *Hepatogastroenterology*. 1998;45:83-89.

683. Yanase M, Ikeda H, Ogata I, et al. Primary smooth muscle tumor of the liver encasing hepatobiliary cystadenoma without mesenchymal stroma. *Am J Surg Pathol*. 1999;23:854-859.
684. Terada T, Nakanuma Y, Ohta T, et al. Mucin-histochemical and immunohistochemical profiles of epithelial cells of several types of hepatic cysts. *Virchows Arch A Pathol Anat Histopathol*. 1991;419:499-504.
685. Maruyama S, Hirayama C, Yamamoto S, et al. Hepatobiliary cystadenoma with mesenchymal stroma in a patient with chronic hepatitis C. *J Gastroenterol*. 2003;38:593-597.
686. Scott FR, More L, Dhillon AP. Hepatobiliary cystadenoma with mesenchymal stroma: expression of oestrogen receptors in formalin-fixed tissue. *Histopathology*. 1995;26:555-558.
687. Grayson W, Teare J, Myburgh JA, Paterson AC. Immunohistochemical demonstration of progesterone receptor in hepatobiliary cystadenoma with mesenchymal stroma. *Histopathology*. 1996;29:461-463.
688. Leger-Ravet MB, Borgonovo G, Amato A, et al. Carcinosarcoma of the liver with mesenchymal differentiation: a case report. *Hepatogastroenterology*. 1996;43:255-259.
689. Lao XM, Chen DY, Zhang YQ, et al. Primary carcinosarcoma of the liver: clinicopathologic features of 5 cases and a review of the literature. *Am J Surg Pathol*. 2007;31:817-826.
690. Balta Z, Sauerbruch T, Hirner A, et al. [Primary neuroendocrine carcinoma of the liver: From carcinoid tumor to small-cell hepatic carcinoma: case reports and review of the literature.]. *Pathologe*. 2008;29:53-60.
691. Cho MS, Lee SN, Sung SH, Han WS. Sarcomatoid hepatocellular carcinoma with hepatoblastoma-like features in an adult. *Pathol Int*. 2004;54:446-450.
692. Wang JH, Dhillon AP, Sankey EA, et al. 'Neuroendocrine' differentiation in primary neoplasms of the liver. *J Pathol*. 1991;163:61-67.
693. Lerut JP, Orlando G, Adam R, et al. The place of liver transplantation in the treatment of hepatic epitheloid hemangioendothelioma: report of the European liver transplant registry. *Ann Surg*. 2007;246:949-957, discussion 957.
694. Ishak KG, Anthony PP, Niederau C, Nakanuma Y. Mesenchymal tumours of the liver. In: Hamilton SR, Aaltonen LA, eds. *Tumours of the Digestive System*. Lyon, France: International Agency for Research on Cancer (IARC); 2000:191-198.
695. Zamboni G, Pea M, Martignoni G, et al. Clear cell "sugar" tumor of the pancreas. A novel member of the family of lesions characterized by the presence of perivascular epithelioid cells. *Am J Surg Pathol*. 1996;20:722-730.
696. Nonomura A, Minato H, Kurumaya H. Angiomyolipoma predominantly composed of smooth muscle cells: problems in histological diagnosis. *Histopathology*. 1998;33:20-27.
697. Nishio J, Iwasaki H, Sakashita N, et al. Undifferentiated (embryonal) sarcoma of the liver in middle-aged adults: smooth muscle differentiation determined by immunohistochemistry and electron microscopy. *Hum Pathol*. 2003;34:246-252.
698. Stocker JT, Ishak KG. Undifferentiated (embryonal) sarcoma of the liver: report of 31 cases. *Cancer*. 1978;42:336-348.
699. Miettinen M, Kahlos T. Undifferentiated (embryonal) sarcoma of the liver. Epithelial features as shown by immunohistochemical analysis and electron microscopic examination. *Cancer*. 1989;64:2096-2103.
700. Aoyama C, Hachitanda Y, Sato JK, et al. Undifferentiated (embryonal) sarcoma of the liver. A tumor of uncertain histogenesis showing divergent differentiation. *Am J Surg Pathol*. 1991;15:615-624.

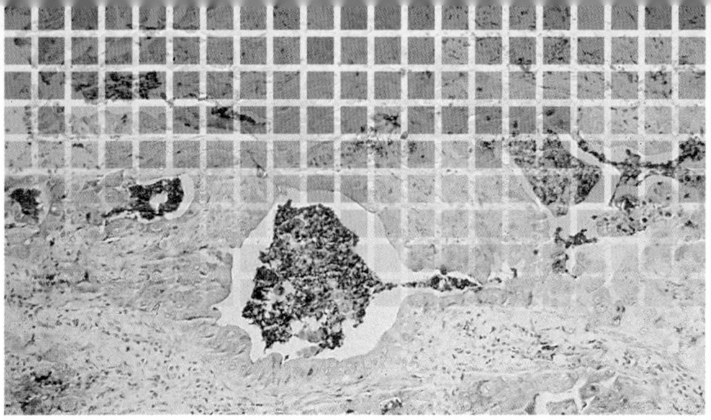

16

Immunohistology of the Prostate, Bladder, Kidney, and Testis

George J. Netto • Jonathan I. Epstein

- Introduction 593
- Immunohistology of the Prostate 593
- Immunohistology of the Urinary Bladder 619
- Immunohistology of Renal Neoplasms 631
- Immunohistology of Testicular Tumors 642

INTRODUCTION

Ancillary techniques, used in the proper setting, can be a great adjunct to light microscopy in obtaining an accurate diagnosis in urologic pathology.

In the past decade, a plethora of molecular biomarkers have been evaluated for their potential role in enhancing our ability to predict disease progression, response to therapy, and survival in prostate cancer (PCa) patients.[1-6] These research efforts have been greatly assisted by the wealth of information garnered from gene expression array studies and by sophisticated bioinformatics tools evaluating the overwhelming datasets generated from genomic, transcriptomic, and proteomic studies. These genomic technologies continue to yield new markers that can in turn be evaluated for clinical utility in a high-throughput manner using immunohistochemistry and fluorescence *in situ* hybridization (FISH)-labeled tissue microarrays and state-of-the-art image analysis systems.[7-10]

In prostate biopsies, immunomarkers that can assist reaching a diagnosis of carcinoma in a small focus of atypical glands are of great utility. The latter has been especially valuable in an organ such as the prostate where a repeat biopsy does not always reach the target focus for additional sampling. The layer of assurance rendered by multiple immunostains used in prostate biopsy is due in part to their amenability to be simultaneously applied in the same section when only limited tissue is available. Ancillary techniques are equally important in helping the pathologist correctly identify many morphologic mimickers of PCa that could lead to a false-positive interpretation. The serious patient care and medico-legal implications of a false-positive diagnosis of PCa are evident.

In recent years the detection and treatment of renal tumors has shifted toward radiologic detection of smaller lesions with an increasing tendency toward a laparoscopic approach for partial nephrectomy, ablative cryotherapy, or radiofrequency ablation. When ablative therapy is contemplated, obtaining a proper classification of renal tumors on a needle biopsy obtained before such therapy is even more crucial given the lack of additional sampling. The increasing number of differentially expressed renal tumor markers has been valuable in such settings. The same is true in morphologically difficult nephrectomy or needle biopsy samples where acceptance into an adjuvant targeted therapy protocol is based on the morphologic type of the renal tumor.

Likewise, newer immunohistochemical (IHC) and molecular markers in bladder and testicular tumors are increasingly used for reaching an accurate diagnosis and classification. The following is a discussion of the utility of immunohistochemical markers, genomic applications, and prognostic aspects of urologic and testicular tumors.

IMMUNOHISTOLOGY OF THE PROSTATE

Biology of Principal Antigens and Antibodies

Many different antibodies are used for the immunohistochemical evaluation of urologic neoplasms. Generally used epithelial, neuroendocrine, and mesenchymal antibodies are discussed in other chapters. In each section we summarize antibodies with particular importance for the neoplasms covered in that section.

Prostate-Specific Antigen

Prostate-specific antigen (PSA) is a serine protease member of the human glandular kallikrein family. PSA is a 34 KD glycoprotein of 237 amino acids with high-sequence homology with human glandular kallikrein 2 (HK2). It is almost exclusively synthesized in the prostate ductal and acinar epithelium. It is found in normal, hyperplastic, and malignant prostate tissue.[11] PSA liquefies the seminal fluid coagulum through proteolysis of the gel-forming proteins, thus releasing spermatozoa. It can reach the serum by diffusion from the luminal cells through the basal cell layer, glandular basement membrane, and extracellular matrix. Measuring total serum PSA levels is currently the mainstay of PCa detection. Numerous studies have shown that patients with PCa have, in general, elevated serum PSA levels. The most commonly used cutoff for PSA is 4 ng/mL. When serum PSA concentrations are 4 to 10 ng/mL, the incidence of cancer detection on prostate biopsy in men with a normal digital rectal examination (DRE) is approximately 25%. With serum PSA levels over 10 ng/mL, the incidence of prostate cancer on biopsy increases to approximately 67%. However, the risk of cancer is proportional to the serum PSA level even at values below 4 ng/mL. As large screening trials have demonstrated, clinically significant cancers occur in men with serum PSA levels of 2.5 to 4.0 ng/mL; thus some experts have proposed lowering the PSA cutoff to 2.5 ng/mL to improve early detection of cancer in younger men.[11]

Once PSA gains access into the circulation, most remains bound to serine protease inhibitors. The three most recognizable inhibitors are α_1 antichymotrypsin (ACT), α_2 macroglobulin, and α_1 protein inhibitor. PSA bound to ACT is the most immunoreactive and is the one clinically most useful in diagnosing prostate cancer. A smaller fraction (5% to 40%) of the measurable serum PSA is free (noncomplexed) PSA. The total serum PSA measured, therefore, reflects both free and complexed PSA. It has been demonstrated that the percent of free PSA can improve the specificity of PSA testing for prostate cancer. A percent of free PSA value of less than 10% is worrisome for cancer. More recently, additional isoforms of free PSA have been discovered, as detailed in a review by Gretzer.[11] PSA is first secreted in the form of a precursor termed pro-PSA. This inactive form of the enzyme constitutes the majority of free PSA in serum in men with prostate cancer, making the relative increase of serum pro-PSA a risk marker of PCa. BPSA ("benign PSA") refers to a cleaved form of PSA from BPH tissue. The ratio of proPSA/BPSA has been proposed as a means of improving the accuracy of diagnosing cancer in men with a low percentage of free PSA levels, who are at relatively high risk of cancer.[9,12]

Serum PSA tests may also be used to monitor patients post therapy to detect early recurrence. Following radical prostatectomy, the serum PSA should drop to undetectable levels. Elevated serum PSA levels following radical prostatectomy (>0.2 ng/mL) indicate recurrent or persistent disease. Following radiotherapy for prostate cancer, serum PSA values will decrease to a nadir, although not to the same extent as those following radical prostatectomy. Three subsequent rises in serum PSA values after radiotherapy indicate treatment failure.

Although PSA expression in extraprostatic tissues and tumors other than PCA has been rarely demonstrated (see Table 16.1), for all practical purposes PSA expression at the IHC level is a specific and sensitive marker of prostatic lineage of differentiation with up to 97.4% sensitivity found in a recent study from our group.[13] Urethral, periurethral, and perianal glands are among normal tissues that have been rarely reported to show PSA reactivity. Extraprostatic neoplasms occasionally expressing PSA include urethral and periurethral adenocarcinoma, cloacogenic carcinoma, pleomorphic adenoma of salivary gland and salivary duct carcinoma, as well as rare mammary carcinomas.[14-16] Although a rare report indicated PSA expression in intestinal-type urachal adenocarcinoma of bladder, we failed to reveal such expression in a recent study of villous adenoma and adenocarcinoma of bladder.[17] The latter is especially important from a differential diagnosis point of view given the topographic proximity of the two organs. Although weaker intensity of PSA expression can be encountered in higher Gleason grade PCa, we were recently able to demonstrate a high degree of PSA immunostain sensitivity (97.4%) in high-grade prostate carcinoma even when TMA sampling was used.[13] Likewise, PSA expression is valuable in defining a prostatic primary site of origin during the evaluation of a poorly differentiated metastatic carcinoma (Table 16.1).

Prostate-Specific Membrane Antigen

Prostate-specific membrane antigen (PSMA) is a type II membrane glycoprotein that is expressed in prostate tissue and to a lesser extent in peripheral and central nervous system, small intestinal, and salivary gland

TABLE 16.1 Prostate-Specific Antigen Immunoreactivity in Extraprostatic Tissues and Tumors

Extraprostatic Tissues
Urethra and periurethral glands (male and female)
Bladder, including cystitis cystica and glandularis
Anal glands (male)
Urachal remnants
Neutrophils
Extraprostatic Tumors
Urethral and periurethral gland adenocarcinoma (female)
Villous adenoma and adenocarcinoma of the bladder
Extramammary Paget disease of the male external genitalia
Pleomorphic adenoma of the salivary glands (male)
Carcinoma of the salivary glands (male)
Breast carcinoma

tissues. PSMA expression has also been documented in endothelial cells of the neovasculature of many solid tumors including renal cell carcinoma.[18-22] In prostate, PSMA is expressed by benign and malignant prostatic epithelial cells with higher-extent staining seen in the latter.[23] It is also expressed by high-grade prostatic intraepithelial carcinoma (PIN).[23] PSMA expression correlates with PCa stage and Gleason grade.[24] The increase in both expression and enzymatic activity of PSMA in aggressive PCa points to a selective advantage imparted on cells expressing PSMA, thereby contributing to the development and progression of PCa.[25] Increased PSMA expression is an independent predictor of PCa recurrence.[25,26] PSMA expression is maintained in hormone-refractory PCa, thus increasing its utility in such settings.[20,27] Several imaging strategies exploited PSMA specificity to PCa and are currently in use for PCa diagnostic imaging.[28-31] Furthermore, PSMA is under investigation as a target of therapy in PCa and other solid tumors given its expression by neovasculature of extraprostatic tumors.[32-34] Cytoplasmic and, to a lesser degree, membranous PSMA expression have been recently documented in 11% of analyzed urinary bladder adenocarcinomas,[17] a fact worth noting when the differential diagnosis includes prostatic and bladder adenocarcinoma.

Prostatic Acid Phosphatase/Prostate-Specific Acid Phosphatase

Prostate-specific acid phosphatase (PSAP) is one of the earlier prostate lineage markers that was exploited for immunolabeling of PCa before the discovery of PSA. Currently, its use as a marker of prostatic differentiation has declined given its relative lack of specificity compared with PSA and the more variable staining of PSAP in higher-grade PCa.[35,36]

Prostein (P501S)

P501S is a 553-amino acid protein that is localized to the Golgi complex. It is expressed in both benign and neoplastic prostate tissues. Typical P501S stain is of perinuclear cytoplasmic (Golgi) location and a speckled pattern. Expression is retained in poorly differentiated and metastatic PCa. P501S demonstrated up to 99% sensitivity in a recent study from our group by Sheridan and colleagues.[37] In rare metastatic lesions, P501S positivity may be encountered in the presence of PSA-negative expression, making it an advantageous addition to a prostate lineage immunopanel. To date, P501S expression has not been shown in extraprostatic carcinomas, making it of great utility in differentiating high-grade PCa from other high-grade carcinomas including colorectal and urothelial carcinoma.[13,17,37-41]

α-Methylacyl Coenzyme A Racemase/P504S

α-Methylacyl coenzyme A racemase (AMACR) enzyme is mainly localized to peroxisomal structures. It plays a critical role in peroxisomal beta oxidation of branched chain fatty acid. In their original detailed immunohistochemical analysis, Luo and colleagues[42] demonstrated that both prostate carcinomas and high-grade PIN consistently revealed a significantly higher expression than matched normal prostate epithelium. Both untreated metastases and hormone refractory prostate metastases cancers generally maintain a strong positive reactivity for AMACR. An overall PCa sensitivity and specificity of 97% and 92%, respectively, have been shown in a multi-institutional study by Jiang and colleagues.[43]

Cytoplasmic AMACR staining, combined with absence of basal cell markers such as the nuclear protein p63 and high-molecular-weight cytokeratins (HMWCKs), has proven to be of greatest utility in providing an added layer of assurance in establishing the diagnosis of PCa on small-needle biopsy foci.[43-46] However, AMACR expression has been repeatedly demonstrated in high-grade PIN and some benign mimics of PCa such as glandular atrophy, partial atrophy, and adenosis. Therefore AMACR is of limited utility as a single marker in resolving the differential diagnosis of PCa in such lesions. Using a panel of immunostains including AMACR, high-molecular-weight cytokeratin, and p63 (positive AMACR immunostaining (Table 16.2) along with negative basal cell markers) is recommended in the interrogation of atypical prostatic glandular foci.[47-54]

High-Molecular-Weight Cytokeratins

HMWCKs are of great utility in highlighting the presence or absence of basal cells in a focus of atypical prostate glands.[55-58] 34βE12 is currently the most widely used clone either individually or as a component of a three-antibody cocktail including a second basal cell marker (e.g., p63, AMACR). Alternatively, CK5/6 can be used as the HMWK marker individually or in combination with p63 and AMACR. A recent study by Abrams and colleagues[59] seems to suggest a superior

TABLE 16.2 Immunoreactivity of α-Methylacyl Coenzyme A Racemase in Benign and Neoplastic Prostate

	Immunoreactive Range (%)	Immunoreactive Glands (%)	Intensity (1-3+)
Benign	8 (0-10)	4.6 (0-24.5)	1+
Atypical adenomatous hyperplasia (AAH)	14 (10-17)	15.1 (1-50)	1+
High-grade prostatic intraepithelial neoplasia	88 (80-100)	21.8 (2.7-5.7)	1+-2+
Cancer	97 (80-100)	35 (6.2-78.2)	2-3+

TABLE 16.3 Immunophenotype of Basal Cell Layer in the Prostate

Biomarker	Function	Findings
Androgen receptors	Nuclear receptors that are necessary for prostatic epithelial growth	Strong immunoreactivity; also present in cancer cells
Prostate-specific antigen	Enzyme that liquefies the seminal coagulum	Present in rare basal cells; mainly in secretory luminal cells
Keratin 34βE12	Keratins 5, 10, 11	Strong immunoreactivity; most commonly used for diagnostic purposes
p63	A member of the p53 gene family	Strong immunoreactivity; most commonly used for diagnostic purposes
S100A6	Calcium-binding protein	Strong immunoreactivity
Epidermal growth factor receptor	Membrane-bound 170 kD glycoprotein that mediates the activity of EGF	Strong immunoreactivity; rare in cancer cells
Glutathione S-transferase gene (GSTP1)	Enzyme that activates electrophilic carcinogens	Strong immunoreactivity; rare in cancer
C-CAM	Epithelial cell adhesion molecule	Strong immunoreactivity; absent in cancer
TGF-β	Growth factor that regulates cell proliferation and differentiation	Strong immunoreactivity; absent in cancer

sensitivity for CK5/6 as an HMWCK in prostate biopsies fixed in "Hollandes" fixative. Following initial examination of hematoxylin/eosin-stained routine sections, the application of such a cocktail to previously prepared unstained intervening sections is recommended in biopsies where establishing the presence or absence of basal cells in a questionable focus will lead to a definitive resolution of a benign or malignant diagnosis, respectively.[60]

p63

The p53 homologue p63 encodes for different isotypes that can either transactivate p53 reporter genes (TAp63) or act as p53-dominant-negatives (ΔNp63). p63 is expressed in the basal cells or myoepithelial cells of many epithelial organs, and its germline inactivation in the mouse results in agenesis of organs such as skin appendages and the breast. In prostate, p63 expression is limited to basal cells and is absent in secretory and neuroendocrine cells.[61] ΔNp63a isotype is the most abundantly represented in normal prostate basal cells. Recent experimental evidence also suggests that the p63 gene is essential for normal stem cell function in the prostate.[62] Several studies have confirmed the clinical utility of p63 immunostain as a prostate basal cell marker with some studies suggesting a slight sensitivity advantage for p63 over HMWCK alone.[63-67] Additionally, the use of basal cell HMWCK and p63 cocktails may reduce the staining variability that may be encountered in basal cells and may further decrease the false-negative and false-positive rates of basal cell labeling by either marker alone (Table 16.3).[65,68]

Finally, given the fact that immunostains for basal cell markers are usually used in a "negative" diagnostic mode in order to show absence of basal cells in PCa, sole reliance on such markers is not advocated and the identification of a combination of major and minor histologic features of PCa is crucial for achieving clinical diagnostic accuracy. In this regard, consideration should be given to the fact that benign prostatic glands from the transition zone are subject to basal cell staining variability, which may result in occasional negative basal cell staining in such benign glands.[65] Furthermore, basal cells can be retained, albeit rarely, in individual glands in otherwise typical acinar PCa focus, and the constellation of diagnostic features is to be relied on in such rare cases. We have recently described an intriguing p63-positive (HMWCK-negative) variant of prostate carcinoma where nuclear p63 staining is seen in secretory PCa cells in a nonbasal distribution.[69]

Diagnostic Immunohistochemistry of Specific Prostate Lesions

IMMUNOHISTOCHEMISTRY IN SMALL FOCUS OF PROSTATE CARCINOMA

The use of immunohistochemical markers to help establish the diagnosis of carcinoma in a morphologically atypical small focus of prostate glands is currently a common laboratory practice. As mentioned earlier, used individually or with two or three markers combined in a panel, HMWCK and/or p63 and/or AMACR offer a great help in assuring absence of basal layer combined with a positive AMACR labeling in such small foci (Fig. 16.1). Such a panel is also of use in distinguishing a small focus of PCa infiltrating adjacent to a high-grade PIN lesion from the glandular outpouching of high-grade

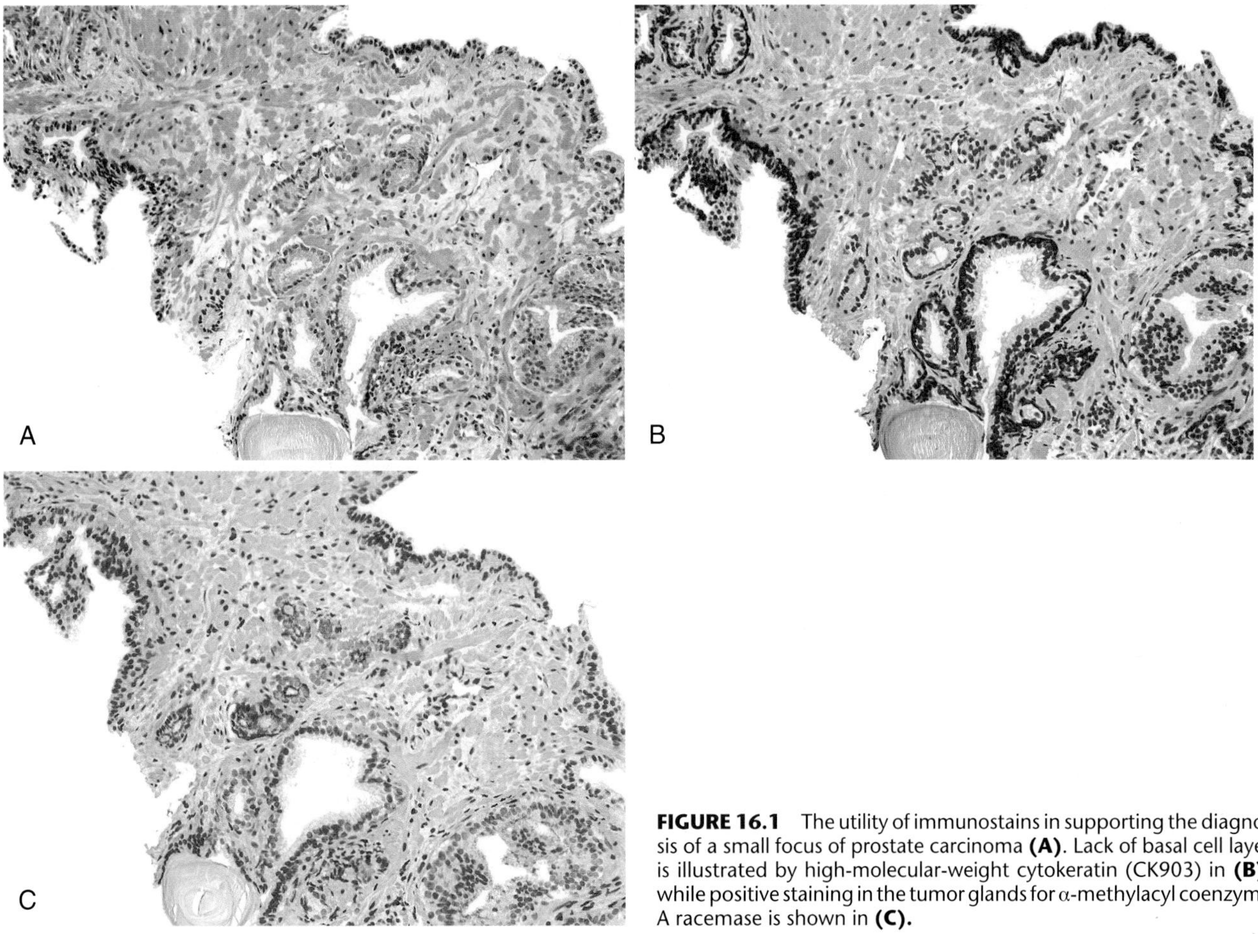

FIGURE 16.1 The utility of immunostains in supporting the diagnosis of a small focus of prostate carcinoma **(A)**. Lack of basal cell layer is illustrated by high-molecular-weight cytokeratin (CK903) in **(B)**, while positive staining in the tumor glands for α-methylacyl coenzyme A racemase is shown in **(C)**.

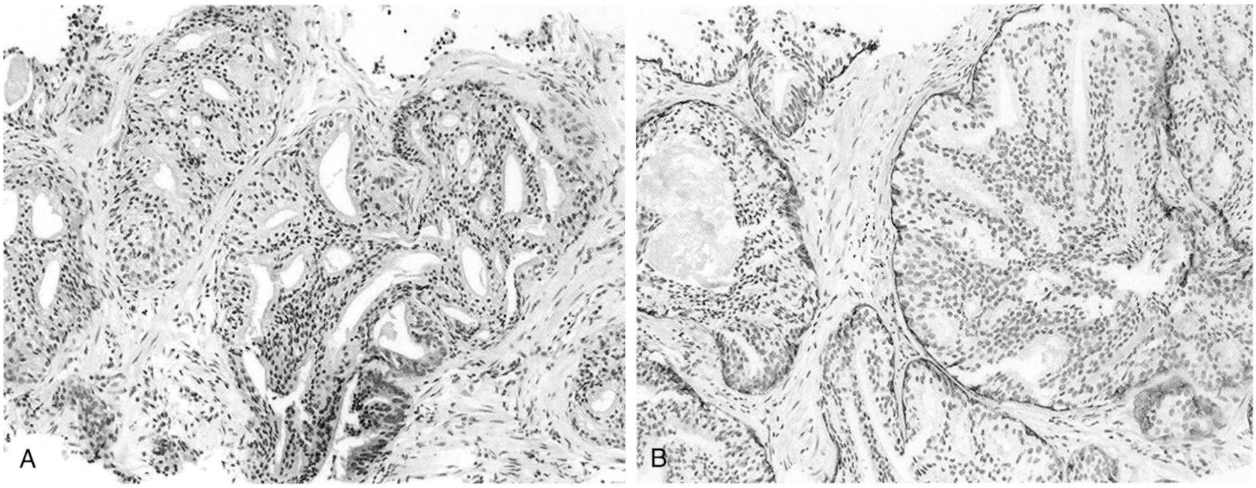

FIGURE 16.2 Cribriform high-grade prostatic intraepithelial neoplasia **(A)** showing preservation of basal layer staining on high-molecular-weight cytokeratin **(B)**.

PIN where an interrupted (patchy) layer of basal cells would still be identified with the aid of immunostains (Figs. 16.2 and 16.3). Fully characterizing and delineating the group of atypical acini in question on the basis of a combination of established H&E morphologic features of malignancy before their interrogation by immunostains are essential for a successful diagnostic approach in PCa. The key H&E morphologic features include small acinar architecture, single-layer lining, straight luminal borders, amphophilic cytoplasm, nuclear

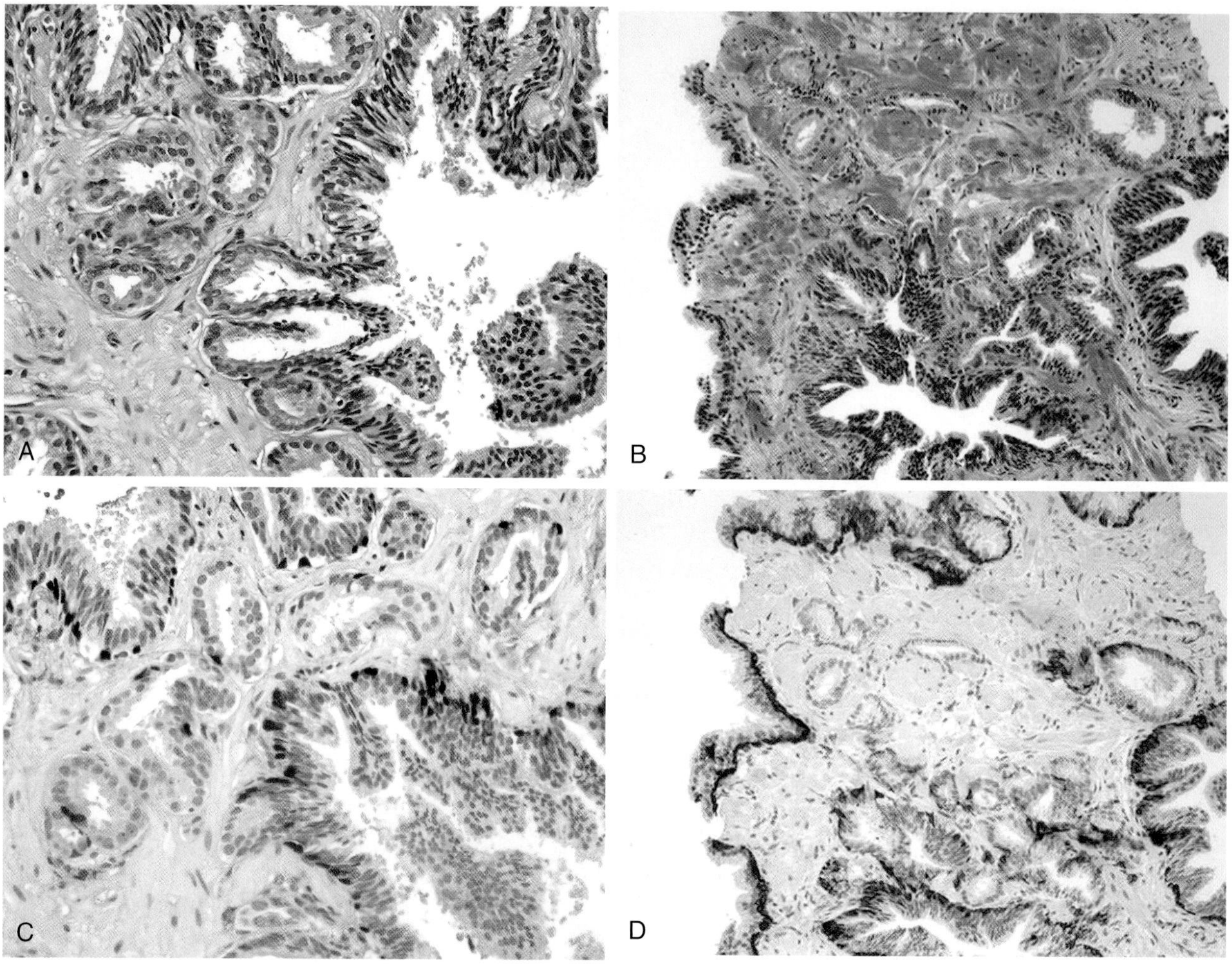

FIGURE 16.3 Atypical glands adjacent to high-grade prostatic intraepithelial neoplasia (PIN) **(A** and **B).** The possibility of glandular outpouchings of PIN could not be excluded given the presence of an interrupted (patchy) layer of basal cells with the aid of immunostains (p63 in **C** and high-molecular-weight cytokeratin in **D**).

enlargement and atypia, presence of prominent nucleoli, wispy or blue mucin content, dense eosinophilic secretions or "cancer" crystalloids, and presence of mucinous fibroplasia. The demonstration of an increasing combination of these morphologic features in the presence of supportive immunostaining pattern will allow for a significant increment in diagnostic confidence when faced with increasingly smaller-size atypical foci on a needle biopsy.[70] If such a confidence level is unobtainable despite the application of immunostains, a diagnosis of "focus of atypical glands suspicious but not diagnostic of malignancy" should be rendered with a recommendation for a close repeat follow-up biopsy in order to rule out malignancy (Fig. 16.4).

Routine initial use of immunostain cocktails as a screening tool before H&E examination (to assist identification of basal cell negative foci) is not advocated for obvious reasons including cost and misallocation of resources and potential detriment to diagnostic accuracy. On the other hand, when used judicially, the role of HMWCK in decreasing diagnostic uncertainty expressed in prostate needle biopsies has been established in several large studies including a College of American Pathology (CAP) Q-probes study of more than 15,000 biopsies.[55-58] In a large study from our center, 34βE12 stains helped establish (14%), confirm (58%), or change (2%) our diagnoses when applied to questionable/atypical foci. In an additional 18% of cases, the diagnosis remained (or became) equivocal despite the use of HMWCK.[55] False-negative staining of basal cells with HMWCK can occur because of various technical reasons including suboptimal antigen retrieval and should be taken into consideration. Finally, it is worthy to note that a low, but existent, false-positive HMWCK immunostaining of PCa cells can be encountered (0.2% to 2.8%)[65,68] characteristically in a non–basal cell distribution pattern (Fig. 16.5). Another complicating issue in interpreting basal cell immunostaining results is the recently described p63-positive (HMWCK-negative) rare variant of PCa as mentioned earlier (Fig. 16.6).[69]

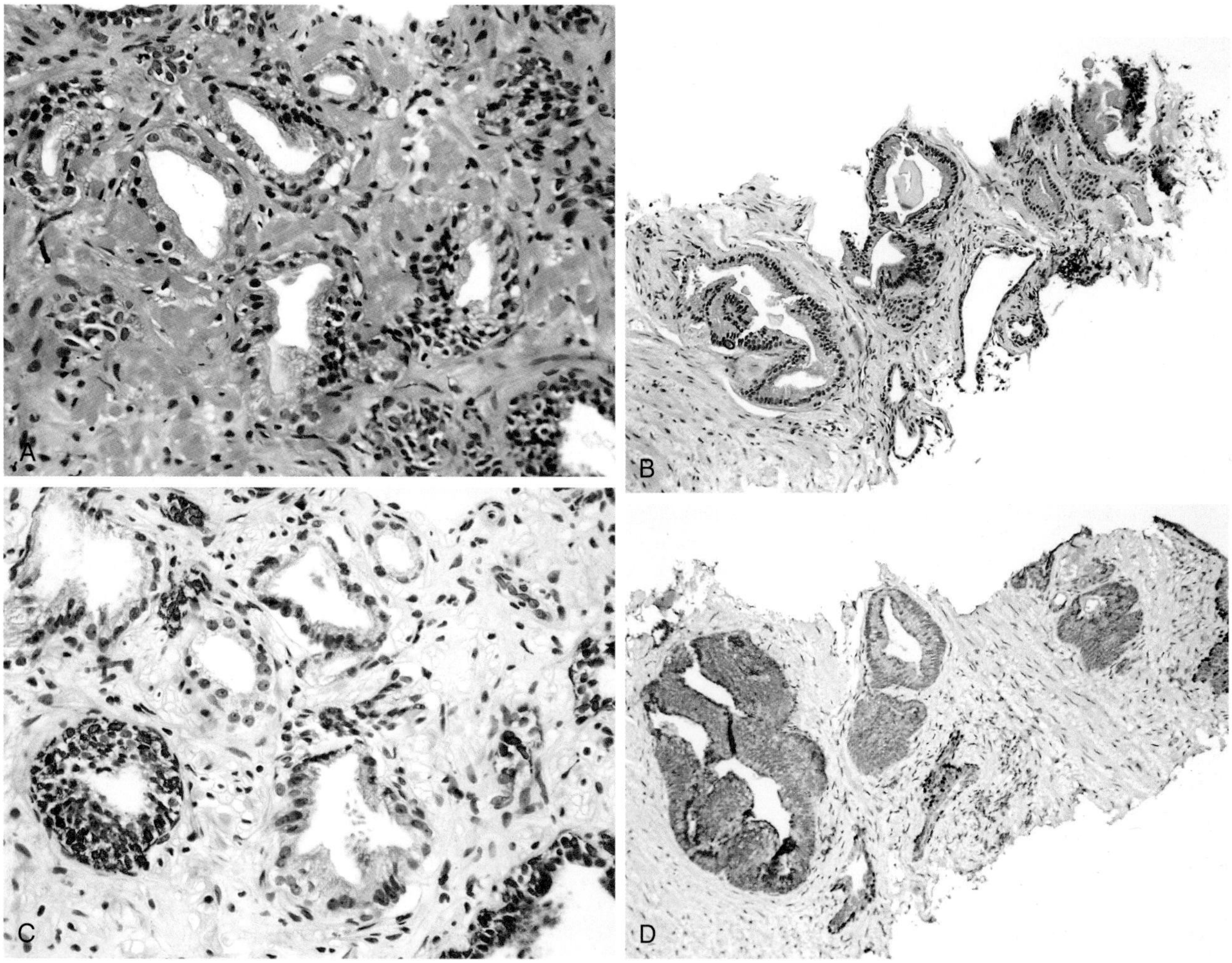

FIGURES 16.4 Prostate adenocarcinoma diagnosis supported by absence of basal layer on immunostains in two groups of atypical glands infiltrating among benign glands **(A** and **B)** using immunostains for HMWCK **(C)** and p63 **(D).**

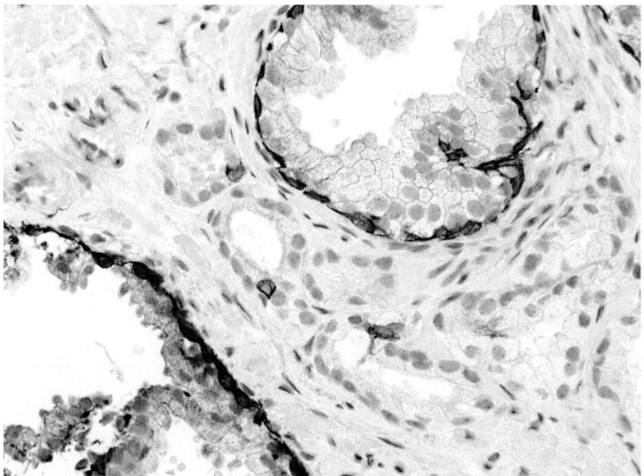

FIGURE 16.5 A focus of prostate adenocarcinoma showing scattered tumor cells with positive expression of high-molecular-weight cytokeratin in a nonbasal distribution. This finding alone should not deter from making a diagnosis of carcinoma if all other features of malignancy are satisfied.

KEY DIAGNOSTIC POINTS

Small Focus of Prostate Carcinoma

- Characteristics are small acinar architecture, single-layer lining, straight luminal borders, amphophilic cytoplasm, nuclear enlargement and atypia, presence of prominent nucleoli, wispy or blue mucin content, dense eosinophilic secretions or "cancer" crystalloids, and presence of mucinous fibroplasia.
- If additional immunostains do not render confidence, "focal atypical glands suspicious for carcinoma" should prompt follow-up biopsy.

BENIGN MIMICS OF PROSTATE ADENOCARCINOMA

Prostatic Atrophy

Partial atrophy (PTAT) and postatrophic hyperplasia (PAH) are the most problematic morphologic variants of atrophy that may mimic PCa. In fact, PTAT is the most common mimic of PCa on needle biopsy. This is mainly

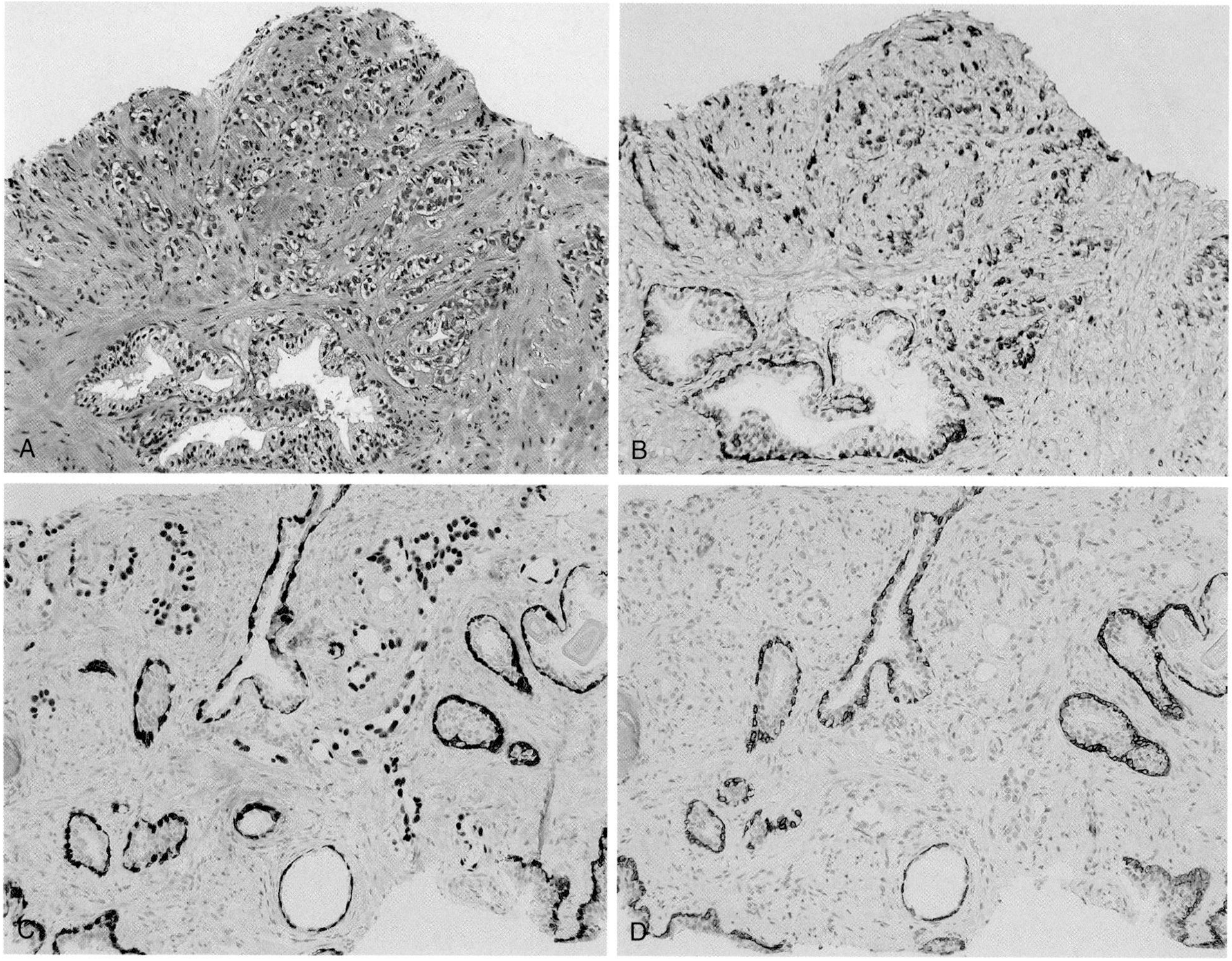

FIGURE 16.6 Rare variant of prostate adenocarcinoma **(A)** showing aberrant expression of p63 (but not high-molecular-weight cytokeratin [HMWCK]). Note nuclear positivity for p63 in tumor glands in **B** (combo p63 and 34βE12) and **C** (p63). The tumor is negative for HMWCK **(D).**

due to the presence of disorganized acini lined by pale cytoplasm with occasional acini retaining full height of cytoplasm and containing slightly enlarged nuclei with notable nucleoli. PTAT foci can morphologically mimic "atrophic" PCa. In difficult PTAT lesions, immunostains for basal cell markers help highlight the presence of basal cells. High-molecular-weight cytokeratins (34βE12, CK5/6) and/or p63 show patchy positivity in basal cells in at least some of the glands (Fig. 16.7). Lack of positivity in some glands should not be misinterpreted as PCa as long as the negative and positive glands share similar cytologic features.[51] It is also important to remember that AMACR can be expressed by some PTAT acini.[71]

Only rarely does one need to resort to immunostains in order to recognize simple atrophy and PAH lesions. The latter two variants of atrophy demonstrate a continuous basal layer on immunostains, and they are usually negative for AMACR (Fig. 16.8).

Adenosis

Adenosis is a common mimic of PCa both on needle biopsy and transurethral resection of the prostate (TURP).[72-74] Given its preferential occurrence in the transition zone, adenosis is more frequently seen in TURP (1.6%) compared with needle biopsy (0.8%). Adenosis is characterized by a nodular proliferation of small glands. Within such a nodule, larger elongated glands with papillary infolding and branching lumina share identical nuclear and cytoplasmic features with the admixed, smaller, more suspicious glands. In contrast, small PCa glands usually stand out cytologically from adjacent benign larger glands. To avoid misinterpretation of adenosis, the constellation of histologic features in a given lesion should outweigh the significance of any one diagnostic feature[75] given the fact that several features are shared between adenosis and PCa. Therefore in difficult cases, IHC for high-molecular-weight cytokeratins can be of great utility to demonstrate the patchy positivity of basal cells in adenosis (Fig. 16.9).[76] Lack of positivity for HMWCK, in some of the glands, should not be misinterpreted as evidence of PCa as long as the negative and positive glands share similar cytologic features. Of note, AMACR can be focally or diffusely expressed in adenosis in up to 10% of cases.[71]

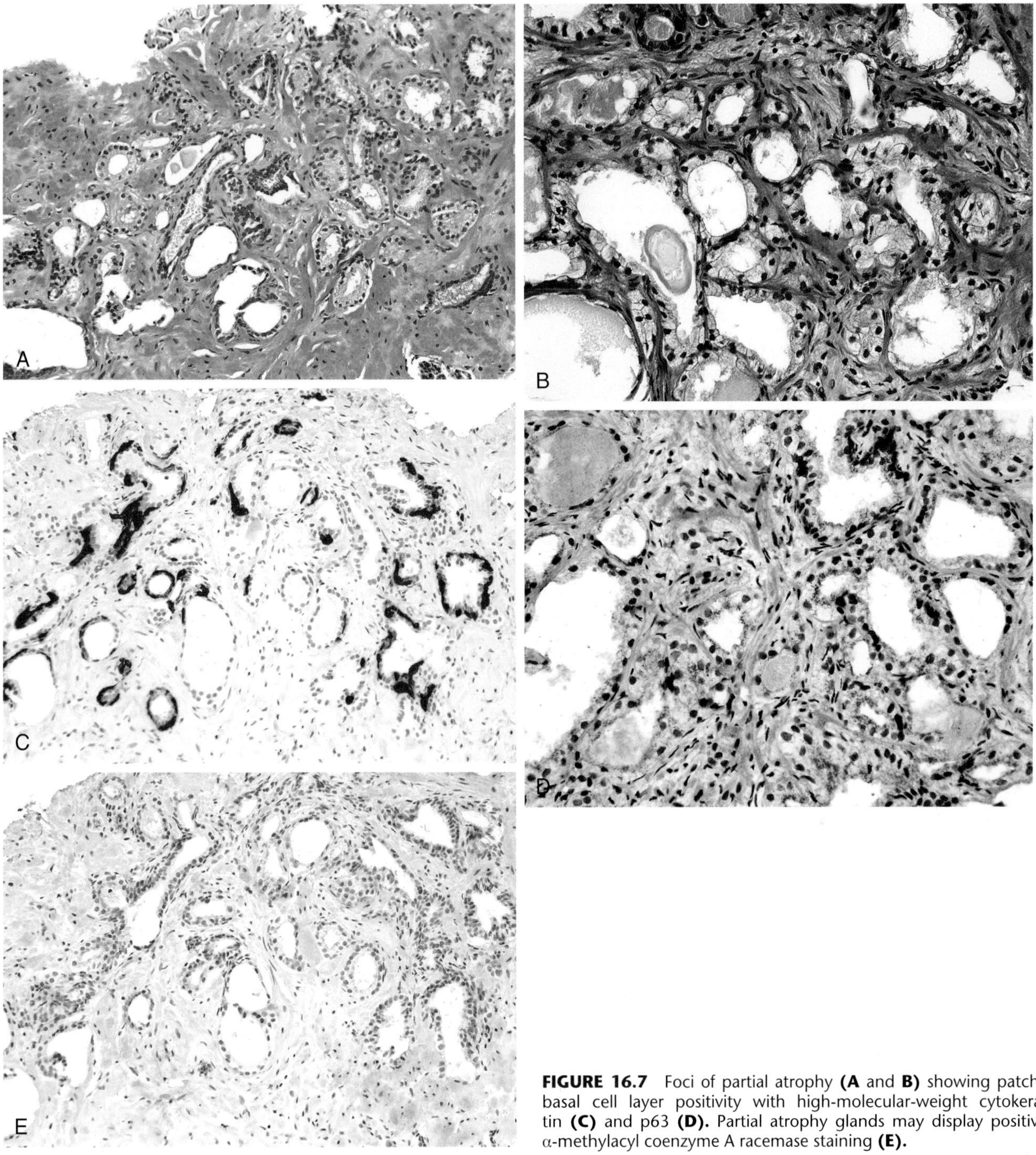

FIGURE 16.7 Foci of partial atrophy **(A** and **B)** showing patchy basal cell layer positivity with high-molecular-weight cytokeratin **(C)** and p63 **(D).** Partial atrophy glands may display positive α-methylacyl coenzyme A racemase staining **(E).**

Sclerosing Adenosis

Sclerosing adenosis is a rare lesion that is mainly encountered in TURP specimens performed for urinary obstruction. Rarely, it may also be sampled on needle biopsy leading to potential overdiagnosis as PCa. Sclerosing adenosis is composed of a relatively well circumscribed proliferation of well-formed glands admixed with single epithelial cells set in a background of dense spindle cell proliferation. The glandular structures are similar to those seen in adenosis. Some glands are surrounded by a distinct eosinophilic hyaline sheathlike collarette. The lining epithelial cells usually lack atypia. Basal cell layer can be appreciated on H&E. Establishing the diagnosis of sclerosing adenosis in examples demonstrating atypical features such as presence of crystalloids, mitotic figures, and prominent nucleoli requires the aid of immunostains. Basal cells and spindle cells are unique in their true myoepithelial differentiation as indicated by coexpression of keratin and muscle-specific actin (Fig. 16.10). The latter is not expressed by basal cells in normal prostate glands.[77-80]

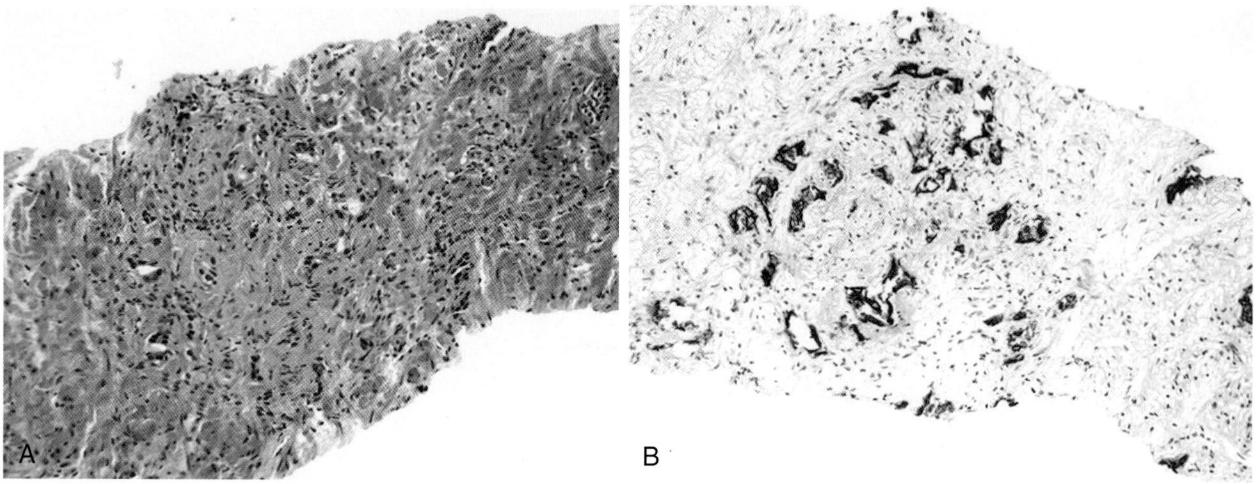

FIGURE 16.8 A focus of prostatic postatrophic hyperplasia **(A)** showing a continuous basal cell layer on high-molecular-weight cytokeratin immunostain **(B).**

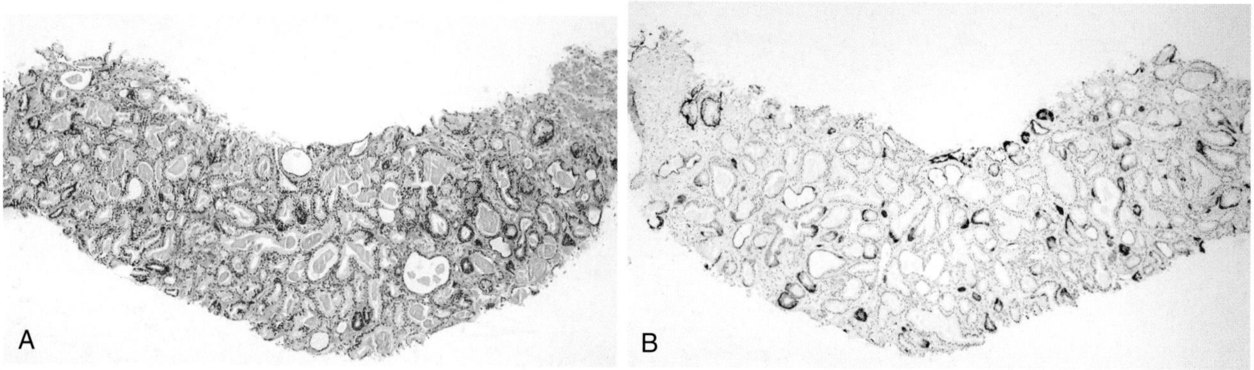

FIGURE 16.9 Prostate gland with a focus of adenosis **(A)** showing patchy staining of basal cells using high-molecular-weight cytokeratin **(B).**

KEY DIAGNOSTIC POINTS

Atrophy, Adenosis, and Sclerosing Adenosis

- Atrophy, adenosis, and sclerosing adenosis may mimic PCa, and basal marker immunostains p63 and 34βE12 may aid in the diagnosis.
- Adenosis and sclerosing adenosis are most commonly seen in transurethral resection of the prostate specimens.

Xanthoma

Prostatic xanthomas are rare but could be potentially misleading lesions in small and distorted needle tissue fragments. Typical low microscopic appearance is that of a small well-circumscribed solid nodule. Examples architecturally set as infiltrative cords and individual cells are more troubling. Xanthoma cells have a uniform appearance and contain abundant foamy cytoplasm and bland nuclei without prominent nucleoli (Fig. 16.11). Mitotic activity is usually lacking.[81] However, mitotic figures are also rare in PCa. Immunostains should be obtained if the possibility of xanthoma is morphologically entertained. Expression of histiocytic markers such as CD68 and lack of cytokeratin (CAM 5.2) staining is supportive of the diagnosis.[82,83]

POST-THERAPY CHANGES IN PROSTATE ADENOCARCINOMA

Antiandrogen Therapy

Currently, luteinizing hormone-releasing hormone (LHRH) agonist (Lupron), typically in association with the antiandrogen flutamide, is the most commonly used form of hormonal therapy in PCa. Both benign and neoplastic prostatic tissue can be significantly altered with hormonal therapy.[84-89] Under hormone deprivation, neoplastic acini usually acquire atrophic appearance and can mimic benign atrophic glands owing to the relative lack of nuclear atypia and absence of prominent nucleoli. At times, treated PCa glands develop pyknotic nuclei with abundant xanthomatous cytoplasm and when present as scattered cells they will closely resemble foamy histiocytes (Fig. 16.12). Immunohistochemistry for prostate-specific antigen (PSA) or pancytokeratin can aid in the diagnosis of carcinoma. Like their untreated counterparts, prostate cancer cells following hormonal therapy demonstrate a lack of high-molecular-weight cytokeratin staining. Following hormonal therapy, there may be a decrease in immunoreactivity with prostate lineage markers such as PSA, P501S, PSMA, and PSAP. However, with the exception of tumors developing focal squamous differentiation, resulting in adenosquamous

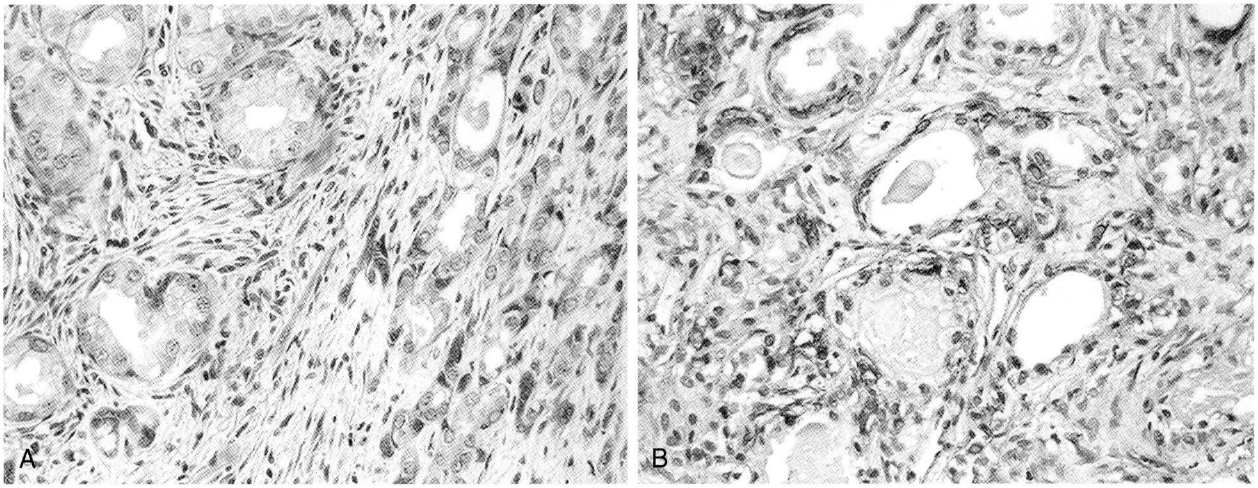

FIGURE 16.10 Sclerosing adenosis of the prostate gland **(A)** showing positive smooth muscle actin staining in myoepithelial cells **(B)**.

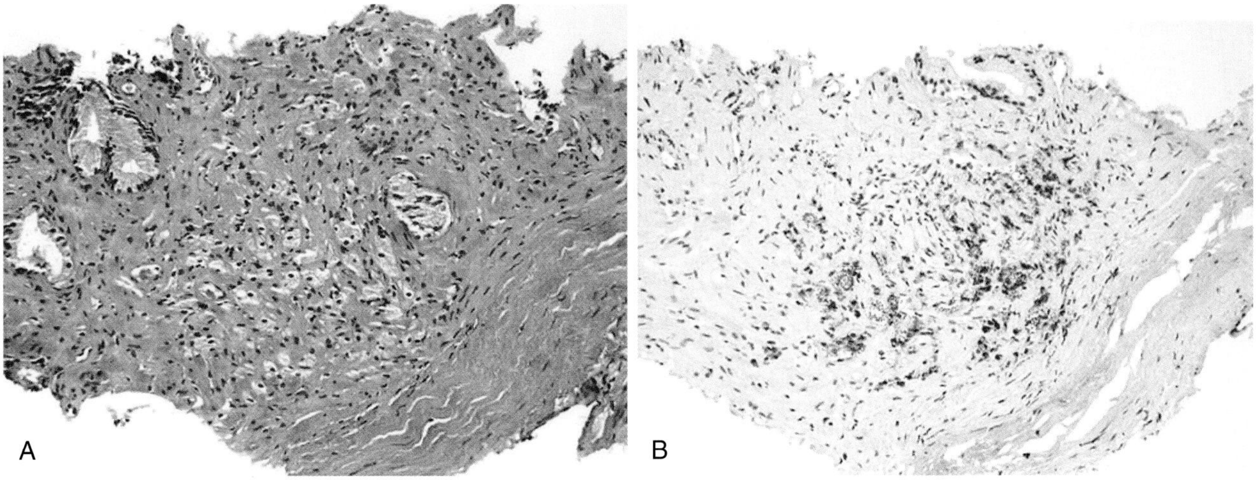

FIGURE 16.11 A focus of xanthoma involving prostate **(A)**. CD68 positivity is shown in **(B)**.

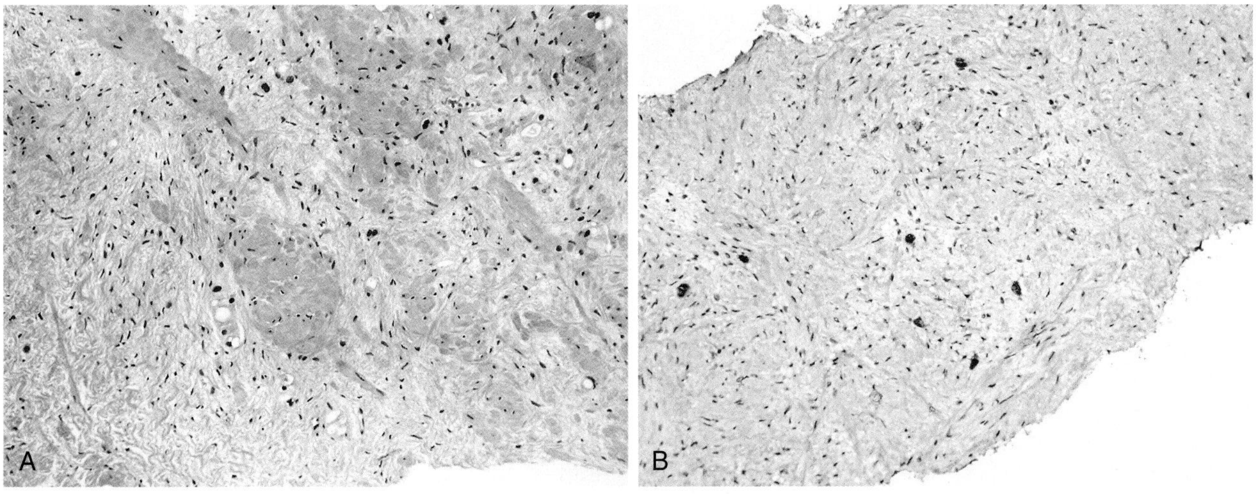

FIGURE 16.12 Prostate adenocarcinoma showing changes of prior hormonal therapy effect **(A)**. α-Methylacyl coenzyme A racemase (AMACR) staining highlights the scattered residual tumor cells lacking basal cell layer (**B,** Combo AMACR and CK 34βE12).

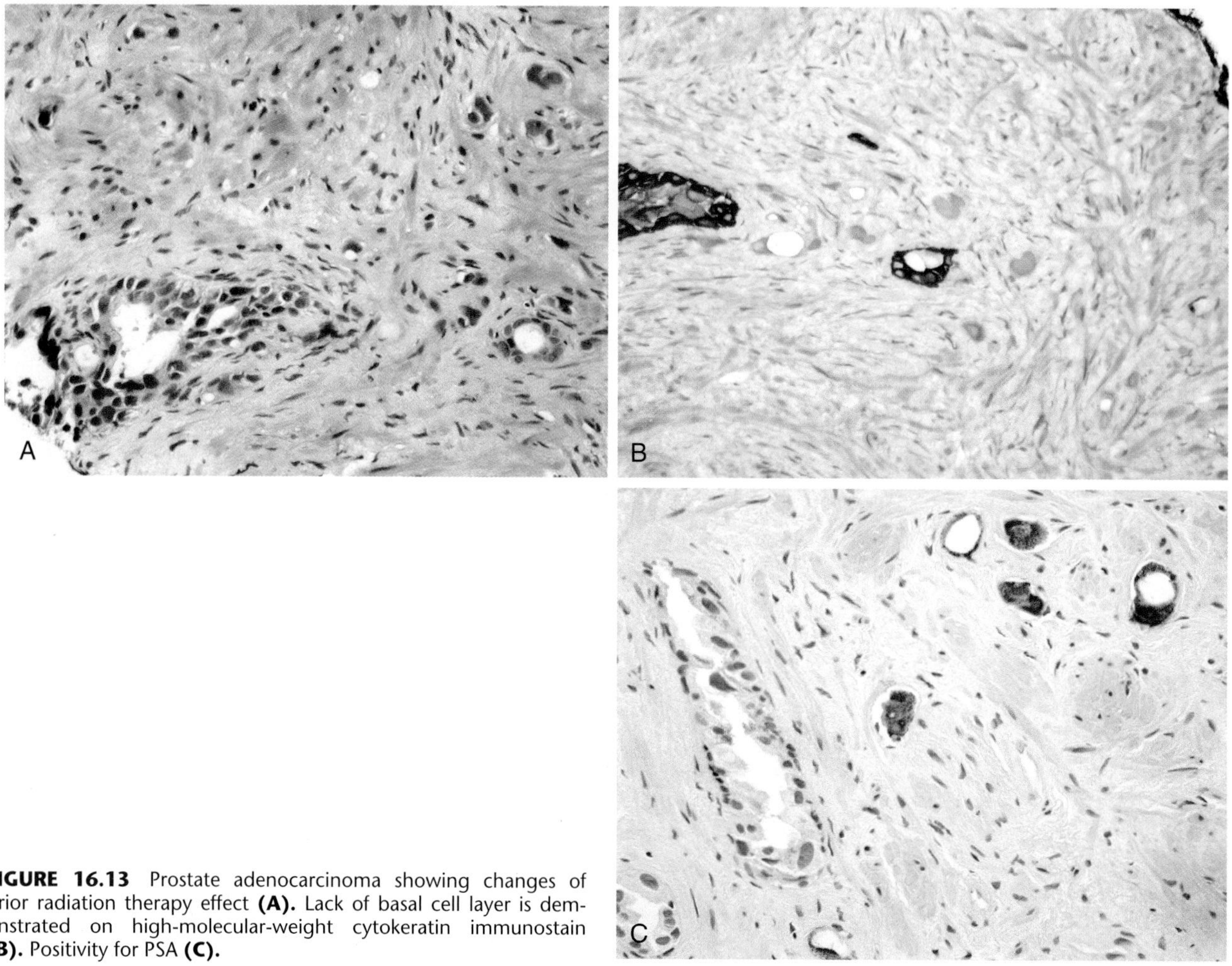

FIGURE 16.13 Prostate adenocarcinoma showing changes of prior radiation therapy effect **(A)**. Lack of basal cell layer is demonstrated on high-molecular-weight cytokeratin immunostain **(B)**. Positivity for PSA **(C)**.

carcinomas, most tumors will maintain at least focal labeling with these antibodies.[90-94] In our laboratory, we find that using a panel of three of the above markers (PSA, PSMA, and P501S) will increase the sensitivity for prostatic differentiation. Finally, it is worth remembering that squamous components of recurrent or metastatic hormone-independent prostatic adenosquamous carcinoma will only rarely and focally be positive for prostate lineage markers such as PSA, PSMA, P501S, and PSAP while diffusely expressing high-molecular-weight cytokeratin in these areas.[90-94]

Radiation Therapy

Besides surgery, external beam radiation and/or interstitial radiotherapy (brachytherapy) are two additional standard treatment options for localized prostate cancer with a curative intent.[95] Radiated non-neoplastic prostatic glands undergo glandular atrophy, squamous metaplasia, and cytologic atypia.[96] The marked epithelial atypia, especially following brachytherapy, tends to persist for several years.[97] The distinction between irradiated nonneoplastic prostatic glands and prostate carcinoma can be difficult, especially if the history of prior treatment is not provided and is not considered by the pathologist. On low magnification radiated benign prostate glands maintain their normal architectural lobular configuration. On higher magnification, there is piling up of the nuclei within irradiated benign glands with recognizable basal cell layer (Fig. 16.13). The finding of scattered markedly atypical nuclei with degenerative, hyperchromatic and smudgy appearance within well-formed acini is typical of radiated benign glands. In contrast, radiated glands of prostatic carcinoma are lined by a single cell layer with typical pyknotic nuclei and foamy cytoplasm. Prostate carcinomas that are sufficiently differentiated to form glands rarely manifest the degree of atypia seen with radiation. In difficult cases, HMWCK can aid in the diagnosis of irradiated prostate by identifying basal cells within benign radiated glands to prevent a false positive interpretation of carcinoma.[98-100]

Another scenario where radiation treatment can introduce diagnostic difficulty is when recurrent or residual prostate cancer displays marked and extensive radiation effect in the form of glands or individual cells with abundant vacuolated cytoplasm acquiring a histiocytic appearance. The nuclei lack apparent nucleoli and are pyknotic with smudged chromatin.[101] Pancytokeratin (AE1/AE3 and CAM5.2) and CD68 markers can be used to illustrate the epithelial nature of treated PCa. In most cases, treated PCa will retain their PSA and PSAP positivity,[101] as well as their expression of AMACR

(P504S).[99,100] However, as mentioned earlier, recurrent or metastatic radiated PCa displaying sarcomatoid, squamous, or adenosquamous phenotype may only focally be positive for prostate lineage markers while expressing HMWCK.[90-94] In evaluating postradiation clinical response, prostate biopsies are obtained 1 year following conclusion of treatment. Negative biopsies portend a good response. Less favorable prognosis is indicated by the presence of residual PCa displaying a typical radiation effect. Residual tumor without demonstrable radiation effect is considered a strong predictor of clinical failure. The expression of proliferation markers (MIB-1 or PCNA) in postradiated cancer has also been shown to correlate with clinical failure.[101,102]

KEY DIAGNOSTIC POINTS

Post-hormonal Therapy Histology

Prostate cancer cells following hormonal therapy demonstrate a lack of high-molecular-weight cytokeratin staining. Following hormonal therapy, there may be a decrease in immunoreactivity with prostate lineage markers such as PSA, P501S, PSMA, and PSAP.

PROSTATIC DUCT CARCINOMA

Less than 1% (0.4% to 0.8%) of prostate cancers show distinctive tall columnar cells in papillary or cribriform structures and are classified as prostatic duct adenocarcinomas.[103-105] Prostatic duct adenocarcinoma can be encountered as a single pattern of tumor differentiation or more frequently found admixed with "usual" acinar differentiation. Prostatic duct adenocarcinomas show a variety of architectural patterns including a papillary exophytic architecture, seen in periurethral location, lined by tall pseudostratified epithelial cells and a cribriform pattern more commonly seen deeper within the tissue formed by back-to-back large glands with slitlike lumen. It is not uncommon to find areas of papillary formation admixed with cribriform patterns. An important point is that ductal adenocarcinomas, as they arise in ducts, may show residual staining for high-molecular-weight cytokeratin staining and p63 (Fig. 16.14).

Prostatic duct adenocarcinomas can invade as single glands lined by tall columnar cells, unlike the cuboidal cells that characterize acinar prostatic carcinoma. The single infiltrating glands of prostatic duct adenocarcinoma may resemble infiltrating colonic adenocarcinoma. The differentiation between prostatic duct adenocarcinoma and secondary involvement of the prostate by colonic adenocarcinoma is usually made by finding more typical prostatic duct adenocarcinoma elsewhere in the biopsy. Rarely in such settings, immunohistochemical demonstration of PSA (or other prostate lineage markers such as P501S) is necessary to identify a prostatic duct adenocarcinoma. Adding β-catenin, CDX2, and villin (all positive in colon cancer) to the immunohistochemistry panel can be of further utility in such a differential.[106,107] Prostatic duct adenocarcinoma on transurethral resection specimens can also mimic papillary urothelial carcinoma. Nuclear features can be helpful in such a differential; nuclei in urothelial carcinoma tend to be more pleomorphic and angulated.[108] PSA and PSAP positivity and negative reactivity for thrombomodulin and uroplakin in prostatic duct adenocarcinoma can be useful.[106,109,110]

NEUROENDOCRINE PROSTATIC NEOPLASMS

It is somewhat controversial whether neuroendocrine differentiation in typical adenocarcinomas worsens prognosis.[111-113] Three studies evaluated the prognostic role of neuroendocrine differentiation in clinically organ-confined prostate adenocarcinoma. No prognostic role was found in the first study, whereas the subsequent larger two, including ours, found only a marginal prognostic role that was not sufficient to be useful clinically.[114-116] In the single study analyzing neuroendocrine differentiation in prostate cancer on needle biopsy, there was no relationship with prognosis.[117] According to the CAP Consensus Statement 1999,[118] neuroendocrine differentiation is still considered a category III prognostic factor not sufficiently studied to demonstrate its prognostic value.

As in other organs, the spectrum of neuroendocrine neoplasms in the prostate include carcinoid tumors, small cell carcinoma, and large cell neuroendocrine carcinoma as defined in the lung by Travis and colleagues.[119]

True carcinoid tumors of the prostate are extremely rare. Recently a total of three such cases have been reported with documented negative immunoreactivity for PSA and PSAP and otherwise typical carcinoid tumor morphology and immunoprofile.[120-122] All three patients presented with normal serum PSA levels and lacked clinical features of carcinoid syndrome.

Several additional cases have been reported where at least focal "carcinoid-like" appearance has been present.[123,124] None of these patients had carcinoid syndrome and all such cases have been positive with antibodies for PSA and PSAP. They have clinically behaved like ordinary prostate carcinomas. A more appropriate designation for these lesions would be "prostatic adenocarcinomas with neuroendocrine differentiation."

The basis for a diagnosis of small cell carcinoma of the prostate is the presence of morphologic features similar to those found in small cell carcinomas of the lung as defined in the 1999 WHO classification criteria.[125-127] In approximately 50% of the cases, the tumors are mixed small cell carcinoma and adenocarcinoma of the prostate. As with other unusual subtypes of prostate cancer, we do not assign a Gleason score to small cell carcinoma, but only to the conventional adenocarcinoma component. Immunohistochemically, the small cell component is positive for one or more neuroendocrine markers (NSE, synaptophysin, chromogranin, CD56) and negative for markers of prostatic differentiation such as PSA, PSMA, P501S, and PSAP. A minority of small cell carcinomas is positive for prostatic markers to varying degrees and may be negative for neuroendocrine markers. In a recent study by Yao and colleagues, strong chromogranin and synaptophysin positivity was present in 61% and 89%,

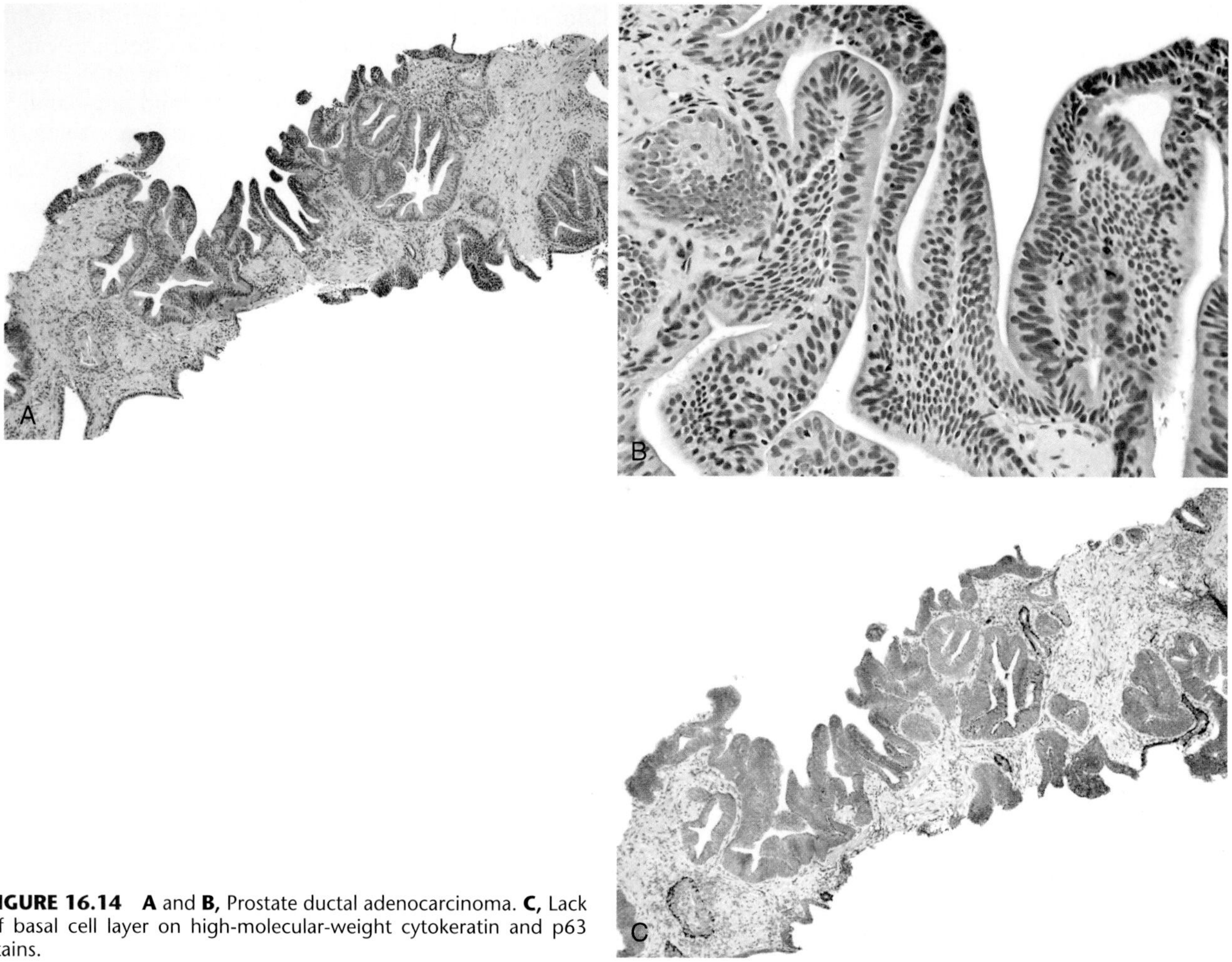

FIGURE 16.14 **A** and **B,** Prostate ductal adenocarcinoma. **C,** Lack of basal cell layer on high-molecular-weight cytokeratin and p63 stains.

respectively, of prostatic small cell carcinoma studied.[127] PSA and PSAP were positive in 17% and 24% of cases, respectively. In 24% and 35% of their cases, positivity was noted for p63 and high-molecular-weight cytokeratin, markers typically negative in prostatic carcinoma, yet expressed in normal basal cells of the prostate. In our recent (and largest) study on small cell carcinoma of the prostate,[40] we found most (88%) small cell carcinoma to be positive for at least one neuroendocrine marker. We also found P501S and prostate-specific membrane antigen were better in identifying the prostatic origin of small cell carcinoma than PSA, although the majority (60%) of prostatic small cell carcinomas were still negative for all three markers (Fig. 16.15). The latter, together with the previously cited heterogeneity of prostatic small cell carcinoma immunophenotype, is consistent with an origin from multipotential transient amplifying cells closely related to stem cells.[127-129]

Ordonez and colleagues[130] originally reported that thyroid transcription factor-1 (TTF-1) was positive in 96% of small cell carcinomas of the lung and negative in all three prostate small cell cancers. Subsequent studies, including ours, demonstrated TTF-1 expression in the majority of small cell carcinoma of prostate, limiting its utility in distinguishing primary small cell carcinoma of the prostate from a metastasis from the lung.[40,127,131]

Small cell carcinoma of the prostate continues to effect a dismal outcome with an average survival of less than a year. There is no difference in prognosis between patients with pure small cell carcinomas or mixed glandular and small cell carcinomas. Tumor immunoprofile does not affect survival. A review by Mackey and colleagues[132] concluded that hormonal manipulation and systemic chemotherapy had little effect on the natural history of prostate small cell carcinoma. Others suggest treatment of small cell carcinoma of the prostate with the same combination chemotherapy used to treat small cell carcinomas in other sites.[133,134] It remains to be seen whether new targeted therapy strategies that are currently under investigation in small cell carcinoma of lung may be applicable to small cell carcinoma of prostate-expressing targets such as c-*kit*, bcl-2, and CD56.

Large cell neuroendocrine carcinoma (LCNEC) of prostate is an extremely rare occurrence. In the largest series on the topic by Evans and colleagues,[135] only one of seven cases was a *de novo* LCNEC with the remaining six representing progression from prior acinar adenocarcinoma following a long-standing hormonal therapy. LCNECs are composed of sheets and ribbons of amphophilic cells with large nuclei, coarse chromatin, and prominent nucleoli. Mitotic activity is brisk and foci of necrosis are common. A minor (<10%) component

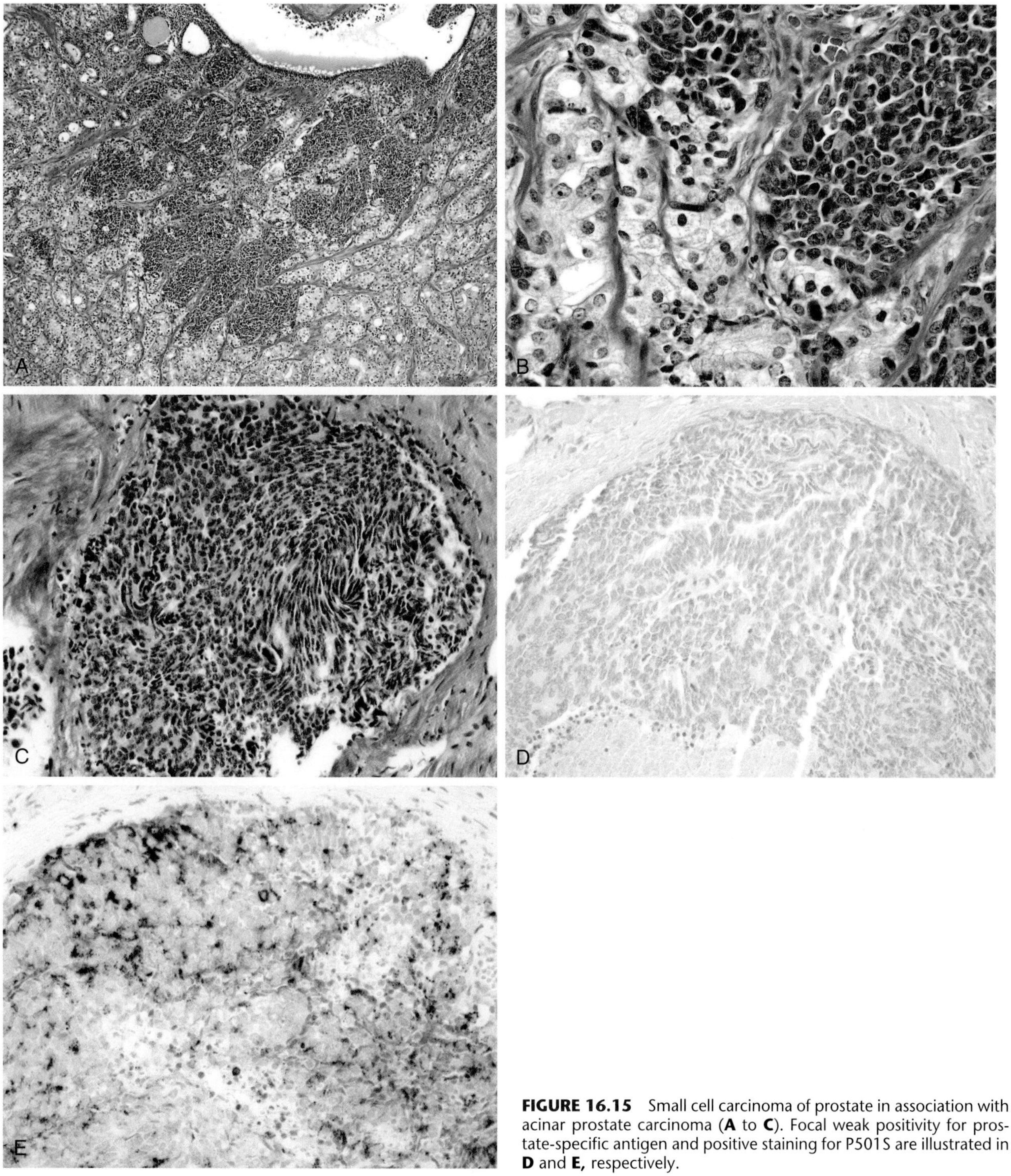

FIGURE 16.15 Small cell carcinoma of prostate in association with acinar prostate carcinoma (**A** to **C**). Focal weak positivity for prostate-specific antigen and positive staining for P501S are illustrated in **D** and **E,** respectively.

of conventional prostate adenocarcinoma showing hormonal deprivation effect was identified in all but the single *de novo* case. The LCNEC component was strongly positive for CD56, CD57, chromogranin A, synaptophysin, and P504S. PSA and PSAP expression was present in the conventional component but was focal or absent in the LCNEC areas. All six patients with available follow-up died with a mean survival of 7 months.

UROTHELIAL CARCINOMA INVOLVING PROSTATE AND PROSTATIC URETHRA

Prostatic involvement by urothelial carcinoma can result from direct invasion of an infiltrating bladder cancer into prostate stroma, as well as through extension of urothelial tumor through intraductal route with or without subsequent stromal invasion of the prostate.[136,137]

In the first scenario (direct bladder wall to prostate invasion) the prognosis of the urothelial carcinoma of the bladder is equivalent in survival to cases of bladder carcinoma with regional lymph node metastases. A common diagnostic problem in this setting is differentiating, in a TURP, between a poorly differentiated urothelial carcinoma of the bladder and a poorly differentiated prostatic adenocarcinoma. Because therapy differs significantly, the distinction between these two entities is crucial. Even in poorly differentiated prostatic carcinomas, there is typically relatively little pleomorphism or mitotic activity compared with poorly differentiated urothelial carcinoma. A subtler finding is that the cytoplasm of prostatic adenocarcinoma is often foamy and pale, imparting a "soft" appearance.

In contrast, urothelial carcinomas may demonstrate hard, glassy eosinophilic cytoplasm or more prominent squamous differentiation. The findings of infiltrating cords of cells or focal cribriform glandular differentiation are other features more typical of prostatic adenocarcinoma. Although the distinction between urothelial carcinoma and prostatic adenocarcinoma on H&E stained sections is valid for almost all cases, we have seen rare cases where prostate adenocarcinoma has had marked pleomorphism identical to urothelial carcinoma. Consequently, in a poorly differentiated tumor involving the bladder and prostate without any glandular differentiation typical of prostate adenocarcinoma, the case should be worked up immunohistochemically given the high stakes of a misdiagnosis. Approximately 95% of poorly differentiated prostatic adenocarcinomas show PSA and PSAP staining, although it may be focal.[138-140] Although some authors demonstrated a superiority of PSA over PSAP in staining prostatic carcinoma, others found poorly differentiated prostatic carcinomas that lacked PSA staining still maintained immunoreactivity to PSAP.[140-142] In our laboratory, PSA has in general been more sensitive. Monoclonal antibodies to PSAP have lower sensitivities than their polyclonal counterparts but are more specific.[143] We have compared PSA staining in a group of poorly differentiated prostatic adenocarcinomas with "poor" PSA staining to newer prostate specific markers including prostate specific membrane antigen (PSMA), P501S (Prostein), and NKX 3.1 (Fig. 16.16).[13] Completely negative staining was seen in 15% (PSA), 12% (PSMA), 17% (P501S), and 5% (NKX 3.1) of the cases. Five percent of the cases were negative for all four markers combined. A similar 5% rate of "false negativity" is found when combining PSA and PSAP stains.[144] Therefore the lack of immunoreactivity to prostate-specific markers in a poorly differentiated tumor within the prostate, especially in small samples, does not exclude the diagnosis of a poorly differentiated prostatic adenocarcinoma. With only a few exceptions, immunoperoxidase staining for PSA and PSAP is specific for prostatic tissue. Situations that can cause diagnostic difficulty include PSA and PSAP within periurethral glands, as well as cystitis cystica and cystitis glandularis in both men and women.[145-147] Other examples of cross-reactive staining include anal glands in men (PSA, PSAP) and urachal remnants (PSA).[148,149] Some intestinal carcinoids and pancreatic islet cell tumors are strongly reactive with antibodies to PSAP yet negative with antibodies to PSA.[150] Periurethral gland carcinomas in women and various salivary gland tumors may also be PSA and PSAP positive.[151,152] Although adenocarcinomas of the bladder, whether as a pure tumor or with mixed urothelial carcinoma, have also been reported to be positive for PSA or PSAP, there has yet to be a case reported positive for both.[153,154] In a poorly differentiated tumor occurring in the bladder and the prostate where the differential diagnosis is between high-grade prostatic adenocarcinoma and urothelial carcinoma, focal strong staining for either marker can be used reliably to make the diagnosis of prostatic adenocarcinoma because PSAP and PSA false positivity have not been convincingly described in urothelial carcinomas.[155,156] In general, various cytokeratins (CK7, CK20, high-molecular-weight cytokeratin) show strong positivity in cases of urothelial carcinoma involving the prostate. Although CK7 and CK20 are more frequently seen in urothelial carcinoma as compared with adenocarcinoma of the prostate, they may also be positive in adenocarcinoma of the prostate, such that in our experience they are not that helpful in this differential diagnosis.[144,157] We and others have found high-molecular-weight cytokeratin to be positive in more than 90% of urothelial carcinomas.[13,158] In contrast, high-molecular-weight cytokeratin is only rarely (8%) expressed, and usually in a small percentage of cells, in adenocarcinoma of the prostate.[13] p63 is another useful marker in differentiating high-grade urothelial carcinoma from prostatic adenocarcinoma. Using tissue microarrays, we found p63 to have a greater specificity, albeit lower sensitivity, for urothelial carcinoma compared with high-molecular-weight cytokeratin (100% specificity and 83% sensitivity) (Fig. 16.17).[13] Other markers that also appear highly specific but only of modest sensitivity for urothelial carcinoma include uroplakin and thrombomodulin (49% to 69% sensitivity).

Currently, biopsies of the prostatic urethra are recommended as a staging procedure in patients undergoing intravesical treatment for superficial bladder tumors. If intraductal urothelial carcinoma is identified on TURP or transurethral biopsy, patients will usually be recommended for radical cystoprostatectomy. The finding of intraductal urothelial carcinoma has also been demonstrated to increase the risk of urethral recurrence following cystoprostatectomy, such that its identification may also result in prophylactic total urethrectomy. Immunohistochemical stains for basal cells (high-molecular-weight cytokeratin, p63) may in some cases only outline the prostatic basal cells and in other cases label the intraductal urothelial carcinoma.

The diagnosis of urothelial carcinoma on prostate needle biopsy is especially difficult. Urothelial carcinoma involving the prostate clinically can mimic prostatic adenocarcinoma in terms of findings on digital rectal examination and ultrasound, along with the potential for an elevated serum PSA level.[159] Histologic features and immunohistochemical studies are therefore essential to establish the correct diagnosis. Urothelial carcinoma

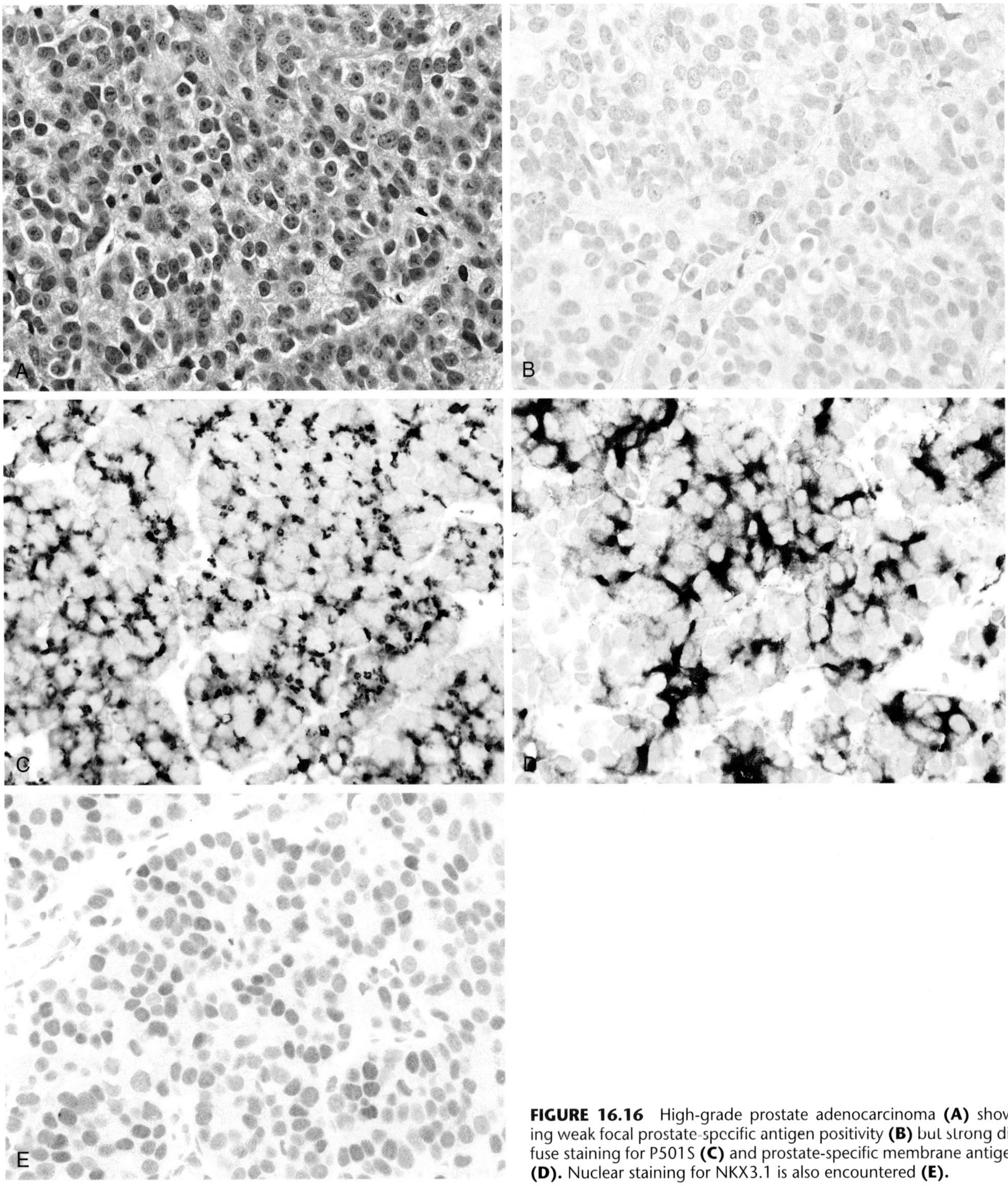

FIGURE 16.16 High-grade prostate adenocarcinoma **(A)** showing weak focal prostate-specific antigen positivity **(B)** but strong diffuse staining for P501S **(C)** and prostate-specific membrane antigen **(D)**. Nuclear staining for NKX3.1 is also encountered **(E)**.

involving the prostate differs from adenocarcinoma of the prostate both architecturally and cytologically. Urothelial carcinoma in the prostate typically forms nests of tumor, whereas poorly differentiated prostate cancer tends to form sheets, individual cells, or cords. Urothelial carcinoma involving the prostate in our study contained areas of necrosis in 43% of cases. Necrosis is an unusual finding in even high-grade adenocarcinoma of the prostate. The presence of an intraductal growth where preexisting benign prostate glands are filled with solid nests of tumor also differs from high-grade prostatic intraepithelial neoplasia, which is composed of flat, tufting, papillary, or cribriform patterns. The presence of squamous differentiation seen in 14% of our cases would also be unusual for adenocarcinoma of the prostate. Cytologically, urothelial carcinomas involving the prostate tend to show greater nuclear pleomorphism, variably prominent nucleoli, and increased mitotic

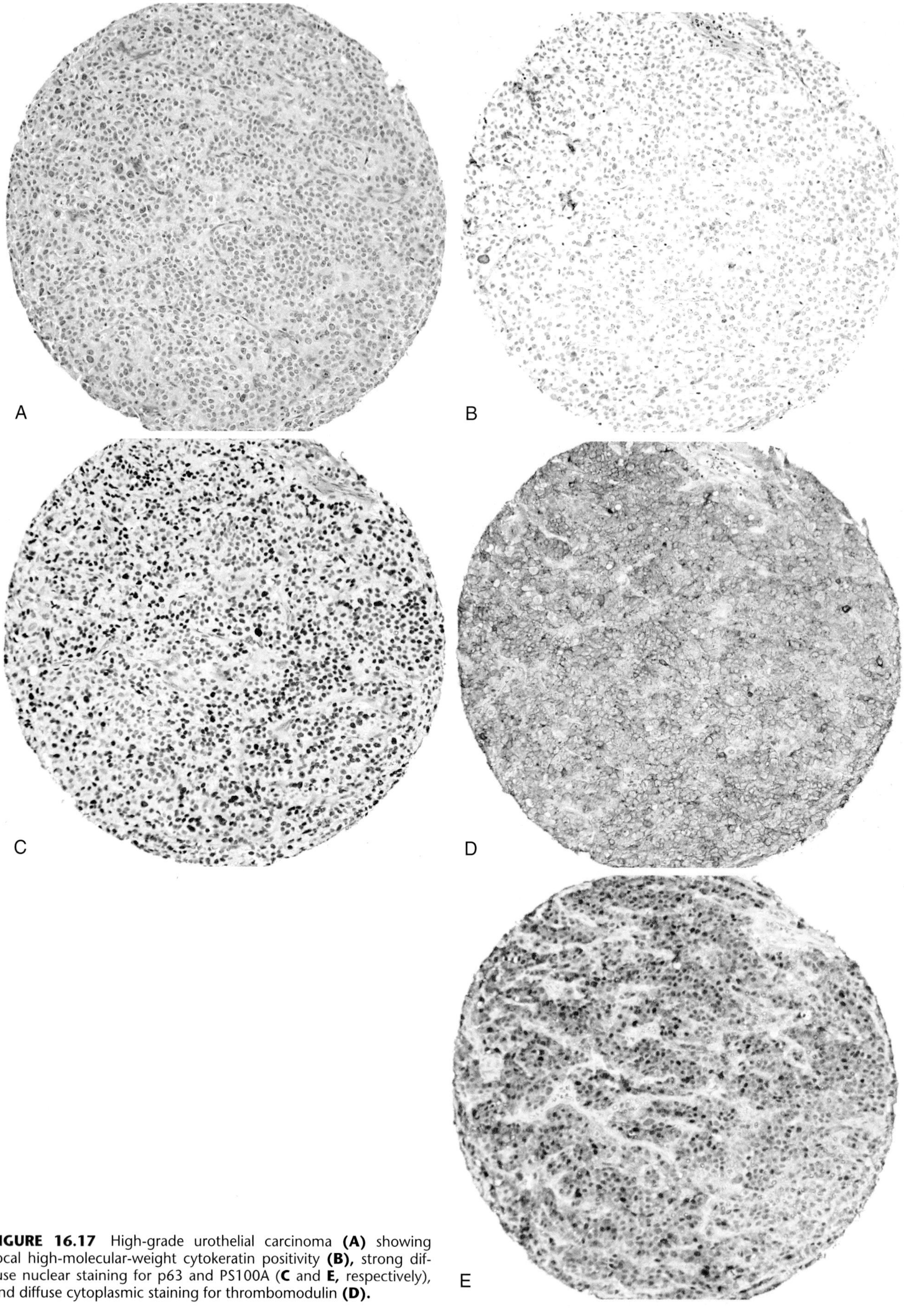

FIGURE 16.17 High-grade urothelial carcinoma **(A)** showing focal high-molecular-weight cytokeratin positivity **(B),** strong diffuse nuclear staining for p63 and PS100A (**C** and **E,** respectively), and diffuse cytoplasmic staining for thrombomodulin **(D).**

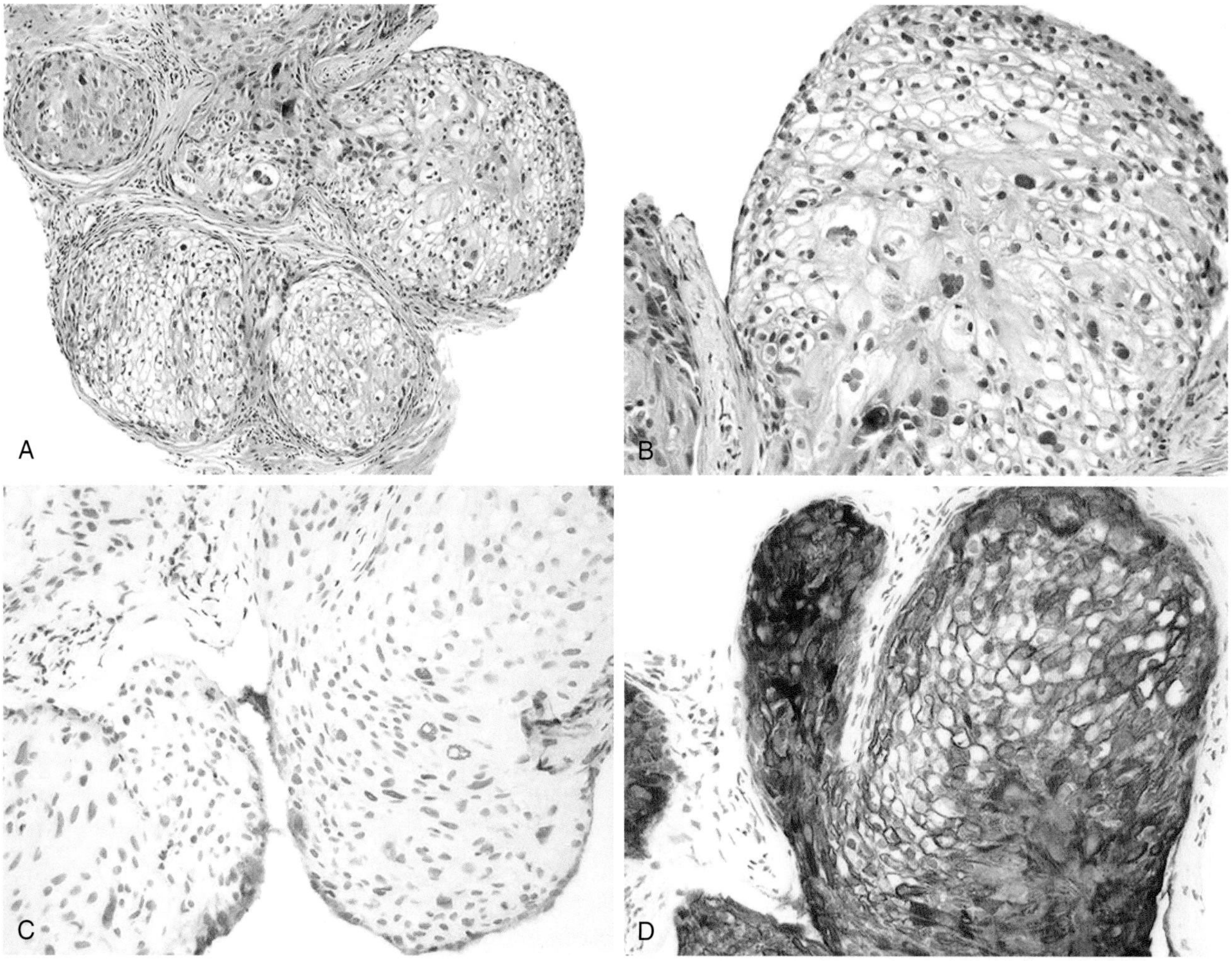

FIGURE 16.18 Intraductal spread of urothelial carcinoma involving prostate gland (**A** and **B**). Urothelial carcinoma undermines secretory prostate epithelial layer as shown on prostate-specific antigen stains **(C)**. The urothelial carcinoma cells react positively with high-molecular-weight cytokeratin **(D)**.

activity compared with even poorly differentiated prostate adenocarcinoma. In high-grade adenocarcinomas of the prostate, nuclei tend to be more uniform from one to another with centrally located prominent eosinophilic nucleoli. Mitotic figures in high-grade prostate cancer are typically not as frequent compared with what is seen in urothelial carcinoma on biopsy. Finally, the presence of stromal inflammation, seen in 76% of our cases of urothelial carcinoma on biopsy, differs from the typical lack of associated inflammation seen with ordinary adenocarcinoma of the prostate (Fig. 16.18).

KEY DIAGNOSTIC POINTS

Prostate Carcinoma versus Urothelial Carcinoma in Prostate

- Distinction is crucial for appropriate therapy.
- Presence of cellular/nuclear pleomorphism, necrosis, squamous differentiation, and intraductal sheet pattern of growth with HMWCK/p63 immunostaining all strongly support urothelial carcinoma.

SECONDARY INVOLVEMENT OF PROSTATE BY COLORECTAL ADENOCARCINOMA

Another source of secondary tumor extension into prostate is the topographically adjacent colorectal tract. Here again, attention to some characteristic morphologic features should raise the possibility of a secondary spread. The presence of goblet/columnar cell differentiation, pseudostratified basally located nuclei, and characteristic "dirty necrosis" is more likely encountered in colorectal carcinoma (CRCa).[106,107,160] One should be cautioned that single infiltrating glands of prostatic duct adenocarcinoma can resemble infiltrating colonic adenocarcinoma. The differentiation between prostatic duct adenocarcinoma and secondary involvement of the prostate by CRCa can be assisted by finding more typical prostatic duct adenocarcinoma elsewhere within the biopsy. An immunohistochemical profile of positive nuclear CDX2 staining, positive nuclear (cytoplasmic staining can occur in PCa) β-catenin and positive staining for CK20 in the face of negative reactivity for PSA, PSMA, and P501S can be used to confirm the diagnosis of CRCa spread.[106,107,160]

TABLE 16.4 Immunohistochemistry of Prostatic Mesenchymal Lesions

	STUMP	SS	Leiomyosarcoma	Rhabdomyosarcoma	IMT	SFT	GIST
CD34	+	+	N	N	N	+	+
SMA	S	N	+	+	+	N	S
Desmin	S	N	+	+	+	N	S
Myogenin	N	N	N	+	N	N	N
c-*kit*	N	N	N	N	S	N	+
ALK-1	N	N	N	N	+	N	N
PR	+	+	S	N	N	S	N

GIST, gastrointestinal stromal tumor; IMT, inflammatory myofibroblastic tumor; N, negative; PR, progesterone receptor; S, sometimes positive; SFT, solitary fibrous tumor; SMA, smooth muscle actin; SS, stromal sarcoma; +, almost always positive.

PROSTATIC MESENCHYMAL TUMORS

As in any other organ, immunostains can be of great utility in resolving a variety of spindle cell mesenchymal lesions occurring in the prostate including benign and malignant smooth muscle neoplasms, peripheral nerve sheath tumors, and rhabdomyosarcoma (Table 16.4).[161,162]

Here we focus our discussion on four lesions that pose a unique differential challenge when encountered in a prostatic biopsy.

Stromal Tumors of Uncertain Malignant Potential and Stromal Sarcomas

Stromal tumors of uncertain malignant potential (STUMPs) are rare but distinct tumors of the specialized prostatic stroma as currently recognized in the 2004 World Health Organization Classification of Tumors of the Urinary System and Male Genital Organs.[163] STUMPs present most commonly with lower urinary tract obstruction, abnormal digital rectal examination, hematuria, hematospermia, palpable rectal mass, or elevated serum PSA levels.[164-166] On gross examination, STUMPs appear as white-tan solid or solid cystic nodules ranging in size from microscopic lesions to large, cystic lesions up to 15 cm in size.

Microscopically, STUMPs present with diverse histologic patterns. Four histologic patterns of STUMP have been described: (1) hypercellular stroma containing scattered atypical degenerative appearing cells; (2) hypercellular stroma consisting of bland fusiform stromal cells with eosinophilic cytoplasm; (3) leaflike hypocellular fibrous stroma covered by benign-appearing prostatic epithelium similar in morphology to a benign phyllodes tumor of the breast; and (4) myxoid stroma containing bland stromal cells and often lacking admixed glands. Some cases exhibit a mixture of these patterns. Immunostains demonstrating STUMPs are positive for CD34 and vimentin and variably positive for smooth muscle actin and desmin (Table 16.4). Not surprisingly, given their presumed derivation from the prostatic stroma, progesterone receptor is frequently found on immunostaining, although estrogen receptor is less commonly positive. C-*kit* and S-100 have been negative in all cases examined, a feature of value in distinguishing STUMP from other spindle cell tumors such as solitary fibrous tumor (SFT) and schwannoma.

Although STUMPs are generally considered to represent a benign neoplastic stromal process, a subset of STUMPs has been associated with stromal sarcoma on a synchronous or metasynchronous biopsy, suggesting a malignant progression in at least some cases.[164] No correlation between the pattern of STUMP and association with stromal sarcoma is apparent.

Stromal sarcoma may arise *de novo* or may exist in association with either a preexisting or concurrent STUMP. Stromal sarcomas either demonstrate a solid growth with storiform, epithelioid, fibrosarcomatous, or patternless patterns or may infiltrate between benign prostatic glands. Less commonly, stromal sarcomas may demonstrate leaflike glands with underlying hypercellular stroma, which are also termed *malignant phyllodes tumors*. Stromal sarcomas have one or more of the following features within the spindle cell component: hypercellularity, cytological atypia, mitotic figures, and necrosis. Stromal sarcomas can be further subclassified into low- and high-grade lesions with high-grade tumors showing moderate to marked pleomorphism and hypercellularity often with increased mitotic activity and occasional necrosis. Immunohistochemical findings in stromal sarcomas are similar to those of STUMPs, with strong vimentin reactivity and positivity for CD34 and progesterone receptor. In a subset of cases studied, pancytokeratin and CAM5.2 stains were negative. Stromal sarcomas can extend out of the prostate and metastasize to distant sites such as bone, lung, abdomen, and retroperitoneum.

The variability of STUMPs' clinical behavior and their occasional association or progression to stromal sarcomas make for a challenging patient management plan. STUMPs warrant close follow-up and consideration of definitive resection in younger individuals. Factors to consider in deciding whether to proceed with definitive resection for STUMPs diagnosed on biopsy include patient age and treatment preference, presence, and size of the lesion on rectal examination or imaging studies, and extent of the lesion on tissue sampling. Expectant management with close clinical follow-up could be considered in an older individual with a limited lesion on biopsy where there is no lesion identified on digital rectal examination or on imaging studies.

Smooth Muscle Neoplasms (Leiomyoma/ Leiomyosarcoma)

Leiomyomas contain well-organized fascicles and may demonstrate degenerative features such as hyalinization and calcification that are not commonly seen in stromal nodules, which are their main differential diagnosis. Large single leiomyomas that are symptomatic are rare.[167,168] Leiomyomas should demonstrate virtually no mitotic activity and minimal if any nuclear atypia, with the exception of occasional scattered degenerative nuclei.

Sarcomas of the prostate account for 0.1% to 0.2% of all malignant prostatic tumors. Leiomyosarcoma is the most common sarcoma of prostate. Lesions range in size from 3 to 21 cm. Microscopically, leiomyosarcomas are hypercellular lesions composed of intersecting bundles of spindled cells with moderate to severe atypia. The vast majority of leiomyosarcomas have been high grade with frequent mitoses and necrosis, although we have encountered a rare low-grade prostatic leiomyosarcoma.[169] Low-grade leiomyosarcomas are distinguished from leiomyomas by a moderate amount of atypia, focal areas of increased cellularity, scattered mitotic figures, and/or a focally infiltrative growth pattern around benign prostate glands at the perimeter. As opposed to some stromal sarcomas, leiomyosarcomas lack admixed normal glands, except entrapped glands at the periphery.

Immunohistochemically, leiomyosarcomas commonly express vimentin, actin, and desmin. Cytokeratin expression is observed in about one quarter of cases. In addition, some leiomyosarcomas have been reported to express progesterone receptor, similar to STUMPs and stromal sarcomas (Table 16.4).[170,171] Leiomyosarcomas have a poor clinical outcome characterized by multiple recurrences. Half to 75% of patients die of their disease within 2 to 5 years. In the study by Sexton and colleagues,[172] variables predictive of a favorable prognosis included presentation with metastasis and complete surgical resection. Optimal treatment requires a multimodal approach rather than surgery alone.

Solitary Fibrous Tumor

There are fewer than 20 reported cases of solitary fibrous tumors (SFTs) involving the prostate.[173] Some older reported cases of hemangiopericytoma of the prostate may also be classified as SFT today. Microscopically, prostatic SFTs appear similar to those identified in extraprostatic sites. Uniform spindled cells with bland nuclei are arranged in a "patternless" pattern in a background of variable ropy collagen and a hemangiopericytomatous appearance.[173] None of the reported prostatic SFTs have behaved in an aggressive fashion. However, on the basis of the behavior of SFTs in other sites and the finding in some prostatic SFTs of hypercellularity, pleomorphism, necrosis, and infiltrative margins, careful long-term clinical follow-up is warranted. Immunohistochemistry generally reveals diffuse reactivity for CD34, vimentin, and bcl-2, although rare SFTs may lack some of these markers (Fig. 16.19). Staining for CD99, β-catenin, p53, smooth muscle actin, and muscle-specific actin have also been reported. These tumors are typically negative for pancytokeratin, S-100, and CD117 (c-*kit*).

Gastrointestinal Stromal Tumors

Although gastrointestinal stromal tumor (GIST) lesions may present as a primary prostatic process on imaging and clinical studies, such cases are typically large masses arising from the rectum or perirectal space that only compress the prostate. Rarely, GISTs may invade the prostate. There is not yet a fully documented example of a GIST arising within the prostate.[174-176] Typically GISTs are not considered in the differential diagnosis of spindle cell lesions of the prostate, although the unique management of these tumors underscores the importance of recognizing them. Unfortunately, several patients have undergone pelvic exenteration, irradiation, and chemotherapy for a misdiagnosis of a GIST as a "pelvic sarcoma."[175] "Prostatic" GISTs present with urinary obstructive symptoms, rectal fullness, and abnormal digital rectal examination.[174-176] Microscopically, they show identical features to lesions within the gastrointestinal tract. GIST is composed of spindled cells with a fascicular growth pattern with occasional epithelioid features and focal dense collagenous stroma (Fig. 16.20). When present, a fascicular or palisading growth pattern and perinuclear vacuoles along with a lack of collagen deposition aids in the discrimination of GIST from SFT and STUMP. Tumors with malignant potential show elevated mitotic rates of greater than 5 per 50 HPF, cytologically malignant features (high cellularity and overlapping nuclei), and/or necrosis. Immunohistochemically, CD117/c-*kit* is uniformly expressed in all cases and CD34 is positive in almost all cases studied. S-100, desmin, and smooth muscle actin are negative. On prostate needle biopsy, before rendering a diagnosis of SFT, schwannoma, leiomyosarcoma, or stromal sarcoma, GIST should be considered in the differential diagnosis. Furthermore, immunostains for CD117 should be performed to verify the diagnosis. CD34 is not discriminatory as it is positive in GISTs, SFTs, and specialized prostatic stromal tumors, and variably positive in schwannomas. It is, however, typically negative in smooth muscle tumors. Strong positive staining for desmin can help discriminate smooth muscle tumors from the other lesions. Similarly, positive immunoreactivity to S-100 may aid in diagnosing neural tumors. Smooth muscle actin is typically expressed in smooth muscle tumors and is variably positive in STUMPs and GISTs and typically negative in SFT and schwannoma.

A subset of patients treated with the c-*kit* tyrosine kinase inhibitor imatinib (Gleevec) following the diagnosis of "prostatic" GIST has demonstrated a subsequent reduction in tumor size.[176]

Genomic and Theranostic Applications

Currently, prostate needle biopsy remains the gold standard for establishing the diagnosis of prostate carcinoma in patients with elevated serum PSA and/or

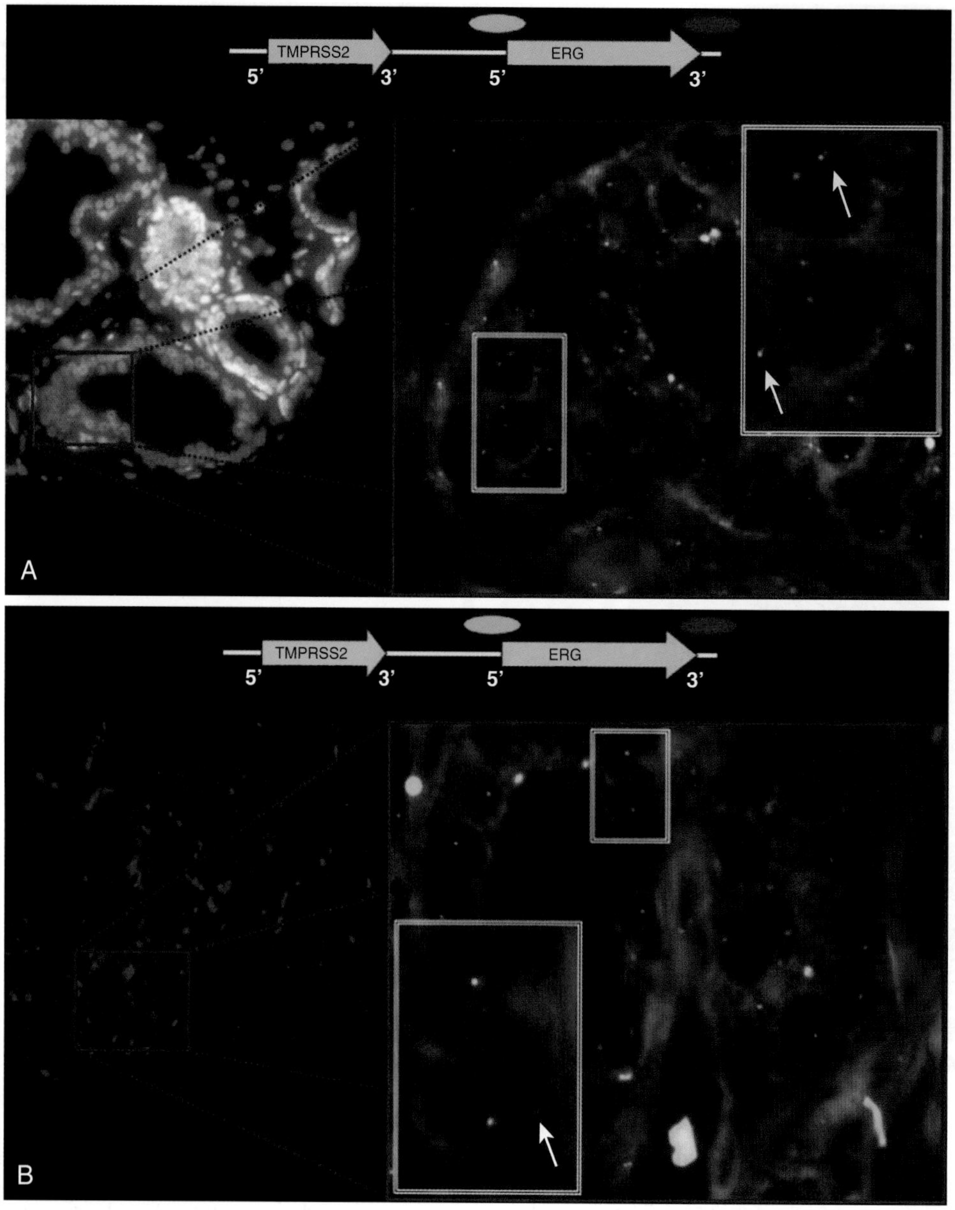

FIGURE 16.21 Fluorescence *in situ* hybridization analysis using ERG split-apart probes. The presence of juxtaposed red and green signals (occasionally forming a yellow signal) indicates lack of TMPRSS2-ERG fusion in the benign glands **(A).** Loss of green signal in one allele indicates the presence of TMPRSS2-ERG fusion by deletion involving the 5′ ERG region as shown in the malignant glands **(B).**

Ki-67 is one of multiple promising markers under study by an NCI-sponsored multi-institutional Inter-Prostate SPORE prospective validation study (including p27 and caveolin-1) that will assess the utility of this marker.

Angiogenesis

The mean number of microscopic blood vessels in tissue is higher in prostate cancer and prostatic intraepithelial neoplasia (PIN) than normal prostate tissue. In a study evaluating microvessel density (MVD) on needle biopsy the authors found MVD, when combined with Gleason score and preoperative PSA, provided improved ability to predict extraprostatic extension at radical prostatectomy.[204] Although microvessel density was significant in the multivariate analysis, Gleason score and serum PSA were much more powerful predictors of extraprostatic disease. Three additional studies revealed a prognostic role for MVD in prostatectomy specimens.[205-207] Others, however, failed to confirm such a role.[208-210] Differences in vascular antibodies used, as well as topography of vessel measurements, could account for the variable results. It appears that microvessel density will have a marginal adjunctive role if any to established current parameters.

Tumor Suppressor Genes and Oncogenes

Among tumor suppressor genes (TSGs), there is mounting evidence to support a role for p53 expression in predicting prognosis in prostate carcinoma. Brewster and colleagues[211] found p53 expression and Gleason score in needle biopsy to be independent predictors of biochemical relapse after radical prostatectomy. Another

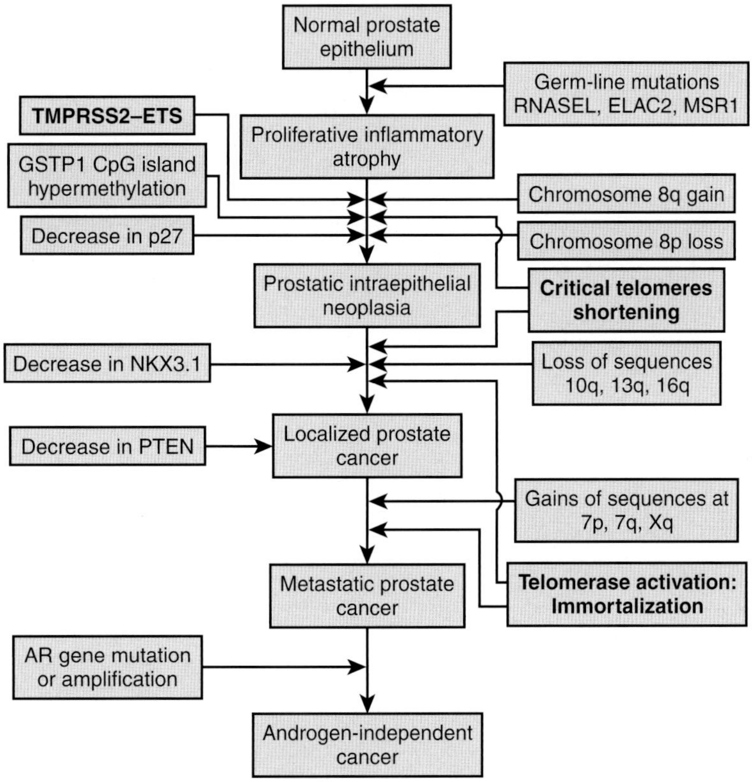

FIGURE 16.22 Somatic genetic alterations involved in the pathogenetic steps of prostate cancer progression.

study found p53 status on prostatectomy but not needle biopsies to be predictive, raising the issue of sampling.[212] Many studies evaluating prostatectomy specimens found p53 to be of prognostic significance independent of grade, stage, and margin status.[202,210,213-218] The results of these studies suggest that p53 evaluation could become a clinically used parameter, at least in prostatectomy specimens, once standardization of cutoffs and immunostaining methodologies are achieved in large prospective studies. The majority of studies of another tumor suppressor gene p27, a cell cycle inhibitor, have also supported a correlation with progression after prostatectomy.[203,219] Less robust evidence exists for the prognostic role of p21,[220] a downstream mediator of p53, PTEN,[221,222] and transcription factors such as NKX3.1.[181,223]

A preponderance of evidence supports a prognostic role for bcl-2[198,211,213,215,217] and myc oncogenes [224,225] as potential adjuncts to histologic prognostic parameters.

Despite great interest in HER2/neu and its potential use as a target of therapy, the data on its relation to prognosis in prostate carcinoma are conflicting with one study by Veltri and colleagues[226,227] showing HER2/neu to be an independent prognosticator and a more recent study using both immunohistochemistry and FISH assessment showing lack of its utility in predicting progression.

Neuroendocrine Differentiation

Two studies have shown neuroendocrine differentiation to be predictive of prognosis in organ-confined prostate carcinoma.[115,116] However, several more recent studies have shown no prognostic role for neuroendocrine differentiation on needle biopsy or prostatectomy.[114,117,228,229]

Morphometry/Karyometry

Nuclear morphometric measurements on needle biopsy have also been demonstrated in limited studies to correlate with prostate cancer prognosis. The same group, however, found lack of correlation in nuclear measurements between needle and corresponding prostatectomy tissue.[230,231] Several studies from our institution have looked at the prognostic role of the integration of multiple nuclear morphometry parameter variables[232,233] and at the potentials of integration of nuclear morphometry parameters with other established factors such as grade and stage. The latter appear to enhance the prediction accuracy of established parameters.[234,235]

Prostatic Lineage Specific Markers

The expression of prostatic markers such as prostate-specific alkaline phosphatase (PSAP) and PSMA[26,236] have been linked to prognosis in an occasional study. The degree of PSA expression does not appear to correlate with progression.[236]

Genomic-Based Approaches

Gene expression profiling studies using cDNA microarrays containing 26,000 genes identified three subclasses of prostate tumors on the basis of distinct patterns of gene expression (Fig. 16.22).[8] High-grade and advanced-stage tumors, as well as tumors associated with recurrence, were disproportionately represented among two of the three subtypes, one of which also included most lymph node metastases. Furthermore, two surrogate genes were differentially expressed among tumor subgroups by immunohistochemistry. These included MUC1, a gene highly expressed in the subgroups with "aggressive" clinicopathological features, and AZGP1, a gene highly expressed in the favorable subgroup. Both were strong predictors of tumor recurrence independent of tumor grade, stage, and preoperative prostate-specific antigen levels. Such a study suggests that prostate tumors can be usefully classified according to their gene expression patterns, and these tumor subtypes may provide a basis for improved prognostication and treatment stratification.

In another study, Tomlins and colleagues[10] used laser-capture microdissection to isolate 101 cell populations to illustrate gene expression profiles of prostate cancer progression from benign epithelium to metastatic disease. By analyzing expression signatures in the context of more than 14,000 "molecular concepts," or sets of biologically connected genes, the authors generated an integrative model of progression. Molecular critical transitions in progression included protein biosynthesis, E26 transformation-specific (ETS) family transcriptional targets, androgen signaling, and cell proliferation. Known prognostic markers such as grade could be ascribed to noted attenuated androgen signaling signature seen in high-grade cancer (Gleason pattern 4), similar to metastatic prostate cancer, which may reflect dedifferentiation and explain the clinical association of grade and prognosis. Taken together, these data show that analyzing gene expression signatures in the context of a compendium of molecular concepts is useful in understanding cancer biology.

At the DNA level, array-based comparative genomic hybridization (array CGH) identified recurrent aberrations,[230] including the following: (1) deletions at 5q21 and 6q15 deletion group associated with favorable outcome group, and (2) an 8p21 (NKX3-1) and 21q22 (resulting in TMPRSS2-ERG fusion) deletion group and 8q24 (MYC) and 16p13 gains, and loss at 10q23 (PTEN) and 16q23 groups correlating with metastatic disease and worse outcome.

Genomic studies suggest that prostate cancers develop via a limited number of alternative preferred genetic pathways. The resultant molecular genetic subtypes provide a new framework for investigating prostate cancer biology and explain in part the clinical heterogeneity of the disease.

EMERGING EARLY DETECTION MARKERS AND TARGETS OF THERAPY

Early detection markers include two major groups. The first group is molecular markers that can be applied to tissue biopsies in order to better stratify at-risk groups. The second group is cancer-associated markers that can be detected in blood, urine, ejaculates, or prostatic massage fluid as a noninvasive diagnostic alternative to needle biopsy.

Only a few studies have used molecular techniques to predict which men with high-grade PIN on needle biopsy are more likely to have cancer on subsequent biopsy. Using fluorescent *in situ* hybridization to assess c-myc, HER2/neu, and the chromosome region of 7q31, Bastacky and colleagues[238] analyzed 11 cases of high-grade PIN with benign repeat biopsies and compared them with 14 cases of high-grade PIN with a subsequent cancer diagnosis. Amplification of HER2/neu was common both in patients with and without cancer on repeat biopsy. Abnormalities in chromosome 7q31 and c-myc were greater in patients with cancer on follow-up. The only other study to address this issue, by Al-Maghrabi and colleagues,[239] analyzed 24 cases of high-grade PIN on needle biopsy with no subsequent diagnosis of cancer and compared them with 20 cases of high-grade PIN with cancer on follow-up. Using fluorescent *in situ* hybridization techniques to analyze chromosomes 4, 7, 8, and 10, there were no statistically significant differences between the two groups. Recently, in two studies,[240,241] the expression of a nuclear matrix protein, early prostate carcinoma antigen "EPCA," in benign biopsies from patients with suspected prostate carcinoma have been suggested to strongly predict the presence of an associated carcinoma. A subsequent study, however, revealed a high false-negative rate of EPCA expression in benign needle biopsies from patients with associated prostate carcinoma on different cores, calling into question the utility of this marker.[242]

Markers of prostate carcinoma detection that can be applied to blood, urine, or prostatic secretion fluid (ejaculate or prostate massage fluids) are of great interest and have been the focus of active research. A serum assay for a second-generation antibody (EPCA-2) has been recently proposed as a noninvasive early detection marker for prostate carcinoma.[243] Markers that have been investigated in the urine or prostatic secretions include gene promoter hypermethylation profile assays[244-247] and DD3 (differential display code 3), also known as PCA3. DD3 is a noncoding RNA that was initially identified by Bussemakers and colleagues[248] as one of the most specific markers of prostate carcinoma. Quantitative real-time reverse transcriptase polymerase chain reaction (RT-PCR) assay detecting DD3 can be applied to blood, urine, or prostatic fluid.[249] These noninvasive detection assays are considered by most authorities to be in the research stage and should undergo statistically robust clinical trials before making their transition into the clinical realm. Likewise, it remains to be seen if RT-PCR–based assays that identify the previously mentioned, newly discovered genetic TMPRSS2-ETS rearrangement that is found in the majority of prostate carcinoma will offer any additional noninvasive detection method.

Finally, several markers are being investigated as potential targets of therapy for prostate cancer.[77-79] The list includes tyrosine kinase receptors (e.g., EGFR), angiogenesis targets (e.g., VEGF),[250] fatty acid synthase (FAS),[251] PI3K/akt/mTOR mammalian target of rapamycin,[252] endothelin receptors,[253,254] and PSMA,[30,255-257] to name a few.

In summary, a wide array of molecular markers discussed in this chapter may be used in the near future as an adjunct to currently established prognostic parameters.

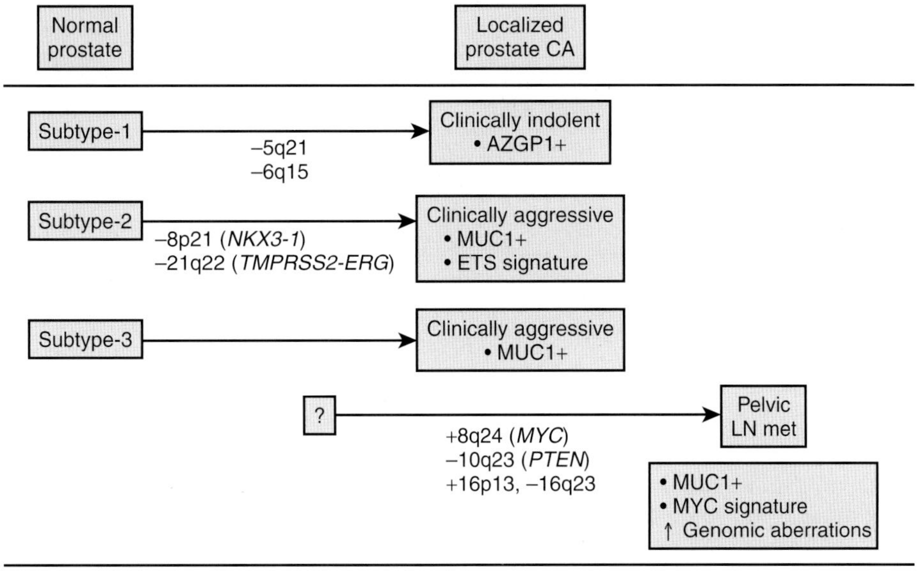

FIGURE 16.23 Biologic markers that can assist in targeting therapy for prostate cancer. *(From Lapointe J, Li C, Giacomini CP, et al. Genomic profiling reveals alternative genetic pathways of prostate tumorigenesis. Cancer Res. 2007;67:8504-8510.)*

Among those, DNA ploidy analysis, proliferation index (Ki-67), and p53 appear to be poised for the earliest transition into the clinical arena. Current research efforts in prostate cancer are also focused on biologic markers that can serve as a target of therapy (Fig. 16.23).

IMMUNOHISTOLOGY OF THE URINARY BLADDER

In 2008 more than 68,810 new cases of urothelial carcinoma (URCa) were diagnosed in the United States, leading to more than 14,100 deaths.[258] The estimated annual incidence worldwide is a staggering 336,000 cases. Bladder cancer is the fourth most common tumor in males and eleventh most common in females. Owing to the high rate of tumor recurrence and the need for frequent cystoscopy, URCa is the cancer with the highest cost per patient with an annual burden of more than 4 billion dollars to our health care system. Nevertheless, URCa presents us with unique challenges and opportunities given urine samples amenable to the application of noninvasive molecular detection methods and the relative ease of delivery of molecular-targeted therapy to a topographically accessible tumor.[163]

Clinically, URCa presents two distinct phenotypes. The first phenotype is superficial (nonmuscle invasive) URCa, representing three fourths of cases. Fifty percent of these superficial tumors will recur as nonmuscle invasive tumors, and only 5% to 10% of progress to muscle invasive disease.

The mainstay of therapy in superficial tumors is transurethral resection biopsy (TURB) with or without intravesical chemotherapy and immune therapy (BCG). The second phenotype is the muscle-invasive URCa representing 20% to 30% of all URCas. Only 15% of muscle-invasive URCas have a prior history of superficial URCa and represent a progression from the superficial phenotype, whereas the majority (80% to 90%) are "primary" *de novo* muscle-invasive URCa. Currently, patients suffering from muscle-invasive, high-grade tumors are destined to a disappointing 50% to 60% overall survival despite aggressive combined treatment modalities including cystectomy and chemotherapy.

Biology of Principal Antigens and Antibodies

CK7/CK20

Cytokeratins (CKs) are a family of intracytoplasmic intermediate filament proteins present in almost all epithelia. Expression of each CK molecule depends on cell type and differentiation status, and therefore specific CKs can be used as markers to identify particular types of epithelial tumors (Table 16.5). CK7 is found in a wide variety of epithelia including the columnar and glandular epithelium of the lung, cervix, and breast, as well as in the bile duct, collecting ducts of the kidney, urothelium, and mesothelium, but not in most gastrointestinal epithelium, hepatocytes, proximal and distal tubules of the kidney, and squamous epithelium. In contrast, CK20 shows relatively restricted expression and is present in gastrointestinal epithelium, Merkel cells of the epidermis, and urothelium.

CK7 expression is observed in the majority of urothelial carcinomas, whereas CK20 expression in urothelial carcinoma has been reported to vary from 15% to 97% in different studies.[259] Bassily and colleagues[260] showed that CK20 is more frequently positive in low-grade tumors (83%) than in high-grade tumors (52%). However, Desai and colleagues[261] showed higher expression in high-grade tumors. Thus most cases of urothelial carcinoma are positive for both CK7 and CK20. This immunoprofile (CK7+/CK20+) is helpful, particularly in the differential diagnosis of metastatic neoplasm of uncertain primary, although other examples of CK7+/CK20+ tumor include carcinomas of extrahepatic bile

TABLE 16.5 Utility of CK7 and CK20 in the Differential Diagnosis of Urothelial Carcinoma

CK7+/CK20+	CK7–/CK20–	CK7+/CK20–	CK7–/CK20+
Urothelial Ca	Hepatocellular carcinoma	Urothelial Ca	Colorectal Ca
Pancreatic carcinoma	RCCa	Breast cancer	Lung non–small cell
Ovarian mucinous Ca	Prostatic Ca	Ovarian serous carcinoma	Primary seminal vesicle Ca
Squamous cell carcinoma		Mesothelioma (all forms)	Prostatic Ca
Neuroendocrine carcinoma		Prostatic Ca	
Endometrial adenocarcinoma			
Prostatic Ca			

duct/gallbladder, pancreatic adenocarcinoma, endocervical adenocarcinoma, mucinous tumors of the ovary and upper gastrointestinal tract, and mucinous bronchioloalveolar adenocarcinoma.[262-265]

More than half of primary adenocarcinomas of the bladder are also positive for both CK7 and CK20.[266] However, given that intestinal-type primary adenocarcinomas of bladder are likely to be CK7–/CK20+, such a panel has only a limited role in the differential diagnosis with secondary bladder involvement by adenocarcinoma of colorectal origin (see later). The utility of the combination of CK7 and CK20 can be further enhanced by the addition of tissue-specific markers such as PSA, PSMA, P501S, and TTF1. For example, prostatic adenocarcinomas that are occasionally CK7+/CK20+ could be distinguished from URCa by their positivity for PSA. Unequivocal strong or extensive PSA positivity should not be encountered in URCa.[13,260]

Several studies suggested a diagnostic role for CK20 expression pattern in distinguishing flat urothelial carcinoma *in situ* (CIS) from reactive urothelial atypia. In reactive non-neoplastic lesions, CK20 expression is usually restricted to surface "umbrella" cells. In contrast, the majority of urothelial dysplasia or carcinoma *in situ* will show at least focal positive transmucosal CK20 expression in all layers of urothelium.[267-269] CK20 staining in conjunction with Ki-67 proliferation index and p53 and p16 expression has also been suggested to be of value in distinguishing reactive atypia from CIS.[268-270] We do not routinely resort to immunostaining in establishing the diagnosis of CIS.

Finally, a role for CK20 expression pattern as a predictor of recurrence in low-grade urothelial neoplasms tumors has been proposed.[271-273]

UROPLAKIN

Uroplakins (UPs) are urothelium-specific transmembrane proteins present in terminally differentiated superficial urothelial cells. Therefore expression of UPs is expected to diminish during urothelial tumorigenesis. The majority of noninvasive and up to two thirds (66%) of advanced invasive and metastatic URCa have been shown to retain UP expression as assessed by UPIII immunohistochemistry.[274-278] Interestingly, in some of these studies loss of UPIII expression was associated with significantly worse prognosis even in patients with advanced disease.[275,277,279] The latter was true on multivariate analysis when established prognostic parameters such as stage and presence of lymph node metastasis were included.[275] Although highly specific for urothelial differentiation, immunohistochemical expression of UPIII is only of moderate degree of sensitivity (as low as 40%)[280] given that UPIII mRNA can often be detected in the absence of UPIII protein.[281] Attesting to their suggested urothelial histogenesis, benign Brenner tumors of the ovary also stain for UPIII.[274,280,282] Interestingly, only a slim minority of malignant Brenner tumors and primary ovarian URCa (6%) stained positive for UPIII in the study by Logani and colleagues.[280]

THROMBOMODULIN

Thrombomodulin (TM), also designated CD141, is an endothelial cell-associated cofactor for thrombin-mediated activator of protein C. TM expression, predominantly as membranous staining, has been found in 69% to 100% of urothelial carcinoma.[13,266,276,283] TM expression is particularly useful in differentiating urothelial carcinoma from high-grade prostatic adenocarcinoma, renal cell carcinoma, and adenocarcinomas of the colon and endometrium in which TM is rarely positive.[13,283] However, it should be kept in mind that TM is also expressed by nonurothelial tumors such as vascular tumors, mesotheliomas, and squamous cell carcinomas.[283] Compared with UPIII, TM has a higher degree of sensitivity but lower specificity as a marker for urothelial carcinoma.

p63

As mentioned in the section on prostate carcinoma, p63, a homologue of the p53 tumor suppressor gene, encodes at least six different proteins with a wide range of biologic functions, including a role in urothelial differentiation. Immunostaining with p63 is normally present in greater than 90% of urothelial layer nuclei. The majority of urothelial carcinomas retain normal expression pattern of p63, but expression may be partially lost in higher-grade invasive URCa.[13,284] However, in a recent study, we found p63 to be superior to TM as a urothelial marker of differentiation in high-grade tumors. p63 in combination with prostate lineage markers is a valuable marker in differentiating URCa from high-grade prostatic adenocarcinoma secondarily invading the bladder.[13]

HIGH-MOLECULAR-WEIGHT CYTOKERATIN

As already mentioned under our discussion on prostate carcinoma, the monoclonal antibody 34βE12 reacts specifically with high-molecular-weight cytokeratins (HMWCKs): CK1, CK5, CK10, and CK14. In addition to its previously mentioned utility in labeling the basal cell layer of prostatic glands, HMWCK is a highly sensitive marker of urothelial differentiation matching the sensitivity of p63 and surpassing that of TM and UPIII.[13,276]

HMWCK is useful in differentiating URCa (+) from PCa (usually −). However, a cautionary note is warranted given that HMWCK labels squamous epithelia including areas of squamous differentiation in post-therapy recurrent PCa lesions. HMWCK positivity that is restricted to areas of squamous differentiation does not exclude the diagnosis of PCa.[92]

Finally, immunohistochemistry for HMWCK has been cited to be helpful in distinguishing urothelial dysplasia (showing only basal staining) from flat urothelial CIS where a transmucosal staining of urothelial layers is expected.[285] Diffuse expression of HMWCK in low-grade papillary urothelial carcinoma has been reported to be a strong predictor of tumor recurrence.[272]

ANAPLASTIC LYMPHOMA KINASE

Anaplastic lymphoma kinase (ALK) is a cytoplasmic membrane tyrosine kinase receptor expressed in anaplastic large cell lymphoma. ALK expression has been detected in about two thirds of inflammatory myofibroblastic tumor (IMT) of the urinary tract, also termed *postoperative spindle cell nodule, inflammatory pseudotumor,* and *pseudosarcomatous fibromyxoid tumor.*[286-289] The ALK gene is located on chromosome 2p23. Rearrangements of the ALK gene through translocations with various gene partners have been identified in inflammatory myofibroblastic tumor from a number of anatomic sites including the urinary bladder. Two recent studies by Montgomery and colleagues[286] and Sukov and colleagues[289] showed 72% and 67% respective rates of ALK gene rearrangement in bladder IMT using split-apart FISH probes strategy. A tighter correlation between positive expression and rearrangement was seen in the study by Sukov and colleagues. Given the close morphologic and immunophenotypic similarities between inflammatory myofibroblastic tumor and malignant spindle cell urinary bladder tumors, demonstration of ALK immunostaining or gene rearrangement by FISH can prevent unnecessary radical surgery.

p53

The tumor suppressor gene p53 orchestrates the transcriptional regulation of cell cycle control elements. p53 mutations represent the most common genetic alterations in human malignancies.[290] A number of studies have revealed p53 mutations in 40% to 60% of invasive bladder cancers and their association with a worse prognosis.[291-295] The altered protein product of mutant p53 gene has an extended half-life leading to its accumulation and detection by immunohistochemical techniques.[296] Staining results may vary because of differences in specimen processing and fixation, and[297] only modest correlation between p53 mutations and p53 protein overexpression has been shown.[298,299] p53 alterations in URCa have also been shown to be predictive of increased sensitivity to chemotherapeutic agents that damage DNA.[300,301]

As mentioned earlier under our discussion of CK20 expression pattern in urothelial CIS, one potential use of p53 immunostaining is differentiating urothelial CIS from reactive urothelial atypia. Strong extensive p53 positivity in greater than 50% of cells is encountered in CIS, whereas reactive urothelium is usually negative or demonstrates only weak patchy p53 nuclear staining (Fig. 16.24).[268]

p16

p16 (CDKN2A) is a tumor suppressor gene that inhibits cyclin D–dependent protein kinases playing a vital role in the regulation of G1-S transition. p16 Gene (9p21) deletions and p16 mutations are frequent in bladder cancer and appear to be more frequent in low-grade superficial tumors compared with higher-grade invasive tumors.[302,303] Several recent studies revealed a significant correlation between loss of p16 expression and progression in noninvasive (pTa) and superficially invasive (pT1) URCa.[296,304]

Yin and colleagues[270] recently showed increased expression of p16 protein in flat urothelial CIS compared with its uniform and weak expression in normal and reactive urothelium, suggesting a potential diagnostic role for p16 immunostaining in such settings.

RETINOBLASTOMA PROTEIN

The retinoblastoma (Rb) gene product was the first tumor suppressor gene identified in human cancer. It encodes a nuclear protein (pRb) that plays a crucial role in cell cycle progression by regulating cell cycle arrest at the G1-S phase. pRb alterations may occur because of Rb gene mutations or loss of p16 that normally phosphorylates pRb. Loss of heterozygosity (LOH) of one Rb gene allele in combination with mutation of the remaining allele is found more frequently in high-grade, muscle-invasive URCa tumors.[305-308] Interestingly, both overexpression and loss of pRb expression have been associated with increased risk for bladder cancer progression.[309] It appears that alterations in pRb and p53 act in a synergistic manner to promote bladder cancer progression.[307,309] Thus pRb immunostaining could be a useful prognostic marker in URCa.[306,307,309,310]

Diagnostic Immunohistochemistry of Specific Bladder Neoplasms

UROTHELIAL CARCINOMA AND VARIANTS

The distinctive morphologic features of noninvasive papillary urothelial neoplasms (papilloma, PUNLMP, low-grade and high-grade noninvasive papillary URCa)

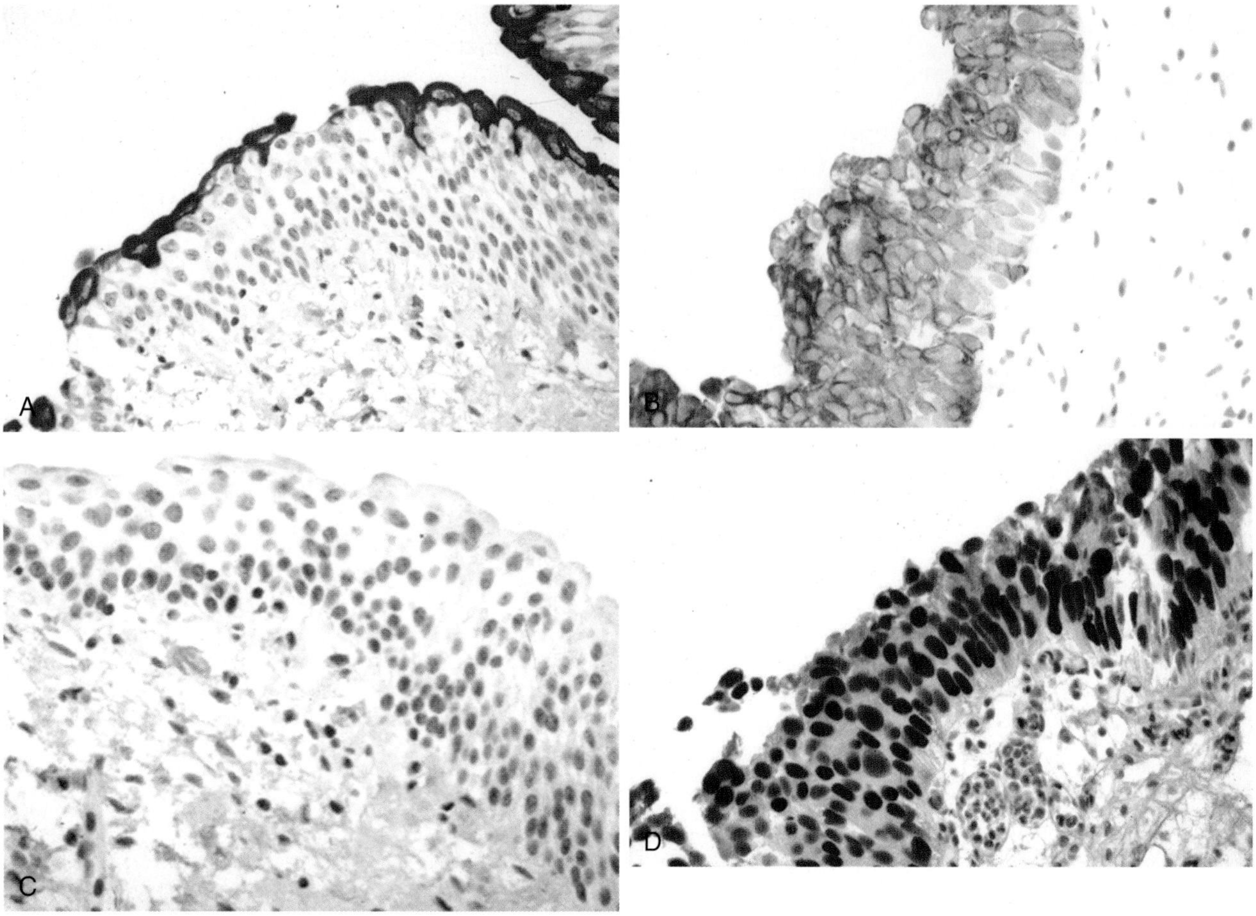

FIGURE 16.24 CK20/p53 staining as an adjunct to differentiate reactive urothelial atypia (**A** and **C**) from urothelial CIS (**B** and **D**). CK20 immunostain (**A** and **B**). p53 immunostain (**C** and **D**).

make their diagnosis easily achieved on H&E sections. Therefore the diagnostic role of immunohistochemistry in urothelial carcinoma is practically limited to (1) distinguishing high-grade invasive URCa from tumors secondarily involving the bladder from adjacent organs or more rarely from distant primary sites; (2) assigning a primary urothelial origin for a metastatic carcinoma of unknown primary; (3) potential utility in distinguishing CIS from reactive urothelial atypia; and (4) establishing the diagnosis in rare variants such as plasmacytoid and sarcomatoid URCa.

Urinary bladder involvement by a secondary tumor either as a metastasis or by direct extension occurs most commonly from colorectal (33%), prostatic (12%), and cervical (11%) sites.[163,311] Less common sources include breast, stomach, lung, and melanoma primaries.

Spread from a colonic or rectal primary could present a diagnostic challenge in bladder transurethral resection (TUR) samples. In fact, such secondary involvement is a more common occurrence than primary adenocarcinoma of the bladder. Differentiating a CRCa spread from "intestinal-type" primary adenocarcinoma of bladder cannot usually be made with certainty. The presence of a background of urothelial intestinal metaplasia with associated glandular dysplasia may favor a primary origin; however, one should consider the possibility of secondary colonization of bladder urothelial mucosa by a well-differentiated CRCa mimicking intestinal metaplasia/dysplasia. In general, a recommendation to clinically rule out spread from a colorectal primary by imaging techniques should be forwarded in order to avoid a potentially unjustifiable radical cystectomy procedure. Immunostains including CDX2, β-catenin, villin, and CK7/CK20 have been shown to be helpful by some authors.[266,312-314] However, some degree of overlap in staining patterns among primary "enteric type" bladder adenocarcinoma and secondary colorectal adenocarcinoma still exist, limiting the utility of these markers on an individual case basis (Fig. 16.25).

The second most common source of secondary tumor involvement of the bladder is prostate carcinoma. Even in cases where a prior known history of PCa is given, superimposed morphologic changes such as squamous differentiation caused by prior hormonal or radiation treatment lead to additional difficulty in distinguishing PCa recurrence from a second primary UCa on a TURP or needle biopsy. As mentioned earlier in the discussion of prostate tumors, poorly differentiated prostate cancers may have enlarged nuclei and prominent nucleoli, yet there is usually little variability in nuclear shape and size in PCa. High-grade URCa often reveals a more pronounced nuclear pleomorphism. URCa tends to grow in nests, even when poorly differentiated, usually lacking the cribriforming and cordlike architecture of PCa.

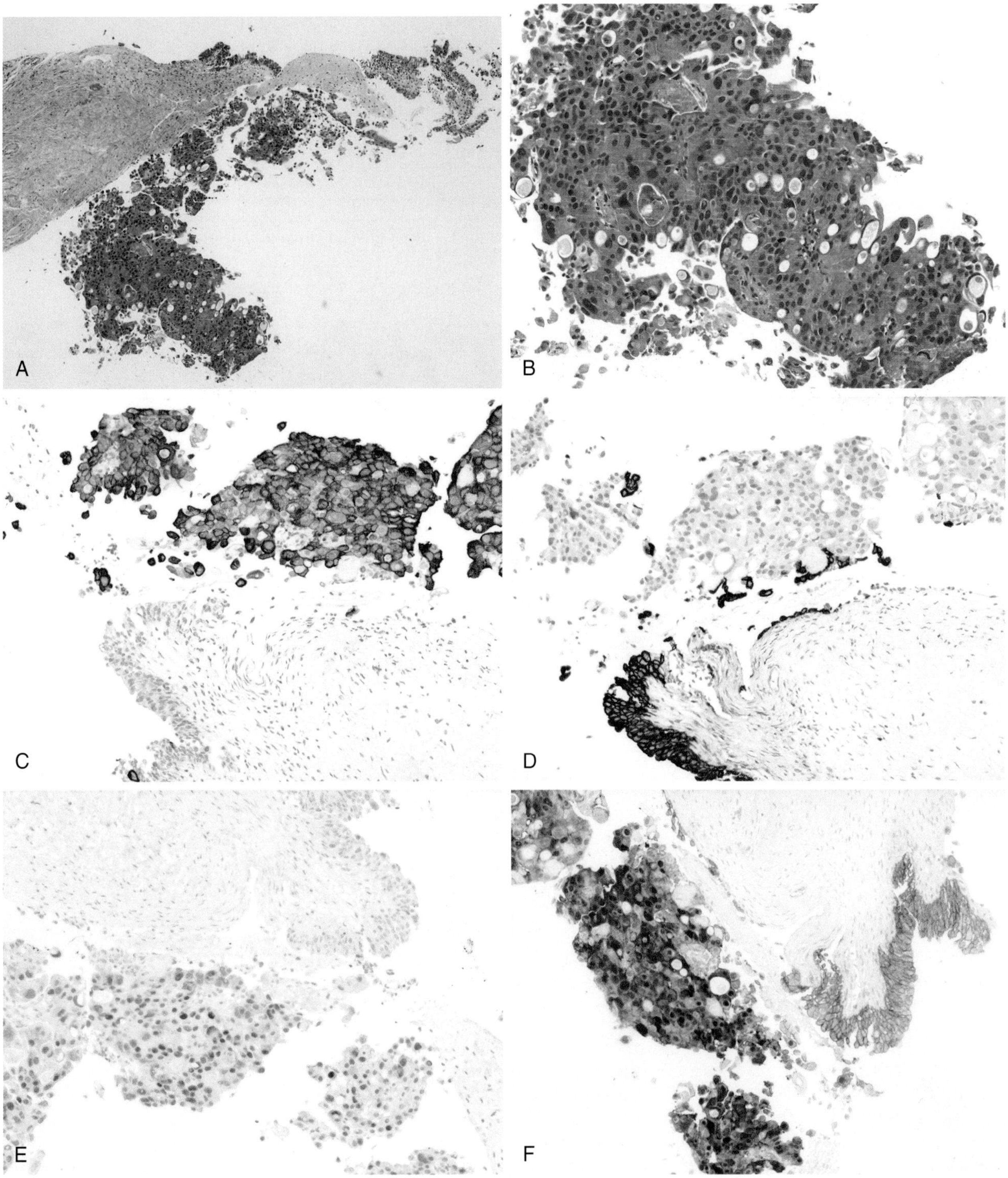

FIGURE 16.25 Rectal adenocarcinoma secondarily involving urinary bladder (**A** and **B**). The tumor is CK20+, CK7−, CDX2+, and β-catenin+ as shown in **C** to **F,** respectively.

However, in the absence of a noninvasive flat or papillary URCa component, it is difficult on limited material to distinguish high-grade prostate carcinoma involving the bladder from primary high-grade infiltrating URCa on routine H&E stained sections. Given the crucial difference in management and prognosis, resorting to immunostains is a must if the distinction cannot be made with absolute certainty on morphologic grounds. As mentioned earlier in the section on prostate, PSA and PSAP have proven to be useful in identifying prostate lineage. However, the sensitivities of PSA and PSAP decrease in poorly differentiated PCa and newer markers such as prostein (P501S), prostate-specific membrane antigen (PSMA), proPSA (pPSA), and NKX3.1[13] may be of added utility. Combining these markers with urothelial lineage markers such as thrombomodulin and

TABLE 16.6 Urothelial and Prostatic Markers in the Differential of High-Grade PCa versus High-Grade URCa

	HMWCK	p63	Thrombo-modulin	PSA	P501S	PSMA	NKX3.1	pPSA
Prostate carcinoma	3/38 (7.9%)	0/38 (0%)	2/38 (5.3%)	37/38 (97.4%)	38/38 (100%)	35/38 (92.1%)	36/38 (94.7%)	36/38 (94.7%)
Urothelial carcinoma	32/35 (91.4%)	29/35 (82.9%)	24/35 (68.6%)	0/35 (0%)	2/35 (5.7%)	0/35 (0%)	0/35 (0%)	0/35 (0%)

Adapted from Chuang AY, DeMarzo AM, Veltri RW, et al. Immunohistochemical differentiation of high-grade prostate carcinoma from urothelial carcinoma. *Am J Surg Pathol.* 2007;31:1246.

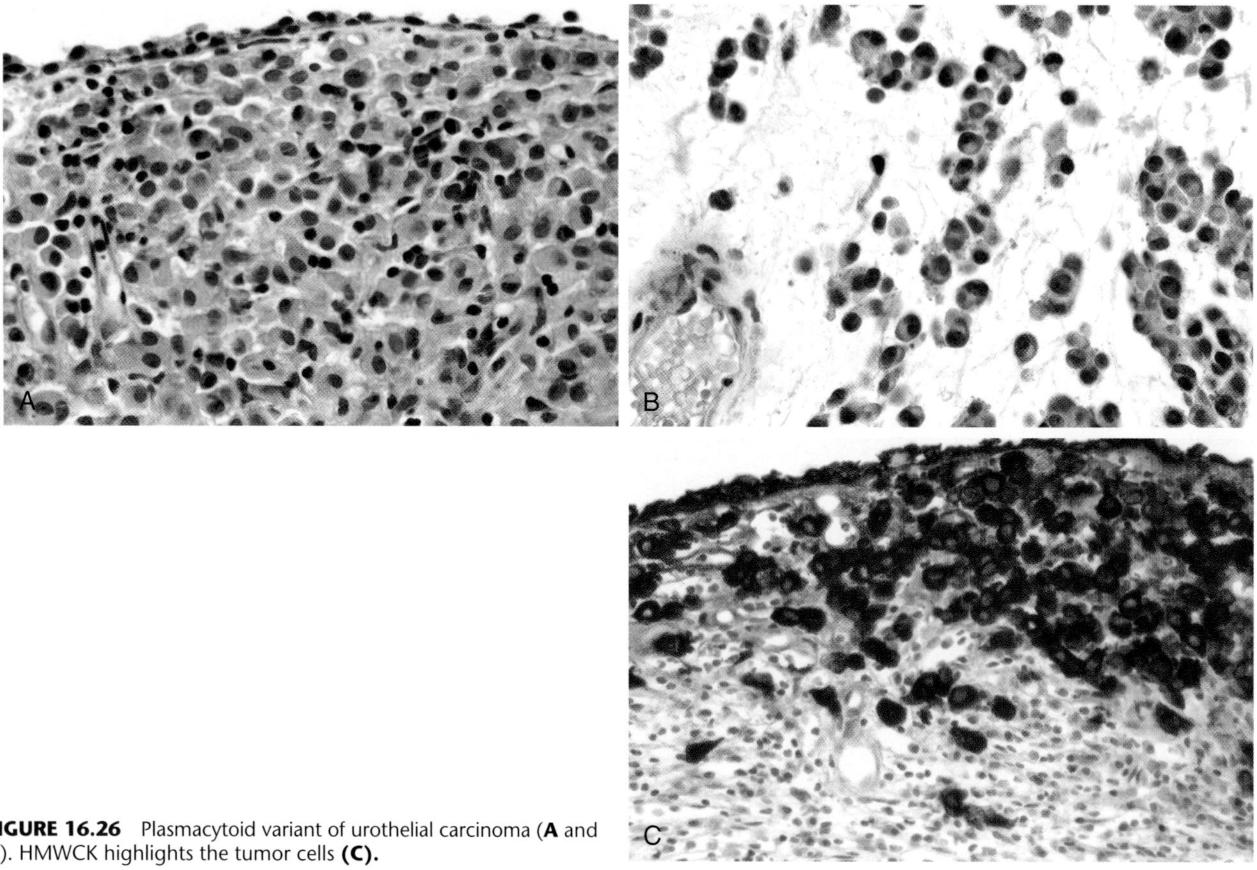

FIGURE 16.26 Plasmacytoid variant of urothelial carcinoma (**A** and **B**). HMWCK highlights the tumor cells **(C).**

uroplakin will further assist resolving a urothelial versus prostatic differential (Table 16.6). It should also be kept in mind that both UPIII and TM are of only moderate sensitivity compared with HMWCK and p63 in labeling URCa. Recent studies have documented HMWCK positivity in more than 90% of URCa.[13,158] HMWCK is only rarely and focally expressed in PCa (8%).[13] p63 has a greater specificity, albeit lower sensitivity for urothelial carcinoma, compared with high-molecular-weight cytokeratin (100% specificity and 83% sensitivity).[13] Finally, in our experience, CK7 and CK20 are of limited utility in this differential given that they may both be positive in a subset of PCa.[144,157]

Among other rare sources of tumors metastasizing to bladder, mammary carcinoma deserves a cautionary note. The possibility of a breast metastasis should be raised when presented with an epithelial infiltration in the form of cords or individual plasmacytoid to signet-ring–shaped cells involving lamia propria without associated overlying papillary urothelial proliferation or CIS. In such cases the differential should also include a rare variant of urothelial carcinoma, namely plasmacytoid variant (Fig. 16.26).[315-319] Obtaining a proper clinical history and the use of immunohistochemistry (estrogen receptor [ER], progesterone receptor [PR], gross cystic disease fluid protein [GCDFP], uroplakin and thrombomodulin) will help reach a proper diagnosis. Finally, positive reactivity for CD138 in the plasmacytoid variant of URCa can lead to misinterpretation as plasma cell dyscrasia if a proper battery of immunostains is not used.

In the workup of metastatic carcinoma of an unknown primary origin, inclusion of CK7, CK20, HMCK, TM, and UPIII is necessary to rule out a urothelial primary origin.

TABLE 16.7 Immunohistochemical Results in Varying Grades and Stages of Urothelial Neoplasms

	UPIII	TM	HMWCK	CK20
LMP (*n* = 14)	12 (86%)	12 (86%)	13 (93%)*	6 (43%)
LG (*n* = 16)	12 (75%)	16 (100%)	10 (63%)	8 (50%)
HG (*n* = 16)	13 (81%)	12 (75%)	11 (69%)†	
INV (*n* = 36)	14 (39%)	22 (61%)	30 (88%)†	17 (50%)
MET (*n* = 25)	13 (52%)	15 (60%)	24 (96%)†	10 (40%)

*Predominantly in basal cells.
†Staining throughout the tumor.
Data from Parker DC, Folpe AL, Bell J, et al. Potential utility of uroplakin III, thrombomodulin, high molecular weight cytokeratin, and cytokeratin 20 in noninvasive, invasive, and metastatic urothelial (transitional cell) carcinomas. *Am J Surg Pathol.* 2003;27:1.

Parker and colleagues,[276] using a panel of four of the latter markers (excluding CK7) in a wide range of 112 urothelial tumors, revealed that expression pattern varied with tumor grade and stage (Table 16.7). Variant morphologic subtypes showed similar staining as conventional urothelial carcinomas. In the same study, tissue microarray analysis showed no UPIII immunoreactivity in tissue cores of nonurothelial tumors, rendering the expression of UPIII in a tumor almost diagnostic of urothelial origin. Although coexpression of TM, HMWCK, and CK20 strongly suggests urothelial origin, none of these markers is as specific as UPIII given that TM is expressed in nonurothelial tumors such as non–small cell lung carcinomas (27%) and rare lymphomas and given that HMWCK is expressed by 43% of non–small cell lung carcinomas and mesotheliomas among others.[276]

Among URCa variants, sarcomatoid carcinoma deserves a special attention given its likelihood to be confused with "true" mesenchymal neoplasms such as leiomyosarcoma, osteosarcoma, and rhabdomyosarcoma. This is especially the case when heterologous elements are displayed and noninvasive papillary or *in situ* urothelial components are not evident. Reactivity for one or more of the following markers—AE1/AE3, CAM5.2, epithelial membrane antigen (EMA), HMWCK, p63, CK7, and/or CK20—supports the diagnosis of sarcomatoid carcinoma. Positive reactivity for actin can be encountered in sarcomatoid carcinoma and should not mislead the observer to a diagnosis of leiomyosarcoma. As discussed later, attention to differentiating sarcomatoid carcinoma from its benign IMT mimic is also crucial.

URINARY BLADDER ADENOCARCINOMA

Primary adenocarcinomas of the bladder are relatively rare. Therefore establishing their diagnosis requires the exclusion of secondary involvement by direct extension or metastatic spread. Bladder adenocarcinoma variants include signet-ring cell carcinomas, urachal adenocarcinomas, and mucinous and enteric adenocarcinomas. Distinguishing a prostate carcinoma extending into bladder from a primary bladder adenocarcinoma has important clinical and management implications. Immunohistochemical markers of prostate lineage are of great utility in this regard. Although the specificity of newer prostate lineage markers has been tested against bladder urothelial carcinoma, the same could not be said about their pattern of reactivity in bladder adenocarcinoma. In a recent immunohistochemistry study evaluating 37 adenocarcinomas of bladder,[17] our group demonstrated that a minority of bladder adenocarcinomas are positive for prostate antigens P501S and PSMA. P501S showed moderate diffuse cytoplasmic staining in 11% of cases including enteric-type and rare mucinous adenocarcinomas.

The granular perinuclear staining pattern of P501S typically seen in prostatic adenocarcinoma was absent in all cases of bladder adenocarcinoma. In addition, PSMA showed diffuse cytoplasmic or membranous staining in (21%) of bladder adenocarcinomas including signet-ring, urachal, mucinous, and enteric-type variants. All cases were negative for PSA and PSAP. Therefore immunoreactivity for P501S and PSMA should be interpreted with caution in such settings (Fig. 16.27). The lack of granular perinuclear staining for P501S and the absence of membranous PSMA staining both favor a bladder adenocarcinoma. Membranous PSMA staining indistinguishable from that seen in prostate cancer is seen in less than 10% of bladder adenocarcinoma.

SMALL CELL CARCINOMA OF URINARY BLADDER

Small cell carcinoma of the bladder involves rare aggressive tumors found either in pure form or more commonly admixed with urothelial CIS, invasive URCa, squamous cell carcinoma, or adenocarcinoma component. Clinically, small cell carcinoma presents with advanced-stage (visceral and bone metastases) and may be associated with paraneoplastic syndromes. In the largest series by Cheng and colleagues,[320] a dismal 5-year survival of 16% was encountered despite adopting a multimodal therapeutic approach including chemotherapy and radical cystectomy. In our experience, immunostains for neuroendocrine markers are only rarely necessary (synaptophysin+, chromogranin+, and CD56+), especially when a non–small cell component is associated. The presence of typical small cell morphology similar to that encountered in the lung counterpart with characteristic brisk mitotic activity and extensive necrosis assists the diagnosis. In cases where the differential diagnosis includes malignant lymphoma or other "small blue cell tumors," pancytokeratins (AE1/AE3 and CAM5.2) in addition to the previously mentioned neuroendocrine markers can help establish the diagnosis.

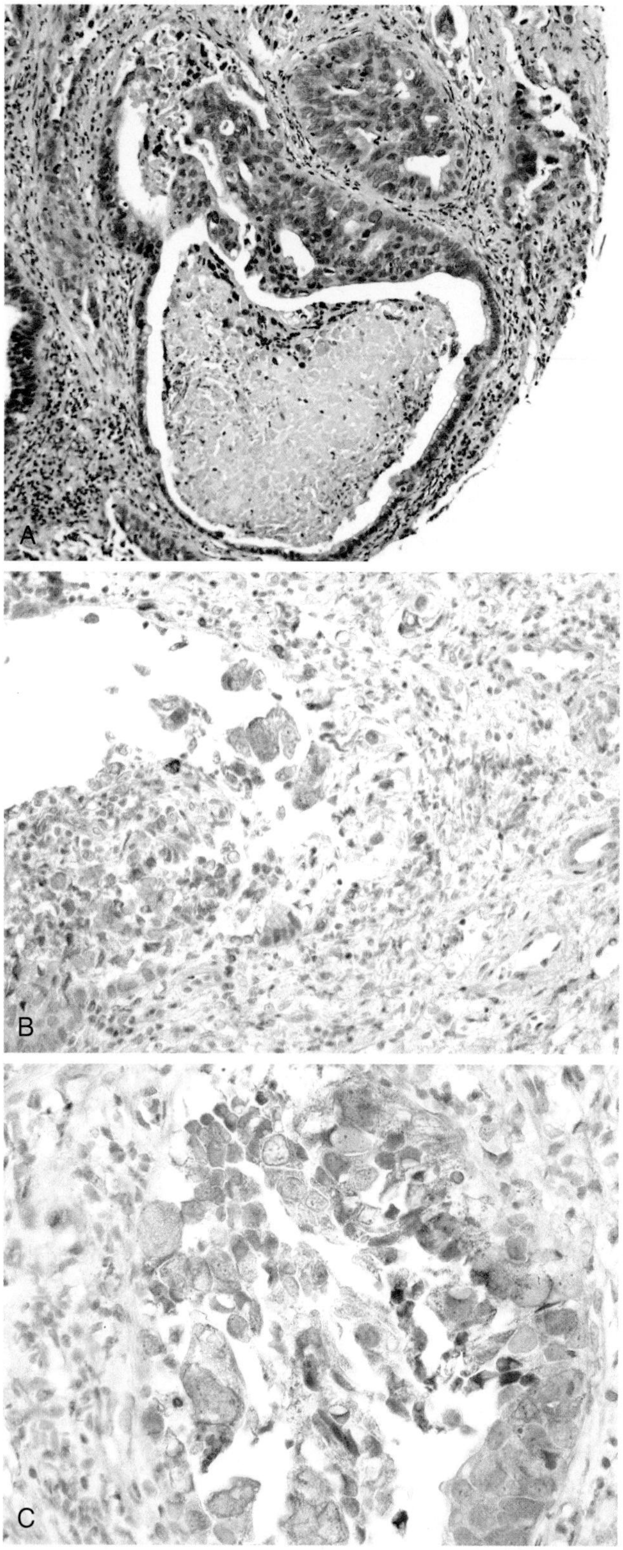

FIGURE 16.27 Primary adenocarcinoma of urinary bladder **(A)** showing cytoplasmic positivity for prostate markers P501S **(B)** and prostate-specific membrane antigen **(C)**.

Small cell carcinoma of bladder has a high number of genomic alterations. Cheng and colleagues,[321-323] in their analysis of a single tumor having areas of both small cell and urothelial carcinoma, revealed genetic evidence that strongly suggests small cell carcinoma can develop from urothelial carcinoma through the acquisition of additional genetic alterations. Deletions are most frequent at 10q, 4q, 5q, and 13q. These regions may carry tumor suppressor genes with relevance for this particular tumor type. Gains at 8q, 5p, 6p, and 20q and amplifications at 1p22-32, 3q26.3, 8q24, and 12q14-21 suggest localization of oncogenes at these loci.[323]

BENIGN MIMICS OF BLADDER CARCINOMA

We limit our discussion here to two of the benign mimickers of bladder tumors: nephrogenic adenoma as a mimic of both urothelial carcinoma and adenocarcinoma and inflammatory myofibroblastic tumor (IMT) as mimic of sarcomatoid carcinoma or sarcomas.

Nephrogenic Adenoma

Typically nephrogenic adenoma (NA) displays tubulopapillary structures lined by a single layer of bland cuboidal epithelial cells with low mitotic activity. Tubular structures are frequently surrounded by distinct ringlike basement membrane and may contain eosinophilic to mucinous secretions. The tubular lining cells frequently display hobnail nuclei. Other tubules can have a flattened lining, thus leading to a false impression of lymphatic structures. Rarely, intracytoplasmic lumina can form in single infiltrating cells that mimic signet ring carcinoma. Finally, rare examples where hyalinized myxoid stroma "suffocates" the compressed tubular structures (termed *fibromyxoid variant of NA*) can be confused with mucinous adenocarcinoma of bladder.[324] When typical, NA is easily recognized in TURB samples. In difficult examples the diagnosis of NA can be supported by their unique positivity for PAX2 and PAX8.[325,326] NA is negative for HMWCK and p63. A word of caution is merited in this setting regarding the fact that clear cell adenocarcinoma of bladder will share the previously mentioned immunophenotype with NA and should be recognized by paying attention to its higher degree of cytologic atypia and mitotic activity. The latter can be further illustrated by their high Ki-67 index compared with NA (Fig. 16.28).[325,326]

KEY DIAGNOSTIC POINTS

Nephrogenic Adenoma

- Lacks immunostaining for HMWCK/p63
- Positive for PAX2 and PAX8
- Lacks malignant cytology of clear cell carcinoma

Inflammatory Myofibroblastic Tumor

An inflammatory myofibroblastic tumor (IMT) of the bladder may arise either spontaneously or as a result of a prior instrumentation of the bladder. IMTs are benign mesenchymal neoplasms composed of a proliferation of relatively monotonous myofibroblastic cells (typical tissue culture appearance) in a richly vascularized background with red blood cell extravasation and lymphoplasmacytic inflammatory infiltrate. Mitotic activity ranges from absent to brisk. Abnormal mitotic figures

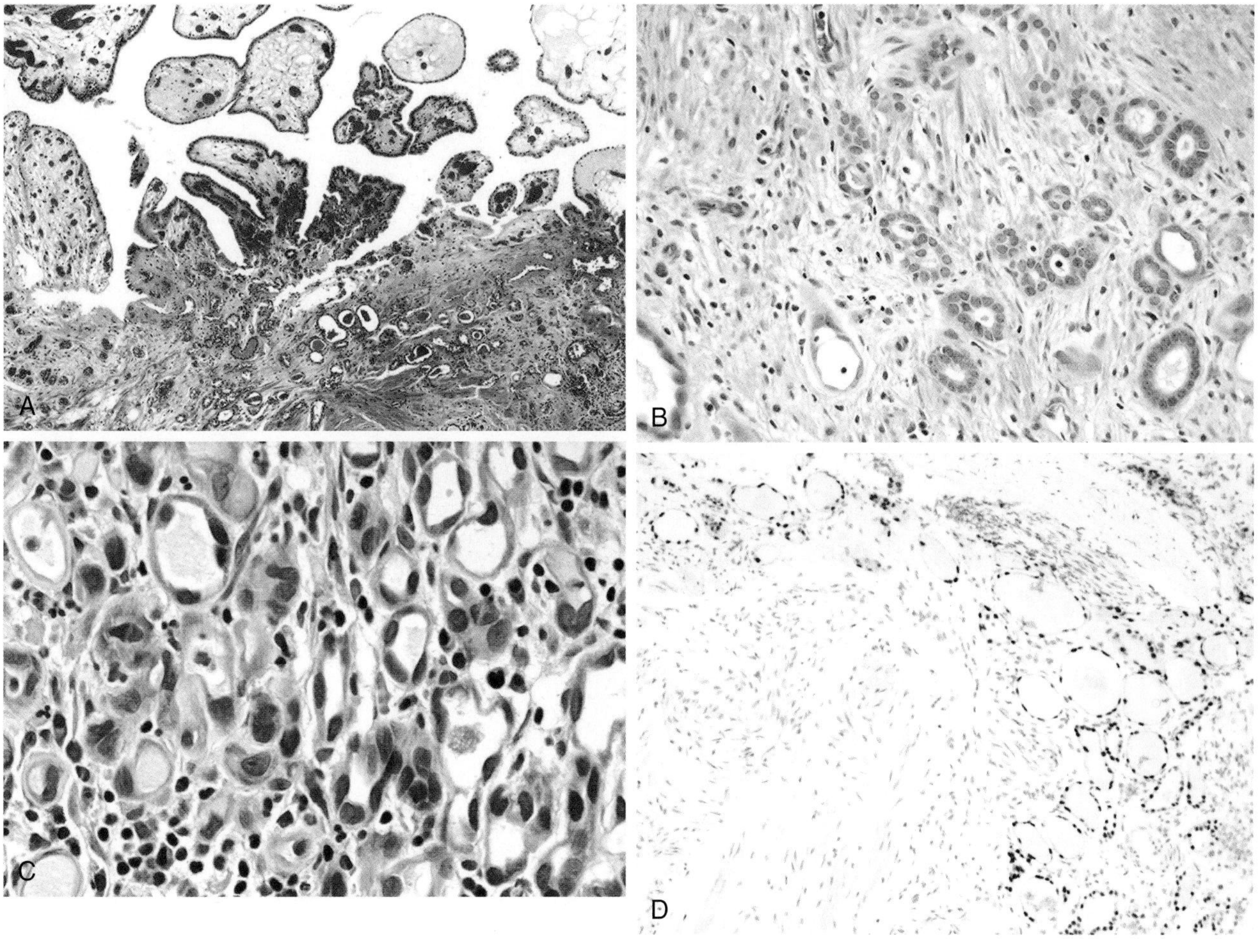

FIGURE 16.28 Nephrogenic adenoma of urinary bladder (**A** to **C**). Nuclear positivity for PAX8 **(D).**

are not present. Although IMTs may occasionally recur (25%), only one case of malignant transformation of IMT has been reported in the genitourinary tract.[286] As mentioned earlier in the section on ALK, two thirds of IMTs contain rearrangement of the anaplastic lymphoma kinase (ALK) gene on chromosome 2p23 with different translocation partners. The latter can be demonstrated by split-apart interphase cytogenetic FISH techniques (Fig. 16.29). The translocation leads to ALK protein overexpression on immunohistochemistry (Fig. 16.30). IMTs are frequently immunoreactive for pancytokeratin CAM5.2, a fact worth remembering when attempting to differentiate IMT from sarcomatoid carcinoma. They are also frequently positive for smooth muscle actin and desmin. The latter may lead to their misinterpretation as leiomyosarcoma. IMT is usually negative for CD34, S100, and CD117 (Table 16.8).

Genomic and Theranostic Applications

In line with the distinct contrasting clinical behavior and prognosis of the two phenotypes of URCa, current molecular evidence is increasingly in support of two distinct pathways of pathogenesis for superficial and invasive urothelial carcinoma. A "linking" progression pathway that would account for the known progression of a subset of superficial URCa into muscle invasive disease has also emerged. Superficial URCa is thought to originate from benign urothelium through hyperplasia with only a small contribution (10% to 15%) to the pool of high-grade noninvasive and subsequently invasive URCa. However, the majority of invasive tumors appear to originate through progression from dysplasia to flat CIS and high-grade, noninvasive URCa where genetic instability leads to accumulation of genetic alterations promoting progression to invasive lesions.[327,328]

Clinically, a significant portion of superficial tumors (pTa and pT1) is deemed to recur after TURB with only a small minority showing ultimate progression into higher-grade, aggressive, deeply invasive tumors.

The superficial URCa pathogenesis pathway is based primarily on alterations in tyrosine kinase receptor FGFR-3 and H-RAS oncogene,[329] whereas the pathogenic pathway for muscle-invasive URCa primarily involves tumor suppressor genes p53, p16, and Rb.[310,327,328] As illustrated in Figure 16.31, p53/Rb alterations are also necessary for the progression of the small portion of superficial lesions to higher-grade, muscle-invasive URCa.

Evidently, prognostic parameters that can accurately predict the subset of superficial tumors that will progress are invaluable for tailoring a more aggressive surveillance and management approach in such a subset.

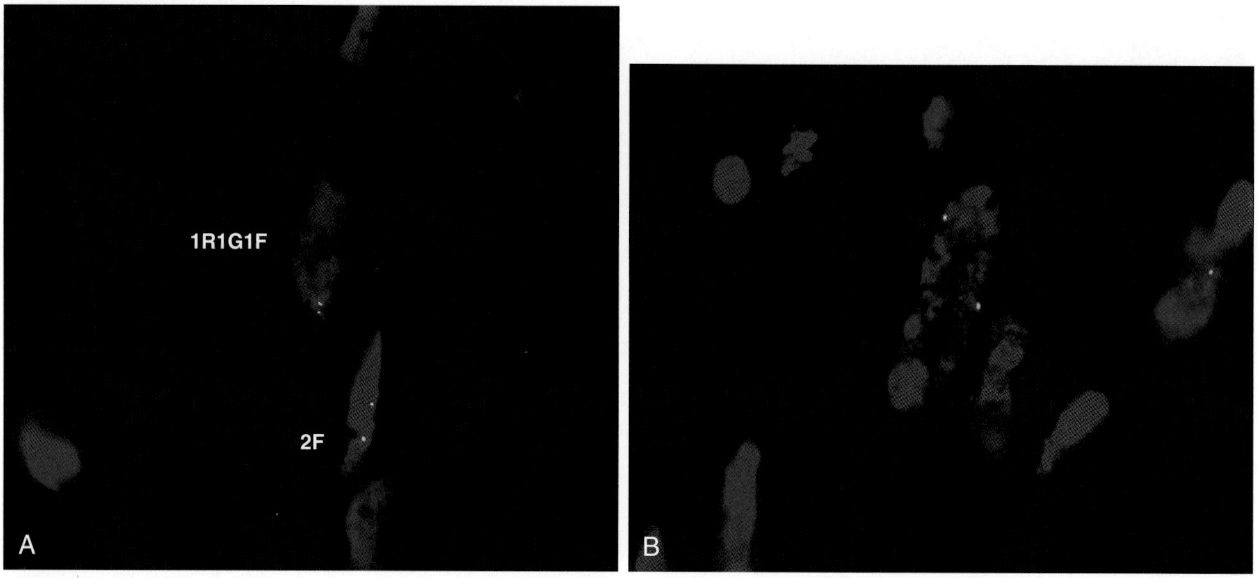

FIGURE 16.29 Interphase fluorescence *in situ* hybridization analysis for ALK-1 gene in inflammatory myofibroblastic tumor using split-apart probes. The presence of a set of one green and one red signal in addition to a juxtaposed red-green (yellow overlap) set indicates a rearrangement in one of the two ALK-1 alleles.

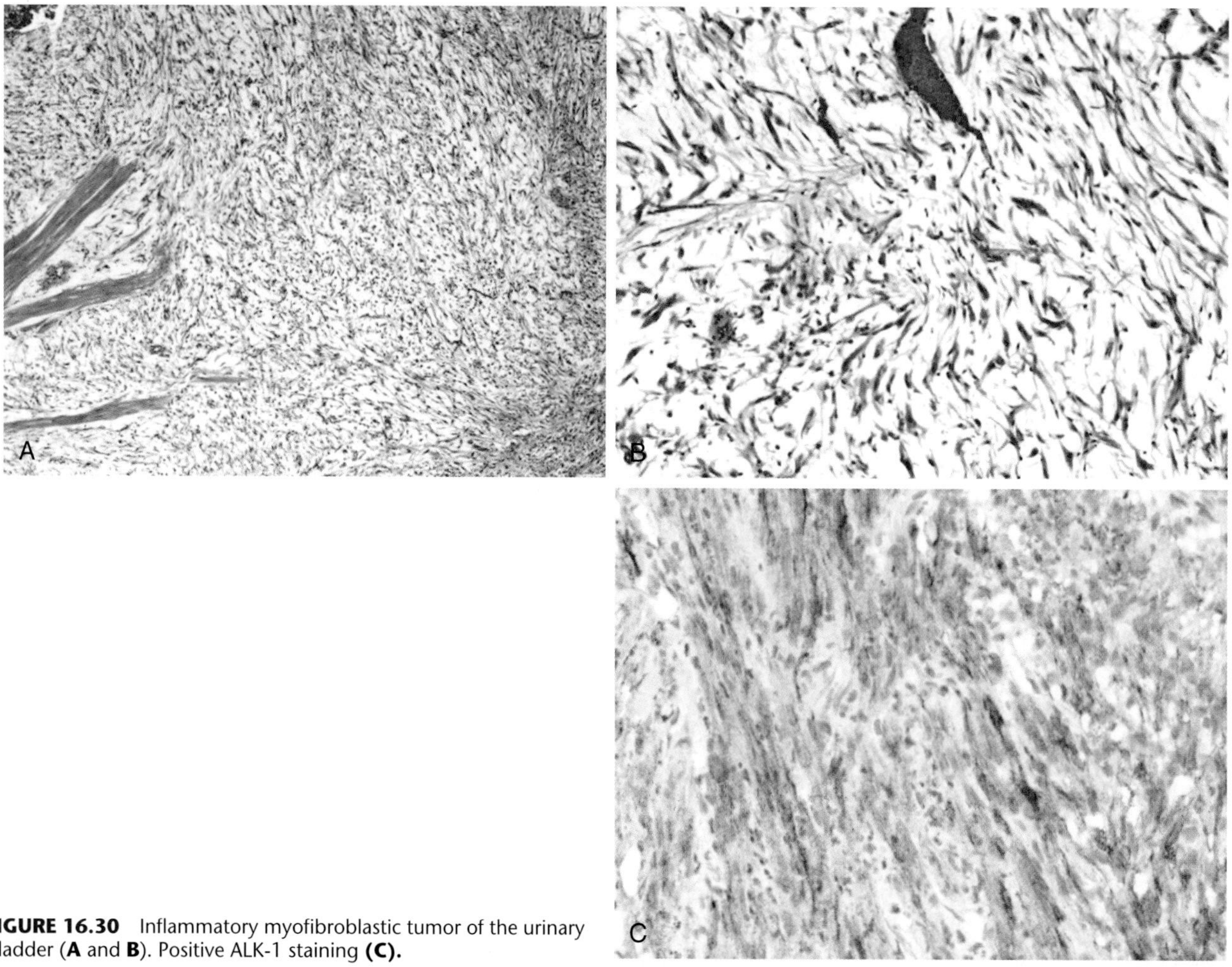

FIGURE 16.30 Inflammatory myofibroblastic tumor of the urinary bladder (**A** and **B**). Positive ALK-1 staining **(C).**

TABLE 16.8 Immunohistochemistry of Spindle Cell Neoplasms of the Urinary Bladder

	IMT	Sarcomatoid URCa	Leiomyosarcoma	Rhabdomyosarcoma
Keratin	+	+	S	N
EMA	N	+	N	N
Vimentin	+	+	+	+
Desmin	+	N	+	+
MSA	+	S	+	+
ALK	S	N	N	N

ALK, anaplastic lymphoma kinase; EMA, epithelial membrane antigen; IMT, inflammatory myofibroblastic tumor; MSA, muscle-specific actin; +, almost always positive; S, sometimes positive; N, negative.

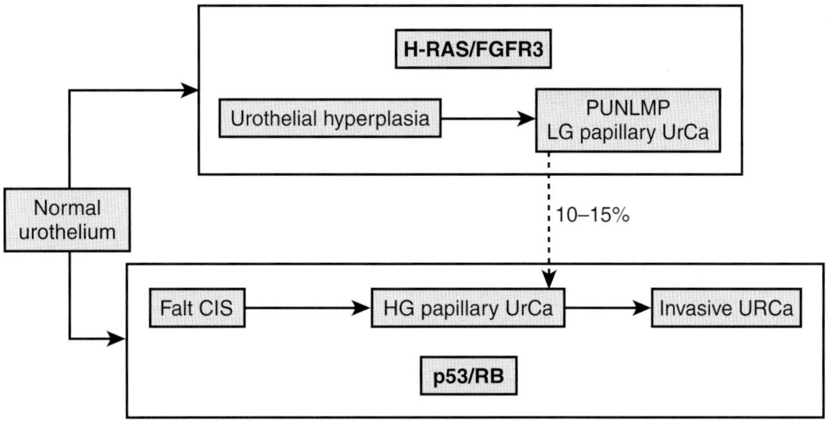

FIGURE 16.31 Divergent molecular pathways in superficial and muscle invasive urothelial carcinoma.

Current established clinicopathologic prognostic parameters in superficial lesions include pTNM stage, WHO/ISUP grade, size of tumor, multifocality and presence of CIS, and frequency and rate of prior recurrences.[330] Sylvester and colleagues[331] recently suggested a scoring system on the basis of the previously mentioned clinicopathologic parameters to improve the ability to predict recurrences and progression in superficial tumors.

Additionally, improved prognostication in muscle-invasive disease is equally crucial to allocation of aggressive therapy protocols, given the current poor outcome (60% 10-year overall survival) in this group of bladder cancer patients.[332] The need is most pressing in this cohort given the paucity and imperfections of current clinicopathologic prognostic parameters in invasive URCa. Our recent understanding of complexed molecular alterations involved in the development and progression of URCa is yielding novel diagnostic and prognostic molecular tools and opening the doors for experimental targeted therapies in bladder cancer.

Beyond Immunohistochemistry: Anatomic Molecular Diagnostic Applications

Chromosome 9 alterations are established to be the earliest events in both pathways of URCa development, setting up the stage for genetic instability that in turn leads to accumulation of subsequent genetic events. Among other common chromosomal gains and deletions, gains of chromosomes 3q, 7p, and 17q and 9p21 deletions (p16 locus) are of special interest given their potential diagnostic value. A multitarget interphase FISH-based urine cytogenetic assay was developed[333] on the basis of these numeric chromosomal alterations. Such a test is now commercially available. The Food and Drug Administration initially approved it for surveillance of URCa recurrence in previously diagnosed URCa patients and subsequently approved it for screening of URCa in high-risk patients with hematuria. The multicolor FISH assay appears to enhance the sensitivity of routine urine cytology analysis and can be used in combination with routine cytology as a reflex testing in cases with atypical cytology. A sensitivity range of 69% to 87% and a specificity range of 89% to 96% have been reported with the multitarget interphase FISH assay. With the exception of one study by Moonen and colleagues,[334] the multitarget FISH urine assay has been shown to be more sensitive than routine cytology. An additional advantage of urine-based FISH testing could be the anticipatory positive category of patients identified by such assay. The latter category refers to patients where FISH assay detects molecular alteration of URCa in urine cells several months before cancer detection by cystoscopy and routine cytology.[325] In the study by Yoder and colleagues,[335] two thirds of the 27% of patients categorized as "anticipatory positive" developed URCa that was detected by cystoscopy up to 29 months later. Such encouraging results point to the great potential of molecular testing in early detection and allocation of vigorous/frequent follow-up cystoscopy to at-risk patients (Fig. 16.32).[326]

As mentioned earlier, the current detailed understanding of the molecular pathways involved in URCa development and progression (Fig. 16.33) has fueled the field of molecular prognostication, theranostics, and targeted therapy in bladder cancer.[292,303,305,336-348]

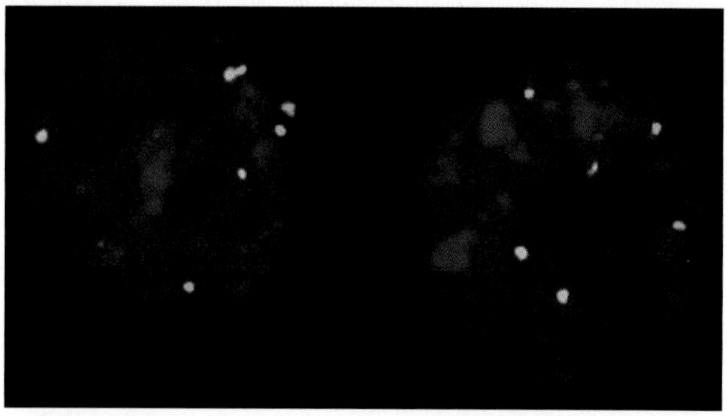

FIGURE 16.32 Interphase fluorescence *in situ* hybridization urine cytology analysis using Vysis UroVision probe sets for chromosomes 3q *(red)*, 7p *(green)*, and 17q *(aqua/blue)* and 9p21 deletions (p16 locus: *gold*). Note polysomy for 17q *(aqua)* and deletion of 9p21 loci (absence of gold signals) in two urothelial carcinoma cells. *(Adapted from Moonen PM, Merkx GF, Peelen P, et al. UroVysion compared with cytology and quantitative cytology in the surveillance of non-muscle-invasive bladder cancer. Eur Urol. 2007;51:1275.)*

A series of recent studies have pointed to the potential prognostic value of receptor tyrosine kinase (RTK) markers such as FGFR-3, EGFR, and other ERB family members (ERBB2/HER2 and ERBB3)[328] in superficial and invasive bladder cancer disease (Table 16.9).

Early studies by Sarkis and colleagues[293,294,349] revealed p53 alterations to be a strong independent predictor of disease progression in URCa (superficial, muscle invasive, and CIS). p53 has also been shown to be predictive of increased sensitivity to chemotherapeutic agents that damage DNA.[300,301] More recent studies have demonstrated a synergistic role for combining p53 evaluation with cell cycle control elements such as pRb, p21, and p27,[346,348] demonstrating the superiority of multimarker approach compared with a prior single-marker approach for prognostication.[293,294,349,350] In a recent study by Shariat and colleagues,[348] superficial URCa patients with tumors on TURB demonstrating synchronous immunohistochemical alterations in all four tested p53, p21, pRb, and p27 markers were at significantly lower likelihood of sustained disease-free survival (DFS) compared with patients with only three

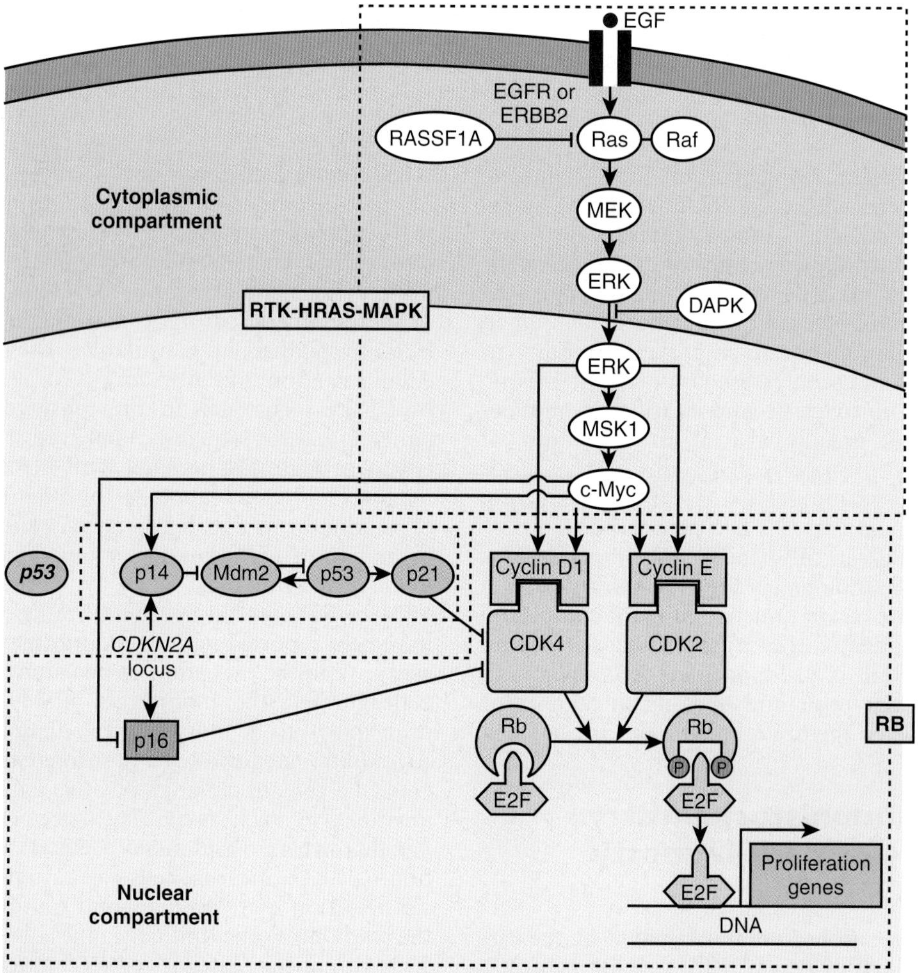

FIGURE 16.33 Molecular pathways in invasive urothelial carcinoma. *(Adapted from Mitra AP, Datar RH, Cote RJ. Molecular pathways in invasive bladder cancer: new insights into mechanisms, progression, and target identification. J Clin Oncol. 2006;24:5552.)*

TABLE 16.9 Potential Molecular Prognostic Markers in Urothelial Carcinoma

Gene	Mode of Activation	Frequency in Tumors	Role in Tumorigenesis	Correlation with Pathway	Relation to Prognosis
HRAS	Mutation	30%-40%	Genesis	LGNP	Good
HRAS	Overexpression	50%	Genesis	ND	Good
FGFR3	Mutation	60%-70%	Genesis	LGNP	Good
ERBB3	Overexpression	ND	Genesis?	LGNP	Good
ERBB4	Overexpression	ND	Genesis?	LGNP	Good
EGFR	Overexpression	50%	Progression	Invasive	Poor
ERBB2	Overexpression	40%-50%	Progression	Invasive	Poor
ERBB2	Amplification	10%	Progression	Invasive	Poor

From Wu Xue-Ru. Urothelial tumorigenesis: a tale of divergent pathways. *Nature Rev Cancer.* 2005;5:713-725.

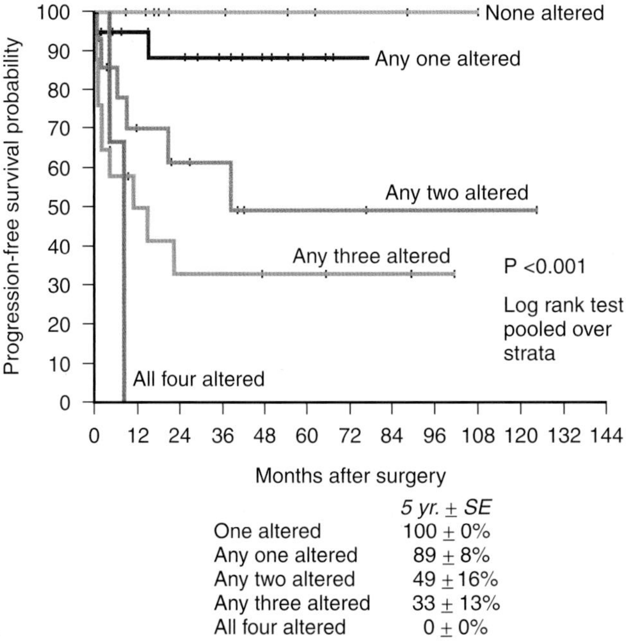

FIGURE 16.34 Synergistic prognostic role of immunohistochemical analysis of four markers (p53, p21, pRb, and p27) in superficial URCa. *(Data from Shariat SF, Ashfaq R, Sagalowsky AI, Lotan Y. Predictive value of cell cycle biomarkers in nonmuscle invasive bladder transitional cell carcinoma. J Urol. 2007;177:481.)*

markers altered. In turn, those with three altered markers did worse than patients with only two altered markers, who in turn had a lower DFS than those with only one marker alteration, as shown in Figure 16.34.[348]

A similar synergistic prognostic role of multiple molecular markers (p53, pRb, and p21) was also demonstrated by Chatterjee and colleagues[346] in patients undergoing cystectomy for invasive URCa using IHC technique.

It is expected, in the near future, that such an approach of prognostication will constitute a new standard of care in URCa patients' management once additional multi-institutional, preferably prospective, trials confirm the previously mentioned findings. An encouraging example is the recent bladder consortium–based multi-institutional trial that confirmed the role of proliferation index (as measured by Ki-67 on IHC) as a prognosticator in URCa.[351]

In the near future, the current clinicopathologic-based prognostic categorization approach will be supplemented by a molecular-based approach as shown in Tables 16.10 and 16.11, respectively.

From a targeted therapy perspective, RTK-HRAS-MAPK (superficial disease) and p53-pRb (muscle-invasive disease) pathogenic pathways, as well as angiogenesis pathway of the tumor microenvironment, offer tremendous new opportunities for future management of URCa. Phase II trials evaluating the role of tyrosine receptor kinase inhibitors (TKI) targeting EGFR with small molecules such as gefitinib and sorafenib or monoclonal antibodies (MoAb) such as cetuximab are under way. Other phase II trials are addressing the role of trastuzumab (Herceptin) (anti HER2 MoAb) and bevacizumab (anti VEGF MoAb) in URCa. Phase I trials testing the safety of p53 or Rb gene intravesical therapy are being evaluated. One strategy example is the intravesical introduction of a wild type p53–loaded, replication-deficient adenovirus (Ad5CMV-TP53) in an ambitious attempt to compensate for the loss of p53 function in invasive URCa.[352-356]

IMMUNOHISTOLOGY OF RENAL NEOPLASMS

Renal carcinoma continues to be a major cause of morbidity and mortality worldwide (Table 16.12). Last year, approximately 54,000 new renal tumor patients were diagnosed and 13,000 deaths were ascribed to renal cancer in the United States. Renal cell carcinoma (RCC) is the seventh most common neoplasm in American males and the ninth most common neoplasm in females. There is a twofold to threefold male predominance of RCC incidence but no obvious racial predilection. Recognized risk factors include tobacco smoking, obesity (body mass index >29 may double the risk of RCC) and acquired or hereditary polycystic diseases. The classic clinical presentation symptom triad of flank pain, hematuria, and palpable mass is no longer the

TABLE 16.10 Risk Categories of URCa According to Current Clincopathologic Parameters

Low (~30%) Recurrence Low (<5%) Progression	Mod-High (>60%) Recurrence Increased (5%-15%) Progression	High (>80%) Recurrence High (>30%) Progression
Low grade	Medium grade	High grade
Stage Ta (mucosal only)	Stage progression Tz to T1	Stage T1 (submucosal invasion)
No dysplasia	Dysplasia	CIS
Negative cytology	Abnormal cytology	Highly suspicious or positive cytology
Solitary	Multifocal	
Primary (first-time tumor)	Recurrent especially within 6 mo or multirecurrent	
Papillary configuration		Sessile-nodular configuration
Size <5 cm	Size >5 cm	
Short disease duration	Long (>4 yr) duration	Very long (>20 yr) duration
Certainty of complete resection	Uncertainty of complete resection	
No prior intravesical therapy	Failed prior intravesical therapy	Lymphovascular invasion

Data from O'Donnell MA. Advances in the management of superficial bladder cancer. *Semin Oncol.* 2007;34:85.

TABLE 16.11 Risk Categories of URCa According to New Molecular Markers

Low Recurrence	Moderate-High Recurrence	High Progression
Proliferation marker low (e.g., Ki-67)	Proliferation marker high, RAS mutation	
Normal DNA ploidy	Abnormal ploidy	Frank DNA aneuploidy
E-cadherin-positive		E-cadherin negative
p53-negative	p53-positive	p53-positive
RB-positive		RB-negative
p21-positive	p21-negative	p21-negative
p14/16-positive	p14/16-negative	
Low VEGF mRNA		High VEGF mRNA

Data from O'Donnell MA. Advances in the management of superficial bladder cancer. *Semin Oncol.* 2007;34:85.

leading form of presentation. Patient presentation as a result of RCC-associated paraneoplastic syndromes due to secreted parathyroid hormone, erythropoietin, prostaglandins, or ACTH is also unusual. This change in clinical presentation is mainly due to a marked increase in incidentally found, smaller RCC lesions during imaging studies performed for a variety of other causes.

The widespread adoption of partial nephrectomy procedures and the introduction of various forms of ablative treatment (cryoablation and radiofrequency ablation) have brought new challenges to the pathologist in terms of the need to render a diagnosis of RCC on small-needle biopsy or during intraoperative consultation. Additionally, the introduction of specific forms of targeted systemic therapy to certain classes of RCC has further emphasized the need for proper classification of RCC on needle biopsy material. Therefore the recent rise in interest in the utilization of ancillary techniques for the diagnosis of RCC comes as no surprise.

The following is a practical discussion of the current use of IHC markers in the diagnosis of RCC followed by exploration of the potential role of molecular markers in the prognostication and prediction of therapy response in this disease.

Biology of Principal Antibodies and Antigens

RENAL CELL CARCINOMA ANTIBODY

Renal cell carcinoma (RCC) antibody binds to a 200 kD glycoprotein (gp200) shown to be expressed in epithelial cells lining normal renal proximal tubule and renal carcinoma cells.[357] Several studies have established the utility of RCC in labeling clear cell and papillary variants of renal carcinoma.[358,359] Avery and colleagues[359] revealed membranous RCC reactivity in up to 85% of clear cell renal cell carcinoma (CCRCC). Almost all tested papillary renal cell carcinomas (PRCC) were also strongly positive for RCC. In contrast, chromophobe renal cell carcinomas (ChRCC) and oncocytomas were completely negative.

TABLE 16.12	Classification of Renal Epithelial Tumors (World Health Organization 2004)
Benign Epithelial Tumors	
Papillary adenoma	
Oncocytoma	
Metanephric adenoma	
Renal Cell Carcinoma	
Clear cell renal cell carcinoma (60%-80%)	
Multilocular cystic renal cell carcinoma	
Papillary renal cell carcinoma (10%-18%)	
Chromophobe renal cell carcinoma (2%-6%)	
Carcinoma of the collecting ducts of Bellini (<1%)	
Medullary carcinoma (<1%)	
Xp11 translocation carcinoma (<1%)	
Mucinous tubular and spindle cell carcinoma (<1%)	
Renal cell carcinoma, unclassified (<1%)	

Data from Eble JN, Sauter G, Epstein JI, Sesterhenn IA: The World Health Organization Classification of Tumours: Pathology and Genetics of Tumours of the Urinary System and Male Genital Organs. Lyon, France: IARC Press; 2004.

CD10

CD10 (common acute lymphocyte leukemia antigen, CALLA) is expressed on the brush border of renal tubular epithelial cells. In the previously cited study by Avery and colleagues,[359] CD10 demonstrated a similar profile to that of RCC antibody with 94% of CCRCC and the majority of PRCC studied showing positivity for CD10. A similar profile was encountered by Bazille and colleagues.[358] Variable CD10 staining has been reported in ChRCC with a negative staining[359] to almost 45% positive CD10 staining rate.[358-360] Around one third of oncocytomas stain positive for CD10.[360]

PAX2/PAX8

PAX2 and PAX8 are members of the paired box (PAX) gene family, which includes nine transcription factors (PAX1-9) involved in the development of several organ systems[361] by preventing terminal differentiation and maintaining a progenitor cell state while inducing cell-lineage commitment. Consequently, PAX gene expression is cell lineage–restricted. (PAX8 is expressed in thyroid, whereas PAX8 and PAX2 are expressed in Wolffian [nephric] ducts and Müllerian ducts.) PAX2 and PAX8 have also been detected in epithelial neoplasms arising in these areas, including renal cell and ovarian tumors.[362,363]

Immunohistochemical expression of PAX2 has been demonstrated in CCRCC, PRCC, and ChRCC subtypes, as well as collecting duct carcinoma and MTSC renal tumors.[364]

Gokden and colleagues[365] showed 85% metastatic CCRCCs had nuclear immunoreactivity for PAX2. The marker, however, is not entirely specific because one third of CCRCC mimics such as parathyroid carcinomas and ovarian clear cell carcinomas also expressed PAX2. Furthermore, PAX2 expression has been demonstrated in other genital tumors such as serous ovarian, endometrioid carcinoma, and epididymal tumors. PAX2 is a reliable marker for nephrogenic adenoma.[326]

PAX8 is structurally and functionally related to PAX2. PAX8 is also expressed in normal and neoplastic tissues of renal tubular cells origin. Immunohistochemical expression of PAX8 has been demonstrated in CCRCC, PRCC, and ChRCC subtypes, as well as collecting duct carcinoma, MTSC, and metastatic renal carcinomas (Fig. 16.35). Like PAX2, PAX8 expression has also been demonstrated in nephrogenic adenoma and clear cell adenocarcinoma of the lower urinary tract.[327] Furthermore, we have recently demonstrated a similar PAX8 expression profile to that of PAX2 in different types of RCC including collecting duct carcinoma.[366,367]

EpCAM

EpCAM, also known as KSA, KS1/4, and 17-1 antigen, is a 34- to 40-kDa glycosylated transmembrane cell surface epithelial protein of 232 amino acids.[368]

Recently, EpCAM has gained interest as a potential therapeutic target owing to its wide-spectrum expression in many epithelial malignancies.[369]

EpCAM is consistently expressed in the distal nephron on normal renal epithelium. Clear cell RCCs show minimal and infrequent EpCAM expression. Almost half of PRCCs are positive for EpCAM, whereas intense and frequent expression is the rule in ChRCC and collecting duct carcinoma.[370] A recent study by Liu and colleagues[360] confirmed the utility of EpCAM in differentiating granular variant of chromophobe renal cell carcinoma (ChRCC) from oncocytoma and CCRCC. EpCAM protein was expressed diffusely (>90% of cells) in all 22 cases of ChRCC analyzed, whereas less than one third of oncocytomas displayed positivity for EpCAM and only in single cells or small cell cluster distribution.[371] Combining EpCAM with other markers such as vimentin, GST-α, CD117, and CK7 can be of utility in resolving the differential diagnosis of ChRCC.

Ksp-CADHERIN

Cadherins are a large family of cell-cell adhesion molecules acting in a homotypic, homophilic manner that play an important role in the maintenance of tissue integrity. In the human kidney, several members of the cadherin family (including E- and N-cadherin, cadherin-6, cadherin-8, and cadherin-11) are expressed in a controlled spatiotemporal pattern. Cadherin-16, also called kidney-specific (Ksp-) cadherin, is exclusively expressed in epithelial cells of the adult kidney. In renal cell carcinomas (RCCs), a complex pattern of cadherin expression is observed.

Thedieck and colleagues[372] revealed loss of Ksp-cadherin in CCRCC. Ksp-cadherin was subsequently proposed to differentiate chromophobe RCC from oncocytoma. However, additional studies failed to reveal any

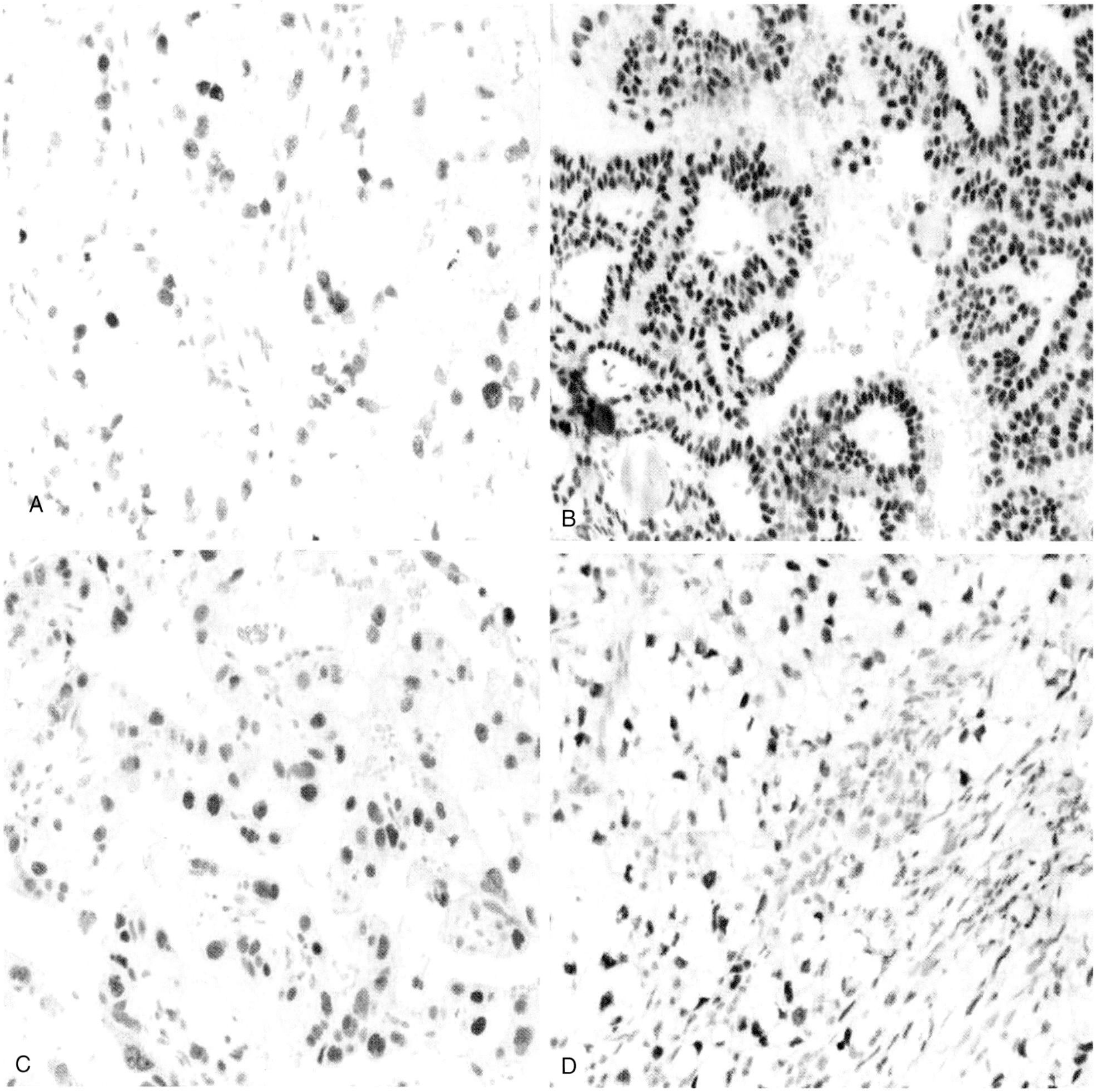

FIGURE 16.35 PAX8 immunoexpression in primary clear cell RCC **(A)**, papillary renal cell carcinoma **(B)**, chromophobe RCC **(C)**, and metastatic clear cell RCC **(D)**.

difference in Ksp-cadherin immunoreactivity between these two tumor types with one study showing Ksp-cadherin at the mRNA and protein levels in approximately 80% of chromophobe RCC and oncocytomas.[373]

CARBONIC ANHYDRASE IX

Carbonic anhydrase IX (CAIX) is an enzyme involved in maintaining intracellular and extracellular pH. In addition, CAIX plays a regulatory role in cell proliferation, oncogenesis, and tumor progression. CAIX expression is von Hippel-Lindau (vHL)-hypoxia inducible factor (HIF) pathway dependent. In normal renal epithelium, expression of CAIX is suppressed by wild type vHL protein. Given loss of vHL gene function in the majority of CCRCC tumors, carbonic anhydrase IX antigen overexpression ensues. Most IHC studies have used clone M75 as the primary CAIX antibody showing diffuse overexpression in CCRCC.[374,375] CAIX expression has also been demonstrated in almost half of PRCCs in a recent study by Gupta and colleagues,[375] whereas other studies including ours revealed only rare PRCC staining (Fig. 16.36).[376] Prognostically, low CAIX expression reportedly indicates poor survival and low response to interleukin therapy in CCRCC. A new commercially available antibody (clone NB100-417) was recently shown by Al Ahmadie and colleagues[374] to have a comparable expression profile. Although carbonic anhydrase IX is of utility in establishing a CCRCC origin of a metastatic carcinoma, it is not entirely specific because

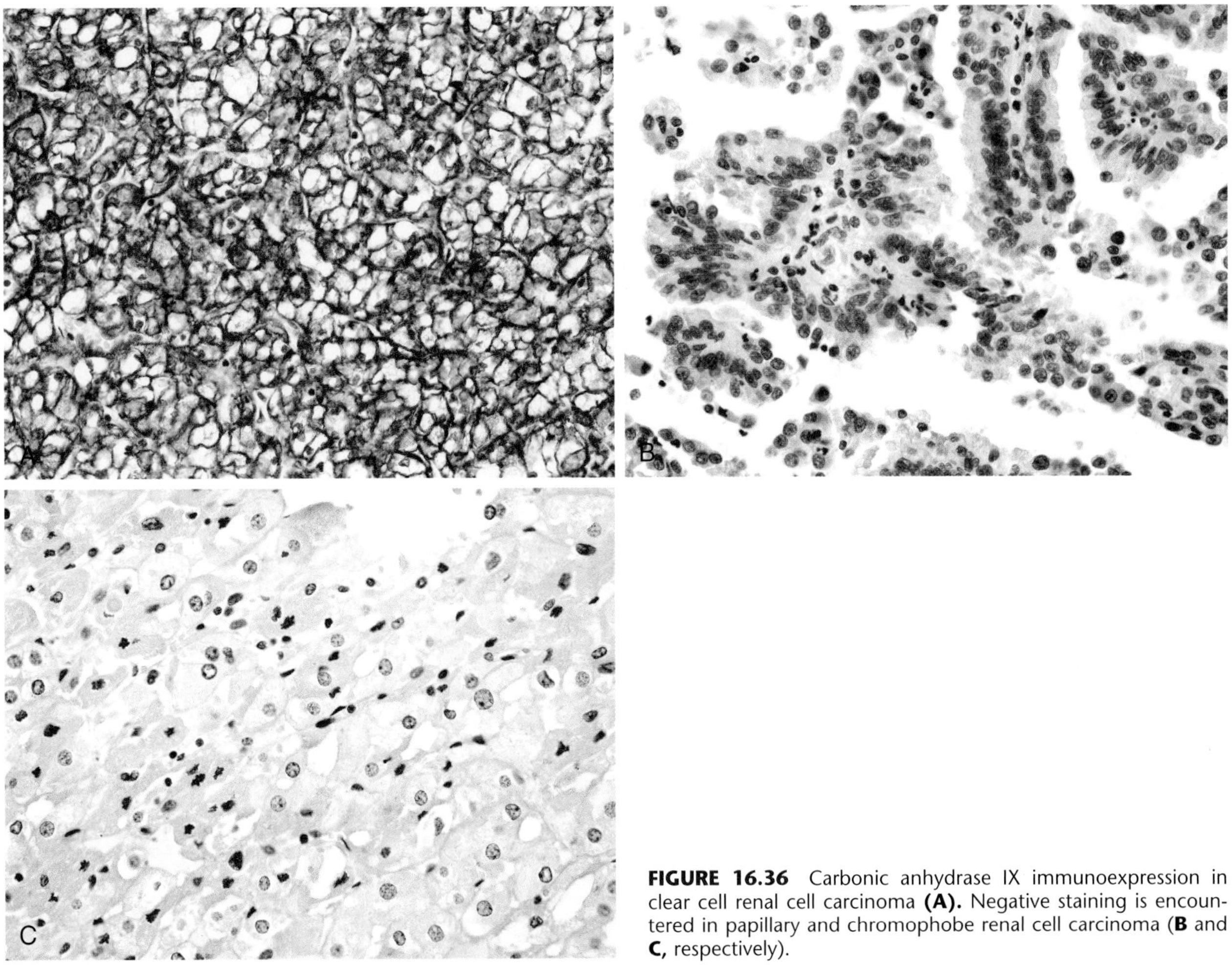

FIGURE 16.36 Carbonic anhydrase IX immunoexpression in clear cell renal cell carcinoma **(A)**. Negative staining is encountered in papillary and chromophobe renal cell carcinoma (**B** and **C**, respectively).

CAIX staining has been demonstrated in normal gastric mucosa and biliary ductules.[377]

GLUTATHIONE-TRANSFERASE-α

Glutathione-transferase alpha (GST-α) protects cells by catalyzing the detoxification of xenobiotics and carcinogens. GST-α was recently found to be of diagnostic value in renal tumors. On the basis of cDNA microarray findings, immunohistochemical studies have so far shown GST-α to be highly expressed in CCRCC (90%) but not in ChRCC or oncocytomas[360,378] and only occasionally in PRCC.

Immunohistology of Specific Renal Tumors

RENAL ONCOCYTOMA

Oncocytomas are benign renal neoplasms characterized by a typical gross mahogany-brown color. Microscopically, the tumor is composed of islands of "oncocytic" cells with coarsely granular eosinophilic cytoplasm set in a typical edematous myxoid focally hyalinized stroma.[379-382] Oncocytomas display round, vesicular, centrally located nuclei with conspicuous nucleoli and occasional marked nuclear polymorphism. A range of architectural features is encountered to include nested, tubular, acinar, cystic, and solid patterns. Variable rates of mitotic activity can be encountered. Areas of necrosis are not seen with the exception of commonly seen central degenerative ischemic change. The diagnosis of oncocytoma should be called into question if an "oncocytic" tumor reveals papillary architecture or areas of bona fide optically clear cytoplasm. An oncoblastic pattern is well recognized in some oncocytomas where the tumor cells become smaller in size with increased nuclear-to-cytoplasmic ratio. The latter does not carry any significant prognostic connotation.[380,381] A cautionary note is warranted when making a diagnosis of oncocytoma on limited material given that other types of renal neoplasms such as PRCC, ChRCC, and CCRCC can display focal "oncocytic" areas that share the granular cytoplasmic appearance of oncocytoma.

Immunohistochemically, oncocytomas are positive for pancytokeratin AE1/AE3 and low-molecular cytokeratin CAM5.2 and are negative for vimentin.[360] C-*kit* (CD117) expression is encountered in more than two thirds of oncocytomas, a feature also shared by chromophobe RCC.[360,383,384] Similarly, Ksp-cadherin is expressed in the majority of both ChRCC and oncocytoma tumors. Unlike chromophobe RCC, oncocytomas are negative for cytokeratin 7, which can be used to differentiate the two types of tumors. Oncocytoma is usually negative for RCC and only occasionally expresses antibody CD10.

Commonly encountered cytogenetic findings in oncocytomas include loss of chromosome Y and chromosome 1.[385-391]

KEY DIAGNOSTIC POINTS

Oncocytoma Immunohistology

- Positive: AE1/AE3, CAM5.2, CD117, Ksp-Cadherin, CD10 (sometimes positive)
- Negative: Vimentin, CAIX, CK7, EpCam, RCC
- Hale's colloidal iron with lumen staining

KEY DIAGNOSTIC POINTS

Renal Oncocytoma

Granular Variant of Chromophobe RCC
- Hale's colloidal iron stain+ in perinuclear location
- CK7+
- EpCam+
- Ksp-Cadherin+

"Oncocytic" Papillary RCC
- CK7+
- CD117−
- Vimentin+
- Ksp-Cadherin−

Clear Cell RCC
- Vimentin+
- CD10+
- RCC+
- CAIX+
- CD117−
- Ksp-Cadherin−

METANEPHRIC ADENOMA

Metanephric adenoma of the kidney is a unique form of renal adenoma characterized by a proliferation of tubular and micropapillary to glomeruloid structures lined by bland cuboidal epithelial cells. The relatively high nuclear-to-cytoplasmic ratio of metanephric adenoma cells and their slightly amphophilic cytoplasmic coloration impart a typical "blue" low-power appearance to the neoplastic nodule. The latter is in contrast to the lighter eosinophilic appearance of its main differential diagnosis entity, namely the solid variant of papillary RCC.[392-395] Like papillary RCC, metanephric adenoma can feature foamy histiocytes in papillary cores and occasional psammomatous calcifications. Helpful immunohistochemical features of the tumor are its positivity for WT1 and negative staining for EMA and CK7, a profile that contrasts with that of solid papillary RCC (WT1−, EMA+, and CK7+) (Fig. 16.37).[392-395]

CLEAR CELL RENAL CELL CARCINOMA

CCRCC is the most common type of renal cell carcinoma,[163] accounting for 70% to 80% of RCC. Microscopically, CCRCCs are composed of cuboidal cells with typical optically cleared cytoplasm arranged in nests, tubules, and acini. CCRCCs are richly vascularized tumors with areas of hemorrhage imparting a "bleeding acini" characteristic morphology. "Granular" RCCs with eosinophilic granular cytoplasm are no longer a unique variant and are included in the CCRCC variant. As discussed later, at the genetic level, similar to their familial counterpart,[396] almost two thirds of sporadic CCRCCs demonstrate partial or complete chromosome 3 loss or mutation on the short arm of chromosome 3p, resulting in the loss of the vHL tumor suppressor gene located at 3p25-26.[163,396] Table 16.13 summarizes the immunohistochemical profile of CCRCC.[380,394,397,398]

KEY DIAGNOSTIC POINTS

Clear Cell Renal Cell Carcinoma

Adrenocortical Carcinoma
- Inhibin+
- Calretinin+
- Epithelial membrane antigen (EMA)−
- CK, AE1/AE3−, CAM 5.2−
- CD10+/−
- RCC−
- Synaptophysin (sometimes positive)

Urothelial Carcinoma of the Renal Pelvis
- HMWCK+
- Cytokeratin 7+
- Cytokeratin 20+
- Uroplakin+
- Thrombomodulin+
- p63+
- Vimentin−

Papillary Renal Cell Carcinoma
- CAIX−
- α-Methyl-CoA-acetyl racemase+
- CK7+

Chromophobe Carcinoma
- Hale's colloidal iron stain perinuclear+
- CD117+
- Cytokeratin 7+
- Vimentin−
- EpCAM+, Ksp-Cadherin+

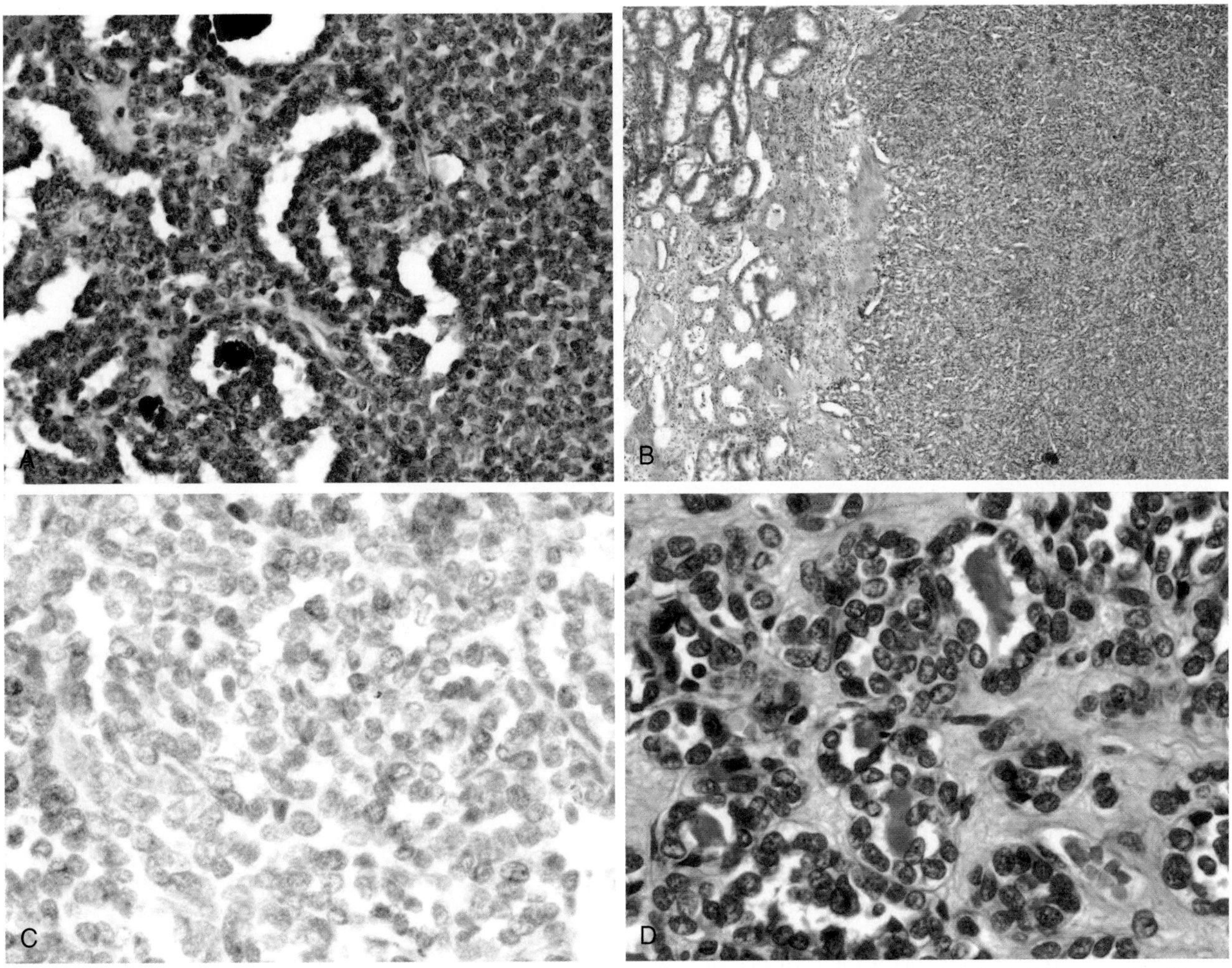

FIGURE 16.37 Metanephric adenoma (**A** and **B**) showing positive nuclear staining for WT1 **(C)** with lack of CK7 expression **(D)**.

TABLE 16.13 Immunohistology of Clear Cell Renal Cell Carcinoma

Positive	Negative
CAM5.2	HMWCK
AE1/AE3	CK7
EMA	CK20
Vimentin	CEA
CAIX	
CD10	
PAX2	
PAX8	

Clear cell RCC is usually positive for low-molecular-weight cytokeratin (LMWCK) such as CAM5.2, cytokeratin 18. CCRCCs are also positive for cytokeratins AE1/AE3 but negative for CK7 and CK20. They are positive for EMA and vimentin.[394,398] Their negative reactivity for high-molecular-weight cytokeratins (HMWCK) such as cytokeratin CK5/6, 34βE12, or CK903 and for p63 are useful features in their differential against upper urinary tract urothelial carcinoma (regularly HMWCK and p63 positive).[394,398]

Of note is that the range of CCRCC reactivity with many of the previously mentioned markers varied among studies, making it necessary to exercise a judicial interpretation of any IHC panel when classifying a renal tumor. Therefore IHC results should always be integrated with the overall morphologic features of a given renal neoplasm.

PAPILLARY RENAL CELL CARCINOMA

Papillary renal cell carcinoma (PRCC) is the second most common subtype of RCC. Microscopically, this subtype of RCC contains characteristic complex papillary formations often accompanied by foamy macrophages infiltrating the fibrovascular cores. Two subtypes of PRCC are recognized: (1) type 1, in which the papillae are lined by a single layer of cells with scant pale cytoplasm and (2) type 2, in which the papillae are lined by pseudostratified cuboidal to columnar epithelial cells with abundant eosinophilic cytoplasm and prominent eosinophilic nucleoli.[399-403] Type 1 tumors are usually of lower Fuhrman nuclear grade and are associated with a more favorable prognosis than type 2 tumors. A solid variant of PRCC

TABLE 16.14	Immunohistology of Papillary Renal Cell Carcinoma
Cytokeratin AE1/A3+	
CAM5.2+	
CK7+	
Vimentin+	
HMWCK–	
AMACR+	
Ulex europaeus lectin–	
CAIX–/+ (sometimes)	
EMA+	
Differential Diagnosis	
Collecting duct carcinoma	
Mucin+	
HMWCK+	
Metanephric adenoma	
EMA–	
WT1+	
CK7–	

AMACR, α-methylacyl coenzyme A racemase; EMA, epithelial membrane antigen; HMWCK, high-molecular-weight cytokeratin.

is well recognized where distinct papillary structures are not easily discernable. Glomeruloid structures and overall cytologic features, together with the presence of typical host infiltrating histiocytes, can point to the diagnosis. As mentioned earlier, the solid variant of PRCC brings up the differential diagnosis of metanephric adenoma. Commonly encountered cytogenetic alterations in RCC include trisomy of chromosomes 7, 17, 3q, 8, 16, and 20 and loss of Y chromosome.[404-406] A subset of sporadic PRCC (12%) exhibits c-met oncogene mutations similar to their familial counterparts in hereditary papillary renal cell carcinoma syndrome (HPRCC).[396] Immunohistochemically,[380,403] the majority of PRCCs are positive for AE1/AE3, vimentin, RCC, and AMACR.[407] Differential EMA immunostaining was found to be useful in differentiating type 1 and type 2 tumors, with polarized expression in type 1 and only rare expression in type 2 (Table 16.14).[399,400]

CHROMOPHOBE RENAL CELL CARCINOMA

Chromophobe renal cell carcinoma (ChromRCC) is composed of characteristic large polygonal cells with cleared to lightly eosinophilic reticulated cytoplasm and distinct "plantlike" cell membranes. Typical perinuclear halos are a unique feature in this type of RCC. Another helpful diagnostic feature is their diffuse cytoplasmic staining with Hale's iron stain. Cytogenetically, ChromRCCs are hypodiploid tumors owing to a commonly present loss of chromosomes 1, 2, 6, 10, 13, 17, and 21 as shown by fluorescence *in situ* hybridization and comparative genomic hybridization analysis.[388-391,408,409]

Ultrastructural and immunohistochemical features of ChromRCC point to differentiation toward the intercalated cells of renal collecting ducts (Table 16.15).[163,358-360,362,383,384,394,410-416]

COLLECTING DUCT CARCINOMA

Collecting duct carcinoma (CDC) of the kidney is a rare but aggressive type of RCC with presumed origin from Bellini's collecting ducts. Previously reported cases of "low-grade collecting duct carcinoma" have been reclassified as mucinous tubular and spindle cell carcinoma (MTSC).

CDC is typically centered in the medulla of the kidney and extends into the cortex. Histologic patterns include tubulopapillary, tubular, solid, and sarcomatoid types. Prominent stromal desmoplasia, angiolymphatic invasion, and host inflammatory response are commonly found. Associated "dysplastic" changes in entrapped non-neoplastic collecting ducts and the presence of intracytoplasmic or luminal mucin secretions in neoplastic glands are also helpful diagnostic features of this type of RCC. Cytogenetic features include loss of chromosome 8p and chromosome 13. Monosomy of chromosomes 1, 6, 14, 15, and 22 are also observed.[386-389]

CDC immunoprofile is that of positive reactivity with pancytokeratins (AE1/AE3), (CAM5.2), and high-molecular-weight keratin (CK19 and 34βE12) (Table 16.16). CDCs are positive for EMA, vimentin, and the lectin *Ulex europaeus* Agglutinin (UEA-1). The diagnosis of CDC carries a poor prognosis with the majority of patients dying of metastatic disease within 2 years of presentation.[358,382,387,394,398,417,418] Recently, we found the combination of PAX8+/p63– phenotype in CDC to be helpful in distinguishing them from URCa of renal pelvis (Fig. 16.38).[367]

MUCINOUS TUBULAR AND SPINDLE CELL CARCINOMA

Mucinous tubular and spindle cell carcinoma (MTSC) is one of the latest types of RCC to be recognized as a distinct variant. Before characterization of MTSC, such tumors were most likely classified as either sarcomatoid variant of RCC or "low-grade CDC."

MTSCs are composed of uniform cuboidal to spindle cells with eosinophilic, focally vacuolated cytoplasm and relatively bland ovoid nuclei. Tumor cells generally form interconnecting tubules with smaller areas of solid growth. The myxoid stroma is a distinguishing feature with mucoid material deposits at times appearing as secretions within tubular or intercellular spaces.

Cytogenetically MTSCs show multiple chromosomal losses (1, –4, –6, –8, –9, –13, –14, –15, and –22). Differentiation toward loop of Henle, distal convoluted tubule, or collecting ducts has been suggested by their overall immunoprofile and ultrastructural features.

MTSCs are low-grade tumors in terms of their biologic behavior with occasional recurrence on record but no known distant metastases or death reported.[419-425] Their relatively good prognosis highlights the importance

TABLE 16.15	Chromophobe Renal Cell Carcinoma: Immunohistochemical Profile
Immunohistochemistry	
Vimentin–	
LMWCK (CAM5.2)+	
Cytokeratin AE1/3+	
Cytokeratin 7+	
HMWCK –/+ (sometimes)	
CD10–	
RCC–	
EMA+	
Parvalbumin+	
CD117+	
Alcian blue+	
EpCAM+	
Ksp-Cadherin+	
Hale's colloidal iron stain+	
Differential Diagnosis	
Oncocytoma	
Cytokeratin 7–	
EpCAM–	
Hale's colloidal iron stain–	
Clear cell renal cell carcinoma	
Vimentin+	
RCC+	
CD10+	
CD117–	
CAIX+	
Hale's colloidal iron stain–	

EMA, epithelial membrane antigen; HMWCK, high-molecular-weight cytokeratin; LMWCK, low-molecular-weight cytokeratin.

TABLE 16.16	Immunohistology of Collecting Duct Carcinoma
Immunohistochemistry	
Vimentin+	
EMA+	
UEA-1+	
CAM5.2+	
AE1/AE3+	
HMWCK+	
Mucin+	
PAX8+	
Differential Diagnosis	
Papillary renal cell carcinoma	
UAE–	
HMWCK–	
Urothelial carcinoma of the renal pelvis	
Vimentin–	
p63+	
Uroplakin+	
Thrombomodulin+	
PAX8–	
HMWCK+	

EMA, epithelial membrane antigen; HMWCK, high-molecular-weight cytokeratin; LMWCK, low-molecular-weight cytokeratin.

of distinguishing these "spindle cell" variants of RCC from the aggressive lethal sarcomatoid phenotype.

Mucinous tubular and spindle cell carcinoma is typically positive for vimentin, CK7, AMACR, and EMA but negative for high-molecular-weight cytokeratin, CD10, and RCC. The presence of some morphologic and immunohistochemical similarities[424] between MTSC and a solid variant of PRCC have led some to suggest a histogenetic relationship between the two subtypes of RCC; however, their distinct cytogenetic and gene expression profile argues against such a relationship (Table 16.17).[408,426]

ANGIOMYOLIPOMA

An angiomyolipoma is a member of the group of tumors containing perivascular epithelioid cells (PECs) referred to as PEComas. Oncogenesis in PEComas is related to the genetic alterations of tuberous sclerosis complex (TSC). Tuberous sclerosis is an autosomal dominant genetic disease owing to losses of TSC1 (9q34) or TSC2 (16p13.3) genes that are involved in the regulation of the Rheb/mTOR/p70S6K pathway. PEComas of the kidney include "classic" angiomyolipoma (AML) and its recognized cystic, epithelioid, and oncocytoma-like variants.[163,427]

"Classic" AMLs are the most common mesenchymal tumors of the kidney. They are composed of variable proportions of adipose cells and spindle and epithelioid smooth muscle cells admixed with and at times appearing to emanate from abnormal thick-walled blood vessels (Fig. 16.39). In patients with TSC, multiple bilateral renal AMLs are found during the third and fourth decades of life. Sporadic AMLs are larger single lesions occurring in older patients.[163]

The epithelioid variant of AML is composed of polygonal epithelioid cells arranged in sheets and usually lacking fat tissue component. Epithelioid AMLs are reactive with HMB45, melan A, tyrosinase and microphthalmia transcription factor, and smooth muscle markers (α-smooth muscle-specific actin). They are negative for epithelial markers including cytokeratins and epithelial membrane antigen. Tumor cells are clear to eosinophilic with at times considerable nuclear atypia and associated necrosis. Epithelioid AMLs have been associated with recurrence and metastasis. However, it

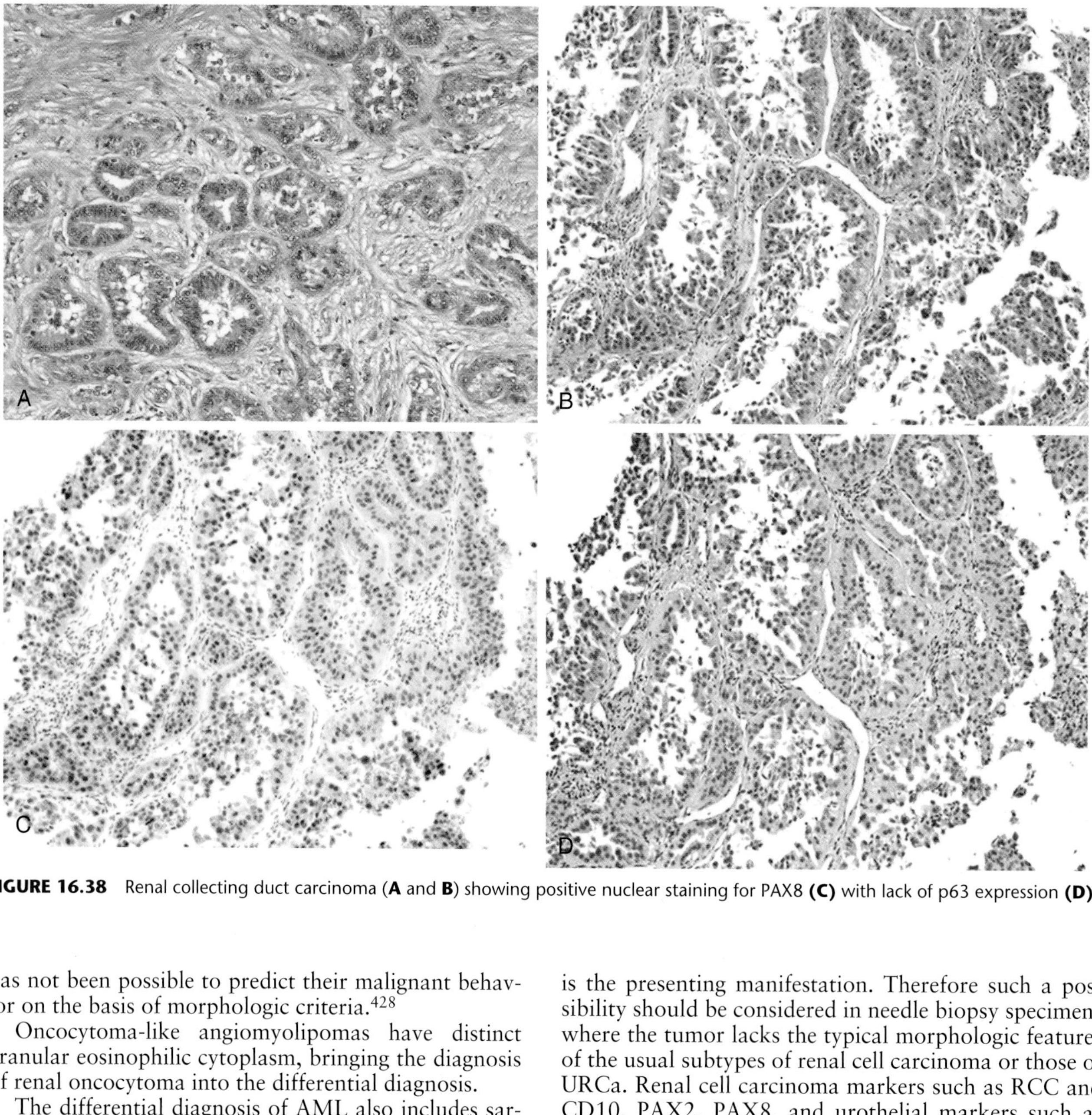

FIGURE 16.38 Renal collecting duct carcinoma (**A** and **B**) showing positive nuclear staining for PAX8 **(C)** with lack of p63 expression **(D)**.

has not been possible to predict their malignant behavior on the basis of morphologic criteria.[428]

Oncocytoma-like angiomyolipomas have distinct granular eosinophilic cytoplasm, bringing the diagnosis of renal oncocytoma into the differential diagnosis.

The differential diagnosis of AML also includes sarcomatoid RCC. This is especially the case with epithelioid AML with significant cytologic atypia. Expression of melanocytic markers and lack of epithelial markers in AML will help differentiate it from sarcomatoid RCC. Rarely, Xp11 translocation carcinoma can enter the differential diagnosis of epithelioid AML. In this regard, expression of some melanocytic markers (HMB45 and Melan A) in rare Xp11 translocation carcinoma should be kept in mind. Positive TFE3 reaction is unique to Xp11 translocation carcinomas (Table 16.18).[429-431]

SECONDARY TUMORS OF KIDNEY

Metastases to the kidney usually occur as part of a widespread dissemination. Renal involvement is frequently bilateral and in a multinodular fashion. Primary carcinoma sources include lung, melanoma, and contralateral kidney and GI tract.[163] Rarely, metastasis to kidney is the presenting manifestation. Therefore such a possibility should be considered in needle biopsy specimens where the tumor lacks the typical morphologic features of the usual subtypes of renal cell carcinoma or those of URCa. Renal cell carcinoma markers such as RCC and CD10, PAX2, PAX8, and urothelial markers such as uroplakin and thrombomodulin can be of some utility only when combined with other tissue lineage–specific markers such as TTF-1 (lung and thyroid) and melanoma markers.

Genomic and Theranostic Applications

Renal tumors are unique among human neoplasms in terms of the tight correlation between their different morphologic phenotypes and underlying genetic alterations. Lessons learned from the relatively rare familial renal cancer syndromes have helped unlock the complex molecular oncogenic mechanisms involved in their sporadic counterparts. As a result, many potential new targets of therapy are now under investigation in the hereto unsuccessful endeavor of treating advanced RCC. The

TABLE 16-17 Immunohistology of MTSC
Immunohistochemistry
CK7+
EMA+
HMWCK–
AMACR+
Vimentin+
Alcian blue+
RCC–
CD10–
Differential Diagnosis
Papillary renal cell carcinoma
CD10+
RCC +
CK7+
EMA+
AMACR+
HMWCK–
Vimentin+

AMACR, α-methylacyl coenzyme A racemase; EMA, epithelial membrane antigen; HMWCK, high-molecular-weight cytokeratin.

following discussion of the molecular basis of von Hippel-Lindau disease (VHL) best illustrates the great therapeutic and theranostic potentials of uncovering the molecular mechanisms of renal oncogenesis.[432]

VHL syndrome is a rare autosomal-dominant familial cancer syndrome (retinal angiomas, hemangioblastomas, pheochromocytomas, CCRCC). VHL syndrome patients are born with a germline VHL mutation affecting all their cellular elements. Inactivation or silencing of the remaining wild-type allele in renal location assists the formation of CCRCC in VHL patients. The fact that similar defects in VHL genes are found to be responsible for approximately 60% of sporadic CCRCC [396,433] greatly widened the implication of our understanding of the molecular mechanisms of VHL inactivation.

VHL can be thought of as a cellular oxygen sensor. Under normoxic conditions, HIF1-α is inhibited by normal VHL protein that assists elimination of HIF1-α.[434] Under hypoxic condition, HIF1-α escapes destruction by VHL and is allowed to exert its crucial role in inducing angiogenesis factors (VEGF), cell growth factors (TGF-α and β), and factors involved in glucose uptake and acid-base balance (GLUT-1 and CAIX, respectively). A defective VHL function in CCRCC leads to abnormal accumulation of HIF1-α even under normal conditions, in turn resulting in the overexpression of the above proteins that are normally inducible only during hypoxia. The overexpressed VEGF, PDGF-B, and TGF-β act on neighboring vascular cells to promote tumor angiogenesis. The augmented tumor vasculature provides additional nutrients and oxygen to promote the growth of tumor cells. Furthermore, TGF-α acts in an autocrine manner on the tumor cells by signaling through the epidermal growth factor receptor, which promotes tumor-cell proliferation and survival.

Several of the above proteins are currently being investigated as targets of therapy for advanced CCRCC.[435-440] A randomized phase 2 trial involving patients with metastatic CCRCC investigated the efficacy of bevacizumab, a humanized anti-VEGF antibody.[441] Although the treatment resulted in only a few months' extension in time to tumor progression, it provided a key "proof of principle" of the efficacy of antiangiogenic therapy. Inhibitors of VEGF receptor tyrosine kinase activity alone and in combination with other tyrosine kinases are also under study. Multitargeted kinase inhibitors sunitinib and sorafenib have shown great promise in phase 2 and phase 3 trials, with at least stabilization of disease in up to 70% of patients with cytokine-refractory disease.

Another growth factor target is TGF-α, which promotes RCC growth through its interaction with EGFR. A human monoclonal antibody against human EGFR (panitumumab [ABX-EGF]), as well as small-molecule inhibitors of the EGFR tyrosine kinase activity (gefitinib and erlotinib), are two strategies being tested to target the TGF-α/EGFR axis.[436,438-440]

Other options being pursued include the use of temsirolimus (CCI-779), a selective inhibitor of the mammalian target of rapamycin. Partial responses were noted in 7% of patients, and minor responses in 26%. The median survival rate was 15 months. The notable activity of the drug in patients with poor prognostic features prompted a phase 3 trial.[437,442]

Finally, agents targeting HIF1-α and CAIX including anti-CAIX radiolabeled monoclonal antibody are also under development.[396,443]

Beyond Immunohistochemistry: Anatomic Molecular Diagnostic Applications

Current established prognostic parameters in RCC include pTNM stage, Fuhrman grade, histologic subtype, and clinical parameters such as ECOG performance status, hemoglobin level, and LDH levels.[382,444,445] Continuous refinements of staging criteria and development of nomograms to integrate the previously mentioned factors promise to yield better prognostic and management discriminators.[446]

A large number of biomarkers are under current intense investigation for their potential utility as prognosticators and/or therapy predictors in RCC.[446-453] Table 16.19 lists some of these markers. Kim and colleagues[448] evaluated a set of immunohistochemical markers including Ki-67, CAIX, CAXII, p53, PTEN, gelsolin, EpCAM, and vimentin in combination with established parameters. Their study suggested a new combined molecular and clinicopathologic prognostic model (CAIX, vimentin, p53, pTNM, ECOG—performance status) to be superior to prior models of clinical and pathologic parameters alone including the commonly used UISS clinical model.

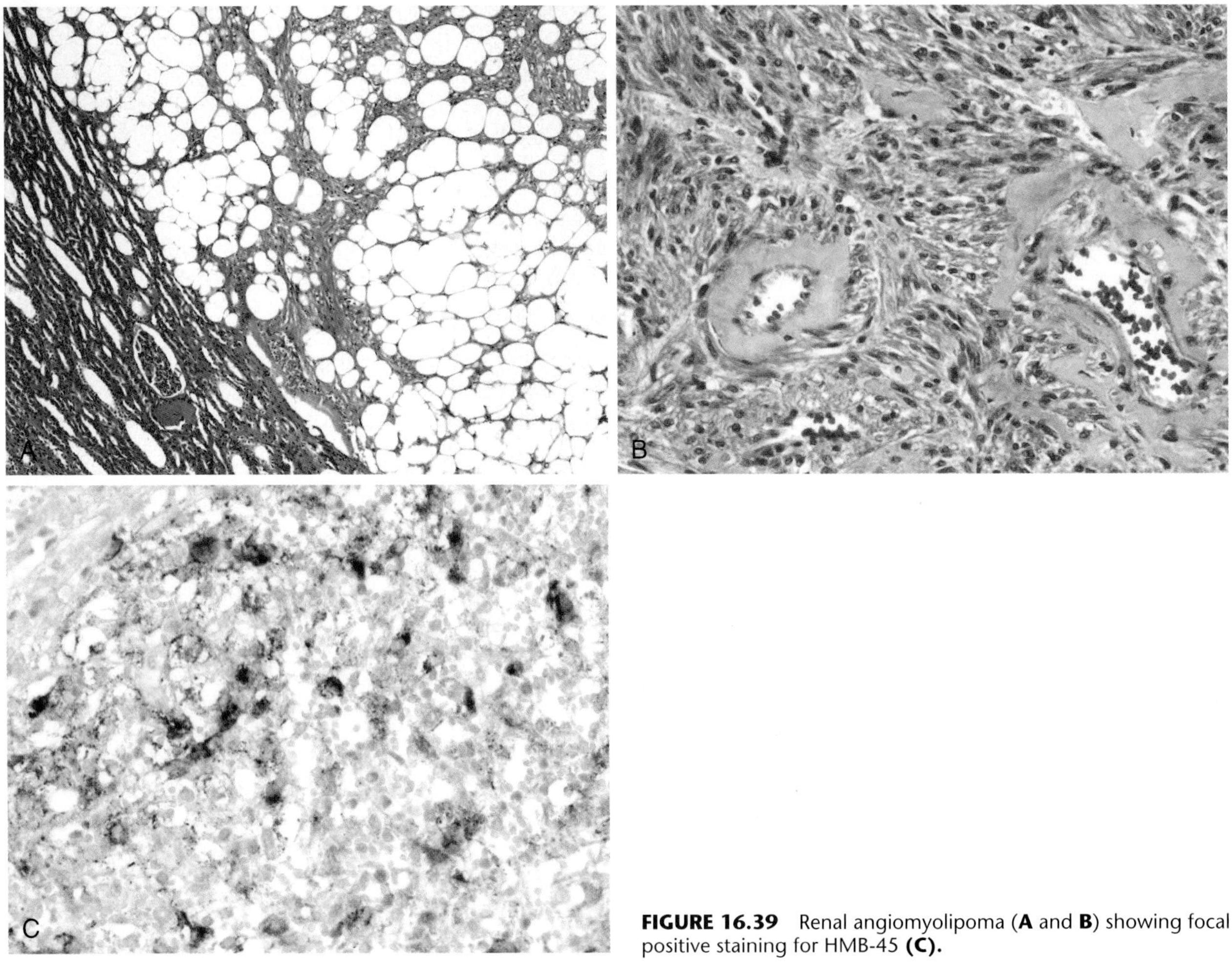

FIGURE 16.39 Renal angiomyolipoma (**A** and **B**) showing focal positive staining for HMB-45 **(C)**.

A promising prognostic role for mTOR pathway members was recently pointed to by Pantuck and colleagues.[454,455] Their study revealed an independent negative prognostic role for PTEN loss and pS6k overexpression. The same study showed increases in pAKT cytoplasmic expression and loss of pAKT nuclear expression to be negative predictors of survival.

A prognostic role for angiogenesis pathway is illustrated in RCC. Bui and colleagues[456] demonstrated that both low expression of CAIX and high Ki-67 proliferation index were independent negative predictors of survival in CCRCC. Interestingly, CAIX overexpression predicted response to IL2 immune therapy in metastatic RCC, a finding also documented in the study by Atkins and colleagues.[442] In another study by Jacobsen and colleagues,[457] VEGF expression appeared to correlate with tumor size and pTNM stage in RCC. The authors found high VEGF expression to be a negative survival prognosticator on univariate but not multivariate analysis. Separately, Kluger and colleagues[449] analyzed tissue microarrays containing 330 CCRCCs and PRCCs using a novel method of automated quantitative analysis of VEGF and VEGF-R expression by fluorescent immunohistochemistry. Unsupervised hierarchical clustering classified tumors by coordinated expression of VEGF and VEGF-Rs. The authors found high expression of VEGF and VEGF-Rs in tumor cells to be associated with poor survival. Finally, a study by Lidgren and colleagues[458] revealed high expression of HIF1-α to be an independent negative prognosticator in CCRCC.

Among cell cycle control molecules, p27 (Kip1) and cyclin D1 appear to have a promising prognostic role in CCRCC. Migita and colleagues[459] found loss of p27 expression to be an independent predictor of poor disease-specific survival. Similar p27 findings were also documented by Hedberg and colleagues.[460,461]

IMMUNOHISTOLOGY OF TESTICULAR TUMORS

Testicular germ-cell tumors (GCTs) are the most common malignancy in men 15 to 44 years of age. In 2008 approximately 500,000 cases were diagnosed worldwide and 8,090 cases were diagnosed in the United States alone. GCT incidence increases after puberty and peaks in the third decade of life. A significant geographic variation in GCT risk is observed—the lifetime risk is estimated to be 0.4% to 0.7% in U.S.-born males and 1% in Nordic European regions, whereas risk is lowest in Asia and the Caribbean. A puzzling steep increase in

TABLE 16.18	Immunohistology of Angiomyolipoma
Immunohistochemistry	
HMB-45+	
Melan-A+	
miTF+	
α-smooth muscle actin+	
Desmin+	
EMA–	
Pancytokeratins–	
RCC–	
CD10–	
PAX2–/PAX8–	
Differential Diagnosis	
Sarcomatoid RCC	
AE1/3+	
CAM5.2+	
CD10+	
RCC+	
EMA+	
α-smooth muscle actin+/–	
Desmin–	
HMB-45–	
Melan-A–	
miTF–	

TABLE 16.19	Current and Future Prognostic Parameters in Renal Cell Carcinoma
Current Prognostic Parameters	
• *Patient factors:* age and gender	
• *Anatomic factors:* pTNM	
• *Histologic factors:* histologic type; Fuhrman grade	
• *Clinical factors:* ECOG performance status, Hgb level, LDH, etc.	
Future Molecular Parameters	
Prediction of Behavior & Prediction/Guidance of Rx	
Hypoxia inducible	
• HIF-1	
• CAIX	
• CAXII	
• CXCR4	
• VEGF/VEGFR-R	
• ILGF1	
Cell adhesion markers	
• EpCAM	
• E-Cadherin	
• A-Catenin	
• Catenin-6	
Proliferation markers	
• Ki-67	
• MCM2	
Cell cycle regulators	
• Cyclin	
• p27	
Apoptosis regulators	
• p53	
• bcl-2	
• Smac/DIABLO	
mTOR pathway	
• PTEN	
• akt	
• pS6k	

incidence in the United States and Northern Europe has been observed up to 2007.

The great advances in our understanding of the biology of GCT and the unparalleled strides in refining the treatment of this group of testicular tumors are among the great success stories in oncologic diseases because only 380 deaths caused by GCT were recorded in the United States in 2008.[258]

Biology of Principal Antigens and Antibodies

OCT4

Among several new markers of GCT, OCT4 is probably of the greatest utility given its great degree of sensitivity and specificity.[462-465] OCT4, also referred to as OCT3/4, OTF3, and POU5F1, is a stem cell transcriptional regulator mapped to chromosome 6p21.3 locus. OCT4 maintains pluripotency in embryonic stem cells and germ cells.[466] As originally demonstrated by Jones and colleagues, OCT4 is a sensitive and specific marker of seminoma and embryonal carcinoma.[467] In their analysis of 91 primary testicular neoplasms, the authors found OCT4 to be expressed in all 51 tested classic seminomas and 53 of 54 embryonal carcinomas (98%). OCT4 staining was diffuse in distribution and nuclear in pattern. Equally important was the finding that none of the tested somatic carcinomas was positive for OCT4 expression. A separate study by the same group also established a great sensitivity of OCT4 for intratubular germ cell neoplasia, unclassified (IGCNU).[468]

CD117 (C-*KIT*)

C-*kit* is a transmembrane glycoprotein receptor tyrosine kinase with homologies to the platelet-derived growth factor (PDGF) and granulocyte-macrophage colony-stimulating factor (GM-CSF) receptors. Intact signal transduction by c-*kit* is crucial for the development and survival of germ cells, hematopoietic stem cells, melanocytes, mast cells, and interstitial cells of Cajal, making it a recent favorite target of molecular therapy. Nikolaou and colleagues[473] revealed CD117 staining (membranous and or cytoplasmic) in 77% of analyzed seminomas and almost 50% of teratomas.

Several studies have demonstrated activating c-*kit* mutations (codons 11 and 17) in seminomas with contradictory conclusions in regard to its association with incidence risk of bilateral seminomas.[469-474]

PODOPLANIN (D2-40/M2A)

Podoplanin is an oncofetal transmembrane mucoprotein expressed by fetal germ cells and testicular GCTs. Monoclonal Ab D2-40 labels podoplanin in a membranous staining pattern. Excellent sensitivity for IGCNU and seminoma including a diffuse staining in metastatic/extratesticular sites has been demonstrated. However, D2-40 has a lower sensitivity for nonseminomatous GCT and will also mark nontesticular neoplasms of lymphatic and vascular endothelial origin and epithelioid mesothelioma.[465]

ACTIVATOR PROTEIN—2γ (Ap-2γ)

This nuclear transcription factor is involved in embryonic morphogenesis and is functionally related to c-*kit* and placental alkaline phosphatase (PLAP) expression. Nuclear staining is demonstrated in IGCNU and seminoma with a high degree of sensitivity. Positivity in nonseminomatous GCT is of lower sensitivity and, like podoplanin, activator protein-2G is also expressed in nontesticular neoplasms such as somatic malignant melanoma and mammary and ovarian carcinomas.[463,464,476-478]

PLACENTA-LIKE ALKALINE PHOSPHATASE

Human alkaline phosphatase activity results from three genetically distinct isoenzymes produced in tissues such as liver, bone, intestine, and placenta.

The placental fraction of alkaline phosphatase is a membrane-bound enzyme of 120 kD, normally synthesized by placental syncytiotrophoblasts and released into maternal circulation after the 12th week of pregnancy. However, it is also produced by many neoplasms and is a useful tumor marker. Physiologically, this enzyme is involved in cellular transport, proliferation and cellular differentiation, and regulation of metabolism and gene transcription.

Despite its common use as a germ cell marker, placenta-like alkaline phosphatase (PLAP) lacks specificity for GCTs and is expressed in gastrointestinal, gynecologic, lung, breast, and urologic tumors among others. Among GCTs, IGCNU, seminoma, and embryonal carcinoma are almost uniformly (>97%) positive for PLAP, whereas a lower rate of positivity is reported with yolk sac tumors (YSTs, 85%), choriocarcinoma, and teratomas (up to 50% positivity rates). PLAP staining pattern is membranous and cytoplasmic.

Normal seminiferous tubules lack PLAP expression, a fact that is exploited in illustration of IGCNU in testicular biopsies from cryptorchid testis, contralateral testis of a germ cell neoplasm, and infertility biopsies.[479,480]

α-FETOPROTEIN

α-Fetoprotein (AFP), a fetal serum protein normally produced by fetal yolk sac, liver, and gastrointestinal epithelium, is elevated in up to 75% of patients with nonseminomatous germ cell tumors (NSGCT) and is expressed by both embryonal carcinoma (ECa) and YST but not pure seminomatous GCT.

Among non-GCTs, AFP is a sensitive serum marker for the diagnosis and surveillance of hepatocellular carcinoma. However, immunohistochemical expression of AFP in HCC tissue is limited to a minority of cases.[163]

HUMAN CHORIONIC GONADOTROPIN

Human chorionic gonadotropin (hCG) is a 37-kD glycoprotein. hCG-β Subunit is synthesized by benign and malignant syncytiotrophoblasts. As a serum marker, β-hCG serves an important role in the diagnosis, staging, therapeutic monitoring, and follow-up of patients with gestational trophoblastic disease and NSGCT testicular tumors. Serum β-hCG is elevated in a majority of the cases of choriocarcinoma (50% to 90%) and in up to 10% of patients with seminoma. In GCTs other than choriocarcinoma, b-hCG is expressed immunohistochemically by associated syncytiotrophoblastic giant cells.[163,481]

HUMAN PLACENTAL LACTOGEN

Human placental lactogen (HPL) is a 22-kD protein with partial homology to growth hormone. HPL is secreted by syncytiotrophoblastic cells in choriocarcinoma and intermediate trophoblasts in a testicular trophoblastic tumor that is a counterpart to a uterine placental site trophoblastic tumor.[481]

INHIBIN A

Inhibin is a 32-kD dimeric (α and β subunits) glycoprotein produced by ovarian granulosa cells, testicular Sertoli cells, and, to a lesser degree, testicular Leydig cells. It inhibits the release of follicle-stimulating hormone from the pituitary-inhibiting folliculogenesis. Inhibin A is a sensitive immunohistochemical marker of ovarian and testicular sex cord-stromal tumors including Leydig cell and Sertoli cell tumors (66% to 90% strong cytoplasmic positivity rate).[482,483] In nontesticular tumors, inhibin A labels benign and malignant adrenal neoplasms while being negative in other carcinomas, melanoma, and hematologic neoplasms. Although not expressed by seminoma cells, a cautionary note is warranted in regard to its expression by accompanying syncytiotrophoblasts.

In fact, inhibin A is a useful immunohistochemical marker for intermediate trophoblasts and

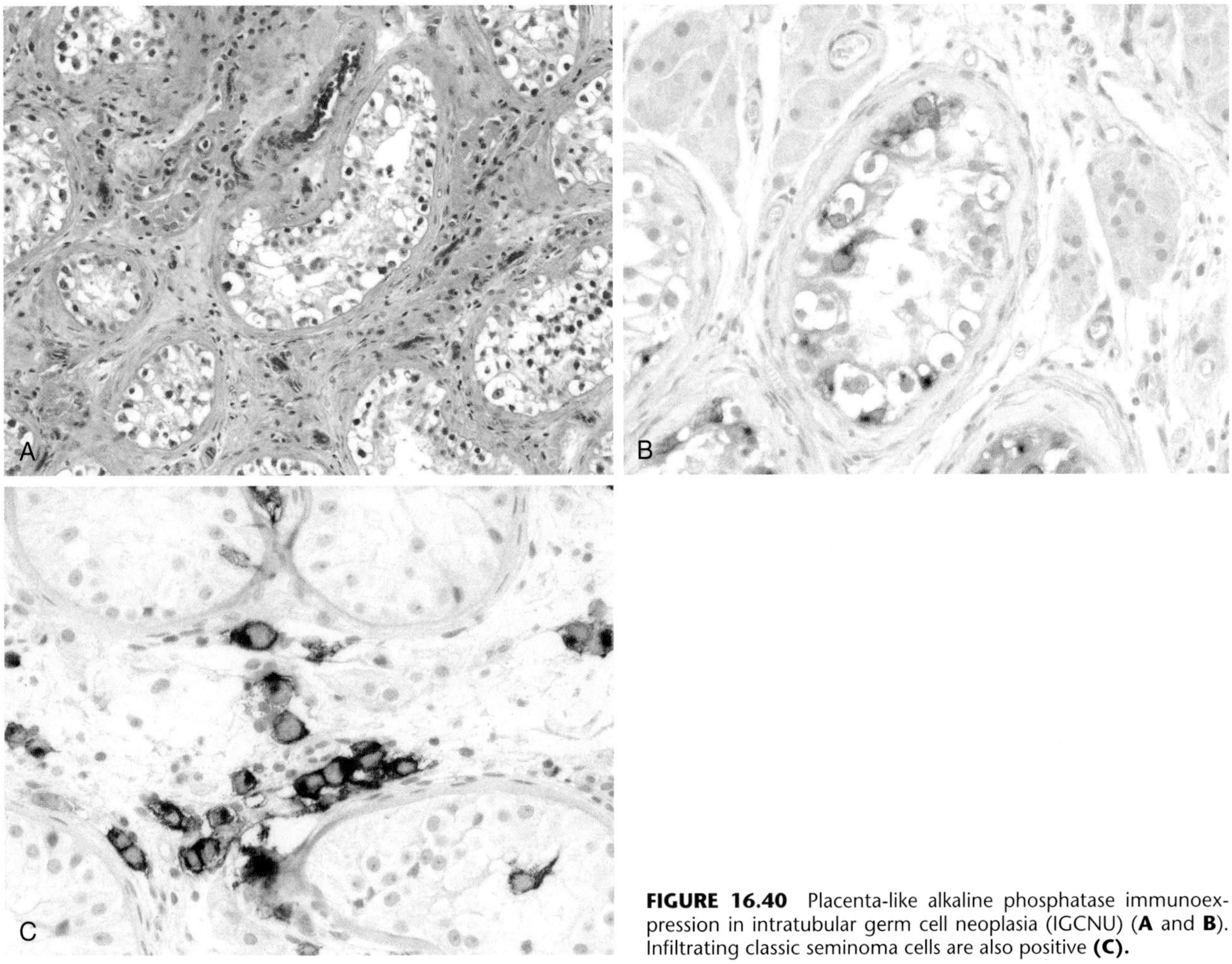

FIGURE 16.40 Placenta-like alkaline phosphatase immunoexpression in intratubular germ cell neoplasia (IGCNU) (**A** and **B**). Infiltrating classic seminoma cells are also positive **(C).**

syncytiotrophoblasts in hydatidiform moles, placental site trophoblastic tumors, and choriocarcinomas.[481,483]

Diagnostic Immunohistochemistry of Specific Testicular Neoplasms

GERM CELL TUMORS

Intratubular Germ Cell Neoplasia

Intratubular germ cell neoplasia, unclassified (IGCNU) type is the precursor of the majority of invasive testicular GCTs with the exception of spermatocytic seminoma and infantile GCTs. Isolated IGCNU can be found in testicular biopsies of cryptorchid testes taken during orchiopexy procedures, as well as biopsies of oligospermic infertility, dysgenetic testes, and contralateral testis of patients with germ cell tumor.

Given the reported higher risk of developing invasive germ cell tumor (up to 50% risk within 5 years) following a diagnosis of IGCNU,[484-487] ancillary techniques should be sought in equivocal cases.

In general, seminiferous tubules involved by IGCNU rarely show spermatogenesis and often have decreased tubular diameter with thickening of their peritubular basement membrane. IGCNU cells are basally located and have enlarged hyperchromatic nuclei with one or more nucleoli, clear cytoplasm containing PAS-positive material (glycogen), and distinct cytoplasmic borders. As mentioned earlier, in such settings, placenta-like alkaline phosphatase (PLAP) is a sensitive and specific marker for IGCNU with up to 98% membranous staining in IGCNU cells in contrast to negative staining in normal spermatogonia and Sertoli cells (Fig. 16.40).[488]

Newer markers of utility include *c-kit* proto-oncogene protein product (CD117) and OCT-4 both with a high degree of sensitivity and specificity for IGCNU.[468,484,486,489,490]

Special attention is warranted in prepubertal testes where occasional spermatogonia can be normally multinucleated and may show nuclear enlargement (giant gonadocytes), thus mimicking IGCNU (Table 16.20).[490]

Immunohistochemistry of Germ Cell Tumors

Proper classification of testicular GCTs is crucial to their management and prognostication. Detailed listing of the histologic types and their proportion in a given testicular tumor is a requirement for adequate surgical pathology reporting. Pure seminomas are treated differently than pure nonseminomatous or mixed seminomatous/NSGCTs. Furthermore, the percentages of different GCT components are to be included in the report.

TABLE 16.20 Immunohistochemistry in IGCNU and Germ-Cell Tumors

Marker	IGCNU	Classic Seminoma	Spermatocytic Seminoma	Embryonal Carcinoma	YST
C-*kit* (CD117)	+	+	S	S	S
OCT3/4	+	+	N	+	N
PLAP	+	+	S	+	+
AE1/AE3	N	N	N	+	+
CD30	N	N	N	+	N
AFP	N	N	N	S	+

+, almost always positive; S, sometimes positive; N, negative.
Modified from Ulbright TM. Germ cell tumors of the gonads: a selective review emphasizing problems in differential diagnosis, newly appreciated, and controversial issues. *Mod Pathol.* 2005;18(Suppl 2):S61.

A 25% cutoff of embryonal carcinoma is considered a negative prognosticator. Therefore in cases where distinction of seminoma from ECa or YST is not certain on H&E sections, immunostains can be of utility and should be used (Table 16.21).

Classic Seminoma versus Nonseminomatous Germ Cell Tumors

Generally, in testicular location, the diagnosis of seminoma is usually achievable on morphologic grounds alone given their characteristic histologic features. The tumor cells have abundant clear cytoplasm, distinct cytoplasmic membranes, round vesicular nuclei, and prominent nucleoli. The fibrous septa separating tumor cell clusters contain lymphoplasmacytic and/or granulomatous infiltrate. Areas of seminoma with increased nuclear atypia, increased apoptotic rate, and increased mitotic activity (especially when combined with sectioning artifactual changes) can mimic ECa. In general, ECa cells display more primitive nuclear features than seminoma and are frequently arranged in tubular and papillary structures. On the other side of the spectrum, given that the tubular and papillary architectural features are not restricted to YSTs, we find the pronounced degree of nuclear anaplasia in ECa to be of help in distinguishing ECa from YST where less primitive nuclear features are usually displayed. Finally, variants of classic seminoma such as tubular/cystic can mimic YSTs.

Although placenta-like alkaline phosphatase, c-*kit*, and OCT-4 are sensitive markers for seminoma,[464,467,473,490-492] all three markers are also positive in ECa, making them of little utility in distinguishing seminoma from ECa. Immunoreactivity for PLAP has been reported in 86% to 97% of embryonal carcinomas and tends to be more intense and focal than in seminomas. OCT4 stains more than 90% of ECa cases. More than 80% of embryonal carcinomas are positive for CD30 (Ki-1, Ber-H2). CD30 immunoreactivity is rarely seen in other germ cell tumors, making it useful in such differential diagnosis. Immunoreactivity for α-fetoprotein and β-hCG may be seen in scattered tumor cells in a minority (21% to 33%) of ECa. Epithelial membrane antigen, CEA, and vimentin are generally negative in ECa (Fig. 16.41).[464,465,467,473,479,489-497]

Although reports on pan cytokeratin (AE1/AE3) expression in seminomas range from 0% to 73% positivity rates, staining is usually weak and seen only in isolated cells or in small clusters. Low-molecular-weight cytokeratin CAM5.2 (CK8 and CK18) have been demonstrated in some seminomas with dotlike staining reported in up to 80% of mediastinal seminomas.[498] In contrast, both pancytokeratins AE1/AE3 and CAM5.2 demonstrate a diffuse and strong staining in nonseminomatous GCT including ECa, YST, choriocarcinoma, and teratomas. For all practical purposes, diffuse and strong reactivity for AE1/AE3 or CAM5.2 should argue against the diagnosis of seminoma, whereas negative staining of AE1/AE3 should support such a diagnosis.

Adding CD30 to AE1/AE3 can further help in differentiating seminoma (CD30 negative) from ECa (CD30 positive).[462,465,473,489-491,498-501]

Negative AE1/AE3, negative α-fetoprotein, and negative β-hCG reactivity in seminoma (except for syncytiotrophoblasts when present) is also helpful in distinguishing it from nonseminomatous YST and choriocarcinoma.[502] PLAP is positive in only half of choriocarcinomas, which also lack OCT4 expression.[464,465,481,490,492-494,503] Finally, in the rare situations where choriocarcinoma foci (including its monophasic cytotrophoblastic variant) are difficult to differentiate from seminoma, YST, or ECa with syncytiotrophoblast, we find demonstrating cytokeratin, β-hCG, inhibin, CEA, and/or HPL positivity in the biphasic syncytia- and cytotrophoblastic proliferation to be helpful (see Tables 16.18 and 16.19).

Extratesticular Primary Germ Cell Tumors and Metastatic Germ Cell Tumors

In extratesticular primary sites (e.g., mediastinal) and in metastatic tumors of unknown origin, distinguishing GCTs from somatic carcinoma is most crucial to prognosis and therapy. Retroperitoneal GCT metastases and metastases to other sites can be encountered in the presence of a completely regressed primary testicular tumor, leading to a low clinical index of suspicion for a GCT.[502] Dense host reaction to a seminoma metastasis combined with negative AE1/AE3 reactivity can also lead to misinterpretation as a lymphoid malignancy. In such settings, adding a germ cell marker such as PLAP, c-*kit*, and OCT4 to an initial IHC panel in the workup of a midline or retroperitoneal mass in a young male is highly recommended. Nevertheless, it is important to remember that PLAP can be positive in non-GCTs (somatic carcinomas).[462,464,465,489,490,492,493,498,503]

TABLE 16.21 Immunohistology of Germ-Cell Tumors
Classic Seminoma
PLAP+
OCT4+
c-*kit*+
AE1/AE3−
CAM5.2−/+
α-fetoprotein−
β-hCG−
Inhibin−
Epithelial membrane antigen−
CD30−
Embryonal Carcinoma
PLAP+
AE1/AE3+
CAM5.2+
OCT4+
CD30+
EMA−
Yolk Sac Tumor
PLAP+/−
Alpha fetoprotein+
AE1/AE3+
CAM5.2+
$Alpha_1$-antitrypsin+/−
CD34+/−
CD30−
EMA−
Choriocarcinoma
β-hCG+ (only in syncytiotrophoblast)
Pancytokeratins (AE1/AE3 and CAM5.2)+
CEA+
EMA+
PLAP+
Inhibin+

Immunoreactivity for PLAP and c-*kit* should be coupled with positive reactivity with germ cell specific markers such as OCT4 to further lend support to a diagnosis of ECa over a somatic malignancy. Negative reactivity for EMA and CD30 positivity would also favor a diagnosis of ECa over a somatic carcinoma in the presence of AE1/AE3 and CAM5.2 pancytokeratin positivity. Although not entirely specific, a profile of AE1/AE3, CAM5.2, PLAP, and AFP positivity with negative CD30 and EMA staining is compatible with YST diagnosis in extratesticular sites.[462,464,465,489,490,492,493,498,503]

Spermatocytic Seminoma

Spermatocytic seminomas (SSs) are unique among GCTs in terms of older age at presentation and their lack of association with other GCTs and the usual risk factors of GCT (cryptorchid testis and dysgeneses). Primary SSs do not occur outside the testis and are considered benign neoplasms with the exception of rare cases that undergo sarcomatous transformation. The differential diagnosis of spermatocytic seminoma includes malignant lymphoma, classic seminoma, and solid embryonal carcinoma.

In difficult cases IHC can play a role. SS are negative for cytokeratins AE1/AE3, AFP, β-hCG, CD30, EMA, and CD45. PLAP is only expressed in rare cases and focally.

CAM5.2 and c-*kit* has been found in 40% of cases of spermatocytic seminoma. Chk2, a regulatory protein in the transition of gonocytes to spermatogonia and from a mitotic phenotype to a meiotic one, and MAGE-A4 (a protein involved in DNA repair) have been found to be positive in more than 90% and 100% of SSs, respectively.[490,493,503-510]

TESTICULAR SEX CORD TUMORS

Leydig Cell Tumor

Immunohistochemistry can occasionally be of value in differentiating Leydig cell tumors from entities such as malacoplakia, malignant lymphoma, plasmacytoma, seminoma, and metastatic carcinoma. Leydig cell tumors are usually diffusely and strongly positive for inhibin. Leydig cell tumors lack PLAP immunoreactivity. Similar to their ovarian counterparts, positive immunoreactivity for a number of antibodies has been found in testicular Leydig cell tumors including CAM5.2 (variable), vimentin, S-100 protein (negative HMB45), and desmin. Immunohistochemical coexpression of inhibin and vimentin with lack of reactivity for epithelial membrane antigen, as well as variable cytokeratin immunoreactivity, supports the diagnosis of Leydig cell tumor over metastatic carcinoma. CD99, a transmembrane glycoprotein encoded by the Mic-2 gene, can be useful in identifying Leydig cell tumors, albeit inferior to inhi bin.[493,494,503,509,511-517]

Sertoli Cell Tumor

Inhibin A is also a sensitive marker of Sertoli cell differentiation (>90% positive). Sertoli cell tumor including its large cell calcifying variant stains variably positive with antibodies to vimentin, cytokeratin, S-100, synaptophysin, chromogranin, and neuron-specific enolase. Cytokeratin immunoreactivity in Sertoli cell tumors is usually stronger than that seen in Leydig cell tumors. Immunoreactivity for PLAP is not seen in Sertoli cell tumors.

Tubular seminoma, which often mimics Sertoli cell tumor architecturally, can be separated from Sertoli cell tumor by its PLAP immunoreactivity and lack of staining for inhibin and cytokeratins. Like Leydig cell tumors, CD99 can be a useful adjunct in identifying Sertoli cell tumors (Table 16.22).[493,494,503,509,511-517]

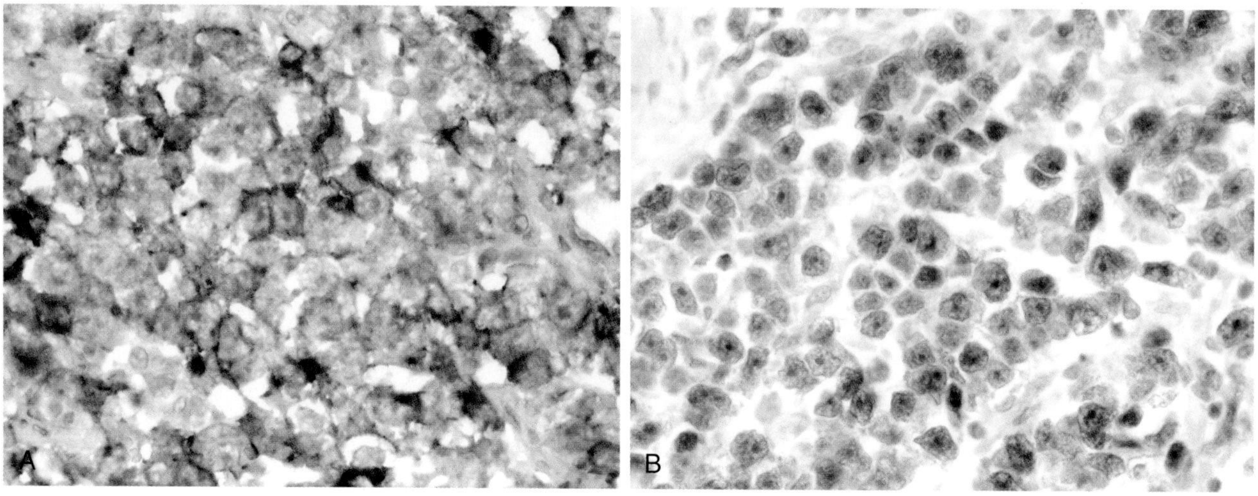

FIGURE 16.41 C-*kit* and OCT4 expression in classic seminoma (**A** and **B**, respectively).

TABLE 16.22 Immunohistology of Testicular Sex Cord Tumors

Leydig Cell Tumor
Inhibin+
Vimentin+
CD99+/–
EMA–
CAM5.2+/–
PLAP–
S-100+
Sertoli Cell Tumor
Inhibin A+
Vimentin+
CAM5.2+/–
PLAP–
S-100+
Synaptophysin+/–
Chromogranin–/+
NSE+
CD99+/–

Secondary Tumors of Testis

Compared with primary tumors, secondary testicular tumors are typically found in an older age group (older than 50 years of age). However, one third of the cases occur before age 40. Prostate carcinoma (50%) dominates the list of primary sources, in large part because of the prior practice of bilateral orchiectomy as part of the hormone deprivation therapy for PCa. Other primary sources, in descending order, include kidney, melanoma, and lung primaries.[163]

Metastatic carcinomas infiltrate the testicular interstitium while usually sparing seminiferous tubules. Rare intratubular growth patterns have been reported, however. Extensive vascular involvement and bilaterality are other features that are more likely to be encountered in metastatic tumors. As mentioned earlier, germ cell markers such as c-*kit*, OCT4 can be used in difficult cases. EMA negativity and CD30 positivity can also be of help in cases where the differential diagnosis includes ECa versus metastatic somatic carcinoma.[490,518,519] Primary and secondary involvement of testes by malignant lymphomas and leukemias can be supported by a panel of lymphoid and hematologic markers including CD45, CD20, CD79a, CD3, CD5, CD33, c-*kit*, and myeloperoxidase.[520,521]

Beyond Immunohistochemistry: Anatomic Molecular Diagnostic Applications

Tremendous advances have been achieved in our understanding of the biology and genetic molecular events involved in the pathogenesis of GCT. Current GCT treatment success rates are the envy of other solid tumor disciplines. Nevertheless, given the young age of affected GCT patient population and the gravity of potential side effects (e.g., secondary malignancy) associated with current treatment protocols, new biomarkers that will help better identify patients in need of such aggressive treatment are invaluable. Likewise, identification of new molecular targets of GCT therapy would be advantageous.[522-526]

As shown in Figure 16.42,[527] during fetal life, following an initiating event in diploid primordial germ cell, loss of imprinting and aneuploidization lead to the formation of the IGCNU precursor lesions. The extensive chromosomal instability in IGCNU leads to further transformation into invasive GCT primarily through loss of DNA and gain of 12p resulting in the development of seminoma. Additional events such as loss of N-myc and c-*kit* activity and activation of pRb, HER2, and p53 result in histogenetic differentiation toward NSGCT.[527,528]

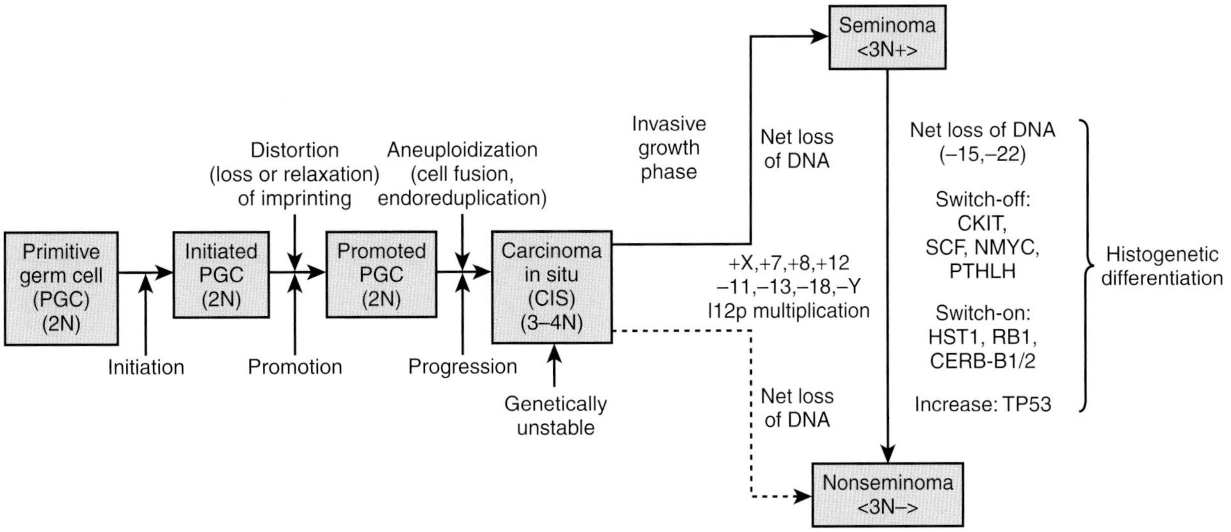

FIGURE 16.42 Proposed model of pathogenetic steps in germ cell tumor. *(Adapted from Sandberg AA, Meloni AM, Suijkerbuijk RF. Reviews of chromosome studies in urological tumors. III. Cytogenetics and genes in testicular tumors. J Urol. 1996;155:1531.)*

Overrepresentation of the chromosome 12p region is a consistently present structural chromosomal aberration in GCT. Isochromosome 12p is present in up to 80% of GCTs including extratesticular tumors. Therefore the identification of isochromosome 12p by interphase FISH-based cytogenetics is occasionally resorted to in cases where the previously mentioned IHC approach fails to resolve the differential diagnosis of GCT versus somatic carcinoma.[529-533]

Among therapy predictive markers, DNA damage detection and apoptosis initiation programs are thought to play a strong role in the exquisite chemosensitivity enjoyed by GCT. Wild type p53 overexpression has been associated with chemosensitivity in GCT, whereas overexpression of MDM2 (p53 inhibitor) was associated with resistance to therapy.[523,534-536] On the other hand, defective mismatch repair pathway leading to microsatellite instability (MSI) has been related to resistance in a subset of cisplatin refractory seminoma. Mayer and colleagues[537,538] illustrated a correlation between IHC loss of MLH1, MSH2, and MSH6 and MSI in 50% of unstable tumors, demonstrating for the first time a positive correlation between MSI and treatment resistance in GCT. In another study, Dimov and colleagues[539] were able to show that a high level of Topo II-α is expressed by most seminomas, embryonal carcinomas, YSTs, and choriocarcinomas, suggesting a possible mechanism for the sensitivity of these components to Topo II-α inhibitors. Interestingly, teratomas with mature and immature elements expressed low levels of Topo II-α, which might have contributed to their relative chemoresistance, further implying that the variable chemoresponsiveness of testicular GCTs could have an underlying molecular basis.[539]

Mazumdar and colleagues[540] recently suggested that a subgroup of embryonal carcinoma (with or without other histologies) with a cluster profile of high Ki-67, low apoptosis, and low p53 had a better survival beyond what would be predicted by their IGCCCG prognostic category, reflecting their increased tendency to respond to treatment.[540]

As mentioned earlier, to date, conflicting results have been found regarding the role of the presence of exon 11 and 17 c-*kit* activating mutations in predicting incidence risk of bilateral seminomas in patients with prior orchiectomy.[469-474]

ACKNOWLEDGMENTS

The authors would like to thank Hiroshi Miyamoto, MD, PhD, and Luciana Schultz, MD, for their valuable assistance.

REFERENCES

1. Srigley JR, Amin M, Boccon-Gibod L, et al. Prognostic and predictive factors in prostate cancer: historical perspectives and recent international consensus initiatives. *Scand J Urol Nephrol.* 2005:(Suppl)(216):8.
2. Schalken JA, Bergh A, Bono A, et al. Molecular prostate cancer pathology: current issues and achievements. *Scand J Urol Nephrol.* 2005:(Suppl)(216):82.
3. Epstein JI, Amin M, Boccon-Gibod L, et al. Prognostic factors and reporting of prostate carcinoma in radical prostatectomy and pelvic lymphadenectomy specimens. *Scand J Urol Nephrol.* 2005:(Suppl)(216):34.
4. DeMarzo AM, Nelson WG, Isaacs WB, Epstein JI. Pathological and molecular aspects of prostate cancer. *Lancet.* 2003;361:955.
5. Amin M, Boccon-Gibod L, Egevad L, et al. Prognostic and predictive factors and reporting of prostate carcinoma in prostate needle biopsy specimens. *Scand J Urol Nephrol.* 2005:(Suppl)(216):20.
6. Nelson WG, De Marzo AM, Isaacs WB. Prostate cancer. *N Engl J Med.* 2003;349:366.
7. Prowatke I, Devens F, Benner A, et al. Expression analysis of imbalanced genes in prostate carcinoma using tissue microarrays. *Br J Cancer.* 2007;96:82.
8. Lapointe J, Li C, Higgins JP, et al. Gene expression profiling identifies clinically relevant subtypes of prostate cancer. *Proc Natl Acad Sci U S A.* 2004;101:811.
9. Khan MA, Sokoll LJ, Chan DW, et al. Clinical utility of proPSA and "benign" PSA when percent free PSA is less than 15%. *Urology.* 2004;64:1160.
10. Tomlins SA, Mehra R, Rhodes DR, et al. Integrative molecular concept modeling of prostate cancer progression. *Nat Genet.* 2007;39:41.

11. Gretzer MB, Partin AW. PSA markers in prostate cancer detection. *Urol Clin North Am.* 2003;30:677.
12. Shen S, Lepor H, Yaffee R, Taneja SS. Ultrasensitive serum prostate specific antigen nadir accurately predicts the risk of early relapse after radical prostatectomy. *J Urol.* 2005;173:777.
13. Chuang AY, DeMarzo AM, Veltri RW, et al. Immunohistochemical differentiation of high-grade prostate carcinoma from urothelial carcinoma. *Am J Surg Pathol.* 2007;31:1246.
14. Kamoshida S, Tsutsumi Y. Extraprostatic localization of prostatic acid phosphatase and prostate-specific antigen: distribution in cloacogenic glandular epithelium and sex-dependent expression in human anal gland. *Hum Pathol.* 1990;21:1108.
15. James GK, Pudek M, Berean KW, et al. Salivary duct carcinoma secreting prostate-specific antigen. *Am J Clin Pathol.* 1996;106:242.
16. Diamandis EP. Prostate specific antigen—new applications in breast and other cancers. *Anticancer Res.* 1996;16:3983.
17. Lane Z, Hansel DE, Epstein JI. Immunohistochemical expression of prostatic antigens in adenocarcinoma and villous adenoma of the urinary bladder. *Am J Surg Pathol.* 2008;32:1322.
18. Chang SS, O'Keefe DS, Bacich DJ, et al. Prostate-specific membrane antigen is produced in tumor-associated neovasculature. *Clin Cancer Res.* 1999;5:2674.
19. Chang SS, Reuter VE, Heston WD, et al. Five different anti-prostate-specific membrane antigen (PSMA) antibodies confirm PSMA expression in tumor-associated neovasculature. *Cancer Res.* 1999;59:3192.
20. Chang SS, Reuter VE, Heston WD, Gaudin PB. Comparison of anti-prostate-specific membrane antigen antibodies and other immunomarkers in metastatic prostate carcinoma. *Urology.* 2001;57:1179.
21. Silver DA, Pellicer I, Fair WR, et al. Prostate-specific membrane antigen expression in normal and malignant human tissues. *Clin Cancer Res.* 1997;3:81.
22. Murphy GP, Elgamal AA, Su SL, et al. Current evaluation of the tissue localization and diagnostic utility of prostate specific membrane antigen. *Cancer.* 1998;83:2259.
23. Marchal C, Redondo M, Padilla M, et al. Expression of prostate specific membrane antigen (PSMA) in prostatic adenocarcinoma and prostatic intraepithelial neoplasia. *Histol Histopathol.* 2004;19:715.
24. Bostwick DG, Pacelli A, Blute M, et al. Prostate specific membrane antigen expression in prostatic intraepithelial neoplasia and adenocarcinoma: a study of 184 cases. *Cancer.* 1998;82:2256.
25. Yao V, Parwani A, Maier C, et al. Moderate expression of prostate-specific membrane antigen, a tissue differentiation antigen and folate hydrolase, facilitates prostate carcinogenesis. *Cancer Res.* 2008;68:9070.
26. Ross JS, Sheehan CE, Fisher HA, et al. Correlation of primary tumor prostate-specific membrane antigen expression with disease recurrence in prostate cancer. *Clin Cancer Res.* 2003;9:6357.
27. Chang SS, Reuter VE, Heston WD, et al. Short term neoadjuvant androgen deprivation therapy does not affect prostate specific membrane antigen expression in prostate tissues. *Cancer.* 2000;88:407.
28. Bander NH. Technology insight: monoclonal antibody imaging of prostate cancer. *Nat Clin Pract Urol.* 2006;3:216.
29. Bander NH, Milowsky MI, Nanus DM, et al. Phase I trial of 177lutetium-labeled J591, a monoclonal antibody to prostate-specific membrane antigen, in patients with androgen-independent prostate cancer. *J Clin Oncol.* 2005;23:4591.
30. Elsasser-Beile U, Wolf P, Gierschner D, et al. A new generation of monoclonal and recombinant antibodies against cell-adherent prostate specific membrane antigen for diagnostic and therapeutic targeting of prostate cancer. *Prostate.* 2006;66:1359.
31. Sodee DB, Sodee AE, Bakale G. Synergistic value of single-photon emission computed tomography/computed tomography fusion to radioimmunoscintigraphic imaging of prostate cancer. *Semin Nucl Med.* 2007;37:17.
32. Mannweiler S, Amersdorfer P, Trajanoski S, et al. Heterogeneity of Prostate-Specific Membrane Antigen (PSMA) Expression in Prostate Carcinoma with Distant Metastasis. *Pathol Oncol Res.* 2009;15:167-172.
33. Milowsky MI, Nanus DM, Kostakoglu L, et al. Vascular targeted therapy with anti-prostate-specific membrane antigen monoclonal antibody J591 in advanced solid tumors. *J Clin Oncol.* 2007;25:540.
34. Olson WC, Heston WD, Rajasekaran AK. Clinical trials of cancer therapies targeting prostate-specific membrane antigen. *Rev Recent Clin Trials.* 2007;2:182.
35. van Dieijen-Visser MP, Delaere KP, Gijzen AH, Brombacher PJ. A comparative study on the diagnostic value of prostatic acid phosphatase (PAP) and prostatic specific antigen (PSA) in patients with carcinoma of the prostate gland. *Clin Chim Acta.* 1988;174:131.
36. Ersev A, Ersev D, Turkeri L, et al. The relation of prostatic acid phosphatase and prostate specific antigen with tumour grade in prostatic adenocarcinoma: an immunohistochemical study. *Prog Clin Biol Res.* 1990;357:129.
37. Sheridan T, Herawi M, Epstein JI, Illei PB. The role of P501S and PSA in the diagnosis of metastatic adenocarcinoma of the prostate. *Am J Surg Pathol.* 2007;31:1351.
38. Kusumi T, Koie T, Tanaka M, et al. Immunohistochemical detection of carcinoma in radical prostatectomy specimens following hormone therapy. *Pathol Int.* 2008;58:687.
39. Osunkoya AO, Netto GJ, Epstein JI. Colorectal adenocarcinoma involving the prostate: report of 9 cases. *Hum Pathol.* 2007;38:1836.
40. Wang W, Epstein JI. Small cell carcinoma of the prostate. A morphologic and immunohistochemical study of 95 cases. *Am J Surg Pathol.* 2008;32:65.
41. Yin M, Dhir R, Parwani AV. Diagnostic utility of p501s (prostein) in comparison to prostate specific antigen (PSA) for the detection of metastatic prostatic adenocarcinoma. *Diagn Pathol.* 2007;2:41.
42. Luo J, Zha S, Gage WR, et al. Alpha-methylacyl-CoA racemase: a new molecular marker for prostate cancer. *Cancer Res.* 2002;62:2220.
43. Jiang Z, Woda BA. Diagnostic utility of alpha-methylacyl CoA racemase (P504S) on prostate needle biopsy. *Adv Anat Pathol.* 2004;11:316.
44. Jiang Z, Wu CL, Woda BA, et al. P504S/alpha-methylacyl-CoA racemase: a useful marker for diagnosis of small foci of prostatic carcinoma on needle biopsy. *Am J Surg Pathol.* 2002;26:1169.
45. Jiang Z, Li C, Fischer A, et al. Using an AMACR (P504S)/34betaE12/p63 cocktail for the detection of small focal prostate carcinoma in needle biopsy specimens. *Am J Clin Pathol.* 2005;123:231.
46. Magi-Galluzzi C, Luo J, Isaacs WB, et al. Alpha-methylacyl-CoA racemase: a variably sensitive immunohistochemical marker for the diagnosis of small prostate cancer foci on needle biopsy. *Am J Surg Pathol.* 2003;27:1128.
47. Kunju LP, Rubin MA, Chinnaiyan AM, Shah RB. Diagnostic usefulness of monoclonal antibody P504S in the workup of atypical prostatic glandular proliferations. *Am J Clin Pathol.* 2003;120:737.
48. Molinie V, Fromont G, Sibony M, et al. Diagnostic utility of a p63/alpha-methyl-CoA-racemase (p504s) cocktail in atypical foci in the prostate. *Mod Pathol.* 2004;17:1180.
49. Zhou M, Aydin H, Kanane H, Epstein JI. How often does alpha-methylacyl-CoA-racemase contribute to resolving an atypical diagnosis on prostate needle biopsy beyond that provided by basal cell markers? *Am J Surg Pathol.* 2004;28:239.
50. Zhou M, Jiang Z, Epstein JI. Expression and diagnostic utility of alpha-methylacyl-CoA-racemase (P504S) in foamy gland and pseudohyperplastic prostate cancer. *Am J Surg Pathol.* 2003;27:772.
51. Farinola MA, Epstein JI. Utility of immunohistochemistry for alpha-methylacyl-CoA racemase in distinguishing atrophic prostate cancer from benign atrophy. *Hum Pathol.* 2004;35:1272.
52. Dorer R, Odze RD. AMACR immunostaining is useful in detecting dysplastic epithelium in Barrett's esophagus, ulcerative colitis, and Crohn's disease. *Am J Surg Pathol.* 2006;30:871.
53. Lin F, Brown RE, Shen T, et al. Immunohistochemical detection of P504S in primary and metastatic renal cell carcinomas. *Appl Immunohistochem Mol Morphol.* 2004;12:153.

54. Sanderson SO, Sebo TJ, Murphy LM, et al. An analysis of the p63/alpha-methylacyl coenzyme A racemase immunohistochemical cocktail stain in prostate needle biopsy specimens and tissue microarrays. *Am J Clin Pathol*. 2004;121:220.
55. Wojno KJ, Epstein JI. The utility of basal cell-specific anti-cytokeratin antibody (34 beta E12) in the diagnosis of prostate cancer. A review of 228 cases. *Am J Surg Pathol*. 1995;19:251.
56. Kahane H, Sharp JW, Shuman GB, et al. Utilization of high molecular weight cytokeratin on prostate needle biopsies in an independent laboratory. *Urology*. 1995;45:981.
57. Oliai BR, Kahane H, Epstein JI. Can basal cells be seen in adenocarcinoma of the prostate?: an immunohistochemical study using high molecular weight cytokeratin (clone 34betaE12) antibody. *Am J Surg Pathol*. 2002;26:1151.
58. Novis DA, Zarbo RJ, Valenstein PA. Diagnostic uncertainty expressed in prostate needle biopsies. A College of American Pathologists Q-probes Study of 15,753 prostate needle biopsies in 332 institutions. *Arch Pathol Lab Med*. 1999;123:687.
59. Abrahams NA, Ormsby AH, Brainard J. Validation of cytokeratin 5/6 as an effective substitute for keratin 903 in the differentiation of benign from malignant glands in prostate needle biopsies. *Histopathology*. 2002;41:35.
60. Humphrey PA. Diagnosis of adenocarcinoma in prostate needle biopsy tissue. *J Clin Pathol*. 2007;60:35.
61. Signoretti S, Waltregny D, Dilks J, et al. p63 is a prostate basal cell marker and is required for prostate development. *Am J Pathol*. 2000;157:1769.
62. Grisanzio C, Signoretti S. P63 in prostate biology and pathology. *J Cell Biochem*. 2008;103:1354.
63. Shah RB, Zhou M, LeBlanc M, et al. Comparison of the basal cell-specific markers, 34betaE12 and p63, in the diagnosis of prostate cancer. *Am J Surg Pathol*. 2002;26:1161.
64. Shah RB, Kunju LP, Shen R, et al. Usefulness of basal cell cocktail (34betaE12 + p63) in the diagnosis of atypical prostate glandular proliferations. *Am J Clin Pathol*. 2004;122:517.
65. Zhou M, Shah R, Shen R, Rubin MA. Basal cell cocktail (34betaE12 + p63) improves the detection of prostate basal cells. *Am J Surg Pathol*. 2003;27:365.
66. Signoretti S, Loda M. Defining cell lineages in the prostate epithelium. *Cell Cycle*. 2006;5:138.
67. Weinstein MH, Signoretti S, Loda M. Diagnostic utility of immunohistochemical staining for p63, a sensitive marker of prostatic basal cells. *Mod Pathol*. 2002;15:1302.
68. Ali TZ, Epstein JI. False positive labeling of prostate cancer with high molecular weight cytokeratin: p63 a more specific immunomarker for basal cells. *Am J Surg Pathol*. 2008; 32:1890-1895.
69. Osunkoya AO, Hansel DE, Sun X, et al. Aberrant diffuse expression of p63 in adenocarcinoma of the prostate on needle biopsy and radical prostatectomy: report of 21 cases. *Am J Surg Pathol*. 2008;32:461.
70. Magi-Galluzzi C, Epstein JI. Threshold for diagnosing prostate cancer over time. *Hum Pathol*. 2003;34:1116.
71. Yang XJ, Wu CL, Woda BA, et al. Expression of alpha-Methylacyl-CoA racemase (P504S) in atypical adenomatous hyperplasia of the prostate. *Am J Surg Pathol*. 2002;26:921.
72. Gaudin PB, Epstein JI. Adenosis of the prostate. Histologic features in needle biopsy specimens. *Am J Surg Pathol*. 1995;19:737.
73. Gaudin PB, Epstein JI. Adenosis of the prostate. Histologic features in transurethral resection specimens. *Am J Surg Pathol*. 1994;18:863.
74. Bostwick DG, Amin MB, Dundore P, et al. Architectural patterns of high-grade prostatic intraepithelial neoplasia. *Hum Pathol*. 1993;24:298.
75. Kramer CE, Epstein JI. Nucleoli in low-grade prostate adenocarcinoma and adenosis. *Hum Pathol*. 1993;24:618.
76. Hedrick L, Epstein JI. Use of keratin 903 as an adjunct in the diagnosis of prostate carcinoma. *Am J Surg Pathol*. 1989;13: 389.
77. Luque RJ, Lopez-Beltran A, Perez-Seoane C, Suzigan S. Sclerosing adenosis of the prostate. Histologic features in needle biopsy specimens. *Arch Pathol Lab Med*. 2003;127:e14.
78. Sakamoto N, Tsuneyoshi M, Enjoji M. Sclerosing adenosis of the prostate. Histopathologic and immunohistochemical analysis. *Am J Surg Pathol*. 1991;15:660.
79. Grignon DJ, Ro JY, Srigley JR, et al. Sclerosing adenosis of the prostate gland. A lesion showing myoepithelial differentiation. *Am J Surg Pathol*. 1992;16:383.
80. Jones EC, Clement PB, Young RH. Sclerosing adenosis of the prostate gland. A clinicopathological and immunohistochemical study of 11 cases. *Am J Surg Pathol*. 1991;15:1171.
81. Nelson RS, Epstein JI. Prostatic carcinoma with abundant xanthomatous cytoplasm. Foamy gland carcinoma. *Am J Surg Pathol*. 1996;20:419.
82. Chuang AY, Epstein JI. Xanthoma of the prostate: a mimicker of high-grade prostate adenocarcinoma. *Am J Surg Pathol*. 2007;31:1225.
83. Sebo TJ, Bostwick DG, Farrow GM, Eble JN. prostatic xanthoma: a mimic of prostatic adenocarcinoma. *Hum Pathol*. 1994;25:386.
84. Balaji KC, Rabbani F, Tsai H, et al. Effect of neoadjuvant hormonal therapy on prostatic intraepithelial neoplasia and its prognostic significance. *J Urol*. 1999;162:753.
85. Tetu B, Srigley JR, Boivin JC, et al. Effect of combination endocrine therapy (LHRH agonist and flutamide) on normal prostate and prostatic adenocarcinoma. A histopathologic and immunohistochemical study. *Am J Surg Pathol*. 1991;15:111.
86. Murphy WM, Soloway MS, Barrows GH. Pathologic changes associated with androgen deprivation therapy for prostate cancer. *Cancer*. 1991;68:821.
87. Smith DM, Murphy WM. Histologic changes in prostate carcinomas treated with leuprolide (luteinizing hormone-releasing hormone effect). Distinction from poor tumor differentiation. *Cancer*. 1994;73:1472.
88. Armas OA, Aprikian AG, Melamed J, et al. Clinical and pathobiological effects of neoadjuvant total androgen ablation therapy on clinically localized prostatic adenocarcinoma. *Am J Surg Pathol*. 1994;18:979.
89. Vailancourt L, Ttu B, Fradet Y, et al. Effect of neoadjuvant endocrine therapy (combined androgen blockade) on normal prostate and prostatic carcinoma. A randomized study. *Am J Surg Pathol*. 1996;20:86.
90. Accetta PA, Gardner WA. Squamous metastases from prostatic adenocarcinoma. *Prostate*. 1982;3:515.
91. Accetta PA, Gardner Jr WA. Adenosquamous carcinoma of prostate. *Urology*. 1983;22:73.
92. Parwani AV, Kronz JD, Genega EM, et al. Prostate carcinoma with squamous differentiation: an analysis of 33 cases. *Am J Surg Pathol*. 2004;28:651.
93. Vernon SE, Williams WD. Pre-treatment and post-treatment evaluation of prostatic adenocarcinoma for prostatic specific acid phosphatase and prostatic specific antigen by immunohistochemistry. *J Urol*. 1983;130:95.
94. Grignon D, Troster M. Changes in immunohistochemical staining in prostatic adenocarcinoma following diethylstilbestrol therapy. *Prostate*. 1985;7:195.
95. Pisansky TM. External-beam radiotherapy for localized prostate cancer. *N Engl J Med*. 2006;355:1583.
96. Bostwick DG, Egbert BM, Fajardo LF. Radiation injury of the normal and neoplastic prostate. *Am J Surg Pathol*. 1982;6:541.
97. Magi-Galluzzi C, Sanderson H, Epstein JI. Atypia in nonneoplastic prostate glands after radiotherapy for prostate cancer: duration of atypia and relation to type of radiotherapy. *Am J Surg Pathol*. 2003;27:206.
98. Brawer MK, Nagle RB, Pitts W, et al. Keratin immunoreactivity as an aid to the diagnosis of persistent adenocarcinoma in irradiated human prostates. *Cancer*. 1989;63:454.
99. Yang XJ, Laven B, Tretiakova M, et al. Detection of alpha-methylacyl-coenzyme A racemase in postradiation prostatic adenocarcinoma. *Urology*. 2003;62:282.
100. Martens MB, Keller JH. Routine immunohistochemical staining for high-molecular weight cytokeratin 34-beta and alpha-methylacyl CoA racemase (P504S) in postirradiation prostate biopsies. *Mod Pathol*. 2006;19:287.
101. Crook JM, Bahadur YA, Robertson SJ, et al. Evaluation of radiation effect, tumor differentiation, and prostate specific antigen staining in sequential prostate biopsies after external beam radiotherapy for patients with prostate carcinoma. *Cancer*. 1997;79:81.

102. Scalzo DA, Kallakury BV, Gaddipati RV, et al. Cell proliferation rate by MIB-1 immunohistochemistry predicts postradiation recurrence in prostatic adenocarcinomas. *Am J Clin Pathol.* 1998;109:163.
103. Bostwick DG, Kindrachuk RW, Rouse RV. Prostatic adenocarcinoma with endometrioid features. Clinical, pathologic, and ultrastructural findings. *Am J Surg Pathol.* 1985;9:595.
104. Greene LF, Farrow GM, Ravits JM, Tomera FM. Prostatic adenocarcinoma of ductal origin. *J Urol.* 1979;121:303.
105. Epstein JI, Woodruff JM. Adenocarcinoma of the prostate with endometrioid features. A light microscopic and immunohistochemical study of ten cases. *Cancer.* 1986;57:111.
106. Hameed O, Humphrey PA. Immunohistochemistry in diagnostic surgical pathology of the prostate. *Semin Diagn Pathol.* 2005;22:88.
107. Owens CL, Epstein JI, Netto GJ. Distinguishing prostatic from colorectal adenocarcinoma on biopsy samples: the role of morphology and immunohistochemistry. *Arch Pathol Lab Med.* 2007;131:599.
108. Grignon DJ. Unusual subtypes of prostate cancer. *Mod Pathol.* 2004;17:316.
109. Mai KT, Collins JP, Veinot JP. Prostatic adenocarcinoma with urothelial (transitional cell) carcinoma features. *Appl Immunohistochem Mol Morphol.* 2002;10:231.
110. Oxley J, Abbott C. Thrombomodulin immunostaining and ductal carcinoma of the prostate. *Histopathology.* 1998;33:391.
111. Bostwick DG, Qian J, Pacelli A, et al. Neuroendocrine expression in node positive prostate cancer: correlation with systemic progression and patient survival. *J Urol.* 2002;168:1204.
112. Abrahamsson PA. Neuroendocrine cells in tumour growth of the prostate. *Endocr Relat Cancer.* 1999;6:503.
113. Abrahamsson PA, Falkmer S, Falt K, Grimelius L. The course of neuroendocrine differentiation in prostatic carcinomas. An immunohistochemical study testing chromogranin A as an "endocrine marker." *Pathol Res Pract.* 1989;185:373.
114. Cohen RJ, Glezerson G, Haffejee Z. Neuro-endocrine cells—a new prognostic parameter in prostate cancer. *Br J Urol.* 1991;68:258.
115. Weinstein MH, Partin AW, Veltri RW, Epstein JI. Neuroendocrine differentiation in prostate cancer: enhanced prediction of progression after radical prostatectomy. *Hum Pathol.* 1996;27:683.
116. Theodorescu D, Broder SR, Boyd JC, et al. Cathepsin D and chromogranin A as predictors of long term disease specific survival after radical prostatectomy for localized carcinoma of the prostate. *Cancer.* 1997;80:2109.
117. Casella R, Bubendorf L, Sauter G, et al. Focal neuroendocrine differentiation lacks prognostic significance in prostate core needle biopsies. *J Urol.* 1998;160:406.
118. Bostwick DG, Grignon DJ, Hammond ME, et al. Prognostic factors in prostate cancer. College of American Pathologists Consensus Statement 1999. *Arch Pathol Lab Med.* 2000;124:995.
119. Travis WD, Linnoila RI, Tsokos MG, et al. Neuroendocrine tumors of the lung with proposed criteria for large-cell neuroendocrine carcinoma. An ultrastructural, immunohistochemical, and flow cytometric study of 35 cases. *Am J Surg Pathol.* 1991;15:529.
120. Murali R, Kneale K, Lalak N, Delprado W. Carcinoid tumors of the urinary tract and prostate. *Arch Pathol Lab Med.* 2006;130:1693.
121. Freschi M, Colombo R, Naspro R, Rigatti P. Primary and pure neuroendocrine tumor of the prostate. *Eur Urol.* 2004;45:166.
122. Tash JA, Reuter V, Russo P. Metastatic carcinoid tumor of the prostate. *J Urol.* 2002;167:2526.
123. Zarkovic A, Masters J, Carpenter L. Primary carcinoid tumour of the prostate. *Pathology.* 2005;37:184.
124. Ghannoum JE, DeLellis RA, Shin SJ. Primary carcinoid tumor of the prostate with concurrent adenocarcinoma: a case report. *Int J Surg Pathol.* 2004;12:167.
125. Ro JY, Tetu B, Ayala AG, Ordonez NG. Small cell carcinoma of the prostate. II. Immunohistochemical and electron microscopic studies of 18 cases. *Cancer.* 1987;59:977.
126. Tetu B, Ro JY, Ayala AG, et al. Small cell carcinoma of the prostate. Part I. A clinicopathologic study of 20 cases. *Cancer.* 1987;59:1803.
127. Yao JL, Madeb R, Bourne P, et al. Small cell carcinoma of the prostate: an immunohistochemical study. *Am J Surg Pathol.* 2006;30:705.
128. Foster CS, Dodson A, Karavana V, et al. Prostatic stem cells. *J Pathol.* 2002;197:551.
129. Uzgare AR, Xu Y, Isaacs JT. In vitro culturing and characteristics of transit amplifying epithelial cells from human prostate tissue. *J Cell Biochem.* 2004;91:196.
130. Ordonez NG. Value of thyroid transcription factor-1 immunostaining in distinguishing small cell lung carcinomas from other small cell carcinomas. *Am J Surg Pathol.* 2000;24:1217.
131. Agoff SN, Lamps LW, Philip AT, et al. Thyroid transcription factor-1 is expressed in extrapulmonary small cell carcinomas but not in other extrapulmonary neuroendocrine tumors. *Mod Pathol.* 2000;13:238.
132. Mackey JR, Au HJ, Hugh J, Venner P. Genitourinary small cell carcinoma: determination of clinical and therapeutic factors associated with survival. *J Urol.* 1998;159:1624.
133. Rubenstein JH, Katin MJ, Mangano MM, et al. Small cell anaplastic carcinoma of the prostate: seven new cases, review of the literature, and discussion of a therapeutic strategy. *Am J Clin Oncol.* 1997;20:376.
134. Amato RJ, Logothetis CJ, Hallinan R, et al. Chemotherapy for small cell carcinoma of prostatic origin. *J Urol.* 1992;147:935.
135. Evans AJ, Humphrey PA, Belani J, et al. Large cell neuroendocrine carcinoma of prostate: a clinicopathologic summary of 7 cases of a rare manifestation of advanced prostate cancer. *Am J Surg Pathol.* 2006;30:684.
136. Chibber PJ, McIntyre MA, Hindmarsh JR, et al. Transitional cell carcinoma involving the prostate. *Br J Urol.* 1981;53:605.
137. Schellhammer PF, Bean MA, Whitmore Jr WF. Prostatic involvement by transitional cell carcinoma: pathogenesis, patterns and prognosis. *J Urol.* 1977;118:399.
138. Svanholm H. Evaluation of commercial immunoperoxidase kits for prostatic specific antigen and prostatic specific acid phosphatase. *Acta Pathol Microbiol Immunol Scand [A].* 1986;94:7.
139. Ellis DW, Leffers S, Davies JS, Ng AB. Multiple immunoperoxidase markers in benign hyperplasia and adenocarcinoma of the prostate. *Am J Clin Pathol.* 1984;81:279.
140. Ford TF, Butcher DN, Masters JR, Parkinson MC. Immunocytochemical localisation of prostate-specific antigen: specificity and application to clinical practice. *Br J Urol.* 1985;57:50.
141. Feiner HD, Gonzalez R. Carcinoma of the prostate with atypical immunohistological features. Clinical and histologic correlates. *Am J Surg Pathol.* 1986;10:765.
142. Keillor JS, Aterman K. The response of poorly differentiated prostatic tumors to staining for prostate specific antigen and prostatic acid phosphatase: a comparative study. *J Urol.* 1987;137:894.
143. Epstein JI. PSAP and PSA as immunohistochemical markers. *Urol Clin North Am.* 1993;20:757.
144. Mhawech P, Uchida T, Pelte MF. Immunohistochemical profile of high-grade urothelial bladder carcinoma and prostate adenocarcinoma. *Hum Pathol.* 2002;33:1136.
145. Nowels K, Kent E, Rinsho K, Oyasu R. Prostate specific antigen and acid phosphatase-reactive cells in cystitis cystica and glandularis. *Arch Pathol Lab Med.* 1988;112:734.
146. Pollen JJ, Dreilinger A. Immunohistochemical identification of prostatic acid phosphatase and prostate specific antigen in female periurethral glands. *Urology.* 1984;23:303.
147. Tepper SL, Jagirdar J, Heath D, Geller SA. Homology between the female paraurethral (Skene's) glands and the prostate. Immunohistochemical demonstration. *Arch Pathol Lab Med.* 1984;108:423.
148. Kamoshida S, Tsutsumi Y. Extraprostatic localization of prostatic acid phosphatase and prostate-specific antigen: distribution in cloacogenic glandular epithelium and sex-dependent expression in human anal gland. *Hum Pathol.* 1990;21:1108.
149. Golz R, Schubert GE. Prostatic specific antigen: immunoreactivity in urachal remnants. *J Urol.* 1989;141:1480.
150. Sobin LH, Hjermstad BM, Sesterhenn IA, Helwig EB. Prostatic acid phosphatase activity in carcinoid tumors. *Cancer.* 1986;58:136.

151. van Krieken JH. Prostate marker immunoreactivity in salivary gland neoplasms. A rare pitfall in immunohistochemistry. *Am J Surg Pathol*. 1993;17:410.
152. Spencer JR, Brodin AG, Ignatoff JM. Clear cell adenocarcinoma of the urethra: evidence for origin within paraurethral ducts. *J Urol*. 1990;143:122.
153. Grignon DJ, Ro JY, Ayala AG, et al. Primary adenocarcinoma of the urinary bladder. A clinicopathologic analysis of 72 cases. *Cancer*. 1991;2165:67.
154. Epstein JI, Kuhajda FP, Lieberman PH. Prostate-specific acid phosphatase immunoreactivity in adenocarcinomas of the urinary bladder. *Hum Pathol*. 1986;17:939.
155. Heyderman E, Brown BM, Richardson TC. Epithelial markers in prostatic, bladder, and colorectal cancer: an immunoperoxidase study of epithelial membrane antigen, carcinoembryonic antigen, and prostatic acid phosphatase. *J Clin Pathol*. 1984;37:1363.
156. Nadji M, Tabei SZ, Castro A, et al. Prostatic-specific antigen: an immunohistologic marker for prostatic neoplasms. *Cancer*. 1981;48:1229.
157. Genega EM, Hutchinson B, Reuter VE, Gaudin PB. Immunophenotype of high-grade prostatic adenocarcinoma and urothelial carcinoma. *Mod Pathol*. 2000;13:1186.
158. Varma M, Morgan M, Amin MB, et al. High molecular weight cytokeratin antibody (clone 34betaE12): a sensitive marker for differentiation of high-grade invasive urothelial carcinoma from prostate cancer. *Histopathology*. 2003;42:167.
159. Oliai BR, Kahane H, Epstein JI. A clinicopathologic analysis of urothelial carcinomas diagnosed on prostate needle biopsy. *Am J Surg Pathol*. 2001;25:794.
160. Lane Z, Epstein JI, Ayub S, Netto GJ. Prostatic adenocarcinoma in colorectal biopsy: clinical and pathologic features. *Hum Pathol*. 2008;39:543.
161. Rames RA, Smith MT. Malignant peripheral nerve sheath tumor of the prostate: a rare manifestion of neurofibromatosis type 1. *J Urol*. 1999;162:165.
162. Raney RB, Anderson JR, Barr FG, et al. Rhabdomyosarcoma and undifferentiated sarcoma in the first two decades of life: a selective review of intergroup rhabdomyosarcoma study group experience and rationale for Intergroup Rhabdomyosarcoma Study V. *J Pediatr Hematol Oncol*. 2001;23:215.
163. Eble JN, Sauter G, Epstein JI, Sesterhenn IA. *The World Health Organization Classification of Tumours: Pathology and Genetics of Tumours of the Urinary System and Male Genital Organs*. Lyon, France: IARC Press; 2004.
164. Gaudin PB, Rosai J, Epstein JI. Sarcomas and related proliferative lesions of specialized prostatic stroma: a clinicopathologic study of 22 cases. *Am J Surg Pathol*. 1998;22:148.
165. Bostwick DG, Hossain D, Qian J, et al. Phyllodes tumor of the prostate: long-term followup study of 23 cases. *J Urol*. 2004;172:894.
166. Herawi M, Epstein JI. Specialized stromal tumors of the prostate: a clinicopathologic study of 50 cases. *Am J Surg Pathol*. 2006;30:694.
167. Michaels MM, Brown HE, Favino CJ. Leiomyoma of prostate. *Urology*. 1974;3:617.
168. Regan JB, Barrett DM, Wold LE. Giant leiomyoma of the prostate. *Arch Pathol Lab Med*. 1987;111:381.
169. Stenram U, Holby LE. A case of circumscribed myosarcoma of the prostate. *Cancer*. 1969;24:803.
170. Kelley TW, Borden EC, Goldblum JR. Estrogen and progesterone receptor expression in uterine and extrauterine leiomyosarcomas: an immunohistochemical study. *Appl Immunohistochem Mol Morphol*. 2004;12:338.
171. Cheville JC, Dundore PA, Nascimento AG, et al. Leiomyosarcoma of the prostate. Report of 23 cases. *Cancer*. 1995;76:1422.
172. Sexton WJ, Lance RE, Reyes AO, et al. Adult prostate sarcoma: the M.D. Anderson Cancer Center Experience. *J Urol*. 2001;166:521.
173. Herawi M, Epstein JI. Solitary fibrous tumor on needle biopsy and transurethral resection of the prostate: a clinicopathologic study of 13 cases. *Am J Surg Pathol*. 2007;31:870.
174. Van der Aa F, Sciot R, Blyweert W, et al. Gastrointestinal stromal tumor of the prostate. *Urology*. 2005;65:388.
175. Madden JF, Burchette JL, Raj GV, et al. Anterior rectal wall gastrointestinal stromal tumor presenting clinically as prostatic mass. *Urol Oncol*. 2005;23:268.
176. Herawi M, Montgomery EA, Epstein JI. Gastrointestinal stromal tumors (GISTs) on prostate needle biopsy: a clinicopathologic study of 8 cases. *Am J Surg Pathol*. 2006;30:1389.
177. Stephenson AJ, Scardino PT, Eastham JA, et al. Preoperative nomogram predicting the 10-year probability of prostate cancer recurrence after radical prostatectomy. *J Natl Cancer Inst*. 2006;98:715.
178. Stephenson AJ, Scardino PT, Eastham JA, et al. Postoperative nomogram predicting the 10-year probability of prostate cancer recurrence after radical prostatectomy. *J Clin Oncol*. 2005;23:7005.
179. Partin AW, Kattan MW, Subong EN, et al. Combination of prostate-specific antigen, clinical stage, and Gleason score to predict pathological stage of localized prostate cancer. A multi-institutional update. *JAMA*. 1997;277:1445.
180. De Marzo AM, DeWeese TL, Platz EA, et al. Pathological and molecular mechanisms of prostate carcinogenesis: implications for diagnosis, detection, prevention, and treatment. *J Cell Biochem*. 2004;91:459.
181. Bethel CR, Faith D, Li X, et al. Decreased NKX3.1 protein expression in focal prostatic atrophy, prostatic intraepithelial neoplasia, and adenocarcinoma: association with gleason score and chromosome 8p deletion. *Cancer Res*. 2006;66:10683.
182. Khan MA, Partin AW. Tissue microarrays in prostate cancer research. *Rev Urol*. 2004;6:44.
183. Tomlins SA, Rhodes DR, Perner S, et al. Recurrent fusion of TMPRSS2 and ETS transcription factor genes in prostate cancer. *Science*. 2005;310:644.
184. Tomlins SA, Mehra R, Rhodes DR, et al. TMPRSS2:ETV4 gene fusions define a third molecular subtype of prostate cancer. *Cancer Res*. 2006;66:3396.
185. Demichelis F, Fall K, Perner S, et al. TMPRSS2:ERG gene fusion associated with lethal prostate cancer in a watchful waiting cohort. *Oncogene*. 2007;26:4596.
186. Lotan TL, Toubaji A, Albadine R, et al. TMPRSS2-ERG gene fusions are infrequent in prostatic ductal adenocarcinomas. *Mod Pathol*. 2009;22(10):1398-1399.
187. Yoshimoto M, Joshua AM, Cunha IW, et al. Absence of TMPRSS2:ERG fusions and PTEN losses in prostate cancer is associated with a favorable outcome. *Mod Pathol*. 2008;21:1451.
188. Fitzgerald LM, Agalliu I, Johnson K, et al. Association of TMPRSS2-ERG gene fusion with clinical characteristics and outcomes: results from a population-based study of prostate cancer. *BMC Cancer*. 2008;8:230.
189. Mao X, Shaw G, James SY, et al. Detection of TMPRSS2:ERG fusion gene in circulating prostate cancer cells. *Asian J Androl*. 2008;10:467.
190. Perner S, Mosquera JM, Demichelis F, et al. TMPRSS2-ERG fusion prostate cancer: an early molecular event associated with invasion. *Am J Surg Pathol*. 2007;31:882.
191. Saramaki OR, Harjula AE, Martikainen PM, et al. TMPRSS2:ERG fusion identifies a subgroup of prostate cancers with a favorable prognosis. *Clin Cancer Res*. 2008;14:3395.
192. Hammond ME, Fitzgibbons PL, Compton CC, et al. College of American Pathologists Conference XXXV: solid tumor prognostic factors-which, how and so what? Summary document and recommendations for implementation. Cancer Committee and Conference Participants. *Arch Pathol Lab Med*. 2000;124:958.
193. Kremer CL, Klein RR, Mendelson J, et al. Expression of mTOR signaling pathway markers in prostate cancer progression. *Prostate*. 2006;66:1203.
194. Sanchez D, Rosell D, Honorato B, et al. Androgen receptor mutations are associated with Gleason score in localized prostate cancer. *BJU Int*. 2006;98:1320.
195. Wikstrom P, Bergh A, Damber JE. Transforming growth factor-beta1 and prostate cancer. *Scand J Urol Nephrol*. 2000;34:85.
196. Wikstrom P, Damber J, Bergh A. Role of transforming growth factor-beta1 in prostate cancer. *Microsc Res Tech*. 2001;52:411.
197. Diaz JI, Mora LB, Austin PF, et al. Predictability of PSA failure in prostate cancer by computerized cytometric assessment of tumoral cell proliferation. *Urology*. 1999;53:931.

198. Keshgegian AA, Johnston E, Cnaan A. Bcl-2 oncoprotein positivity and high MIB-1 (Ki-67) proliferative rate are independent predictive markers for recurrence in prostate carcinoma. *Am J Clin Pathol*. 1998;110:443.
199. Bubendorf L, Tapia C, Gasser TC, et al. Ki67 labeling index in core needle biopsies independently predicts tumor-specific survival in prostate cancer. *Hum Pathol*. 1998;29:949.
200. Bettencourt MC, Bauer JJ, Sesterhenn IA, et al. Ki-67 expression is a prognostic marker of prostate cancer recurrence after radical prostatectomy. *J Urol*. 1996;156:1064.
201. Cheng L, Pisansky TM, Sebo TJ, et al. Cell proliferation in prostate cancer patients with lymph node metastasis: a marker for progression. *Clin Cancer Res*. 1999;5:2820.
202. Stapleton AM, Zbell P, Kattan MW, et al. Assessment of the biologic markers p53, Ki-67, and apoptotic index as predictive indicators of prostate carcinoma recurrence after surgery. *Cancer*. 1998;82:168.
203. Vis AN, van Rhijn BW, Noordzij MA, et al. Value of tissue markers p27(kip1), MIB-1, and CD44s for the pre-operative prediction of tumour features in screen-detected prostate cancer. *J Pathol*. 2002;197:148.
204. Bostwick DG, Wheeler TM, Blute M, et al. Optimized microvessel density analysis improves prediction of cancer stage from prostate needle biopsies. *Urology*. 1996;48:47.
205. Silberman MA, Partin AW, Veltri RW, Epstein JI. Tumor angiogenesis correlates with progression after radical prostatectomy but not with pathologic stage in Gleason sum 5 to 7 adenocarcinoma of the prostate. *Cancer*. 1997;79:772.
206. Strohmeyer D, Rossing C, Strauss F, et al. Tumor angiogenesis is associated with progression after radical prostatectomy in pT2/pT3 prostate cancer. *Prostate*. 2000;42:26.
207. Strohmeyer D, Strauss F, Rossing C, et al. Expression of bFGF, VEGF and c-met and their correlation with microvessel density and progression in prostate carcinoma. *Anticancer Res*. 2004;24:1797.
208. Gettman MT, Bergstralh EJ, Blute M, et al. Prediction of patient outcome in pathologic stage T2 adenocarcinoma of the prostate: lack of significance for microvessel density analysis. *Urology*. 1998;51:79.
209. Gettman MT, Pacelli A, Slezak J, et al. Role of microvessel density in predicting recurrence in pathologic Stage T3 prostatic adenocarcinoma. *Urology*. 1999;54:479.
210. Krupski T, Petroni GR, Frierson Jr HF, Theodorescu JU. Microvessel density, p53, retinoblastoma, and chromogranin A immunohistochemistry as predictors of disease-specific survival following radical prostatectomy for carcinoma of the prostate. *Urology*. 2000;55:743.
211. Brewster SF, Oxley JD, Trivella M, et al. Preoperative p53, bcl-2, CD44 and E-cadherin immunohistochemistry as predictors of biochemical relapse after radical prostatectomy. *J Urol*. 1999;161:1238.
212. Stackhouse GB, Sesterhenn IA, Bauer JJ, et al. p53 and bcl-2 immunohistochemistry in pretreatment prostate needle biopsies to predict recurrence of prostate cancer after radical prostatectomy. *J Urol*. 1999;2040:162.
213. Bauer JJ, Sesterhenn IA, Mostofi FK, et al. Elevated levels of apoptosis regulator proteins p53 and bcl-2 are independent prognostic biomarkers in surgically treated clinically localized prostate cancer. *J Urol*. 1996;156:1511.
214. Bauer JJ, Sesterhenn IA, Mostofi KF, et al. p53 nuclear protein expression is an independent prognostic marker in clinically localized prostate cancer patients undergoing radical prostatectomy. *Clin Cancer Res*. 1995;1:1295.
215. Moul JW, Bettencourt MC, Sesterhenn IA, et al. Protein expression of p53, bcl-2, and KI-67 (MIB-1) as prognostic biomarkers in patients with surgically treated, clinically localized prostate cancer. *Surgery*. 1996;120:159.
216. Osman I, Drobnjak M, Fazzari M, et al. Inactivation of the p53 pathway in prostate cancer: impact on tumor progression. *Clin Cancer Res*. 1999;2082:5.
217. Theodorescu D, Broder SR, Boyd JC, et al. p53, bcl-2 and retinoblastoma proteins as long-term prognostic markers in localized carcinoma of the prostate. *J Urol*. 1997;158:131.
218. Kuczyk MA, Serth J, Bokemeyer C, et al. The prognostic value of p53 for long-term and recurrence-free survival following radical prostatectomy. *Eur J Cancer*. 1998;34:679.
219. Cheng L, Lloyd RV, Weaver AL, et al. The cell cycle inhibitors p21WAF1 and p27KIP1 are associated with survival in patients treated by salvage prostatectomy after radiation therapy. *Clin Cancer Res*. 1896;2000:6.
220. Lacombe L, Maillette A, Meyer F, et al. Expression of p21 predicts PSA failure in locally advanced prostate cancer treated by prostatectomy. *Int J Cancer*. 2001;95:135.
221. Schmitz M, Grignard G, Margue C, et al. Complete loss of PTEN expression as a possible early prognostic marker for prostate cancer metastasis. *Int J Cancer*. 2006.
222. Yoshimoto M, Cutz JC, Nuin PA, et al. Interphase FISH analysis of PTEN in histologic sections shows genomic deletions in 68% of primary prostate cancer and 23% of high-grade prostatic intraepithelial neoplasias. *Cancer Genet Cytogenet*. 2006;169:128.
223. Aslan G, Irer B, Tuna B, et al. Analysis of NKX3.1 expression in prostate cancer tissues and correlation with clinicopathologic features. *Pathol Res Pract*. 2006;202:93.
224. Gurel B, Iwata T, Koh CM, et al. Nuclear MYC protein overexpression is an early alteration in human prostate carcinogenesis. *Mod Pathol*. 2008;21:1156.
225. Gurel B, Iwata T, Koh CM, et al. Molecular alterations in prostate cancer as diagnostic, prognostic, and therapeutic targets. *Adv Anat Pathol*. 2008;15:319.
226. Veltri RW, Partin AW, Epstein JE, et al. Quantitative nuclear morphometry, Markovian texture descriptors, and DNA content captured on a CAS-200 Image analysis system, combined with PCNA and HER-2/neu immunohistochemistry for prediction of prostate cancer progression. *J Cell Biochem (Suppl)*. 1994;19:249.
227. Ross JS, Sheehan CE, Hayner-Buchan AM, et al. Prognostic significance of HER-2/neu gene amplification status by fluorescence in situ hybridization of prostate carcinoma. *Cancer*. 1997;79:2162.
228. McWilliam LJ, Manson C, George NJ. Neuroendocrine differentiation and prognosis in prostatic adenocarcinoma. *Br J Urol*. 1997;80:287.
229. Shariff AH, Ather MH. Neuroendocrine differentiation in prostate cancer. *Urology*. 2006;68:2.
230. Zhang YH, Kanamaru H, Oyama N, et al. Prognostic value of nuclear morphometry on needle biopsy from patients with prostate cancer: is volume-weighted mean nuclear volume superior to other morphometric parameters? *Urology*. 2000;55:377.
231. Zhang YH, Kanamaru H, Oyama N, et al. Comparison of nuclear morphometric results between needle biopsy and surgical specimens from patients with prostate cancer. *Urology*. 1999;54:763.
232. Veltri RW, Miller MC, Partin AW, et al. Ability to predict biochemical progression using Gleason score and a computer-generated quantitative nuclear grade derived from cancer cell nuclei. *Urology*. 1996;48:685.
233. Khan MA, Walsh PC, Miller MC, et al. Quantitative alterations in nuclear structure predict prostate carcinoma distant metastasis and death in men with biochemical recurrence after radical prostatectomy. *Cancer*. 2003;98:2583.
234. Partin AW, Steinberg GD, Pitcock RV, et al. Use of nuclear morphometry, Gleason histologic scoring, clinical stage, and age to predict disease-free survival among patients with prostate cancer. *Cancer*. 1992;70:161.
235. Potter SR, Miller MC, Mangold LA, et al. Genetically engineered neural networks for predicting prostate cancer progression after radical prostatectomy. *Urology*. 1999;54:791.
236. Hammond ME, Sause WT, Martz KL, et al. Correlation of prostate-specific acid phosphatase and prostate-specific antigen immunocytochemistry with survival in prostate carcinoma. *Cancer*. 1989;63:461.
237. Lapointe J, Li C, Giacomini CP, Salari K, et al. Genomic profiling reveals alternative genetic pathways of prostate tumorigenesis. *Cancer Res*. 2007;67:8504.
238. Bastacky S, Cieply K, Sherer C, et al. Use of interphase fluorescence in situ hybridization in prostate needle biopsy specimens with isolated high-grade prostatic intraepithelial neoplasia as a predictor of prostate adenocarcinoma on follow-up biopsy. *Hum Pathol*. 2004;35:281.

239. Al-Maghrabi J, Vorobyova L, Toi A, et al. Identification of numerical chromosomal changes detected by interphase fluorescence in situ hybridization in high-grade prostate intraepithelial neoplasia as a predictor of carcinoma. *Arch Pathol Lab Med*. 2002;126:165.
240. Dhir R, Vietmeier B, Arlotti J, et al. Early identification of individuals with prostate cancer in negative biopsies. *J Urol*. 2004;171:1419.
241. Uetsuki H, Tsunemori H, Taoka R, et al. Expression of a novel biomarker, EPCA, in adenocarcinomas and precancerous lesions in the prostate. *J Urol*. 2005;174:514.
242. Hansel DE, DeMarzo AM, Platz EA, et al. Early prostate cancer antigen expression in predicting presence of prostate cancer in men with histologically negative biopsies. *J Urol*. 2007;177:1736.
243. Paul B, Dhir R, Landsittel D, et al. Detection of prostate cancer with a blood-based assay for early prostate cancer antigen. *Cancer Res*. 2005;65:4097.
244. Bastian PJ, Ellinger J, Wellmann A, et al. Diagnostic and prognostic information in prostate cancer with the help of a small set of hypermethylated gene loci. *Clin Cancer Res*. 2005;11:4097.
245. Bastian PJ, Nakayama M, De Marzo AM, Nelson WG. GSTP1 CpG island hypermethylation as a molecular marker of prostate cancer. *Urologe A*. 2004;43:573.
246. Bastian PJ, Palapattu GS, Lin X, et al. Preoperative serum DNA GSTP1 CpG island hypermethylation and the risk of early prostate-specific antigen recurrence following radical prostatectomy. *Clin Cancer Res*. 2005;11:4037.
247. Bastian PJ, Yegnasubramanian S, Palapattu GS, et al. Molecular biomarker in prostate cancer: the role of CpG island hypermethylation. *Eur Urol*. 2004;46:698.
248. Bussemakers MJ, van Bokhoven A, Verhaegh GW, et al. DD3: a new prostate-specific gene, highly overexpressed in prostate cancer. *Cancer Res*. 1999;59:5975.
249. de Kok JB, Verhaegh GW, Roelofs RW, et al. DD3(PCA3), a very sensitive and specific marker to detect prostate tumors. *Cancer Res*. 2002;62:2695.
250. Kantoff P. Recent progress in management of advanced prostate cancer. *Oncology (Williston Park)*. 2005;19:631.
251. Pizer ES, Pflug BR, Bova GS, et al. Increased fatty acid synthase as a therapeutic target in androgen-independent prostate cancer progression. *Prostate*. 2001;47:102.
252. Wu L, Birle DC, Tannock IF. Effects of the mammalian target of rapamycin inhibitor CCI-779 used alone or with chemotherapy on human prostate cancer cells and xenografts. *Cancer Res*. 2005;65:2825.
253. Jimeno A, Carducci M. Atrasentan: a rationally designed targeted therapy for cancer. *Drugs Today (Barc)*. 2006;42:299.
254. Jimeno A, Carducci M. Atrasentan: a novel and rationally designed therapeutic alternative in the management of cancer. *Expert Rev Anticancer Ther*. 2005;5:419.
255. Aggarwal S, Singh P, Topaloglu O, et al. A dimeric peptide that binds selectively to prostate-specific membrane antigen and inhibits its enzymatic activity. *Cancer Res*. 2006;66:9171.
256. Ikegami S, Yamakami K, Ono T, et al. Targeting gene therapy for prostate cancer cells by liposomes complexed with anti-prostate-specific membrane antigen monoclonal antibody. *Hum Gene Ther*. 2006;17:997.
257. Jayaprakash S, Wang X, Heston WD, Kozikowski AP. Design and synthesis of a PSMA inhibitor-doxorubicin conjugate for targeted prostate cancer therapy. *Chem Med Chem*. 2006;1:299.
258. Jemal A, Siegel R, Ward E, et al. Cancer statistics, 2008. *CA Cancer J Clin*. 2008;58:71.
259. Jiang J, Ulbright TM, Younger C, et al. Cytokeratin 7 and cytokeratin 20 in primary urinary bladder carcinoma and matched lymph node metastasis. *Arch Pathol Lab Med*. 2001;125:921.
260. Bassily NH, Vallorosi CJ, Akdas G, et al. Coordinate expression of cytokeratins 7 and 20 in prostate adenocarcinoma and bladder urothelial carcinoma. *Am J Clin Pathol*. 2000;113:383.
261. Desai S, Lim SD, Jimenez RE, et al. Relationship of cytokeratin 20 and CD44 protein expression with WHO/ISUP grade in pTa and pT1 papillary urothelial neoplasia. *Mod Pathol*. 2000;13:1315.
262. Cabibi D, Licata A, Barresi E, et al. Expression of cytokeratin 7 and 20 in pathological conditions of the bile tract. *Pathol Res Pract*. 2003;199:65.
263. Matros E, Bailey G, Clancy T, et al. Cytokeratin 20 expression identifies a subtype of pancreatic adenocarcinoma with decreased overall survival. *Cancer*. 2006;106:693.
264. Vang R, Gown AM, Barry TS, et al. Cytokeratins 7 and 20 in primary and secondary mucinous tumors of the ovary: analysis of coordinate immunohistochemical expression profiles and staining distribution in 179 cases. *Am J Surg Pathol*. 2006;30:1130.
265. Saad RS, Cho P, Silverman JF, Liu Y. Usefulness of Cdx2 in separating mucinous bronchioloalveolar adenocarcinoma of the lung from metastatic mucinous colorectal adenocarcinoma. *Am J Clin Pathol*. 2004;122:421.
266. Wang HL, Lu DW, Yerian LM, et al. Immunohistochemical distinction between primary adenocarcinoma of the bladder and secondary colorectal adenocarcinoma. *Am J Surg Pathol*. 2001;25:1380.
267. Harnden P, Eardley I, Joyce AD, Southgate J. Cytokeratin 20 as an objective marker of urothelial dysplasia. *Br J Urol*. 1996;78:870.
268. McKenney JK, Desai S, Cohen C, Amin MB. Discriminatory immunohistochemical staining of urothelial carcinoma in situ and non-neoplastic urothelium: an analysis of cytokeratin 20, p53, and CD44 antigens. *Am J Surg Pathol*. 2001;25:1074.
269. Yin H, He Q, Li T, Leong AS. Cytokeratin 20 and Ki-67 to distinguish carcinoma in situ from flat non-neoplastic urothelium. *Appl Immunohistochem Mol Morphol*. 2006;14:260.
270. Yin M, Bastacky S, Parwani AV, et al. P16ink4 immunoreactivity is a reliable marker for urothelial carcinoma in situ. *Hum Pathol*. 2008;39:527.
271. Burger M, Denzinger S, Hartmann A, et al. Mcm2 predicts recurrence hazard in stage Ta/T1 bladder cancer more accurately than CK20, Ki67 and histological grade. *Br J Cancer*. 2007;96:1711.
272. Ramos D, Navarro S, Villamon R, et al. Cytokeratin expression patterns in low-grade papillary urothelial neoplasms of the urinary bladder. *Cancer*. 2003;97:1876.
273. Barbisan F, Santinelli A, Mazzucchelli R, et al. Strong immunohistochemical expression of fibroblast growth factor receptor 3, superficial staining pattern of cytokeratin 20, and low proliferative activity define those papillary urothelial neoplasms of low malignant potential that do not recur. *Cancer*. 2008;112:636.
274. Kaufmann O, Volmerig J, Dietel M. Uroplakin III is a highly specific and moderately sensitive immunohistochemical marker for primary and metastatic urothelial carcinomas. *Am J Clin Pathol*. 2000;113:683.
275. Ohtsuka Y, Kawakami S, Fujii Y, et al. Loss of uroplakin III expression is associated with a poor prognosis in patients with urothelial carcinoma of the upper urinary tract. *BJU Int*. 2006;97:1322.
276. Parker DC, Folpe AL, Bell J, et al. Potential utility of uroplakin III, thrombomodulin, high molecular weight cytokeratin, and cytokeratin 20 in noninvasive, invasive, and metastatic urothelial (transitional cell) carcinomas. *Am J Surg Pathol*. 2003;27:1.
277. Huang HY, Shariat SF, Sun TT, et al. Persistent uroplakin expression in advanced urothelial carcinomas: implications in urothelial tumor progression and clinical outcome. *Hum Pathol*. 2007;38:1703.
278. Moll R, Wu XR, Lin JH, Sun TT. Uroplakins, specific membrane proteins of urothelial umbrella cells, as histological markers of metastatic transitional cell carcinomas. *Am J Pathol*. 1995;147:1383.
279. Matsumoto K, Satoh T, Irie A, et al. Loss expression of uroplakin III is associated with clinicopathologic features of aggressive bladder cancer. *Urology*. 2008;72:444.
280. Logani S, Oliva E, Amin MB, et al. Immunoprofile of ovarian tumors with putative transitional cell (urothelial) differentiation using novel urothelial markers: histogenetic and diagnostic implications. *Am J Surg Pathol*. 2003;27:1434.
281. Olsburgh J, Harnden P, Weeks R, et al. Uroplakin gene expression in normal human tissues and locally advanced bladder cancer. *J Pathol*. 2003;199:41.
282. Ogawa K, Johansson SL, Cohen SM. Immunohistochemical analysis of uroplakins, urothelial specific proteins, in ovarian Brenner tumors, normal tissues, and benign and neoplastic lesions of the female genital tract. *Am J Pathol*. 1999;155:1047.

283. Ordonez NG. Thrombomodulin expression in transitional cell carcinoma. *Am J Clin Pathol.* 1998;110:385.
284. Comperat E, Camparo P, Haus R, et al. Immunohistochemical expression of p63, p53 and MIB-1 in urinary bladder carcinoma. A tissue microarray study of 158 cases. *Virchows Arch.* 2006;448:319.
285. Helpap B, Kollermann J. Assessment of basal cell status and proliferative patterns in flat and papillary urothelial lesions: a contribution to the new WHO classification of the urothelial tumors of the urinary bladder. *Hum Pathol.* 2000;31:745.
286. Montgomery EA, Shuster DD, Burkart AL, et al. Inflammatory myofibroblastic tumors of the urinary tract: a clinicopathologic study of 46 cases, including a malignant example inflammatory fibrosarcoma and a subset associated with high-grade urothelial carcinoma. *Am J Surg Pathol.* 2006;30:1502.
287. Cook JR, Dehner LP, Collins MH, et al. Anaplastic lymphoma kinase (ALK) expression in the inflammatory myofibroblastic tumor: a comparative immunohistochemical study. *Am J Surg Pathol.* 2001;25:1364.
288. Tsuzuki T, Magi-Galluzzi C, Epstein JI. ALK-1 expression in inflammatory myofibroblastic tumor of the urinary bladder. *Am J Surg Pathol.* 2004;28:1609.
289. Sukov WR, Cheville JC, Carlson AW, et al. Utility of ALK-1 protein expression and ALK rearrangements in distinguishing inflammatory myofibroblastic tumor from malignant spindle cell lesions of the urinary bladder. *Mod Pathol.* 2007;20:592.
290. Sengupta S, Harris CC. p53: traffic cop at the crossroads of DNA repair and recombination. *Nat Rev Mol Cell Biol.* 2005;6:44.
291. Fujimoto K, Yamada Y, Okajima E, et al. Frequent association of p53 gene mutation in invasive bladder cancer. *Cancer Res.* 1992;52:1393.
292. Miyamoto H, Kubota Y, Shuin T, et al. Analyses of p53 gene mutations in primary human bladder cancer. *Oncol Res.* 1993;5:245.
293. Sarkis AS, Bajorin DF, Reuter VE, et al. Prognostic value of p53 nuclear overexpression in patients with invasive bladder cancer treated with neoadjuvant MVAC. *J Clin Oncol.* 1995;13:1384.
294. Sarkis AS, Dalbagni G, Cordon-Cardo C, et al. Association of P53 nuclear overexpression and tumor progression in carcinoma in situ of the bladder. *J Urol.* 1994;152:388.
295. Lianes P, Orlow I, Zhang ZF, et al. Altered patterns of MDM2 and TP53 expression in human bladder cancer. *J Natl Cancer Inst.* 1994;86:1325.
296. Brunner A, Verdorfer I, Prelog M, et al. Large-scale analysis of cell cycle regulators in urothelial bladder cancer identifies p16 and p27 as potentially useful prognostic markers. *Pathobiology.* 2008;75:25.
297. McShane LM, Aamodt R, Cordon-Cardo C, et al. Reproducibility of p53 immunohistochemistry in bladder tumors. National Cancer Institute, Bladder Tumor Marker Network. *Clin Cancer Res.* 2000;6:1854.
298. Watanabe J, Nishiyama H, Okubo K, et al. Clinical evaluation of p53 mutations in urothelial carcinoma by IHC and FASAY. *Urology.* 2004;63:989.
299. Salinas-Sanchez AS, Atienzar-Tobarra M, Lorenzo-Romero JG, et al. Sensitivity and specificity of p53 protein detection by immunohistochemistry in patients with urothelial bladder carcinoma. *Urol Int.* 2007;79:321.
300. Garcia del Muro X, Condom E, Vigues F, et al. p53 and p21 Expression levels predict organ preservation and survival in invasive bladder carcinoma treated with a combined-modality approach. *Cancer.* 2004;100:1859-1867.
301. Tzai TS, Tsai YS, Chow NH. The prevalence and clinicopathologic correlate of p16INK4a, retinoblastoma and p53 immunoreactivity in locally advanced urinary bladder cancer. *Urol Oncol.* 2004;22:112.
302. Orlow I, Lacombe L, Hannon GJ, et al. Deletion of the p16 and p15 genes in human bladder tumors. *J Natl Cancer Inst.* 1995;87:1524.
303. Miyamoto H, Kubota Y, Fujinami K, et al. Infrequent somatic mutations of the p16 and p15 genes in human bladder cancer: p16 mutations occur only in low-grade and superficial bladder cancers. *Oncol Res.* 1995;7:327.
304. Kruger S, Mahnken A, Kausch I, Feller AC. P16 immunoreactivity is an independent predictor of tumor progression in minimally invasive urothelial bladder carcinoma. *Eur Urol.* 2005;47:463.
305. Miyamoto H, Shuin T, Torigoe S, et al. Retinoblastoma gene mutations in primary human bladder cancer. *Br J Cancer.* 1995;71:831.
306. Cordon-Cardo C, Wartinger D, Petrylak D, et al. Altered expression of the retinoblastoma gene product: prognostic indicator in bladder cancer. *J Natl Cancer Inst.* 1992;84:1251.
307. Cordon-Cardo C. p53 and RB: simple interesting correlates or tumor markers of critical predictive nature? *J Clin Oncol.* 2004;22:975.
308. Cairns P, Proctor AJ, Knowles MA. Loss of heterozygosity at the RB locus is frequent and correlates with muscle invasion in bladder carcinoma. *Oncogene.* 1991;6:2305.
309. Cote RJ, Dunn MD, Chatterjee SJ, et al. Elevated and absent pRb expression is associated with bladder cancer progression and has cooperative effects with p53. *Cancer Res.* 1998;58:1090.
310. Kubota Y, Miyamoto H, Noguchi S, et al. The loss of retinoblastoma gene in association with c-myc and transforming growth factor-beta 1 gene expression in human bladder cancer. *J Urol.* 1995;154:371.
311. Bates AW, Baithun SI. Secondary neoplasms of the bladder are histological mimics of nontransitional cell primary tumours: clinicopathological and histological features of 282 cases. *Histopathology.* 2000;36:32.
312. Raspollini MR, Nesi G, Baroni G, et al. Immunohistochemistry in the differential diagnosis between primary and secondary intestinal adenocarcinoma of the urinary bladder. *Appl Immunohistochem Mol Morphol.* 2005;13:358.
313. Jacobs LB, Brooks JD, Epstein JI. Differentiation of colonic metaplasia from adenocarcinoma of urinary bladder. *Hum Pathol.* 1997;28:1152.
314. Silver SA, Epstein JI. Adenocarcinoma of the colon simulating primary urinary bladder neoplasia. A report of nine cases. *Am J Surg Pathol.* 1993;17:171.
315. Fritsche HM, Burger M, Denzinger S, et al. Plasmacytoid urothelial carcinoma of the bladder: histological and clinical features of 5 cases. *J Urol.* 1923;2008:180.
316. McKenney JK, Amin MB. The role of immunohistochemistry in the diagnosis of urinary bladder neoplasms. *Semin Diagn Pathol.* 2005;22:69.
317. Patriarca C, Di Pasquale M, Giunta P, Bergamaschi F. CD138-positive plasmacytoid urothelial carcinoma of the bladder. *Int J Surg Pathol.* 2008;16:215.
318. Ro JY, Shen SS, Lee HI, et al. Plasmacytoid transitional cell carcinoma of urinary bladder: a clinicopathologic study of 9 cases. *Am J Surg Pathol.* 2008;32:752.
319. Sato K, Ueda Y, Kawamura K, et al. Plasmacytoid urothelial carcinoma of the urinary bladder: A case report and immunohistochemical study. *Pathol Res Pract.* 2009;205:189-194.
320. Cheng L, Pan CX, Yang XJ, et al. Small cell carcinoma of the urinary bladder: a clinicopathologic analysis of 64 patients. *Cancer.* 2004;101:957.
321. Cheng L, Huang WB, Chen J. Recent advances in pathology and molecular genetics of small cell carcinoma of the urinary bladder. *Zhonghua Bing Li Xue Za Zhi.* 2007;36:700.
322. Cheng L, Jones TD, McCarthy RP, et al. Molecular genetic evidence for a common clonal origin of urinary bladder small cell carcinoma and coexisting urothelial carcinoma. *Am J Pathol.* 2005;166:1533.
323. Terracciano L, Richter J, Tornillo L, et al. Chromosomal imbalances in small cell carcinomas of the urinary bladder. *J Pathol.* 1999;189:230.
324. Hansel DE, Nadasdy T, Epstein JI. Fibromyxoid nephrogenic adenoma: a newly recognized variant mimicking mucinous adenocarcinoma. *Am J Surg Pathol.* 2007;31:1231.
325. Tong GX, Melamed J, Mansukhani M, et al. PAX2: a reliable marker for nephrogenic adenoma. *Mod Pathol.* 2006;19:356.
326. Tong GX, Weeden EM, Hamele-Bena D, et al. Expression of PAX8 in nephrogenic adenoma and clear cell adenocarcinoma of the lower urinary tract: evidence of related histogenesis? *Am J Surg Pathol.* 2008;32:1380.

327. Mitra AP, Datar RH, Cote RJ. Molecular pathways in invasive bladder cancer: new insights into mechanisms, progression, and target identification. *J Clin Oncol.* 2006;24:5552.
328. Wu XR. Urothelial tumorigenesis: a tale of divergent pathways. *Nat Rev Cancer.* 2005;5:713.
329. Oxford G, Theodorescu D. The role of Ras superfamily proteins in bladder cancer progression. *J Urol* 2003;170:1987.
330. O'Donnell MA. Advances in the management of superficial bladder cancer. *Semin Oncol.* 2007;34:85.
331. Sylvester RJ, van der Meijden AP, Oosterlinck W, et al. Predicting recurrence and progression in individual patients with stage Ta T1 bladder cancer using EORTC risk tables: a combined analysis of 2596 patients from seven EORTC trials. *Eur Urol.* 2006;49:466.
332. Stein JP, Lieskovsky G, Cote R, et al. Radical cystectomy in the treatment of invasive bladder cancer: long-term results in 1,054 patients. *J Clin Oncol.* 2001;19:666.
333. Skacel M, Fahmy M, Brainard JA, et al. Multitarget fluorescence in situ hybridization assay detects transitional cell carcinoma in the majority of patients with bladder cancer and atypical or negative urine cytology. *J Urol.* 2003;169:2101.
334. Moonen PM, Merkx GF, Peelen P, et al. UroVysion compared with cytology and quantitative cytology in the surveillance of non-muscle-invasive bladder cancer. *Eur Urol.* 2007;51:1275.
335. Yoder BJ, Skacel M, Hedgepeth R, et al. Reflex UroVysion testing of bladder cancer surveillance patients with equivocal or negative urine cytology: a prospective study with focus on the natural history of anticipatory positive findings. *Am J Clin Pathol.* 2007;127:295.
336. Rabbani F, Koppie TM, Charytonowicz E, et al. Prognostic significance of p27(Kip1) expression in bladder cancer. *BJU Int.* 2007;100:259.
337. Sanchez-Carbayo M, Socci ND, Lozano J, et al. Defining molecular profiles of poor outcome in patients with invasive bladder cancer using oligonucleotide microarrays. *J Clin Oncol.* 2006;24:778.
338. Sanchez-Carbayo M, Socci ND, Charytonowicz E, et al. Molecular profiling of bladder cancer using cDNA microarrays: defining histogenesis and biological phenotypes. *Cancer Res.* 2002;62:6973.
339. Sanchez-Carbayo M, Cordon-Cardo C. Applications of array technology: identification of molecular targets in bladder cancer. *Br J Cancer.* 2003;2172:89.
340. Sanchez-Carbayo M, Cordon-Cardo C. Molecular alterations associated with bladder cancer progression. *Semin Oncol.* 2007;34:75.
341. Rotterud R, Nesland JM, Berner A, Fossa SD. Expression of the epidermal growth factor receptor family in normal and malignant urothelium. *BJU Int.* 2005;95:1344.
342. Lascombe I, Clairotte A, Fauconnet S, et al. N-cadherin as a novel prognostic marker of progression in superficial urothelial tumors. *Clin Cancer Res.* 2006;12:2780.
343. Ioachim E, Michael MC, Salmas M, et al. Thrombospondin-1 expression in urothelial carcinoma: prognostic significance and association with p53 alterations, tumour angiogenesis and extracellular matrix components. *BMC Cancer.* 2006;6:140.
344. Highshaw RA, McConkey DJ, Dinney CP. Integrating basic science and clinical research in bladder cancer: update from the first bladder Specialized Program of Research Excellence (SPORE). *Curr Opin Urol.* 2004;14:295.
345. Clairotte A, Lascombe I, Fauconnet S, et al. Expression of E-cadherin and alpha-, beta-, gamma-catenins in patients with bladder cancer: identification of gamma-catenin as a new prognostic marker of neoplastic progression in T1 superficial urothelial tumors. *Am J Clin Pathol.* 2006;125:119.
346. Chatterjee SJ, Datar R, Youssefzadeh D, et al. Combined effects of p53, p21, and pRb expression in the progression of bladder transitional cell carcinoma. *J Clin Oncol.* 2004;22:1007.
347. Beekman KW, Bradley D, Hussain M. New molecular targets and novel agents in the treatment of advanced urothelial cancer. *Semin Oncol.* 2007;34:154.
348. Shariat SF, Ashfaq R, Sagalowsky AI, Lotan Y. Predictive value of cell cycle biomarkers in nonmuscle invasive bladder transitional cell carcinoma. *J Urol.* 2007;177:481.
349. Sarkis AS, Dalbagni G, Cordon-Cardo C, et al. Nuclear overexpression of p53 protein in transitional cell bladder carcinoma: a marker for disease progression. *J Natl Cancer Inst.* 1993;85:53.
350. Dalbagni G, Presti Jr JC, Reuter VE, et al. Molecular genetic alterations of chromosome 17 and p53 nuclear overexpression in human bladder cancer. *Diagn Mol Pathol.* 1993;2:4.
351. Margulis V, Lotan Y, Karakiewicz PI, et al. Multi-institutional validation of the predictive value of Ki-67 labeling index in patients with urinary bladder cancer. *J Natl Cancer Inst.* 2009;101:114.
352. Bellmunt J, Hussain M, Dinney CP. Novel approaches with targeted therapies in bladder cancer. Therapy of bladder cancer by blockade of the epidermal growth factor receptor family. *Crit Rev Oncol Hematol* 2003; 46(Suppl):S85.
353. Black PC, Agarwal PK, Dinney CP. Targeted therapies in bladder cancer—an update. *Urol Oncol.* 2007;25:433.
354. Black PC, Dinney CP. Bladder cancer angiogenesis and metastasis—translation from murine model to clinical trial. *Cancer Metastasis Rev.* 2007;26:623.
355. Wallerand H, Reiter RR, Ravaud A. Molecular targeting in the treatment of either advanced or metastatic bladder cancer or both according to the signalling pathways. *Curr Opin Urol.* 2008;18:524.
356. Wallerand H, Robert G, Bernhard JC, et al. Targeted therapy for locally advanced and/or metastatic bladder cancer. *Prog Urol.* 2008;18:407.
357. Yoshida SO, Imam A. Monoclonal antibody to a proximal nephrogenic renal antigen: immunohistochemical analysis of formalin-fixed, paraffin-embedded human renal cell carcinomas. *Cancer Res.* 1989;49:1802.
358. Bazille C, Allory Y, Molinie V, et al. Immunohistochemical characterisation of the main histologic subtypes of epithelial renal tumours on tissue-microarrays. Study of 310 cases. *Ann Pathol.* 2004;24:395.
359. Avery AK, Beckstead J, Renshaw AA, Corless CL. Use of antibodies to RCC and CD10 in the differential diagnosis of renal neoplasms. *Am J Surg Pathol.* 2000;24:203.
360. Liu L, Qian J, Singh H, et al. Immunohistochemical analysis of chromophobe renal cell carcinoma, renal oncocytoma, and clear cell carcinoma: an optimal and practical panel for differential diagnosis. *Arch Pathol Lab Med.* 2007;131:1290.
361. Mansouri A, Hallonet M, Gruss P. Pax genes and their roles in cell differentiation and development. *Curr Opin Cell Biol.* 1996;8:851.
362. Mazal PR, Exner M, Haitel A, et al. Expression of kidney-specific cadherin distinguishes chromophobe renal cell carcinoma from renal oncocytoma. *Hum Pathol.* 2005;36:22.
363. Mazal PR, Stichenwirth M, Koller A, et al. Expression of aquaporins and PAX-2 compared to CD10 and cytokeratin 7 in renal neoplasms: a tissue microarray study. *Mod Pathol.* 2005;18:535.
364. Daniel L, Lechevallier E, Giorgi R, et al. Pax-2 expression in adult renal tumors. *Hum Pathol.* 2001;32:282.
365. Gokden N, Gokden M, Phan DC, McKenney JK. The utility of PAX-2 in distinguishing metastatic clear cell renal cell carcinoma from its morphologic mimics: an immunohistochemical study with comparison to renal cell carcinoma marker. *Am J Surg Pathol.* 2008;32:1462.
366. Jadallah S, Albadine R, Sharma RB, Netto GJ. PAX-8 Expression in Clear Cell, Papillary and Chromophobe RCC and Urothelial Carcinoma of Renal Pelvis. *Mod Pathol.* 2009;22:174A.
367. Netto GJ, Wang W, Brownlee NA, et al. PAX-8(+)/p63(-) Immunostaining Pattern in Renal Collecting Duct Carcinoma (CDC): A Helpful Immunoprofile in the Differential Diagnosis of CDC vs Urothelial Carcinoma od Upper Urinary Tract. *Mod Pathol.* 2009;22:186A.
368. Calabrese G, Crescenzi C, Morizio E, et al. Assignment of TACSTD1 (alias TROP1, M4S1) to human chromosome 2p21 and refinement of mapping of TACSTD2 (alias TROP2, M1S1) to human chromosome 1p32 by in situ hybridization. *Cytogenet Cell Genet.* 2001;92:164.

369. Shetye J, Christensson B, Rubio C, et al. The tumor-associated antigens BR55-2, GA73-3 and GICA 19-9 in normal and corresponding neoplastic human tissues, especially gastrointestinal tissues. *Anticancer Res.* 1989;9:395.
370. Seligson DB, Pantuck AJ, Liu X, et al. Epithelial cell adhesion molecule (KSA) expression: pathobiology and its role as an independent predictor of survival in renal cell carcinoma. *Clin Cancer Res.* 2004;10:2659.
371. Went P, Dirnhofer S, Salvisberg T, et al. Expression of epithelial cell adhesion molecule (EpCam) in renal epithelial tumors. *Am J Surg Pathol.* 2005;29:83.
372. Thedieck C, Kuczyk M, Klingel K, et al. Expression of Ksp-cadherin during kidney development and in renal cell carcinoma. *Br J Cancer.* 2005;92:2010.
373. Adley BP, Gupta A, Lin F, et al. Expression of kidney-specific cadherin in chromophobe renal cell carcinoma and renal oncocytoma. *Am J Clin Pathol.* 2006;126:79.
374. Al-Ahmadie HA, Alden D, et al. Carbonic anhydrase IX expression in clear cell renal cell carcinoma: an immunohistochemical study comparing 2 antibodies. *Am J Surg Pathol.* 2008;32:377.
375. Gupta R, Balzer B, Picken M, et al. Diagnostic implications of transcription factor Pax 2 protein and transmembrane enzyme complex carbonic anhydrase IX immunoreactivity in adult renal epithelial neoplasms. *Am J Surg Pathol.* 2009;33:241.
376. Illei PB, Albadine R, Sharma R, Netto GJ. Immunohistochemical analysis of hypoxia inducible protein 2 (HIG2), KSP-cadherin and carbonic anhydrase IX (CAIX) expression in papillary, clear cell and chromophobe renal cell carcinoma. *Mod Pathol.* 2009;22:174A.
377. Uemura H, Nakagawa Y, Yoshida K, et al. MN/CA IX/G250 as a potential target for immunotherapy of renal cell carcinomas. *Br J Cancer.* 1999;81:741.
378. Grignon DJ, Abdel-Malak M, Mertens WC, et al. Glutathione S-transferase expression in renal cell carcinoma: a new marker of differentiation. *Mod Pathol.* 1994;7:186.
379. Perez-Ordonez B, Hamed G, Campbell S, et al. Renal oncocytoma: a clinicopathologic study of 70 cases. *Am J Surg Pathol.* 1997;21:871.
380. Reuter VE. The pathology of renal epithelial neoplasms. *Semin Oncol.* 2006;33:534.
381. Reuter VE. Renal tumors exhibiting granular cytoplasm. *Semin Diagn Pathol.* 1999;16:135.
382. Amin MB, Amin MB, Tamboli P, et al. Prognostic impact of histologic subtyping of adult renal epithelial neoplasms: an experience of 405 cases. *Am J Surg Pathol.* 2002;26:281.
383. Huo L, Sugimura J, Tretiakova MS, et al. C-kit expression in renal oncocytomas and chromophobe renal cell carcinomas. *Hum Pathol.* 2005;36:262.
384. Pan CC, Chen PC, Chiang H. Overexpression of KIT (CD117) in chromophobe renal cell carcinoma and renal oncocytoma. *Am J Clin Pathol.* 2004;121:878.
385. Al-Saleem T, Cairns P, Dulaimi EA, et al. The genetics of renal oncocytosis: a possible model for neoplastic progression. *Cancer Genet Cytogenet.* 2004;152:23.
386. Paner GP, Lindgren V, Jacobson K, et al. High incidence of chromosome 1 abnormalities in a series of 27 renal oncocytomas: cytogenetic and fluorescence in situ hybridization studies. *Arch Pathol Lab Med.* 2007;131:81.
387. Sibony M, Vieillefond A. Non clear cell renal cell carcinoma. 2008 update in renal tumor pathology. *Ann Pathol.* 2008;28:381.
388. Storkel S. Epithelial tumors of the kidney. Pathological subtyping and cytogenetic correlation. *Urologe A.* 1999;38:425.
389. Verdorfer I, Hobisch A, Hittmair A, et al. Cytogenetic characterization of 22 human renal cell tumors in relation to a histopathological classification. *Cancer Genet Cytogenet.* 1999;111:61.
390. Barocas DA, Mathew S, DelPizzo JJ, et al. Renal cell carcinoma sub-typing by histopathology and fluorescence in situ hybridization on a needle-biopsy specimen. *BJU Int.* 2007;99:290.
391. Furge KA, Lucas KA, Takahashi M, et al. Robust classification of renal cell carcinoma based on gene expression data and predicted cytogenetic profiles. *Cancer Res.* 2004;64:4117.
392. Argani P. Metanephric neoplasms: the hyperdifferentiated, benign end of the Wilms tumor spectrum? *Clin Lab Med.* 2005;25:379.
393. Olgac S, Hutchinson B, Tickoo SK, Reuter VE. Alpha-methylacyl-CoA racemase as a marker in the differential diagnosis of metanephric adenoma. *Mod Pathol.* 2006;19:218.
394. Skinnider BF, Folpe AL, Hennigar RA, et al. Distribution of cytokeratins and vimentin in adult renal neoplasms and normal renal tissue: potential utility of a cytokeratin antibody panel in the differential diagnosis of renal tumors. *Am J Surg Pathol.* 2005;29:747.
395. Galmiche L, Vasiliu V, Poiree S, et al. Diagnosis of renal metanephric adenoma: relevance of immunohistochemistry and biopsy. *Ann Pathol.* 2007;27:365.
396. Cohen HT, McGovern FJ. Renal-cell carcinoma. *N Engl J Med.* 2005;353:2477.
397. Reuter VE, Presti Jr JC. Contemporary approach to the classification of renal epithelial tumors. *Semin Oncol.* 2000;27:124.
398. Skinnider BF, Amin MB. An immunohistochemical approach to the differential diagnosis of renal tumors. *Semin Diagn Pathol.* 2005;22:51.
399. Leroy X, Zini L, Leteurtre E, et al. Morphologic subtyping of papillary renal cell carcinoma: correlation with prognosis and differential expression of MUC1 between the two subtypes. *Mod Pathol.* 2002;15:1126.
400. Langner C, Ratschek M, Rehak P, et al. Expression of MUC1 (EMA) and E-cadherin in renal cell carcinoma: a systematic immunohistochemical analysis of 188 cases. *Mod Pathol.* 2004;17:180.
401. Delahunt B, Eble JN. Papillary renal cell carcinoma: a clinicopathologic and immunohistochemical study of 105 tumors. *Mod Pathol.* 1997;10:537.
402. Renshaw AA, Corless CL. Papillary renal cell carcinoma. Histology and immunohistochemistry. *Am J Surg Pathol.* 1995;19:842.
403. Renshaw AA, Zhang H, Corless CL, et al. Solid variants of papillary (chromophil) renal cell carcinoma: clinicopathologic and genetic features. *Am J Surg Pathol.* 1997;21:1203.
404. Corless CL, Aburatani H, Fletcher JA, et al. Papillary renal cell carcinoma: quantitation of chromosomes 7 and 17 by FISH, analysis of chromosome 3p for LOH, and DNA ploidy. *Diagn Mol Pathol.* 1996;5:53.
405. Kattar MM, Grignon DJ, Wallis T, et al. Clinicopathologic and interphase cytogenetic analysis of papillary (chromophilic) renal cell carcinoma. *Mod Pathol.* 1997;10:1143.
406. Henke RP, Erbersdobler A. Numerical chromosomal aberrations in papillary renal cortical tumors: relationship with histopathologic features. *Virchows Arch.* 2002;440:604.
407. Tretiakova MS, Sahoo S, Takahashi M, et al. Expression of alpha-methylacyl-CoA racemase in papillary renal cell carcinoma. *Am J Surg Pathol.* 2004;28:69.
408. Couturier J. Genomic classification of renal cell tumors in adults. *Ann Pathol.* 2008;28:402.
409. Meyer PN, Cao Y, Jacobson K, et al. Chromosome 1 analysis in chromophobe renal cell carcinomas with tissue microarray (TMA)-facilitated fluorescence in situ hybridization (FISH) demonstrates loss of 1p/1 which is also present in renal oncocytomas. *Diagn Mol Pathol.* 2008;17:141.
410. Adley BP, Papavero V, Sugimura J, et al. Diagnostic value of cytokeratin 7 and parvalbumin in differentiating chromophobe renal cell carcinoma from renal oncocytoma. *Anal Quant Cytol Histol.* 2006;28:228.
411. Abrahams NA, MacLennan GT, Khoury JD, et al. Chromophobe renal cell carcinoma: a comparative study of histological, immunohistochemical and ultrastructural features using high throughput tissue microarray. *Histopathology.* 2004;45:593.
412. Amin MB, Paner GP, Alvarado-Cabrero I, et al. Chromophobe renal cell carcinoma: histomorphologic characteristics and evaluation of conventional pathologic prognostic parameters in 145 cases. *Am J Surg Pathol.* 2008;32:1822.
413. Pan CC, Chen PC, Ho DM. The diagnostic utility of MOC31, BerEP4, RCC marker and CD10 in the classification of renal cell carcinoma and renal oncocytoma: an immunohistochemical analysis of 328 cases. *Histopathology.* 2004;45:452.
414. Rao Q, Zhou XJ, Shi QL, et al. Expression of Ksp-cadherin in renal epithelial neoplasm and its clinicopathologic significance. *Zhonghua Bing Li Xue Za Zhi.* 2007;36:15.

415. Shen SS, Krishna B, Chirala R, et al. Kidney-specific cadherin, a specific marker for the distal portion of the nephron and related renal neoplasms. *Mod Pathol*. 2005;18:933.
416. Tickoo SK, Amin MB, Zarbo RJ. Colloidal iron staining in renal epithelial neoplasms, including chromophobe renal cell carcinoma: emphasis on technique and patterns of staining. *Am J Surg Pathol*. 1998;22:419.
417. Nese N, Paner GP, Mallin K, et al. Renal cell carcinoma: assessment of key pathologic prognostic parameters and patient characteristics in 47,909 cases using the National Cancer Data Base. *Ann Diagn Pathol*. 2009;13:1.
418. Srigley JR, Eble JN. Collecting duct carcinoma of kidney. *Semin Diagn Pathol*. 1998;15:54.
419. Brandal P, Lie AK, Bassarova A, et al. Genomic aberrations in mucinous tubular and spindle cell renal cell carcinomas. *Mod Pathol*. 2006;19:186.
420. Cossu-Rocca P, Eble JN, Delahunt B, et al. Renal mucinous tubular and spindle carcinoma lacks the gains of chromosomes 7 and 17 and losses of chromosome Y that are prevalent in papillary renal cell carcinoma. *Mod Pathol*. 2006;19:488.
421. Furge KA, Dykema K, Petillo D, et al. Combining differential expression, chromosomal and pathway analyses for the molecular characterization of renal cell carcinoma. *Can Urol Assoc J*. 2007;1:S21.
422. Kuroda N, Hes O, Michal M, et al. Mucinous tubular and spindle cell carcinoma with Fuhrman nuclear grade 3: a histological, immunohistochemical, ultrastructural and FISH study. *Histol Histopathol*. 2008;23:1517.
423. Owens CL, Argani P, Ali SZ. Mucinous tubular and spindle cell carcinoma of the kidney: cytopathologic findings. *Diagn Cytopathol*. 2007;35:593.
424. Paner GP, Srigley JR, Radhakrishnan A, et al. Immunohistochemical analysis of mucinous tubular and spindle cell carcinoma and papillary renal cell carcinoma of the kidney: significant immunophenotypic overlap warrants diagnostic caution. *Am J Surg Pathol*. 2006;30:13.
425. Trabelsi A, Stita W, Yacoubi MT, et al. Renal mucinous tubular and spindle cell carcinoma. *Can Urol Assoc J*. 2008;2:635.
426. Argani P, Netto GJ, Parwani AV. Papillary renal cell carcinoma with low-grade spindle cell foci: a mimic of mucinous tubular and spindle cell carcinoma. *Am J Surg Pathol*. 2008;32:1353.
427. Martignoni G, Pea M, Reghellin D, et al. PEComas: the past, the present and the future. *Virchows Arch*. 2008;452:119.
428. Eble JN, Amin MB, Young RH. Epithelioid angiomyolipoma of the kidney: a report of five cases with a prominent and diagnostically confusing epithelioid smooth muscle component. *Am J Surg Pathol*. 1997;21:1123.
429. Kato I, Inayama Y, Yamanaka S, et al. Epithelioid angiomyolipoma of the kidney. *Pathol Int*. 2009;59:38.
430. Argani P, Aulmann S, Karanjawala Z, et al. Melanotic Xp11 translocation renal cancers: a distinctive neoplasm with overlapping features of PEComa, carcinoma, and melanoma. *Am J Surg Pathol*. 2009;33(4):609-619.
431. Argani P, Hawkins A, Griffin CA, et al. A distinctive pediatric renal neoplasm characterized by epithelioid morphology, basement membrane production, focal HMB45 immunoreactivity, and t(6;11)(p21.1;q12) chromosome translocation. *Am J Pathol*. 2001;158(6):2089-2096.
432. Linehan WM, Pinto PA, Srinivasan R, et al. Identification of the genes for kidney cancer: opportunity for disease-specific targeted therapeutics. *Clin Cancer Res*. 2007;13:671s.
433. Kim WY, Kaelin WG. Role of VHL gene mutation in human cancer. *J Clin Oncol*. 2004;22:4991.
434. Iliopoulos O, Levy AP, Jiang C, et al. Negative regulation of hypoxia-inducible genes by the von Hippel-Lindau protein. *Proc Natl Acad Sci U S A*. 1996;93:10595.
435. Kroog GS, Motzer RJ. Systemic therapy for metastatic renal cell carcinoma. *Urol Clin North Am*. 2008;35:687.
436. Motzer RJ, Bukowski RM, Figlin RA, et al. Prognostic nomogram for sunitinib in patients with metastatic renal cell carcinoma. *Cancer*. 2008;113:1552.
437. Bhatia S, Thompson JA. Temsirolimus in patients with advanced renal cell carcinoma: an overview. *Adv Ther*. 2009.
438. Patard JJ, Pouessel D, Bensalah K, Culine S. Targeted therapy in renal cell carcinoma. *World J Urol*. 2008;26:135.
439. Patard JJ, Pouessel D, Culine S. New therapies in renal cell carcinoma. *Curr Opin Support Palliat Care*. 2007;1:174.
440. Patard JJ, Thuret R, Raffi A, et al. Treatment with Sunitinib enabled complete resection of massive lymphadenopathy not previously amenable to excision in a patient with renal cell carcinoma. *Eur Urol*. 2008; Sept 18:Epub ahead of print.
441. Yang JC, Haworth L, Sherry RM, et al. A randomized trial of bevacizumab, an anti-vascular endothelial growth factor antibody, for metastatic renal cancer. *N Engl J Med*. 2003;349:427.
442. Atkins M, Regan M, McDermott D, et al. Carbonic anhydrase IX expression predicts outcome of interleukin 2 therapy for renal cancer. *Clin Cancer Res*. 2005;11:3714.
443. Steffens MG, Boerman OC, de Mulder PH, et al. Phase I radioimmunotherapy of metastatic renal cell carcinoma with 131I-labeled chimeric monoclonal antibody G250. *Clin Cancer Res*. 1999;5:3268s.
444. Patard JJ, Leray E, Rioux-Leclercq N, et al. Prognostic value of histologic subtypes in renal cell carcinoma: a multicenter experience. *J Clin Oncol*. 2005;23:2763.
445. Cheville JC, Lohse CM, Zincke H, et al. Comparisons of outcome and prognostic features among histologic subtypes of renal cell carcinoma. *Am J Surg Pathol*. 2003;27:612.
446. Lane BR, Kattan MW. Prognostic models and algorithms in renal cell carcinoma. *Urol Clin North Am*. 2008;35:613.
447. Kim HL, Seligson D, Liu X, et al. Using tumor markers to predict the survival of patients with metastatic renal cell carcinoma. *J Urol*. 2005;173:1496.
448. Kim HL, Seligson D, Liu X, et al. Using protein expressions to predict survival in clear cell renal carcinoma. *Clin Cancer Res*. 2004;10:5464.
449. Kluger HM, Siddiqui SF, Angeletti C, et al. Classification of renal cell carcinoma based on expression of VEGF and VEGF receptors in both tumor cells and endothelial cells. *Lab Invest*. 2008;88:962.
450. Hager M, Haufe H, Kemmerling R, et al. Increased activated Akt expression in renal cell carcinomas and prognosis. *J Cell Mol Med*. 2008.
451. Eichelberg C, Junker K, Ljungberg B, Moch H. Diagnostic and prognostic molecular markers for renal cell carcinoma: a critical appraisal of the current state of research and clinical applicability. *Eur Urol*. 2009; B, Jan 13:Epub ahead of print.
452. Djordjevic G, Mozetic V, Mozetic DV, et al. Prognostic significance of vascular endothelial growth factor expression in clear cell renal cell carcinoma. *Pathol Res Pract*. 2007;203:99.
453. Bensalah K, Pantuck AJ, Crepel M, et al. Prognostic variables to predict cancer-related death in incidental renal tumours. *BJU Int*. 2008;102:1376.
454. Pantuck AJ, Seligson DB, Klatte T, et al. Prognostic relevance of the mTOR pathway in renal cell carcinoma: implications for molecular patient selection for targeted therapy. *Cancer*. 2007;109:2257.
455. Pantuck AJ, Thomas G, Belldegrun AS, Figlin RA. Mammalian target of rapamycin inhibitors in renal cell carcinoma: current status and future applications. *Semin Oncol*. 2006;33:607.
456. Bui MH, Seligson D, Han KR, et al. Carbonic anhydrase IX is an independent predictor of survival in advanced renal clear cell carcinoma: implications for prognosis and therapy. *Clin Cancer Res*. 2003;9:802.
457. Jacobsen J, Grankvist K, Rasmuson T, et al. Expression of vascular endothelial growth factor protein in human renal cell carcinoma. *BJU Int*. 2004;93:297.
458. Lidgren A, Hedberg Y, Grankvist K, et al. The expression of hypoxia-inducible factor 1alpha is a favorable independent prognostic factor in renal cell carcinoma. *Clin Cancer Res*. 2005;11:1129.
459. Migita T, Oda Y, Naito S, Tsuneyoshi M. Low expression of p27(Kip1) is associated with tumor size and poor prognosis in patients with renal cell carcinoma. *Cancer*. 2002;94:973.
460. Hedberg Y, Davoodi E, Ljungberg B, et al. Cyclin E and p27 protein content in human renal cell carcinoma: clinical outcome and associations with cyclin D. *Int J Cancer*. 2002;102:601.
461. Hedberg Y, Ljungberg B, Roos G, Landberg G. Expression of cyclin D1, D3, E, and p27 in human renal cell carcinoma analysed by tissue microarray. *Br J Cancer*. 2003;88:1417.

462. Cheng L. Establishing a germ cell origin for metastatic tumors using OCT4 immunohistochemistry. *Cancer*. 2004;101:206.
463. Biermann K, Klingmuller D, Koch A, et al. Diagnostic value of markers M2A, OCT3/4, AP-2gamma, PLAP and c-KIT in the detection of extragonadal seminomas. *Histopathology*. 2006;49:290.
464. Iczkowski KA, Butler SL, Shanks JH, et al. Trials of new germ cell immunohistochemical stains in 93 extragonadal and metastatic germ cell tumors. *Hum Pathol*. 2008;39:275.
465. Sung MT, Jones TD, Beck SD, et al. OCT4 is superior to CD30 in the diagnosis of metastatic embryonal carcinomas after chemotherapy. *Hum Pathol*. 2006;37:662.
466. Looijenga LH, Stoop H, de Leeuw HP, et al. POU5F1 (OCT3/4) identifies cells with pluripotent potential in human germ cell tumors. *Cancer Res*. 2003;63:2244.
467. Jones TD, Ulbright TM, Eble JN, et al. OCT4 staining in testicular tumors: a sensitive and specific marker for seminoma and embryonal carcinoma. *Am J Surg Pathol*. 2004;28:935.
468. Jones TD, Ulbright TM, Eble JN, Cheng L. OCT4: A sensitive and specific biomarker for intratubular germ cell neoplasia of the testis. *Clin Cancer Res*. 2004;10:8544.
469. Biermann K, Goke F, Nettersheim D, et al. c-KIT is frequently mutated in bilateral germ cell tumours and down-regulated during progression from intratubular germ cell neoplasia to seminoma. *J Pathol*. 2007;213:311.
470. Coffey J, Linger R, Pugh J, et al. Somatic KIT mutations occur predominantly in seminoma germ cell tumors and are not predictive of bilateral disease: report of 220 tumors and review of literature. *Genes Chromosomes Cancer*. 2008;47:34.
471. Kemmer K, Corless CL, Fletcher JA, et al. KIT mutations are common in testicular seminomas. *Am J Pathol*. 2004;164:305.
472. Leroy X, Augusto D, Leteurtre E, Gosselin B. CD30 and CD117 (c-kit) used in combination are useful for distinguishing embryonal carcinoma from seminoma. *J Histochem Cytochem*. 2002;50:283.
473. Nikolaou M, Valavanis C, Aravantinos G, et al. Kit expression in male germ cell tumors. *Anticancer Res*. 2007;27:1685.
474. Willmore-Payne C, Holden JA, Chadwick BE, Layfield LJ. Detection of c-kit exons 11- and 17-activating mutations in testicular seminomas by high-resolution melting amplicon analysis. *Mod Pathol*. 2006;19:1164.
475. Lau SK, Weiss LM, Chu PG. D2-40 immunohistochemistry in the differential diagnosis of seminoma and embryonal carcinoma: a comparative immunohistochemical study with KIT (CD117) and CD30. *Mod Pathol*. 2007;20:320.
476. Hoei-Hansen CE, Nielsen JE, Almstrup K, et al. Transcription factor AP-2gamma is a developmentally regulated marker of testicular carcinoma in situ and germ cell tumors. *Clin Cancer Res*. 2004;10:8521.
477. Hong SM, Frierson Jr HF, Moskaluk CA. AP-2gamma protein expression in intratubular germ cell neoplasia of testis. *Am J Clin Pathol*. 2005;124:873.
478. Pauls K, Jager R, Weber S, et al. Transcription factor AP-2gamma, a novel marker of gonocytes and seminomatous germ cell tumors. *Int J Cancer*. 2005;115:470.
479. Manivel JC, Jessurun J, Wick MR, Dehner LP. Placental alkaline phosphatase immunoreactivity in testicular germ-cell neoplasms. *Am J Surg Pathol*. 1987;11:21.
480. Javadpour N. The role of biologic tumor markers in testicular cancer. *Cancer*. 1980;45:1755.
481. Ulbright TM, Young RH, Scully RE. Trophoblastic tumors of the testis other than classic choriocarcinoma: "monophasic" choriocarcinoma and placental site trophoblastic tumor: a report of two cases. *Am J Surg Pathol*. 1997;21:282.
482. McCluggage WG, Shanks JH, Whiteside C, et al. Immunohistochemical study of testicular sex cord-stromal tumors, including staining with anti-inhibin antibody. *Am J Surg Pathol*. 1998;22:615.
483. McCluggage WG, Ashe P, McBride H, et al. Localization of the cellular expression of inhibin in trophoblastic tissue. *Histopathology*. 1998;32:252.
484. Skakkebaek NE. Carcinoma in situ of the testis: frequency and relationship to invasive germ cell tumours in infertile men. *Histopathology*. 2002;41(3A):5-18.
485. Ulbright TM. Testis risk and prognostic factors. The pathologist's perspective. *Urol Clin North Am*. 1999;26:611.
486. van Casteren NJ, de Jong J, Stoop H, et al. Evaluation of testicular biopsies for carcinoma in situ: immunohistochemistry is mandatory. *Int J Androl*. 2008.
487. Akre O, Pettersson A, Richiardi L. Risk of contralateral testicular cancer among men with unilaterally undescended testis: a meta analysis. *Int J Cancer*. 2009;124:687.
488. Burke AP, Mostofi FK. Intratubular malignant germ cells in testicular biopsies: clinical course and identification by staining for placental alkaline phosphatase. *Mod Pathol*. 1988;1:475.
489. Cheng L, Sung MT, Cossu-Rocca P, et al. OCT4: biological functions and clinical applications as a marker of germ cell neoplasia. *J Pathol*. 2007;211:1.
490. Ulbright TM. Germ cell tumors of the gonads: a selective review emphasizing problems in differential diagnosis, newly appreciated, and controversial issues. *Mod Pathol*. 2005;18(Suppl) 2:S61.
491. Liu DL, Lu YP, Shi HY, et al. Expression of CD117 in human testicular germ cell tumors and its diagnostic value for seminoma and nonseminoma. *Zhonghua Nan Ke Xue*. 2008;14:38.
492. Iczkowski KA, Butler SL. New immunohistochemical markers in testicular tumors. *Anal Quant Cytol Histol*. 2006;28:181.
493. Emerson RE, Ulbright TM. The use of immunohistochemistry in the differential diagnosis of tumors of the testis and paratestis. *Semin Diagn Pathol*. 2005;22:33.
494. Emerson RE, Ulbright TM. Morphological approach to tumours of the testis and paratestis. *J Clin Pathol*. 2007;60:866.
495. de Jong J, Looijenga LH. Stem cell marker OCT3/4 in tumor biology and germ cell tumor diagnostics: history and future. *Crit Rev Oncog*. 2006;12:171.
496. Carano KS, Soslow RA. Immunophenotypic analysis of ovarian and testicular Mullerian papillary serous tumors. *Mod Pathol*. 1997;10:414.
497. Wick MR, Swanson PE, Manivel JC. Placental-like alkaline phosphatase reactivity in human tumors: an immunohistochemical study of 520 cases. *Hum Pathol*. 1987;18:946.
498. Suster S, Moran CA, Dominguez-Malagon H, Quevedo-Blanco P. Germ cell tumors of the mediastinum and testis: a comparative immunohistochemical study of 120 cases. *Hum Pathol*. 1998;29:737.
499. Cheville JC, Rao S, Iczkowski KA, et al. Cytokeratin expression in seminoma of the human testis. *Am J Clin Pathol*. 2000;113:583.
500. Hittmair A, Rogatsch H, Hobisch A, et al. CD30 expression in seminoma. *Hum Pathol*. 1996;27:1166.
501. Koshida K, Wahren B. Placental-like alkaline phosphatase in seminoma. *Urol Res*. 1990;18:87.
502. Balzer BL, Ulbright TM. Spontaneous regression of testicular germ cell tumors: an analysis of 42 cases. *Am J Surg Pathol*. 2006;30:858.
503. Ulbright TM. The most common, clinically significant misdiagnoses in testicular tumor pathology, and how to avoid them. *Adv Anat Pathol*. 2008;15:18.
504. Bomeisl PE, MacLennan GT. Spermatocytic seminoma. *J Urol*. 2007;177:734.
505. Chung PW, Bayley AJ, Sweet J, et al. Spermatocytic seminoma: a review. *Eur Urol*. 2004;45:495.
506. Decaussin M, Borda A, Bouvier R, et al. Spermatocytic seminoma. A clinicopathological and immunohistochemical study of 7 cases. *Ann Pathol*. 2004;24:161.
507. Dundr P, Pesl M, Povysil C, et al. Anaplastic variant of spermatocytic seminoma. *Pathol Res Pract*. 2007;203:621.
508. Looijenga LH, Hersmus R, Gillis AJ, et al. Genomic and expression profiling of human spermatocytic seminomas: primary spermatocyte as tumorigenic precursor and DMRT1 as candidate chromosome 9 gene. *Cancer Res*. 2006;66:290.
509. Ulbright TM, Young RH. Seminoma with tubular, microcystic, and related patterns: a study of 28 cases of unusual morphologic variants that often cause confusion with yolk sac tumor. *Am J Surg Pathol*. 2005;29:500.
510. Rajpert-De Meyts E, Jacobsen GK, Bartkova J, et al. The immunohistochemical expression pattern of Chk2, p53, p19INK4d, MAGE-A4 and other selected antigens provides new evidence for the premeiotic origin of spermatocytic seminoma. *Histopathology*. 2003;42:217.

511. Billings SD, Roth LM, Ulbright TM. Microcystic Leydig cell tumors mimicking yolk sac tumor: a report of four cases. *Am J Surg Pathol.* 1999;23:546.
512. Comperat E, Tissier F, Boye K, et al. Non-Leydig sex-cord tumors of the testis. The place of immunohistochemistry in diagnosis and prognosis. A study of twenty cases. *Virchows Arch.* 2004;444:567.
513. Gilcrease MZ, Delgado R, Albores-Saavedra J. Testicular Sertoli cell tumor with a heterologous sarcomatous component: immunohistochemical assessment of Sertoli cell differentiation. *Arch Pathol Lab Med.* 1998;122:907.
514. Gordon MD, Corless C, Renshaw AA, Beckstead J. CD99, keratin, and vimentin staining of sex cord-stromal tumors, normal ovary, and testis. *Mod Pathol.* 1998;11:769.
515. Groisman GM, Dische MR, Fine EM, Unger PD. Juvenile granulosa cell tumor of the testis: a comparative immunohistochemical study with normal infantile gonads. *Pediatr Pathol.* 1993;13:389.
516. Young RH, Koelliker DD, Scully RE. Sertoli cell tumors of the testis, not otherwise specified: a clinicopathologic analysis of 60 cases. *Am J Surg Pathol.* 1998;22:709.
517. Zukerberg LR, Young RH, Scully RE. Sclerosing Sertoli cell tumor of the testis. A report of 10 cases. *Am J Surg Pathol.* 1991;15:829.
518. Ulbright TM, Young RH. Metastatic carcinoma to the testis: a clinicopathologic analysis of 26 nonincidental cases with emphasis on deceptive features. *Am J Surg Pathol.* 2008;32:1683.
519. Al-Abbadi MA, Hattab EM, Tarawneh MS, et al. Primary testicular diffuse large B-cell lymphoma belongs to the nongerminal center B-cell-like subgroup: a study of 18 cases. *Mod Pathol.* 2006;19:1521.
520. Ferry JA, Harris NL, Young RH, et al. Malignant lymphoma of the testis, epididymis, and spermatic cord. A clinicopathologic study of 69 cases with immunophenotypic analysis. *Am J Surg Pathol.* 1994;18:376.
521. Ferry JA, Young RH, Scully RE. Testicular and epididymal plasmacytoma: a report of 7 cases, including three that were the initial manifestation of plasma cell myeloma. *Am J Surg Pathol.* 1997;21:590.
522. Ulbright TM, Orazi A, de Riese W, et al. The correlation of P53 protein expression with proliferative activity and occult metastases in clinical stage I non-seminomatous germ cell tumors of the testis. *Mod Pathol.* 1994;7:64.
523. Baltaci S, Orhan D, Turkolmez K, et al. P53, bcl-2 and bax immunoreactivity as predictors of response and outcome after chemotherapy for metastatic germ cell testicular tumours. *BJU Int.* 2001;87:661.
524. Bartkova J, Bartek J, Lukas J, et al. P53 Protein Alterations in Human Testicular Cancer Including Pre-Invasive Intratubular Germ-Cell Neoplasia. *Int J Cancer.* 1991;49:196.
525. Berney DM, Shamash J, Gaffney J, et al. DNA topoisomerase I and II expression in drug resistant germ cell tumours. *Br J Cancer.* 2002;87:624.
526. Kersemaekers AM, Mayer F, Molier M, et al. Role of P53 and MDM2 in treatment response of human germ cell tumors. *J Clin Oncol.* 2002;20:1551.
527. Sandberg AA, Meloni AM, Suijkerbuijk RF. Reviews of chromosome studies in urological tumors. III. Cytogenetics and genes in testicular tumors. *J Urol.* 1996;155:1531.
528. Suijkerbuijk RF, Sinke RJ, Meloni AM, et al. Overrepresentation of chromosome 12p sequences and karyotypic evolution in i(12p)-negative testicular germ-cell tumors revealed by fluorescence in situ hybridization. *Cancer Genet Cytogenet.* 1993;70:85.
529. Cheng L, Zhang S, MacLennan GT, et al. Interphase fluorescence in situ hybridization analysis of chromosome 12p abnormalities is useful for distinguishing epidermoid cysts of the testis from pure mature teratoma. *Clin Cancer Res.* 2006;12:5668.
530. Looijenga LH, Zafarana G, Grygalewicz B, et al. Role of gain of 12p in germ cell tumour development. *APMIS.* 2003;111:161.
531. Reuter VE. Origins and molecular biology of testicular germ cell tumors. *Mod Pathol.* 2005;18:(suppl)2:S51.
532. Rosenberg C, Van Gurp RJ, Geelen E, et al. Overrepresentation of the short arm of chromosome 12 is related to invasive growth of human testicular seminomas and nonseminomas. *Oncogene.* 2000;19:5858.
533. Wehle D, Yonescu R, Long PP, et al. Fluorescence in situ hybridization of 12p in germ cell tumors using a bacterial artificial chromosome clone 12p probe on paraffin-embedded tissue: clinical test validation. *Cancer Genet Cytogenet.* 2008;183:99.
534. Eid H, Geczi L, Magori A, et al. Drug resistance and sensitivity of germ cell testicular tumors: evaluation of clinical relevance of MDR1/Pgp, p53, and metallothionein (MT) proteins. *Anticancer Res.* 1998;18:3059.
535. Eid H, Institoris E, Geczi L, Bodrogi I, Bak M. Mdm-2 Expression in Human Testicular Germ-Cell Tumors and its Clinical Value. *Anticancer Res.* 1999;19:3485.
536. Eid H, Van der Looij M, Institoris E, et al. Is p53 expression, detected by immunohistochemistry, an important parameter of response to treatment in testis cancer? *Anticancer Res.* 1997;17:2663.
537. Mayer F, Gillis AJ, Dinjens W, et al. Microsatellite instability of germ cell tumors is associated with resistance to systemic treatment. *Cancer Res.* 2002;62:2758.
538. Mayer F, Stoop H, Scheffer GL, et al. Molecular determinants of treatment response in human germ cell tumors. *Clin Cancer Res.* 2003;9:767.
539. Dimov ND, Zynger DL, Luan C, et al. Topoisomerase II alpha expression in testicular germ cell tumors. *Urology.* 2007;69:955.
540. Mazumdar M, Bacik J, Tickoo SK, et al. Cluster analysis of p53 and Ki67 expression, apoptosis, alpha-fetoprotein, and human chorionic gonadotrophin indicates a favorable prognostic subgroup within the embryonal carcinoma germ cell tumor. *J Clin Oncol.* 2003;21:2679.

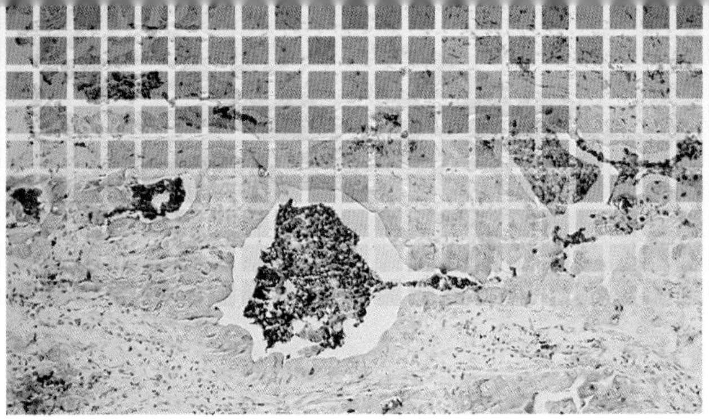

17

Immunohistology of Pediatric Neoplasms

Cheryl M. Coffin • Jessica M. Comstock • Jeremy C. Wallentine

Introduction 662
Biology of the Antigens and Antibodies 662
Diagnostic Immunohistochemistry of Specific Tumors 663
Summary 683

INTRODUCTION

Solid neoplasms of childhood and adolescence comprise a diverse group of diagnostically challenging entities with the basic morphologic themes of small round blue cell and spindle cell neoplasms. Immunohistochemistry and molecular diagnostic tests have greatly improved the ability to classify these neoplasms.[1-4] Use of ancillary diagnostic techniques has become increasingly important in diagnosis, evaluation of recurrent or metastatic disease, and, in some, cases prognostic classification. The importance of close communication among a multidisciplinary team including oncologists, surgeons, radiologists, radiation oncologists, medical geneticists, and pathologists must be emphasized. In addition, ancillary diagnostic tests must be interpreted in the context of the light microscopic findings, and specimen adequacy is a critical factor. Immunohistochemistry is a valuable tool but has significant pitfalls in specific instances.[5,6] Tissue fixation, necrosis, focality of marker expression, artifactual changes on small specimens such as core needle biopsies, and other technical factors may influence the immunohistochemical results. Techniques such as flow cytometry for leukemias and lymphomas,[7] electron microscopy,[8-12] and molecular testing[13-15] may be necessary to support the diagnosis or provide prognostic information. Therefore tumor protocols for handling specimens and procuring tissues can provide important guidelines for pathologic evaluation.[16-21]

This chapter discusses the diagnostic evaluation, immunohistochemical findings, and genomic and prognostic aspects of pediatric and adolescent solid neoplasms including neuroblastoma (NB) and related neuroblastic tumors, rhabdomyosarcoma (RMS), Ewing's sarcoma/primitive neuroectodermal tumor (EWS/PNET), desmoplastic small round cell tumor (DSRCT), malignant rhabdoid tumor (MRT), Wilms' tumor (WT), and osteosarcoma (OS). In many cases the combination of the clinical and radiologic presentation and the light microscopic appearance are sufficient for diagnosis. In other cases the tumor may have a predominantly round or spindle cell pattern, which leads to a differential diagnosis that depends on the clinical, radiologic, and morphologic findings. For example, a tumor in an infant with an adrenal mass, elevated serum and urine catecholamine levels, and the microscopic finding of neuroblasts in a background of neuropil with calcification and thin fibrovascular septa can be confidently diagnosed as NB. On the other hand, a primitive RMS may require immunohistochemistry or even molecular analysis to reach a diagnosis. The decision about when to order special tests depends on the complexity of the tumor and the individual pathologist's experience. An initial limited panel of immunohistochemistry is often the first step toward refining or confirming the diagnosis. If this results in unexpected or contradictory findings, another more comprehensive panel may then be obtained and cytogenetic or molecular genetic testing can be considered. In any case, use of a panel of immunohistochemical stains rather than over-reliance on a single antibody is an important diagnostic principle.

BIOLOGY OF THE ANTIGENS AND ANTIBODIES

Principal Antibodies

Many different antibodies are used for the immunohistochemical evaluation of pediatric solid neoplasms. The more generally used antibodies are discussed in other chapters. This section summarizes antibodies with particular importance for the neoplasms covered in this chapter such as myogenic transcriptional regulatory proteins, CD99, the FLI-1 protein, the Wilms' tumor-1 (WT1) protein, and the hSNF5/INI1 protein. All of these antibodies reflect specific genomic activity related to this group of tumors.

MYOGENIC REGULATORY PROTEINS

Myogenin (myf-4), Myo-D1, myf-5, and mrf-4-herculin/myf-6 comprise a family of myogenic transcriptional regulatory proteins that are involved in skeletal muscle differentiation and are expressed earlier than structural proteins such as desmin or actin. Myogenin and Myo-D1 are expressed in RMS, even those that are less differentiated and lack definitive morphologic evidence of rhabdomyoblastic differentiation such as strap cells with cross striations.[22-24] Numerous studies have demonstrated the specificity of myogenin and Myo-D1 as a marker for RMS.[22-28] This contrasts with muscle specific actin and desmin, which can be found in many different neoplasms including skeletal muscle, smooth muscle, and fibroblastic-myofibroblastic tumors. Cytoplasmic staining for Myo-D1 can be observed in nonmyogenous tumors such as NB, so it is important to adhere strictly to the requirement for nuclear staining for interpretation of Myo-D1 stains. Tumors that display skeletal muscle differentiation such as WT, ectomesenchymoma, and malignant peripheral nerve sheath tumor with divergent differentiation can show reactivity for myogenic transcriptional regulatory proteins.[29] Non-neoplastic skeletal muscle fiber nuclei can stain positively for myogenin.[27] Different patterns of staining for myogenin in different subtypes of RMS have been observed.[30]

CD99 (P30/32 MIC2)

This group of antibodies detects a transmembrane glycoprotein that is the product of the pseudoautosomal mic2-gene on chromosome Xp22-pter,[31] and chromosome Yq11-pter.[32] CD99, as detected with a variety of antibodies including O13, 12E7, and HBA-71, is expressed by 85% to 95% of EWS/PNET and demonstrates strong membranous staining in this context.[31,33,34] Absence of staining for CD99 may be an indication to perform additional studies such as further immunohistochemical stains, molecular analysis, or electron microscopy to support the diagnosis of EWS/PNET and exclude other small round blue cell tumors. CD99 is also positive in acute lymphoblastic leukemia/lymphoblastic lymphoma, acute myelogenous leukemia, granulocytic sarcoma, mesenchymal chondrosarcoma, synovial sarcoma, vascular tumors, and other malignancies.[35-40] There has been some speculation that antigen retrieval techniques may result in increased expression of CD99 in a variety of tumors.[39] Caution is warranted in distinguishing between EWS/PNET and acute lymphoblastic leukemia/lymphoma in similar tumors because of the immunohistochemical overlap, especially in cases with unusual clinical presentations.[35,41] CD99 is especially useful in the distinction between EWS/PNET and NB.[42] The potential for many different types of tumors to express CD99 emphasizes the importance of a panel of antibodies in differential diagnosis of small round cell tumors.

FLI-1

The FLI-1 protein is overexpressed in EWS/PNETs, which contain the *EWS-FLI1/1* fusion gene, owing to the translocation t(11;22)(q24;q12).[43] Nuclear FLI-1 immunoreactivity is found in approximately 70% of EWS/PNET but is also observed in nearly 90% of lymphoblastic lymphomas and in vascular tumors.[44,45] This antibody is useful as part of a panel for evaluation of potential EWS/PNET, when the overlap with lymphoblastic lymphomas and vascular neoplasms is considered.

WT1

An antibody to the carboxy-terminal (C-terminal) region of the *WT* gene (WT1) is useful in recognition of desmoplastic small round cell tumor. DSRCT shows strong nuclear staining with a C-terminal WT1 antibody.[46-48] WT and RMS can also show nuclear reactivity for WT1.[37,47,48] We have observed occasional examples of other small round cell tumors including EWS/PNET, with reactivity for WT1, so further evaluation of this antibody will be necessary.

hSNF5/INI1

MRT (atypical teratoid/rhabdoid tumor) frequently demonstrates deletion and mutation of the *hSNF5/INI1* gene, with decreased or absent INI1 protein expression. An antibody to INI1 can be used to assess *INI1* loss, characterized by absence of immunoreactivity in contrast to functional *INI1* with positive immunoreactivity in normal tissues and other neoplasms.[49] Like MRT of the kidney and extrarenal soft tissues, atypical teratoid/rhabdoid tumors of the central nervous system showed absence of nuclear staining for INI1 in a recent study.[49-51]

Antibody Specifications

Table 17.1 illustrates the optimized antibodies commonly used in the evaluation of these tumors.

DIAGNOSTIC IMMUNOHISTOCHEMISTRY OF SPECIFIC TUMORS

Neuroblastoma and Neuroblastic Tumors

NB, ganglioneuroblastoma, and ganglioneuroma are members of the family of neuroblastic tumors of the adrenal gland and sympathetic nervous system, which are derived from migrating neuroectodermal tumors

TABLE 17.1 Key Pathologic, Immunohistochemical, and Genetic Features of Selected Pediatric Neoplasms

Diagnosis	Histopathology	Immunophenotype	Genetic Aberrations
Neuroblastoma	SRCs in sheets or nests with variable mitoses, karyorrhexis, neuropil, rosettes, fibrovascular septa, and schwannian stroma.	NSE, synaptophysin, chromogranin, neurofilament, CD57, CD56, PGP9.5.	*MYCN* amplification; deletion of chromosomes 1p or 11q.
Rhabdomyosarcoma	Alveolar: alveolar or solid architecture. SRCs with variable rhabdomyoblastic differentiation, giant rhabdomyoblastic cells, clear cells.	Alveolar: myogenin, Myo-D1, desmin, muscle-specific actin.	t(2;13)(q35;q14) with *PAX3/FKHR* fusion. t(1;13)(p36;q14) with *PAX7/FKHR* fusion.
	Embryonal: primitive spindled, stellate, round, and polygonal cells in variably myxoid background. Variable rhabdomyoblasts, strap cells, multinucleated cells, and myotube forms.	Embryonal: myogenin, Myo-D1, muscle-specific actin, desmin.	Loss of heterozygosity at 11p15.5 and other nonspecific abnormalities.
Ewing's sarcoma/ PNET	SRCs in sheets with round nuclei, fine chromatin, scanty cytoplasm. Variable rosettes, prominent nucleoli, spindle cells, necrosis.	Vimentin, CD99, synaptophysin, Fli-1.	t(11;22)(q24;q12) with *EWS/FLI-1* fusion. t(21;22)(q22;q12) with *EWS/ERG* fusion. t(7;22)(p22;q12) with *EWS/ETV1* fusion. t(17;22)(q12;q12) with *EWS/E1AF* fusion. t(2;22)(q33;q12)with *EWS/FEV* fusion. Other translocations.
Desmoplastic small round cell tumor	SRCs in nests with prominent stromal desmoplasia, central necrosis, variable cystic degeneration, and epithelial differentiation.	Polyphenotypic: cytokeratins, epithelial membrane antigen, vimentin, desmin, WT1 (C-terminus), CD99.	t(11;22)(p13;q12) with *EWS/WT1* fusion.
Malignant rhabdoid tumor	Polygonal or SRCs in sheets or trabeculae with large, vesicular nuclei, prominent central nucleoli, abundant eccentric cytoplasm, frequent mitoses. Globoid, hyaline, eosinophilic cytoplasmic inclusion.	Polyphenotypic: vimentin cytokeratin, epithelial membrane antigen. Variable CD99, synaptophysin, S-100 protein, muscle-specific actin. Absence of INI1.	Deletion or mutation of *HSNF5/INI1 (SMARCB1)* on chromosome 22q11.
Wilms' tumor	Triphasic blastemal, epithelial, and stromal components. Blastemal cells small, round or oval, in nodules or serpentine patterns. Epithelial component primitive rosette-like to tubular or papillary. Mesenchymal component fibrous, myoid, adipose, chondroid, osseous, neural.	Blastemal: vimentin, desmin. Epithelial: cytokeratin. Mesenchymal: variable according to differentiation pattern.	Various abnormalities including mutations of *WT1* at 11p13 and *WT2* at 11p15; numeric and structural karyotypic abnormalities of chromosomes 1, 11, 13, 14, 16, 17, 19, and 22.
Osteosarcoma	Anaplastic, pleomorphic cells with morphologic spectrum, osteoid, bone formation.	Heterogeneous, without a specific immunophenotype.	Nonspecific numeric and structural abnormalities.

NSE, Neuron-specific enolase; PNET, primitive neuroectodermal tumor; SRCs, small round cells.

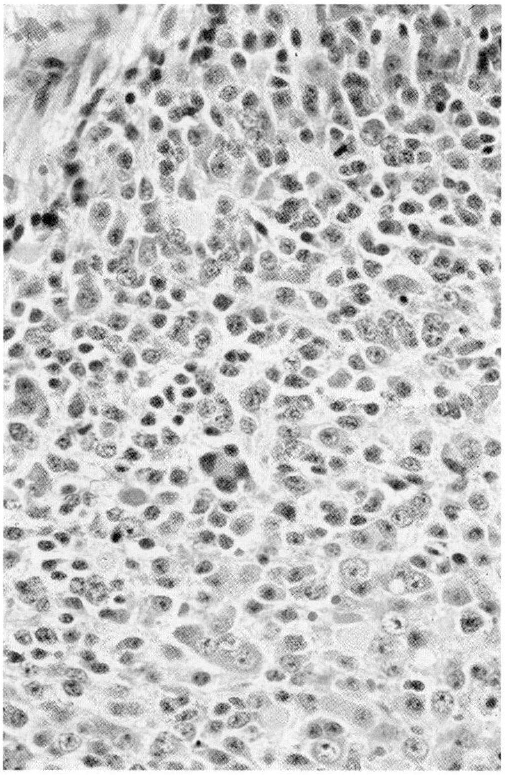

FIGURE 17.1 Neuroblastoma with differentiation consists of small round blue cells and occasional larger cells with more vesicular nuclei and more abundant eosinophilic cytoplasm (hematoxylin-eosin, ×200).

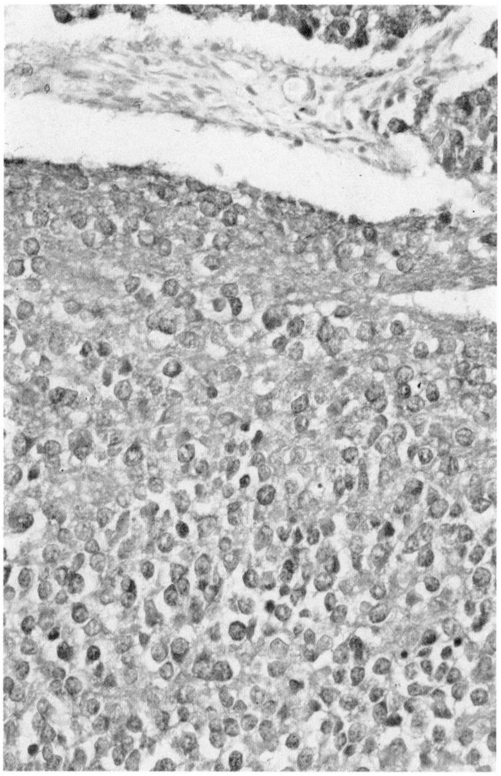

FIGURE 17.2 Neuron-specific enolase shows diffuse cytoplasmic reactivity in neuroblastoma (immunoperoxidase, ×400).

of the neural crest.[52] The specific types of neuroblastic tumors are designated according to the degree of neuroblastic differentiation and schwannian stromal development. The current terminology has been defined by the International Neuroblastoma Pathology Committee as NB, ganglioneuroblastoma (intermixed schwannian stroma-rich), ganglioneuroma, and ganglioneuroblastoma, nodular (composite schwannian stroma-rich/stroma-dominant, and stroma-poor).[21,53] Neuroblastic tumors are the most common solid extracranial malignant neoplasm of the first 2 years of life, and most occur in the first decade. The most common site is the adrenal gland, followed by the abdominal, thoracic, cervical, and pelvic regions in areas where sympathetic ganglia are found. The macroscopic appearance varies according to the amount of schwannian stroma, degree of differentiation, and extent of necrosis and hemorrhage.

Classic NB is a cellular neuroblastic tumor without a prominent schwannian stroma and consists of small blue cells with varying degrees of rosette formation, fibrillar neuropil background, fibrovascular stroma, and differentiating neuroblasts with or without recognizable ganglion cells (Fig. 17.1).[21,53] Ganglioneuroblastoma has two subtypes, intermixed and nodular. The intermixed type of ganglioneuroblastoma contains foci of neuroblastic elements similar to NB within a schwannian stroma, which comprises more than 50% of the volume of the tumor. Nodular ganglioneuroblastoma, in contrast, contains one or more grossly visible neuroblastic nodules in a tumor with a dominant appearance of intermixed ganglioneuroblastoma or ganglioneuroma. Ganglioneuroma is composed predominantly of schwannian stroma with individually distributed mature ganglion cells with or without sparse differentiating neuroblasts and immature ganglion cells.

Although NB has a neuronal phenotype, it does not have a specific immunohistochemical profile. Neuroblasts are reactive for a variety of markers that characterize neuronal differentiation including neuron-specific enolase (Fig.17.2), CD57, CD56, protein gene product 9.5 (PGP 9.5), GD2 (a ganglioside on human NB cell membranes), NB84 (an antibody to NB cell lines), synaptophysin (Fig. 17.3), chromogranin, and neurofilament protein.[21,53-58] Some of these markers are highly sensitive but nonspecific such as neuron-specific enolase, CD57, CD56, and PGP9.5. On the other hand, the more specific markers such as synaptophysin, chromogranin, and neurofilament protein are less sensitive. Endocrine markers may occasionally be found in neuroblastic tumors, especially in the context of secretory diarrhea associated with vasoactive intestinal peptide production in a neuroblastic tumor. The schwannian stroma may be reactive for S-100 protein, and favorable histology NBs typically have more prominent S-100 protein stromal staining.[59] The neuronal markers may also be more strongly positive and more frequently positive in more differentiated NB but do not contribute to prognostic categorization.[60] Markers that are nonreactive in

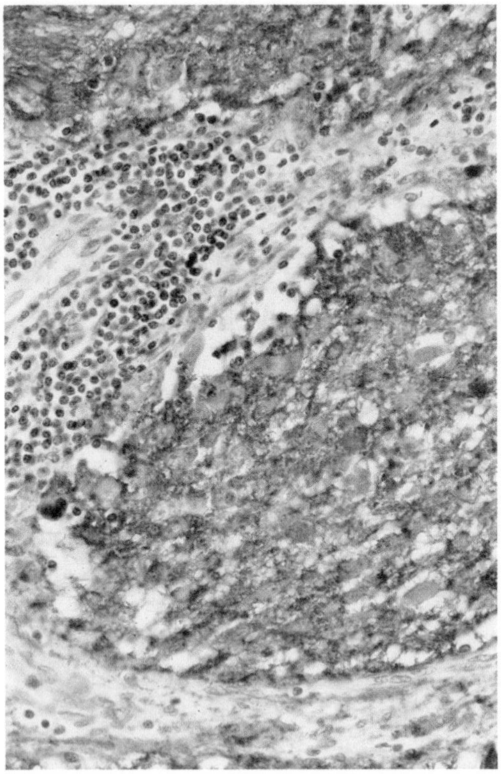

FIGURE 17.3 Synaptophysin shows strong cytoplasmic reactivity in neuroblastoma (immunoperoxidase, ×400).

NB and therefore useful for differential diagnosis from other small blue cell malignant neoplasms include desmin, myogenic markers such as myogenin and Myo-D1, vimentin, leukocyte common antigen, and CD99. Reactivity for leukocyte common antigen (CD45) can be used to distinguish chronic inflammation from neuroblastoma in small biopsies, post-treatment specimens, or other problematic cases.[55] Evaluation of neuronal markers can also be useful for detection of bone marrow metastases.[61] A potential pitfall in distinction from anaplastic large cell lymphoma and some examples of RMS is the presence of reactivity for ALK-1 in more than 90% of NB.[62]

KEY DIAGNOSTIC POINTS

Neuroblastoma and Neuroblastic Tumors

- TRK-A expression in NB correlates with favorable prognosis and has an inverse correlation with *MYCN* amplification.
- Other markers such as CD44 and proliferation markers may be useful in the future for prognostic categorization.
- Neuroblastic tumors are typically nonreactive for vimentin, desmin, specific myogenic markers such as myogenin and Myo-D1, keratins, and CD99.
- A potential pitfall in the distinction of neuroblastic tumors from anaplastic large cell lymphoma and some examples of RMS is the presence of reactivity for ALK-1 in more than 90% of NB.

Undifferentiated and poorly differentiated NB without obvious ganglion cells or schwannian differentiation may be extremely difficult to distinguish from other small blue cell tumors, particularly EWS/PNET, leukemia/lymphoma, RMS, and MRT. Judicious use of myogenic markers and hematolymphoid markers helps to identify RMS, leukemias, and lymphomas. NBs are typically negative for vimentin and CD99, which permit distinction from EWS/PNET.[54] MRT displays reactivity for vimentin, keratins, and epithelial membrane antigen, in addition to other mesenchymal markers, which aid in the distinction from NB.[63]

KEY DIFFERENTIAL DIAGNOSIS

Neuroblastoma and Neuroblastic Tumors

- Neuroblastic tumors express neuronal markers of varying sensitivity and specificity: neuron-specific enolase, leu-7, protein gene product 9.5, synaptophysin, chromogranin, and other markers.
- S-100 protein expression may be seen in the schwannian stroma of differentiating neuroblastoma, ganglioneuroblastoma, and ganglioneuroma.

GENOMIC APPLICATIONS

This group of antibodies is used in the diagnostic sense and detects the transmembrane glycoprotein that is the product of the pseudoautosomal mic2-gene on chromosome Xp22.32-pter and chromosome Yq11-pter.[32] CD99 is the expression product of the mic-2 gene, and its absence is a diagnostic indication to perform additional studies in order to exclude other small round blue cell tumors.

THERANOSTIC APPLICATIONS

A variety of immunohistochemical markers have been assessed for prognostic utility. Proliferation markers are more highly expressed in more advanced neuroblastic tumors with unfavorable prognostic features, and their absence may be associated with longer survival. These markers include Ki-67 and REPP 86.[64-66] The cell surface glycoprotein, CD44, is expressed in favorable histology NB and nonexpression is associated with unfavorable histology.[67-69] Conflicting results have been published about the prognostic significance of c-*kit* expression.[70,71] Expression of apoptotic markers bcl-2 and bax proteins appear to be related to the chemotherapeutic response and may be useful future prognostic markers.[72] There is also a potential role for evaluating matrix metalloproteinase expression and its specific tissue inhibitor metalloproteinases for prognostic purposes.[73] It is well known that high levels of TRK-A expression with or without TRK-C expression are associated with favorable histology and favorable outcome and that unfavorable tumors express TRK-B and its ligand BDNF.[52,74-80]

The DNA index is a prognostic marker in patients younger than 2 years old who have disseminated NB, with triploidy being favorable and near-diploidy being unfavorable.[81] Deletion or rearrangement of chromosome 1p36 is the most common karyotypic abnormality and seems to predict an increased risk of relapse in patients with localized tumors.[4,74,75,81] *MYCN* amplification is associated with unfavorable outcome and is an important molecular prognostic marker.[82-84]

Recently, an international consensus panel has proposed initial criteria for neuroblastoma risk stratification, called the International Neuroblastoma Risk Group (INRG) classification system.[81] Preliminary elements include age at diagnosis dichotomized around 18 months, stage before treatment, and *MYCN* amplification status. The INRG criteria are still in development, so whether immunohistochemical markers will be included is unclear.

BEYOND IMMUNOHISTOCHEMISTRY: ANATOMIC MOLECULAR DIAGNOSTIC APPLICATIONS

A variety of cytogenetic and molecular genetic abnormalities have been described in NB, but none has diagnostic specificity.[74,75]

MYCN amplification status can be measured by fluorescent *in situ* hybridization (FISH) or polymerase chain reaction (PCR) on formalin-fixed paraffin-embedded tissue.[85] Loss of 11q and gain of 17q copies may herald a more aggressive phenotype.[81] Other recent reports have emphasized molecular and cytogenetic analysis for ploidy,[86,87] structural and numerical chromosomal aberrations,[88] multidrug transporter gene *MRP1* expression,[89] and gene expression signatures[90] as having potential prognostic utility, but these are not yet in widespread clinical use.

Rhabdomyosarcoma

RMS is the most common soft tissue sarcoma of childhood and accounts for 5% to 10% of solid tumors in children and approximately half of pediatric soft tissue sarcomas.[18,91,92] This primitive malignancy recapitulates the phenotypic and biologic features of embryonic skeletal muscle. Histologic subtypes of pediatric and adolescent RMS are defined in the International Classification of RMS.[91,93-95] The World Health Organization (WHO) has adopted this classification,[96] and also includes pleomorphic RMS, which is principally a neoplasm of adulthood, in the current classification scheme. Although RMS of all types displays evidence of skeletal muscle differentiation, it frequently occurs in areas that do not contain skeletal muscle. Clinically RMS shows a bimodal age distribution, with more than half of cases occurring in the first decade of life and a second peak in adolescence. The greatest proportion of embryonal RMS occurs in children younger than 5 years of age, and alveolar RMS occurs at all ages. The most frequent sites of embryonal RMS are the head and neck and genitourinary tract, whereas alveolar RMS has a predilection for the extremities.[96] Most RMSs form a poorly circumscribed, fleshy, pale gray–tan mass, but certain subtypes have distinctive macroscopic features. Spindle cell RMS forms a firm fibrous mass with a whorled cut surface resembling smooth muscle tumors. Botryoid RMS has a polypoid appearance with clusters of small sessile or pedunculated nodules covered by an epithelial surface.[96]

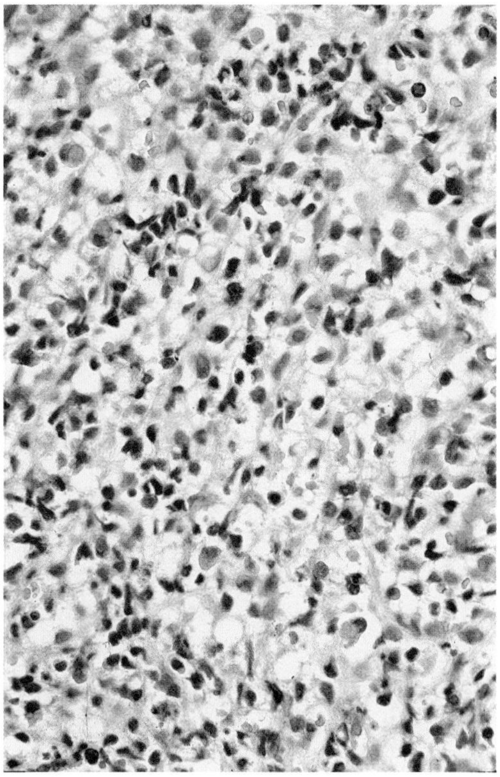

FIGURE 17.4 Embryonal rhabdomyosarcoma consists of small, round, polygonal, and elongated tumor cells with variable amounts of eosinophilic cytoplasm and hyperchromatic nuclei (hematoxylin-eosin, ×200).

Histologic subtypes of pediatric and adolescent RMS are defined in the International Classification of RMS,[91,93-95] which is included in the WHO classification. The major subtypes are botryoid, spindle cell, embryonal (not otherwise specified), and alveolar RMS. Embryonal RMS without further distinguishing features accounts for 49% of RMS and displays a range of morphology from primitive mesenchymal cells to highly differentiated neoplastic muscle cells with rhabdomyoblastic, strap cell, and myotube appearances (Fig. 17.4). At the less-differentiated end of the histologic spectrum, the cells are fusiform or stellate with scant cytoplasm and minimal nuclear and cytoplasmic maturation. This more primitive pattern of embryonal RMS creates challenges in histologic differential diagnosis. Botryoid embryonal RMS accounts for 6% of RMS and is distinguished by a cambial layer of condensed tumor cells beneath the epithelium, with variable differentiation and degree of myogenesis. Spindle cell embryonal RMS accounts for 3% of RMS and consists of elongated spindle cells with a fascicular, storiform, or whorled pattern and variable amounts of collagen between cells. This subtype mimics leiomyosarcoma.

Both botryoid and spindle RMS are favorable histologic-prognostic subtypes, whereas embryonal RMS, not otherwise designated, has an intermediate prognosis. Alveolar RMS accounts for 31% of RMS and is an unfavorable histologic-prognostic subtype. The classic alveolar pattern is characterized by anastomosing fibrovascular septa lined by tumor cells and with round and occasional multinucleated tumor cells with myogenic cytoplasm dispersed within the alveolar spaces (Fig. 17.5). The common theme among the subtypes of alveolar RMS is a round cell tumor morphology with some variation in cell size, little differentiation toward rhabdomyoblasts and strap cells, and round or oval nuclei with a smooth, distinct nuclear membrane, coarse chromatin, and indistinct or multiple nucleoli. The microalveolar and solid variants of alveolar RMS and focal areas of an alveolar architecture in tumors with a predominantly embryonal pattern create challenges in recognition of alveolar RMS. Anaplastic features may be seen in both embryonal and alveolar RMS and further define an unfavorable histologic-prognostic group, although anaplasia has not yet been incorporated into the International Classification of RMS.[94,96-98]

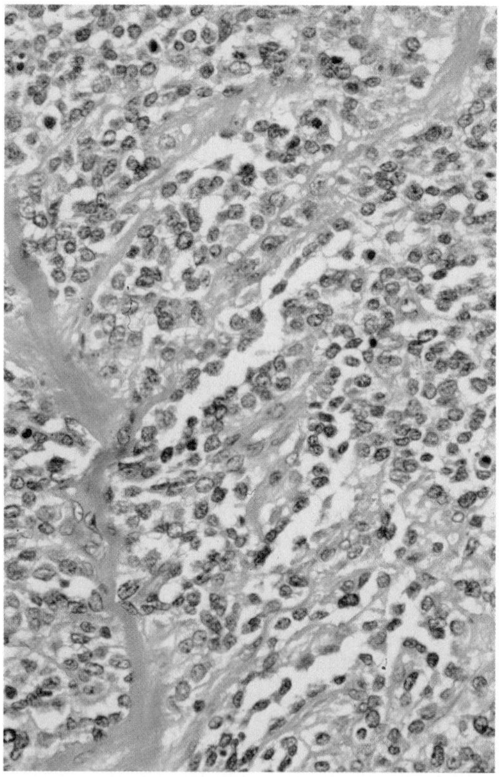

FIGURE 17.5 Alveolar rhabdomyosarcoma displays fibrovascular septa lined by small, round tumor cells surrounding spaces with dispersed individual tumor cells (hematoxylin-eosin, ×200).

The immunohistochemical profile of RMS is illustrated in Figure 17.6, compiled from several series.[22-27,99,100] The typical immunohistochemical profile includes reactivity for vimentin, myogenin, Myo-D1, muscle-specific actin, and desmin. Early immunohistochemical studies emphasized a panel of actin, myosin, creatine kinase, alpha-actinin, myoglobin, and tropomyosin.[101,102] Of these markers, only myoglobin is specific for skeletal muscle differentiation. Although myoglobin is highly specific, it is identified immunohistochemically in less than half of RMS.[103-106] Desmin (Figs. 17.7 and 17.8) and muscle-specific actin (Figs. 17.9 and 17.10) are sensitive markers but are not entirely specific and can be found in smooth muscle and myofibroblastic proliferations.[105-111] Polyclonal desmin is more sensitive for RMS than monoclonal desmin.[94] Fetal heavy-chain myosin is found in a significant proportion of RMS but is seldom used because of its lack of specificity.[111] The extent of differentiation of RMS also influences the immunohistochemical pattern, with more differentiated tumors showing a higher proportion of positivity for myoglobin, muscle-specific actin, and desmin.[99,100,106] Reactivity also varies depending on whether tissues are formalin-fixed, alcohol-fixed, or frozen.[105]

Availability of antibodies to myogenic transcription factors myogenin (also called myf-4) and Myo-D1 has greatly improved the ability to demonstrate a skeletal muscle phenotype in suspected RMS. Myogenin and Myo-D1 are myogenic transcriptional regulatory proteins

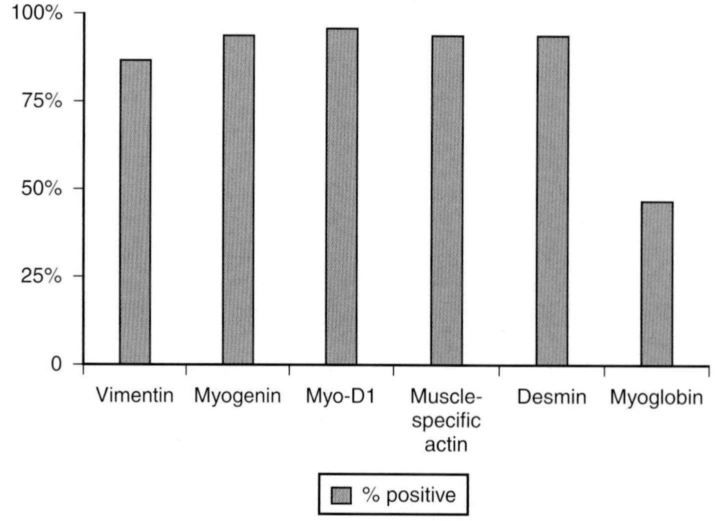

FIGURE 17.6 An immunohistogram of rhabdomyosarcoma.

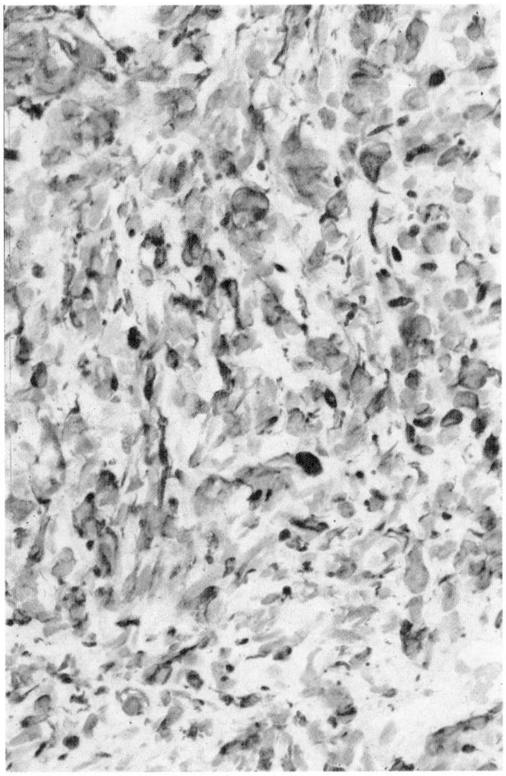

FIGURE 17.7 Desmin displays cytoplasmic reactivity in embryonal rhabdomyosarcoma and highlights elongated straplike cells (immunoperoxidase, ×200).

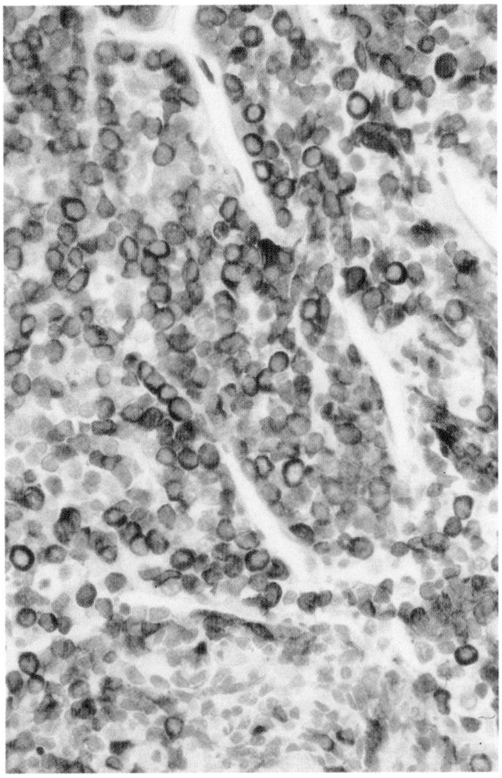

FIGURE 17.8 Desmin displays strong cytoplasmic reactivity in alveolar rhabdomyosarcoma (immunoperoxidase, ×400).

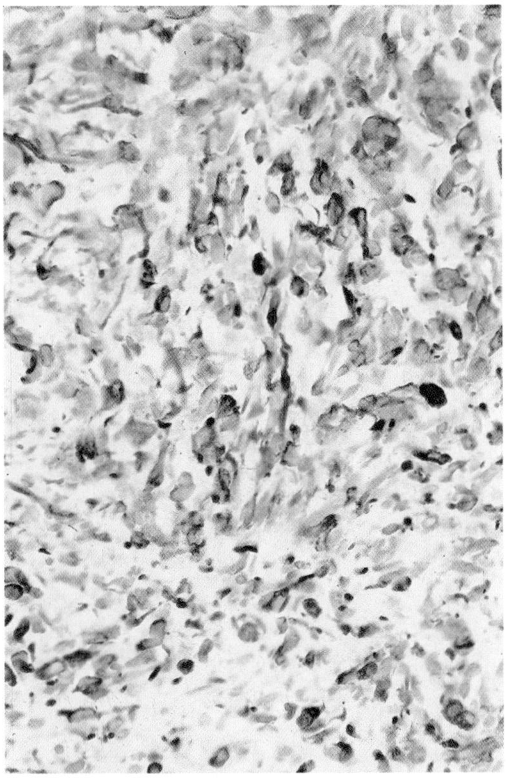

FIGURE 17.9 Muscle-specific actin displays cytoplasmic reactivity and highlights spindled and rhabdomyoblastic cells in embryonal rhabdomyosarcoma (immunoperoxidase, ×400).

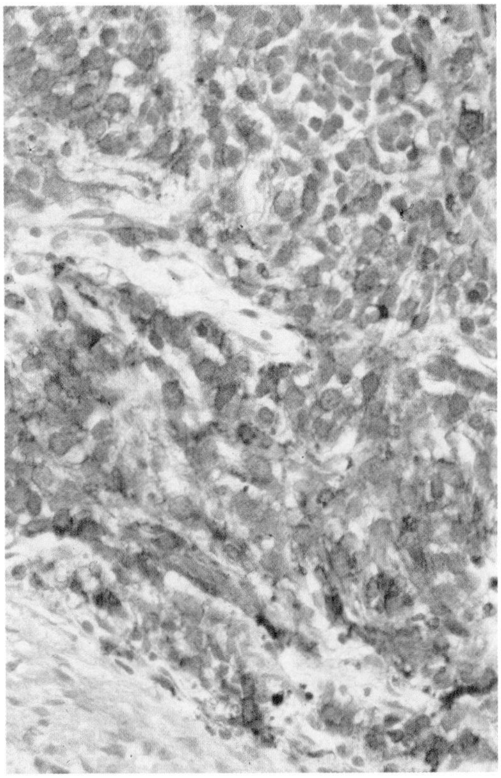

FIGURE 17.10 Muscle-specific actin demonstrates diffuse cytoplasmic reactivity in alveolar rhabdomyosarcoma (immunoperoxidase, ×400).

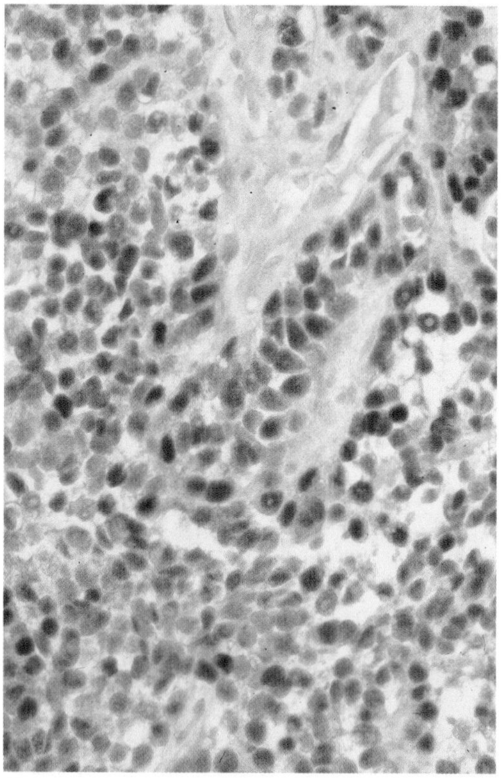

FIGURE 17.11 Myogenin decorates nuclei and highlights the architecture of alveolar rhabdomyosarcoma (immunoperoxidase, ×400).

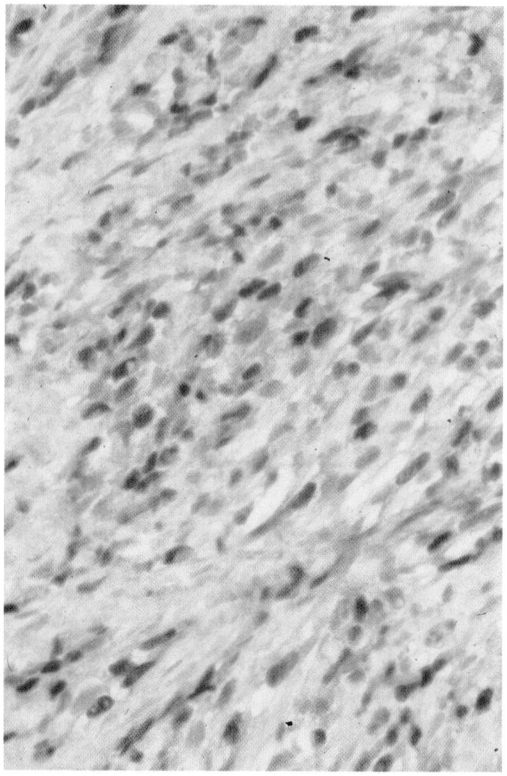

FIGURE 17.12 Myogenin stains variably in proportions of nuclei in embryonal rhabdomyosarcoma (immunoperoxidase, ×400).

expressed early in skeletal muscle differentiation and display a nuclear staining pattern in RMS. They are sensitive and specific for RMS.[22-24,26-28] In a recent series of 956 cases, myogenin and Myo-D1 each had a sensitivity of 97% and specificity of 90% and 91%, respectively.[112] These transcriptional regulatory proteins are more sensitive than myoglobin and more specific than desmin and muscle-specific actin. Myogenin displays strong diffuse nuclear positivity in alveolar RMS (Fig. 17.11) but varies in intensity and distribution in embryonal RMS (Fig. 17.12).[22,24,26,27] Myo-D1 is predominantly a nuclear stain in RMS (Fig. 17.13) but may also decorate the cytoplasm of rhabdomyoblasts and other types of tumor cells.[25] Myogenin is considered technically superior to Myo-D1 for immunohistochemistry because of a tendency for high background and cytoplasmic staining with Myo-D1 antibodies.[22,27] However, the variability of staining patterns in RMS subtypes must be kept in mind as a potential source of false-negative staining in a small specimen. False-negative staining can also occur when mercury-based fixatives are used or if unstained slides are stored at room temperature before immunohistochemical staining is performed.[112] Although both myogenin and Myo-D1 can be detected by reverse transcriptase polymerase chain reaction (RT-PCR), myogenin detection by this technique appears to be more specific for RMS than Myo-D1 detection.[113]

Various other immunohistochemical markers have been identified in RMS and can lead to diagnostic pitfalls if interpreted out of the context of the histologic and

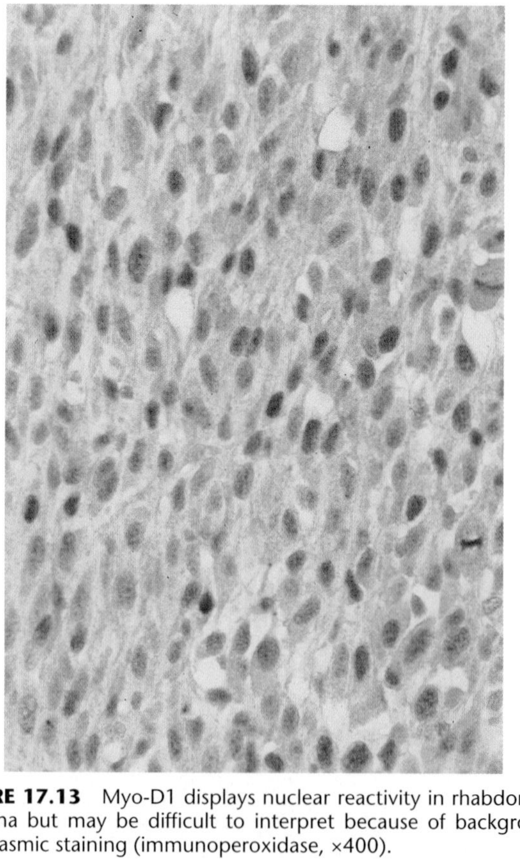

FIGURE 17.13 Myo-D1 displays nuclear reactivity in rhabdomyosarcoma but may be difficult to interpret because of background cytoplasmic staining (immunoperoxidase, ×400).

immunohistochemical findings. CD99, smooth muscle actin, ALK-1, cytokeratin, 68-kD neurofilament protein, and S-100 protein have all been observed in relatively small proportions of RMS.[22,24,105,114-116] Although placental alkaline phosphatase and cytoplasmic reactivity for WT1 are found in a high proportion of RMS, they are nonspecific in this context.[117,118] WT1 reactivity in RMS is cytoplasmic, whereas the pattern of diagnostic WT1 staining in WT is nuclear.

A panel approach to the immunohistochemical evaluation of a potential RMS is most useful, with use of myogenin, Myo-D1, muscle-specific actin, and desmin[18,27,100] to detect a skeletal muscle phenotype. Muscle-specific actin and desmin reactivity are also seen in smooth muscle tumors, fibromatoses, WT, ectomesenchymoma, EWS/PNET, MRT, myositis ossificans, malignant fibrous histiocytoma, and embryonal sarcoma of the liver but are generally nonreactive in NB and retinoblastoma.[105,107,108] Although myogenin and Myo-D1 are specific for skeletal muscle differentiation, tumors with rhabdomyomatous or rhabdomyoblastic features such as rhabdomyomatous WT, ectomesenchymoma, and malignant peripheral nerve sheath tumor with divergent differentiation, as well as fetal, atrophic, and regenerating skeletal muscle, can display reactivity for these markers.[22,26,27] Both myogenin and Myo-D1 are typically nonreactive in NB, EWS/PNET, fibroblastic-myofibroblastic tumors, smooth muscle tumors, alveolar soft part sarcoma, synovial sarcoma, MRT, DSRCT, NB, esthesioneuroblastoma, hematopoietic tumors, and carcinomas.[22,24,26,27]

KEY DIAGNOSTIC POINTS

Rhabdomyosarcoma

- RMSs are classified into embryonal, alveolar, spindle cell, and botryoid subtypes according to the International Classification of RMS, and many can be recognized by light microscopy alone.
- The immunohistochemical profile of RMS includes the myogenic transcriptional regulatory proteins myogenin and Myo-D1, as well as muscle-specific actin, desmin, and myoglobin.
- Myogenin and Myo-D1 are the most sensitive and specific markers for RMS, but their patterns and distribution of reactivity can vary among different RMS subtypes.
- In problematic cases, detection of translocations by RT-PCR or FISH can be useful in recognition of alveolar RMS, but a characteristic genetic abnormality has not yet been identified for embryonal RMS.
- Aberrant reactivity for cytokeratin, CD99, and other markers in RMS is a potential diagnostic pitfall.

GENOMIC APPLICATIONS

Aside from the immunohistochemical detection of muscle-specific transcription factors as described earlier, no other genomic–immunohistochemical diagnostic applications are currently available. The PAX-FKHR chimeric transcripts are, to date, not detectable by immunohistochemistry.

THERANOSTIC APPLICATIONS

Prognostic immunohistochemical markers for RMS include p53 and proliferation markers. A high-proliferation index as detected by immunohistochemistry for proliferating cell nuclear antigen (PCNA) or Mib-1 (Ki-67) is associated with lower survival, higher relapse, and greater disease progression.[119,120] p53 overexpression seems to be associated with a higher Mib-1 labeling index and is associated with a poor prognosis.[121,122] Anaplastic RMS also displays p53 reactivity.[98] Some investigators have advocated categorization of RMS according to genotype because of the prognostic associations with *PAX-FKHR* translocations or their absence.[123]

BEYOND IMMUNOHISTOCHEMISTRY: ANATOMIC MOLECULAR DIAGNOSTIC APPLICATIONS

In recent years, cytogenetic and molecular genetic studies have become critical in the evaluation of RMS and its subtypes.[13,14,94-96,98] Alveolar RMS can display one of two translocations involving the *PAX* genes, with different prognostic implications.[124] The t(2;13)(q35;q14) with the chimeric product *PAX 3-FKHR* is the more common translocation, occurs in 55% of cases, and is associated with a poorer prognosis. The t(1;13)(p36;q14) with the chimeric product *PAX 7-FKHR* is the less common type, is found in 22% of cases, and identifies a lower-risk subgroup. However, up to 30% of alveolar RMS will not display either translocation, and these behave similarly to embryonal RMS.[125] The translocations can be identified by conventional cytogenetics, RT-PCR, or FISH. Embryonal RMS can display a variety of cytogenetic abnormalities including loss of heterozygosity at chromosome 11p15.5 and a possible tumor-related locus on 11q, but a specific genetic abnormality to characterize embryonal RMS has not yet been identified.

Ewing's Sarcoma/Primitive Neuroectodermal Tumor

EWS/PNET is a primitive round cell sarcoma with varying degrees of neuroectodermal differentiation.[126,127] In the past the diagnoses of EWS and PNET were separated on the basis of light microscopic, electron microscopic, and immunohistochemical features of neuroectodermal differentiation, but in recent years it has been recognized that EWS/PNET is a single entity with a shared clinical course, prognosis, and groups of molecular genetic abnormalities. This unified concept of EWS/PNET has been codified in the current WHO Classification of Tumors of Soft Tissue and Bones.[126]

EWS/PNET is the second most common bone and soft tissue sarcoma in children and occurs more frequently in bone, although extraskeletal EWS/PNET accounts for 15% or more of cases.[128] There is a predilection for males. In bone, EWS/PNET tends to arise in long bones, pelvis, and ribs.[126] It can also occur in superficial or deep soft tissues, as a disseminated neoplasm

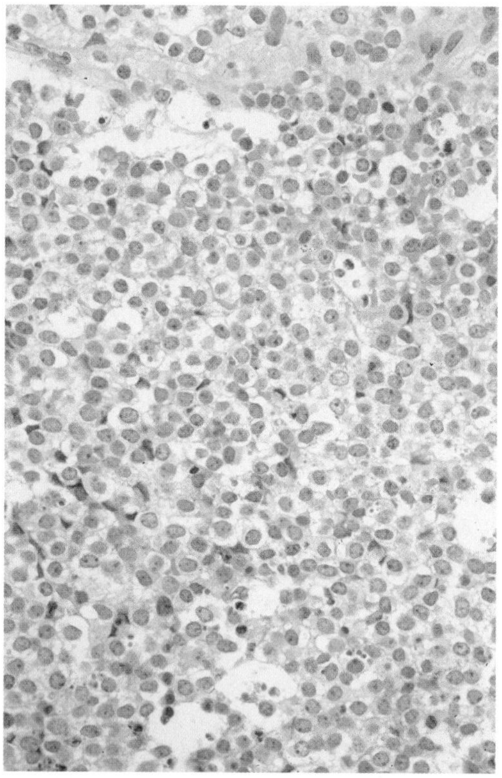

FIGURE 17.14 Ewing's sarcoma/primitive neuroectodermal tumor displays cohesive sheets of small- to medium-sized round cells with round to oval nuclei, fine chromatin, scant clear cytoplasm, and indistinct cell borders (hematoxylin-eosin, ×200).

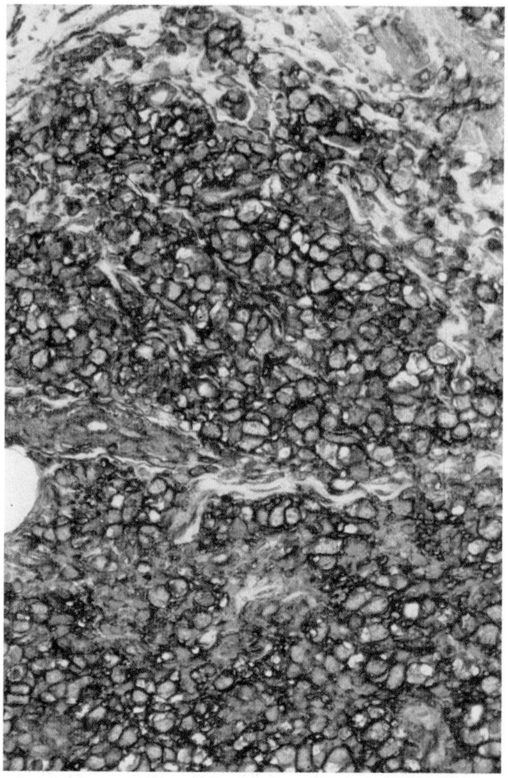

FIGURE 17.16 CD99 (O13) reactivity in Ewing's sarcoma/primitive neuroectodermal tumor typically shows a strong membranous and cytoplasmic staining pattern (immunoperoxidase ×400).

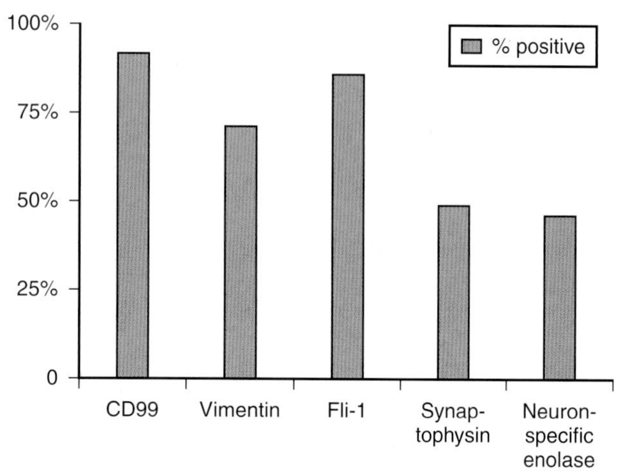

FIGURE 17.15 An immunohistogram of Ewing's sarcoma/primitive neuroectodermal tumor.

without obvious primary site, or in organs such as the kidney.[128-132] EWS/PNET occurs throughout life, and age is no limit to the diagnosis. The peak age incidence is during the second decade of life, and most patients are younger than 20 years of age at diagnosis. The tumor is a tan-gray and frequently a necrotic, hemorrhagic mass. Occasional cases are associated with a peripheral nerve.[126]

The histologic spectrum of EWS/PNET ranges from a neoplasm composed of uniform small round cells with round nuclei, fine chromatin, scant cytoplasm, and indistinct cell borders to a neoplasm with larger, more irregular cells with irregular nuclear contours, pseudorosettes, a nesting pattern, and even spindle cell morphology (Fig. 17.14). Geographic zones of necrosis are frequently observed, with preserved perivascular clusters of tumor cells. Ultrastructurally, EWS/PNET shows a similar spectrum from relatively undifferentiated mesenchymal cells to neural differentiation. Tumor cells typically contain intermediate filaments, have cell junctions including desmosomes, and may contain abundant glycogen, dense core granules, and neurotubules.[8,133,134]

The immunohistochemical profile of EWS/PNET is illustrated in Figure 17.15, compiled from several series.[41,135-137] The typical immunohistochemical profile includes reactivity for vimentin, CD99 (O13, HBA-71, mic-2), and variable reactivity for neuron-specific enolase, CD57, synaptophysin, and cytokeratin. Rare cases stain positively for desmin and glial fibrillary acidic protein, but EWS/PNET does not typically stain for leukocyte common antigen or actins.[31,55,136] Expression of neural markers does not correlate with outcome.[135] CD99 typically displays a membranous staining pattern (Fig. 17.16) and was initially thought to be a highly specific marker for EWS/PNET. However, it is now recognized that although its sensitivity ranges from 84% to 100% in EWS/PNET, the specificity is limited.[33,34,40,42,138] CD99 is an antibody to a cell

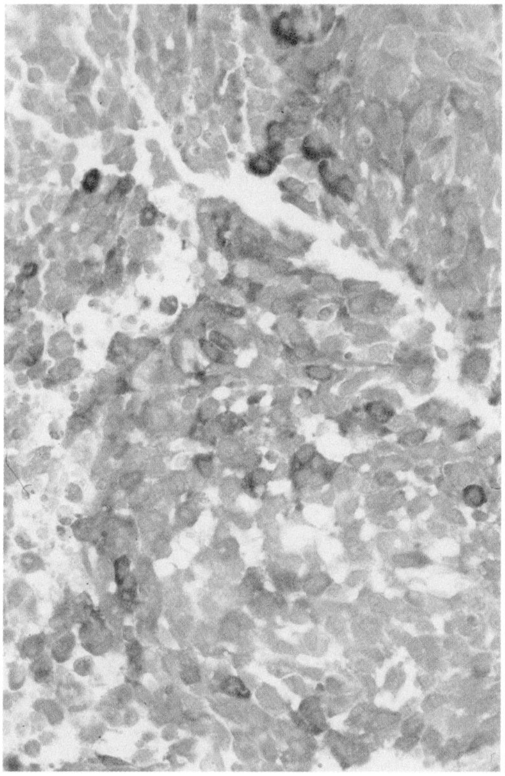

FIGURE 17.17 Neuron-specific enolase is frequently positive in Ewing's sarcoma/primitive neuroectodermal tumor but can be seen in many other tumors (immunoperoxidase, ×400).

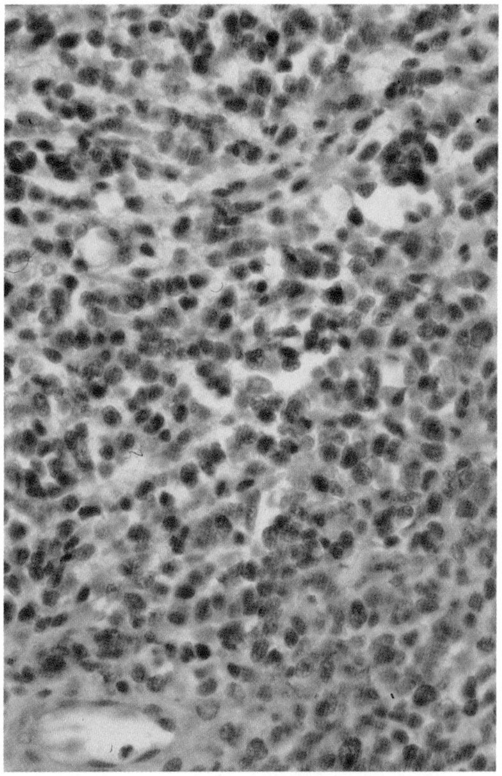

FIGURE 17.18 FLI-1 protein expression with nuclear reactivity is found in Ewing's sarcoma/primitive neuroectodermal tumor but can also be observed in other small round blue cell tumors, particularly lymphoblastic lymphoma (immunoperoxidase, ×400).

surface antigen but is not related to the translocations involving the *EWS* gene. Other CD99 positive tumors that mimic EWS/PNET include RMS, glial tumors, neuroendocrine tumors, some carcinomas, lymphoblastic lymphoma, other primitive hematolymphoid neoplasms, WT, uterine sarcomas, clear cell sarcoma of the kidney, teratoma, synovial sarcoma, osteosarcoma, and mesenchymal chondrosarcoma.[33,34,40,139,140] Fortunately, the blastemal elements of WT are not CD99 positive. A significant diagnostic challenge is distinction of lymphoblastic lymphoma from EWS/PNET because both can be reactive for CD99 in a membranous and cytoplasmic pattern.[33,141] A combination of immunohistochemical reactivity for TdT, CD43, CD34, CD10, CD79a, and gene rearrangement studies can distinguish lymphoblastic lymphoma from EWS/PNET.[41,141] Vimentin is reactive in a high proportion of EWS/PNET but in less than 25% of lymphoblastic lymphoma. However, neuron-specific enolase is not a reliable discriminator between the two tumors (Fig. 17.17).

A translocation involving the *EWS* gene on chromosome 22q12 and other partners, most frequently the *FLI-1* gene on chromosome 11q24, is typical for EWS/PNET, and there are several different subtypes of *EWS/FLI-1* fusion transcripts.[142-147] Other fusion partners for EWS include ERG, ETV1, E1AF, FEV, and other genes. The genetic abnormalities are detectable by conventional cytogenetics, FISH, and RT-PCR.[13,14,148-151] Overexpression of the FLI-1 protein resulting from the translocation between the *EWS* and *FLI-1* genes is observed in 71% to 100% of EWS/PNET.[44,45,140] Only nuclear FLI-1 staining is considered positive for EWS/PNET (Fig. 17.18). Unfortunately a number of other mimics of EWS/PNET can also exhibit FLI-1 reactivity by immunohistochemistry including lymphoblastic lymphoma in nearly 90% of cases, myeloid neoplasms, DSRCT, malignant melanoma, Merkel cell carcinoma, synovial sarcoma, some carcinomas, and vascular neoplasms such as benign hemangiomas, angiosarcoma, epithelioid hemangioendothelioma, glomus tumor, and Kaposi sarcoma. Although the literature suggests that FLI-1 immunoreactivity is not observed in RMS, we have seen a number of cases of RMS, particularly the alveolar subtype, with FLI-1 reactivity. When the morphology is characteristic, the diagnosis of EWS/PNET can be made on the basis of light microscopy and immunohistochemical reactivity for CD99 and FLI-1, with absence of lymphoblastic, epithelial, and myogenic markers.[152] Others have advocated for more routine use of RT-PCR for unequivocal identification of EWS/PNET,[139] but current evidence indicates that genetic confirmation is not required unless unusual morphologic variants of EWS/PNET such as epithelioid, spindle cell, or desmin-positive tumors are encountered.[149,152,153] Recently, a group of Ewing-like sarcomas has been identified with a translocation involving chromosomes 4 and 19 with a *CIC* and *DUX4* gene fusion, and these rare tumors have pathologic features identical to Ewing's sarcoma with

EWS gene rearrangements.[154] This emphasizes that even with the advances of the past several decades, the understanding of this group of tumors remains incomplete.

KEY DIAGNOSTIC POINTS

Ewing's Sarcoma/Primitive Neuroectodermal Tumor

- EWS/PNET shows a morphologic spectrum from a primitive small round cell tumor to a predominantly round cell neoplasm with a lobular architecture and pseudorosette formation.
- The characteristic immunohistochemical profile includes reactivity for vimentin, CD99, and FLI-1, with variable immunohistochemical reactivity for neural markers.
- EWS/PNET has a variety of cytogenetic abnormalities involving the *EWS* gene, and the most common is a translocation involving chromosomes 11 and 22 with an *EWS/FLI-1* gene fusion.
- FLI-1 protein expression is typical for cases of EWS/PNET with a translocation involving the *EWS* gene on chromosome 22 and the *FLI-1* gene on chromosome 11, but nuclear FLI-1 reactivity is not entirely specific.
- Immunohistochemistry can be used to distinguish EWS/PNET from RMS and other small blue cell tumor mimics, with the recognition that neither CD99 nor FLI-1 is completely specific for EWS/PNET in this context and that a diagnostic panel of muscle markers is necessary.
- Strong CD99 staining in primitive hematolymphoid neoplasms, especially lymphoblastic lymphoma, is a potentially serious diagnostic trap that can be avoided by use of immunohistochemistry and molecular analyses.
- In problematic cases, cytogenetic and molecular genetic tests can be useful in differential diagnosis.

GENOMIC APPLICATIONS

Overexpression of the FLI-1 protein resulting from the translocation between the *EWS* and *FLI-1* genes is observed in 71% to 100% of EWS/PNET, but the nuclear expression is not specific to the EWS/PNET group of tumors. In these circumstances, it is critical to include the clinical assessment of the patient along with other markers in the diagnostic panel.

THERANOSTIC APPLICATIONS

Prognostic and biologic immunohistochemical markers for EWS/PNET include p53 and p16. Overexpression of p53 by immunohistochemistry has been associated with a poor outcome.[155,156] Loss of p16 may be associated with more aggressive clinical behavior.[157] Although immunohistochemical staining for c-*kit* can be strong and diffuse in some cases of EWS/PNET, its therapeutic and genetic significance is not yet clear.[158] There is no prognostic significance of neural differentiation or neural marker expression by light microscopy, immunohistochemistry, or ultrastructure.[136,159-161] Some evidence suggests that a type 1 *EWS/FLI-1* fusion transcript may signify an improved survival among patients with localized disease.[162]

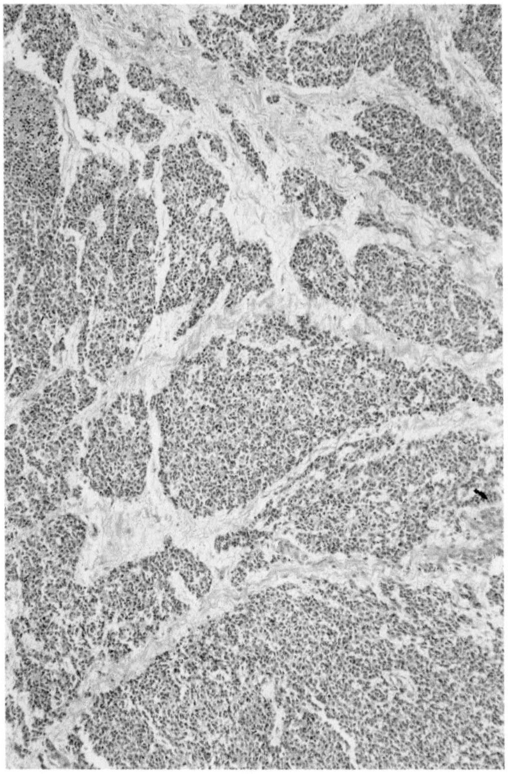

FIGURE 17.19 Desmoplastic small round cell tumor displays round and polygonal tumor cells arranged in geographic nests separated by a fibrous stroma (hematoxylin-eosin, ×100).

BEYOND IMMUNOHISTOCHEMISTRY: ANATOMIC MOLECULAR DIAGNOSTIC APPLICATIONS

The translocations involving the *EWS* gene on chromosome 22q12 and other partners, most frequently the *FLI-1* gene on chromosome 11q24, are typical for EWS/PNET, and there are several different subtypes of *EWS/FLI-1* fusion transcripts.[142-147] Other fusion partners for EWS include ERG, ETV1, E1AF, FEV, and other genes. The genetic abnormalities are detectable by conventional cytogenetics, FISH, and RT-PCR.

Desmoplastic Small Round Cell Tumor

DSRCT is an aggressive, polyphenotypic, malignant tumor occurring predominantly in children and young adults, with a male predominance and an age range spanning the first through fifth decades.[163-167] Typically DSRCT presents as widespread tumor nodules in the abdominal serosa, but it also occurs in the thoracic cavity, paratesticular region, head and neck, central nervous system, extremities, and solid organs.[168-173] Grossly the tumor forms bulky multinodular masses with smooth bosselated surfaces.[174,175]

The classic microscopic appearance consists of small round tumor cells arranged in nests and aggregates separated by a dense collagenized to fibromyxoid stroma (Fig. 17.19).[174] The tumor cells can vary in appearance from round to rhabdoid to clear. Central necrosis and

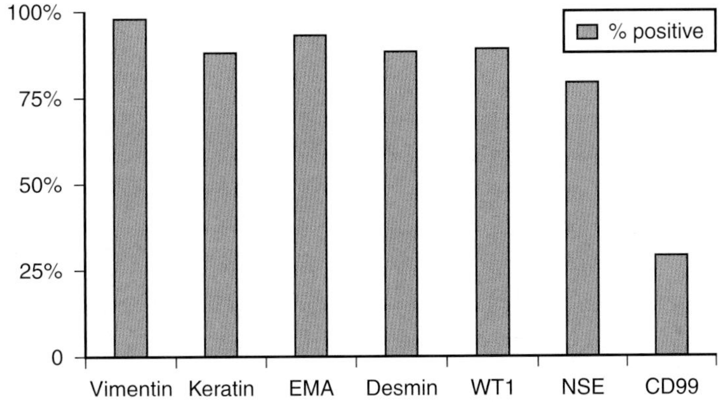

FIGURE 17.20 An immunohistogram of desmoplastic small round cell tumor.

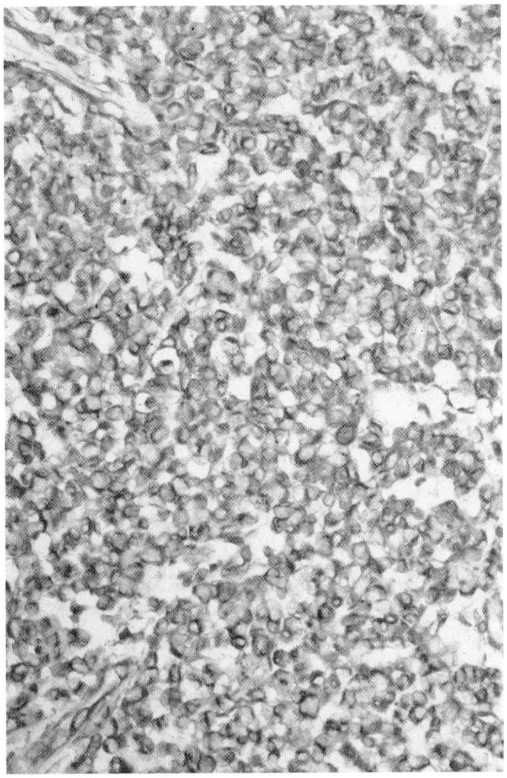

FIGURE 17.21 Vimentin displays diffuse cytoplasmic reactivity in desmoplastic small round cell tumor (immunoperoxidase, ×400).

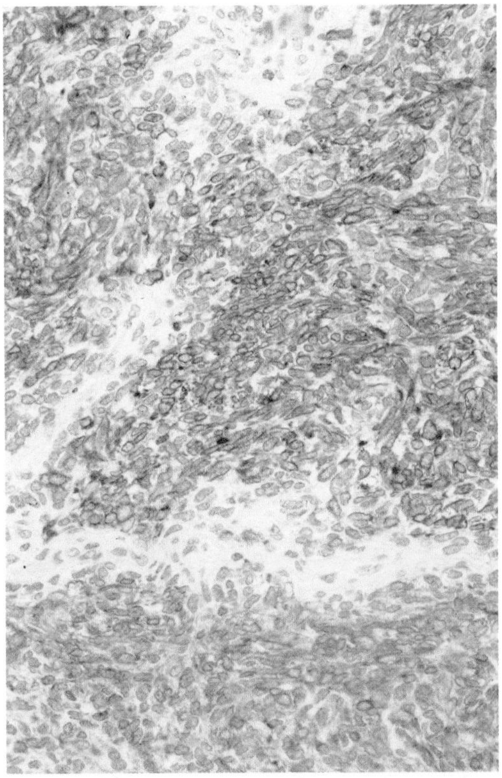

FIGURE 17.22 Cytokeratin demonstrates cytoplasmic reactivity in desmoplastic small round cell tumor (immunoperoxidase, ×200).

cystic degeneration may be seen. Variations in histologic patterns include rosette formation, focal epithelial differentiation, a myxoid or hypervascular stroma, and frequent mitoses. Cytoplasmic intermediate filaments in varying amounts are demonstrated by electron microscopy and may correspond to the rhabdoid phenotype displayed in some examples of DSRCT.[11]

DSRCT has a distinctive immunohistochemical profile with coexpression of epithelial and mesenchymal markers. Vimentin, cytokeratin, epithelial membrane antigen, desmin, neuron-specific enolase, and WT1 reactivity are characteristic. The immunohistochemical profile compiled from seven published series is shown in Figure 17.20.[37,46-48,164,174,176] Nearly all cases express vimentin (Fig. 17.21), and both keratin (Fig. 17.22) and epithelial membrane antigen (Fig. 17.23) are expressed in approximately 90% of cases. Although some series have indicated that CAM 5.2 cytokeratin may be more sensitive than AE1/AE3 cytokeratin,[37] other investigators have found similar frequencies of positivity for these two keratin markers.[48] Desmin staining (Fig. 17.24) may be diffuse cytoplasmic or dotlike. Nuclear reactivity for WT1, using an antibody to the C-terminal region of the WT1 protein, is found in nearly 90% of cases (Fig. 17.25). Many other tumors can display cytoplasmic staining for WT1.[177] CD99 is expressed in less than 30% of DSRCT and usually lacks the well-defined membranous pattern observed in EWS/PNET. Neuron-specific enolase is present in 79% of DSRCT, but other neural markers such as synaptophysin, chromogranin, neurofilament, glial fibrillary acidic protein, and S-100 protein are typically absent or seldom

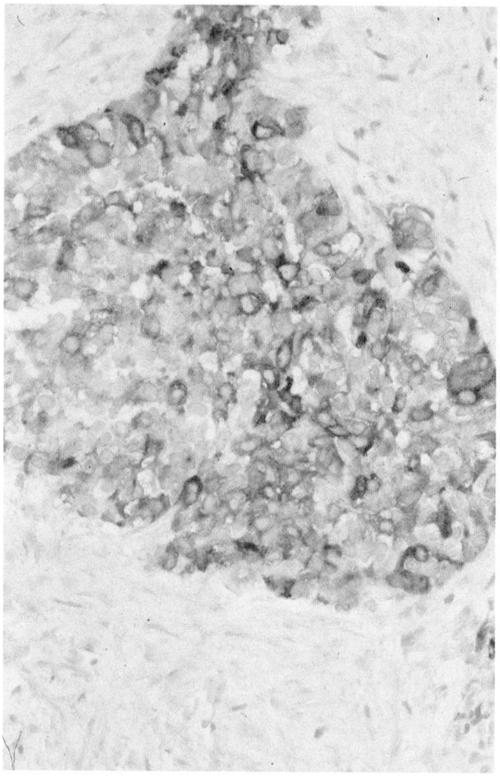

FIGURE 17.23 Epithelial membrane antigen demonstrates cytoplasmic and membranous reactivity in desmoplastic small round cell tumor (immunoperoxidase, ×400).

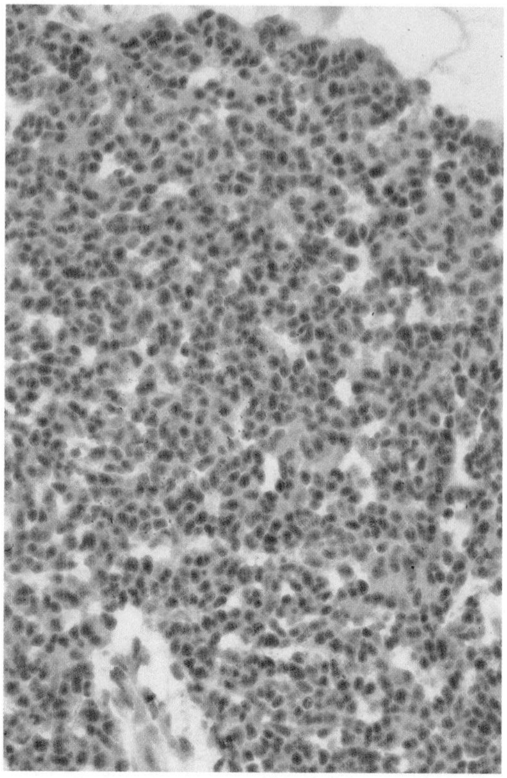

FIGURE 17.25 WT1 using an antibody to the C-terminus shows diffuse nuclear reactivity in desmoplastic small round cell tumor (immunoperoxidase, ×400).

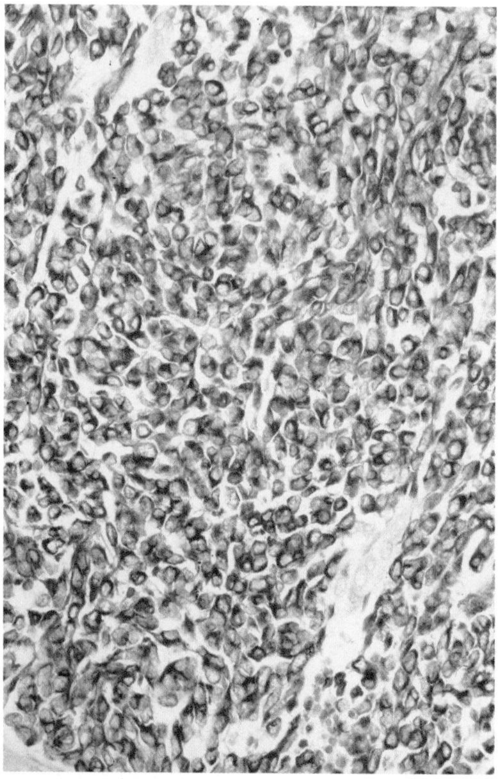

FIGURE 17.24 Desmin shows diffuse strong cytoplasmic reactivity in desmoplastic small round cell tumor (immunoperoxidase, ×400).

expressed.[37,47,48,164,174,176] In addition, only rare, if any, examples of DSRCT show immunoreactivity for smooth muscle actin, muscle specific actin, or myoglobin and myogenin. Myo-D1 is not expressed. Potential diagnostic pitfalls include expression of CD57, CD15, Ca125, Ber-EP4, MOC31, placental alkaline phosphatase, and HER2.[37,176] Sporadic cases have been reported with expression of calretinin and c-*kit*.[37]

DSRCT harbors a characteristic translocation, t(11;22)(p13;q12), with an *EWS-WT1* gene fusion. This can be detected by tumor karyotype and RT-PCR.[145,148-152,178] *In situ* hybridization to detect an EWS gene rearrangement, but without identification of the translocation partner, is a useful diagnostic adjunct.[179-181] In diagnostically difficult cases or unusual clinical settings, FISH or RT-PCR to search for the t(11;22)(p13;q12) translocation and the *EWS-WT1* gene rearrangement support the diagnosis of DSRCT.[182-188] The translocation results in overexpression of the WT1 protein, which can be detected by immunohistochemistry with antibodies to the C-terminal of WT1, resulting in nuclear staining.[46,47,183]

DIFFERENTIAL DIAGNOSES

Although immunohistochemistry is helpful for confirmation of the diagnosis of DSRCT, there is overlap with other small neoplasms with polyphenotypic features including occasional cases of EWS/PNET, WT, MRT, and synovial sarcoma. RMS is distinguished by the presence of staining for myogenin and Myo-D1, despite the overlap in staining between RMS and DSRCT for desmin, myoglobin, and muscle-specific actin. Blastema-predominant WT could pose a challenge in differential diagnosis if epithelial components are not identified, but in such cases molecular or cytogenetic tests can be useful in the distinction from DSRCT. Synovial sarcoma typically has different morphologic features than DSRCT and has a distinctive translocation between chromosomes X and 18 in addition to strong immunohistochemical expression of bcl-2. MRT is another polyphenotypic small cell malignancy and lacks WT1 staining and the *EWS/WT1* gene fusion, in addition to having its own genetic abnormality involving the *INI1* gene. Recently two spindle cell tumors with an *EWS-WT1* transcript and a favorable clinical course have been reported, raising the question of a variant of DSRCT, a variant of leiomyosarcoma, or a unique entity among mesenchymal tumors.[189]

Upregulation of autocrine and paracrine growth factors such as transforming growth factor beta-1, platelet-derived growth factor receptor alpha, platelet-derived growth factor-AB chains, insulin-like growth factor 2, and connective tissue growth factor have been demonstrated by immunohistochemistry in DSRCT.[190,191] The diagnostic, therapeutic, and prognostic significance of these findings has yet to be determined.

KEY DIAGNOSTIC POINTS

Desmoplastic Small Round Cell Tumor

- Coexpression of vimentin, cytokeratin, epithelial membrane antigen, desmin, and WT1 support the diagnosis of DSRCT.
- Molecular or cytogenetic confirmation of the *EWS-WT1* gene fusion supports the diagnosis of DSRCT.
- WT1 nuclear staining and lack of a membranous staining pattern for CD99 help to distinguish DSRCT from EWS/PNET.
- Absence of staining for the myogenic regulatory proteins myogenin and Myo-D1 help to distinguish DSRCT from RMS and both tumors can be immunoreactive for desmin, myoglobin, and actin.
- Presence of WT1 staining and the *EWS-WT1* gene fusion distinguish DSRCT from malignant rhabdoid tumor, which is another polyphenotypic small cell malignant neoplasm.

Malignant Rhabdoid Tumor

MRT is a highly aggressive neoplasm of infancy and childhood with a tendency for widespread metastases.[192-194] Originally described in the kidney[194-196] and central nervous system,[197,198] the clinicopathologic spectrum of MRT is now known to include other organs, extrarenal soft tissue, and a congenital disseminated form.[63,193,199,200] Familial cases with involvement of the central nervous system and other sites have been reported.[192,201] Although most tumors occur in children, rare examples of true MRT have been observed in

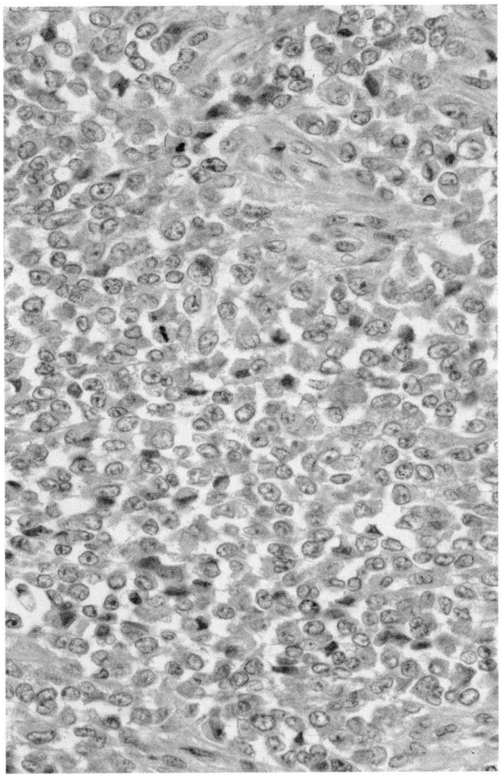

FIGURE 17.26 Malignant rhabdoid tumor consists of sheets of round cells with vesicular nuclei, prominent nucleoli, and variable amounts of eosinophilic cytoplasm with occasional large cytoplasmic eosinophilic globules (hematoxylin-eosin, ×200).

adults. There is no gender predilection. These primitive tumors are polyphenotypic and their name is derived from the rhabdoid appearance of the tumor cells. The gross appearance is a soft gray or tan mass with focal hemorrhage and necrosis.

The histopathologic appearance of MRT is a densely cellular neoplasm composed of sheets or cords of cells with large vesicular round or oval nuclei, prominent central eosinophilic nucleoli, and abundant eccentric eosinophilic cytoplasm (Fig. 17.26). Histologic variability is typical, and some cases have smaller numbers of characteristic rhabdoid cells or display a primitive small blue cell pattern, a myxoid background, a lack of cellular cohesion, increased collagen deposition between bands of tumor cells, and scattered non-neoplastic osteoclast-like giant cells. Occasionally cases have focal epithelial areas. Mitoses are frequent. Electron microscopy reveals cytoplasmic whorls of intermediate filaments, which correspond to the eosinophilic globules of cytoplasm in the classic rhabdoid cells.

Immunohistochemistry is an invaluable adjunct technique because of the potential for many different neoplasms to display a rhabdoid appearance. Figure 17.27 shows an immunohistogram of the most frequently found markers in MRT, compiled from four series.[90,193,197,200] MRT is typically a polyphenotypic neoplasm with coexpression of vimentin (Fig. 17.28); at least one epithelial marker such as cytokeratin (Fig. 17.29) or epithelial membrane antigen (Fig. 17.30); neuroectodermal markers such as neuron-specific enolase, synaptophysin

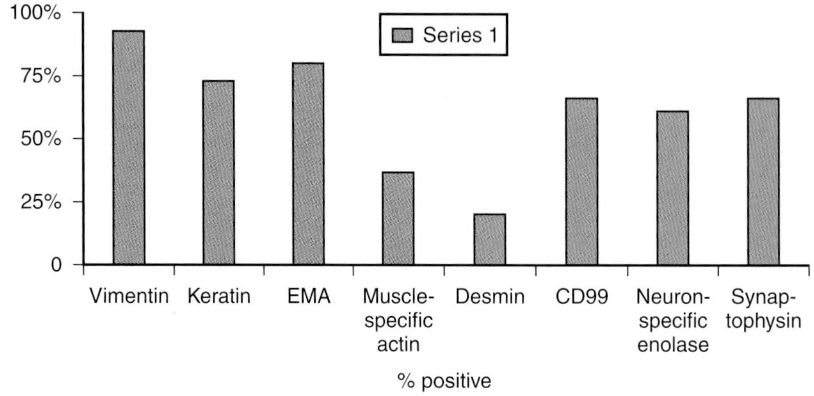

FIGURE 17.27 An immunohistogram of malignant rhabdoid tumor.

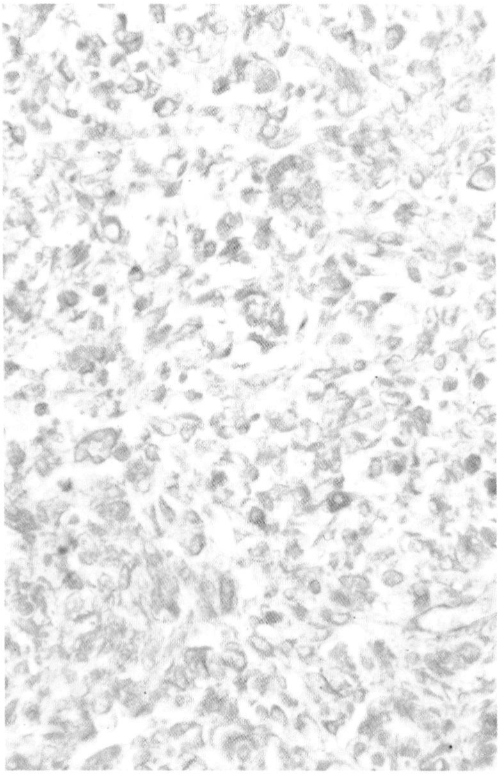

FIGURE 17.28 Vimentin displays cytoplasmic reactivity in malignant rhabdoid tumor (immunoperoxidase, ×400).

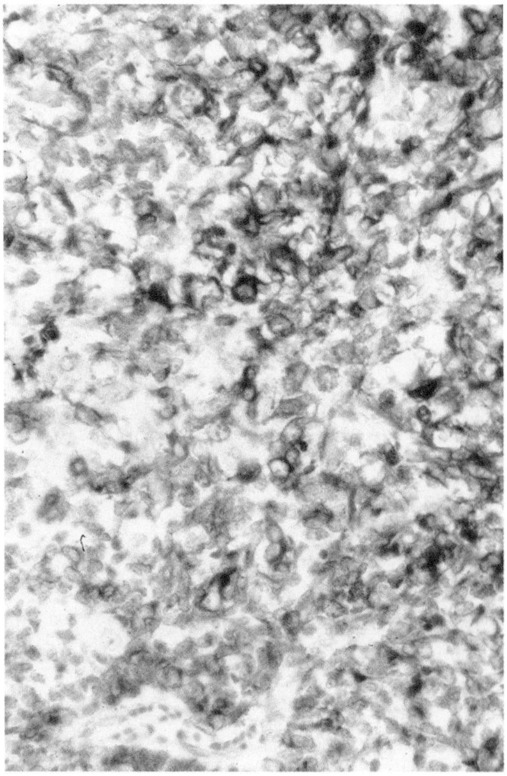

FIGURE 17.29 CAM 5.2 cytokeratin shows variable cytoplasmic reactivity in malignant rhabdoid tumor (immunoperoxidase, ×400).

(Fig. 17.31), or CD99; and mesenchymal markers such as muscle-specific actin (Fig. 17.32) and S-100 protein.[90,193,197,200] Other markers that may be identified include smooth muscle actin, carcinoembryonic antigen, glial fibrillary acidic protein, and neurofilament.[197,200] However, myogenin, myoglobin, HMB45, chromogranin, and CD34 are typically absent.[200] The rhabdoid eosinophilic cytoplasmic inclusion contains filaments comprising both vimentin and cytokeratin 8, and malignant rhabdoid tumor has been found to have mutations of the human cytokeratin gene.[202]

Immunohistochemical analyses for the INI1 protein in MRT of the central nervous system, kidney, and extrarenal soft tissue have shown that absence of INI1 immunostaining (Fig. 17.33) correlates well with deletion and mutation of *hSNF5/INI1* gene.[49-51]

Recent studies have shown that central nervous system MRT expresses insulin-like growth factor-2, insulin-like growth factor receptor type 1, and cathepsin D,[203] but not beta-catenin.[204] Definitive pathologic-prognostic features beyond the diagnosis of MRT have not been identified.

The polyphenotypic immunohistochemical profile of MRT presents challenges in the differential diagnosis, particularly with DSRCT, RMS, choroid plexus carcinoma, and epithelioid sarcoma. In particular, the absence of INI1 protein in proximal-type epithelioid sarcoma, in a subset of central nervous system primitive neuroectodermal tumors without a rhabdoid phenotype and in renal medullary carcinoma, suggests the existence of a wider family of *hSNF5/INI1*-deficient tumors.[50,205-208] The lack of expression of INI1 protein

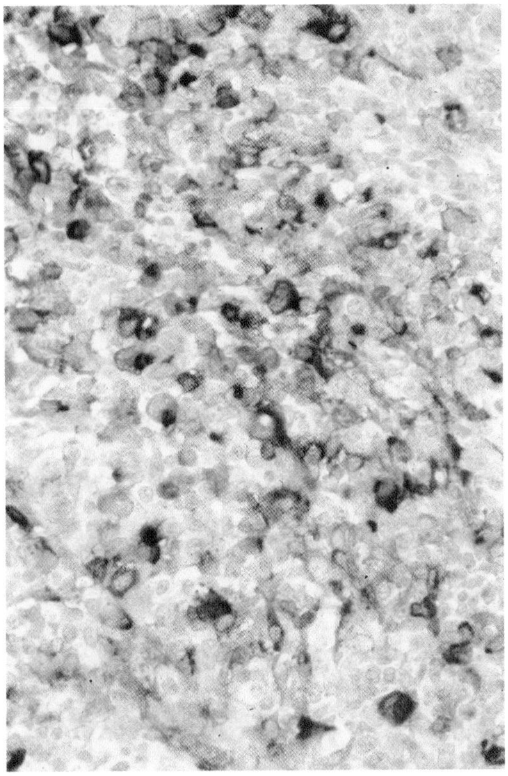

FIGURE 17.30 Epithelial membrane antigen shows focal strong cytoplasmic reactivity in malignant rhabdoid tumor (immunoperoxidase, ×400).

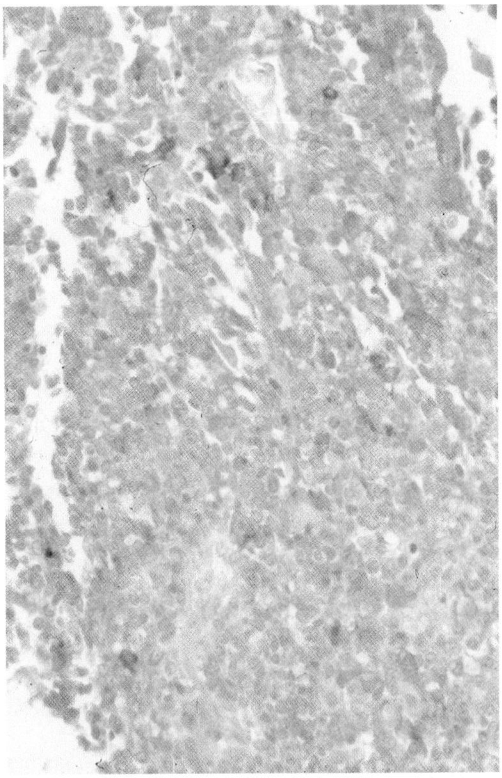

FIGURE 17.31 Weak synaptophysin reactivity is present in the cytoplasm of malignant rhabdoid tumor but may show weak staining (immunoperoxidase, ×400).

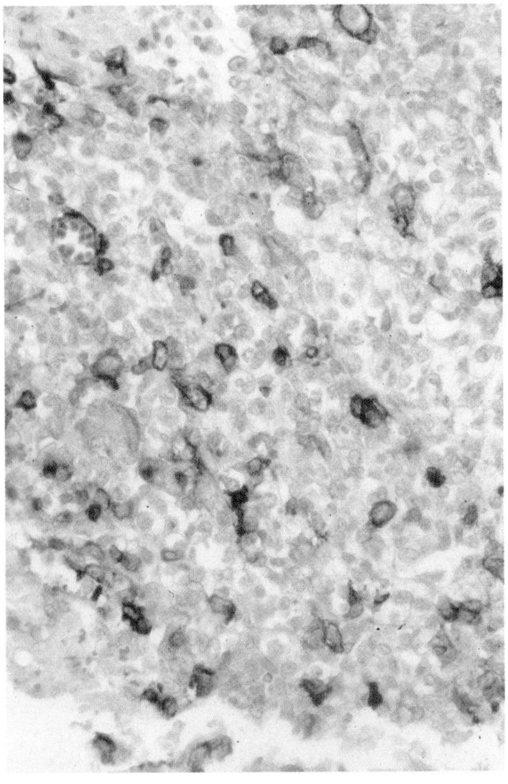

FIGURE 17.32 Muscle-specific actin demonstrates focal cytoplasmic reactivity in malignant rhabdoid tumor (immunoperoxidase, ×400).

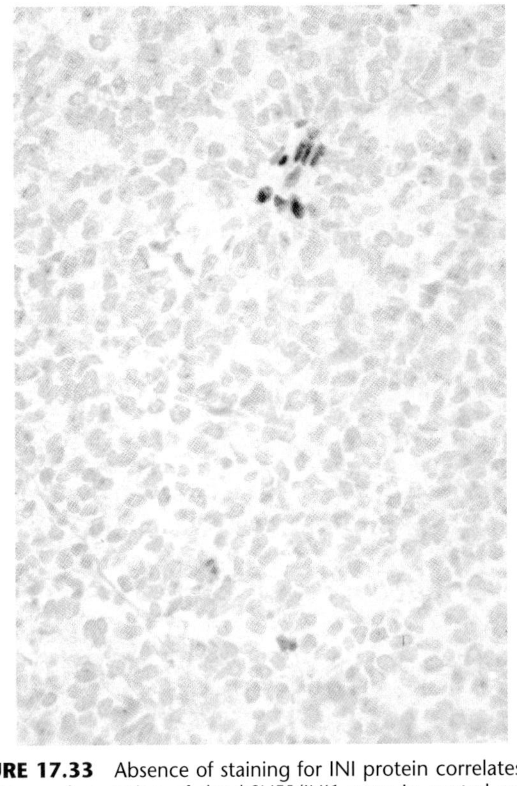

FIGURE 17.33 Absence of staining for INI protein correlates with deletion and mutation of the *hSNF5/INI1* gene in central nervous system, malignant rhabdoid tumor (immunoperoxidase, ×400).

in MRT contrasts with other similar neoplasms, and analysis of specific markers of skeletal muscle differentiation such as myogenin and Myo-D1 is helpful in the differential diagnosis. In questionable cases, cytogenetic and molecular genetic analysis can be used as a diagnostic adjunct.

KEY DIAGNOSTIC POINTS

Malignant Rhabdoid Tumor

- MRT is a highly aggressive, polyphenotypic malignant neoplasm with a tendency for widespread metastases or a disseminated presentation.
- The proportion of rhabdoid cells within MRT varies and there is a histopathologic spectrum that mimics EWS/PNET, medulloblastoma, RMS, DSRCT, epithelioid sarcoma, and other primitive malignant neoplasms.
- MRT characteristically shows diffuse reactivity for vimentin, focal reactivity for at least one epithelial marker, and variable expression of mesenchymal and neuroectodermal markers.
- Absence of INI1 protein expression is useful for recognition of MRT and its distinction from other neoplasms, which lack *INI1* deletions or mutations and show INI1 immunoreactivity.
- Molecular genetics analysis to identify abnormalities of chromosome 22q11 provides additional support for the diagnosis of MRT.

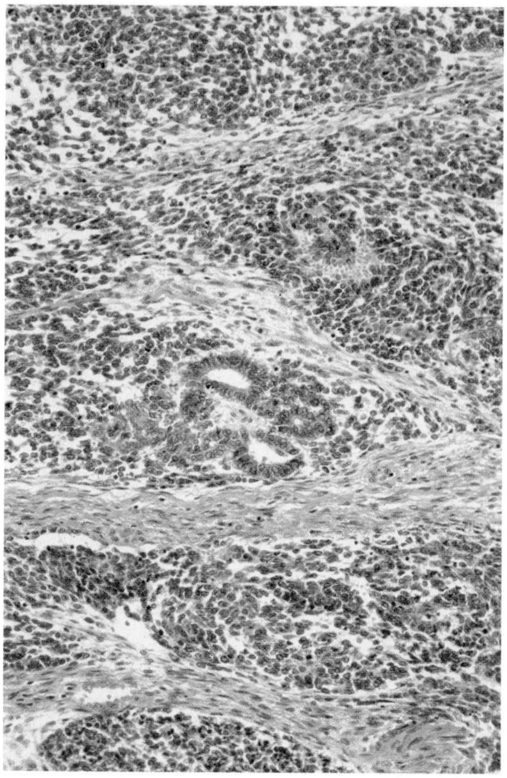

FIGURE 17.34 Wilms' tumor displays characteristic triphasic histology of epithelial differentiation with tubules, sheets of primitive round blastemal cells, and a nondescript fibrous stroma (hematoxylin-eosin, ×200).

GENOMIC APPLICATIONS

Mutations and homozygous deletions of the *INI1(hSNF5)* gene result in the absence of INI1 protein expression and are useful for recognition of MRT and its distinction from other neoplasms, which lack *INI1* deletions or mutations and do show INI1 immunoexpression.

BEYOND IMMUNOHISTOCHEMISTRY: ANATOMIC MOLECULAR DIAGNOSTIC APPLICATIONS

Regardless of location, about 70% of MRTs harbor deletions or mutations of the *hSNF5/INI1* gene at chromosome 22q11.2.[63,209-211] The spectrum of cytogenetic abnormalities includes monosomy 22, deletion of 22q11, translocations involving chromosome 22q11.2, and mutations and homozygous deletions of the *INI1(hSNF5)* gene.[192,212-214] An additional 20% to 25% of MRTs have a loss-of-function event with reduced expression of INI1 at the RNA or protein level.[211] FISH is useful for detection of deletions.[215]

Wilms' Tumor

WT, or nephroblastoma, is the most common pediatric renal neoplasm. Ninety-eight percent occur before 10 years of age, and there is no sex predilection. It is derived from nephrogenic blastemal cells and thus can exhibit a wide range of histologic appearances that replicate the developing kidney and display divergent differentiation.[17,216] Most WT are unicentric, but 7% are multicentric and 5% are bilateral. The rounded mass is sharply circumscribed and has a solid, soft, tan or gray cut surface.

The classic histologic pattern of WT consists of triphasic elements including blastemal, epithelial, and stromal components (Fig. 17.34). Proportions of these three elements vary, and biphasic or monophasic lesions may be encountered. Blastemal cells are small, round or oval, and densely packed in diffuse nodular or serpentine patterns. The epithelial component ranges from primitive tubular forms with a rosette-like appearance to more obvious tubular or papillary structures. Heterologous epithelial elements include mucinous and squamous epithelium. Stromal differentiation includes nondescript fibrous tissue, smooth muscle, skeletal muscle, adipose tissue, cartilage, bone, and neural tissue including ganglion cells, nerve, and neuroglia.[216,217] Pathologic evaluation for WT has been standardized with both the National Wilms' Tumor Study in North America and the SIOP Protocols in Europe.[17,20,218] Nuclear anaplasia occurs in about 5% of WT and is characterized by multipolar, polyploid cells with marked nuclear enlargement and hyperchromasia. The histologic pattern most likely to cause diagnostic difficulty is the blastemal pattern, which simulates many other small round cell neoplasms. The monomorphous sheets of blue blastemal cells can appear dyscohesive. The differential diagnosis includes lymphoma, EWS/PNET, NB, DSRCT, and RMS.

WTs do not exhibit a specific immunophenotype. The blastemal component is typically reactive for vimentin and usually shows desmin reactivity (Fig. 17.35).[216,219]

Other muscle markers such as myogenin and Myo-D1 are absent from blastemal foci but can be positive in areas of skeletal muscle differentiation. Nuclear staining for WT1 is positive in blastemal areas and in foci of early epithelial differentiation (Fig. 17.36).[220] More mature areas of epithelial differentiation such as tubules are typically reactive for cytokeratin (Fig. 17.37), CD56, and CD57.[220] Blastema is also focally positive for neuron-specific enolase and cytokeratin, but not for CD99.[216] Neural differentiation in WT is associated with reactivity for neuron-specific enolase, chromogranin, and synaptophysin, but staining for glial fibrillary acidic protein and S-100 protein is variable.[217,221] The absence of CD99 reactivity helps to distinguish blastemal predominant WT from EWS/PNET. Generally, the most important clue to the correct diagnosis of WT is the clinical history of a renal mass in a young child and the presence of a mixture of blastemal, epithelial, and mesenchymal components.

Specific genetic loci have been implicated in Wilms' tumorigenesis including the *WT1* tumor suppressor gene at chromosome 11p13, *WT2* at chromosome 11p15, and loci at chromosomes 1p13 and 16q.[216,222,223] A variety of nonspecific cytogenetic aberrations have been reported in anaplastic WT.[224]

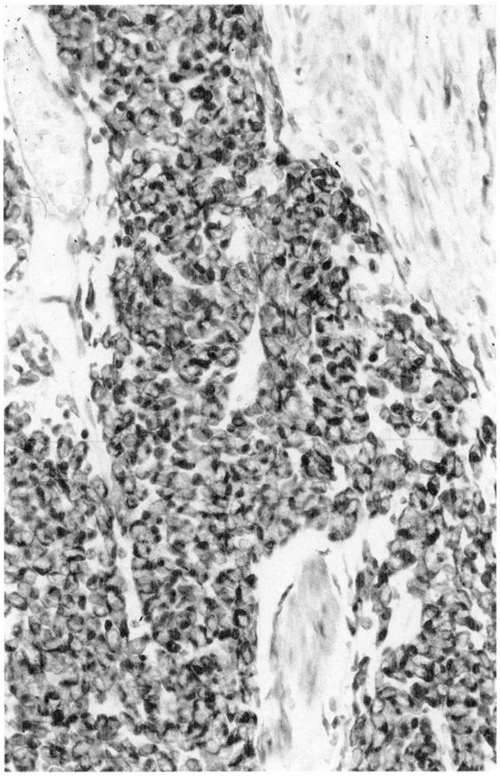

FIGURE 17.35 Desmin shows strong cytoplasmic reactivity in a blastemal area of Wilms' tumor (immunoperoxidase, ×400).

KEY DIAGNOSTIC POINTS

Wilms' Tumor

- WT can usually be diagnosed in a combination of classic histologic findings combined with clinical information about age and site of the tumor.
- Blastemal predominant WT, especially in small biopsy specimens, mimics other small blue cell tumors.
- Muscle markers such as myogenin and Myo-D1 are not expressed in blastemal predominant WT and serve as a useful differential diagnostic tool in desmin-positive, blastemal-predominant WTs. CD99 expression is also a useful distinguishing feature of EWS/PNET, in contrast to blastemal predominant WT.
- Pitfalls in the diagnosis of WT versus other kidney tumors include primary renal EWS/PNET, small cell synovial sarcoma, leukemia/lymphoma, and metastatic alveolar RMS.

THERANOSTIC APPLICATIONS

Potentially prognostically significant immunohistochemical markers have been identified for WT and include p53, CD44, growth factors, proliferative markers, angiogenic markers, and apoptotic markers. *p53* mutations are found in 73% to 100% of anaplastic WTs (225) (Figs. 17.38 and 17.39), and some evidence suggests that p53 expression is associated with advanced disease and relapse, although this point is controversial.[226,227] It is also thought that deregulation of apoptosis with increased expression of bcl-2 may influence outcome.[228] Blastemal expression of CD44 isoforms correlates with stage, progression, and death.[229] Transforming growth factor alpha and epidermal growth factor receptor are thought to assist clinical progression through promotion of proliferation and transformation.[230] Higher PCNA expression is associated with advanced stage and death.[231]

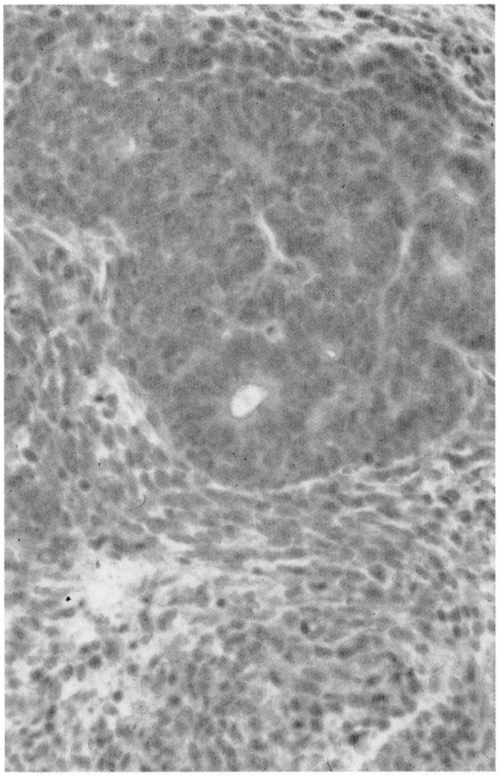

FIGURE 17.36 WT1 shows nuclear reactivity in blastemal and primitive epithelial areas of Wilms' tumor (immunoperoxidase, ×400).

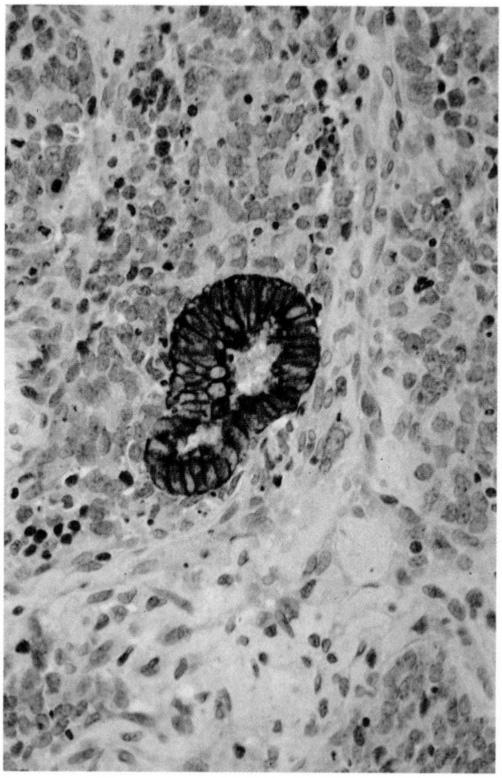

FIGURE 17.37 Cytokeratin highlights an area of tubular epithelial differentiation in Wilms' tumor (immunoperoxidase, ×400).

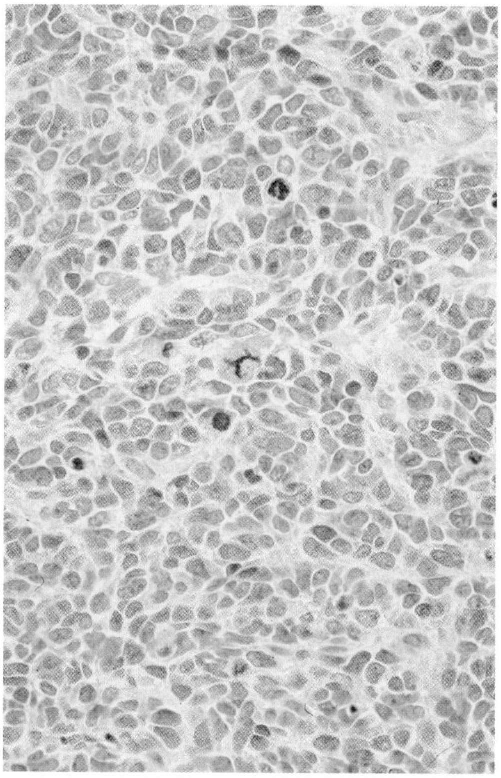

FIGURE 17.38 Anaplastic Wilms' tumor is characterized by enlarged, hyperchromatic nuclei with atypical mitoses (hematoxylin-eosin, ×400).

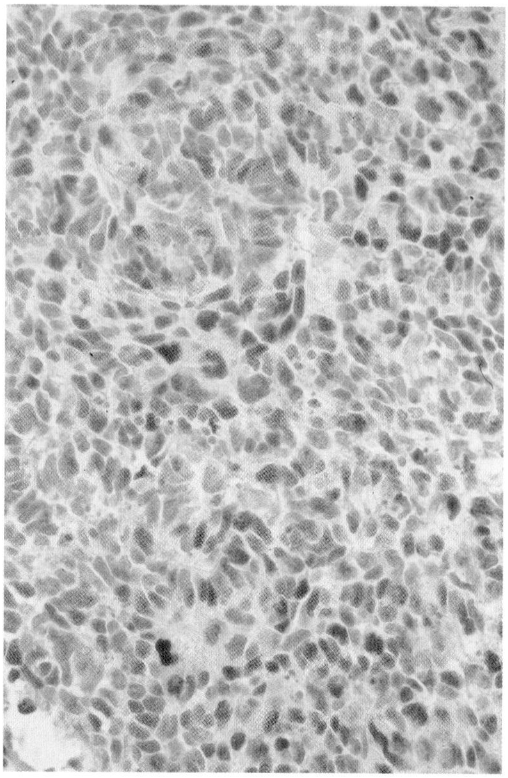

FIGURE 17.39 Nuclear reactivity for p53 is present in anaplastic Wilms' tumor and is associated with p53 mutation (immunoperoxidase, ×400).

Expression of vascular endothelial growth factor and its receptor FLT-1 is associated with a poor prognosis.[232]

Osteosarcoma

OS is the most common primary bone malignancy, and the classic type is a high-grade neoplasm in which tumor cells characteristically produce osteoid.[233,234] Although OS is primarily a malignancy of the young, with a peak in the second decade of life and 60% occurrence in patients younger than 25 years old, approximately 30% of cases occur in individuals older than 40 years of age. Males are more often affected than females, especially in the younger age range. The most frequent sites are the long bones of the appendicular skeleton, with a tumor origin in the metaphysis or diaphysis. The mass is large, fleshy, or hard and contains variable amounts of calcification, bone, and cartilage.

Microscopically, OS is composed of anaplastic pleomorphic cells with a morphologic spectrum including spindle, round, ovoid, epithelioid, plasmacytoid, clear, and multinucleated cells. Usually more than one cell type is present in individual OS. Osteoid is required for the diagnosis. Variable bone formation, cartilage, and fibrous tissue may also be encountered. Histologic subtypes of conventional OS include osteoblastic, chondroblastic, and fibroblastic patterns.[234] Ultrastructural studies have also demonstrated multiple cell types including osteoblastic, osteoclastic, chondroblastic, and fibroblastic features.[235]

There is no specific immunophenotype for OS, and it is immunohistochemically heterogenous, with expression of osteocalcin, cytokeratin, epithelial membrane antigen, desmin, smooth muscle actin, type 4 collagen, S-100 protein, factor 13, and even CD99 in varying proportions of cases.[236,237] Immunohistochemistry is useful for the differential diagnostic distinction of osteosarcomatous mimics such as sarcomatoid carcinoma, other sarcomas like synovial sarcoma, lymphoma, and malignant melanoma. The presence of reactivity for CD99 is a potential diagnostic pitfall, especially if the OS has a predominantly small round cell pattern. Cyclo-oxygenase 2 (COX 2) expression in high-grade chondroblastic osteosarcoma may be useful in the distinction from osteoblastoma.[238]

Complex cytogenetic abnormalities are often detected in osteosarcomas and are nonspecific.[234] The most significant pathologic-prognostic indicator in osteosarcoma is the extent of necrosis after chemotherapy.[239-243] Various potentially prognostically or biologically significant immunohistochemical markers have been investigated. Although there is some controversy about the genetic basis and significance of cytoplasmic versus nuclear patterns of immunoreactivity for HER2/ERB B2,[244-246] it now appears that immunohistochemical expression of HER2-ERB B2 is associated with a poor prognosis and increased risk of lung metastases.[247-250] Other potential poor prognostic markers include ephrin,[251] ezrin,[252] cytochrome P450 CYP 3A4/5,[253] WT1,[254] chemokine receptor CXC R4,[205] VEGF,[205] drug-related genes IMPDH2 and FTL,[255] p-glycoprotein,[247,256,257] p53,[247,258,259] and proliferative markers such as Ki-67 and PCNA.[39,258,259] Data about the prognostic significance of survivin expression are conflicting.[260,261] Bone morphogenic proteins 7 and 8 are highly expressed, and cytoplasmic and nuclear beta-catenin accumulations have been observed, but these markers do not have known prognostic significance.[262,263]

KEY DIAGNOSTIC POINTS

Osteosarcoma

- OS is an immunohistochemically heterogenous neoplasm and lacks a characteristic immunohistochemical profile.
- The presence of osteoid is the key distinguishing feature of OS.
- Expression of cytokeratin, epithelial membrane antigen, CD99, and S-100 protein are potential diagnostic pitfalls in the distinction from metastatic or sarcomatoid carcinoma, EWS/PNET, synovial sarcoma, malignant melanoma, and other malignancies.

SUMMARY

In conclusion, the availability of more specific and more sensitive immunohistochemical markers has enabled pathologists to categorize pediatric tumors, especially small blue cell tumors and spindle cell tumors, more accurately (Table 17.1). As therapeutic protocols for these tumors become more specific, precise diagnoses become even more imperative. Immunohistochemistry is only one of the tools available to pathologists to categorize solid tumors of childhood and adolescence, with cytogenetic and molecular analysis, flow cytometry, and electron microscopy of great use for selected cases. The ready availability, ease of use, and cost-effectiveness of immunohistochemistry make it an important diagnostic tool in pediatric surgical pathology. An awareness of reactivity patterns, sensitivity, specificity, and potential diagnostic pitfalls is essential.

REFERENCES

1. Ordonez NG. Application of immunocytochemistry in the diagnosis of soft tissue sarcomas: a review and update. *Adv Anat Pathol.* 1998;5:67-85.
2. Parham DM. Immunohistochemistry of childhood sarcomas: old and new markers. *Mod Pathol.* 1993;6:133-138.
3. Coindre JM. Immunohistochemistry in the diagnosis of soft tissue tumours. *Histopathology*. 2003;43:1-16.
4. Meis-Kindblom JM, Stenman G, Kindblom LG. Differential diagnosis of small round cell tumors. *Semin Diagn Pathol.* 1996;13:213-241.
5. Leong AS. Pitfalls in diagnostic immunohistology. *Adv Anat Pathol.* 2004;11:86-93.
6. Sebire NJ, Ramsay AD, Levitt G, et al. Aberrant immunohistochemical expression in nonrhabdomyosarcoma soft tissue sarcomas of infancy: retrospective review of clinical material. *Pediatr Dev Pathol.* 2002;5:579-586.
7. Zutter MM, Hess JL. Guidelines for the diagnosis of leukemia or lymphoma in children. *Am J Clin Pathol.* 1998;109:S9-22.
8. Mierau GW, Berry PJ, Orsini EN. Small round cell neoplasms: can electron microscopy and immunohistochemical studies accurately classify them? *Ultrastruct Pathol.* 1985;9:99-111.
9. Mierau GW, Berry PJ, Malott RL, Weeks DA. Appraisal of the comparative utility of immunohistochemistry and electron microscopy in the diagnosis of childhood round cell tumors. *Ultrastruct Pathol.* 1996;20:507-517.
10. Mierau GW, Weeks DA, Hicks MJ. Role of electron microscopy and other special techniques in the diagnosis of childhood round cell tumors. *Hum Pathol.* 1998;29:1347-1355.
11. Peydro-Olaya A, Llombart-Bosch A, Carda-Batalla C, Lopez-Guerrero JA. Electron microscopy and other ancillary techniques in the diagnosis of small round cell tumors. *Semin Diagn Pathol.* 2003;20:25-45.
12. Brahmi U, Srinivasan R, Komal HS, et al. Comparative analysis of electron microscopy and immunocytochemistry in the cytologic diagnosis of malignant small round cell tumors. *Acta Cytol.* 2003;47:443-449.
13. Kushner BH, LaQuaglia MP, Cheung NK, et al. Clinically critical impact of molecular genetic studies in pediatric solid tumors. *Med Pediatr Oncol.* 1999;33:530-535.
14. McManus AP, Gusterson BA, Pinkerton CR, Shipley JM. The molecular pathology of small round-cell tumours—relevance to diagnosis, prognosis, and classification. *J Pathol.* 1996;178:116-121.
15. de Alava E. Molecular pathology in sarcomas. *Clin Transl Oncol.* 2007;9:130-144.
16. Askin FB, Perlman EJ. Neuroblastoma and peripheral neuroectodermal tumors. *Am J Clin Pathol.* 1998;109:S23-S30.
17. Qualman SJ, Bowen J, Amin MB, et al. Protocol for the examination of specimens from patients with Wilms tumor (nephroblastoma) or other renal tumors of childhood. *Arch Pathol Lab Med.* 2003;127:1280-1289.
18. Qualman SJ, Bowen J, Parham DM, et al. Protocol for the examination of specimens from patients (children and young adults) with rhabdomyosarcoma. *Arch Pathol Lab Med.* 2003;127:1290-1297.
19. Coffin CM, Dehner LP. Pathologic evaluation of pediatric soft tissue tumors. *Am J Clin Pathol.* 1998;109:S38-S52.
20. Boccon-Gibod LA. Pathological evaluation of renal tumors in children: international society of pediatric oncology approach. *Pediatr Dev Pathol.* 1998;1:243-248.
21. Shimada H, Ambros IM, Dehner LP, et al. Terminology and morphologic criteria of neuroblastic tumors: recommendations by the International Neuroblastoma Pathology Committee. *Cancer.* 1999;86:349-363.

22. Wang NP, Marx J, McNutt MA, Rutledge JC, Gown AM. Expression of myogenic regulatory proteins (myogenin and MyoD1) in small blue round cell tumors of childhood. *Am J Pathol.* 1995;147:1799-1810.
23. Dias P, Parham DM, Shapiro DN, et al. Myogenic regulatory protein (MyoD1) expression in childhood solid tumors: diagnostic utility in rhabdomyosarcoma. *Am J Pathol.* 1990;137:1283-1291.
24. Cui S, Hano H, Harada T, et al. Evaluation of new monoclonal anti-MyoD1 and anti-myogenin antibodies for the diagnosis of rhabdomyosarcoma. *Pathol Int.* 1999;49:62-68.
25. Engel ME, Mouton SC, Emms M. Paediatric rhabdomyosarcoma: MyoD1 demonstration in routinely processed tissue sections using wet heat pretreatment (pressure cooking) for antigen retrieval. *J Clin Pathol.* 1997;50:37-39.
26. Kumar S, Perlman E, Harris CA, et al. Myogenin is a specific marker for rhabdomyosarcoma: an immunohistochemical study in paraffin-embedded tissues. *Mod Pathol.* 2000;13:988-993.
27. Cessna MH, Zhou H, Perkins SL, et al. Are myogenin and myoD1 expression specific for rhabdomyosarcoma? A study of 150 cases, with emphasis on spindle cell mimics. *Am J Surg Pathol.* 2001;25:1150-1157.
28. Sebire NJ, Malone M. Myogenin and MyoD1 expression in paediatric rhabdomyosarcomas. *J Clin Pathol.* 2003;56:412-416.
29. Dias P, Parham DM, Shapiro DN, et al. Monoclonal antibodies to the myogenic regulatory protein MyoD1: epitope mapping and diagnostic utility. *Cancer Res.* 1992;52:6431-6439.
30. Dias P, Chen B, Dilday B, et al. Strong immunostaining for myogenin in rhabdomyosarcoma is significantly associated with tumors of the alveolar subclass. *Am J Pathol.* 2000;156:399-408.
31. Stevenson AJ, Chatten J, Bertoni F, Miettinen M. (p30/32^{MIC2}) Neuroectodermal/Ewing's sarcoma antigen as an immunohistochemical marker: review of more than 600 tumors and the literature experience. *Appl Immunohistochem.* 1994;2:231-240.
32. Perlman EJ, Dickman PS, Askin FB, et al. Ewing's sarcoma—routine diagnostic utilization of MIC2 analysis: a Pediatric Oncology Group/Children's Cancer Group Intergroup Study. *Hum Pathol.* 1994;25:304-307.
33. Weidner N, Tjoe J. Immunohistochemical profile of monoclonal antibody O13: antibody that recognizes glycoprotein p30/32MIC2 and is useful in diagnosing Ewing's sarcoma and peripheral neuroepithelioma. *Am J Surg Pathol.* 1994;18:486-494.
34. Ambros IM, Ambros PF, Strehl S, et al. MIC2 is a specific marker for Ewing's sarcoma and peripheral primitive neuroectodermal tumors. Evidence for a common histogenesis of Ewing's sarcoma and peripheral primitive neuroectodermal tumors from MIC2 expression and specific chromosome aberration. *Cancer.* 1991;67:1886-1893.
35. Ramani P, Rampling D, Link M. Immunocytochemical study of 12E7 in small round-cell tumours of childhood: an assessment of its sensitivity and specificity. *Histopathology.* 1993;23:557-561.
36. Riopel M, Dickman PS, Link MP, Perlman EJ. MIC2 analysis in pediatric lymphomas and leukemias. *Hum Pathol.* 1994;25:396-399.
37. Zhang PJ, Goldblum JR, Pawel BR, et al. Immunophenotype of desmoplastic small round cell tumors as detected in cases with EWS-WT1 gene fusion product. *Mod Pathol.* 2003;16:229-235.
38. Granter SR, Renshaw AA, Fletcher CD, et al. CD99 reactivity in mesenchymal chondrosarcoma. *Hum Pathol.* 1996;27:1273-1276.
39. Folpe AL, Schmidt RA, Chapman D, Gown AM. Poorly differentiated synovial sarcoma: immunohistochemical distinction from primitive neuroectodermal tumors and high-grade malignant peripheral nerve sheath tumors. *Am J Surg Pathol.* 1998;22:673-682.
40. Fellinger EJ, Garin-Chesa P, Triche TJ, et al. Immunohistochemical analysis of Ewing's sarcoma cell surface antigen p30/32MIC2. *Am J Pathol.* 1991;139:317-325.
41. Ozdemirli M, Fanburg-Smith JC, Hartmann DP, et al. Differentiating lymphoblastic lymphoma and Ewing's sarcoma: lymphocyte markers and gene rearrangement. *Mod Pathol.* 2001;14:1175-1182.
42. Pappo AS, Douglass EC, Meyer WH, et al. Use of HBA 71 and anti-beta 2-microglobulin to distinguish peripheral neuroepithelioma from neuroblastoma. *Hum Pathol.* 1993;24:880-885.
43. Nilsson G, Wang M, Wejde J, et al. Detection of EWS/FLI-1 by immunostaining. An adjunctive tool in diagnosis of Ewing's sarcoma and primitive neuroectodermal tumor on cytological samples and paraffin-embedded archival material. *Sarcoma.* 1999;3:25-32.
44. Folpe AL, Hill CE, Parham DM, et al. Immunohistochemical detection of FLI-1 protein expression: a study of 132 round cell tumors with emphasis on CD99-positive mimics of Ewing's sarcoma/primitive neuroectodermal tumor. *Am J Surg Pathol.* 2000;24:1657-1662.
45. Rossi S, Orvieto E, Furlanetto A, et al. Utility of the immunohistochemical detection of FLI-1 expression in round cell and vascular neoplasm using a monoclonal antibody. *Mod Pathol.* 2004;17:547-552.
46. Hill DA, Pfeifer JD, Marley EF, et al. WT1 staining reliably differentiates desmoplastic small round cell tumor from Ewing sarcoma/primitive neuroectodermal tumor. An immunohistochemical and molecular diagnostic study. *Am J Clin Pathol.* 2000;114:345-353.
47. Barnoud R, Sabourin JC, Pasquier D, et al. Immunohistochemical expression of WT1 by desmoplastic small round cell tumor: a comparative study with other small round cell tumors. *Am J Surg Pathol.* 2000;24:830-836.
48. Lae ME, Roche PC, Jin L, et al. Desmoplastic small round cell tumor: a clinicopathologic, immunohistochemical, and molecular study of 32 tumors. *Am J Surg Pathol.* 2002;26:823-835.
49. Judkins AR, Mauger J, Ht A, et al. Immunohistochemical analysis of hSNF5/INI1 in pediatric CNS neoplasms. *Am J Surg Pathol.* 2004;28:644-650.
50. Sigauke E, Rakheja D, Maddox DL, et al. Absence of expression of SMARCB1/INI1 in malignant rhabdoid tumors of the central nervous system, kidneys and soft tissue: an immunohistochemical study with implications for diagnosis. *Mod Pathol.* 2006;19:717-725.
51. Hoot AC, Russo P, Judkins AR, et al. Immunohistochemical analysis of hSNF5/INI1 distinguishes renal and extra-renal malignant rhabdoid tumors from other pediatric soft tissue tumors. *Am J Surg Pathol.* 2004;28:1485-1491.
52. Schwab M, Shimada H, Joshi V, Brodeur GM. Neuroblastic tumors of adrenal gland and sympathetic nervous system. In: Kleihues P, Cavenee WK, eds. *World Health Organization Classification of Tumours. Tumours of the Nervous System.* Lyon, France: IARC Press; 2000.
53. Shimada H, Ambros IM, Dehner LP, et al. The International Neuroblastoma Pathology Classification (the Shimada system). *Cancer.* 1999;86:364-372.
54. Miettinen M, Chatten J, Paetau A, Stevenson A. Monoclonal antibody NB84 in the differential diagnosis of neuroblastoma and other small round cell tumors. *Am J Surg Pathol.* 1998;22:327-332.
55. Parham DM. Neuroectodermal and neuroendocrine tumors principally seen in children. *Am J Clin Pathol.* 2001;115(Suppl):S113-S128.
56. Wick MR. Immunohistology of neuroendocrine and neuroectodermal tumors. *Semin Diagn Pathol.* 2000;17:194-203.
57. Joshi VV. Peripheral neuroblastic tumors: pathologic classification based on recommendations of international neuroblastoma pathology committee (modification of Shimada classification). *Pediatr Dev Pathol.* 2000;3:184-199.
58. Carter RL, al-Sams SZ, Corbett RP, Clinton S. A comparative study of immunohistochemical staining for neuron-specific enolase, protein gene product 9.5 and S-100 protein in neuroblastoma, Ewing's sarcoma and other round cell tumours in children. *Histopathology.* 1990;16:461-467.
59. Shimada H, Aoyama C, Chiba T, Newton Jr WA. Prognostic subgroups for undifferentiated neuroblastoma: immunohistochemical study with anti-S-100 protein antibody. *Hum Pathol.* 1985;16:471-476.
60. Brook FB, Raafat F, Eldeeb BB, Mann JR. Histologic and immunohistochemical investigation of neuroblastomas and correlation with prognosis. *Hum Pathol.* 1988;19:879-888.

61. Moss TJ, Reynolds CP, Sather HN, et al. Prognostic value of immunocytologic detection of bone marrow metastases in neuroblastoma. *N Engl J Med.* 1991;324:219-226.
62. Lamant L, Pulford K, Bischof D, et al. Expression of the ALK tyrosine kinase gene in neuroblastoma. *Am J Pathol.* 2000;156:1711-1721.
63. White FV, Dehner LP, Belchis DA, et al. Congenital disseminated malignant rhabdoid tumor: a distinct clinicopathologic entity demonstrating abnormalities of chromosome 22q11. *Am J Surg Pathol.* 1999;23:249-256.
64. Mejia C, Navarro S, Pellin A, et al. Prognostic significance of cell proliferation in human neuroblastoma: comparison with other prognostic factors. *Oncol Rep.* 2003;10:243-247.
65. Krams M, Hero B, Berthold F, et al. Proliferation marker KI-S5 discriminates between favorable and adverse prognosis in advanced stages of neuroblastoma with and without MYCN amplification. *Cancer.* 2002;94:854-861.
66. Krams M, Heidebrecht HJ, Hero B, et al. Repp86 expression and outcome in patients with neuroblastoma. *J Clin Oncol.* 2003;21:1810-1818.
67. Munchar MJ, Sharifah NA, Jamal R, Looi LM. CD44s expression correlated with the International Neuroblastoma Pathology Classification (Shimada system) for neuroblastic tumours. *Pathology.* 2003;35:125-129.
68. Comito MA, Savell VH, Cohen MB. CD44 expression in neuroblastoma and related tumors. *J Pediatr Hematol Oncol.* 1997;19:292-296.
69. Combaret V, Gross N, Lasset C, et al. Clinical relevance of CD44 cell-surface expression and N-myc gene amplification in a multicentric analysis of 121 pediatric neuroblastomas. *J Clin Oncol.* 1996;14:25-34.
70. Krams M, Parwaresch R, Sipos B, et al. Expression of the c-kit receptor characterizes a subset of neuroblastomas with favorable prognosis. *Oncogene.* 2004;23:588-595.
71. Vitali R, Cesi V, Nicotra MR, et al. c-Kit is preferentially expressed in MYCN-amplified neuroblastoma and its effect on cell proliferation is inhibited in vitro by STI-571. *Int J Cancer.* 2003;106:147-152.
72. Gallo G, Giarnieri E, Bosco S, et al. Aberrant bcl-2 and bax protein expression related to chemotherapy response in neuroblastoma. *Anticancer Res.* 2003;23:777-784.
73. Ara T, Fukuzawa M, Kusafuka T, et al. Immunohistochemical expression of MMP-2, MMP-9, and TIMP-2 in neuroblastoma: association with tumor progression and clinical outcome. *J Pediatr Surg.* 1998;33:1272-1278.
74. Brodeur GM, Maris JM, Yamashiro DJ, et al. Biology and genetics of human neuroblastomas. *J Pediatr Hematol Oncol.* 1997;19:93-101.
75. Brodeur GM, Nakagawara A, Yamashiro DJ, et al. Expression of TrkA, TrkB and TrkC in human neuroblastomas. *J Neurooncol.* 1997;31:49-55.
76. Nakagawara A, Arima-Nakagawara M, Scavarda NJ, et al. Association between high levels of expression of the TRK gene and favorable outcome in human neuroblastoma. *N Engl J Med.* 1993;328:847-854.
77. Nakagawara A, Liu XG, Ikegaki N, et al. Cloning and chromosomal localization of the human TRK-B tyrosine kinase receptor gene (NTRK2). *Genomics.* 1995;25:538-546.
78. Kramer K, Gerald W, LeSauteur L, et al. Prognostic value of TrkA protein detection by monoclonal antibody 5C3 in neuroblastoma. *Clin Cancer Res.* 1996;2:1361-1367.
79. Kramer K, Gerald W, LeSauteur L, et al. Monoclonal antibody to human Trk-A: diagnostic and therapeutic potential in neuroblastoma. *Eur J Cancer.* 1997;33:2090-2091.
80. Tanaka T, Hiyama E, Sugimoto T, et al. trk A gene expression in neuroblastoma. The clinical significance of an immunohistochemical study. *Cancer.* 1995;76:1086-1095.
81. Maris JM, Hogarty MD, Bagatell R, Cohn SL. Neuroblastoma. *Lancet.* 2007;369:2106-2120.
82. Brodeur GM. Molecular pathology of human neuroblastomas. *Semin Diagn Pathol.* 1994;11:118-125.
83. Brodeur GM. Molecular basis for heterogeneity in human neuroblastomas. *Eur J Cancer.* 1995;31A:505-510.
84. Brodeur GM. Neuroblastoma: biological insights into a clinical enigma. *Nat Rev Cancer.* 2003;3:203-216.
85. Layfield LJ, Willmore-Payne C, Shimada H, Holden JA. Assessment of NMYC amplification: a comparison of FISH, quantitative PCR monoplexing and traditional blotting methods used with formalin-fixed, paraffin-embedded neuroblastomas. *Anal Quant Cytol Histol.* 2005;27:5-14.
86. George RE, London WB, Cohn SL, et al. Hyperdiploidy plus nonamplified MYCN confers a favorable prognosis in children 12 to 18 months old with disseminated neuroblastoma: a Pediatric Oncology Group study. *J Clin Oncol.* 2005;23:6466-6473.
87. Spitz R, Betts DR, Simon T, et al. Favorable outcome of triploid neuroblastomas: a contribution to the special oncogenesis of neuroblastoma. *Cancer Genet Cytogenet.* 2006;167:51-56.
88. Spitz R, Hero B, Ernestus K, Berthold F. FISH analyses for alterations in chromosomes 1, 2, 3, and 11 define high-risk groups in neuroblastoma. *Med Pediatr Oncol.* 2003;41:30-35.
89. Haber M, Smith J, Bordow SB, et al. Association of high-level MRP1 expression with poor clinical outcome in a large prospective study of primary neuroblastoma. *J Clin Oncol.* 2006;24:1546-1553.
90. Asgharzadeh S, Pique-Regi R, Sposto R, et al. Prognostic significance of gene expression profiles of metastatic neuroblastomas lacking MYCN gene amplification. *J Natl Cancer Inst.* 2006;98:1193-1203.
91. Asmar L, Gehan EA, Newton WA, et al. Agreement among and within groups of pathologists in the classification of rhabdomyosarcoma and related childhood sarcomas. Report of an international study of four pathology classifications. *Cancer.* 1994;74:2579-2588.
92. Miller RW, Young Jr JL, Novakovic B. Childhood cancer. *Cancer.* 1995;75:395-405.
93. Newton Jr WA, Gehan EA, Webber BL, et al. Classification of rhabdomyosarcomas and related sarcomas. Pathologic aspects and proposal for a new classification—an Intergroup Rhabdomyosarcoma Study. *Cancer.* 1995;76:1073-1085.
94. Qualman SJ, Coffin CM, Newton WA, et al. Intergroup Rhabdomyosarcoma Study: update for pathologists. *Pediatr Dev Pathol.* 1998;1:550-561.
95. Coffin CM. The new international rhabdomyosarcoma classification, its progenitors, and considerations beyond morphology. *Adv Anat Pathol.* 1997;4:1-16.
96. Parham D, Barr FG. Pathology and Genetics of Tumors of Soft Tissue and Bone. In: Fletcher CD, Unni KK, Mertens F, eds. *World Health Organization Classification of Tumours.* Lyon, France: IARC Press; 2002:146-152.
97. Kodet R, Newton Jr WA, Hamoudi AB, et al. Childhood rhabdomyosarcoma with anaplastic (pleomorphic) features. A report of the Intergroup Rhabdomyosarcoma Study. *Am J Surg Pathol.* 1993;17:443-453.
98. Parham DM. Pathologic classification of rhabdomyosarcomas and correlations with molecular studies. *Mod Pathol.* 2001;14:506-514.
99. Kodet R. Rhabdomyosarcoma in childhood. An immunohistological analysis with myoglobin, desmin and vimentin. *Pathol Res Pract.* 1989;185:207-213.
100. Coffin CM, Rulon J, Smith L, et al. Pathologic features of rhabdomyosarcoma before and after treatment: a clinicopathologic and immunohistochemical analysis. *Mod Pathol.* 1997;10:1175-1187.
101. Tsokos M. The role of immunocytochemistry in the diagnosis of rhabdomyosarcoma. *Arch Pathol Lab Med.* 1986;110:776-778.
102. Scupham R, Gilbert EF, Wilde J, Wiedrich TA. Immunohistochemical studies of rhabdomyosarcoma. *Arch Pathol Lab Med.* 1986;110:818-821.
103. Brooks JJ. Immunohistochemistry of soft tissue tumors. Myoglobin as a tumor marker for rhabdomyosarcoma. *Cancer.* 1982;50:1757-1763.
104. Leader M, Patel J, Collins M, Henry K. Myoglobin: an evaluation of its role as a marker of rhabdomyosarcomas. *Br J Cancer.* 1989;59:106-109.
105. Parham DM, Webber B, Holt H, et al. Immunohistochemical study of childhood rhabdomyosarcomas and related neoplasms. Results of an Intergroup Rhabdomyosarcoma study project. *Cancer.* 1991;67:3072-3080.
106. Carter RL, McCarthy KP, Machin LG, et al. Expression of desmin and myoglobin in rhabdomyosarcomas and in developing skeletal muscle. *Histopathology.* 1989;15:585-595.

107. Schmidt RA, Cone R, Haas JE, Gown AM. Diagnosis of rhabdomyosarcomas with HHF35, a monoclonal antibody directed against muscle actins. *Am J Pathol.* 1988;131:19-28.
108. Azumi N, Ben-Ezra J, Battifora H. Immunophenotypic diagnosis of leiomyosarcomas and rhabdomyosarcomas with monoclonal antibodies to muscle-specific actin and desmin in formalin-fixed tissue. *Mod Pathol.* 1988;1:469-474.
109. Dodd S, Malone M, McCulloch W. Rhabdomyosarcoma in children: a histological and immunohistochemical study of 59 cases. *J Pathol.* 1989;158:13-18.
110. Dias P, Kumar P, Marsden HB, et al. Evaluation of desmin as a diagnostic and prognostic marker of childhood rhabdomyosarcomas and embryonal sarcomas. *Br J Cancer.* 1987;56:361-365.
111. Eusebi V, Ceccarelli C, Gorza L, et al. Immunocytochemistry of rhabdomyosarcoma. The use of four different markers. *Am J Surg Pathol.* 1986;10:293-299.
112. Morotti RA, Nicol KK, Parham DM, et al. An immunohistochemical algorithm to facilitate diagnosis and subtyping of rhabdomyosarcoma: the Children's Oncology Group experience. *Am J Surg Pathol.* 2006;30:962-968.
113. Michelagnoli MP, Burchill SA, Cullinane C, et al. Myogenin—a more specific target for RT-PCR detection of rhabdomyosarcoma than MyoD1. *Med Pediatr Oncol.* 2003;40:1-8.
114. Cessna MH, Zhou H, Sanger WG, et al. Expression of ALK1 and p80 in inflammatory myofibroblastic tumor and its mesenchymal mimics: a study of 135 cases. *Mod Pathol.* 2002;15:931-938.
115. Miettinen M, Rapola J. Immunohistochemical spectrum of rhabdomyosarcoma and rhabdomyosarcoma-like tumors. Expression of cytokeratin and the 68-kD neurofilament protein. *Am J Surg Pathol.* 1989;13:120-132.
116. Coindre JM, de Mascarel A, Trojani M, et al. Immunohistochemical study of rhabdomyosarcoma. Unexpected staining with S100 protein and cytokeratin. *J Pathol.* 1988;155:127-132.
117. Goldsmith JD, Pawel B, Goldblum JR, et al. Detection and diagnostic utilization of placental alkaline phosphatase in muscular tissue and tumors with myogenic differentiation. *Am J Surg Pathol.* 2002;26:1627-1633.
118. Carpentieri DF, Nichols K, Chou PM, et al. The expression of WT1 in the differentiation of rhabdomyosarcoma from other pediatric small round blue cell tumors. *Mod Pathol.* 2002;15:1080-1086.
119. Tokuc G, Dogan O, Ayan I, et al. Prognostic value of proliferating cell nuclear antigen immunostaining in pediatric rhabdomyosarcomas. *Acta Paediatr Jpn.* 1998;40:573-579.
120. San Miguel-Fraile P, Carrillo-Gijon R, Rodriguez-Peralto JL, Badiola IA. Prognostic significance of DNA ploidy and proliferative index (MIB-1 index) in childhood rhabdomyosarcoma. *Am J Clin Pathol.* 2004;121:358-365.
121. Ayan I, Dogan O, Kebudi R, et al. Immunohistochemical detection of p53 protein in rhabdomyosarcoma: association with clinicopathological features and outcome. *J Pediatr Hematol Oncol.* 1997;19:48-53.
122. Takahashi Y, Oda Y, Kawaguchi K, et al. Altered expression and molecular abnormalities of cell-cycle-regulatory proteins in rhabdomyosarcoma. *Mod Pathol.* 2004;17:660-669.
123. Davicioni E, Finckenstein FG, Shahbazian V, et al. Identification of a PAX-FKHR gene expression signature that defines molecular classes and determines the prognosis of alveolar rhabdomyosarcomas. *Cancer Res.* 2006;66:6936-6946.
124. Sorensen PH, Lynch JC, Qualman SJ, et al. PAX3-FKHR and PAX7-FKHR gene fusions are prognostic indicators in alveolar rhabdomyosarcoma: a report from the children's oncology group. *J Clin Oncol.* 2002;20:2672-2679.
125. Barr FG, Qualman SJ, Macris MH, et al. Genetic heterogeneity in the alveolar rhabdomyosarcoma subset without typical gene fusions. *Cancer Res.* 2002;62:4704-4710.
126. Ushigome S, Machinami R, Sorensen PH. Ewing sarcoma/primitive neuroectodermal tumour (PNET). In: Fletcher CD, Unni KK, Mertens F, eds. *Pathology and Genetics of Tumours of Soft Tissue and Bone. World Health Organization Classification of Tumours.* Lyon, France: IARC Press; 2002:298-300.
127. Khoury JD. Ewing sarcoma family of tumors. *Adv Anat Pathol.* 2005;12:212-220.
128. Coffin CM, Dehner LP. Peripheral neurogenic tumors of the soft tissues in children and adolescents: a clinicopathologic study of 139 cases. *Pediatr Pathol.* 1989;9:387-407.
129. de Alava E, Gerald WL. Molecular biology of the Ewing's sarcoma/primitive neuroectodermal tumor family. *J Clin Oncol.* 2000;18:204-213.
130. Hasegawa SL, Davison JM, Rutten A, et al. Primary cutaneous Ewing's sarcoma: immunophenotypic and molecular cytogenetic evaluation of five cases. *Am J Surg Pathol.* 1998;22:310-318.
131. Marley EF, Liapis H, Humphrey PA, et al. Primitive neuroectodermal tumor of the kidney—another enigma: a pathologic, immunohistochemical, and molecular diagnostic study. *Am J Surg Pathol.* 1997;21:354-359.
132. Lawlor ER, Mathers JA, Bainbridge T, et al. Peripheral primitive neuroectodermal tumors in adults: documentation by molecular analysis. *J Clin Oncol.* 1998;16:1150-1157.
133. Moll R, Lee I, Gould VE, et al. Immunocytochemical analysis of Ewing's tumors. Patterns of expression of intermediate filaments and desmosomal proteins indicate cell type heterogeneity and pluripotential differentiation. *Am J Pathol.* 1987;127:288-304.
134. Llombart-Bosch A, Lacombe MJ, Peydro-Olaya A, et al. Malignant peripheral neuroectodermal tumours of bone other than Askin's neoplasm: characterization of 14 new cases with immunohistochemistry and electron microscopy. *Virchows Arch A Pathol Anat Histopathol.* 1988;412:421-430.
135. Shanfeld RL, Edelman J, Willis JE, et al. Immunohistochemical analysis of neural markers in peripheral primitive neuroectodermal tumors (pPNET) without light microscopic evidence of neural differentiation. *Appl Immunohistochem.* 1997;5:78-86.
136. Fellinger EJ, Garin-Chesa P, Glasser DB, et al. Comparison of cell surface antigen HBA71 (p30/32MIC2), neuron-specific enolase, and vimentin in the immunohistochemical analysis of Ewing's sarcoma of bone. *Am J Surg Pathol.* 1992;16:746-755.
137. Gu M, Antonescu CR, Guiter G, et al. Cytokeratin immunoreactivity in Ewing's sarcoma: prevalence in 50 cases confirmed by molecular diagnostic studies. *Am J Surg Pathol.* 2000;24:410-416.
138. Hamilton G, Fellinger EJ, Schratter I, Fritsch A. Characterization of a human endocrine tissue and tumor-associated Ewing's sarcoma antigen. *Cancer Res.* 1988;48:6127-6131.
139. Scotlandi K, Serra M, Manara MC, et al. Immunostaining of the p30/32MIC2 antigen and molecular detection of EWS rearrangements for the diagnosis of Ewing's sarcoma and peripheral neuroectodermal tumor. *Hum Pathol.* 1996;27:408-416.
140. Olsen SH, Thomas DG, Lucas DR. Cluster analysis of immunohistochemical profiles in synovial sarcoma, malignant peripheral nerve sheath tumor, and Ewing sarcoma. *Mod Pathol.* 2006;19:659-668.
141. Lucas DR, Bentley G, Dan ME, et al. Ewing sarcoma vs lymphoblastic lymphoma. A comparative immunohistochemical study. *Am J Clin Pathol.* 2001;115:11-17.
142. Kumar S, Pack S, Kumar D, et al. Detection of EWS-FLI-1 fusion in Ewing's sarcoma/peripheral primitive neuroectodermal tumor by fluorescence in situ hybridization using formalin-fixed paraffin-embedded tissue. *Hum Pathol.* 1999;30:324-330.
143. Fritsch MK, Bridge JA, Schuster AE, et al. Performance characteristics of a reverse transcriptase-polymerase chain reaction assay for the detection of tumor-specific fusion transcripts from archival tissue. *Pediatr Dev Pathol.* 2003;6:43-53.
144. Dagher R, Pham TA, Sorbara L, et al. Molecular confirmation of Ewing sarcoma. *J Pediatr Hematol Oncol.* 2001;23:221-224.
145. Sandberg AA, Bridge JA. Updates on cytogenetics and molecular genetics of bone and soft tissue tumors: Ewing sarcoma and peripheral primitive neuroectodermal tumors. *Cancer Genet Cytogenet.* 2000;123:1-26.
146. Delattre O, Zucman J, Melot T, et al. The Ewing family of tumors—a subgroup of small-round-cell tumors defined by specific chimeric transcripts. *N Engl J Med.* 1994;331:294-299.
147. Wang L, Bhargava R, Zheng T, et al. Undifferentiated small round cell sarcomas with rare EWS gene fusions: identification of a novel EWS-SP3 fusion and of additional cases with the EWS-ETV1 and EWS-FEV fusions. *J Mol Diagn.* 2007;9:498-509.
148. Antonescu CR. The role of genetic testing in soft tissue sarcoma. *Histopathology.* 2006;48:13-21.

149. Folpe AL, Goldblum JR, Rubin BP, et al. Morphologic and immunophenotypic diversity in Ewing family tumors: a study of 66 genetically confirmed cases. *Am J Surg Pathol.* 2005;29:1025-1033.
150. Lazar A, Abruzzo LV, Pollock RE, et al. Molecular diagnosis of sarcomas: chromosomal translocations in sarcomas. *Arch Pathol Lab Med.* 2006;130:1199-1207.
151. Lewis TB, Coffin CM, Bernard PS. Differentiating Ewing's sarcoma from other round blue cell tumors using a RT-PCR translocation panel on formalin-fixed paraffin-embedded tissues. *Mod Pathol.* 2007;20:397-404.
152. Folpe AL, Goldblum JR, Rubin BP, et al. When can Ewing sarcoma/primitive neuroectodermal tumor (ES/PNET) be diagnosed without genetic confirmation? A study of 62 proven cases. *Mod Pathol.* 2004;17(Suppl 1):13A.
153. Jambhekar NA, Bagwan IN, Ghule P, et al. Comparative analysis of routine histology, immunohistochemistry, reverse transcriptase polymerase chain reaction, and fluorescence in situ hybridization in diagnosis of Ewing family of tumors. *Arch Pathol Lab Med.* 2006;130:1813-1818.
154. Kawamura-Saito M, Yamazaki Y, Kaneko K, et al. Fusion between CIC and DUX4 up-regulates PEA3 family genes in Ewing-like sarcomas with t(4;19)(q35;q13) translocation. *Hum Mol Genet.* 2006;15:2125-2137.
155. Amir G, Issakov J, Meller I, et al. Expression of p53 gene product and cell proliferation marker Ki-67 in Ewing's sarcoma: correlation with clinical outcome. *Hum Pathol.* 2002;33:170-174.
156. de Alava E, Antonescu CR, Panizo A, et al. Prognostic impact of P53 status in Ewing sarcoma. *Cancer.* 2000;89:783-792.
157. Maitra A, Roberts H, Weinberg AG, Geradts J. Aberrant expression of tumor suppressor proteins in the Ewing family of tumors. *Arch Pathol Lab Med.* 2001;125:1207-1212.
158. Smithey BE, Pappo AS, Hill DA. C-kit expression in pediatric solid tumors: a comparative immunohistochemical study. *Am J Surg Pathol.* 2002;26:486-492.
159. Daugaard S, Kamby C, Sunde LM, et al. Ewing's sarcoma. A retrospective study of histological and immunohistochemical factors and their relation to prognosis. *Virchows Arch A Pathol Anat Histopathol.* 1989;414:243-251.
160. Parham DM, Hijazi Y, Steinberg SM, et al. Neuroectodermal differentiation in Ewing's sarcoma family of tumors does not predict tumor behavior. *Hum Pathol.* 1999;30:911-918.
161. Pinto A, Grant LH, Hayes FA, et al. Immunohistochemical expression of neuron-specific enolase and Leu 7 in Ewing's sarcoma of bone. *Cancer.* 1989;64:1266-1273.
162. de Alava E, Kawai A, Healey JH, et al. EWS-FLI1 fusion transcript structure is an independent determinant of prognosis in Ewing's sarcoma. *J Clin Oncol.* 1998;16:1248-1255.
163. Ordonez NG, Zirkin R, Bloom RE. Malignant small-cell epithelial tumor of the peritoneum coexpressing mesenchymal-type intermediate filaments. *Am J Surg Pathol.* 1989;13:413-421.
164. Gerald WL, Miller HK, Battifora H, et al. Intra-abdominal desmoplastic small round-cell tumor. Report of 19 cases of a distinctive type of high-grade polyphenotypic malignancy affecting young individuals. *Am J Surg Pathol.* 1991;15:499-513.
165. Gonzalez-Crussi F, Crawford SE, Sun CC. Intraabdominal desmoplastic small-cell tumors with divergent differentiation. Observations on three cases of childhood. *Am J Surg Pathol.* 1990;14:633-642.
166. Livaditi E, Mavridis G, Soutis M, et al. Diffuse intraabdominal desmoplastic small round cell tumor: a ten-year experience. *Eur J Pediatr Surg.* 2006;16:423-427.
167. Saab R, Khoury JD, Krasin M, et al. Desmoplastic small round cell tumor in childhood: the St. Jude Children's Research Hospital experience. *Pediatr Blood Cancer.* 2007;49:274-279.
168. Kawano N, Inayama Y, Nagashima Y, et al. Desmoplastic small round-cell tumor of the paratesticular region: report of an adult case with demonstration of EWS and WT1 gene fusion using paraffin-embedded tissue. *Mod Pathol.* 1999;12:729-734.
169. Parkash V, Gerald WL, Parma A, et al. Desmoplastic small round cell tumor of the pleura. *Am J Surg Pathol.* 1995;19:659-665.
170. Tison V, Cerasoli S, Morigi F, et al. Intracranial desmoplastic small-cell tumor. Report of a case. *Am J Surg Pathol.* 1996;20:112-117.
171. Backer A, Mount SL, Zarka MA, et al. Desmoplastic small round cell tumour of unknown primary origin with lymph node and lung metastases: histological, cytological, ultrastructural, cytogenetic and molecular findings. *Virchows Arch.* 1998;432:135-141.
172. Collardeau-Frachon S, Ranchere-Vince D, Delattre O, et al. Primary desmoplastic small round cell tumor of the kidney: a case report in a 14-year-old girl with molecular confirmation. *Pediatr Dev Pathol.* 2007;10:320-324.
173. Wang LL, Perlman EJ, Vujanic GM, et al. Desmoplastic small round cell tumor of the kidney in childhood. *Am J Surg Pathol.* 2007;31:576-584.
174. Gerald WL, Ladanyi M, de Alava E, et al. Clinical, pathologic, and molecular spectrum of tumors associated with t(11;22)(p13;q12): desmoplastic small round-cell tumor and its variants. *J Clin Oncol.* 1998;16:3028-3036.
175. Ordonez NG. Desmoplastic small round cell tumor: I: a histopathologic study of 39 cases with emphasis on unusual histological patterns. *Am J Surg Pathol.* 1998;22:1303-1313.
176. Ordonez NG. Desmoplastic small round cell tumor: II: an ultrastructural and immunohistochemical study with emphasis on new immunohistochemical markers. *Am J Surg Pathol.* 1998;22:1314-1327.
177. Nakatsuka S, Oji Y, Horiuchi T, et al. Immunohistochemical detection of WT1 protein in a variety of cancer cells. *Mod Pathol.* 2006;19:804-814.
178. Chang F. Desmoplastic small round cell tumors: cytologic, histologic, and immunohistochemical features. *Arch Pathol Lab Med.* 2006;130:728-732.
179. Waugh MS, Dash RC, Turner KC, Dodd LG. Desmoplastic small round cell tumor: using FISH as an ancillary technique to support cytologic diagnosis in an unusual case. *Diagn Cytopathol.* 2007;35:516-520.
180. Yamaguchi U, Hasegawa T, Morimoto Y, et al. A practical approach to the clinical diagnosis of Ewing's sarcoma/primitive neuroectodermal tumour and other small round cell tumours sharing EWS rearrangement using new fluorescence in situ hybridisation probes for EWSR1 on formalin fixed, paraffin wax embedded tissue. *J Clin Pathol.* 2005;58:1051-1056.
181. Zhang J, Dalton J, Fuller C. Epithelial marker-negative desmoplastic small round cell tumor with atypical morphology: definitive classification by fluorescence in situ hybridization. *Arch Pathol Lab Med.* 2007;131:646-649.
182. Antonescu CR, Gerald WL, Magid MS, Ladanyi M. Molecular variants of the EWS-WT1 gene fusion in desmoplastic small round cell tumor. *Diagn Mol Pathol.* 1998;7:24-28.
183. Barnoud R, Delattre O, Peoc'h M, et al. Desmoplastic small round cell tumor: RT-PCR analysis and immunohistochemical detection of the Wilms' tumor gene WT1. *Pathol Res Pract.* 1998;194:693-700.
184. de Alava E, Ladanyi M, Rosai J, Gerald WL. Detection of chimeric transcripts in desmoplastic small round cell tumor and related developmental tumors by reverse transcriptase polymerase chain reaction. A specific diagnostic assay. *Am J Pathol.* 1995;147:1584-1591.
185. Gerald WL, Rosai J, Ladanyi M. Characterization of the genomic breakpoint and chimeric transcripts in the EWS-WT1 gene fusion of desmoplastic small round cell tumor. *Proc Natl Acad Sci U S A.* 1995;92:1028-1032.
186. Ladanyi M, Gerald W. Fusion of the EWS and WT1 genes in the desmoplastic small round cell tumor. *Cancer Res.* 1994;54:2837-2840.
187. Ladanyi M. The emerging molecular genetics of sarcoma translocations. *Diagn Mol Pathol.* 1995;4:162-173.
188. Leuschner I, Radig K, Harms D. Desmoplastic small round cell tumor. *Semin Diagn Pathol.* 1996;13:204-212.
189. Alaggio R, Rosolen A, Sartori F, et al. Spindle cell tumor with EWS-WT1 transcript and a favorable clinical course: a variant of DSCT, a variant of leiomyosarcoma, or a new entity? Report of two pediatric cases. *Am J Surg Pathol.* 2007;31:454-459.
190. Froberg K, Brown RE, Gaylord H, Manivel C. Intra-abdominal desmoplastic small round cell tumor: immunohistochemical evidence for up-regulation of autocrine and paracrine growth factors. *Ann Clin Lab Sci.* 1998;28:386-393.

191. Rachfal AW, Luquette MH, Brigstock DR. Expression of connective tissue growth factor (CCN2) in desmoplastic small round cell tumour. *J Clin Pathol.* 2004;57:422-425.
192. Schofield D. Extrarenal rhabdoid tumour. In: Fletcher CDM, Unni KK, FM, eds. *Pathology and Genetics of Tumours of Soft Tissue and Bone. World Health Organization Classification of Tumours.* Lyon, France: IARC Press; 2002:219-220.
193. Kodet R, Newton Jr WA, Sachs N, et al. Rhabdoid tumors of soft tissues: a clinicopathologic study of 26 cases enrolled on the Intergroup Rhabdomyosarcoma Study. *Hum Pathol.* 1991;22:674-684.
194. Tsuneyoshi M, Daimaru Y, Hashimoto H, Enjoji M. Malignant soft tissue neoplasms with the histologic features of renal rhabdoid tumors: an ultrastructural and immunohistochemical study. *Hum Pathol.* 1985;16:1235-1242.
195. Beckwith JB, Palmer NF. Histopathology and prognosis of Wilms tumors: results from the First National Wilms' Tumor Study. *Cancer.* 1978;41:1937-1948.
196. Tsokos M, Kouraklis G, Chandra RS, et al. Malignant rhabdoid tumor of the kidney and soft tissues. Evidence for a diverse morphological and immunocytochemical phenotype. *Arch Pathol Lab Med.* 1989;113:115-120.
197. Rorke LB, Packer RJ, Biegel JA. Central nervous system atypical teratoid/rhabdoid tumors of infancy and childhood: definition of an entity. *J Neurosurg.* 1996;85:56-65.
198. Burger PC, Yu IT, Tihan T, et al. Atypical teratoid/rhabdoid tumor of the central nervous system: a highly malignant tumor of infancy and childhood frequently mistaken for medulloblastoma: a Pediatric Oncology Group study. *Am J Surg Pathol.* 1998;22:1083-1092.
199. Parham DM, Weeks DA, Beckwith JB. The clinicopathologic spectrum of putative extrarenal rhabdoid tumors. An analysis of 42 cases studied with immunohistochemistry or electron microscopy. *Am J Surg Pathol.* 1994;18:1010-1029.
200. Fanburg-Smith JC, Hengge M, et al. Extrarenal rhabdoid tumors of soft tissue: a clinicopathologic and immunohistochemical study of 18 cases. *Ann Diagn Pathol.* 1998;2:351-362.
201. Gessi M, Giangaspero F, Pietsch T. Atypical teratoid/rhabdoid tumors and choroid plexus tumors: when genetics "surprise" pathology. *Brain Pathol.* 2003;13:409-414.
202. Shiratsuchi H, Saito T, Sakamoto A, et al. Mutation analysis of human cytokeratin 8 gene in malignant rhabdoid tumor: a possible association with intracytoplasmic inclusion body formation. *Mod Pathol.* 2002;15:146-153.
203. Ogino S, Cohen ML, Abdul-Karim FW. Atypical teratoid/rhabdoid tumor of the CNS: cytopathology and immunohistochemistry of insulin-like growth factor-II, insulin-like growth factor receptor type 1, cathepsin D, and Ki-67. *Mod Pathol.* 1999;12:379-385.
204. Saito T, Oda Y, Itakura E, et al. Expression of intercellular adhesion molecules in epithelioid sarcoma and malignant rhabdoid tumor. *Pathol Int.* 2001;51:532-542.
205. Oda Y, Yamamoto H, Tamiya S, et al. CXCR4 and VEGF expression in the primary site and the metastatic site of human osteosarcoma: analysis within a group of patients, all of whom developed lung metastasis. *Mod Pathol.* 2006;19:738-745.
206. Bourdeaut F, Freneaux P, Thuille B, et al. hSNF5/INI1-deficient tumours and rhabdoid tumours are convergent but not fully overlapping entities. *J Pathol.* 2007;211:323-330.
207. Haberler C, Laggner U, Slavc I, et al. Immunohistochemical analysis of INI1 protein in malignant pediatric CNS tumors: Lack of INI1 in atypical teratoid/rhabdoid tumors and in a fraction of primitive neuroectodermal tumors without rhabdoid phenotype. *Am J Surg Pathol.* 2006;30:1462-1468.
208. Oda Y, Tsuneyoshi M. Extrarenal rhabdoid tumors of soft tissue: clinicopathological and molecular genetic review and distinction from other soft-tissue sarcomas with rhabdoid features. *Pathol Int.* 2006;56:287-295.
209. Biegel JA, Burk CD, Parmiter AH, Emanuel BS. Molecular analysis of a partial deletion of 22q in a central nervous system rhabdoid tumor. *Genes Chromosomes Cancer.* 1992;5:104-108.
210. Schofield DE, Beckwith JB, Sklar J. Loss of heterozygosity at chromosome regions 22q11-12 and 11p15.5 in renal rhabdoid tumors. *Genes Chromosomes Cancer.* 1996;15:10-17.
211. Biegel JA. Molecular genetics of atypical teratoid/rhabdoid tumor. *Neurosurg Focus.* 2006;20:E11.
212. Uno K, Takita J, Yokomori K, et al. Aberrations of the hSNF5/INI1 gene are restricted to malignant rhabdoid tumors or atypical teratoid/rhabdoid tumors in pediatric solid tumors. *Genes Chromosomes Cancer.* 2002;34:33-41.
213. Sevenet N, Lellouch-Tubiana A, Schofield D, et al. Spectrum of hSNF5/INI1 somatic mutations in human cancer and genotype-phenotype correlations. *Hum Mol Genet.* 1999;8:2359-2368.
214. Sevenet N, Sheridan E, Amram D, et al. Constitutional mutations of the hSNF5/INI1 gene predispose to a variety of cancers. *Am J Hum Genet.* 1999;65:1342-1348.
215. Bruch LA, Hill DA, Cai DX, et al. A role for fluorescence in situ hybridization detection of chromosome 22q dosage in distinguishing atypical teratoid/rhabdoid tumors from medulloblastoma/central primitive neuroectodermal tumors. *Hum Pathol.* 2001;32:156-162.
216. Perlman E, Grosfeld JL, Togashi K, Boccon-Gibod L. Pathology and Genetics of Tumors of the Urinary System and Male Genital Organs. In: Eble JN, Sauter G, Epstein JI, Sesterhenn IA, eds. *World Health Organization Classification of Tumours.* Lyon, France: IARC Press; 2004:48-52.
217. Hussong JW, Perkins SL, Huff V, et al. Familial Wilms' tumor with neural elements: characterization by histology, immunohistochemistry, and genetic analysis. *Pediatr Dev Pathol.* 2000;3:561-567.
218. Vujanic GM, Sandstedt B, Harms D, et al. Revised International Society of Paediatric Oncology (SIOP) working classification of renal tumors of childhood. *Med Pediatr Oncol.* 2002;38:79-82.
219. Folpe AL, Patterson K, Gown AM. Antibodies to desmin identify the blastemal component of nephroblastoma. *Mod Pathol.* 1997;10:895-900.
220. Muir TE, Cheville JC, Lager DJ. Metanephric adenoma, nephrogenic rests, and Wilms' tumor: a histologic and immunophenotypic comparison. *Am J Surg Pathol.* 2001;25:1290-1296.
221. Magee F, Mah RG, Taylor GP, Dimmick JE. Neural differentiation in Wilms' tumor. *Hum Pathol.* 1987;18:33-37.
222. Coppes MJ, Haber DA, Grundy PE. Genetic events in the development of Wilms' tumor. *N Engl J Med.* 1994;331:586-590.
223. Fukuzawa R, Heathcott RW, Sano M, et al. Myogenesis in Wilms' tumors is associated with mutations of the WT1 gene and activation of Bcl-2 and the Wnt signaling pathway. *Pediatr Dev Pathol.* 2004;7:125-137.
224. Stock C, Ambros IM, Lion T, et al. Genetic changes of two Wilms tumors with anaplasia and a review of the literature suggesting a marker profile for therapy resistance. *Cancer Genet Cytogenet.* 2002;135:128-138.
225. el Bahtimi R, Hazen-Martin DJ, Re GG, et al. Immunophenotype, mRNA expression, and gene structure of p53 in Wilms' tumors. *Mod Pathol.* 1996;9:238-244.
226. Sredni ST, de Camargo B, Lopes LF, et al. Immunohistochemical detection of p53 protein expression as a prognostic indicator in Wilms tumor. *Med Pediatr Oncol.* 2001;37:455-458.
227. D'Angelo MF, Kausik SJ, Sebo TJ, et al. p53 immunopositivity in histologically favorable Wilms tumor is not related to stage at presentation or to biological aggression. *J Urol.* 2003;169:1815-1817.
228. Ghanem MA, Van der Kwast TH, Den Hollander JC, et al. The prognostic significance of apoptosis-associated proteins BCL-2, BAX and BCL-X in clinical nephroblastoma. *Br J Cancer.* 2001;85:1557-1563.
229. Ghanem MA, Van Steenbrugge GJ, Van Der Kwast TH, et al. Expression and prognostic value Of CD44 isoforms in nephroblastoma (Wilms tumor). *J Urol.* 2002;168:681-686.
230. Ghanem MA, Van Der Kwast TH, Den Hollander JC, et al. Expression and prognostic value of epidermal growth factor receptor, transforming growth factor-alpha, and c-erb B-2 in nephroblastoma. *Cancer.* 2001;92:3120-3129.
231. Skotnicka-Klonowicz G, Kobos J, Los E, et al. Prognostic value of proliferating cell nuclear antigen in Wilms' tumour in children. *Eur J Surg Oncol.* 2002;28:67-71.
232. Ghanem MA, van Steenbrugge GJ, Sudaryo MK, et al. Expression and prognostic relevance of vascular endothelial growth factor (VEGF) and its receptor (FLT-1) in nephroblastoma. *J Clin Pathol.* 2003;56:107-113.

233. Klein MJ, Siegal GP. Osteosarcoma: anatomic and histologic variants. *Am J Clin Pathol.* 2006;125:555-581.
234. Raymond AK. Conventional osteosarcoma. In: Fletcher CDM, Unni KK, Merten F, eds. *Pathology and Genetics of Tumours of Soft Tissue and Bone.* World Health Organization Classification of Tumours. Lyon, France: IARC Press; 2002:264-270.
235. Ferguson RJ, Yunis EJ. The ultrastructure of human osteosarcoma: a study of nine cases. *Clin Orthop.* 1978:234-246.
236. Okada K, Hasegawa T, Yokoyama R, et al. Osteosarcoma with cytokeratin expression: a clinicopathological study of six cases with an emphasis on differential diagnosis from metastatic cancer. *J Clin Pathol.* 2003;56:742-746.
237. Hasegawa T, Hirose T, Kudo E, et al. Immunophenotypic heterogeneity in osteosarcomas. *Hum Pathol.* 1991;22:583-590.
238. Hosono A, Yamaguchi U, Makimoto A, et al. Utility of immunohistochemical analysis for cyclo-oxygenase 2 in the differential diagnosis of osteoblastoma and osteosarcoma. *J Clin Pathol.* 2007;60:410-414.
239. Bacci G, Bertoni F, Longhi A, et al. Neoadjuvant chemotherapy for high-grade central osteosarcoma of the extremity. Histologic response to preoperative chemotherapy correlates with histologic subtype of the tumor. *Cancer.* 2003;97:3068-3075.
240. Coffin CM, Lowichik A, Zhou H. Treatment effects in pediatric soft tissue and bone tumors: practical considerations for the pathologist. *Am J Clin Pathol.* 2005;123:75-90.
241. Hauben EI, Weeden S, Pringle J, et al. Does the histological subtype of high-grade central osteosarcoma influence the response to treatment with chemotherapy and does it affect overall survival? A study on 570 patients of two consecutive trials of the European Osteosarcoma Intergroup. *Eur J Cancer.* 2002;38:1218-1225.
242. Lowichik A, Zhou H, Pysher TJ, et al. Therapy associated changes in childhood tumors. *Adv Anat Pathol.* 2000;7:341-359.
243. Picci P, Bacci G, Campanacci M, et al. Histologic evaluation of necrosis in osteosarcoma induced by chemotherapy. Regional mapping of viable and nonviable tumor. *Cancer.* 1985;56:1515-1521.
244. Kilpatrick SE, Geisinger KR, King TS, et al. Clinicopathologic analysis of HER-2/neu immunoexpression among various histologic subtypes and grades of osteosarcoma. *Mod Pathol.* 2001;14:1277-1283.
245. Akatsuka T, Wada T, Kokai Y, et al. ErbB2 expression is correlated with increased survival of patients with osteosarcoma. *Cancer.* 2002;94:1397-1404.
246. Tsai JY, Aviv H, Benevenia J, et al. HER-2/neu and p53 in osteosarcoma: an immunohistochemical and fluorescence in situ hybridization analysis. *Cancer Invest.* 2004;22:16-24.
247. Ferrari S, Bertoni F, Zanella L, et al. Evaluation of P-glycoprotein, HER-2/ErbB-2, p53, and Bcl-2 in primary tumor and metachronous lung metastases in patients with high-grade osteosarcoma. *Cancer.* 2004;100:1936-1942.
248. Gorlick R, Huvos AG, Heller G, et al. Expression of HER2/erbB-2 correlates with survival in osteosarcoma. *J Clin Oncol.* 1999;17:2781-2788.
249. Onda M, Matsuda S, Higaki S, et al. ErbB-2 expression is correlated with poor prognosis for patients with osteosarcoma. *Cancer.* 1996;77:71-78.
250. Zhou H, Randall RL, Brothman AR, et al. Her-2/neu expression in osteosarcoma increases risk of lung metastasis and can be associated with gene amplification. *J Pediatr Hematol Oncol.* 2003;25:27-32.
251. Varelias A, Koblar SA, Cowled PA, et al. Human osteosarcoma expresses specific ephrin profiles: implications for tumorigenicity and prognosis. *Cancer.* 2002;95:862-869.
252. Kim MS, Song WS, Cho WH, et al. Ezrin expression predicts survival in stage IIB osteosarcomas. *Clin Orthop Relat Res.* 2007;459:229-236.
253. Dhaini HR, Thomas DG, Giordano TJ, et al. Cytochrome P450 CYP3A4/5 expression as a biomarker of outcome in osteosarcoma. *J Clin Oncol.* 2003;21:2481-2485.
254. Srivastava A, Fuchs B, Zhang K, et al. High WT1 expression is associated with very poor survival of patients with osteogenic sarcoma metastasis. *Clin Cancer Res.* 2006;12:4237-4243.
255. Fellenberg J, Bernd L, Delling G, et al. Prognostic significance of drug-regulated genes in high-grade osteosarcoma. *Mod Pathol.* 2007;20:1085-1094.
256. Serra M, Scotlandi K, Reverter-Branchat G, et al. Value of P-glycoprotein and clinicopathologic factors as the basis for new treatment strategies in high-grade osteosarcoma of the extremities. *J Clin Oncol.* 2003;21:536-542.
257. Pakos EE, Ioannidis JP. The association of P-glycoprotein with response to chemotherapy and clinical outcome in patients with osteosarcoma. A meta-analysis. *Cancer.* 2003;98:581-589.
258. Nakashima H, Nishida Y, Sugiura H, et al. Telomerase, p53 and PCNA activity in osteosarcoma. *Eur J Surg Oncol.* 2003;29:564-567.
259. Junior AT, de Abreu Alves F, Pinto CA, et al. Clinicopathological and immunohistochemical analysis of twenty-five head and neck osteosarcomas. *Oral Oncol.* 2003;39:521-530.
260. Trieb K, Lehner R, Stulnig T, et al. Survivin expression in human osteosarcoma is a marker for survival. *Eur J Surg Oncol.* 2003;29:379-382.
261. Wang W, Luo H, Wang A. Expression of survivin and correlation with PCNA in osteosarcoma. *J Surg Oncol.* 2006;93:578-584.
262. Haydon RC, Deyrup A, Ishikawa A, et al. Cytoplasmic and/or nuclear accumulation of the beta-catenin protein is a frequent event in human osteosarcoma. *Int J Cancer.* 2002;102:338-342.
263. Sulzbacher I, Birner P, Trieb K, et al. The expression of bone morphogenetic proteins in osteosarcoma and its relevance as a prognostic parameter. *J Clin Pathol.* 2002;55:381-385.

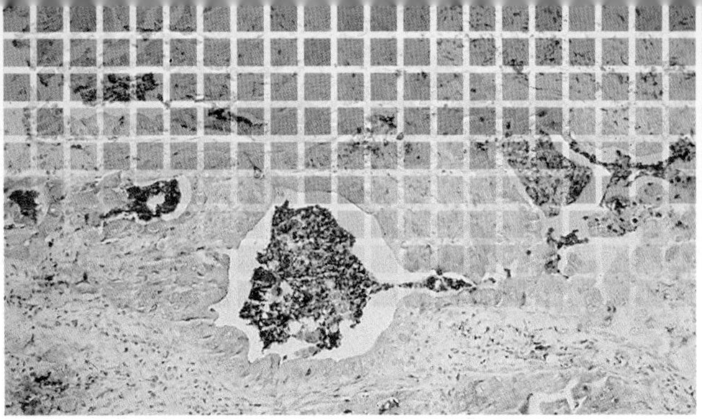

18

Immunohistology of the Female Genital Tract

Joseph T. Rabban • Robert A. Soslow • Charles Z. Zaloudek

- Introduction 690
- Vulva, Vagina, and Cervix 690
- Uterus and Gestational Trophoblastic Disease 699
- Ovary 721
- Mesothelioma 742

INTRODUCTION

In this chapter we will focus on the use of immunohistochemistry in the setting of diagnostic gynecologic pathology. This chapter is divided into four sections: vulva, vagina, and cervix; uterus; gestational trophoblastic disease; and ovary, fallopian tube, and peritoneum. The first part of each section includes a description of the properties and applications of the antibodies that are most useful in diagnostic work. A table of commonly used antibodies is provided for reference (Table 18.1). In the second part of each section, we will discuss the use of immunohistochemistry for the resolution of diagnostic problems or for the diagnosis of gynecologic lesions. Each section also includes a discussion of aspects of molecular pathology as it can be used to supplement or in some cases substitute for immunohistochemical analysis.

The focus of this chapter is on diagnostic immunohistochemistry, but we wish to emphasize that antibodies must be used and stains interpreted in conjunction with careful assessment of routine H&E-stained slides and clinicopathologic correlation.

VULVA, VAGINA, AND CERVIX

Immunohistochemical Markers

Most of the antibodies used in the lower gynecologic tract are also used in other anatomic locations and are described in applicable sections in the text. The most commonly used antibody in the lower gynecologic tract is p16; therefore we will discuss it in detail in the following section.

p16

p16 is a tumor suppressor protein that is a cyclin-dependent kinase inhibitor and is essential in regulating the cell cycle. p16 inactivates cyclin-dependent kinases that phosphorylate Rb; therefore p16 can decelerate the cell cycle. Rb phosphorylation status in turn influences expression of p16. In human papilloma virus (HPV) infection, the HPV oncogenes E6 and E7 can inactivate pRB and thus lead to p16 overexpression.[1] Therefore, p16 overexpression is a surrogate biomarker of HPV infection (in particular high-risk HPV types), which makes it useful in evaluating HPV-associated squamous and glandular neoplasia of the lower gynecologic tract.[2-9] As discussed later in this chapter, the intensity and distribution of p16 is important in interpretation as well as in nuclear versus cytoplasmic localization. HPV-independent mechanisms of p16 overexpression also exist, so one may observe p16 expression in tumors that do not necessarily harbor HPV infection, such as ovarian serous carcinoma.[10]

Vulva and Vagina

VULVAR PAGET DISEASE

Vulvar Paget disease is a vulvar intraepidermal adenocarcinoma that may be of primary or metastatic origin. Four diagnostic issues arise when evaluating vulvar Paget disease: 1) determining site of origin, 2) excluding diagnostic mimics, and 3) assessing margin status, and 4) assessing for stromal invasion. Unlike Paget disease of the breast, primary vulvar Paget disease is not commonly associated with an underlying adenocarcinoma but is typically a pure intraepidermal tumor. Primary vulvar Paget disease expresses CK7, GCDFP, and CEA (Fig. 18.1), but not CDX2, S-100, HMB45, or estrogen/progesterone receptors;[11-15] rare cases express CK20.[16] HER2/neu is typically expressed.[17] Questionable cells near surgical margins can be evaluated by CK7 since normal epidermis is CK7 negative. Small foci of stromal invasion may also be highlighted by CK7 (Fig. 18.1D); p53 expression may be associated with risk of stromal invasion.[18] Secondary vulvar Paget disease most commonly represents spread of primary urinary tract or colorectal adenocarcinoma. The immunophenotype reflects that of the primary tumor: vulvar Paget disease of colorectal origin expresses CK20, CDX2, and CEA; vulvar Paget disease of urothelial origin may express CK20, uroplakin, and thrombomodulin.[13,14,19-21] Rare colorectal cases may express GCDFP, so a panel approach is advised rather than reliance on a single marker.

Vulvar melanoma and vulvar intraepithelial neoplasia (VIN) may rarely exhibit features that mimic vulvar Paget disease. Primary Paget disease tumor cells do not express the melanocytic markers S-100 or HMB45.[14,22,23] Pagetoid VIN does not express GCDFP but may express CK7; better markers of pagetoid VIN are high molecular weight keratin, p16, and p63.[24-26]

TABLE 18.1 Commonly Used Antibodies in Gynecologic Pathology

Antibody	Vendor	Dilution	Pattern
AFP	Dako	1:80	Cytoplasmic
CA125	Signet	1:500	Cytoplasmic/membrane
Caldesmon	Dako	1:200	Cytoplasmic
Calretinin	Zymed	1:200	Cytoplasmic/nuclear
CEA-monoclonal	Dako	1:2	Cytoplasmic/luminal
CD10	Novocastra	1:160	Cytoplasmic/membrane
CD30	Dako	1:100	Cytoplasmic
CD56	Zymed	1:100	Cytoplasmic
CD99	Signet	1:200	Membrane
CD117/*c-kit*	Dako	1:50	Cytoplasmic
CDX2	BioGenex	1:100	Nuclear
Chromogranin	BioGenex	1:200	Cytoplasmic
CK7	Dako	1:500	Cytoplasmic
CK20	Dako	1:100	Cytoplasmic
D2-40	Dako	1:50	Cytoplasmic/membrane
Desmin	Cell Marque	undiluted	Cytoplasmic
EMA	Dako	1:240	Membrane/cytoplasmic
Estrogen receptor (SP1)	Lab Vision	1:50	Nuclear
GCFP15	Signet	1:20	Cytoplasmic
Glypican 3	BioMosaics	undiluted	Cytoplasmic
hCG	Biomeda	1:40	Cytoplasmic
High molecular weight keratin/34βE12	Enzo	1:2	Cytoplasmic
HMB45	Enzo	1:8	Cytoplasmic
HNF-1β	Santa Cruz	1:300	Nuclear
HPL	Dako	1:20,000	Cytoplasmic
Keratin AE1/AE3	Dako	1:100	Cytoplasmic
Inhibin	Serotec	1:100	Cytoplasmic
MIB1	Dako	1:1000	Nuclear
MLH1	BD Pharmingen	1:100	Nuclear
MSH2	Oncogene	1:100	Nuclear
MSH6	BD Transduction	1:100	Nuclear
Myogenin	Dako	1:200	Nuclear

Continued

TABLE 18.1 Commonly Used Antibodies in Gynecologic Pathology, cont'd

Antibody	Vendor	Dilution	Pattern
Oct-4	Cell Marque	1:2	Nuclear
p16	MTM Lab	undiluted	Nuclear/cytoplasmic
p53	Novocastra	1:300	Nuclear
p57	Lab Vision	1:400	Nuclear
p63	Lab Vision	1:100	Nuclear
PLAP	BioGenex	1:2	Cytoplasmic
PMS2	BD Pharmingen	1:150	Nuclear
Progesterone receptor	Dako	1:250	Nuclear
S-100	Dako	1:2000	Cytoplasmic
Smooth muscle actin, alpha	Dako	1:800	Cytoplasmic
Smooth muscle myosin	Dako	1:200	Cytoplasmic
Synaptophysin	Dako	1:150	Cytoplasmic
Vimentin	Zymed	1:1600	Cytoplasmic
WT1	Dako	1:200	Nuclear

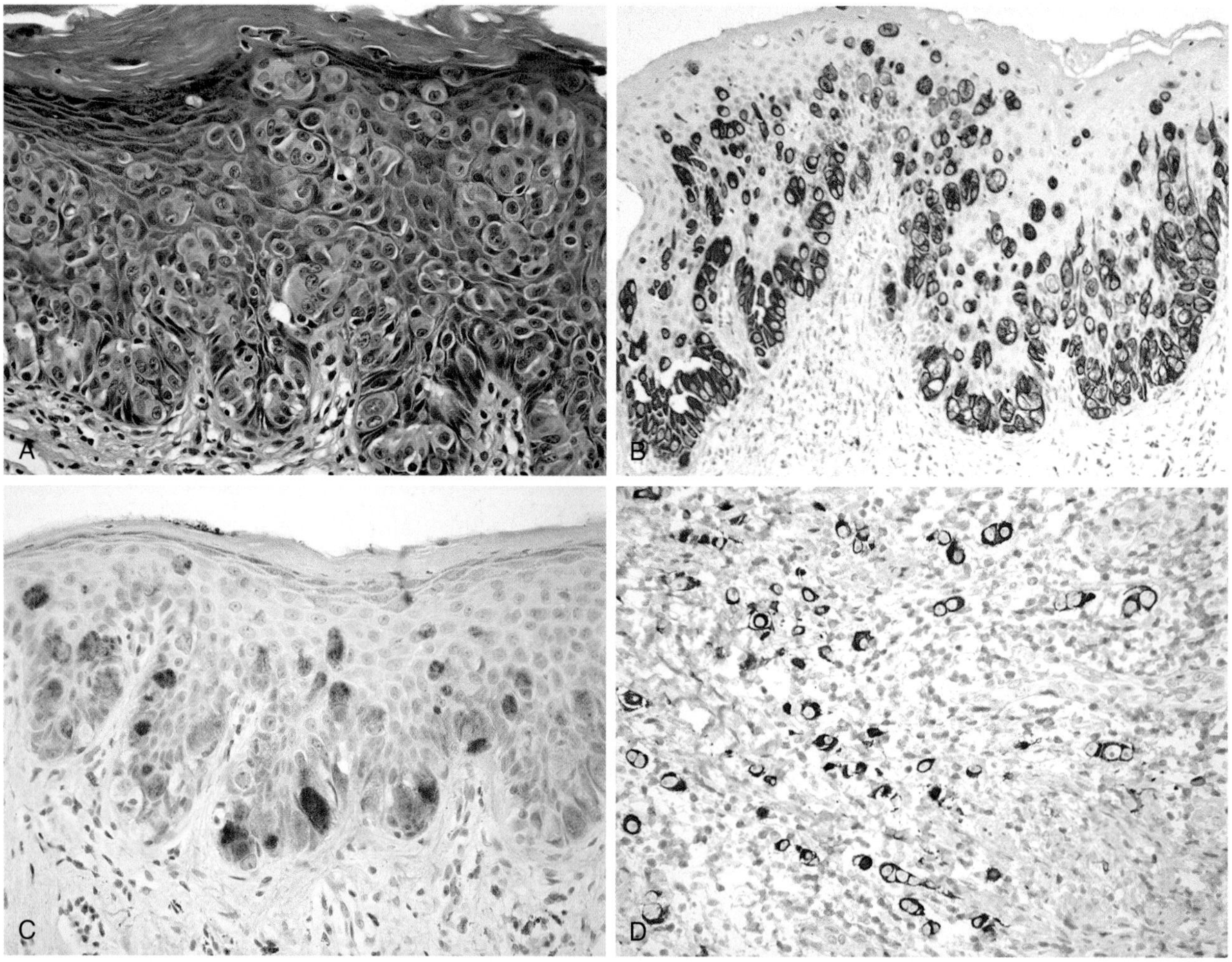

FIGURE 18.1 Primary vulvar Paget disease **(A)**. (H&E.) Tumor cells express CK7 **(B)** and GCDFP **(C)**, but normal epithelium does not. Occult stromal invasion can be highlighted by CK7 **(D)** when inflammation obscures the epidermal-dermal junction.

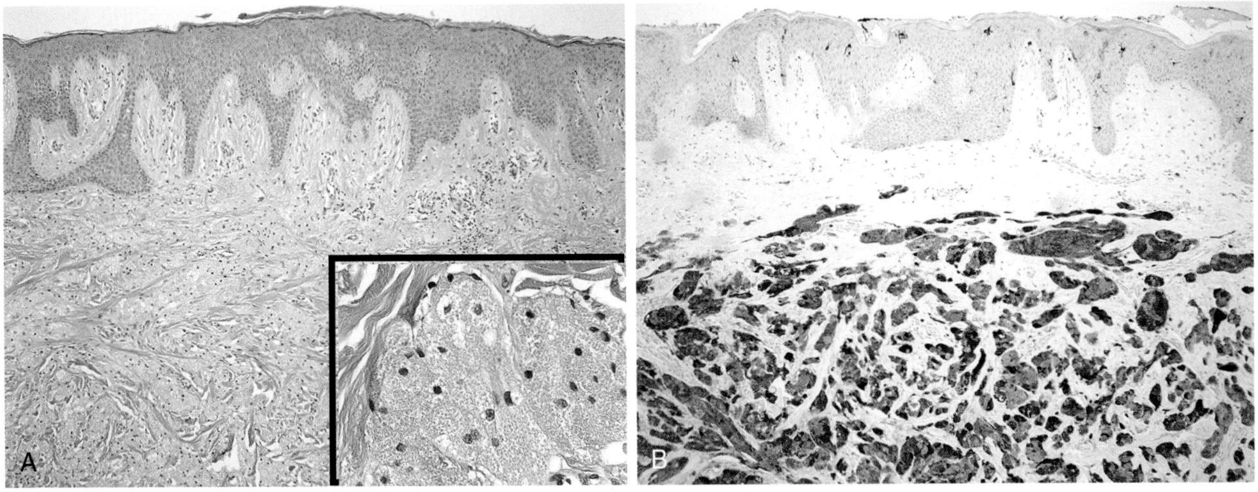

FIGURE 18.2 Vulvar granular cell tumor **(A)**. (H&E.) Tumor cells (inset A) express S-100 **(B)**, calretinin, and inhibin (not shown).

KEY DIAGNOSTIC POINTS

Vulvar Paget Disease

- Primary vulvar Paget disease is typically positive for CK7 and GCDFP, and negative for CK20 and CDX2.
- Secondary vulvar Paget disease of colorectal or urothelial origin shows similar immunophenotype as the tumor at the primary site.
- A panel approach is advised because overlap of individual markers may occur rarely.
- Pagetoid vulvar intraepithelial neoplasia (VIN) is distinguished by expression of HMWK, p16, and p63.
- Pagetoid melanoma is distinguished by expression of S-100 and HMB45.

VULVOVAGINAL MESENCHYMAL LESIONS

Though uncommon, a broad array of mesenchymal lesions may arise in the vulva or vagina. Among these, aggressive angiomyxoma is a mesenchymal neoplasm with a propensity for deep infiltrative growth and local recurrence that should be distinguished from its benign mimics, which include fibroepithelial polyp, angiomyofibroblastoma, cellular angiofibroma, myxoid leiomyoma, and nodular fasciitis. The relatively bland morphology of all these entities can make diagnosis problematic. Immunostains are of minimal value because almost all will express vimentin, ER, PR, and, to a variable extent, desmin, actin, and CD34.[27] Cellular angiofibroma stands out in that it lacks actin and desmin expression.[28,29] Gastrointestinal stromal tumors (GIST) may rarely arise primarily in this location and mimic smooth muscle tumors; as in conventional GIST, CD117 and CD34 expression are characteristic.[30] Proximal type epithelioid sarcoma of vulva is distinguished by expression of keratin and EMA.[31] Rhabdomyosarcoma of the lower genital tract is distinguished by expression of desmin and myogenin, though regenerating, reactive, and entrapped non-neoplastic skeletal muscle may also express myogenic markers.[32,33]

Recent study of the cytogenetics of aggressive angiomyxoma has identified that gene rearrangements in HMGA2, an architectural transcription factor encoded on chromosome 12q15, are common. Limited studies suggest that nuclear immunoexpression of HMGA2 is present in about 50% of aggressive angiomyxomas and in a minority of vulvar smooth muscle tumors.[34-37] This antibody is not widely used, and larger studies in the mimics of AA are required; however it may potentially emerge as a useful tool.

KEY DIAGNOSTIC POINTS

Vulvar Mesenchymal Lesions

- Classification of vulvar mesenchymal lesions is primarily based on morphologic criteria.
- Most entities, including aggressive angiomyxoma, express vimentin, ER, PR, desmin, actin, and CD34.
- Cellular angiofibroma lacks desmin and actin.
- CD117 may help distinguish vaginal GISTs that mimic smooth muscle tumors.

VULVAR GRANULAR CELL TUMOR

Granular cell tumors may occasionally arise in the vulva. Their appearance is similar to tumors at other anatomic sites. They are thought to derive from peripheral nerve sheath and express S-100 protein, inhibin, and calretinin (Fig. 18.2).[38,39] The diagnosis is usually straightforward but occasionally the differential may include melanoma, histiocytes, or even a decidual reaction.

VULVAR PAPILLARY SQUAMOUS LESIONS

The main differential diagnosis for papillary squamous lesions of the vulva includes condyloma, fibroepithelial polyp, and squamous papilloma. Vulvar condyloma demonstrates papillomatosis, acanthosis, parakeratosis, and dyskeratosis but often lacks koilocytes, which makes the differential difficult in occasional cases. MIB1 is useful in this context. In normal vulvar epithelium, fibroepithelial polyp, and squamous papilloma, MIB1 is confined to parabasal cells; in condyloma, MIB1 expression occurs in the middle and upper third of epithelium (Fig. 18.3).[40-43] Vulvar seborrheic keratosis may show increased MIB1 expression, and focal p16 expression has been reported in rare cases; HPV type 6 has been detected in some vulvar seborrheic keratoses.[44] As discussed later in the section on MIB1 expression in the cervix, caution is advised in interpreting specimens with tangential sectioning or sub-optimal orientation since MIB1 expression by normal parabasal cells could appear to be located in upper layers of epithelium.

VULVAR INTRAEPITHELIAL NEOPLASIA

Similar to cervical squamous lesions associated with high-risk HPV, immunostains can assist in distinguishing vulvar dysplasia (vulvar intraepithelial neoplasia, VIN) from its benign mimics as well as identifying the unusual variant of simplex (differentiated) VIN. Normal and atrophic vulvar epithelium contain minimal MIB1 expression in parabasal cells, whereas the common type of high-grade VIN (undifferentiated or bowenoid type) shows expression in the middle and upper epithelial layers. p16 expression in high-grade VIN is similar, although some cases may be negative.[45,46] The expression patterns are similar to those seen in cervical squamous intraepithelial lesion. Simplex (differentiated) VIN is characterized by nuclear atypia and brisk mitoses confined to the basal zone and is typically not associated with HPV; therefore, p16 is usually absent.[46,47] Instead, simplex VIN may harbor p53 gene mutations; hence, p53 immunoexpression is present (Fig. 18.4).[48,49] Caution is warranted, however, because benign lesions such as lichen sclerosis may be focally p53-positive; staining should be interpreted in context of the morphologic findings.[50]

Cervix

MESONEPHRIC REMNANTS

Mesonephric duct remnants may be found in the deep wall of cervix specimens. Sometimes, hyperplasia may be pronounced and raise concern for minimal deviation type endocervical adenocarcinoma. Apical expression of CD10 is common in these remnants, as is expression by the intraluminal secretions. CD10, however, is not pathognomonic for mesonephric differentiation because some endocervical and endometrial adenocarcinomas may express CD10. Minimal deviation type endocervical adenocarcinoma, however, lacks CD10 expression.[51] Variable expression of p16 is reported in mesonephric remnants and may lead to misinterpretation as endocervical adenocarcinoma; however, MIB1 is not increased. ER, PR, and CEA are generally negative. The immunophenotype is similar in mesonephric adenocarcinoma as well.[51-53]

CERVICAL SQUAMOUS INTRAEPITHELIAL LESIONS

The main diagnostic roles for immunohistochemistry in evaluation of cervical squamous intraepithelial lesions (SILs) are distinguishing dysplasia from benign mimics and evaluating cauterized margins. Grading dysplasia remains an issue for morphologic criteria. The markers used most widely are MIB1 and p16. We will briefly discuss emerging data on novel markers. MIB1 helps distinguish benign squamous lesions from SIL but is less helpful in distinguishing low-grade squamous intraepithelial lesions (LSILs) from high-grade squamous intraepithelial lesions (HSILs). Parabasal cells of normal cervical squamous epithelium express MIB1, as do parabasal cells of immature squamous metaplasia, atrophy, and transitional cell metaplasia (Fig. 18.5). In well-developed HSIL, full-thickness MIB1 expression occurs. Lesser degrees of dysplasia will also demonstrate MIB1 expression in cells above the basal layer to varying degrees (Fig. 18.6).[54-57] Proper tissue orientation is critical to interpreting MIB1 because it depends on understanding the relationship between the basal layer and upper layers of epithelium. Tangential sectioning, sub-optimal orientation, or artifactual loss of the outer layer of epithelium may lead to difficulty in determining whether a MIB1-positive cell is part of the basal layer or higher.

p16 expression is seen in most high-risk HPV-associated squamous lesions;[2,5,58] absent or occasional focal weak expression is seen in normal, inflamed, and atrophic cervical epithelium, as well as in transitional cell metaplasia. In HSIL, diffuse strong p16 staining of nuclei and cytoplasm occurs from the upper two thirds to entire full thickness of the epithelium, though not all cases are positive (Fig. 18.7).[2,5,59] In LSIL, p16 expression is variable and typically limited to the lower half of the epithelium. p16 positivity in LSIL appears to be a function of whether high-risk HPV is present, and it has been suggested that it is a marker of progression to HSIL.[2,5,58,59] p16 immunoexpression has been studied in comparison to *in situ* hybridization assays for high risk HPV. While HPV *in situ* hybridization exhibits excellent specificity and may be useful to further evaluate cases of focal p16 positivity, diffuse strong p16 immunoexpression appears to be a more sensitive marker and, in conjunction with its wider availability and easier interpretation, better suited as a first step in evaluating questionable morphology.[60]

Recent studies suggest potential value for novel markers of cell-cycle regulation, including minichromosome maintenance protein 2 (MCM2) and DNA topoisomerase II alpha (TOP 2A), which are involved in early steps of DNA replication and are overexpressed in HPV infection. Antibodies to a cocktail of the two, ProEx C, show promise. Recent work suggests that a combination of ProEx C and p16 may improve detection of SIL. In one study comparing the two, p16 alone detected 76.5% of LSIL, ProEx C detected 94.1%, and the use of both detected 100%.[61] Stain intensity and distribution for ProEx C was greater than that for p16. In the same study, ProEx C detected 78.6% of HSIL while p16 alone detected 100%. Normal ectocervix expresses ProEx C in one or two basal layers, a caveat to using this marker. Another recent study examining HSIL and difficult mimics of HSIL, including metaplastic and reactive epithelium, reported better specificity for ProEx C combined with p16 than for p16 or MIB1 alone.[62] Larger scale studies may define a role for ProEx C as a useful adjunct to p16.

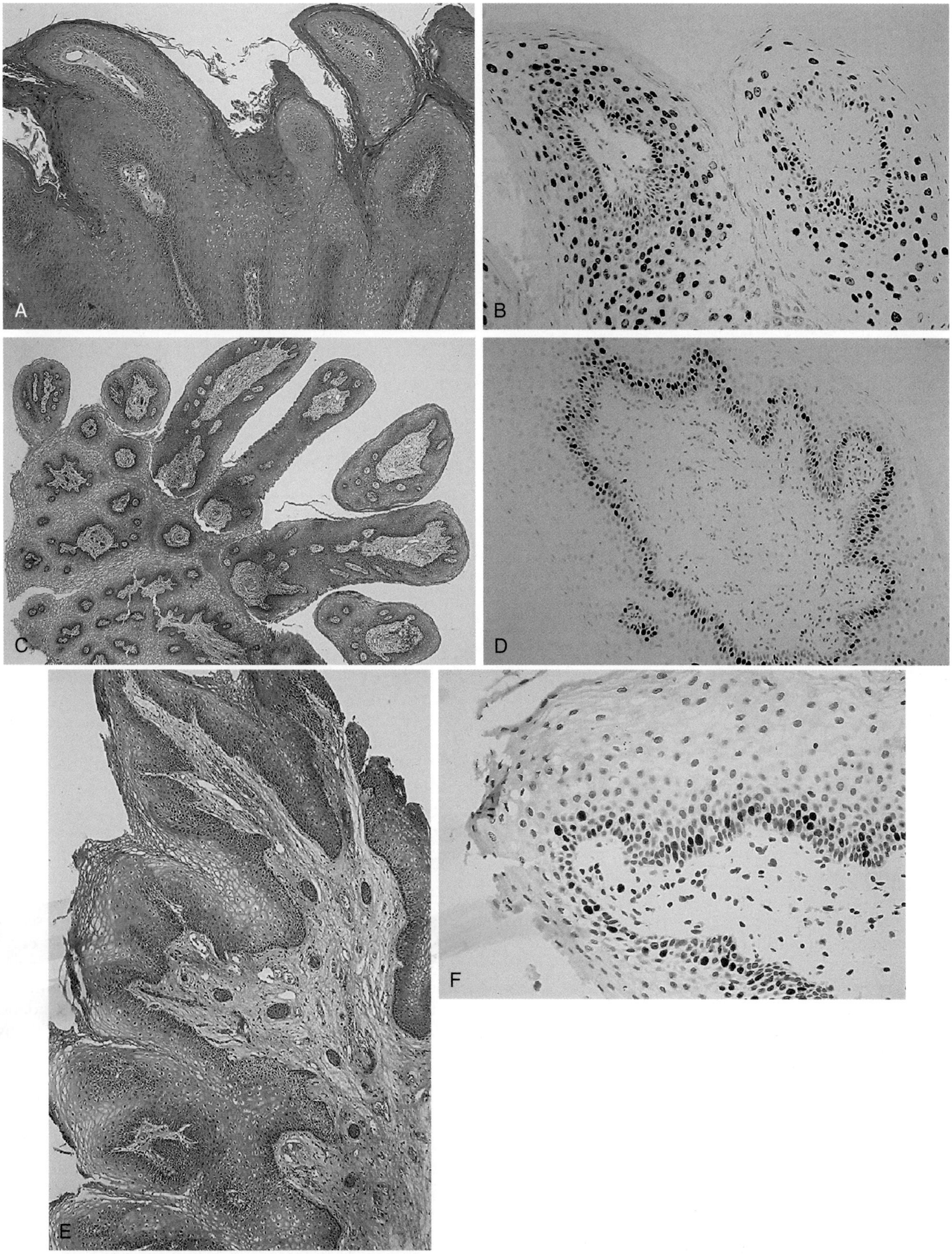

FIGURE 18.3 In exophytic vulvar lesions, MIB1 is expressed above the basal layer in condyloma **(A, B)** but is confined to parabasal cells in squamous papilloma **(C, D)** and in fibroepithelial polyp **(E, F)**.

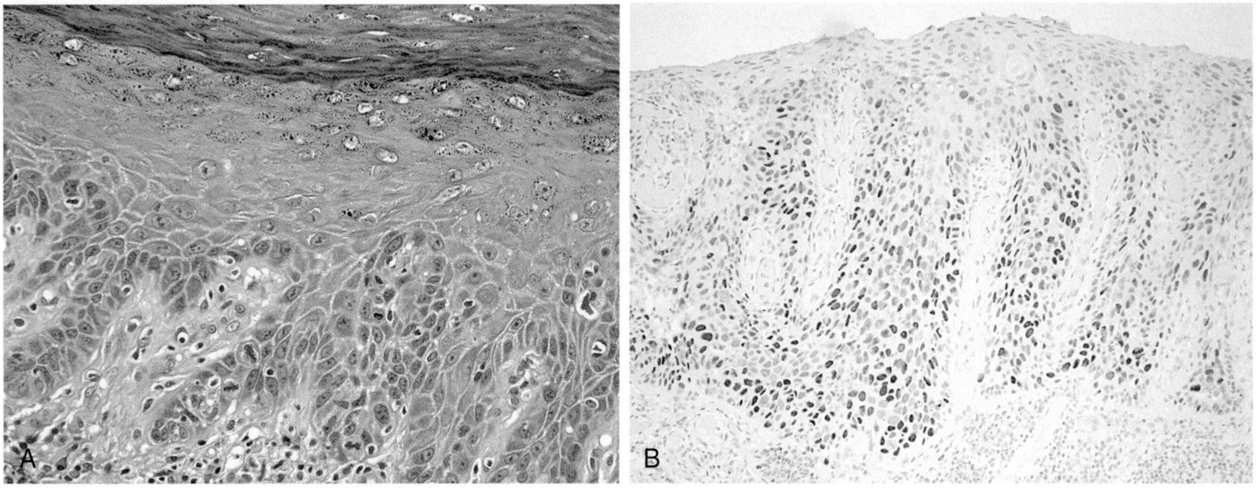

FIGURE 18.4 Simplex (differentiated) VIN consists of nuclear atypia and brisk mitoses confined to the basal zone **(A)**. (H&E.) Tumor cells express p53 **(B)** and MIB1 (not shown) but typically not p16.

KEY DIAGNOSTIC POINTS

Cervical Squamous Intraepithelial Lesions

- MIB1 expression in the upper layers of epithelium distinguishes HSIL from benign mimics, as does diffuse p16 expression.
- Tangential sectioning or loss of the outer layer of epithelium may make interpretation of MIB1 difficult because it is expressed in the parabasal cells of benign cervical epithelium.

ENDOCERVICAL ADENOCARCINOMA *IN SITU*

Two diagnostic issues arise with endocervical adenocarcinoma *in situ*: 1) distinguishing it from benign mimics and 2) assessing for stromal invasion. Immunohistochemistry can help with the former but not the latter. The constellation of nuclear enlargement, hyperchromasia, crowding, atypia, mitoses, and cribriform growth define endocervical adenocarcinoma *in situ*. Tubal metaplasia, microglandular hyperplasia, endometriosis, and inflammatory changes may sometimes harbor one or more of these features. Endocervical adenocarcinoma *in situ* expresses increased MIB1, p16 (diffuse, strong), and monoclonal CEA, but not ER, PR, vimentin, or BCL-2 (Fig. 18.8). Tubal metaplasia and endometriosis show cytoplasmic BCL-2 but no increase in MIB1 or CEA; p16 is either negative or focal and weak. Microglandular hyperplasia also lacks increased MIB1, p16, and CEA.[3,6,7,63-66]

KEY DIAGNOSTIC POINTS

Endocervical Adenocarcinoma in Situ

- Endocervical adenocarcinoma (AIS) is distinguished from endocervical glandular metaplasias, hyperplasia, and endometriosis by increased MIB1 and by strong diffuse p16 and CEA expression.

INVASIVE ENDOCERVICAL ADENOCARCINOMA

The main diagnostic role for immunohistochemistry in invasive endocervical adenocarcinoma is distinguishing it from endometrial adenocarcinoma. No single immunostain is accurate, and even a panel of several immunostains is not perfect. Correlation with clinical and radiologic findings is paramount. Generally endocervical adenocarcinoma expresses monoclonal CEA and p16 but does not express vimentin, ER, or PR, whereas low-grade endometrial endometrioid adenocarcinoma shows the converse profile. CEA expression is cytoplasmic and at luminal borders, while p16 is a diffuse strong nuclear and cytoplasmic pattern (Fig. 18.9). CEA can be positive in endometrial adenocarcinoma, though usually in a weak, luminal pattern. p16 can also be expressed in endometrioid adenocarcinoma, sometimes in a weak patchy pattern but occasionally in a strong diffuse pattern.[67-71] Because of this potential overlap and because of importance of staining pattern and intensity, caution is advised in interpreting small samplings. p16 is also positive in uterine serous carcinoma, though the morphology of serous carcinoma typically allows for distinction from endocervical adenocarcinoma.[72] Rarely, endocervical microglandular hyperplasia may mimic endometrial mucinous adenocarcinoma; increased MIB1 and positive vimentin distinguish the latter from the former. Both entities lack CEA and have variable ER and PR expression; therefore, these stains are not helpful.[73]

KEY DIAGNOSTIC POINTS

Invasive Endocervical Adenocarcinoma

- Primary endocervical adenocarcinoma is usually positive for p16 and CEA and negative for vimentin and ER, while primary endometrial adenocarcinoma is usually the converse.
- Overlap exists in this profile; therefore, clinical and radiologic findings should be the ultimate indicator of origin of adenocarcinoma involving the cervix.

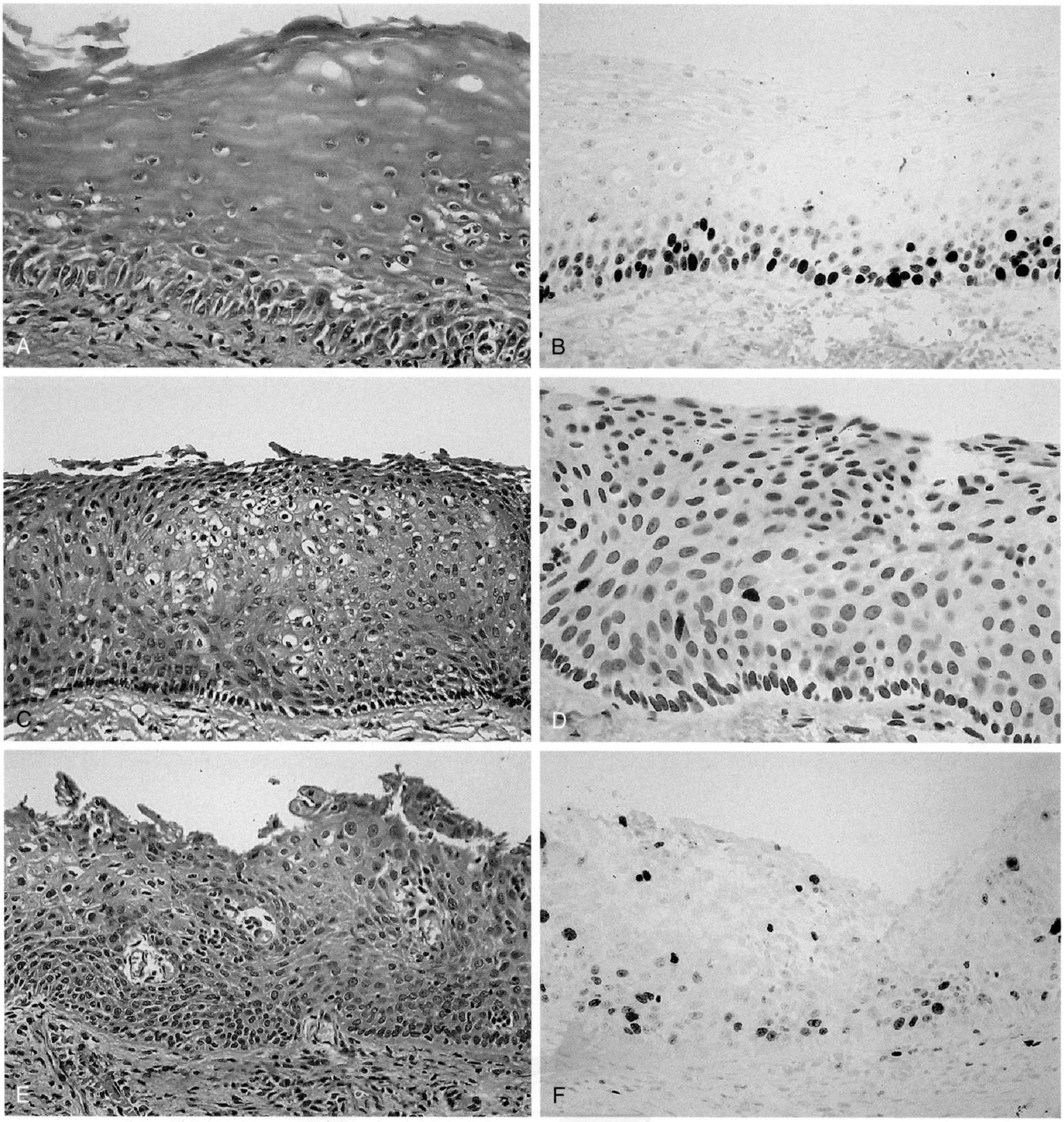

FIGURE 18.5 MIB1 expression is confined to the parabasal cells of normal cervix **(A, B)**, postmenopausal atrophy **(C, D)**, and inflamed squamous metaplasia **(E, F)**.

INTESTINAL-TYPE ENDOCERVICAL ADENOCARCINOMA

Intestinal-type endocervical adenocarcinoma and AIS contain goblet cells and intestinal type epithelium and may be mistaken for spread of primary intestinal adenocarcinoma. The intestinal marker CDX2 is expressed in intestinal type endocervical adenocarcinoma and AIS as well as in some non-intestinal types (Fig. 18.10). Therefore CDX2 does not help define site of origin. Instead, CK7, CK20, and p16 should be used. Whereas primary endocervical adenocarcinoma expresses CK7 and p16 but not CK20, the converse applies to primary colorectal adenocarcinoma involving the cervix.[74,75]

MINIMAL DEVIATION ENDOCERVICAL ADENOCARCINOMA

Diagnosis of minimal deviation endocervical adenocarcinoma can be challenging since the cytologic and architectural features of this tumor can be subtle. Robust forms of lobular or diffuse endocervical glandular hyperplasia or deep endocervical glands may mimic minimal deviation adenocarcinoma. A subtle type of endocervical

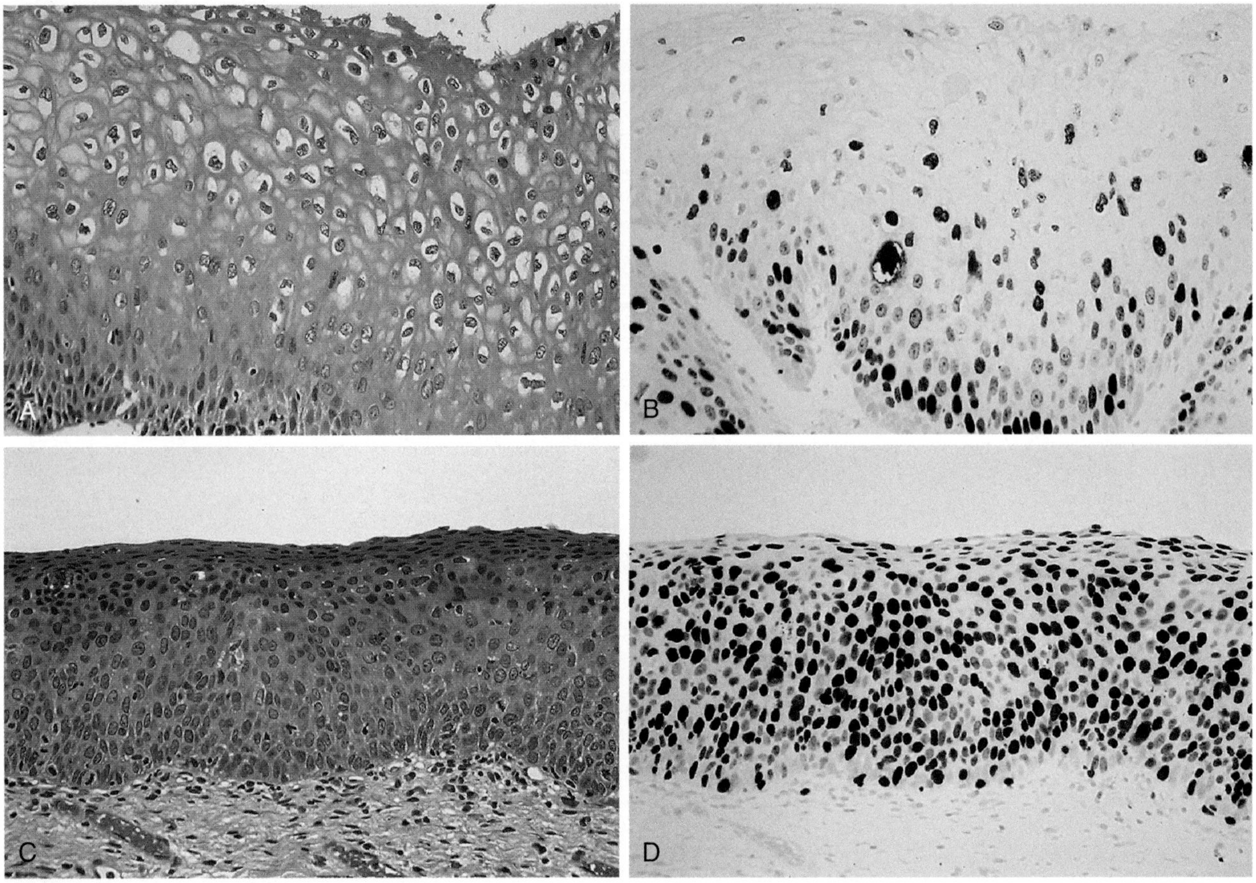

FIGURE 18.6 MIB1 is expressed variably in the mid and upper layers of cervical low-grade squamous intraepithelial lesion **(A, B)** and diffusely throughout the full thickness of cervical high-grade squamous intraepithelial lesion **(C, D)**.

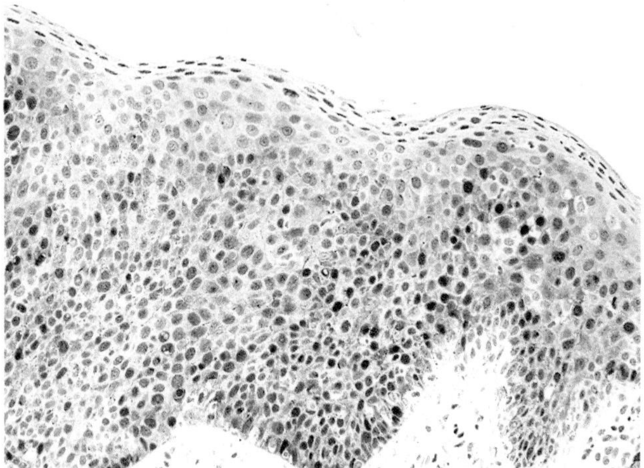

FIGURE 18.7 In high-grade squamous intraepithelial lesion, p16 shows diffuse strong nuclear and cytoplasmic expression throughout the lesion.

spread of endometrial adenocarcinoma may also mimic it. Immunostains are of limited value. CEA can be positive in some but not all minimal deviation adenocarcinoma (Fig. 18.11) as can MIB1 and p53; therefore the stains are not informative if negative. p16 is not helpful because most cases are not HPV associated.[63,76-78]

ADENOID CYSTIC CARCINOMA

This tumor is similar to its counterpart in salivary glands in both morphology and immunophenotype and may arise in the cervix or vulvovaginal soft tissue. It is a dual-cell population tumor growing in cribriform, tubular, and/or solid patterns. The major cell type is a basaloid polygonal cell with modified myoepithelial features, and it is positive for p63 and smooth muscle actin. The minor cell type is an epithelial cell forming tiny ductules that may be inconspicuous. These cells express keratin and CD117. Distinction from basaloid squamous carcinoma is based on the distinct morphology of adenoid cystic carcinoma because overlap exists in immunostains: p63 is diffusely expressed in basaloid squamous carcinoma, as opposed to adenoid cystic carcinoma, in which p63 is confined to basaloid cells and not epithelium of the ductules; CD117 can be expressed at low levels in basaloid squamous carcinoma.[79-83]

ADENOID BASAL CARCINOMA

This uncommon tumor of bland basaloid cells without mitoses is arranged in palisaded clusters and nests, and it grows in an infiltrative, scattered pattern in the cervical stroma. Squamous metaplasia can occur. The tumor may coexist with other tumors such as squamous cell carcinoma, adenoid cystic carcinoma, or neuroendocrine carcinoma. The basaloid cells express keratin, p63, and p16 (Fig. 18.12).[84-86]

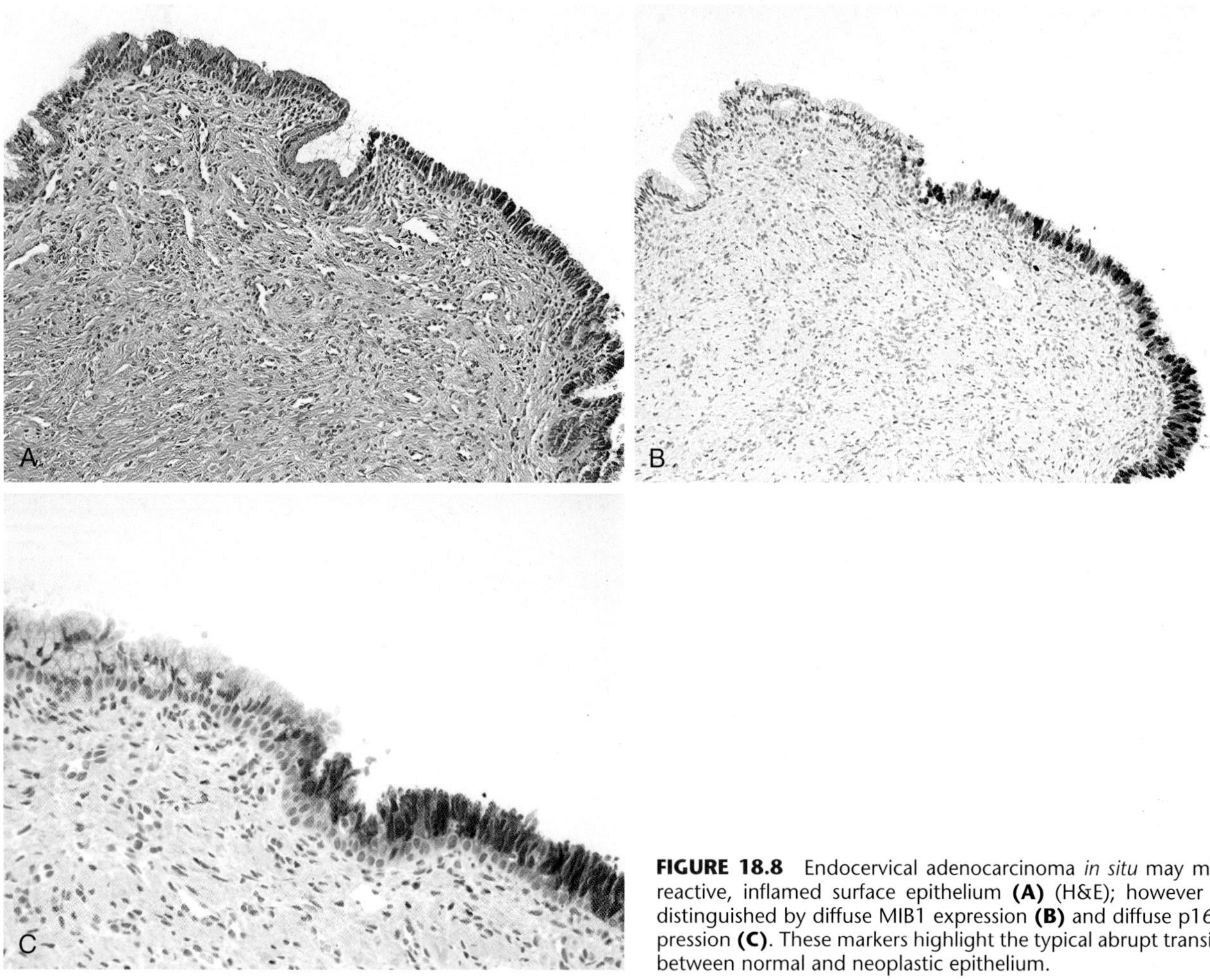

FIGURE 18.8 Endocervical adenocarcinoma *in situ* may mimic reactive, inflamed surface epithelium **(A)** (H&E); however it is distinguished by diffuse MIB1 expression **(B)** and diffuse p16 expression **(C)**. These markers highlight the typical abrupt transition between normal and neoplastic epithelium.

NEUROENDOCRINE CARCINOMAS

Small cell carcinoma of the cervix is an aggressive tumor that should be distinguished from small cell squamous carcinoma and lymphoma. Though morphologic features are often sufficient, immunohistochemistry can help if the sample is small or questionable. Most small cell carcinomas will express at least one neuroendocrine marker such as synaptophysin, chromogranin, or CD56 (Fig. 18.13).[87,88] p16 tends to be present as well, which may create diagnostic problems in distinguishing small cell carcinoma from small cell squamous cell carcinoma.[89-91] In such cases, the useful marker is p63, which is negative in small cell carcinoma.[92] A similar immunophenotype is reported for large cell neuroendocrine carcinoma. TTF-1 can be positive in primary cervical neuroendocrine tumors and therefore is not necessarily a marker of pulmonary origin.[93,94]

Theranostic Applications

Recent studies suggest that cervical LSIL that express p16 diffusely may be more likely to progress to HSIL than those that are p16-negative.[95-97] In these studies, p16-positive LSIL progression rates range from 36% to 62.2%, while p16-negative LSIL progression rates range from 4% to 28.6%. p16 is not a perfect predictor in this setting, however, since some p16-positive LSIL may regress while some p16-negative LSIL may progress.[96,97] The prognostic value of p16 may be enhanced by use of an additional marker, the HPV capsidic protein HPV-L1 (L1). L1 is expressed in the early productive phase of cervical carcinogenesis and diminishes in the later phase of proliferation, correlating with onset of p16 overexpression. Early data suggests that L1 expression diminishes with progression from LSIL to HSIL and may enhance the value of p16 in stratifying behavior of LSIL.[98]

UTERUS AND GESTATIONAL TROPHOBLASTIC DISEASE

Immunohistochemical Markers

EPITHELIAL MARKERS (CYTOKERATINS AND EMA)

Expression of cytokeratins (AE1/AE3 and CAM5.2) is usually sufficient to confirm epithelial differentiation in tumors of most organ systems. However, in the uterus, cytokeratin expression is not limited to epithelial cells. Both endometrial stromal and smooth muscle cells have been shown to have focal cytokeratin expression,

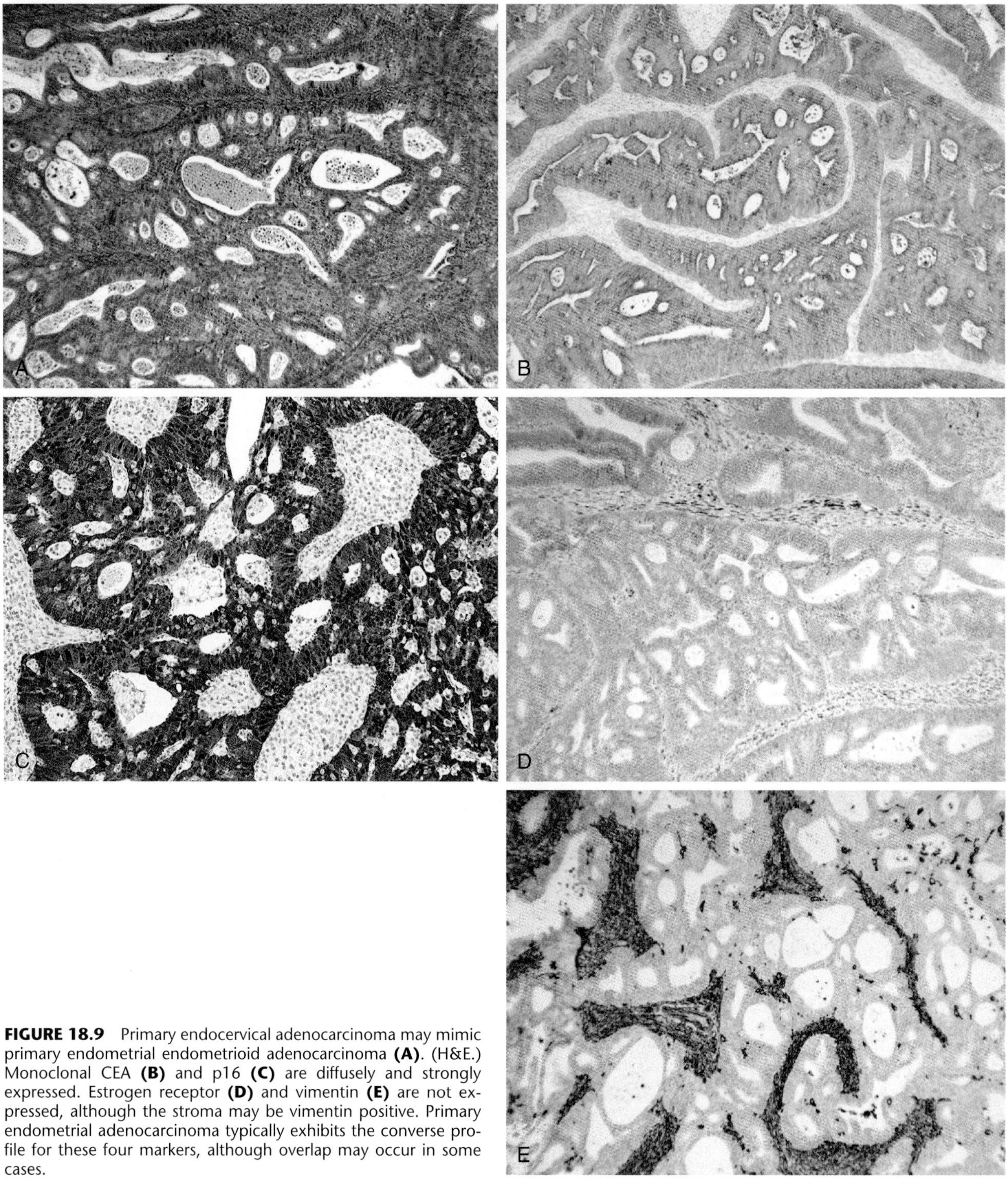

FIGURE 18.9 Primary endocervical adenocarcinoma may mimic primary endometrial endometrioid adenocarcinoma **(A)**. (H&E.) Monoclonal CEA **(B)** and p16 **(C)** are diffusely and strongly expressed. Estrogen receptor **(D)** and vimentin **(E)** are not expressed, although the stroma may be vimentin positive. Primary endometrial adenocarcinoma typically exhibits the converse profile for these four markers, although overlap may occur in some cases.

although it is much weaker than in epithelial cells.[99-101] There is usually no expression of epithelial membrane antigen (EMA) in these tumors.[99-101] Cytokeratin expression can be particularly evident in the sarcomatous portion of carcinosarcomas (malignant mixed müllerian tumor [MMMT]), which frequently coexpresses cytokeratins in addition to mesenchymal markers.[102,103] Other commonly used epithelial markers include CK7 and CK20.

VIMENTIN

Vimentin, an intermediate filament, is expressed in mesenchymal tissues, normal proliferative endometrial epithelial cells, and in the majority of endometrial carcinomas.[104,105] The coexpression of vimentin and low molecular weight cytokeratin can aid in the differential diagnosis of an endocervical versus an endometrial adenocarcinoma.

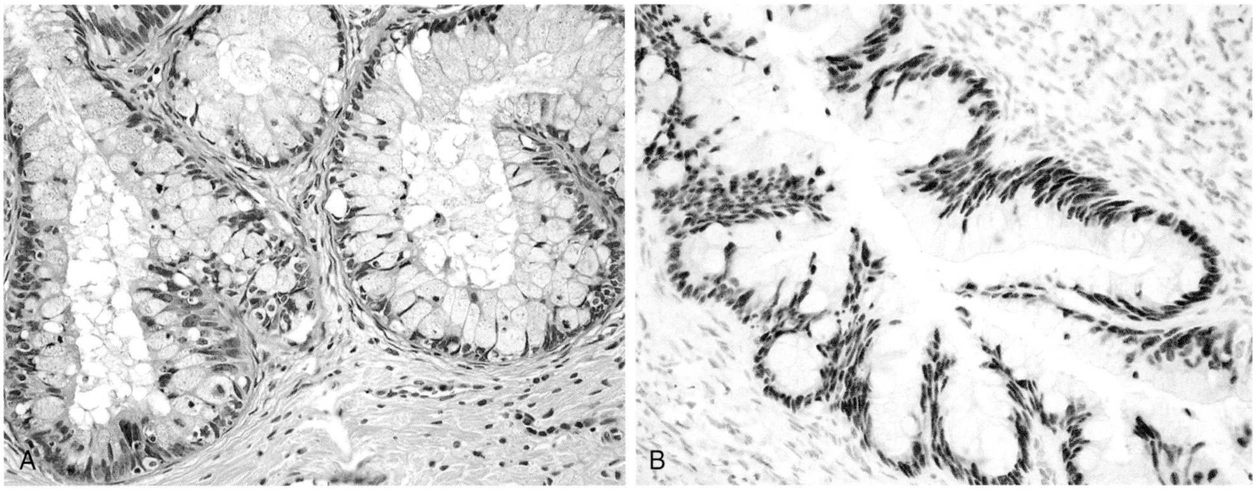

FIGURE 18.10 Intestinal-type endocervical adenocarcinoma with prominent goblet cells **(A)** (H&E) may resemble primary intestinal adenocarcinomas that spread to the cervix. CDX2 **(B)** is expressed in the nuclei of this variant of endocervical adenocarcinoma and therefore should not be used to determine site of origin. CK7, CK20, and p16 should be used instead.

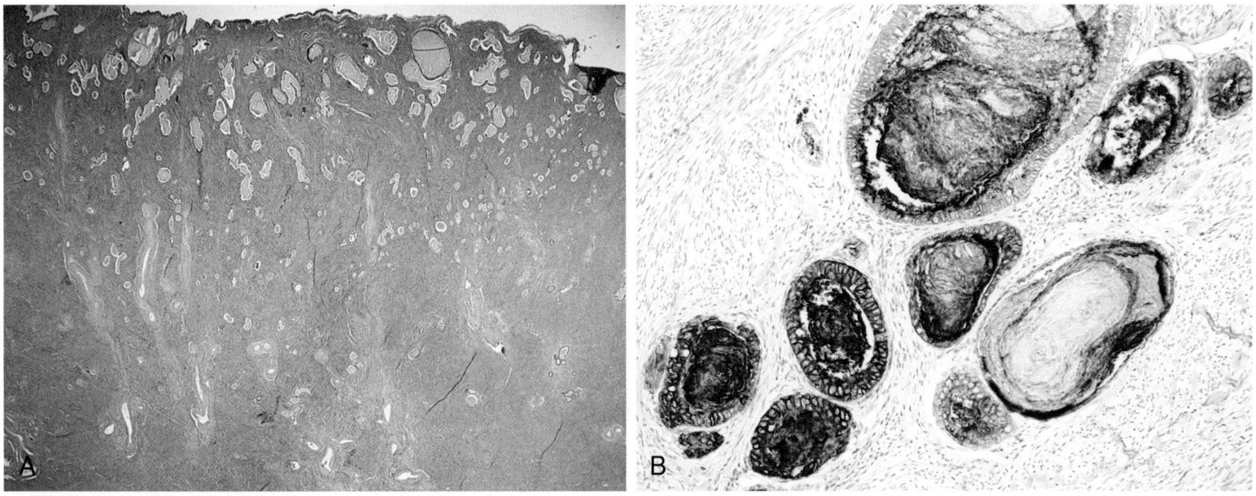

FIGURE 18.11 Minimal deviation endocervical adenocarcinoma consists of a deeply invasive, haphazardly infiltrative proliferation of bland endocervical glands that, in a small tissue sampling, may mimic endocervical glandular hyperplasia or mesonephric remnants **(A)**. (H&E.) Some cases may express CEA **(B)**, which is not expressed by its benign mimics.

p53

Overexpression of the p53 tumor suppressor protein is seen in more than 80% of uterine serous carcinomas and in their putative precursor lesion, endometrial intraepithelial carcinoma (EIC).[106-108] The most commonly used antibodies against the p53 protein recognize both mutated and wild-type 53, but only mutated *p53* gene products result in diffuse and strong *over*expression of p53 in the setting of serous endometrial carcinoma. An immunohistochemical assay for p53 allows us to recognize the abnormal p53 protein that results from *p53* gene mutation because it accumulates in tumor cell nuclei, likely because of decreased degradation and/or stabilization. The pattern of staining is dramatic: More than 75% of the tumor cells stain with strong intensity, and there is an abrupt cutoff with the adjacent uninvolved atrophic endometrium. Complex atypical hyperplasia and FIGO grade 1 endometrioid adenocarcinomas rarely demonstrate p53 immunoreactivity, and when present, the pattern is weak and focal.[109-112] There is increasing expression of p53 in endometrioid adenocarcinomas with increasing grade, and some FIGO grade 3 endometrioid adenocarcinomas will stain intensely.[109,111-113]

There has also been recent work in defining markers that could act as a counterbalance to p53. These include antibodies against antigens associated with endometrioid differentiation: ER, PR,[111,114-116] β-catenin,[117,118] and PTEN.[119-124]

ER and PR expression is seen in a wide range of nonuterine tissues and in both benign and malignant tumors. Of note, ER and PR expression is moderate to strong in endometrioid carcinomas, but is not expressed or only weakly expressed in clear cell carcinomas.[125-127] ER and

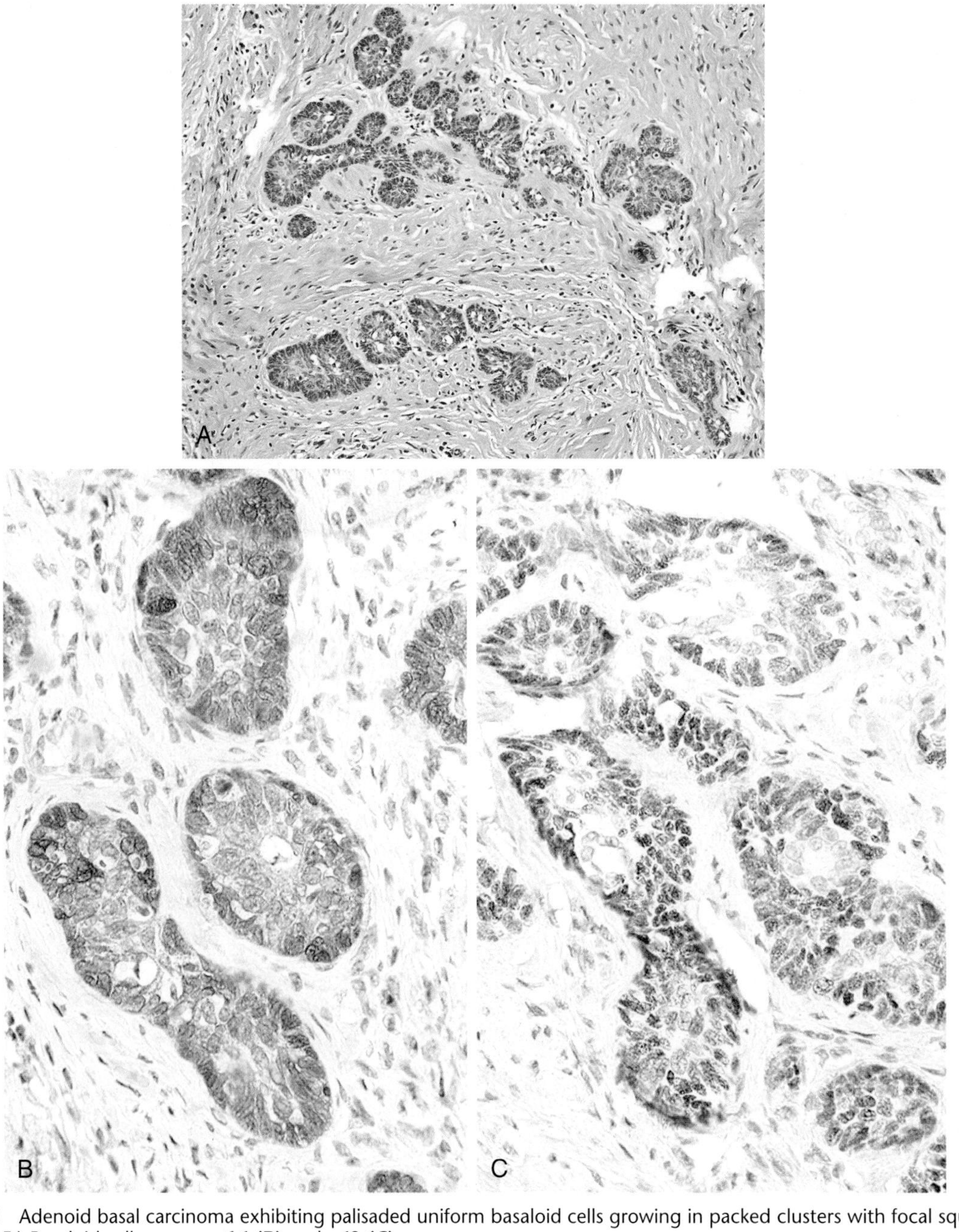

FIGURE 18.12 Adenoid basal carcinoma exhibiting palisaded uniform basaloid cells growing in packed clusters with focal squamous metaplasia **(A)**. (H&E.) Basaloid cells express p16 **(B)** and p63 **(C)**.

PR expression is just as weak in poorly differentiated endometrioid carcinomas as it is in serous and clear cell carcinomas.[114-116,127]

β-CATENIN AND *PTEN*

β-catenin is involved in cell adhesion and, as a component of the Wnt signal transduction pathway, becomes translocated to the nucleus when mutated or stabilized by another factor. Nuclear β-catenin expression is seen in as many as 50% of endometrioid adenocarcinomas[118,124,128-130] and is rarely, if ever, seen in serous carcinomas.[118,124] *PTEN,* the phosphatase and tensin homologue deleted on chromosome 10, is a tumor suppressor gene involved in the genesis of 40% to 75% of endometrioid adenocarcinomas.[119-124,131] In contrast to p53, in which expression is up-regulated in most cases of *p53* mutation, *PTEN* mutation results in immunohistochemical loss compared to normal tissues. *PTEN* loss has only rarely been documented in serous carcinomas.[119-124,131]

MUSCLE MARKERS

The muscle actins (MSA and SMSA), desmin, and h-caldesmon are useful in identifying smooth muscle cells. Normal endometrial stromal cells express vimentin and muscle actins, but they generally lack expression

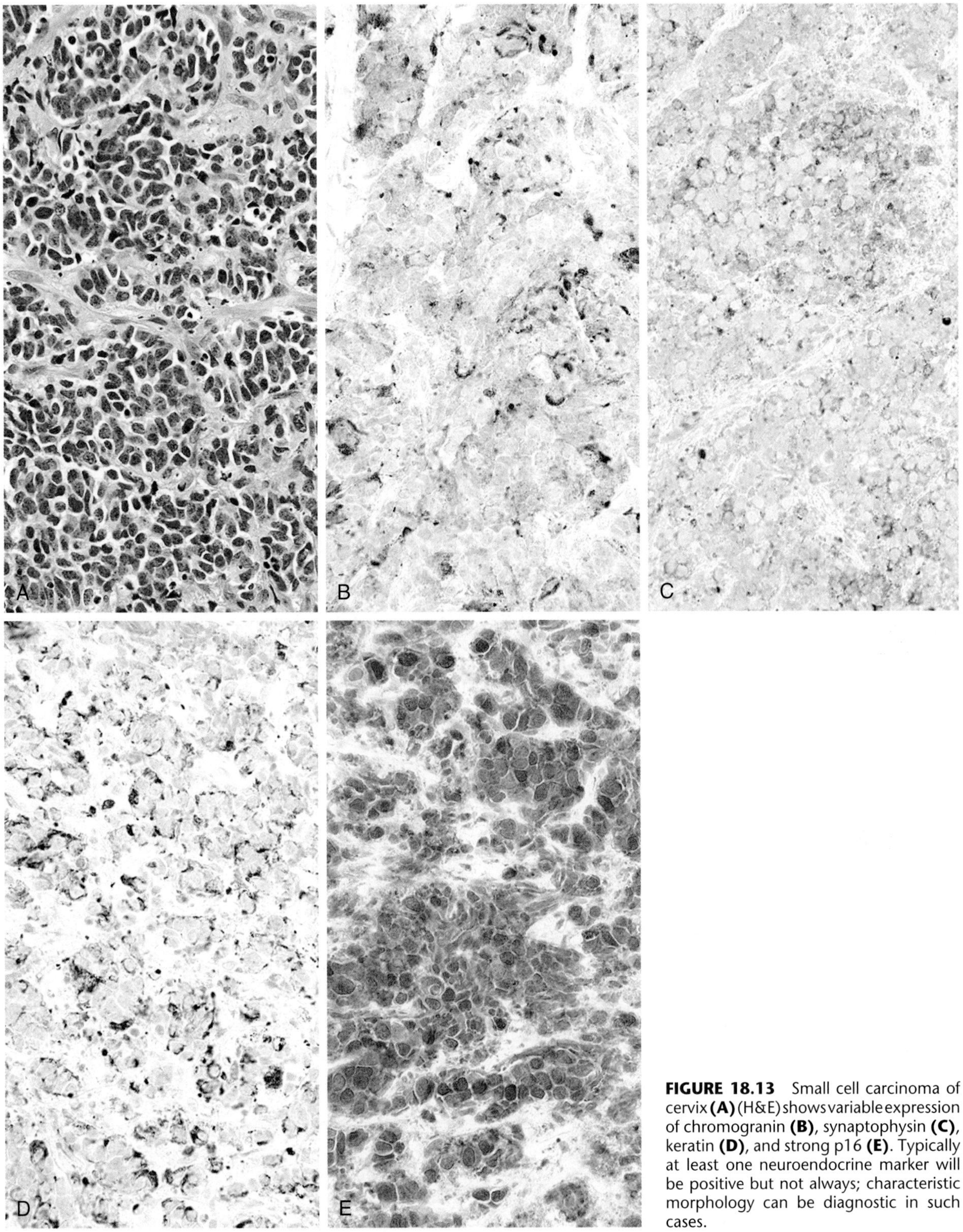

FIGURE 18.13 Small cell carcinoma of cervix **(A)** (H&E) shows variable expression of chromogranin **(B)**, synaptophysin **(C)**, keratin **(D)**, and strong p16 **(E)**. Typically at least one neuroendocrine marker will be positive but not always; characteristic morphology can be diagnostic in such cases.

of cytokeratins and epithelial membrane antigen.[100] Some authors have found desmin expression in normal endometrial stromal cells and endometrial stromal neoplasms, but others have found it to be a reliable indicator for differentiating smooth muscle from endometrial stromal cells.[101,132,133] h-caldesmon, a more specific marker of smooth muscle differentiation than MSA, SMSA, and desmin, has been used to discriminate between endometrial stromal neoplasms and those showing smooth muscle differentiation.[134,135] h-caldesmon (and other muscle markers) can also be expressed in portions of endometrial stromal neoplasms showing smooth muscle differentiation. Sex-cord–like elements in uterine mesenchymal tumors show immunohistochemical evidence of sex-cord differentiation with inhibin (a peptide hormone normally expressed by ovarian granulosa cells),[136] but they also frequently express smooth muscle actin and sometimes desmin.[136-139] Antidesmin antibodies, and more specifically myogenin and Myo-D1, can be used to highlight rhabdomyoblastic differentiation in carcinosarcomas. However, in the absence of malignant heterologous elements, distinction of carcinosarcoma from poorly differentiated carcinoma using immunohistochemistry is frequently impossible as their immunophenotypes overlap.[140]

CD10 AND WT1

CD10, also known as common acute lymphoblastic leukemia antigen, is now recognized to mark neoplastic and non-neoplastic endometrial stromal cells.[138,141,142] Potential uses therefore fall into two categories: distinguishing adenomyosis from invasive endometrial cancer and distinguishing endometrial stromal neoplasms from smooth muscle neoplasms. There are many complexities, however, with the use of antibodies against CD10. These include frequent expression in myometrium surrounding invading endometrial cancer cells, expression in occasional smooth muscle neoplasms, and loss of expression in endometrial stromal neoplasms with divergent differentiation. WT1, the Wilms' tumor suppressor gene product, is expressed in endometrial stroma and endometrial stromal neoplasms as well as in smooth muscle tumors. WT1 immunoreactivity does not discriminate between these two categories of tumors.[143]

Endometrial Carcinoma (Table 18.2)

ENDOMETRIOID ADENOCARCINOMA

Endometrioid adenocarcinoma is a neoplasm that recapitulates non-neoplastic endometrium in most cases. That is, the tumor is typically formed of endometrioid tubules, at least focally, and demonstrates the same range of cytoplasmic changes and metaplasias seen in non-neoplastic endometrium. The immunophenotype, in general, is similar to that of its precursor, complex atypical hyperplasia. As with other common adenocarcinomas, endometrioid adenocarcinoma expresses pan-cytokeratins, EMA, and the glycoprotein associated markers CA125, Ber-EP4,[144] and B72.3,[145,146] among others. Expression of carcinoembryonic antigen (CEA), which is uncommon, is almost always limited to apical membranes, although tumors showing extensive mucinous differentiation may express this antigen more diffusely.[68-70,104,127,147] There is much less striking CEA expression in endometrioid carcinoma when compared to endocervical, pulmonary, and gastrointestinal carcinomas. Most endometrioid adenocarcinomas express low molecular weight cytokeratins, and those showing squamous differentiation or morules express high molecular weight cytokeratins as well.[148] Nearly all endometrioid adenocarcinomas are CK7-positive and CK20-negative.[68,149] Occasional mucinous varieties express CDX2.[150,151] Unusually for adenocarcinomas, endometrioid tumors are well-known for their frequently strong expression of vimentin.[68,152,153]

TABLE 18.2 Key Differential Diagnosis: Primary Uterine Carcinomas

	ER/PR	p53, p16 (overexpression)	Ki-67 (% tumor cells positive)
Endometrioid	+++*	+	+*
Serous	+	+++	+++
Clear cell	N	+	++

*Except in FIGO grade 3 endometrioid adenocarcinoma, about 50% of which express significant ER and PR; these also tend to be more proliferative than grade 1 and 2 carcinomas.
+ Rarely positive (or Ki-67 low).
++ Frequently positive (or Ki-67 intermediate).
+++ Almost always positive (or Ki-67 high).
N, Negative.

Recent advances in our understanding of the molecular pathogenesis of endometrioid adenocarcinoma have led to the study of proteins featured in the relevant pathways (Fig. 18.14). These include ER, PR, p53, β-catenin, p16, PTEN, and the DNA mismatch repair proteins (MMR proteins) MLH1, MSH2, MSH6, and PMS2. The preponderance of FIGO grade 1 and 2 endometrioid adenocarcinomas express ER and PR, and approximately 50% of FIGO grade 3 endometrioid adenocarcinomas without serous, clear cell, or undifferentiated features express these markers as well.[111,116,124,126,127,154] p53 overexpression (intense expression in greater than 75% of tumor cell nuclei) resulting from *p53* mutation and accumulation of mutant p53 protein is encountered in a minority of FIGO grade 2 and 3 adenocarcinomas, and the numbers become even smaller when tumors with serous, clear cell, or undifferentiated features are excluded.[106-108,111-113,124,125] That is not to say, however, that p53 expression (as opposed to *over*expression defined above) is uncommon in endometrioid carcinomas; in fact, it is very common to find weak expression in less than 50% of endometrioid carcinoma tumor cell nuclei. As a consequence of *CTNNB1* mutation, β-catenin expression in tumor cell nuclei and cytoplasm (as opposed to cell membranes alone) is found in perhaps 33% of FIGO grade 1 and 2 adenocarcinomas, especially those showing squamous or morular metaplasia.[118,124] p16 is occasionally expressed in endometrioid carcinomas, and this appears related to grade; a minority of grade 1 and 2 adenocarcinomas express p16 in scattered tumor cells, whereas more diffuse and intense staining is seen in occasional grade 3 adenocarcinomas.[127,155] A diffuse, strong, "every-cell" expression pattern is exceptional in endometrioid adenocarcinomas. *PTEN* is frequently mutated in endometrioid adenocarcinomas, and expression of this gene is sometimes silenced via hypermethylation of its promoter.[119-124,131] However, detecting these abnormalities with immunohistochemistry is challenging.[124,156] Although imperfect, the 6H2.1

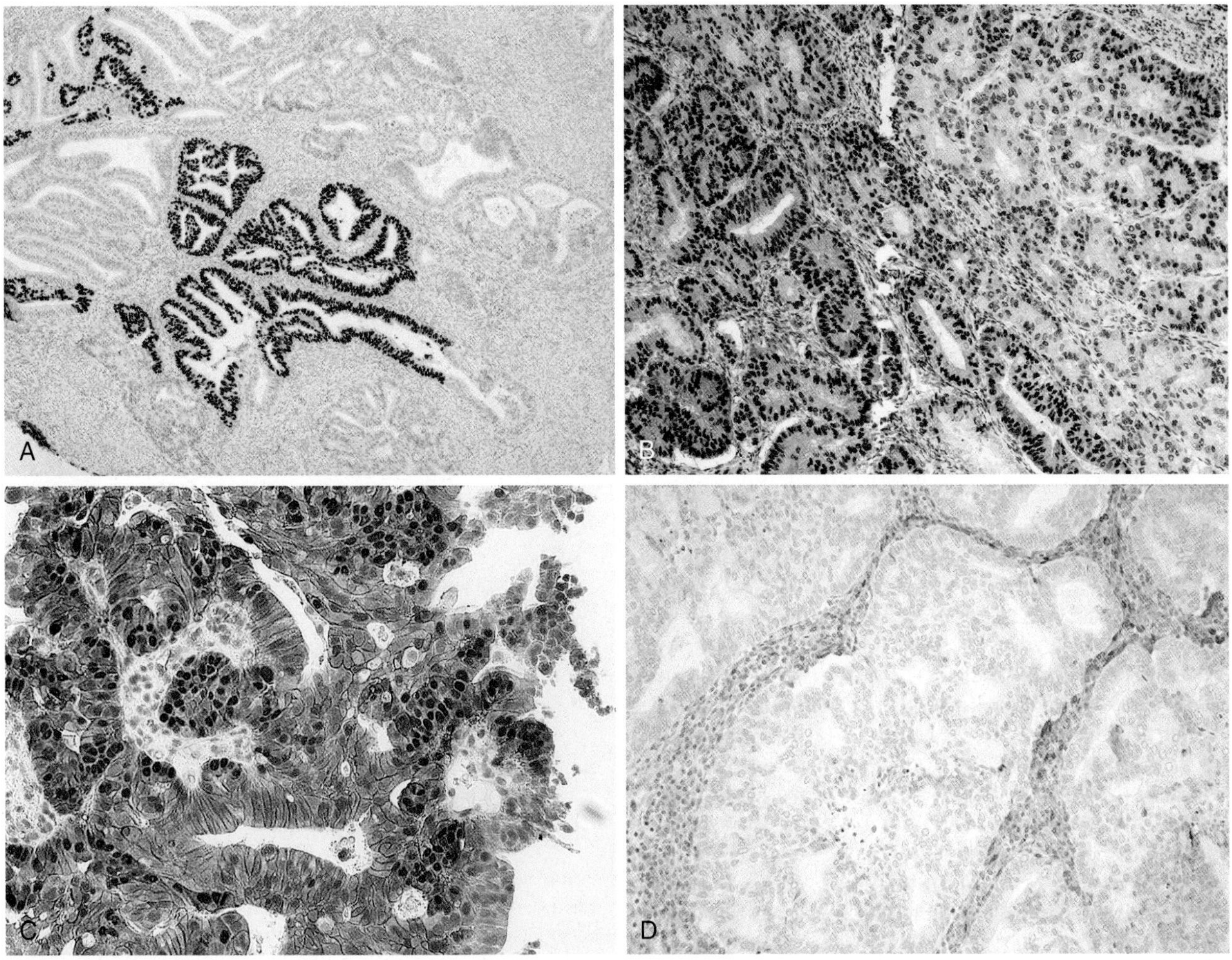

FIGURE 18.14 Markers of emerging importance in distinguishing uterine endometrioid carcinoma and uterine serous carcinoma include p53, β-catenin, and PTEN. While serous carcinomas characteristically overexpress p53 **(A)**, endometrioid adenocarcinomas, especially when gland-forming, frequently express estrogen receptors **(B)**, commonly show at least focal nuclear and cytoplasmic staining with anti–β-catenin **(C)**, and lose expression of PTEN **(D)**.

antibody appears to allow recognition of PTEN protein *loss;* correct interpretation of PTEN immunostains involves the identification of an intact positive internal control (the cytoplasm and sometimes nuclei of endometrial stroma and non-neoplastic endometrial glands) *and* expression loss in at least 90% of tumor cells. DNA MMR proteins are found to be lacking in tumor cell nuclei by immunohistochemistry in up to 33% of endometrioid adenocarcinomas;[157-160] this results from MLH1 promoter hypermethylation in most cases or mutation of *MLH1*, *MSH2*, *MSH6*, or *PMS2* in the rest. Interpreting DNA MMR protein immunohistochemistry is similar to the PTEN story; only complete expression loss in the setting of a valid positive internal control is considered interpretable. Valid internal controls include non-neoplastic endometrial stroma and glands with reproducibly stained nuclei. Almost as a rule, expression loss, when present, occurs in couplets (MLH1 with PMS2 and MSH2 with MSH6).

More detailed discussion of ER, PR, p53, and DNA MMR can be found in the "Theranostic Applications" section. Finally, it should be noted that while many endometrioid adenocarcinomas of endometrium resemble endometrioid ovarian carcinomas, there are some subtle differences. We will discuss these differences in the "Ovary" section.

KEY DIAGNOSTIC POINTS

Endometrioid Carcinomas

- Endometrioid carcinomas typically express CK7, CA125, ER, PR, and vimentin, while they are usually negative for CEA and CK20.
- p53 and p16 are only occasionally overexpressed.
- Nuclear β-catenin expression and loss of PTEN and DNA MMR proteins are seen in significant minorities.

ENDOMETRIAL SEROUS CARCINOMA

It is easy to recognize endometrial serous carcinoma when it is tumor forming and present in its characteristic papillary form with bizarre tumor cell nuclei. However, endometrial serous carcinoma can be difficult to diagnose correctly when glandular, clear cell, or solid forms predominate; the tumor is admixed with an endometrioid or clear cell neoplasm; it is intraepithelial and apparently confined to an endometrial polyp; or there is uncertainty regarding the possibility of endocervical, ovarian, tubal, or peritoneal primaries. However, what constitutes the morphologic and immunophenotypic threshold at which serous and endometrioid carcinomas can be meaningfully and reproducibly separated is currently being debated. Despite important immunophenotypic differences that distinguish between clear-cut examples of serous, clear cell, and endometrioid carcinomas of the endometrium, discussed subsequently, these tumors share notable similarities. Like endometrioid carcinomas, endometrial serous carcinomas commonly express pan-cytokeratins, EMA, CA125, Ber-EP4, B72.3, CK7, and vimentin, while they are usually negative for CK20 and lack diffuse, strong cytoplasmic expression of CEA. Their immunophenotype resembles that of its putative precursor, intraepithelial serous carcinoma (endometrial intraepithelial carcinoma).[106,161,162] The existence of so-called *serous dysplasia* has also been suggested.[163,164] This lesion demonstrates some of the morphologic and immunohistochemical features of serous carcinoma, and it is thought to precede the development of intraepithelial serous carcinoma and accompany it in some cases.

It is not surprising that the expression of proteins discussed in reference to molecular pathways essential to endometrioid carcinogenesis differs significantly in serous carcinoma (Figs. 18.14, 18.15, and 18.16). Approximately 90% of endometrial serous carcinomas show p53 overexpression (intense expression in greater than 75% of tumor cell nuclei) as a result of *p53* mutation and the consequent accumulation of mutant protein.[106-108,112,113] The majority of remaining tumors, most of which show absolutely no p53 expression, harbor *p53* mutations that result in a truncated p53 protein or a protein with conformational changes that cannot be detected using commercially available antibodies.[107] Proliferative activity, approximated with a Ki-67 labeling index, is extremely high, with rates that mimic p53 overexpression patterns (i.e., greater than 75% of tumor cell nuclei).[111] The typical serous carcinoma lacks diffuse ER and PR expression,[111,114-116,124] although many carcinomas with hybrid endometrioid/serous features and admixtures of endometrioid and serous components may express considerable amounts of ER.[165] PR probably is expressed even less frequently than ER. p16 is almost always highly expressed in an "every-cell" pattern."[127,155] In contrast to most endocervical carcinomas, this does not imply HPV infection; rather, it may reflect disturbances in the cell cycle that favor hyperproliferative activity. Abnormalities involving the *CTNNB1* (β-catenin), *PTEN,* and MMR pathways are very rare in endometrial serous carcinomas; this means that nuclear β-catenin expression and loss of PTEN, MLH1, MSH2, MSH6, and PMS2 are almost never encountered. One possible exception includes the extraordinary occurrence of endometrial serous carcinoma in the setting of hereditary non-polyposis colorectal carcinoma (HNPCC) with loss of MSH2 and MSH6. More detailed discussions of ER, PR, p53, and DNA MMR can be found in the "Theranostic Applications" section.

Finally, it should be noted that while many serous adenocarcinomas of endometrium resemble ovarian serous carcinomas, there are some important differences. We will discuss these differences in the "Ovary" section. The most important of these is infrequent WT1 expression in endometrial serous carcinomas (seen in at most 20% to 30% of such cases) and the very common diffuse nuclear expression of WT1 in ovarian, tubal, and primary peritoneal examples (at least 70% to 80% of such cases).[166-168]

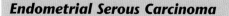

KEY DIAGNOSTIC POINTS

Endometrial Serous Carcinoma

- Serous carcinomas express CK7, CA125, and vimentin, while they are usually negative for CEA and CK20, just like endometrioid carcinomas.
- Unlike endometrioid carcinomas, they typically overexpress p53 and p16 and show extremely high proliferative indices with Ki-67; most examples have low-level expression of ER and low-level or absent PR.

CLEAR CELL CARCINOMA

Clear cell carcinoma is increasingly strictly defined, which means that endometrioid and serous carcinomas composed of cells showing cytoplasmic clearing should not be diagnosed as clear cell carcinomas.[169] Like endometrioid and serous carcinomas, clear cell carcinomas usually express pan-cytokeratins, EMA, CA125, Ber-EP4, B72.3, CK7, and vimentin, while they are usually negative for CK20 and WT1 and lack diffuse, strong cytoplasmic expression of CEA.

Clear cell carcinomas are typically ER- and PR-negative and show rates of p53, p16, and Ki-67 expression that are intermediate between endometrioid and serous carcinomas.[125-127] A typical example might show 10% of tumor cells labeling with anti-PR and perhaps 30% of cells in a given tumor marking with Ki-67. Notably, p53 overexpression (as defined earlier in this section) and proliferative rates that mimic serous carcinomas are generally not seen in clear cell carcinoma. Although it is conceivable that some clear cell carcinomas might show abnormalities in *CTNNB1* (β-catenin) and *PTEN* pathways,[170,171] insufficient numbers of well-characterized cases have been studied, and it is thought that abnormalities would largely be lacking. It is increasingly recognized that clear cell carcinoma of the endometrium might represent a manifestation of HNPCC;[172] as such, there are rare clear cell carcinomas with loss of MSH2 and MSH6, related to mutations in the corresponding genes. Finally, it is likely that hepatocyte nuclear factor-1β (HNF-1β) is uniformly expressed in the vast majority of endometrial clear cell carcinomas, thus providing a candidate marker linking endometrial and ovarian clear cell carcinoma (see the "Ovary" section).[173]

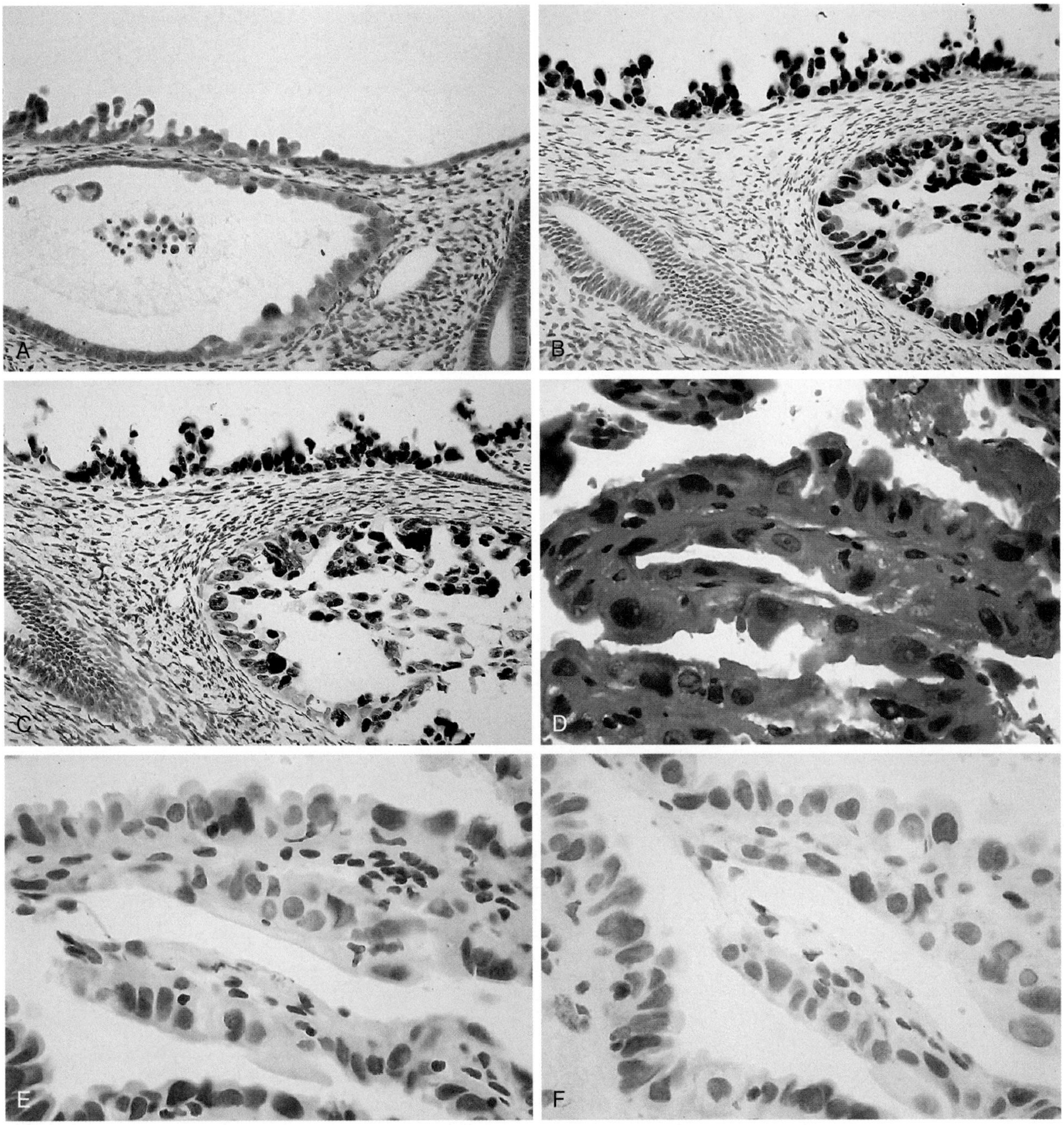

FIGURE 18.15 p53 and Ki-67 can be useful for distinguishing endometrial surface metaplastic and degenerative changes from endometrial intraepithelial carcinoma (EIC). EIC **(A-C)** contrasts with metaplastic-degenerative change **(D-F)** by virtue of uniform and intense nuclear expression for p53 (**B** versus **E**) and Ki-67 (**C** versus **F**) in EIC.

KEY DIAGNOSTIC POINTS

Clear Cell Carcinomas

- Clear cell carcinomas express CK7, CA125, and vimentin, while they are usually negative for CEA and CK20, just like endometrioid and serous carcinomas.
- Unlike serous carcinomas, p53 and p16 overexpression is rare; unlike typical endometrioid carcinomas, ER and PR expression is low or absent.
- Loss of DNA MMR protein expression can be encountered.
- Nuclear expression HNF-1β may emerge as a specific marker for endometrial and ovarian clear cell carcinoma.

OTHER HISTOLOGIC SUBTYPES OF ENDOMETRIAL CARCINOMA AND SECONDARY CARCINOMAS, INCLUDING METASTASES (TABLE 18.3)

Endometrial carcinomas with mucinous, squamous, transitional, neuroendocrine, and undifferentiated features have been described, but information about the immunophenotype of squamous cell, transitional cell, and small cell carcinomas (excluding case reports and small series) is hard to obtain. Data concerning the immunophenotype of mucinous carcinoma center mainly on its distinction from microglandular hyperplasia and endocervical adenocarcinoma, which we have discussed earlier in this chapter.

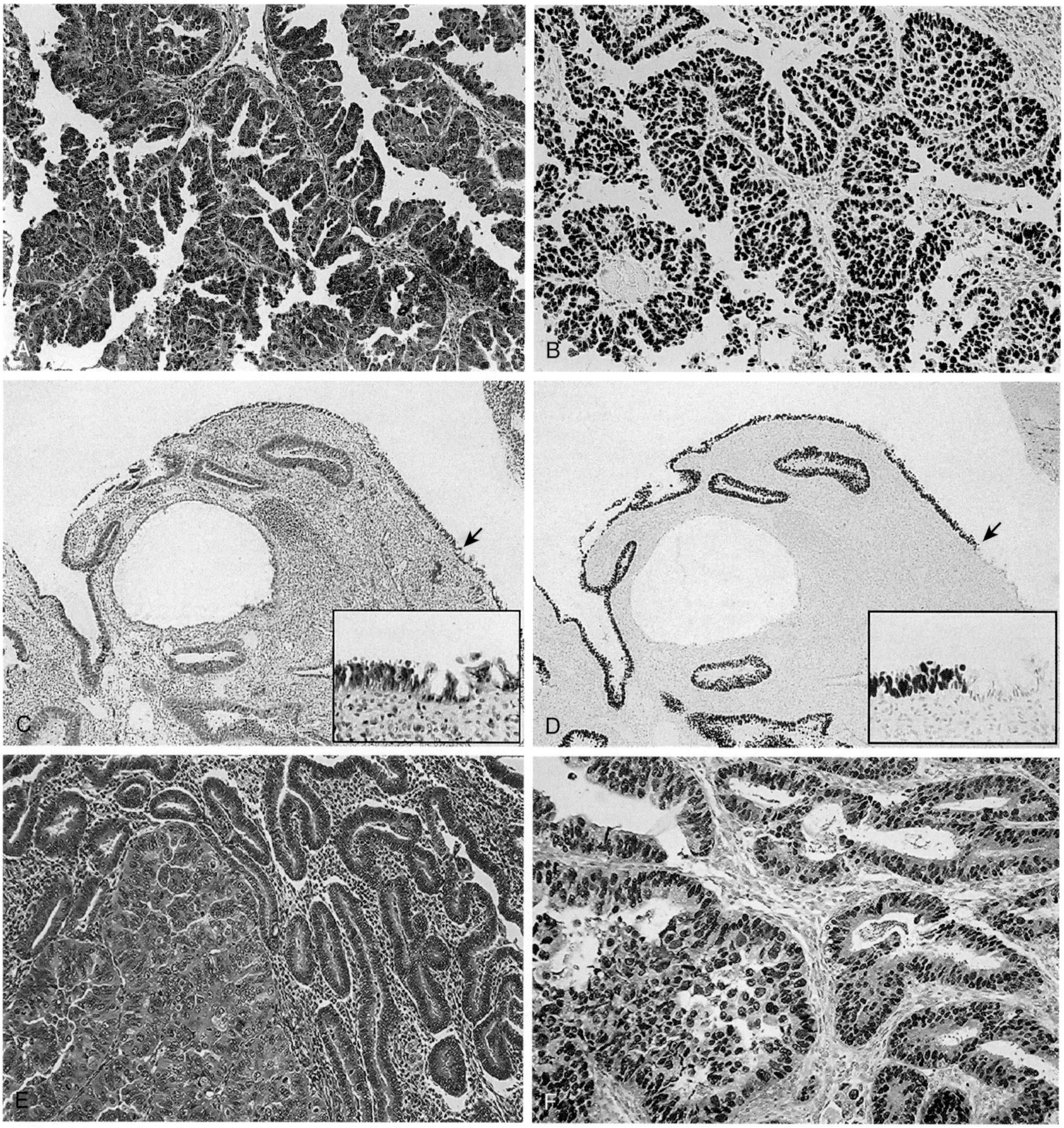

FIGURE 18.16 p53 immunohistochemical staining can be used when the differential diagnosis includes uterine serous carcinoma (USC) and uterine endometrioid carcinoma (UEC). USC shows diffuse and intense nuclear immunoreactivity for p53 **(A, B)**, as does the USC precursor EIC **(C, D)**. Not infrequently, USC can demonstrate a glandular architectural pattern **(E)**. Diffuse and intense p53 immunoreactivity in glandular USC **(F)** can provide support for this entity when simple atypical hyperplasia and endometrioid adenocarcinoma are considerations.

Neuroendocrine Carcinomas

Extrapolating data from the cervical and pulmonary literature, assorted case reports, and reviews,[174-176] it appears that small cell and large cell neuroendocrine carcinomas involving endometrium would express chromogranin, synaptophysin, neuron-specific enolase, and CD56 in a significant number of cases. The extent to which these endometrial neuroendocrine carcinomas can express TTF-1 and p16 has not been studied extensively.[176-178] It should be noted, however, that conventional endometrioid carcinomas can contain significant subpopulations of neuroendocrine cells, which can be a pitfall when using immunohistochemistry alone to diagnose small cell and large cell neuroendocrine carcinomas. Significant neuroendocrine marker expression (e.g., greater than 20% of tumor cells) should be present before classifying a large cell neoplasm as definitively neuroendocrine, especially when it does not exhibit compelling features of neuroendocrine differentiation on an H&E-stained slide. Small cell carcinoma, however, can be diagnosed

TABLE 18.3 Key Differential Diagnosis: Adenocarcinomas Involving Uterus

	ER/PR	WT1	CK20	CEA	TTF-1
Endometrioid of endometrium	+++[2]	N	N	N[4]	N[3]
Serous of endometrium	+	+	N	N	N[3]
Serous of ovary[1]	++	+++	N	N	N[3]
Endocervix	N	N	N	+++	N[3]
Breast	++	N[3]	N	+	N
Colorectal	N	N	+++	+++	N
Pulmonary	N[3]	N[3]	N[3]	+++	+++

[1]Includes ovarian, peritoneal, and tubal serous carcinomas.
[2]Except in FIGO grade 3 endometrioid adenocarcinoma, about 50% of which express significant ER and PR.
[3]Rare examples have been reported positive.
[4]Luminal membrane positivity is expected, but a diffuse, cytoplasmic reaction is not.
+ Rarely positive.
++ Frequently positive.
+++ Almost always positive.
N, Negative.

without immunohistochemical support for neuroendocrine differentiation if the features are absolutely classic and entities in the differential diagnosis have been excluded.

Undifferentiated Carcinomas

The immunophenotype of undifferentiated and dedifferentiated endometrial carcinomas, as defined by Silva and colleagues, has been explored in recent publications.[179,180] It should be noted, however, that these tumors probably constitute only one clinical and morphologic manifestation of undifferentiation. Other varieties undoubtedly exist. Compared to typical endometrioid adenocarcinomas, the undifferentiated components of Silva's tumors tend to show relative loss of cytokeratin, ER, and PR expression when juxtaposed with the typical endometrioid component. EMA expression, however, appears to be retained in most examples. It is interesting to note, furthermore, that although they are rare, a disproportionate number of undifferentiated and de-differentiated endometrial carcinomas have been reported to show abnormal expression of DNA MMR proteins,[181] which suggests that some may represent a manifestation of HNPCC.[182]

Mixed Epithelial Carcinomas

Mixed epithelial carcinoma (i.e., mixed endometrioid and serous carcinoma) can be diagnosed when at least two histologically distinctive elements are present and each constitutes at least 10% of the tumor. The elements should be obvious, separable, and characteristic to diagnose a mixed tumor. Immunohistochemical stains, when performed, should demonstrate that the immunophenotypes of each component are distinctive as well. Mixed epithelial carcinomas should not be diagnosed when the overall morphology is a hybrid of features generally encountered in different endometrial cancer subtypes. This point was addressed in a recent abstract where the immunophenotype of the different components of tumors diagnosed as mixed endometrioid and serous carcinomas were found to be similar.[183] This supported the idea that these tumors were, in fact, not composed of two disparate cancer types.

Metastatic Carcinomas

Data regarding the sources of secondary or metastatic carcinomas to the endometrium are limited, but it is estimated that lobular breast cancers, high-grade serous ovarian and tubal carcinomas, HPV-associated endocervical adenocarcinomas, and typical colorectal adenocarcinomas probably constitute at least 90% of such cases.

ENDOMETRIAL CARCINOMA STAGING

Myometrial Invasion

It has been proposed that studying CD10 expression could help to distinguish invasive endometrial cancer from adenocarcinomas that colonize adenomyosis.[184,185] Since CD10 expression is characteristic of endometrial stroma and not myometrial smooth muscle, the theory goes that CD10 expression surrounding adenocarcinoma in the myometrium would support adenomyosis over invasive carcinoma. Unfortunately, there are at least two problems with this idea. It turns out that many invasive adenocarcinomas are surrounded by a rim of tissue that expresses CD10, such that the appearance mimics the endometrial stroma that one expects in adenomyosis. A less common problem involves metaplastic stroma. In occasional endometrial cancers, endometrial stroma supporting endometrial cancer undergoes metaplasia to a smooth muscle or fibroblastic phenotype, similar to the stroma that is characteristic of endometrial polyps. This metaplastic stroma frequently expresses CD10 only weakly or focally. Therefore, absent CD10 staining does not entirely exclude the presence of endometrial stroma and adenomyosis.

Lymphovascular Invasion (LVI)

It has been shown that LVI is an important determinant of lymph node metastasis, but the extent to which it associates with other features of high-risk endometrial cancer means that it usually doesn't feature as an independent indicator of prognosis. Although assessment of LVI is not required for stage assignment, a surgical pathology report lacking this information is generally considered incomplete. Vascular endothelial markers, such as CD34 and CD31, and the lymphatic endothelial marker podoplanin (D2-40) have been used to verify the presence of a vascular space containing a tumor embolus, but the contribution of these tests with respect to their association with lymph node metastases and prognosis has not been extensively studied in endometrial cancer.[186-189] IHC for these endothelial markers should therefore be considered essentially untested for practical (diagnostic) purposes in endometrial cancer.

Lymph Node Metastasis and Sentinel Lymph Node Evaluation

Cytokeratin immunostains are occasionally used to detect microscopic deposits of occult carcinoma cells in lymph nodes. Carcinomas demonstrating the microcystic, elongated, and fragmented pattern (MELF) of myometrial invasion are frequently associated with lymphovascular invasion[190] and deposits of carcinoma in lymph nodes that resemble histiocytes—this is an obvious application of the use of keratin stains to confirm epithelial differentiation and the presence of rare, single tumor cells in lymph node sinuses.[191] Keratin stains have also been studied in the setting of sentinel lymph node evaluation, but this is currently experimental.[192]

SYNCHRONOUS ENDOMETRIAL AND OVARIAN, TUBAL, AND PERITONEAL CARCINOMAS

Immunohistochemical evaluation is unnecessary for the two categories of endometrial and ovarian tumors that can be recognized as highly likely to be synchronous. The first is a non-invasive or minimally invasive well-differentiated endometrioid carcinoma of endometrium with coincident complex atypical hyperplasia and a well-differentiated endometrioid carcinoma of ovary with coincident endometriosis or endometrioid adenofibromatous tumor, but without ovarian surface involvement. The second concerns endometrial and ovarian tumors of obviously different grades and histologic types. At the other end of the spectrum are the obviously metastatic tumors: deeply invasive, high-grade endometrial carcinomas with multiple ovarian tumor nodules, including ovarian surface deposits; the occasional, huge ovarian, tubal, or peritoneal carcinoma with multifocal, small "drop-metastases" along a cycling endometrium; and an endometrial serous carcinoma, arising in an endometrial polyp with intraepithelial serous carcinoma along with a serous carcinoma involving ovary, fallopian tube, and peritoneum. It is not debatable that the former two scenarios represent metastasis from one organ to another, but whether the latter situation is an example of metastasis from endometrium to ovary is up for discussion. Both evidence of monoclonality[193] and immunohistochemical substantiation of endometrial serous differentiation support the idea that the latter situation is one where an endometrial serous carcinoma metastasized to extrauterine organs.[194] In a paper published by Anderson,[194] the authors studied WT1 immunohistochemistry in two groups of patients, one with peritoneal carcinomatosis and no endometrial disease and another with peritoneal carcinomatosis and serous carcinomas in endometrial polyps. Peritoneal tumors in the first group were almost always WT1-positive (supporting ovarian, tubal, or peritoneal serous carcinoma), but the endometrial and peritoneal tumors in the second group were almost always WT1-negative (supporting endometrial serous carcinoma). Therefore, given the appropriate context, WT1 immunostains can be used to determine the *likelihood* that a given serous carcinoma is endometrial or extrauterine in origin. However, since as many as 20% to 30% of endometrial serous carcinomas have been reported to be WT1-positive and 20% to 30% of ovarian, tubal, and peritoneal carcinomas have been reported to be WT1-negative, it is imprudent to claim that this test offers unqualified support for one situation over another.[166-168,195]

Scenarios other than the ones previously described are common, and it is unfortunate because it can be difficult or impossible to determine whether the tumors are synchronous. Regarding contributions from immunohistochemistry for sorting through these challenging cases, Prat's group studied *CTNNB1* mutations and β-catenin expression in a group of patients with both endometrial and ovarian tumors.[196] They found that tumors reported to be synchronous were more likely than metastatic carcinomas to express β-catenin in tumor cell nuclei. Although these data are intriguing, practitioners should be cautious when basing their diagnoses solely on the status of this test result.

TABLE 18.4 Key Differential Diagnosis: Primary Uterine Mesenchymal Tumors

	CD10	Desmin/ h-caldesmon	Cytokeratin
Smooth muscle, spindled	+	+++	+
Smooth muscle, epithelioid	+	++	++
Endometrial stromal*	+++	N	+

*Includes the mesenchymal component of müllerian adenosarcoma without stromal overgrowth.
+ Rarely positive.
++ Frequently positive.
+++ Almost always positive.
N, Negative.

Uterine Mesenchymal Tumors (Tables 18.4 and 18.5)

LEIOMYOMA AND LEIOMYOSARCOMA

Uterine smooth muscle tumors, particularly those composed of spindled cells, characteristically express smooth muscle actin, muscle-specific actin, desmin, h-caldesmon, and vimentin.[134,135] Leiomyosarcomas also commonly express WT1,[197] BCL-2,[198-200] ER, PR,[201-204] and CD10.[138] Less frequently assayed uterine smooth muscle–associated markers include histone deacetylase 8 (HDAC8)[205] and oxytocin receptors.[206] Note that cytokeratin expression can be found in up to 25% to 30% of cases, particularly epithelioid varieties,[138,207] although it is usually patchy in distribution, while up to 25% to 30% of epithelioid and myxoid leiomyosarcomas fail to demonstrate appreciable expression of smooth muscle-associated markers.[138] Although leiomyosarcomas express more p53 and MIB1 than leiomyomas, and less BCL-2, ER, and PR, this immunohistochemical panel is not clinically useful because the results have shown a broad gradient of expression in leiomyomas, atypical smooth muscle tumors, and leiomyosarcomas,

TABLE 18.5 Key Differential Diagnosis: Epithelioid Uterine Tumors

	Cytokeratin	Desmin	Inhibin	S100
Carcinoma	+++	N	N	+
Epithelioid smooth muscle	++	++	N	+
Trophoblastic	+++	N	++	
Melanoma	N	+	+	+++

+ Rarely positive.
++ Frequently positive.
+++ Almost always positive.
N, Negative.

instead of sharp cutoff points that facilitate quantitation.[199,202,208-211]

The mitosis marker, anti-phosphohistone H3 (PHH3) is emerging as an attractive alternative to MIB1.[212] This marker is detectable specifically during mitotic chromatin condensation; it should therefore be preferable to MIB1 for estimating proliferative activity. It is also reportedly useful for separating bizarre nuclear forms and apoptotic bodies from true mitotic figures.[212] Additional studies will more clearly define the diagnostic utility of this marker.

KEY DIAGNOSTIC POINTS

Leiomyosarcomas

- Uterine leiomyosarcoma is composed of spindle cells that typically express smooth muscle actin and desmin, although desmin expression is sometimes lacking. It may express CD10.
- Uterine leiomyosarcomas frequently express cytokeratins in a patchy distribution.
- Uterine epithelioid leiomyosarcomas frequently express cytokeratins and lack desmin expression.
- Uterine myxoid leiomyosarcomas frequently fail to express desmin.
- Assays for p53, MIB1, BCL-2, ER, and PR are not currently used for diagnostic purposes in this setting.

ENDOMETRIAL STROMAL NODULE AND LOW-GRADE ENDOMETRIAL STROMAL SARCOMA

Endometrial stromal neoplasms, both nodules and sarcomas, almost always express CD10, ER, PR, and WT1 (Fig. 18.17).[138,141-143,213,214] Many also express β-catenin.[215-217] They frequently express smooth muscle actin,[100,101,138,214] cytokeratin,[99,214] or androgen receptors patchily.[218] They only unusually express desmin[100,135,219,220] and CD34 (unpublished observation) in varieties where the constituent cells resemble non-neoplastic proliferative endometrial stroma. Diffuse desmin and h-caldesmon expression supports smooth muscle differentiation and disqualifies categorization as an endometrial stromal tumor except in rare cases.

Several endometrial stromal tumor variants have been described (Fig. 18.18). These include the smooth muscle variant (also referred to as *mixed endometrial stromal* and *smooth muscle tumor* or *stromomyoma*),[133,220] fibromyxoid variant,[132,220] sex cord variant, and variants including endometrioid glands or epithelioid cells.[221,222] The key to understanding the immunophenotype of these tumors is that variant or metaplastic elements often lose the phenotype of endometrial stroma and acquire the phenotype of the corresponding metaplastic element.[220] Therefore, the smooth muscle in a smooth muscle variant of endometrial stromal nodule expresses muscle markers (Fig. 18.18B) and is frequently CD10-negative.[138,220] The endometrioid glands in a low-grade endometrial stromal sarcoma, glandular variant, will express epithelial markers, such as EMA. Similarly, the sex cord component of an endometrial stromal nodule, sex cord variant, might express inhibin and lose CD10 expression.[136] Hybrid forms also exist, further complicating interpretation. For example, some stromal neoplasms with sex cord features contain elements that coexpress muscle markers and cytokeratins.[138] With the exception of the fibroblastic variant, in which CD10 expression can be muted, all other variants should have at least remnants of a proliferation that resembles non-neoplastic proliferative-phase endometrial stroma and retains CD10, ER, and PR expression. A negative CD34 result, particularly in a tumor with fibroblastic features, can be useful in the discrimination of metastatic stromal sarcoma and solitary fibrous tumor, which is CD34-positive.[214]

KEY DIAGNOSTIC POINTS

Endometrial Stromal Tumors

- Endometrial stromal tumors are typically CD10, ER, and PR positive and lack staining for desmin, h-caldesmon, and CD34.
- If confronted with a possible endometrial stromal tumor variant, concentrate the examination on components that resemble proliferative phase endometrial stroma.
- Expression of CD10 without h-caldesmon and/or desmin in these areas supports an endometrial stromal component.

CARCINOSARCOMA

The diagnosis of carcinosarcoma (MMMT) requires clearly defined and separable carcinomatous and sarcomatous components. If they are not *clearly* defined on H&E examination, a diagnosis of carcinosarcoma is difficult or impossible to substantiate. Often, immunohistochemical study of an apparently undifferentiated neoplasm whose differential diagnosis includes carcinoma and sarcoma reveals a confusing immunophenotype-coexpression of epithelial and mesenchymal markers or a complementary expression of both in areas that are morphologically similar.[102,103] It is reasonable to consider a diagnosis of carcinosarcoma if there are geographic zones that express cytokeratins exclusively

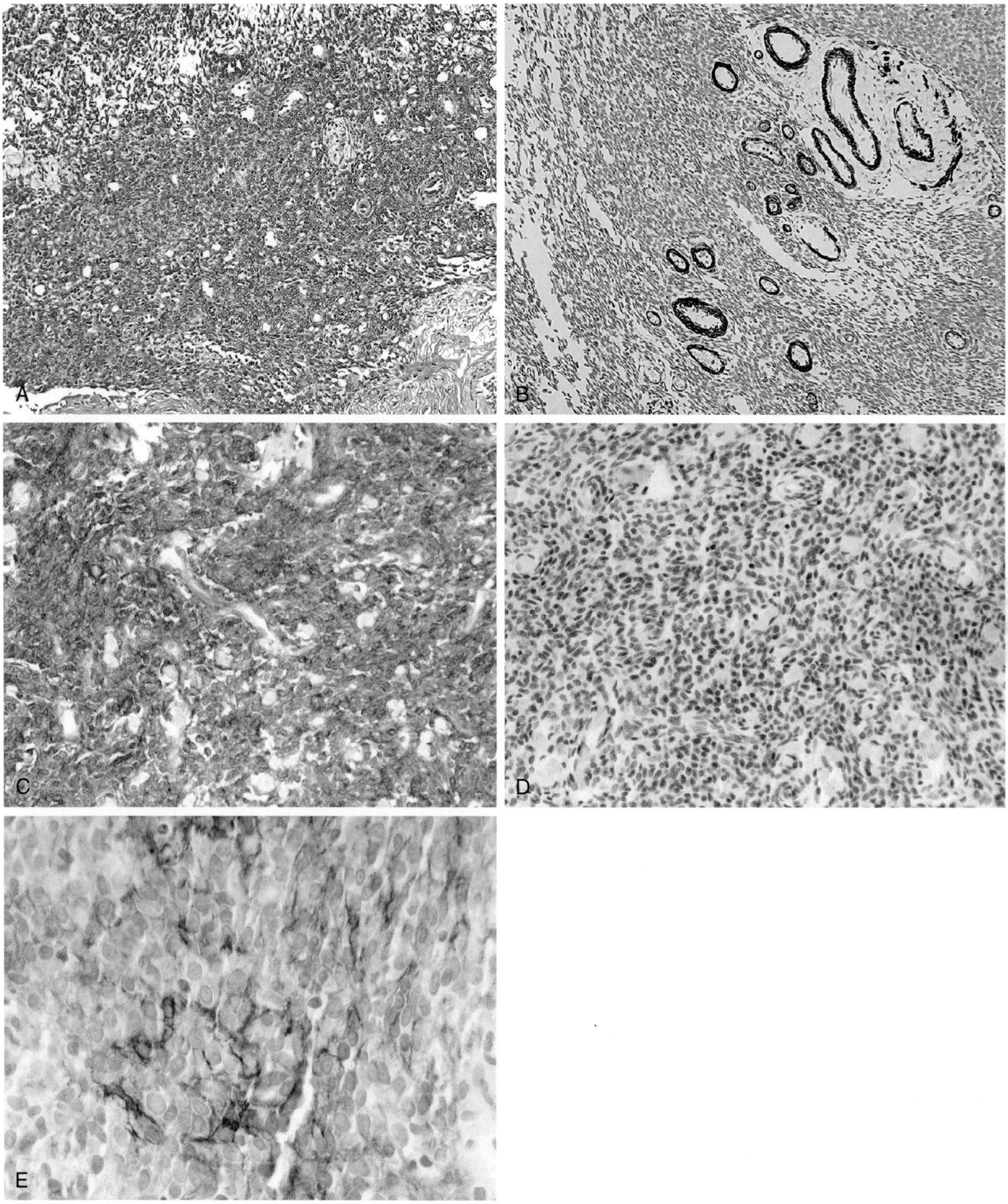

FIGURE 18.17 Endometrial stromal tumors (nodules and sarcomas) and cellular leiomyomas can show significant morphologic similarity. Although desmin reactivity can frequently distinguish these entities, h-caldesmon antibody appears to be more specific for smooth muscle differentiation. **A** shows an endometrial stromal sarcoma that is not immunoreactive for h-caldesmon **(B)**. Endometrial stromal sarcomas nearly always express CD10 **(C)** and estrogen **(D)** and progesterone receptors. Several histologic mimics of metastatic endometrial stromal sarcoma, including solitary fibrous tumor, can express progesterone receptors and CD10 **(E)** as well. Although many endometrial stromal sarcomas express CD10 strongly and diffusely, many express CD10 in a patchy pattern, which overlaps with that seen in solitary fibrous tumor and hemangiopericytoma, both tumors with a staghorn vascular pattern. ***C-E*** *from Bhargava R, Shia J, Hummer AJ, et al. Distinction of endometrial stromal sarcomas from "hemangiopericytomatous" tumors using a panel of immunohistochemical stains. Mod Pathol. 2005;18:40-47.*

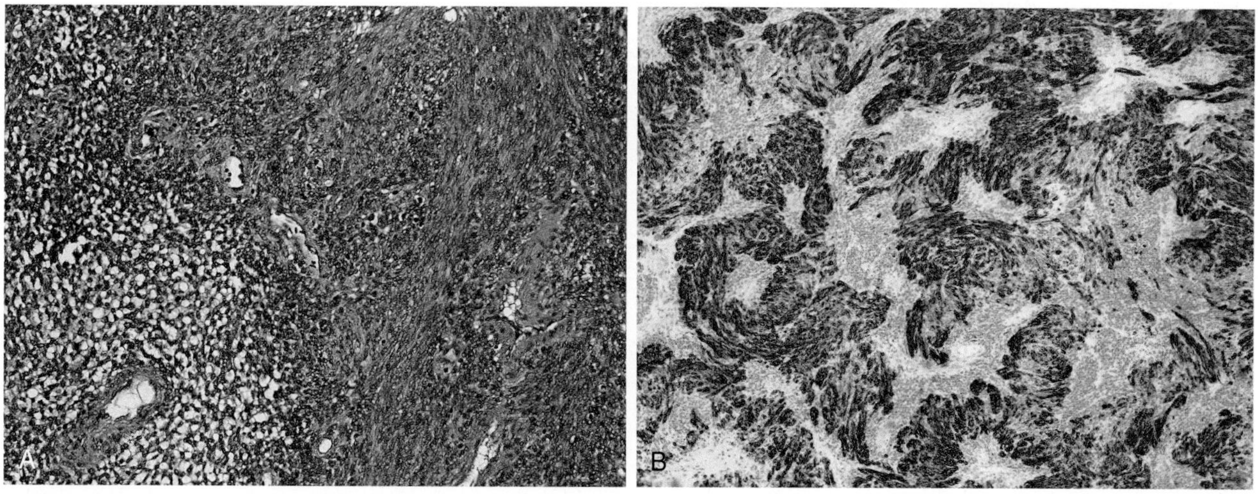

FIGURE 18.18 Immunohistochemistry can be used to evaluate endometrial stromal neoplasms with smooth muscle differentiation. Areas resembling endometrial stroma (**A**, left) contrast with areas resembling smooth muscle (**A**, right). CD10 marks endometrial stromal cells, while muscle markers, such as h-caldesmon, mark zones showing smooth muscle differentiation. **(B)** Endometrial stromal neoplasms are generally diagnosed when conventional-appearing endometrial stroma is present; the diagnosis should not be abandoned solely because of divergent differentiation, such as smooth muscle differentiation, illustrated here.

and separate, distinct zones that express mesenchymal markers exclusively, but other patterns of immunoreactivity are probably not informative.

Despite previous arguments to the contrary, the presence of heterologous elements, particularly rhabdomyoblasts, likely heralds highly aggressive behavior in the context of carcinosarcoma. This was recently reported in a study of surgically staged patients with FIGO stage I carcinosarcoma.[223] A myogenin or Myo-D1 immunostain is therefore recommended for establishing skeletal muscle differentiation when it is suspected and cross-striations are not evident.

Rare case reports exist of carcinosarcomas harboring yolk sac tumor[224] or neuroectodermal elements (including primitive, peripheral neuroectodermal tumor).[225,226] When it has been studied, the immunophenotype of these components has been similar to that described in tumors outside the context of carcinosarcoma.

MÜLLERIAN ADENOSARCOMA

The immunophenotype of this tumor closely parallels that of endometrial stromal neoplasms when stromal overgrowth is not present. The mesenchymal component of müllerian adenosarcomas without stromal overgrowth typically expresses ER, PR, androgen receptors, CD10, and WT1, while significant minorities also express smooth muscle actin and even pan-cytokeratins (Fig. 18.19).[201,227-229] Cases demonstrating stromal overgrowth generally lose strong and diffuse ER, PR, CD10, and WT1 expression.[229] Tumors containing heterologous elements exhibit an immunophenotype that is similar to eutopic tumors; therefore, the mesenchymal component of an adenosarcoma with rhabdomyoblastic differentiation would be expected to express desmin, myogenin, and myoD1. As with carcinosarcoma, recent work suggests that the presence of rhabdomyoblastic differentiation portends a poor prognosis.[230] The proliferative index, estimated with a Ki-67 immunostain, increases with mitotic rate and the presence of sarcomatous stromal overgrowth.[229]

OTHER MESENCHYMAL TUMORS

Undifferentiated Sarcoma

As is the case with undifferentiated carcinomas, undifferentiated sarcomas are an extraordinarily heterogeneous collection of different tumors. The undifferentiated endometrial sarcoma (of which many examples were considered high-grade endometrial stromal sarcoma) is the best known member of this group. Despite this, the criteria for diagnosing this tumor and its immunophenotype are not well understood. Some examples might represent de-differentiation from a low-grade endometrial stromal sarcoma.[217] Immunohistochemistry has been studied in a small series of such cases. CD10 and PR expression were noted to be lost when compared to the differentiated components in most cases.

Should a pleomorphic tumor with diffuse smooth muscle actin expression be classified as leiomyosarcoma? Should a high-grade spindle cell tumor without diffuse desmin expression be classified as undifferentiated sarcoma? Unfortunately, the criteria that separate this tumor from morphologically similar ones and the answers to these questions are unclear. Regardless, there are some practical points worth discussing. Undifferentiated carcinoma (primary or metastatic), leiomyosarcoma, adenosarcoma with stromal overgrowth, melanoma, lymphoma, and leukemia should be considered before a diagnosis of undifferentiated uterine sarcoma is established. An immunohistochemical panel including antibodies against cytokeratin, EMA, S100, LCA, CD43, CD30, and a muscle marker should be helpful with respect to excluding carcinoma, melanoma, lymphoma, and leukemia. Diffuse strong keratin expression supports carcinoma, and diffuse muscle marker expression without keratin immunoreactivity supports a

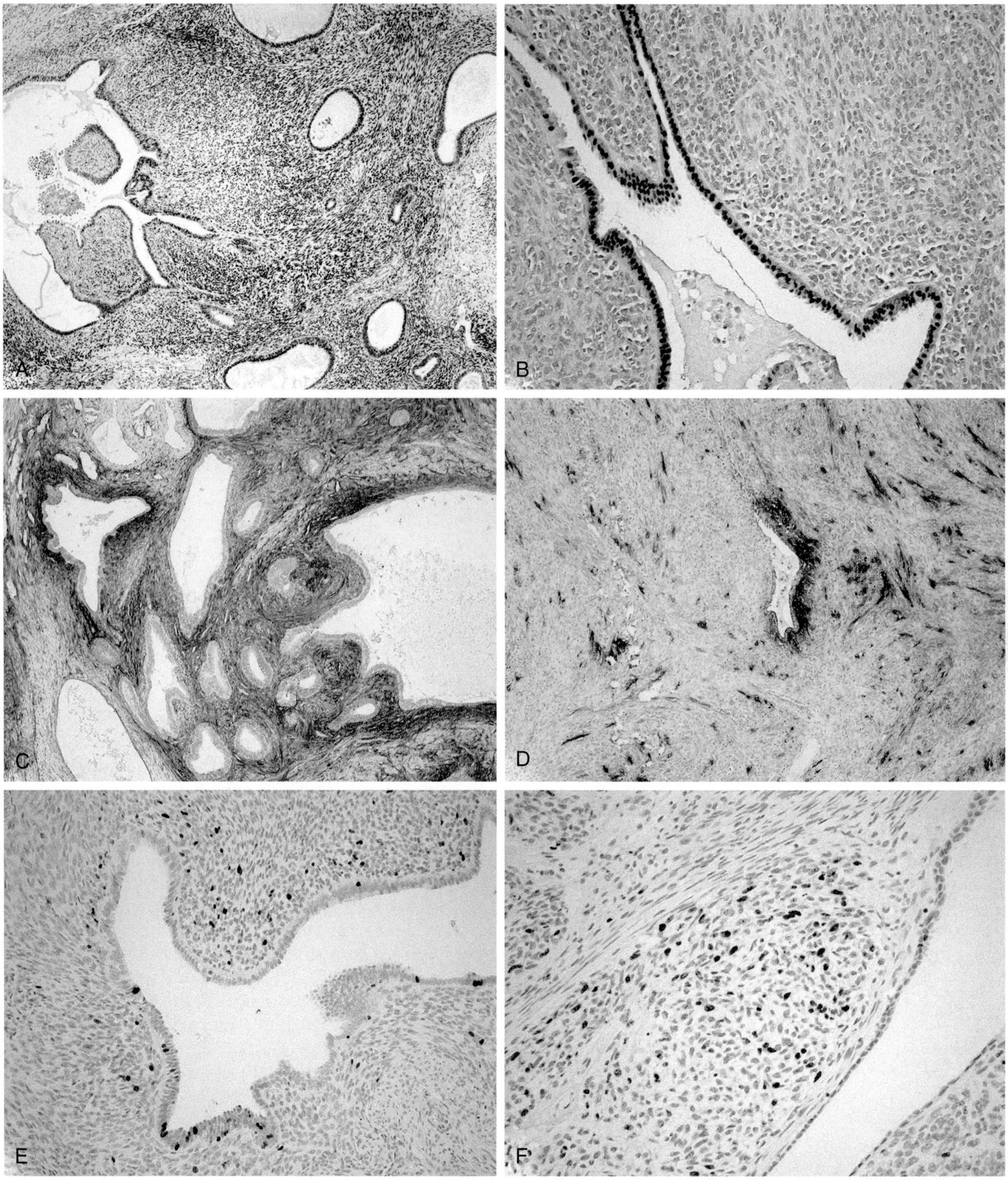

FIGURE 18.19 The immunophenotype of müllerian adenosarcoma with and without stromal overgrowth differs. Expression of PR **(A, B)** and CD10 **(C, D)** is significantly more diffuse in adenosarcomas without stromal overgrowth **(A, C)** than adenosarcomas with stromal overgrowth **(B, D)**. Note that epithelial expression of ER is retained in this adenosarcoma with stromal overgrowth **(B)**. Most adenosarcomas without stromal overgrowth show a proliferative index with MIB1 of less than 5% overall, but the proliferative index is also generally elevated in periglandular cuffs **(E)**. The proliferative index in adenosarcomas with stromal overgrowth almost always exceeds 5% **(F)**. *From Soslow RA, Ali A, Oliva E. Mullerian adenosarcomas: An immunophenotypic analysis of 35 cases. Am J Surg Pathol. 2008;32:1013-1021.*

sarcoma with a myogenous phenotype. Focal but strong EMA expression in a tumor that closely resembles the undifferentiated carcinoma described by Silva and colleagues would also support that entity.[179,180] Most of these tumors are composed of a diffuse, sheetlike proliferation of small- to intermediate-sized round cells that resemble lymphoma, plasmacytoma, or rhabdoid tumor; they do not show glandular or squamous differentiation and do not contain pleomorphic spindled cells. If clinical correlation is unsatisfactory and the immunophenotype is not contributory, a diagnosis of "undifferentiated malignant neoplasm" should be considered. It is worthwhile to discuss with the contributing gynecologist the extent of immunohistochemical workup needed for surgical planning and the consideration of adjuvant therapy. It is usually more efficient to scrutinize the tumor in a very well-sampled hysterectomy specimen than to spend time and resources using immunohistochemistry on a scant endometrial biopsy specimen. An important exception to this rule is the need to exclude metastasis and lymphoma/leukemia before hysterectomy, if at all possible.

Perivascular Epithelioid Cell Tumors

Perivascular epithelioid cell tumors (PEComas), described to occasionally arise in the uterus,[231-233] belong to a group of tumors with histologic appearances that overlap with those of epithelioid smooth muscle tumors, especially those with clear cytoplasm. PEComas are related to other tuberous sclerosis-associated proliferations (e.g., lymphangioleiomyomatosis and angiomyolipoma) and are composed of specialized or hybrid muscle cells that coexpress muscle markers and some of those associated with melanocytic differentiation, namely HMB45 and Melan-A. Uterine smooth muscle neoplasms can occasionally express HMB45 and/or Melan-A but only in a very restricted distribution.[234,235] PEComas, which are frequently but not always desmin-negative, tend to show much stronger expression of these melanoma-associated markers. It is not known whether or not important clinical differences exist between uterine PEComas and conventional uterine epithelioid smooth muscle tumors. Only rare patients with uterine PEComas have been found to have the tuberous sclerosis complex.[231]

Uterine Tumor Resembling Ovarian Sex Cord Tumor (UTROSCT)

As the name implies, uterine tumor resembling ovarian sex cord tumors (UTROSCTs) contain elements that are reminiscent of Sertoliform tubules or aggregates of granulosa cells.[236] From a morphologic perspective, the differential diagnosis usually concerns an epithelioid smooth muscle tumor, an endometrial stromal tumor with sex cord differentiation or, rarely, an adenocarcinoma. Tumors showing any appreciable endometrial stromal tumor-like features are usually assigned to that category (i.e., endometrial stromal tumor with sex cord–like differentiation) and are not regarded as UTROSCTs. UTROSCTs are probably polyphenotypic tumors that frequently coexpress cytokeratins, muscle markers, and inhibin.[136-139,205] Therefore, this profile should theoretically contrast with that of carcinoma and endometrial stromal and smooth muscle tumors.

Gastrointestinal Stromal Tumor

Although only one primary uterine gastrointestinal stromal tumor (GIST) has been reported,[237] rectal examples may occasionally be mistaken for fibroids. Spindle cell examples would then suggest leiomyoma or perhaps even leiomyosarcoma, and epithelioid varieties could mimic an epithelioid smooth muscle tumor, carcinoma, or even a PEComa or UTROSCT. The successful treatment of GISTs and chronic myelogenous leukemia with imatinib mesylate (Gleevec) has resulted in a great deal of interest in c-kit expression in neoplasms for which good adjuvant therapy does not exist. In several studies, uterine smooth muscle and endometrial stromal neoplasms were negative or rarely immunoreactive for c-*kit*,[138,238,239] although others have shown c-*kit* positivity in leiomyosarcomas and carcinosarcomas.[239-241] Importantly, in one study, immunohistochemical expression of c-*kit* was found in leiomyosarcomas and carcinosarcomas, but *without* activating mutations of the *c-kit* gene.[240] We therefore believe that it is wasteful to analyze uterine smooth muscle tumors and endometrial stromal neoplasms with c-*kit* antibodies for determining candidacy for treatment with Gleevec. However, immunohistochemical stains for c-*kit* along with CD34 are indicated when the differential diagnosis includes both a gynecologic smooth muscle neoplasm and a gastrointestinal stromal tumor.

Inflammatory Myofibroblastic Tumor

This is a very rare, possibly benign uterine tumor that is characterized by a cytologically bland and largely mitotically inactive proliferation of spindle cells in a myxoid matrix.[242] The main differential diagnostic considerations include myxoid leiomyoma and leiomyosarcoma and endometrial stromal neoplasm with myxoid stroma. All inflammatory myofibroblastic tumors reported in the largest series were ALK-positive, which is similar to what has been described to occur in other sites.[242] All uterine mesenchymal neoplasms studied were ALK-negative, including smooth muscle and endometrial stromal tumors and carcinosarcomas.

Gestational Trophoblastic Disease

A number of different trophoblastic lesions occur in the uterus. Some of these are benign, non-neoplastic proliferations, such as placental site reactions and placental site nodules. Hydatiform mole usually has a benign clinical evolution after therapy, but it can give rise to recurrent or progressive gestational trophoblastic disease. Malignant trophoblastic tumors include choriocarcinoma, placental site trophoblastic tumor, and epithelioid trophoblastic tumor. The various types of trophoblastic cells have distinctive immunophenotypes, so it is possible to use immunohistochemistry to assist in the diagnosis of trophoblastic lesions. Trophoblastic lesions include hydatidiform mole (partial, complete, and invasive), choriocarcinoma, placental site trophoblastic tumor, epithelioid trophoblastic tumor, exaggerated placental site, and placental site nodule. Immunohistochemistry is rarely used for the diagnosis of hydatidiform moles, although there is an emerging role for p57, as discussed in the following section.

Trophoblasts, including cytotrophoblasts, intermediate trophoblasts, and syncytiotrophoblasts, stain strongly and diffusely with cytokeratins (AE1/AE3),[243] while inhibin,[248,245] CD10,[52,246] CK18,[247,248] and hydroxyl-d-5-steroid dehydrogenase (HSD3B1) are

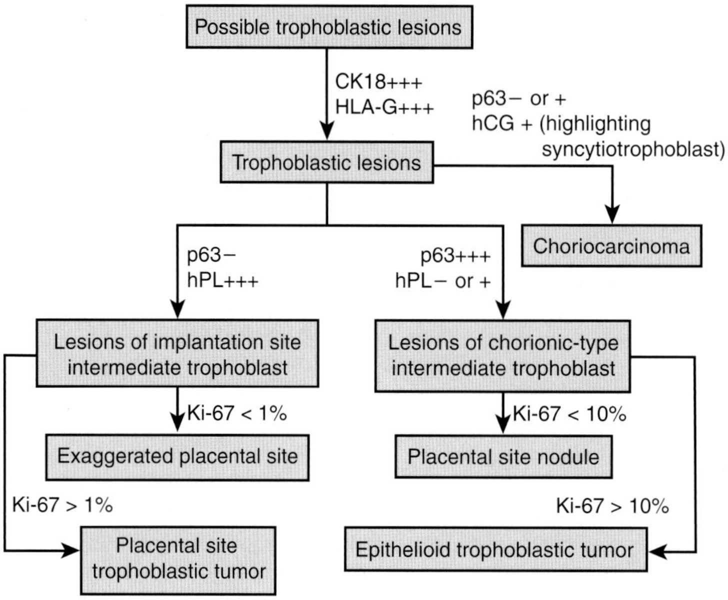

FIGURE 18.20 An algorithm using a panel of immunohistochemical markers is useful for the differential diagnosis of trophoblastic lesions. The algorithm begins with immunostaining with CK18 and HLA-G antibodies. If they are both diffusely positive, the lesion is trophoblastic. If p63 is selectively stained in mononucleate trophoblasts and hCG is selectively stained in syncytiotrophoblast, the lesion is a choriocarcinoma. If p63 is negative and hPL is diffusely positive, the lesion is either an exaggerated placental site or a PSTT. These lesions can be distinguished based on the Ki-67 labeling index. If p63 is diffusely positive and only focally positive for hPL, the lesion is either PSN or ETT. These lesions can be distinguished based on the Ki-67 labeling index (+++, diffusely positive; +, focally positive; –, negative). *From Shih IM, Kurman RJ. p63 expression is useful in the distinction of epithelioid trophoblastic and placental site trophoblastic tumors by profiling trophoblastic subpopulations. Am J Surg Pathol. 2004;28:1177-1183.*

good pan-trophoblastic markers.[247,249] Mel-CAM (also known as CD146), a membrane glycoprotein of the immunoglobulin gene superfamily involved in cell-to-cell interaction,[250] is a good general marker of intermediate trophoblasts, as is HLA-G.[251] Syncytiotrophoblasts stain strongly with human chorionic gonadotropin (hCG) as do some intermediate trophoblasts of implantation site type.[252] Human placental lactogen (hPL) marks intermediate trophoblasts of the implantation site type and it also stains syncytiotrophoblasts.[252] Placental alkaline phosphatase (PLAP) is expressed in intermediate cells and syncytiotrophoblastic cells as well,[253] but the intermediate trophoblasts marked here are of chorionic type.[252,254] Chorionic type intermediate trophoblasts also express p63.[248] Cytotrophoblasts express β-catenin.[255-257]

The trophogram is a diagram developed by Ie-Ming Shih and colleagues that provides diagnostic help for trophoblastic lesions using a decision tree format (Fig. 18.20).[248,249] First, trophoblastic lesions express CK18, HSD3B1, and HLA-G diffusely. hCG expression in numerous syncytiotrophoblasts intimately admixed with mononuclear trophoblasts favors choriocarcinoma. For lesions without numerous syncytiotrophoblasts, hPL expression without p63 favors a lesion composed of implantation site intermediate trophoblasts (exaggerated placental site versus placental site trophoblastic tumor [PSTT]); p63 expression with variable hPL favors a lesion composed of chorionic-type intermediate trophoblast (placental site nodule versus epithelioid trophoblastic tumor [ETT]). Ki-67 labeling of less than 1% favors exaggerated placental site reaction over PSTT, and Ki-67 labeling of less than 8% to 10% favors placental site nodule over ETT.

COMPLETE HYDATIDIFORM MOLE

The morphologic criteria for distinguishing complete hydatidiform moles from mimickers are robust, particularly when the tissue is derived from a second trimester conceptus. Detection of abnormal gestations in the first trimester has led to diagnostic difficulties, however, because increased villous size and trophoblastic proliferation are less pronounced than in tissue derived from more advanced gestations. Complete moles diagnosed in the first trimester have been referred to as "early" complete hydatidiform moles. Immunohistochemical evaluation with antibodies against the p57 protein, a maternally transcribed gene product, has emerged as a useful adjunct to morphologic, flow cytometric, and cytogenetic study of molar tissue. Whereas p57 protein is expressed in intermediate trophoblasts of complete moles, partial moles, and non-molar abortuses, only complete hydatidiform moles lack p57 expression in cytotrophoblasts and villous stromal cells.[258-262] Subtle, but reproducible, morphologic differences between early complete moles and other entities in the differential have been reported.[263,264]

Using ancillary diagnostic techniques, including cytogenetics and assays for DNA ploidy (see the "Genomic Applications" section), it has become evident that many early complete hydatidiform moles have historically been misdiagnosed as non-molar abortuses or partial moles. This has led to the mistaken impression that the development of choriocarcinoma from partial mole is a common event. In fact, choriocarcinoma almost never follows partial mole when it is diagnosed correctly; early complete moles, in contrast, remain a common source from which choriocarcinoma evolves.

PLACENTAL SITE NODULE

Placental site nodules are composed of mitotically inactive intermediate trophoblastic cells of chorionic type within a nodular, hyalinized stroma. Lesional cells express pan-trophoblastic markers as well as the chorionic intermediate trophoblast-associated markers PLAP and p63. The Ki-67 index in a placental site nodule is less than 10% to 15%.[265]

EXAGGERATED PLACENTAL SITE

This lesion, actually an exuberant, non-neoplastic physiologic finding that frequently accompanies molar pregnancies, is composed mostly of implantation site intermediate trophoblasts. The constituent cells express human placental lactogen (hPL) and HLA-G.[251] The Ki-67 index in an exaggerated placental site reaction is less than 10% to 15%.[266]

PLACENTAL SITE TROPHOBLASTIC TUMOR (PSTT)

This tumor is composed of neoplastic implantation site intermediate trophoblasts that infiltrate myometrium. hPL and HLA-G are typically expressed. Placental site trophoblastic tumors have an index of 14% (+/– 7%).[266] PSTTs can also contain scattered hCG-expressing syncytiotrophoblasts, but they are rare and haphazardly situated, not intimately admixed with mononuclear trophoblasts as is typical of choriocarcinoma. Biopsy or curettage material may suggest the presence of PSTT or placental site nodule. Both the immunophenotype and proliferative index of these lesions differ, with preferential expression of hPL and HLA-G in PSTT, as opposed to PLAP and p63 in placental site nodule.[248,249]

EPITHELIOID TROPHOBLASTIC TUMOR (ETT)

This tumor is composed of chorionic site intermediate trophoblasts that tend to arise in the cervix where they have a rounded contour and a pushing pattern of stromal of stromal infiltration.[267] PLAP and p63 are expressed, but hPL and HLA-G are not.[248,249] Owing to its frequently cervical location and its epithelioid, eosinophilic appearance, this tumor can be confused with squamous carcinoma. ETT shares expression of p63 with squamous cell carcinoma, but ETT expresses the trophoblast-associated markers inhibin, CD10,[244,267] CK18,[248] and HSD3B1.[248] ETTs lack the p16 expression that is typical of HPV-associated squamous neoplasms.[268]

CHORIOCARCINOMA

It was previously thought that choriocarcinomas were biphasic neoplasms composed of mononuclear cytotrophoblasts and multinucleate syncytiotrophoblasts. While it is certainly still the case that these tumors have a biphasic appearance with H&E stains, they are actually triphasic using markers that recognize cytotrophoblasts, intermediate trophoblasts, and syncytiotrophoblasts.[257] Cytotrophoblasts, which show nuclear labeling with antibodies against β-catenin, represent a small minority of the mononuclear cells; most of the mononuclear cells in choriocarcinomas are actually intermediate trophoblasts.[257]

The main differential diagnostic entities to consider with a tumor that resembles gestational choriocarcinoma include germinal choriocarcinoma, complete hydatidiform mole with sparse villi, epithelioid and placental site trophoblastic tumors, and carcinomas containing trophoblastic elements. Germinal choriocarcinoma without admixture of other germ cell elements is so rare in women that it really is not a viable diagnostic consideration. The trophoblastic proliferation associated with a complete mole may be histologically indistinguishable from choriocarcinoma, but it is not clear whether immunohistochemical differences exist. Therefore, with the exception of the rare choriocarcinomas that arise in non-molar placentas and those that coexist with a non-molar twin, choriocarcinoma cannot be diagnosed confidently when villi are present.

Choriocarcinomas and tumors composed of intermediate trophoblasts may resemble one another when syncytiotrophoblasts are few; this is particularly problematic when presented with tissue from choriocarcinomas previously exposed to chemotherapeutic agents.[269] Serum hCG levels are likely to be very helpful because choriocarcinomas (even those relatively deficient in syncytiotrophoblasts) are frequently associated with higher serum levels than is the case with intermediate trophoblastic tumors. As expected, an hCG immunostain would mark syncytiotrophoblasts that are almost always more numerous in choriocarcinoma as compared to placental site and epithelioid trophoblastic tumors.[252] An hCG immunostain would also be expected to highlight the characteristic morphologic relationship of syncytiotrophoblasts and mononuclear trophoblasts in choriocarcinoma, in which the multinucleated cells envelop the mononuclear cells. A MIB1 immunostain is likely to be even more helpful when syncytiotrophoblasts are very few in number; the proliferative rate is usually 15% to 25% in tumors derived from intermediate trophoblasts, while it frequently exceeds 70% in choriocarcinoma.[266] Based on current data, study with immunohistochemistry is not useful for the separation of gestational choriocarcinoma from a carcinoma that contains trophoblastic elements, which can be seen in cervical squamous carcinoma and transitional cell carcinoma of the bladder, in addition to others (See Table 18.4).[270,271] Syncytiotrophoblasts encountered in occasional pleomorphic carcinomas express hCG as well.

Genomic Applications

DNA MISMATCH REPAIR PROTEINS

As discussed earlier in the chapter, DNA MMR proteins are found to be lacking in tumor cell nuclei by immunohistochemistry in up to one third of endometrioid

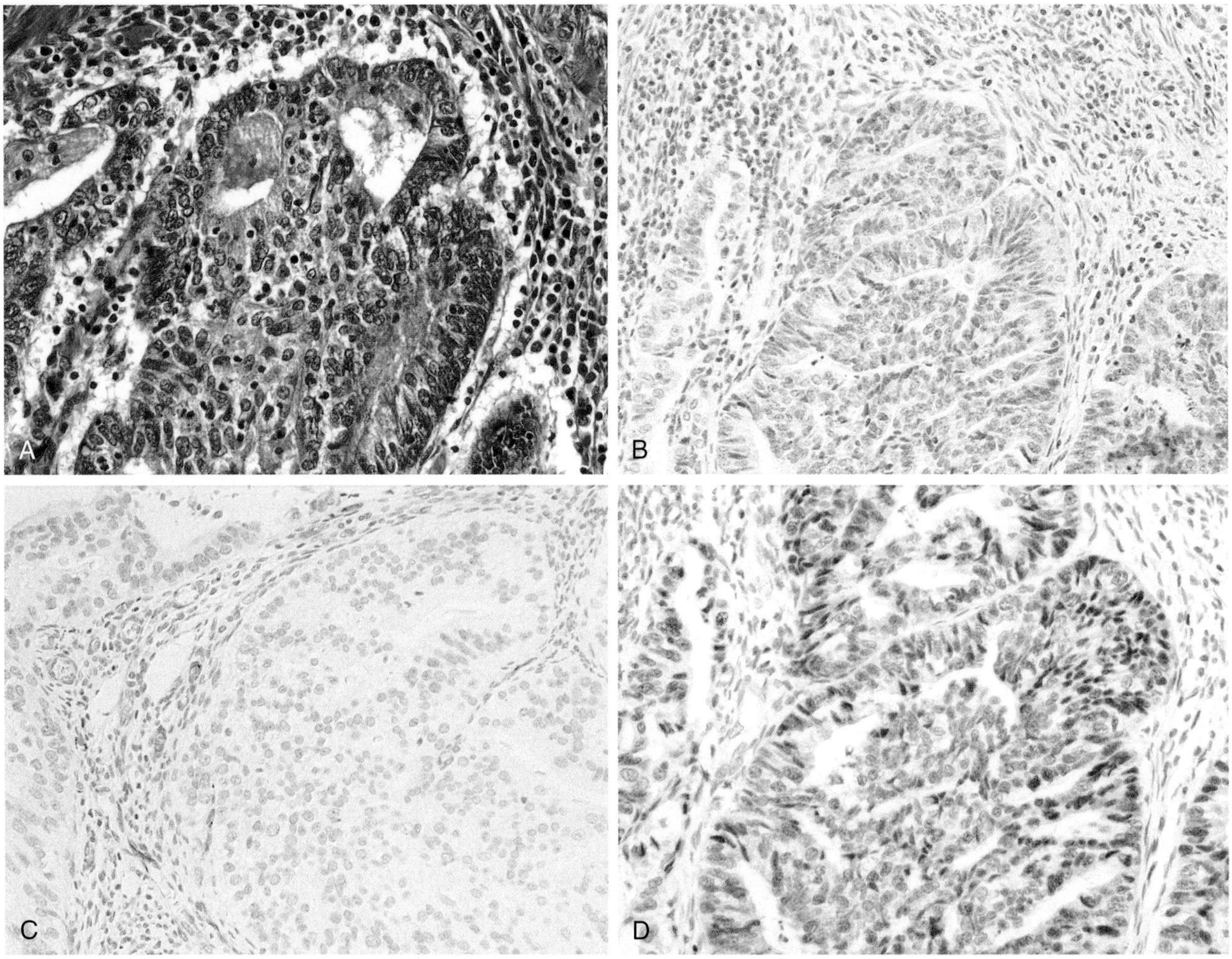

FIGURE 18.21 DNA mismatch repair protein expression in endometrial carcinoma. An endometrioid adenocarcinoma (H&E, **A**) showing negative staining for PMS2 **(B)**, focal weak positive nuclear staining for MLH1 **(C)**, and positive nuclear staining for MSH2 **(D)**. Note inset in **(B)** showing positive nuclear labeling in stromal cells that serves as a positive internal control. *From Modica I, Soslow RA, Black D, et al. Utility of immunohistochemistry in predicting microsatellite instability in endometrial carcinoma. Am J Surg Pathol. 2007;31:744-751.*

adenocarcinomas;[157-160] this results from MLH1 promoter hypermethylation in most cases and from mutation of *MLH1, MSH2, MSH6,* or *PMS2* in the remaining cases (Fig. 18.21). Mutation of one of these genes (not loss of expression alone) indicates that the affected patient is part of an HNPCC kindred.[272-274] Therefore, DNA MMR protein immunohistochemistry can serve as a screen for HNPCC, but it is not a diagnostic test.

In an effort to define a target endometrial cancer population in which the DNA MMR stains might be informative, several institutions have begun testing for DNA MMR abnormalities in endometrial carcinomas that occur in women younger than 50 years of age and in older women whose tumors exhibit morphologic features that have been reported to covary with high levels of microsatellite instability (MSI-H).[182] Such morphologic features, although not specific and currently considered of debatable significance, include dense peritumoral lymphocytes and tumor-infiltrating lymphocytes (greater than 40 TILs per 10 high power fields) and biphasic tumors with the appearance of a collision tumor, such as the de-differentiated carcinoma described earlier in the chapter.[180,182,275] Most HNPCC tumors are endometrioid, but a proportion of endometrial clear cell carcinomas may also belong to this group.[172,181] The preliminary data from a study investigating the feasibility and utility of testing such patients' tumors for DNA MMR expression indicate disproportionate representation of tumors lacking MSH2 and MSH6 expression,[182] indirectly indicating mutation in either of the corresponding genes and membership in an HNPCC kindred.[276] Tumors lacking MLH1 and PMS2 are also well represented, but additional testing is required in this scenario to determine whether loss of expression is due to epigenetic mechanisms (i.e., a sporadic tumor) or a mutation.[277,278] Any patient with an abnormal immunohistochemical result is currently referred for a comprehensive genetics evaluation that might include MSI testing and, when indicated, methylation and mutational analysis of the candidate genes. These techniques are discussed later in "Beyond Immunohistochemistry: Anatomic Molecular Diagnostic Applications to Diagnosis."

Almost as a rule, expression loss, when present, occurs in couplets (MLH1 with PMS2 and MSH2 with MSH6). Only complete expression loss in the setting of a valid positive internal control is considered interpretable. Valid internal controls include non-neoplastic endometrial stroma and glands with reproducibly stained nuclei. Care should be taken to ensure that the lesion being assessed is adenocarcinoma, not hyperplasia.[160] It is also extremely important that the immunohistochemical methodology and interpretation of stains be performed with the strictest guidelines in mind, as performing and interpreting the MLH1 stain, in particular, is very tricky.[160] Interpreting an MLH1 stain as negative in the absence of a valid positive internal control, as discussed previously, is a rather common occurrence. Common pitfalls in interpreting these stains are discussed in a review by Shia and associates.[279] In a series studied by Modica and colleagues,[160] IHC with MLH1 and MSH2 antibodies had a sensitivity of 69% and a specificity of 100% in detecting MSI-H. Addition of PMS2 and MSH6 antibodies improved the sensitivity to 91% but decreased the specificity to 83%. The decreased specificity was primarily due to loss of MSH6, which is known to be found occasionally in endometrial carcinomas that are MSI-low or MSI-stable. It has been proposed that a simple panel including only MSH6 and PMS2 could allow recognition of all colorectal carcinoma mutation carriers,[279] but this has not yet been tested in endometrial carcinoma patients.

The ethical and regulatory issues regarding reflexive IHC testing for DNA MMR protein expression are currently unresolved. Some institutions require specific patient consent for IHC testing, whereas others have added general statements regarding genetic testing in standard surgical consent forms. Yet others do not currently require any patient consent, the idea being that IHC testing in this setting is not a direct test of a patient's genome. If this approach is chosen, it is recommended that all involved pathologists, gynecologic oncologists, and geneticists agree to the medical necessity of performing the test and arrange a chain of command that guarantees that all targeted patient material is tested and that all applicable patients are referred for the appropriate counseling.

Theranostic Applications

ENDOMETRIAL CARCINOMA

p53, ER, and PR

Although stage and grade are still considered the most important prognostic indices in endometrial cancer, much has been written about using immunohistochemistry to predict prognosis. Of possible relevance is immunohistochemical overexpression of p53. Several studies have now documented that overexpression of p53 is a negative prognostic indicator in endometrial cancer.[195,280-282] It is possible that ER and PR expression is also of therapeutic and even prognostic relevance here, as it has recently been shown that tumors overexpressing p53 while coexpressing ER and PR are less aggressive than those without ER and PR expression.[165] This observation was understood to mean that occasional high-grade endometrial carcinomas represent tumors that have progressed or transformed from ER- and PR-positive low-grade endometrioid carcinomas that acquire p53 mutations. Clinicians commonly request ER and PR testing for metastatic or recurrent endometrial carcinoma when therapy with hormonal agents, particularly high-dose progestins, is considered.

HER2/neu

A large percentage of uterine serous carcinomas overexpress HER2/neu,[283-287] but there is an imperfect correlation with *HER2/neu* gene amplification. Several studies have reported a relationship between HER2 neu overexpression and poor clinical outcomes. The Gynecologic Oncology Group (GOG) attempted to study the efficacy of trastuzumab (GOG 181B), but the results of this have not yet been published.

UTERINE SARCOMA

ER, PR, p53, MIB1, *c-kit*, p16

As independent variables, expression of ER, PR, p53, and MIB1 has a prognostic significance in leiomyosarcoma[199,202,204,208,209,211]; however, these lose significance in multivariate models in which stage remains the most important prognostic factor. In several studies, uterine smooth muscle and endometrial stromal neoplasms were negative or rarely immunoreactive for c-*kit*,[138,238,239] although others have shown c-*kit* positivity in leiomyosarcomas and carcinosarcomas.[240,241] Importantly, in one study immunohistochemical expression of c-*kit* was found in leiomyosarcomas and carcinosarcomas, but *without* activating mutations of the *c-kit* gene.[240] We therefore believe it is wasteful to analyze uterine smooth muscle tumors and endometrial stromal neoplasms with c-*kit* antibodies for determining candidacy for treatment with Gleevec. Finally, a number of recent publications have called attention to the significance of p16 expression in atypical uterine smooth muscle tumors, although the mechanisms underlying p16 overexpression in uterine sarcomas has not been elucidated.[288-291] Among uterine leiomyomas, smooth muscle tumors of uncertain malignant potential (STUMPs) and leiomyosarcomas, p16 expression is found mostly in leiomyosarcomas and in a subset of STUMPs, some of which behave in a malignant fashion. The implication is that STUMPS that overexpress p16 might be at higher risk of relapse compared to those that are p16-negative. This remains to be studied in greater detail.

Retrospective data suggest that progestational agents are a beneficial adjuvant therapy, so clinicians frequently request ER and PR testing for low-grade sarcomas such as endometrial stromal sarcomas and adenosarcomas. This is actually unnecessary in most cases because more than 90% of these tumors express ER and PR when they are histologically low grade and when (in the case of adenosarcoma) stromal overgrowth is lacking.[229]

Beyond Immunohistochemistry: Anatomic Molecular Diagnostic Applications to Diagnosis

DNA MMR GENES AND ASSOCIATED ASSAYS (FIG. 18.22)

Assays for microsatellite instability (MSI), methylation of the *MLH1* promoter, and sequencing of DNA mismatch repair (DNA MMR) genes are used to determine whether endometrial cancer patients whose tumors lack expression of one or more of the DNA MMR proteins are part of an HNPCC/Lynch syndrome kindred. Mutation of one of the commonly assayed DNA MMR genes (*MLH1, MSH2, MSH6, PMS2*) confirms a clinical diagnosis of HNPCC/Lynch syndrome, but the test is cumbersome, time-consuming, and expensive. MSI analysis can be used to identify patients at risk for HNPCC, but MSI does not distinguish genetic (heritable) and epigenetic (not heritable) mechanisms that lead to high-frequency MSI (MSI-H). Because assays that detect methylation of the *MLH1* promoter can recognize epigenetic mechanisms that lead to MSI-H, one can derive information, albeit indirect, regarding DNA MMR mutation if both MSI and methylation assays are performed.[181] A patient whose tumor is MSI-H but lacks *MLH1* promoter methylation will likely have HNPCC, whereas one whose tumor is MSI-H with *MLH1* promoter methylation probably does not. Many patients display the clinical manifestations of the syndrome without a known mutation; it is assumed that these patients have uncharacterized mutations in one of these four genes or in other genes. Some of these presumed mutations do not lead to detectable MSI-H. Many uncharacterized mutations are thought to involve *MSH6*. Immunohistochemistry is a reasonable screen for these.

IHC loss of MSH2 with MSH6 usually indicates a mutation in either *MSH2* or *MSH6*.[276] Paradoxically, recent data suggest that sequencing studies and microsatellite instability analysis may be unnecessary and even potentially misleading when IHC shows loss of MSH2 and/or MSH6.[279] Many MSH6 mutations are as yet uncharacterized and cannot be identified using sequencing. Also, mutations in *MSH6*, encountered in larger proportions of HNPCC-associated endometrial cancers as compared to HNPCC-associated colon cancers, result in lower rates of MSI-H when compared to mutations in *MSH2* or *MLH1*. *MSH6* mutations could therefore potentially be missed on MSI analysis alone.[276,292-294]

However, when MLH1 and/or PMS2 are lost using IHC, additional testing is warranted. In these instances, a methylation assay can be informative. The presence of *MLH1* promoter methylation is usually sufficient to indicate that a given endometrial cancer is sporadic, not HNPCC defining. Absence of *MLH1* promoter methylation coupled with immunohistochemical loss of MLH1 and/or PMS2 are together highly suspicious for HNPCC.[181] The *MLH1* and *PMS2* genes can then be sequenced to detect a mutation, which would confirm HNPCC. However, only a minority of patients whose tumors lack MLH1 and/or PMS2 have HNPCC.[181] A discussion of the relevant immunohistochemical features and regulatory complexities surrounding IHC testing can be found earlier in the text.

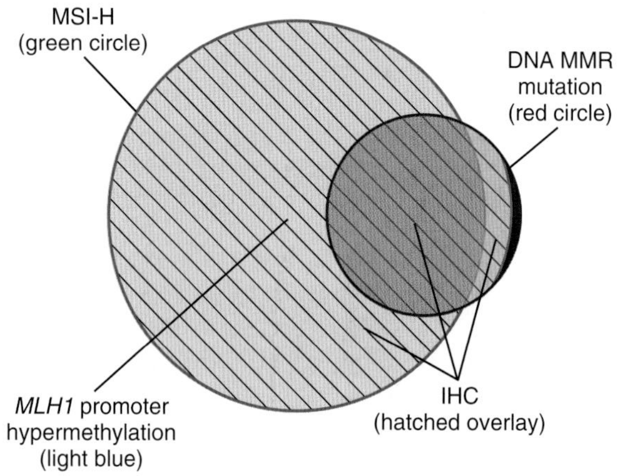

FIGURE 18.22 Relationship between DNA mismatch repair gene mutation, microsatellite instability, and DNA mismatch repair immunohistochemistry in endometrial carcinoma. Endometrial carcinoma patients with hereditary non-polyposis colorectal cancer/Lynch syndrome have mutations in one of the DNA MMR genes, represented by the area inside the red circle. In endometrial cancer, mutations in MSH2 or MSH6 far outnumber those involving MLH1. Approximately 80% of cases with gene mutations can be indirectly detected with microsatellite instability testing, indicated by the area inside the green circle (MSI-H). MSI testing, however, is not specific for DNA MMR gene mutation, as most MSI-H cases, indicated by areas shaded light green, arise secondary to MLH1 promoter hypermethylation, not gene mutation. These patients have MSI-H cancers that are sporadic, and the affected patients do not have hereditary non-polyposis colorectal cancer/Lynch syndrome. MSI testing is also somewhat insensitive for gene mutations in general and MSH6 mutations specifically (i.e., it does not recognize all mutated cases). These cases are represented by the sliver of grey shading within the red circle between the green and blue lines. Abnormalities with immunohistochemical testing for DNA MMR expression (IHC; areas underneath the hatched overlay) detect a greater percentage of gene mutation cases than does MSI testing, including many MSH6 mutated cases, but, similar to MSI testing, IHC recognizes many sporadic cases as well. Finally, there are rare mutations that cannot be recognized by either MSI or IHC testing (red sliver outside the blue line).

JAZF1-JJAZ1 Translocation

The translocation between chromosome 7p15 and 17q21 gives rise to a fusion gene containing contributions from 2 genes with prominent zinc finger motifs: *JAZF1* and *JJAZ1*.[295] This translocation has been documented in approximately 50% of low-grade endometrial stromal sarcomas and endometrial stromal nodules.[295-300] Endometrial stromal tumors with typical morphologic features and the smooth muscle variant are more frequently composed of cells that harbor this abnormality when compared with tumors showing fibroblastic differentiation.[301] RT-PCR to detect the fusion gene product[295,297,298] and FISH for the gene rearrangement[299,300] are assays used to identify this aberration. t(7;17) is apparently specific for tumors in the endometrial stromal category, as this has not yet been described in other tumor types.

GESTATIONAL TROPHOBLASTIC DISEASE

Studies for DNA ploidy, including computer-assisted image analysis of Feulgen stains, and cytogenetics, including fluorescent *in situ* hybridization (FISH), have been used to distinguish between non-molar abortuses and partial hydatidiform mole and between partial and complete hydatidiform moles. In contrast to partial moles, which are almost always triploid, non-molar abortuses and complete moles are usually diploid. Some complete moles are tetraploid[301] and some non-molar abortuses are triploid.[302] In the case of a triploid conceptus, distinguishing between diandric triploidy and digynic triploidy is important, as partial moles are specifically diandric.[303] That is, partial moles contain 2 sets of paternal chromosomes and 1 set of maternal chromosomes.

OVARY

Ovarian neoplasms can be divided into four main categories: primary epithelial tumors, sex cord–stromal tumors, germ cell tumors, and other types of tumors. The latter includes a wide variety of primary and metastatic tumors, including mesenchymal neoplasms, lymphoma and leukemia, and metastatic epithelial tumors. Tumors of the fallopian tube are primarily epithelial, and resemble their ovarian counterparts. A detailed classification of ovarian and tubal tumors is presented in the WHO fascicle *Pathology and Genetics of Tumours of the Breast and Female Genital Organs*.[304] Ovarian and tubal neoplasms can usually be correctly diagnosed using routine H&E-stained sections. Each of the main categories of tumors has distinctive immunohistochemical features, however, and immunohistochemistry is often useful to establish or confirm a diagnosis. Ovarian tumors are relatively uncommon, so pathologists often have little experience with them. Immunohistochemical stains can be used to suggest or support a diagnosis. Immunohistochemistry is an important aid in the classification of poorly differentiated neoplasms, and it is essential for the diagnosis and classification of some metastatic or systemic tumors that involve the ovary.

Immunohistochemical Markers

A relatively small number of antibodies are sufficient for the diagnosis of most ovarian and tubal tumors. These core antibodies are listed in the following paragraphs. Additional antibodies are sometimes helpful and are discussed where appropriate in subsequent sections.

CYTOKERATIN

Keratins are intermediate filament proteins that contribute to the cytoskeleton of epithelial cells. As they are present in all epithelial cells, immunostains for cytokeratins are useful as a screening test to identify a neoplasm as being of epithelial type. Human cytokeratins have been classified according to their molecular weights and isoelectric pHs in the catalog published by Moll and colleagues.[305] Twenty epithelial cytokeratin polypeptides have been identified. Some of these have specific tissue distributions that can be exploited for the differential diagnosis of tumors. For screening purposes, a wide spectrum antibody that recognizes many different cytokeratins is most valuable. We use a cocktail of AE1/AE3 and CAM5.2.

CYTOKERATIN 7

Cytokeratin 7 (CK7) is a type II basic low molecular weight cytokeratin that is found in simple epithelia in a variety of organs, including all epithelia in the female genital tract.[305,306] Epithelial tumors of the ovary and fallopian tube all exhibit cytoplasmic and/or membrane staining for CK7.[307-309] This characteristic staining pattern of female genital tract tumors can be used, usually in combination with staining for other keratins such as CK20, to differentiate primary female genital tract adenocarcinomas from adenocarcinomas arising in other organs.[149,310] A panel of immunostains needs to be evaluated because some primary ovarian neoplasms fail to stain for CK7 and a proportion of metastatic carcinomas in the ovary are CK7-positive.[311]

CYTOKERATIN 20

Cytokeratin 20 (CK20) is a type I acidic low molecular weight cytokeratin that was initially described in 1992.[312] It is found in normal tissues of the stomach, intestine, urothelium, and in Merkel cells. It is found in most adenocarcinomas of the large and small intestines, in mucinous tumors of the ovary, and in Merkel cell carcinomas, and it is frequently present in urothelial carcinoma and in adenocarcinomas of the stomach, pancreas, and bile ducts.[310,313] It is a useful marker for primary mucinous tumors of the ovary and for various types of metastases that are found in the ovaries.[314-316] Most primary non-mucinous epithelial tumors are CK20-negative.

ANTI-ADENOCARCINOMA ANTIBODIES

Antibodies that are reactive against adenocarcinoma, but nonreactive with mesothelial cells, are used in a panel for the differential diagnosis between adenocarcinoma and mesothelioma. The antibodies that have been used for this purpose include CD15, Ber-EP4, monoclonal carcinoembryonic antigen (mCEA), and MOC 31. CD15 (LeuM1) is used mainly in hematopathology as it is reactive in neutrophils, histiocytes, immunoblasts, and classic Reed-Sternberg cells, but it also stains various adenocarcinomas. Positive staining is reported in about one third to two thirds of ovarian serous carcinomas and in a higher percentage of endometrioid and clear cell adenocarcinomas.[317,318] Staining can be either granular and cytoplasmic or membranous. Ber-EP4 is a monoclonal antibody directed against glycoproteins on epithelial cells that shows diffuse strong membrane staining in nearly all serous carcinomas of the ovary and peritoneum.[317,319] Monoclonal CEA is rarely positive in ovarian cancers, with the exception of mucinous adenocarcinomas, which are typically CEA-positive.[317,319-326] Areas of squamous differentiation in endometrioid adenocarcinoma can also show staining for CEA. Polyclonal CEA appears to be less specific than monoclonal CEA and stains a somewhat greater percentage of ovarian carcinomas. B72.3 is a monoclonal antibody against a tumor related glycoprotein (TAG-72).[327] It is usually positive in carcinomas of the ovary, exhibiting a granular cytoplasmic staining pattern.[317,319,328] This stain can be difficult to interpret, because there is often background staining of mucin and other secretions. MOC 31 is a monoclonal antibody against a glycoprotein that shows strong membrane staining in most cases of ovarian cancer.[317] All of these antibodies are negative or only rarely immunoreactive in mesothelioma. In general, Ber-EP4, MOC-31, and B72.3 are more sensitive for detection of ovarian surface epithelial tumors than LeuM1 and CEA.

CA125

CA125 is a high molecular weight glycoprotein recognized by the monoclonal antibody OC 125, which has intracellular, transmembrane, and extracellular domains.[329-331] The OC 125 and M11 binding sites are located in the extracellular domain.[329] CA125 is commonly expressed by primary non-mucinous epithelial ovarian cancers, but can also be expressed by various other gynecologic cancers, including tumors of the cervix, endometrium, and fallopian tube, and by certain non-gynecologic cancers, including those of the pancreas, breast, colon, lung, and thyroid.[332-334] Normal endometrium expresses CA125 and can be used as a positive control.[335] Mesothelioma can also be immunoreactive for CA125.[328] Evaluation for the expression of CA125 (OC125) is of limited value because female genital surface epithelial proliferations, metastatic carcinomas from extragenital sites, and mesothelial proliferations can all express CA125.[332,336]

INHIBIN

Inhibin is a dimeric 32-kD glycoprotein hormone that participates in the regulation of the pituitary-gonadal feedback system.[337-340] Inhibins secreted in the ovary consist of an α-subunit linked to one of two β-subunits. In inhibin A an α-subunit is linked to a β-A subunit; in inhibin B an α-subunit is linked to a β-B subunit. The monoclonal antibody in general use for immunohistochemistry recognizes inhibin A. Inhibin is a sensitive and relatively specific marker of sex cord–stromal tumors of the ovary, and its main use in gynecologic pathology is in the differential diagnosis of such tumors.[341-346] Luteinized stromal cells that are sometimes present around carcinomas can express inhibin,[341,343,347] which can lead to the erroneous interpretation that a carcinoma expresses inhibin. In general, inhibin expression in carcinomas is encountered uncommonly, and when it is, the pattern is only exceptionally strong and diffuse.[341,343,347-349] Adrenal cortical neoplasms also commonly express inhibin.[350-355]

CALRETININ

Calretinin is a 29-kD calcium-binding protein that was initially detected in the central nervous system.[356] It belongs to the same family of EF-hand proteins as the S-100 proteins.[357,358] Subsequent studies revealed that calretinin is present in benign mesothelial cells and mesothelioma, and it is now the most widely used marker for mesothelioma. Staining is both cytoplasmic and nuclear, with nuclear staining required for specificity for mesothelioma. Calretinin is also present in mast cells, schwannoma, granular cell tumor, adrenal cortical tumors, and, of particular interest to gynecologic pathologists, in sex cord–stromal tumors of the ovary. Calretinin stains a broader range of sex cord–stromal tumors than inhibin, and it is a more sensitive but less specific marker of such tumors.[346,359-361] It is typically used in an immunohistochemical panel that also includes inhibin.

WT1

The Wilms' tumor gene, WT1, is located on chromosome 11 at 11p13. It functions in the development of the genitourinary tract and is thought to have a tumor suppressor function.[362] The Wilms' tumor gene product is a DNA binding protein that is localized in the nucleus. Positive nuclear staining is observed in Wilms' tumor,[363] desmoplastic small round cell tumor,[364-366] and mesothelioma.[367,368] WT1 is expressed in the ovarian surface epithelium, in inclusion cysts, and in normal tubal epithelium.[369] There is expression in serous carcinoma of the ovary, fallopian tube, and peritoneum,[368] but expression in serous carcinoma of the endometrium tends to be limited. Both polyclonal and monoclonal antibodies to WT1 are available. The sensitivity for staining of serous carcinoma is high, with nuclear staining in more than 90% of cases reported in some studies.[167,367] Other ovarian tumors reported to express WT1 include transitional cell carcinoma, small cell carcinoma of hypercalcemic type, and some sex cord–stromal tumors.[346,370,371]

PLACENTAL ALKALINE PHOSPHATASE

Placental alkaline phosphatase (PLAP) is a marker for malignant germ cell tumors, especially dysgerminoma and embryonal carcinoma. However, positive staining is also seen in some epithelial tumors, especially serous carcinomas.[372,373] PLAP is a useful marker for dysgerminoma and neoplasms that contain related cells,[374] such as gonadoblastoma.[375] Absence of PLAP expression is unusual in dysgerminoma, but expression of PLAP does not prove that a tumor is a dysgerminoma as nondysgerminomatous germ cell tumors and some carcinomas also express PLAP.

CD117

The CD117 protein is a transmembrane, tyrosine kinase growth factor receptor that is the product of *c-kit* gene expression. It is present in a variety of normal human cell types, including breast epithelium, germ cells, melanocytes, immature myeloid cells, and mast cells.[376,377] Staining for CD117 occurs in a variety of tumor types, although strong staining is present mainly in mast cell disease and gastrointestinal stromal tumors, for which

CD117 is the preferred marker.[376,378-380] A minority of serous ovarian carcinomas stain strongly for CD117.[376] In ovarian pathology, CD117 is most useful as a marker of dysgerminoma, which shows diffuse strong membrane staining in nearly all cases.[377,381,382] CD117 does not stain embryonal carcinoma, and is thus a more specific marker of dysgerminoma than is PLAP. Since metastatic melanoma can occasionally mimic dysgerminoma, it is worth noting that melanoma is occasionally CD117-positive, although usually with a cytoplasmic staining pattern.

Oct-4

Oct-4, also known as POU5F1, is a nuclear transcription factor that is necessary for maintenance of the pluripotentiality of stem cells and primordial germ cells.[383] There is positive staining in the nuclei of such pluripotential germ cell tumors as dysgerminoma and embryonal carcinoma and for *in situ* germ cell neoplasia such as intratubular germ cell neoplasia in the testis and gonadoblastoma in dysgenetic gonads.[384,385] Other types of germ cell tumors are negative. Oct-4 has proven to be an excellent immunostain, as staining is generally strong and diffuse, and interpretation is usually straightforward even in small samples, or samples with crush artifact or necrosis. In one study, staining for Oct-4 was noted in the germ cells in dysgenetic gonads in children up to at least the age of 14 months.[386] Therefore, positive staining of germ cells in a dysgenetic gonad from a young patient should not be taken as an indication of germ cell neoplasia unless a tumor with clear cut features of a gonadoblastoma, germinoma, or embryonal carcinoma is present. NANOG is another stem cell marker that stains pluripotential germ cell tumors such as dysgerminoma in a manner similar to Oct-4.[387] NANOG has not been as widely used in diagnostic pathology as Oct-4.

ALPHA-FETOPROTEIN

Alpha-fetoprotein (AFP) is an oncofetal glycoprotein that is expressed in yolk sac tumor and its variants, including hepatoid and endometrioid yolk sac tumor.[388-394] Other ovarian tumors that are frequently AFP-positive are the rare ovarian hepatoid carcinoma,[395-397] metastatic hepatocellular carcinoma,[396,398] and Sertoli-Leydig cell tumors with heterologous hepatocytic differentiation.[399-401] Among ovarian germ cell tumors, AFP expression is almost entirely confined to yolk sac tumors,[390,402] although focal expression can be seen in embryonal carcinoma and in hepatic or enteric tissues in teratomas.[403-407] Rarely, AFP-positive yolk sac tumors have been reported to arise from somatic adenocarcinomas such as endometrioid adenocarcinoma.[224,408] For the most part, however, AFP expression in an ovarian tumor is indicative of a yolk sac tumor given the appropriate morphologic context.

HUMAN CHORIONIC GONADOTROPIN

Human chorionic gonadotropin is a glycoprotein hormone secreted by syncytiotrophoblastic cells. Like other glycoprotein hormones, it consists of an α-chain linked to a β-chain by disulfide bonds. The α-chain is identical to that in follicle-stimulating hormone, luteinizing hormone, and thyroid-stimulating hormone. The β-chain is unique, and it is to this chain that antibodies used for immunohistochemistry are directed. In germ cell tumors, hCG expression is limited to syncytiotrophoblastic cells and some intermediate trophoblastic cells. Primary ovarian tumors that contain syncytiotrophoblastic cells, including choriocarcinoma and some dysgerminomas and embryonal carcinomas, express hCG.[407,409-411] Rare poorly differentiated carcinomas show choriocarcinomatous differentiation, and the syncytiotrophoblastic cells in such tumors express hCG.[412] In addition, occasional carcinomas that lack syncytiotrophoblastic cells have also been reported to express hCG.[413,414]

S-100 PROTEIN

S-100 protein is a multigenic family of small acidic EF-hand calcium binding proteins initially discovered in brain extract.[415-417] Melanoma is nearly always strongly S-100 positive, so staining for S-100 is a practical way to screen for primary or metastatic ovarian melanoma.[418] S-100 can also be identified in a variety of other neoplasms, including some carcinomas,[419,420] peripheral nerve sheath tumors, and tumors that contain myoepithelial cells, and in the dendritic cells that frequently accompany neoplasms. Sex cord–stromal tumors, including granulosa cell tumors,[421] Sertoli cell tumors,[422] and tumors in the fibroma-thecoma group, occasionally show positive staining for S-100. A diagnosis of melanoma can be confirmed by positive staining with antibodies against HMB45 or melan-A (A103) in cases in which the diagnosis remains unclear.[423-425] HMB45 and melan-A are more specific for melanoma than is S-100, but they are less sensitive.[426] HMB45 is also expressed in lymphangioleiomyomatosis, angiomyolipoma, and PEComa,[232,427-433] and melan-A can be expressed in luteinized cells, Leydig cells, and ectopic adrenal tissue.[349,434,435]

CD45

CD45, also known as leukocyte common antigen (LCA), is a family of transmembrane protein tyrosine phosphatases. It is expressed on the surface of all hematopoietic cells except erythroid and megakaryocytic cells. Commercially available monoclonal antibodies effectively mark lymphoid cells, both benign and malignant, and are therefore useful for screening tumors to determine whether they might be hematopoietic neoplasms.[436] Staining is usually membranous. Plasma cell neoplasms tend to stain weakly or not to stain at all, and there is variable staining of myeloid leukemic cells. If a neoplasm is suspected of being of hematopoietic type, numerous additional markers are available to further characterize it, as discussed in detail in the chapters on lymphomas (Chapters 5 and 6).

MARKERS OF NEUROENDOCRINE DIFFERENTIATION

Markers of neuroendocrine differentiation are helpful in the diagnosis of primary and metastatic neuroendocrine carcinomas, primitive neuroectodermal tumors, and

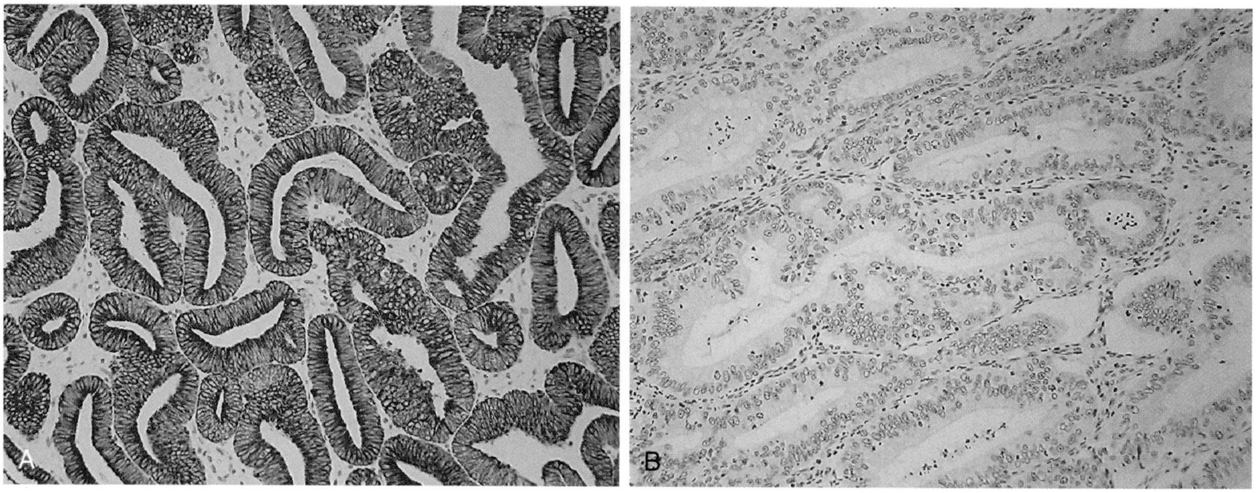

FIGURE 18.23 Cytokeratin subsets in primary epithelial tumors. **(A)** Primary epithelial tumors usually exhibit diffuse strong staining for CK7, like this endometrioid adenocarcinoma. **(B)** Except for mucinous tumors, primary epithelial tumors do not stain for CK20.

for identification of primary and secondary carcinoid tumors. The antibodies used for this purpose are discussed in detail in the chapter on endocrine neoplasms (Chapter 10). Chromogranin and synaptophysin are the most specific markers of neuroendocrine differentiation in general use. Neuron-specific enolase (NSE) and CD56 (neural cell adhesion molecule; NCAM) are less specific but are more sensitive and are used for screening purposes.

Epithelial Tumors

Epithelial tumors are by far the most common ovarian neoplasms. They account for 60% of all ovarian tumors and about 95% of all malignant tumors. Most tumors of the fallopian tube are epithelial. Keratin antibodies are helpful in the diagnosis of epithelial tumors. Broad-spectrum antikeratins, such as AE1/AE3, can be used to confirm the epithelial nature of a tumor. While the epithelial nature of low- to intermediate-grade carcinomas is usually obvious, ovarian cancers are often poorly differentiated, and some are difficult to recognize as carcinomas. Positive staining for keratin and EMA suggests that a tumor is a carcinoma. Antibodies against specific keratins have become indispensable in the evaluation of ovarian tumors. Immunoreactivity for CK7 is characteristic of epithelial tumors of the female genital tract, including those of the ovary and fallopian tube. Nearly 100% of primary epithelial tumors of the ovary and tube are CK7-positive (Fig. 18.23A),[149,307-309,316] so lack of staining for CK7 suggests the possibility of a metastasis. Antibodies to CK20 are also of assistance in the evaluation of ovarian and tubal tumors. Except for mucinous tumors of intestinal type, stains for CK20 are generally negative in primary epithelial tumors (Fig. 18.23B). Primary ovarian epithelial tumors are generally CK7-positive and CK20-negative, so the immunophenotype CK7-negative, CK20-positive suggests a metastatic tumor in the ovary, especially one from the intestine or appendix.

SEROUS TUMORS

Most Useful Antibodies: CK7, WT1

Like other primary epithelial tumors of the ovary, serous tumors exhibit positive staining for CK7 and negative staining for CK20 (Table 18.6).[307,309] Keratin stains can be used to highlight foci of microinvasion in borderline serous tumors.[437] There is typically positive staining of the cell membranes with CA125 in serous carcinoma (Fig. 18.24).[326] Stains for estrogen and progesterone receptors are positive in up to 50% of serous carcinomas.[438] There is strong positive nuclear staining for p53 in 30% to 50% of serous carcinomas.[167,438-440] Small foci of intraepithelial carcinoma on the surface of the ovary or in the fallopian tube can sometimes be highlighted with this stain. Benign and borderline serous tumors, including micropapillary borderline tumors, are p53-negative. Low-grade serous carcinoma, which appears to evolve via a different pathway than high-grade serous carcinoma, is significantly less likely than high-grade serous carcinoma to express p53.[441] Positive nuclear staining for the Wilms' tumor gene product WT1 is generally observed in serous carcinoma of the ovary, fallopian tube, and peritoneum, although the extent and intensity of staining is variable (Fig. 18.25).[167,325,367,442-444] Staining is also observed in borderline serous tumors.[441,443] Serous carcinoma of the endometrium tends to lack staining for WT1[166] or to stain only weakly and focally,[167] so absence of staining for WT1 and strong staining for p53 suggests that a metastatic serous carcinoma is more likely to be of endometrial than ovarian origin. Of note, sex cord–stromal tumors of the ovary are also reported to exhibit nuclear staining for WT1.[346] PAX2 and PAX8 are transcription factors that are involved in the development of the müllerian system, and both are expressed as positive nuclear staining in a significant percentage of serous carcinomas.[445,446] Staining for PAX8 is not specific for serous carcinoma, as other types of epithelial tumors also show positive staining.

TABLE 18.6 Primary vs. Metastatic Adenocarcinoma

	CK7	CK20	CDX2	DPC4	CK17	mCEA
Primary mucinous	+	+	S	+	N	+
Primary endometrioid	+	N	N	+	N	N
Metastatic colorectal	N	+	+	+	N	+
Metastatic pancreas	S	S	N	N (50%)	S	+

CK7, cytokeratin 7; CK20, cytokeratin 20; DPC4, deleted in pancreas cancer 4; CK17, cytokeratin 17; mCEA, monoclonal carcinoembryonic antigen.
+ almost always positive; S, sometimes positive; N, negative.

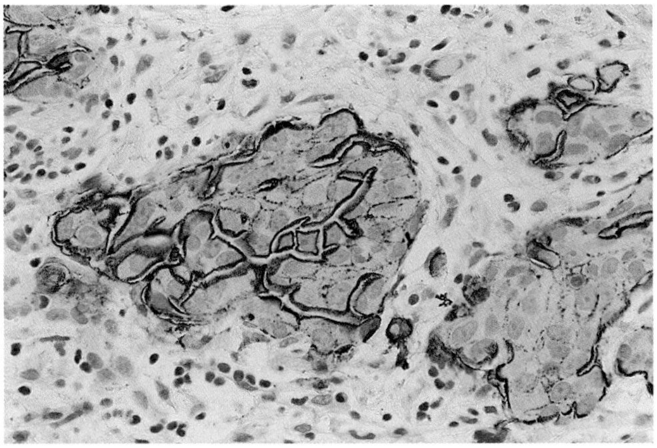

FIGURE 18.24 Many non-mucinous ovarian epithelial tumors, particularly serous tumors, exhibit positive staining for CA125. This microscopic serous carcinoma, found in a woman with a family history of ovarian cancer, illustrates the typical strong membranous staining pattern.

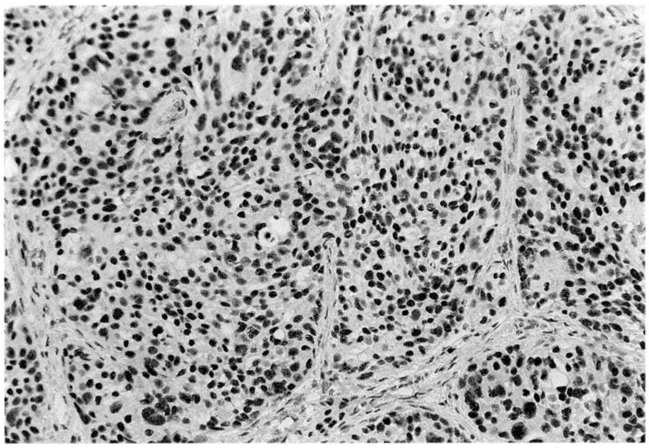

FIGURE 18.25 Positive staining for WT1 in serous carcinoma. Strong staining of most tumor cell nuclei is a characteristic finding in serous carcinoma of the ovary.

MUCINOUS TUMORS

Most Useful Antibodies: CK7, CK20

Immunohistochemistry can play an important role in the diagnosis and classification of mucinous tumors of the ovary. Two types of primary mucinous tumors occur in the ovary. Tumors composed of cells with an intestinal phenotype are most common, but a minority of mucinous tumors has an endocervical-like or seromucinous phenotype. These two types of mucinous tumors have different immunophenotypes, and immunostains can be used to differentiate between the two types. Immunostains for cytokeratin or epithelial membrane antigen can help identify foci of microinvasion.

Intestinal-type mucinous tumors are diffusely and strongly positive for CK7 (Fig. 18.26A).[316,447,448] The majority are also immunoreactive for CK20.[149,447] Staining for CK20 tends to be patchy, and the extent and intensity of staining is variable in primary mucinous tumors of the ovary (Fig. 18.26B).[448] Some pathologists advocate that using a high threshold for a positive result will improve the reproducibility of results (i.e., >25% or >50% of tumor cells stained); if this practice is adopted, only 40% to 50% of ovarian mucinous carcinomas will be designated as CK20-positive.[309,325] *CDX* genes encode homeobox nuclear transcription factors that are involved in the proliferation and differentiation of intestinal epithelial cells. Diffuse strong nuclear staining for CDX2 is present in normal intestine and in most colorectal adenocarcinomas and their ovarian metastases.[449-451] Diffuse strong positive staining for CDX2 is observed in only a minority of primary mucinous tumors of the ovary.[311,447,452-454] Non-mucinous ovarian tumors are CDX2 negative. Strong positive staining for CK7 coupled with variable or negative staining for CK20 and CDX2 typically differentiates a primary mucinous tumor from metastatic colorectal adenocarcinoma, as the latter typically is CK7-negative and shows diffuse strong positive staining for CK20 and CDX2 (see Table 18.6).[149,307,309,310,326] Occasional mucinous tumors that arise in the ovary in association with a benign cystic teratoma have a lower intestinal tract phenotype (CK7-negative and CK20- and CDX2-positive).[455] These tumors are often associated with pseudomyxoma ovarii. If a metastasis from a lower intestinal tract carcinoma can be excluded, such tumors are acceptable as primary ovarian mucinous neoplasms with an aberrant immunophenotype. It is important to remember that occasional primary and metastatic tumors show aberrant cytokeratin staining patterns. In particular, rectal adenocarcinomas can be CK7-positive, and occasional primary mucinous tumors of the ovary are CK7-negative.[448,456] Immunostains for polyclonal and monoclonal carcinoembryonic antigen (CEA) show staining of luminal mucin, the apical cell borders, and the cytoplasm of the tumor cells.[325,457] Immunostains for villin intensely stain the apical border of the tumor cells in most cases.[449] Chromogranin and synaptophysin stains reveal scattered basal endocrine cells among

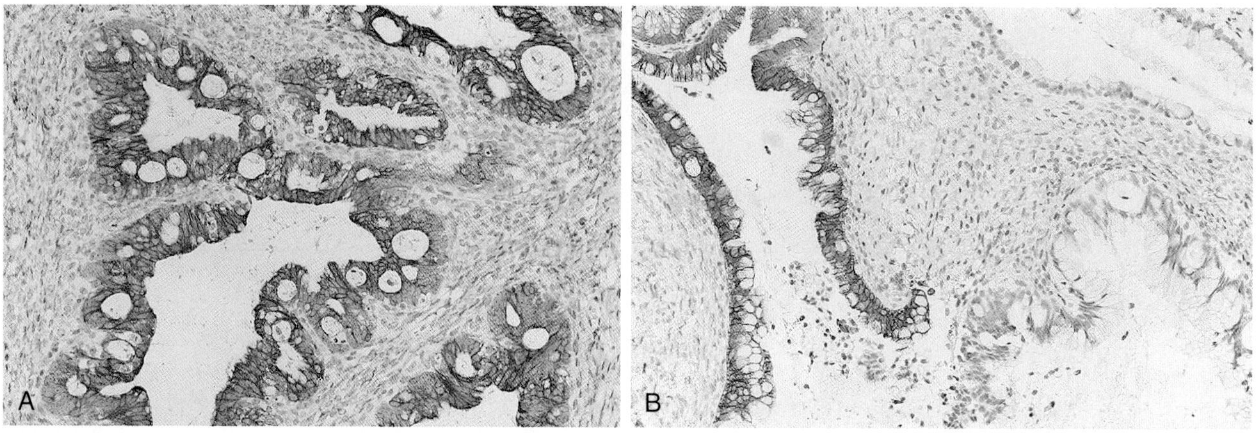

FIGURE 18.26 Cytokeratin subsets in primary intestinal-type mucinous tumors. **(A)** Like other primary epithelial tumors, intestinal-type mucinous tumors generally show strong positive staining for CK7. **(B)** In contrast to other primary epithelial tumors, intestinal-type mucinous tumors are generally CK20 positive. Staining for CK20 tends to be patchy, as seen here, and can be less intense than is observed in metastatic colorectal adenocarcinoma, which is typically CK7-negative and CK20-positive.

the columnar tumor cells. The epithelium in mucinous tumors is inhibin-negative, but pericystic stromal cells are often partly or completely luteinized and strongly positive for inhibin. Intestinal mucinous tumors are usually negative for estrogen and progesterone receptors.[458]

Several additional immunostains are useful for the evaluation of mucinous tumors of the ovary. Stains for the mucin gene product MUC5A and for the pancreas cancer tumor suppressor gene product Dpc4 are generally positive in mucinous carcinoma of the ovary.[316] Mutation of Dpc4 occurs in about 50% of pancreatic adenocarcinomas, and results in loss of staining for the protein. About 40% of pancreas adenocarcinomas are CK17-positive, but ovarian mucinous tumors rarely stain for this marker.[325] Thus, lack of staining for Dpc4 and/or positive staining for CK17 suggests that a mucinous tumor in the ovary may be metastatic from the pancreas.

Pseudomyxoma peritonei can occur in patients with mucinous tumors involving ovary. The ovarian tumors have a varied appearance, ranging from benign cystadenomas to adenocarcinomas, although most resemble borderline mucinous tumors of intestinal type. Clinicopathologic and molecular studies suggest that in most instances pseudomyxoma peritonei is secondary to a tumor of the gastrointestinal tract, especially one of the appendix, and that the ovarian tumors represent secondary involvement of the ovaries by a metastatic neoplasm. Immunohistochemical stains tend to support this impression, as most tumors lack staining for CK7 and show positive staining for the intestinal mucin MUC2.[448,459,460]

Mural nodules are occasionally detected in the walls of mucinous tumors. The mucinous tumors can be benign, borderline, or carcinoma. Three types of mural nodules have been described: anaplastic carcinoma,[461,462] sarcoma,[463] and sarcoma-like reactive spindle cell proliferations.[464,465] Anaplastic carcinoma is an obviously malignant proliferation that expresses cytokeratin, usually in a strong and diffuse pattern, and which often coexpresses vimentin.[466,467] Sarcomatous mural nodules are malignant spindle or epithelioid cell proliferations that express vimentin, but not cytokeratin.[468] Sarcoma-like nodules have a varied morphology, but usually cytologic atypia and mitotic activity are less than in malignant nodules. Some of these benign proliferations show limited, usually weak and focal, expression of cytokeratin in addition to vimentin.[465,469]

Seromucinous (endocervical-like) tumors have a different immunophenotype than intestinal-type mucinous tumors. They are CK7-positive (Fig. 18.27A) but, in contrast with intestinal-type mucinous tumors, they are CK20-negative (Fig. 18.27B) and CDX2-negative regardless of what threshold is selected for a positive result.[447] Seromucinous tumors tend to be CEA-negative, except that the eosinophilic indifferent cells that are found in borderline seromucinous tumors can exhibit strong staining for CEA.[457] Seromucinous tumors frequently exhibit positive nuclear staining for estrogen and progesterone receptors and positive cytoplasmic staining for vimentin.[458,470]

ENDOMETRIOID TUMORS

Most Useful Antibodies: CK7, CK20, CDX2, Cytokeratin Cocktail, EMA, Inhibin

Benign, borderline, and malignant endometrioid tumors occur in the ovary. Benign and borderline endometrioid tumors are mainly adenofibromatous neoplasms, although rare borderline endometrioid tumors are papillary or glandular. All endometrioid tumors have a similar immunophenotype, and as endometrioid carcinomas comprise the vast majority of endometrioid tumors in the ovary, we will focus this discussion on them. Endometrioid carcinoma is CK7-positive, and it is negative or at most weakly and focally positive for CK20 (see Fig. 18.23).[451] About 33% of endometrioid carcinomas show perinuclear or basal cytoplasmic staining for vimentin.[104] Among the epithelial tumors, endometrioid neoplasms are most likely (38% in one series) to show nuclear and cytoplasmic staining for β-catenin,[174] and a majority of these have β-catenin mutations.[471] Carcinomas with β-catenin mutations tend to be low grade,

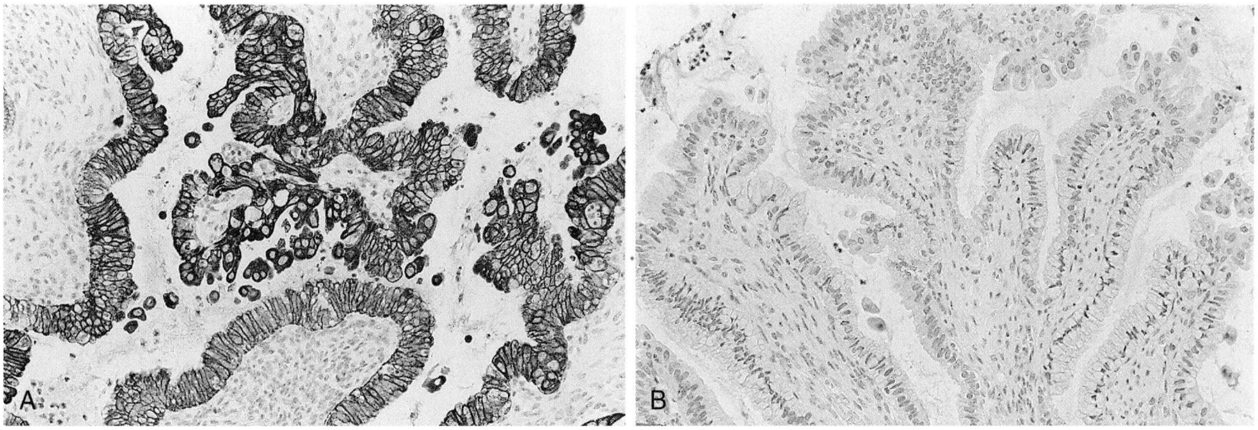

FIGURE 18.27 Cytokeratin subsets in primary endocervical-type mucinous tumors (seromucinous tumors). This type of mucinous tumor has a typical müllerian immunophenotype. **(A)** Endocervical-type mucinous tumors show diffuse strong staining for CK7. **(B)** In contrast to intestinal-type mucinous tumors, endocervical-type mucinous tumors are CK20-negative.

to exhibit morular or squamous differentiation, to be low stage, and to have a favorable prognosis. Borderline endometrioid tumors, particularly those with morules, appear to be particularly likely to show nuclear staining for β-catenin.[472] Staining is present in the nuclei and cytoplasm of a variable percentage of glandular tumor cells and tends to be particularly prominent in the nuclei of cells in morules or foci of squamous differentiation.[473] Most epithelial tumors, including endometrioid tumors, show membrane staining with β-catenin. Only nuclear staining, which is more common in endometrioid tumors than in other types of epithelial neoplasms, is associated with β-catenin mutation. Nuclear staining can be difficult to identify in cases with intense membrane staining. Morules and foci of squamous differentiation also show nuclear staining for CDX2 and cytoplasmic staining for CD10; staining is more likely to be present and more intense in morules.[473] As performed in our laboratory, staining for CDX2 tends to be faint, and it is not likely to be confused with the strong staining seen in metastatic colorectal adenocarcinoma.

Some endometrioid carcinomas exhibit growth patterns that mimic sex cord–stromal tumors such as Sertoli cell tumors, Sertoli-Leydig cell tumors, or granulosa cell tumors. Sertoliform variants of endometrioid carcinoma are the most common of these. Immunohistochemical stains help to differentiate these variants of endometrioid carcinoma from sex cord–stromal tumors, as endometrioid carcinoma is EMA-positive (Fig. 18.28), exhibits positive nuclear staining for estrogen and progesterone receptors, and does not stain for inhibin or calretinin (Table 18.7).[474,475] In contrast, sex cord–stromal tumors may stain for cytokeratin, but they are negative for EMA and they show cytoplasmic staining for inhibin and cytoplasmic and nuclear staining for calretinin.[348]

Metastatic colorectal adenocarcinoma can mimic endometrioid carcinoma. Diffuse strong staining for CK7 is characteristic of endometrioid carcinoma. On the other hand, metastatic colorectal adenocarcinoma tends to show diffuse strong cytoplasmic staining for CK20 and nuclear staining for CDX2, both of which are negative in endometrioid carcinoma, except, as

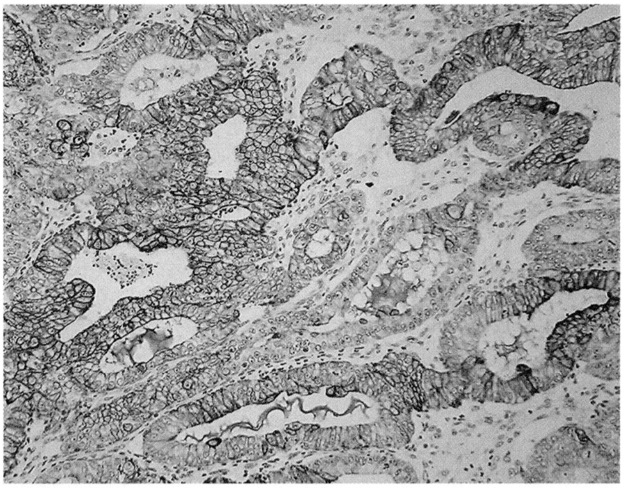

FIGURE 18.28 Endometrioid carcinoma, including its Sertoliform variant, shows diffuse strong staining for epithelial membrane antigen (EMA). Sertoli cell and Sertoli-Leydig cell tumors are EMA negative.

noted earlier in the chapter, in morules and foci of squamous differentiation (see Table 18.6).[307,451] There is no cytoplasmic staining for carcinoembryonic antigen in glandular areas of endometrioid carcinoma, although there can be focal staining in areas of squamous differentiation.[104] Metastatic cervical adenocarcinoma can also mimic endometrioid adenocarcinoma. The cervical primary adenocarcinoma is sometimes only minimally invasive, and the possibility of ovarian metastasis is often not suspected. Metastatic cervical adenocarcinoma exhibits histologic features that suggest the correct diagnosis; the tumor is glandular and the tumor cells are columnar with hyperchromatic fusiform nuclei, pale cytoplasm, and mitotic figures in the upper poles of the columnar tumor cells. Immunostains are usually necessary to confirm the diagnosis. Positive immunostaining for carcinoembryonic antigen, p16, and a positive molecular test for HPV (*in situ* hybridization or PCR) support a diagnosis of metastatic cervical adenocarcinoma.[476] Staining for p16 must be strong and diffuse (nearly all tumor cells positive) to be indicative of

TABLE 18.7 Endometrioid Carcinoma vs. Sex Cord Stromal Tumors

	Cytokeratin	EMA	Inhibin	Calretinin
Endometrioid carcinoma	+	+	N	N
Granulosa cell tumor	S	N	+	+
Sertoli-Leydig cell tumor	+	N	+	+
Sertoli cell tumor	+	N	+	+

EMA, epithelial membrane antigen.
+ almost always positive; S, sometimes positive; N, negative.

metastatic cervical adenocarcinoma, as primary ovarian carcinomas, including endometrioid adenocarcinomas, can show lesser degrees of staining.[477,478]

Carcinosarcoma, adenosarcoma, and endometrioid stromal sarcoma are classified as types of endometrioid tumors of the ovary.[304] Accurate diagnosis of these tumors can require identification of an epithelial component or correct identification of various mesenchymal cell types. In carcinosarcoma and adenosarcoma, immunohistochemical testing for cytokeratin or EMA can help the pathologist identify an epithelial component in a predominantly mesenchymal neoplasm.[479,480] Immunostains for desmin and myogenin are useful to confirm the presence of rhabdomyoblasts, and chondroid elements are often S-100-positive. Endometrioid stromal sarcoma exhibits a distinctive positive staining reaction for CD10,[141] while sex cord–stromal tumors, with which it may be confused, are typically positive for inhibin and calretinin. Endometrioid stromal sarcomas that contain foci of epithelioid or sex cord–like differentiation pose particular diagnostic problems, since these can express inhibin or calretinin.[481] In addition to diffuse staining for CD10, endometrioid stromal sarcomas tend to show strong positive staining for estrogen and progesterone receptors.

CLEAR CELL CARCINOMA

Most Useful Antibodies: CK7, CK20, Hepatocyte Nuclear Factor-1β, WT1, EMA, Glypican-3, Alpha-Fetoprotein, CD10

Clear cell carcinoma shows the typical pattern of immunoreactivity seen in other primary epithelial tumors of the ovary. The tumor cells stain for cytokeratin, CK7 (Fig. 18.29A), high molecular weight keratin, and epithelial membrane antigen.[126,482] They also stain for CD15 (Fig. 18.29B) but usually not for CK20.[126] Variable results have been noted with stains for estrogen and progesterone receptors, but in more recent reports clear cell carcinoma has shown no or minimal staining for ER and PR.[440,482] Recently, hepatocyte nuclear factor-1beta (HNF-1β) has emerged as a sensitive and specific marker for clear cell tumors, particularly clear cell carcinoma.[173,440,483] Diffuse strong nuclear staining for HNF-1beta is observed in more than 80% of clear cell carcinomas (Fig. 18.30). A panel that includes HNF-1beta, WT1, and ER has proven effective in resolving the common differential diagnosis of clear cell carcinoma vs. serous carcinoma. HNF-1beta is likely to be positive in clear cell carcinoma, while WT1 and ER are likely to be positive in serous carcinoma. The osteopontin gene is a target of HNF-1beta protein, and clear cell carcinomas that express HNF-1beta also tend to show cytoplasmic and membrane staining for osteopontin.[484] Diffuse positive nuclear staining for p53 has been reported by some authors,[126] but not by others.[485,486] Our experience is that staining for p53, when present, is usually irregular in distribution and less intense than is observed in serous carcinoma, where nuclear staining tends to be strong and diffuse when present. This can be exploited in cases in which differentiation between clear cell and serous carcinoma is a problem, as diffuse strong nuclear staining for p53 favors serous carcinoma. Clear cell carcinoma frequently contains waxy eosinophilic hyaline material in the stroma between glands or in papillae. This material, which is not observed in other types of epithelial tumors, is thought to be basement membrane material because it stains positively for laminin and type IV collagen.[487,488]

In the past, clear cell carcinoma and yolk sac tumor were thought to comprise a single tumor type (mesonephroma). Yolk sac tumor still poses a differential diagnostic problem in some cases, as there is a degree of overlap in the histologic appearance of these tumors. Knowledge of the patient's age, the clinical setting, and the serum AFP level can assist with the differential diagnosis. Clear cell carcinoma generally does not stain for AFP, but yolk sac tumor is usually at least focally AFP-positive (Table 18.8).[318] Glypican-3 is a recently introduced marker that shows cytoplasmic and membrane staining in most yolk sac tumors, but only rarely stains clear cell carcinoma.[394] Clear cell carcinoma stains strongly for CD15 and EMA, and these are typically negative or weakly positive in yolk sac tumor.[392] CK7 staining has been reported to be absent in yolk sac tumor of the ovary,[318] although we observed it in about 33% of yolk sac tumors of the testis and others have reported it in ovarian yolk sac tumors.[393] Clear cell carcinoma is almost always CK7-positive, however, so lack of staining for CK7 favors a diagnosis of yolk sac tumor.

The clear cell variant of renal cell carcinoma can mimic a primary clear cell carcinoma of the ovary. Primary clear cell carcinoma is CK7-positive, whereas metastatic clear cell renal cell carcinoma is rarely CK7-positive.[482] Another useful stain for differentiating between these tumors is CD10,[52] which is negative in primary clear cell carcinoma of the ovary, but shows positive staining, often with membrane accentuation, in metastatic clear cell renal cell carcinoma. Additional stains that are more likely to be positive in clear cell carcinoma include high molecular weight keratin, CA125, estrogen receptor, and progesterone receptor.[489] On the other hand, positive staining for the renal cell carcinoma antigen (RCC) favors metastatic renal cell carcinoma.[482] The most useful panel includes CK7, CD10, and RCC.[482] Diffuse strong positive staining for CK7

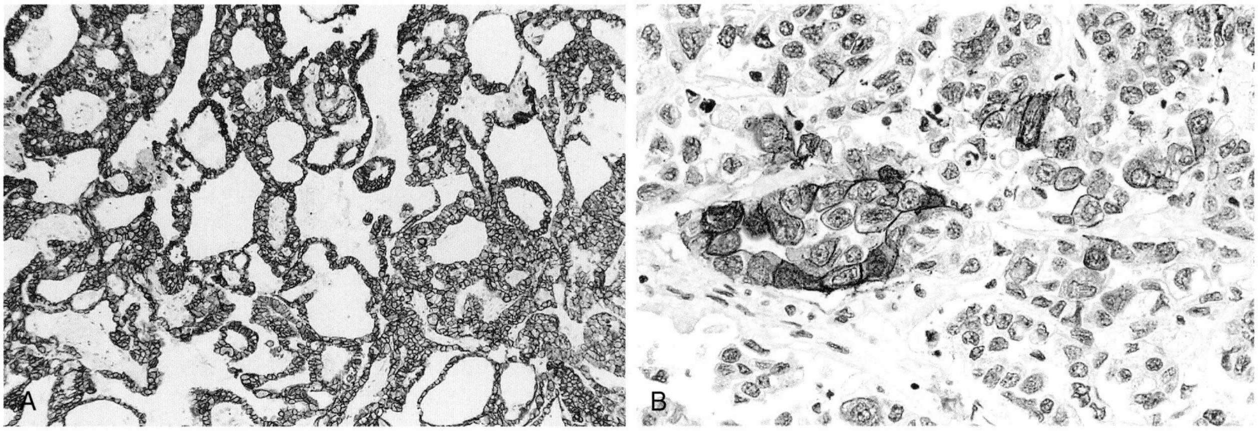

FIGURE 18.29 Clear cell carcinoma. **(A)** CK7 is diffusely and strongly positive in clear cell carcinoma. **(B)** Although its primary use is in hematopathology, CD15 stains some adenocarcinomas, including clear cell carcinoma. Yolk sac tumor, an important differential diagnostic consideration, is typically CK7- and CD15-negative.

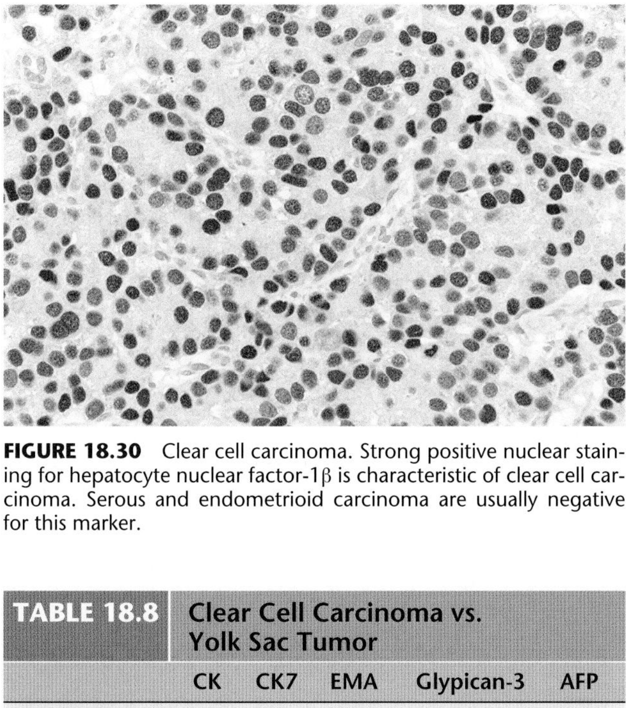

FIGURE 18.30 Clear cell carcinoma. Strong positive nuclear staining for hepatocyte nuclear factor-1β is characteristic of clear cell carcinoma. Serous and endometrioid carcinoma are usually negative for this marker.

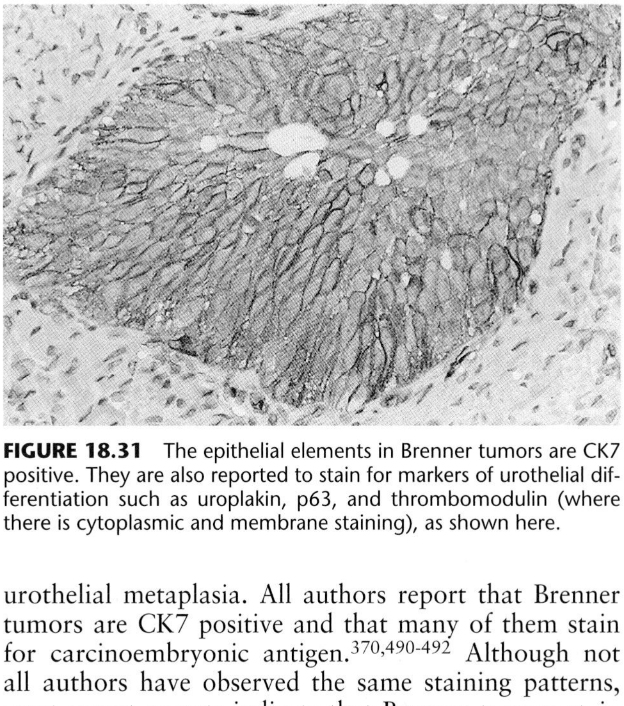

FIGURE 18.31 The epithelial elements in Brenner tumors are CK7 positive. They are also reported to stain for markers of urothelial differentiation such as uroplakin, p63, and thrombomodulin (where there is cytoplasmic and membrane staining), as shown here.

TABLE 18.8 Clear Cell Carcinoma vs. Yolk Sac Tumor

	CK	CK7	EMA	Glypican-3	AFP
Clear cell carcinoma	+	+	+	N	N
Yolk sac tumor	+	N	N	+	+

CK, cytokeratin; CK7, cytokeratin 7; EMA, epithelial membrane antigen; AFP, alpha-fetoprotein.
+, almost always positive; N, negative.

and absence of staining for CD10 and RCC favor primary clear cell carcinoma of the ovary.

BRENNER AND TRANSITIONAL CELL TUMORS

Most Useful Antibodies: CK7, CK20, WT1

Recent studies show similarities between the immunophenotypes of Brenner tumor epithelium and urothelium, suggesting that the transitional cell appearance of the epithelium in Brenner tumors represents true urothelial metaplasia. All authors report that Brenner tumors are CK7 positive and that many of them stain for carcinoembryonic antigen.[370,490-492] Although not all authors have observed the same staining patterns, most recent reports indicate that Brenner tumors stain like urothelium, being positive for CK7, uroplakin III,[493] and thrombomodulin (Fig. 18.31), and, in some studies, for CK20.[491,494] Some authors have been unable to detect immunostaining for such markers of urothelial cells as CK20 and thrombomodulin.[490,492] There is positive nuclear staining for p63 in urothelium and urothelial carcinoma of the bladder, and benign and borderline Brenner tumors show diffuse strong nuclear staining for p63 supporting a urothelial phenotype.[495] Although the number of cases studied is limited, p63 appears to be a good marker for Brenner tumors, since they are p63-positive while other types of ovarian tumors are p63-negative. Borderline and malignant Brenner tumors express urothelial markers less often than benign Brenner tumors.[370] Transitional cell carcinoma of the ovary has the same immunohistochemical features as other types of surface epithelial carcinomas, particularly serous carcinomas, and its immunophenotype is different from that of transitional cell carcinoma of urothelial type. Transitional cell carcinoma of the ovary expresses CK7 and CA125; rarely expresses urothelial markers such as CK13, CK20, uroplakin III, thrombomodulin, or p63; and frequently expresses WT1.[370,491,492,495,496] Like other nonmucinous types of ovarian epithelial tumors, transitional cell carcinoma expresses mesothelin, while transitional cell carcinoma of urothelial type does not.[497] A staining panel that includes CK7, CK20, thrombomodulin, p63, and WT1 can be helpful in the differential diagnosis between primary transitional cell carcinoma of the ovary and metastatic transitional cell carcinoma from the bladder. As performed in our laboratory, however, uroplakin III lacks sensitivity and we no longer rely on it in diagnostic work.

OTHER EPITHELIAL TUMORS

Most Useful Antibodies: CK, EMA, CK7, CD56, Synaptophysin, Chromogranin, WT1

The immunophenotype of primary undifferentiated/poorly differentiated carcinoma is not well defined. Our experience is that high-grade carcinomas stain for general epithelial markers such as cytokeratin and EMA. These stains can help differentiate poorly differentiated carcinomas from carcinosarcoma and various poorly differentiated non-epithelial neoplasms, such as lymphomas.

Two types of small cell carcinoma occur in the ovary. Small cell carcinoma of neuroendocrine type can arise in the ovary as a pure tumor but most often it is admixed with a more common type of primary epithelial neoplasia, such as mucinous or endometrioid carcinoma. Small cell carcinoma of the lung can also metastasize to the ovary. Small cell carcinoma of neuroendocrine type, whether primary or metastatic, is typically immunoreactive for such general neuroendocrine markers as NSE (Fig. 18.32) and CD56. Some examples stain for synaptophysin and/or chromogranin. These tumors sometimes show limited staining for cytokeratin, which can exhibit a dot or cytoplasmic rim pattern of staining that is highly suggestive of small cell carcinoma. Extrapulmonary small cell carcinomas can be immunoreactive for thyroid transcription factor-1 (TTF-1), so positive staining for TTF-1 does not necessarily indicate that a small cell carcinoma in the ovary is metastatic from the lung. Most sex cord–stromal tumors, including granulosa cell tumors, show positive staining for CD56,[498,499] so staining for this marker is not, by itself, indicative of small cell carcinoma.

A second type of small cell carcinoma, small cell carcinoma of the hypercalcemic type, also occurs in the ovary. This is a highly malignant neoplasm of the ovary that occurs mainly in young women. About two thirds of patients have hypercalcemia. The nature of this tumor has been controversial, but recent studies suggest that it is best grouped with the epithelial tumors. Immunohistochemical stains reveal an epithelial phenotype, as most tumors show staining for EMA and a significant proportion are cytokeratin-positive.[371,500-502] Recent studies have revealed staining for WT1, CD10, and p53 in a significant percentage of cases.[177,374] Other stains that are nonspecific, but that are frequently positive, are vimentin, NSE and chromogranin, and CD99.[500,502] Occasional tumors stain for parathyroid hormone–related protein or parathyroid hormone,[501] but the cause of the hypercalcemia that accompanies small cell carcinoma has yet to be elucidated. Absence of staining for inhibin, generally weak staining for calretinin, and frequent positive staining for EMA help to differentiate small cell carcinoma from juvenile granulosa cell tumor and suggest that small cell carcinoma is not a sex cord–stromal neoplasm.[344,361,371,500] We have observed a distinctive immunoprofile in cases of small cell carcinoma that helps support this diagnosis: weak focal staining for cytokeratin, weak focal staining for EMA, weak staining for p53 in about 50% of tumor cell nuclei, and strong diffuse nuclear staining for WT1.

Other primary and metastatic small round cell tumors that enter into the differential diagnosis of ovarian small cell carcinoma include lymphoma, melanoma,[418,503,504] desmoplastic small round cell tumor,[505-507] Ewing's sarcoma/primitive neuroectodermal tumor (ES/PNET),[508] and primary and metastatic round cell sarcomas, including embryonal and alveolar rhabdomyosarcomas.[509-511] Antibodies that are useful for the differential diagnosis of these tumors include CD45 and related markers for lymphoma (Fig. 18.33); S-100, HMB45, and related markers for melanoma; cytokeratin, desmin, FLI-1, WT1 (only with a polyclonal antibody that detects the c-terminal portion of the protein), and NSE for desmoplastic small round cell tumor (Fig. 18.34); CD99 and FLI-1 for ES/PNET; and desmin and myogenin for rhabdomyosarcoma.

KEY DIAGNOSTIC POINTS

Epithelial Tumors

- All common primary epithelial tumors of the ovary express CK7.
- If an epithelial tumor is CK7 negative, consider a metastasis or one of the rare types of primary epithelial tumors.
- Serous carcinoma and transitional cell carcinoma are commonly WT1 positive.
- Most primary ovarian tumors are negative for CK20 and CDX2. The exception is the intestinal type of mucinous ovarian tumor, which is positive for CK7, and variably positive for CK20 and CDX2.

Sex Cord–Stromal Tumors

Tumors derived from the sex cords or ovarian mesenchyme compose 5% to 12% of all ovarian neoplasms.[512,513] Benign tumors in the fibroma-thecoma group are relatively common. Other sex cord–stromal tumors and mesenchymal tumors are rare. The most common malignant sex cord– stromal tumor is granulosa cell tumor, which composes 1% of 2% of all malignant ovarian tumors. There are two types of granulosa cell tumors: an adult type that occurs mainly in postmenopausal

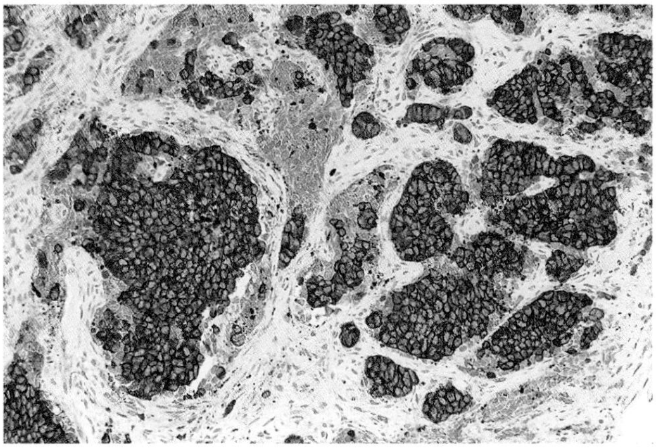

FIGURE 18.32 Small cell carcinoma of neuroendocrine type. This tumor arose in association with an endometrioid adenocarcinoma. The tumor cells are strongly positive for NSE.

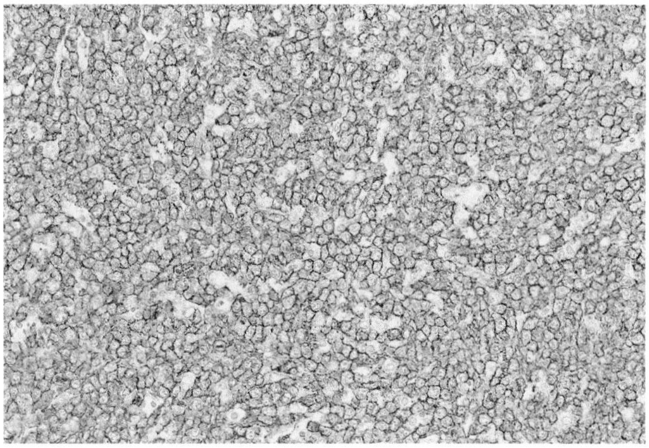

FIGURE 18.33 Lymphoma of the ovary. This diffusely infiltrative tumor proved to be a large cell lymphoma of B-cell type; an immunostain for CD20, a B-cell marker, shows strong staining of the membranes of every tumor cell.

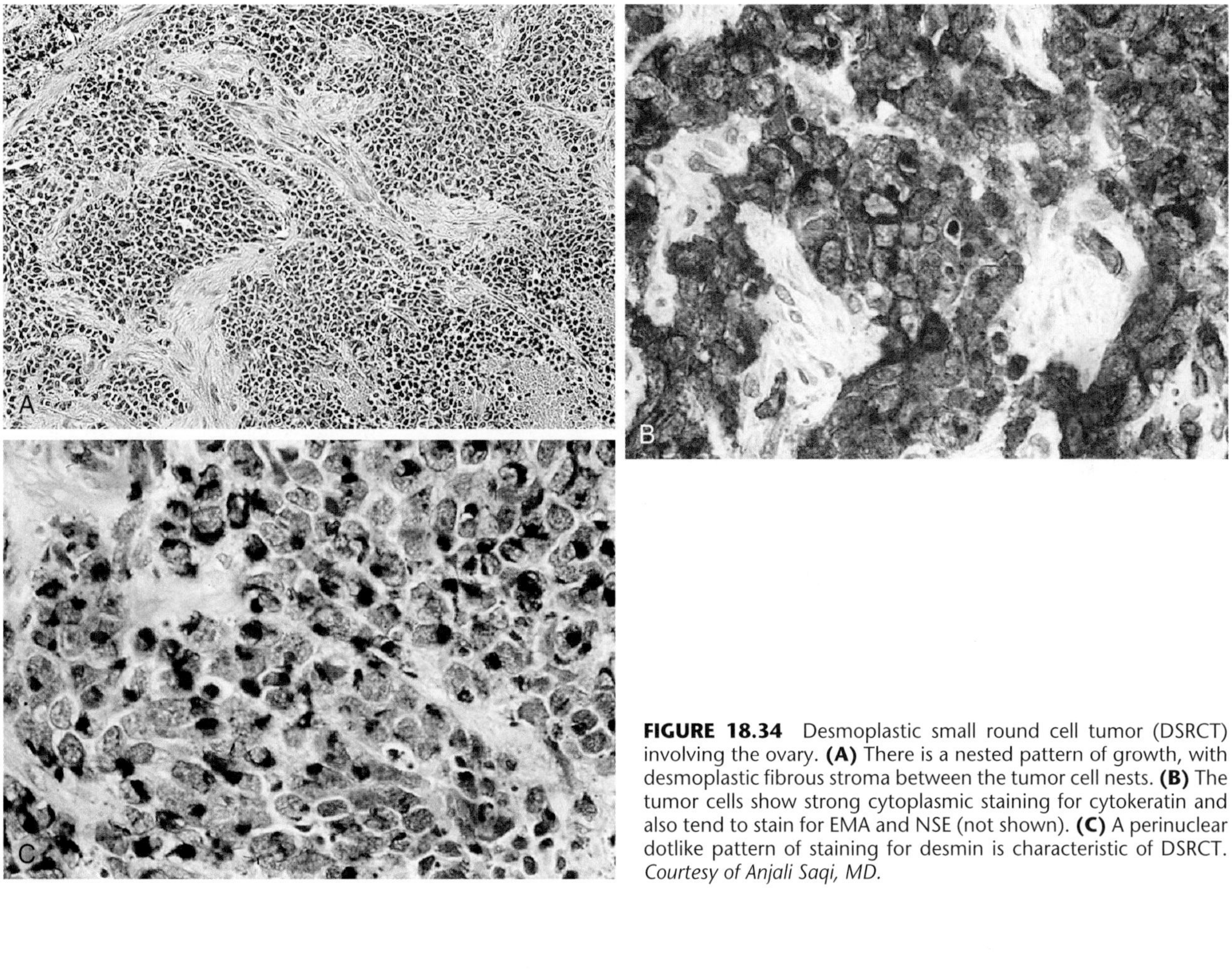

FIGURE 18.34 Desmoplastic small round cell tumor (DSRCT) involving the ovary. **(A)** There is a nested pattern of growth, with desmoplastic fibrous stroma between the tumor cell nests. **(B)** The tumor cells show strong cytoplasmic staining for cytokeratin and also tend to stain for EMA and NSE (not shown). **(C)** A perinuclear dotlike pattern of staining for desmin is characteristic of DSRCT. *Courtesy of Anjali Saqi, MD.*

women and a juvenile type that occurs mainly in children. Other sex cord–stromal tumors that commonly cause diagnostic problems and require immunohistochemical testing include Sertoli-Leydig cell tumors, Sertoli cell tumors, sex cord tumors with annular tubules, Leydig cell tumors, and unclassified steroid cell tumors.

Several antibodies have proven to be invaluable for the diagnosis of sex cord–stromal tumors. These include inhibin and calretinin, which are positive in most sex cord–stromal tumors and EMA, which is almost always negative in these tumors, a finding that excludes various types of carcinoma from the differential diagnosis. Inhibin is the most specific marker for sex cord–stromal tumors.[341,342,344,345,347,348,435,500,514] Calretinin is more sensitive, staining more tumors and tumor types, but it is less specific as it also stains mesotheliomas and about 20% of epithelial neoplasms.[360,361,435] Staining for inhibin tends to be patchy and of variable intensity. Ovarian stromal cells and most types of sex cord–stromal tumors show positive staining for CD56 and WT1.[499] Staining for CD56 is membranous, cytoplasmic, or both, and staining for WT1 is nuclear. In many sex cord–stromal tumors, CD99 is positive and the cells stain in a membranous pattern. Leydig cell and steroid cell tumors tend to stain strongly for Melan-A (MART-1). CD10 is expressed in many types of sex cord–stromal tumors, but expression is usually focal and weak.[515] We have not found CD10 to be particularly useful in the diagnosis of sex cord–stromal tumors. Finally, steroidogenic factor-1 (SF-1) is reported to stain most types of sex cord–stromal tumors.[516] Our standard panel for the diagnosis of sex cord–stromal tumors uses inhibin, calretinin, and often EMA. The other markers mentioned above are useful on occasion, depending on the differential diagnosis under consideration. In our laboratory, staining for WT1 tends to be weak, while CD56 can be difficult to interpret because of strong staining of the background stroma in some tumors. SF-1 is reportedly positive in a high percentage of cases, but with weaker and more limited staining than is observed with other markers.[516]

FIBROMA, THECOMA, AND RELATED TUMORS

Most Useful Antibodies: Inhibin, Calretinin, CD56

A fibroma is a benign stromal tumor in which spindle-shaped stromal cells grow in abundant collagenous stroma. Immunohistochemistry is rarely performed on fibromas because their appearance on H&E-stained slides is usually distinctive. Fibromas and related tumors such as cellular fibromas and fibrosarcomas stain only infrequently for inhibin but most are calretinin-positive.[344,346,361] They show patchy and weak to moderate staining for CD56 and WT1.[517] Staining for CD56 tends to be cytoplasmic rather than membranous, as is typical in most other types of sex cord–stromal cells.[499]

A thecoma is a benign spindle cell stromal tumor that differs from a fibroma in that it is often hormonally active, usually secreting estrogen. There are morphologic differences as well, as the tumor cells in a thecoma tend to be plump, with clear or vacuolated cytoplasm, and there is less collagen in the background stroma than is present in a fibroma. A thecoma is usually positive for both inhibin and calretinin.[342-344,346,361] Strong positive staining for inhibin favors classifying a stromal tumor as a thecoma rather than as a fibroma. Stains for myoid markers, such as smooth muscle actin, are often positive as well.[517,518]

A sclerosing stromal tumor is a benign hormonally inactive stromal tumor of the ovary.[519,520] The histologic appearance is variegated, with cellular, spindle cell zones alternating with paucicellular fibrous zones. Scattered throughout are branched dilated blood vessels with a hemangiopericytoma-like appearance. The tumor cells adjacent to the vessels are often polygonal and vaguely myoid in appearance. The tumor cells are vimentin-positive, and they often stain for smooth muscle actin, with staining for SMA concentrated in the plump cells in perivascular regions of the tumor.[521-523] Immunostains for inhibin and calretinin are positive in more than 50% of sclerosing stromal tumors.[344,361,521] Several authors have correlated the high vascularity observed in these tumors with staining for vascular endothelial growth factor (VEGF) in tumor cells.[520,524] Stains for vascular markers such as CD31 and CD34 highlight the prominent branched vessels.[521]

GRANULOSA CELL TUMORS

Most Useful Antibodies: CK, EMA, Inhibin, Calretinin, CD99

There are two types of granulosa cell tumors of the ovary. The adult type is most common. It is an indolent neoplasm of low malignant potential; most patients survive, but granulosa cell tumors can spread beyond the ovary, recur, and cause death.[525,526] Recurrences tend to be late and in some cases are detected more than 20 years after primary therapy.[527] Microscopically, the tumor cells are small and uniform with darkly stained nuclei and scanty cytoplasm. The mitotic rate is typically very low. The tumor can often be recognized by the distinctive arrangement of tumor cells in insular, microfollicular, trabecular, and diffuse patterns. Immunohistochemical staining for inhibin and calretinin is helpful in establishing a diagnosis of granulosa cell tumor (Table 18.9).[342,344,348,349,360,361,500,528] Both inhibin and calretinin are typically strongly positive, with diffuse staining for calretinin and either diffuse or patchy staining for inhibin (Fig. 18.35A).[341] These stains are not specific, since other types of sex cord–stromal tumors also show positive staining, and occasional carcinomas show weak staining. Immunostains for low molecular weight cytokeratins are positive, often in a patchy pattern, in occasional tumors (Fig. 18.35B),[421,529,530] but granulosa cell tumors are EMA-negative.[421] Other immunostains that are often positive include CD56, WT1, steroidogenic factor-1 (SF-1), smooth muscle actin, S-100, and CD99.[346,348,421,499,516,539,531-533] Stains for hormone receptors are frequently positive. Staining for progesterone receptors tends to be stronger and more extensive than staining for estrogen receptors, but neither is positive in some tumors.[534]

The tumor that is most often mistaken for a granulosa cell tumor is a poorly differentiated carcinoma, either primary in the ovary or metastatic to it. Carcinomas exhibit features that are not found in granulosa cell tumors such as bilaterality, high nuclear grade, and a high mitotic index. In addition, immunohistochemistry can help to establish the correct diagnosis; as carcinomas are usually strongly and diffusely positive for keratin and EMA, they often stain for subsets of keratin such as CK7 or CK20, and they are negative for inhibin and calretinin. Carcinoid tumors can also mimic granulosa cell tumors, particularly when they grow in insular, microglandular, or diffuse patterns. Clues to the correct diagnosis include the presence of other teratomatous elements and tumor cells with coarse, clumped nuclear chromatin and granular cytoplasm. Their

TABLE 18.9 Differential Diagnosis of Granulosa Cell Tumor

	I	CR	CK	EMA	LCA	CD99	CGR/SYN
Granulosa cell tumor	+	+	S	N	N	+	N
Carcinoma	N	N	+	+	N	N	N
Carcinoid	N	N	+	+	N	N	+
Lymphoma	N	N	N	N	+	S	N
Small cell carcinoma	N	S	S	S	N	S	S

I, inhibin; CR, calretinin; CK, cytokeratin; EMA, epithelial membrane antigen; LCA, leukocyte common antigen; CGR, chromogranin; SYN, synaptophysin.
+, almost always positive; S sometimes positive; N, negative.

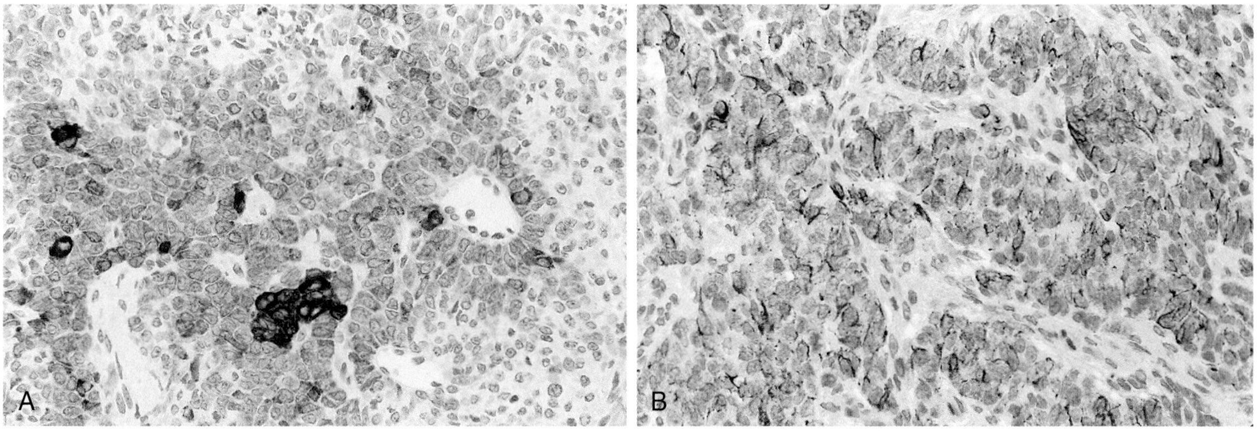

FIGURE 18.35 Adult-type granulosa cell tumor. **(A)** Immunostains for inhibin are positive in granulosa cell tumors, but staining is variable in intensity and distribution. As shown here, some cells show strong cytoplasmic staining, while in other cells staining is weak or absent. **(B)** Staining for cytokeratin is variable in granulosa cell tumors. There is patchy moderate cytoplasmic staining in this example, but many granulosa cell tumors are cytokeratin negative.

immunophenotype differs from granulosa cell tumor as carcinoids tend to be strongly and diffusely positive for keratin, negative for inhibin and calretinin, and they stain for markers of neuroendocrine differentiation such as synaptophysin or chromogranin.

The second type of granulosa cell tumor that occurs in the ovary is the juvenile granulosa cell tumor.[535,536] It occurs mainly in children and young women, but it can occur at any age, including in postmenopausal women.[537] Juvenile granulosa cell tumor has a favorable prognosis when confined to the ovary, but its histologic appearance can be alarming. The tumor cells are large, with atypical nuclei that can contain prominent nucleoli. The cytoplasm is abundant and is often luteinized. Mitotic figures tend to be frequent. The tumor cells grow in macrofollicular or diffuse patterns. The immunophenotype is similar to that of adult type granulosa cell tumor. The tumor cells stain for inhibin and calretinin,[343,344,348] and they usually show strong membrane staining for CD99 (Fig. 18.36).[348] SF-1, WT1, and CD56 also are usually positive.[499] Staining for cytokeratin is present in some tumors. Immunohistochemistry can help differentiate juvenile granulosa cell tumor from small cell carcinoma of the hypercalcemic type (see Table 18.9). Juvenile granulosa cell tumor is inhibin-positive, while small cell carcinoma does not stain for inhibin.[344,500] Small cell carcinoma stains more intensely for cytokeratin, and a majority of small cell carcinomas are EMA positive.[371,500] Most sex cord–stromal tumors are EMA-negative, but juvenile granulosa cell tumor can be immunoreactive for EMA[346,538]; staining is usually weak and focal. Staining for calretinin can be present in small cell carcinoma, but it is usually weaker than in juvenile granulosa cell tumor.[371] There are conflicting results in the literature regarding staining of small cell carcinoma for CD99, with some authors reporting no staining and others staining in about half of the cases.[371,500] Although small cell carcinoma can be CD99-negative, nearly all juvenile granulosa cell tumors are CD99-positive.

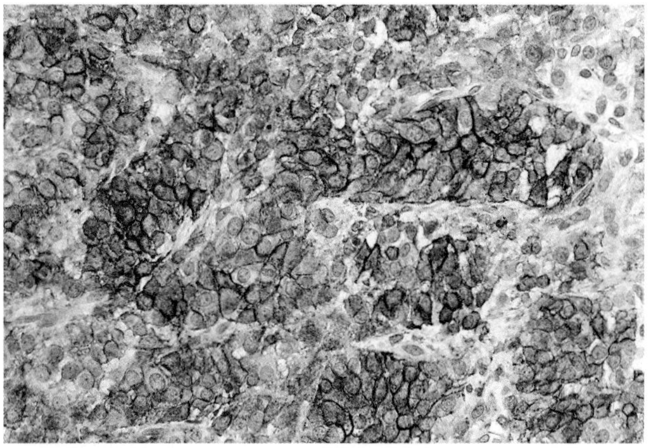

FIGURE 18.36 Juvenile granulosa cell tumor. Strong membrane staining for CD99 is present in nearly all juvenile granulosa cell tumors.

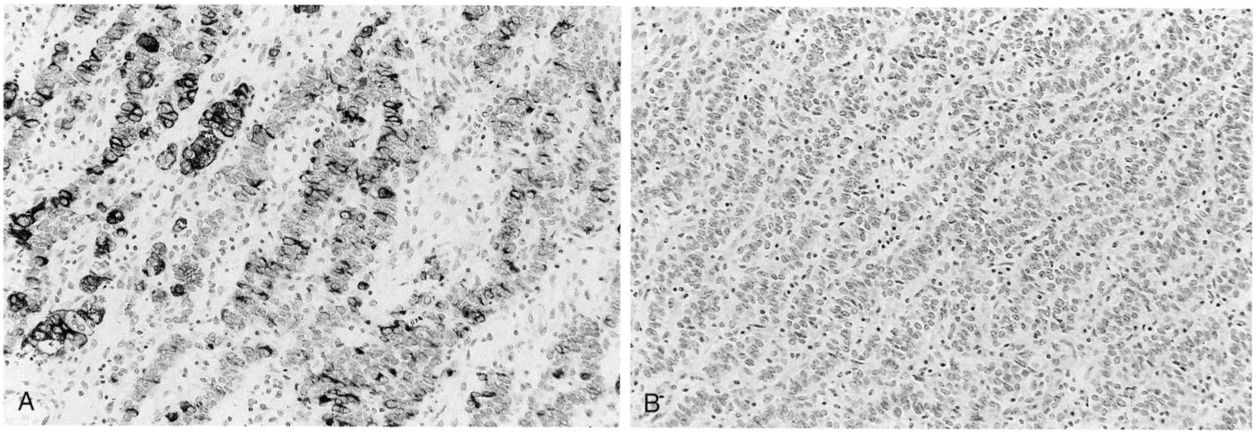

FIGURE 18.37 Sertoli-Leydig cell tumor. The Sertoli cell cords and tubules can be difficult to identify. **(A)** Staining for cytokeratin can be helpful; positive cytoplasmic staining in Sertoli cells growing in cords or tubules, as shown here, is characteristic. **(B)** Sertoli cell cords and tubules are EMA negative. The lack of staining for EMA in Sertoli cords and tubules contrasts with positive staining for both cytokeratin and EMA in sertoliform variants of endometrioid carcinoma (illustrated in Figure 18.28).

SERTOLI-LEYDIG CELL TUMOR

Most Useful Antibodies: CK, EMA, Inhibin, Calretinin

Sertoli-Leydig cell tumors occur mainly in young women, and about half are virilizing.[539] In well-differentiated variants, Sertoli cells line well formed tubules that grow in a fibrous stroma that contains clusters of polygonal Leydig cells.[540,541] Immature stromal and Sertoli cells are not present. The more common intermediate and poorly differentiated Sertoli-Leydig cell tumors contain variably mature Sertoli cells growing in trabeculae or nests or lining round or retiform tubules.[540,542-544] The stroma is cellular and immature, and Leydig cells, present either singly or in clusters, are present in most tumors. Most patients present with tumors confined to the ovary and have a favorable prognosis.

Immunohistochemical stains are important in the diagnosis of Sertoli-Leydig cell tumors because the various cell types can be difficult to recognize and because other tumor types, especially the Sertoliform variant of endometrioid carcinoma, share some histologic features with Sertoli-Leydig cell tumors. Sertoli cells stain for cytokeratin, which highlights tubules and delineates cords, nests, and sheets of immature Sertoli cells, but they are EMA-negative (Fig. 18.37).[346,348,545,546] The stromal cells and Leydig cells are cytokeratin- and EMA-negative. Inhibin and calretinin are usually positive in Sertoli-Leydig cell tumors, although staining can be patchy and is strongest in the Leydig cells.[337,341-344,359,361,435,500,533] Sertoli cells tend to show strong membrane staining with CD99.[532] Sertoli cells can also exhibit strong nuclear staining for WT1, a finding that is also seen in various types of adenocarcinoma that can enter into the differential diagnosis of Sertoli-Leydig cell tumor.[435] Staining for estrogen and/or progesterone receptors is present in some Sertoli-Leydig cell tumors.[534] Staining for estrogen receptors is likely to be stronger and more diffuse than staining for progesterone receptors.

Heterologous elements are present in about 20% of Sertoli-Leydig cell tumors, and immunostains can help with their identification and classification. Gastrointestinal type epithelium is the most common heterologous element;[547] it stains for cytokeratin and EMA but is negative for inhibin. Cells that are immunoreactive for chromogranin, serotonin, and various peptides such as corticotropin, somatostatin, and calcitonin are often present in the heterologous enteric epithelium.[548] Rarely, Sertoli-Leydig cell tumors exhibit foci of heterologous hepatoid differentiation that secrete α-fetoprotein (Fig. 18.38).[399,401] The hepatoid cells stain for low molecular weight cytokeratins (cytokeratins 8/18), with anti-hepatocyte antibody, and for α-fetoprotein, but not for inhibin. Heterologous carcinoid differentiation is chromogranin- and/or synaptophysin-positive. Foci of heterologous rhabdomyoblastic differentiation, a poor prognostic finding, stain for desmin and, usually, myogenin.[549]

The uncommon Sertoliform variant of endometrioid carcinoma is generally cytokeratin- and EMA-positive and lacks staining for inhibin or calretinin. Positive staining for inhibin and calretinin and lack of staining for EMA helps to differentiate between a Sertoli-Leydig cell tumor and the Sertoliform variant of endometrioid carcinoma (see Table 18.7).[474,545,546,550] Rare Sertoli-Leydig cell tumors with pseudoendometrioid tubules almost invariably contain at least focal areas of more typical Sertoli-Leydig cell tumor morphology, and the pseudoendometrioid tubules show positive staining for inhibin and calretinin, and lack staining for EMA.[551]

SERTOLI CELL TUMOR

Most Useful Antibodies: CK, EMA, Inhibin, Calretinin

Sertoli cell tumors are rare benign neoplasms in which Sertoli cells line tubules or grow in trabeculae.[418,552] They lack the primitive stroma and Leydig cells that are present in Sertoli-Leydig cell tumors. Oxyphilic and lipid-rich variants have been described,[553] and Sertoli cell tumors can contain areas of diffuse growth. Immunohistochemistry can help to confirm the diagnosis and to differentiate a Sertoli cell tumor from such differential diagnostic considerations as Sertoliform endometrioid

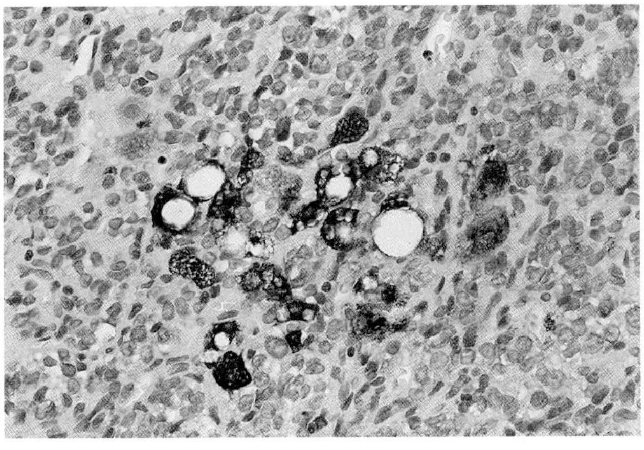

FIGURE 18.38 Sertoli-Leydig cell tumor. This tumor shows focal heterologous hepatic differentiation in which the hepatocytic cells show strong cytoplasmic staining for AFP; they also stained with anti-hepatocyte antibody.

carcinoma and metastatic carcinoma. Sertoli cell tumors exhibit positive staining for vimentin and cytokeratin but they do not stain for epithelial membrane antigen.[422] They are inhibin- and calretinin-positive, and most also stain for CD99.[361,422] Sertoliform endometrioid carcinomas stain not only for cytokeratin but also for EMA, and they are usually inhibin- and calretinin-negative.[474,475,545,550,554,555]

SEX CORD TUMOR WITH ANNULAR TUBULES

Most Useful Antibodies: CK, EMA, Inhibin, Calretinin

The sex cord tumor with annular tubules (SCTAT) is an unclassified sex cord–stromal tumor that occurs in two clinical settings. About 33% of patients with SCTAT have Peutz-Jeghers syndrome and small, often microscopic tumors that are usually multifocal and bilateral. The remaining 66% of patients do not have the Peutz-Jeghers syndrome; they have larger unilateral tumors that can be hormonally active and can recur or metastasize. Regardless of the clinical setting, the tumors are composed of columnar cells with basal nuclei that line closed annular tubules that often surround cores of eosinophilic hyaline material. The SCTAT has an immunophenotype that is similar to that of other sex cord–stromal tumors: they stain for vimentin, cytokeratin, inhibin, and calretinin[343,344,346,556] and do not stain for epithelial membrane antigen. The hyaline material in the eosinophilic cores and stroma has been shown to be basement membrane material by ultrastructural study. It stains, at least in some cases, for laminin and type IV collagen.

LEYDIG CELL TUMOR

Most Useful Antibodies: CK, EMA, Inhibin, Calretinin

Leydig cell tumors are benign ovarian tumors that frequently secrete sufficient testosterone to cause symptoms that lead to their discovery at a small size. They are composed of polygonal Leydig cells with vesicular nuclei, often conspicuous nucleoli, and abundant eosinophilic or pale vacuolated cytoplasm. The cytoplasm characteristically contains eosinophilic hyaline globules or rod-shaped inclusions. The latter are known as crystalloids of Reinke, and their presence is diagnostic of a Leydig cell tumor. Most Leydig cell tumors develop in the hilum of the ovary and are sometimes called hilus cell tumors. Nonhilar Leydig cell tumors and stromal Leydig cell tumors are difficult to diagnose because crystalloids of Reinke are required for their positive identification, and these can only be found in about 50% of cases. Immunohistochemical stains are usually not required for the diagnosis of a Leydig cell tumor, and they do not help to differentiate Leydig cell tumors from other sex cord–stromal tumors and tumor-like conditions that enter into the differential diagnosis, such as luteinized thecoma, unclassified steroid cell tumors, and luteoma of pregnancy. Leydig cells stain for inhibin, calretinin, and melan-A, and they are usually negative for keratin and epithelial membrane antigen.[359]

STEROID CELL TUMOR

Most Useful Antibodies: CK, EMA, Inhibin, Calretinin

Steroid cell tumors tend to be large unilateral neoplasms. Many are hormonally active and secrete testosterone or other hormones. Microscopically, they are composed of large polygonal cells with abundant cytoplasm. Some cells have clear, vacuolated cytoplasm and resemble adrenal cortical cells. Others have dense eosinophilic cytoplasm and resemble Leydig cells, except for the absence of crystalloids of Reinke. Both cell types can be present in a steroid cell tumor, but one or the other cell type can predominate. Large size, marked nuclear atypia, and a high mitotic index correlate with malignant behavior. Steroid cell tumors are typically immunoreactive for inhibin, calretinin, and melan A.[341,344,435,516,557] Steroid cell tumors tend to show positive staining for steroidogenic factor-1 (SF-1), but staining for CD99 is weak and variable and most tumors lack staining for WT1. Most steroid cell tumors are vimentin-positive, and 40% to 50% stain for cytokeratin.[558] Stains for EMA are negative.

KEY DIAGNOSTIC POINTS

Sex Cord–Stromal Tumors

- Sex cord–stromal tumors can be either positive or negative for CK.
- Sex cord–stromal tumors are almost always EMA negative. Positive staining for EMA suggests an epithelial tumor, either primary or metastatic, that is mimicking a sex cord–stromal tumor.
- Inhibin is a relatively specific marker for sex cord–stromal tumors.
- Calretinin is a more sensitive, but less specific marker for sex cord–stromal tumors than inhibin.
- Other markers for sex cord–stromal tumors include CD56, WT1, and SF-1.

Germ Cell Tumors

Germ cell tumors can be grouped into three main categories. The first includes the common benign cystic teratoma, which accounts for most of the germ cell tumors observed in general practice, and a less common solid mature variant. These tumors tend to be grossly and microscopically distinctive, and they contain skin and skin appendages as well as benign tissues derived from other germ cell layers. Glial tissue is often conspicuous. Immunohistochemistry is rarely required for the diagnosis of simple benign teratomas. The second group includes variants of benign cystic teratoma in which one line of differentiation predominates or completely overgrows the teratoma, resulting in a monodermal teratoma. Tumors in this category include struma ovarii, carcinoid tumors, and malignant tumors such as carcinomas and melanomas that have arisen in a benign cystic teratoma. Immunohistochemistry is useful in the diagnosis of tumors in this category. The third main group comprises the malignant germ cell tumors: dysgerminoma, immature teratoma, yolk sac tumor, embryonal carcinoma, choriocarcinoma, polyembryoma, and mixed germ cell tumors that contain two or more of the pure types. These are rare tumors that tend to occur in young patients. Treatment is by conservative surgery, often followed by chemotherapy. Accurate diagnosis is essential to assure proper management, and immunostains are often used to confirm the diagnosis. The stains most often used for the diagnosis of malignant germ cell tumors include CD117, placental alkaline phosphatase (PLAP), Oct-4, D2-40, α-fetoprotein, glypican-3, CD30, hCG, broad-spectrum antikeratins such as AE1/AE3, and EMA. We will discuss these stains in the following paragraphs.

DYSGERMINOMA

Most Useful Antibodies: CK, EMA, PLAP, CD117, Oct-4, D2-40, hCG

Dysgerminoma is the ovarian analogue of testicular seminoma. It consists of large polygonal tumor cells with round vesicular nuclei with conspicuous nucleoli. The cells have abundant clear or eosinophilic cytoplasm, and the cell membranes tend to be well defined. The tumor cells grow in nests and sheets divided by fibrous trabeculae. Lymphocytes are present in variable numbers in the fibrous trabeculae and among the tumor cells, and sarcoid-like granulomas are commonly present. Dysgerminoma shows cytoplasmic and membrane staining for placental alkaline phosphatase (PLAP) and membrane staining for CD117 (c-*kit*)(Fig. 18.39).[374,382,387] Staining for CD117 is especially helpful because other tumors in the differential diagnosis, such as embryonal carcinoma and yolk sac tumor, do not show the membranous pattern of CD117 staining that is characteristic of dysgerminoma (Table 18.10).[318] Dysgerminoma and embryonal carcinoma, like seminoma and embryonal carcinoma of the testis, exhibit strong nuclear staining for the stem cell–related proteins Oct-4 and NANOG.[384,347] Oct-4 is more widely used and is an excellent marker for dysgerminoma, showing strong positive nuclear staining in almost every case (Fig. 18.40). Most other types of germ cell tumors, such as yolk sac tumor and choriocarcinoma, lack staining for Oct-4. As previously noted, embryonal carcinoma is positive. Clear cell carcinoma, which enters the differential diagnosis of dysgerminoma in some cases, shows focal staining (<10% of tumor cells) in a minority of cases.[384] D2-40 (podoplanin), widely used to mark lymphovascular endothelial cells and mesothelioma, shows diffuse strong positive cytoplasmic and membrane staining in dysgerminoma. Embryonal carcinoma is usually negative for D2-40, or shows only limited staining.[559] Dysgerminoma can show patchy positive staining for cytokeratin, often in a rimlike or dotlike cytoplasmic pattern.[560] Diffuse strong staining such as that seen in other germ cell tumors and in epithelial tumors does not occur. Stains for EMA and CD30 are negative, as are stains for S-100 protein, lymphoid markers, and neuroendocrine markers. About 5% of dysgerminomas contain syncytiotrophoblastic giant cells (STGCs) that show strong cytoplasmic staining for cytokeratin and hCG (Fig. 18.41).[411]

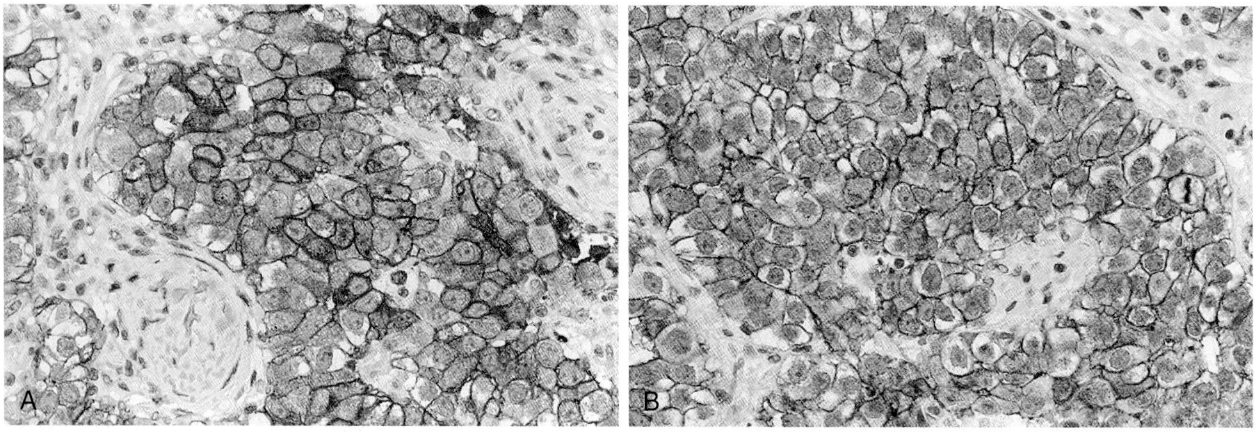

FIGURE 18.39 Dysgerminoma shows **(A)** strong cytoplasmic and membrane staining for placental alkaline phosphatase (PLAP) and **(B)** strong membrane staining for CD117 (c-*kit*).

TABLE 18.10 Differential Diagnosis of Dysgerminoma

	PLAP	CD117	Oct-4	CK	CD30	S-100	LCA	MPO
Dysgerminoma	+	+	+	N	N	N	N	N
Embryonal carcinoma	+	N	+	+	+	N	N	N
Yolk sac tumor	+	N	N	+	N	N	N	N
Lymphoma	N	N	N	N	N	N	+	N
Granulocytic sarcoma	N	+	N	N	N	N	+	+
Melanoma	N	N	N	N	N	+	N	N

PLAP, placental alkaline phosphatase; CD117 (c-*kit),* membrane staining; CK, cytokeratin, rare dysgerminomas show weak staining, with AE1/AE3 embryonal carcinoma shows membrane staining and yolk sac tumor cytoplasmic staining; LCA, leukocyte common antigen; MPO, myeloperoxidase.
+, almost always positive; N, negative.

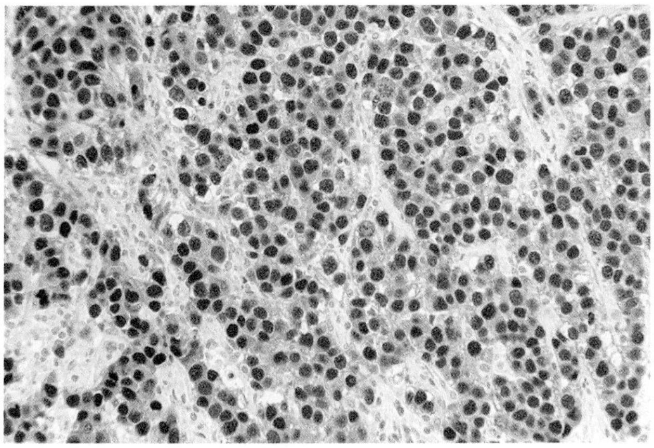

FIGURE 18.40 Dysgerminoma. Strong nuclear staining for Oct-4, as shown here, is characteristic of dysgerminoma. In the ovary, the only other tumor types that stain for this marker are embryonal carcinoma and the germ cells in gonadoblastoma.

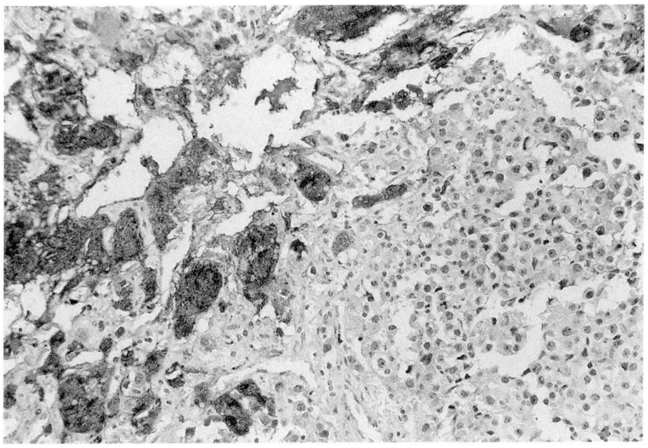

FIGURE 18.41 Dysgerminoma. The patient had an elevated serum beta-hCG, and the tumor contained many syncytiotrophoblastic giant cells. These show diffuse strong cytoplasmic staining for hCG (left), while the dysgerminoma cells are hCG-negative (right).

YOLK SAC TUMOR

Most Useful Antibodies: CK AE1/AE3, CK7, EMA, Alpha Fetoprotein, Glypican-3

Yolk sac tumor is an uncommon malignant germ cell tumor that grows in a confusing variety of histologic patterns. Immunohistochemical staining can help establish the diagnosis. The most useful stain is for α-fetoprotein, as positive staining for AFP is a characteristic of yolk sac tumor (Fig. 18.42).[388] Staining for α-fetoprotein is variable and often patchy; diffuse strong staining is not seen in every tumor.[318] Nevertheless, more than 75% of yolk sac tumors show positive cytoplasmic staining for α-fetoprotein. Secretory material in gland lumens and the hyaline globules that are often seen in yolk sac tumors can also stain for α-fetoprotein. Positive staining for AFP is particularly helpful in the identification of some of the rare variants of yolk sac tumor, such as the endometrioid and glandular variants. Hepatoid yolk sac tumor is AFP-positive and also shows positive cytoplasmic staining with anti-hepatocyte antibody.[396] This can help with the diagnosis of this rare variant of yolk sac tumor, but positive staining does not differentiate hepatoid yolk sac tumor from hepatoid carcinoma of the ovary or from metastatic hepatocellular carcinoma, as these also show positive staining. Glypican-3 shows strong positive cytoplasmic staining in more than 95% of yolk sac tumors, and it has emerged as an additional positive confirmatory stain for the diagnosis.[394] Glypican-3 rarely stains clear cell carcinoma, but, like AFP, it is positive in tumors with hepatoid features, including hepatoid yolk sac tumor, hepatoid carcinoma, and metastatic hepatocellular carcinoma.[394] Yolk sac tumor is positive for broad-spectrum cytokeratins. Yolk sac tumor shows diffuse cytoplasmic staining with AE1/AE3 (Fig. 18.43), as opposed to the membrane staining seen in embryonal carcinoma. This difference can be exploited for differential diagnostic purposes (see Table 18.10). Yolk sac tumor usually does not stain for EMA or CD15,[394,402] and it is reported to be CK7-negative.[318] When only small foci of yolk sac tumor are present, they often fail to stain for AFP, although they usually mark with cytokeratin and/or glypican-3. Immunostains for placental alkaline phosphatase are often positive, but they are nonspecific because other types of germ cell tumors and some epithelial tumors are also positive.[402] The extracellular hyaline material in yolk sac tumors is laminin-positive. Immunostains for hCG are negative except for positive cytoplasmic staining in the STGCs that are occasionally present in yolk sac tumors.

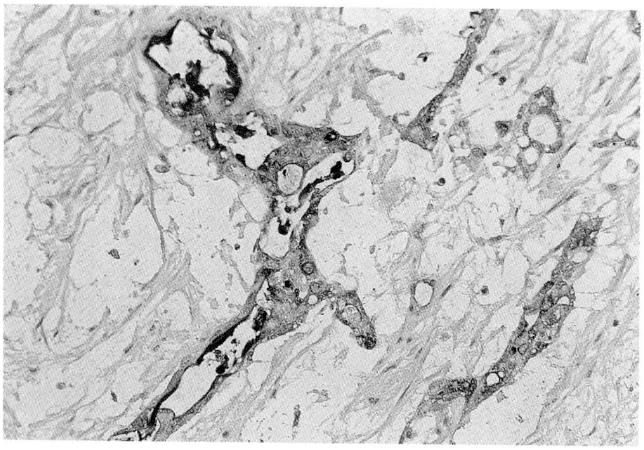

FIGURE 18.42 Yolk sac tumor, showing positive staining for AFP. Weak to moderate patchy staining, as shown here, is characteristic. Diffuse strong staining for AFP is unusual.

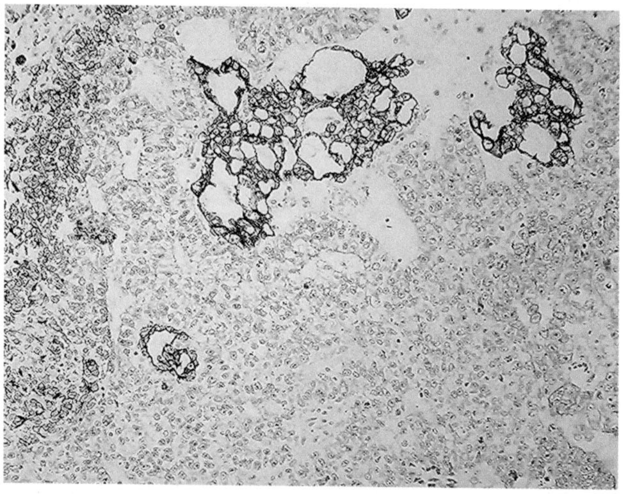

FIGURE 18.43 Mixed germ cell tumor. An immunostain for cytokeratin AE1/AE3 helps to delineate the various elements. Foci of yolk sac tumor (top) show strong cytoplasmic staining for keratin. The surrounding dysgerminoma is keratin negative.

EMBRYONAL CARCINOMA

Most Useful Antibodies: CK AE1/AE3, EMA, CD30, Oct-4

Although it is a relatively common form of germ cell neoplasia in the testis, embryonal carcinoma is rare in the ovary. It occurs most often as a constituent of a mixed germ cell tumor, mixed with yolk sac tumor or other tumor types, but it can occur in pure form. Immunostains are helpful to confirm the diagnosis and delineate areas of embryonal carcinoma from yolk sac tumor, which can be difficult in routine H&E-stained sections. Embryonal carcinoma is keratin-positive. We find staining with cytokeratin AE1/AE3 useful as it shows staining of tumor cell membranes with little if any staining in tumor cell cytoplasm. This contrasts with the cytoplasmic pattern of staining seen in yolk sac tumor. The two most characteristic immunohistochemical features of embryonal carcinoma are diffuse strong nuclear staining for Oct-4 and diffuse strong membrane staining for CD30 (Fig. 18.44). Embryonal carcinoma and dysgerminoma are the only two types of germ cell tumors that stain for Oct-4, and embryonal carcinoma is the only one that stains for CD30. Diffuse positive staining for cytokeratin and CD30 and absence of staining for CD117 differentiates embryonal carcinoma from dysgerminoma. Immunostains for placental alkaline phosphatase (PLAP) are frequently positive. Embryonal carcinoma does not stain for epithelial membrane antigen. Based on limited testing of ovarian tumors and staining of testicular ones, embryonal carcinoma shows no or at most limited staining of the tumor cells for D2-40,[559] which is strongly positive in dysgerminoma. Syncytiotrophoblastic giant cells are commonly present in embryonal carcinoma. These show strong homogeneous cytoplasmic staining for keratin, and they are positive for hCG. Patchy staining for α-fetoprotein is noted in some embryonal carcinomas. It is unclear whether this represents staining of embryonal carcinoma cells, staining of cells showing early functional differentiation toward yolk sac tumor, or a difficult-to-recognize component of yolk sac tumor.

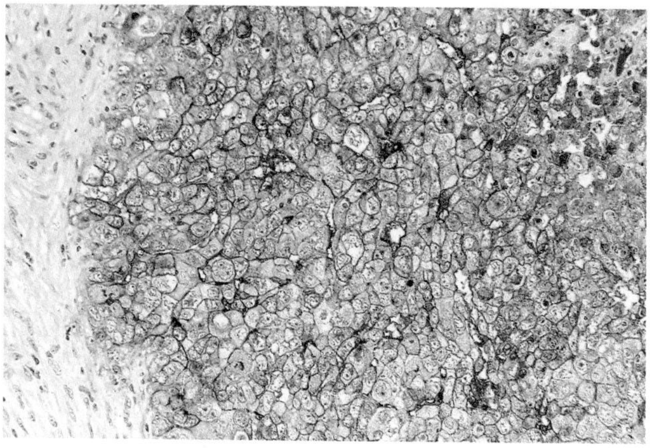

FIGURE 18.44 Embryonal carcinoma. An immunostain for CD30 shows strong membrane staining, characteristic of embryonal carcinoma. Staining for cytokeratin AE1/AE3 shows a similar membrane pattern in embryonal carcinoma, as compared to a cytoplasmic pattern of staining in yolk sac tumor (see Figure 18.43).

CHORIOCARCINOMA

Most Useful Antibodies: CK AE1/AE3, hCG

Choriocarcinoma rarely occurs in pure form in the ovary; it is usually present as a constituent of a mixed germ cell tumor. Choriocarcinoma is characterized by an admixture of cytotrophoblastic, intermediate trophoblastic, and syncytiotrophoblastic cells. There is positive staining for hCG in the cytoplasm of the syncytiotrophoblastic giant cells but not in cytotrophoblastic or intermediate trophoblastic cells. Stains for hCG can be somewhat difficult to interpret owing to high background staining most likely caused by hCG in the serum. Inhibin can also be used as a marker for syncytiotrophoblastic cells and has the advantage of low background staining.[244,245,561,562] It is worth noting that CD10 stains trophoblastic cells.[563] All trophoblastic

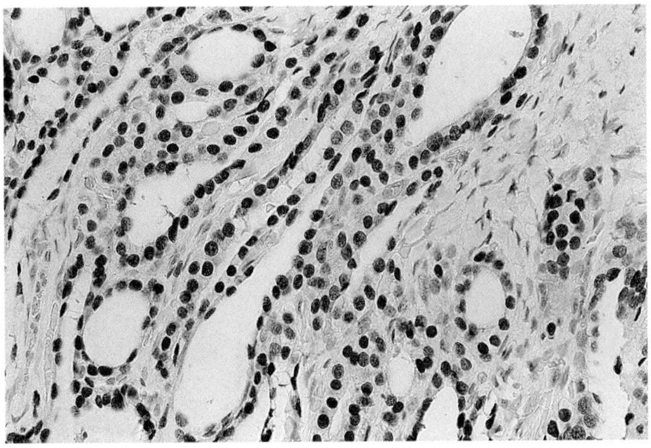

FIGURE 18.45 Struma ovarii is a form of monodermal teratoma in which thyroid tissue predominates. The thyroid cells show strong nuclear staining for thyroid transcription factor 1 (TTF-1), as shown here. The tumor cell cytoplasm and the colloid also stain positively for thyroglobulin.

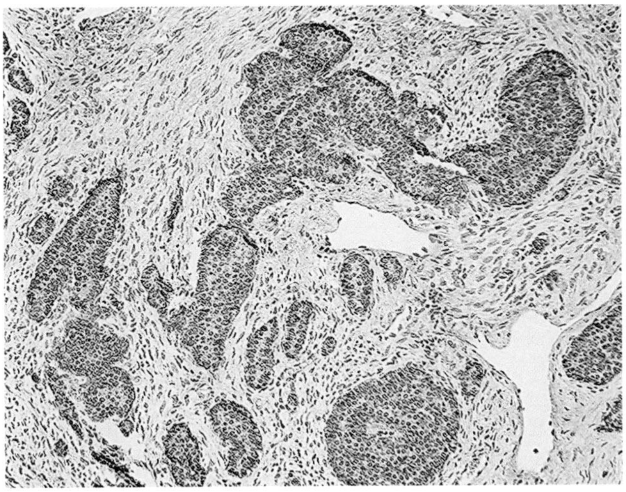

FIGURE 18.46 Carcinoid tumors in the ovary can be found with other tissues as a component of a teratoma. They can also be primary in the ovary but not associated with other teratomatous tissues, in which case they are viewed as monodermal teratomas. Finally, they can be metastatic from the appendix, small intestine, or other sites. Regardless of their origin, they show cytoplasmic staining for chromogranin, as shown here, and for synaptophysin.

cells are positive for cytokeratin, but negative for epithelial membrane antigen. The syncytiotrophoblastic giant cells have abundant cytoplasm that shows diffuse strong staining for cytokeratin, thereby making them easy to identify even at low magnification. While choriocarcinoma is most often present as a component of a mixed germ cell tumor or in pure form, rare ovarian carcinomas with choriocarcinomatous differentiation have been reported.[416,564]

TERATOMAS

Most Useful Antibodies: Depends on Specific Type of Teratoma

Immunohistochemistry usually plays little role in the evaluation of mature and immature teratomas. Glial tissue can be abundant, and its identity can be confirmed by staining for glial fibrillary acidic protein (GFAP) if necessary. Staining for the proliferation marker Ki-67 (MIB1) can be of assistance in the differential diagnosis between mature and immature teratoma. The ependymal rosettes that can be found in mature teratomas show low proliferative activity, while the neuroepithelial tubules that occur in immature teratomas show high proliferative activity. Recently, glial cell line-derived neurotrophic factor receptor α 1 (GFR alpha-1) has been shown to exhibit strong membranous staining in immature neuroectodermal cells in immature teratoma, and it has been proposed that it might be helpful in identifying areas of immaturity.[565] Increased serum levels of α-fetoprotein are detected in some patients who have an immature teratoma. Immunohistochemical staining in such cases shows α-fetoprotein staining in endodermal glandlike vesicles, immature enteric epithelium, and hepatic cells.[403,566]

There is a greater role for immunohistochemistry in the diagnosis of monodermal teratomas. Some examples of struma ovarii are largely cystic and contain few follicles[567]; grow in unusual patterns or are composed of cells with clear or eosinophilic cytoplasm[568]; or resemble thyroid adenomas or carcinomas.[569] In such cases it may be necessary to identify thyroglobulin in the tumor cell cytoplasm and colloid or TTF-1 in the tumor cell nuclei (Fig. 18.45) to confirm the diagnosis.[567,568] Various types of carcinoid tumors, which may or may not be associated with other teratomatous elements, occur in the ovary. The types of carcinoids that occur in the ovary include insular, trabecular, strumal, and mucinous carcinoids. Carcinoid tumors can mimic other ovarian tumors, so immunohistochemical stains help to establish the correct diagnosis. Insular and trabecular carcinoids can resemble sex cord–stromal tumors, such as granulosa cell tumors, Sertoli cell tumors, or Sertoli-Leydig cell tumors. However, in carcinoids, diffuse strong positive staining for cytokeratin and for the neuroendocrine markers chromogranin and synaptophysin (Fig. 18.46) plus a lack of staining for inhibin and calretinin can establish the correct diagnosis. A variety of peptide hormones, such as serotonin, can also be identified in carcinoids.[570] Strumal carcinoids show partial thyroid differentiation and can be mistaken for cellular or malignant struma ovarii. Positive staining for thyroglobulin in the parts of the tumor showing thyroid differentiation and positive staining for chromogranin and synaptophysin in the carcinoid component serve to confirm the diagnosis.[571-573] Some strumal carcinoids exhibit positive staining for calcitonin, and most have the interesting characteristic of staining for prostatic acid phosphatase (PSAP), although they do not stain for prostate-specific antigen (PSA).[571,572] In addition, strumal carcinoids that are associated with a severe constipation syndrome show positive staining for protein YY.[574] Mucinous carcinoids tend to exhibit positive staining for chromogranin, synaptophysin, and/or serotonin, and their immunophenotype can help differentiate them from various types of primary and metastatic mucinous neoplasms.[575] We have observed that primary insular and mucinous carcinoids express CDX2, so staining for CDX2 cannot be used to determine whether a carcinoid in the ovary is primary or metastatic.[576] Primary ovarian carcinoids other than strumal carcinoids lack staining for TTF-1, and they do not stain for CK7.[576] Only mucinous carcinoids show staining for CK20.

GONADOBLASTOMA

Gonadoblastoma contains a mixture of primitive germ cells and sex cord cells, typically arranged around cores of hyaline material. In some cases an invasive malignant germ cell tumor, usually a germinoma, arises in the gonadoblastoma. Immunohistochemical stains reveal that the germ cells stain for placental alkaline phosphatase, CD117, and Oct-4 and that the sex cord cells stain for vimentin, cytokeratin, and inhibin.[344,384,514,577,578] The hyaline material that is intermixed with the tumor cells will stain for laminin, which indicates that it is basement membrane material.[578]

KEY DIAGNOSTIC POINTS

Germ Cell Tumors

- PLAP can be positive in most types of malignant germ cell tumors, but it also can stain epithelial neoplasms.
- Oct-4, CD117, and D2-40 are the most useful markers for dysgerminoma.
- Oct-4 and CD30 are the most useful markers for embryonal carcinoma.
- Alpha-fetoprotein and glypican-3 are the most useful markers for yolk sac tumor.
- Cytokeratin AE1/AE3 stains many malignant germ cell tumors, and the pattern of staining can help with classification.
- EMA is negative in most malignant germ cell tumors.

METASTATIC TUMORS

Metastases to the ovary are common; they are usually of epithelial type and account for as many as 10% of malignant ovarian tumors in some series. The most common primary sites of tumors that metastasize to the ovary are the gastrointestinal tract, particularly the large intestine, the stomach, and the appendix; the breast; the female genital tract, including the endometrium and the cervix; and the pancreas, although tumors of any type and from any site can on occasion give rise to ovarian metastases.[579] The differentiation of a primary surface epithelial tumor of the ovary from an extragenital primary tumor can be difficult, especially when the surgeon or pathologist, or both, do not know the patient's clinical history. Morphologic clues are useful, but there are many instances in which the histopathologic appearance is misleading; immunohistochemistry can be particularly valuable in such cases. Immunohistochemistry is most helpful in identifying metastases from nongenital sites. Differentiation between a primary ovarian tumor and a metastasis from another genital primary site, such as the endometrium, is more difficult, and immunohistochemical staining may not be helpful.

Among common epithelial tumors, serous neoplasms are usually readily recognized as primary neoplasms and are only infrequently mimicked by metastases. On the other hand, metastatic adenocarcinomas commonly mimic both mucinous and endometrioid tumors. In a recent report, 77% of mucinous ovarian cancers were metastatic.[580] Primary mucinous and endometrioid tumors tend to be unilateral, and primary mucinous tumors are usually larger than 10 cm in diameter.[580] Small mucinous tumors and bilateral tumors that are thought to be of mucinous or endometrioid type should be evaluated for the possibility that they represent metastases.[581] This rule of thumb applies not only to obviously invasive tumors (carcinomas) but also to apparently borderline tumors. Metastatic mucinous adenocarcinomas from the appendix, colon, pancreas, and gallbladder can on occasion show remarkable morphologic overlap with borderline mucinous and endometrioid tumors. Evaluation of tumors that might represent metastases from these sites should include antibodies against CK7, CK20, and CDX2 (see Table 18.6). Primary ovarian carcinomas are almost invariably diffusely and strongly positive for CK7, and, although there are exceptions,[448] metastatic colorectal carcinomas are usually entirely negative (Fig. 18.47A) or show only minimal staining.[582] Tumors from the rectum and appendix are somewhat more likely to show staining for CK7,[316,583] and biliary tract tumors are almost invariably CK7-positive.[584,585] Metastatic colorectal tumors are usually diffusely and strongly positive for CK20 and CDX2 (Fig. 18.47B and 18.48).[582] Carcinomas of the biliary tract and pancreas stain variably for CK20. Endometrioid carcinoma does not stain for CK20 or CDX2. Primary mucinous carcinoma is CK20-positive, and it can stain for CDX2, but the staining for both of these markers is typically weaker and more focal than is observed in metastatic colorectal carcinoma.[448,454] Thus, the immunophenotypes CK7+ CK20– and CK7+ CK20+ CDX2+ favor an ovarian primary tumor, and the immunophenotype CK7– CK20+ CDX2+ strongly favors a metastasis.[315,454,586] Another antibody that may be of utility is Dpc4 (Smad4), a nuclear factor that is absent in about 50% of pancreatic adenocarcinomas.[316] We will discuss the use of these antibodies in the "Mucinous Tumors" section.

Metastatic adenocarcinoma from the stomach tends to be bilateral and of the signet ring cell (Krukenberg tumor) or poorly differentiated type, although gland formation is present in some tumors and rare tumors are composed entirely of intestinal-type glands.[587] Signet ring cells are rare in primary ovarian tumors,[588,589] so their presence indicates that the tumor is almost certainly metastatic, with stomach being the most likely primary site.[590] Metastatic stomach cancer tends to be CK7-positive (56% of cases in one study), and a substantial proportion of cases (33%) are also positive for CK20.[586] Morphology can therefore be more important than immunohistochemistry in establishing the correct diagnosis.

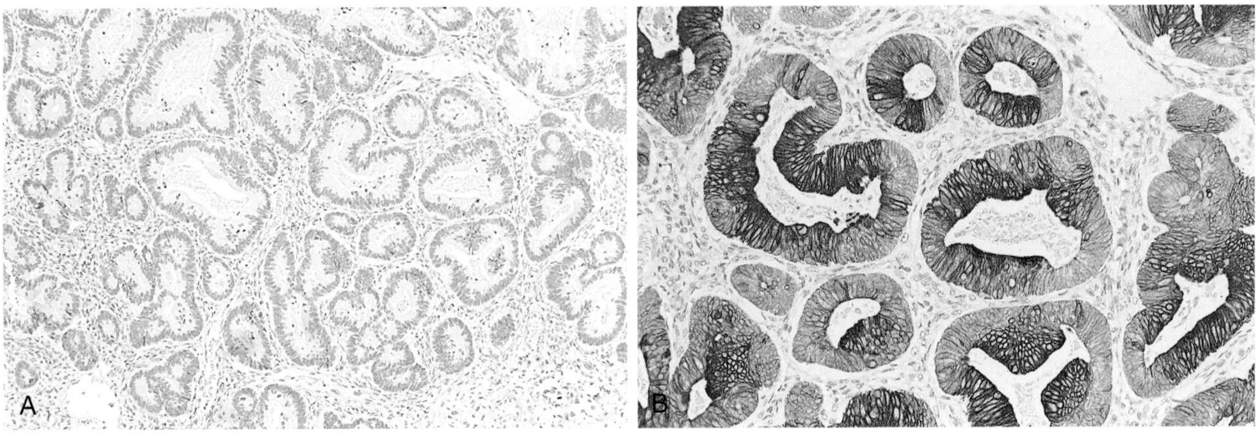

FIGURE 18.47 Colorectal adenocarcinoma is the tumor that most often metastasizes to the ovary. Metastatic colorectal adenocarcinoma is **(A)** typically CK7-negative but **(B)** it shows diffuse strong staining for CK20.

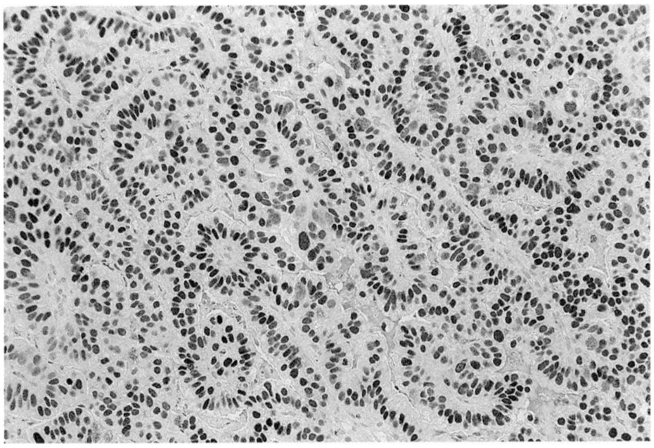

FIGURE 18.48 Metastatic adenocarcinoma from the appendix, showing diffuse strong nuclear staining for the transcription factor CDX2, a useful marker for metastatic intestinal and appendiceal adenocarcinoma. Some primary mucinous carcinomas of the ovary stain for CDX2, but staining is often weaker or patchier than is seen in metastatic intestinal carcinomas.

Metastases from the pancreas, biliary tract, and even the gastrointestinal tract can occasionally mimic clear cell carcinoma;[591] these can also be evaluated with antibodies against CK7, CK20, and Dpc4. Pancreatic ductal adenocarcinoma shows a variable staining pattern for CK7 and CK20, and in some cases its staining pattern overlaps that of primary mucinous carcinoma of the ovary. Primary ovarian carcinomas are not known to show loss of staining for Dpc4, so this finding is very helpful in identifying metastatic pancreatic ductal adenocarcinoma. Pancreatic acinar adenocarcinoma is rare, but it can metastasize to the ovary.[592] The tumor cells have granular eosinophilic cytoplasm and are arranged in acini. Positive staining for trypsin and chymotrypsin facilitates recognition of this type of metastatic adenocarcinoma. Metastatic clear cell carcinoma of the kidney can also mimic primary ovarian clear cell carcinoma, but this is a rare diagnostic problem as renal tumors usually do not metastasize to the ovaries. Metastatic renal cell carcinoma of clear cell type is CK7-negative, but it shows strong membrane staining with antibodies to CD10 and renal cell carcinoma antigen (RCC). Primary clear cell carcinoma is CK7-positive, CD10-negative, and RCC-negative. Finally, when transitional cell tumors do not contain a benign Brenner component, distinction from a metastatic urothelial tumor is important. Primary ovarian transitional cell carcinoma is CK7-positive. While metastatic urothelial carcinoma is also CK7-positive, it can stain for CK20, thrombomodulin, or uroplakin, with the latter results differentiating it from ovarian transitional cell carcinoma. Transitional cell carcinoma is WT1-positive and more likely than urothelial carcinoma to stain for estrogen and progesterone receptors.

Other carcinomas that metastasize to the ovary and for which immunohistochemistry is helpful in the differential diagnosis include breast, lung, and thyroid. Breast cancer only rarely poses a differential diagnostic problem because the patient is usually known to have a history of a breast neoplasm,[593,594] and the morphology of metastatic breast cancer differs from that of most ovarian cancers. However, some breast cancers, particularly those with a micropapillary appearance, can be difficult to differentiate from a primary ovarian carcinoma.[595] There is considerable overlap in the immunophenotype of breast and ovarian cancer. Both are CK7-positive and CK20-negative, and they may show staining for estrogen and progesterone receptors. Some breast cancers show staining for gross cystic disease fluid protein 15 (GCDFP15), making this a potentially useful stain for differentiating between breast and ovarian cancers.[308,596] In our practice, and as noted in reports by others,[321] GCDFP15 lacks sensitivity, thus it has not proven to be particularly useful as a marker of metastatic breast cancer. We find mammaglobin to be a more useful marker for metastatic breast cancer.[597] WT1 is more commonly expressed by serous ovarian cancer than by metastatic breast carcinoma. CA125 is also more likely to stain primary ovarian carcinomas, but there is staining in a significant minority of breast cancers. An immunohistochemical panel that includes WT1, CA125, mammaglobin, and GCDFP15 generally helps resolve the differential diagnosis between metastatic breast cancer and primary ovarian cancer. PAX8 may also be useful in this differential diagnosis, as it is reported to stain all types of ovarian cancer except for mucinous, and to be negative in breast cancer.[446]

Thyroid transcription factor-1 is a nuclear transcription factor. Staining for TTF-1 is specific for tumors of the thyroid and lung. Thyroid tumors occasionally metastasize to the ovaries, and their nature can be confirmed by positive staining for TTF-1 as well as for thyroglobulin or calcitonin,[598] depending upon their histologic type. Adenocarcinoma and small cell carcinoma of the lung also stain for TTF-1 in a high percentage of cases, and staining for this marker can be helpful when a lung primary is considered for a metastatic tumor in the ovary.[598-600] TTF-1 positivity is confirmatory of lung origin for metastatic adenocarcinoma. Nonpulmonary small cell carcinomas can also stain for TTF-1,[93,601,602] so a positive TTF-1 stain does not prove that a small cell carcinoma in the ovary is metastatic from the lung; it could be primary or metastatic from some other site.[603] Clinicopathologic correlation is necessary to establish the primary site.

Metastases from other genital tract sites can be difficult to differentiate from primary ovarian neoplasms. Morphologic criteria have been developed for deciding whether tumors in the endometrium and ovary are separate synchronous primaries or an endometrial primary with ovarian metastases.[196] For most tumor types, immunohistochemistry is not helpful in resolving this diagnostic dilemma, since endometrioid and clear cell endometrial and ovarian neoplasms have similar immunophenotypes. Immunohistochemistry may be helpful in the evaluation of serous carcinomas because while a high proportion of ovarian primary tumors show strong nuclear staining for WT1, most[166,443] but not all[167] authors have found that staining is detected in a much lower proportion of endometrial serous carcinomas. Thus, lack of staining for WT1 favors an endometrial primary with ovarian metastasis. Endocervical adenocarcinomas occasionally metastasize to the ovaries where they can mimic a primary endometrioid or mucinous adenocarcinoma.[476,604] Cervical tumors that metastasize to the ovaries are often deeply invasive, but metastases can arise from surprisingly superficial cervical adenocarcinomas. Cervical adenocarcinomas are often CEA-positive and, owing to the involvement of human papilloma virus infection in their pathogenesis, they are often p16-positive (see the section entitled "Cervix"). Positive staining for CEA and diffuse strong staining for p16 in an ovarian tumor with an endometrioid appearance is compatible with a metastasis from the cervix; in this context a positive result is strong cytoplasmic and/or nuclear staining in more than 75% of tumor cells.[477] When metastatic cervical adenocarcinoma mimics an ovarian mucinous carcinoma, staining for CEA is not helpful because ovarian mucinous adenocarcinoma is also CEA-positive, but staining for p16 is compatible with metastatic cervical adenocarcinoma. Some have found p16 to be of value in identifying metastatic cervical adenocarcinomas in the ovary and have observed little staining in primary ovarian neoplasms.[477] Others have reported staining of a substantial percentage of primary endometrioid and mucinous carcinomas, all of which were negative for HPV DNA.[478] These conflicting results indicate that the use of p16 staining to determine whether an ovarian neoplasm is metastatic from the cervix requires further investigation.

Virtually any type of tumor, including soft tissue tumors and hematopoietic neoplasms such as lymphoma and leukemia, can involve the ovaries, either primarily or as metastases from a distant site. Many of these have specific immunohistochemical features, as detailed elsewhere in this book, which can be used to assist in their diagnosis.

KEY DIAGNOSTIC POINTS

Metastatic Tumors

- 5% to 10% of malignant ovarian tumors are metastases.
- Colorectal adenocarcinoma is the most frequent metastasis, and it can mimic endometrioid and mucinous adenocarcinoma of the ovary.
- The most useful stains for identifying metastases in the ovary are CK7, CK20, and CDX2.
- Primary ovarian carcinomas are usually CK7-positive, CK20-negative, and CDX2-negative except for mucinous carcinoma, which is CK7-positive, and variably positive for CK20 and CDX2.
- Metastatic tumors are usually, but not always, CK7-negative.
- Metastases from colorectal adenocarcinoma are usually, but not always, CK20-positive.
- Other antibodies can be useful in the identification of metastases, as detailed above.

MESOTHELIOMA

Serous tumors involving the ovaries and peritoneal surfaces can clinically and even pathologically raise the possibility of mesothelioma. While uncommon, peritoneal mesothelioma occurs in women and occasionally in children,[605] and rarely it can be confined to the ovaries.[606-608] Peritoneal mesotheliomas tend to be of the epithelioid type; sarcomatoid and mixed mesotheliomas are uncommon.[609] A deciduoid variant of mesothelioma, in which the tumor cells are large with abundant cytoplasm, was initially described in the peritoneum with some cases occurring in young women.[610-612] The differential diagnosis between peritoneal mesothelioma and serous carcinoma typically requires immunohistochemical analysis. Currently, a panel of immunohistochemical stains is performed (Table 18.11),[317,319] including stains that are usually positive in mesothelioma and negative in serous carcinoma, such as calretinin, D2-40, and h-caldesmon,[613] and stains that are generally positive in serous carcinoma but negative in mesothelioma, such as Ber-EP4, MOC-31, and ER (Fig. 18.49).[614-616] A small percentage of mesotheliomas show positive staining, usually focal, for Ber-EP4 or MOC-31.[617] It is worth noting that some of the stains used to evaluate pleural mesotheliomas are less useful in evaluating peritoneal mesotheliomas. CD15 is positive in only a minority of serous carcinomas, CEA is rarely positive in serous car-

TABLE 18.11 Peritoneal Mesothelioma vs. Serous Carcinoma

	CR	CK5/6	D2-40	Ber-EP4	MOC-31	ER	WT1
Mesothelioma	+	+	+	N	N	N	+
Serous carcinoma	N	N	N	+	+	+	+

CR, calretinin; CK5/6, cytokeratin 5/6; ER, estrogen receptors.
+, almost always positive; N, negative.

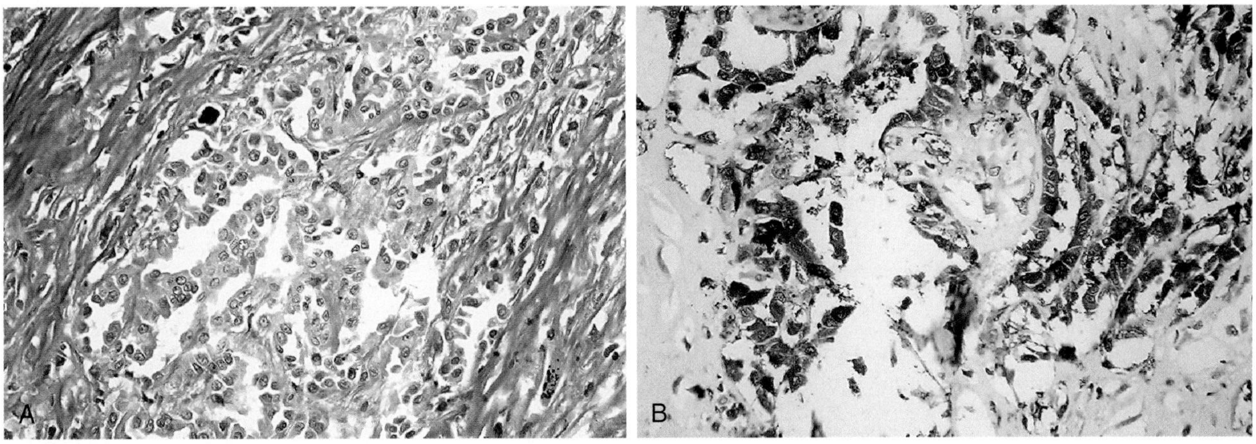

FIGURE 18.49 Mesothelioma. **(A)** A tubular growth pattern and the cuboidal appearance of the tumor cells usually differentiate mesothelioma from serous carcinoma, but in some cases the histologic patterns overlap. **(B)** Mesothelioma shows strong cytoplasmic and nuclear staining for calretinin, as shown here.

cinoma, and WT1 is typically positive in both mesothelioma and serous carcinoma; therefore, none of these antibodies are used in the immunohistochemical panel.

Fallopian Tube and Broad Ligament

Tumors of the fallopian tube and broad ligament are much less common than ovarian neoplasms. Most occur in the fallopian tube, and epithelial tumors are by far the most common.[618] Benign and borderline tumors are rare; most fallopian tube tumors are carcinomas. The same types of carcinoma that occur in the ovary also occur in the fallopian tube. Certain types that are relatively common in the ovary, such as clear cell carcinoma and mucinous carcinoma, rarely arise in the tube. The most common histologic type of tubal carcinoma is serous carcinoma. Endometrioid carcinoma is the second most common, and most of the remaining cases are transitional cell and undifferentiated carcinomas. In one large series, the frequency of the various types of carcinoma was 50% serous, 25% endometrioid, 11% transitional, 8% undifferentiated, 4% mixed cell types, and 2% clear cell.[619] Other studies have reported a higher proportion of serous carcinomas.[620-622] The immunohistochemical features of fallopian tube carcinomas are similar to those of their ovarian counterparts, which are discussed earlier in the chapter. Serous carcinoma of the fallopian tube, the most frequent type, has the same immunophenotype as serous carcinoma of the ovary, with most tumors showing positive immunostaining for WT1, p53, CK7, and CA125.

In recent years, studies of risk reducing salpingo-oophorectomy specimens from women with BRCA mutations have shown that incidentally discovered intraepithelial and invasive carcinomas, almost invariably of serous type, are found mainly in the fallopian tubes rather than the ovaries.[623-625] Detection of small grossly invisible carcinomas in these patients requires sectioning of all tissue. Intraepithelial carcinoma is characterized by marked nuclear atypia, nuclear stratification and disorder, and mitotic activity (Fig. 18.50A). Small invasive carcinomas form masses of malignant cells in the tubal mucosa. The neoplasms, which are preferentially located in the fimbriae of the tubes,[626] typically show diffuse strong nuclear staining for p53 and MIB1, as well as WT1 (Fig. 18.50B). The p53 and MIB1 stains help delineate the neoplasms, often highlighting subtle foci of intraepithelial carcinoma that can then be confirmed by careful evaluation of routine H&E-stained sections. A possible precursor of intraepithelial carcinoma, the so-called *p53 signature lesion,* is p53-positive but lacks the atypia and proliferative activity present in intraepithelial carcinoma.[627,628] Staining for MIB1 differentiates the signature lesion from intraepithelial carcinoma, since staining is low in the former while most nuclei are positive in the latter.

Serial sectioning studies of the fallopian tube have shown that intraepithelial and invasive carcinomas, usually of serous type, are far more frequent than was previously appreciated. Serous neoplasia is frequently present in the fallopian tube in women with serous carcinoma of the ovaries or peritoneum, and it has been proposed that many carcinomas involving these sites represent metastases from a carcinoma of the fallopian tube rather than primary neoplasms.[629] Alternatively, this could be an example of multifocal tumorigenesis.[630]

There are two tumor types that occur preferentially in the region of the tube and broad ligament and that

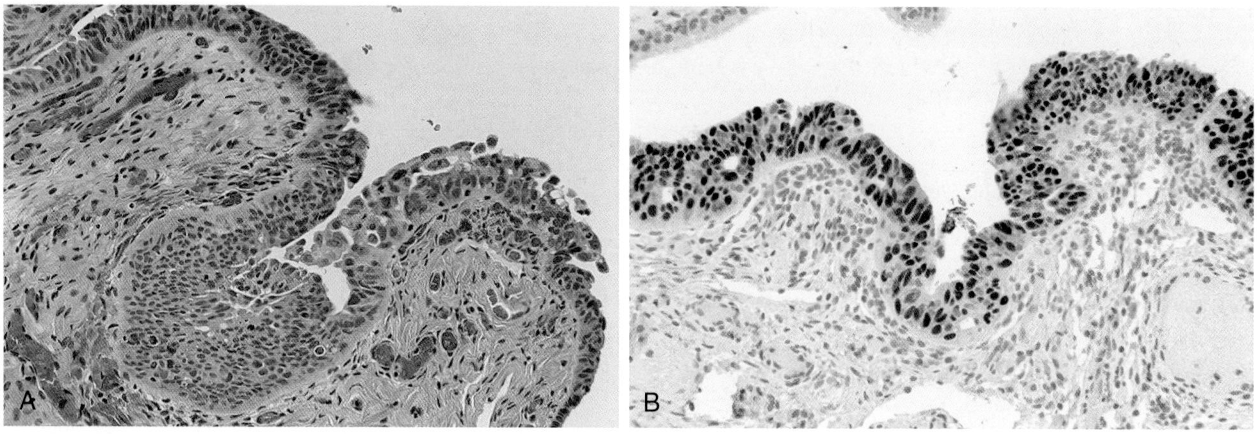

FIGURE 18.50 Tubal intraepithelial carcinoma (TIC). **(A)** The columnar tubal lining cells have stratified enlarged, hyperchromatic atypical nuclei. Intraepithelial carcinoma, shown here **(B)**, and invasive serous carcinoma typically show diffuse strong nuclear staining for p53, which helps to confirm the diagnosis and to identify small inconspicuous foci of TIC. TIC is strongly positive for the proliferation marker MIB1, which shows a similar pattern of staining to that shown here.

rarely occur in the ovary. The first is the adenomatoid tumor, and the second is the female adnexal tumor of Wolffian origin (FATWO).

ADENOMATOID TUMOR

Most Useful Antibodies: CK, Calretinin

Adenomatoid tumor is the most common benign tumor of the fallopian tube.[631] These are generally viewed as being of mesothelial origin, although origin from submesothelial mesenchymal cells has also been considered.[632-634] Adenomatoid tumors are small neoplasms that are usually only 1 to 2 cm in diameter. Microscopically, they grow as cords and tubules lined by cuboidal cells with eosinophilic cytoplasm or as glandlike cystic spaces lined by flattened cells. Some tumor cells have prominent cytoplasmic vacuoles; these are sometimes mistaken for signet ring cells. The epithelial elements can have a somewhat infiltrative appearance raising the differential diagnosis of adenocarcinoma. The gross circumscription, the bland cytology, and the lack of mitotic activity are features that distinguish adenomatoid tumors from malignant neoplasms. Immunohistochemical studies indicate that adenomatoid tumors are of mesothelial origin. Immunostains for cytokeratin, calretinin, and CK5/6 and WT1 are positive.[635,636] Stains that mark epithelial tumors, such as Ber-EP4, CEA, and B72.3 are usually negative or at most weakly and focally positive.[637] In one study of uterine adenomatoid tumors, there was a high frequency of staining for Ber-EP4,[144] which is inconsistent with other reports and experience with mesothelioma in general.

FEMALE ADNEXAL TUMOR OF WOLFFIAN ORIGIN

Most Useful Antibodies: CK7, EMA, Inhibin, Calretinin, CD10

The female adnexal tumor of Wolffian origin (FATWO) is a distinctive tumor that arises in the broad ligament, attached to the mesosalpinx, or, rarely, in the ovary.[638-640] It may be derived from mesonephric remnants, which are common in the area. Most adnexal tumors of Wolffian origin are found in middle aged women and are benign. Rare malignant variants show increased mitotic activity or cytologic atypia, overgrowth of spindle cells or lymphovascular space invasion, or they may unexpectedly metastasize.

The FATWO is a solid neoplasm that ranges from 2 to 20 cm in diameter. It is composed of uniform polygonal or spindled epithelial cells that grow in diffuse, trabecular, tubular, retiform, and microcystic patterns. The nuclei are uniform and darkly stained, and mitotic figures and cytologic atypia are typically absent. The main differential diagnostic considerations are a variant of endometrioid carcinoma of the fallopian tube[641-643] and a sex cord–stromal tumor such as a granulosa cell tumor or a Sertoli cell tumor. The immunophenotype is similar to that of the rete ovarii, and it overlaps between that of an epithelial tumor and a sex cord–stromal tumor.[644] The FATWO is CK-positive, but most are EMA-negative.[644-646] Immunostains for inhibin and calretinin are frequently positive.[344,644] The FATWO is CD10-positive, showing cytoplasmic staining, which helps to differentiate it from other diagnostic considerations.[490]

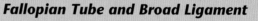

KEY DIAGNOSTIC POINTS

Fallopian Tube and Broad Ligament

- Epithelial tumors of the tube and peritubal region resemble ovarian tumors and have similar immunophenotypic features.
- No stains differentiate between primary tumors of the ovary and those of the fallopian tube.
- Staining for cytokeratin and calretinin helps with the identification of adenomatoid tumors.
- The immunophenotype of the FATWO overlaps with that of epithelial and sex cord–stromal tumors, but positive cytoplasmic staining for CD10 may help differentiate it. Lack of staining for EMA and positive staining for inhibin differentiate the FATWO from an endometrioid carcinoma variant.

Genomic Applications

As extensively discussed in previous sections of this chapter, women with Lynch syndrome (hereditary nonpolyposis colon cancer syndrome, HNPCC) have an increased risk of developing various types of cancer. The most frequent cancers in this patient population are endometrial adenocarcinoma and colorectal adenocarcinoma. The pathology of HNPCC associated endometrial cancers has been studied,[181,647] and criteria have been developed for selecting endometrial cancer patients for screening for HNPCC, based on their personal and family histories and on the morphology of their endometrial cancers. As discussed earlier in this chapter, histologic features often found in HNPCC-associated endometrial cancers include the presence of a dense peritumoral lymphocytic infiltrate, frequent tumor infiltrating lymphocytes (>40/10 high power fields), and a biphasic tumor appearance in which there is a combination of well-differentiated and undifferentiated areas.[275,647] HNPCC is caused by mutation of one of the mismatch repair genes: *MLH1, PMS2, MSH2,* or *MSH6*. Definitive testing requires molecular analyses, but screening for possible mutations can be performed using immunohistochemistry, as antibodies are available that detect the presence of the various mismatch repair proteins. If a mutation has occurred, the corresponding mismatch repair protein is not produced, and staining for that protein is absent.[160] Staining is nuclear and is somewhat variable from area to area on the slide; a positive result is complete absence of nuclear staining in all tumor cells on the slide, with a positive internal control (positive staining in the nuclei in normal tissues, no staining in tumor cell nuclei). Generally, loss of *MLH1* results in loss of *PMS2,* and loss of *MSH2* results in loss of *MSH6* as well. On the other hand, a mutation in *PMS2* or *MSH6* will result in loss of the corresponding protein only. Interpretation is further complicated by the fact that loss of *MLH1* can be due not only to mutation of the gene, but also, more commonly, to hypermethylation of the *MLH1* gene promoter. Immunohistochemical staining for the mismatch repair proteins is a screening test, and women with a positive result are usually referred for genetic counseling and possible molecular testing to identify a mutation of one of the mismatch repair genes or hypermethylation of the *MLH1* gene promoter. Immunohistochemical testing for MMR proteins is of value not only for selecting patients for further testing, but also for deciding which gene needs to be tested first. Testing can commence with the gene for which staining is lost, and it may not be necessary to test for mutations in all four genes.

Endometrial cancer is the most common gynecologic cancer in women with Lynch syndrome, and about 12% of women with the syndrome will develop ovarian cancer.[648] The same types of testing that are performed on endometrial cancer specimens can also be performed on ovarian tumors. Unfortunately, in contrast with the substantial body of knowledge that exists about endometrial cancers developing in affected women, little is known about the ovarian cancers that they develop. For example, we do not know what histologic types of cancers they develop, and there are no histologic criteria for selecting cases for screening by immunostaining for MMR proteins. At this time, we stain ovarian cancers for MMR proteins only when asked by the clinician or when a suggestive personal or family history exists based on evaluation of pathology history, the electronic medical record, or information on the pathology requisition. One might suspect that women with synchronous endometrial and ovarian cancers (two Lynch syndrome–associated cancers) would have a high likelihood of having the syndrome and that their tumors should be routinely tested for loss of one of the MMR proteins. However, one study of women with synchronous cancers did not find a high frequency of microsatellite instability in the endometrial or ovarian tumors.[649] In another study, no low-risk women (those with no personal or family history) had mutations of MLH1 or MSH2.[650] Thus, it appears that routine screening of women with synchronous endometrial and ovarian cancers using immunohistochemistry for MMR proteins is not warranted, and only women with a suggestive clinical history should be tested.

Theranostic Applications

Clinical and routine pathologic findings are of prognostic significance in tumors of the ovary and fallopian tube. Pathologic stage is the most significant prognostic factor. The tumor grade and tumor type are of some importance, and immunohistochemistry can provide assistance in the accurate classification of ovarian tumors, as detailed earlier in the chapter. No immunohistochemical stain has been identified that is generally accepted to have independent prognostic significance in ovarian or fallopian tube cancer, and we do not routinely perform any immunostains for such a purpose. A variety of markers have been tested in ovarian and tubal neoplasms, including p53, BCL-2, and BAX.[651,652] In general, standard clinical-pathologic parameters have provided more significant prognostic information than immunohistochemistry.[653] The authors of a recent study concluded that the various histologic types of ovarian cancer are different diseases, and that they should not be grouped together, as is usually done, in assessing the prognostic value of various biomarkers.[654] Immunohistochemical studies have suffered from problems such as variable definitions of a positive result, use of different antibodies, and variations in fixation and testing parameters. We presently view immunohistochemical testing for biomarkers as research tools rather than as validated clinical tests used in predicting prognosis or response to therapy.

Beyond Immunohistochemistry: Diagnostic Applications of Molecular Pathology

As discussed earlier in this chapter, Lynch syndrome or hereditary nonpolyposis colon cancer syndrome (HNPCC) is a cancer predisposition syndrome caused by mutation of a mismatch repair gene. Immunohistochemistry can be used to screen for mutations in mismatch repair genes. Molecular testing for microsatellite instability (MSI) likewise can serve as a screening test for mutation of a mismatch repair gene, since a mutation results in a microsatellite-unstable phenotype. Several methods are available for MSI testing, and most involve a polymerase chain reaction–based (PCR-based) process. Our laboratory uses a fluorescent multiplex assay.[655] Tumors with microsatellite-instability are usually classified as MSI-high (MSI-H) or MSI-low (MSI-L) depending on the number of positive microsatellite markers detected by molecular testing. Unlike immunohistochemistry, MSI testing does not identify which mismatch repair gene might be abnormal. Like immunohistochemistry, it also does not determine whether an abnormality of MLH1 is due to a mutation in the gene or hypermethylation of the gene promoter. So, if a tumor shows MSI, or there is an abnormality of MLH1 by immunohistochemistry, the next step in molecular testing is usually to assess for methylation of the MLH1 promoter. This can be accomplished using PCR-based methods and non–PCR-based methods. If methylation is detected, the abnormality is likely due to an epigenetic phenomenon, not mutation of the gene, and the patient is unlikely to have HNPCC. If methylation of the promoter is not detected, the next step is to sequence the MMR genes. Knowledge of the pattern of immunostaining for MMR proteins is helpful at this point, as assay of the MMR genes can commence with the one that shows loss of protein by immunohistochemistry. Identification of a mutation in one of the MMR genes confirms that the patient has Lynch syndrome. While immunohistochemical and molecular testing for abnormalities of the MMR genes and proteins is important, mutations in these genes account for only 1% of ovarian cancer cases, and a survey of patients with endometrial cancer revealed that only about 2% are due to MMR gene abnormalities.

A more common problem is mutation of one of the *BRCA* genes, *BRCA1* or *BRCA2*. Women with germline *BRCA* mutations have a high risk of developing breast and ovarian cancer.[656] Mutation of the *BRCA1* gene, located on chromosome 17 (17q12-21), accounts for about 70% of hereditary ovarian cancer cases and about 7% of ovarian cancer cases overall. Women with a *BRCA1* mutation have a 36% to 40% risk of developing ovarian cancer by age 70, with most cancers developing after age 40. The *BRCA2* gene is located on chromosome 13 (13q12-13), and women with mutations of this gene have a 10% to 27% risk of developing ovarian cancer by age 70, with most cancers developing after age 50. *BRCA2* mutations account for about 2% of ovarian cancers. Women with *BRCA* mutations also have a high risk of developing breast cancer. There are no immunohistochemical tests for abnormalities of the *BRCA* genes, nor are there any simple screening tests, so identification of a mutation requires molecular testing. If the patient belongs to a kindred with a specific known mutation, one can test for that mutation. Some mutations are common in specific populations, such as women of Ashkenazi Jewish heritage, and one can test for the known mutations.[657] Otherwise, full sequencing of both genes is necessary to identify abnormalities. Genetic counseling and testing for *BRCA* mutations have become increasingly important, as women with such mutations are often offered risk-reducing surgery, usually bilateral laparoscopic salpingo-oophorectomy, as a means of eliminating their risk of developing ovarian cancer. Clinical studies of women with *BRCA* mutations or strong family histories of ovarian cancer have shown that prophylactic bilateral salpingo-oophorectomy is highly effective in reducing the risk of pelvic cancer, and that the risk of breast cancer is also reduced.[658,659] Not all cancers are prevented, because some women have developed primary peritoneal cancer after prophylactic bilateral salpingo-oophorectomy. Thorough pathologic study of prophylactic salpingo-oophorectomy specimens has revealed occult intraepithelial or invasive carcinoma, usually of serous type, in 5% to 10% of patients who underwent the procedure. Interestingly, occult cancers occur more often in the fallopian tubes than in the ovaries.[623-626,660]

Molecular pathologic studies of epithelial tumors of the ovary are an area of extensive research and will doubtless result in additional tests that help in the diagnosis, treatment, and prognosis of ovarian cancer. At the present time, however, the two areas discussed earlier in this section are the only ones with wide clinical applications. Molecular pathologic studies of germ cell and sex cord–stromal tumors are less established, mainly because these tumors are rare. Abnormalities of chromosome 12p, usually an isochromosome 12p, are frequent in some germ cell tumors, particularly dysgerminoma. These abnormalities can be detected by fluorescence *in situ* hybridization (FISH) as well as by standard genetic analysis. In one study, chromosome12p abnormalities were detected by FISH in 81% of dysgerminomas.[661] This type of testing can be used for diagnostic purposes; however, as the diagnosis is usually readily established by routine light microscopy with or without the use of immunohistochemistry, FISH is rarely performed. Moreover, a test for chromosome 12p abnormalities is not readily available.

REFERENCES

1. Sano T, Oyama T, Kashiwabara K, et al. Expression status of p16 protein is associated with human papillomavirus oncogenic potential in cervical and genital lesions. *Am J Pathol.* 1998;153:1741-1748.
2. Agoff SN, Lin P, Morihara J, et al. p16(INK4a) expression correlates with degree of cervical neoplasia: A comparison with Ki-67 expression and detection of high-risk HPV types. *Mod Pathol.* 2003;16:665-673.
3. Ishikawa M, Fujii T, Masumoto N, et al. Correlation of p16INK4A overexpression with human papillomavirus infection in cervical adenocarcinomas. *Int J Gynecol Pathol.* 2003;22:378-385.
4. Keating JT, Cviko A, Riethdorf S, et al. Ki-67, cyclin E, and p16INK4 are complimentary surrogate biomarkers for human papilloma virus-related cervical neoplasia. *Am J Surg Pathol.* 2001;25:884-891.
5. Klaes R, Benner A, Friedrich T, et al. p16INK4a immunohistochemistry improves interobserver agreement in the diagnosis of cervical intraepithelial neoplasia. *Am J Surg Pathol.* 2002;26:1389-1399.
6. Negri G, Egarter-Vigl E, Kasal A, et al. p16INK4a is a useful marker for the diagnosis of adenocarcinoma of the cervix uteri and its precursors: An immunohistochemical study with immunocytochemical correlations. *Am J Surg Pathol.* 2003;27:187-193.

7. Riethdorf L, Riethdorf S, Lee KR, et al. Human papillomaviruses, expression of p16, and early endocervical glandular neoplasia. *Hum Pathol.* 2002;33:899-904.
8. Tringler B, Gup CJ, Singh M, et al. Evaluation of p16INK4a and pRb expression in cervical squamous and glandular neoplasia. *Hum Pathol.* 2004;35:689-696.
9. O'Neill CJ, McCluggage WG. p16 expression in the female genital tract and its value in diagnosis. *Adv Anat Pathol.* 2006;13:8-15.
10. Armes JE, Lourie R, de SM, et al. Abnormalities of the RB1 pathway in ovarian serous papillary carcinoma as determined by overexpression of the p16(INK4A) protein. *Int J Gynecol Pathol.* 2005;24:363-368.
11. Zeng HA, Cartun R, Ricci Jr A. Potential diagnostic utility of CDX-2 immunophenotyping in extramammary Paget's disease. *Appl Immunohistochem Mol Morphol.* 2005;13:342-346.
12. Battles OE, Page DL, Johnson JE. Cytokeratins, CEA, and mucin histochemistry in the diagnosis and characterization of extramammary Paget's disease. *Am J Clin Pathol.* 1997;108:6-12.
13. Goldblum JR, Hart WR. Vulvar Paget's disease: A clinicopathologic and immunohistochemical study of 19 cases. *Am J Surg Pathol.* 1997;21:1178-1187.
14. Nowak MA, Guerriere-Kovach P, Pathan A, et al. Perianal Paget's disease: Distinguishing primary and secondary lesions using immunohistochemical studies including gross cystic disease fluid protein-15 and cytokeratin 20 expression. *Arch Pathol Lab Med.* 1998;122:1077-1081.
15. Olson DJ, Fujimura M, Swanson P, et al. Immunohistochemical features of Paget's disease of the vulva with and without adenocarcinoma. *Int J Gynecol Pathol.* 1991;10:285-295.
16. Crawford D, Nimmo M, Clement PB, et al. Prognostic factors in Paget's disease of the vulva: A study of 21 cases. *Int J Gynecol Pathol.* 1999;18:351-359.
17. Brummer O, Stegner HE, Bohmer G, et al. HER-2/neu expression in Paget disease of the vulva and the female breast. *Gynecol Oncol.* 2004;95:336-340.
18. Zhang C, Zhang P, Sung CJ, et al. Overexpression of p53 is correlated with stromal invasion in extramammary Paget's disease of the vulva. *Hum Pathol.* 2003;34:880-885.
19. Ohnishi T, Watanabe S. The use of cytokeratins 7 and 20 in the diagnosis of primary and secondary extramammary Paget's disease. *Br J Dermatol.* 2000;142:243-247.
20. Brown HM, Wilkinson EJ. Uroplakin-III to distinguish primary vulvar Paget disease from Paget disease secondary to urothelial carcinoma. *Hum Pathol.* 2002;33:545-548.
21. Lopez-Beltran A, Luque RJ, Moreno A, et al. The pagetoid variant of bladder urothelial carcinoma in situ A clinicopathological study of 11 cases. *Virchows Arch.* 2002;441:148-153.
22. Diaz de Leon E, Carcangiu ML, Prieto VG, et al. Extramammary Paget disease is characterized by the consistent lack of estrogen and progesterone receptors but frequently expresses androgen receptor. *Am J Clin Pathol.* 2000;113:572-575.
23. Glasgow BJ, Wen DR, Al-Jitawi S, et al. Antibody to S-100 protein aids the separation of pagetoid melanoma from mammary and extramammary Paget's disease. *J Cutan Pathol.* 1987;14:223-226.
24. Armes JE, Lourie R, Bowlay G, et al. Pagetoid squamous cell carcinoma in situ of the vulva: Comparison with extramammary Paget disease and nonpagetoid squamous cell neoplasia. *Int J Gynecol Pathol.* 2008;27:118-124.
25. Raju RR, Goldblum JR, Hart WR. Pagetoid squamous cell carcinoma in situ (pagetoid Bowen's disease) of the external genitalia. *Int J Gynecol Pathol.* 2003;22:127-135.
26. Williamson JD, Colome MI, Sahin A, et al. Pagetoid bowen disease: A report of 2 cases that express cytokeratin 7. *Arch Pathol Lab Med.* 2000;124:427-430.
27. McCluggage WG. Recent developments in vulvovaginal pathology. *Histopathology.* 2008.
28. Iwasa Y, Fletcher CD. Cellular angiofibroma: Clinicopathologic and immunohistochemical analysis of 51 cases. *Am J Surg Pathol.* 2004;28:1426-1435.
29. McCluggage WG, Ganesan R, Hirschowitz L, et al. Cellular angiofibroma and related fibromatous lesions of the vulva: Report of a series of cases with a morphological spectrum wider than previously described. *Histopathology.* 2004;45:360-368.
30. Lam MM, Corless CL, Goldblum JR, et al. Extragastrointestinal stromal tumors presenting as vulvovaginal/rectovaginal septal masses: A diagnostic pitfall. *Int J Gynecol Pathol.* 2006;25:288-292.
31. Guillou L, Wadden C, Coindre JM, et al. Proximal-type" epithelioid sarcoma, a distinctive aggressive neoplasm showing rhabdoid features. Clinicopathologic, immunohistochemical, and ultrastructural study of a series. *Am J Surg Pathol.* 1997;21:130-146.
32. Cessna MH, Zhou H, Perkins SL, et al. Are myogenin and myoD1 expression specific for rhabdomyosarcoma? A study of 150 cases, with emphasis on spindle cell mimics. *Am J Surg Pathol.* 2001;25:1150-1157.
33. Morotti RA, Nicol KK, Parham DM, et al. An immunohistochemical algorithm to facilitate diagnosis and subtyping of rhabdomyosarcoma: the Children's Oncology Group experience. *Am J Surg Pathol.* 2006;30:962-968.
34. Medeiros F, Erickson-Johnson MR, Keeney GL, et al. Frequency and characterization of HMGA2 and HMGA1 rearrangements in mesenchymal tumors of the lower genital tract. *Genes Chromosomes Cancer.* 2007;46:981-990.
35. Medeiros F, Oliveira AM, Lloyd R. HMGA2 expression as a biomarker for aggressive angiomyxoma. *Mod Pathol.* 2008;21:214A.
36. Nucci MR, Weremowicz S, Neskey DM, et al. Chromosomal translocation t(8;12) induces aberrant HMGIC expression in aggressive angiomyxoma of the vulva. *Genes Chromosomes Cancer.* 2001;32:172-176.
37. Rabban JT, Dal CP, Oliva E. HMGA2 rearrangement in a case of vulvar aggressive angiomyxoma. *Int J Gynecol Pathol.* 2006;25:403-407.
38. Horowitz IR, Copas P, Majmudar B. Granular cell tumors of the vulva. *Am J Obstet Gynecol.* 1995;173:1710-1713.
39. Le BH, Boyer PJ, Lewis JE, et al. Granular cell tumor: Immunohistochemical assessment of inhibin-alpha, protein gene product 9.5, S100 protein, CD68, and Ki-67 proliferative index with clinical correlation. *Arch Pathol Lab Med.* 2004;128:771-775.
40. Brustmann H, Naude S. Expression of topoisomerase II alpha, Ki-67, proliferating cell nuclear antigen, p53, and argyrophilic nucleolar organizer regions in vulvar squamous lesions. *Gynecol Oncol.* 2002;86:192-199.
41. Pirog EC, Chen YT, Isacson C. MIB-1 immunostaining is a beneficial adjunct test for accurate diagnosis of vulvar condyloma acuminatum. *Am J Surg Pathol.* 2000;24:1393-1399.
42. Scurry J, Beshay V, Cohen C, et al. Ki67 expression in lichen sclerosus of vulva in patients with and without associated squamous cell carcinoma. *Histopathology.* 1998;32:399-404.
43. van Hoeven KH, Kovatich AJ. Immunohistochemical staining for proliferating cell nuclear antigen, BCL2, and Ki-67 in vulvar tissues. *Int J Gynecol Pathol.* 1996;15:10-16.
44. Bai H, Cviko A, Granter S, et al. Immunophenotypic and viral (human papillomavirus) correlates of vulvar seborrheic keratosis. *Hum Pathol.* 2003;34:559-564.
45. Riethdorf S, Neffen EF, Cviko A, et al. p16INK4A expression as biomarker for HPV 16-related vulvar neoplasias. *Hum Pathol.* 2004;35:1477-1483.
46. Santos M, Montagut C, Mellado B, et al. Immunohistochemical staining for p16 and p53 in premalignant and malignant epithelial lesions of the vulva. *Int J Gynecol Pathol.* 2004;23:206-214.
47. Ruhul QM, Xu C, Steinhoff MM, et al. Simplex (differentiated) type VIN: Absence of p16INK4 supports its weak association with HPV and its probable precursor role in non-HPV related vulvar squamous cancers. *Histopathology.* 2005;46:718-720.
48. Mulvany NJ, Allen DG. Differentiated intraepithelial neoplasia of the vulva. *Int J Gynecol Pathol.* 2008;27:125-135.
49. Yang B, Hart WR. Vulvar intraepithelial neoplasia of the simplex (differentiated) type: A clinicopathologic study including analysis of HPV and p53 expression. *Am J Surg Pathol.* 2000;24:429-241.
50. Liegl B, Regauer S. p53 immunostaining in lichen sclerosus is related to ischaemic stress and is not a marker of differentiated vulvar intraepithelial neoplasia (d-VIN). *Histopathology.* 2006;48:268-274.

51. McCluggage WG, Oliva E, Herrington CS, et al. CD10 and calretinin staining of endocervical glandular lesions, endocervical stroma and endometrioid adenocarcinomas of the uterine corpus: CD10 positivity is characteristic of, but not specific for, mesonephric lesions and is not specific for endometrial stroma. *Histopathology.* 2003;43:144-150.
52. Ordi J, Romagosa C, Tavassoli FA, et al. CD10 expression in epithelial tissues and tumors of the gynecologic tract: A useful marker in the diagnosis of mesonephric, trophoblastic, and clear cell tumors. *Am J Surg Pathol.* 2003;27:178-186.
53. Silver SA, Devouassoux-Shisheboran M, Mezzetti TP, et al. Mesonephric adenocarcinomas of the uterine cervix: A study of 11 cases with immunohistochemical findings. *Am J Surg Pathol.* 2001;25:379-387.
54. Mittal K, Mesia A, Demopoulos RI. MIB-1 expression is useful in distinguishing dysplasia from atrophy in elderly women. *Int J Gynecol Pathol.* 1999;18:122-124.
55. Kruse AJ, Baak JP, Helliesen T, et al. Evaluation of MIB-1-positive cell clusters as a diagnostic marker for cervical intraepithelial neoplasia. *Am J Surg Pathol.* 2002;26:1501-1507.
56. McCluggage WG, Buhidma M, Tang L, et al. Monoclonal antibody MIB1 in the assessment of cervical squamous intraepithelial lesions. *Int J Gynecol Pathol.* 1996;15:131-136.
57. Pirog EC, Baergen RN, Soslow RA, et al. Diagnostic Accuracy of Cervical Low-Grade Squamous Intraepithelial Lesions Is Improved With MIB-1 Immunostaining. *Am J Surg Pathol.* 2002;26:70-75.
58. Klaes R, Friedrich T, Spitkovsky D, et al. Overexpression of p16(INK4A) as a specific marker for dysplastic and neoplastic epithelial cells of the cervix uteri. *Int J Cancer.* 2001;92:276-284.
59. Benevolo M, Mottolese M, Marandino F, et al. Immunohistochemical expression of p16(INK4a) is predictive of HR-HPV infection in cervical low-grade lesions. *Mod Pathol.* 2006;19:384-391.
60. Kong CS, Balzer BL, Troxell ML, et al. p16INK4A immunohistochemistry is superior to HPV in situ hybridization for the detection of high-risk HPV in atypical squamous metaplasia. *Am J Surg Pathol.* 2007;31:33-43.
61. Shi J, Liu H, Wilkerson M, et al. Evaluation of p16INK4a, minichromosome maintenance protein 2, DNA topoisomerase II alpha, ProEX C, and p16INK4a/ProEX C in cervical squamous intraepithelial lesions. *Hum Pathol.* 2007;38:1335-1344.
62. Pinto AP, Schlecht NF, Woo TY, et al. Biomarker (ProEx C, p16(INK4A), and MiB-1) distinction of high-grade squamous intraepithelial lesion from its mimics. *Mod Pathol.* 2008;21:1067-1074.
63. Cina SJ, Richardson MS, Austin RM, et al. Immunohistochemical staining for Ki-67 antigen, carcinoembryonic antigen, and p53 in the differential diagnosis of glandular lesions of the cervix. *Mod Pathol.* 1997;10:176-180.
64. Marques T, Andrade LA, Vassallo J. Endocervical tubal metaplasia and adenocarcinoma in situ: Role of immunohistochemistry for carcinoembryonic antigen and vimentin in differential diagnosis. *Histopathology.* 1996;28:549-550.
65. Cameron RI, Maxwell P, Jenkins D, et al. Immunohistochemical staining with MIB1, bcl2 and p16 assists in the distinction of cervical glandular intraepithelial neoplasia from tubo-endometrial metaplasia, endometriosis and microglandular hyperplasia. *Histopathology.* 2002;41:313-321.
66. McCluggage WG, Maxwell P, McBride HA, et al. Monoclonal antibodies Ki-67 and MIB1 in the distinction of tuboendometrial metaplasia from endocervical adenocarcinoma and adenocarcinoma in situ in formalin-fixed material. *Int J Gynecol Pathol.* 1995;14:209-216.
67. Ansari-Lari MA, Staebler A, Zaino RJ, et al. Distinction of endocervical and endometrial adenocarcinomas: Immunohistochemical p16 expression correlated with human papillomavirus (HPV) DNA detection. *Am J Surg Pathol.* 2004;28:160-167.
68. Castrillon DH, Lee KR, Nucci MR. Distinction between endometrial and endocervical adenocarcinoma: An immunohistochemical study. *Int J Gynecol Pathol.* 2002;21:4-10.
69. Kamoi S, Al-Juboury MI, Akin MR, et al. Immunohistochemical staining in the distinction between primary endometrial and endocervical adenocarcinomas: Another viewpoint. *Int J Gynecol Pathol.* 2002;21:217-223.
70. McCluggage WG, Sumathi VP, McBride HA, et al. A panel of immunohistochemical stains, including carcinoembryonic antigen, vimentin, and estrogen receptor, aids the distinction between primary endometrial and endocervical adenocarcinomas. *Int J Gynecol Pathol.* 2002;21:11-15.
71. McCluggage WG, Jenkins D. p16 immunoreactivity may assist in the distinction between endometrial and endocervical adenocarcinoma. *Int J Gynecol Pathol.* 2003;22:231-235.
72. O'Neill CJ, McBride HA, Connolly LE, et al. High-grade ovarian serous carcinoma exhibits significantly higher p16 expression than low-grade serous carcinoma and serous borderline tumour. *Histopathology.* 2007;50:773-779.
73. Qiu W, Mittal K. Comparison of morphologic and immunohistochemical features of cervical microglandular hyperplasia with low-grade mucinous adenocarcinoma of the endometrium. *Int J Gynecol Pathol.* 2003;22:261-265.
74. McCluggage WG, Shah R, Connolly LE, et al. Intestinal-type cervical adenocarcinoma in situ and adenocarcinoma exhibit a partial enteric immunophenotype with consistent expression of CDX2. *Int J Gynecol Pathol.* 2008;27:92-100.
75. Sullivan LM, Smolkin ME, Frierson Jr HF, et al. Comprehensive Evaluation of CDX2 in Invasive Cervical Adenocarcinomas: Immunopositivity in the Absence of Overt Colorectal Morphology. *Am J Surg Pathol.* 2008;32(11):1608-1612.
76. Gilks CB, Young RH, Aguirre P, et al. Adenoma malignum (minimal deviation adenocarcinoma) of the uterine cervix. A clinicopathological and immunohistochemical analysis of 26 cases. *Am J Surg Pathol.* 1989;13:717-729.
77. Mikami Y, Kiyokawa T, Hata S, et al. Gastrointestinal immunophenotype in adenocarcinomas of the uterine cervix and related glandular lesions: A possible link between lobular endocervical glandular hyperplasia/pyloric gland metaplasia and "adenoma malignum". *Mod Pathol.* 2004;17:962-972.
78. Xu JY, Hashi A, Kondo T, et al. Absence of human papillomavirus infection in minimal deviation adenocarcinoma and lobular endocervical glandular hyperplasia. *Int J Gynecol Pathol.* 2005;24:296-302.
79. Mino M, Pilch BZ, Faquin WC. Expression of KIT (CD117) in neoplasms of the head and neck: An ancillary marker for adenoid cystic carcinoma. *Mod Pathol.* 2003;16:1224-1231.
80. Grayson W, Taylor LF, Cooper K. Adenoid cystic and adenoid basal carcinoma of the uterine cervix: Comparative morphologic, mucin, and immunohistochemical profile of two rare neoplasms of putative "reserve cell" origin. *Am J Surg Pathol.* 1999;23:448-458.
81. Grayson W, Cooper K. A reappraisal of "basaloid carcinoma" of the cervix, and the differential diagnosis of basaloid cervical neoplasms. *Adv Anat Pathol.* 2002;9:290-300.
82. Emanuel P, Wang B, Wu M, et al. p63 Immunohistochemistry in the distinction of adenoid cystic carcinoma from basaloid squamous cell carcinoma. *Mod Pathol.* 2005;18:645-650.
83. Ferry JA, Scully RE. "Adenoid cystic" carcinoma and adenoid basal carcinoma of the uterine cervix. A study of 28 cases. *Am J Surg Pathol.* 1988;12:134-144.
84. Russell MJ, Fadare O. Adenoid basal lesions of the uterine cervix: Evolving terminology and clinicopathological concepts. *Diagn Pathol.* 2006;1:18.
85. Cviko A, Briem B, Granter SR, et al. Adenoid basal carcinomas of the cervix: A unique morphological evolution with cell cycle correlates. *Hum Pathol.* 2000;31:740-744.
86. Parwani AV, Smith Sehdev AE, Kurman RJ, et al. Cervical adenoid basal tumors comprised of adenoid basal epithelioma associated with various types of invasive carcinoma: Clinicopathologic features, human papillomavirus DNA detection, and P16 expression. *Hum Pathol.* 2005;36:82-90.
87. Albores-Saavedra J, Latif S, Carrick KS, et al. CD56 reactivity in small cell carcinoma of the uterine cervix. *Int J Gynecol Pathol.* 2005;24:113-117.
88. Gilks CB, Young RH, Gersell DJ, et al. Large cell neuroendocrine carcinoma of the uterine cervix: A clinicopathologic study of 12 cases. *Am J Surg Pathol.* 1997;21:905-914.
89. Horn LC, Lindner K, Szepankiewicz G, et al. p16, p14, p53, and cyclin D1 expression and HPV analysis in small cell carcinomas of the uterine cervix. *Int J Gynecol Pathol.* 2006;25:182-186.

90. Masumoto N, Fujii T, Ishikawa M, et al. P16 overexpression and human papillomavirus infection in small cell carcinoma of the uterine cervix. *Hum Pathol.* 2003;34:778-783.
91. Wang HL, Lu DW. Detection of human papillomavirus DNA and expression of p16, Rb, and p53 proteins in small cell carcinomas of the uterine cervix. *Am J Surg Pathol.* 2004; 28:901-908.
92. Wang TY, Chen BF, Yang YC, et al. Histologic and immunophenotypic classification of cervical carcinomas by expression of the p53 homologue p63: A study of 250 cases. *Hum Pathol.* 2001;32:479-486.
93. Agoff SN, Lamps LW, Philip AT, et al. Thyroid transcription factor-1 is expressed in extrapulmonary small cell carcinomas but not in other extrapulmonary neuroendocrine tumors. *Mod Pathol.* 2000;13:238-242.
94. McCluggage WG, Sargent A, Bailey A, et al. Large cell neuroendocrine carcinoma of the uterine cervix exhibiting TTF1 immunoreactivity. *Histopathology.* 2007;51:405-407.
95. Guimaraes MC, Goncalves MA, Soares CP, et al. Immunohistochemical expression of p16INK4a and bcl-2 according to HPV type and to the progression of cervical squamous intraepithelial lesions. *J Histochem Cytochem.* 2005;53:509-516.
96. Hariri J, Oster A. The negative predictive value of p16INK4a to assess the outcome of cervical intraepithelial neoplasia 1 in the uterine cervix. *Int J Gynecol Pathol.* 2007; 26:223-228.
97. Negri G, Vittadello F, Romano F, et al. p16INK4a expression and progression risk of low-grade intraepithelial neoplasia of the cervix uteri. *Virchows Arch.* 2004;445:616-620.
98. Negri G, Bellisano G, Zannoni GF, et al. p16 ink4a and HPV L1 immunohistochemistry is helpful for estimating the behavior of low-grade dysplastic lesions of the cervix uteri. *Am J Surg Pathol.* 2008;32:1715-1720.
99. Farhood AI, Abrams J. Immunohistochemistry of endometrial stromal sarcoma. *Hum Pathol.* 1991;22:224-230.
100. Franquemont DW, Frierson Jr HF, Mills SE. An immunohistochemical study of normal endometrial stroma and endometrial stromal neoplasms. Evidence for smooth muscle differentiation. *Am J Surg Pathol.* 1991;15:861-870.
101. Oliva E, Young RH, Clement PB, et al. Cellular benign mesenchymal tumors of the uterus: A comparative morphologic and immunohistochemical analysis of 33 highly cellular leiomyomas and six endometrial stromal nodules, two frequently confused tumors. *Am J Surg Pathol.* 1995;19:757-768.
102. Bitterman P, Chun B, Kurman RJ. The significance of epithelial differentiation in mixed mesodermal tumors of the uterus. A clinicopathological and immunohistochemical study. *Am J Surg Pathol.* 1990;14:317-328.
103. George E, Manivel JC, Dehner LP, et al. Malignant mixed mullerian tumors: An immunohistochemical study of 47 cases, with histogenetic considerations and clinical correlation. *Hum Pathol.* 1991;22:215-223.
104. Dabbs DJ, Sturtz K, Zaino RJ. The immunohistochemical discrimination of endometrioid adenocarcinomas. *Hum Pathol.* 1996;27:172-177.
105. Dabbs DJ, Geisinger KR, Norris HT. Intermediate filaments in endometrial and endocervical carcinomas. The diagnostic utility of vimentin patterns. *Am J Surg Pathol.* 1986;10:568-576.
106. Sherman ME, Bur ME, Kurman RJ. p53 in endometrial cancer and its putative precursors: Evidence for diverse pathways of tumorigenesis. *Hum Pathol.* 1995;26:1268-1274.
107. Tashiro H, Isacson C, Levine R, et al. p53 gene mutations are common in uterine serous carcinoma and occur early in their pathogenesis. *Am J Pathol.* 1997;150:177-185.
108. Zheng WX, Khurana R, Farahmand S, et al. p53 immunostaining as a significant adjunct diagnostic method for uterine surface carcinoma—Precursor of uterine papillary serous carcinoma. *Am J Surg Pathol.* 1998;22:1463-1473.
109. Kohler MF, Kerns B-JM, Humphrey PA, et al. Mutation and overexpression of p53 in early-stage epithelial ovarian cancer. *Obstet Gynecol.* 1993;81:643-650.
110. Yu CC, Wilkinson N, Brito MJ, et al. Patterns of immunohistochemical staining for proliferating cell nuclear antigen and p53 in benign and neoplastic human endometrium. *Histopathology.* 1993;23:367-371.
111. Lax SF, Pizer ES, Ronnett BM, et al. Comparison of estrogen and progesterone receptor, Ki-67, and p53 immunoreactivity in uterine endometrioid carcinoma and endometrioid carcinoma with squamous, mucinous, secretory, and ciliated cell differentiation. *Hum Pathol.* 1998;29:924-931.
112. Lax SF, Kendall B, Tashiro H, et al. The frequency of p53, K-ras mutations, and microsatellite instability differs in uterine endometrioid and serous carcinoma—Evidence of distinct molecular genetic pathways. *Cancer.* 2000;88:814-824.
113. Soslow RA, Shen PU, Chung MH, et al. Distinctive p53 and mdm2 immunohistochemical expression profiles suggest different pathogenetic pathways in poorly differentiated endometrial carcinoma. *Int J Gynecol Pathol.* 1998;17:129-134.
114. Carcangiu ML, Chambers JT, Voynick IM, et al. Immunohistochemical evaluation of estrogen and progesterone receptor content in 183 patients with endometrial carcinoma. Part I: Clinical and histologic correlations. *Am J Clin Pathol.* 1990; 94:247-254.
115. Chambers JT, Carcangiu ML, Voynick IM, et al. Immunohistochemical evaluation of estrogen and progesterone receptor content in 183 patients with endometrial carcinoma. Part II: Correlation between biochemical and immunohistochemical methods and survival. *Am J Clin Pathol.* 1990;94:255-260.
116. Soslow RA, Shen PU, Chung MH, et al. Cyclin D1 expression in high-grade endometrial carcinomas—Association with histologic subtype. *Int J Gynecol Pathol.* 2000;19:329-334.
117. Nei H, Saito T, Yamasaki H, et al. Nuclear localization of beta-catenin in normal and carcinogenic endometrium. *Mol Carcinog.* 1999;25:207-218.
118. Schlosshauer PW, Ellenson LH, Soslow RA. Beta-catenin and E-cadherin expression patterns in high-grade endometrial carcinoma are associated with histological subtype. *Mod Pathol.* 2002;15:1032-1037.
119. Risinger JI, Hayes AK, Berchuck A, et al. PTEN/MMAC1 mutations in endometrial cancers. *Cancer Res.* 1997;57:4736-4738.
120. Tashiro H, Blazes MS, Wu R, et al. Mutations in PTEN are frequent in endometrial carcinoma but rare in other common gynecological malignancies. *Cancer Res.* 1997;57:3935-3940.
121. Obata K, Morland SJ, Watson RH, et al. Frequent PTEN/MMAC mutations in endometrioid but not serous or mucinous epithelial ovarian tumors. *Cancer Res.* 1998;58:2095-2097.
122. Simpkins SB, Peiffer-Schneider S, Mutch DG, et al. PTEN mutations in endometrial cancers with 10q LOH: Additional evidence for the involvement of multiple tumor suppressors. *Gynecol Oncol.* 1998;71:391-395.
123. Yokoyama Y, Wan X, Shinohara A, et al. Expression of PTEN and PTEN pseudogene in endometrial carcinoma. *Int J Mol Med.* 2000;6:47-50.
124. Darvishian F, Hummer AJ, Thaler HT, et al. Serous endometrial cancers that mimic endometrioid adenocarcinomas: A clinicopathologic and immunohistochemical study of a group of problematic cases. *Am J Surg Pathol.* 2004;28:1568-1578.
125. Lax SF, Pizer ES, Ronnett BM, et al. Clear cell carcinoma of the endometrium is characterized by a distinctive profile of p53, Ki-67, estrogen, and progesterone receptor expression. *Hum Pathol.* 1998;29:551-558.
126. Vang R, Whitaker BP, Farhood AI, et al. Immunohistochemical analysis of clear cell carcinoma of the gynecologic tract. *Int J Gynecol Pathol.* 2001;20:252-259.
127. Reid-Nicholson M, Iyengar P, Hummer AJ, et al. Immunophenotypic diversity of endometrial adenocarcinomas: Implications for differential diagnosis. *Mod Pathol.* 2006;19:1091-1100.
128. Fukuchi T, Sakamoto M, Tsuda H, et al. Beta-catenin mutation in carcinoma of the uterine endometrium. *Cancer Res.* 1998;58:3526-3528.
129. Schlosshauer PW, Pirog EC, Levine RL, et al. Mutational analysis of the CTNNB1 and APC genes in uterine endometrioid carcinoma. *Mod Pathol.* 2000;13:1066-1071.
130. Saegusa M, Hamano M, Kuwata T, et al. Up-regulation and nuclear localization of beta-catenin in endometrial carcinoma in response to progesterone therapy. *Cancer Sci.* 2003;94:103-111.
131. Bussaglia E, Del Rio E, Matias-Guiu X, et al. PTEN mutations in endometrial carcinomas: A molecular and clinicopathologic analysis of 38 cases. *Hum Pathol.* 2000;31:312-317.

132. Oliva E, Young RH, Clement PB, et al. Myxoid and fibrous endometrial stromal tumors of the uterus: A report of 10 cases. *Int J Gynecol Pathol.* 1999;18:310-319.
133. Oliva E, Clement PB, Young RH, et al. Mixed endometrial stromal and smooth muscle tumors of the uterus—A clinicopathologic study of 15 cases. *Am J Surg Pathol.* 1998;22:997-1005.
134. Nucci MR, O'Connell JT, Huettner PC, et al. h-Caldesmon expression effectively distinguishes endometrial stromal tumors from uterine smooth muscle tumors. *Am J Surg Pathol.* 2001;25:455-463.
135. Rush DS, Tan JY, Baergen RN, et al. h-caldesmon, a novel smooth muscle-specific antibody, distinguishes between cellular leiomyoma and endometrial stromal sarcoma. *Am J Surg Pathol.* 2001;25:253-258.
136. Baker RJ, Hildebrandt RH, Rouse RV, et al. Inhibin and CD99 (MIC2) expression in uterine stromal neoplasms with sex-cord-like elements. *Hum Pathol.* 1999;30:671-679.
137. Krishnamurthy S, Jungbluth AA, Busam KJ, et al. Uterine tumors resembling ovarian sex-cord tumors have an immunophenotype consistent with true sex-cord differentiation. *Am J Surg Pathol.* 1998;22:1078-1082.
138. Oliva E, Young RH, Amin MB, et al. An immunohistochemical analysis of endometrial stromal and smooth muscle tumors of the uterus—A study of 54 cases emphasizing the importance of using a panel because of overlap in immunoreactivity for individual antibodies. *Am J Surg Pathol.* 2002;26:403-412.
139. Czernobilsky B. Uterine tumors resembling ovarian sex cord tumors: An update. *Int J Gynecol Pathol.* 2008;27:229-235.
140. Meis JM, Lawrence WD. The immunohistochemical profile of malignant mixed müllerian tumor. Overlap with endometrial adenocarcinoma. *Am J Clin Pathol.* 1990;94:1-7.
141. Chu PG, Arber DA, Weiss LM, et al. Utility of CD10 in distinguishing between endometrial stromal sarcoma and uterine smooth muscle tumors: An immunohistochemical comparison of 34 cases. *Mod Pathol.* 2001;14:465-471.
142. McCluggage WG, Sumathi VP, Maxwell P. CD10 is a sensitive and diagnostically useful immunohistochemical marker of normal endometrial stroma and of endometrial stromal neoplasms. *Histopathology.* 2001;39:273-278.
143. Sumathi VP, Al-Hussaini M, Connolly LE, et al. Endometrial stromal neoplasms are immunoreactive with WT-1 antibody. *Int J Gynecol Pathol.* 2004;23:241-247.
144. Otis CN. Uterine adenomatoid tumors: Immunohistochemical characteristics with emphasis on Ber-EP4 immunoreactivity and distinction from adenocarcinoma. *Int J Gynecol Pathol.* 1996;15:146-151.
145. Thor A, Viglione MJ, Muraro R, et al. Monoclonal antibody B72.3 reactivity with human endometrium: A study of normal and malignant tissues. *Int J Gynecol Pathol.* 1987;6:235-247.
146. Hareyama H, Sakuragi N, Makinoda S, et al. Serum and tissue measurements of CA72-4 in patients with endometrial carcinoma. *J Clin Pathol.* 1996;49:967-970.
147. Dallenbach-Hellweg G, Lang-Averous G, Hahn U. The value of immunohistochemistry in the differential diagnosis of endometrial carcinomas. *APMIS.* 1991;23(Suppl):91-99.
148. Yaziji H, Gown AM. Immunohistochemical analysis of gynecologic tumors. *Int J Gynecol Pathol.* 2001;20:64-78.
149. Wang NP, Zee S, Zarbo RJ, et al. Coordinate expression of cytokeratins 7 and 20 defines unique subsets of carcinomas. *Appl Immunohistochem.* 1995;3:99-107.
150. Wani Y, Notohara K, Saegusa M, et al. Aberrant Cdx2 expression in endometrial lesions with squamous differentiation: important role of Cdx2 in squamous morula formation. *Hum Pathol.* 2008;39:1072-1079.
151. Park KJ, Bramlage MP, Ellenson LH, et al. Immunoprofile of adenocarcinomas of the endometrium, endocervix, and ovary with mucinous differentiation. *Appl Immunohistochem Mol Morphol.* 2009;17:8-11.
152. Bonazzi del Poggetto C, Virtanen I, Lehto VP, et al. Expression of intermediate filaments in ovarian and uterine tumors. *Int J Gynecol Pathol.* 1983;1:359-366.
153. Azumi N, Battifora H. The distribution of vimentin and keratin in epithelial and nonepithelial neoplasms. A comprehensive immunohistochemical study on form. *Am J Clin Pathol.* 1987;88:286-296.
154. Koshiyama M, Konishi I, Wang DP, et al. Immunohistochemical analysis of p53 protein over-expression in endometrial carcinomas: Inverse correlation with sex steroid receptor status. *Virchows Arch A Pathol Anat Histopathol.* 1993;423:265-271.
155. Chiesa-Vottero AG, Malpica A, Deavers MT, et al. Immunohistochemical overexpression of p16 and p53 in uterine serous carcinoma and ovarian high-grade serous carcinoma. *Int J Gynecol Pathol.* 2007;26:328-333.
156. Pallares J, Bussaglia E, Martinez-Guitarte JL, et al. Immunohistochemical analysis of PTEN in endometrial carcinoma: A tissue microarray study with a comparison of four commercial antibodies in correlation with molecular abnormalities. *Mod Pathol.* 2005;18:719-727.
157. De Leeuw WJF, Dierssen J, Vasen HFA, et al. Prediction of a mismatch repair gene defect by microsatellite instability and immunohistochemical analysis in endometrial tumours from HNPCC patients. *J Pathol.* 2000;192:328-335.
158. Peiro G, Diebold J, Lohse P, et al. Microsatellite instability, loss of heterozygosity, and loss of hMLH1 and hMSH2 protein expression in endometrial carcinoma. *Hum Pathol.* 2002;33:347-354.
159. Vasen HF, Hendriks Y, de Jong AE, et al. Identification of HNPCC by molecular analysis of colorectal and endometrial tumors. *Dis Markers.* 2004;20:207-213.
160. Modica I, Soslow RA, Black D, et al. Utility of immunohistochemistry in predicting microsatellite instability in endometrial carcinoma. *Am J Surg Pathol.* 2007;31:744-751.
161. Sherman ME, Bitterman P, Rosenshein NB, et al. Uterine serous carcinoma: A morphologically diverse neoplasm with unifying clinicopathologic features. *Am J Surg Pathol.* 1992;16:600-610.
162. Ambros RA, Sherman ME, Zahn CM, et al. Endometrial intraepithelial carcinoma: A distinctive lesion specifically associated with tumors displaying serous differentiation. *Hum Pathol.* 1995;26:1260-1267.
163. Liang SX, Chambers SK, Cheng L, et al. Endometrial glandular dysplasia: A putative precursor lesion of uterine papillary serous carcinoma. Part II: molecular features. *Int J Surg Pathol.* 2004;12:319-331.
164. Zheng W, Liang SX, Yu H, et al. Endometrial glandular dysplasia: A newly defined precursor lesion of uterine papillary serous carcinoma. Part I: morphologic features. *Int J Surg Pathol.* 2004;12:207-223.
165. Alkushi A, Clarke BA, Akbari M, et al. Identification of prognostically relevant and reproducible subsets of endometrial adenocarcinoma based on clustering analysis of immunostaining data. *Mod Pathol.* 2007;20:1156-1165.
166. Goldstein NS, Uzieblo A. WT1 immunoreactivity in uterine papillary serous carcinomas is different from ovarian serous carcinomas. *Am J Clin Pathol.* 2002;117:541-545.
167. Acs G, Pasha T, Zhang PJ. WT1 is differentially expressed in serous, endometrioid, clear cell, and mucinous carcinomas of the peritoneum, fallopian tube, ovary, and endometrium. *Int J Gynecol Pathol.* 2004;23:110-118.
168. Egan JA, Ionescu MC, Eapen E, et al. Differential expression of WT1 and p53 in serous and endometrioid carcinomas of the endometrium. *Int J Gynecol Pathol.* 2004;23:119-122.
169. Silva EG, Young RH. Endometrioid neoplasms with clear cells: A report of 21 cases in which the alteration is not of typical secretory type. *Am J Surg Pathol.* 2007;31:1203-1208.
170. An HJ, Logani S, Isacson C, et al. Molecular characterization of uterine clear cell carcinoma. *Mod Pathol.* 2004;17:530-537.
171. Catasus L, Bussaglia E, Rodrguez I, et al. Molecular genetic alterations in endometrioid carcinomas of the ovary: Similar frequency of beta-catenin abnormalities but lower rate of microsatellite instability and PTEN alterations than in uterine endometrioid carcinomas. *Hum Pathol.* 2004;35:1360-1368.
172. Carcangiu ML, Dorji T, Radice P, et al. HNPCC-related endometrial carcinomas show a high frequency of non-endometrioid types and of high FIGO grade endometrioid carcinomas. *Mod Pathol.* 2006;19:173A.
173. Yamamoto S, Tsuda H, Aida S, et al. Immunohistochemical detection of hepatocyte nuclear factor 1beta in ovarian and endometrial clear-cell adenocarcinomas and nonneoplastic endometrium. *Hum Pathol.* 2007;38:1074-1080.

174. Huntsman DG, Clement PB, Gilks CB, et al. Small-cell carcinoma of the endometrium: A clinicopathological study of sixteen cases. *Am J Surg Pathol.* 1994;18:364-375.
175. Katahira A, Akahira J, Niikura H, et al. Small cell carcinoma of the endometrium: Report of three cases and literature review. *Int J Gynecol Cancer.* 2004;14:1018-1023.
176. Mulvany NJ, Allen DG. Combined large cell neuroendocrine and endometrioid carcinoma of the endometrium. *Int J Gynecol Pathol.* 2008;27:49-57.
177. Carlson JW, Nucci MR, Brodsky J, et al. Biomarker-assisted diagnosis of ovarian, cervical and pulmonary small cell carcinomas: The role of TTF-1, WT-1 and HPV analysis. *Histopathology.* 2007;51:305-312.
178. Siami K, McCluggage WG, Ordonez NG, et al. Thyroid transcription factor-1 expression in endometrial and endocervical adenocarcinomas. *Am J Surg Pathol.* 2007;31:1759-1763.
179. Altrabulsi B, Malpica A, Deavers MT, et al. Undifferentiated carcinoma of the endometrium. *Am J Surg Pathol.* 2005;29:1316-1321.
180. Silva EG, Deavers MT, Bodurka DC, et al. Association of low-grade endometrioid carcinoma of the uterus and ovary with undifferentiated carcinoma: A new type of dedifferentiated carcinoma? *Int J Gynecol Pathol.* 2006;25:52-58.
181. Broaddus RR, Lynch HT, Chen LM, et al. Pathologic features of endometrial carcinoma associated with HNPCC: A comparison with sporadic endometrial carcinoma. *Cancer.* 2006;106:87-94.
182. Garg K, Kauff N, Hansen J, et al. IHC for DNA-MMR in EEC in a selected group of patients. *Mod Pathol.* 2008;21:205A.
183. Albannai RA, Alkushi A, Gilks CB. Serous and endometrioid components of mixed endometrial adenocarcinoma show similar immunostaining profiles. *Mod Pathol.* 2009;21:194A.
184. Nascimento AF, Hirsch MS, Cviko A, et al. The role of CD10 staining in distinguishing invasive endometrial adenocarcinoma from adenocarcinoma involving adenomyosis. *Mod Pathol.* 2003;16:22-27.
185. Srodon M, Klein WM, Kurman RJ. CD10 immunostaining does not distinguish endometrial carcinoma invading myometrium from carcinoma involving adenomyosis. *Am J Surg Pathol.* 2003;27:786-789.
186. Tsuruchi N, Kaku T, Kamura T, et al. The prognostic significance of lymphovascular space invasion in endometrial cancer when conventional hemotoxylin and eosin staining is compared to immunohistochemical staining. *Gynecol Oncol.* 1995;57:307-312.
187. Alexander-Sefre F, Salvesen HB, Ryan A, et al. Molecular assessment of depth of myometrial invasion in stage I endometrial cancer: A model based on K-ras mutation analysis. *Gynecol Oncol.* 2003;91:218-225.
188. Lim CS, Alexander-Sefre F, Allam M, et al. Clinical value of immunohistochemically detected lymphovascular space invasion in early stage cervical carcinoma. *Ann Surg Oncol.* 2008;15:2581-2588.
189. Ali A, Black D, Soslow RA. Difficulties in assessing the depth of myometrial invasion in endometrial carcinoma. *Int J Gynecol Pathol.* 2007;26:115-123.
190. Murray SK, Young RH, Scully RE. Unusual epithelial and stromal changes in myoinvasive endometrioid adenocarcinoma: A study of their frequency, associated diagnostic problems, and prognostic significance. *Int J Gynecol Pathol.* 2003;22:324-333.
191. McKenney JK, Kong CS, Longacre TA. Endometrial adenocarcinoma associated with subtle lymph-vascular space invasion and lymph node metastasis: A histologic pattern mimicking intravascular and sinusoidal histiocytes. *Int J Gynecol Pathol.* 2005;24:73-78.
192. Frumovitz M, Bodurka DC, Broaddus RR, et al. Lymphatic mapping and sentinel node biopsy in women with high-risk endometrial cancer. *Gynecol Oncol.* 2007;104:100-103.
193. Baergen RN, Warren CD, Isacson C, et al. Early uterine serous carcinoma: Clonal origin of extrauterine disease. *Int J Gynecol Pathol.* 2001;20:214-219.
194. Euscher ED, Malpica A, Deavers MT, et al. Differential expression of WT-1 in serous carcinomas in the peritoneum with or without associated serous carcinoma in endometrial polyps. *Am J Surg Pathol.* 2005;29:1074-1078.
195. Dupont J, Wang X, Marshall DS, et al. Wilms Tumor Gene (WT1) and p53 expression in endometrial carcinomas: A study of 130 cases using a tissue microarray. *Gynecol Oncol.* 2004;94:449-455.
196. Irving JA, Catasus L, Gallardo A, et al. Synchronous endometrioid carcinomas of the uterine corpus and ovary: Alterations in the beta-catenin (CTNNB1) pathway are associated with independent primary tumors and favorable prognosis. *Hum Pathol.* 2005;36:605-619.
197. Coosemans A, Nik SA, Caluwaerts S, et al. Upregulation of Wilms' tumour gene 1 (WT1) in uterine sarcomas. *Eur J Cancer.* 2007;43:1630-1637.
198. Zhai YL, Nikaido T, Toki T, et al. Prognostic significance of bcl-2 expression in leiomyosarcoma of the uterus. *Br J Cancer.* 1999;80:1658-1664.
199. Leiser AL, Anderson SE, Nonaka D, et al. Apoptotic and cell cycle regulatory markers in uterine leiomyosarcoma. *Gynecol Oncol.* 2006;101:86-91.
200. Iwasa Y, Haga H, Konishi I, et al. Prognostic factors in uterine carcinosarcoma—A clinicopathologic study of 25 patients. *Cancer.* 1998;82:512-519.
201. Sutton GP, Stehman FB, Michael H, et al. Estrogen and progesterone receptors in uterine sarcomas. *Obstet Gynecol.* 1986;68:709-714.
202. Zhai YL, Kobayashi Y, Mori A, et al. Expression of steroid receptors, Ki-67, and p53 in uterine leiomyosarcomas. *Int J Gynecol Pathol.* 1999;18:20-28.
203. Mittal K, Demopoulos RI. MIB-1 (Ki-67), p53, estrogen receptor, and progesterone receptor expression in uterine smooth muscle tumors. *Hum Pathol.* 2001;32:984-987.
204. Leitao MM, Soslow RA, Nonaka D, et al. Tissue microarray immunohistochemical expression of estrogen, progesterone, and androgen receptors in uterine leiomyomata and leiomyosarcoma. *Cancer.* 2004;101:1455-1462.
205. de Leval L, Waltregny D, Boniver J, et al. Use of histone deacetylase 8 (HDAC8), a new marker of smooth muscle differentiation, in the classification of mesenchymal tumors of the uterus. *Am J Surg Pathol.* 2006;30:319-327.
206. Loddenkemper C, Mechsner S, Foss HD, et al. Use of oxytocin receptor expression in distinguishing between uterine smooth muscle tumors and endometrial stromal sarcoma. *Am J Surg Pathol.* 2003;27:1458-1462.
207. Rizeq MN, Van de Rijn M, Hendrickson MR, et al. A comparative immunohistochemical study of uterine smooth muscle neoplasms with emphasis on the epithelioid variant. *Hum Pathol.* 1994;25:671-677.
208. Blom R, Guerrieri C, Stal O, et al. Leiomyosarcoma of the uterus: A clinicopathologic, DNA flow cytometric, p53, and mdm-2 analysis of 49 cases. *Gynecol Oncol.* 1998;68:54-61.
209. Nordal RR, Kristensen GB, Stenwig AE, et al. Immunohistochemical analysis of p53 protein in uterine sarcomas. *Gynecol Oncol.* 1998;70:45-48.
210. Leitao MM, Soslow RA, Baergen RN, et al. Mutation and expression of the TP53 gene in early stage epithelial ovarian carcinoma. *Gynecol Oncol.* 2004;93:301-306.
211. Anderson SE, Nonaka D, Chuai S, et al. p53, epidermal growth factor, and platelet-derived growth factor in uterine leiomyosarcoma and leiomyomas. *Int J Gynecol Cancer.* 2006;16:849-853.
212. Toledo G, Growdon WB, Palmeri ML, et al. Utility of the mitosis marker anti-phosphohistone H3 (PHH3) in precise and rapid evaluation of mitotic index in leiomyomas with bizarre nuclei. *Mod Pathol.* 2008;21:226A-227A.
213. Agoff SN, Grieco VS, Garcia R, et al. Immunohistochemical distinction of endometrial stromal sarcoma and cellular leiomyoma. *Appl Immunohistochem Mol Morphol.* 2001;9:164-169.
214. Bhargava R, Shia J, Hummer AJ, et al. Distinction of endometrial stromal sarcomas from "hemangiopericytomatous" tumors using a panel of immunohistochemical stains. *Mod Pathol.* 2005;18:40-47.
215. Ng TL, Gown AM, Barry TS, et al. Nuclear beta-catenin in mesenchymal tumors. *Mod Pathol.* 2005;18:68-74.
216. Jung CK, Jung JH, Lee A, et al. Diagnostic use of nuclear beta-catenin expression for the assessment of endometrial stromal tumors. *Mod Pathol.* 2008;21:756-763.

217. Kurihara S, Oda Y, Ohishi Y, et al. Endometrial stromal sarcomas and related high-grade sarcomas: Immunohistochemical and molecular genetic study of 31 cases. *Am J Surg Pathol.* 2008;32:1228-1238.
218. Moinfar F, Regitnig P, Tabrizi AD, et al. Expression of androgen receptors in benign and malignant endometrial stromal neoplasms. *Virchows Arch.* 2004;444:410-414.
219. Devaney K, Tavassoli FA. Immunohistochemistry as a diagnostic aid in the interpretation of unusual mesenchymal tumors of the uterus. *Mod Pathol.* 1991;4:225-231.
220. Yilmaz A, Rush DS, Soslow RA. Endometrial stromal sarcomas with unusual histologic features: A report of 24 primary and metastatic tumors emphasizing fibroblastic and smooth muscle differentiation. *Am J Surg Pathol.* 2002;26:1142-1150.
221. Clement PB, Scully RE. Endometrial stromal sarcomas of the uterus with extensive glandular differentiation: A report of three cases that caused problems in differential diagnosis. *Int J Gynecol Pathol.* 1992;11:163-173.
222. Oliva E, Clement PB, Young RH. Epithelioid endometrial and endometrioid stromal tumors: A report of four cases emphasizing their distinction from epithelioid smooth muscle tumors and other oxyphilic uterine and extrauterine tumors. *Int J Gynecol Pathol.* 2002;21:48-55.
223. Ferguson SE, Tornos C, Hummer A, et al. Prognostic features of surgical stage I uterine carcinosarcoma. *Am J Surg Pathol.* 2007;31:1653-1661.
224. Nogales FF, Bergeron C, Carvia RE, et al. Ovarian endometrioid tumors with yolk sac tumor component, an unusual form of ovarian neoplasm—Analysis of six cases. *Am J Surg Pathol.* 1996;20:1056-1066.
225. Ehrmann RL, Weidner N, Welch WR, et al. Malignant mixed müllerian tumor of the ovary with prominent neuroectodermal differentiation (teratoid carcinosarcoma). *Int J Gynecol Pathol.* 1990;9:272-282.
226. Fukunaga M, Nomura K, Endo Y, et al. Carcinosarcoma of the uterus with extensive neuroectodermal differentiation. *Histopathology.* 1996;29:565-570.
227. Mikami Y, Hata S, Kiyokawa T, et al. Expression of CD10 in malignant müllerian mixed tumors and adenosarcomas: An immunohistochemical study. *Mod Pathol.* 2002;15:923-930.
228. Amant F, Steenkiste E, Schurmans K, et al. Immunohistochemical expression of CD10 antigen in uterine adenosarcoma. *Int J Gynecol Cancer.* 2004;14:1118-1121.
229. Soslow RA, Ali A, Oliva E. Mullerian adenosarcomas: An immunophenotypic analysis of 35 cases. *Am J Surg Pathol.* 2008;32:1013-1021.
230. Tedeschi A, Di Mezza G, D'Amico O, et al. A case of pelvic actinomycosis presenting as cutaneous fistula. *Eur J Obstet Gynecol Reprod Biol.* 2003;108:103-105.
231. Vang R, Kempson RL. Perivascular epithelioid cell tumor ("PEComa") of the uterus: A subset of HMB-45-positive epithelioid mesenchymal neoplasms with an uncertain relationship to pure smooth muscle tumors. *Am J Surg Pathol.* 2002;26:1-13.
232. Folpe AL, Mentzel T, Lehr HA, et al. Perivascular epithelioid cell neoplasms of soft tissue and gynecologic origin: a clinicopathologic study of 26 cases and review of the literature. *Am J Surg Pathol.* 2005;29:1558-1575.
233. Fadare O. Perivascular epithelioid cell tumors (PEComas) and smooth muscle tumors of the uterus. *Am J Surg Pathol.* 2007;31:1454-1455.
234. Silva EG, Deavers MT, Bodurka DC, et al. Uterine epithelioid leiomyosarcomas with clear cells: Reactivity with HMB-45 and the concept of PEComa. *Am J Surg Pathol.* 2004;28:244-249.
235. Oliva E, Wang WL, Branton P, et al. Expression of melanocytic ("PEComa") markers in smooth muscle tumors of the uterus: An immunohistochemical analysis of 86 cases. *Mod Pathol.* 2006;19:191A.
236. Clement PB, Scully RE. Uterine tumors resembling ovarian sex-cord tumors. A clinicopathologic analysis of 14 cases. *Am J Clin Pathol.* 1976;66:512-525.
237. Wingen CB, Pauwels PA, Debiec-Rychter M, et al. Uterine gastrointestinal stromal tumour (GIST). *Gynecol Oncol.* 2005;97:970-972.
238. Klein WM, Kurman RJ. Lack of expression of c-kit protein (CD117) in mesenchymal tumors of the uterus and ovary. *Int J Gynecol Pathol.* 2003;22:181-184.
239. Winter III WE, Seidman JD, Krivak TC, et al. Clinicopathological analysis of c-kit expression in carcinosarcomas and leiomyosarcomas of the uterine corpus. *Gynecol Oncol.* 2003;91:3-8.
240. Rushing RS, Shajahan S, Chendil D, et al. Uterine sarcomas express KIT protein but lack mutation(s) in exon 11 or 17 of c-KIT. *Gynecol Oncol.* 2003;91:9-14.
241. Wang L, Felix JC, Lee JL, et al. The proto-oncogene c-kit is expressed in leiomyosarcomas of the uterus. *Gynecol Oncol.* 2003;90:402-406.
242. Rabban JT, Zaloudek CJ, Shekitka KM, Tavassoli FA. Inflammatory myofibroblastic tumor of the uterus: a clinicopathologic study of 6 cases emphasizing distinction from aggressive mesenchymal tumors. *Am J Surg Pathol.* 2005;29:1348-1355.
243. Daya D, Sabet L. The use of cytokeratin as a sensitive and reliable marker for trophoblastic tissue. *Am J Clin Pathol.* 1991;95:137-141.
244. Shih IM, Kurman RJ. Immunohistochemical localization of inhibin-alpha in the placenta and gestational trophoblastic lesions. *Int J Gynecol Pathol.* 1999;18:144-150.
245. Kommoss F, Schmidt D, Coerdt W, et al. Immunohistochemical expression analysis of inhibin-alpha and -beta subunits in partial and complete moles, trophoblastic tumors, and endometrial decidua. *Int J Gynecol Pathol.* 2001;20:380-385.
246. Ino K, Suzuki T, Uehara C, et al. The expression and localization of neutral endopeptidase 24.11/CD10 in human gestational trophoblastic diseases. *Lab Invest.* 2000;80:1729-1738.
247. Mao TL, Kurman RJ, Jeng YM, et al. HSD3B1 as a novel trophoblast-associated marker that assists in the differential diagnosis of trophoblastic tumors and tumorlike lesions. *Am J Surg Pathol.* 2008;32:236-242.
248. Shih IM, Kurman RJ. p63 Expression is useful in the distinction of epithelioid trophoblastic and placental site trophoblastic tumors by profiling trophoblastic subpopulations. *Am J Surg Pathol.* 2004;28:1177-1183.
249. Shih I. Trophogram, an immunohistochemistry-based algorithmic approach, in the differential diagnosis of trophoblastic tumors and tumorlike lesions. *Ann Diagn Pathol.* 2007;11:228-234.
250. Shih IM, Kurman RJ. Expression of melanoma cell adhesion molecule in intermediate trophoblast. *Lab Invest.* 1996;75:377-388.
251. Singer G, Kurman RJ, McMaster MT, et al. HLA-G immunoreactivity is specific for intermediate trophoblast in gestational trophoblastic disease and can serve as a useful marker in differential diagnosis. *Am J Surg Pathol.* 2002;26:914-920.
252. Kurman RJ, Young RH, Norris HJ, et al. Immunocytochemical localization of placental lactogen and chorionic gonadotropin in the normal placenta and trophoblastic tumors, with emphasis on intermediate trophoblast and the placental site trophoblastic tumor. *Int J Gynecol Pathol.* 1984;3:101-121.
253. Huettner PC, Gersell DJ. Placental site nodule: A clinicopathologic study of 38 cases. *Int J Gynecol Pathol.* 1994;13:191-198.
254. Yeh IT, O'Connor DM, Kurman RJ. Vacuolated cytotrophoblast: A subpopulation of trophoblast in the chorion laeve. *Placenta.* 1989;10:429-438.
255. Li HW, Cheung AN, Tsao SW, et al. Expression of e-cadherin and beta-catenin in trophoblastic tissue in normal and pathological pregnancies. *Int J Gynecol Pathol.* 2003;22:63-70.
256. Wong SC, Chan AT, Chan JK, et al. Nuclear beta-catenin and Ki-67 expression in choriocarcinoma and its pre-malignant form. *J Clin Pathol.* 2006;59:387-392.
257. Mao TL, Kurman RJ, Huang CC, et al. Immunohistochemistry of choriocarcinoma: An aid in differential diagnosis and in elucidating pathogenesis. *Am J Surg Pathol.* 2007;31:1726-1732.
258. Castrillon DH, Sun DQ, Weremowicz S, et al. Discrimination of complete hydatidiform mole from its mimics by immunohistochemistry of the paternally imprinted gene product p57KIP2. *Am J Surg Pathol.* 2001;25:1225-1230.
259. Fisher RA, Hodges MD, Rees HC, et al. The maternally transcribed gene p57(KIP2) (CDNK1C) is abnormally expressed in both androgenetic and biparental complete hydatidiform moles. *Hum Mol Genet.* 2002;11:3267-3272.
260. Fukunaga M. Immunohistochemical characterization of p57(KIP2) expression in early hydatidiform moles. *Hum Pathol.* 2002;33:1188-1192.

261. Genest DR, Dorfman DM, Castrillon DH. Ploidy and imprinting in hydatidiform moles. Complementary use of flow cytometry and immunohistochemistry of the imprinted gene product p57KIP2 to assist molar classification. *J Reprod Med.* 2002;47:342-346.
262. Hoffner L, Dunn J, Esposito N, et al. P57KIP2 immunostaining and molecular cytogenetics: Combined approach aids in diagnosis of morphologically challenging cases with molar phenotype and in detecting androgenetic cell lines in mosaic/chimeric conceptions. *Hum Pathol.* 2008;39:63-72.
263. Keep D, Zaragoza MV, Hassold T, et al. Very early complete hydatidiform mole. *Hum Pathol.* 1996;27:708-713.
264. Kim MJ, Kim KR, Ro JY, et al. Diagnostic and pathogenetic significance of increased stromal apoptosis and incomplete vasculogenesis in complete hydatidiform moles in very early pregnancy periods. *Am J Surg Pathol.* 2006;30:362-369.
265. Shih IM, Seidman JD, Kurman RJ. Placental site nodule and characterization of distinctive types of intermediate trophoblast. *Hum Pathol.* 1999;30:687-694.
266. Shih IM, Kurman RJ. Ki-67 labeling index in the differential diagnosis of exaggerated placental site, placental site trophoblastic tumor, and choriocarcinoma: A double immunohistochemical staining technique using Ki-67 and Mel-CAM antibodies. *Hum Pathol.* 1998;29:27-33.
267. Shih IM, Kurman RJ. Epithelioid trophoblastic tumor—A neoplasm distinct from choriocarcinoma and placental site trophoblastic tumor simulating carcinoma. *Am J Surg Pathol.* 1998;22:1393-1403.
268. Mao TL, Seidman JD, Kurman RJ, et al. Cyclin E and p16 immunoreactivity in epithelioid trophoblastic tumor—An aid in differential diagnosis. *Am J Surg Pathol.* 2006;30:1105-1110.
269. Mazur MT. Metastatic gestational choriocarcinoma. Unusual pathologic variant following therapy. *Cancer.* 1989;63:1370-1377.
270. Bacchi CE, Coelho KI, Goldberg J. Expression of beta-human chorionic gonadotropin (beta-hCG) in non-trophoblastic elements of transitional cell carcinoma of the bladder: Possible relationship with the prognosis. *Rev Paul Med.* 1993;111:412-416.
271. Hameed A, Miller DS, Muller CY, et al. Frequent expression of beta-human chorionic gonadotropin (beta-hCG) in squamous cell carcinoma of the cervix. *Int J Gynecol Pathol.* 1999;18:381-386.
272. Lynch HT, Smyrk TC, Watson P, et al. Genetics, natural history, tumor spectrum, and pathology of hereditary nonpolyposis colorectal cancer: An updated review. *Gastroenterology.* 1993;104:1535-1549.
273. Lynch HT, Lanspa S, Smyrk T, et al. Hereditary nonpolyposis colorectal cancer (Lynch syndromes I & II). Genetics, pathology, natural history, and cancer control. *Part I. Cancer Genet Cytogenet.* 1991;53:143-160.
274. Lynch HT, Smyrk T. An update on Lynch syndrome. *Curr Opin Oncol.* 1998;10:349-356.
275. Shia J, Black D, Hummer AJ, et al. Routinely assessed morphological features correlate with microsatellite instability status in endometrial cancer. *Hum Pathol.* 2008;39:116-125.
276. Lu KH, Schorge JO, Rodabaugh KJ, et al. Prospective determination of prevalence of Lynch syndrome in young women with endometrial cancer. *J Clin Oncol.* 2007;25:5158-5164.
277. Simpkins SB, Bocker T, Swisher EM, et al. MLH1 promoter methylation and gene silencing is the primary cause of microsatellite instability in sporadic endometrial cancers. *Hum Mol Genet.* 1999;8:661-666.
278. Buttin BM, Powell MA, Mutch DG, et al. Increased risk for hereditary nonpolyposis colorectal cancer-associated synchronous and metachronous malignancies in patients with microsatellite instability-positive endometrial carcinoma lacking MLH1 promoter methylation. *Clin Cancer Res.* 2004;10:481-490.
279. Shia J. Immunohistochemistry versus microsatellite instability testing for screening colorectal cancer patients at risk for hereditary nonpolyposis colorectal cancer syndrome. Part I. The utility of immunohistochemistry. *J Mol Diagn.* 2008;10:293-300.
280. Ito K, Watanabe K, Nasim S, et al. Prognostic significance of p53 overexpression in endometrial cancer. *Cancer Res.* 1994;54:4667-4670.
281. Sung CJ, Zheng Y, Quddus MR, et al. p53 as a significant prognostic marker in endometrial carcinoma. *Int J Gynecol Cancer.* 2000;10:119-127.
282. Alkushi A, Lim P, Coldman A, et al. Interpretation of p53 immunoreactivity in endometrial carcinoma: Establishing a clinically relevant cut-off level. *Int J Gynecol Pathol.* 2004;23:129-137.
283. Santin AD, Bellone S, Gokden M, et al. Overexpression of HER-2/neu in uterine serous papillary cancer. *Clin Cancer Res.* 2002;8:1271-1279.
284. Lax SF. Molecular genetic pathways in various types of endometrial carcinoma: From a phenotypical to a molecular-based classification. *Virchows Arch.* 2004;444:213-223.
285. Slomovitz BM, Broaddus RR, Burke TW, et al. Her-2/neu overexpression and amplification in uterine papillary serous carcinoma. *J Clin Oncol.* 2004;22:3126-3132.
286. Santin AD, Bellone S, Van SS, et al. Determination of HER2/neu status in uterine serous papillary carcinoma: Comparative analysis of immunohistochemistry and fluorescence in situ hybridization. *Gynecol Oncol.* 2005;98:24-30.
287. Odicino FE, Bignotti E, Rossi E, et al. HER-2/neu overexpression and amplification in uterine serous papillary carcinoma: Comparative analysis of immunohistochemistry, real-time reverse transcription-polymerase chain reaction, and fluorescence in situ hybridization. *Int J Gynecol Cancer.* 2008;18:14-21.
288. Bodner-Adler B, Bodner K, Czerwenka K, et al. Expression of p16 protein in patients with uterine smooth muscle tumors: An immunohistochemical analysis. *Gynecol Oncol.* 2005;96:62-66.
289. O'Neill CJ, McBride HA, Connolly LE, et al. Uterine leiomyosarcomas are characterized by high p16, p53 and MIB1 expression in comparison with usual leiomyomas, leiomyoma variants and smooth muscle tumours of uncertain malignant potential. *Histopathology.* 2007;50:851-858.
290. Atkins KA, Arronte N, Darus CJ, et al. The Use of p16 in enhancing the histologic classification of uterine smooth muscle tumors. *Am J Surg Pathol.* 2008;32:98-102.
291. Gannon BR, Manduch M, Childs TJ. Differential Immunoreactivity of p16 in Leiomyosarcomas and Leiomyoma Variants. *Int J Gynecol Pathol.* 2008;27:68-73.
292. Goodfellow PJ, Buttin BM, Herzog TJ, et al. Prevalence of defective DNA mismatch repair and MSH6 mutation in an unselected series of endometrial cancers. *Proc Natl Acad Sci U S A.* 2003;100:5908-5913.
293. Ollikainen M, Abdel-Rahman WM, Moisio AL, et al. Molecular analysis of familial endometrial carcinoma: A manifestation of hereditary nonpolyposis colorectal cancer or a separate syndrome? *J Clin Oncol.* 2005;23:4609-4616.
294. Hampel H, Frankel W, Panescu J, et al. Screening for Lynch syndrome (hereditary nonpolyposis colorectal cancer) among endometrial cancer patients. *Cancer Res.* 2006;66:7810-7817.
295. Koontz JI, Soreng AL, Nucci M, et al. Frequent fusion of the JAZF1 and JJAZ1 genes in endometrial stromal tumors. *Proc Natl Acad Sci U S A.* 2001;98:6348-6353.
296. Micci F, Walter CU, Teixeira MR, et al. Cytogenetic and molecular genetic analyses of endometrial stromal sarcoma: Nonrandom involvement of chromosome arms 6p and 7p and confirmation of JAZF1/JJAZ1 gene fusion in t(7;17). *Cancer Genet Cytogenet.* 2003;144:119-124.
297. Huang HY, Ladanyi M, Soslow RA. Molecular detection of JAZF1-JJAZ1 gene fusion in endometrial stromal neoplasms with classic and variant histology: Evidence for genetic heterogeneity. *Am J Surg Pathol.* 2004;28:224-232.
298. Hrzenjak A, Moinfar F, Tavassoli FA, et al. JAZF1/JJAZ1 gene fusion in endometrial stromal sarcomas: Molecular analysis by reverse transcriptase-polymerase chain reaction optimized for paraffin-embedded tissue. *J Mol Diagn.* 2005;7:388-395.
299. Nucci MR, Harburger D, Koontz J, et al. Molecular analysis of the JAZF1-JJAZ1 gene fusion by RT-PCR and fluorescence in situ hybridization in endometrial stromal neoplasms. *Am J Surg Pathol.* 2007;31:65-70.
300. Oliva E, de Leval L, Soslow RA, et al. High frequency of JAZF1-JJAZ1 gene fusion in endometrial stromal tumors with smooth muscle differentiation by interphase FISH detection. *Am J Surg Pathol.* 2007;31:1277-1284.

301. Fukunaga M. Immunohistochemical characterization of p57Kip2 expression in tetraploid hydropic placentas. *Arch Pathol Lab Med.* 2004;128:897-900.
302. Lage JM, Mark SD, Roberts DJ, et al. A flow cytometric study of 137 fresh hydropic placentas: Correlation between types of hydatidiform moles and nuclear DNA ploidy. *Obstet Gynecol.* 1992;79:403-410.
303. Zaragoza MV, Surti U, Redline RW, et al. Parental origin and phenotype of triploidy in spontaneous abortions: Predominance of diandry and association with the partial hydatidiform mole. *Am J Hum Genet.* 2000;66:1807-1820.
304. Tavassoli FA, Devilee P, International Agency for Research on Cancer, et al. *Pathology and genetics of tumours of the breast and female genital organs.* Lyon: International Agency for Research on Cancer; 2003.
305. Moll R, Franke WW, Schiller DL, et al. The catalog of human cytokeratins: Patterns of expression in normal epithelia, tumors and cultured cells. *Cell.* 1982;31:11-24.
306. Moll R, Levy R, Czernobilsky B, et al. Cytokeratins of normal epithelia and some neoplasms of the female genital tract. *Lab Invest.* 1983;49:599-610.
307. Berezowski K, Stastny JF, Kornstein MJ. Cytokeratins 7 and 20 and carcinoembryonic antigen in ovarian and colonic carcinoma. *Mod Pathol.* 1996;9:426-429.
308. Lagendijk JH, Mullink H, Van Diest PJ, et al. Immunohistochemical differentiation between primary adenocarcinomas of the ovary and ovarian metastases of colonic and breast origin. Comparison between a statistical and an intuitive approach. *J Clin Pathol.* 1999;52:283-290.
309. Cathro HP, Stoler MH. Expression of cytokeratins 7 and 20 in ovarian neoplasia. *Am J Clin Pathol.* 2002;117:944-951.
310. Chu P, Wu E, Weiss LM. Cytokeratin 7 and cytokeratin 20 expression in epithelial neoplasms: A survey of 435 cases. *Mod Pathol.* 2000;13:962-972.
311. Raspollini MR, Amunni G, Villanucci A, et al. Utility of CDX-2 in distinguishing between primary and secondary (intestinal) mucinous ovarian carcinoma: An immunohistochemical comparison of 43 cases. *Appl Immunohistochem Mol Morphol.* 2004;12:127-131.
312. Moll R, Lowe A, Laufer J, et al. Cytokeratin 20 in human carcinomas. A new histodiagnostic marker detected by monoclonal antibodies. *Am J Pathol.* 1992;140:427-447.
313. Miettinen M. Keratin 20: Immunohistochemical marker for gastrointestinal, urothelial, and Merkel cell carcinomas. *Mod Pathol.* 1995;8:384-388.
314. Wauters CC, Smedts F, Gerrits LG, et al. Keratins 7 and 20 as diagnostic markers of carcinomas metastatic to the ovary. *Hum Pathol.* 1995;26:852-855.
315. Loy TS, Calaluce RD, Keeney GL. Cytokeratin immunostaining in differentiating primary ovarian carcinoma from metastatic colonic adenocarcinoma. *Mod Pathol.* 1996;9:1040-1044.
316. Ji H, Isacson C, Seidman JD, et al. Cytokeratins 7 and 20, Dpc4, and MUC5AC in the distinction of metastatic mucinous carcinomas in the ovary from primary ovarian mucinous tumors: Dpc4 assists in identifying metastatic pancreatic carcinomas. *Int J Gynecol Pathol.* 2002;21:391-400.
317. Ordonez NG. Role of immunohistochemistry in distinguishing epithelial peritoneal mesotheliomas from peritoneal and ovarian serous carcinomas. *Am J Surg Pathol.* 1998;22:1203-1214.
318. Ramalingam P, Malpica A, Silva EG, et al. The use of cytokeratin 7 and EMA in differentiating ovarian yolk sac tumors from endometrioid and clear cell carcinomas. *Am J Surg Pathol.* 2004;28:1499-1505.
319. Attanoos RL, Webb R, Dojcinov SD, et al. Value of mesothelial and epithelial antibodies in distinguishing diffuse peritoneal mesothelioma in females from serous papillary carcinoma of the ovary and peritoneum. *Histopathology.* 2002;40:237-244.
320. Charpin C, Bhan AK, Zurawski VRJ, et al. Carcinoembryonic antigen (CEA) and carbohydrate determinant 19-9 (CA 19-9) localization in 121 primary and metastatic ovarian tumors: An immunohistochemical study with the use of monoclonal antibodies. *Int J Gynecol Pathol.* 1982;1:231-245.
321. Brown RW, Campagna LB, Dunn JK, et al. Immunohistochemical identification of tumor markers in metastatic adenocarcinoma. A diagnostic adjunct in the determination of primary site. *Am J Clin Pathol.* 1997;107:12-19.
322. Lagendijk JH, Mullink H, Van Diest PJ, et al. Tracing the origin of adenocarcinomas with unknown primary using immunohistochemistry: Differential diagnosis between colonic and ovarian carcinomas as primary sites. *Hum Pathol.* 1998;29:491-497.
323. Ulfig N. Calcium-binding proteins in the human developing brain. *Adv Anat Embryol Cell Biol.* 2002;165:1-92:III-IX.
324. Chou YY, Jeng YM, Kao HL, et al. Differentiation of ovarian mucinous carcinoma and metastatic colorectal adenocarcinoma by immunostaining with beta-catenin. *Histopathology.* 2003;43:151-156.
325. Goldstein NS, Bassi D, Uzieblo A. WT1 is an integral component of an antibody panel to distinguish pancreaticobiliary and some ovarian epithelial neoplasms. *Am J Clin Pathol.* 2001;116:246-252.
326. Multhaupt HAB, Arenas-Elliott CP, Warhol MJ. Comparison of glycoprotein expression between ovarian and colon adenocarcinomas. *Arch Pathol Lab Med.* 1999;123:909-916.
327. Thor A, Gorstein F, Ohuchi N, et al. Tumor-associated glycoprotein (TAG-72) in ovarian carcinomas defined by monoclonal antibody B72.3. *J Natl Cancer Inst.* 1986;76:995-1006.
328. Bollinger DJ, Wick MR, Dehner LP, et al. Peritoneal malignant mesothelioma versus serous papillary adenocarcinoma. A histochemical and immunohistochemical comparison. *Am J Surg Pathol.* 1989;13:659-670.
329. O'Brien TJ, Beard JB, Underwood LJ, et al. The CA 125 gene: An extracellular superstructure dominated by repeat sequences. *Tumor Biol.* 2001;22:348-366.
330. O'Brien TJ, Beard JB, Underwood LJ, et al. The CA 125 gene: A newly discovered extension of the glycosylated N-terminal domain doubles the size of this extracellular superstructure. *Tumor Biol.* 2002;23:154-169.
331. Bast Jr RC, Xu FJ, Yu YH, et al. CA 125: The past and the future. *Int J Biol Markers.* 1998;13:179-187.
332. Loy TS, Quesenberry JT, Sharp SC. Distribution of CA 125 in adenocarcinomas: An immunohistochemical study of 481 cases. *Am J Clin Pathol.* 1992;98:175-179.
333. Koelma IA, Nap M, Rodenburg CJ, et al. The value of tumour marker CA 125 in surgical pathology. *Histopathology.* 1987;11:287-294.
334. Keen CE, Szakacs S, Okon E, et al. CA125 and thyroglobulin staining in papillary carcinomas of thyroid and ovarian origin is not completely specific for site of origin. *Histopathology.* 1999;34:113-117.
335. Nap M, Vitali A, Nustad K, et al. Immunohistochemical characterization of 22 monoclonal antibodies against the CA125 antigen: 2nd report from the ISOBM TD-1 workshop. *Tumor Biol.* 1996;17:325-331.
336. Leake J, Woolas RP, Daniel J, et al. Immunocytochemical and serological expression of CA 125: A clinicopathological study of 40 malignant ovarian epithelial tumours. *Histopathology.* 1994;24:57-64.
337. Zheng W, Senturk BZ, Parkash V. Inhibin immunohistochemical staining: A practical approach for the surgical pathologist in the diagnoses of ovarian sex cord-stromal tumors. *Adv Anat Pathol.* 2003;10:27-38.
338. Rivier C, Meunier H, Roberts V, et al. Inhibin: Role and secretion in the rat. *Recent Prog Horm Res.* 1990;46:231-257.
339. Vale W, Rivier C, Hsueh A, et al. Chemical and biological characterization of the inhibin family of protein hormones. *Recent Prog Horm Res.* 1988;44:1-34.
340. Welt CK. The physiology and pathophysiology of inhibin, activin and follistatin in female reproduction. *Curr Opin Obstet Gynecol.* 2002;14:317-323.
341. Rishi M, Howard LN, Bratthauer GL, et al. Use of monoclonal antibody against human inhibin as a marker for sex cord stromal tumors of the ovary. *Am J Surg Pathol.* 1997;21:583-589.
342. Costa MJ, Ames PF, Walls J, et al. Inhibin immunohistochemistry applied to ovarian neoplasms: A novel, effective, diagnostic tool. *Hum Pathol.* 1997;28:1247-1254.
343. Hildebrandt RH, Rouse RV, Longacre TA. Value of inhibin in the identification of granulosa cell tumors of the ovary. *Hum Pathol.* 1997;28:1387-1395.
344. Kommoss F, Oliva E, Bhan AK, et al. Inhibin expression in ovarian tumors and tumor-like lesions: An immunohistochemical study. *Mod Pathol.* 1998;11:656-664.
345. McCluggage WG. Value of inhibin staining in gynecological pathology. *Int J Gynecol Pathol.* 2001;20:79-85.

346. Deavers MT, Malpica A, Liu J, et al. Ovarian sex cord-stromal tumors: An immunohistochemical study including a comparison of calretinin and inhibin. *Mod Pathol.* 2003;16:584-590.
347. Pelkey TJ, Frierson HFJ, Mills SE, et al. The diagnostic utility of inhibin staining in ovarian neoplasms. *Int J Gynecol Pathol.* 1998;17:97-105.
348. Matias-Guiu X, Pons C, Prat J. Mullerian inhibiting substance, alpha-inhibin, and CD99 expression in sex cord-stromal tumors and endometrioid ovarian carcinomas resembling sex cord-stromal tumors. *Hum Pathol.* 1998;29:840-845.
349. Yao DX, Soslow RA, Hedvat CV, et al. Melan-A (A103) and inhibin expression in ovarian neoplasms. *Appl Immunohistochem Mol Morphol.* 2003;11:244-249.
350. McCluggage WG, Burton J, Maxwell P, et al. Immunohistochemical staining of normal, hyperplastic, and neoplastic adrenal cortex with a monoclonal antibody against alpha inhibin. *J Clin Pathol.* 1998;51:114-116.
351. Pelkey TJ, Frierson HFJ, Mills SE, et al. The alpha subunit of inhibin in adrenal cortical neoplasia. *Mod Pathol.* 1998;11:516-524.
352. Chivite A, MatiasGuiu X, Pons C, et al. Inhibin A expression in adrenal neoplasms—A new immunohistochemical marker for adrenocortical tumors. *Appl Immunohistochem.* 1998;6:42-49.
353. Cho EY, Ahn GH. Immunoexpression of inhibin alpha-subunit in adrenal neoplasms. *Appl Immunohistochem Mol Morphol.* 2001;9:222-228.
354. Jorda M, De MB, Nadji M. Calretinin and inhibin are useful in separating adrenocortical neoplasms from pheochromocytomas. *Appl Immunohistochem Mol Morphol.* 2002;10:67-70.
355. Zhang PJ, Genega EM, Tomaszewski JE, et al. The role of calretinin, inhibin, melan-A, BCL-2, and C-kit in differentiating adrenal cortical and medullary tumors: An immunohistochemical study. *Mod Pathol.* 2003;16:591-597.
356. Rogers JH. Calretinin: A gene for a novel calcium-binding protein expressed principally in neurons. *J Cell Biol.* 1987;105:1343-1353.
357. Tos AP, Doglioni C. Calretinin: A novel tool for diagnostic immunohistochemistry. *Adv Anat Pathol.* 1998;5:61-66.
358. Rogers J, Khan M, Ellis J. Calretinin and other CaBPs in the nervous system. *Adv Exp Med Biol.* 1990;269:195-203.
359. Cao QJ, Jones JG, Li M. Expression of calretinin in human ovary, testis, and ovarian sex cord-stromal tumors. *Int J Gynecol Pathol.* 2001;20:346-352.
360. McCluggage WG, Maxwell P. Immunohistochemical staining for calretinin is useful in the diagnosis of ovarian sex cord-stromal tumours. *Histopathology.* 2001;38:403-408.
361. Movahedi-Lankarani S, Kurman RJ. Calretinin, a more sensitive but less specific marker than alpha-inhibin for ovarian sex cord-stromal neoplasms—An immunohistochemical study of 215 cases. *Am J Surg Pathol.* 2002;26:1477-1483.
362. Lee SB, Haber DA. Wilms tumor and the WT1 gene. *Exp Cell Res.* 2001;264:74-99.
363. Charles AK, Mall S, Watson J, et al. Expression of the Wilms' tumour gene WT1 in the developing human and in paediatric renal tumours: an immunohistochemical study. *Mol Pathol.* 1997;50:138-144.
364. Ordonez NG. Desmoplastic small round cell tumor II: An ultrastructural and immunohistochemical study with emphasis on new immunohistochemical markers. *Am J Surg Pathol.* 1998;22:1314-1327.
365. Hill DA, Pfeifer JD, Marley EF, et al. WT1 staining reliably differentiates desmoplastic small round cell tumor from Ewing sarcoma/primitive neuroectodermal tumor—An immunohistochemical and molecular diagnostic study. *Am J Clin Pathol.* 2000;114:345-353.
366. Lae ME, Roche PC, Jin L, et al. Desmoplastic small round cell tumor—A clinicopathologic, immunohistochemical, and molecular study of 32 tumors. *Am J Surg Pathol.* 2002;26:823-835.
367. Hwang H, Quenneville L, Yaziji H, et al. Wilms tumor gene product: Sensitive and contextually specific marker of serous carcinomas of ovarian surface epithelial origin. *Appl Immunohistochem Mol Morphol.* 2004;12:122-126.
368. Ordonez NG. Value of thyroid transcription factor-1, E-cadherin, BG8, WT1, and CD44S immunostaining in distinguishing epithelial pleural mesothelioma from pulmonary and nonpulmonary adenocarcinoma. *Am J Surg Pathol.* 2000; 24:598-606.
369. Shimizu M, Toki T, Takagi Y, et al. Immunohistochemical detection of the Wilms' tumor gene (WT1) in epithelial ovarian tumors. *Int J Gynecol Pathol.* 2000;19:158-163.
370. Logani S, Oliva E, Amin MB, et al. Immunoprofile of ovarian tumors with putative transitional cell (urothelial) differentiation using novel urothelial markers: Histogenetic and diagnostic implications. *Am J Surg Pathol.* 2003;27:1434-1441.
371. McCluggage WG, Oliva E, Connolly LE, et al. An immunohistochemical analysis of ovarian small cell carcinoma of hypercalcemic type. *Int J Gynecol Pathol.* 2004;23:330-336.
372. Nakopoulou L, Stefanaki K, Janinis J, et al. Immunohistochemical expression of placental alkaline phosphatase and vimentin in epithelial ovarian neoplasms. *Acta Oncol.* 1995;34:511-515.
373. Nouwen EJ, Hendrix PG, Dauwe S, et al. Tumor markers in the human ovary and its neoplasms. A comparative immunohistochemical study. *Am J Pathol.* 1987;126:230-242.
374. Lifschitz-Mercer B, Walt H, Kushnir I, et al. Differentiation potential of ovarian dysgerminoma: An immunohistochemical study of 15 cases. *Hum Pathol.* 1995;26:62-66.
375. Hustin J, Gillerot Y, Collette J, et al. Placental alkaline phosphatase in developing normal and abnormal gonads and in germ-cell tumours. *Virchows Arch A Pathol Anat Histopathol.* 1990;417:67-72.
376. Arber DA, Tamayo R, Weiss LM. Paraffin section detection of the c-kit gene product (CD117) in human tissues: Value in the diagnosis of mast cell disorders. *Hum Pathol.* 1998;29:498-504.
377. Gibson PC, Cooper K. CD117 (KIT): A diverse protein with selective applications in surgical pathology. *Adv Anat Pathol.* 2002;9:65-69.
378. Sarlomo-Rikala M, Kovatich AJ, Barusevicius A, et al. CD117: A sensitive marker for gastrointestinal stromal tumors that is more specific than CD34. *Mod Pathol.* 1998;11:728-734.
379. Miettinen M, Sarlomo-Rikala M, Lasota J. Gastrointestinal stromal tumors: Recent advances in understanding of their biology. *Hum Pathol.* 1999;30:1213-1220.
380. Lee JR, Joshi V, Griffin Jr JW, et al. Gastrointestinal autonomic nerve tumor—Immunohistochemical and molecular identity with gastrointestinal stromal tumor. *Am J Surg Pathol.* 2001;25:979-987.
381. Leroy X, Augusto D, Leteurtre E, et al. CD30 and CD117 (c-kit) used in combination are useful for distinguishing embryonal carcinoma from seminoma. *J Histochem Cytochem.* 2002;50:283-285.
382. Sever M, Jones TD, Roth LM, et al. Expression of CD117 (c-kit) receptor in dysgerminoma of the ovary: Diagnostic and therapeutic implications. *Mod Pathol.* 2005;18:1411-1416.
383. Cheng L, Sung MT, Cossu-Rocca P, et al. OCT4: biological functions and clinical applications as a marker of germ cell neoplasia. *J Pathol.* 2007;211:1-9.
384. Cheng L, Thomas A, Roth LM, et al. OCT4: A novel biomarker for dysgerminoma of the ovary. *Am J Surg Pathol.* 2004;28:1341-1346.
385. De Jong J, Stoop H, Dohle GR, et al. Diagnostic value of OCT3/4 for pre-invasive and invasive testicular germ cell tumours. *J Pathol.* 2005;206:242-249.
386. Rajpert-DeMeyts E, Hanstein R, Jorgensen N, et al. Developmental expression of POU5F1 (OCT-3/4) in normal and dysgenetic human gonads. *Hum Reprod.* 2004;19:1338-1344.
387. Hoei-Hansen CE, Kraggerud SM, Abeler VM, et al. Ovarian dysgerminomas are characterised by frequent KIT mutations and abundant expression of pluripotency markers. *Mol Cancer.* 2007;6:12.
388. Harms D, Janig U. Germ cell tumours of childhood. Report of 170 cases including 59 pure and partial yolk-sac tumours. *Virchows Arch A.* 1986;409:223-239.
389. Clement PB, Young RH, Scully RE. Endometrioid-like variant of ovarian yolk sac tumor. A clinicopathological analysis of eight cases. *Am J Surg Pathol.* 1987;11:767-778.
390. Kurman RJ, Norris HJ. Endodermal sinus tumor of the ovary. A clinical and pathologic analysis of 71 cases. *Cancer.* 1976;38:2404-2419.
391. Prat J, Bhan AK, Dickersin GR, et al. Hepatoid yolk sac tumor of the ovary (endodermal sinus tumor with hepatoid differentiation): A light microscopic, ultrastructural and immunohistochemical study of seven cases. *Cancer.* 1982;50:2355-2368.

392. Zirker TA, Silva EG, Morris M, et al. Immunohistochemical differentiation of clear-cell carcinoma of the female genital tract and endodermal sinus tumor with the use of alpha-fetoprotein and Leu-M1. *Am J Clin Pathol.* 1989;91:511-514.
393. Devouassoux-Shisheboran M, Schammel DP, Tavassoli FA. Ovarian hepatoid yolk sac tumours: Morphological, immunohistochemical and ultrastructural features. *Histopathology.* 1999;34:462-469.
394. Esheba GE, Pate LL, Longacre TA. Oncofetal protein glypican-3 distinguishes yolk sac tumor from clear cell carcinoma of the ovary. *Am J Surg Pathol.* 2008;32:600-607.
395. Ishikura H, Scully RE. Hepatoid carcinoma of the ovary. A newly described tumor. *Cancer.* 1987;60:2775-2784.
396. Pitman MB, Triratanachat S, Young RH, et al. Hepatocyte paraffin 1 antibody does not distinguish primary ovarian tumors with hepatoid differentiation from metastatic hepatocellular carcinoma. *Int J Gynecol Pathol.* 2004;23:58-64.
397. Tochigi N, Kishimoto T, Supriatna Y, et al. Hepatoid carcinoma of the ovary: A report of three cases admixed with a common surface epithelial carcinoma. *Int J Gynecol Pathol.* 2003;22:266-271.
398. Young RH, Gersell DJ, Clement PB, et al. Hepatocellular carcinoma metastatic to the ovary: A report of three cases discovered during life with discussion of the differential diagnosis of hepatoid tumors of the ovary. *Hum Pathol.* 1992;23:574-580.
399. Gagnon S, Tëtu B, Silva EG, et al. Frequency of alpha-fetoprotein production by Sertoli-Leydig cell tumors of the ovary: An immunohistochemical study of eight cases. *Mod Pathol.* 1989;2:63-67.
400. Hammad A, Jasnosz KM, Olson PR. Expression of alpha-fetoprotein by ovarian Sertoli-Leydig cell tumors—Case report and review of the literature. *Arch Pathol Lab Med.* 1995;119:1075-1079.
401. Mooney EE, Nogales FF, Tavassoli FA. Hepatocytic differentiation in retiform Sertoli-Leydig cell tumors: distinguishing a heterologous element from Leydig cells. *Hum Pathol.* 1999;30:611-617.
402. Niehans GA, Manivel JC, Copland GT, et al. Immunohistochemistry of germ cell and trophoblastic neoplasms. *Cancer.* 1988;62:1113-1123.
403. Perrone T, Steeper TA, Dehner LP. Alpha-fetoprotein localization in pure ovarian teratoma. An immunohistochemical study of 12 cases. *Am J Clin Pathol.* 1987;88:713-717.
404. Kurman RJ, Norris HJ. Embryonal carcinoma of the ovary: A clinicopathologic entity distinct from endodermal sinus tumor resembling embryonal carcinoma of the adult testis. *Cancer.* 1976;38:2420-2433.
405. Ueda G, Abe Y, Yoshida M, et al. Embryonal carcinoma of the ovary: A six-year survival. *Int J Gynaecol Obstet.* 1990;31:287-292.
406. Nakashima N, Fukatsu T, Nagasaka T, et al. The frequency and histology of hepatic tissue in germ cell tumors. *Am J Surg Pathol.* 1987;11:682-692.
407. Furumoto M. Cellular localization of AFP, hCG and its free subunits, and SP1 in embryonal carcinoma of the testis and ovary. *Pathol Res Pract.* 1981;173:12-21.
408. Lopez JM, Malpica A, Deavers MT, et al. Ovarian yolk sac tumor associated with endometrioid carcinoma and mucinous cystadenoma of the ovary. *Ann Diagn Pathol.* 2003; 7:300-305.
409. Kurman RJ, Scardino PT, McIntire KR, et al. Cellular localization of alpha-fetoprotein and human chorionic gonadotropin in germ cell tumors of the testis using an indirect immunoperoxidase technique. *Cancer.* 1977;40:2136-2151.
410. Hustin J, Reuter AM, Franchimont P. Immunohistochemical localization of HCG and its subunits in testicular germ cell tumours. *Virchows Arch A Pathol Anat Histopathol.* 1985;406:333-338.
411. Zaloudek CJ, Tavassoli FA, Norris HJ. Dysgerminoma with syncytiotrophoblastic giant cells: A histologically and clinically distinctive subtype of dysgerminoma. *Am J Surg Pathol.* 1981;5:361-367.
412. Oliva E, Andrada E, Pezzica E, et al. Ovarian carcinomas with choriocarcinomatous differentiation. *Cancer.* 1993;72:2441-2446.
413. Matias-Guiu X, Prat J. Ovarian tumors with functioning stroma. An immunohistochemical study of 100 cases with human chorionic gonadotropin monoclonal and polyclonal antibodies. *Cancer.* 1990;65:2001-2005.
414. Mohabeer J, Buckley CH, Fox H. An immunohistochemical study of the incidence and significance of human chorionic gonadotrophin synthesis by epithelial ovarian neoplasms. *Gynecol Oncol.* 1983;16:78-84.
415. Donato R. S100: A multigenic family of calcium-modulated proteins of the EF-hand type with intracellular and extracellular functional roles. *Int J Biochem Cell Biol.* 2001;33:637-668.
416. Donato R. Intracellular and extracellular roles of S100 proteins. *Microsc Res Tech.* 2003;60:540-551.
417. Heizmann CW, Fritz G, Schafer BW. S100 proteins: Structure, functions and pathology. *Front Biosci.* 2002;7:d1356-d1368.
418. Gupta D, Deavers MT, Silva EG, et al. Malignant melanoma involving the ovary: A clinicopathologic and immunohistochemical study of 23 cases. *Am J Surg Pathol.* 2004;28:771-780.
419. Drier JK, Swanson PE, Cherwitz DL, et al. S100 protein immunoreactivity in poorly differentiated carcinomas. Immunohistochemical comparison with malignant melanoma. *Arch Pathol Lab Med.* 1987;111:447-452.
420. Herrera GA, Turbat-Herrera EA, Lott RL. S-100 protein expression by primary and metastatic adenocarcinomas. *Am J Clin Pathol.* 1988;89:168-176.
421. Costa MJ, DeRose PB, Roth LM, et al. Immunohistochemical phenotype of ovarian granulosa cell tumors: Absence of epithelial membrane antigen has diagnostic value. *Hum Pathol.* 1994;25:60-66.
422. Oliva E, Alvarez T, Young RH. Sertoli cell tumors of the ovary: A clinicopathologic and immunohistochemical study of 54 cases. *Am J Surg Pathol.* 2005;29:143-156.
423. Jungbluth AA, Busam KJ, Gerald WL, et al. A103—An anti-Melan-A monoclonal antibody for the detection of malignant melanoma in paraffin-embedded tissues. *Am J Surg Pathol.* 1998;22:595-602.
424. Bacchi CE, Bonetti F, Pea M, et al. HMB-45: A review. *Appl Immunohistochem.* 1996;4:73-85.
425. Gown AM, Vogel AM, Hoak D, et al. Monoclonal antibodies specific for melanocytic tumors distinguish subpopulations of melanocytes. *Am J Pathol.* 1986;123:195-203.
426. Wick MR, Swanson PE, Rocamora A. Recognition of malignant melanoma by monoclonal antibody HMB-45. An immunohistochemical study of 200 paraffin-embedded cutaneous tumors. *J Cutan Pathol.* 1988;15:201-207.
427. Hoon V, Thung SN, Kaneko M, et al. HMB-45 reactivity in renal angiomyolipoma and lymphangioleiomyomatosis. *Arch Pathol Lab Med.* 1994;118:732-734.
428. Gyure KA, Hart WR, Kennedy AW. Lymphangiomyomatosis of the uterus associated with tuberous sclerosis and malignant neoplasia of the female genital tract: A report of two cases. *Int J Gynecol Pathol.* 1995;14:344-351.
429. Longacre TA, Hendrickson MR, Kapp DS, et al. Lymphangioleiomyomatosis of the uterus simulating high-stage endometrial stromal sarcoma. *Gynecol Oncol.* 1996;63:404-410.
430. Anderson AE, Yang X, Young RH. Epithelioid angiomyolipoma of the ovary: A case report and literature review. *Int J Gynecol Pathol.* 2002;21:69-73.
431. Makhlouf HR, Ishak KG, Shekar R, et al. Melanoma markers in angiomyolipoma of the liver and kidney—A comparative study. *Arch Pathol Lab Med.* 2002;126:49-55.
432. Stone CH, Lee MW, Amin MB, et al. Renal angiomyolipoma—Further immunophenotypic characterization of an expanding morphologic spectrum. *Arch Pathol Lab Med.* 2001;125:751-758.
433. Matsui K, Tatsuguchi A, Valencia J, et al. Extrapulmonary lymphangioleiomyomatosis (LAM): Clinicopathologic features in 22 cases. *Hum Pathol.* 2000;31:1242-1248.
434. Busam KJ, Iversen K, Coplan KA, et al. Immunoreactivity for A103, an antibody to Melan-A (MART-1), in adrenocortical and other steroid tumors. *Am J Surg Pathol.* 1998;22:57-63.
435. Deavers MT, Malpica A, Ordonez NG, et al. Ovarian steroid cell tumors: An immunohistochemical study including a comparison of calretinin with inhibin. *Int J Gynecol Pathol.* 2003;22:162-167.

436. Weiss LM, Chang KL. CD 45: A review. *Appl Immunohistochem*. 1993;1:166-181.
437. Hanselaar AG, Vooijs GP, Mayall B, et al. Epithelial markers to detect occult microinvasion in serous ovarian tumors. *Int J Gynecol Pathol*. 1993;12:20-27.
438. Halperin R, Zehavi S, Hadas E, et al. Immunohistochemical comparison of primary peritoneal and primary ovarian serous papillary carcinoma. *Int J Gynecol Pathol*. 2001;20:341-345.
439. Geisler JP, Geisler HE, Wiemann MC, et al. Quantification of p53 in epithelial ovarian cancer. *Gynecol Oncol*. 1997;66:435-438.
440. Köbel M, Kalloger SE, Carrick J, et al. A limited panel of immunomarkers can reliably distinguish between clear cell and high-grade serous carcinoma of the ovary. *Am J Surg Pathol*. 2009;33:14-21.
441. O'Neill CJ, Deavers MT, Malpica A, et al. An immunohistochemical comparison between low-grade and high-grade ovarian serous carcinomas: Significantly higher expression of p53, MIB1, BCL2, HER-2/neu, and C-KIT in high-grade neoplasms. *Am J Surg Pathol*. 2005;29:1034-1041.
442. Hashi A, Yuminamochi T, Murata S, et al. Wilms tumor gene immunoreactivity in primary serous carcinomas of the fallopian tube, ovary, endometrium, and peritoneum. *Int J Gynecol Pathol*. 2003;22:374-377.
443. Al Hussaini M, Stockman A, Foster H, et al. WT-1 assists in distinguishing ovarian from uterine serous carcinoma and in distinguishing between serous and endometrioid ovarian carcinoma. *Histopathology*. 2004;44:109-115.
444. Waldstrom M, Grove A. Immunohistochemical expression of wilms tumor gene protein in different histologic subtypes of ovarian carcinomas. *Arch Pathol Lab Med*. 2005;129:85-88.
445. Tong GX, Chiriboga L, Hamele-Bena D, et al. Expression of PAX2 in papillary serous carcinoma of the ovary: Immunohistochemical evidence of fallopian tube or secondary Müllerian system origin? *Mod Pathol*. 2007;20:856-863.
446. Nonaka D, Chiriboga L, Soslow RA. Expression of pax8 as a useful marker in distinguishing ovarian carcinomas from mammary carcinomas. *Am J Surg Pathol*. 2008;32:1566-1571.
447. Lin X, Lindner JL, Silverman JF, et al. Intestinal type and endocervical-like ovarian mucinous neoplasms are immunophenotypically distinct entities. *Appl Immunohistochem Mol Morphol*. 2008;16:453-458.
448. Vang R, Gown AM, Barry TS, et al. Cytokeratins 7 and 20 in primary and secondary mucinous tumors of the ovary: Analysis of coordinate immunohistochemical expression profiles and staining distribution in 179 cases. *Am J Surg Pathol*. 2006;30:1130-1139.
449. Werling RW, Yaziji H, Bacchi CE, et al. CDX2, a highly sensitive and specific marker of adenocarcinomas of intestinal origin: An immunohistochemical survey of 476 primary and metastatic carcinomas. *Am J Surg Pathol*. 2003;27:303-310.
450. Moskaluk CA, Zhang H, Powell SM, et al. Cdx2 protein expression in normal and malignant human tissues: An immunohistochemical survey using tissue microarrays. *Mod Pathol*. 2003;16:913-919.
451. Groisman GM, Meir A, Sabo E. The value of Cdx2 immunostaining in differentiating primary ovarian carcinomas from colonic carcinomas metastatic to the ovaries. *Int J Gynecol Pathol*. 2004;23:52-57.
452. Tornillo L, Moch H, Diener PA, et al. CDX-2 immunostaining in primary and secondary ovarian carcinomas. *J Clin Pathol*. 2004;57:641-643.
453. Logani S, Oliva E, Arnell PM, et al. Use of novel immunohistochemical markers expressed in colonic adenocarcinoma to distinguish primary ovarian tumors from metastatic colorectal carcinoma. *Mod Pathol*. 2005;18:19-25.
454. Vang R, Gown AM, Wu LS, et al. Immunohistochemical expression of CDX2 in primary ovarian mucinous tumors and metastatic mucinous carcinomas involving the ovary: Comparison with CK20 and correlation with coordinate expression of CK7. *Mod Pathol*. 2006;19:1421-1428.
455. Vang R, Gown AM, Zhao C, et al. Ovarian mucinous tumors associated with mature cystic teratomas: Morphologic and immunohistochemical analysis identifies a subset of potential teratomatous origin that shares features of lower gastrointestinal tract mucinous tumors more commonly encountered as secondary tumors in the ovary. *Am J Surg Pathol*. 2007;31:854-869.
456. Zhang PJ, Shah M, Spiegel GW, et al. Cytokeratin 7 immunoreactivity in rectal adenocarcinomas. *Appl Immunohistochem Mol Morphol*. 2003;11:306-310.
457. Rutgers JL, Bell DA. Immunohistochemical characterization of ovarian borderline tumors of intestinal and mullerian types. *Mod Pathol*. 1992;5:367-371.
458. Vang R, Gown AM, Barry TS, et al. Immunohistochemistry for estrogen and progesterone receptors in the distinction of primary and metastatic mucinous tumors in the ovary: An analysis of 124 cases. *Mod Pathol*. 2006;19:97-105.
459. Ronnett BM, Shmookler BM, Diener-West M, et al. Immunohistochemical evidence supporting the appendiceal origin of pseudomyxoma peritonei in women. *Int J Gynecol Pathol*. 1997;16:1-9.
460. O'Connell JT, Tomlinson JS, Roberts AA, et al. Pseudomyxoma peritonei is a disease of MUC2-expressing goblet cells. *Am J Pathol*. 2002;161:551-564.
461. Prat J, Young RH, Scully RE. Ovarian mucinous tumors with foci of anaplastic carcinoma. *Cancer*. 1982;50:300-304.
462. Provenza C, Young RH, Prat J. Anaplastic carcinoma in mucinous ovarian tumors: A clinicopathologic study of 34 cases emphasizing the crucial impact of stage on prognosis, their histologic spectrum, and overlap with sarcomalike mural nodules. *Am J Surg Pathol*. 2008;32:383-389.
463. Prat J, Scully RE. Sarcomas in ovarian mucinous tumors. A report of two cases. *Cancer*. 1979;44:1327-1331.
464. Prat J, Scully RE. Ovarian mucinous tumors with sarcoma-like mural nodules. A report of seven cases. *Cancer*. 1979;44:1332-1344.
465. Bague S, Rodriguez IM, Prat J. Sarcoma-like mural nodules in mucinous cystic tumors of the ovary revisited—A clinicopathologic analysis of 10 additional cases. *Am J Surg Pathol*. 2002;26:1467-1476.
466. Nichols GE, Mills SE, Ulbright TM, et al. Spindle cell mural nodules in cystic ovarian mucinous tumors: A clinicopathologic and immunohistochemical study of five cases. *Am J Surg Pathol*. 1991;15:1055-1062.
467. Chan YF, Ho HC, Yau SM, et al. Ovarian mucinous tumor with mural nodules of anaplastic carcinoma. *Gynecol Oncol*. 1989;35:112-119.
468. Baergen RN, Rutgers JL. Mural nodules in common epithelial tumors of the ovary. *Int J Gynecol Pathol*. 1994;13:62-71.
469. Matias-Guiu X, Aranda I, Prat J. Immunohistochemical study of sarcoma-like mural nodules in a mucinous cystadenocarcinoma of the ovary. *Virchows Arch A Pathol Anat Histopathol*. 1991;419:89-92.
470. Lee KR, Nucci MR. Ovarian mucinous and mixed epithelial carcinomas of mullerian (endocervical-like) type: A clinicopathologic analysis of four cases of an uncommon variant associated with endometriosis. *Int J Gynecol Pathol*. 2003;22:42-51.
471. Sarrio D, Moreno-Bueno G, Sanchez-Estevez C, et al. Expression of cadherins and catenins correlates with distinct histologic types of ovarian carcinomas. *Hum Pathol*. 2006;37:1042-1049.
472. Oliva E, Sarrio D, Brachtel EF, et al. High frequency of beta-catenin mutations in borderline endometrioid tumours of the ovary. *J Pathol*. 2006;208:708-713.
473. Houghton O, Connolly LE, McCluggage WG. Morules in endometrioid proliferations of the uterus and ovary consistently express the intestinal transcription factor CDX2. *Histopathology*. 2008;53:156-165.
474. Ordi J, Schammel DP, Rasekh L, et al. Sertoliform endometrioid carcinomas of the ovary: A clinicopathologic and immunohistochemical study of 13 cases. *Mod Pathol*. 1999;12:933-940.
475. Misir A, Sur M. Sertoliform endometrioid carcinoma of the ovary: A potential diagnostic pitfall. *Arch Pathol Lab Med*. 2007;131:979-981.
476. Elishaev E, Gilks CB, Miller D, et al. Synchronous and metachronous endocervical and ovarian neoplasms: Evidence supporting interpretation of the ovarian neoplasms as metastatic endocervical adenocarcinomas simulating primary ovarian surface epithelial neoplasms. *Am J Surg Pathol*. 2005;29:281-294.
477. Vang R, Gown AM, Farinola M, et al. p16 expression in primary ovarian mucinous and endometrioid tumors and metastatic adenocarcinomas in the ovary: Utility for identification of metastatic HPV-related endocervical adenocarcinomas. *Am J Surg Pathol*. 2007;31:653-663.

478. Wentzensen N, du Bois AD, Kommoss S, et al. No metastatic cervical adenocarcinomas in a series of p16INK4a-positive mucinous or endometrioid advanced ovarian carcinomas: An analysis of the AGO Ovarian Cancer Study Group. *Int J Gynecol Pathol.* 2008;27:18-23.
479. Dellers EA, Valente PT, Edmonds PR, et al. Extrauterine mixed mesodermal tumors: An immunohistochemical study. *Arch Pathol Lab Med.* 1991;115:918-920.
480. De Brito PA, Silverberg SG, Orenstein JM. Carcinosarcoma (malignant mixed Müllerian (mesodermal) tumor) of the female genital tract: Immunohistochemical and ultrastructural analysis of 28 cases. *Hum Pathol.* 1993;24:132-142.
481. Chang KL, Crabtree GS, Lim-Tan SK, et al. Primary extrauterine endometrial stromal neoplasms: A clinicopathologic study of 20 cases and a review of the literature. *Int J Gynecol Pathol.* 1993;12:282-296.
482. Cameron RI, Ashe P, O'Rourke DM, et al. A panel of immunohistochemical stains assists in the distinction between ovarian and renal clear cell carcinoma. *Int J Gynecol Pathol.* 2003;22:272-276.
483. Kato N, Sasou S, Motoyama T. Expression of hepatocyte nuclear factor-1beta (HNF-1beta) in clear cell tumors and endometriosis of the ovary. *Mod Pathol.* 2006;19:83-89.
484. Kato N, Motoyama T. Overexpression of osteopontin in clear cell carcinoma of the ovary: Close association with HNF-1beta expression. *Histopathology.* 2008;52:682-688.
485. Ho ES, Lai CR, Hsieh YT, et al. p53 mutation is infrequent in clear cell carcinoma of the ovary. *Gynecol Oncol.* 2001;80:189-193.
486. Shimizu M, Nikaido T, Toki T, et al. Clear cell carcinoma has an expression pattern of cell cycle regulatory molecules that is unique among ovarian adenocarcinomas. *Cancer.* 1999;85:669-677.
487. Kwon TJ, Ro JY, Tornos C, et al. Reduplicated basal lamina in clear-cell carcinoma of the ovary: An immunohistochemical and electron microscopic study. *Ultrastruct Pathol.* 1996; 20:529-536.
488. Mikami Y, Hata S, Melamed J, et al. Basement membrane material in ovarian clear cell carcinoma: Correlation with growth pattern and nuclear grade. *Int J Gynecol Pathol.* 1999; 18:52-57.
489. Nolan LP, Heatley MK. The value of immunocytochemistry in distinguishing between clear cell carcinoma of the kidney and ovary. *Int J Gynecol Pathol.* 2001;20:155-159.
490. Ordonez NG, Mackay B. Brenner tumor of the ovary: A comparative immunohistochemical and ultrastructural study with transitional cell carcinoma of the bladder. *Ultrastruct Pathol.* 2000;24:157-167.
491. Riedel I, Czernobilsky B, Lifschitz-Mercer B, et al. Brenner tumors but not transitional cell carcinomas of the ovary show urothelial differentiation: Immunohistochemical staining of urothelial markers, including cytokeratins and uroplakins. *Virchows Arch Int J Pathol.* 2001;438:181-191.
492. Soslow RA, Rouse RV, Hendrickson MR, et al. Transitional cell neoplasms of the ovary and urinary bladder: A comparative immunohistochemical analysis. *Int J Gynecol Pathol.* 1996;15:257-265.
493. Kaufmann O, Volmerig J, Dietel M. Uroplakin III is a highly specific and moderately sensitive immunohistochemical marker for primary and metastatic urothelial carcinomas. *Am J Clin Pathol.* 2000;113:683-687.
494. Ogawa K, Johansson SL, Cohen SM. Immunohistochemical analysis of uroplakins, urothelial specific proteins, in ovarian Brenner tumors, normal tissues, and benign and neoplastic lesions of the female genital tract. *Am J Pathol.* 1999; 155:1047-1050.
495. Liao XY, Xue WC, Shen DH, et al. p63 expression in ovarian tumours: A marker for Brenner tumours but not transitional cell carcinomas. *Histopathology.* 2007;51:477-483.
496. Ordonez NG. Transitional cell carcinomas of the ovary and bladder are immunophenotypically different. *Histopathology.* 2000;36:433-438.
497. Ordonez NG. Application of mesothelin immunostaining in tumor diagnosis. *Am J Surg Pathol.* 2003;27:1418-1428.
498. Ohishi Y, Kaku T, Oya M, et al. CD56 expression in ovarian granulosa cell tumors, and its diagnostic utility and pitfalls. *Gynecol Oncol.* 2007;107:30-38.
499. McCluggage WG, McKenna M, McBride HA. CD56 is a sensitive and diagnostically useful immunohistochemical marker of ovarian sex cord-stromal tumors. *Int J Gynecol Pathol.* 2007;26:322-327.
500. Riopel MA, Perlman EJ, Seidman JD, et al. Inhibin and epithelial membrane antigen immunohistochemistry assist in the diagnosis of sex cord-stromal tumors and provide clues to the histogenesis of hypercalcemic small cell carcinomas. *Int J Gynecol Pathol.* 1998;17:46-53.
501. Young RH, Oliva E, Scully RE. Small cell carcinoma of the ovary, hypercalcemic type: A clinicopathological analysis of 150 cases. *Am J Surg Pathol.* 1994;18:1102-1116.
502. Aguirre P, Thor AD, Scully RE. Ovarian small cell carcinoma. Histogenetic considerations based on immunohistochemical and other findings. *Am J Clin Pathol.* 1989;92:140-149.
503. Young RH, Scully RE. Malignant melanoma metastatic to the ovary: A clinicopathologic analysis of 20 cases. *Am J Surg Pathol.* 1991;15:849-860.
504. McCluggage WG, Bissonnette JP, Young RH. Primary malignant melanoma of the ovary: A report of 9 definite or probable cases with emphasis on their morphologic diversity and mimicry of other primary and secondary ovarian neoplasms. *Int J Gynecol Pathol.* 2006;25:321-329.
505. Young RH, Eichhorn JH, Dickersin GR, et al. Ovarian involvement by the intra-abdominal desmoplastic small round cell tumor with divergent differentiation: A report of three cases. *Hum Pathol.* 1992;23:454-464.
506. Zaloudek C, Miller TR, Stern JL. Desmoplastic small cell tumor of the ovary: A unique polyphenotypic tumor with an unfavorable prognosis. *Int J Gynecol Pathol.* 1995;14:260-265.
507. Fang X, Rodabaugh K, Penetrante R, et al. Desmoplastic small round cell tumor (DSRCT) with ovarian involvement in 2 young women. *Appl Immunohistochem Mol Morphol.* 2008;16:94-99.
508. Kawauchi S, Fukuda T, Miyamoto S, et al. Peripheral primitive neuroectodermal tumor of the ovary confirmed by CD99 immunostaining, karyotypic analysis, and RT-PCR for EWS/FLI-1 chimeric mRNA. *Am J Surg Pathol.* 1998;22:1417-1422.
509. Young RH, Scully RE. Alveolar rhabdomyosarcoma metastatic to the ovary. A report of two cases and a discussion of the differential diagnosis of small cell malignant tumors of the ovary. *Cancer.* 1989;64:899-904.
510. Nielsen GP, Oliva E, Young RH, et al. Primary ovarian rhabdomyosarcoma: A report of 13 cases. *Int J Gynecol Pathol.* 1998;17:113-119.
511. Paler RJ, Felix JC. Desmin, myoglobin, and muscle-specific actin immunohistochemical staining in a case of embryonal rhabdomyosarcoma of the ovary. *Appl Immunohistochem Mol Morphol.* 1999;7:237-241.
512. Katsube Y, Berg JW, Silverberg SG. Epidemiologic pathology of ovarian tumors: A histopathologic review of primary ovarian neoplasms diagnosed in the Denver Standard Metropolitan Statistical Area, 1 July-31 December 1969 and 1 July-31 December 1979. *Int J Gynecol Pathol.* 1982;1:3-16.
513. Koonings PP, Campbell K, Mishell Jr DR, et al. Relative frequency of primary ovarian neoplasms: A 10-year review. *Obstet Gynecol.* 1989;74:921-926.
514. Stewart CJR, Jeffers MD, Kennedy A. Diagnostic value of inhibin immunoreactivity in ovarian gonadal stromal tumours and their histological mimics. *Histopathology.* 1997;31:67-74.
515. Oliva E, Garcia-Miralles N, Vu Q, et al. CD10 expression in pure stromal and sex cord-stromal tumors of the ovary: An immunohistochemical analysis of 101 cases. *Int J Gynecol Pathol.* 2007;26:359-367.
516. Zhao C, Vinh TN, McManus K, et al. Identification of the most sensitive and robust immunohistochemical markers in different categories of ovarian sex cord-stromal tumors. *Am J Surg Pathol.* 2009;33:354-366.
517. He H, Luthringer DJ, Hui P, et al. Expression of CD56 and WT1 in ovarian stroma and ovarian stromal tumors. *Am J Surg Pathol.* 2008;32:884-890.
518. Tiltman AJ, Haffajee Z. Sclerosing stromal tumors, thecomas, and fibromas of the ovary: An immunohistochemical profile. *Int J Gynecol Pathol.* 1999;18:254-258.
519. Chalvardjian A, Scully RE. Sclerosing stromal tumors of the ovary. *Cancer.* 1973;31:664-670.

520. Kawauchi S, Tsuji T, Kaku T, et al. Sclerosing stromal tumor of the ovary. A clinicopathologic, immunohistochemical, ultrastructural, and cytogenetic analysis with special reference to its vasculature. *Am J Surg Pathol.* 1998;22:83-92.
521. Sabah M, Leader M, Kay E. The problem with KIT: Clinical implications and practical difficulties with CD117 immunostaining. *Appl Immunohistochem Mol Morphol.* 2003;11:56-61.
522. Saitoh A, Tsutsumi Y, Osamura RY, et al. Sclerosing stromal tumor of the ovary. Immunohistochemical and electron microscopic demonstration of smooth-muscle differentiation. *Arch Pathol Lab Med.* 1989;113:372-376.
523. Shaw JA, Dabbs DJ, Geisinger KR. Sclerosing stromal tumor of the ovary: An ultrastructural and immunohistochemical analysis with histogenetic considerations. *Ultrastruct Pathol.* 1992;16:363-377.
524. Ishioka S, Sagae S, Saito T, et al. A case of a sclerosing stromal ovarian tumor that expresses VEGF. *J Obstet Gynaecol Res.* 2000;26:35-38.
525. Fox H. Pathologic prognostic factors in early stage adult-type granulosa cell tumors of the ovary. *Int J Gynecol Cancer.* 2003;13:1-4.
526. Schumer ST, Cannistra SA. Granulosa cell tumor of the ovary. *J Clin Oncol.* 2003;21:1180-1189.
527. Hines JF, Khalifa MA, Moore JL, et al. Recurrent granulosa cell tumor of the ovary 37 years after initial diagnosis: A case report and review of the literature. *Gynecol Oncol.* 1996; 60:484-488.
528. Shah VI, Freites NO, Maxwell P, et al. Inhibin is more specific than calretinin as an immunohistochemical marker for differentiating sarcomatoid granulosa cell tumour of the ovary from other spindle cell neoplasms. *J Clin Pathol.* 2003; 56:221-224.
529. Gitsch G, Kohlberger P, Steiner A, et al. Expression of cytokeratins in granulosa cell tumors and ovarian carcinomas. *Arch Gynecol Obstet.* 1992;251:193-197.
530. Otis CN, Powell JL, Barbuto D, et al. Intermediate filamentous proteins in adult granulosa cell tumors: An immunohistochemical study of 25 cases. *Am J Surg Pathol.* 1992;16:962-968.
531. Choi YL, Kim HS, Ahn G. Immunoexpression of inhibin alpha subunit, inhibin/activin betaA subunit and CD99 in ovarian tumors. *Arch Pathol Lab Med.* 2000;124:563-569.
532. Gordon MD, Corless C, Renshaw AA, et al. CD99, keratin, and vimentin staining of sex cord-stromal tumors, normal ovary, and testis. *Mod Pathol.* 1998;11:769-773.
533. Cathro HP, Stoler MH. The utility of calretinin, inhibin, and WT1 immunohistochemical staining in the differential diagnosis of ovarian tumors. *Hum Pathol.* 2005;36:195-201.
534. Farinola MA, Gown AM, Judson K, et al. Estrogen receptor alpha and progesterone receptor expression in ovarian adult granulosa cell tumors and Sertoli-Leydig cell tumors. *Int J Gynecol Pathol.* 2007;26:375-382.
535. Young RH, Dickersin GR, Scully RE. Juvenile granulosa cell tumor of the ovary. A clinicopathological analysis of 125 cases. *Am J Surg Pathol.* 1984;8:575-596.
536. Zaloudek CJ, Norris HJ. Granulosa tumors of the ovary in children: A clinical and pathologic study of 32 cases. *Am J Surg Pathol.* 1982;6:503-512.
537. Rakheja D, Sharma S. Pathologic quiz case—Cystic and solid ovarian tumor in a 43-year-old woman—Pathologic diagnosis: Cystic juvenile-type granulosa cell tumor of the ovary in an adult. *Arch Pathol Lab Med.* 2002;126:1123-1124.
538. McCluggage WG. Immunoreactivity of ovarian juvenile granulosa cell tumours with epithelial membrane antigen. *Histopathology.* 2005;46:235-236.
539. Young RH. Sertoli-Leydig cell tumors of the ovary: Review with emphasis on historical aspects and unusual forms. *Int J Gynecol Pathol.* 1993;12:141-147.
540. Zaloudek C, Norris HJ. Sertoli-Leydig tumors of the ovary. A clinicopatholgic study of 64 intermediate and poorly differentiated neoplasms. *Am J Surg Pathol.* 1984;8:405-418.
541. Young RH, Scully RE. Well-differentiated ovarian Sertoli-Leydig cell tumors: A clinicopathological analysis of 23 tumors. *Int J Gynecol Pathol.* 1984;3:277-290.
542. Young RH, Scully RE. Ovarian Sertoli-Leydig cell tumors. A clinicopathological analysis of 207 cases. *Am J Surg Pathol.* 1985;9:543-569.
543. Young RH, Scully RE. Ovarian Sertoli-Leydig cell tumors with a retiform pattern—A problem in diagnosis: A report of 25 cases. *Am J Surg Pathol.* 1983;7:755-771.
544. Mooney EE, Nogales FF, Bergeron C, et al. Retiform Sertoli-Leydig cell tumours: Clinical, morphological and immunohistochemical findings. *Histopathology.* 2002;41:110-117.
545. Guerrieri C, Franlund B, Malmstrom H, et al. Ovarian endometrioid carcinomas simulating sex cord-stromal tumors: A study using inhibin and cytokeratin 7. *Int J Gynecol Pathol.* 1998;17:266-271.
546. McCluggage WG, Young RH. Ovarian sertoli-leydig cell tumors with pseudoendometrioid tubules (pseudoendometrioid sertoli-leydig cell tumors). *Am J Surg Pathol.* 2007;31:592-597.
547. Young RH, Prat J, Scully RE. Ovarian Sertoli-Leydig cell tumors with heterologous elements. I. Gastrointestinal epithelium and carcinoid: A clinicopathologic analysis of 36 cases. *Cancer.* 1982;50:2448-2456.
548. Aguirre P, Scully RE, DeLellis RA. Ovarian heterologous Sertoli-Leydig cell tumors with gastrointestinal-type epithelium. An immunohistochemical analysis. *Arch Pathol Lab Med.* 1986;110:528-533.
549. Prat J, Young RH, Scully RE. Ovarian Sertoli-Leydig cell tumors with heterologous elements. II. Cartilage and skeletal muscle. A clinicopathologic analysis of twelve cases. *Cancer.* 1982;50:2465-2475.
550. Roth LM, Liban E, Czernobilsky B. Ovarian endometrioid tumors mimicking Sertoli and Sertoli-Leydig cell tumors: Sertoliform variant of endometrioid carcinoma. *Cancer.* 1982;50:1322-1331.
551. McCluggage WG, Young RH. Ovarian sertoli-leydig cell tumors with pseudoendometrioid tubules (pseudoendometrioid sertoli-leydig cell tumors). *Am J Surg Pathol.* 2007;31:592-597.
552. Young RH, Scully RE. Ovarian Sertoli cell tumors. A report of 10 cases. *Int J Gynecol Pathol.* 1984;2:349-363.
553. Ferry JA, Young RH, Engel G, et al. Oxyphilic Sertoli cell tumor of the ovary: A report of three cases, two in patients with the Peutz-Jeghers syndrome. *Int J Gynecol Pathol.* 1994;13:259-266.
554. Aguirre P, Thor AD, Scully RE. Ovarian endometrioid carcinomas resembling sex cord-stromal tumors. An immunohistochemical study. *Int J Gynecol Pathol.* 1989;8:364-373.
555. Young RH, Prat J, Scully RE. Ovarian endometrioid carcinomas resembling sex cord-stromal tumors. A clinicopathologic analysis of 13 cases. *Am J Surg Pathol.* 1982;6:513-522.
556. Benjamin E, Law S, Bobrow LG. Intermediate filaments cytokeratin and vimentin in ovarian sex cord-stromal tumours with correlative studies in adult and fetal ovaries. *J Pathol.* 1987;152:253-263.
557. Stewart GJR, Nandini CL, Richmond JA. Value of A103 (melan-A) immunostaining in the differential diagnosis of ovarian sex cord stromal tumours. *J Clin Pathol.* 2000;53:206-211.
558. Seidman JD, Abbondanzo SL, Bratthauer GL. Lipid cell (steroid cell) tumor of the ovary: Immunophenotype with analysis of potential pitfall due to endogenous biotin-like activity. *Int J Gynecol Pathol.* 1995;14:331-338.
559. Lau SK, Weiss LM, Chu PG. D2-40 immunohistochemistry in the differential diagnosis of seminoma and embryonal carcinoma: A comparative immunohistochemical study with KIT (CD117) and CD30. *Mod Pathol.* 2007;20:320-325.
560. Cossu-Rocca P, Jones TD, Roth LM, et al. Cytokeratin and CD30 expression in dysgerminoma. *Hum Pathol.* 2006;37: 1015-1021.
561. McCluggage WG, Ashe P, McBride H, et al. Localization of the cellular expression of inhibin in trophoblastic tissue. *Histopathology.* 1998;32:252-256.
562. Pelkey TJ, Frierson HFJ, Mills SE, et al. Detection of the alpha-subunit of inhibin in trophoblastic neoplasia. *Hum Pathol.* 1999;30:26-31.
563. Oliva E, Musulen E, Prat J, et al. Transitional cell carcinoma of the renal pelvis with symptomatic ovarian metastases. *Int J Surg Pathol.* 1995;2:231-236.
564. Hirabayashi K, Yasuda M, Osamura RY, et al. Ovarian nongestational choriocarcinoma mixed with various epithelial malignancies in association with endometriosis. *Gynecol Oncol.* 2006;102:111-117.

565. Bing Z, Pasha TL, Lal P, et al. Expression of glial cell line-derived neurotropic factor receptor alpha-1 in immature teratomas. *Am J Clin Pathol.* 2008;130:892-896.
566. Nogales FF, Avila IR, Concha A, et al. Immature endodermal teratoma of the ovary: Embryologic correlations and immunohistochemistry. *Hum Pathol.* 1993;24:364-370.
567. Szyfelbein WM, Young RH, Scully RE. Cystic struma ovarii: A frequently unrecognized tumor: A report of 20 cases. *Am J Surg Pathol.* 1994;18:785-788.
568. Szyfelbein WM, Young RH, Scully RE. Struma ovarii simulating ovarian tumors of other types. A report of 30 cases. *Am J Surg Pathol.* 1995;19:21-29.
569. Devaney K, Snyder R, Norris HJ, et al. Proliferative and histologically malignant struma ovarii: A clinicopathologic study of 54 cases. *Int J Gynecol Pathol.* 1993;12:333-343.
570. Sporrong B, Falkmer S, Robboy SJ, et al. Neurohormonal peptides in ovarian carcinoids: An immunohistochemical study of 81 primary carcinoids and of intraovarian metastases from six mid-gut carcinoids. *Cancer.* 1982;49:68-74.
571. Sidhu J, Sánchez RL. Prostatic acid phosphatase in strumal carcinoids of the ovary: An immunohistochemical study. *Cancer.* 1993;72:1673-1678.
572. Stagno PA, Petras RE, Hart WR. Strumal carcinoids of the ovary. An immunohistologic and ultrastructural study. *Arch Pathol Lab Med.* 1987;111:440-446.
573. Snyder RR, Tavassoli FA. Ovarian strumal carcinoid: Immunohistochemical, ultrastructural, and clinicopathologic analysis. *Int J Gynecol Pathol.* 1986;5:187-201.
574. Matsuda K, Maehama T, Kanazawa K. Strumal carcinoid tumor of the ovary: A case exhibiting severe constipation associated with PYY. *Gynecol Oncol.* 2002;87:143-145.
575. Baker PM, Oliva E, Young RH, et al. Ovarian mucinous carcinoids including some with a carcinomatous component—A report of 17 cases. *Am J Surg Pathol.* 2001;25:557-568.
576. Rabban JT, Lerwill MF, McCluggage WG, et al. Primary ovarian carcinoid tumors may express CDX-2: A potential pitfall in distinction from metastatic intestinal carcinoid tumors involving the ovary. *Int J Gynecol Pathol.* 2009;28:41-48.
577. Hussong J, Crussi FG, Chou PM. Gonadoblastoma: Immunohistochemical localization of Müllerian-inhibiting substance, inhibin, WT-1, and p53. *Mod Pathol.* 1997;10:1101-1105.
578. Roth LM, Eglen DE. Gonadoblastoma. Immunohistochemical and ultrastructural observations. *Int J Gynecol Pathol.* 1989;8:72-81.
579. Moore RG, Chung M, Granai CO, et al. Incidence of metastasis to the ovaries from nongenital tract primary tumors. *Gynecol Oncol.* 2004;93:87-91.
580. Seidman JD, Kurman RJ, Ronnett BM. Primary and metastatic mucinous adenocarcinomas in the ovaries: Incidence in routine practice with a new approach to improve intraoperative diagnosis. *Am J Surg Pathol.* 2003;27:985-993.
581. Yemelyanova AV, Vang R, Judson K, et al. Distinction of primary and metastatic mucinous tumors involving the ovary: Analysis of size and laterality data by primary site with reevaluation of an algorithm for tumor classification. *Am J Surg Pathol.* 2008;32:128-138.
582. Lewis MR, Deavers MT, Silva EG, et al. Ovarian involvement by metastatic colorectal adenocarcinoma: Still a diagnostic challenge. *Am J Surg Pathol.* 2006;30:177-184.
583. Ronnett BM, Kurman RJ, Shmookler BM, et al. The morphologic spectrum of ovarian metastases of appendiceal adenocarcinomas—A clinicopathologic and immunohistochemical analysis of tumors often misinterpreted as primary ovarian tumors or metastatic tumors from other gastrointestinal sites. *Am J Surg Pathol.* 1997;21:1144-1155.
584. Khunamornpong S, Siriaunkgul S, Suprasert P, et al. Intrahepatic cholangiocarcinoma metastatic to the ovary: A report of 16 cases of an underemphasized form of secondary tumor in the ovary that may mimic primary neoplasia. *Am J Surg Pathol.* 2007;31:1788-1799.
585. Khunamornpong S, Lerwill MF, Siriaunkgul S, et al. Carcinoma of extrahepatic bile ducts and gallbladder metastatic to the ovary: A report of 16 cases. *Int J Gynecol Pathol.* 2008; 27:366-379.
586. Park SY, Kim HS, Hong EK, et al. Expression of cytokeratins 7 and 20 in primary carcinomas of the stomach and colorectum and their value in the differential diagnosis of metastatic carcinomas to the ovary. *Hum Pathol.* 2002;33:1078-1085.
587. Lerwill MF, Young RH. Ovarian metastases of intestinal-type gastric carcinoma: A clinicopathologic study of 4 cases with contrasting features to those of the Krukenberg tumor. *Am J Surg Pathol.* 2006;30:1382-1388.
588. McCluggage WG, Young RH. Primary ovarian mucinous tumors with signet ring cells: Report of 3 cases with discussion of so-called primary Krukenberg tumor. *Am J Surg Pathol.* 2008;32:1373-1379.
589. Reichert RA. Primary ovarian adenofibromatous neoplasms with mucin-containing signet-ring cells: A report of 2 cases. *Int J Gynecol Pathol.* 2007;26:165-172.
590. Kiyokawa T, Young RH, Scully RE. Krukenberg tumors of the ovary: A clinicopathologic analysis of 120 cases with emphasis on their variable pathologic manifestations. *Am J Surg Pathol.* 2006;30:277-299.
591. Young RH, Hart WR. Metastatic intestinal carcinomas simulating primary ovarian clear cell carcinoma and secretory endometrioid carcinoma—A clinicopathologic and immunohistochemical study of five cases. *Am J Surg Pathol.* 1998;22:805-815.
592. Vakiani E, Young RH, Carcangiu ML, et al. Acinar cell carcinoma of the pancreas metastatic to the ovary: A report of 4 cases. *Am J Surg Pathol.* 2008;32:1540-1545.
593. Gagnon Y, Tëtu B. Ovarian metastases of breast carcinoma. A clinicopathologic study of 59 cases. *Cancer.* 1989;64:892-898.
594. Young RH, Carey RW, Robboy SJ. Breast carcinoma masquerading as primary ovarian neoplasm. *Cancer.* 1981;48:210-212.
595. Moritani S, Ichihara S, Hasegawa M, et al. Serous papillary adenocarcinoma of the female genital organs and invasive micropapillary carcinoma of the breast. Are WT1, CA125, and GCDFP-15 useful in differential diagnosis? *Hum Pathol.* 2008;39:666-671.
596. Monteagudo C, Merino MJ, LaPorte N, et al. Value of gross cystic disease fluid protein-15 in distinguishing metastatic breast carcinomas among poorly differentiated neoplasms involving the ovary. *Hum Pathol.* 1991;22:368-372.
597. Kanner WA, Galgano MT, Stoler MH, et al. Distinguishing breast carcinoma from Müllerian serous carcinoma with mammaglobin and mesothelin. *Int J Gynecol Pathol.* 2008;27:491-495.
598. Lau SK, Luthringer DJ, Eisen RN. Thyroid transcription factor-1: A review. *Appl Immunohistochem Mol Morphol.* 2002;10:97-102.
599. Howell NR, Zheng W, Cheng L, et al. Carcinomas of ovary and lung with clear cell features: can immunohistochemistry help in differential diagnosis? *Int J Gynecol Pathol.* 2007; 26:134-140.
600. Irving JA, Young RH. Lung Carcinoma Metastatic to the Ovary: A clinicopathologic study of 32 cases emphasizing their morphologic spectrum and problems in differential diagnosis. *Am J Surg Pathol.* 2005;29:997-1006.
601. Kaufmann O, Dietel M. Expression of thyroid transcription factor-1 in pulmonary and extrapulmonary small cell carcinomas and other neuroendocrine carcinomas of various primary sites. *Histopathology.* 2000;36:415-420.
602. Ordonez NG. Value of thyroid transcription factor-1 immunostaining in distinguishing small cell lung carcinomas from other small cell carcinomas. *Am J Surg Pathol.* 2000;24:1217-1223.
603. Cheuk W, Kwan MY, Suster S, et al. Immunostaining for thyroid transcription factor 1 and cytokeratin 20 aids the distinction of small cell carcinoma from Merkel cell carcinoma, but not pulmonary from extrapulmonary small cell carcinomas. *Arch Pathol Lab Med.* 2001;125:228-231.
604. Ronnett BM, Yemelyanova AV, Vang R, et al. Endocervical adenocarcinomas with ovarian metastases: Analysis of 29 cases with emphasis on minimally invasive cervical tumors and the ability of the metastases to simulate primary ovarian neoplasms. *Am J Surg Pathol.* 2008;32:1835-1853.
605. Moran CA, Albores-Saavedra J, Suster S. Primary peritoneal mesotheliomas in children: A clinicopathological and immunohistochemical study of eight cases. *Histopathology.* 2008; 52:824-830.

606. Goldblum J, Hart WR. Localized and diffuse mesotheliomas of the genital tract and peritoneum in women—A clinicopathologic study of nineteen true mesothelial neoplasms, other than adenomatoid tumors, multicystic mesotheliomas, and localized fibrous tumors. *Am J Surg Pathol.* 1995;19:1124-1137.
607. Clement PB, Young RH, Scully RE. Malignant mesotheliomas presenting as ovarian masses—A report of nine cases, including two primary ovarian mesotheliomas. *Am J Surg Pathol.* 1996;20:1067-1080.
608. Kerrigan SAJ, Turnnir RT, Clement PB, et al. Diffuse malignant epithelial mesotheliomas of the peritoneum in women—A clinicopathologic study of 25 patients. *Cancer.* 2002;94:378-385.
609. Baker PM, Clement PB, Young RH. Malignant peritoneal mesothelioma in women: A study of 75 cases with emphasis on their morphologic spectrum and differential diagnosis. *Am J Clin Pathol.* 2005;123:724-737.
610. Nascimento AG, Keeney GL, Fletcher CDM. Deciduoid peritoneal mesothelioma: An unusual phenotype affecting young females. *Am J Surg Pathol.* 1994;18:439-445.
611. Orosz Z, Nagy P, Szentirmay Z, et al. Epithelial mesothelioma with deciduoid features. *Virchows Arch.* 1999;434:263-266.
612. Shanks JH, Harris M, Banerjee SS, et al. Mesotheliomas with deciduoid morphology—A morphologic spectrum and a variant not confined to young females. *Am J Surg Pathol.* 2000;24:285-294.
613. Comin CE, Saieva C, Messerini L. h-caldesmon, calretinin, estrogen receptor, and Ber-EP4: A useful combination of immunohistochemical markers for differentiating epithelioid peritoneal mesothelioma from serous papillary carcinoma of the ovary. *Am J Surg Pathol.* 2007;31:1139-1148.
614. Barnetson RJ, Burnett RA, Downie I, et al. Immunohistochemical analysis of peritoneal mesothelioma and primary and secondary serous carcinoma of the peritoneum: Antibodies to estrogen and progesterone receptors are useful. *Am J Clin Pathol.* 2006;125:67-76.
615. Ordonez NG. Value of estrogen and progesterone receptor immunostaining in distinguishing between peritoneal mesotheliomas and serous carcinomas. *Hum Pathol.* 2005;36:1163-1167.
616. Ordonez NG. Value of immunohistochemistry in distinguishing peritoneal mesothelioma from serous carcinoma of the ovary and peritoneum: A review and update. *Adv Anat Pathol.* 2006;13:16-25.
617. Ordonez NG. The diagnostic utility of immunohistochemistry and electron microscopy in distinguishing between peritoneal mesotheliomas and serous carcinomas: A comparative study. *Mod Pathol.* 2006;19:34-48.
618. Young RH. Neoplasms of the fallopian tube and broad ligament: A selective survey including historical perspective and emphasising recent developments. *Pathology.* 2007;39:112-124.
619. Alvarado-Cabrero I, Young RH, Vamvakas EC, et al. Carcinoma of the fallopian tube: A clinicopathological study of 105 cases with observations on staging and prognostic factors. *Gynecol Oncol.* 1999;72:367-379.
620. Baekelandt M, Nesbakken AJ, Kristensen GB, et al. Carcinoma of the fallopian tube—Clinicopathologic study of 151 patients treated at the Norwegian Radium Hospital. *Cancer.* 2000;89:2076-2084.
621. Piura B, Rabinovich A. Primary carcinoma of the fallopian tube: Study of 11 cases. *Eur J Obstet Gynecol Reprod Biol.* 2000;91:169-175.
622. di Re E, Grosso G, Raspagliesi F, et al. Fallopian tube cancer: Incidence and role of lymphatic spread. *Gynecol Oncol.* 1996;62:199-202.
623. Callahan MJ, Crum CP, Medeiros F, et al. Primary fallopian tube malignancies in BRCA-positive women undergoing surgery for ovarian cancer risk reduction. *J Clin Oncol.* 2007;25:3985-3990.
624. Carcangiu ML, Peissel B, Pasini B, et al. Incidental carcinomas in prophylactic specimens in BRCA1 and BRCA2 germ-line mutation carriers, with emphasis on fallopian tube lesions: Report of 6 cases and review of the literature. *Am J Surg Pathol.* 2006;30:1222-1230.
625. Finch A, Shaw P, Rosen B, et al. Clinical and pathologic findings of prophylactic salpingo-oophorectomies in 159 BRCA1 and BRCA2 carriers. *Gynecol Oncol.* 2006;100:58-64.
626. Medeiros F, Muto MG, Lee Y, et al. The tubal fimbria is a preferred site for early adenocarcinoma in women with familial ovarian cancer syndrome. *Am J Surg Pathol.* 2006;30:230-236.
627. Folkins AK, Jarboe EA, Saleemuddin A, et al. A candidate precursor to pelvic serous cancer (p53 signature) and its prevalence in ovaries and fallopian tubes from women with BRCA mutations. *Gynecol Oncol.* 2008;109:168-173.
628. Jarboe E, Folkins A, Nucci MR, et al. Serous carcinogenesis in the fallopian tube: A descriptive classification. *Int J Gynecol Pathol.* 2008;27:1-9.
629. Kindelberger DW, Lee Y, Miron A, et al. Intraepithelial carcinoma of the fimbria and pelvic serous carcinoma: Evidence for a causal relationship. *Am J Surg Pathol.* 2007;31:161-169.
630. Bannatyne P, Russell P. Early adenocarcinoma of the fallopian tubes. A case for multifocal tumorigenesis. *Diagn Gynecol Obstet.* 1981;3:49-60.
631. Youngs LA, Taylor HB. Adenomatoid tumors of the uterus and fallopian tube. *Am J Clin Pathol.* 1967;48:537-545.
632. Stephenson TJ, Mills PM. Adenomatoid tumours: An immunohistochemical and ultrastructural appraisal of their histogenesis. *J Pathol.* 1986;148:327-335.
633. Salazar H, Kanbour A, Burgess F. Ultrastructure and observations on the histogenesis of mesotheliomas, "adenomatoid tumors," of the female genital tract. *Cancer.* 1972;29:141-152.
634. Mai KT, Yazdi HM, Perkins DG, et al. Adenomatoid tumor of the genital tract: Evidence of mesenchymal cell origin. *Pathol Res Pract.* 1999;195:605-610.
635. Nogales FF, Isaac MA, Hardisson D, et al. Adenomatoid tumors of the uterus: An analysis of 60 cases. *Int J Gynecol Pathol.* 2002;21:34-40.
636. Schwartz EJ, Longacre TA. Adenomatoid tumors of the female and male genital tracts express WT1. *Int J Gynecol Pathol.* 2004;23:123-128.
637. Delahunt B, Eble JN, King D, et al. Immunohistochemical evidence for mesothelial origin of paratesticular adenomatoid tumour. *Histopathology.* 2000;36:109-115.
638. Kariminejad MH, Scully RE. Female adnexal tumor of probable Wolffian origin: A distinctive pathologic entity. *Cancer.* 1973;31:671-677.
639. Young RH, Scully RE. Ovarian tumors of probable Wolffian origin: A report of 11 cases. *Am J Surg Pathol.* 1983;7:125-136.
640. Tavassoli FA, Andrade R, Merino M. Retiform wolffian adenoma. In: Fenoglio-Preiser CM, Wolffe M, Rilke F, eds. *Progress in surgical pathology.* vol. XI. New York: Field and Wood Medical Publishers; 1990:121-136.
641. Daya D, Young RH, Scully RE. Endometrioid carcinoma of the fallopian tube resembling an adnexal tumor of probable Wolffian origin: A report of six cases. *Int J Gynecol Pathol.* 1992;11:122-130.
642. Karpuz V, Berger SD, Burkhardt K, et al. A case of endometrioid carcinoma of the fallopian tube mimicking an adnexal tumor of probable Wolffian origin. *APMIS.* 1999;107:550-554.
643. Fukunaga M, Bisceglia M, Dimitri L. Endometrioid carcinoma of the fallopian tube resembling a female adnexal tumor of probable wolffian origin. *Adv Anat Pathol.* 2004;11:269-272.
644. Devouassoux-Shisheboran M, Silver SA, Tavassoli FA. Wolffian adnexal tumor, so-called female adnexal tumor of probable Wolffian origin (FATWO): Immunohistochemical evidence in support of a Wolffian origin. *Hum Pathol.* 1999;30:856-863.
645. Rahilly MA, Williams ARW, Krausz T, et al. Female adnexal tumour of probable Wolffian origin: A clinicopathological and immunohistochemical study of three cases. *Histopathology.* 1995;26:69-74.
646. Tiltman AJ, Allard U. Female adnexal tumours of probable Wolffian origin: An immunohistochemical study comparing tumours, mesonephric remnants and paramesonephric derivatives. *Histopathology.* 2001;38:237-242.
647. van den Bos M, van den Hoven M, Jongejan E, et al. More differences between HNPCC-related and sporadic carcinomas from the endometrium as compared to the colon. *Am J Surg Pathol.* 2004;28:706-711.
648. Lu KH, Dinh M, Kohlmann W, et al. Gynecologic cancer as a "sentinel cancer" for women with hereditary nonpolyposis colorectal cancer syndrome. *Obstet Gynecol.* 2005;105:569-574.

649. Shannon C, Kirk J, Barnetson R, et al. Incidence of microsatellite instability in synchronous tumors of the ovary and endometrium. *Clin Cancer Res*. 2003;9:1387-1392.
650. Soliman PT, Broaddus RR, Schmeler KM, et al. Women with synchronous primary cancers of the endometrium and ovary: Do they have Lynch syndrome? *J Clin Oncol*. 2005;23:9344-9350.
651. Ziolkowska-Seta I, Madry R, Kraszewska E, et al. TP53, BCL-2 and BAX analysis in 199 ovarian cancer patients treated with taxane-platinum regimens. *Gynecol Oncol*. 2009;112:179-184.
652. Darcy KM, Brady WE, McBroom JW, et al. Associations between p53 overexpression and multiple measures of clinical outcome in high-risk, early stage or suboptimally-resected, advanced stage epithelial ovarian cancers A Gynecologic Oncology Group study. *Gynecol Oncol*. 2008;111:487-495.
653. Palmer JE, Sant Cassia LJ, Irwin CJ, et al. P53 and bcl-2 assessment in serous ovarian carcinoma. *Int J Gynecol Cancer*. 2008;18:241-248.
654. Kobel M, Kalloger SE, Boyd N, et al. Ovarian carcinoma subtypes are different diseases: implications for biomarker studies. *PLoS Med*. 2008;5:e232.
655. Bacher JW, Flanagan LA, Smalley RL, et al. Development of a fluorescent multiplex assay for detection of MSI-High tumors. *Dis Markers*. 2004;20:237-250.
656. Narod SA, Foulkes WD. BRCA1 and BRCA2: 1994 and beyond. *Nat Rev Cancer*. 2004;4:665-676.
657. Levine DA, Argenta PA, Yee CJ, et al. Fallopian tube and primary peritoneal carcinomas associated with BRCA mutations. *J Clin Oncol*. 2003;21:4222-4227.
658. Kauff ND, Satagopan JM, Robson ME, et al. Risk-reducing salpingo-oophorectomy in women with a BRCA1 or BRCA2 mutation. *N Engl J Med*. 2002;346:1609-1615.
659. Rebbeck TR, Lynch HT, Neuhausen SL, et al. Prophylactic oophorectomy in carriers of BRCA1 or BRCA2 mutations. *N Engl J Med*. 2002;346:1616-1622.
660. Agoff SN, Mendelin JE, Grieco VS, et al. Unexpected gynecologic neoplasms in patients with proven or suspected BRCA-1 or -2 mutations: Implications for gross examination, cytology, and clinical follow-up. *Am J Surg Pathol*. 2002;26:171-178.
661. Cossu-Rocca P, Zhang S, Roth LM, et al. Chromosome 12p abnormalities in dysgerminoma of the ovary: A FISH analysis. *Mod Pathol*. 2006;19:611-615.

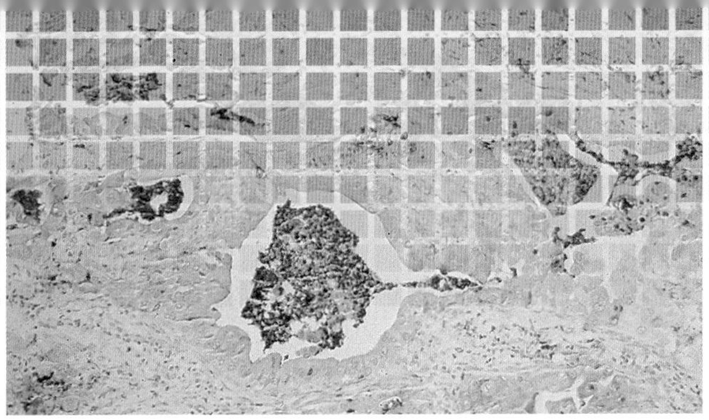

19

Immunohistology of the Breast

Rohit Bhargava • Nicole N. Esposito • David J. Dabbs

Introduction 763

Myoepithelial Cells and Assessment of Stromal Invasion 763

Immunohistochemistry of Papillary Lesions 770

Proliferative Ductal Epithelial Lesions and *In Situ* Carcinomas 771

Tumor Type Identification by Immunohistochemistry 773

Paget Disease of the Breast 785

Detection of Lymphatic Space Invasion 787

Sentinel Lymph Node Examination 787

Systemic Metastasis of Breast Carcinoma 790

Fibroepithelial Tumors 791

Theranostic Applications 796

Genomic Applications: Breast Cancer Molecular Classification and Immunogenomics 802

Other Tumor Markers 807

Summary 809

INTRODUCTION

Perhaps the most frequent use of diagnostic immunohistochemistry (IHC) in the surgical pathology laboratory is for breast biopsies by virtue of the volume and sheer difficulty of cases. In addition to IHC being used for diagnostic problems with breast biopsies, the latter lend themselves to the frequent use of IHC for prognostic and predictive tests. In addition, the diagnosis of breast carcinoma in the metastatic setting remains a challenge even today.

In this chapter we will address diagnostic issues involving stromal invasion, papillary lesions, atypical proliferative lesions, discrimination of ductal and lobular neoplasia, identification of breast tumor types, Paget disease of the breast, fibroepithelial lesions, and metastatic breast carcinoma. The diagnostic section is followed by theranostic applications in breast cancer and a discussion regarding immunogenomics.

MYOEPITHELIAL CELLS AND ASSESSMENT OF STROMAL INVASION

Although epithelial lesions of the breast are the most frequent lesions encountered by the surgical pathologist, they also cause the greatest concern in differential diagnosis of benign versus malignant lesions. The lesion categories that typically need to be differentiated include non-neoplastic proliferative lesions versus malignant lesions (sclerosing adenosis and invasive carcinoma); *in situ* carcinoma versus invasive malignancy (lobular or ductal); and pseudo-invasive lesions versus invasive malignancies (adenosis, radial scar, sclerosing papillary tumors).[1,2] In addition, atypical ductal epithelial hyperplasia (ADH), papillary lesions, and microinvasive carcinoma (invasive focus less than or equal to 1 mm) lend themselves to IHC clarification in many instances.

In all of these diagnostic situations, the presence of myoepithelial cells (MECs) in intimate relationship with the epithelial cells of the lesion determines the difference between *in situ* and invasive disease and between benign pseudo-invasive lesions and invasive carcinoma. Microglandular adenosis, a distinct non-organoid benign form of adenosis, is the only known exception to this statement (discussed later in the chapter). The presence of MECs that envelop ductal-lobular epithelium (situated on the epithelial basal lamina) has always been the important criterion that separates invasive from noninvasive neoplasms.[3-8] Myoepithelial cells can be visualized rather easily in normal breast ductules and acini, but when these structures dilate and fill with proliferating cells or are compressed, it is impossible to visualize them on H&E stain. Smooth muscle actin (SMA), calponin, smooth-muscle myosin heavy chain (SMMHC), and the nuclear marker p63 are more sensitive and specific to cytoplasmic components of MECs and have replaced the antibodies of yesteryear to S-100 protein and high molecular weight keratin (HMWK) (Table 19.1).

Antibodies to S-100 protein are not sensitive or specific for MEC, and they stain MEC in an erratic manner.[9-12] In addition, the recent use of antibodies to maspin and CD10 has been tempered by the fact that

TABLE 19.1 Antibodies for Myoepithelial Cells (MECs) in the Breast

Antibody	Localization	MEC	Myofibroblast	Microvasculature	Carcinoma
S-100	Cytoplasm	Weak	Variable	Negative	Variable
SMA	Cytoplasm	Strong	Moderate	Strong	Rare
Calponin	Cytoplasm	Strong	Weak-moderate	Strong	Rare
SMMHC	Cytoplasm	Strong	Rare	Strong	Negative
p63	Nucleus	Strong	Negative	Negative	Rare nuclei

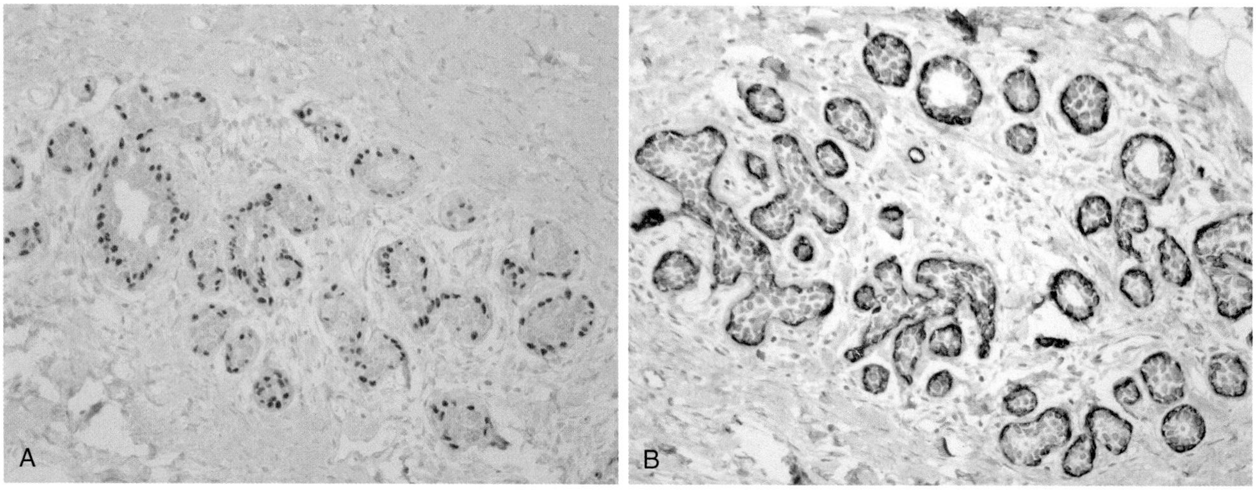

FIGURE 19.1 p63 **(A)** and smooth-muscle myosin heavy chain **(B)** stain myoepithelial cells (MEC) of a breast lobule.

they stain a variety of cell types, including luminal cells of the terminal duct lobular unit and tumor cells.[13-17]

Cytokeratin cocktail antibodies can be used to identify MECs (in addition to CK14 and CK17).[18] However, because of the proximity of MECs to acinar cells, differentiation is difficult because these cocktails also immunostain acinar cells. Anti–smooth muscle actins react with stromal myofibroblasts in addition to MECs[19-22] and thus are not specific for MECs. The cross-reaction with myofibroblasts makes it difficult to identify MECs specifically, especially for ductal carcinoma *in situ* (DCIS) cases in which periductal stromal desmoplasia may exist.

Although anti–smooth muscle actin (Dako, Carpinteria, Calif) and muscle-specific actin HHF-35 (Enzo, Farmingdale, NY) stain MECs in the majority of benign breast lesions, there is a substantial cross-reaction with stromal myofibroblasts, especially with SMA. Calponin and SMMHC are two antibodies that are more specific for MECs.[23-25] SMMHC is a structural component (200 kD) unique to smooth muscle cells, which functions within the hexagonal array of the thick-thin filament contractile apparatus.[26] Calponin, a 34-kD polypeptide, modulates actomyosin adenosine triphosphatase (ATPase) activity in the smooth muscle contractile apparatus and is unique to smooth muscle.[23,25,27] In their analysis of 85 breast lesions, Werling and colleagues found that (1) calponin and SMMHC always detected MEC in benign lesions and (2) SMMHC stained myofibroblasts in 8% of cases compared to calponin, which stained 76% of cases.[24] It is also our experience that SMMHC and calponin are excellent antibodies, but calponin does stain stromal myofibroblasts to a greater extent than SMMHC.

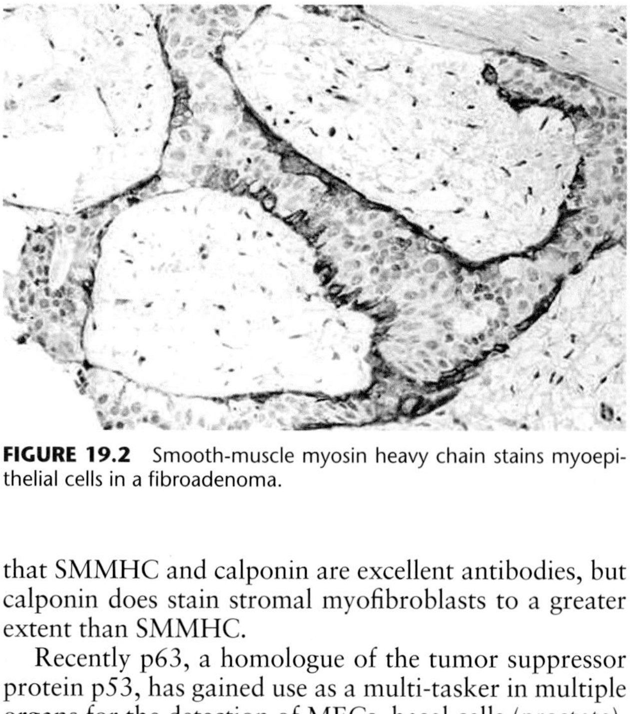

FIGURE 19.2 Smooth-muscle myosin heavy chain stains myoepithelial cells in a fibroadenoma.

Recently p63, a homologue of the tumor suppressor protein p53, has gained use as a multi-tasker in multiple organs for the detection of MECs, basal cells (prostate), and myoepithelial differentiation (breast metaplastic carcinoma and salivary gland tumors) and as a marker for squamous differentiation.[24,28,29] The advantage of p63 in the diagnosis of stromal invasion is that it is present only in the nucleus, which renders it most specific for

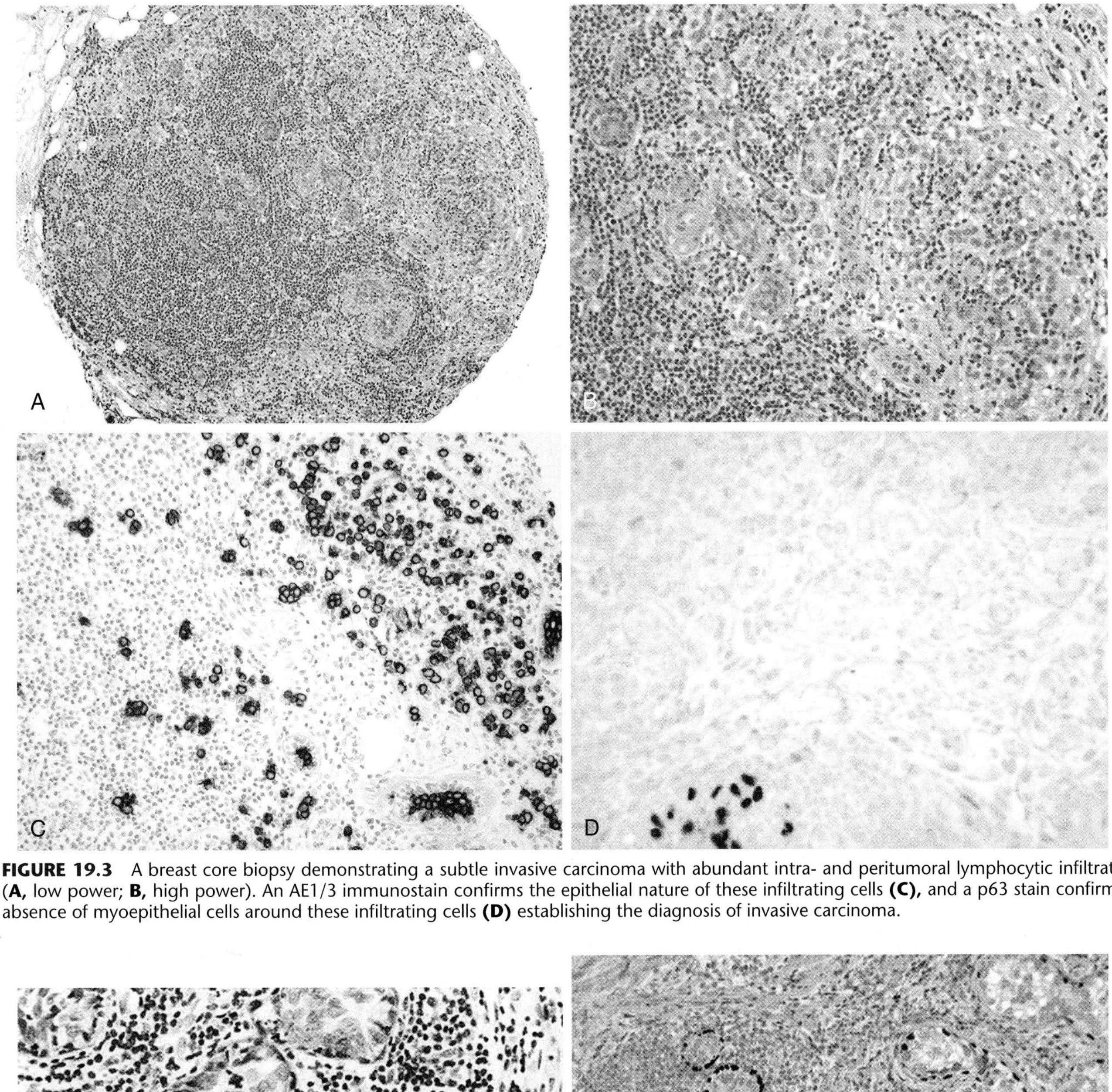

FIGURE 19.3 A breast core biopsy demonstrating a subtle invasive carcinoma with abundant intra- and peritumoral lymphocytic infiltrate (**A,** low power; **B,** high power). An AE1/3 immunostain confirms the epithelial nature of these infiltrating cells **(C),** and a p63 stain confirms absence of myoepithelial cells around these infiltrating cells **(D)** establishing the diagnosis of invasive carcinoma.

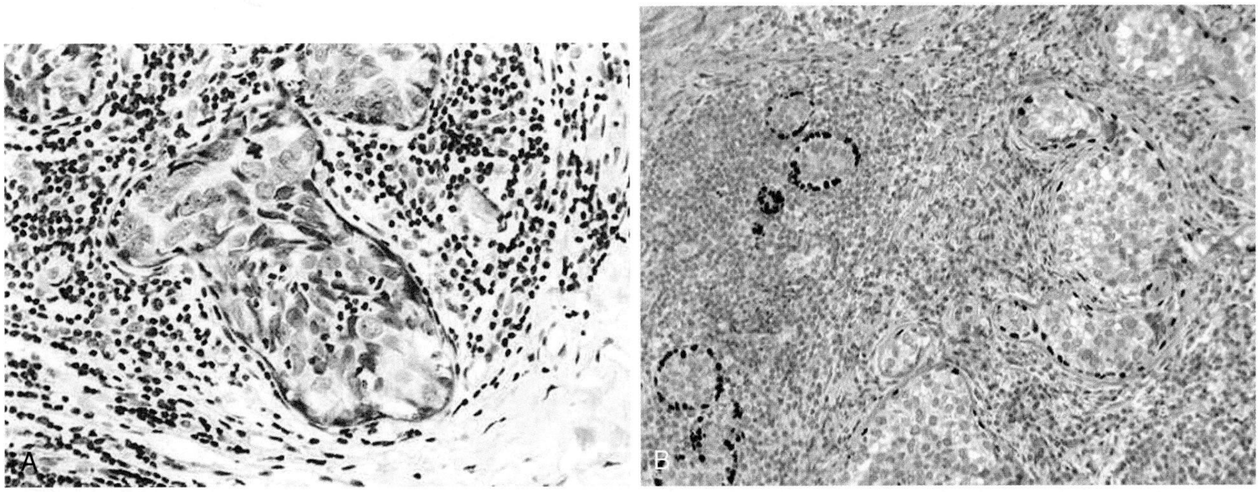

FIGURE 19.4 DCIS is heavily obscured with lymphocytes, but smooth-muscle myosin heavy chain clearly reflects the presence of myoepithelial cells **(A)**. Another case in which myoepithelial cells are easy to see with p63 in spite of heavy lymphoid infiltrate on core biopsy, which confirms a lack of invasion **(B)**.

MEC in the breast, and it does not stain myofibroblasts. Some have used a cocktail of dual-staining for SMMHC and p63. In our experience, using SMMHC and p63 is optimal for discerning MEC on difficult breast biopsies, especially diagnostic core biopsies (Figs. 19.1 to 19.5). Distinguishing DCIS from invasive carcinoma on core biopsy can be crucial, as almost all patients with invasive carcinoma will have a sentinel lymph node biopsy.

An important pitfall to note is that around 5% of DCIS cases (especially the DCIS in the background of papillary lesion) completely lack MEC using any antibody (Fig. 19.6). In these situations, critical appraisal of the histologic section is crucial to arrive at the correct diagnosis. It is also important to remember that p63 nuclear immunostaining results in apparent "gaps" of immunostaining because staining of cytoplasm of the MEC does not occur (Fig. 19.7). Any nuclear staining around nests of tumor cells can be construed as evidence of the presence of MEC. Special care must be taken to exclude nuclear staining of tumor cells around the periphery of neoplastic ducts, as p63 stains tumoral cells in approximately 10% to 15% of cases (see Fig. 19.7).

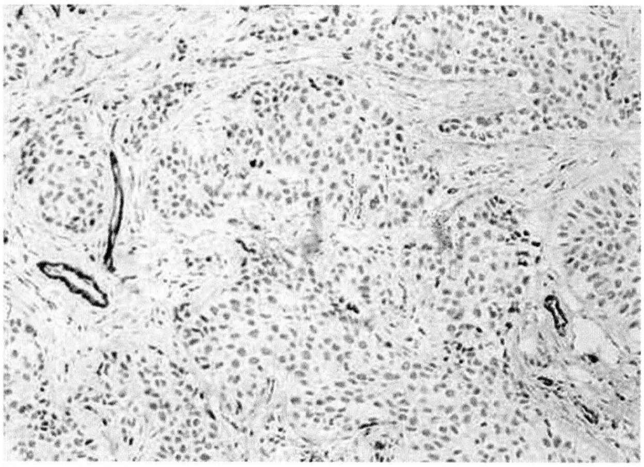

FIGURE 19.5 This infiltrative-appearing breast core biopsy is clearly invasive carcinoma, as seen with complete lack of smooth-muscle myosin heavy chain. A blood vessel serves as positive internal control.

Lesions that are especially difficult to diagnose on core biopsies include carcinoma *in situ* versus invasive carcinoma in the presence of prominent periductal stromal desmoplasia ("regressive changes") or heavy lymphoid infiltrates; lobular growth of rounded sheets of tumor cells (to the pathologist's eye, invasion is "all or none"); infiltrating cribriform carcinoma; sclerosing adenosis (with or without DCIS involvement); cancerization of lobules; radial scars with stromal elastosis-desmoplasia; tubular carcinoma; and sclerosing papillary lesion. The optimal MEC antibodies needed to attack these difficult cases include both SMMHC and p63 (Figs. 19.8 to 19.12).[30]

A significant pitfall for misinterpretation of MEC antibodies such as calponin and even SMMHC is that

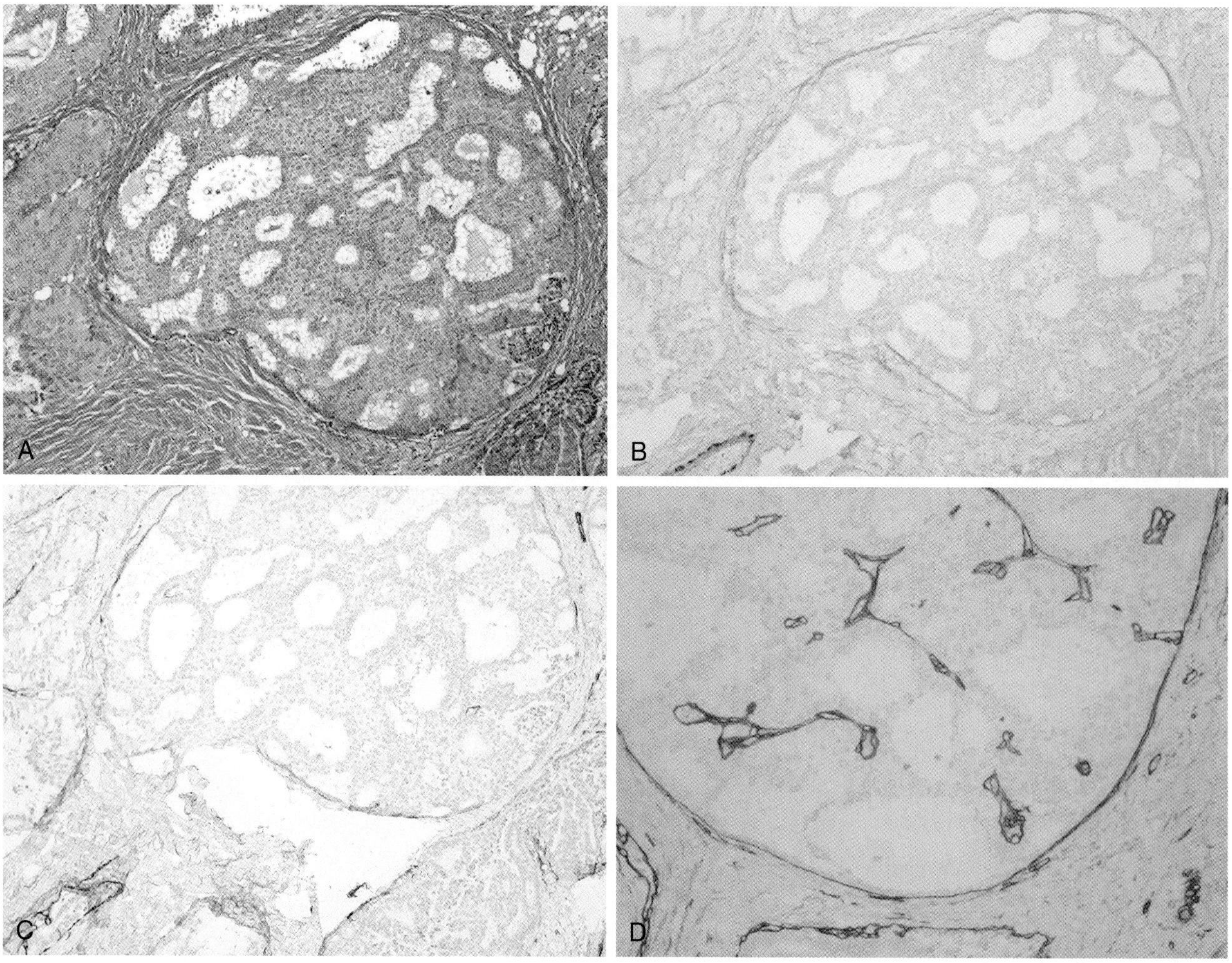

FIGURE 19.6 Approximately 5% of morphologically identifiable DCIS may not show myoepithelial cells. This case of cribriform and papillary DCIS **(A)** shows lack of staining with p63 **(B)** and smooth-muscle myosin heavy chain **(C)**. Collagen type IV demonstrates strong continuous staining around tumor nests confirming the *in situ* nature of the lesion **(D)**.

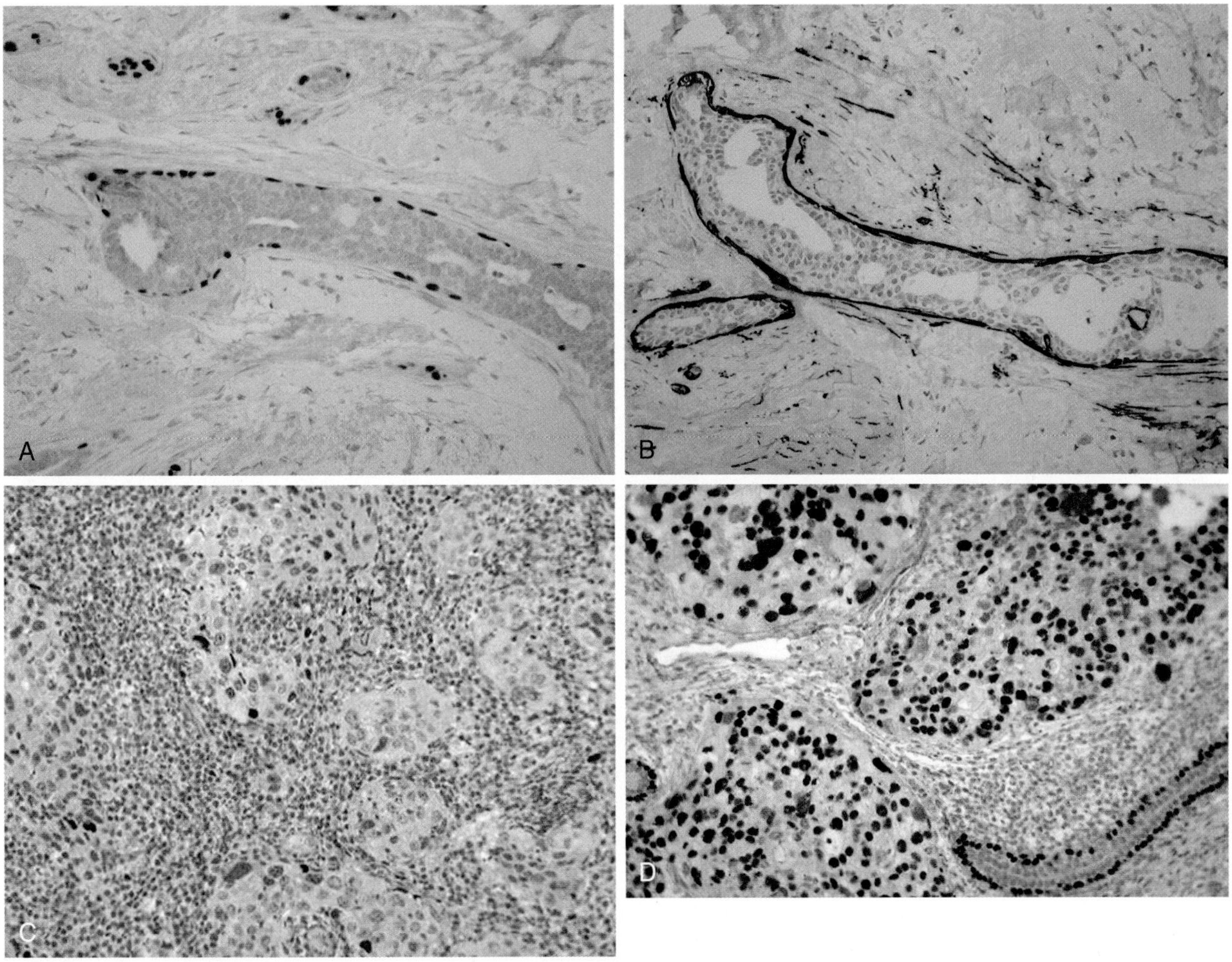

FIGURE 19.7 Pitfalls of p63 and smooth-muscle myosin heavy chain. A p63 stain demonstrates apparent gaps in staining around the luminal epithelium of a duct within a radial scar **(A)**. Same duct shows intense continuous staining with smooth-muscle myosin heavy chain, but myofibroblastic cells in the background are also positive **(B)**. A p63 stain on core biopsy shows staining of few tumor cells **(C)**. A rare example of diffuse p63 staining of tumor cells **(D)**.

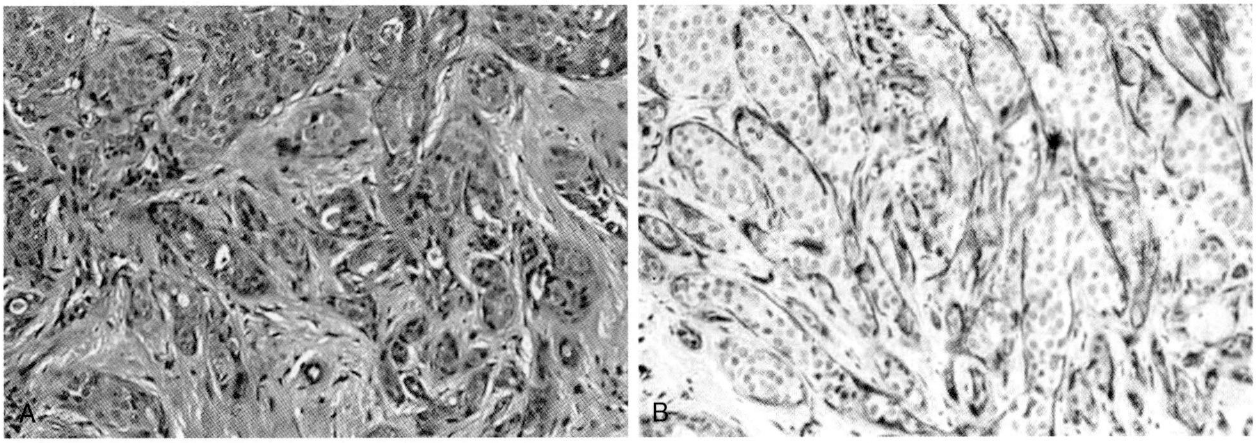

FIGURE 19.8 Sclerosing adenosis may simulate carcinoma **(A)** but demonstrates envelopment of cell nests by myoepithelial cells with smooth-muscle myosin heavy chain immunostaining **(B)**.

these antibodies may immunostain the microvasculature around tumor nests. Initial examination of such a case with SMMHC will reveal immunostaining hugging the tumor nests, suggesting the presence of MECs (Fig. 19.13). Examination at higher magnification will reveal the microvasculature around the tumor nests. When one then examines the p63, it is negative (see Fig. 19.13).

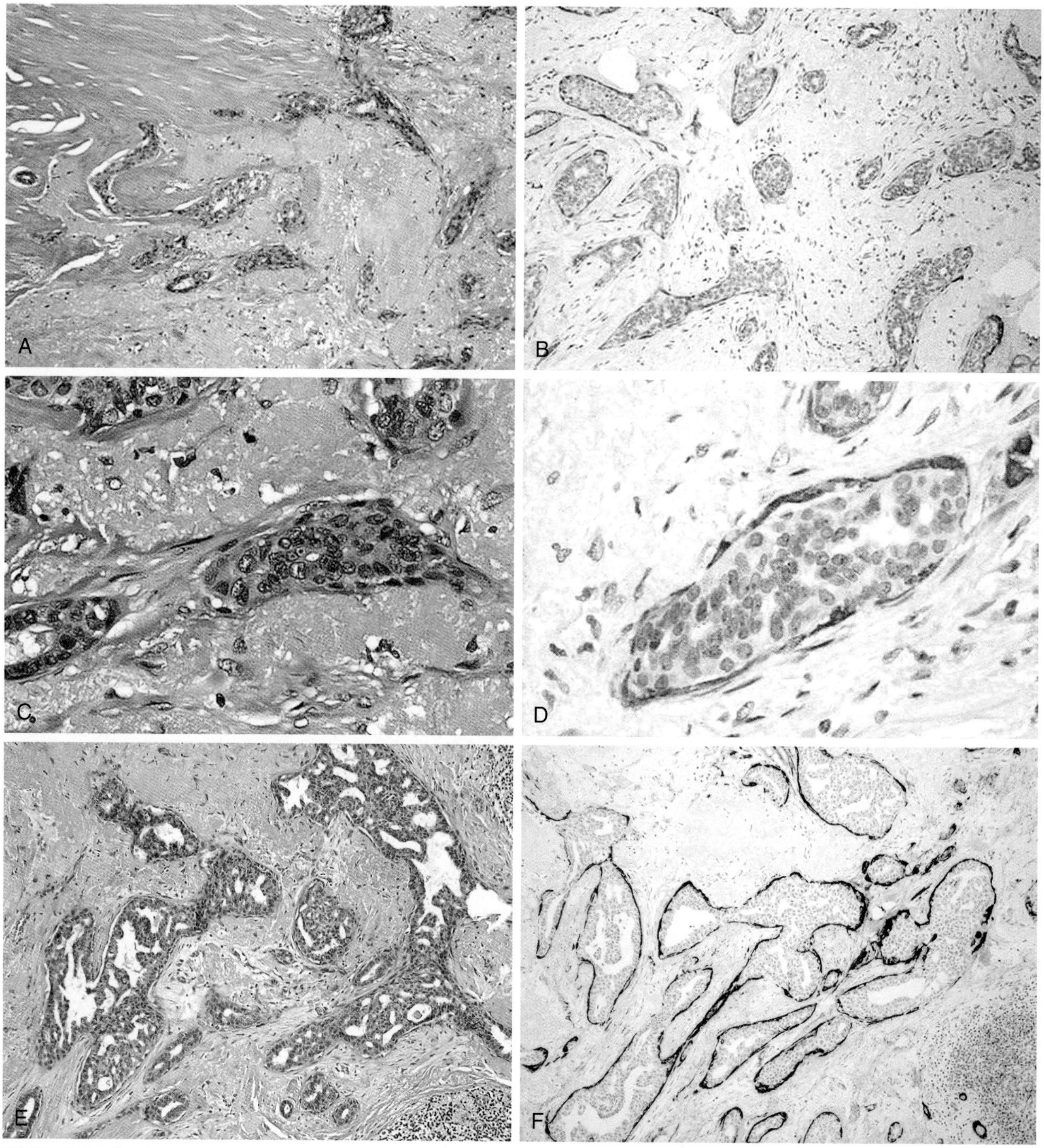

FIGURE 19.9 Simulating cancer, this case of radial scar shows prominent elastosis **(A, C)**, but it also shows strong smooth-muscle myosin heavy chain staining of myoepithelial cells, which is indicative of a benign process **(B, D)**. Another case of radial scar **(E)** shows strong smooth-muscle myosin heavy stain staining in the periphery of the ducts **(F)**, which is indicative of a benign process.

Immunohistochemistry for MEC is useful to help discriminate the three dominant benign lesions of the breast: sclerosing adenosis, microglandular adenosis (MGA), and tubular carcinoma (Table 19.2), but a detailed morphologic study of the lesion is essential.[31,32] The MECs are seen by IHC in all forms of adenosis except the microglandular form, the only benign lesion that is known not to contain MECs. In addition to the distinct non-organoid morphology of MGA, tubular adenosis—described by Lee and colleagues—may mimic both MGA and carcinoma but differs from MGA by containing MECs.[32] Microglandular adenosis is positive with S-100 protein, whereas sclerosing adenosis and tubular carcinomas are S-100 negative.

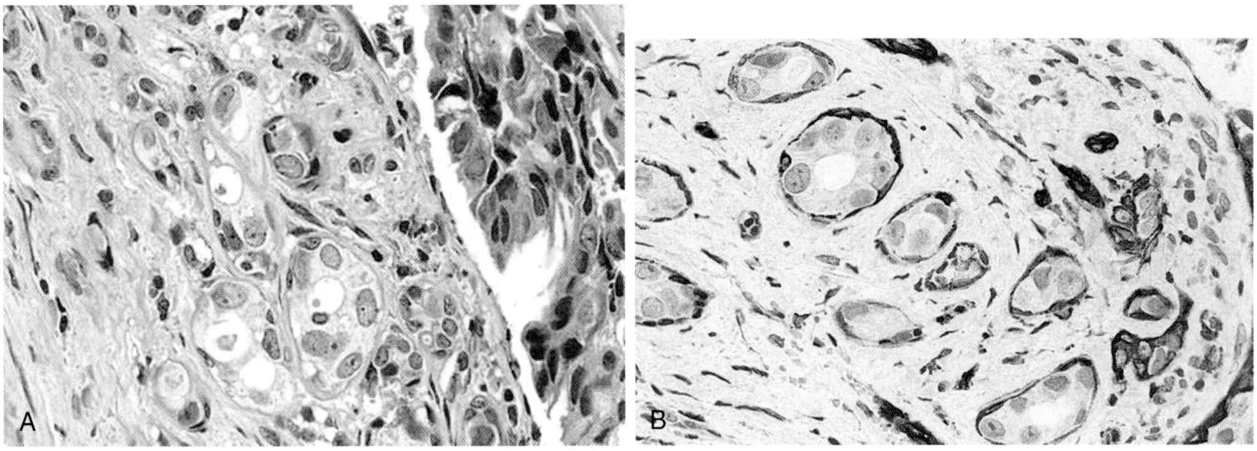

FIGURE 19.10 Carcinoma *in situ* involving sclerosing adenosis is always frightful to look at **(A)**, but the diagnosis is confirmed with smooth-muscle myosin heavy chain documenting the presence of myoepithelial cells **(B)**.

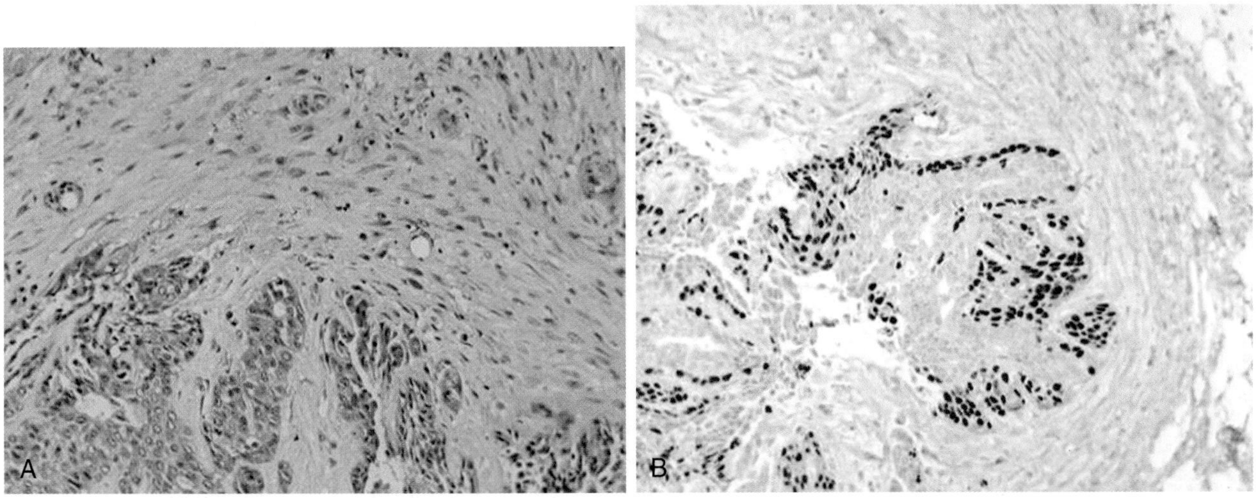

FIGURE 19.11 Edge of sclerosing papillary lesion **(A)**. A p63 stain confirms absence of invasion **(B)**.

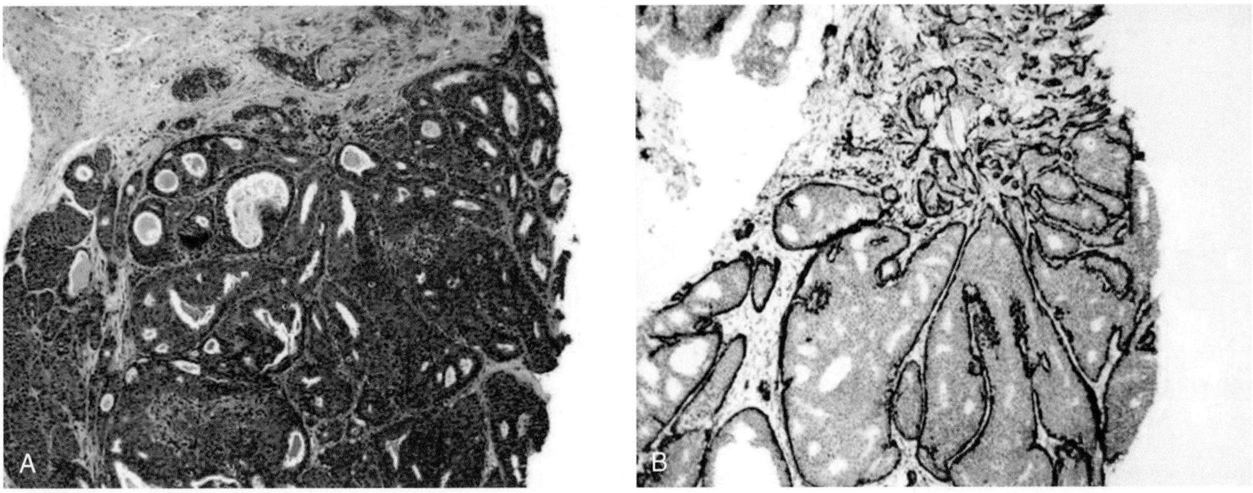

FIGURE 19.12 Cribriform growth pattern—is this *in situ* or invasive **(A)**? A smooth-muscle myosin heavy chain immunostain confirms the diagnosis of DCIS **(B)**.

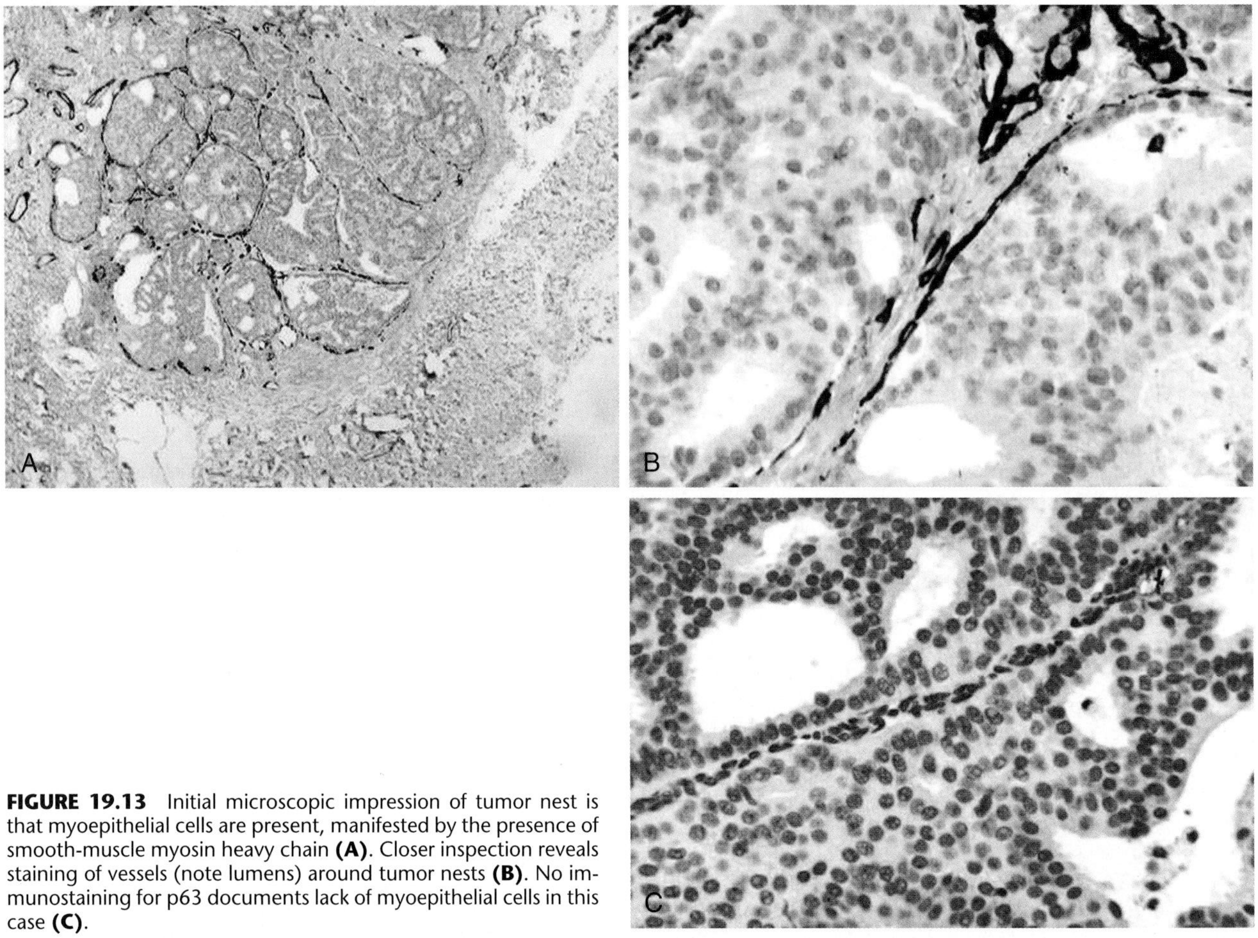

FIGURE 19.13 Initial microscopic impression of tumor nest is that myoepithelial cells are present, manifested by the presence of smooth-muscle myosin heavy chain **(A)**. Closer inspection reveals staining of vessels (note lumens) around tumor nests **(B)**. No immunostaining for p63 documents lack of myoepithelial cells in this case **(C)**.

KEY DIAGNOSTIC POINTS

Myoepithelial Cell Antibodies for Stromal Invasion

- The presence of MEC enveloping proliferating and sclerosing breast lesions is indicative of a benign or noninvasive process.
- A combination of cytoplasmic SMMHC and nuclear p63 antibodies is the best discriminator for the presence of MECs, especially in desmoplastic-sclerotic proliferations.
- MEC antibodies may be confirmatory for diagnosing microinvasive carcinoma provided that the lesion is no greater than 1 mm and has a jagged invasive configuration, stromal response, single invasive cells, or a combination of the three.
- Microglandular adenosis is SMMHC-negative, p63-negative, S-100–positive.
- A pitfall is immunostaining of vascular walls with SMMHC; also, p63 occasionally stains neoplastic cells.

IMMUNOHISTOCHEMISTRY OF PAPILLARY LESIONS

Papillary lesions range from benign papilloma to atypical papilloma to papillary carcinoma (*in situ* and invasive). There are several reports on the use of myoepithelial cell markers to distinguish between different categories.[12,33-35] A papillary lesion could be classified as a papilloma if there is a uniform layer of myoepithelial cells in the proliferating intraluminal component of the lesion, whereas the absence of myoepithelial cells would be suggestive of a papillary carcinoma.[34] Some papillomas show the features of an "atypical papilloma," areas in which there is atypical ductal epithelial hyperplasia that overgrows the papilloma.[36] These atypical areas lack MECs by immunoperoxidase examination.[37] Atypical papillomas and papillary carcinoma *in situ* also lose high molecular weight keratin immunostaining with 34βE12 and CK5/6.[38] The distinction between a papilloma, atypical papilloma, and papillary DCIS (either *de novo* or DCIS involving papilloma) is quite straightforward in the majority of cases and can be made using morphology and IHC staining (Fig. 19.14). The more difficult and confusing area is the distinction between an *in situ* lesion and an invasive carcinoma. The *in situ* papillary carcinoma has been referred to by different names in the literature. The term *intracystic papillary carcinoma* has been used for a single mass-forming cystic lesion with malignant papillary proliferation.[39] The term *papillary ductal carcinoma in situ* has been used for more diffuse lesions.[40] The use of myoepithelial cell markers to assess invasion in these lesions has yielded variable results. In an immunohistochemical study of papillary breast lesions, Hill and Yeh found a consistent

TABLE 19.2 Differential Diagnosis of Tubular Carcinoma, Microglandular Adenosis, Tubular Adenosis, and Sclerosing Adenosis

Diagnosis	Histology	MECs	Collagen IV	Other IHC
Tubular carcinoma	Invasive teardrop-shape tubules, apical snouts, desmoplasia	Absent	Absent	EMA+, ER/PR+
Microglandular adenosis	Round glands in fat lined by flat to cuboidal epithelium; inspissated secretions within glands	Absent	Present	S-100+, EMA–, ER/PR–, GCDFP15–
Tubular adenosis	Tubules sectioned longitudinally and lack lobulocentric distribution	Present	Present	S-100–
Sclerosing adenosis	Lobular growth pattern, epithelial cell atrophy, and lobular fibrosis	Present (relative abundance)	Present	S-100–

staining pattern in cases originally diagnosed as papilloma or invasive papillary carcinoma, but found variable staining in cases diagnosed as intra-ductal papillary carcinomas.[33] Of the nine intra-ductal papillary carcinomas in their series, four cases showed unequivocal basal myoepithelial cells by IHC, one showed partial discontinuous staining, and four were predominantly negative for basal myoepithelial cells. The authors found that lesions originally classified as intra-ductal papillary carcinoma but that lacked basal myoepithelial cells by IHC were uniformly large, expansile, papillary lesions with pushing borders and a fibrotic rim. The authors hypothesized that such lesions form a part of the spectrum of progression intermediate between *in situ* and invasive disease and suggested that these lesions be termed *encapsulated papillary carcinomas.*[33] Collins and colleagues also favored such designation.[41] In some recent reviews of papillary lesions, an attempt has been made to classify the lesions in a uniform fashion using morphology and IHC. The papillary lesions are now classified as papilloma, papilloma with atypical ductal epithelial hyperplasia (atypical papilloma), papilloma with DCIS, papillary DCIS, intracystic papillary carcinoma (encysted or encapsulated papillary carcinoma), solid-papillary carcinoma, and invasive papillary carcinoma.[37,42]

The problem in diagnosis arises from the fact that intracystic and solid-papillary carcinomas have the morphology of an *in situ* lesion, but most lesions lack the presence of MECs around the periphery (Fig. 19.15). Since type IV collagen is an integral component of the basal lamina (BL) that envelops normal and proliferative benign lesions, we recently studied its expression in intracystic papillary carcinoma and compared it to expression in a variety of papillary lesions and invasive carcinoma. We found continuous strong collagen type IV staining around the periphery of intracystic papillary carcinomas (Fig. 19.16), which was similar to benign lesions and DCIS, but generally a weak and discontinuous-type staining around invasive carcinomas.[43] Our results are very similar to a previous study regarding the usefulness of collagen type IV, published several years ago.[44] This pattern of staining supports the *in situ* nature of intracystic papillary carcinomas. Moreover, the clinical behavior of these lesions is more akin to *in situ* disease[39,45-47]; thus, intracystic papillary carcinomas and solid-papillary carcinomas with absence of basal myoepithelial cells around the periphery should still be considered as a variant of *in situ* carcinoma for practical purposes. However, it is extremely important to analyze the resection specimen on these lesions in entirety by histologic evaluation owing to the frequent presence of frank invasion (into the fat beyond the fibrotic rim) in the periphery of these lesions. We believe that the presence of these minute foci of invasive carcinoma are responsible for the occasional metastatic disease reported with intracystic papillary carcinomas.[48] Table 19.3 summarizes the MEC staining pattern for each papillary lesion.

KEY DIAGNOSTIC POINTS

Myoepithelial Cell Antibodies in Papillary Lesions

- The MECs are present in the proliferative cellular component of a papilloma but are absent in the area of atypical ductal epithelial hyperplasia or DCIS.
- MECs are uniformly present around the periphery of the lesion in a papilloma, atypical papilloma, and papilloma with DCIS and are often present around papillary DCIS; however, they are often absent at the periphery in intracystic and solid-papillary carcinomas.
- Caution is advised in diagnosing invasion based on MEC antibodies in a papillary lesion on a core biopsy. Recommend complete excision for assessing invasion.

PROLIFERATIVE DUCTAL EPITHELIAL LESIONS AND *IN SITU* CARCINOMAS

Differences in cytokeratin expression have been described between hyperplasia and DCIS.[49,50] The 34βE12 antibody recognizes CK1, CK5, CK10, and CK14; these keratins are typically found in duct-derived epithelium and squamous epithelium. Normal breast MECs and luminal cells express 34βE12, as does proliferative duct epithelium of the usual type (Fig. 19.17). The expression is generally lost in atypical ductal epithelial hyperplasia.[51] DCIS is largely negative for 34βE12 in 81% to 100% of cases (see Fig. 19.17) but may show some positive cells. Most cases of DCIS are uniformly

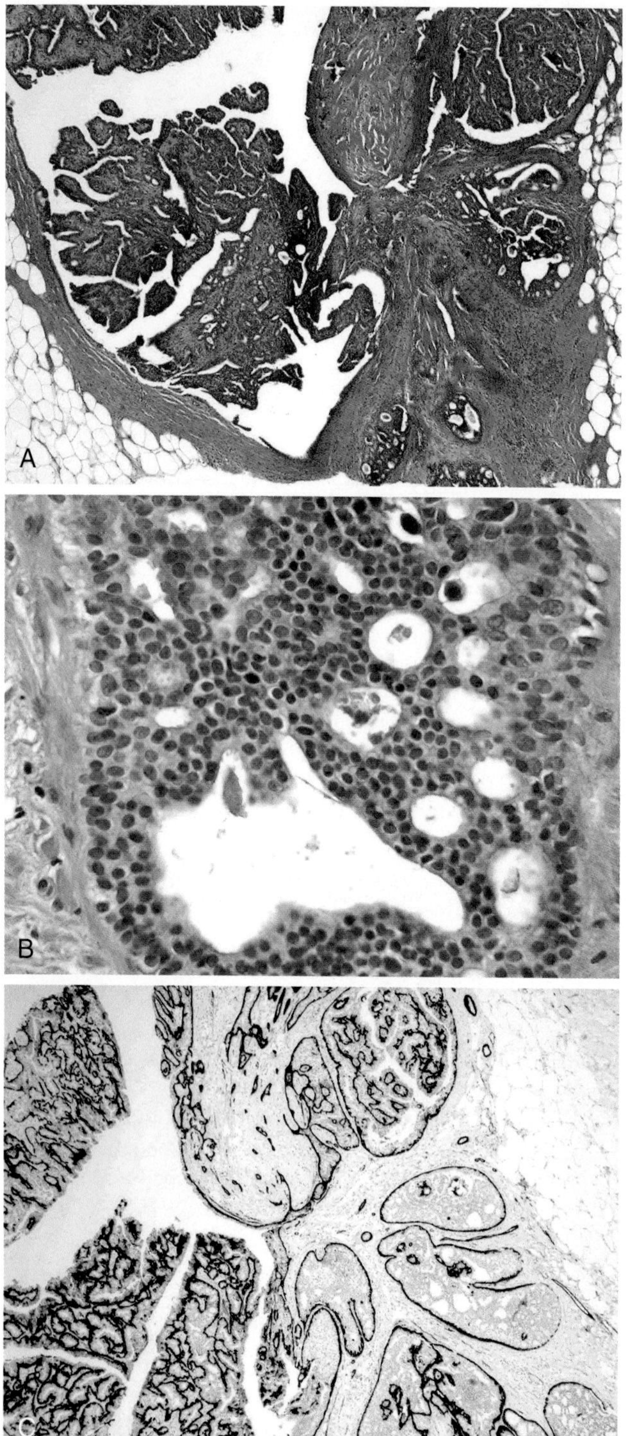

FIGURE 19.14 A low-power view of an intraductal papilloma with monomorphic cellular proliferation at the bottom right **(A)**. A high-power view demonstrates the presence of DCIS in a papilloma **(B)**. A lack of smooth-muscle myosin heavy chain immunostaining in this morphologically abnormal area confirms the diagnosis of DCIS involving papilloma **(C)**.

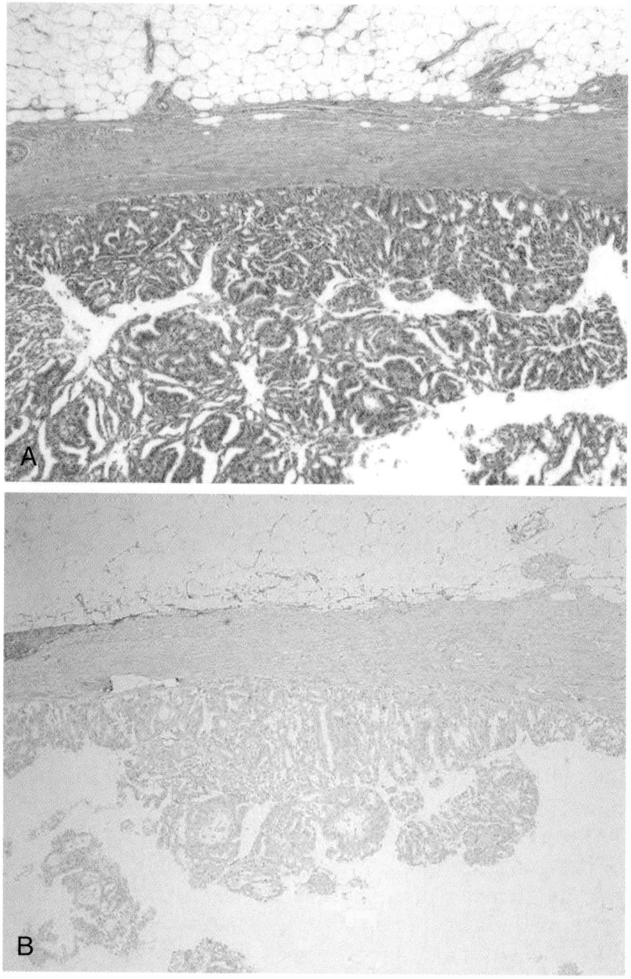

FIGURE 19.15 An intracystic (encapsulated) papillary carcinoma **(A)**, with lack of p63 staining at the periphery of the lesion **(B)**.

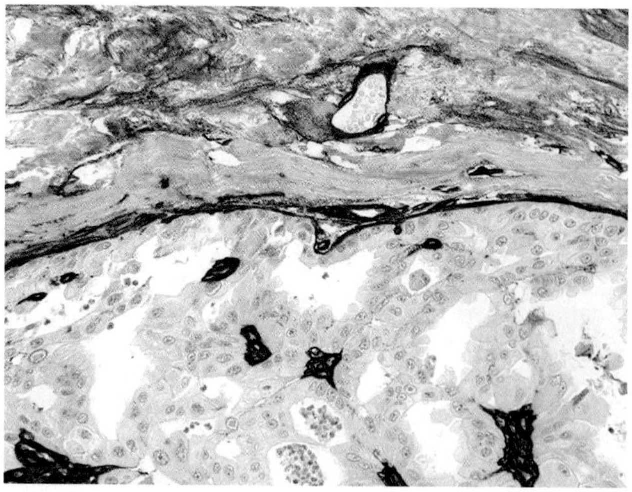

FIGURE 19.16 Another case of intracystic (encapsulated) papillary carcinoma demonstrating strong continuous collagen type IV staining.

positive for CAM5.2, which reflects a shift away from high molecular weight keratins to the more simple keratins 8 and 18. The 34βE12 immunostaining profile for DCIS and ADH is very similar and cannot be used to help distinguish DCIS from ADH. It can, however, aid in histomorphology when separating DCIS from florid ductal epithelial hyperplasia (DEH) in difficult cases. Clone D5/16B4 antibody CK5/6 is more specific for the DCIS morphology as it is largely completely negative in DCIS.[51]

TABLE 19.3 Distribution of Myoepithelial Cells and Clinical Behavior in Papillary Lesions of the Breast

Papillary Lesion	Myoepithelial Cells	Clinical Behavior
Papilloma	Present within and around ducts	Benign
Papilloma with ADH/DCIS or papillary DCIS	Reduced/absent within, present around ducts	Risk for invasive malignancy
Encapsulated papillary carcinoma	Absent within, rare +/– around ducts	Similar to DCIS, unless frankly invasive
Solid papillary carcinoma	Absent within, rare +/– around ducts	Similar to DCIS, unless frankly invasive

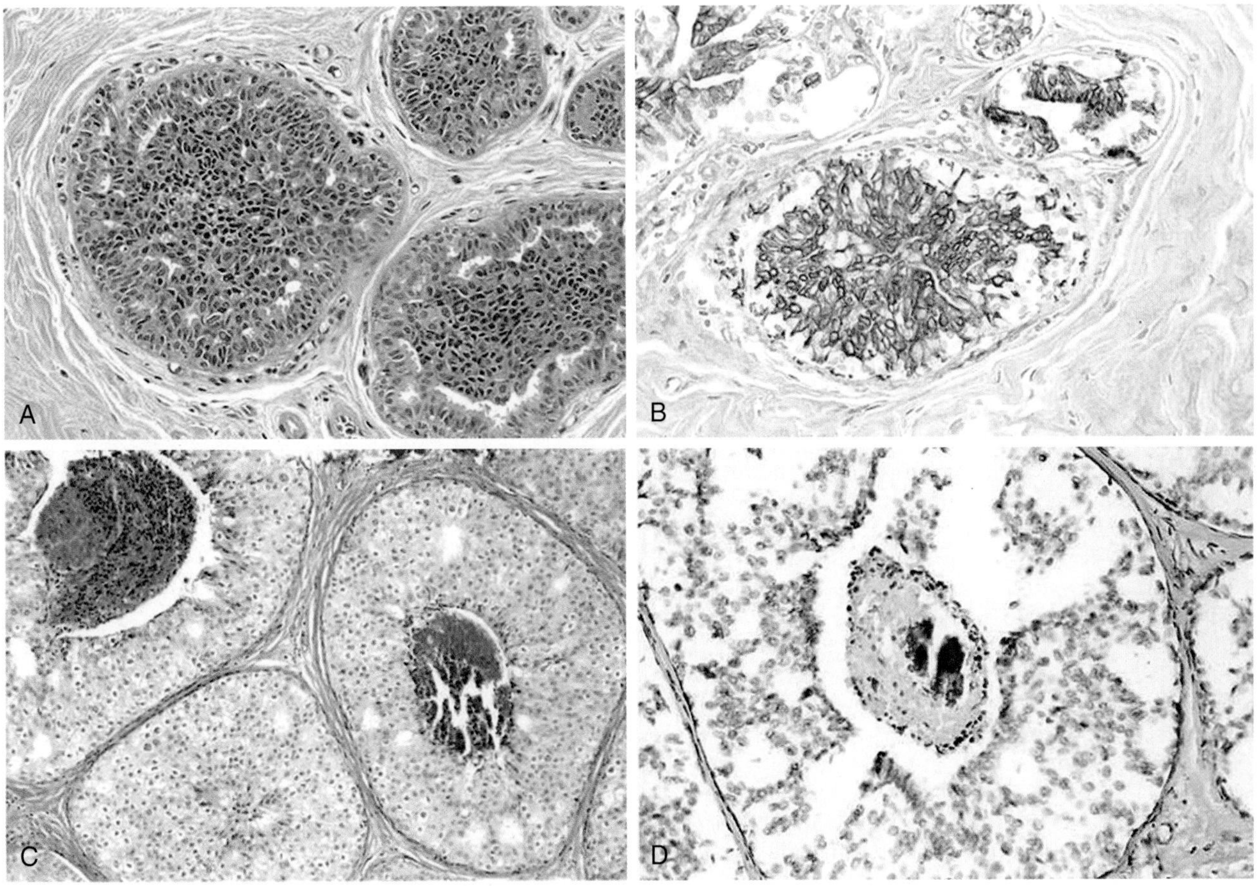

FIGURE 19.17 This case of florid duct hyperplasia **(A)** demonstrates strongly positive reactivity to keratin 903 (34βE12) **(B)**. In contrast to ductal hyperplasia, DCIS **(C)** is negative with keratin 903 **(D)**.

Papillary proliferations can be especially challenging. Fortunately, the same cytokeratin patterns of immunostaining hold up for the differential diagnosis of *in situ* papillary carcinoma versus florid hyperplasia.[38]

KEY DIAGNOSTIC POINTS

Keratins in Proliferative and in Situ Lesions

- Cytokeratin antibody 34βE12 and CK5/6 routinely intensely stain florid ductal hyperplasia of the breast, which may be useful in separating florid DEH in ducts or papillomas from ADH/DCIS.
- Both ADH and DCIS lack 34βE12 or CK5/6 antibody staining and cannot be distinguished by IHC.

TUMOR TYPE IDENTIFICATION BY IMMUNOHISTOCHEMISTRY

Cell Adhesion: Ductal versus Lobular Carcinoma

Based on cell cohesiveness, the two broad categories of breast carcinoma (invasive and *in situ*) are ductal and lobular types. Ductal carcinoma *in situ* increases the risk of invasive malignancy at the local site. Lobular carcinoma *in situ* is considered a marker of generalized increased risk of invasive malignancy, although some recent data suggest precursor properties for lobular carcinoma *in situ*.[52-61] Invasive ductal carcinomas are often unifocal lesions compared to invasive lobular carcinomas, which are often multifocal or more extensive than what is estimated on clinical and mammographic examination.[62-64] Distant metastases from ductal carcinoma preferentially involve lung and brain, whereas metastases from lobular carcinoma more often involve the peritoneum, bone, bone marrow, and visceral organs of gastrointestinal and gynecologic tracts.[65-68] In spite of all of these differences, with the combined multimodality therapy there appears to be no difference in disease-free or overall survival between ductal and lobular carcinomas.[63,69,70] However, there are enough significant differences in patient pre-operative evaluation and subsequent treatment that an accurate diagnosis is warranted at the time of core biopsy. At some breast cancer centers, a pre-operative (before lumpectomy or mastectomy) magnetic resonance image (MRI) of the breast is performed to evaluate the extent of disease with a core biopsy diagnosis of invasive lobular carcinoma,[62,64,71,72] the rationale being that margins are difficult to obtain from the surgeon's viewpoint. This probably has merit in selected patients pertaining to breast reconstruction. A core biopsy diagnosis of ductal versus lobular carcinoma is also important if the patient will be treated by neo-adjuvant chemotherapy. Although there are scant data on the subject, a few studies have indicated response only in a subset of ductal cancers with no or minimal effect on lobular cancers.[73-76] Therefore, pathologists have to strive to give the best diagnosis possible for current management and also for the future as specific therapies become available.

Strong E-cadherin (ECAD) membranous staining has been long used to define ductal carcinomas.[13,77,78] Ductal carcinomas (*in situ* or invasive) retain membranous ECAD because they do not show homozygous mutation/silencing of the *ECAD* gene.[79-81] Either mutation of the *ECAD* gene leads to a mutant protein that loses its adhesive properties, or there is not enough protein to function as an adhesive molecule.

The *ECAD* gene, *CDH1*, is large and located on 16q22.1. The ECAD protein has an intracytoplasmic portion, an intramembranous portion, and an extracellular domain. Cell-to-cell adhesion through ECAD is also critically dependent on the subplasmalemmal cytoplasmic catenin complexes (alpha, beta, gamma, and p120 isoforms) that link ECAD to the actin cytoskeleton of the cell. Abnormalities of the catenins or *ECAD* gene expression can result in a variety of immunohistochemical ECAD pathologies. Lobular carcinomas studied at the genetic level have often shown E-cadherin mutation that accounts for the loss of cohesiveness of the tumor cells.[79,80] The majority of these mutations have been found in combination with loss of heterozygosity (LOH) of the wild-type *ECAD* locus (16q22.1), a hallmark of classic tumor suppressor genes. Immunohistochemically, this correlates with either a complete absence of the ECAD protein or abnormal localization (apical or perinuclear). This abnormal localization may be dependent on the type of mutation.[82] Truncation mutations produce an ECAD product that is inept at binding to neighboring cells, resulting in a histologic pattern of widely dyshesive cells that are completely negative for ECAD by IHC (e.g., classic infiltrating lobular carcinoma) (Fig. 19.18). Loss of membrane staining may be associated with a granular cytoplasmic immunostaining (Fig. 19.19A, B) that represents cytoplasmic solubilization of a portion of the truncated protein. Proximal truncation mutations may result in the inability of ECAD to bind to the catenin complex, resulting in a short ECAD represented

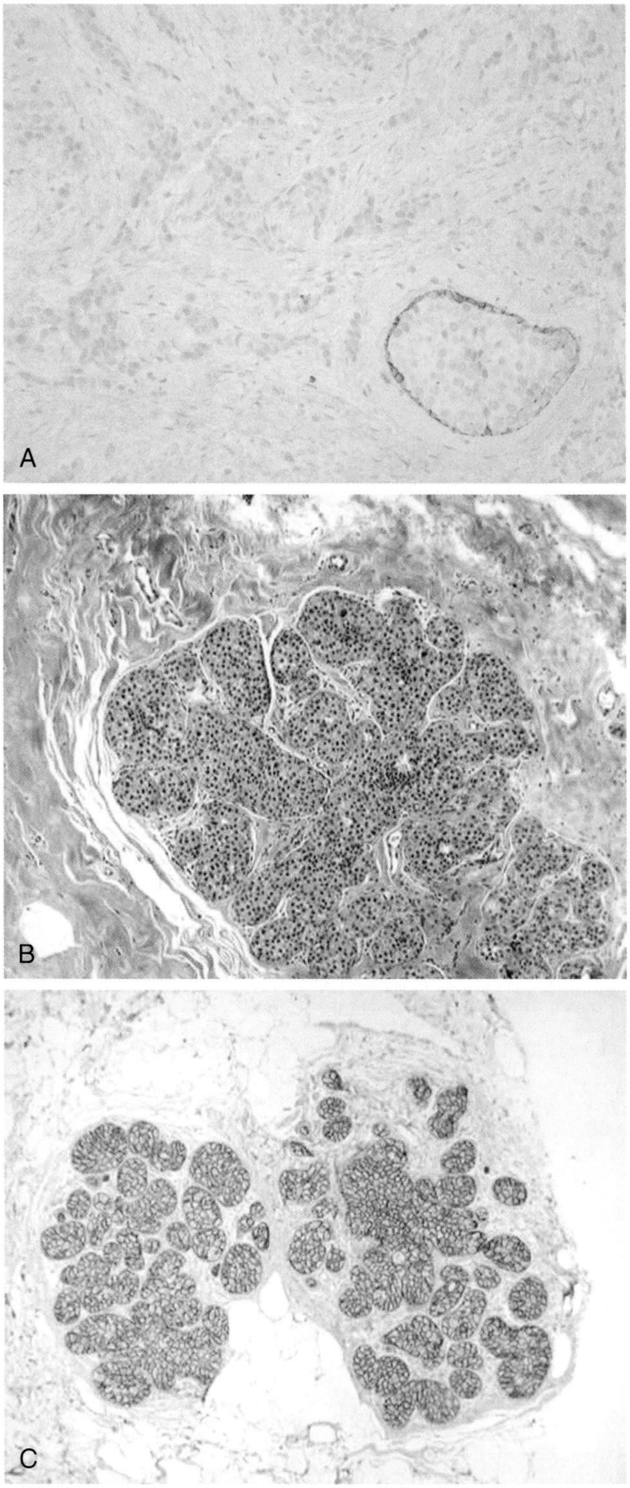

FIGURE 19.18 A classic invasive and *in situ* lobular carcinoma demonstrating complete lack of ECAD staining **(A)**. Note the staining of myoepithelial cells with ECAD **(A)**. The growth pattern of *in situ* carcinoma is indeterminate for cell type **(B)**, but positive membranous staining for ECAD indicates lobular involvement by DCIS **(C)**.

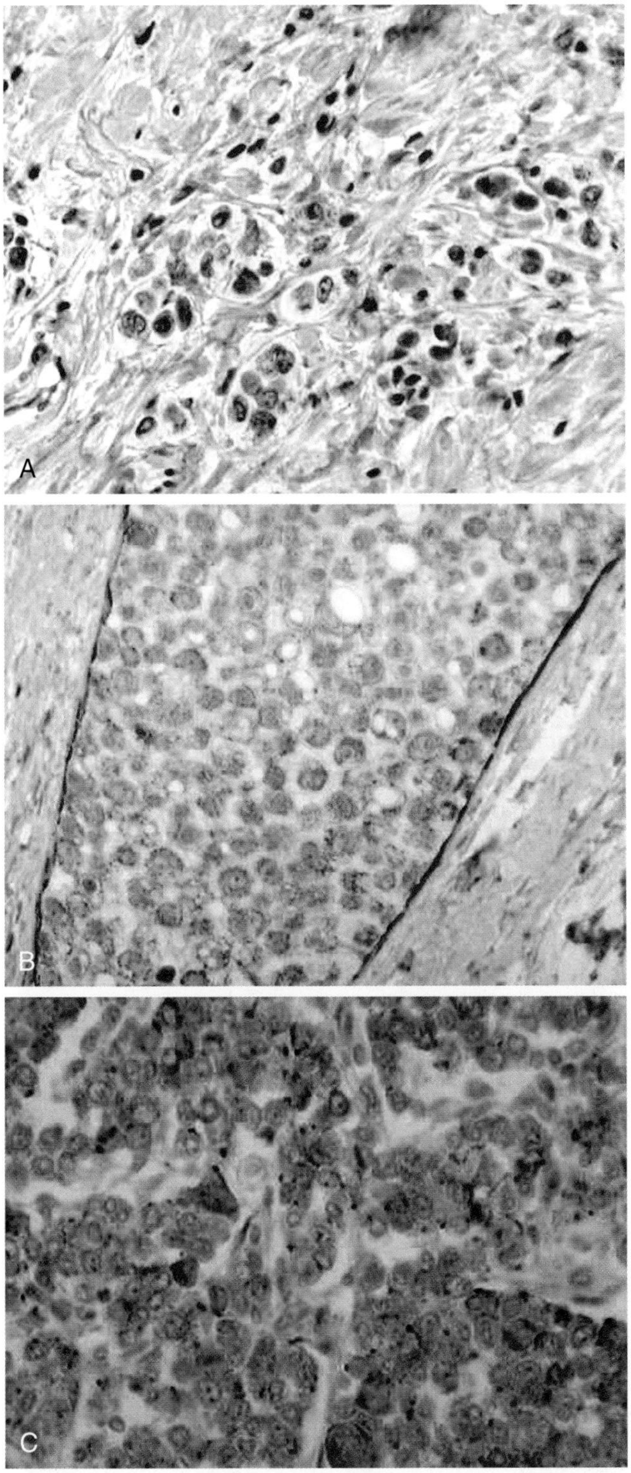

FIGURE 19.19 Aberrant staining with ECAD: Cytoplasmic ECAD staining in invasive lobular carcinoma **(A)** and lobular carcinoma *in situ* **(B)**. An example of dotlike ECAD staining in invasive carcinoma is seen in **C**.

by focal or dot-like membrane immunostaining (see Fig. 19.19C). Patients with focal staining of LCIS cells with ECAD may have an ipsilateral risk of carcinoma akin to DCIS.[83] Mutations in the catenin complex can also lead to dysfunctional ECAD and loss of membrane staining.[84,85] While deletions of the *CDH1* gene as a result of LOH are seen in ductal carcinomas, they are not early events and are not usually associated with the point mutations seen in lobular neoplasia.

In the majority of cases, ECAD staining is unequivocal (positive or negative) and can be solely used in distinguishing ductal from lobular carcinomas. In a minority of cases (approximately 15%), the stain may be difficult to interpret. Another stain that could be used in such situations is p120. This stain represents p120 catenin, which binds with ECAD on the internal aspect of the cell membrane to form the cadherin-catenin complex (Fig. 19.20A). The complex is essential for the formation of intercellular tight junctions. It is composed of an external domain of calcium-dependent ECAD and an internal domain of ECAD to which is bound α-catenin, β-catenin, and p120 catenin.[86-90] α-Catenin and β-catenin are complexed with the carboxy-terminal cytoplasmic tail of ECAD, whereas the p120 catenin is anchored to ECAD in a juxta-membranous site.[91] p120 is actively involved in the status of cell motility, ECAD trafficking, ECAD turnover, promotion of cell junction formation, and regulation of the actin cytoskeleton.[92] The binding of p120 to ECAD stabilizes the complex and increases the half-life of membrane ECAD by slowing the normal turnover of ECAD that occurs by cellular endocytosis.[93] p120 that is bound to ECAD exists in equilibrium with a small cytoplasmic pool of p120. When ECAD is absent, the cytoplasmic pool of p120 increases.[94] Therefore, in normal ducts and ductal carcinomas, p120 shows a membranous pattern of staining (see Fig. 19.20B, C). In stark contrast, lobular carcinomas (with absent or non-functional e-cadherin) show a strong cytoplasmic p120 immunoreactivity (see Fig. 19.20D, E). This positive cytoplasmic staining for lobular carcinoma is much easier to interpret than ECAD negative staining.[43] A combination of E-cadherin and p120 drastically reduces the number of ambiguous diagnoses and better delineates (or diagnoses with increased confidence) the category of mixed ductal and lobular carcinoma (see Fig. 19.20F). These mixed carcinomas compose not more than 10% of all breast carcinomas and probably arise owing to "late" ECAD inactivation within a ductal carcinoma.[95] In contrast, loss of ECAD protein occurs very early in lobular carcinogenesis.[96] Lack of E-cadherin staining and strong p120 cytoplasmic staining are observed in all morphologically characterized invasive and *in situ* lobular carcinomas and atypical lobular hyperplasias (Fig. 19.21). Additionally, lack of ECAD within minimal epithelial proliferation in the breast terminal duct lobular unit defines atypical lobular hyperplasia and distinguishes it from mild ductal hyperplasia. This distinction is important because patients with ALH are typically referred to a risk clinic. Also, some recent studies have advocated surgical excision with core needle biopsy diagnosis of atypical lobular hyperplasia.[54,97] The IHC stains support the notion that the term *lobular hyperplasia* has no significance in breast pathology.

Not only do immunohistochemical and molecular methods aid with diagnostic issues, but to some extent they also demand that one considers the morphology that has been learned in a new light. All invasive breast carcinomas that infiltrate in a "single-file" pattern with

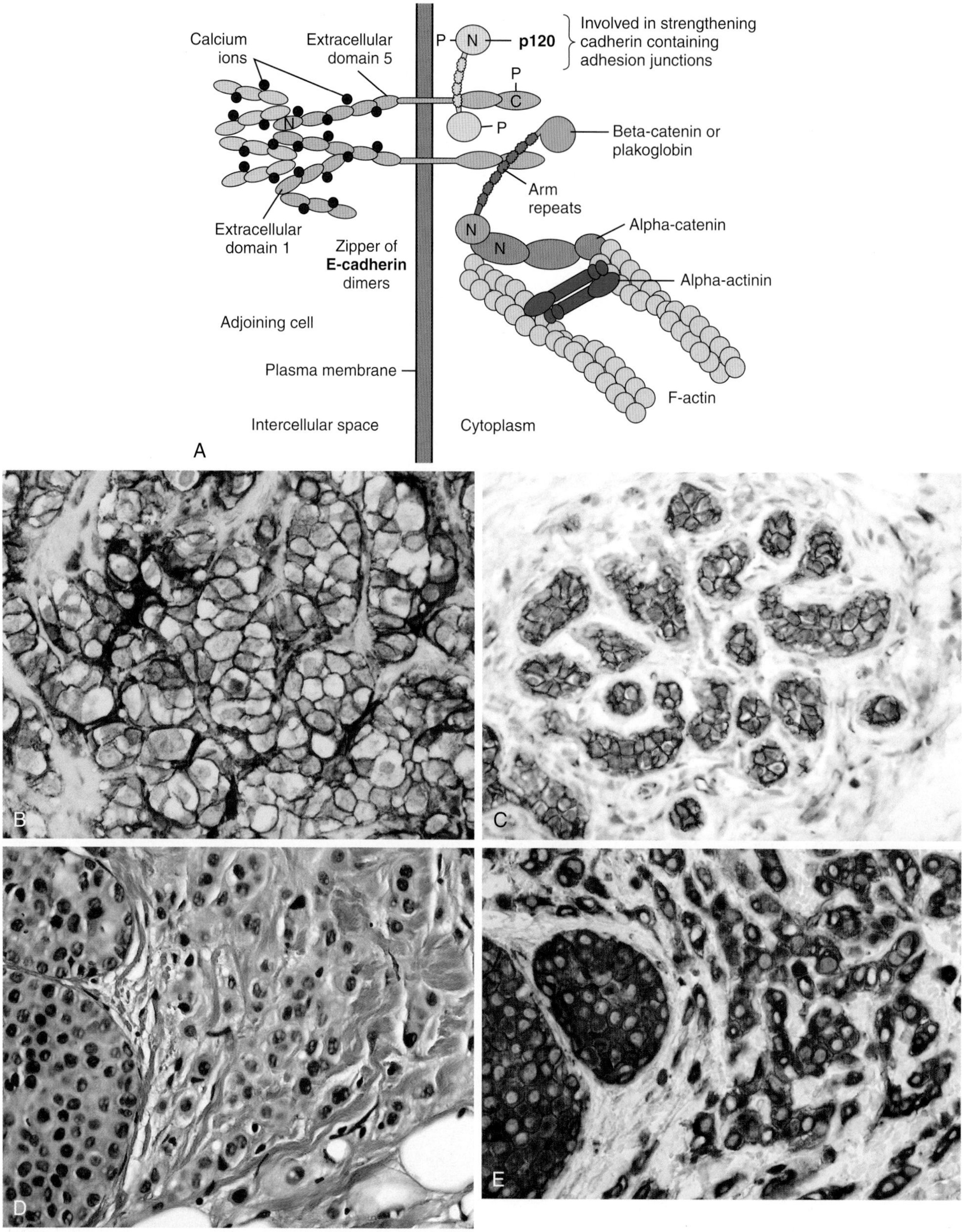

FIGURE 19.20 Diagrammatic representation of ECAD relationship to p120 **(A)**. The dynamic biology of ECAD-p120 can be illustrated using a dual ECAD (brown)-p120 (red) stain **(B** and **C)**. In this example of invasive ductal carcinoma, strong membranous reactivity (reddish-brown) is identified for both ECAD and p120 **(B)**. Similar reddish-brown membranous staining is identified in acinar cells within this lobule **(C)**. An example of invasive and *in situ* lobular carcinoma **(D)** demonstrates strong cytoplasmic immunoreactivity for p120 using a single color stain **(E)**.

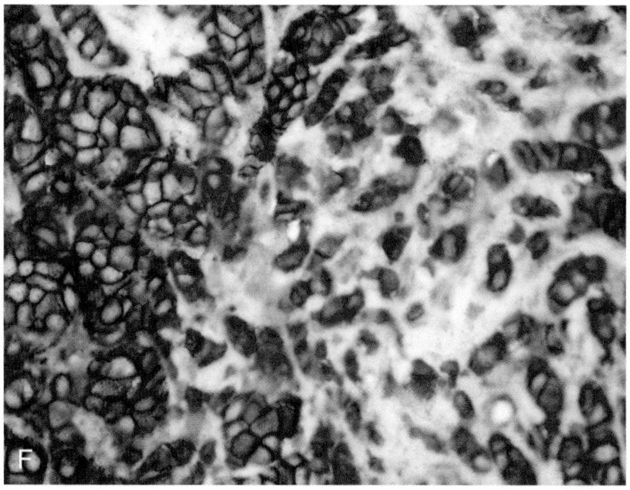

FIGURE 19.20, cont'd A dual ECAD-p120 stain demonstrates membranous ECAD and p120 (reddish-brown) immunoreactivity in the ductal component with lack of ECAD (absence of brown staining) but strong cytoplasmic p120 (red) staining in this example of mixed ductal and lobular carcinoma **(F).**

a low nuclear grade are not lobular carcinomas, as invasive ductal carcinomas also have this pattern.

The morphologic assessment of a ductal or lobular phenotype is not without controversy, and it has limitations. The classic infiltrating lobular carcinoma (ILC) is composed of small cells with bland cytology and some plasmacytoid features. The growth pattern is completely dyshesive. Breast tissue can appear normal grossly (as well as on the mammogram) yet show widespread dyshesive carcinoma of the classic type. These tumors are uniformly ECAD negative and associated with specific patterns of systemic metastases.[98] Invasive ductal carcinomas (IDC) can also show patterns seen in ILC (e.g., single-filing of tumor cells, targetoid patterns, and regional dyshesiveness). Such patterns may be confusing but are readily resolved with ECAD immunostaining. There are subgroups of morphologically indeterminate lobular/ductal phenotypes. ECAD separates these groups distinctly in most cases and demonstrates the existence of mixed lobular-ductal phenotypes in a minority of cases.[99-101] ECAD stains myoepithelial cells, a pitfall for misinterpretation of LCIS as DCIS (see Fig. 19.18A).

The morphologic reproducibility of distinguishing IDC from ILC and LCIS from DCIS is less than optimal. There can be substantial variation in the interpretation of ILC versus IDC and LCIS versus DCIS. For this reason alone, ECAD and similarly p120 IHC could be justified to aid in correctly classifying these lesions.

KEY DIAGNOSTIC POINTS

Ductal versus Lobular Carcinoma

- ECAD stain is a useful diagnostic adjunct in cases with indeterminate morphology.
- p120 further enhances diagnostic accuracy because it is a positive stain for lobular carcinoma.
- Lobular lesions are characteristically negative for ECAD and demonstrate intense cytoplasmic immunoreactivity for p120.
- Normal ducts and ductal lesions demonstrate membranous staining for ECAD and p120.

Lobular Carcinoma Variants and Former Lobular Variants

PLEOMORPHIC LOBULAR CARCINOMA

Bassler in 1980[102] as well as Weidner,[103] Eusebi,[104] and Reis-Filho[105] have detailed the genetic, immunohistologic, and clinical features sufficiently to recognize invasive pleomorphic lobular carcinoma (PLC) and pleomorphic lobular carcinoma *in situ* (PLCIS) as a distinct clinicopathologic entity.[106-109] Based on cell cohesiveness, PLC and PLCIS are basically a subtype of lobular carcinoma. The histologically recognizable PLC and PLCIS are almost always ECAD negative (or show aberrant staining) and demonstrate strong cytoplasmic immunoreactivity for p120.[110] Histologically, they show grade 3 nuclei with a dyshesive pattern of growth in both *in situ* and infiltrating varieties (Fig. 19.22). The *in situ* component may be discovered on mammograms as calcifications. The core biopsies demonstrate *in situ* dyshesive grade 3 nuclei with some cases showing comedonecrosis and calcification. Recently a comprehensive analysis of 26 PLCs revealed a closer association between PLC and classic lobular carcinoma than between PLC and ductal carcinoma.[111] The authors used IHC, array comparative genomic hybridization (aCGH), fluorescence *in situ* hybridization (FISH), and chromogenic *in situ* hybridization (CISH) to analyze 26 cases of PLC, 16 cases of classic lobular carcinoma, and 34 cases of IDC. Comparative analysis of aCGH data suggested that the molecular features of PLC (ER+, PR+, E-cadherin–, 1q+, 11q–, 16p+, and 16q–) were more closely related to those of classic ILC than IDC. However, PLCs also showed some molecular alterations that are more typical of high-grade IDC than ILC: p53+ and HER+ in some cases; 8q+, 17q24-q25+, 13q–; and amplification of 8q24, 12q14, 17q12, and 20q13. Some of these IDC-like alterations may be responsible for the aggressive biology of PLC.

Sneige and colleagues studied 24 cases of PLCIS by immunohistochemistry and found them to be universally positive for ER (100%).[112] They also showed frequent p53 reactivity (25%) and moderate to high proliferative activity. *HER2* positivity was seen in 4%

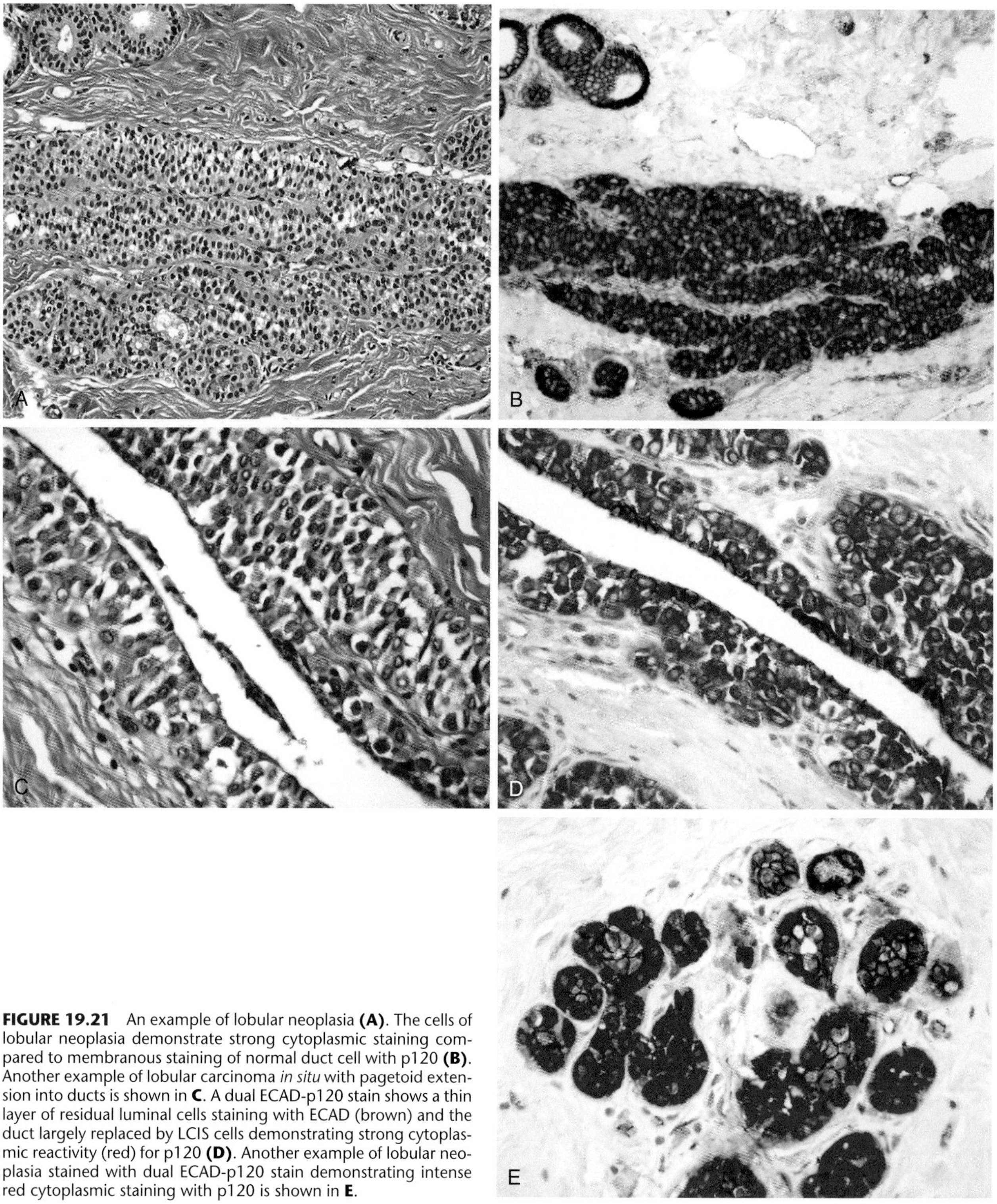

FIGURE 19.21 An example of lobular neoplasia **(A)**. The cells of lobular neoplasia demonstrate strong cytoplasmic staining compared to membranous staining of normal duct cell with p120 **(B)**. Another example of lobular carcinoma *in situ* with pagetoid extension into ducts is shown in **C**. A dual ECAD-p120 stain shows a thin layer of residual luminal cells staining with ECAD (brown) and the duct largely replaced by LCIS cells demonstrating strong cytoplasmic reactivity (red) for p120 **(D)**. Another example of lobular neoplasia stained with dual ECAD-p120 stain demonstrating intense red cytoplasmic staining with p120 is shown in **E**.

of cases. Fourteen cases were associated with PLC that showed similar IHC profile. Our experience with PLC and PLCIS is also very similar. Although *HER2* overexpression/amplification may be seen in PLCs, the *HER2* positivity rate is not very high, as previously reported.[108] Also, PLCs are ER positive in the majority of cases, albeit expression levels may vary from case to case. Because there is a high likelihood for developing invasive carcinoma in the vicinity of PLCIS, these lesions should be managed similar to DCIS.

Tubulolobular Carcinoma

Described originally by Fisher in 1977 as a lobular growth pattern with tiny tubules and single-filing characteristic of lobular carcinoma, the prognosis of

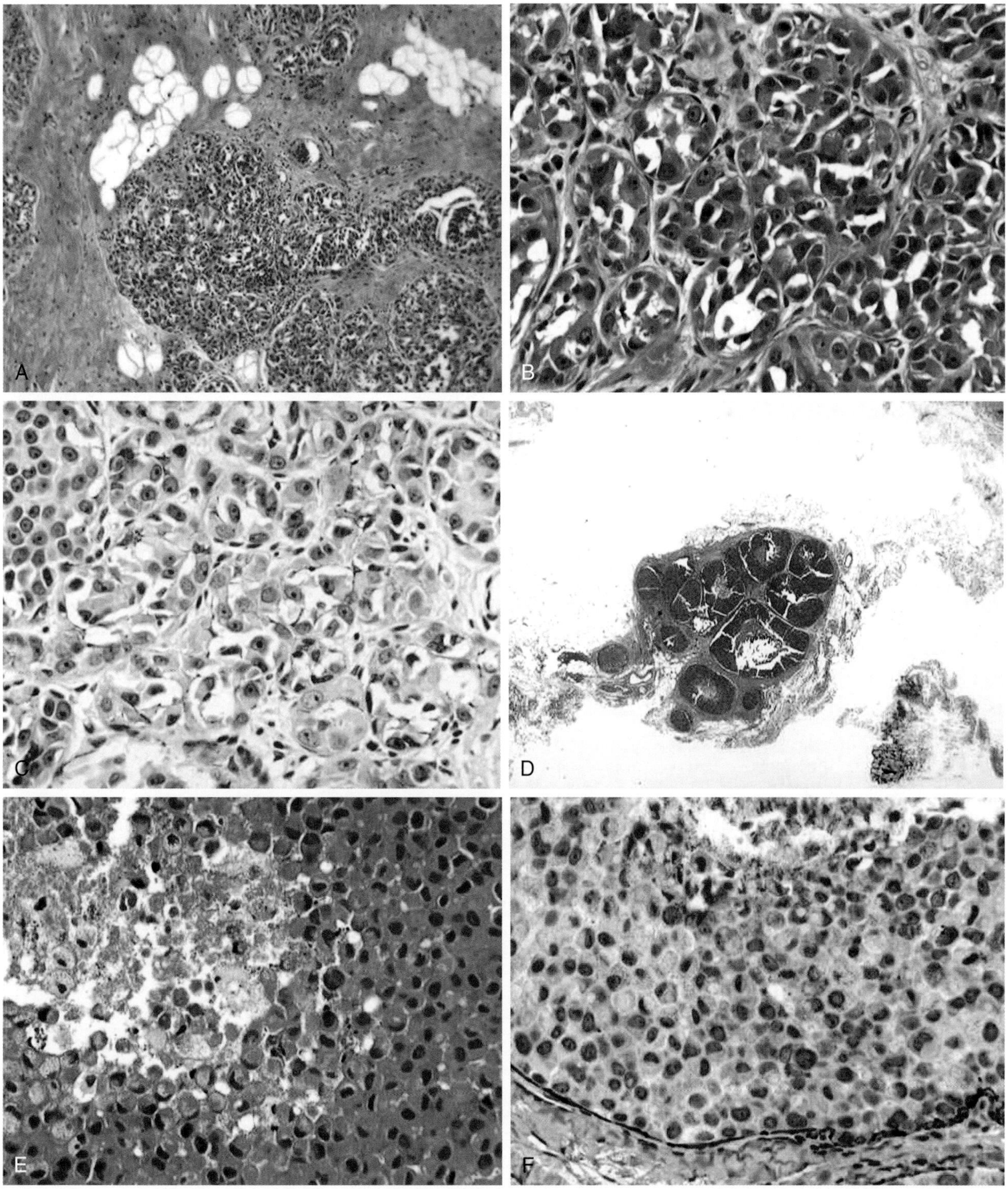

FIGURE 19.22 Pleomorphic LCIS (PLCIS) in lobular arrangement showing nuclear grade 3 and prominent nucleoli **(A** and **B)**. PLCIS is ECAD-negative **(C)**. Shown is low magnification of PLCIS with comedonecrosis and calcification simulating DCIS **(D)**. Note the dyshesion and plasmacytoid cellular features characteristic of PLCIS **(E)**. ECAD is negative in PLCIS and positive in myoepithelial cells **(F)**.

tubulolobular carcinoma was described as intermediate between that of pure tubular carcinoma and infiltrating lobular carcinoma.[113,114] This lesion had been categorized as a variant of ILC because of the small cells and characteristic ILC pattern of single-filing and targetoid infiltration.

Wheeler as well as Esposito recently documented uniform membranous ECAD immunostaining in the tubules and lobular-appearing components (Fig. 19.23).[115,116] Both Wheeler and Esposito discovered that pure LCIS and mixed LCIS/DCIS predominate in these lesions. Uniform membranous ECAD immunoreactivity in tubulolobular carcinoma supports ductal differentiation of the tumor cells.

Histiocytoid Carcinoma

The term *histiocytoid breast carcinoma* (HBC) was coined by Hood and colleagues because the tumor cells resembled histiocytes.[117] In 1983, Filotico described a case of lobular-appearing carcinoma with histiocytic features.[118] Subsequent reports assumed that this variant was of lobular type by virtue of the characteristic infiltrating pattern. Until recently, published immunohistologic studies on this rare entity were unavailable. Gupta and coworkers[119] reported on the largest series and found that 8 of 11 cases lacked ECAD and 8 of 11 had LCIS. Three cases had ECAD; the authors concluded that the histiocytic appearance and lack of distinct clinical features were insufficient to ascribe a distinct entity of histiocytoid carcinoma. The current evidence suggests that HBC is a morphologic pattern that can be observed in ductal, lobular, and apocrine tumors and may not be a distinct entity by itself.[120]

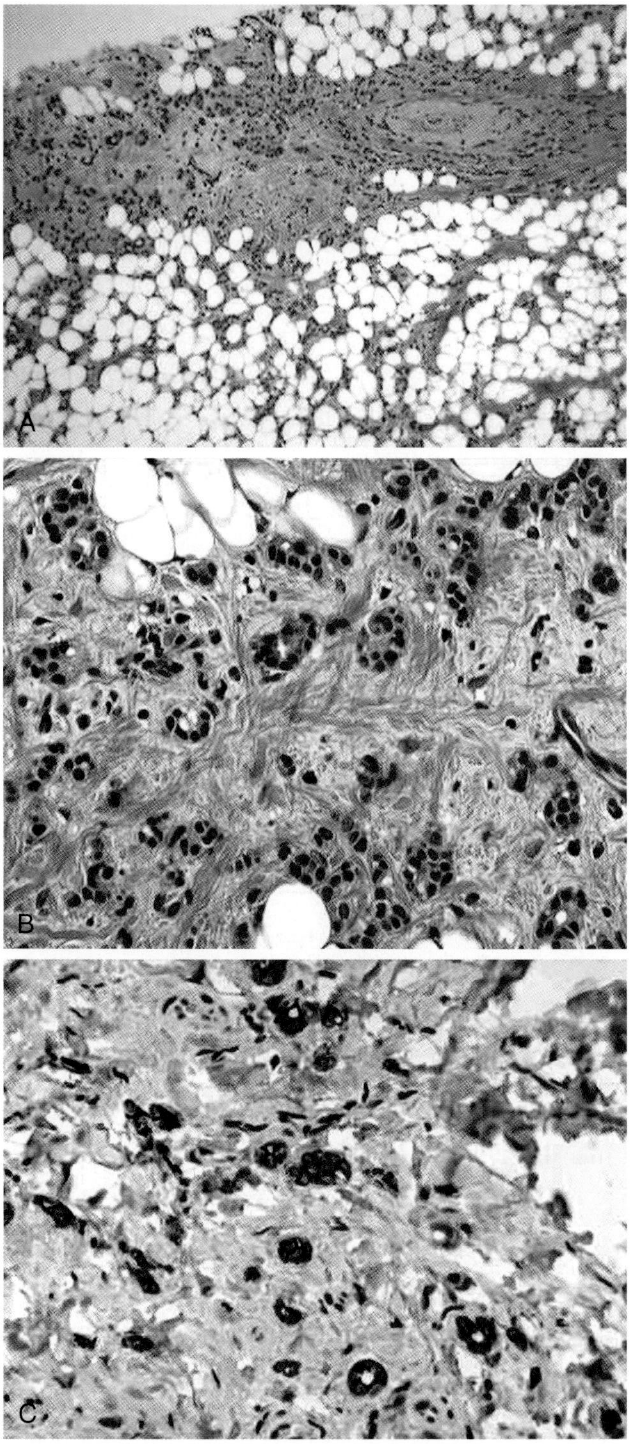

FIGURE 19.23 Pattern of infiltration of tubulolobular carcinoma (TLC) is similar to lobular carcinoma **(A)**. Tiny tubules populate the tumor, which otherwise simulates lobular carcinoma **(B)**. ECAD is positive in tiny tubules and single cells **(C)**.

Immunohistochemistry for Identifying Special Types of Breast Carcinomas

INVASIVE MICROPAPILLARY CARCINOMA: USE OF EMA

Tight clusters of neoplastic cells surrounded by clear spaces characterize the invasive micropapillary carcinoma.[121,122] The cell clusters are devoid of fibrovascular cores (unlike papillary carcinoma) and often display tubular structures in the center. The stroma is typically described as "spongy" with little or no desmoplasia of the surrounding tissue.[121,122] Some ductal carcinomas of "no special type" (NST) also show clear spaces around neoplastic cells, which are likely due to retraction of intervening fibrotic stroma and should not be confused with micropapillary morphology. Fortunately, the distinction between true micropapillary carcinoma and NST carcinoma with retraction artifact can be easily made by EMA (or MUC1) stain.[121,123,124] Ductal carcinoma of NST shows apical or cytoplasmic staining with EMA. In contrast, invasive micropapillary carcinomas show accentuation of the basal surface (stroma facing) of the neoplastic cells (Fig. 19.24). This reverse polarity of neoplastic cells is a characteristic feature of invasive micropapillary carcinoma. The distinction between a ductal NST and micropapillary carcinoma may not be clinically very significant because stage for stage, there is no significant difference between the two entities. However, micropapillary morphology (even when small) is highly predictive of lymph node metastases, and these tumors also more commonly tend to involve the skin and chest wall.[125-129] The incidence of axillary lymph node metastasis has been reported to be as high as 95%.[130] Therefore, we believe that a confident diagnosis of a true micropapillary carcinoma based on a core biopsy can help the surgeon plan appropriate management, such as paying special attention to and performing a clinical exam of the axilla, performing fine-needle aspiration if axillary nodes are slightly enlarged (but not definitely suspicious), and requesting an intra-operative frozen section even if the lymph node is grossly negative.

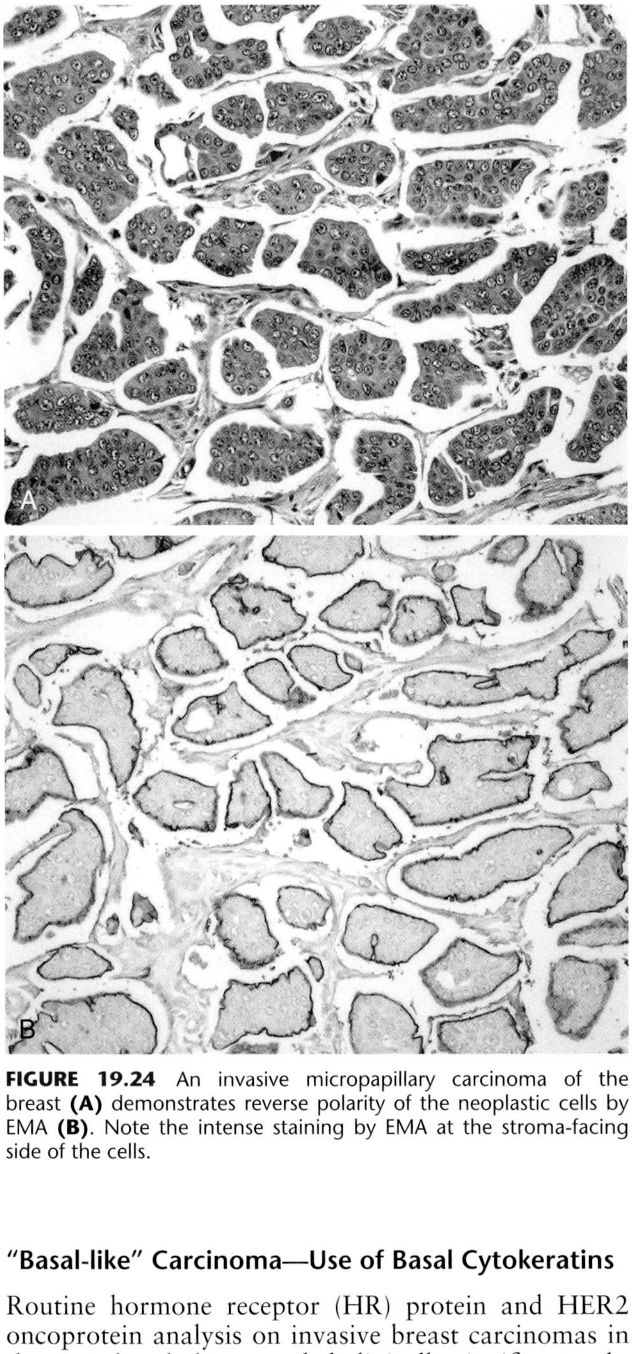

FIGURE 19.24 An invasive micropapillary carcinoma of the breast **(A)** demonstrates reverse polarity of the neoplastic cells by EMA **(B)**. Note the intense staining by EMA at the stroma-facing side of the cells.

"Basal-like" Carcinoma—Use of Basal Cytokeratins

Routine hormone receptor (HR) protein and HER2 oncoprotein analysis on invasive breast carcinomas in the past decade has revealed clinically significant subgroups. One such group is that of "triple negative" tumors (i.e., tumors that are negative for all three biomarkers [ER, PR, and HER2]). These tumors have been known to be clinically aggressive, and therapeutic options are limited because they are not amenable to HR-based therapy or HER2-targeted therapy. The so-called basal-like breast carcinomas constitute at least 85% of the triple negative tumors. The basal-like subtype was initially recognized by gene-expression profiling studies.[131,132] Basal-like carcinomas are histologically characterized by high Nottingham grade, geographic necrosis, good circumscription, and mild to moderate host lymphocytic response.[133] These tumors generally show reduced (not absent) E-cadherin membranous expression but strong membranous p120 immunoreactivity (unpublished data). Therefore, we consider them as subtypes of ductal carcinomas. Basal-like carcinomas are characteristically triple negative and show expression of basal-type cytokeratin (CK5/6, CK14, CK17), EGFR, vimentin, and p53.[133,134] Often, a panel of basal-type cytokeratins and EGFR in triple-negative tumors is used to identify basal-like carcinomas (Fig. 19.25). The immunomarkers used to identify the basal-like variant is an example of genomic application of immunohistochemistry. This details fundamental immunohistologic profiles, used as surrogate markers, that reflect a genomic profile. We have recently shown that antibody to CK5 (clone XM26) is much more sensitive (but equally specific) than CK5/6 (clone D5/16B4) for identifying basal-like breast carcinomas.[135] Our immunohistochemical studies have also confirmed the existence of *in situ* carcinoma of basal phenotype.[136,137] Gene-expression studies have consistently identified basal-like carcinomas to have poor prognosis.[132,138,139] These tumors occur in both pre- and post-menopausal patients; however, identifying basal-like carcinoma in a young pre-menopausal patient may suggest the presence of hereditary breast and ovarian carcinoma syndrome.[140] Although there are no specific chemotherapeutic drugs currently available to treat these patients, data are emerging that it is important to recognize these tumors as therapies become more refined.

KEY DIAGNOSTIC POINTS

Expression Profile of Basal-like Carcinomas

- CK5 is superior to CK5/6 in sensitivity and is comparable in specificity for identifying basal-like tumors by IHC.
- A recommended panel for detection of basal-like triple negative tumors is ER/PR/HER2–, CK5+, EGFR+/–, CK14+/–, and CK17+/–.

Metaplastic Carcinoma—Use of Keratins, Melanoma, and Vascular Markers

Metaplastic carcinoma comprises a group of heterogeneous neoplasms that exhibit pure epithelial or mixed epithelial and mesenchymal phenotypes.[141,142] Diagnosis is not problematic when there is a recognizable component of metaplastic carcinoma (i.e., an obvious adenocarcinoma, adenosquamous or squamous cell carcinoma, or osseous or chondroid differentiation). The most problematic cases are those that predominantly show spindle cell morphology without an obvious epithelial or DCIS component (Fig. 19.26). This is usually the issue on a core biopsy rather than on an excision specimen. IHC stains can be helpful in this situation.[141] A panel composed of multiple keratin stains (CAM5.2, AE1/3, 34βE12, CK5, and CK7) and EMA is more useful than a single keratin.[143] Another sensitive and specific marker for metaplastic carcinoma is p63, and it should always be included in the panel.[144,145] Vimentin expression in the tumor does not exclude a

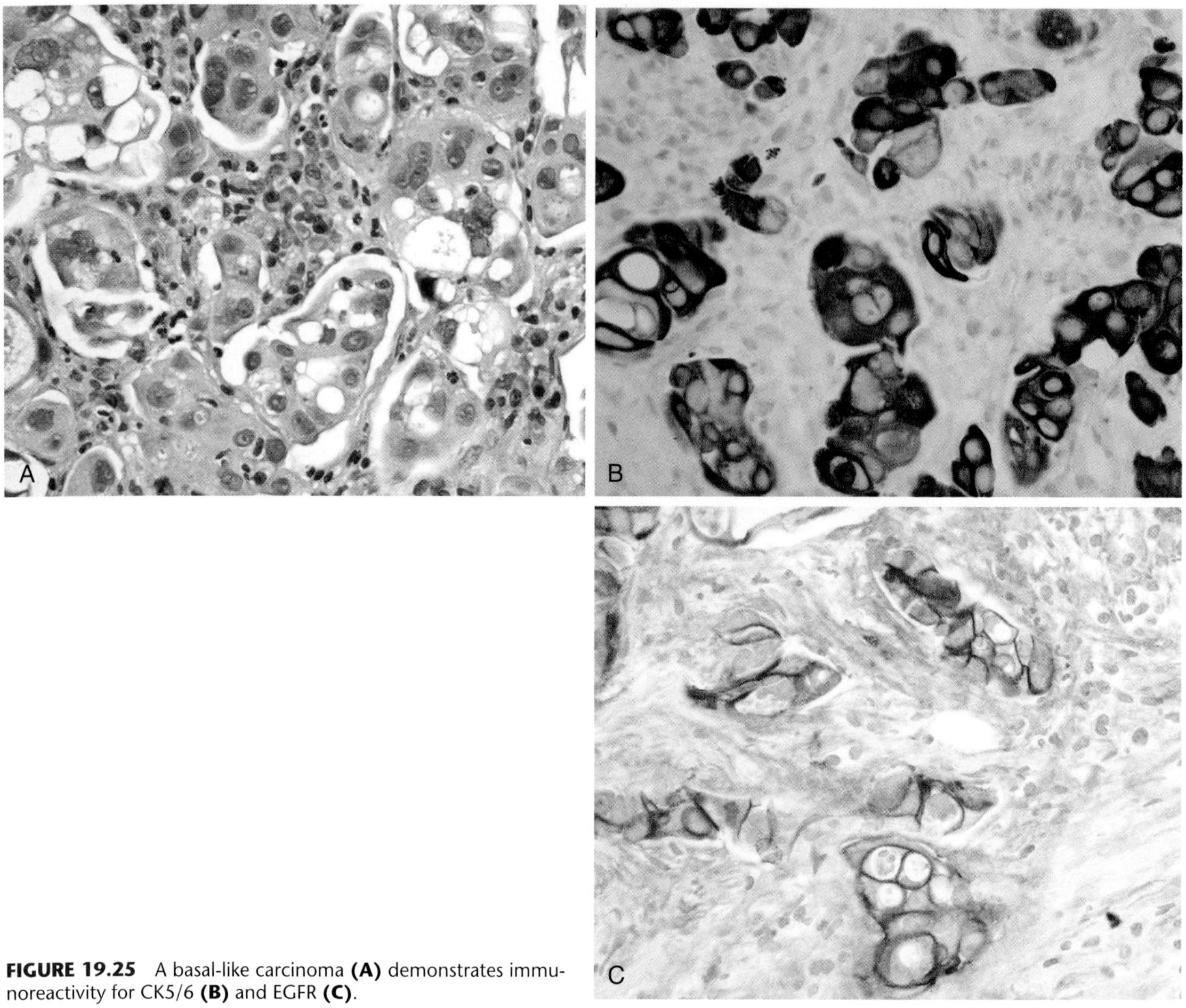

FIGURE 19.25 A basal-like carcinoma **(A)** demonstrates immunoreactivity for CK5/6 **(B)** and EGFR **(C)**.

spindle cell carcinoma.[143,146,147] Vimentin expression has been found in 50% of hormone-independent cell lines and is actually expected because metaplastic carcinomas are usually negative for receptors.[148] If all the keratins, EMA, and p63 fail to show any immunoreactivity on a core biopsy, complete excision of the lesion should be recommended. In many cases, an epithelial component is present only focally. Although every effort should be made to prove an atypical spindle cell lesion to be a metaplastic carcinoma, it is important not to forget that melanomas and angiosarcomas can also occur in the breast. At least two melanoma markers should be performed. S100 is a very sensitive melanoma marker but has been reported to stain 20% to 50% of metaplastic breast carcinomas and therefore is not the best stain for this differential diagnosis.[149,150] Strong keratin reactivity or multiple keratin positivity would also exclude a melanoma. However, CAM5.2 positivity alone is not enough to exclude a melanoma unless it is strong and diffuse.[151,152] Another significant malignant lesion with which metaplastic carcinoma can be confused is an angiosarcoma. These tumors may occur after radiation treatment or *de novo*. It is obvious to think about angiosarcoma in a malignant spindle or epithelioid lesion of the breast if there has been a prior history of radiation treatment. However, in absence of such a clinical history, the lesion should be extensively examined by means of available IHC stains. More than one vascular marker should be used owing to the heterogeneous expression of vascular markers.[153] Of the three commonly used vascular markers (CD31, CD34, and Factor VIII), CD31 is generally considered the most specific vascular endothelial marker, but occasional weak staining of carcinomas has been described.[154] We have also seen equivocal staining of carcinoma cells with CD31, likely because of neovascularization within the tumor. It is a diagnostic pitfall, especially in small samples. A diagnosis of a *de novo* primary angiosarcoma of the breast should be made only if there is unequivocal IHC staining for vascular markers, negative staining for p63 and high molecular weight keratins, and appropriate histologic findings in the lesion. In summary, a malignant spindle cell lesion is a metaplastic carcinoma unless proven otherwise. A panel composed of multiple keratins, EMA,

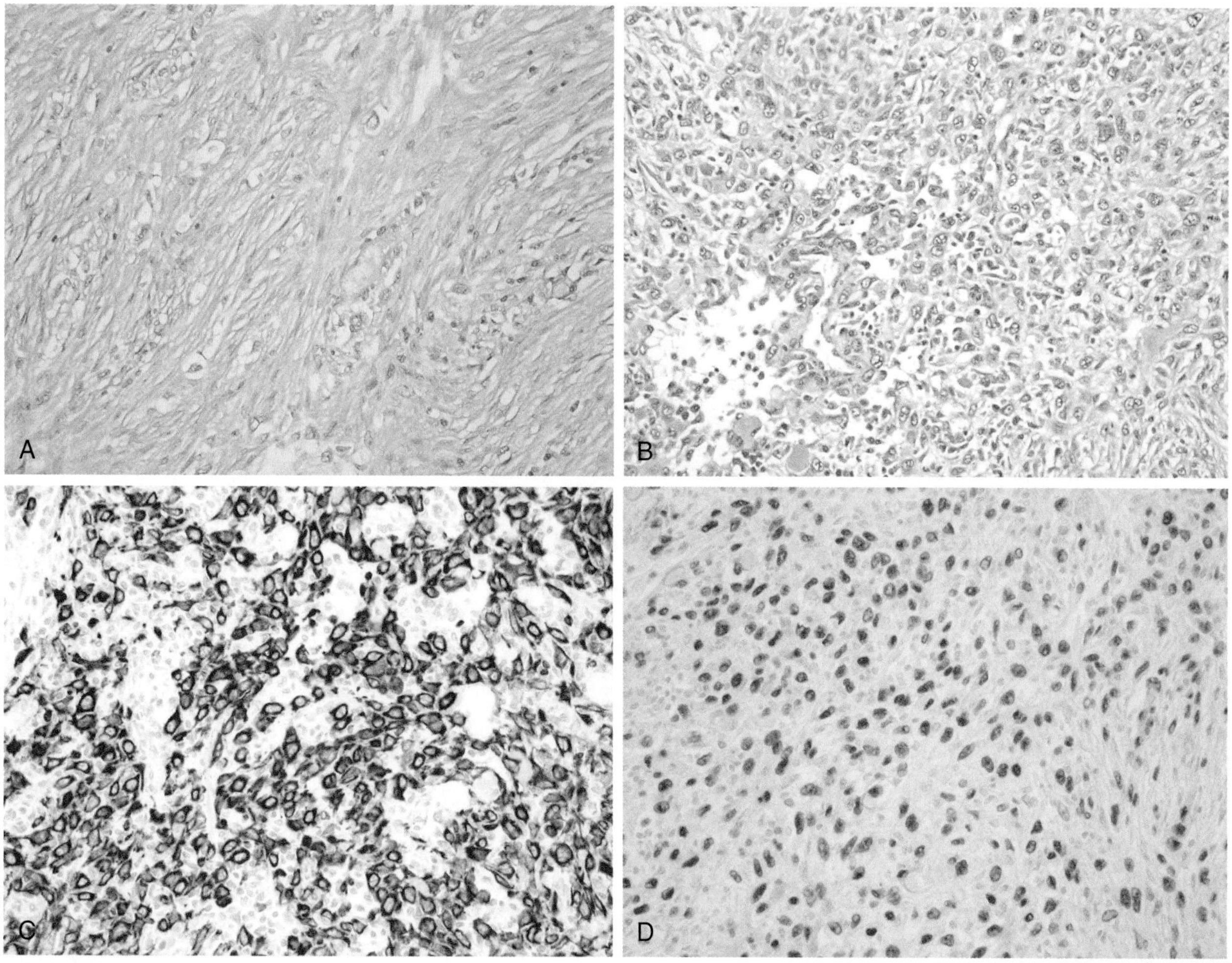

FIGURE 19.26 This predominantly spindle cell neoplasm **(A)** showed only a focal area of epithelioid malignant cells **(B)**. The tumor was completely negative for AE1/3 and CAM5.2 but demonstrated staining for basal cytokeratins (CK5/6, CK14, CK17) and p63 (**C** and **D**, respectively), supporting the diagnosis of spindle cell metaplastic carcinoma.

p63, melanoma, and vascular markers is required in the workup of a malignant spindle cell lesion.

Other Spindle Cell Neoplasms (Myoepithelial and Mesenchymal Tumors)

Tumors of the breast in which MEC differentiation predominates include adenomyoepithelioma, myoepithelioma, and myoepithelial cell carcinoma (MECC).[155-158] Although the majority of adenomyoepitheliomas are benign, occasional tumors may exhibit aggressive behavior in the form of carcinoma or myoepithelial carcinoma.[159,160] The typical immunostaining pattern of the myoepithelial components of these tumors is strong cytoplasmic staining for 34βE12, CK5, and nuclear p63. Tumor cells are typically positive with S-100 protein (90%) and may be positive with muscle markers such as calponin (86%), desmin (14%), and alpha-smooth muscle actin (36%).[155,157] Occasional cells exhibit immunostaining with glial fibrillary acidic protein (GFAP). The presence of smooth muscle markers and immunostaining for GFAP is more in keeping with pure myoepithelial differentiation as opposed to metaplastic carcinomas (discussed earlier in the chapter), which are largely negative for these markers.[161,162] Expression of smooth muscle actin is very non-specific and is not a definitive marker for muscle differentiation. Metaplastic carcinomas of the breast (carcinosarcoma, spindle cell carcinoma, and sarcomatoid carcinoma) have an immunoprofile very similar to myoepithelial differentiation, as they regularly coexpress weak cytoplasmic CAM5.2 for low molecular weight keratins; strong cytoplasmic immunostaining for high molecular weight keratin 34βE12, CK5/6 or CK5, and vimentin; and nuclear immunostaining for p63 (90%).[144] However, findings for GFAP and smooth-muscle myosin heavy chain are largely negative. Immunostaining with the muscle markers is most indicative of a pure myoepithelial neoplasm as opposed to a metaplastic carcinoma. The immunoprofile of metaplastic carcinoma is shared to a great degree with myoepithelial neoplasms, with some investigators suggesting that the myoepithelial cell is the progenitor cell for metaplastic carcinomas.[149,150,163,164] Leibl recently demonstrated that the newly discovered experimental myoepithelial markers CD29 and 14-3-3 sigma stain metaplastic carcinomas,

TABLE 19.4 Metaplastic Carcinoma versus Spindle Cell Sarcoma of the Breast

Diagnosis	CK5/6	34βE12	P63	GFAP	S-100	HHF-35
Metaplastic carcinoma	+	+	+	N	N	S
Myoepithelial carcinoma	+	S	+	S	+	+
Fibrosarcoma	N	N	N	N	N	R-N
Myosarcoma	N	N	R-N	N	N	+
MPNST	N	N	N	N	S	N
Synovial sarcoma	N	N	N	N	R-N	N

+, almost always positive; S, sometimes positive; R, rare; N, negative.
GFAP, glial fibrillary acidic protein; MPNST, malignant peripheral nerve sheath tumor.

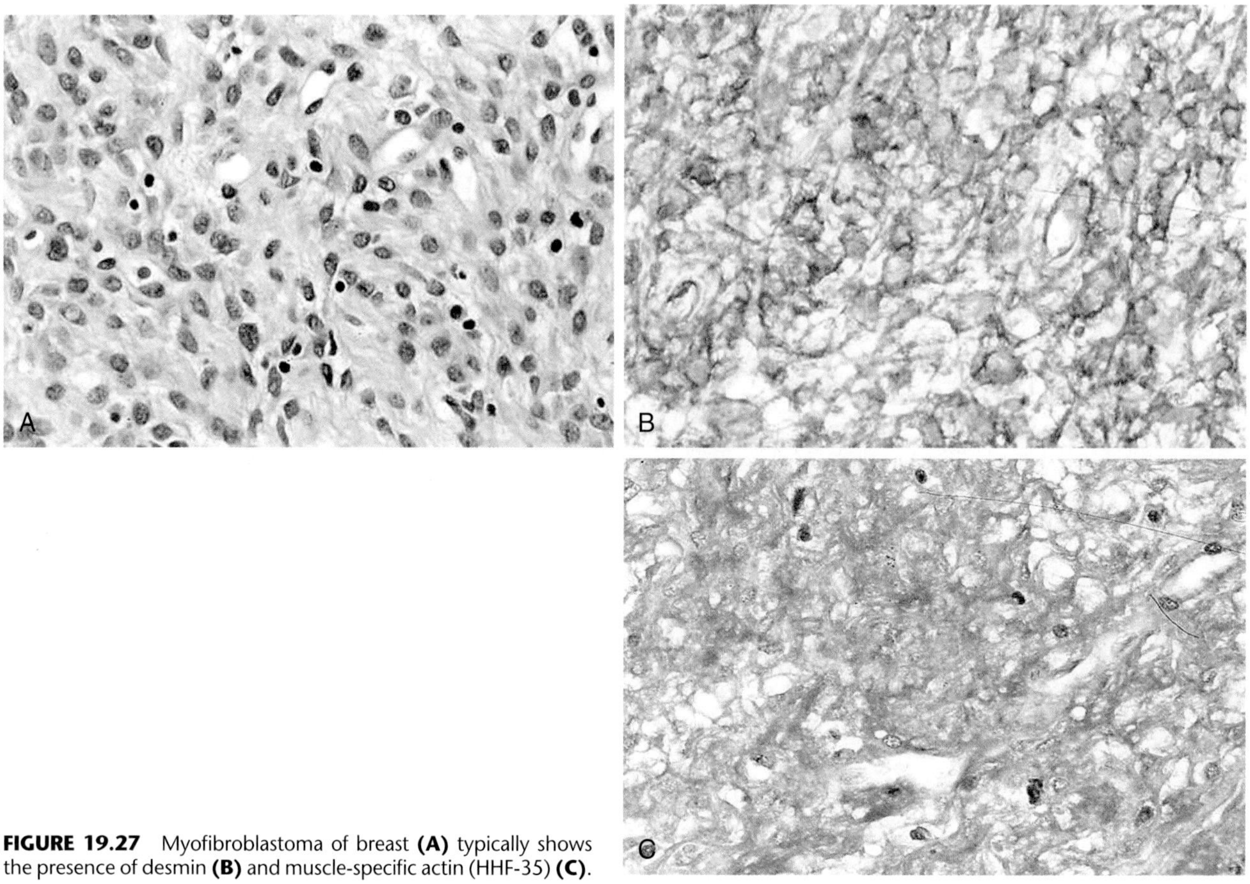

FIGURE 19.27 Myofibroblastoma of breast **(A)** typically shows the presence of desmin **(B)** and muscle-specific actin (HHF-35) **(C)**.

supplying further evidence of the myoepithelial nature of these tumors.[150] The literature suggests that using the term *myoepithelial carcinoma* versus *metaplastic carcinoma* is a matter of semantics and may not have any clinical significance.

Myoepithelial tumors need to be separated from the rare primary spindle cell sarcoma of the breast, which may include fibrosarcoma (vimentin-positive), leiomyosarcoma, and rhabdomyosarcoma (positive for muscle markers); synovial sarcoma (CK7+ and CK19+);[165] malignant nerve sheath tumors (S-100+ and vimentin+); and malignant fibrous histiocytomas (vimentin+). Although each of these tumors may have characteristic light-microscopic features, immunostaining patterns may be useful in the diagnostic distinction (Table 19.4). Primary liposarcomas (S-100+) of breast are rare tumors that may arise in a pre-existing phyllodes tumor (CD34+ stroma).

The rare myofibroblastoma of the breast (Fig. 19.27) is distinguished immunohistochemically from myoepithelial tumors by lack of immunostaining for keratins, S-100 protein, and SMMHC.[166-168] The myofibroblastoma may also demonstrate CD34+ cells. In contrast, fibromatosis involving the breast is negative for CD34 but may demonstrate abnormal (nuclear) localization of β-catenin.[149,169]

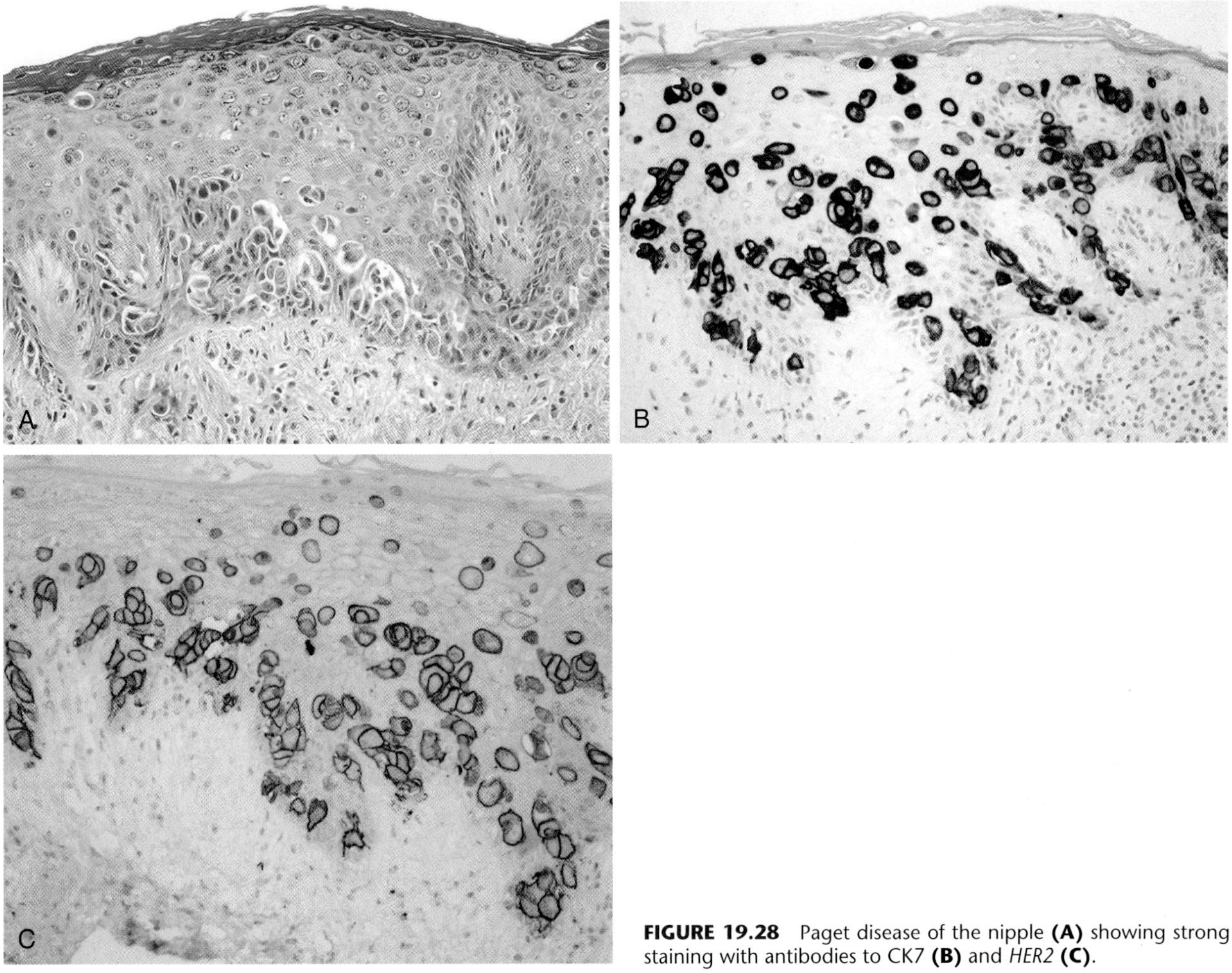

FIGURE 19.28 Paget disease of the nipple **(A)** showing strong staining with antibodies to CK7 **(B)** and *HER2* **(C)**.

KEY DIAGNOSTIC POINTS

Tumor Type Identification by IHC

- Micropapillary carcinomas can be confidently identified using EMA (or MUC1), which demonstrates reverse polarity of the tumor cells.
- Basal-like carcinomas are triple negative and show immunoreactivity for basal cytokeratins and EGFR.
- CK5 (clone XM26) is the most sensitive stain for identifying basal-like breast carcinomas.
- Basal cytokeratins along with p63 are also very sensitive markers for identifying spindle cell metaplastic carcinomas.
- Although muscle differentiation in myoepithelial carcinomas separates them from spindle cell metaplastic carcinomas, they likely represent two different spectra of one entity.
- Adenomyoepitheliomas are biphasic tumors that resemble (are a variant of) intraductal papilloma at one extreme and show pure spindle cell myoepithelioma at the other extreme.
- Non-carcinomatous spindle cell proliferation in a breast core biopsy sample includes fibromatosis, myofibroblastoma, stromal component of phyllodes tumor, or rare primary sarcomas.

PAGET DISEASE OF THE BREAST

Paget disease occurs in mammary and extramammary (EM) forms. Paget disease of the breast is almost always indicative of an underlying breast carcinoma, which may be *in situ* or invasive, whereas EM Paget disease may be an indicator of metastatic carcinoma.

Paget disease of the breast is manifested as CK7-positive malignant cells infiltrating the epidermis of the nipple. Tumor cells are conspicuous by their infiltrative "shotgun" pattern, large size, abundant cytoplasm, signet-ring forms, and, sometimes, mucin positivity (Fig. 19.28).

The majority of the underlying breast carcinomas are ductal in nature.[170,171] For a nipple/areola biopsy or a cases in which underlying carcinoma cannot be documented, the differential diagnosis for Paget disease includes melanoma and squamous cell carcinoma *in situ* (Bowen disease). The single best stain for this differential diagnosis is CK7, which is positive in almost all cases of Paget disease (see Fig. 19.28). Cells of Paget disease are also positive for HER2 (in approximately 80% to 90% of cases).[172-175] This correlates to the IHC expression of underlying breast carcinoma, which is often an HER2-positive high-grade DCIS with comedonecrosis.[176] Additional stains that can be positive in Paget disease

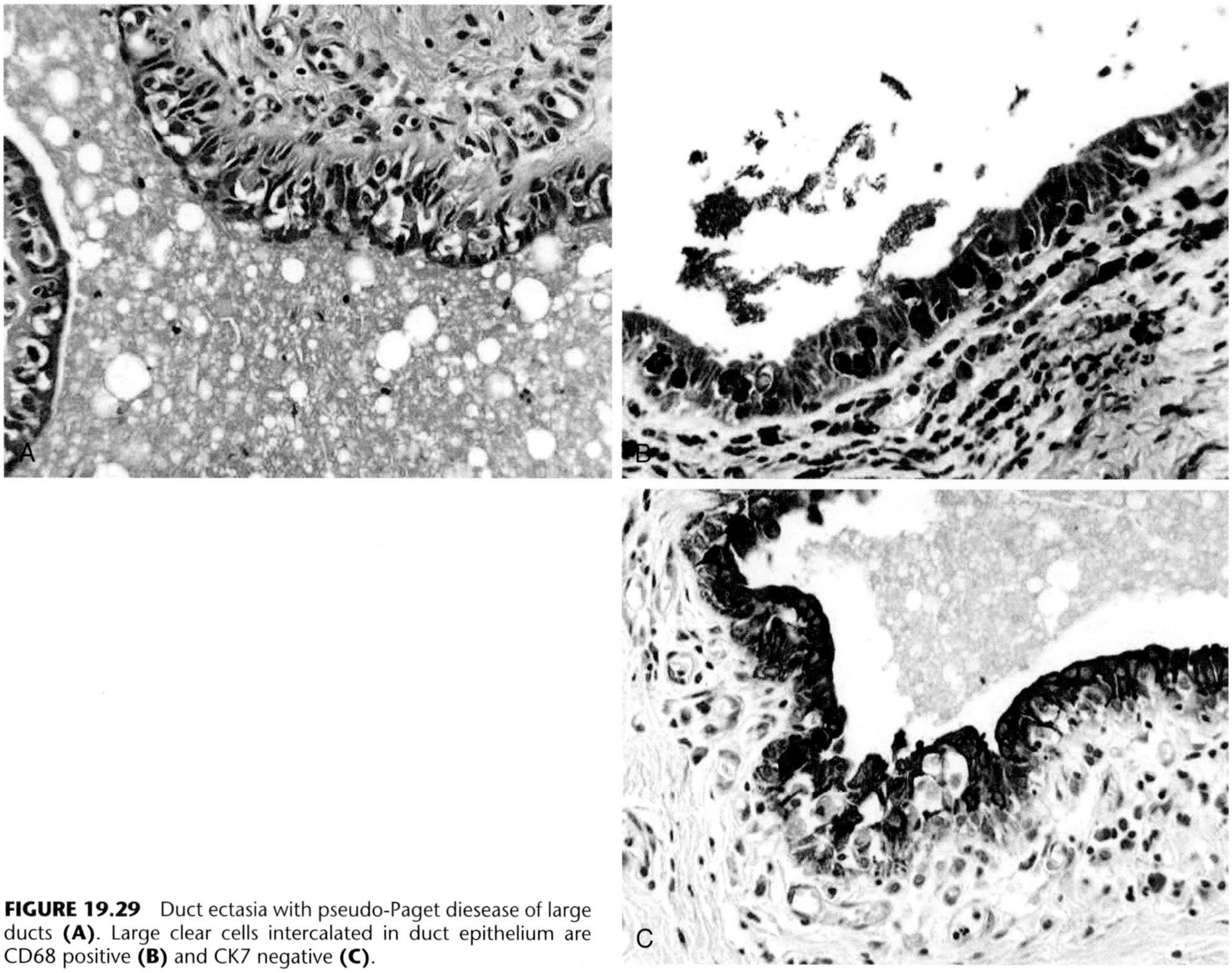

FIGURE 19.29 Duct ectasia with pseudo-Paget diesease of large ducts **(A)**. Large clear cells intercalated in duct epithelium are CD68 positive **(B)** and CK7 negative **(C)**.

are gross cystic disease fluid protein-15 (GCDFP15+), polyclonal carcinoembryonic antigen (pCEA+), and hormone receptors.[177] However, it is important to remember that estrogen receptors (ERs) and progesterone receptors (PRs) are not good markers of Paget disease. Although Paget disease is a manifestation of underlying breast carcinoma, most often the carcinoma is a DCIS with comedonecrosis, and these tumors are frequently negative for HRs.[178] If the possibility of a melanoma is entertained, then at least two melanoma markers should be used because S-100 can be positive in about 18% of Paget disease cases.[179] However, it should be noted that malignant melanoma on the nipple is extraordinarily rare. Pagetoid squamous carcinoma (Bowen disease) of the breast is rare, and it can be distinguished from Paget disease. Cells of Bowen disease are negative for CK7, and one can confirm the squamous nature of the cells by CK5/6 and p63 stains, while Paget shows reverse result for these antibodies.

Toker cells are CK7 positive and may be present in the skin of the normal nipple,[180] but generally they are inconspicuous compared with Paget cells, are cytologically bland, and do not cause diagnostic problems. It has been suggested that Toker cells may be the origin of intraepithelial Paget cells, based on similarity of immunophenotypes.[181] In cases of florid papillomatosis of the nipple, some CK7-positive cells may be found in the epidermis, a pitfall to be aware of in diagnosing Paget disease of the nipple.[182] In addition, the intraepidermal portion of nipple ducts can be a pitfall in the diagnosis of intraepidermal CK7-positive cells.[183]

Pseudo-Paget disease may on occasion be seen in the major ducts. Large histiocytes infiltrate the epithelium and impart a picture simulating Paget disease. These large cells are CK7 negative and strongly positive for CD68 (Fig. 19.29).

KEY DIAGNOSTIC POINTS

Mammary Paget Disease

- Most often positive in Paget disease: CK7, HER2
- Other positive but less helpful stains: GCDFP15, pCEA, ER, PR
- Pitfall: CK7-positive cells in the epidermis in cases of florid nipple duct papillomatosis; Toker cells or intraepithelial extension of lactiferous duct cells
- Pagetoid Bowen disease: CK7-negative, CK5-positive, and p63-positive
- Melanoma: Keratin-negative; positive for melanoma markers

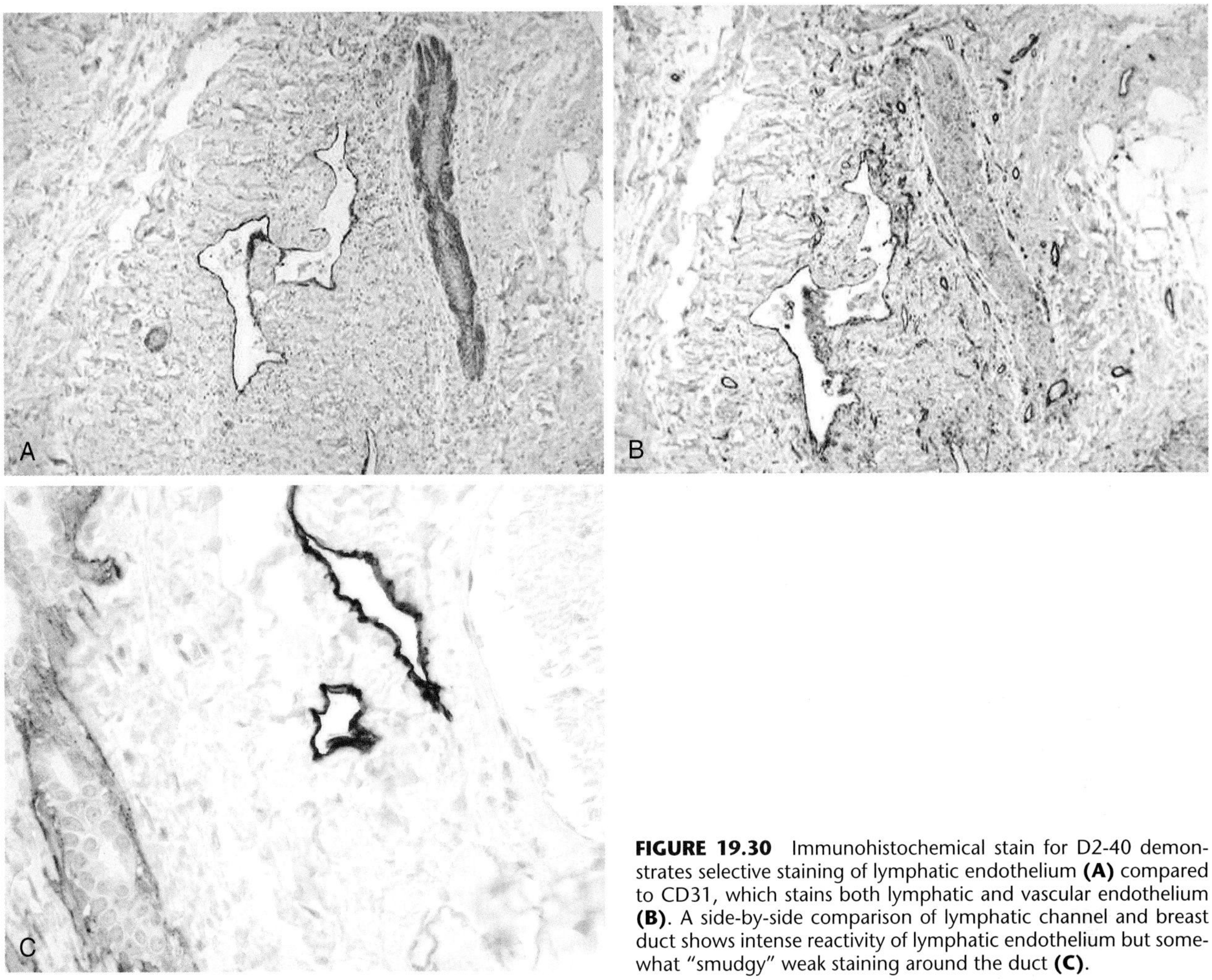

FIGURE 19.30 Immunohistochemical stain for D2-40 demonstrates selective staining of lymphatic endothelium **(A)** compared to CD31, which stains both lymphatic and vascular endothelium **(B)**. A side-by-side comparison of lymphatic channel and breast duct shows intense reactivity of lymphatic endothelium but somewhat "smudgy" weak staining around the duct **(C)**.

DETECTION OF LYMPHATIC SPACE INVASION

Lympho-vascular space invasion in breast carcinoma is an independent predictor of axillary lymph node metastasis, which in turn is one of the most important prognostic factors in breast carcinoma.[184-187] One recent study has shown that peritumoral lymphatic space invasion (and not blood vessel invasion) was determinant of lymph node metastasis.[188] In addition, identification of tumor emboli within dermal lymphatics is also important for correlation purposes in cases of inflammatory carcinomas.[189-191]

The pitfalls of interpretation of lymphatic channels in paraffin-embedded breast tissue are well known. Retraction artifacts, ducts with misplaced epithelium, and artifactual displacement of cells commonly complicate the interpretation of biopsy samples. A recently available antibody, D2-40, shows high sensitivity and specificity for normal lymphatic channels in a variety of tissues.[192,193] D2-40 stains the lymphatic endothelium crisply and intensely but does not stain the normal vascular endothelium (Fig. 19.30).[194] It is highly sensitive and specific in identifying lymphatic space invasion.[192] In the breast, D2-40 stains lymphatic channels with a crisp, intense membrane staining of lymphatic endothelium. D2-40 shows a smudgy immunostaining pattern with myoepithelial cells and reactive stromal myofibroblasts. This is a pitfall because the faint to occasionally moderate staining around the periphery of a small duct may be mistaken for lymphatic space invasion; however, it is important to remember that lymphatic vessels are stained very intensely with D2-40 (see Fig. 19.30C).

SENTINEL LYMPH NODE EXAMINATION

Historically, complete axillary lymph node dissections had been performed with lumpectomy or mastectomy primarily for staging purposes, providing information that was used to determine adjuvant chemotherapy. The complete axillary lymph node dissection (CALND) may not change the course of the disease, although with removal of involved axillary nodes, the control of local recurrence in the axilla is easier. The morbidity associated with this procedure is substantial in terms of limitation of arm motion, arm pain, and chronic lymphedema.

The concept of a sentinel lymph node (SLN) was spawned by Cabanas[195] in his study of penile carcinoma.

The pioneering studies of sentinel lymph node metastasis (SLNM) originated with the study of melanoma patients; the goal was to spare these patients the morbidity of large regional lymph node dissections. Patients with melanomas who had SLN surgery were found to have a relatively orderly progression of lymph node metastases, with the sentinel lymph node receiving the initial deposits of metastatic cells, followed by metastases in more distal lymph node groups.[196] The same rationale is now being used for breast cancer patients. The SLN is identified by injecting a radioisotope and blue dye before planned surgical excision. The SLN, identified by a combination of visual inspection for blue dye and intraoperative scanning for radioactivity, is harvested and submitted for pathologic study. The rationale is that for patients who are SLN negative, a further morbid procedure of axillary cleanout is unnecessary, but for SLN-positive patients, an axillary dissection is indicated for proper staging and possibly to provide better control for local recurrence. The controversy in this approach arises from several valid questions:

1. What is the natural history of micrometastatic (MM) disease in the axilla?
2. Is MM SLN disease an obligate pathway to clinically manifested local recurrence in the axilla?
3. Is MM SLN disease an indication for adjuvant chemotherapy?
4. How should the excised SLN be examined pathologically?
5. Does MM SLN disease affect overall survival?
6. What biologic parameters of MM disease can predict the behavior of the disease in an individual patient?
7. Is it possible to recognize "benign transport" of epithelial elements in an SLN?

These are interesting and provocative questions for the care of the breast cancer patient. The American Joint Commission on Cancer defines micrometastasis as a cluster of cells that are no larger than 2 mm. Recent studies with more than 10 years of follow-up conclude that micrometastases are associated with a small but statistically significant decrease in tumor-free survival and overall survival when compared with truly node-negative cases,[197] but they are not an independent prognostic factor. The size of the metastatic deposit, taken together with tumor size and other factors, may additionally stratify patients at risk for further disease.

In most institutions, SLN biopsy with lumpectomy or mastectomy as indicated has become the standard of care.[198] The vast majority of SLN metastases are found in the first three SLNs that are submitted.[199]

Sentinel Lymph Node Immunohistochemistry

For the surgical pathologist, the appropriate triage and examination of the SLN is of utmost importance, but even here some controversy exists. When the SLN mapping procedure began to be the standard of care a few years ago, the SLNs were examined histologically by multiple levels and cytokeratin stains on at least two levels. Since then, more experience has been gained with the procedure and the reporting of SLNs. It was soon realized that the majority of micrometastases (metastases between 0.2 and 2 mm) can be identified by H&E alone, and IHC for cytokeratin stains generally highlight isolated tumor cells (tumor cell aggregates ≤0.2 mm).[200] Although the exact clinical significance of isolated tumor cells, and even micrometastases, remains uncertain, studies have shown that they both are associated with non-sentinel lymph node positivity in approximately 10% of cases, especially when the tumor size is larger than 1 cm (pT stage 1C or more).[201-204] If the primary breast carcinoma is of ductal type, it would be difficult (not impossible) to identify isolated tumor cells by H&E stain, and most pathologists would agree that they would be able to identify micrometastases (Fig. 19.31A). Therefore, cytokeratin stains on a SLN do not add any significant information beyond H&E staining in a primary ductal cancer. However, there are significant differences when the primary breast tumor shows a lobular morphology. Owing to single cell infiltration, small (micro)metastases of lobular carcinoma (especially the classic type) in a lymph node are extremely difficult to identify (see Fig. 19.31B, C). Occasionally, cytokeratin stains would identify macrometastases not readily apparent on H&E stain.[205] Cserni and colleagues have recently reported that sentinel node positivity detected by IHC in lobular carcinomas was associated with further nodal metastases in 12 of 50 (24%) cases.[205] Therefore, it is not unreasonable to do cytokeratin stains on SLNs in cases of lobular carcinoma and to save some resources in cases of ductal carcinoma.

When performing cytokeratin immunostaining of SLNs, one should use a cocktail such as AE1/AE3;[206] CAM5.2 is less desirable because of the manner in which it stains dendritic cells in the lymph node.[207] Micrometastatic cells occur in small clusters less than 2 mm in diameter within the lymph node or subcapsular sinus, and they need to be distinguished from the dendritic appearance of the interstitial reticulum cells of the lymph node, which are also keratin positive.[208] Studies with larger numbers of patients are needed to discern if the site of lymph node micrometastasis (peripheral sinus versus parenchyma of lymph node) is clinically significant.

Aggregates of breast epithelial cells in the subcapsular sinus of axillary lymph nodes have been described by Carter and associates[209] as occurring as a result of "mechanical transport" after a breast biopsy. Some impugn the core biopsy itself or the breast massage that follows isotope/dye injection as sources of mechanical displacement of cells into the SLN.[210,211] Solitary keratin-positive cells may be transported to the SLN, and the histologic feature often associated with true benign transport is the association of CK-positive cells with altered red blood cells and hemosiderin and macrophages (Fig. 19.32). Diaz[212] described benign epithelial tissue in skin dermal lymphatics and an SLN from a patient with pure DCIS. This lends morphologic documentation to the concept of benign mechanical transport. The distinction between benign transport and true

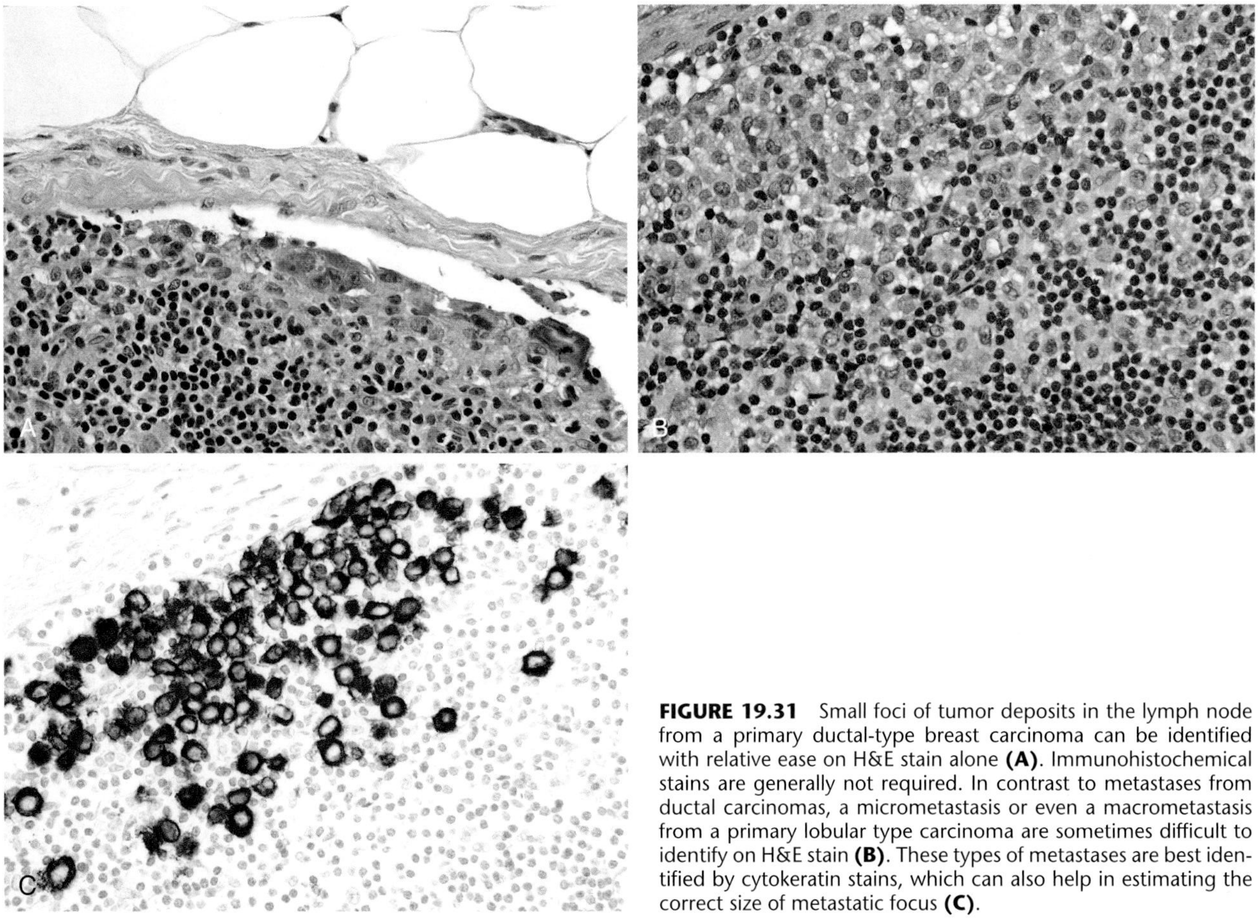

FIGURE 19.31 Small foci of tumor deposits in the lymph node from a primary ductal-type breast carcinoma can be identified with relative ease on H&E stain alone **(A)**. Immunohistochemical stains are generally not required. In contrast to metastases from ductal carcinomas, a micrometastasis or even a macrometastasis from a primary lobular type carcinoma are sometimes difficult to identify on H&E stain **(B)**. These types of metastases are best identified by cytokeratin stains, which can also help in estimating the correct size of metastatic focus **(C)**.

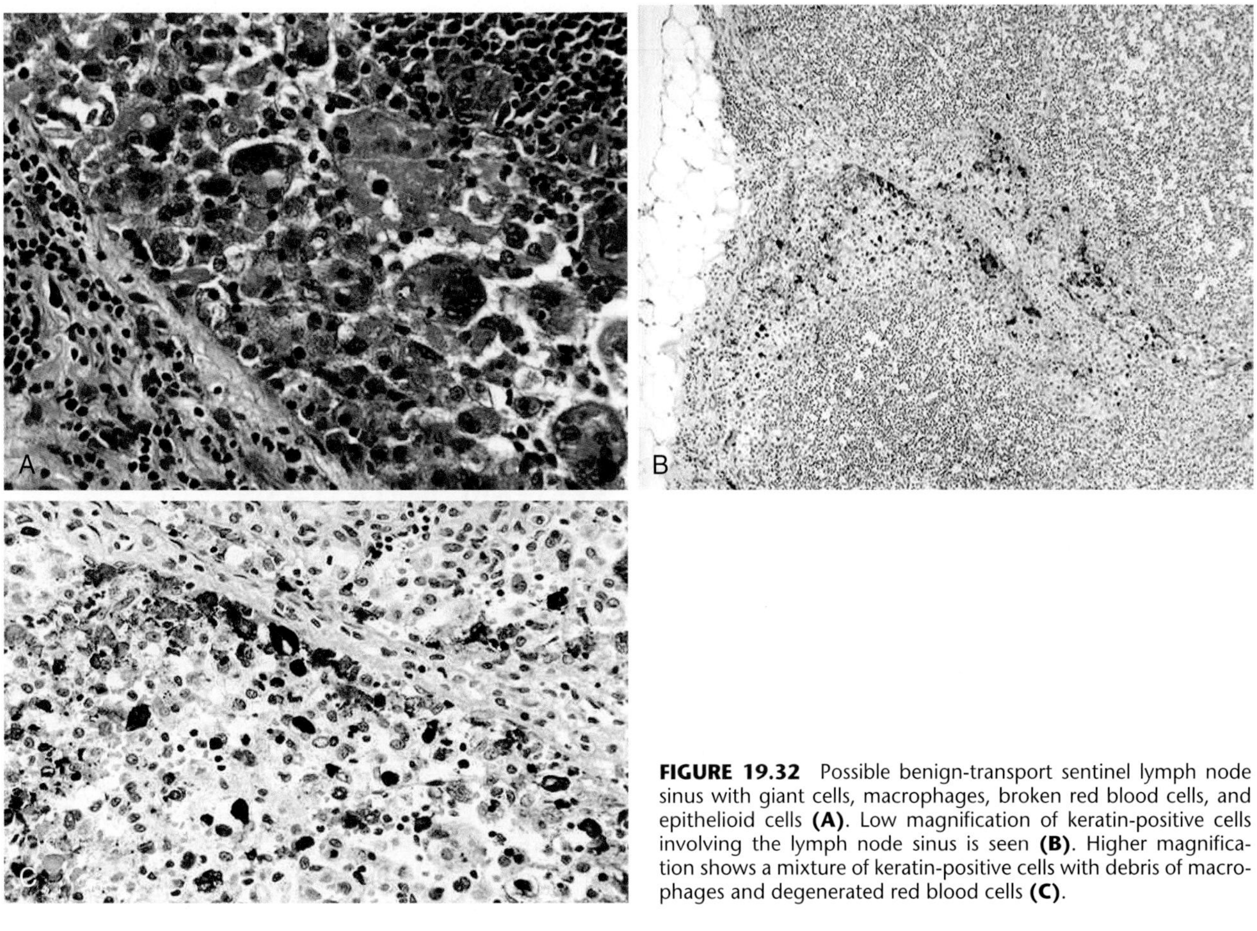

FIGURE 19.32 Possible benign-transport sentinel lymph node sinus with giant cells, macrophages, broken red blood cells, and epithelioid cells **(A)**. Low magnification of keratin-positive cells involving the lymph node sinus is seen **(B)**. Higher magnification shows a mixture of keratin-positive cells with debris of macrophages and degenerated red blood cells **(C)**.

metastasis is easy if the cells in the lymph node appear benign, but there is no objective way to distinguish benign transport from true metastasis when the cells appear cytologically malignant.

Intra-operative Molecular Testing of Sentinel Lymph Node

Recently, a few studies have shown the usefulness of intra-operative molecular tests in determining metastatic disease.[213,214] These are reverse transcriptase polymerase chain reaction (RT-PCR) assays, which use a completely closed system and are fully automated from RNA extraction to final interpretation. One such assay, the GeneSearch Breast Lymph Node (BLN) Assay (Veridex LLC, Warren, NJ), was recently approved by United States Food and Drug Administration (FDA) for axillary lymph node testing. The GeneSearch BLN assay is composed of a sample preparation kit, all reagents required for performing RT-PCR, and protocol software to be used with the Cepheid SmartCycler System (Sunnyvale, Calif). According to the company, the test has been optimized for detecting metastatic disease larger than 0.2 mm. The test analyzes the expression of CK19 and mammaglobin genes. Some recent studies have shown high sensitivity, specificity, and positive and negative predictive values for the test.[214-217] Overall, this molecular assay is very much comparable to the frozen section examination, permanent sections, and even IHC. However, just like any other test, one should be aware of the false-positive and false-negative test results as well as the usefulness and pitfalls of a particular test. Since molecular tests are not morphologic assays, one has to be extremely careful with any sources of contamination. A cutting bench metastasis (floater) can be easily recognized on an H&E-stained slide as such, but it will give a false-positive result by RT-PCR and there will be no definite way to identify this as an error. The SLNs identified in the axillary tail may contain a minute amount of breast tissue in the surrounding adipose tissue, which may also give a false-positive result. Therefore, lymph nodes should be completely trimmed of the adipose tissue before they are sectioned for molecular analysis. Moreover, fat interferes with the assay itself, and this could be an issue when the sentinel lymph node is diffusely replaced by adipose tissue. Occasionally a benign epithelial inclusion (> 0.2 mm) within the lymph node is a source of a false-positive result (Fig. 19.33). Given the significance of the treatment decision based on a positive sentinel lymph node result (complete axillary lymph node dissection that cannot be undone) and several sources of false-positive results with molecular tests, we believe that currently there are insufficient data to replace the morphologic methods with molecular assay. At present, we suggest that a positive molecular result should be confirmed by morphologic analysis, either by frozen or by permanent sections, before a final decision is made. In contrast, a negative result is highly valuable given the very high negative predictive value of the molecular tests.

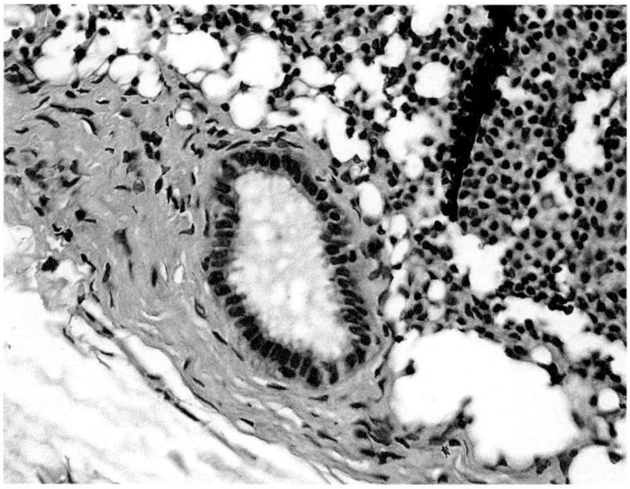

FIGURE 19.33 A benign epithelial glandular inclusion in an axillary lymph node as shown here may result in a false-positive molecular test for assessing micrometastatic disease.

KEY DIAGNOSTIC POINTS

Sentinel Lymph Node Micrometastatic Disease

- Section the lymph node perpendicular to the long axis at 2-mm intervals; examine with H&E and AE1/3 as indicated.
- For primary ductal carcinomas, AE1/3 keratin stain can be avoided.
- Always perform AE1/3 for lobular carcinomas as even large tumor aggregates may be missed on H&E examination alone.
- The SLN procedure has been adopted as a standard of care in many institutions.
- Ninety-seven percent of all SLN metastases will be found in the first three SLN when multiple SLNs are submitted.
- Intra-operative molecular tests are comparable to morphologic examination, but potential sources of false-positive results exist.
- Molecular tests have very high negative predictive value that could be very useful for individual patient management.

SYSTEMIC METASTASIS OF BREAST CARCINOMA

The diagnosis of breast carcinoma at a metastatic site requires a careful histologic examination, a review of all prior case material, and immunohistologic evaluation of tumor cells. For a patient with a prior history of breast cancer, it is valuable to know if it shows a ductal or lobular morphology. In a majority of cases, comparison to a prior tumor is helpful in making the correct diagnosis. Immunohistologic evaluation is required mainly in cases of carcinoma of unknown origin.[218] CK7 and CK20 have been generally used in this evaluation to narrow the differential diagnosis.[219,220] Breast carcinomas are generally CK7 positive and CK20 negative; however, a similar cytokeratin profile is seen in lung and gynecological tract carcinomas.

GCDFP15 has been used for several years as the most specific marker of breast carcinoma;[221,222] however, its sensitivity in formalin-fixed paraffin-embedded tissue is less than optimal.[221] Originally described by Pearlman and colleagues[223] and Haagensen and associates,[224] the prolactin-inducing protein identified by Murphy and coworkers[225] has the same amino acid sequence as GCDFP15 and is found in abundance in breast cystic fluid and any cell type that has apocrine features.[222,226] The latter (apocrine features), in addition to breast, includes acinar structures in salivary glands, apocrine glands, and sweat glands, and in Paget disease of skin, vulva, and prostate.[222,227-230] Homologous-appearing carcinomas of the breast, skin adnexa, and salivary glands demonstrate a great deal of overlap immunostaining with GCDFP15.[231] Aside from these immunoreactivities, most other carcinomas show no appreciable immunostaining. Breast carcinoma metastatic to the skin (or locally recurrent) may be difficult to distinguish from skin adnexal tumors.[232] In a study of the overlapping morphologic features of breast, salivary gland, and skin adnexal tumors, Wick and associates found that GCDFP15 was infrequently found in eccrine sweat gland carcinomas, a paucity of CEA was found in breast carcinomas, and ERs were largely absent in salivary duct carcinomas.[233]

The positive predictive value and specificity for detection of breast carcinoma with GCDFP15 have been reported to be up to 99%.[222] The sensitivity for the GCDFP15 antibodies has been reported to be as high as 75% for tumors with apocrine differentiation,[222,232] but the overall sensitivity is 55%, and only 23% for tumors without apocrine differentiation.[232] The sensitivity is even worse when it comes to core biopsy, since the pattern of staining for GCDFP15 is often patchy.

Because the specificity of GCDFP15 antibodies for breast carcinoma is so high, this antibody is often used in a screening panel in the appropriate clinical situation, often for a woman with metastasis of unknown primary or a new lung mass in a patient with a history of breast cancer. Others have demonstrated the utility and specificity of GCDFP15 antibodies in the distinction of breast carcinoma metastatic in the lung.[234-236] However, a recent study by Striebel and associates demonstrated GCDFP15 immunoreactivity in 11 of 211 (5.2%) lung adenocarcinomas.[237] This study again stresses the importance of a panel rather than an individual stain in determining site of origin of a metastatic tumor. On a similar note, WT1 (a specific marker of ovarian serous carcinoma) nuclear expression is seen in a subset of breast carcinoma that demonstrates mucinous differentiation. However, the expression is generally weak to moderate in contrast to ovarian serous carcinoma, in which expression is generally strong and diffuse.[238]

ERs and PRs may be helpful in cases with a history of receptor-positive breast cancer; however, a large proportion of gynecological tumors are positive for HRs. Hormone receptors have also been reported to be positive in non-breast and non-gynecological sites.[239-241]

Recently, mammaglobin has been described to be a more sensitive marker than GCDFP15 for diagnosis of breast carcinoma.[242,243] The mammaglobin gene is a member of the uteroglobin family that encodes a glycoprotein associated with breast epithelial cells. The immunostaining pattern is cytoplasmic, analogous to GCDFP15. If the weak equivocal staining is disregarded (as it is not helpful in determining site of origin in "real life"), the sensitivity of mammaglobin is 50% to 60% compared to <30% for GCDFP15. We have seen that even in cases that are positive for both GCDFP15 and mammaglobin, the percentage of cells and intensity of staining is much higher with mammaglobin than with GCDFP15 (Fig. 19.34).[244] Some initial studies have suggested association of mammaglobin staining with HR positivity, but we have not found such an association. Therefore, mammaglobin may be useful in identifying breast tumors that are negative or low (patchy) positive for receptors. The drawback of using mammaglobin is its lack of specificity. It is noteworthy that mammaglobin stains a substantial number (approximately 40%) of endometrioid carcinomas and occasional melanomas.[244] With respect to distinction of breast carcinoma from skin adnexal tumor or ductal salivary gland tumor, both mammaglobin and GCDFP15 are unreliable because these tumors have a similar IHC profile.[233,241] In spite of some non-specificity, we believe that a combination of GCDFP15 and mammaglobin is better than GCDFP15 alone in diagnosis of metastatic breast cancer.

KEY DIAGNOSTIC POINTS

Metastatic Breast Carcinoma

- Diagnostic confirmation requires the use of a panel.
- The usual breast carcinoma immunoprofile is CK7+, GCDFP15+, mammaglobin+, ER+, CK20–, TTF-1–, and WT1–.
- GCDFP15 is the most specific marker of breast carcinoma; however, weak/equivocal staining is not helpful in the workup for a tumor of unknown origin.
- Mammaglobin is a more sensitive marker of breast carcinoma than GCDFP15.
- Mammaglobin also stains up to 40% of cases of endometrioid adenocarcinomas and some rare melanomas.
- Salivary gland carcinomas and skin adnexal carcinomas have overlap staining with GCDFP15 and mammaglobin.
- Up to 30% of breast carcinomas may be negative for both GCDFP15 and mammaglobin.

FIBROEPITHELIAL TUMORS

Fibroadenomas and phyllodes tumors comprise the vast majority of fibroepithelial tumors of the breast, though mammary hamartomas and periductal stromal tumor are also considered in this category.

Fibroadenomas do not require immunohistochemical assessment because the diagnosis is made on its classic histologic findings in the majority of cases. IHC may be useful in the so-called myoid hamartoma, which

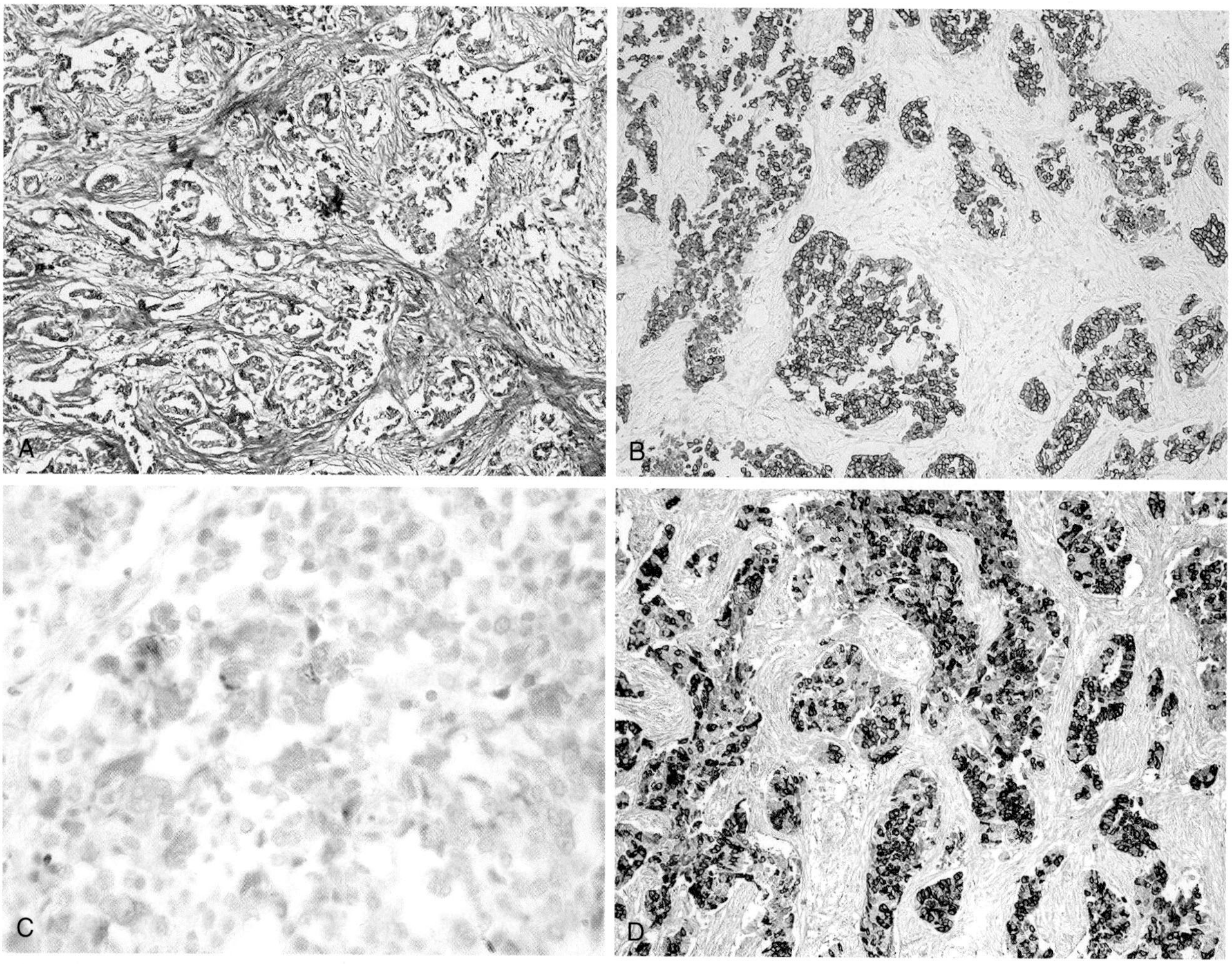

FIGURE 19.34 Adenocarcinoma involving abdominal wall **(A)**. The tumor cells were strongly and diffusely positive for CK7 **(B)** and patchy positive for GCDFP15 **(C)** and showed diffuse strong staining for mammaglobin **(D)**. In spite of negative receptor status, the morphology and IHC profile were consistent with the patient's known history of breast carcinoma from several years previously.

some authors regard as a variant of fibroadenoma, or in adenosis tumor with myoid metaplasia, which may be regarded as a variant of mammary hamartoma. These tumors show positive stromal immunoreactivity for smooth muscle actin, desmin, and vimentin and are negative for S-100.[245,246]

Phyllodes Tumor

Phyllodes tumors are characterized histologically by a double-layered epithelial component arranged in cleft-like ducts compressed by a variably cellular spindled-cell stroma, the latter of which has been proven by clonal analysis to be the neoplastic compartment.[247] Several classification schemes exist and are based on assessment of the tumor stroma. Most of these schemes divide phyllodes tumors into benign, borderline/low-grade malignant, and malignant/high-grade malignant categories.[248] Immunohistochemical reports have shown that regardless of grade, the majority will express CD34 in the stromal compartment, which is consistent with fibroblastic or myofibroblastic differentiation and is supported by ultrastructural studies.[249-251] Additionally, ERs and PRs are variably expressed in phyllodes tumors, but their expression is limited to the non-neoplastic epithelial compartment and is negative in the neoplastic stromal cells (with the exception of ER-beta, which has been shown to be expressed by the stroma of phyllodes tumors as well as by fibroadenomas).[252,253]

Subclassification of phyllodes tumors is usually not diagnostically challenging. Benign phyllodes tumors are histologically akin to cellular intracanalicular fibroadenomas but with stromal heterogeneity and/or 1 to 3 mitoses per 10 high-power field (HPF). Malignant phyllodes tumors are akin to sarcomas with stromal expansion, pleomorphism, and mitotic rates of >10 per 10 HPF, and borderline tumors lie somewhere in between. Numerous immunohistochemical studies have nevertheless shown correlation of biomarker expression with tumor grade. Studies targeting Ki-67 (a nuclear antigen expressed in non-G0 proliferating cells) with the monoclonal antibody MIB-1 have shown progressively increased expression with tumor grade. In published reports, Ki-67 labeling indexes range from 1% to 5% in benign tumors, 6% to 16% in borderline tumors, and 12% to 50% in malignant tumors (Fig. 19.35).[254-257] Similarly, tumor suppressor gene *p53* is increasingly expressed with tumor grade, though less consistently

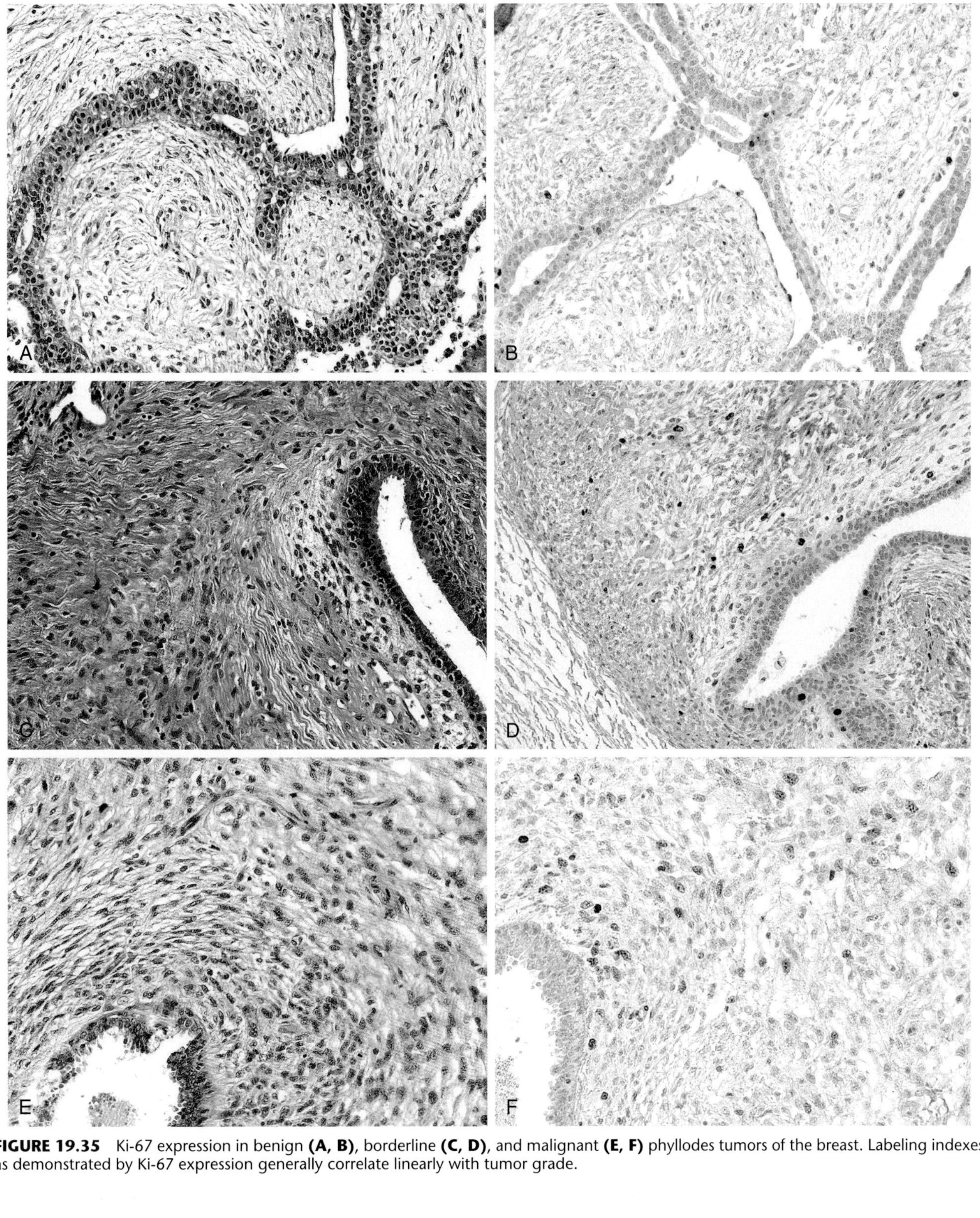

FIGURE 19.35 Ki-67 expression in benign **(A, B)**, borderline **(C, D)**, and malignant **(E, F)** phyllodes tumors of the breast. Labeling indexes as demonstrated by Ki-67 expression generally correlate linearly with tumor grade.

than Ki-67.[257-260] More recently, the expression of proteins with targeted therapy implications in phyllodes tumors have been explored. Chen and coworkers first reported c-*kit* expression in the stroma of phyllodes tumors in 2000 and found c-*kit* expression to be preferentially expressed in histologically malignant phyllodes tumors.[261] Since then, several additional studies have reported increased c-*kit* expression in malignant phyllodes tumors compared to benign and/or borderline tumors.[262-264] However, it is doubtful whether or not c-*kit* expression in these tumors infers susceptibility to the KIT-receptor tyrosine kinase inhibitor imatinib mesylate, as activating c-*kit* mutations have yet to be reported. Of interest is a recent study by Djordjevic and Hanna that suggests c-*kit* expression in fibroepithelial tumors to be related to the presence of mast cells. The

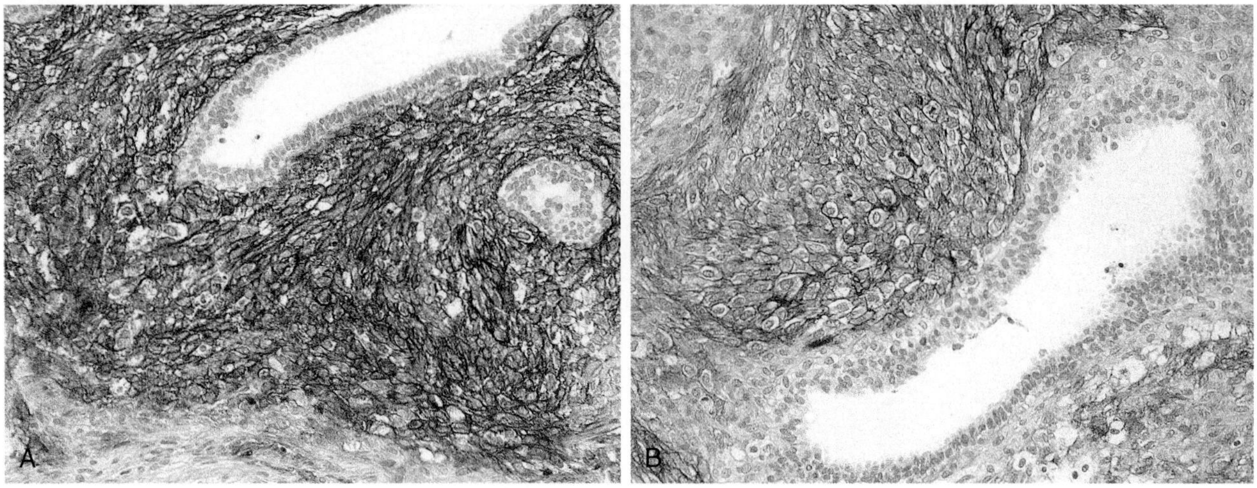

FIGURE 19.36 EGFR expression in two malignant phyllodes tumors **(A, B)**. EGFR expression has been shown to be more common in malignant phyllodes tumors and usually corresponds to polysomy 7 rather than EGFR amplification.

authors have argued against any appreciable true stromal-cell c-*kit* staining in fibroepithelial tumors.[265] Epidermal growth factor receptor (EGFR) has also recently been studied in phyllodes tumors, with most reports correlating increased stromal expression with tumor grade as well as chromosome 7 polysomy (Fig. 19.36).[259,266,267]

Prognostication solely based on histologic categories, however, has proved problematic in some cases, as histologically benign phyllodes tumors may recur as higher-grade tumors with associated metastases, and many histologically malignant tumors neither recur nor metastasize.[268-270] Thus the primary aim of most immunohistochemical studies has been to correlate biomarker expression with recurrence or patient outcome rather than diagnostic category. Unfortunately, most reports have failed to do so and are conflicting. For example, one study reported an inverse relationship between Ki-67 expression and overall survival in multivariate analysis of 117 phyllodes tumors, whereas others have not corroborated this finding.[254,256,262,271] Similarly, although p53 expression appears to correlate with tumor grade as noted earlier, it has failed to consistently predict tumor recurrence.[257,260,272] The potential prognostic value of EGFR is yet to be determined given the modest body of literature that exists on the subject to date.

Overall, studies aimed at developing better prognostic markers in phyllodes tumors have suffered from low sample size, a lack of patient follow-up data, and lack of reproducibility. The most significant consistently reported variables in the prediction of phyllodes tumor behavior remain histologic characteristics, in particular the presence of stromal overgrowth and adequate surgical resection margins.[256,273-279]

Fibroadenoma versus Phyllodes Tumor: IHC and Molecular Approach

The main diagnostic dilemma involving fibroepithelial lesions of the breast is probably differentiating cellular fibroadenomas from benign phyllodes tumors, since there is a great deal of histologic overlap. Several immunohistochemical studies aiming to resolve this issue, largely focused on proliferative markers, have thus been performed.

Jacobs and colleagues found significantly higher stromal proliferation indices, such as Ki-67 and topoisomerase II-alpha, in phyllodes tumors compared to fibroadenomas on core needle biopsy.[280] In this report, however, Ki-67 index ranged from 0.4% to 4.4% (average 1.6%) in fibroadenomas and from 0% to 18% (average 6%) in benign phyllodes tumors. Thus, the margin of error in determination of the proliferation index is relatively small. Given the subjectivity involved in its estimation, it may not be entirely reliable in distinguishing between the two (Fig. 19.37). Similarly, another immunohistochemical study of MIB1 expression in fibroepithelial lesions concluded that Ki-67 indexes could not reliably differentiate between fibroadenomas and benign phyllodes tumors with low mitotic rates.[281]

Molecular and chromosomal-based assays have also attempted to differentiate phyllodes tumors from fibroadenomas. Whereas studies of fibroadenoma have shown a much lower frequency of chromosomal alterations compared to phyllodes tumor, differentiation of the two based on karyotypic analysis alone is not optimal since chromosomal changes are only observed in a small proportion of phyllodes tumors. In addition, the most common abnormality reported—gain of 1q—has also been reported in fibroadenomas.[282-285] A study examining mutations on a global scale using single-nucleotide polymorphism arrays (SNPs) reported at least one occurrence of loss of heterozygosity (LOH) in benign phyllodes tumors, whereas fibroadenomas most often had no LOH or very low fractional allelic losses (FALs).[286] However, cases designated as benign phyllodes tumors in this study included those with mitotic rates of up to 5/10 HPF, which are thus more than likely to be borderline tumors by conventional criteria. Inclusion of such cases in the "benign" category likely inflated the FALs of the benign phyllodes study group.

One final detail of note is that the studies by Noguchi and associates on clonality showed fibroadenomas to be polyclonal and phyllodes tumors to be monoclonal in origin.[247,287] In contrast to most classification systems, this finding strongly suggests that fibroadenomas represent a hyperplastic rather than a neoplastic process. In support of this finding is the related fibroadenomatoid nodule, which is generally accepted to be a hyperplastic lesion and is essentially histologically identical to fibroadenomas but smaller and unencapsulated. Additionally, fibroadenomas are hormonally responsive, supporting the concept that they are hyperplastic in origin. However, whether clonal analysis can consistently and reliably differentiate between benign phyllodes tumors and fibroadenomas has not been adequately studied to date.

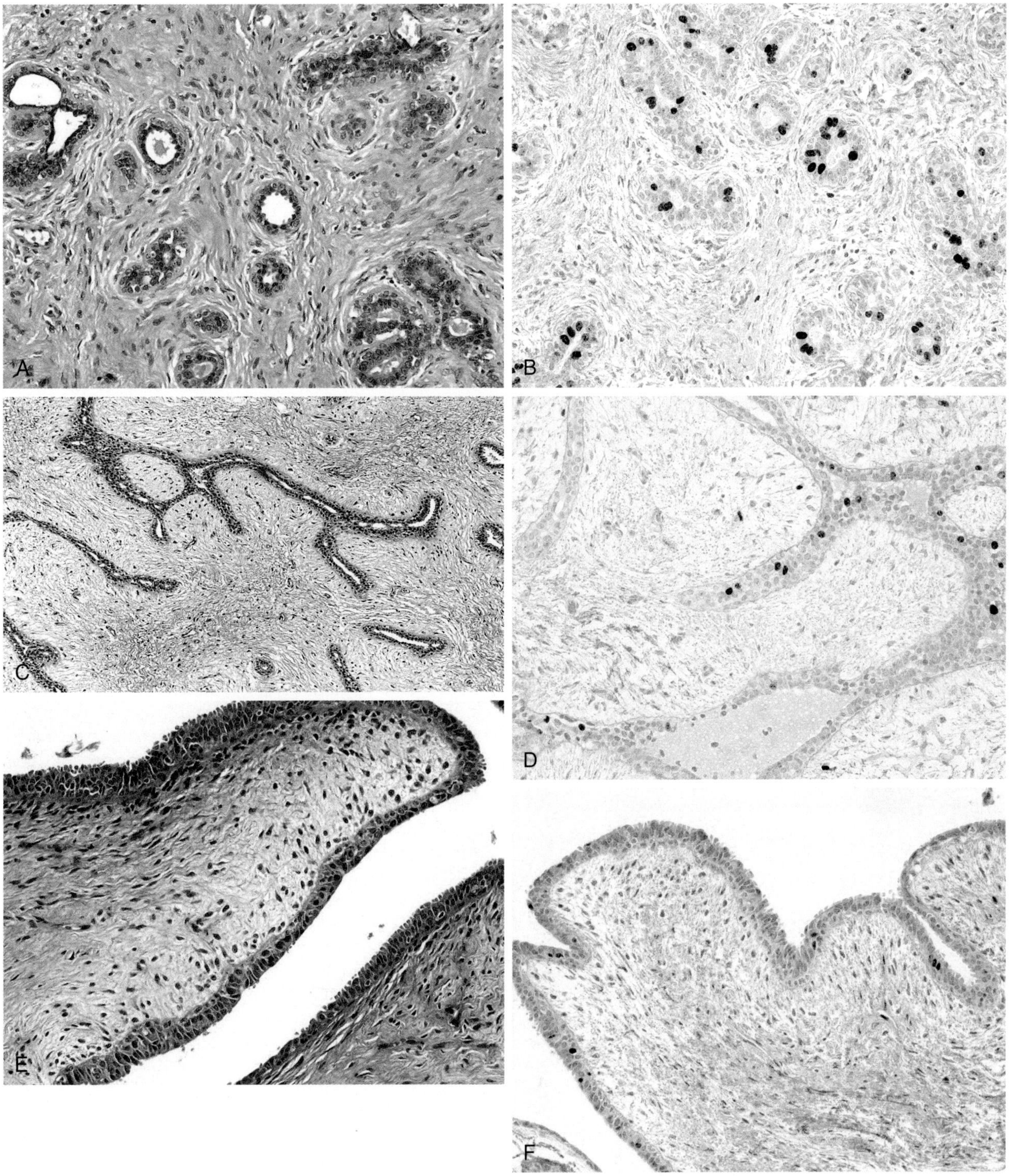

FIGURE 19.37 Proliferative activity in fibroadenomas versus benign phyllodes tumors. The fibroadenoma depicted in **(A)** and **(B)** shows no Ki-67 positive stromal cells, whereas that depicted in **(C)** and **(D)** shows focal (~1%) Ki-67 stromal cell immunoreactivity. Note the numerous positive ductal epithelial cells. Similarly, a benign phyllodes tumor may show minimal or no proliferative activity with Ki-67 as shown in **(E-H)**.

Continued

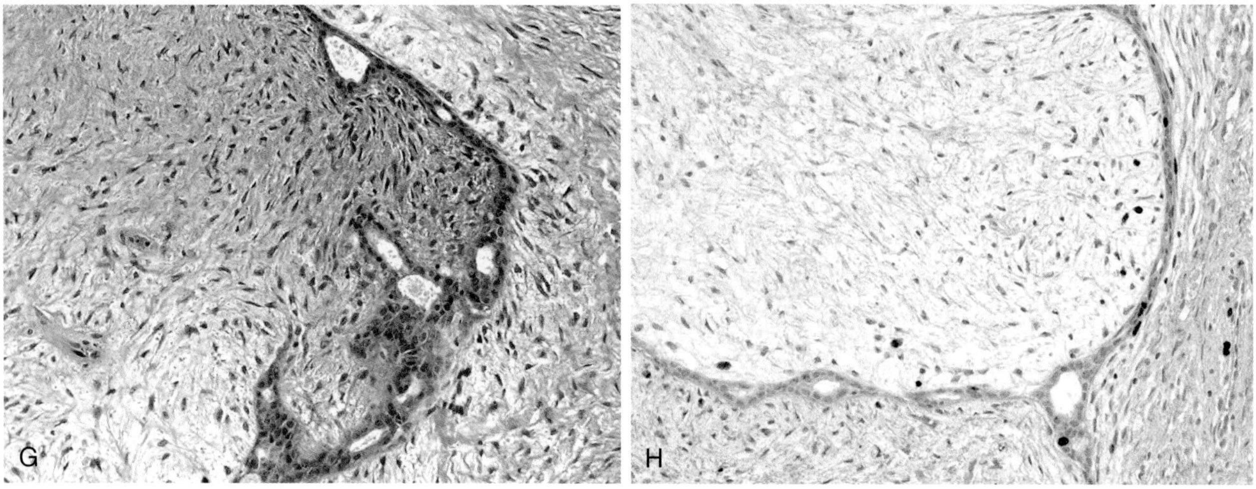

FIGURE 19.37, cont'd

Periductal Stromal Tumor

Periductal stromal tumor was initially described by Burga and Tavassoli as a distinct entity from phyllodes tumors that was histologically identical but lacked the intracanalicular or leaflike pattern.[288] Like phyllodes tumors, however, the stromal cells express CD34, and thus some have proposed that they are best regarded as a phyllodes tumor variant that lacks the classic leaflike architecture rather than a distinct entity.[169,288]

KEY DIAGNOSTIC POINTS

Fibroepithelial Tumors

- Phyllodes tumor stroma is CD34 positive, a finding that is useful in the workup of spindle cell lesion in a core biopsy.
- Ki-67 may supplement grading of phyllodes tumor in addition to morphology and counting of mitotic figures.
- Ki-67 proliferation index does not reliably distinguish between fibroadenoma and phyllodes tumor.
- Molecular analyses in distinguishing fibroadenomas from phyllodes tumors have also been inconclusive.
- Periductal stromal tumor is likely a variant of phyllodes tumor; it also has a CD34-positive stroma.

THERANOSTIC APPLICATIONS

Paraffin-embedded tissue, which is used for the primary morphologic diagnosis of breast carcinoma, also lends itself to a variety of antibody tests. These tests not only shed a great deal of light on the biology of the disease but also serve as a cutting-edge medium for the development of tests that may have an impact on how the disease is treated.

Pathologic features of breast carcinoma that have prognostic value include the following:

- Tumor size
- Lymph node status
- Histologic type of tumor
- Nuclear grade
- Mitotic activity
- ERs and PRs
- *HER2*

These parameters, which should be included in each pathologist's surgical pathology report, have been thoroughly studied and found to have significant predictive value for the patient's clinical course and response to therapy. Immunohistochemical stains for ERs, PRs, and HER2 are the most common stains performed for prognostic and predictive information. We have come a long way from ligand-binding assays to IHC for analyzing ER and PR. ER and PR ligand-binding assays have been validated by long-term follow-up for clinical use, with established cut-offs for positive results. Although there are several studies with excellent correlation between the two tests,[289-291] over the years there have been concerns about the quality, reproducibility, and accuracy of IHC in studying markers that predict response to targeted therapy.[292-294] When interpreting these results, one should carefully take into account the pre-analytical and analytical factors that affect IHC results.[295-297]

In this section, we will discuss the IHC tests that are performed routinely, in that they may have direct, immediate therapeutic implications.

Needle biopsy of the breast and fine needle aspiration (FNA) cytologic techniques are the most common methods of making the diagnosis of breast carcinoma. All of the diagnostic and prognostic tests (SMMHC, muscle-specific actin, ER, PR, MIB-1, p53, HER2/neu, and so on) can be applied to these small core-biopsy specimens and yield reliable results.[298-303] Of all the tests on core biopsy specimens, only progesterone gives a substantial number of false-negative results because of the wide heterogeneity of immunoperoxidase staining in tissue.[303] However, caution is advised in performing prognostic assays (ER, PR, HER2) on FNA material. Apart from pre-analytical factors related to fixation, one cannot be absolutely sure about the presence of invasive carcinoma in the cytology material and may erroneously report ER, PR, HER2 on *in situ* carcinoma.

HER2/neu

The *ERBB2* (*HER2*) gene was originally called *NEU* as it was first derived from rat neuro/glioblastoma cell lines. Coussens and coworkers named it *HER2* because its primary sequence was very similar to human epidermal growth factor receptor (*EGFR* or *ERBB* or *ERBB1*).[304] Semba and colleagues independently identified an ERBB-related but distinct gene that they named *ERBB2*.[305] Di Fiore and associates indicated that both *NEU* and *HER2* were the same as *ERBB2*.[306] Akiyama and coworkers precipitated the *ERBB2* gene product from adenocarcinoma cells and demonstrated it to be a 185-kD glycoprotein with tyrosine kinase activity.[307] In 1987, two years after discovery of the gene, the clinical significance of *HER2* gene amplification was shown in breast cancer.[308] We now know that approximately 15% to 20% of breast cancers demonstrate *HER2* gene amplification or protein overexpression.[309,310] In the absence of adjuvant systemic therapy, *HER2*-positive breast cancer patients have a worse prognosis (i.e., a higher rate of recurrence and mortality), which clearly demonstrates the prognostic significance of this gene. An even more important aspect of determining *HER2* status is its role as a predictive factor. *HER2* positivity is predictive of response to anthracycline- and taxane-based therapy, whereas the benefits derived from non-anthracyclines and non-taxane therapy may be inferior.[311-315]

It is also important to note that *HER2*-positive tumors generally show relative resistance to all endocrine therapies; however, this effect may be more toward selective endocrine receptor modulators such as tamoxifen and less likely toward estrogen depletion therapies such as aromatase inhibitors.[316,317] Most important, the availability of *HER2*-targeted therapy brought this biomarker to the forefront of theranostic testing for breast cancer. Trastuzumab is a humanized monoclonal antibody to HER2 that was approved by the FDA in 1998 for use in metastatic breast cancer. Trastuzumab improves response rates, time to progression, and survival when used alone or in combination with chemotherapy in the treatment of metastatic breast cancer. Although approved for use in metastatic cancer, several prospective randomized clinical trials have shown large therapeutic benefits from trastuzumab in early stage breast cancers.[318-321] The same paradigm has also shifted to neo-adjuvant chemotherapy using trastuzumab in *HER2*-positive tumors.

Given the enormous therapeutic benefit derived from trastuzumab in *HER2*-positive tumors, it is absolutely critical that an accurate determination of *HER2* status be made on each case. Owing to its prognostic and predictive value, *HER2* status should be determined on all newly diagnosed invasive breast cancers, which is now also recommended according to the recently released American Society of Clinical Oncology/College of American Pathologists (ASCO/CAP) guidelines.[322] These guidelines provide a detailed review of literature and recommendations for optimal *HER2* testing. The issues ensuring reliable *HER2* testing can be divided into three categories: pre-analytic, analytic, and post-analytic. All three issues are equally important and require a commitment to continuous quality improvement.

Pre-analytic

This mainly relates to time of fixation and type of fixative used. Since most studies with clinical outcome have been performed using formalin-fixed paraffin-embedded tissue, the current ASCO/CAP recommendation is the use of 10% neutral buffered formalin with the tissue fixed for 6 (excluding time in processor) to 48 hours. If an alternative fixative or fixation method is used, it has to be validated with standard fixation before it is implemented in clinical testing. Although the guidelines stress more regarding over-fixation, we believe under-fixation seems to be the real problem with *HER2* testing. The antigen can be retrieved by various methodologies and the enzymatic digestion times for *in situ* hybridization can be altered if the tissue is over-fixed, but nothing can be done if the tissue is under-fixed. Over-fixation may become an issue with alcohol fixation, which can lead to antigen diffusion, but it is generally not an issue with formalin fixation. We have validated tissue fixation times up to 96 hours for performing HRs and *HER2* testing on breast carcinoma at our institution.

The effect of under-fixation on biomarker testing has been nicely shown by Goldstein and colleagues, using ER as an example.[323] Using semi-quantitative IHC, the authors demonstrated that with 40 minutes of standard antigen retrieval, tissues fixed for less than 6 hours had very low "Q score" for ER, and the "Q score" plateaued at 8 hours to 7 days. It should also be noted that ASCO/CAP guidelines for fixation times were addressed to resection specimens, but there is no reason to believe that these cannot be applied to needle core biopsies. As a matter of fact, the guidelines should remain the same irrespective of the size of the specimen. This is because tissue permeation (which is roughly 1 mm/hour) is not equal to fixation. It is true that formalin will permeate core biopsy samples faster and make it harder for sectioning, but actual fixation or chemical reaction of aldehyde cross-linking takes time and is independent of specimen size.

Analytic

This refers to the actual testing protocol, including IHC equipment, reagents, competency of the staff performing IHC, use of appropriate controls, and finally the type of antibody used. The last issue, the type of antibody used, deserves special mention. The very first clinical trial assay for assessing the effect of trastuzumab on metastatic breast cancer used CB11 and 4D5 antibodies for determining HER2 status. In these studies, only patients with 2+ or 3+ scores were eligible to receive trastuzumab. Retrospective analyses have revealed therapeutic benefit in cases with a 3+ score or *HER2* amplification by FISH.[324] Only 24% of 2+ cases showed amplification by FISH. At the time of FDA approval of trastuzumab, a polyclonal antibody (HercepTest, Dako USA, Carpinteria, Calif.) was compared with the clinical trial assay antibody CB11 using the same scoring criteria. HercepTest received FDA approval based on its 79% concordance with CB11. It was soon realized and shown by numerous studies that HercepTest had a slightly higher false-positive rate than other monoclonal antibodies (CB11, TAB250) when compared with FISH.[325,326] Several antibodies are still used, but all IHC 2+ cases are sent for reflex FISH testing, which in most cases resolves the clinical dilemma about *HER2* status. Recently, a more reliable rabbit monoclonal antibody, 4B5, has become available. In a recent study, Powell and coworkers showed that rabbit monoclonal 4B5 demonstrates sharper membrane staining with less cytoplasmic and stromal background staining than CB11.[327] The major advantage of 4B5 was its excellent inter-laboratory reproducibility (kappa of 1.0).

Post-analytic

This involves interpretation criteria, reporting methods, and quality assurance measures, including competency of the interpreting pathologist.

The literature regarding HER2 IHC testing would suggest that 2+ score is the most problematic;[328-330] however, we believe the 3+ score that is often misinterpreted has grave clinical consequences. Nowadays, most laboratories would do FISH for HER2 gene copy number assessment when the IHC score is 2+ but would skip *HER2* FISH testing for 0, 1+, or 3+ scores.[331-333] There is ample data that HER2 FISH has great correlation with response to trastuzumab treatment.[334,335] Therefore, a 2+ HER2 IHC score coupled with *HER2* FISH has no adverse clinical consequences. In contrast, a false-positive HER2 IHC 3+ score would result in inappropriate (ineffective, expensive, and potentially harmful) therapy. Utmost care should be exercised in interpreting HER2 IHC results, especially when the staining intensity is strong 2+ or weak 3+.

The ASCO/CAP guidelines recently modified the criteria by changing the number of positive cells for a 3+ score from 10% to 30%.[322] Although the numerical change appears large, this will have a negligible practical effect. We do not deny the presence of HER2 IHC heterogeneity, but it is exceedingly rare in strongly positive cases. HER2 heterogeneity with respect to IHC is much more common in weakly positive cases in which the score ranges from 1+ to 2+. Because a small percentage of cells may show intense staining owing to edge artifacts, the change in criteria attempts to reduce the number of 3+ false-positives. Moreover, scoring these cases (those with 11% to 30% strongly staining cells) as 2+, which are now called *equivocal* per guidelines, will result in additional confirmation by FISH if they are true positives. Image analysis systems could be further used to achieve consistency in interpretation. However, these instruments should be calibrated and undergo regular maintenance just like any other laboratory equipment. Apart from judging the HER2 score, it is also important to effectively communicate it to the treating physician. A standardized template could be used that states the time tissue was fixed, controls used, antibody used, and the HER2 IHC score with description of staining. An example of such a template is shown in Fig. 19.38.

HER2 IHC TEMPLATE

HER2 immunohistochemistry: Using appropriate formalin fixed (6–48 hours) controls and tissue test block, ...antibody (clone, vendor information) is used to assess HER2 status and is interpreted as follows:

0 (negative): No staining is observed or membranous staining is observed in less than 10% of the tumor cells.

1+ (negative): A faint/barely perceptible staining is detected in more than 10% of the tumor cells. The cells are stained in part of their membrane.

2+ (equivocal): A weak to moderate complete membrane staining is observed in more than 10% of the tumor cells. HER2 FISH is being performed and will be subsequently reported.

3+ (positive): A strong complete membrane staining is observed in more than 30% of the tumor cells.

FIGURE 19.38 Template for reporting HER2 immunohistochemical results.

Finally, a quality assurance program should be in place for the laboratories that perform *HER2* testing. Quality control procedures for HER2 IHC should include the laboratory statistics of percentage of positive cases and the percentage of IHC cases that are amplified by FISH. Periodic laboratory assessment of these correlations is essential for quality reporting. Rigorous adherence to quality, tissue fixation times, control tissues/cell lines, and improved inter-observer interpretation agreement or image-assisted analysis are preferable.[336-338] ASCO/CAP guidelines recommend participation in a proficiency testing program that is specific to each method used.

KEY DIAGNOSTIC POINTS

HER2 IHC

- Owing to its predictive value, *HER2* is currently the most important theranostic test for breast cancer.
- Accurate assessment of *HER2* status is critical, and the lessons learned from *HER2* testing can be applied for future biomarker assessment.
- Tissues should be fixed in 10% neutral buffered formalin for at least 6 hours for accurate assessment.
- Choice of antibody may vary but should be mentioned in the report.
- Scoring criteria should be rigidly followed so that there are no 3+ false-positives.
- All 2+ cases should go for reflex FISH testing.
- Continuous quality measures should be in place for any laboratory performing *HER2* testing.

HER2 FISH

FISH is a molecular cytogenetic technique that uses fluorescent probes to detect specific DNA sequences on the chromosome. In the case of *HER2* FISH, a *HER2* probe is used to identify *HER2* gene amplification. The probe could be a single-color *HER2* probe or a dual-color probe with one sequence labeled for the *HER2* gene and another for the chromosome 17 centromere (chromosome enumeration probe 17 or CEP 17) on which the *HER2* gene resides. For a single-color probe, an absolute *HER2* gene copy number determines amplification; for the dual-color probe, a ratio of *HER2* to CEP17 is used to define amplification. DNA is a more robust molecule than protein, and therefore *HER2* gene amplification studies could be performed on a wide variety of samples. However, owing to the significance of this test result and to avoid any variability, the ASCO/CAP guidelines recommend pre-analytic conditions similar to those required for HER2 IHC. In the available literature, *HER2* FISH has a better track record than *HER2* IHC in predicting response to trastuzumab. This may be due to several factors, including tissue fixation, criteria used to define positivity, wide number of antibodies used, and subjectivity in interpreting HER2 IHC test result compared to FISH. However, after years of experience in both *HER2* IHC and FISH, the current ASCO/CAP guidelines demand 95% concordance (of negative and unequivocal positive results) between the two methods.[322] This seems like a high number, but theoretically it is not unreasonable because *HER2* gene amplification almost always results in HER2 protein overexpression.

For many genes, there are alternative ways of protein overexpression, but the *HER2* gene is unique in the sense that its gene amplification is very tight coupled with protein overexpression. In the past few years, it has also been realized that just like IHC, a FISH assay may also give equivocal results. Until recently, *HER2* gene amplification was defined as a *HER2*/CEP17 ratio of 2 or higher, and lack of amplification was defined as a ratio less than 2. This was also the cut-off used for the clinical trial assay. Using the cut-off value of 2 makes sense, but it has been realized over the years that there is variability in interpretation when the value is around 2.[339] Therefore, the recently released ASCO/CAP guidelines recommended that a ratio of 1.8 to 2.2 should be considered as *equivocal* for *HER2* gene amplification.[322] A ratio less than 1.8 is negative for amplification, and a ratio greater than 2.2 is positive for amplification. If a lab is using a single-color probe to define gene amplification, then a positive result is an average *HER2* gene copy number greater than 6, a negative result is an average *HER2* number less than 4, and an equivocal result is a *HER2* number of 4 to 6.

Apart from its better prediction value than IHC, FISH is also very useful when the *HER2* IHC test result is equivocal, that is, with an IHC 2+ score.[340] An IHC 2+ score is seen in up to 25% of all breast cancers.[341] It is now standard of care to use FISH for these IHC 2+ cases to determine if they show gene amplification. We reviewed FISH results on all IHC 2+ cases (186 cases) in the past year at our institution and found that a majority (~80%) of these cases do not show amplification (i.e., a *HER2*/CEP 17 ratio of less than 1.8). An equal number of cases (10% in each category) demonstrated equivocal (ratio of 1.8 to 2.2) or true amplification (ratio >2.2). However, it was extremely unusual (even in cases with ratio above 2.2) for IHC 2+ cases to show large *HER2* gene clusters, which is characteristic of IHC 3+ cases. Although FISH is useful for clinical decision-making in these cases, it appears that *HER2* IHC 2+ cases may be biologically different form *HER2* IHC 3+ cases. Our review also showed that some of these *HER2* non-amplified, IHC 2+ cases contained more than three copies of *HER2* and CEP 17, indicative of polyploidy/aneuploidy for chromosome 17, as reported previously.[330,342] Another caveat for a *HER2*-equivocal FISH result is whether FISH was performed on a core biopsy or a resection specimen. Recently, Striebel and associates showed that evaluating *HER2* status by FISH on a larger tumor sample (resection specimen) affects patient management if the core biopsy shows an equivocal FISH result, indicating genetic heterogeneity in tumors showing low-level *HER2* gene copy numbers.[343]

In spite of its usefulness, there are some limitations to FISH assay, mainly related to dark-field fluorescence microscopy and lack of morphologic details (Table 19.5). To overcome some of these limitations, chromogenic *in situ* hybridization (CISH) method has gained popularity. A range of studies comparing FISH and CISH show average to cent percent concordance.[344-347] CISH uses diaminobenzidine (DAB) as chromogen and therefore results in brown signals. This method combines the expertise of an immunohistochemistry and cytogenetic laboratory. This may be the reason for lack of wide acceptance for CISH, which we believe can improve with automation. Some pathologists also feel uncomfortable interpreting *HER2* CISH slides when there are between two and eight gene signals per nucleus because the signals may not be very discrete, especially when one is looking under a 40X objective using bright-field microscopy. Silver *in situ* hybridization (SISH) has been developed specifically to overcome this problem. SISH uses an enzyme-linked probe to deposit silver ions from the solution to the target site to provide a dense, punctate, high-resolution black stain that is readily distinguished from other commonly used stains. It appears that these innovative *in situ* hybridization assays will become more widely available and will be more acceptable to laboratories if the assays are automated and do not interfere with the current workflow. Since FISH slides are evaluated under a 100X oil immersion lens, the amount of tumor analyzed is fairly limited. An added advantage of these other *in situ* hybridization assays would be to examine the tumor for heterogeneity with respect to *HER2* gene copy number.

KEY DIAGNOSTIC POINTS

HER2 FISH

- All IHC 2+ cases should be referred for reflex FISH testing.
- The pre-analytic variables are similar to IHC testing.
- FISH interpretation also has an equivocal category (*HER2*:CEP17 ratio of 1.8 to 2.2 or an average *HER2* gene copy number between 4 and 6).
- Alternate *in situ* hybridization assays, especially SISH, may become more widely available and acceptable.
- Continuous quality measures should be in place for any laboratory performing *HER2* FISH testing.

TABLE 19.5 Benefits and Limitations of Immunohistochemistry and *In situ* Hybridization Assays

	Immunohistochemistry	FISH	CISH/SISH
Availability of the test	Widely available	Available at major labs	Available at major labs
Microscopy	Brightfield	Fluorescent	Brightfield
Training for interpretation	No special training required	Special training required	Minimal training required
Amount of tumor analyzed with ease	Large tumor area can be analyzed	Generally a small tumor area is analyzed	Large tumor area can be analyzed
Morphology	Morphology well preserved	Morphology not well preserved	Morphology well preserved
Turnaround time	4-6 hours	3 days	2 days with CISH; 4-6 hours with SISH
Average time for interpretation	<1 minute	20 minutes	1-2 minutes
Number of equivocal results	Approximately 25%	<5%	<5% (but limited experience)
Cost	Relatively inexpensive	Expensive	Intermediate
Automation	Possible	Possible	Possible; available with SISH

FISH, Fluorescence *in situ* hybridization; CISH, chromogenic *in situ* hybridization (generally DAB as chromogen); SISH, silver *in situ* hybridization.

Hormone Receptors

Recognition that estrogen ablation had an impact on groups of patients with breast cancer[348] and that clinical responsiveness correlated with the expression of the ER were seminal events in the treatment of patients with breast cancer.

ERs and PRs bind hormones that exert their effects in the nucleus. Nuclear immunostaining for both receptor proteins can be demonstrated in normal breast acini, which serve as internal controls for the testing procedure. Nuclear staining in normal breast tissue is heterogeneous and varies with the menstrual cycle.[349] One effect of estrogen is to induce the PR; thus the coordinate expression of both hormones in the same cell reflects the fidelity of the ER/PR axis in the cell. In carcinomas of the breast, most PR-positive tumors are also ER positive and ER negative. PR-positive tumors account for <5% of all breast cancers. This percentage is dependent on having adequate formalin fixation as well as the clone of PR antibody. In general, patients with positive PRs have a significantly longer disease-free survival than patients who are PR negative.[350-357]

Since the early 1990s, the IHC assay determination of ER/PR levels has replaced the dextran-coated charcoal (DCC) method, also called the *ligand binding assay* (LBA). The DCC method, the gold standard for many years, suffers significant drawbacks: (1) tumor sampling error; (2) heavy reliance on obtaining tissue immediately on termination of the blood supply to the tumor, usually in the operating room; (3) normal tissue contamination; and (4) analytic error. Some advantages of the IHC method include (1) histologic documentation of the tumor tissue to be assayed; (2) appreciation of the heterogeneity of ERs and PRs in tumor cell nuclei; (3) rapid assessment of tissue for ERs and PRs by direct visualization, semiquantitative methods, or both; (4) rapid turnaround time; (5) lower cost; and (6) ability to use minute quantities of tissue.

Despite the widespread use of IHC for HR determination, the lack of standardization of pre-analytic and analytic variables, scoring schemes, and threshold for determining HR positivity remains a concern. All pre-analytic, analytic, and post-analytic issues discussed for *HER2* apply similarly for HR reporting.

A critically important, recently published paper by the ad hoc committee on improved standardization for HR testing (Consensus Recommendations on Estrogen Receptor Testing in Breast Cancer by Immunohistochemistry[358]) has undoubtedly influenced ASCO/CAP group. This paper details the fundamental recommendations that a laboratory should follow in order to assure consistent and reliable results for HR testing by IHC. While the details can be found in the paper (and in Table 1.4), the essentials include the following.

1. Prompt fixation of breast tissue, with both resections and core biopsies requiring 8 to 72 hours of 10% neutral buffered formalin fixation with processing by conventional (not microwave-enhanced) tissue processors.
2. Only 10% neutral phosphate buffered formalin is recommended, even for fine-needle aspirate specimens where ER and PR are to be assayed by IHC. Formalin should always be newly replenished in the processor, and processor fluids should not exceed 37°C.
3. *In vitro* diagnostic kits should be used that utilize one of these ER clones: 6F11, 1D5 or SP1.
4. Positive and negative controls, internal and external, should be used on each run.
5. A positive cut-off of 1% should be adopted under nuclear expression, and results should be semiquantitated with the percentage of cells staining and their intensity.

This is the most important document on HR testing published to date in the United States. The recommendations are critically important for optimal patient results.

Recently, ASCO/CAP guidelines on HR testing adopted all the recommendations of the ad hoc committee.

Pre-analytic

Most laboratories currently perform HR analysis on core biopsy samples. There has been some misconception regarding formalin exposure time on smaller samples. As mentioned earlier, permeation and fixation are not synonymous. Fixation is a chemical reaction that takes time; therefore both small and large tissues need to be fixed for a similar amount of time. However, larger resection specimens need to be sectioned for efficient permeation of formalin. Impact of formalin fixation time on ER staining has been elegantly shown by Goldstein and colleagues.[323] The authors studied tissue sections from 24 known strongly ER-positive tumors that were fixed for 3, 6, 8, and 12 hours and for 1, 2, and 7 days. They used a semi-quantitative score (Q score with a range of 0 to 7) to determine ER expression. With 40 minutes of antigen retrieval, the mean Q score at 3 hours was 2.46 and reached a plateau of 6.70 at 8 hours. The mean Q score at 7 days was 6.60. However, with 25 minutes of antigen retrieval, the mean Q score at 3 hours was 1.75; it progressively increased with time to 6.62 at 10 hours, and then it declined with time to 3.79 at 7 days. This classic example shows that (1) optimum formalin exposure time for ER determination is 8 hours, and (2) antigen can be retrieved with increasing retrieval times for over-exposed tissue, but an under-fixed tissue is completely useless for biomarker study.

Analytic

Another issue of concern for HR and other biomarker testing is the use of rapid or alternate processors. It is strongly recommended that breast cancer specimens be processed in conventional processors. If alternate processors or alternate solutions are being used, the procedures need to be validated for ER results against similar samples that are processed in conventional processors. There also appears to be a need for documenting the type of fixative and the formalin exposure time on pathology reports. Having the fixation time for each breast tissue sample might prove valuable for interpreting and troubleshooting aberrant and/or unexpected ER results. Another important issue is the choice of antibody. Currently, the literature is mostly available for three different antibody clones—1D5, 6F11, and SP1—for ER. Most studies suggest a high degree of concordance among these antibodies; however, subtle differences are present depending on the cut-off value for a positive result. All commercially available antibodies for ER assessment in breast carcinoma target only ER-alpha isoform. Although another isoform ER-beta exists, its role in breast cancer is not well defined.[359] There are currently conflicting data concerning its potential role as a prognostic or predictive factor.[360-363] Unlike ER-alpha, ER-beta expression is seen in a variety of tissues other than breast and female pelvic organs.[364,365] Additionally, similar to *HER2* or any other biomarker assay, controls should ideally be placed on each test slide.

Post-analytic

An equally important component for HR assays is the post-analytic (interpretation) portion of the tests; however, scoring schemes and threshold for determining HR positivity remain a concern. A critically important statement from the NIH Consensus Conference of December 2000 states, "Any nuclear expression of HRs should be regarded as a positive result and render a patient eligible for hormonal therapy."[366] This pronouncement is also supported by studies performed by Pertschuk and colleagues and by Cheang and coworkers, in which both documented a cut-off of greater than 1% of cells for the 1D5 and SP1 ER antibody clones, respectively.[367,368] This has enormous ramifications for treatment purposes. Given the previous statement, the remaining question is: Is quantitation of HR by IHC therapeutically important?

Quantitation of HR results is important if evidence shows that patients with high HR levels have different responses to anti-HR therapy compared to those with low levels. The issue at hand is proper validation of the HR IHC test against clinical outcomes and tests that demonstrate the linear relationship between HR level and clinical outcome.

Quantitative results of the IHC method correlate closely with biochemical results and are predictive of prognosis.[369-372] Few studies have examined whether the presence of ER predicts an endocrine response. In the studies that have been undertaken, the number of patients has been small.[368] In a study using ER1D5, Veronese and colleagues found that immunostaining was predictive of response to tamoxifen in 65 homogeneously treated patients and was a discriminator for relapse-free and overall survival.[373] Barnes and coworkers and Goulding and colleagues confirmed that ER by IHC correlated better than the DCC method, and the results were strongly related to patient outcome, regardless of the method of immunoscoring.[374,375]

The effect of quantitation and establishing that ER is a continuous variable (and not bimodal) was clearly shown by Harvey and coworkers in 1999 using the *Allred score* (Fig. 19.39) in their series of 1982 primary breast cancer cases.[290] An Allred score of 0, 2, 3, 4, 5, 6, 7, and 8 was seen in 26%, 3%, 6%, 10%, 16%, 19%, 16%, and 4% cases, respectively. The authors demonstrated that there was a linear correlation between Allred score and ER content, as measured by LBA. This study also showed differences in disease-free survival based on the Allred score. Even the current reverse transcriptase polymerase chain reaction (RT-PCR) assay for HR has shown a broad dynamic range of HRs that are present in tumor cells.[376,377] These tests do not demonstrate a bimodal distribution of HR results, as suggested by a few studies.[378,379] Although the data from the NSABP-B14 clinical trial showed that the level of ER expression (as measured by RT-PCR) has little prognostic significance in the absence of endocrine therapy, the expression level has clinical significance when patients are treated with tamoxifen. When the tamoxifen-treated cohort was examined, patients in the top two tertiles showed benefit, whereas the lower

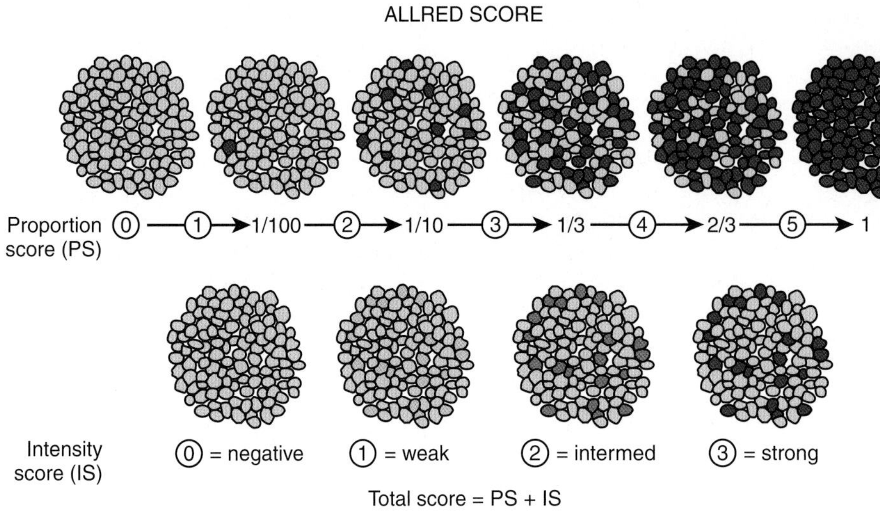

FIGURE 19.39 Semiquantitative scoring method for hormone receptors known as *Allred score. (Adapted from Harvey et al. J Clin Oncol. 1999;17:1474-1481.)*

tertile showed the same outcome as the placebo control group. The results suggest that the benefit from tamoxifen was limited to patients with a higher level of expression.[380]

Therefore, in addition to a positive or negative ER/PR result, we report a percentage of tumor cells staining with 0, 1+, 2+, and 3+ intensity, which is helpful in calculating the modified H-score. The score is given as the sum of the percent staining multiplied by an ordinal value corresponding to the intensity level (0 = none, 1 = weak, 2 = moderate, 3 = strong). With four intensity levels, the resulting score ranges from 0 (no staining in the tumor) to 300 (diffuse intense staining of the tumor). Since the likelihood of benefit correlates with the amount of HR protein in tumor cells, we recommend using a semi-quantitative criterion in addition to a positive/negative test result, which clearly states the percentage and intensity of ER and PR staining within tumor cells. An example of our reporting template is shown in Figure 19.40.

Regarding PR IHC, Press and colleagues compared 12 different PR antibodies. They found that PgR636 and PgR1294 stained the highest percentage of breast carcinomas known to be positive by the biochemical assay (95% to 98%), and they exhibited the highest concordance with the biochemical assay (88% to 90%).[381] Later, Mohsin and associates performed clinical validation of the PR by IHC.[382] Using a positive result of 1% of cells with PR clone 1294 (Dako USA) and the Allred scoring system, the authors demonstrated that PR was better than the ligand binding assay in predicting disease-free and overall survival.

Progesterone nuclear staining by the IHC method is more heterogeneous than ER and may be a cause of false-negative results, especially in core biopsies[303] or needle aspirates. We have seen similar results on some core biopsies; as a result, if a negative ER and PR result on a core biopsy specimen is obtained, one should repeat the test on the excisional breast specimen.

The sensitivity and specificity of other PR antibodies, namely 1A6 and the more recently available rabbit monoclonal antibody (1E2), are similar to previously used antibodies. There are two isoforms for PR (PRA and PRB), and both are recognized by the commercially available antibodies. Our preliminary data indicate that there are far fewer ER-negative/PR-positive cases with the 1E2 clone (1% of cases) compared to clone 1A6 (5% to 6%).

KEY DIAGNOSTIC POINTS

Hormone Receptors

- Pre-analytic, analytic, and post-analytic factors can significantly alter hormone receptor results.
- Clinically validated studies for ER clones SP1, 1D5, and 6F11 are available, and all demonstrate a positive cut-off value of greater than 1% of cells staining, linked to the response to tamoxifen.
- Some form of semi-quantitation (H-score, Q score, Allred score) should be performed on all positive cases, as it is therapeutically important.
- Hormone receptor analysis should be repeated on a resection specimen if the tumor was double negative on core biopsy sample.

GENOMIC APPLICATIONS: BREAST CANCER MOLECULAR CLASSIFICATION AND IMMUNOGENOMICS

Advances in molecular genetic techniques in the new millennium have transformed the way breast cancer has been studied. Gene microarray techniques that first analyzed hematologic malignancies[383] have been applied to several solid cancers. The breakthrough for breast cancer microarray studies came in 2000, when Perou and coworkers reported molecular classification of breast cancer using gene expression analysis on DNA microarrays.[131]

ER AND PR IMMUNOHISTOCHEMICAL REPORT

Using formalin fixed tissues (8–72 hours) and appropriate positive and negative controls, the test for the presence of these hormone receptor proteins is performed by the immunoperoxidase method. A positive ER or PR tumor shows ≥1% nuclear immunostaining and the semiquantitation immunostaining raw data are indicated below.

The ER and PR histologic score (modified H-score) is calculated as the sum of intensity (I) of staining times the proportion (P) of cells staining [HS = Sum P(I)] and has a dynamic range of 0 to 300.

	Result	H score	Raw immunostaining semiquantitation
ER:	_____	______	(0 ___%; 1+ ___%; 2+ ___%; 3+ ___%)
PR:	_____	______	(0 ___%; 1+ ___%; 2+ ___%; 3+ ___%)

Antigen/Antibody	Clone	Vendor
ER	....	....
PR	....	....

FIGURE 19.40 Template for reporting hormone receptors results using the modified H-score method.

Molecular Classification ("Intrinsic" Gene Set)

Perou and colleagues used a cDNA microarray to study 8102 human genes on 65 surgical specimens (36 invasive ductal carcinomas, 2 lobular carcinomas, 1 DCIS, 1 fibroadenoma, 3 normal breast tissues).[131] Of the 36 invasive ductal carcinomas, 20 tumors had samples obtained before and after doxorubicin chemotherapy, and 2 additional tumors were paired with lymph nodes. These paired samples were a unique feature of their study design: In spite of chemotherapy and a time interval of 16 weeks between them, these paired samples clustered together in the hierarchical clustering algorithm. These findings implied that each tumor is unique and has a distinct gene expression signature. It also implied that type and number of non-epithelial cells in carcinoma remain fairly constant and do not interfere in expression analysis. Therefore, the authors selected a subset of 496 genes that showed significantly greater variation in expression between different tumors than between paired samples of the same tumor. This subset was called the *intrinsic* gene set because it consisted of genes whose expression patterns were characteristic of an individual tumor, as opposed to those that vary as a function of tissue sampling. The same investigative group further extended the analyses to 115 carcinoma samples to reveal 5 distinct classes of breast carcinoma with prognostic significance.[132,140] These were termed *luminal A, luminal B* (which likely also includes the initially described luminal C), *ERBB2, basal-like,* and *normal breast–like.* The luminal tumors were named as such owing to the high expression of genes normally expressed by luminal epithelium of the breast. These luminal tumors also expressed ER and ER-related genes (*LIV1, GATA3, HNF3A*, X-box binding protein 1), with luminal A tumors showing highest expression of ER. Luminal B tumors expressed ER cluster genes at a lower level but also expressed some unique genes (*GGH, LAPTMB4, NSEP1, CCNE1*) whose coordinated function is unknown. The three other subtypes constitute the ER-negative group.

As the name implies, ERBB2 tumors are characterized by expression of genes in the *ERBB2* (or *HER2*) amplicon at 17q22.24. Basal-like tumors are named as such because they express genes expressed by the basal cells (myoepithelial cells) of the breast. Therefore, basal-like tumors are characterized by expression of keratin genes *KRT5* and *KRT17.* The normal breast–like group has been described to express genes known to be expressed by adipose tissue and other non-epithelial cell types. These tumors were also shown to express basal epithelial genes. However, more recently it is argued that this was likely an artificial category due to poorly sampled tumor tissue.[384] Over the years, the validity of this classification system has been tested with respect to overall and relapse free survival.[140] Basal-like and ERBB2 tumors have shown the worst outcome, luminal A tumors have shown the best, and luminal B outcome is intermediate.

Given the simplicity and the clinical relevance of the molecular classification, it appears that immunohistochemical markers can be used to identify molecular subtypes in routine diagnostic use. A few studies have detailed the use of IHC in identifying a particular molecular subtype.[133,134,138] It is true that analyzing a few biomarkers by IHC cannot be directly compared to a classification that analyzes gene expression of hundreds and thousands of genes. It is also true, however, that we have gained enough experience over a number of years in analyzing some key biomarkers that can predict a molecular class with almost 100% accuracy. A tumor that demonstrates 3+ IHC staining for HER2 and is completely negative for ER and PR almost certainly belongs to the molecular class ERBB2. However, we also realize that a 100% concordance cannot be achieved between the molecular classification (using intrinsic gene set) and IHC criteria, but a working formulation for use in routine pathology practice is feasible. Our proposed criteria based on a morpho-immunohistologic study of 205 consecutive breast cancers are shown in Table 19.6.[385,386]

Our hypothesis echoes that of Cheang and coworkers,[387] but we have sub-divided the luminal category into luminal A (LUMA), luminal B (LUMB), luminal A-*HER2* hybrid (LAHH), and luminal B-*HER2* hybrid (LBHH) based on ER expression level and *HER2* positivity. Additionally, Cheang and associates have used CK5/6 and EGFR in identifying basal-like carcinomas and have shown that basal-like carcinomas have significantly worse prognosis compared to triple-negative (TN) tumors that are also negative for CK5/6 and EGFR.[387] However, it remains to be seen if the choice of these antibodies in defining basal-phenotype is accurate. We have shown that CK5 (clone XM26) is much more sensitive (but equally specific) than CK5/6 in identifying basal-like carcinomas.[135] Moreover, the criteria for defining EGFR positivity are variable.[134,388] Unlike HER2, EGFR staining in breast carcinomas is often variable and patchy. It is estimated that the molecularly defined basal-like group constitutes approximately 80% of the immunohistochemically defined TN group. The initial

TABLE 19.6 Molecular Classes and Corresponding IHC Categories

Molecular Class (Intrinsic Gene Set)	Proposed IHC Categories	Criteria Used for Proposed Categories	Corresponding Categories*
Luminal A	LUMA	ER score 200 or higher, *HER2–*	Luminal
Luminal B	LUMB	ER score 11-199 or PR score >10, *HER2–*	Luminal
Basal-like	TN-basal TN-non-basal	ER and PR score 10 or less, *HER2–*; CK5+ for basal; CK5– for non-basal	TNP; Core Basal if positive for CK5/6 or EGFR; 5NP if negative for CK5/6 and EGFR
ERBB2	ERBB2	ER and PR score 10 or less, *HER2+*	HER2+/ER–/PR–
? Luminal C	LAHH	ER score 200 or higher, *HER2+*	Luminal/HER2+
? Luminal C	LBHH	ER score 11-199 or PR score >10, *HER2+*	Luminal/HER2+

*Categories from Cheang MC, Voduc D, Bajdik C, et al. Basal-like breast cancer defined by five biomarkers has superior prognostic value than triple-negative phenotype. *Clin Cancer Res.* 2008;14:1368-1376.

LUMA, luminal A; LUMB, luminal B; TN, triple negative; LAHH, luminal A-*HER2* hybrid; LBHH, luminal B-*HER2* hybrid; TNP, triple negative phenotype; 5NP, five negative phenotype. ER/PR scored using modified H-score method with a dynamic range of 0-300 (see Figure 19.40). *HER2* considered positive if 3+ by IHC or unequivocally amplified by FISH.

gene expression studies have shown the expression of *KRT5* and *KRT17* genes in basal-like tumors, but there is lack of evidence if *KRT6* is overexpressed. Therefore it remains to be settled as to which IHC antibodies best predict the basal-like molecular subtype, but it appears that if a panel is used then it should include CK5.

Using the simple IHC criteria (see Table 19.6), we have examined the morphology of over 200 consecutive breast carcinoma cases at our institution. The LUMA tumors (corresponding molecular class luminal A) are the most well-differentiated and comprise 55% of all tumors. They contain tumors of both ductal and lobular types. Although the largest segment is that of no special type (NST) ductal carcinoma, the group also consists of several special types of breast carcinomas with good prognosis, such as tubular, mucinous, cribriform, and papillary types. The lobular tumors contain both classic and pleomorphic variants.

The LUMB tumors (corresponding molecular class luminal B) constitute 16% of all breast tumors. They comprise both ductal and lobular types and are generally moderately differentiated. The lobular LUMB tumors also contain both classic and pleomorphic types.

The ERBB2 (same corresponding molecular class) tumors constitute a mere 4% of all tumors. These tumors generally lack tubule formation and show high-grade pleomorphic nuclei. However, a mitosis score of 3 is seen in less than one quarter of all HER2-positive tumors. Therefore, the Nottingham score is generally 7 or 8. The interesting part, however, is the overwhelming presence of apocrine differentiation in ERBB2 tumors. The ERBB2 tumors also show some morphologic features (such as necrosis and intratumoral lymphoid infiltrate) classically ascribed to TN tumors.

The TN (molecular class basal-like) constitutes approximately 16% of all breast tumors. Morphologically, they show three dominant patterns: sheetlike growth (~50%), ductal NST (~40%), or apocrine carcinomas (~10%). These tumors may also show spindle cell metaplastic features. The sheetlike growth pattern was recently described by Livasy and colleagues as the classic morphologic pattern for basal-like tumors.[133] In addition to a sheetlike growth pattern, the classic form of these tumors demonstrates highly pleomorphic nuclei, two to five mitotic figures in each high-power field, geographic necrosis, and lympho-plasmacytic infiltrate. The morphologic description is somewhat reminiscent of medullary carcinomas, but if Ridolfi's strict criteria are applied, only a few cases would qualify as medullary.[389] When we examined the expression of basal cytokeratin CK5, reactivity was seen in 73% (11/15) of cases of tumors with sheetlike growth pattern, in 62% (8/13) of cases of ductal NST, and in 75% (3/4) of apocrine carcinomas. The average Ki-67 LI was highest (71.3%) in a tumors with a sheetlike growth pattern, slightly lower (58.5%) in ductal NST, and lowest (27%) in apocrine carcinomas.

LAHH and LBHH tumors (likely molecular class luminal C) account for approximately 9% of all breast tumors. Morphologically, they are moderately differentiated tumors and predominantly of the ductal, no special type. However, some pleomorphic lobular carcinomas also fall into these groups if they are HER2 positive. Average PR expression is generally higher in LAHH tumors compared to LBHH tumors. Some LBHH tumors may also show a certain degree of apocrine differentiation.

The molecular classification using an "intrinsic" gene set was derived mainly from analyzing IDC of no special type, but there is no reason to believe that it cannot be applied to other morphologic tumor types. As a matter of fact, Weigelt and coworkers recently reported molecular characterization of the various histologic subtypes of breast cancer.[390] In this study, the molecular classes (luminal, ERBB2, and basal-like) correlated with immunohistochemical surrogate markers ER, PR, and HER2 protein expression profile (i.e. the TN adenoid cystic, medullary, and metaplastic tumors) clustered with the usual type of basal-like carcinomas and the ER+/*HER2* negative tumors (e.g., tubular, mucinous and classic lobular carcinomas) clustered together as luminal tumors.

To further examine the validity of immunohistochemical surrogate markers for molecular classification in a clinical setting, we have examined HR metrics and HER2 for 359 tumors treated with standard neoadjuvant chemotherapy (NACT) at our institution. Of these 359 tumors treated with NACT, 111 (30.7%) were LUMA, 73 (20.4%) were LUMB, 79 (22%) were TN, 57 (16%) were ERBB2, 15 (4.2%) were LAHH, and 24 (6.7%) were LBHH. Complete pathologic response was identified in 33% of ERBB2, 30.3% in TN, 8.3% of LBHH, 1.8% of LUMA, 1.4% of LUMB, and 0% of LAHH tumors ($p < 0.0001$).[386] These data are very much comparable to other studies that have used gene expression profiling to predict pathologic complete response.[391] Therefore, we believe that these simple IHC criteria can be used in routine practice to provide important clinical information.

Apart from the intrinsic gene set–based expression analysis of breast cancer, several other expression studies using different models were published recently. These models include 70-gene profile, wound response, Rotterdam signature, recurrence score, and two-gene ratio.

Seventy-Gene Profile (Mammaprint)

The 70-gene good versus poor outcome model was developed by van de Vijver and coworkers and van't Veer and colleagues.[392,393] The authors used oligonucleotide array to identify genes that predict prognosis in breast cancer. They estimated that an odds ratio for metastasis among tumors with "good prognosis" gene signature as compared to "poor prognosis" gene signature was approximately 15 using a cross-validation procedure. The poor prognosis signature consisted of genes regulating cell cycle, invasion, metastasis, and angiogenesis. They further studied 295 cases of breast cancers from young patients, including pT1 and pT2 cases with (n=144) or without (n=151) lymph node metastasis. Of the 295 cases, 180 showed poor prognosis and 115 showed good prognosis profile. The mean (SE) overall 10-year survival rates were 54.6% (+/–4.4%) and 94.5% (+/–2.6%), respectively. The estimated hazard ratio for distant metastases with the poor prognosis signature as compared to the group with the good prognosis signature was 5.1. This ratio remained significant when the groups were analyzed with respect to lymph node status. This assay has now formed the basis of a commercial test called MammaPrint (Agendia BV, Amsterdam, Netherlands).[394] The test was recently cleared by the United States FDA for clinical use; however, ASCO/CAP guidelines conclude that more evidence is required in order to advocate use in clinical practice.[395] Another problem with the test is that fresh frozen tissue containing at least 30% of the invasive tumor is required, and it must reach the company listed in their kit within five days of obtaining the tissue.[322]

Wound Response Gene Set

The wound response model for predicting breast cancer prognosis was described by Chang and associates.[396] The authors used the same set of 295 cases used for validating the 70-gene expression profile. Breast cancer samples showed predominant expression of either serum-induced or serum-repressed genes, allowing the investigators to assign each sample to the activated or quiescent wound-response signature. Patients with the activated wound-response signature (126/295, 42.7%) had a significantly decreased distant metastasis–free probability and overall survival in univariate analysis. Even when the analysis was extended to different pathologic subsets, such as pT1 tumors, lymph node–positive tumors, and lymph node–negative tumors, the results remained the same (i.e., patients with tumors showing an activated wound-response signature had a significantly worse distant metastasis–free probability and overall survival compared to those with a quiescent wound signature). Based on this study and the authors' prior studies on other epithelial tumors, they concluded that physiologic response to a wound is frequently activated in common human epithelial tumors and confers an increased risk of metastasis and cancer progression.

Seventy-Six Gene Profile (Rotterdam Assay)

The Rotterdam signature is also known as the 76-gene profile/assay. The test has been developed at the Erasmus University Medical Center in Rotterdam, Netherlands, in collaboration with Veridex LLC (Warren, NJ). Using the Affymetrix Human U133a GeneChips, Wang and colleagues analyzed the expression of 22,000 transcripts in a series of 286 lymph node–negative patients who had not received adjuvant systemic treatment.[397] Of these 286 tumors, 115 tumors were used as a training set to identify 76 genes (60 genes for ER-positive and 16 genes for ER-negative) whose expression levels correlated with distant metastasis within 5 years. Although genes involved in cell death, cell proliferation, and transcriptional regulation were found in both groups of patients stratified by ER status, the 60 genes selected for the ER-positive group and the 16 selected for the ER-negative group had no overlap.

The remaining 171 tumors were used as the testing set; the 76-gene profile was highly informative in identifying patients who developed distant metastases within 5 years (hazard ratio 5.67 [95% CI 2.59 to 12.4]). This signature showed 93% sensitivity and 48% specificity. When this testing set of 171 patients was divided into 84 pre-menopausal and 87 post-menopausal patients, the 76-gene profile was still a strong prognostic factor for the development of metastasis. Similar results were obtained when 79 patients with pT1C tumors were analyzed. The Rotterdam assay was further validated in a multicenter study of lymph node–negative patients.[398] The developmental history of the 76-gene profile is very similar to the 70-gene profile, but the two tests are directed at different patient population. The 76-gene profile has been developed for lymph node–negative patients irrespective of hormone status and patient age. However, like the 70-gene profile, the Rotterdam assay is an oligonucleotide array–based test that will require fresh/frozen tissue for analysis. It is also interesting to note that there is only a 3-gene overlap between the Mammaprint and the Rotterdam assay. At present, a commercial assay based on 76-gene profile is not available but is under development by Veridex (Warren, NJ).

Recurrence Score Model (Onco*type* DX)

Recurrence score model is better known as Onco*type* DX, which is a commercially available RT-PCR based assay that provides a recurrence score (RS) and has been shown to provide prognostic and predictive information in ER-positive, lymph node–negative breast cancers.[399] The test analyzes the expression of 21 genes (16 cancer-related and 5 control genes) to give a distant disease RS ranging from 0 to 100. The RS was created using training sets and a proprietary analytic method. The Onco*type* DX RS was originally validated in 668 lymph node–negative, ER-positive breast cancer patients receiving tamoxifen in NSABP trial B-14. A multivariate analysis of patient age, tumor size, tumor grade, *HER2* status, HR status, and RS demonstrated that only tumor grade and recurrence score were significant predictors of distant recurrence. The RS was also significantly correlated with the relapse-free interval and overall survival. The RS was subsequently validated as a predictive marker for response to chemotherapy and tamoxifen in 651 patients on NSABP B-20 and 645 patients on NSABP B-14.[400] The 16 genes analyzed by the test can be categorized as the estrogen group (ER, PGR, BCL2, SCUBE2); the *HER2* group (GRB7, *HER2*), the proliferation group (Ki67, STK15, Survivin, CCNB1, MYBL2), the invasion group (MMP11, CTSL2), and others (GSTM1, CD68, BAG1).

Since the ER, PR, and *HER2* genes are already analyzed by either protein expression or gene amplification (and pathologists analyze morphologic expression of proliferation genes by mitotic count), we examined the relationship between traditional histopathologic variables and the RS in our pilot series of 42 cases. We found that recurrence score significantly correlated with tubule formation, nuclear grade, mitotic count, ER immunohistochemical score, PR immunohistochemical score, and *HER2*/neu status, and that the equation RS = 13.424 + 5.420 (nuclear grade) + 5.538 (mitotic count) – 0.045 (ER immunohistochemical score) – 0.030 (PR immunohistochemical score) + 9.486 (HER2/neu) predicts the recurrence score with an R^2 of 0.66, indicating that the full model accounts for 66% of the data variability.[401]

Two Gene Ratio and Molecular Grade Index (H/I index and MGI)

The two gene ratio model analyzes the expression of *HOXB13* and *IL17BR* genes. In the initial cohort of 60 tamoxifen-treated patients, Ma and coworkers identified the *HOXB13* gene (a homeodomain-containing protein) and the *IL17BR* gene (interleukin 17 receptor B), which were significantly associated with clinical outcome.[402] The authors hypothesized that a two-gene expression index (*HOXB13:IL17BR*) might be a novel biomarker for predicting treatment outcome in tamoxifen monotherapy. They further tested their hypothesis on 852 formalin-fixed, paraffin-embedded primary breast cancers from 566 untreated and 286 tamoxifen-treated breast cancer patients using real-time quantitative RT-PCR technique.[403] They found that expression of *HOXB13* was associated with shorter recurrence-free survival (p = .008), and expression of *IL17BR* was associated with longer recurrence-free survival (P < .0001). In ER+ patients, the *HOXB13:IL17BR (H/I)* index predicted clinical outcome independently of treatment, but more strongly in node-negative patients. In spite of these validation assays, a comparative study of five-gene expression–based assays, Fan and coworkers found concordance between four tests (intrinsic gene set, recurrence score, 70-gene profile, and wound response gene set) but not with a two gene ratio. Therefore, to improvise on the two gene ratio test, the same group of investigators recently described a molecular grade index (MGI) by selecting five cell-cycle–related genes to be used concurrently with H/I index to improve risk stratification.[404] Using their previously published gene expression database on pre-invasive and invasive lesions that showed differential gene expression within higher-grade and lower-grade lesions,[405] the investigators selected five genes (*BUB1B, CENPA, NEK2, RACGAP1,*and *RRM2*) based on functional annotation, tumor grade, and clinical outcome. A numerical score was created using these five genes and called the *MGI*. The prognostic performance of the MGI was tested using two independent publicly available microarray data sets to predict clinical outcome. The five-gene MGI was also compared to the 97-gene genomic grade index (GGI) previously described by Sotiriou and colleagues and found to be equivalent.[406] Interestingly, the five genes of the MGI were part of the 97-gene GGI.

Ma and associates developed an RT-PCR–based assay for calculating MGI so that the assay could be easily applied to FFPE tissues. They further described the complementary value of MGI and H/I in stratifying patients into risk groups (similar to Onco*type* DX) to determine 10-year distant metastasis–free survival probability.[404] One primary reason that MGI and H/I are complementary is that high proliferation rate (high MGI) and a decreased cell death (high *HOXB13:IL17BR*) promote aggressive tumor growth in a synergistic manner.

Gene expression studies have improved our understanding of breast carcinoma, but it is difficult to integrate all these data into our current practice. It seems that the intrinsic gene set–based classification is simple to follow and that key biomarkers assessment by IHC can predict the molecular class with high confidence. Other gene expression–based assays may be used in special circumstances when clinical decision-making is not so straightforward using conventional parameters.

These gene expression models are summarized in Table 19.7.

TABLE 19.7 Gene Expression Models Described for Use in Breast Carcinoma

Expression Models	Test Purpose	Method	Classes	Specimen	Test Name
Intrinsic gene set	Molecular classification for all breast carcinomas	c-DNA microarray	Luminal A Luminal B ERBB2 Basal-like Normal breast-like	Fresh/frozen	NA
Seventy-gene profile	Prognostic for young breast cancer patients, pT1 or pT2 tumors	Oligonucleotide microarray	Good prognosis versus Poor prognosis	Fresh/frozen	Mammaprint (Agendia BV, The Netherlands)
Wound response	Prognostic; improved risk stratification	Oligonucleotide microarray	Quiescent versus Activated	Fresh/frozen	NA
Seventy-six gene profile	Prognostic for lymph node negative irrespective of HR status	Oligonucleotide microarray	Good prognosis versus Poor prognosis	Fresh/frozen	Rotterdam Assay-in development by Veridex, Warren, NJ)
Recurrence score (RS)	Prognostic and predictive use in ER+, lymph node negative tumors	RT-PCR quantitative	Low risk Intermediate High risk	FFPE acceptable	onco*type* DX (Genomic Health Inc., Redwood City, CA)
Two gene ratio*	Prognostic use in ER+, lymph node negative tumors	RT-PCR quantitative	Low versus High ratio	FFPE acceptable	Theros H/I (bioTheranostics, San Diego, CA)
Five gene index*	Objective measurement of tumor grade and chemotherapy prediction in ER+ tumors	RT-PCR quantitative	High or low	FFPE acceptable	Theros MGI (bioTheranostics, San Diego, CA)

*Two gene ratio (Theros H/I) is now tested in combination with five gene index (Theros MGI) as a combined assay called Theros breast cancer index to stratify patients into low, intermediate, and high risk for distant metastasis.
NA, not available; HR, hormone receptor; RT-PCR, reverse transcriptase polymerase chain reaction; FFPE, formalin-fixed paraffin-embedded; MGI, molecular grade index.

OTHER TUMOR MARKERS

p53

p53 is a tumor suppressor gene and is commonly mutated in several human cancers. In routine diagnostic surgical pathology, mutation status is assessed based on p53 expression by IHC. In some tumor types, such as bladder carcinomas, it has been shown that diffuse strong p53 expression by IHC correlates with *p53* mutation by molecular techniques.[407,408] The commonly used antibody clone DO7 recognizes both the wild-type and mutant p53 proteins. However, since the mutant protein has a longer half life than the wild-type protein, the mutant protein is more diffusely and intensely stained on IHC. Therefore, weak or patchy staining with p53 antibodies should be considered a negative result. Some of the confusion regarding p53 staining in breast and other cancers stems from interpretation. In any event, p53 staining has been associated with poor prognosis in breast carcinoma. With our continued improvement in understanding breast carcinoma, we now know that a large majority of tumors that demonstrate strong p53 immunoreactivity or show *p53* mutations belong to the basal subtype.[140] The clinical usefulness of *p53* mutation analysis or diffuse strong immunoreactivity in non-basal tumors has not been well studied. However, a recent study showed that *p53* gene abnormalities, as defined by sequencing, were associated with worse prognosis and that *p53* mutations/deletions were particularly prognostic in node-negative, ER-positive patients.[409] However, the present data are insufficient to recommend use of *p53* measurements for management of patients with breast cancer, as per the 2007 ASCO/CAP guidelines for testing in breast cancer.[322,395]

Ki-67

Numerous studies have been published regarding proliferation activity of breast carcinomas, many of which date back to the pre-expression profiling era. Investigators have used either flow cytometry to determine S-phase fraction or immunohistochemistry to study expression of proliferating cell nuclear antigen (PCNA) or Ki-67.[410,411] Numerous studies have shown a good correlation between different methodologies. Many studies have analyzed Ki-67 LI and have shown a high LI to be a poor prognostic factor in breast cancer.[412,413] However, different cut-off points have been used to define the high proliferation index, and different techniques have been used to determine the labeling index. Therefore, it is somewhat difficult to compare these studies and likely explains the reluctance to universally accept Ki-67 LI as a prognostic marker in breast cancer. Colozza and coworkers thoroughly reviewed 132 articles including 159,516 patients in regard to the prognostic and predictive value of Ki-67 and other proliferation markers (cyclin D, cyclin E, p27, p21, TK, and topoisomerase II-alpha).[414] The authors appropriately pointed out that all studies concerning these markers are level IV or III evidence at best. (Level I or II is required for use in clinical practice.) This demonstrates the difficulty in interpreting the literature owing to lack of standardization of assay reagents, procedures, and scoring. Therefore, the authors recommended not using these markers in routine clinical practice, a view also endorsed by the 2007 ASCO in their guidelines for testing in breast cancer.[395]

In spite of this argument, it is interesting to note that the very first gene-expression profiling study not only revealed "molecular portraits" but also identified genes responsible for the biologic differences between the tumor types.[131,415] One of the largest distinct gene clusters identified by expression profiling consisted of proliferation genes and included both PCNA and Ki-67. Since then, no study has primarily focused on the issue of Ki-67 LI and its correlation to all the molecular classes. Therefore, we examined the Ki-67 LI using image analysis in ~200 consecutive breast carcinomas divided into molecular class using IHC criteria (detailed in the Immunogenomics section earlier in the chapter). It was interesting to note that the average Ki-67 labeling index was highest in TN tumors and that most tumors showed an index above 50%.[385] The ERBB2 tumors were a distant second (average Ki-67 LI of 28%), followed by HR-positive tumors (LBHH>LAHH=LUMB>LUMA). Although the mean Ki-67 LI was low in HR-positive tumors, not all tumors had low Ki-67 LI and showed a wide range. This difference in proliferation activity coupled with quantitative difference in ER expression has been exploited in the development of a commercial assay (Onco*type* Dx) for predicting breast cancer prognosis and treatment.[399] Although it is not the most robust prognostic or predictive marker, Ki-67 LI is an additional piece of information that may be used in clinical decision-making provided the physician understands the limitations of the test and the test result.

EGFR

The epidermal growth factor receptor (EGFR, HER-1, c-erbB-1) is one of the four transmembrane growth factor receptor proteins that share similarities in structure and function. Using a criterion similar to assessing HER2 IHC expression, EGFR over-expression in breast carcinoma is seen in less than 10% of all tumors.[388] The best correlation of EGFR-increased gene copy number is with 3+ IHC score. Breast tumors that show EGFR expression/over-expression are generally negative for steroid HRs. With our current understanding of breast carcinoma molecular classification, EGFR expression would be predominantly seen in basal-like breast carcinomas. Therefore, it has been proposed to use EGFR along with CK5/6 in identifying basal-like carcinomas.[134,387] It seems like EGFR does have a diagnostic use in breast pathologic examination. As far as prognostic and predictive value are concerned, the role of EGFR IHC is unknown. As per our understanding from lung carcinoma studies, the tumors that are responsive to small-molecule tyrosine kinase inhibitors demonstrate mutations in exon 19 and 21 of EGFR. Such mutations have not been identified in breast carcinomas.[388,416] In colon carcinoma, use of an EGFR inhibitor (cetuximab) was initially based on EGFR expression. However, subsequent studies have found no correlation between EGFR expression and response to cetuximab. Whether cetuximab therapy would have a role in breast cancer (especially basal-like) remains to be seen.[417,418] Until further clinical trials and additional studies are performed, the role of EGFR is limited to diagnostic use only.

uPA and PAI-1

Urokinase plasminogen activator (uPA)/plasminogen activator inhibitor (PAI-1) are part of the plasminogen activating system, which includes the receptor for uPA and other inhibitors (PAI-2 and PAI-3). This system has been shown experimentally to be associated with invasion, angiogenesis, and metastasis.[419] Low levels of both markers are associated with a sufficiently low risk of recurrence (especially in HR-positive women who will receive adjuvant endocrine therapy) that chemotherapy will only contribute minimal additional benefit. Furthermore, Cytoxan-, methotrexate-, and 5-fluorouracil-based adjuvant chemotherapy provides substantial benefit, compared with observation alone, in patients with high risk of recurrence as determined by high levels of uPA and PAI-1. Although any technique (IHC, RT-PCR, or ELISA) could be used to determine levels of uPA and PAI-1, the outcome is best correlated with ELISA.[420-422] Unfortunately, IHC results do not reliably predict outcomes, and the prognostic value of ELISA using smaller tissue specimens, such as tissue collected by core biopsy, has not been validated.[423] We believe that the clinical utility of this test is limited, as availability of 300 mg of fresh or frozen breast tumor would be a severe impediment in this era of mammographic and MRI detection of cancers.

FOXA1

FOXA1 is a forkhead family transcription factor that segregates with genes that characterize the luminal subtypes in DNA microarray analyses.[424] Using genome-wide analysis, Laganiere and colleagues identified 153 promoters bound by ER-alpha in the breast cancer cell line MCF-7 in the presence of estradiol.[425] One of the promoters identified was for FOXA1, whose expression correlated with expression of ER-alpha. Laganiere and colleagues further found that ablation of FOXA1 expression in MCF-7 cells suppressed ER-alpha binding to the prototypic TFF1 promoter (which contains a FOXA1 binding site), hindered the induction of TFF1 expression by estradiol, and prevented hormone-induced reentry into the cell cycle. The practical utility of FOXA1 was assessed by Badve and coworkers, who showed positive correlation between FOXA1 expression and ER/PR expression by immunohistochemistry.[424] Another immunohistochemical study by Thorat and associates demonstrated a positive correlation between FOXA1 expression and ER-alpha ($p<0.0001$), PR ($p<0.0001$), and luminal subtype ($p<0.0001$) and a negative correlation with basal subtype ($p<0.0001$), proliferation markers, and high histologic grade ($p = 0.0327$).[426] Although FOXA1 was a significant predictor of overall survival in univariate analysis in this study, only nodal status and ER expression were significant predictors of overall survival on multivariate analyses. FOXA1 has also been proposed as a clinical/immunohistochemical marker to identify luminal A molecular subtype,[427] but data are currently limited on this subject.

GATA3

GATA binding protein 3 (GATA3) is a transcriptional activator highly expressed by the luminal epithelial cells in the breast. It is involved in growth and differentiation. Gene expression profiling has shown that GATA-3 is highly expressed in the luminal A subtype of breast cancer.[140,384] In an immunohistochemical study of 139 breast cancers, Mehra and coworkers showed that low GATA3 expression was associated with higher histologic grade ($P < 0.001$), positive nodes ($P = 0.002$), larger tumor size ($P = 0.03$), negative ER and PR ($P < 0.001$ for both), and HER2/neu overexpression ($P = 0.03$).[428] Patients whose tumors expressed low GATA3 had significantly shorter overall and disease-free survival when compared with those whose tumors had high GATA3 levels.[428] In a much larger series of 3119 breast cancer cases, Voduc and associates showed somewhat similar findings; however, they also clarified some of the issues.[429] In their study, GATA-3 was almost exclusively expressed in ER-positive patients and was also associated with lower tumor grade, older age at diagnosis, and the absence of HER2 overexpression. GATA-3 was a marker of good prognosis and predicted for superior breast cancer-specific survival, relapse-free survival, and overall survival in univariate analysis.[429] However, in multivariate models including patient age, tumor size, histologic grade, nodal status, ER status, and HER2 status, GATA-3 was not independently prognostic for these same outcomes. Furthermore, in the subgroups of ER-positive patients treated with or without tamoxifen, GATA-3 was again nonprognostic for all outcomes.[429]

Both FOXA1 and GATA-3 are molecular markers that are highly associated with ER expression, but they do not seem to have prognostic value independent of ER. Additional clinical validation studies are required before their use can be recommended in routine practice.

We will not discuss several other prognostic/predictive markers published in the literature (nm23, cathepsin D, microvascular density, PS2, p-glycoprotein, BCL-2, fibroblast growth factor, transforming growth factor-beta, insulin-like growth factor network, androgen receptor, matrix metalloproteinase) because of limited clinical utility at the time of this writing.

SUMMARY

Immunohistochemistry is a critical tool for diagnostic, theranostic, and genomic applications in breast pathology. We believe as more and more targeted therapy is applied in breast cancer, pathologists will be under pressure to analyze additional biomarkers. We also predict that pathologists will have to reconcile not only with morphology and IHC but also with additional molecular tests that clinicians are going to use in the future.

REFERENCES

1. Joshi MG, Lee AK, Pedersen CA, et al. The role of immunocytochemical markers in the differential diagnosis of proliferative and neoplastic lesions of the breast. *Mod Pathol.* 1996;9:57-62.
2. Rudland PS, Leinster SJ, Winstanley J, et al. Immunocytochemical identification of cell types in benign and malignant breast diseases: Variations in cell markers accompany the malignant state. *J Histochem Cytochem.* 1993;41:543-553.
3. Ahmed A. The myoepithelium in human breast carcinoma. *J Pathol.* 1974;113:129-135.
4. Bussolati G. Actin-rich (myoepithelial) cells in lobular carcinoma in situ of the breast. *Virchows Arch B Cell Pathol Incl Mol Pathol.* 1980;32:165-176.
5. Bussolati G, Botta G, Gugliotta P. Actin-rich (myoepithelial) cells in ductal carcinoma *in situ* of the breast. *Virchows Arch B Cell Pathol Incl Mol Pathol.* 1980;34:251-259.
6. Bussolati G, Botto Micca FB, Eusebi V, et al. Myoepithelial cells in lobular carcinoma in situ of the breast: A parallel immunocytochemical and ultrastructural study. *Ultrastruct Pathol.* 1981;2:219-230.
7. Gould VE, Jao W, Battifora H. Ultrastructural analysis in the differential diagnosis of breast tumors. The significance of myoepithelial cells, basal lamina, intracytoplasmic lumina and secretory granules. *Pathol Res Pract.* 1980;167:45-70.
8. Gusterson BA, Warburton MJ, Mitchell D, et al. Distribution of myoepithelial cells and basement membrane proteins in the normal breast and in benign and malignant breast diseases. *Cancer Res.* 1982;42:4763-4770.
9. Dwarakanath S, Lee AK, Delellis RA, et al. S-100 protein positivity in breast carcinomas: A potential pitfall in diagnostic immunohistochemistry. *Hum Pathol.* 1987;18:1144-1148.
10. Jarasch ED, Nagle RB, Kaufmann M, et al. Differential diagnosis of benign epithelial proliferations and carcinomas of the breast using antibodies to cytokeratins. *Hum Pathol.* 1988;19:276-289.
11. Nagle RB, Bocker W, Davis JR, et al. Characterization of breast carcinomas by two monoclonal antibodies distinguishing myoepithelial from luminal epithelial cells. *J Histochem Cytochem.* 1986;34:869-881.

12. Raju UB, Lee MW, Zarbo RJ, et al. Papillary neoplasia of the breast: Immunohistochemically defined myoepithelial cells in the diagnosis of benign and malignant papillary breast neoplasms. *Mod Pathol.* 1989;2:569-576.
13. Acs G, Lawton TJ, Rebbeck TR, et al. Differential expression of E-cadherin in lobular and ductal neoplasms of the breast and its biologic and diagnostic implications. *Am J Clin Pathol.* 2001;115:85-98.
14. Lele SM, Graves K, Gatalica Z. Immunohistochemical detection of maspin is a useful adjunct in distinguishing radial sclerosing lesion from tubular carcinoma of the breast. *Appl Immunohistochem Mol Morphol.* 2000;8:32-36.
15. Mohsin SK, Zhang M, Clark GM, et al. Maspin expression in invasive breast cancer: Association with other prognostic factors. *J Pathol.* 2003;199:432-435.
16. Navarro Rde L, Martins MT, de Araujo VC. Maspin expression in normal and neoplastic salivary gland. *J Oral Pathol Med.* 2004;33:435-440.
17. Umekita Y, Yoshida H. Expression of maspin is up-regulated during the progression of mammary ductal carcinoma. *Histopathology.* 2003;42:541-545.
18. Bocker W, Bier B, Freytag G, Brommelkamp B, et al. An immunohistochemical study of the breast using antibodies to basal and luminal keratins, alpha-smooth muscle actin, vimentin, collagen IV and laminin. Part II: Epitheliosis and ductal carcinoma in situ. *Virchows Arch A Pathol Anat Histopathol.* 1992;421:323-330.
19. Bose S, Derosa CM, Ozzello L. Immunostaining of type IV collagen and smooth muscle actin as an aid in the diagnosis of breast lesions. *Breast J.* 1999;5:194-201.
20. Gottlieb C, Raju U, Greenwald KA. Myoepithelial cells in the differential diagnosis of complex benign and malignant breast lesions: An immunohistochemical study. *Mod Pathol.* 1990;3:135-140.
21. Gugliotta P, Sapino A, Macri L, et al. Specific demonstration of myoepithelial cells by anti-alpha smooth muscle actin antibody. *J Histochem Cytochem.* 1988;36:659-663.
22. Raymond WA, Leong AS. Assessment of invasion in breast lesions using antibodies to basement membrane components and myoepithelial cells. *Pathology.* 1991;23:291-297.
23. Gimona M, Herzog M, Vandekerckhove J, Small JV. Smooth muscle specific expression of calponin. *FEBS Lett.* 1990;274: 159-162.
24. Werling RW, Hwang H, Yaziji H, et al. Immunohistochemical distinction of invasive from noninvasive breast lesions: A comparative study of p63 versus calponin and smooth muscle myosin heavy chain. *Am J Surg Pathol.* 2003;27:82-90.
25. Winder SJ, Walsh MP. Calponin: Thin filament-linked regulation of smooth muscle contraction. *Cell Signal.* 1993;5:677-686.
26. Titus MA. Myosins. *Curr Opin Cell Biol.* 1993;5:77-81.
27. Strasser P, Gimona M, Moessler H, et al. Mammalian calponin. Identification and expression of genetic variants. *FEBS Lett.* 1993;330:13-18.
28. Barbareschi M, Pecciarini L, Cangi MG, et al. p63, a p53 homologue, is a selective nuclear marker of myoepithelial cells of the human breast. *Am J Surg Pathol.* 2001;25:1054-1060.
29. Kaufmann O, Fietze E, Mengs J, et al. Value of p63 and cytokeratin 5/6 as immunohistochemical markers for the differential diagnosis of poorly differentiated and undifferentiated carcinomas. *Am J Clin Pathol.* 2001;116:823-830.
30. Bhargava R, Dabbs DJ. Use of immunohistochemistry in diagnosis of breast epithelial lesions. *Adv Anat Pathol.* 2007;14: 93-107.
31. Eusebi V, Foschini MP, Betts CM, et al. Microglandular adenosis, apocrine adenosis, and tubular carcinoma of the breast. An immunohistochemical comparison. *Am J Surg Pathol.* 1993;17:99-109.
32. Lee KC, Chan JK, Gwi E. Tubular adenosis of the breast. A distinctive benign lesion mimicking invasive carcinoma. *Am J Surg Pathol.* 1996;20:46-54.
33. Hill CB, Yeh IT. Myoepithelial cell staining patterns of papillary breast lesions: From intraductal papillomas to invasive papillary carcinomas. *Am J Clin Pathol.* 2005;123:36-44.
34. Papotti M, Eusebi V, Gugliotta P, et al. Immunohistochemical analysis of benign and malignant papillary lesions of the breast. *Am J Surg Pathol.* 1983;7:451-461.
35. Saddik M, Lai R. CD44s as a surrogate marker for distinguishing intraductal papilloma from papillary carcinoma of the breast. *J Clin Pathol.* 1999;52:862-864.
36. Raju U, Vertes D. Breast papillomas with atypical ductal hyperplasia: A clinicopathologic study. *Hum Pathol.* 1996;27:1231-1238.
37. Collins LC, Schnitt SJ. Papillary lesions of the breast: Selected diagnostic and management issues. *Histopathology.* 2008;52:20-29.
38. Rabban JT, Koerner FC, Lerwill MF. Solid papillary ductal carcinoma in situ versus usual ductal hyperplasia in the breast: A potentially difficult distinction resolved by cytokeratin 5/6. *Hum Pathol.* 2006;37:787-793.
39. Carter D, Orr SL, Merino MJ. Intracystic papillary carcinoma of the breast. After mastectomy, radiotherapy or excisional biopsy alone. *Cancer.* 1983;52:14-19.
40. Carter D. Intraductal papillary tumors of the breast: A study of 78 cases. *Cancer.* 1977;39:1689-1692.
41. Collins LC, Carlo VP, Hwang H, et al. Intracystic papillary carcinomas of the breast: A reevaluation using a panel of myoepithelial cell markers. *Am J Surg Pathol.* 2006;30:1002-1007.
42. Mulligan AM, O'Malley FP. Papillary lesions of the breast: A review. *Adv Anat Pathol.* 2007;14:108-119.
43. Esposito NN, Dabbs DJ, Bhargava R. Are encapsulated papillary carcinomas of the breast *in situ* or invasive? A basement membrane study of 27 cases. *Am J Clin Pathol.* 2009;131:228-242.
44. Barsky SH, Siegal GP, Jannotta F, et al. Loss of basement membrane components by invasive tumors but not by their benign counterparts. *Lab Invest.* 1983;49:140-147.
45. Leal C, Costa I, Fonseca D, et al. Intracystic (encysted) papillary carcinoma of the breast: A clinical, pathological, and immunohistochemical study. *Hum Pathol.* 1998;29:1097-1104.
46. Lefkowitz M, Lefkowitz W, Wargotz ES. Intraductal (intracystic) papillary carcinoma of the breast and its variants: A clinicopathological study of 77 cases. *Hum Pathol.* 1994;25:802-809.
47. Solorzano CC, Middleton LP, Hunt KK, et al. Treatment and outcome of patients with intracystic papillary carcinoma of the breast. *Am J Surg.* 2002;184:364-368.
48. Mulligan AM, O'Malley FP. Metastatic potential of encapsulated (intracystic) papillary carcinoma of the breast: A report of 2 cases with axillary lymph node micrometastases. *Int J Surg Pathol.* 2007;15:143-147.
49. Masood S, Sim SJ, Lu L. Immunohistochemical differentiation of atypical hyperplasia vs. carcinoma in situ of the breast. *Cancer Detect Prev.* 1992;16:225-235.
50. Moinfar F, Man YG, Lininger RA, et al. Use of keratin 35betaE12 as an adjunct in the diagnosis of mammary intraepithelial neoplasia-ductal type—benign and malignant intraductal proliferations. *Am J Surg Pathol.* 1999;23:1048-1058.
51. Lacroix-Triki M, Mery E, Voigt JJ, et al. Value of cytokeratin 5/6 immunostaining using D5/16 B4 antibody in the spectrum of proliferative intraepithelial lesions of the breast. A comparative study with 34betaE12 antibody. *Virchows Arch.* 2003; 442:548-554.
52. Chuba PJ, Hamre MR, Yap J, et al. Bilateral risk for subsequent breast cancer after lobular carcinoma- *in situ*: Analysis of surveillance, epidemiology, and end results data. *J Clin Oncol.* 2005;23:5534-5541.
53. Crisi GM, Mandavilli S, Cronin E, et al. Invasive mammary carcinoma after immediate and short-term follow-up for lobular neoplasia on core biopsy. *Am J Surg Pathol.* 2003;27:325-333.
54. Elsheikh TM, Silverman JF. Follow-up surgical excision is indicated when breast core needle biopsies show atypical lobular hyperplasia or lobular carcinoma in situ: A correlative study of 33 patients with review of the literature. *Am J Surg Pathol.* 2005;29:534-543.
55. Fisher ER, Costantino J, Fisher B, et al. Pathologic findings from the National Surgical Adjuvant Breast Project (NSABP) Protocol B-17. Five-year observations concerning lobular carcinoma in situ. *Cancer.* 1996;78:1403-1416.
56. Fisher ER, Land SR, Fisher B, et al. Pathologic findings from the National Surgical Adjuvant Breast and Bowel Project: Twelve-year observations concerning lobular carcinoma in situ. *Cancer.* 2004;100:238-244.

57. Leonard GD, Swain SM. Ductal carcinoma in situ, complexities and challenges. *J Natl Cancer Inst*. 2004;96:906-920.
58. Li CI, Malone KE, Saltzman BS, et al. Risk of invasive breast carcinoma among women diagnosed with ductal carcinoma in situ and lobular carcinoma in situ, 1988-2001. *Cancer*. 2006;106:2104-2112.
59. Maluf H, Koerner F. Lobular carcinoma in situ and infiltrating ductal carcinoma: frequent presence of DCIS as a precursor lesion. *Int J Surg Pathol*. 2001;9:127-131.
60. Winchester DP, Jeske JM, Goldschmidt RA. The diagnosis and management of ductal carcinoma *in situ* of the breast. *CA Cancer J Clin*. 2000;50:184-200.
61. Cangiarella J, Guth A, Axelrod D, et al. Is surgical excision necessary for the management of atypical lobular hyperplasia and lobular carcinoma in situ diagnosed on core needle biopsy?: A report of 38 cases and review of the literature. *Arch Pathol Lab Med*. 2008;132:979-983.
62. Bedrosian I, Mick R, Orel SG, et al. Changes in the surgical management of patients with breast carcinoma based on preoperative magnetic resonance imaging. *Cancer*. 2003;98:468-473.
63. Molland JG, Donnellan M, Janu NC, et al. Infiltrating lobular carcinoma—A comparison of diagnosis, management and outcome with infiltrating duct carcinoma. *Breast*. 2004;13: 389-396.
64. Munot K, Dall B, Achuthan R, et al. Role of magnetic resonance imaging in the diagnosis and single-stage surgical resection of invasive lobular carcinoma of the breast. *Br J Surg*. 2002;89:1296-1301.
65. Borst MJ, Ingold JA. Metastatic patterns of invasive lobular versus invasive ductal carcinoma of the breast. *Surgery*. 1993;114:637-641; discussion 641-642.
66. Harris M, Howell A, Chrissohou M, et al. A comparison of the metastatic pattern of infiltrating lobular carcinoma and infiltrating duct carcinoma of the breast. *Br J Cancer*. 1984;50:23-30.
67. Jain S, Fisher C, Smith P, et al. Patterns of metastatic breast cancer in relation to histological type. *Eur J Cancer*. 1993;29A:2155-2157.
68. Tham YL, Sexton K, Kramer R, et al. Primary breast cancer phenotypes associated with propensity for central nervous system metastases. *Cancer*. 2006;107:696-704.
69. Arpino G, Bardou VJ, Clark GM, et al. Infiltrating lobular carcinoma of the breast: Tumor characteristics and clinical outcome. *Breast Cancer Res*. 2004;6:R149-R156.
70. Mersin H, Yildirim E, Gulben K, et al. Is invasive lobular carcinoma different from invasive ductal carcinoma? *Eur J Surg Oncol*. 2003;29:390-395.
71. Kneeshaw PJ, Turnbull LW, Smith A, et al. Dynamic contrast enhanced magnetic resonance imaging aids the surgical management of invasive lobular breast cancer. *Eur J Surg Oncol*. 2003;29:32-37.
72. Schelfout K, Van Goethem M, Kersschot E, et al. Preoperative breast MRI in patients with invasive lobular breast cancer. *Eur Radiol*. 2004;14:1209-1216.
73. Cocquyt VF, Blondeel PN, Depypere HT, et al. Different responses to preoperative chemotherapy for invasive lobular and invasive ductal breast carcinoma. *Eur J Surg Oncol*. 2003;29:361-367.
74. Cristofanilli M, Gonzalez-Angulo A, Sneige N, et al. Invasive lobular carcinoma classic type: Response to primary chemotherapy and survival outcomes. *J Clin Oncol*. 2005;23:41-48.
75. Mathieu MC, Rouzier R, Llombart-Cussac A, et al. The poor responsiveness of infiltrating lobular breast carcinomas to neoadjuvant chemotherapy can be explained by their biological profile. *Eur J Cancer*. 2004;40:342-351.
76. Tubiana-Hulin M, Stevens D, Lasry S, et al. Response to neoadjuvant chemotherapy in lobular and ductal breast carcinomas: A retrospective study on 860 patients from one institution. *Ann Oncol*. 2006;17:1228-1233.
77. Gamallo C, Palacios J, Suarez A, et al. Correlation of E-cadherin expression with differentiation grade and histological type in breast carcinoma. *Am J Pathol*. 1993;142:987-993.
78. Moll R, Mitze M, Frixen UH, et al. Differential loss of E-cadherin expression in infiltrating ductal and lobular breast carcinomas. *Am J Pathol*. 1993;143:1731-1742.
79. Berx G, Cleton-Jansen AM, Nollet F, et al. E-cadherin is a tumour/invasion suppressor gene mutated in human lobular breast cancers. *Embo J*. 1995;14:6107-6115.
80. Berx G, Cleton-Jansen AM, Strumane K, et al. E-cadherin is inactivated in a majority of invasive human lobular breast cancers by truncation mutations throughout its extracellular domain. *Oncogene*. 1996;13:1919-1925.
81. Vos CB, Cleton-Jansen AM, Berx G, et al. E-cadherin inactivation in lobular carcinoma in situ of the breast: An early event in tumorigenesis. *Br J Cancer*. 1997;76:1131-1133.
82. Handschuh G, Candidus S, Luber B, et al. Tumour-associated E-cadherin mutations alter cellular morphology, decrease cellular adhesion and increase cellular motility. *Oncogene*. 1999;18:4301-4312.
83. Goldstein NS, Kestin LL, Vicini FA. Clinicopathologic implications of E-cadherin reactivity in patients with lobular carcinoma in situ of the breast. *Cancer*. 2001;92:738-747.
84. De Leeuw WJ, Berx G, Vos CB, et al. Simultaneous loss of E-cadherin and catenins in invasive lobular breast cancer and lobular carcinoma in situ. *J Pathol*. 1997;183:404-411.
85. Gonzalez MA, Pinder SE, Wencyk PM, et al. An immunohistochemical examination of the expression of E-cadherin, alpha- and beta/gamma-catenins, and alpha2- and beta1-integrins in invasive breast cancer. *J Pathol*. 1999;187:523-529.
86. Aberle H, Schwartz H, Kemler R. Cadherin-catenin complex: Protein interactions and their implications for cadherin function. *J Cell Biochem*. 1996;61:514-523.
87. Aghib DF, McCrea PD. The E-cadherin complex contains the src substrate p120. *Exp Cell Res*. 1995;218:359-369.
88. Gooding JM, Yap KL, Ikura M. The cadherin-catenin complex as a focal point of cell adhesion and signalling: New insights from three-dimensional structures. *Bioessays*. 2004;26:497-511.
89. Piepenhagen PA, Nelson WJ. Defining E-cadherin-associated protein complexes in epithelial cells: Plakoglobin, beta- and gamma-catenin are distinct components. *J Cell Sci*. 1993;104(Pt 3):751-762.
90. Reynolds AB, Daniel J, McCrea PD, et al. Identification of a new catenin: The tyrosine kinase substrate p120cas associates with E-cadherin complexes. *Mol Cell Biol*. 1994;14:8333-8342.
91. Yap AS, Niessen CM, Gumbiner BM. The juxtamembrane region of the cadherin cytoplasmic tail supports lateral clustering, adhesive strengthening, and interaction with p120ctn. *J Cell Biol*. 1998;141:779-789.
92. Shibamoto S, Hayakawa M, Takeuchi K, et al. Association of p120, a tyrosine kinase substrate, with E-cadherin/catenin complexes. *J Cell Biol*. 1995;128:949-957.
93. Davis MA, Ireton RC, Reynolds AB. A core function for p120-catenin in cadherin turnover. *J Cell Biol*. 2003;163:525-534.
94. Noren NK, Liu BP, Burridge K, et al. p120 catenin regulates the actin cytoskeleton via Rho family GTPases. *J Cell Biol*. 2000;150:567-580.
95. Berx G, Van Roy F. The E-cadherin/catenin complex: An important gatekeeper in breast cancer tumorigenesis and malignant progression. *Breast Cancer Res*. 2001;3:289-293.
96. Berx G, Nollet F, van Roy F. Dysregulation of the E-cadherin/catenin complex by irreversible mutations in human carcinomas. *Cell Adhes Commun*. 1998;6:171-184.
97. Karabakhtsian RG, Johnson R, Sumkin J, Dabbs DJ. The clinical significance of lobular neoplasia on breast core biopsy. *Am J Surg Pathol*. 2007;31:717-723.
98. Goldstein NS. Does the level of E-cadherin expression correlate with the primary breast carcinoma infiltration pattern and type of systemic metastases? *Am J Clin Pathol*. 2002;118:425-434.
99. Goldstein NS, Bassi D, Watts JC, et al. E-cadherin reactivity of 95 noninvasive ductal and lobular lesions of the breast. Implications for the interpretation of problematic lesions. *Am J Clin Pathol*. 2001;115:534-542.
100. Jacobs TW, Pliss N, Kouria G, et al. Carcinomas in situ of the breast with indeterminate features: Role of E-cadherin staining in categorization. *Am J Surg Pathol*. 2001;25:229-236.
101. Lehr HA, Folpe A, Yaziji H, et al. Cytokeratin 8 immunostaining pattern and E-cadherin expression distinguish lobular from ductal breast carcinoma. *Am J Clin Pathol*. 2000;114:190-196.
102. Bassler R, Kronsbein H. Disseminated lobular carcinoma—a predominantly pleomorphic lobular carcinoma of the whole breast. *Pathol Res Pract*. 1980;166:456-470.

103. Weidner N, Semple JP. Pleomorphic variant of invasive lobular carcinoma of the breast. *Hum Pathol.* 1992;23:1167-1171.
104. Eusebi V, Magalhaes F, Azzopardi JG. Pleomorphic lobular carcinoma of the breast: An aggressive tumor showing apocrine differentiation. *Hum Pathol.* 1992;23:655-662.
105. Reis-Filho JS, Simpson PT, Jones C, et al. Pleomorphic lobular carcinoma of the breast: Role of comprehensive molecular pathology in characterization of an entity. *J Pathol.* 2005;207: 1-13.
106. Bentz JS, Yassa N, Clayton F. Pleomorphic lobular carcinoma of the breast: Clinicopathologic features of 12 cases. *Mod Pathol.* 1998;11:814-822.
107. Frolik D, Caduff R, Varga Z. Pleomorphic lobular carcinoma of the breast: Its cell kinetics, expression of oncogenes and tumour suppressor genes compared with invasive ductal carcinomas and classical infiltrating lobular carcinomas. *Histopathology.* 2001;39:503-513.
108. Middleton LP, Palacios DM, Bryant BR, et al. Pleomorphic lobular carcinoma: Morphology, immunohistochemistry, and molecular analysis. *Am J Surg Pathol.* 2000;24:1650-1656.
109. Radhi JM. Immunohistochemical analysis of pleomorphic lobular carcinoma: Higher expression of p53 and chromogranin and lower expression of ER and PgR. *Histopathology.* 2000;36:156-160.
110. Dabbs DJ, Kaplai M, Chivukula M, et al. The spectrum of morphomolecular abnormalities of the E-cadherin/catenin complex in pleomorphic lobular carcinoma of the breast. *Appl Immunohistochem Mol Morphol.* 2007;15:260-266.
111. Simpson PT, Reis-Filho JS, Lambros MB, et al. Molecular profiling pleomorphic lobular carcinomas of the breast: Evidence for a common molecular genetic pathway with classic lobular carcinomas. *J Pathol.* 2008;215:231-244.
112. Sneige N, Wang J, Baker BA, et al. Clinical, histopathologic, and biologic features of pleomorphic lobular (ductal-lobular) carcinoma in situ of the breast: A report of 24 cases. *Mod Pathol.* 2002;15:1044-1050.
113. Fisher ER, Gregorio RM, Redmond C, et al. Tubulolobular invasive breast cancer: A variant of lobular invasive cancer. *Hum Pathol.* 1977;8:679-683.
114. Green I, McCormick B, Cranor M, et al. A comparative study of pure tubular and tubulolobular carcinoma of the breast. *Am J Surg Pathol.* 1997;21:653-657.
115. Esposito NN, Chivukula M, Dabbs DJ. The ductal phenotypic expression of the E-cadherin/catenin complex in tubulolobular carcinoma of the breast: An immunohistochemical and clinicopathologic study. *Mod Pathol.* 2007;20:130-138.
116. Wheeler DT, Tai LH, Bratthauer GL, et al. Tubulolobular carcinoma of the breast: An analysis of 27 cases of a tumor with a hybrid morphology and immunoprofile. *Am J Surg Pathol.* 2004;28:1587-1593.
117. Hood CI, Font RL, Zimmerman LE. Metastatic mammary carcinoma in the eyelid with histiocytoid appearance. *Cancer.* 1973;31:793-800.
118. Filotico M, Trabucco M, Gallone D, et al. Histiocytoid carcinoma of the breast. A problem of differential diagnosis for the pathologist. Report of a case. *Pathologica.* 1983;75:429-433.
119. Gupta D, Croitoru CM, Ayala AG, et al. E-cadherin immunohistochemical analysis of histiocytoid carcinoma of the breast. *Ann Diagn Pathol.* 2002;6:141-147.
120. Reis-Filho JS, Fulford LG, Freeman A, et al. Pathologic quiz case: A 93-year-old woman with an enlarged and tender left breast. Histiocytoid variant of lobular breast carcinoma. *Arch Pathol Lab Med.* 2003;127:1626-1628.
121. Luna-More S, Gonzalez B, Acedo C, et al. Invasive micropapillary carcinoma of the breast. A new special type of invasive mammary carcinoma. *Pathol Res Pract.* 1994;190:668-674.
122. Siriaunkgul S, Tavassoli FA. Invasive micropapillary carcinoma of the breast. *Mod Pathol.* 1993;6:660-662.
123. Li YS, Kaneko M, Sakamoto DG, et al. The reversed apical pattern of MUC1 expression is characteristics of invasive micropapillary carcinoma of the breast. *Breast Cancer.* 2006;13: 58-63.
124. Nassar H, Pansare V, Zhang H, et al. Pathogenesis of invasive micropapillary carcinoma: Role of MUC1 glycoprotein. *Mod Pathol.* 2004;17:1045-1050.
125. Guo X, Chen L, Lang R, et al. Invasive micropapillary carcinoma of the breast: Association of pathologic features with lymph node metastasis. *Am J Clin Pathol.* 2006;126:740-746.
126. Nassar H. Carcinomas with micropapillary morphology: Clinical significance and current concepts. *Adv Anat Pathol.* 2004;11:297-303.
127. Nassar H, Wallis T, Andea A, et al. Clinicopathologic analysis of invasive micropapillary differentiation in breast carcinoma. *Mod Pathol.* 2001;14:836-841.
128. Pettinato G, Manivel CJ, Panico L, et al. Invasive micropapillary carcinoma of the breast: Clinicopathologic study of 62 cases of a poorly recognized variant with highly aggressive behavior. *Am J Clin Pathol.* 2004;121:857-866.
129. Walsh MM, Bleiweiss IJ. Invasive micropapillary carcinoma of the breast: Eighty cases of an underrecognized entity. *Hum Pathol.* 2001;32:583-589.
130. Paterakos M, Watkin WG, Edgerton SM, et al. Invasive micropapillary carcinoma of the breast: A prognostic study. *Hum Pathol.* 1999;30:1459-1463.
131. Perou CM, Sorlie T, Eisen MB, et al. Molecular portraits of human breast tumours. *Nature.* 2000;406:747-752.
132. Sorlie T, Perou CM, Tibshirani R, et al. Gene expression patterns of breast carcinomas distinguish tumor subclasses with clinical implications. *Proc Natl Acad Sci U S A.* 2001;98:10869-10874.
133. Livasy CA, Karaca G, Nanda R, et al. Phenotypic evaluation of the basal-like subtype of invasive breast carcinoma. *Mod Pathol.* 2006;19:264-271.
134. Nielsen TO, Hsu FD, Jensen K, et al. Immunohistochemical and clinical characterization of the basal-like subtype of invasive breast carcinoma. *Clin Cancer Res.* 2004;10:5367-5374.
135. Bhargava R, Beriwal S, McManus K, et al. CK5 is more sensitive than CK5/6 in identifying "basal-like" phenotype of breast carcinoma. *Am J Clin Pathol.* 2008;130:724-730.
136. Bryan BB, Schnitt SJ, Collins LC. Ductal carcinoma in situ with basal-like phenotype: A possible precursor to invasive basal-like breast cancer. *Mod Pathol.* 2006;19:617-621.
137. Dabbs DJ, Chivukula M, Carter G, et al. Basal phenotype of ductal carcinoma in situ: Recognition and immunohistologic profile. *Mod Pathol.* 2006;19:1506-1511.
138. Carey LA, Perou CM, Livasy CA, et al. Race, breast cancer subtypes, and survival in the Carolina Breast Cancer Study. *JAMA.* 2006;295:2492-2502.
139. van de Rijn M, Perou CM, Tibshirani R, et al. Expression of cytokeratins 17 and 5 identifies a group of breast carcinomas with poor clinical outcome. *Am J Pathol.* 2002;161: 1991-1996.
140. Sorlie T, Tibshirani R, Parker J, et al. Repeated observation of breast tumor subtypes in independent gene expression data sets. *Proc Natl Acad Sci U S A.* 2003;100:8418-8423.
141. Carter MR, Hornick JL, Lester S, et al. Spindle cell (sarcomatoid) carcinoma of the breast: A clinicopathologic and immunohistochemical analysis of 29 cases. *Am J Surg Pathol.* 2006;30:300-309.
142. Davis WG, Hennessy B, Babiera G, et al. Metaplastic sarcomatoid carcinoma of the breast with absent or minimal overt invasive carcinomatous component: A misnomer. *Am J Surg Pathol.* 2005;29:1456-1463.
143. Adem C, Reynolds C, Adlakha H, et al. Wide spectrum screening keratin as a marker of metaplastic spindle cell carcinoma of the breast: An immunohistochemical study of 24 patients. *Histopathology.* 2002;40:556-562.
144. Koker MM, Kleer CG. p63 expression in breast cancer: A highly sensitive and specific marker of metaplastic carcinoma. *Am J Surg Pathol.* 2004;28:1506-1512.
145. Tse GM, Tan PH, Chaiwun B, et al. p63 is useful in the diagnosis of mammary metaplastic carcinomas. *Pathology.* 2006;38:16-20.
146. Ellis IO, Bell J, Ronan JE, et al. Immunocytochemical investigation of intermediate filament proteins and epithelial membrane antigen in spindle cell tumours of the breast. *J Pathol.* 1988;154:157-165.
147. Wargotz ES, Norris HJ. Metaplastic carcinomas of the breast. III. Carcinosarcoma. *Cancer.* 1989;64:1490-1499.

148. Sommers CL, Walker Jones D, Heckford SE, et al. Vimentin rather than keratin expression in some hormone-independent breast cancer cell lines and in oncogene-transformed mammary epithelial cells. *Cancer Res.* 1989;49:4258-4263.
149. Dunne B, Lee AH, Pinder SE, et al. An immunohistochemical study of metaplastic spindle cell carcinoma, phyllodes tumor and fibromatosis of the breast. *Hum Pathol.* 2003;34:1009-1015.
150. Leibl S, Gogg-Kammerer M, Sommersacher A, et al. Metaplastic breast carcinomas: Are they of myoepithelial differentiation?: Immunohistochemical profile of the sarcomatoid subtype using novel myoepithelial markers. *Am J Surg Pathol.* 2005;29:347-353.
151. Miettinen M, Franssila K. Immunohistochemical spectrum of malignant melanoma. The common presence of keratins. *Lab Invest.* 1989;61:623-628.
152. Zarbo RJ, Gown AM, Nagle RB, et al. Anomalous cytokeratin expression in malignant melanoma: One- and two-dimensional western blot analysis and immunohistochemical survey of 100 melanomas. *Mod Pathol.* 1990;3:494-501.
153. Pusztaszeri MP, Seelentag W, Bosman FT. Immunohistochemical expression of endothelial markers CD31, CD34, von Willebrand factor, and Fli-1 in normal human tissues. *J Histochem Cytochem.* 2006;54:385-395.
154. Miettinen M, Lindenmayer AE, Chaubal A. Endothelial cell markers CD31, CD34, and BNH9 antibody to H- and Y-antigens—Evaluation of their specificity and sensitivity in the diagnosis of vascular tumors and comparison with von Willebrand factor. *Mod Pathol.* 1994;7:82-90.
155. Chen PC, Chen CK, Nicastri AD, et al. Myoepithelial carcinoma of the breast with distant metastasis and accompanied by adenomyoepitheliomas. *Histopathology.* 1994;24:543-548.
156. Foschini MP, Eusebi V. Carcinomas of the breast showing myoepithelial cell differentiation. A review of the literature. *Virchows Arch.* 1998;432:303-310.
157. Thorner PS, Kahn HJ, Baumal R, et al. Malignant myoepithelioma of the breast. An immunohistochemical study by light and electron microscopy. *Cancer.* 1986;57:745-750.
158. Young RH, Clement PB. Adenomyoepithelioma of the breast. A report of three cases and review of the literature. *Am J Clin Pathol.* 1988;89:308-314.
159. Schurch W, Potvin C, Seemayer TA. Malignant myoepithelioma (myoepithelial carcinoma) of the breast: An ultrastructural and immunocytochemical study. *Ultrastruct Pathol.* 1985;8:1-11.
160. Tavassoli FA. Myoepithelial lesions of the breast. Myoepitheliosis, adenomyoepithelioma, and myoepithelial carcinoma. *Am J Surg Pathol.* 1991;15:554-568.
161. Hornick JL, Fletcher CD. Myoepithelial tumors of soft tissue: A clinicopathologic and immunohistochemical study of 101 cases with evaluation of prognostic parameters. *Am J Surg Pathol.* 2003;27:1183-1196.
162. Hornick JL, Fletcher CD. Cutaneous myoepithelioma: A clinicopathologic and immunohistochemical study of 14 cases. *Hum Pathol.* 2004;35:14-24.
163. Popnikolov NK, Ayala AG, Graves K, et al. Benign myoepithelial tumors of the breast have immunophenotypic characteristics similar to metaplastic matrix-producing and spindle cell carcinomas. *Am J Clin Pathol.* 2003;120:161-167.
164. Reis-Filho JS, Milanezi F, Paredes J, et al. Novel and classic myoepithelial/stem cell markers in metaplastic carcinomas of the breast. *Appl Immunohistochem Mol Morphol.* 2003;11:1-8.
165. Smith TA, Machen SK, Fisher C, et al. Usefulness of cytokeratin subsets for distinguishing monophasic synovial sarcoma from malignant peripheral nerve sheath tumor. *Am J Clin Pathol.* 1999;112:641-648.
166. Damiani S, Miettinen M, Peterse JL, et al. Solitary fibrous tumour (myofibroblastoma) of the breast. *Virchows Arch.* 1994;425:89-92.
167. Julien M, Trojani M, Coindre JM. [Myofibroblastoma of the breast. Report of 8 cases]. *Ann Pathol.* 1994;14:143-147.
168. Wargotz ES, Weiss SW, Norris HJ. Myofibroblastoma of the breast. Sixteen cases of a distinctive benign mesenchymal tumor. *Am J Surg Pathol.* 1987;11:493-502.
169. Lee AH. Recent developments in the histological diagnosis of spindle cell carcinoma, fibromatosis and phyllodes tumour of the breast. *Histopathology.* 2008;52:45-57.
170. Chaudary MA, Millis RR, Lane EB, et al. Paget's disease of the nipple: A ten year review including clinical, pathological, and immunohistochemical findings. *Breast Cancer Res Treat.* 1986;8:139-146.
171. Yim JH, Wick MR, Philpott GW, et al. Underlying pathology in mammary Paget's disease. *Ann Surg Oncol.* 1997;4:287-292.
172. Anderson JM, Ariga R, Govil H, et al. Assessment of Her-2/Neu status by immunohistochemistry and fluorescence in situ hybridization in mammary Paget disease and underlying carcinoma. *Appl Immunohistochem Mol Morphol.* 2003;11:120-124.
173. Haerslev T, Krag Jacobsen G. Expression of cytokeratin and erbB-2 oncoprotein in Paget's disease of the nipple. An immunohistochemical study. *APMIS.* 1992;100:1041-1047.
174. Lammie GA, Barnes DM, Millis RR, et al. An immunohistochemical study of the presence of c-erbB-2 protein in Paget's disease of the nipple. *Histopathology.* 1989;15:505-514.
175. Wolber RA, Dupuis BA, Wick MR. Expression of c-erbB-2 oncoprotein in mammary and extramammary Paget's disease. *Am J Clin Pathol.* 1991;96:243-247.
176. Meissner K, Riviere A, Haupt G, et al. Study of neu-protein expression in mammary Paget's disease with and without underlying breast carcinoma and in extramammary Paget's disease. *Am J Pathol.* 1990;137:1305-1309.
177. Tani EM, Skoog L. Immunocytochemical detection of estrogen receptors in mammary Paget cells. *Acta Cytol.* 1988;32:825-828.
178. Fu W, Lobocki CA, Silberberg BK, et al. Molecular markers in Paget disease of the breast. *J Surg Oncol.* 2001;77:171-178.
179. Gillett CE, Bobrow LG, Millis RR. S100 protein in human mammary tissue—Immunoreactivity in breast carcinoma, including Paget's disease of the nipple, and value as a marker of myoepithelial cells. *J Pathol.* 1990;160:19-24.
180. Lundquist K, Kohler S, Rouse RV. Intraepidermal cytokeratin 7 expression is not restricted to Paget cells but is also seen in Toker cells and Merkel cells. *Am J Surg Pathol.* 1999;23:212-219.
181. Marucci G, Betts CM, Golouh R, et al. Toker cells are probably precursors of Paget cell carcinoma: A morphological and ultrastructural description. *Virchows Arch.* 2002;441:117-123.
182. Zeng Z, Melamed J, Symmans PJ, et al. Benign proliferative nipple duct lesions frequently contain CAM 5.2 and anti-cytokeratin 7 immunoreactive cells in the overlying epidermis. *Am J Surg Pathol.* 1999;23:1349-1355.
183. Yao DX, Hoda SA, Chiu A, et al. Intraepidermal cytokeratin 7 immunoreactive cells in the non-neoplastic nipple may represent interepithelial extension of lactiferous duct cells. *Histopathology.* 2002;40:230-236.
184. Bader AA, Tio J, Petru E, et al. T1 breast cancer: Identification of patients at low risk of axillary lymph node metastases. *Breast Cancer Res Treat.* 2002;76:11-17.
185. Barth A, Craig PH, Silverstein MJ. Predictors of axillary lymph node metastases in patients with T1 breast carcinoma. *Cancer.* 1997;79:1918-1922.
186. Chadha M, Chabon AB, Friedmann P, et al. Predictors of axillary lymph node metastases in patients with T1 breast cancer. A multivariate analysis. *Cancer.* 1994;73:350-353.
187. Gajdos C, Tartter PI, Bleiweiss IJ. Lymphatic invasion, tumor size, and age are independent predictors of axillary lymph node metastases in women with T1 breast cancers. *Ann Surg.* 1999;230:692-696.
188. Van den Eynden GG, Van der Auwera I, Van Laere SJ, et al. Distinguishing blood and lymph vessel invasion in breast cancer: A prospective immunohistochemical study. *Br J Cancer.* 2006;94:1643-1649.
189. Amparo RS, Angel CD, Ana LH, et al. Inflammatory breast carcinoma: Pathological or clinical entity? *Breast Cancer Res Treat.* 2000;64:269-273.
190. Bonnier P, Charpin C, Lejeune C, et al. Inflammatory carcinomas of the breast: A clinical, pathological, or a clinical and pathological definition? *Int J Cancer.* 1995;62:382-385.
191. Le MG, Arriagada R, Contesso G, et al. Dermal lymphatic emboli in inflammatory and noninflammatory breast cancer: A French-Tunisian joint study in 337 patients. *Clin Breast Cancer.* 2005;6:439-445.

192. Kahn HJ, Marks A. A new monoclonal antibody, D2-40, for detection of lymphatic invasion in primary tumors. *Lab Invest.* 2002;82:1255-1257.
193. Kaiserling E. [Immunohistochemical identification of lymph vessels with D2-40 in diagnostic pathology]. *Pathologe.* 2004;25:362-374.
194. Kahn HJ, Bailey D, Marks A. Monoclonal antibody D2-40, a new marker of lymphatic endothelium, reacts with Kaposi's sarcoma and a subset of angiosarcomas. *Mod Pathol.* 2002;15:434-440.
195. Steinhoff MM. Axillary node micrometastases: Detection and biologic significance. *Breast J.* 1999;5:325-329.
196. Mansi JL, Gogas H, Bliss JM, et al. Outcome of primary-breast-cancer patients with micrometastases: A long-term follow-up study. *Lancet.* 1999;354:197-202.
197. Nasser IA, Lee AK, Bosari S, et al. Occult axillary lymph node metastases in "node-negative" breast carcinoma. *Hum Pathol.* 1993;24:950-957.
198. Bass SS, Lyman GH, McCann CR, et al. Lymphatic mapping and sentinel lymph node biopsy. *Breast J.* 1999;5:288-295.
199. Dabbs DJ, Johnson R. The optimal number of sentinel lymph nodes for focused pathologic examination. *Breast J.* 2004;10:186-189.
200. Klevesath MB, Bobrow LG, Pinder SE, et al. The value of immunohistochemistry in sentinel lymph node histopathology in breast cancer. *Br J Cancer.* 2005;92:2201-2205.
201. Dabbs DJ, Fung M, Landsittel D, et al. Sentinel lymph node micrometastasis as a predictor of axillary tumor burden. *Breast J.* 2004;10:101-105.
202. den Bakker MA, van Weeszenberg A, de Kanter AY, et al. Non-sentinel lymph node involvement in patients with breast cancer and sentinel node micrometastasis; too early to abandon axillary clearance. *J Clin Pathol.* 2002;55:932-935.
203. Kamath VJ, Giuliano R, Dauway EL, et al. Characteristics of the sentinel lymph node in breast cancer predict further involvement of higher-echelon nodes in the axilla: A study to evaluate the need for complete axillary lymph node dissection. *Arch Surg.* 2001;136:688-692.
204. Mignotte H, Treilleux I, Faure C, et al. Axillary lymph-node dissection for positive sentinel nodes in breast cancer patients. *Eur J Surg Oncol.* 2002;28:623-626.
205. Cserni G, Bianchi S, Vezzosi V, et al. The value of cytokeratin immunohistochemistry in the evaluation of axillary sentinel lymph nodes in patients with lobular breast carcinoma. *J Clin Pathol.* 2006;59:518-522.
206. Czerniecki BJ, Scheff AM, Callans LS, et al. Immunohistochemistry with pancytokeratins improves the sensitivity of sentinel lymph node biopsy in patients with breast carcinoma. *Cancer.* 1999;85:1098-1103.
207. Doglioni C, Dell'Orto P, Zanetti G, et al. Cytokeratin-immunoreactive cells of human lymph nodes and spleen in normal and pathological conditions. An immunocytochemical study. *Virchows Arch A Pathol Anat Histopathol.* 1990;416:479-490.
208. Iuzzolino P, Bontempini L, Doglioni C, et al. Keratin immunoreactivity in extrafollicular reticular cells of the lymph node. *Am J Clin Pathol.* 1989;91:239-240.
209. Carter BA, Jensen RA, Simpson JF, et al. Benign transport of breast epithelium into axillary lymph nodes after biopsy. *Am J Clin Pathol.* 2000;113:259-265.
210. Diaz NM, Cox CE, Ebert M, et al. Benign mechanical transport of breast epithelial cells to sentinel lymph nodes. *Am J Surg Pathol.* 2004;28:1641-1645.
211. Diaz NM, Vrcel V, Centeno BA, et al. Modes of benign mechanical transport of breast epithelial cells to axillary lymph nodes. *Adv Anat Pathol.* 2005;12:7-9.
212. Diaz NM, Mayes JR, Vrcel V. Breast epithelial cells in dermal angiolymphatic spaces: A manifestation of benign mechanical transport. *Hum Pathol.* 2005;36:310-313.
213. Hughes SJ, Xi L, Raja S, et al. A rapid, fully automated, molecular-based assay accurately analyzes sentinel lymph nodes for the presence of metastatic breast cancer. *Ann Surg.* 2006;243:389-398.
214. Viale G, Dell'Orto P, Biasi MO, et al. Comparative evaluation of an extensive histopathologic examination and a real-time reverse-transcription-polymerase chain reaction assay for mammaglobin and cytokeratin 19 on axillary sentinel lymph nodes of breast carcinoma patients. *Ann Surg.* 2008;247:136-142.
215. Blumencranz P, Whitworth PW, Deck K, et al. Scientific Impact Recognition Award. Sentinel node staging for breast cancer: Intraoperative molecular pathology overcomes conventional histologic sampling errors. *Am J Surg.* 2007;194:426-432.
216. Mansel RE, Goyal A, Douglas-Jones A, et al. Detection of breast cancer metastasis in sentinel lymph nodes using intra-operative real time GeneSearch BLN Assay in the operating room: Results of the Cardiff study. *Breast Cancer Res Treat.* 2009;115:595-600.
217. Martin Martinez MD, Veys I, Majjaj S, et al. Clinical validation of a molecular assay for intra-operative detection of metastases in breast sentinel lymph nodes. *Eur J Surg Oncol.* 2009;35:387-392.
218. DeYoung BR, Wick MR. Immunohistologic evaluation of metastatic carcinomas of unknown origin: An algorithmic approach. *Semin Diagn Pathol.* 2000;17:184-193.
219. Rubin BP, Skarin AT, Pisick E, et al. Use of cytokeratins 7 and 20 in determining the origin of metastatic carcinoma of unknown primary, with special emphasis on lung cancer. *Eur J Cancer Prev.* 2001;10:77-82.
220. Tot T. Adenocarcinomas metastatic to the liver: the value of cytokeratins 20 and 7 in the search for unknown primary tumors. *Cancer.* 1999;85:171-177.
221. Perry A, Parisi JE, Kurtin PJ. Metastatic adenocarcinoma to the brain: An immunohistochemical approach. *Hum Pathol.* 1997;28:938-943.
222. Wick MR, Lillemoe TJ, Copland GT, Swanson PE, Manivel JC, Kiang DT. Gross cystic disease fluid protein-15 as a marker for breast cancer: immunohistochemical analysis of 690 human neoplasms and comparison with alpha-lactalbumin. *Hum Pathol.* 1989;20:281-287.
223. Pearlman WH, Gueriguian JL, Sawyer ME. A specific progesterone-binding component of human breast cyst fluid. *J Biol Chem.* 1973;248:5736-5741.
224. Haagensen Jr DE, Mazoujian G, Holder Jr WD, et al. Evaluation of a breast cyst fluid protein detectable in the plasma of breast carcinoma patients. *Ann Surg.* 1977;185:279-285.
225. Murphy LC, Lee-Wing M, Goldenberg GJ, et al. Expression of the gene encoding a prolactin-inducible protein by human breast cancers in vivo: Correlation with steroid receptor status. *Cancer Res.* 1987;47:4160-4164.
226. Mazoujian G, Parish TH, Haagensen Jr DE. Immunoperoxidase localization of GCDFP-15 with mouse monoclonal antibodies versus rabbit antiserum. *J Histochem Cytochem.* 1988;36:377-382.
227. Mazoujian G, Margolis R. Immunohistochemistry of gross cystic disease fluid protein (GCDFP-15) in 65 benign sweat gland tumors of the skin. *Am J Dermatopathol.* 1988;10:28-35.
228. Mazoujian G, Pinkus GS, Davis S, et al. Immunohistochemistry of a gross cystic disease fluid protein (GCDFP-15) of the breast. A marker of apocrine epithelium and breast carcinomas with apocrine features. *Am J Pathol.* 1983;110:105-112.
229. Swanson PE, Pettinato G, Lillemoe TJ, et al. Gross cystic disease fluid protein-15 in salivary gland tumors. *Arch Pathol Lab Med.* 1991;115:158-163.
230. Viacava P, Naccarato AG, Bevilacqua G. Spectrum of GCDFP-15 expression in human fetal and adult normal tissues. *Virchows Arch.* 1998;432:255-260.
231. Ormsby AH, Snow JL, Su WP, et al. Diagnostic immunohistochemistry of cutaneous metastatic breast carcinoma: A statistical analysis of the utility of gross cystic disease fluid protein-15 and estrogen receptor protein. *J Am Acad Dermatol.* 1995;32:711-716.
232. Mazoujian G, Bodian C, Haagensen Jr DE, et al. Expression of GCDFP-15 in breast carcinomas. Relationship to pathologic and clinical factors. *Cancer.* 1989;63:2156-2161.
233. Wick MR, Ockner DM, Mills SE, et al. Homologous carcinomas of the breasts, skin, and salivary glands. A histologic and immunohistochemical comparison of ductal mammary carcinoma, ductal sweat gland carcinoma, and salivary duct carcinoma. *Am J Clin Pathol.* 1998;109:75-84.
234. Fiel MI, Cernaianu G, Burstein DE, et al. Value of GCDFP-15 (BRST-2) as a specific immunocytochemical marker for breast carcinoma in cytologic specimens. *Acta Cytol.* 1996;40:637-641.

235. Kaufmann O, Deidesheimer T, Muehlenberg M, et al. Immunohistochemical differentiation of metastatic breast carcinomas from metastatic adenocarcinomas of other common primary sites. *Histopathology*. 1996;29:233-240.
236. Raab SS, Berg LC, Swanson PE, et al. Adenocarcinoma in the lung in patients with breast cancer. A prospective analysis of the discriminatory value of immunohistology. *Am J Clin Pathol*. 1993;100:27-35.
237. Striebel JM, Dacic S, Yousem SA. Gross cystic disease fluid protein-(GCDFP-15): expression in primary lung adenocarcinoma. *Am J Surg Pathol*. 2008;32:426-432.
238. Domfeh AB, Carley AL, Striebel JM, et al. WT1 immunoreactivity in breast carcinoma: Selective expression in pure and mixed mucinous subtypes. *Mod Pathol*. 2008;21:1217-1223.
239. Dabbs DJ, Landreneau RJ, Liu Y, et al. Detection of estrogen receptor by immunohistochemistry in pulmonary adenocarcinoma. *Ann Thorac Surg*. 2002;73:403-405; discussion 406.
240. Nash JW, Morrison C, Frankel WL. The utility of estrogen receptor and progesterone receptor immunohistochemistry in the distinction of metastatic breast carcinoma from other tumors in the liver. *Arch Pathol Lab Med*. 2003;127:1591-1595.
241. Wallace ML, Longacre TA, Smoller BR. Estrogen and progesterone receptors and anti-gross cystic disease fluid protein 15 (BRST-2) fail to distinguish metastatic breast carcinoma from eccrine neoplasms. *Mod Pathol*. 1995;8:897-901.
242. Ciampa A, Fanger G, Khan A, et al. Mammaglobin and CRxA-01 in pleural effusion cytology: Potential utility of distinguishing metastatic breast carcinomas from other cytokeratin 7-positive/cytokeratin 20-negative carcinomas. *Cancer*. 2004;102: 368-372.
243. Han JH, Kang Y, Shin HC, et al. Mammaglobin expression in lymph nodes is an important marker of metastatic breast carcinoma. *Arch Pathol Lab Med*. 2003;127:1330-1334.
244. Bhargava R, Beriwal S, Dabbs DJ. Mammaglobin vs GCDFP-15: An immunohistologic validation survey for sensitivity and specificity. *Am J Clin Pathol*. 2007;127:103-113.
245. Garfein CF, Aulicino MR, Leytin A, et al. Epithelioid cells in myoid hamartoma of the breast: A potential diagnostic pitfall for core biopsies. *Arch Pathol Lab Med*. 1996;120:676-680.
246. Mathers ME, Shrimankar J. Lobular neoplasia within a myoid hamartoma of the breast. *Breast J*. 2004;10:58-59.
247. Noguchi S, Motomura K, Inaji H, et al. Clonal analysis of fibroadenoma and phyllodes tumor of the breast. *Cancer Res*. 1993;53:4071-4074.
248. Pietruszka M, Barnes L. Cystosarcoma phyllodes: A clinicopathologic analysis of 42 cases. *Cancer*. 1978;41:1974-1983.
249. Aranda FI, Laforga JB, Lopez JI. Phyllodes tumor of the breast. An immunohistochemical study of 28 cases with special attention to the role of myofibroblasts. *Pathol Res Pract*. 1994;190:474-481.
250. Auger M, Hanna W, Kahn HJ. Cystosarcoma phylloides of the breast and its mimics. An immunohistochemical and ultrastructural study. *Arch Pathol Lab Med*. 1989;113:1231-1235.
251. Yeh IT, Francis DJ, Orenstein JM, et al. Ultrastructure of cystosarcoma phyllodes and fibroadenoma. A comparative study. *Am J Clin Pathol*. 1985;84:131-136.
252. Sapino A, Bosco M, Cassoni P, et al. Estrogen receptor-beta is expressed in stromal cells of fibroadenoma and phyllodes tumors of the breast. *Mod Pathol*. 2006;19:599-606.
253. Umekita Y, Yoshida H. Immunohistochemical study of hormone receptor and hormone-regulated protein expression in phyllodes tumour: Comparison with fibroadenoma. *Virchows Arch*. 1998;433:311-314.
254. Kleer CG, Giordano TJ, Braun T, et al. Pathologic, immunohistochemical, and molecular features of benign and malignant phyllodes tumors of the breast. *Mod Pathol*. 2001;14: 185-190.
255. Kuenen-Boumeester V, Henzen-Logmans SC, Timmermans MM, et al. Altered expression of p53 and its regulated proteins in phyllodes tumours of the breast. *J Pathol*. 1999;189:169-175.
256. Niezabitowski A, Lackowska B, Rys J, et al. Prognostic evaluation of proliferative activity and DNA content in the phyllodes tumor of the breast: Immunohistochemical and flow cytometric study of 118 cases. *Breast Cancer Res Treat*. 2001;65:77-85.
257. Shpitz B, Bomstein Y, Sternberg A, et al. Immunoreactivity of p53, Ki-67, and c-erbB-2 in phyllodes tumors of the breast in correlation with clinical and morphologic features. *J Surg Oncol*. 2002;79:86-92.
258. Millar EK, Beretov J, Marr P, et al. Malignant phyllodes tumours of the breast display increased stromal p53 protein expression. *Histopathology*. 1999;34:491-496.
259. Suo Z, Nesland JM. Phyllodes tumor of the breast: EGFR family expression and relation to clinicopathological features. *Ultrastruct Pathol*. 2000;24:371-381.
260. Tse GM, Putti TC, Kung FY, et al. Increased p53 protein expression in malignant mammary phyllodes tumors. *Mod Pathol*. 2002;15:734-740.
261. Chen CM, Chen CJ, Chang CL, et al. CD34, CD117, and actin expression in phyllodes tumor of the breast. *J Surg Res*. 2000;94:84-91.
262. Esposito NN, Mohan D, Brufsky A, et al. Phyllodes tumor: A clinicopathologic and immunohistochemical study of 30 cases. *Arch Pathol Lab Med*. 2006;130:1516-1521.
263. Sawyer EJ, Poulsom R, Hunt FT, et al. Malignant phyllodes tumours show stromal overexpression of c-myc and c-kit. *J Pathol*. 2003;200:59-64.
264. Tse GM, Putti TC, Lui PC, et al. Increased c-kit (CD117) expression in malignant mammary phyllodes tumors. *Mod Pathol*. 2004;17:827-831.
265. Djordjevic B, Hanna WM. Expression of c-kit in fibroepithelial lesions of the breast is a mast cell phenomenon. *Mod Pathol*. 2008;21:1238-1245.
266. Kersting C, Kuijper A, Schmidt H, et al. Amplifications of the epidermal growth factor receptor gene (egfr) are common in phyllodes tumors of the breast and are associated with tumor progression. *Lab Invest*. 2006;86:54-61.
267. Tse GM, Lui PC, Vong JS, et al. Increased epidermal growth factor receptor (EGFR) expression in malignant mammary phyllodes tumors. *Breast Cancer Res Treat*. 2009;114:441-448.
268. Inoshita S. Phyllodes tumor (cystosarcoma phyllodes) of the breast. A clinicopathologic study of 45 cases. *Acta Pathol Jpn*. 1988;38:21-33.
269. Khan SA, Badve S. Phyllodes tumors of the breast. *Curr Treat Options Oncol*. 2001;2:139-147.
270. Shabahang M, Franceschi D, Sundaram M, et al. Surgical management of primary breast sarcoma. *Am Surg*. 2002;68:673-677; discussion 677.
271. Kuijper A, de Vos RA, Lagendijk JH, et al. Progressive deregulation of the cell cycle with higher tumor grade in the stroma of breast phyllodes tumors. *Am J Clin Pathol*. 2005;123:690-698.
272. Feakins RM, Mulcahy HE, Nickols CD, et al. p53 expression in phyllodes tumours is associated with histological features of malignancy but does not predict outcome. *Histopathology*. 1999;35:162-169.
273. Asoglu O, Ugurlu MM, Blanchard K, et al. Risk factors for recurrence and death after primary surgical treatment of malignant phyllodes tumors. *Ann Surg Oncol*. 2004;11:1011-1017.
274. Ben Hassouna J, Damak T, Gamoudi A, et al. Phyllodes tumors of the breast: A case series of 106 patients. *Am J Surg*. 2006;192:141-147.
275. Chen WH, Cheng SP, Tzen CY, et al. Surgical treatment of phyllodes tumors of the breast: Retrospective review of 172 cases. *J Surg Oncol*. 2005;91:185-194.
276. Cheng SP, Chang YC, Liu TP, et al. Phyllodes tumor of the breast: The challenge persists. *World J Surg*. 2006;30:1414-1421.
277. Hawkins RE, Schofield JB, Fisher C, et al. The clinical and histologic criteria that predict metastases from cystosarcoma phyllodes. *Cancer*. 1992;69:141-147.
278. Kapiris I, Nasiri N, A'Hern R, et al. Outcome and predictive factors of local recurrence and distant metastases following primary surgical treatment of high-grade malignant phyllodes tumours of the breast. *Eur J Surg Oncol*. 2001;27:723-730.
279. Tan PH, Jayabaskar T, Chuah KL, et al. Phyllodes tumors of the breast: The role of pathologic parameters. *Am J Clin Pathol*. 2005;123:529-540.
280. Jacobs TW, Chen YY, Guinee Jr DG, et al. Fibroepithelial lesions with cellular stroma on breast core needle biopsy: Are there predictors of outcome on surgical excision? *Am J Clin Pathol*. 2005;124:342-354.

281. Umekita Y, Yoshida H. Immunohistochemical study of MIB1 expression in phyllodes tumor and fibroadenoma. *Pathol Int.* 1999;49:807-810.
282. Lae M, Vincent-Salomon A, Savignoni A, et al. Phyllodes tumors of the breast segregate in two groups according to genetic criteria. *Mod Pathol.* 2007;20:435-444.
283. Lu YJ, Birdsall S, Osin P, et al. Phyllodes tumors of the breast analyzed by comparative genomic hybridization and association of increased 1q copy number with stromal overgrowth and recurrence. *Genes Chromosomes Cancer.* 1997;20:275-281.
284. Ojopi EP, Rogatto SR, Caldeira JR, et al. Comparative genomic hybridization detects novel amplifications in fibroadenomas of the breast. *Genes Chromosomes Cancer.* 2001;30:25-31.
285. Polito P, Cin PD, Pauwels P, et al. An important subgroup of phyllodes tumors of the breast is characterized by rearrangements of chromosomes 1q and 10q. *Oncol Rep.* 1998;5:1099-1102.
286. Wang ZC, Buraimoh A, Iglehart JD, et al. Genome-wide analysis for loss of heterozygosity in primary and recurrent phyllodes tumor and fibroadenoma of breast using single nucleotide polymorphism arrays. *Breast Cancer Res Treat.* 2006;97:301-309.
287. Noguchi S, Aihara T, Motomura K, et al. Demonstration of polyclonal origin of giant fibroadenoma of the breast. *Virchows Arch.* 1995;427:343-347.
288. Burga AM, Tavassoli FA. Periductal stromal tumor: A rare lesion with low-grade sarcomatous behavior. *Am J Surg Pathol.* 2003;27:343-348.
289. Cheng L, Binder SW, Fu YS, et al. Demonstration of estrogen receptors by monoclonal antibody in formalin-fixed breast tumors. *Lab Invest.* 1988;58:346-353.
290. Harvey JM, Clark GM, Osborne CK, et al. Estrogen receptor status by immunohistochemistry is superior to the ligand-binding assay for predicting response to adjuvant endocrine therapy in breast cancer. *J Clin Oncol.* 1999;17:1474-1481.
291. McCarty Jr KS, Miller LS, Cox EB, et al. Estrogen receptor analyses. Correlation of biochemical and immunohistochemical methods using monoclonal antireceptor antibodies. *Arch Pathol Lab Med.* 1985;109:716-721.
292. Allred DC, Harvey JM, Berardo M, et al. Prognostic and predictive factors in breast cancer by immunohistochemical analysis. *Mod Pathol.* 1998;11:155-168.
293. Diaz LK, Sneige N. Estrogen receptor analysis for breast cancer: Current issues and keys to increasing testing accuracy. *Adv Anat Pathol.* 2005;12:10-19.
294. Press MF, Sauter G, Bernstein L, et al. Diagnostic evaluation of HER-2 as a molecular target: An assessment of accuracy and reproducibility of laboratory testing in large, prospective, randomized clinical trials. *Clin Cancer Res.* 2005;11:6598-6607.
295. Shi SR, Liu C, Taylor CR. Standardization of immunohistochemistry for formalin-fixed, paraffin-embedded tissue sections based on the antigen retrieval technique: From experiments to hypothesis. *J Histochem Cytochem.* 2007;55:105-109.
296. Taylor CR. Standardization in immunohistochemistry: The role of antigen retrieval in molecular morphology. *Biotech Histochem.* 2006;81:3-12.
297. Goldstein NS, Hewitt SM, Taylor CR, et al. Recommendations for improved standardization of immunohistochemistry. *Appl Immunohistochem Mol Morphol.* 2007;15:124-133.
298. Jacobs TW, Siziopikou KP, Prioleau JE, et al. Do prognostic marker studies on core needle biopsy specimens of breast carcinoma accurately reflect the marker status of the tumor? *Mod Pathol.* 1998;11:259-264.
299. Keshgegian AA, Inverso K, Kline TS. Determination of estrogen receptor by monoclonal antireceptor antibody in aspiration biopsy cytology from breast carcinoma. *Am J Clin Pathol.* 1988;89:24-29.
300. Marrazzo A, Taormina P, Leonardi P, et al. Immunocytochemical determination of estrogen and progesterone receptors on 219 fine-needle aspirates of breast cancer. A prospective study. *Anticancer Res.* 1995;15:521-526.
301. Masood S. Estrogen and progesterone receptors in cytology: A comprehensive review. *Diagn Cytopathol.* 1992;8:475-491.
302. Masood S, Dee S, Goldstein JD. Immunocytochemical analysis of progesterone receptors in breast cancer. *Am J Clin Pathol.* 1991;96:59-63.
303. Zidan A, Christie Brown JS, Peston D, et al. Oestrogen and progesterone receptor assessment in core biopsy specimens of breast carcinoma. *J Clin Pathol.* 1997;50:27-29.
304. Coussens L, Yang-Feng TL, Liao YC, et al. Tyrosine kinase receptor with extensive homology to EGF receptor shares chromosomal location with neu oncogene. *Science.* 1985;230:1132-1139.
305. Semba K, Kamata N, Toyoshima K, et al. A v-erbB-related protooncogene, c-erbB-2, is distinct from the c-erbB-1/epidermal growth factor-receptor gene and is amplified in a human salivary gland adenocarcinoma. *Proc Natl Acad Sci U S A.* 1985;82:6497-6501.
306. Di Fiore PP, Pierce JH, Kraus MH, et al. erbB-2 is a potent oncogene when overexpressed in NIH/3T3 cells. *Science.* 1987;237:178-182.
307. Akiyama T, Sudo C, Ogawara H, et al. The product of the human c-erbB-2 gene: A 185-kilodalton glycoprotein with tyrosine kinase activity. *Science.* 1986;232:1644-1646.
308. Slamon DJ, Clark GM, Wong SG, et al. Human breast cancer: Correlation of relapse and survival with amplification of the HER-2/neu oncogene. *Science.* 1987;235:177-182.
309. Owens MA, Horten BC, Da Silva MM. *HER2* amplification ratios by fluorescence in situ hybridization and correlation with immunohistochemistry in a cohort of 6556 breast cancer tissues. *Clin Breast Cancer.* 2004;5:63-69.
310. Yaziji H, Goldstein LC, Barry TS, et al. HER-2 testing in breast cancer using parallel tissue-based methods. *JAMA.* 2004;291:1972-1977.
311. Hayes DF, Thor AD, Dressler LG, et al. *HER2* and response to paclitaxel in node-positive breast cancer. *N Engl J Med.* 2007;357:1496-1506.
312. Konecny GE, Thomssen C, Luck HJ, et al. Her-2/neu gene amplification and response to paclitaxel in patients with metastatic breast cancer. *J Natl Cancer Inst.* 2004;96:1141-1151.
313. Menard S, Valagussa P, Pilotti S, et al. Response to cyclophosphamide, methotrexate, and fluorouracil in lymph node-positive breast cancer according to *HER2* overexpression and other tumor biologic variables. *J Clin Oncol.* 2001;19:329-335.
314. Pritchard KI, Shepherd LE, O'Malley FP, et al. *HER2* and responsiveness of breast cancer to adjuvant chemotherapy. *N Engl J Med.* 2006;354:2103-2111.
315. Thor AD, Berry DA, Budman DR, et al. erbB-2, p53, and efficacy of adjuvant therapy in lymph node-positive breast cancer. *J Natl Cancer Inst.* 1998;90:1346-1360.
316. Ellis MJ, Coop A, Singh B, et al. Letrozole is more effective neoadjuvant endocrine therapy than tamoxifen for ErbB-1- and/or ErbB-2-positive, estrogen receptor-positive primary breast cancer: Evidence from a phase III randomized trial. *J Clin Oncol.* 2001;19:3808-3816.
317. Konecny G, Pauletti G, Pegram M, et al. Quantitative association between HER-2/neu and steroid hormone receptors in hormone receptor-positive primary breast cancer. *J Natl Cancer Inst.* 2003;95:142-153.
318. Joensuu H, Kellokumpu-Lehtinen PL, Bono P, et al. *N Engl J Med.* 2006;354:809-820.
319. Piccart-Gebhart MJ, Procter M, Leyland-Jones B, et al. Trastuzumab after adjuvant chemotherapy in *HER2*-positive breast cancer. *N Engl J Med.* 2005;353:1659-1672.
320. Romond EH, Perez EA, Bryant J, et al. Trastuzumab plus adjuvant chemotherapy for operable *HER2*-positive breast cancer. *N Engl J Med.* 2005;353:1673-1684.
321. Smith I, Procter M, Gelber RD, et al. 2-year follow-up of trastuzumab after adjuvant chemotherapy in *HER2*-positive breast cancer: A randomised controlled trial. *Lancet.* 2007;369:29-36.
322. Wolff AC, Hammond ME, Schwartz JN, et al. American Society of Clinical Oncology/College of American Pathologists guideline recommendations for human epidermal growth factor receptor 2 testing in breast cancer. *J Clin Oncol.* 2007;25:118-145.
323. Goldstein NS, Ferkowicz M, Odish E, et al. Minimum formalin fixation time for consistent estrogen receptor immunohistochemical staining of invasive breast carcinoma. *Am J Clin Pathol.* 2003;120:86-92.

324. Slamon DJ, Leyland-Jones B, Shak S, et al. Use of chemotherapy plus a monoclonal antibody against *HER2* for metastatic breast cancer that overexpresses *HER2*. *N Engl J Med*. 2001;344:783-792.
325. Egervari K, Szollosi Z, Nemes Z. Immunohistochemical antibodies in breast cancer *HER2* diagnostics. A comparative immunohistochemical and fluorescence in situ hybridization study. *Tumour Biol*. 2008;29:18-27.
326. Gouvea AP, Milanezi F, Olson SJ, et al. Selecting antibodies to detect *HER2* overexpression by immunohistochemistry in invasive mammary carcinomas. *Appl Immunohistochem Mol Morphol*. 2006;14:103-108.
327. Powell WC, Hicks DG, Prescott N, et al. A new rabbit monoclonal antibody (4B5) for the immunohistochemical (IHC) determination of the *HER2* status in breast cancer: Comparison with CB11, fluorescence in situ hybridization (FISH), and interlaboratory reproducibility. *Appl Immunohistochem Mol Morphol*. 2007;15:94-102.
328. Acs G, Wang L, Raghunath PN, et al. Role of different immunostaining patterns in HercepTest interpretation and criteria for gene amplification as determined by fluorescence in situ hybridization. *Appl Immunohistochem Mol Morphol*. 2003;11:222-229.
329. Bhargava R, Naeem R, Marconi S, et al. Tyrosine kinase activation in breast carcinoma with correlation to HER-2/neu gene amplification and receptor overexpression. *Hum Pathol*. 2001;32:1344-1350.
330. Perez EA, Roche PC, Jenkins RB, et al. *HER2* testing in patients with breast cancer: Poor correlation between weak positivity by immunohistochemistry and gene amplification by fluorescence in situ hybridization. *Mayo Clin Proc*. 2002;77:148-154.
331. Garcia-Caballero T, Menendez MD, Vazquez-Boquete A, et al. HER-2 status determination in breast carcinomas. A practical approach. *Histol Histopathol*. 2006;21:227-236.
332. Tsuda H, Akiyama F, Terasaki H, et al. Detection of HER-2/neu (c-erb B-2) DNA amplification in primary breast carcinoma. Interobserver reproducibility and correlation with immunohistochemical HER-2 overexpression. *Cancer*. 2001;92:2965-2974.
333. Tubbs RR, Pettay JD, Roche PC, et al. Discrepancies in clinical laboratory testing of eligibility for trastuzumab therapy: Apparent immunohistochemical false-positives do not get the message. *J Clin Oncol*. 2001;19:2714-2721.
334. Chorn N. Accurate identification of *HER2*-positive patients is essential for superior outcomes with trastuzumab therapy. *Oncol Nurs Forum*. 2006;33:265-272.
335. Mass RD, Press MF, Anderson S, et al. Evaluation of clinical outcomes according to *HER2* detection by fluorescence in situ hybridization in women with metastatic breast cancer treated with trastuzumab. *Clin Breast Cancer*. 2005;6:240-246.
336. Cell Markers and Cytogenetics Committees College of American Pathologists. Clinical laboratory assays for HER-2/neu amplification and overexpression: Quality assurance, standardization, and proficiency testing. *Arch Pathol Lab Med*. 2002;126:803-808.
337. Rhodes A, Borthwick D, Sykes R, et al. The use of cell line standards to reduce HER-2/neu assay variation in multiple European cancer centers and the potential of automated image analysis to provide for more accurate cut points for predicting clinical response to trastuzumab. *Am J Clin Pathol*. 2004;122:51-60.
338. Zarbo RJ, Hammond ME. Conference summary, Strategic Science symposium. Her-2/neu testing of breast cancer patients in clinical practice. *Arch Pathol Lab Med*. 2003;127:549-553.
339. Persons DL, Tubbs RR, Cooley LD, et al. HER-2 fluorescence in situ hybridization: Results from the survey program of the College of American Pathologists. *Arch Pathol Lab Med*. 2006;130:325-331.
340. Chivukula M, Bhargava R, Brufsky A, et al. Clinical importance of *HER2* immunohistologic heterogeneous expression in core-needle biopsies vs resection specimens for equivocal (immunohistochemical score 2+) cases. *Mod Pathol*. 2008;21:363-368.
341. Lal P, Salazar PA, Hudis CA, et al. HER-2 testing in breast cancer using immunohistochemical analysis and fluorescence in situ hybridization: A single-institution experience of 2,279 cases and comparison of dual-color and single-color scoring. *Am J Clin Pathol*. 2004;121:631-636.
342. Bose S, Mohammed M, Shintaku P, et al. Her-2/neu gene amplification in low to moderately expressing breast cancers: Possible role of chromosome 17/Her-2/neu polysomy. *Breast J*. 2001;7:337-344.
343. Striebel JM, Bhargava R, Horbinski C, et al. The equivocally amplified *HER2* FISH result on breast core biopsy: Indications for further sampling do affect patient management. *Am J Clin Pathol*. 2008;129:383-390.
344. Bhargava R, Lal P, Chen B. Chromogenic in situ hybridization for the detection of HER-2/neu gene amplification in breast cancer with an emphasis on tumors with borderline and low-level amplification: Does it measure up to fluorescence in situ hybridization? *Am J Clin Pathol*. 2005;123:237-243.
345. Gupta D, Middleton LP, Whitaker MJ, et al. Comparison of fluorescence and chromogenic in situ hybridization for detection of HER-2/neu oncogene in breast cancer. *Am J Clin Pathol*. 2003;119:381-387.
346. Isola J, Tanner M, Forsyth A, Cooke TG, Watters AD, Bartlett JM. Interlaboratory comparison of HER-2 oncogene amplification as detected by chromogenic and fluorescence in situ hybridization. *Clin Cancer Res*. 2004;10:4793-4798.
347. Tanner M, Gancberg D, Di Leo A, et al. Chromogenic in situ hybridization: A practical alternative for fluorescence in situ hybridization to detect HER-2/neu oncogene amplification in archival breast cancer samples. *Am J Pathol*. 2000;157:1467-1472.
348. Beatson GT. On the treatment of inoperable cases of carcinoma of the mamma: Suggestions for a new method of treatment, with illustrative cases. *CA Cancer J Clin*. 1983;33:108-121.
349. Jacquemier JD, Hassoun J, Torrente M, et al. Distribution of estrogen and progesterone receptors in healthy tissue adjacent to breast lesions at various stages—Immunohistochemical study of 107 cases. *Breast Cancer Res Treat*. 1990;15:109-117.
350. Brdar B, Graf D, Padovan R, et al. Estrogen and progesterone receptors as prognostic factors in breast cancer. *Tumori*. 1988;74:45-52.
351. Castagnetta L, Traina A, Carruba G, et al. The prognosis of breast cancer patients in relation to the oestrogen receptor status of both primary disease and involved nodes. *Br J Cancer*. 1992;66:167-170.
352. Clark GM, McGuire WL. Steroid receptors and other prognostic factors in primary breast cancer. *Semin Oncol*. 1988;15:20-25.
353. Clark GM, McGuire WL, Hubay CA, et al. Progesterone receptors as a prognostic factor in Stage II breast cancer. *N Engl J Med*. 1983;309:1343-1347.
354. Crowe JP, Hubay CA, Pearson OH, et al. Estrogen receptor status as a prognostic indicator for stage I breast cancer patients. *Breast Cancer Res Treat*. 1982;2:171-176.
355. Lesser ML, Rosen PP, Senie RT, et al. Estrogen and progesterone receptors in breast carcinoma: Correlations with epidemiology and pathology. *Cancer*. 1981;48:299-309.
356. Pichon MF, Pallud C, Hacene K, et al. Prognostic value of progesterone receptor after long-term follow-up in primary breast cancer. *Eur J Cancer*. 1992;28A:1676-1680.
357. Reiner A, Reiner G, Spona J, et al. Histopathologic characterization of human breast cancer in correlation with estrogen receptor status. A comparison of immunocytochemical and biochemical analysis. *Cancer*. 1988;61:1149-1154.
358. Yaziji H, Taylor CR, Goldstein NS, et al. Consensus recommendations on estrogen receptor testing in breast cancer by immunohistochemistry. *Appl Immunohistochem Molec Morphol*. 2008;16:513-520.
359. Tong D, Schuster E, Seifert M, et al. Expression of estrogen receptor beta isoforms in human breast cancer tissues and cell lines. *Breast Cancer Res Treat*. 2002;71:249-255.
360. Esslimani-Sahla M, Simony-Lafontaine J, Kramar A, et al. Estrogen receptor beta (ER beta) level but not its ER beta cx variant helps to predict tamoxifen resistance in breast cancer. *Clin Cancer Res*. 2004;10:5769-5776.
361. Hopp TA, Weiss HL, Parra IS, et al. Low levels of estrogen receptor beta protein predict resistance to tamoxifen therapy in breast cancer. *Clin Cancer Res*. 2004;10:7490-7499.
362. Speirs V, Parkes AT, Kerin MJ, et al. Coexpression of estrogen receptor alpha and beta: Poor prognostic factors in human breast cancer? *Cancer Res*. 1999;59:525-528.

363. Stefanou D, Batistatou A, Briasoulis E, et al. Estrogen receptor beta (ERbeta) expression in breast carcinomas is not correlated with estrogen receptor alpha (ERalpha) and prognosis: The Greek experience. *Eur J Gynaecol Oncol*. 2004;25:457-461.
364. Matsuyama S, Ohkura Y, Eguchi H, et al. Estrogen receptor beta is expressed in human stomach adenocarcinoma. *J Cancer Res Clin Oncol*. 2002;128:319-324.
365. Pais V, Leav I, Lau KM, et al. Estrogen receptor-beta expression in human testicular germ cell tumors. *Clin Cancer Res*. 2003;9:4475-4482.
366. National Institutes of Health Consensus Development Conference statement: Adjuvant therapy for breast cancer, November 1-3, 2000. *J Natl Cancer Inst Monogr*. 2001;5-15.
367. Cheang MC, Treaba DO, Speers CH, et al. Immunohistochemical detection using the new rabbit monoclonal antibody SP1 of estrogen receptor in breast cancer is superior to mouse monoclonal antibody 1D5 in predicting survival. *J Clin Oncol*. 2006;24: 5637-5644.
368. Pertschuk LP, Feldman JG, Kim YD, et al. Estrogen receptor immunocytochemistry in paraffin embedded tissues with ER1D5 predicts breast cancer endocrine response more accurately than H222Sp gamma in frozen sections or cytosol-based ligand-binding assays. *Cancer*. 1996;77:2514-2519.
369. Charpin C, Andrac L, Habib MC, et al. Immunodetection in fine-needle aspirates and multiparametric (SAMBA) image analysis. Receptors (monoclonal antiestrogen and antiprogesterone) and growth fraction (monoclonal Ki67) evaluation in breast carcinomas. *Cancer*. 1989;63:863-872.
370. Esteban JM, Kandalaft PL, Mehta P, et al. Improvement of the quantification of estrogen and progesterone receptors in paraffin-embedded tumors by image analysis. *Am J Clin Pathol*. 1993;99:32-38.
371. Layfield LJ, Saria EA, Conlon DH, et al. Estrogen and progesterone receptor status determined by the Ventana ES 320 automated immunohistochemical stainer and the CAS 200 image analyzer in 236 early-stage breast carcinomas: Prognostic significance. *J Surg Oncol*. 1996;61:177-184.
372. McClelland RA, Finlay P, Walker KJ, et al. Automated quantitation of immunocytochemically localized estrogen receptors in human breast cancer. *Cancer Res*. 1990;50: 3545-3550.
373. Veronese SM, Barbareschi M, Morelli L, et al. Predictive value of ER1D5 antibody immunostaining in breast cancer: A paraffin-based retrospective study of 257 cases. *Appl Immunohistochem*. 1993;3:85-90.
374. Barnes DM, Harris WH, Smith P, et al. Immunohistochemical determination of oestrogen receptor: Comparison of different methods of assessment of staining and correlation with clinical outcome of breast cancer patients. *Br J Cancer*. 1996;74:1445-1451.
375. Goulding H, Pinder S, Cannon P, et al. A new immunohistochemical antibody for the assessment of estrogen receptor status on routine formalin-fixed tissue samples. *Hum Pathol*. 1995;26:291-294.
376. Baehner FL, Maddala T, Alexander C, et al. A Kaiser-Permanente population-based study of ER and PR expression by the standard method, immunohistochemistry (IHC), compared to a new method, quantitative reverse transcription polymerase chain reaction (RT-PCR). *ASCO Breast Cancer Symposium*. 2007; Abstract 88.
377. Cronin M, Pho M, Dutta D, et al. Measurement of gene expression in archival paraffin-embedded tissues: Development and performance of a 92-gene reverse transcriptase-polymerase chain reaction assay. *Am J Pathol*. 2004;164:35-42.
378. Collins LC, Botero ML, Schnitt SJ. Bimodal frequency distribution of estrogen receptor immunohistochemical staining results in breast cancer: An analysis of 825 cases. *Am J Clin Pathol*. 2005;123:16-20.
379. Nadji M, Gomez-Fernandez C, Ganjei-Azar P, et al. Immunohistochemistry of estrogen and progesterone receptors reconsidered: Experience with 5,993 breast cancers. *Am J Clin Pathol*. 2005;123:21-27.
380. Baehner FL, Watson D, Shak S, et al. Quantitative RT-PCR analysis of ER and PR by Oncotype DX indicates distinct and different associations with prognosis and prediction of tamoxifen benefit. *29th Annual San Antonio Breast Cancer Symposium*. 2006; Abstract 45.
381. Press M, Spaulding B, Groshen S, et al. Comparison of different antibodies for detection of progesterone receptor in breast cancer. *Steroids*. 2002;67:799-813.
382. Mohsin SK, Weiss H, Havighurst T, et al. Progesterone receptor by immunohistochemistry and clinical outcome in breast cancer: A validation study. *Mod Pathol*. 2004;17:1545-1554.
383. Golub TR, Slonim DK, Tamayo P, et al. Molecular classification of cancer: Class discovery and class prediction by gene expression monitoring. *Science*. 1999;286:531-537.
384. Sorlie T. Molecular classification of breast tumors: Toward improved diagnostics and treatments. *Methods Mol Biol*. 2007;360:91-114.
385. Bhargava R, Striebel J, Beriwal S, et al. Prevalence, morphologic features and proliferation indices of breast carcinoma molecular classes using immunohistochemical surrogate markers. *J Clin Exp Pathol*. 2009;2:444-455.
386. Bhargava R, Beriwal S, Dabbs DJ, et al. Immunohistochemical surrogate markers of breast cancer molecular classes predict response to neoadjuvant chemotherapy: A single institutional experience with 359 cases. *Cancer*. in press.
387. Cheang MC, Voduc D, Bajdik C, et al. Basal-like breast cancer defined by five biomarkers has superior prognostic value than triple-negative phenotype. *Clin Cancer Res*. 2008;14:1368-1376.
388. Bhargava R, Gerald WL, Li AR, et al. EGFR gene amplification in breast cancer: Correlation with epidermal growth factor receptor mRNA and protein expression and HER-2 status and absence of EGFR-activating mutations. *Mod Pathol*. 2005;18:1027-1033.
389. Ridolfi RL, Rosen PP, Port A, Kinne D, Mike V. Medullary carcinoma of the breast: A clinicopathologic study with 10 year follow-up. *Cancer*. 1977;40:1365-1385.
390. Weigelt B, Horlings H, Kreike B, et al. Refinement of breast cancer classification by molecular characterization of histological special types. *J Pathol*. 2008;216:141-150.
391. Rouzier R, Perou CM, Symmans WF, et al. Breast cancer molecular subtypes respond differently to preoperative chemotherapy. *Clin Cancer Res*. 2005;11:5678-5685.
392. van de Vijver MJ, He YD, van't Veer LJ, et al. A gene-expression signature as a predictor of survival in breast cancer. *N Engl J Med*. 2002;347:1999-2009.
393. van't Veer LJ, Dai H, van de Vijver MJ, et al. Gene expression profiling predicts clinical outcome of breast cancer. *Nature*. 2002;415:530-536.
394. Glas AM, Floore A, Delahaye LJ, et al. Converting a breast cancer microarray signature into a high-throughput diagnostic test. *BMC Genomics*. 2006;7:278.
395. Harris L, Fritsche H, Mennel R, et al. American Society of Clinical Oncology 2007 update of recommendations for the use of tumor markers in breast cancer. *J Clin Oncol*. 2007;25:5287-5312.
396. Chang HY, Nuyten DS, Sneddon JB, et al. Robustness, scalability, and integration of a wound-response gene expression signature in predicting breast cancer survival. *Proc Natl Acad Sci U S A*. 2005;102:3738-3743.
397. Wang Y, Klijn JG, Zhang Y, et al. Gene-expression profiles to predict distant metastasis of lymph-node-negative primary breast cancer. *Lancet*. 2005;365:671-679.
398. Foekens JA, Atkins D, Zhang Y, et al. Multicenter validation of a gene expression-based prognostic signature in lymph node-negative primary breast cancer. *J Clin Oncol*. 2006;24:1665-1671.
399. Paik S, Shak S, Tang G, et al. A multigene assay to predict recurrence of tamoxifen-treated, node-negative breast cancer. *N Engl J Med*. 2004;351:2817-2826.
400. Paik S, Tang G, Shak S, et al. Gene expression and benefit of chemotherapy in women with node-negative, estrogen receptor-positive breast cancer. *J Clin Oncol*. 2006;24:3726-3734.

401. Flanagan MB, Dabbs DJ, Brufsky AM, et al. Histopathologic variables predict Oncotype DX recurrence score. *Mod Pathol.* 2008;21:1255-1261.
402. Ma XJ, Wang Z, Ryan PD, et al. A two-gene expression ratio predicts clinical outcome in breast cancer patients treated with tamoxifen. *Cancer Cell.* 2004;5:607-616.
403. Ma XJ, Hilsenbeck SG, Wang W, et al. The HOXB13:IL17BR expression index is a prognostic factor in early-stage breast cancer. *J Clin Oncol.* 2006;24:4611-4619.
404. Ma XJ, Salunga R, Dahiya S, et al. A five-gene molecular grade index and HOXB13:IL17BR are complementary prognostic factors in early stage breast cancer. *Clin Cancer Res.* 2008;14:2601-2608.
405. Ma XJ, Salunga R, Tuggle JT, et al. Gene expression profiles of human breast cancer progression. *Proc Natl Acad Sci U S A.* 2003;100:5974-5979.
406. Sotiriou C, Wirapati P, Loi S, et al. Gene expression profiling in breast cancer: Understanding the molecular basis of histologic grade to improve prognosis. *J Natl Cancer Inst.* 2006;98: 262-272.
407. Gao JP, Uchida T, Wang C, et al. Relationship between p53 gene mutation and protein expression: Clinical significance in transitional cell carcinoma of the bladder. *Int J Oncol.* 2000;16: 469-475.
408. Salinas-Sanchez AS, Atienzar-Tobarra M, Lorenzo-Romero JG, et al. Sensitivity and specificity of p53 protein detection by immunohistochemistry in patients with urothelial bladder carcinoma. *Urol Int.* 2007;79:321-327.
409. Olivier M, Langerod A, Carrieri P, et al. The clinical value of somatic TP53 gene mutations in 1,794 patients with breast cancer. *Clin Cancer Res.* 2006;12:1157-1167.
410. Caly M, Genin P, Ghuzlan AA, et al. Analysis of correlation between mitotic index, MIB1 score and S-phase fraction as proliferation markers in invasive breast carcinoma. Methodological aspects and prognostic value in a series of 257 cases. *Anticancer Res.* 2004;24:3283-3288.
411. Gonzalez-Vela MC, Garijo MF, Fernandez F, et al. MIB1 proliferation index in breast infiltrating carcinoma: Comparison with other proliferative markers and association with new biological prognostic factors. *Histol Histopathol.* 2001;16:399-406.
412. Molino A, Micciolo R, Turazza M, et al. Ki-67 immunostaining in 322 primary breast cancers: Associations with clinical and pathological variables and prognosis. *Int J Cancer.* 1997;74:433-437.
413. Nakagomi H, Miyake T, Hada M, et al. Prognostic and Therapeutic implications of the MIB-1 Labeling Index in Breast Cancer. *Breast Cancer.* 1998;5:255-259.
414. Colozza M, Azambuja E, Cardoso F, et al. Proliferative markers as prognostic and predictive tools in early breast cancer: Where are we now? *Ann Oncol.* 2005;16:1723-1739.
415. Perou CM, Jeffrey SS, van de Rijn M, et al. Distinctive gene expression patterns in human mammary epithelial cells and breast cancers. *Proc Natl Acad Sci U S A.* 1999;96:9212-9217.
416. Reis-Filho JS, Pinheiro C, Lambros MB, et al. EGFR amplification and lack of activating mutations in metaplastic breast carcinomas. *J Pathol.* 2006;209:445-453.
417. Gholam D, Chebib A, Hauteville D, et al. Combined paclitaxel and cetuximab achieved a major response on the skin metastases of a patient with epidermal growth factor receptor-positive, estrogen receptor-negative, progesterone receptor-negative and human epidermal growth factor receptor-2-negative (triple-negative) breast cancer. *Anticancer Drugs.* 2007;18:835-837.
418. Modi S, D'Andrea G, Norton L, et al. A phase I study of cetuximab/paclitaxel in patients with advanced-stage breast cancer. *Clin Breast Cancer.* 2006;7:270-277.
419. Duffy MJ. Urokinase plasminogen activator and its inhibitor, PAI-1, as prognostic markers in breast cancer: from pilot to level 1 evidence studies. *Clin Chem.* 2002;48:1194-1197.
420. Foekens JA, Schmitt M, van Putten WL, et al. Plasminogen activator inhibitor-1 and prognosis in primary breast cancer. *J Clin Oncol.* 1994;12:1648-1658.
421. Look MP, van Putten WL, Duffy MJ, et al. Pooled analysis of prognostic impact of urokinase-type plasminogen activator and its inhibitor PAI-1 in 8377 breast cancer patients. *J Natl Cancer Inst.* 2002;94:116-128.
422. Visscher DW, Sarkar F, LoRusso P, et al. Immunohistologic evaluation of invasion-associated proteases in breast carcinoma. *Mod Pathol.* 1993;6:302-306.
423. Schmitt M, Sturmheit AS, Welk A, et al. Procedures for the quantitative protein determination of urokinase and its inhibitor, PAI-1, in human breast cancer tissue extracts by ELISA. *Methods Mol Med.* 2006;120:245-265.
424. Badve S, Turbin D, Thorat MA, et al. FOXA1 expression in breast cancer—Correlation with luminal subtype A and survival. *Clin Cancer Res.* 2007;13:4415-4421.
425. Laganiere J, Deblois G, Lefebvre C, et al. From the Cover: Location analysis of estrogen receptor alpha target promoters reveals that FOXA1 defines a domain of the estrogen response. *Proc Natl Acad Sci U S A.* 2005;102:11651-11656.
426. Thorat MA, Marchio C, Morimiya A, et al. Forkhead box A1 expression in breast cancer is associated with luminal subtype and good prognosis. *J Clin Pathol.* 2008;61:327-332.
427. Badve S, Nakshatri H. Oestrogen receptor-positive breast cancer: Towards bridging histopathologic and molecular classifications. *J Clin Pathol.* 2009;62:6-12.
428. Mehra R, Varambally S, Ding L, et al. Identification of GATA3 as a breast cancer prognostic marker by global gene expression meta-analysis. *Cancer Res.* 2005;65:11259-11264.
429. Voduc D, Cheang M, Nielsen T. GATA-3 expression in breast cancer has a strong association with estrogen receptor but lacks independent prognostic value. *Cancer Epidemiol Biomarkers Prev.* 2008;17:365-373.

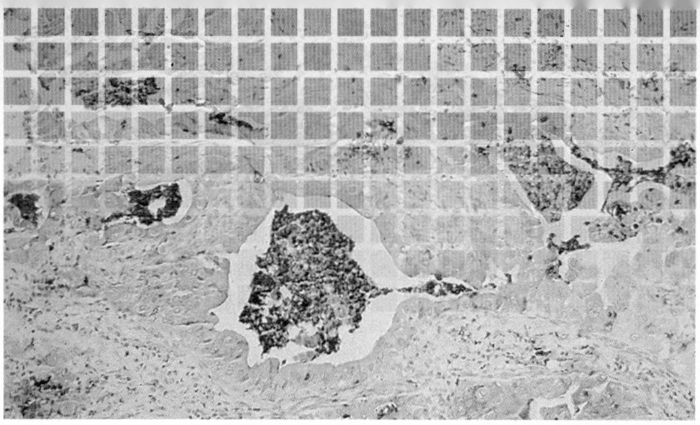

20

Immunohistology of the Nervous System

Paul E. McKeever

Clinical and Radiographic Perspective of Lesions 821
Non-neoplastic Brain Lesions 824
Tumors 831
Cysts 875
Dementias 876
Demyelination 878
Epilepsy 879
Pitfalls in Diagnosis 881

In this chapter we will focus on the diagnostic immunohistochemistry (IHC) of nervous system diseases. Concise information about pathologic entities is provided in Tables 20.2 to 20.13 and the algorithms in Boxes 20.1 and 20.2. A suspected specific disease can be checked directly in the individual table in which its structural, immunohistochemical, and topographic features are listed, or, if you prefer, you can use the algorithms. The text and figures elaborate on these features.[1-3]

Features of unknown diseases may be found in individual algorithms and tables to assist diagnosis. For example, for a mass, specific tables in the chapter summarize differential features of the mass, as follows:

- Fibrillar cells: Table 20.5; Figures 20.8, 20.9, and 20.15
- Epithelioid cells: Table 20.6; Figures 20.1, 20.19, and 20.36
- More than one type of cell: Table 20.7; Figure 20.31
- Small anaplastic cells: Table 20.8; Figures 20.21 and 20.38 to 20.41
- Syncytial cells: Table 20.9; Figure 20.46

The above features are evident on cytologic and histologic preparations.[3,4]

Box 20.1 focuses on the differential diagnosis of clear cell lesions. Box 20.2 displays the differential IHC of epithelioid tumors. Box 20.3 displays the differential of "blue tumors."

Immunohistochemical stains that are particularly useful for diagnosis of nervous system diseases are listed in alphabetical order in Table 20.1.

IHC should always be controlled. I prefer selecting a specimen with all of the following items: (1) the lesion of interest; (2) the tissue with regions that should react positively to the stain; and (3) the tissue with regions that should react negatively to the stain. Regions 2 and 3 serve as internal standard tissue controls.[1,5] For example, a specimen being stained with glial fibrillary acidic protein (GFAP) could contain regions of gliosis (positive control) and vessels (negative control) in the same block. This is better than using a separate tissue control block (STCB) that probably was neither fixed nor treated exactly the same as the one in question. These differences remain when a section of STCB is put on the same slide with the specimen and are aggravated if additional heat is needed to make both sections stick onto one slide.

Although normal and reactive tissues retain their expected immunophenotype, individual neoplasms may not stain for a marker generally representative of their type.[5,6] Because of this, a positive immunostaining result is more meaningful than a negative result. We will emphasize the positive features in this chapter.

If a lesion is not identified immediately, a differential diagnosis may be constructed for which a group of appropriate IHC stains is described in the text, algorithms, and tables. The following example describes the application of this approach to an actual case.

Figure 20.1 shows a cerebral tumor from the lumbosacral region of a middle-aged woman. The H&E–stained slide reveals a neoplasm with mainly epithelioid cells and a few clear cells, and abundant round to oval nuclei with fine chromatin (Table 20.6; see Fig. 20.1A). Its IHC is focally positive to epithelial membrane antigen (EMA) (see Fig. 20.1B). Boxes 20.1 and 20.2 show carcinoma, chordoma, craniopharyngioma, pituitary adenoma, and meningioma to be EMA positive. This tumor is negative for cytokeratin (CK) CAM5.2 (see Fig. 20.1C), so it does not fit the immunohistochemical

TABLE 20.1 Immunohistochemical Stains Used for Nervous Tissue

Primary Antibody/Source/Dilution*	Principal Lesions and Tissue Components	Antigen Rescue*
A6 (CD45RO)/Zymed/1:50	T lymphocytes	Mw 15 min in citrate, pH 6.0
Chromogranin A/Dr. Lloyd/1:160	Pituitary adenoma; paraganglioma; neuroendocrine tumors	Mw 15 min in citrate, pH 6.0
Collagen type IV/Dako/1:8	Fibrosis; abscess; sarcoma; teratoma; fibrous cyst and vessel walls; dura	Ventana protease 1, 16 min
CAM5.2 cytokeratin/BD/1:10	Carcinoma; craniopharyngioma; chordoma; epithelia	Ventana protease 2, 16 min
EMA/Dako/1:50	Carcinoma; meningioma; craniopharyngioma; chordoma; epithelia	Mw 15 min in citrate, pH 6.0
GFAP/Dako/1:6400	Gliosis; gliomas; CNS parenchyma	Ventana protease 2, 16 min
HV antigen/Dako/1:1000	Herpes simplex encephalitis; CMV; herpes zoster	None
JCV/SV40 viral antigen/Lee Biomolecular/1:500	PML	None
KP1 (CD68)/Dako/1:1600	Macrophages	Mw 15 min in citrate, pH 6.0
L26 (CD20)/Dako/1:500	B lymphocytes; B lymphoma	Mw 15 min in citrate, pH 6.0
MIB1/Immunotech/1:25	Proliferating cells	Mw 15 min in citrate, pH 6.0
NF/Dako/1:50	Ganglion cell tumors; neurofibroma; PNET; Alzheimer disease; CNS parenchyma	Mw 15 min in citrate, pH 6.0
Prealbumin/Dako/1:500	Choroid plexus tumors	None
S-100 protein/Dako/1:500	Gliomas; PNET; melanoma; schwannoma; neurofibroma; neuronal and chondroid tumors; chordoma; CNS; PNS	None
Synaptophysin/BioGenex/1:600	Neuronal and pineal tumors; PNET; medulloblastoma	Mw 10 min in citrate, pH 6.0
Toxoplasma/BioGenex/neat	Toxoplasmosis	None
Vimentin/Dako/1:800	Many cells; excessive in meningiomas	Mw 15 min in citrate, pH 6.0

*Data modified from McKeever PE. New methods of brain tumor analysis. In: Mena H, Sandberg G, eds. Dr. Kenneth M. Earle Memorial Neuropathology Review. Washington, DC: Armed Forces Institute of Pathology, 2004, with the expert advice and careful assistance of the immunohistology staff of the Immunoperoxidase Laboratory, Department of Pathology, University of Michigan Medical School.

CMV, cytomegalovirus; CNS, central nervous system; EMA, epithelial membrane antigen; GFAP, glial fibrillary acidic protein; HV, herpesvirus; NF, neurofilament; PML, progressive multifocal leukoencephalopathy; PNET, primitive neuroectodermal tumor; PNS, peripheral nervous system; Mw, microwave starting in cold buffer for time noted.

profile of carcinoma, chordoma, or craniopharyngioma. It is negative for chromogranin A (see Fig. 20.1D) and negative for hormones of pituitary adenomas. (It was also found to be negative for GFAP, synaptophysin, and HMB45.) Table 20.6, which summarizes the differential diagnosis for epithelioid cells, confirms the immunohistochemical profile for meningioma and notes common features and locations. The tumor in the example was observed to have rare whorls and to involve the spinal meninges. In comparison with descriptions of meningiomas in the text, the cells were epithelioid and only focally syncytial. The clear cells were not prominent and lacked the cytoplasmic glycogen found in the clear cell variant. The tumor was as a meningothelial meningioma with prominent epithelioid appearance.[1,3]

Brain biopsies for non-neoplastic diseases often require IHC combined with additional studies such as microbiologic culture, polymerase chain reaction (PCR), Western blot, or electron microscopy (EM).[7-9] Specialized centers are available to assist interpretations of these.[9-13]

CLINICAL AND RADIOGRAPHIC PERSPECTIVE OF LESIONS

Major categories of lesions of the brain, spinal cord, and meninges—such as solitary and multiple masses, cysts, vascular malformations, and abscesses—are likely to be recognized clinically through the use of computed tomography (CT), magnetic resonance imaging (MRI), or angiography. New methods of using flow voids with CT or MRI have provided non-invasive evaluations of vessels like MRA. MRI can be targeted on specific CNS chemicals like choline and NAA to help identify tumor tissue. Diffusion-weighted MRIs can differentiate tissues by their water movement in three dimensions.[14]

Multiple lesions can be produced by degenerative, vascular, and infectious diseases, or by neoplasms. Regarding neoplasms, the *M-rule* for differential diagnosis of common multiple central nervous system (CNS) neoplasms includes metastases, malignant lymphoma, melanoma, and medulloblastoma.[13]

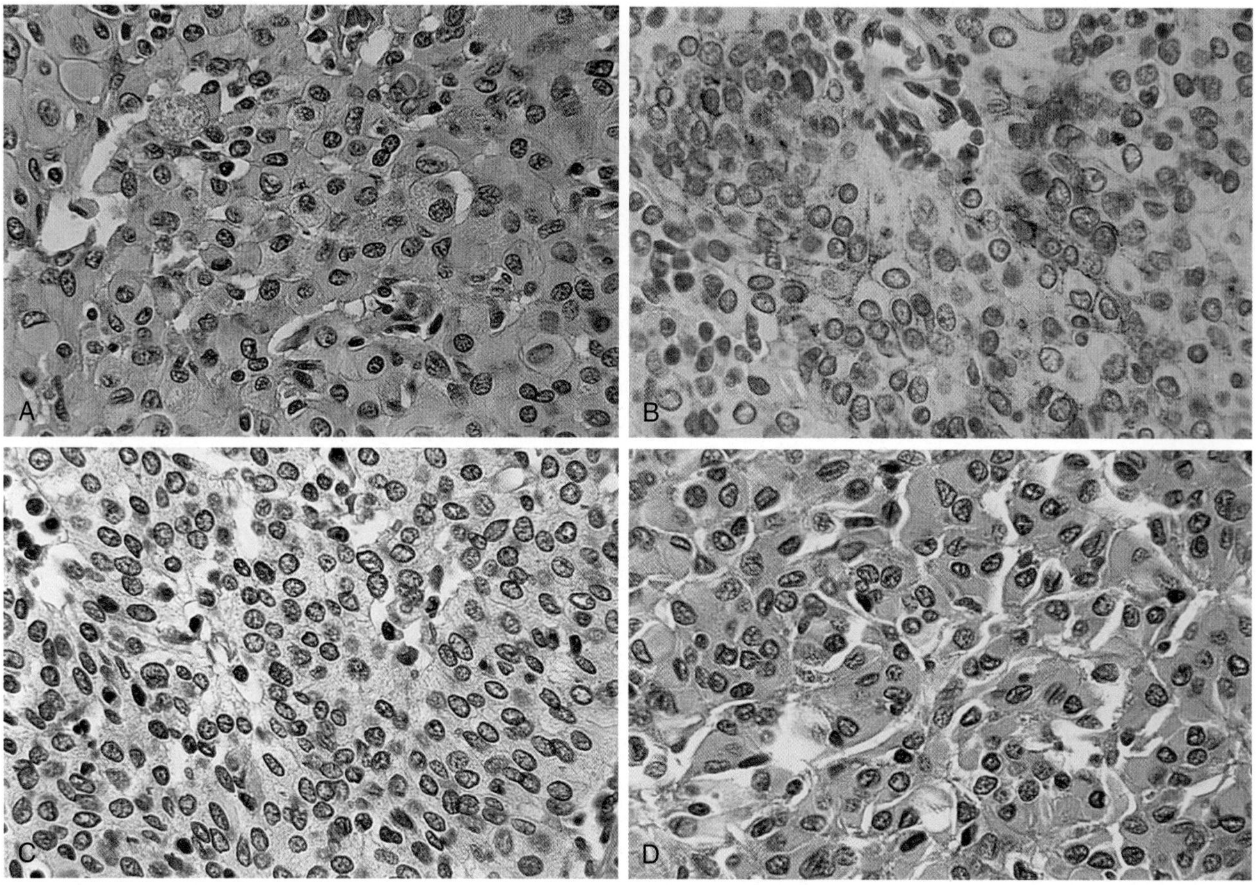

FIGURE 20.1 This actual case illustrates how the algorithms (see Boxes 20.1 and 20.2), tables, and text assist interpretation from initial impression to final diagnosis. **(A)** Large mass is from the lumbosacral region of a middle-aged woman (H&E). It is focally positive for epithelial membrane antigen (EMA) **(B)**, negative for CAM5.2 **(C)**, and negative for chromogranin A (CgA) **(D)**. It also reacted positively to vimentin and negatively to glial fibrillary acidic protein (GFAP) and synaptophysin *(not shown)*. This tumor is a meningothelial meningioma with prominent epithelioid cells. *From McKeever PE. New methods of brain tumor analysis. In: Mena H, Sandberg G, eds. Dr. Kenneth M. Earle Memorial Neuropathology Review. Washington, DC: Armed Forces Institute of Pathology, 2004.*

TABLE 20.2 Differential Diagnosis of Cells Infiltrating CNS Parenchyma

	Differential Features		
Diagnosis	**Structures**	**Antibody**	**Locations***
Gliosis[a]	Cells fibrillar; uncrowded; round/oval nuclei	GFAP in stellate glial processes	CNS
Macrophages	Cells and nuclei round to elongated; cell content reflects injury	KP1; α-ACT	CNS; meninges
Encephalitis/cerebritis	Perivascular mixture of inflammatory cells	LCA; L26; A6; κ and λ Ig; α-ACT; KP1; microorganism	CNS gray matter/CNS
Hemorrhage	RBCs or macrophages with hemosiderin	Fibrin; KP1	Deep cerebrum; cerebellum; CNS
Margin of gliomas[b]	Cells fibrillar; angular nuclei indent each other; (mitoses)[b,c]	GFAP	CNS
Lymphoma	Perivascular non-cohesive small round cells	LCA; L26; A6; κ and λ Ig	Deep cerebrum; CNS; meninges

*Most common or most specific location is listed first.

[a]Nonspecific reaction to injury.

[b]Suspicion of margin of glioma on frozen section should be followed by a request for another, more central biopsy. Mitoses suggest margin of a high-grade glioma.

[c]Parentheses around a differential feature indicate an uncommon feature that is very useful in differential diagnosis when found.

CNS, central nervous system; GFAP, glial fibrillary acid protein; α-ACT, alpha-antichymotrypsin; Ig, immunoglobulin; LCA, leukocyte common antigen; RBC, red blood cell.

Modified from McKeever PE, Blaivas M. The brain, spinal cord, and meninges. In: Sternberg SS, ed. Diagnostic Surgical Pathology. 2nd ed. New York, NY: Raven Press; 1994:409-492.

<table>
<tr><th colspan="4">Immunohistochemical stain response</th><th>Margin</th><th>Entity</th></tr>
<tr><td rowspan="7">GFAP+</td><td rowspan="7">EMA–</td><td rowspan="2"></td><td rowspan="2"></td><td>Diffuse</td><td>Oligodendroglioma</td></tr>
<tr><td></td><td>PXA</td></tr>
<tr><td>Syn–</td><td rowspan="3">KP1–</td><td rowspan="3">Sharp</td><td>Clear cell ependymoma</td></tr>
<tr><td rowspan="2">Syn+</td><td>DNT</td></tr>
<tr><td>Central neurocytoma</td></tr>
<tr><td rowspan="4">Syn–</td><td rowspan="2">KP1+</td><td rowspan="2"></td><td>Demyelination</td></tr>
<tr><td>Infarct</td></tr>
<tr><td rowspan="2">GFAP–</td><td rowspan="2">EMA+</td><td rowspan="3">KP1–</td><td rowspan="3">Sharp</td><td>Clear cell meningioma</td></tr>
<tr><td>Renal cell carcinoma</td></tr>
<tr><td></td><td>EMA–</td><td></td><td>Hemangioblastoma</td></tr>
</table>

DNT, dysembryoplastic neuroepithelial tumor; EMA, epithelial membrane antigen; GFAP, glial fibrillary acidic protein; PXA, pleomorphic xanthoastrocytoma; Syn, synaptophysin.
Modified from Gokden M, Roth KA, Garroll SL, et al. Clear cell neoplasms and pseudoneoplastic lesions of the central nervous system. *Semin Diagn Pathol.* 1997; 14:253–269.

BOX 20.1 Differential diagnoses of clear cell lesions. Unmarked boxes reflect neoplasms for which the feature or the immunohistochemical stain response is not decisive.

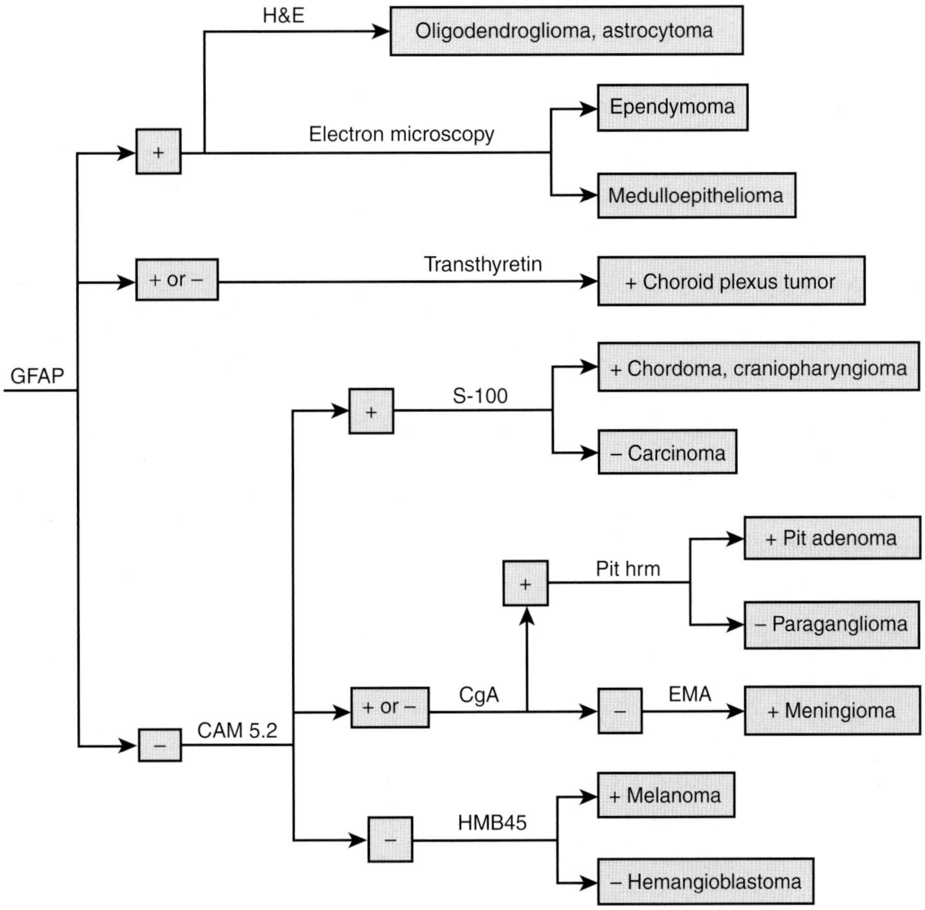

BOX 20.2 Immunohistochemical diagnosis of epithelioid cell tumors.

TABLE 20.3 Biopsies Directed toward a Neurologic Symptom or Specific Disease

	Confirmatory Features of Suspected Disease		
Symptom/Suspected Disease*	**Structures**	**Antibody**	**Locations[a]**
Herpes simplex encephalitis	Encephalitis (Table 20.2); Cowdry A amphophilic nuclear inclusions of 90-100 nm target capsids	HSV	Temporal or basilar frontal lobe(s); CNS; frequently bilateral
Toxoplasmosis	Necrosis containing 3-5 μm tachyzoites; (cysts); (inflammation)[b]	Toxoplasma	CNS; frequent multiple lesions
Progressive multifocal leukoencephalopathy	Demyelination; bizarre glia; amphophilic nuclear inclusions of 15-25 nm or 30-40 nm diameter filaments or spheres	JCV/SV40; myelin; neurofilament; KP1	Cerebral white matter; CNS
Dementia/Creutzfeldt-Jakob disease	Cytoplasmic vacuoles indenting nuclei; gliosis	PrP; GFAP	Bilateral cerebral cortex; gray matter
Small vessel disease	Vasculitis or arterial sclerosis or congophilic angiopathy	A6; L26; CD31; amyloid; muscle actin; elastin	Cerebrum; CNS; frequent multiple lesions
Dementia/Alzheimer disease	Argyrophilic plaques; neurofibrillary tangles of bihelical filaments	Neurofilament; tau; ubiquitin; Alz-50	Bilateral cerebral cortex
Demyelination	Loss of myelin; gliosis; Gitter cells; with or without axonal preservation	Myelin; neurofilament; KP1	Cerebral white matter; CNS
Epilepsy	Low-grade glioma or ganglioglioma; gliosis; or vascular malformation	GFAP; neurofilament; elastin	Cerebral cortex

*The order of tabulated lesions follows the order of discussion in text.
[a]Most common or most specific location is listed first.
[b]Parentheses around a differential feature indicate an uncommon feature that is very useful in differential diagnosis when found.
CNS, central nervous system; GFAP, glial fibrillary acid protein; HSV, herpes simplex virus.
Modified from McKeever PE, Blaivas M. The brain, spinal cord, and meninges. In: Sternberg SS, ed. Diagnostic Surgical Pathology. 2nd ed. New York, NY: Raven Press; 1994:409-492.

Depending upon its age, the tomographic density of hemorrhage is often sufficiently unique to identify hemorrhage as a major component of a lesion. Calcifications and relationships with the skull are resolved well on CT. Gray and white matter, edema, and melanin are better seen on MRI. Vascular abnormalities are frequently defined by MRA, or, if needed, angiographically.

Non-neoplastic lesions are often evaluated by a neurologist. Thus, a major neurologic symptom (e.g., pain, weakness, or visual loss) or category of neurologic disease (e.g., dementia) may focus the differential diagnosis (Table 20.3).

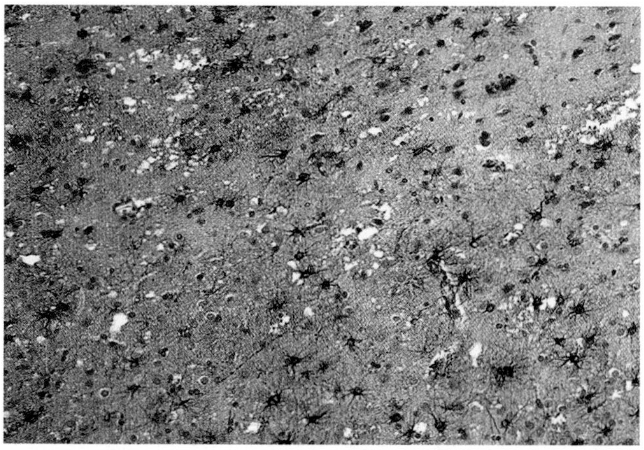

FIGURE 20.2 GFAP stain of gliosis. This gliosis is in the cerebral cortex from a patient with Creutzfeldt-Jakob disease (CJD). The glia are reactive and stellate with abundant brown cytoplasmic GFAP, which is quite different from the remote gliosis illustrated in the case of long-standing seizures (see Fig. 20.31B). The coalescing vacuoles are a feature of CJD but not of gliosis in general. (Anti-GFAP with H&E.)

NON-NEOPLASTIC BRAIN LESIONS

Reactive Changes

GLIOSIS

Gliosis is a reaction of the CNS to injury of the brain or spinal cord. Although subtle changes occur earlier, gliosis is usually appreciated by two to three weeks after an injury. Nearly any injury of the CNS can cause gliosis, so its presence is not diagnostic of a specific pathologic entity (see Table 20.2).[15]

Anti-GFAP immunostain (Fig. 20.2) highlights the dark-brown intense immunoreactivity, relatively low nuclear to cytoplasmic ratio, and the separation of astrocytes in gliosis. When it is critical to distinguish gliosis from normal brain, an age- and site-matched control slide of normal CNS can be stained concurrently. Both the number and the density of GFAP-positive cells and cellular processes should be greater in the specimen than in the normal control.

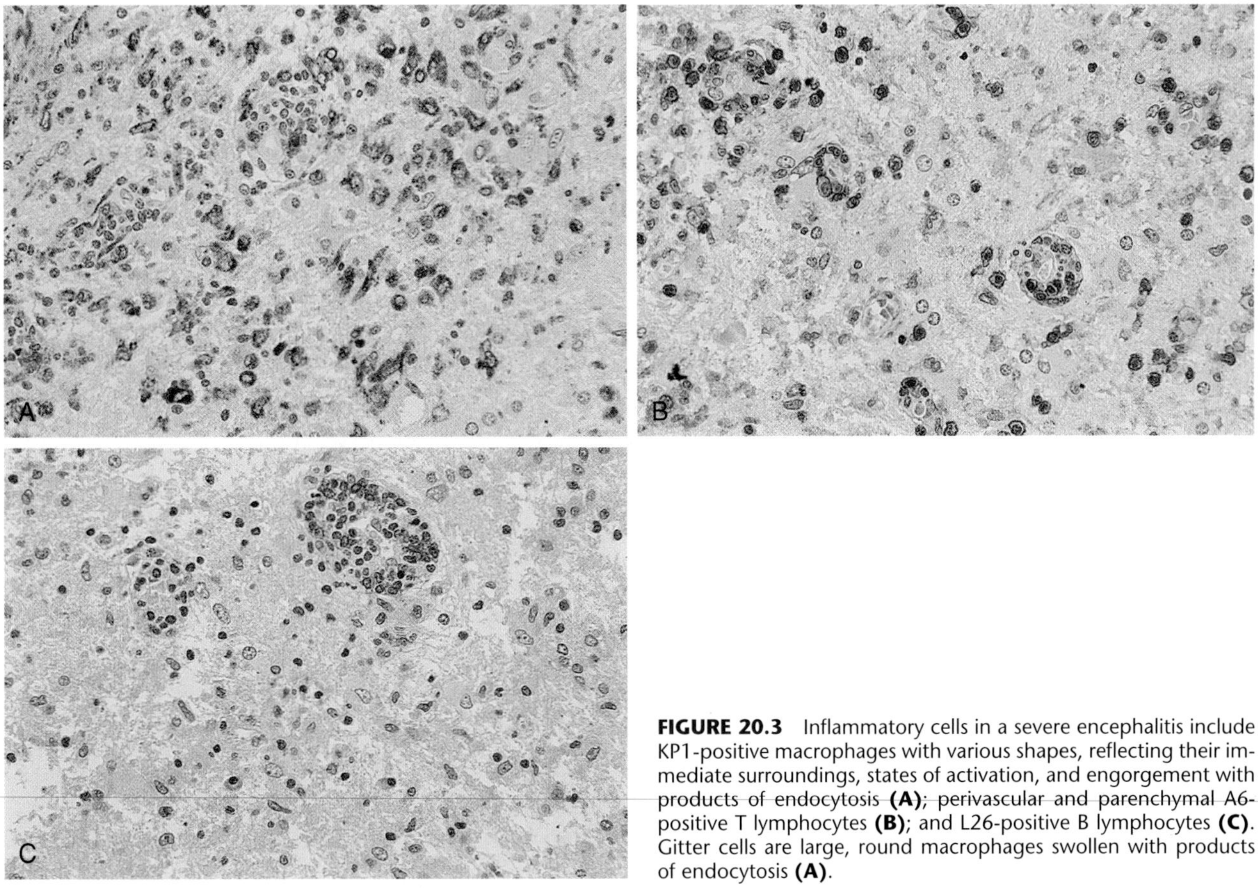

FIGURE 20.3 Inflammatory cells in a severe encephalitis include KP1-positive macrophages with various shapes, reflecting their immediate surroundings, states of activation, and engorgement with products of endocytosis **(A)**; perivascular and parenchymal A6-positive T lymphocytes **(B)**; and L26-positive B lymphocytes **(C)**. Gitter cells are large, round macrophages swollen with products of endocytosis **(A)**.

The GFAP stain helps distinguish gliosis from glioma (see Table 20.2). GFAP-positive cells are uniformly spaced apart in gliosis (see Fig. 20.2). This spacing of individual reactive astrocytes is more uniform than that found in the margin of an infiltrative glioma (see Gliomas section later in the chapter). The nuclear to cytoplasmic ratio of gliosis is less than that of a glioma.[3]

MACROPHAGES

After three days, phagocytic macrophages may be seen in any destruction or irritation (Fig. 20.3A; see Tables 20.2 and 20.3). Macrophages are rich in enzymes such as alpha-antichymotrypsin and muramidase, and they possess markers of mononuclear phagocytic cells and thus react with antibodies CD68 (KP1) and MAC387. All of these features can be stained using IHC. Around hemorrhages or traumatic lesions, macrophages contain iron-positive hemosiderin.

Encephalitis simply means brain inflammation. Many things cause it—from a virus to surgical implants.[13]

In cerebritis, meningitis, or encephalitis, the macrophages are pleomorphic cells. Some are thin, and others are loaded with debris (see Fig. 20.3). They may contain yeast and other organisms. Macrophages swollen plump by phagocytosis within the CNS are called *granular* or *Gitter cells*. They are large and round with a foamy cytoplasm filled with lipid droplets (Fig. 20.4; see Fig. 20.3A). Macrophages that are small cells with scant cytoplasm participate in the chronic inflammatory infiltrate centered on blood vessels in encephalitides; in glial nodules; around dying neurons (neuronophagia); and in other inflammatory, demyelinating, and degenerative processes.[3,16] CD68 stains them well (see Fig. 20.3A).

Perivascular Inflammation

Perivascular inflammation consists of small round cells with high nuclear to cytoplasmic ratios. These can be mistaken for lymphoma and for neuroectodermal clusters, which are particularly common in brains of children. Leukocyte common antigen (LCA;CD45/45R), CD3 epsilon, CD5, CD20, and CD79 alpha markers distinguish the inflammation by highlighting polyclonal reactive lymphocytes (see Fig. 20.3B and C).

Irritation of the CNS elicits inflammation around blood vessels.[17] CD68-positive macrophages ingest the irritant or injured cellular constituents and move them to the perivascular space.[16] In the absence of classic lymph nodes in the brain, this perivascular region is where cells that respond to antigen intermingle. Depending on the severity and duration of illness, the perivascular inflammation varies substantially.[3] Old hemorrhage exemplifies a minimal response characterized mainly by perivascular macrophages laden with hemosiderin (see Table 20.2). Surgical wounds and implants cause substantial reactions. Viral or allergic encephalitis produces a maximal response with abundant perivascular macrophages and many CD3 epsilon–positive T lymphocytes.[3]

Some diseases affect mainly veins, such as perivenous encephalitis (PVE). Others affect small arteries, such as

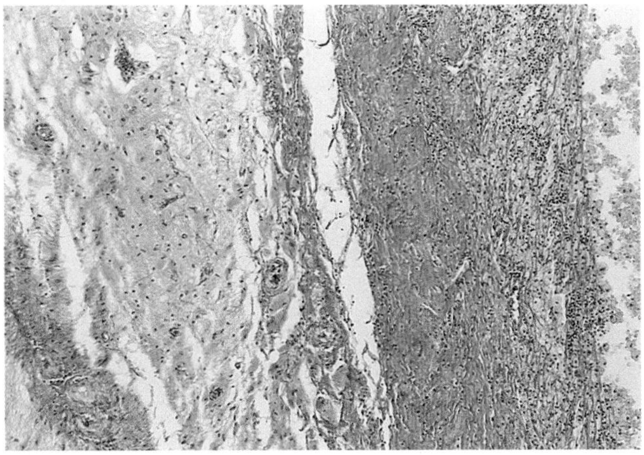

FIGURE 20.4 This specimen from a brain abscess shows an inflammatory lesion with a distinctive wall of collagen-stained cyan with Masson's trichrome stain. Brain around this wall *(orange side)* contains highly reactive (gemistocytic) astrocytes. Toward the center of the abscess *(gray side)* are leukocytes and swollen macrophages.

cerebral autosomal dominant arteriopathy with subcortical infarcts and leukoencephalopathy (CADASIL). Unlike PVE, CADASIL has little or no inflammation (see Small Vessel Disease section later in the chapter). Affected vessels may be distinguished with anti–smooth muscle actin or myosin, because cerebral arteries have a thicker circumferential layer of spindle-shaped smooth muscle cells than cerebral veins.

FIBROSIS

Fibrosis is rare in brain tissue. It occurs around abscesses (see Fig. 20.4), in granulomas, and in desmoplastic and sarcomatous tumors. Fibrosis is more common in meninges. Meningeal fibrosis develops after traumatic injuries, meningitis, vasculitis involving meningeal vessels, and radiation therapy and as a desmoplastic response to a tumor.

Various constituents of fibrosis can be detected with immunohistochemical stains: collagen, fibronectin, and laminin.[18] Type IV collagen works best for most brain and meningeal tissues.[3] For routine identification of fibrosis, standard tinctorial stains rival immunohistochemical stains (see Fig. 20.4).

KEY DIAGNOSTIC POINTS

Reactive Changes

- Gliosis is the usual slow reaction to brain injury.
- GFAP, the single most important brain immunostain, highlights the low n:c ratios, stellate processes, and evenly separated reactive astrocytes in gliosis.
- PMN, macrophages, and lymphocytes react to brain injury in a way similar to the reaction to systemic injury. Without lymph nodes in brain, their interactions are less obvious and their clusters are perivascular.
- Common systemically, fibrosis is rare in brain tissue.

Infectious Diseases

Infections may produce meningitis, cerebritis, abscess, encephalitis, or encephalopathy.[19] Except for encephalopathy, inflammation is a prominent feature. It proceeds from acute to chronic phases much like a systemic infection. Infection must be distinguished from lymphoma. Infections cause polyclonal inflammation and often show a prominent T-cell component that stains with immunohistochemical markers, including CD45R0, CD3 epsilon, and CD5 (see Table 20.1). Mature, EMA-positive plasma cells signify inflammation when present. On the other hand, large neoplastic cells with malignant nuclei in primary brain lymphomas are usually B cells that stain with CD20 or CD79 alpha (see the Hematopoietic and Lymphoid Neoplasms section later in the chapter). We will describe each histopathologic type of infection here and follow with discussions of the organisms that cause each type.

HISTOPATHOLOGY

Meningitis is an inflammation of the meninges that cover the brain and spinal cord. Leptomeningitis affects the thin meninges: the pia and arachnoid. Pachymeningitis affects the thick dura and is less common than leptomeningitis in non-surgical cases. Organisms access the meninges by local extension from sinuses or from the blood stream. The perivascular space in the CNS is an extension of the subarachnoid space. Persistent meningitis travels along this space, where it can cause cerebritis or an abscess.

Cerebritis is focal inflammation of brain parenchyma (*myelitis* in the spinal cord). Cerebritis precedes abscess formation but requires an early biopsy to be seen (see Tables 20.2 and 20.10). The inflammatory infiltrate is composed of neutrophils, macrophages, lymphocytes, and plasma cells, with or without parenchymal necrosis. Septic cerebritis is usually caused by bacterial agents, most often streptococci or staphylococci, and less commonly by gram-negative organisms, such as *Escherichia coli*, *Pseudomonas*, and *Haemophilus influenzae*. Cerebritis also occurs around neoplasms, ruptured vascular malformations, infarcts, and traumatic lesions.

Granulomatous forms of meningitis and cerebritis are seen in tuberculosis and other mycobacterial infections; fungal, parasitic, or spirochetal infections; idiopathic conditions, such as sarcoidosis, systemic lupus erythematosus, Wegener's and lymphomatoid granulomatoses; and histiocytosis X.

Some diagnoses are made through biopsy and culture, and others are made through clinical correlation.[13,20,21]

An *abscess* combines features of inflammation and fibrosis in response to a suppurative microorganism, often bacterial or fungal. A mixture of polymorphonuclear leukocytes, polyclonal T and B lymphocytes, macrophages, and plasma cells (with or without necrosis) confirms inflammation. Polymorphism of inflammatory components can be verified in difficult cases with CD45RO and CD20 immunohistochemical stains for polyclonal T and B lymphocytes, CD68 for macrophages, and EMA for plasma cells (see Tables 20.1 and 20.10).

The wall of a brain abscess consists of a lining of CD31-positive and CD34-positive vascular tissue and collagen surrounded by highly GFAP-positive reactive gliosis. Adjacent brain is edematous. Because collagen is rare within the CNS, its presence is an important diagnostic feature of an abscess (see Table 20.10). Collagen may be difficult to distinguish from fibrillary gliosis on a slide stained with H&E. It can be confirmed histochemically with Masson's trichrome stain or immunohistochemically with staining for collagen (see Fig. 20.4 and Table 20.1).

Encephalitis is inflammation of brain tissue (see Fig. 20.3). It is often caused by viral or rickettsial organisms that produce a more diffuse inflammation than cerebritis.[7] Most viral infections are self limited and cause only meningitis or mild meningoencephalitis. The entities emphasized here require surgical attention and are more serious.

Encephalopathy (which translates as "brain suffering") that is caused by infection may show little or no inflammation. This is especially true for the spongiform encephalopathies caused by prions, such as Creutzfeldt-Jakob disease (CJD).[9] Brain cell death followed by gliosis is the common feature of the encephalopathies. A *leukoencephalopathy* ("*white* brain suffering") targets white matter. A *myelopathy* ("cord-medulla suffering") generally targets the spinal cord.

ORGANISMS

Every brain biopsy specimen should be handled in such a way that if inflammation is found at surgery, it will be possible to culture the tissue for bacteria, mycobacteria, and fungi and to use special stains, immunostaining techniques, and electron microscopy. This author's experience has been that for organisms that grow *in vitro*, microbiologic culture is preferable to histochemical stains, IHC, or polymerase chain reaction (PCR) assay if sampling of the lesion is uniform. Prior antibiotic treatment or non-uniform sampling of focal infection affects individual cases.

Fungal, bacterial, and parasitic infections are increasingly common in immunocompromised hosts. The common organisms are *Cryptococcus neoformans, Listeria monocytogenes, Aspergillus fumigatus,* and conventional bacteria such as *H. influenzae, Streptococcus pneumoniae, Staphylococcus epidermidis,* and *Pseudomonas*. Cryptococcal meningitis is the most common form of fungal meningitis, but brain inflammation may be minimal in its presence. Chronic infections with these organisms produce granulomas. The organisms can be cultured or found with special stains, such as periodic acid-Schiff (PAS) and Gomori's methenamine silver (GMS), but immunohistochemical analysis with specific reagents is an option for organisms refractory to culture.[3,13,21] Species identification can be accomplished with immunostaining.[21]

Tuberculosis can involve any region of the CNS and its coverings. The disease usually causes granulomatous inflammation with or without caseating necrosis, meningitis, or arteritis. The extensive time required to grow mycobacteria invites preliminary testing with IHC, PCR assay, or acid-fast stains.[20]

Syphilis is rising in incidence, predominantly among immunocompromised patients, and contributing to the differential diagnosis of granulomatous inflammation. The responsible organism, *Treponema pallidum,* is refractory to culture. Silver stains for it also stain brain, which produces background staining that confounds detection. IHC offers an alternative and more specific test.[22]

The most common parasitic infection of the CNS is *neurocysticercosis,* which prevails in developing countries. If a brain cyst contains a typical cysticercus with a characteristic invaginated scolex, the disorder can be identified without IHC. Immunohistochemical analysis using cerebrospinal fluid (CSF) from proven cases as the source of primary antibody is available for mangled or degenerated organisms in cases for which the glycocalyx remains to be found.[23] *Schistosomiasis* infects the brain and spinal cord. It can be highlighted with the readily available immunohistochemical stain for standard high molecular weight cytokeratin.[24] Because there is little CK in brain, bits of organism stand out. This is one example of using a surrogate IHC marker when a more specific marker is not readily available. Whenever possible, the more specific marker is preferable.

Whipple's disease rarely causes a primary brain disease without gastrointestinal symptoms.[13] The causative bacillus is *Tropheryma whippelii.* The diagnosis can be made on brain biopsy specimen evaluated by light microscopy with immunoperoxidase staining for group B streptococci.[25] Histologic features include PAS-positive, diastase-resistant rods in macrophages, microgranulomas, perivascular CD3 epsilon and CD20 positive lymphocytes, and microglia reactive for CD68.

Lyme disease is caused by a tick-borne spirochete, *Borrelia burgdorferi.* It involves CNS and can be detected in CSF.[26]

The most common cause of non-epidemic encephalitis, and the most often found on biopsy, is *Herpes simplex* virus (HSV) (see Table 20.3).[27] The process is usually but not always localized to the temporal and frontal lobes. The earliest lesion is an area of vascular engorgement with ischemic changes in neurons, positive for HSV on immunoperoxidase technique performed on routine paraffin-embedded tissue. Perivascular inflammation is characteristic, composed predominantly of CD45R0-positive and CD20-positive lymphocytes mixed with CD68-positive macrophages and accompanied by varying degrees of focal necrosis and hemorrhage. Intranuclear inclusion bodies are consistent with HSV but may be produced by many viruses, such as cytomegalovirus, varicella-zoster, JC virus, and simian virus 40 (SV40).[7]

Cowdry type A bodies of HSV are not easy to demonstrate in small brain-biopsy specimens. This argues for sensitive and specific methods of identification such as *in situ* hybridization (ISH), PCR, and IHC.[3,28] Electron microscopy may demonstrate viral particles within the nuclei or cytoplasm but is less sensitive and less specific. Culture and sequential serologic CSF evaluations are slow but are still the most accurate methods of diagnosis for many viral CNS infections, including HSV.

Enterovirus (e.g., Coxsackievirus, echovirus) and arbovirus infections (e.g., Eastern equine, St. Louis,

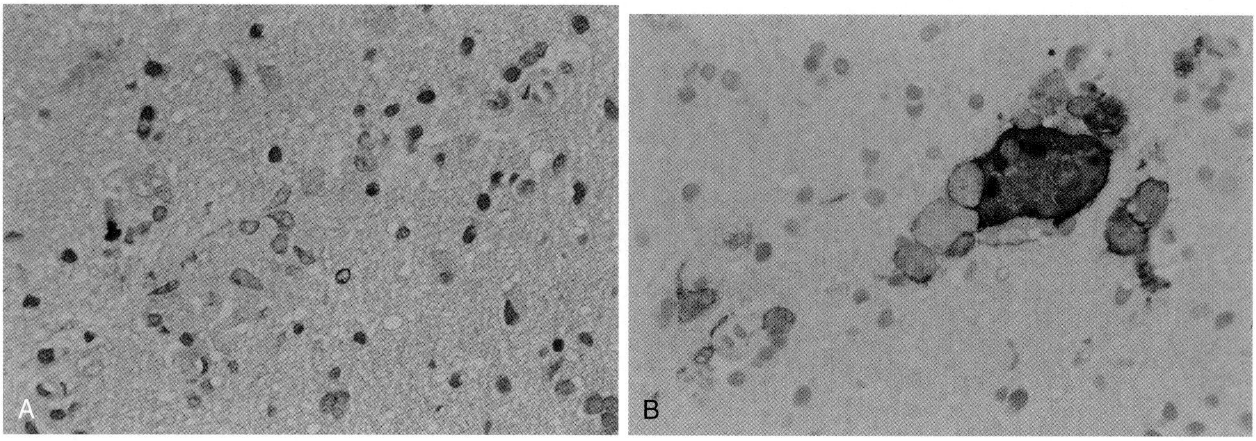

FIGURE 20.5 Multinucleated giant cells formed from coalescence of macrophages have cytoplasm less fibrillar than surrounding brain and tapered nuclei with light chromatin. They are elusive on H&E stain **(A)**, but obvious upon IHC staining for HIV p24 antigen **(B)**. *Courtesy of Dr. Clayton Wiley, University of Pittsburgh, Pittsburgh, Pa.*

West Nile) lack characteristic inclusions. West Nile virus is an arbovirus. With mosquito and bird vectors and hosts, it has caused human infection.[3] Its transmission by blood transfusion and organ transplantation has been documented. Some cases are fatal.

The findings include patchy meningitis, encephalitis, and poliomyelitis with variable involvement of the cerebrum, thalamus, basal ganglia, brainstem, and cerebellum. CD3 epsilon and CD68 highlight perivascular inflammation with evidence of meningoencephalitis, microglial nodules, and neuronophagia. The anterior horn cells are targeted in some patients.[3]

Rabies produces round or oval eosinophilic 1- to 7-μm cytoplasmic inclusions.[29] Immunostains and PCR assay are available for diagnosis.[13]

Subacute sclerosing panencephalitis and milder encephalitis are caused by measles virus. Focal lymphocytic inflammation in the leptomeninges and perivascular spaces, with many CD4-positive cells, patchy GFAP-positive fibrillary astrocytosis, and occasional microglial nodules, involves the cerebral cortex. Diffuse mononuclear inflammation, gliosis, and loss of myelin occur in subcortical white matter. Inclusion bodies are Cowdry type A and may be seen on H&E–stained slides; their specific identification requires IHC.[30]

Acquired Immunodeficiency Syndrome

CNS lesions in AIDS reflect the entire spectrum of neuropathologic disease, beginning with cerebritis, meningitis, encephalitis, and vascular disease and ending with degenerative-metabolic changes and neoplasia. The lesions have been summarized in several detailed reviews.[8,31] Diseases either are directly caused by human immunodeficiency virus (HIV) or are secondary opportunistic diseases resulting from immunosuppression. CNS diseases were extremely common in the early era of AIDS, with neurologic symptoms at clinical presentation and CNS abnormalities noted in more than 50% of patients. Highly active antiretroviral therapy (HAART) has altered the disease course, such that fewer CNS complications occur.[31]

PRIMARY MANIFESTATIONS OF HUMAN IMMUNODEFICIENCY VIRUS

HIV encephalitis can be reliably diagnosed by histologic evaluation. The hallmark of HIV encephalitis is multinucleated giant cells in both parenchyma and around vessels. They are mixed with macrophages and microglia, and they form multiple foci of various sizes within the white matter, deep gray matter, and cortex. Immunohistochemical detection of HIV p23 and p24 antigen and ISH are useful (Fig. 20.5).[3]

HIV leukoencephalopathy is characterized by diffuse damage to the white matter with loss of myelin, reactive astrogliosis, multinucleated cells, and macrophages. IHC or ISH helps confirm the association of HIV with the process. Leukoencephalopathy occasionally manifests as marked vacuolar myelin swelling. This finding is more common in the spinal cord, however, where it forms multiple foci of vacuolar myelopathy that resemble combined systems degeneration without pernicious anemia.

Still another manifestation of HIV infection, lymphocytic meningitis, is remarkable for heavy lymphocytic infiltrates within the leptomeninges and perivascular spaces. HIV cerebral vasculitis and granulomatous angiitis may occur with lymphocytic or lymphoplasmahistiocytic multinucleated giant cell infiltration of cerebral vessel walls, occasionally accompanied by necrosis.[3]

Since the onset of HAART, a new form of HIV encephalitis with severe leukoencephalopathy and intensive perivascular macrophage and lymphocyte infiltrates has been described. It may be a response of the revived immune system.[31]

INFECTIONS SECONDARY TO AIDS

Opportunistic infections are common in patients with AIDS but may also be found in other immunodeficient patients. *Toxoplasmosis* is the most common of these infections. It manifests as a necrotizing encephalomyelitis

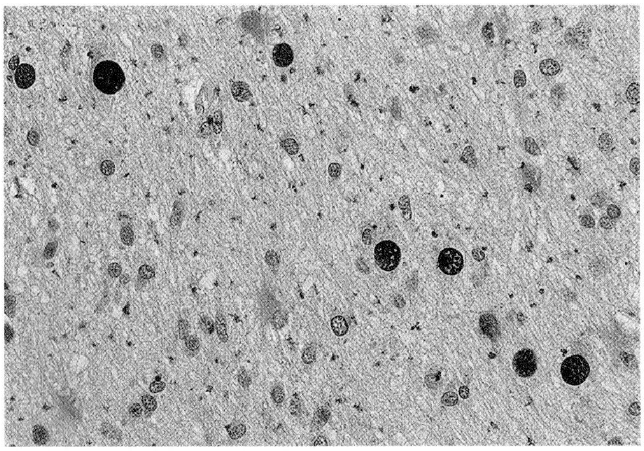

FIGURE 20.6 Progressive multifocal leukoencephalopathy (PML). The patient, a young woman, had systemic lupus erythematosus, which was treated with high-dose anti-inflammatory and cytotoxic agents. Immunohistochemical detection of JC viral antigen in swollen oligodendroglial nuclei stained brown. Negative, smaller, round oligodendroglial and elongated astrocytic nuclei counterstained purple with hematoxylin. *Courtesy of Dr. Riccardo Valdez, University of Michigan, Ann Arbor, Mich.*

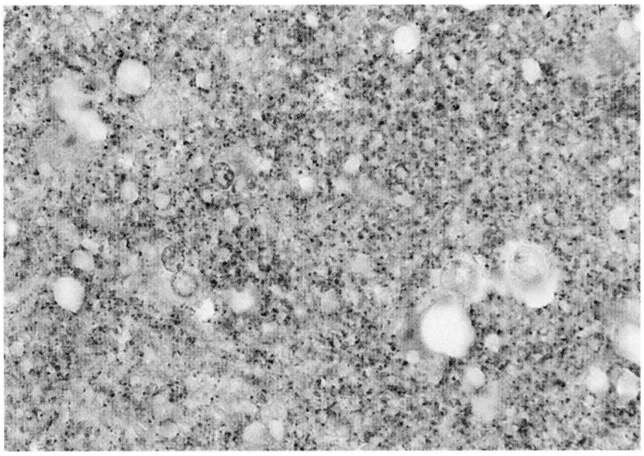

FIGURE 20.7 Creutzfeldt-Jakob disease (CJD). Biopsy specimen from the cerebral frontal lobe of an elderly man who had displayed progressive behavioral and memory changes for a few weeks. Patches of vacuoles and synaptic depletion can be seen in the cortical gray matter. Each tiny brown dot is a synapse in the neuropil stained with synaptophysin. Vacuoles in neuronal cytoplasm indent their nuclei. (Anti-synaptophysin with hematoxylin counterstain.)

characterized by discrete lesions that contain free trophozoites or cysts filled with parasites at the periphery of the necrotic foci.[32] Immunoperoxidase or immunofluorescence stains pinpoint the organism, which is not easily found on routine H&E–stained sections.[33]

Cytomegalovirus (CMV) infection follows toxoplasmosis in frequency and varies from virtually no associated inflammation to severe necrotizing meningoencephalitis and ependymitis.[34] Immunohistochemistry, ISH, and PCR assay are useful for detecting the virus in paraffin-embedded tissue if bizarre giant cells with nuclear inclusions are not evident.[35]

Severe encephalitis results from coinfection with HIV and JCV.[36] Tuberculosis and neurosyphilis affect patients with AIDS.[37,38] Microscopic examination reveals focal lymphoplasmacytic inflammatory infiltrates in a predominantly perivascular arrangement. Exotic CNS infections in patients with AIDS include amebic encephalitis, trypanosomiasis, and strongyloidiasis.[13,39]

PROGRESSIVE MULTIFOCAL LEUKOENCEPHALOPATHY

Progressive multifocal leukoencephalopathy (PML) is a disease manifested as multiple discrete foci of destruction of myelin with relative preservation of axons, often with no other evidence of inflammation. Radiographically, it may simulate multiple sclerosis or a mass. It is caused by DNA papovavirus (predominantly JC papovavirus [JCP] and rarely SV40 virus) in immunodeficient patients (see Table 20.3). JCP has nothing in common with prions. Common underlying diseases are leukemia and AIDS. PML also occurs in patients with various types of carcinoma, tuberculosis, systemic lupus erythematosus, and sarcoidosis or after the immunosuppression associated with organ transplantation.

Brain biopsy may show a destructive process within the white matter, with multiple lipid-laden macrophages, frequent large glial nuclei with a ground-glass appearance, and many large, unusual glia with pleomorphic and hyperchromatic nuclei. Perivascular infiltrates of mature lymphocytes are prominent in some cases. The pathology of JCV infection is similar in patients with and without AIDS. However, in patients with AIDS, bizarre astrocytes are less common and perivascular inflammatory cells are more common.[13]

Glial nuclei are filled with virions in this disease. PML should be differentiated from multiple sclerosis, other demyelinating disorders, and astrocytic neoplasia. Random distribution of rather uniformly distorted astrocytes among multiple lipid-laden macrophages is helpful in differentiating this lesion from an astrocytic neoplasm. Bizarre astrocytes and abnormal oligodendrocytes with large nuclei containing inclusion bodies are characteristic. Diagnosis of PML is confirmed by electron microscopy; ISH; immunostaining (Fig. 20.6); or PCR assay for JCV, SV40, and BK virus.[40,41]

KEY DIAGNOSTIC POINTS
Infectious Diseases

- Lesions found to be inflammatory at biopsy should be sent sterile from the OR to the microbiology laboratory for cultures. Cultures are more sensitive than tissue stains for nearly all microorganisms that grow *in vitro*.
- A variety of serologic and tissue-based assays including IHC, ISH, special stains, EM, and PCR are available. These should be selected individually on the basis of clinical situation and suspected organisms.

Spongiform Encephalopathies

Spongiform encephalopathies are characterized by vacuoles (spongiform change) in the gray matter.[3] Vacuoles vary in size up to 30 μm in diameter and larger (Fig. 20.7). They are in the neuropil and cellular perikaryon.

Their neuroanatomic distribution varies among specific diseases and in individual cases. Lack of inflammation is usual. Specimens in which a spongiform encephalopathy is suspected should be processed as described later (see Dementias section).

The spongiform encephalopathies include CJD, the much-publicized mad cow disease, scrapie, kuru, Gerstmann-Sträussler-Scheinker (GSS) syndrome, and fatal familial insomnia.[3,8,42-44] They are caused by infectious proteins called *prions,* modified forms of normal counterpart proteins. Hereditary prion diseases, such as familial fatal insomnia, GSS syndrome, and familial CJD, have germline mutations that produce prions. Infectious prion diseases, such as mad cow disease, scrapie, kuru, and spontaneous CJD, are transmitted by intimate contact with prions. Like catalysts, these pathogenic prions propagate by inducing their ubiquitous normal counterparts to refold into the pathogenic conformation. As this cycle continues, a growing percentage of normal counterpart proteins is converted to the pathogenic configuration.

Prions are very difficult to inactivate. Agents that completely denature protein, such as bleach and strong alkali or acid (see the Dementias section later in the chapter) are effective, but ultraviolet light, routine formalin fixative, and standard disinfectants fail to eradicate prions.

CJD was a common diagnosis in one evaluation of cerebral biopsy specimens for dementia.[42] Vacuoles in the neuropil and perikaryon of neurons are regionally and temporally variable in CJD (see Figs. 20.2 and 20.6). If not prominent, vacuoles can be overlooked or mistaken for artifacts.[9] Spongiform changes usually diminish in late-stage disease (see Table 20.3). In contrast, GFAP-positive gliosis gradually increases (see Fig. 20.2). Immunostaining with anti-prion protein (PrP) antiserum is a useful tool in the identification of isoforms of this protein for the rapid diagnosis of CJD.[45] Definitive diagnosis can be achieved by Western blot analysis for prion proteins resistant to digestion by proteinase K enzyme.[9]

In 1996, the European Union banned imports of British beef following the mysterious deaths of young "fast food" enthusiasts in 1995 from an atypical variant of CJD. These deaths and the deaths of cattlemen with bovine spongiform encephalopathy (BSE) in their herds were highly publicized.[3,46] Thus emerged mad cow disease. Microscopic plaques that stain immunohistochemically for prion protein are the most striking and consistent neuropathologic features of this atypical variant of CJD.[46] They are even more distinctive when surrounded by spongiform change.

Cerebrovascular Diseases

Hemorrhage into brain tissue has many causes and often accompanies other lesions within the CNS. The major role of IHC is to identify certain causes of hemorrhage such as amyloid and neoplasm. Amyloid angiopathy is a common cause of spontaneous intracerebral hemorrhage in the elderly (see Table 20.3). Immunohistochemical staining with an antibody to β/A4 protein is more sensitive than Congo red stain in demonstrating the extent of vascular amyloid.[47]

Most neoplasms that cause brain hemorrhages are metastatic. Melanoma, renal cell carcinoma, choriocarcinoma (Chapters 7, 8, 16, and 18), leukemia, and glioblastoma tend to hemorrhage. Glioblastoma contains GFAP-positive cellular processes, vimentin-positive vascular proliferations, and an MIB1 proliferation index that is high among gliomas (see the Grading Malignant Potential section later in the chapter). Carcinomas express cytokeratins.

Hemorrhages in patients with hypertension often occur within the cerebral hemispheres, especially in the lateral areas of the basal ganglia.[48] Coagulopathy is an important cause of intracerebral hemorrhage, including drug-induced coagulopathy. Saccular aneurysms occasionally rupture into the brain, but radiography reveals their nature. Embolism is an important cause of hemorrhagic cerebral infarcts.[49] Sinus thrombosis followed by venous infarction may occur, usually as a complication of a pre-existing infectious or inflammatory disease.[3]

Non-traumatic subarachnoid hemorrhages are usually due to rupture of a saccular aneurysm, most often located at a branch of a major artery or the circle of Willis. Their source is radiographically apparent.

A subdural hematoma may follow a traumatic event and is seen in elderly patients as well as in patients with systemic cancer and brain tumors.[50] Membranes are formed on both sides of the hematoma; membrane formation requires several weeks to complete. The membrane on the dural side is usually two to five vimentin-positive fibroblasts thick in a 5-day-old subdural hematoma. It eventually becomes as thick as normal dura with new collagen that reacts with immunohistochemical stains for type IV collagen and fibronectin.

SMALL VESSEL DISEASE

Brain biopsy specimens obtained in search of "small vessel disease" may require sectioning through the entire block of tissue to yield diagnostic material. Excessively involved vessels may not be recognizable, but CD31 shows them by highlighting their endothelial cells (see Table 20.3); it is the endothelial marker of choice for its sensitivity and specificity.[50] Involvement of small cerebral veins that have few spindle-shaped smooth muscle cells (SMC) compared with arteries of the same diameter with more SMCs can be assessed with anti–smooth muscle actin or myosin.[51] Causes are often cryptogenic in isolated angiitis of the CNS.[52] Systemic vasculitides that may affect brain are associated with lupus erythematosus; drugs, including cocaine, heroin, and amphetamines; infection, including zoster-varicella virus and meningovascular syphilis; toxins; granulomatous disease; Wegener disease; relapsing polychondritis; and Behçet disease.[7,13,15,53,54] IHC can aid in the identification of microorganisms and the classification of inflammatory cell types.

CADASIL affects small arteries.[55] It is a rare disorder resulting from *Notch3* gene mutations (chromosome 19).[13] Characteristic vascular changes can be identified in brain, skin, and muscle biopsy specimens. By light microscopy, the affected vessels have a thickened appearance, and basophilic granular material is seen by H&E stain. This material is PAS positive. It displaces

TABLE 20.4 Vascular Malformation

Type	Location	Histology
AVM	Cerebral hemispheres; brainstem; cerebellum	Veins and arteries with often poorly formed elastic membrane; gliotic brain tissue
Venous malformation	CNS; spinal leptomeninges	Veins and gliotic or normal brain tissue; no arteries
Capillary telangiectasia	Pons; brainstem; CNS	Thin-walled dilated capillaries within brain parenchyma
Cavernous angioma	CNS	Clusters of abnormal, often fibrotic or hyalinized vessels with elastic lamina and without intervening brain tissue

AVM, arteriovenous malformation; CNS, central nervous system.
Modified from McKeever PE, Blaivas M. The brain, spinal cord, and meninges. In: Sternberg SS, ed. Diagnostic Surgical Pathology. 2nd ed. New York, NY: Raven Press; 1994:409-492.

the smooth muscle cells, best seen with an IHC stain for smooth muscle actin. EM reveals the presence of dark granular osmophilic deposits. IHC for Notch3 protein deposition is available.[55]

VASCULAR MALFORMATION

The following five types of vascular malformations are recognized:[3,56]

- Capillary telangiectasia
- Cavernous angioma
- Arteriovenous malformation (AVM)
- Venous malformation
- Sturge-Weber disease (cerebrofacial or cerebrotrigeminal angiomatosis)

Although they may occur anywhere in the CNS, AVMs have a predilection for the cerebral hemispheres (Table 20.4). Elastic stains identify medium to large arteries and their abnormal counterparts. In AVMs, these stains often show abnormal vessels with focal loss or duplication of elastin. There is a monoclonal antielastin antibody, but special stains like Movat's pentachrome stain are usually used.[3]

Abnormal smooth muscle layers can be highlighted with muscle actin. Cerebral veins are reported to have a thinner circumferential layer of smooth muscle cells than cerebral arteries, and these different features exist in vascular malformations.[57] IHC can be used to identify and localize vascular collagen, fibronectin, myofibroblasts (vimentin and muscle actin), and endothelial cells (CD31).

TUMORS

Different neoplasms of brain predominate in adults and in children. More pediatric neoplasms occur in the posterior fossa than in the anterior fossa, and the opposite is true of adult neoplasms.

Grading Malignant Potential

The World Health Organization (WHO) has established uniform terminology and grading of brain tumors according to histologic criteria.[2] Starting with the most "benign" as grade I, numerical grades II, III, and IV represent increasing malignancy. The numerical grades assigned by the WHO classification are included in parentheses after the tumor names in headings in this section of the chapter. The most important aids to assessing grade of malignancy provided by IHC are as follows:[3,58]

1. Cell type identification with markers (Tables 20.5-20.11)
2. Identification of vascular proliferations with vimentin; CD31, CD34, *Ulex europaeus* (Ulex), and factor VIII endothelial markers; and smooth muscle actin
3. Proliferation markers such as molecular immunology Borstel 1 (MIB1) to supplement mitotic activity in assessing the growth potential (Fig. 20.8)

A rule of thumb for grading is that primary brain tumors without mitotic activity and with a distinct margin tend to be grade I, whereas infiltrating tumors tend to be grade II and higher. Neurofilament (NF) and synaptophysin stains aid assessment of tumor infiltration by staining pre-existing axons (especially in white matter) and pre-existing synapses (in gray matter). With a good hematoxylin nuclear counterstain, infiltrating neoplastic cells are evident with such stains.[59] Eosin can be applied in addition to hematoxylin if needed.

Proliferation markers show nuclear antigens that appear during one or more proliferative phases of the cell cycle. A labeling index (LI), also known as a proliferation index (PI), can be derived from them.[60,61] The LI of any of the proliferation antigens is the number of antigen-positive cells divided by the total number of cells in sampled microscopic areas of the tumor. Histologic grading of astrocytomas correlates with LI.[61]

MIB1 is an antibody that detects proliferating cells in various phases of the cell cycle. Properly standardized, MIB1 LI helps to predict patient outcome.[62-64] Proper standardization with tissue processed in the same laboratory from a group of tumors is needed to glean the best prognostic information from the labeling index of an individual patient's tumor. Laboratories vary in their range of staining and LI assessments, limiting the value of comparison with published data.

PCNA is an auxiliary protein to DNA polymerase.[65] This author favors MIB1 over PCNA for distinct staining and reproducible LI.[61]

Apoptosis is the programmed death of cells. One can determine from cytologic and cytochemical assays an apoptotic index that is analogous to the LI for proliferation mentioned earlier in this chapter. The balance between cell proliferation and cell death affects tumor growth.[66]

Tumor progression in gliomas is associated with an increase in the grade of malignancy, resulting in a

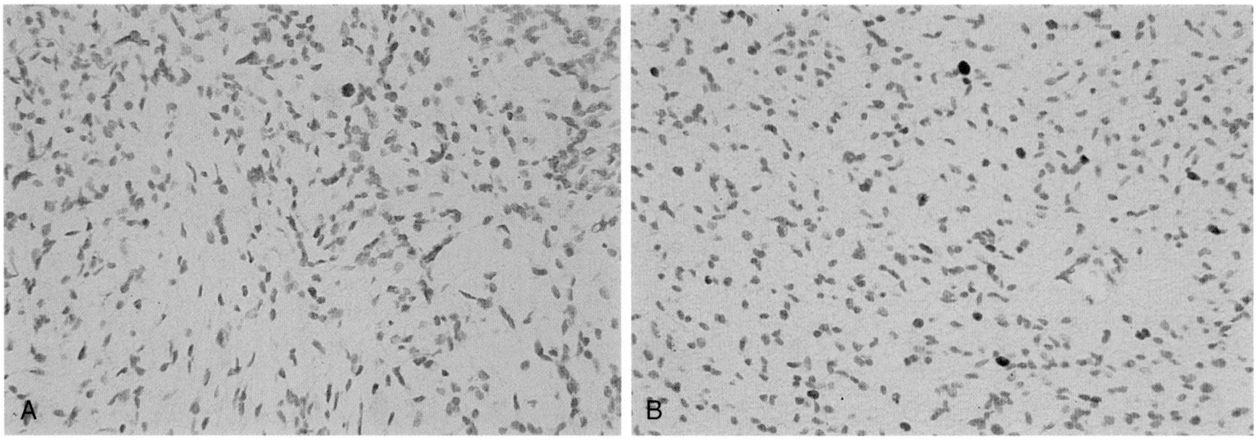

FIGURE 20.8 Diffuse fibrillary astrocytomas, grade II. MIB1 antibody distinguishes long and short survivals in patients with grade II astrocytoma. **(A)** Specimen with few brown MIB1-positive nuclei was taken from a patient who survived more than 8 years. **(B)** Specimen with many MIB1-positive nuclei was taken from a patient who survived less than 6 months. Hematoxylin counterstain colors MIB1-negative nuclei purple. *From McKeever PE, Strawderman MS, Yamini B, et al. MIB-1 proliferation index predicts survival among patients with grade II astrocytoma. J Neuropathol Exp Neurol. 1998;57:931-936.*

poorer prognosis. Cyclin-dependent kinase 4 inhibitor (CDKN2/p16) is a cell cycle regulatory protein that has been demonstrated to be inactivated by mutations, deletions, or transcriptional silencing during pathogenesis of a variety of human malignancies. CDKN2/p16 immunocytochemistry may identify those low-grade gliomas that are likely to progress and to have poor outcome and that thus would need more aggressive therapy.[67] Various other genes and their immunoreactive proteins are altered during glioma tumor progression; they have been reviewed elsewhere.[1,2]

Gliomas

Glioma is a term that describes astrocytoma, glioblastoma, ependymoma, oligodendroglioma, and their various subtypes and combinations. An important general rule is that gliomas tend to contain GFAP and to lack collagen, reticulin, and fibronectin in their parenchyma, distinguishing them from non-glial neoplasms.[68,69] Uncommon variants like xanthoastrocytomas may have parenchymal reticulin (see Tables 20.1 and 20.5). However, oligodendroglioma cells are more variable in their GFAP expression, and they uniformly express only glial proteins of low specificity, such as Leu7 and S-100 protein.[3] Gliomas lack widespread cytokeratin (CK) in their parenchyma but have been misinterpreted because of cross-reactivity between some anti-CK antibodies and GFAP (see Fig. 20.8).[5]

Clinical needs are expanding the pathologist's role in the interpretation of gliomas. For example, the effectiveness of procarbazine-CCNU-vincristine (PCV) chemotherapy for gliomas with an oligodendroglial component, especially malignant gliomas with 1p or 19q chromosomal deletions,[70] has increased the value of recognizing these tumors. Also, postoperative systemic thromboses are a major complication of brain tumor surgery. The pathologist may be able to identify patients likely to encounter this difficulty by reporting the tumors (usually malignant gliomas) that contain thrombosed vessels.[71]

The histologic term *low-grade* as applied to astrocytomas and other gliomas does not necessarily imply a benign neoplasm or even a favorable prognosis. A benign designation, which implies that once removed the glioma will not recur, is frequently encountered only among WHO grade I astrocytomas, gangliogliomas, and ependymomas. Even these tumors need to be in favorable locations where they can be completely resected, thus giving the patient a good chance for cure.[13] A general tendency that seems to be emerging from studies of the molecular biology of gliomas is that grade I gliomas and gliomas that do not infiltrate brain tend to not overexpress p53 gene product and not overexpress epidermal growth factor receptors (EGFR).[72,73] In contrast, high-grade and infiltrative gliomas tend to overexpress at least one of these.[2,73]

TUMOR AND TUMOR MARGIN

It is important to recognize two types of specimens of glioma (Fig. 20.9). The first type is the *tumor* itself (Tables 20.5 to 20.8), which has cellular density exceeding that of surrounding brain (see Fig. 20.9B). This tumor nidus is optimal for histopathologic classification.[74,75]

The second type of specimen is brain tissue infiltrated by the *margin* of the glioma and is a product of the infiltrative nature of many gliomas.[3] Immunohistochemical stains for brain neuroanatomic components are very helpful in identifying this brain tissue. NF protein localizes axons in white matter, where axons are neuroanatomically oriented in parallel, and also in gray matter.[59] The extent that glioma cells infiltrate this axonal meshwork in brain tissue is evident from the hematoxylin counterstain in immunohistochemical preparations (Fig. 20.10). Synaptophysin stains a finely pixelated "carpet" of synapses in gray matter; glioma cells disrupt this carpet.

If only the margin is available for examination, it is often impossible to determine the histologic grade and type of glioma, giving rise to an infiltrative margin of neoplastic glia. Further from the glioma itself, neoplastic glia in CNS parenchyma are difficult to distinguish from gliosis (Fig. 20.11; see Fig. 20.9A). Nonetheless, GFAP can help

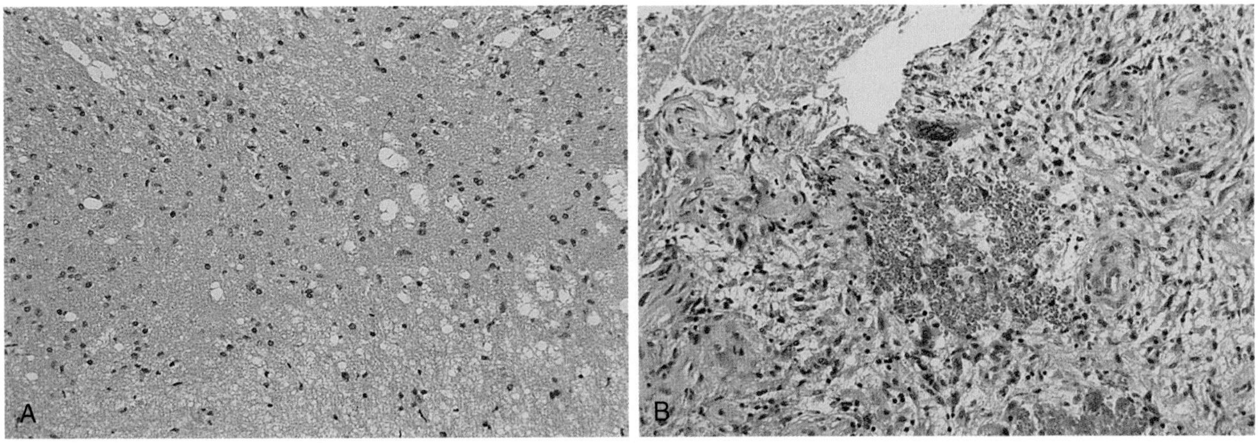

FIGURE 20.9 Stereotactic biopsy specimens of a left temporoparietal mass in an elderly woman. The first specimen shows gliosis and rare neoplastic glia, classification and grade uncertain **(A)**. The last of several more specimens shows glioblastoma with highly pleomorphic fibrillar cells, mitotic spindles, vascular proliferation, and necrosis **(B)**. *From McKeever PE. New methods of brain tumor analysis. In: Mena H, Sandberg G, eds. Dr. Kenneth M. Earle Memorial Neuropathology Review. Washington, DC: Armed Forces Institute of Pathology, 2004.*

identify gliosis by showing excess cytoplasmic GFAP and regular spacing between cells in gliosis (see Fig. 20.2).

KEY DIAGNOSTIC POINTS

Gliomas

- Proper surgical sampling is needed for accurate classification and grading of diffuse or heterogeneous gliomas. Intraoperative consultation of pathologist and surgeon optimizes sampling.
- Most grade II to IV gliomas infiltrate CNS tissue, which makes total resection difficult to impossible. Exceptions include certain ependymomas and xanthoastrocytomas.
- The proliferation marker MIB1 augments grading and prediction of patient outcome.

ASTROCYTOMAS

Astrocytomas are among the most fibrillar of CNS neoplasms, more fibrillar than other gliomas except tanycytic ependymomas and subependymomas (see Table 20.5). Astrocytomas nearly always contain GFAP (Fig. 20.12A; see Fig. 20.8A), although the amount is variable. GFAP is the single most important immunohistochemical marker distinguishing astrocytomas from nearly all nonglial neoplasms.[3] Nerve sheath tumors occasionally show focal GFAP, in substantially lesser amounts than the fibrillary astrocytomas that resemble them. Many astrocytomas express vimentin, and when they do, this feature distinguishes them from vimentin-negative oligodendrogliomas.[13]

Pilocytic Astrocytoma (WHO Grade I)

Pilocytic means "composed of hair cells," which is a major feature of the pilocytic astrocytoma. Parallel bundles of elongated, fibrillar, cytoplasmic processes resemble mats of hair (see Fig. 20.12A).[76] These hairlike processes contain large amounts of glial fibrils, which stain well with immunoperoxidase for GFAP (see Table 20.5).

A diagnosis of pilocytic astrocytoma is about the only good news within the group of astrocytomas. This tumor has a better prognosis than its diffuse counterparts, especially when it occurs in the cerebellum rather than its other common location near the third ventricle.[77,78] It is critical to distinguish pilocytic astrocytoma from fibrillary grade II astrocytoma, which has a poorer prognosis. Even the better prognosis is tempered because adequate surgical removal of a pilocytic astrocytoma depends on its location, and some pilocytic astrocytomas develop as multicentric disease. The 10-year survival of patients with supratentorial tumors is 100% after gross total resection and 74% after subtotal resection or biopsy.[79] Pilocytic astrocytomas rarely manifest malignant degeneration, which is indicated by hypercellularity, mitoses, and necrosis.

Pilocytic astrocytomas have a well-demarcated MRI appearance; some have discrete margins, but many incorporate elements of brain at their margins. However, diffuse grade II astrocytomas (see discussion later in this section) infiltrate brain to a much greater extent than pilocytic astrocytomas.[80] The extent of microscopic infiltration can be evaluated by comparing (1) GFAP staining in serial sections to identify the edge of the highly GFAP-positive tumor and (2) NF protein staining to identify axons at the edge of the tumor. Pilocytic astrocytomas show few axons in their margins, but grade II astrocytomas show many. A nearly even mix of axons and neoplastic cells signals a grade II astrocytoma.

Most, but not all, pilocytic astrocytomas occur in children or young adults. They are most abundant in the posterior fossa and around the third ventricle, thalamus, hypothalamus, neurohypophysis, and optic nerve. Cerebral hemispheric pilocytic astrocytomas are less common, but it is important to recognize them to ensure appropriate treatment.[81]

Rosenthal fibers (RFs) are highly eosinophilic hyaline structures. They are round, oval, or beaded, and they have slightly irregular margins.[3] Their beaded appearance results from their formation within glial processes. In comparison with erythrocytes, they are

TABLE 20.5 Differential Diagnosis of a Mass of Fibrillar Cells

	Differential Features		
Diagnosis*	Structures	Antibody[a]	Locations[b]
Fibrosis	Spindle cells of meningeal or perivascular origin	Type IV collagen (+); vimentin (+)	Meninges; CNS
Granuloma	Like fibrosis with "whorls" and inflammation	Microorganisms (Table 20.1)	Basal meninges; CNS
Pilocytic astrocytoma	Hypercellularity; hairlike fibrillarity; Rosenthal fibers; microcysts	GFAP (+); S-100; alpha B-crystalline	Cerebellum; thalamus/ hypothalamus; optic nerve; CNS
Astrocytoma	Hypercellularity; angular nuclei cluster and indent one another; infiltrates CNS	GFAP (S); S-100	Cerebrum; brainstem; spinal cord; CNS
Anaplastic astrocytoma	Increase in above features; mitoses	GFAP (S); S-100	Cerebrum; brainstem; CNS
Gemistocytic astrocytoma	Hypercellularity; cells swollen with hyaline pink cytoplasm and eccentric pleomorphic nuclei; infiltrates CNS	GFAP (S)	Cerebrum
Giant cell astrocytoma	Giant astrocytes with thick fibrils; large round/oval nuclei	GFAP (S)	Lateral ventricle; subependymal
Astroblastoma	Perivascular rosettes with expanded glial cell processes	Nonfibrillar GFAP (S)	Cerebrum; CNS
Pleomorphic xanthoastrocytoma	Pleomorphic cells are often vacuolated	GFAP (S); type IV collagen (S)	Leptomeninges; cerebral cortex
Ependymoma	Hypercellularity; ependymal or perivascular rosettes, or both; round/oval nuclei; cilia; and basal bodies	GFAP (+)	Cerebrum; cerebellum; spinal cord; CNS
Tanycytic ependymoma/ subependymoma	Combination of astrocytoma and ependymoma; round/oval nuclei cluster among fibrillar mats	GFAP (+)	Spinal cord; fourth ventricle; subependymal; CNS
Anaplastic ependymoma	Preceding features with mitoses; necrosis	GFAP (S); S-100	Cerebrum; cerebellum
Glioblastoma multiforme	Regions of coagulation necrosis; mitoses; pleomorphism; endothelial proliferation	GFAP (S); S-100	Cerebrum; CNS
Gliosarcoma	Glioblastoma plus fibrosarcoma intermixed	GFAP (S); fibronectin; type IV collagen (S); laminin; vimentin (S)	Cerebrum
Ganglion cell tumors	Binucleated and pleomorphic neurons; diagnosis depends on gliomatous and neuroblastic elements	GFAP (S); synaptophysin(S); PGP9.5; neurofilament (S); type IV collagen	Cerebrum; CNS
Central neurocytoma	Round cells and nuclei; thin fibrils near vessels	Synaptophysin (+); neurofilament (R)	Septum pellucidum; lateral ventricles
Pineocytoma	Normal pineal structures	Synaptophysin (+); neurofilament (R)	Pineal
Polar spongioblastoma	Rhythmic palisades of fibrillary cells		Cerebrum; CNS
Fibroblastic meningioma	Spindle cells; interdigitating cell processes and desmosomes; (thick collagen); (whorls)[c]	Vimentin (+); EMA (S); S-100 (R)	Falx, tentorium; meninges; choroid plexus
Fibrosarcoma/maligant fibrous histiocytoma	Hypercellular; pleomorphic spindle cells and nuclei; mitoses; necrosis	Vimentin; collagen	Meninges; CNS

TABLE 20.5 Differential Diagnosis of a Mass of Fibrillar Cells, cont'd

	Differential Features		
Diagnosis*	**Structures**	**Antibody[a]**	**Locations[b]**
Schwannoma	Verocay bodies; Antoni A and B; thin pericellular basement membrane	S-100 (+); Leu7; type IV collagen; GFAP (R)	Eighth cranial nerve; spinal roots; PNS
Neurofibroma	Multiple cell types spread axons	Neurofilament (R); EMA; S-100 (+); Leu7	Spinal root; PNS; cranial nerve
Histiocytosis	Sheetlike pattern of macrophages, fibroblasts, and leukocytes	α-ACT; S-100 (S)	Parasellar; CNS; systemic
Melanoma	Anaplasia, mitoses, necrosis	HMB45 (S); S-100 (+)	CNS/meninges; frequent multiple metastases; systemic

*The order of tabulated lesions follows the order of discussion in text.
[a]Key to staining results: +, almost always strong, diffuse positivity; *S,* sometimes or focally positive; *R,* rare cells may be positive.
[b]Most common or most specific location is listed first.
[c]Parentheses around a differential feature indicate an uncommon feature that is very useful in differential diagnosis when found.
α-ACT, alpha-antichymotrypsin; CNS, central nervous system; EMA, epithelial membrane antigen; GFAP, glial fibrillary acid protein; PNS, peripheral nervous system.
Modified from McKeever PE, Blaivas M. The brain, spinal cord, and meninges. In: Sternberg SS, ed. Diagnostic Surgical Pathology. 2nd ed. New York, NY: Raven Press; 1994:409-492.

TABLE 20.6 Differential Diagnosis of a Mass of Epithelioid Cells

	Differential Features		
Diagnosis*	**Structures**	**Antibody[a]**	**Locations[b]**
Gitter cells/ xanthogranuloma	Crowded macrophages engorged with lipid vacuoles; eccentric nucleus; noncohesive cells	α-ACT (S); KP1 (+); muramidase (S)	CNS
Ependymoma/ malignant ependymoma	Structures of ependymoma or malignant ependymoma plus epithelioid cells	GFAP (S); cytokeratin (R); EMA (R)	Cerebellum; cerebrum; spinal cord; CNS
Myxopapillary ependymoma	Cuboidal/columnar epithelium on hyaline fibrovascular papillae; variable fibrillarity	GFAP (S)	Regions of the filum terminale
Oligodendroglioma	Round cells and nuclei with prominent perinuclear halos; nests of cells between delicate vessels	Leu7 (+); S-100 (+); GFAP (R)	Cerebrum; CNS
Anaplastic oligodendroglioma	Above features with mitoses and pleomorphism	Leu7 (S); S-100 (S); GFAP (R)	Cerebrum; CNS
Choroid plexus papilloma	Large mass with structure of choroid plexus	Laminin (+); cytokeratin (+); transthyretin (S); synaptophysin; IGF-II	Fourth ventricle; lateral ventricle; CP angle; choroid plexus
Choroid plexus carcinoma	Above features with anaplasia and mitoses; (necrosis)[c]	Cytokeratin (+); CD44; synaptophysin; transthyretin (R)	Preceding locations
Medulloepithelioma	Columnar epithelium with basement membrane on both surfaces; fibrovascular base for papillae and tubules	GFAP; nestin	Deep cerebrum; cauda equina; CNS
Meningioma	Whorls; psammoma bodies; interdigitating cell processes and desmosomes; (thick collagen)[c]	Vimentin (+); EMA (S; S-100 (R)	Falx, tentorium; meninges; choroid plexus; (extracranial)[c]
Chordoma	Masses or cords of physaliphorous cells	Cytokeratin (+); S-100 (+); EMA (+); vimentin (+)	Cauda equina; clivus; spinal canal

Continued

TABLE 20.6 Differential Diagnosis of a Mass of Epithelioid Cells, cont'd

	Differential Features		
Diagnosis*	Structures	Antibody[a]	Locations[b]
Craniopharyngioma	Squamous; adamantinomatous	Cytokeratin (+)	Suprasellar; sellar
Carcinoma	Distinct margin with CNS; anaplasia; mitoses; necrosis	Cytokeratin (+); EMA (S)	Cerebrum; cerebellum; meninges; CNS; frequent multiple masses; systemic
Melanoma	Anaplasia; mitoses, necrosis	HMB45 (S); S-100 (+)	Preceding locations

*The order of tabulated lesions follows the order of discussion in text.
[a]Key to staining results: +, almost always strong, diffuse positivity; *S*, sometimes or focally positive; *R*, rare cells may be positive.
[b]Most common or most specific location is listed first.
[c]Parentheses around a differential feature indicate an uncommon feature that is very useful in differential diagnosis when found.
α-ACT, alpha-antichymotrypsin; CNS, central nervous system; CP; cerebellopontine; EMA, epithelial membrane antigen; GFAP, glial fibrillary acidic protein; IGF-II, insulin-like growth factor II.
Modified from McKeever PE, Blaivas M. The brain, spinal cord, and meninges. In: Sternberg SS, ed. Diagnostic Surgical Pathology. 2nd ed. New York, NY: Raven Press; 1994:409-492.

TABLE 20.7 Differential Diagnosis of a Mass of Conspicuously Different Cells

	Differential Features		
Diagnosis*	Structures	Antibody[a]	Locations[b]
Oligoastrocytoma	Mixture of astrocytoma (Table 20.5) and oligodendroglioma (Table 20.6)	GFAP (S); Leu7 (+); S-100 (+)	Cerebrum; CNS
Anaplastic oligoastrocytoma	Above features with mitoses and pleomorphism	GFAP (S); Leu7 (S); S-100 (S)	Cerebrum; CNS
Glioblastoma/gliosarcoma with epithelial metaplasia	Structures of glioblastoma/gliosarcoma (Table 20.5) plus epithelial regions	GFAP (S); S-100 (S); cytokeratin (S); EMA (S)	Cerebrum; CNS
Ganglion cell tumors	Binucleated and pleomorphic neurons plus glioma (Table 20.5) plus fibrosis plus inflammation	GFAP (S); synaptophysin (S); PGP9.5; neurofilament (R); type IV collagen (R)	Cerebrum, CNS
Desmoplastic medulloblastoma	Regions of medulloblastoma and fibrosis	Synaptophysin; S-100; type IV collagen; neurofilament (R); GFAP (R)	Lateral cerebellum; CNS; meninges; (extra-axial)[c]
Transitional meningioma	Regions of fibrous (Table 20.5) and syncytial (Table 20.9) meningioma	Vimentin (+); EMA (S); S-100 (R)	Falx; tentorium; meninges; choroid plexus
Hemangioblastoma	Multivacuolated stromal cells between many capillaries; hypervascularity; (fibrillarity is frozen section artifact)[c]	CD31 (S); factor VIII (S); NSE (S)	Cerebellum; spinal cord; CNS
Desmoplastic carcinoma	Regions of carcinoma (Table 20.6) and fibrosis (Table 20.5); occasional inflammation	Cytokeratin (S); EMA (S)	Cerebrum; cerebellum; meninges; CNS; frequent multiple masses; systemic
Melanoma	Regions of fibrillar and epithelioid melanoma (Tables 20.5, 20.6)	HMB45 (S); S-100 (+)	Cerebrum; cerebellum; meninges; CNS; frequently multiple masses; systemic

*The order of tabulated lesions follows the order of discussion in text.
[a]Key to staining results: +, almost always strong, diffuse positivity; *S*, sometimes or focally positive; or mixed cell populations; *R*, rare cells may be positive.
[b]Most common or most specific location is listed first.
[c]Parentheses around a differential feature indicate an uncommon feature that is very useful in differential diagnosis when found.
CNS, central nervous system; EMA, epithelial membrane antigen; GFAP, glial fibrillary acidic protein; NSE, neuron-specific enolase.
Modified from McKeever PE, Blaivas M. The brain, spinal cord, and meninges. In: Sternberg SS, ed. Diagnostic Surgical Pathology. 2nd ed. New York, NY: Raven Press; 1994:409-492.

TABLE 20.8 Differential Diagnosis of a Mass of Small, Crowded Anaplastic Cells

Diagnosis	Differential Features: Structures	Antibody*	Locations[a]
Ependymoblastoma	Like PNET; ribbons/cords of cells; true ependymal rosettes	Vimentin (S); GFAP (R)	Cerebrum; cerebellum
Medulloblastoma/ pineoblastoma/ neuroblastoma/PNET	Slight fibrillarity; (Homer-Wright rosettes); (palisades); "carrot" nuclei; (neural or glial foci)[b]	Synaptophysin (+); PGP9.5; S-100; neurofilament (R); GFAP (R)	Cerebellum; brainstem; pineal; CNS; (extra-axial)[b]
Rhabdomyosarcoma/ medullomyoblastoma	Like PNET; muscle striations	Desmin (S); muscle-specific actin	Pineal; cerebellum; CNS
Atypical teratoid-rhabdoid tumor	Like PNET; more cytoplasm	Vimentin (+); GFAP (S); cytokeratin (S); EMA (S); synaptophysin (R); chromogranin (R)	Cerebellum; brain
Hemangiopericytoma	Hypercellularity; thick pericellular matrix; mitoses	Vimentin (+)	Falx, tentorium meninges; (extracranial)[b]
Lymphoma	Noncohesive round cells; vascular wall invasion	L26 (+); LCA (S); monoclonal κ and λ Ig	Deep cerebrum; CNS; meninges; may be multiple
Small cell carcinoma	Cohesive cells; (epithelioid); (desmosomes)[b]	Cytokeratin (+); EMA; synaptophysin (S)	CNS; meninges; frequent multiple masses; systemic

*Key to staining results: +, almost always strong, diffuse positivity; *S*, sometimes or focally positive; *R*, rare cells may be positive.
[a]Most common or most specific location is listed first.
[b]Parentheses around a differential feature indicate an uncommon feature that is very useful in differential diagnosis when found.
CNS, central nervous system; EMA, epithelial membrane antigen; GFAP, glial fibrillary acidic protein; Ig, immunoglobulin; LCA, leukocyte common antigen; PNET, primitive neuroectodermal tumor.
Modified from McKeever PE, Blaivas M. The brain, spinal cord, and meninges. In: Sternberg SS, ed. Diagnostic Surgical Pathology. 2nd ed. New York, NY: Raven Press; 1994:409-492.

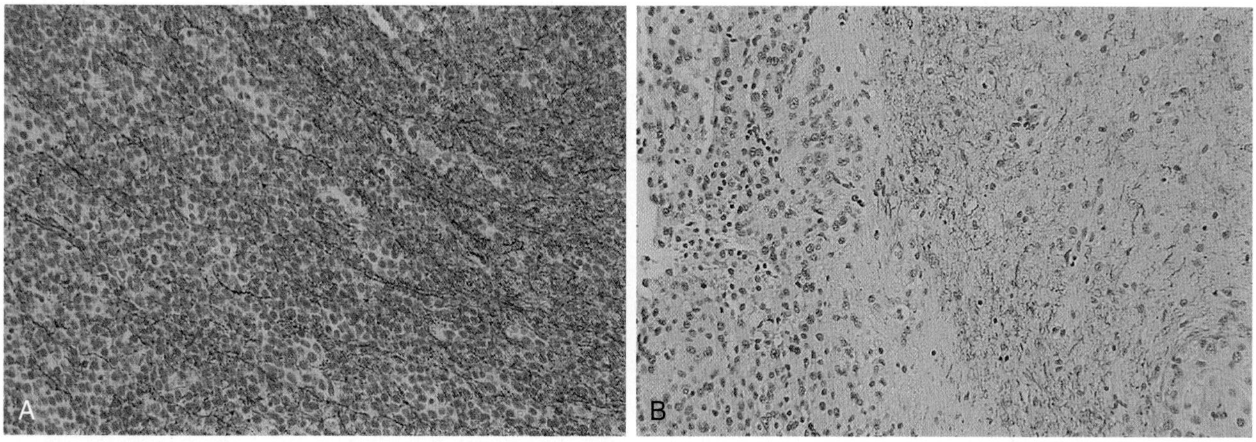

FIGURE 20.10 (A) The neurofilament (NF) immunohistochemical stain highlights axons in brain, facilitating evaluation of glioma infiltration into brain tissue. Crowded round and elongated nuclei of a grade II oligoastrocytoma (stained purple with hematoxylin) diffusely infiltrate between long brown axonal constituents of the underlying brain tissue. **(B)** In contrast, this pleomorphic xanthoastrocytoma (PXA) does not infiltrate between individual brown axons, and its margin with cerebral cortex is distinct. Other features of the PXA (its pleomorphic cells and nuclei and its lipid vacuoles) may be seen without IHC (see Fig. 20.16). *From McKeever PE. New methods of brain tumor analysis. In: Mena H, Sandberg G, eds. Dr. Kenneth M. Earle Memorial Neuropathology Review. Washington, DC: Armed Forces Institute of Pathology, 2004.*

pink rather than orange and have greater variation in size and shape. Although RFs assist in distinguishing the pilocytic astrocytoma from other variants, they are of no value in differentiating astrocytomas from gliosis because they occur in both abnormalities.

IHC reveals that RFs contain alpha B–crystallin, stain with ubiquitin, and are centrally GFAP negative (see Fig. 20.12A). Alpha B–crystallin is a lens protein in the small heat-shock protein family. When abundant, RFs are easily appreciated on H&E stain. IHC is most needed when they are scarce. The ideal marker for scarce RFs would be both sensitive and specific. Ubiquitin is sensitive and not specific. Alpha B–crystallin is only slightly more specific and less sensitive than ubiquitin (see Fig. 20.12). My experience is that ubiquitin is best for screening for scarce RF, but these should be confirmed with either alpha B–crystallin or H&E stain. Structural features and color on H&E are often sufficient to identify RFs.

Eosinophilic granular bodies (EGB) are eosinophilic droplets of protein often found in pilocytic astrocytomas.

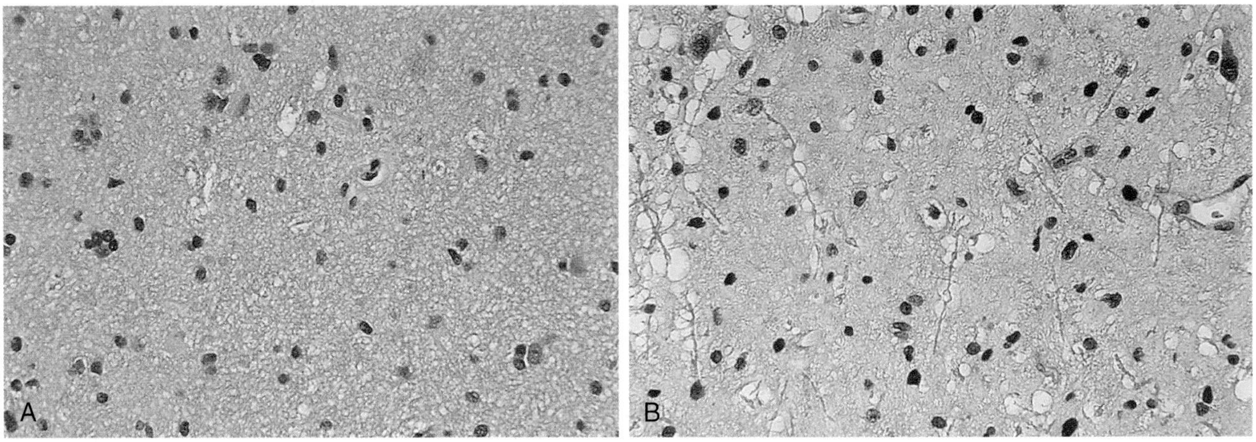

FIGURE 20.11 Gliosis and non-neoplastic perineuronal oligodendroglia **(A)** near a metastatic carcinoma (*not shown*) appear similar to the margin of a grade II fibrillary astrocytoma **(B)** distant from its nidus. Nuclei are more pleomorphic and hyperchromatic in **B.** (Compare with lighter nuclei in capillary endothelium at sides of panels.) (H&E.) *From McKeever PE. New methods of brain tumor analysis. In: Mena H, Sandberg G, eds. Dr. Kenneth M. Earle Memorial Neuropathology Review. Washington, DC: Armed Forces Institute of Pathology, 2004.*

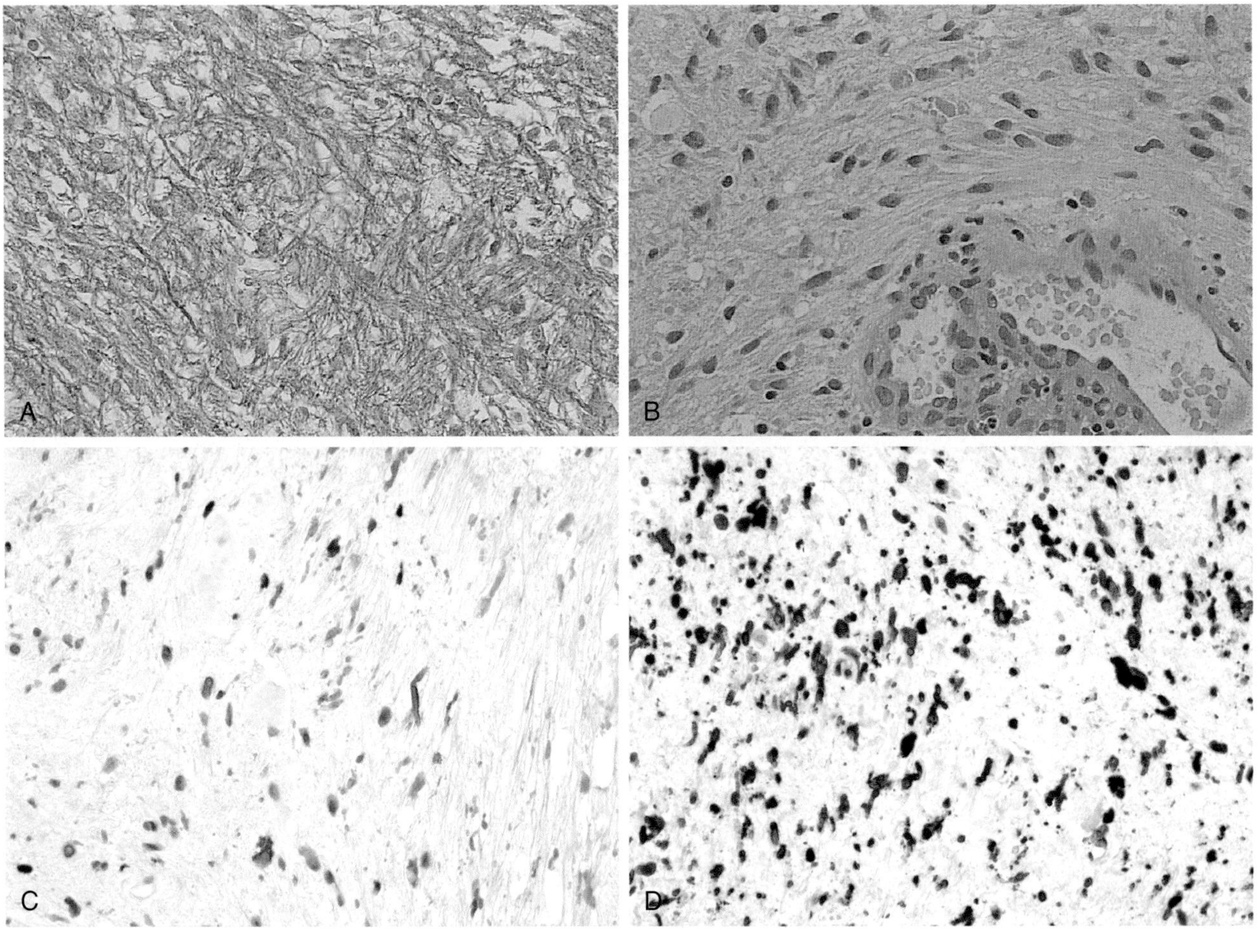

FIGURE 20.12 This tumor was in the cerebellar midline of a young man with headaches and vomiting. **(A)** Pilocytic astrocytoma features numerous brown GFAP-positive cytoplasmic processes. Pale gray, refractile globules, some with brown GFAP-positive rims, are Rosenthal fibers (RFs). The GFAP-negative RF resides in astrocytic processes. **(B)** Pale gray RFs in this tumor mingle with pink, periodic acid-Schiff (PAS)–positive protein droplets (PAS with diastase). Both are less uniform in diameter than the light brown intravascular erythrocytes. **(C)** The specific marker alpha–B-crystallin is specific for RFs but not very sensitive. Although glial fibrils and purple nuclear chromatin are appropriately negative, many RFs show little or no brown staining. **(D)** The sensitive marker ubiquitin stains all RFs in this nearby section from the same block as panel **(C)**. Although not evident here, ubiquitin sometimes stains nuclei. Structural features including elongated beading of RFs within longitudinal sections of astrocytic processes and absence of chromatin distinguish the RFs. *From McKeever PE. New methods of brain tumor analysis. In: Mena H, Sandberg G, eds. Dr. Kenneth M. Earle Memorial Neuropathology Review. Washington, DC: Armed Forces Institute of Pathology, 2004.*

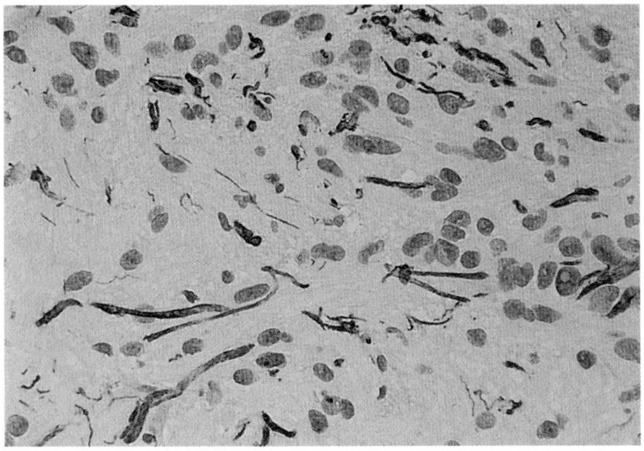

FIGURE 20.13 Pleomorphism of blue nuclei as well as crowding, touching, and indentation occurs in this diffuse grade II astrocytoma. These nuclei infiltrate between pre-existing axons stained brown with anti-NF protein stain. Diffuse infiltration of brain distinguishes most grade II and higher astrocytomas from grade I tumors. (Immunoperoxidase anti-NF protein with hematoxylin.) *From McKeever PE. Neurofilament (NF) and synaptophysin stains reveal diagnostic and prognostic patterns of interaction between normal and neoplastic tissues. Presented at the Annual Meeting of the Histochemical Society, Bethesda, Md, March 24, 2000.*

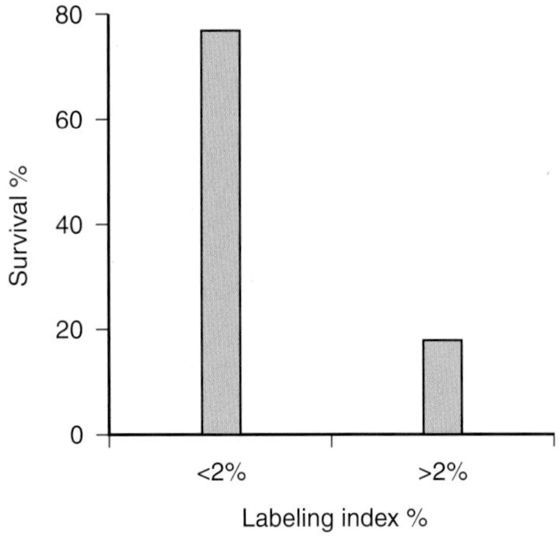

FIGURE 20.14 Probabilities of survival of patients with grade II astrocytomas in which mean MIB1 labeling indices were ≤2% and >2%. *Bars represent data from McKeever PE, Strawderman MY, Yamini B, et al. MIB-1 proliferation index predicts survival among patients with grade II astrocytoma. J Neuropathol Exp Neurol. 1998;57:931-936.*

These protein droplets are usually smaller and more aggregated than RFs. They are usually intracellular but occasionally are extracellular and up to 40 μm in diameter. They are PAS positive (see Fig. 20.12B). Both EGB and RFs are immunoreactive with alpha B–crystallin, which also is reported to stain cortical Lewy bodies, other astrocytomas, schwannomas, hemangioblastomas, and chordomas.[13,82]

Observations of subtypes of S-100 protein suggest that they distinguish pilocytic astrocytomas from WHO grade II to IV astrocytomas.[83] Pilocytic astrocytomas do not overexpress p53 protein.[72] They tend to lack EGFR abnormalities.[84] These features may have future diagnostic use.

Cystic cerebellar pilocytic astrocytomas resemble hemangioblastomas, which may have focally GFAP-positive cells and a GFAP-positive cyst wall. Unlike hemangioblastoma, the mural nodule of a pilocytic astrocytoma contains highly fibrillar and abundantly GFAP-positive neoplastic astrocytes without clear vacuoles from lipids. CD31 and other endothelial cell markers show less abundant capillaries in the astrocytoma than in the hemangioblastoma.

Diffuse Astrocytoma (Low-Grade Astrocytoma; WHO Grade II)

The fibrillary astrocytoma is more common than the protoplasmic astrocytoma.[74] Fibrillary astrocytomas are a mixture of cellular processes (fibrils) and nuclei of greater angularity and density than normal or reactive astrocytes (Fig. 20.13; see Fig. 20.11B). They contain more intracytoplasmic fibrils, and their cellular processes are longer than those in protoplasmic astrocytomas. Thus, only the fibrillary astrocytoma stains well with phosphotungstic acid hematoxylin (PTAH), which stains fibrillar protein arrays, whereas both astrocytomas contain GFAP that can be stained immunohistochemically.[13]

The term *diffuse* appropriately describes an astrocytoma whose margin gradually diminishes in cellularity. Within the extensive margin, neoplastic cells intermingle with brain parenchyma (see Fig. 20.13). NF staining highlights parallel axons of white matter infiltrated by neoplastic astrocytes. Diffuse invasion of brain may also be evident as formation of secondary structures of Scherer, which are described in the Gliosis versus Glioma section later in the chapter.

The diffuse nature of the growth and infiltration of low-grade astrocytomas demonstrates why they are so seldom cured despite their relatively benign histologic features. Postoperative survival is highly variable but usually is 3 to 10 years. The extreme variation in prognosis among grade II diffuse astrocytomas places a premium on better measures of outcome for individual patients. A low MIB1 LI identifies patients with good prognosis (Fig. 20.14; see Fig. 20.8).[63] It is possible that p53 overexpression is associated with tumor progression to glioblastomas.[85]

The variety of chromosomal abnormalities in astrocytomas includes losses in chromosomes 13, 22, X, and Y and gains in chromosome 7.[1,5] These changes can be detected with fluorescent and immunohistochemically enhanced ISH procedures.[86]

Gemistocytic Astrocytoma (WHO Grade II)

Gemistocytes are cells swollen with hyaline, pink cytoplasm that is reactive for GFAP (Fig. 20.15A; see Table 20.5). Their hyperchromatic and angulated nuclei are at the rim of the cells, producing a bizarre caricature of a reactive astrocyte. Astrocytomas with at least 20% gemistocytes may be considered gemistocytic astrocytomas. Gemistocytic astrocytomas are considered more aggressive than their non-gemistocytic counterparts. Whereas gemistocytic astrocytomas are particularly likely to progress to a higher grade, those without high-grade

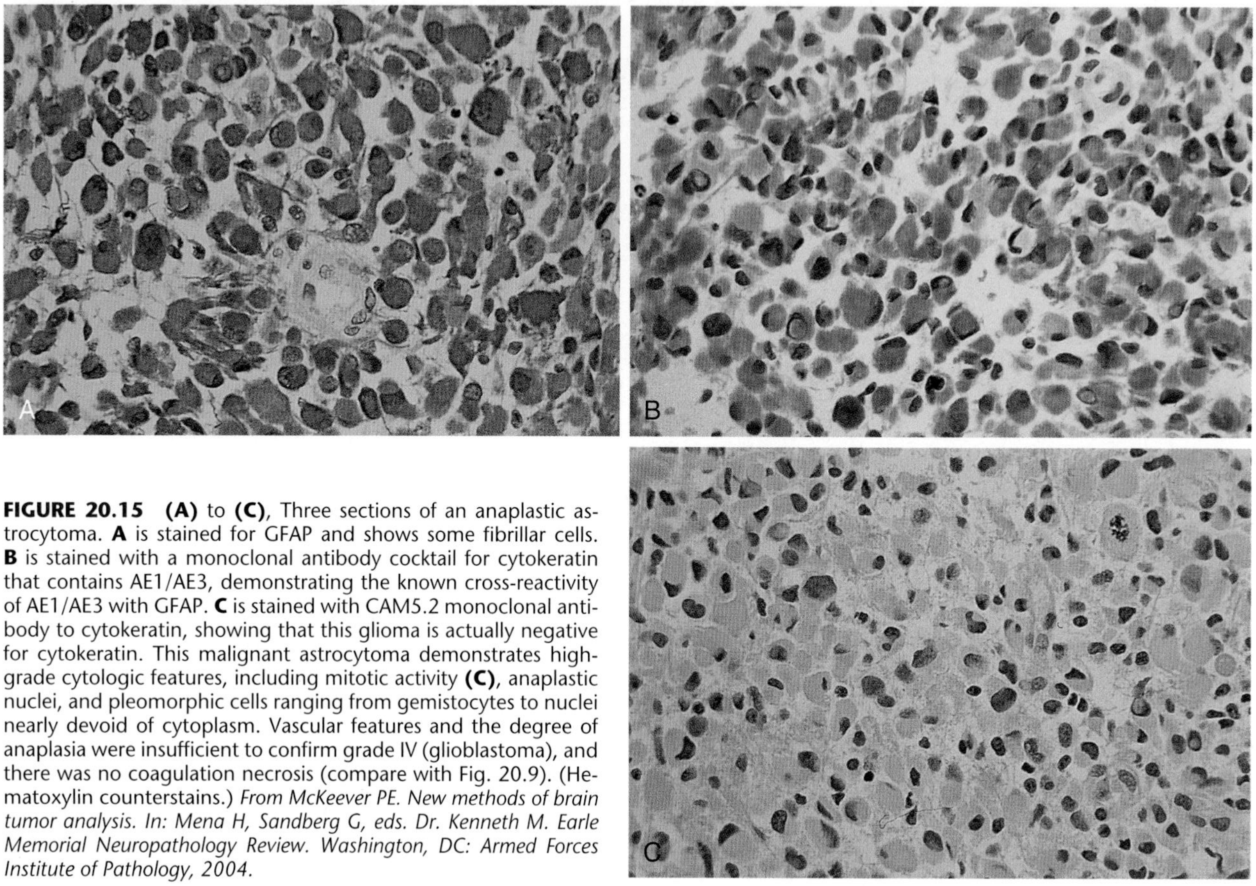

FIGURE 20.15 **(A)** to **(C)**, Three sections of an anaplastic astrocytoma. **A** is stained for GFAP and shows some fibrillar cells. **B** is stained with a monoclonal antibody cocktail for cytokeratin that contains AE1/AE3, demonstrating the known cross-reactivity of AE1/AE3 with GFAP. **C** is stained with CAM5.2 monoclonal antibody to cytokeratin, showing that this glioma is actually negative for cytokeratin. This malignant astrocytoma demonstrates high-grade cytologic features, including mitotic activity **(C)**, anaplastic nuclei, and pleomorphic cells ranging from gemistocytes to nuclei nearly devoid of cytoplasm. Vascular features and the degree of anaplasia were insufficient to confirm grade IV (glioblastoma), and there was no coagulation necrosis (compare with Fig. 20.9). (Hematoxylin counterstains.) *From McKeever PE. New methods of brain tumor analysis. In: Mena H, Sandberg G, eds. Dr. Kenneth M. Earle Memorial Neuropathology Review. Washington, DC: Armed Forces Institute of Pathology, 2004.*

features are considered grade II astrocytomas prior to progression.[2]

Gemistocytic astrocytomas are distinguished from oligodendrogliomas with microgemistocytes by their more angulated and pleomorphic nuclei and their longer GFAP-positive cellular processes; from gangliogliomas by their lack of synaptophysin-positive neoplastic neurons; and from subependymal giant cell tumors by their smaller and more angulated nuclei and greater tendency to infiltrate brain.

Anaplastic Astrocytoma (WHO Grade III)

The anaplastic designation emphasizes the high grade of malignancy of the anaplastic astrocytoma. Features shared by high-grade gliomas are mitotic activity as well as increases in cellular density, nuclear pleomorphism (see Fig. 20.15), and nuclear hyperchromatism. Anaplastic astrocytomas retain GFAP-positive cellular processes and GFAP reactivity around their anaplastic nuclei (see Fig. 20.15A); this important feature distinguishes them from reactive astrocytes trapped in other tumors. Their MIB1 LIs are intermediate among gliomas.[61]

The combined lack of foci of coagulation necrosis and lack of conspicuous vascular proliferation in an astrocytic glioma distinguish anaplastic astrocytomas from glioblastomas (see Table 20.5).[2] Average survival of patients with anaplastic astrocytoma is slightly more than 2 years. In pediatric patients, a low MIB1 L1 identifies a group of patients who have a better prognosis.[87]

Other Variants of Astrocytoma

Subependymal giant cell astrocytoma (GCA or SEGA) has a distinctive location, histology, and association with tuberous sclerosis (TS).[88] The suppressor gene product associated with TS, tuberin, is predictably lost in GCA associated with TS.[89] The tumor arises from the medial portion of the floor of the lateral ventricle in the region where the subependymal nodules of giant astrocytes in TS (called "candle guttering") are frequently found (see Table 20.5). It is composed of giant astrocytes with large nuclei and prominent nucleoli (Fig. 20.16). Although these tumors are pleomorphic, most nuclei lack sharp angulations, and the giant cells are not crowded. These cells may contain glial filaments variably positive for GFAP (see Fig. 20.16A).

IHC has revealed partial neuronal differentiation in some GCAs (see Fig. 20.16B), complicating their classification as astrocytomas (versus gangliogliomas). These giant astrocytes and their characteristically thick cytoplasmic processes have a tendency to form disoriented fascicles. It is very important to recognize this histologic entity, because (1) their pleomorphism is at variance with their relatively benign behavior and WHO grade I and (2) many GCAs are associated with TS.[3]

Astroblastoma is rare.[2] Astroblastic rosettes resemble perivascular pseudo-rosettes of ependymomas, except that the astroblastic processes remain thick the entire distance from cell body to adventitia of the vessel. Foot processes may even thicken near the adventitia.

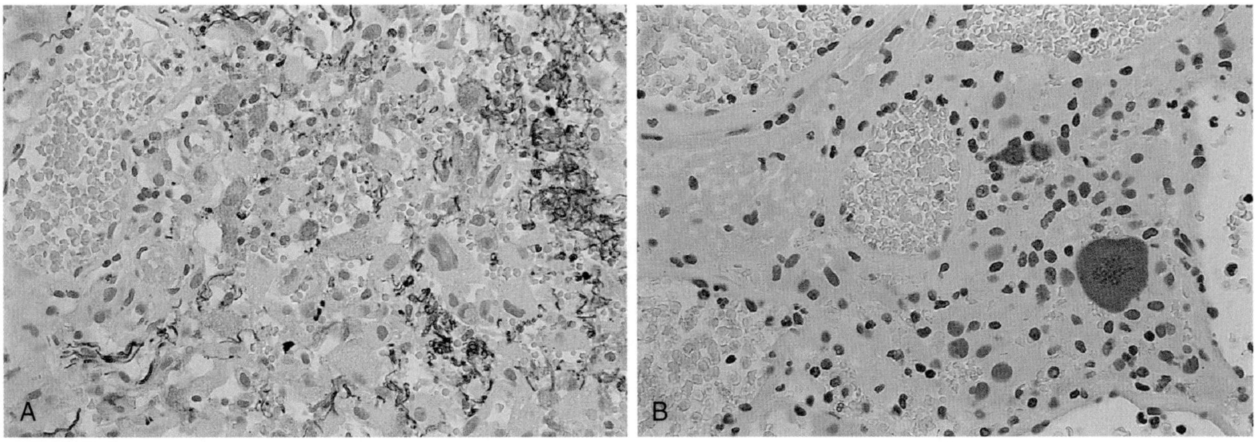

FIGURE 20.16 Giant cell astrocytoma. **(A)** Huge cells with large nuclei and nucleoli and abundant, finely granular cytoplasm variably reactive for GFAP mingle with bundles of thick, dark brown GFAP-positive cellular processes that are part of the tumor. Despite their size, most nuclei and nucleoli lack sharp edges. **(B)** Nuclei have delicately stippled chromatin and rare mitoses. There are a few NF-positive and many NF-negative cells in this subependymal giant cell astrocytoma. One neoplastic cell has a mitosis and shows NF reactivity. This is a rare indication of the neoplastic nature of this cell type. This tumor grew from the septum pellucidum of a 20-year-old woman with tuberous sclerosis. (Immunoperoxidase anti-GFAP with hematoxylin.) *From McKeever PE. New methods of brain tumor analysis. In: Mena H, Sandberg G, eds. Dr. Kenneth M. Earle Memorial Neuropathology Review. Washington, DC: Armed Forces Institute of Pathology, 2004.*

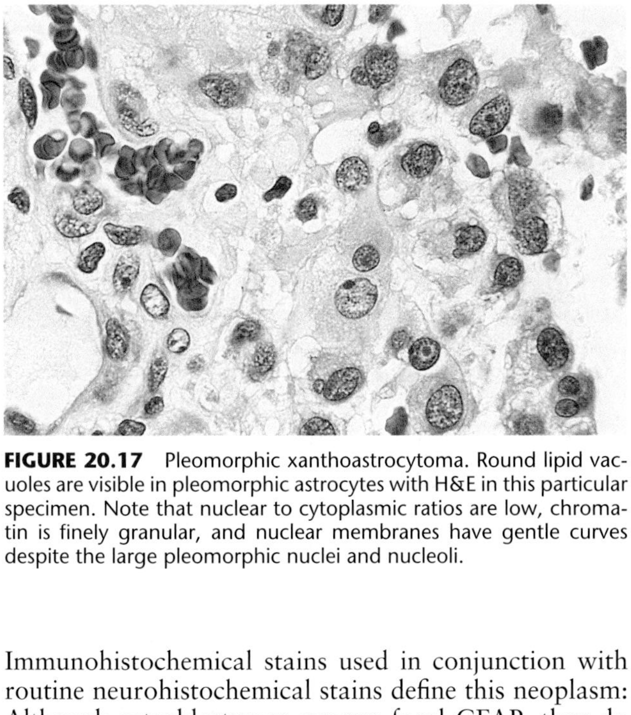

FIGURE 20.17 Pleomorphic xanthoastrocytoma. Round lipid vacuoles are visible in pleomorphic astrocytes with H&E in this particular specimen. Note that nuclear to cytoplasmic ratios are low, chromatin is finely granular, and nuclear membranes have gentle curves despite the large pleomorphic nuclei and nucleoli.

Immunohistochemical stains used in conjunction with routine neurohistochemical stains define this neoplasm: Although astroblastomas express focal GFAP, they do not stain with PTAH. This dichotomy may be due to expression of a nonfibrillar form of the GFAP molecule different from the fibrils of ependymoma and astrocytoma that stain for both.

Pleomorphic xanthoastrocytoma is a supratentorial astrocytoma that often involves both the leptomeninges and cerebral cortex (see Table 20.5).[90] It has a more distinct margin with brain than most astrocytomas (see Fig. 20.10B). Its fibrillarity and its pleomorphic, hyaline, lipid-laden, and multinucleated cells are clues to its diagnosis (Fig. 20.17). Intracellular lipid content and protein granular degeneration vary from abundant to absent in individual tumors.

Pleomorphic xanthoastrocytoma (PXA) may assume a clear cell appearance and thus may require identification by a panel of immunohistochemical reagents (see Box 20.1).[91] Astrocytes are identified from their characteristic strongly GFAP-positive cells, often with coexpression of alpha$_1$-antitrypsin. Sparse lipid droplets are conspicuously negative for GFAP. These cells may be surrounded by reticulin fibers and basement membranes positive for type IV collagen, breaking a general rule that glioma cells lack reticulin. Neuronal elements occur in some tumors, suggesting that a pleomorphic xanthoastrocytoma may be the glial portion of a ganglioglioma.[92] The grade II PXA has been confused with the grade IV glioblastoma. Both are very pleomorphic. One must look for low MIB1, virtual lack of mitoses, EGBs, little invasion (see the Pilocytic Astrocytoma section earlier in this chapter), and little or no overexpression of EGFR or p53 to distinguish the PXA from diffuse astrocytomas, and especially from glioblastomas (Fig.20.18).[93,94]

KEY DIAGNOSTIC POINTS

Astrocytomas

- GFAP with a good hematoxylin counterstain is the most important IHC stain to show neoplastic nuclei surrounded by GFAP, and fibrillar GFAP-positive processes of astrocytomas.
- Neurofilaments stain both tests for a ganglionic tumor component (see the Neuronal Tumors section later in this chapter) and often show axons of brain tissue that existed before the tumor.[58] The latter helps assess infiltration by neoplastic cells.
- Non-infiltrating astrocytomas that lack both p53 and EGFR overexpression tend to be grade I tumors.
- MIB1 is important in assessing proliferation, particularly among astrocytomas with inconspicuous mitoses.

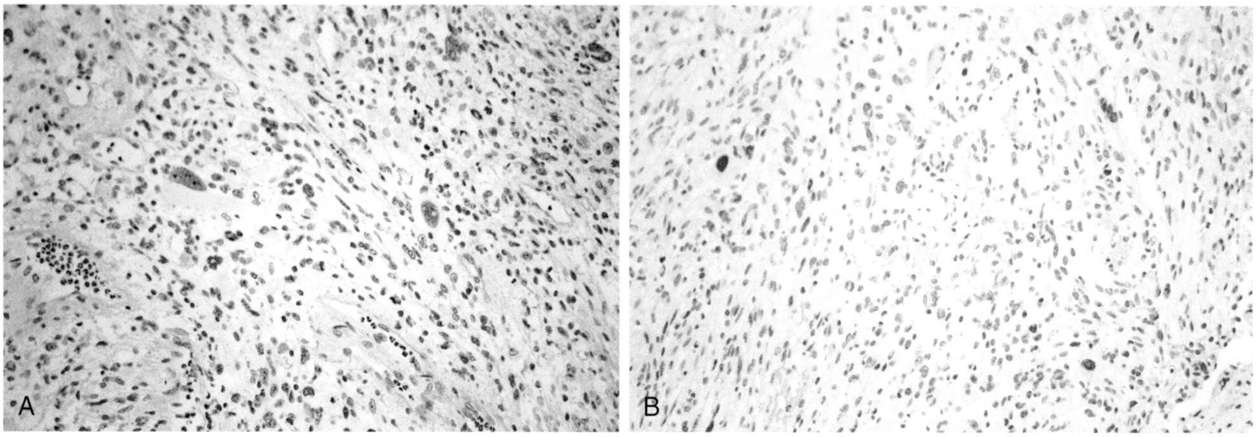

FIGURE 20-18 This pleomorphic xanthoastrocytoma does not overexpress epidermal growth factor receptors **(A)**. Rare cells overexpress p53 **(B)**.

Theranostic Applications

Among groups of patients with grade II astrocytomas, MIB1 distinguishes tumors with good prognosis by their low LI (see Fig. 20.7A).[63] MIB1 LI differentiates between grade II and grade III gliomas.[64]

About 33% to 50% of diffuse astrocytomas have p53 abnormalities, which makes p53 mutations and/or overexpression an early change in astrocytomas that progress to higher grades.[95] These p53 abnormalities may be useful in distinguishing between astrocytomas and oligodendrogliomas.

Beyond Immunohistochemistry: Anatomic Molecular Diagnostic Applications

About 5% of gliomas are familial.[96] A fraction of these is associated with Li-Fraumeni syndrome (LFS), a germline mutation of the *p53* gene on the short arm of chromosome 17 (17p13). Data suggest that about 1% of gliomas occur in patients with LFS.[97] More than 50% of these are astrocytic gliomas, including astrocytoma grades 2 to 4 (diffuse low-grade astrocytoma through glioblastoma).[2] Clinical situations that should arouse suspicion of LFS in a glioma patient include any second neoplasm in this patient, a family history of sarcoma or choroid plexus tumor, or a young (<45 years) close blood relative of the patient with a cancer, lymphoma, or brain tumor.[98-101]

EPENDYMOMAS

Ependymomas are an excellent example of how IHC highlights structural features important to their interpretation.

The cellular conformations of ependymomas vary between fibrillar and epithelial, posing special problems of differentiation not only from other gliomas but also from carcinomas and meningiomas (see Tables 20.5 and 20.6). These latter differentiations are facilitated if one recalls that even epithelioid ependymomas frequently stain with anti-GFAP, have distinctive ultrastructure, and often contain at least a few cells with fibrillar processes (Fig. 20.19; see Boxes 20.1 and 20.2). The anti-GFAP stain highlights these fibrillar processes, greatly facilitating their identification (see Fig. 20.19A and B). A good place to look for these fibrillar processes is around vessels.

In contrast to nonglial neoplasms, aggregated ependymoma cells in tumor parenchyma lack a basement membrane. Immunostaining shows no collagen or fibronectin in these aggregates.[68] Low-grade ependymomas have round and oval nuclei with finely dispersed chromatin. These nuclei distinguish them from virtually all brain tumors other than meningiomas.[3]

One should look for rosettes to confirm suspicion of an ependymoma (see Tables 20.5 and 20.6). Perivascular rosettes are most useful because they occur in nearly all ependymomas. They have a fibrillar zone that is at least three erythrocyte diameters wide around central vessels. Anti-GFAP stains the fibrillar zone, making a subtle zone easier to find (see Fig. 20.19B). The processes taper to become very thin as they radiate from the cells to the vascular adventitia, distinguishing them from the thick processes of astroblastic formations. True ependymal rosettes are characteristic, but some samples of ependymoma lack them. The ependymal rosette consists of ependymal cells spaced around a lumen (Fig. 20.20). Cilia often protrude into the lumen from the ependymal lining. Some tumors show expanded ependymal rosettes, and others have long ependymal linings that do not close into rosettes.[3]

Many ependymomas have a relatively discrete margin with brain compared with other gliomas. This margin is revealed best in white matter with the NF immunohistochemical stain, which shows an abrupt border between the NF-positive axons abundant in white matter and the NF-negative ependymoma. Synaptophysin shows a corresponding distinct border between positively reacting neuropil and negatively reacting tumor.[59]

Electron microscopy is better than IHC for difficult ependymomas (see Fig. 20.19C). It shows cilia, basal bodies, cytoplasmic inclusions of microvilli, and elongated intercellular junctions.

Rare ependymomas have sparse CK or EMA immunoreactivity on their most differentiated epithelium. However, even these have much less CAM5.2 than choroid plexus papillomas and carcinomas. CAM5.2 is recommended to distinguish them.

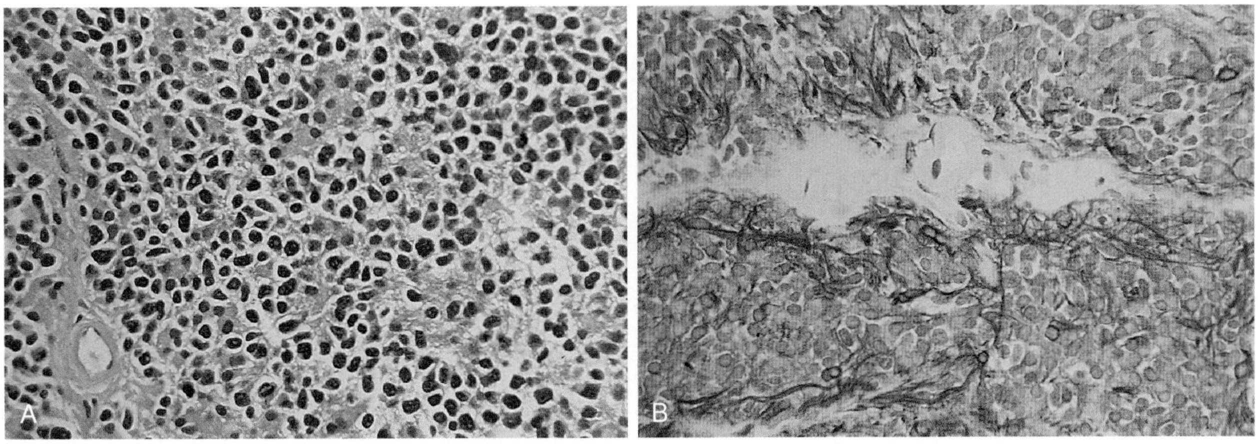

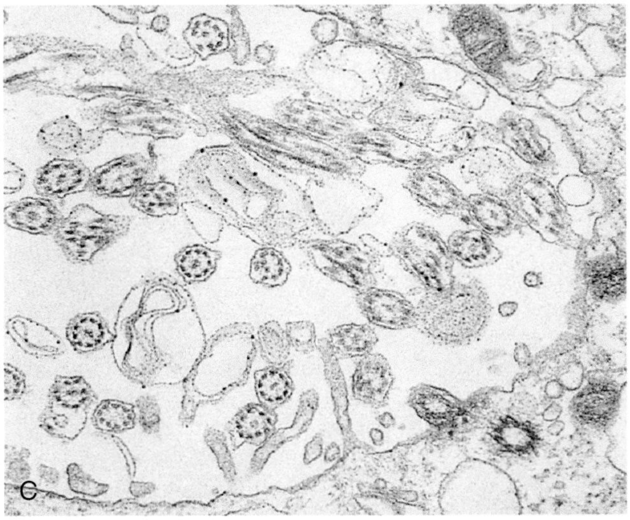

FIGURE 20.19 **(A)** and **(B)**, Sections of a tumor. **(A)** This tumor is composed of epithelioid cells. (H&E.) **(B)** The tumor is GFAP positive, and this stain highlights slight fibrillarity near the appropriately GFAP-negative vessels. **(C)** Electron microscopy reveals cilia and basal bodies of ependymoma. Structural but not ultrastructural features of this clear cell ependymoma mimic oligodendroglioma. *From McKeever PE. New methods of brain tumor analysis. In: Mena H, Sandberg G, eds. Dr. Kenneth M. Earle Memorial Neuropathology Review. Washington, DC: Armed Forces Institute of Pathology, 2004.*

The general features of ependymoma just described are useful in identifying the variants of ependymoma discussed in this section, except where specifically excluded.

Low-Grade Ependymoma

The low-grade designation is often dropped from the name for this group of tumors, which are referred to simply as *ependymomas*. The features just described and the nuclear features of low-grade ependymomas distinguish them from other tumors. Nuclei of ependymomas are typically round or oval with prominent light and dark regions stained with hematoxylin (see Figs. 20.19A and 20.20). In the parenchyma away from rosettes, nuclei tend to be more uniformly crowded than nuclei in low-grade astrocytomas and less crowded than in medulloblastomas and primitive neuroectodermal tumors (Fig. 20.19; see Figs. 20.8, 20.11, and 20.21).

Epithelioid ependymomas occasionally have remarkably distinct margins with brain that imitate margins of nonglial neoplasms (see Box 20.2). Anti-GFAP stain for glial filaments is extremely helpful in differentiating these ependymomas from carcinomas, pituitary adenomas, craniopharyngiomas, and meningiomas (see Fig. 20.19B and Table 20.6). The stain accentuates fibrillar cellular processes, which distinguish the ependymoma.[3]

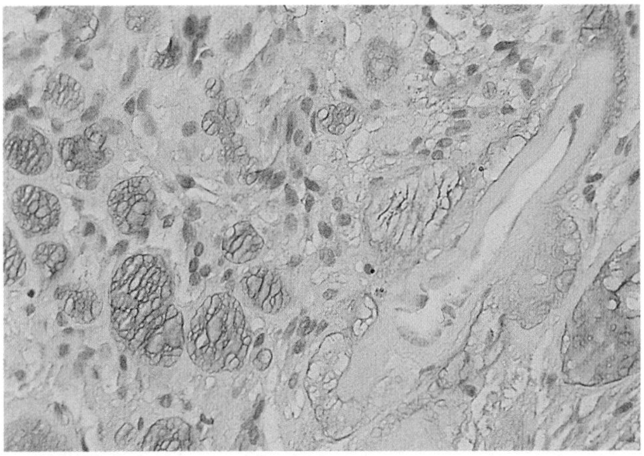

FIGURE 20.20 Myxopapillary ependymoma. This tumor originated in the cauda equina of a middle-aged woman who had experienced knee pain for several years. It has epithelioid cells and blue-tinged mucin both in the center of vague ependymal rosettes and in the perivascular space. (Alcian blue and nuclear fast red.) *From McKeever PE, Blaivas M. The brain, spinal cord, and meninges. In: Sternberg SS, ed. Diagnostic Surgical Pathology. 2nd ed. New York, NY: Raven Press; 1994:409-492.*

Papillary ependymomas closely resemble choroid plexus papillomas. Solid regions of ependymoma parenchyma where GFAP-positive neoplastic cells grow on one another rather than on fibrovascular stroma can be appreciated from their lack of collagen and fibronectin with immunohistochemical staining.[3] Histologic grade is less predictive of survival in ependymoma than in astrocytoma.[13] Radiographic evidence of residual disease after surgery predicts markedly reduced survival, putting a premium on correct intraoperative diagnosis and total removal of the tumor. In infratentorial ependymomas, expression of large amounts of GFAP is associated with better prognosis.[102]

Clear Cell Ependymoma

Clear cell ependymoma resembles oligodendroglioma and central neurocytoma (Figs. 20.22A and 20.23A; see Fig. 20.19A). It is an epithelioid ependymoma that also has clear perinuclear halos. Immunohistochemical staining for GFAP may reveal ependymal features such as perivascular fibrils (see Fig. 20.19B). The clear cell appearance of these ependymomas requires a panel of immunohistochemical reagents or, often, electron microscopy to differentiate them from other clear cell tumors (see Fig. 20.19C and Box 20.1).[91]

Tanycytic Ependymoma

Tanycytic ependymomas are found within the brain and particularly the spinal cord. Their round to oval nuclei with distinctly light and dark regions of chromatin resemble those in ependymoma. Their abundant GFAP-positive cellular processes resemble those in astrocytomas. They form structures replete with nuclei next to zones of fibrillar cellular processes. These structures are distinguished from Verocay bodies by their diffuse, extensive GFAP positivity and their lack of type IV collagen. They are not limited to surrounding GFAP-negative vessels such as the perivascular rosettes of other ependymomas. The margins of tanycytic ependymomas with surrounding parenchyma tend to be discrete, to exclude NF-positive axons of spinal cord tracts, and to be potentially resectable. Diffuse astrocytoma cells infiltrate between NF-positive axons.[3,59]

Subependymoma (WHO Grade I)

The subependymoma protrudes from the wall of a ventricle into the ventricular space.[3] Its histologic and immunohistochemical features closely resemble those of tanycytic ependymoma (see Table 20.5). It is usually benign.

Myxopapillary Ependymoma (WHO Grade I; Rarely Grade II)

The myxopapillary ependymoma (MXPE) appears the least glial in H&E-stained slides. It is nearly always found in the region of the filum terminale, cauda equina, sacrum, and adjacent extravertebral soft tissues (see Fig. 20.20 and Table 20.6). This ependymoma differs from others in its amount of mucin production. Its hallmark is parenchymal and perivascular mucin produced by ependymal cells (see Fig. 20.20). MXPE is often papillary but may be solid.

Although the differential features described in the general discussion of ependymomas can be useful, the peculiar morphology and growth of MXPEs pose unique problems. Individual tumors vary dramatically between epithelial and fibrillar cells. The most difficult variants of MXPE to recognize are those that are nearly all myxoid or all epithelial. The highly myxoid variety may produce cords of cells in a mucoid matrix resembling chordoma, a neoplasm found in the same location. Presence of GFAP is the key immunohistochemical feature distinguishing MXPE from chordoma.

Fibrillary MXPE may be confused with fibrous meningioma and schwannoma. The epithelial and papillary variants may resemble carcinoma or meningioma.[3] A positive GFAP stain response differentiates the MXPE from GFAP-negative carcinoma and meningioma. MXPE lacks type IV collagen and fibronectin-positive basement membranes around each cell, which is a feature of schwannoma (Fig. 20.24A).

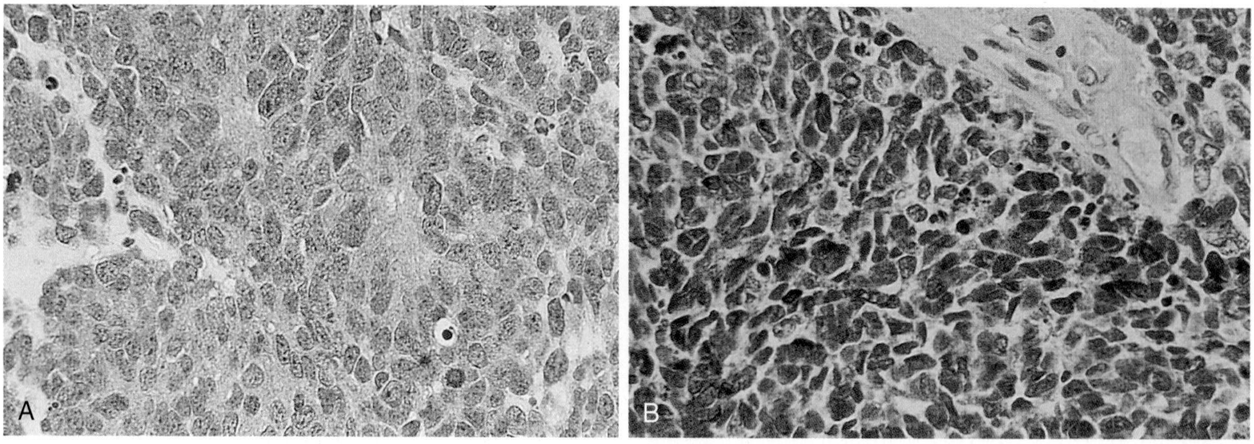

FIGURE 20.21 One medulloblastoma with well-differentiated Homer Wright rosettes, from the posterior fossa of a girl of elementary school age, was positive for both NF **(A)** and synaptophysin (*not shown*). Another, less well differentiated medulloblastoma, from the posterior fossa of a boy of the same age, was synaptophysin positive **(B)** and NF negative (*not shown*). Synaptophysin highlights the sparse fibrillar cellular processes. *From McKeever PE. New methods of brain tumor analysis. In: Mena H, Sandberg G, eds. Dr. Kenneth M. Earle Memorial Neuropathology Review. Washington, DC: Armed Forces Institute of Pathology, 2004.*

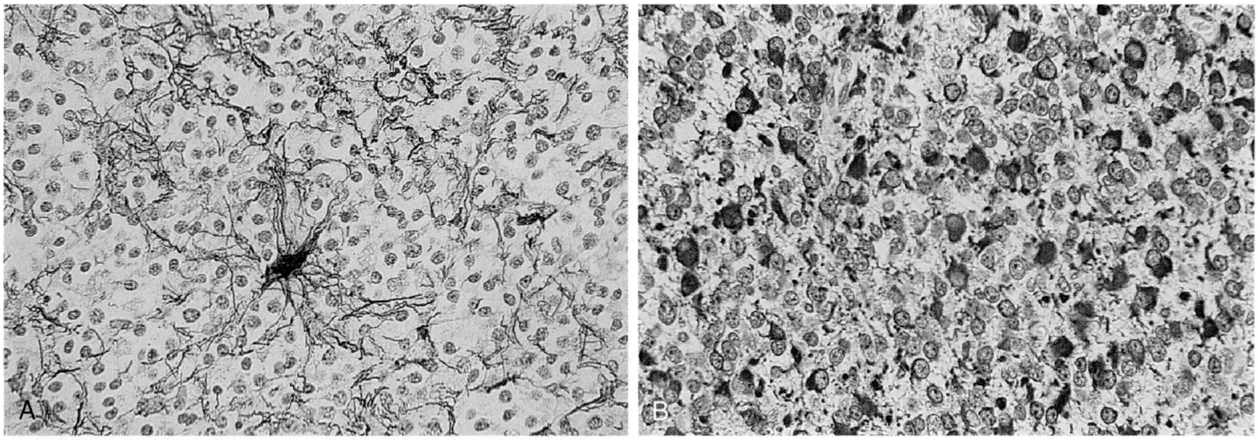

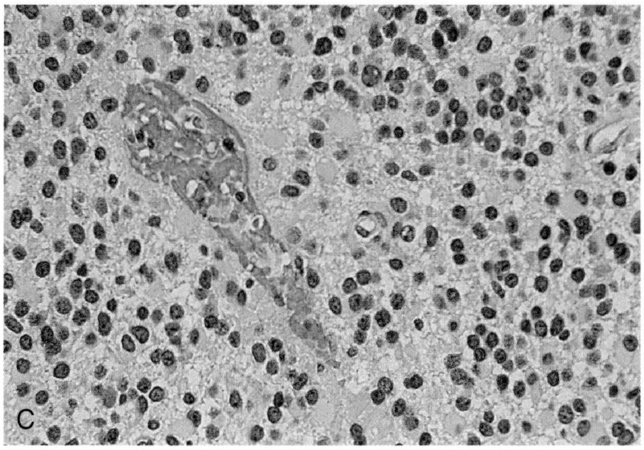

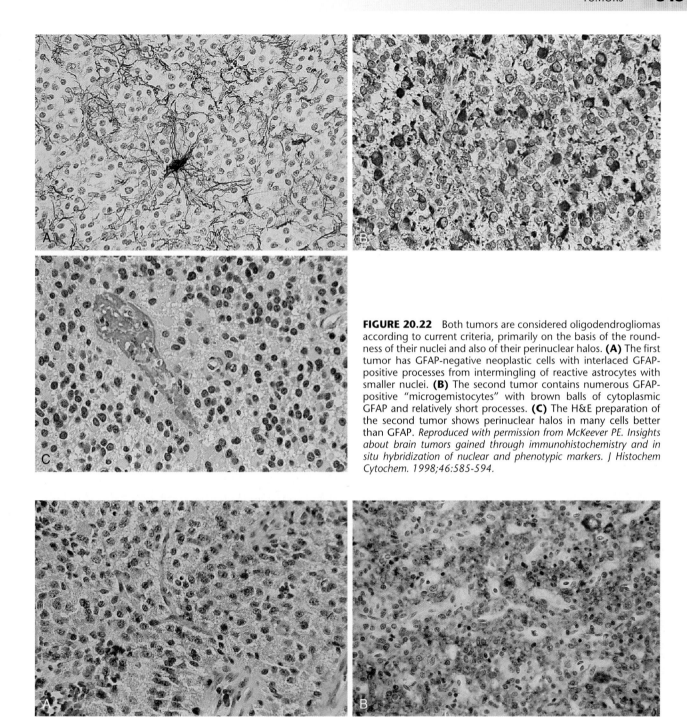

FIGURE 20.22 Both tumors are considered oligodendrogliomas according to current criteria, primarily on the basis of the roundness of their nuclei and also of their perinuclear halos. **(A)** The first tumor has GFAP-negative neoplastic cells with interlaced GFAP-positive processes from intermingling of reactive astrocytes with smaller nuclei. **(B)** The second tumor contains numerous GFAP-positive "microgemistocytes" with brown balls of cytoplasmic GFAP and relatively short processes. **(C)** The H&E preparation of the second tumor shows perinuclear halos in many cells better than GFAP. *Reproduced with permission from McKeever PE. Insights about brain tumors gained through immunohistochemistry and in situ hybridization of nuclear and phenotypic markers. J Histochem Cytochem. 1998;46:585-594.*

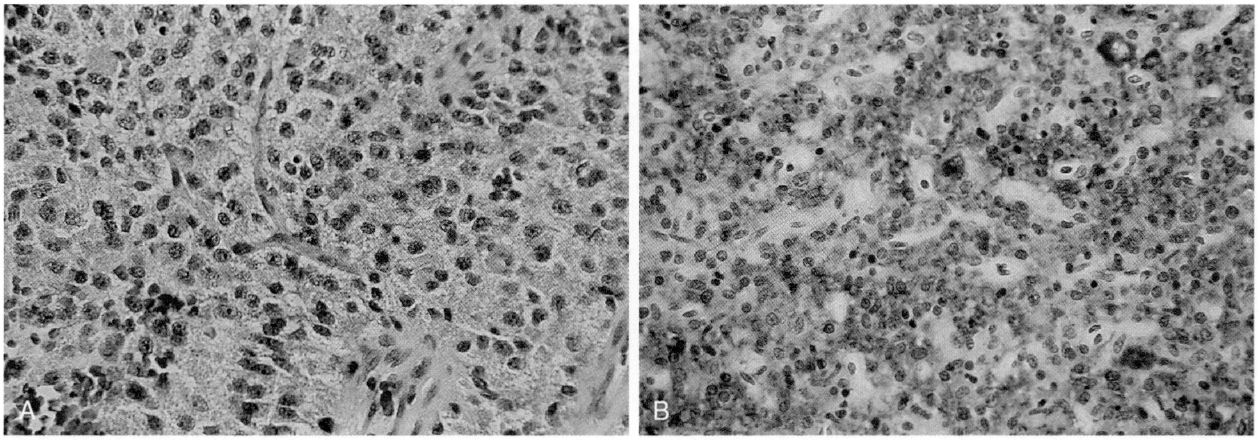

FIGURE 20.23 Central neurocytoma. **(A)** The fibrillar perivascular zone and round cells with halos around round nuclei imitate features of ependymoma and oligodendroglioma. (H&E.) **(B)** Neoplastic cells ubiquitously express synaptophysin. *Reproduced with permission from McKeever PE. Insights about brain tumors gained through immunohistochemistry and in situ hybridization of nuclear and phenotypic markers. J Histochem Cytochem. 1998;46:585-594.*

In contrast to metastatic carcinoma, MXPEs lack malignant cytology, have a lower MIB1 LI, and are focally fibrillar.[7] Paragangliomas may mimic MXPEs, but MXPEs lack chromogranin A and express GFAP.

Anaplastic Ependymoma (Malignant Ependymoma; WHO Grade III)

Anaplastic ependymomas are ependymomas with malignant features, including conspicuous mitotic activity, nuclear and cellular pleomorphism, multinucleated and giant cells, high cellular density, necrosis, and vascular proliferation (see Tables 20.5 and 20.6).[3]

Histopathologic features of malignancy do not accurately predict poor survival.[13] This problem may eventually be solved by IHC. The combination of increased vimentin expression and decreased GFAP expression may predict poor survival in infratentorial anaplastic ependymomas.[102] Anaplastic ependymomas are more likely to overexpress p53 or EGFR protein than low-grade ependymomas.[73]

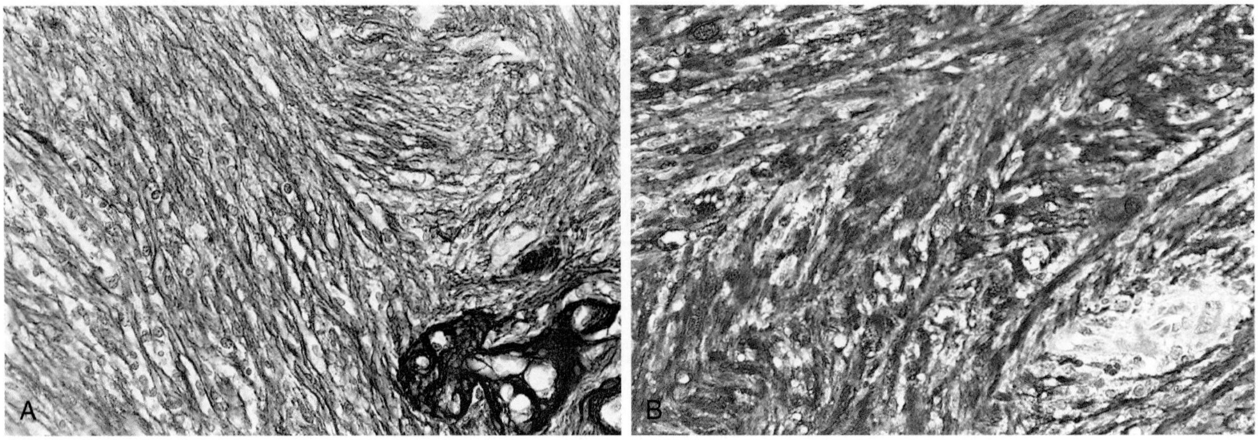

FIGURE 20.24 Schwannoma of a peripheral nerve in the brachial plexus of a young man. **(A)** Type IV collagen-positive basement membranes surround each tumor cell in compact Antoni A tissue. Darker brown vessel in corner of figure has more collagen. **(B)** Nuclei and cytoplasm are abundantly immunoreactive for S-100 protein, but vessel in corner is not.

OLIGODENDROGLIOMA

The oligodendroglioma and particularly its anaplastic counterpart have been found to respond to PCV chemotherapy. This feature has put a premium on the recognition of both tumors.[2] The pure oligodendroglioma differs from other gliomas, except for a few ependymomas, in having an epithelioid rather than a fibrillar appearance (see Table 20.6). This appearance is most evident within the central portion of the neoplasm, which is most crowded with neoplastic cells.[3] Perinuclear halos are an important feature of formalin-fixed paraffin sections of oligodendroglioma (see Fig. 20.22). Well-differentiated oligodendrogliomas have remarkably round and regular nuclei centrally placed within cells, which thereby resemble fried eggs. Their vessels are usually numerous, fine, CD31-positive capillaries that sometimes segregate the parenchyma into small lobules.[13]

Microgemistocytes have been considered oligodendroglial and are distinguished by their round nuclei and short processes from gemistocytic astrocytoma cells. Microgemistocytes have a ball of cytoplasmic GFAP immunoreactivity near their nucleus and shorter cellular processes than gemistocytic astrocytes and astrocytomas (see Fig. 20.22B).

The epithelioid appearance of pure oligodendrogliomas imitates that of true epithelial neoplasms (see Fig. 20.22C and Table 20.6).[58] Suprasellar oligodendrogliomas may be mistaken for pituitary adenomas (see Box 20.2). Oligodendrogliomas may be confused with meningotheliomatous or clear cell meningiomas, or with lipoid metaplasia in meningiomas. Anaplastic oligodendrogliomas simulate metastatic carcinoma, particularly renal cell carcinoma. GFAP-positive tumor cells (see Fig. 20.22B) distinguish the oligodendroglioma from these other tumors, but not all oligodendrogliomas have GFAP-positive neoplastic cells. In their absence, the tumor margin with brain is key (see Box 20.1). All types of oligodendroglioma, including oligoastrocytoma, have diffuse margins (see Fig. 20.10A). It is also helpful to find reactive astrocytes widely dispersed within an oligodendroglioma (see Fig. 20.22A), a pattern not seen in meningioma.

Even macroscopically discrete oligodendrogliomas show a more diffuse margin with brain than adenomas, carcinomas, and meningiomas. Either NF or synaptophysin used as a brain tissue marker[59] or the presence of GFAP-positive gliosis delineates a sharp margin with brain in these other tumors, even carcinomas that engulf chunks of brain (Figs. 20.25 and 20.26B). Among these tumors, secondary structures are seen only with the oligodendroglioma (see the sections on Astrocytomas and Gliomas). Precise localization of the biopsy specimens is helpful, because oligodendrogliomas do not originate from the adenohypophysis or dura and rarely invade them. A panel of immunostains for chromogranin and pituitary hormones can identify adenomas, but there is no specific marker for oligodendroglia that withstands paraffin embedding. The discovery of such a marker would be a major contribution to neuropathology.

The broad specificity of Leu7 and S-100 limit their use for immunohistochemical analysis of oligodendroglioma. However, an oligodendroglioma invading the meninges can be differentiated from a syncytial meningioma by its positivity with the Leu7 monoclonal antibody, because meningiomas are typically Leu7 negative. The expression of synaptophysin by up to 18% of oligodendrogliomas[105] should be noted so that they are not confused with central neurocytomas (CNs) and dysembryoplastic neuroepithelial tumors (DNTs). Both CNs and DNTs have distinct margins with brain, which is in contrast to the diffuse margin of oligodendroglioma.

Oligoastrocytoma (Mixed Oligodendroglioma-Astrocytoma; WHO Grade II)

The oligoastrocytoma is a mixed glioma composed of both astrocytoma and oligodendroglioma, as described in the respective sections on these tumors (see Fig. 20.10A). Much less common than oligoastrocytoma, mixed gliomas may have a component of ependymoma.[13]

Difficulties are encountered in the attempt to determine whether individual tumors contain a mixture of both oligodendroglial and astrocytic elements and whether both elements are neoplastic. Each element must be conspicuous for this diagnosis. Oligodendroglioma cells must be distinguished from infiltrating macrophages with lipid. The former have neoplastic nuclei and lack immunohistochemical macrophage markers like KP1 (see Figs. 20.3A and 20.22A).

The astrocytic component can be assessed for neoplastic cells with hematoxylin on H&E and/or GFAP stains. The purpose of GFAP is to reveal neoplastic nuclei in cells with long cellular processes. If necessary, GFAP staining can be reduced to avoiding hiding the purple nuclei in brown. For automatic stainers, the primary anti-GFAP antibody can be titrated to a dilution that shows a discernible light brown. In manual staining, either this titrating can be done, or the diaminobenzidine (DAB) substrate can be used for less than half the usual time. Regular-strength hematoxylin counterstain then reveals nuclear details without interference from a dark brown immunohistochemical reaction product, which somehow obscures nuclei even though glial fibrils are cytoplasmic. A good nuclear counterstain should always be used with immunohistochemical analysis of brain lesions. Indistinct cell borders and infiltrations in brain require the counterstain for orientation. The counterstain provides important information about cell type and reactive versus neoplastic cells.

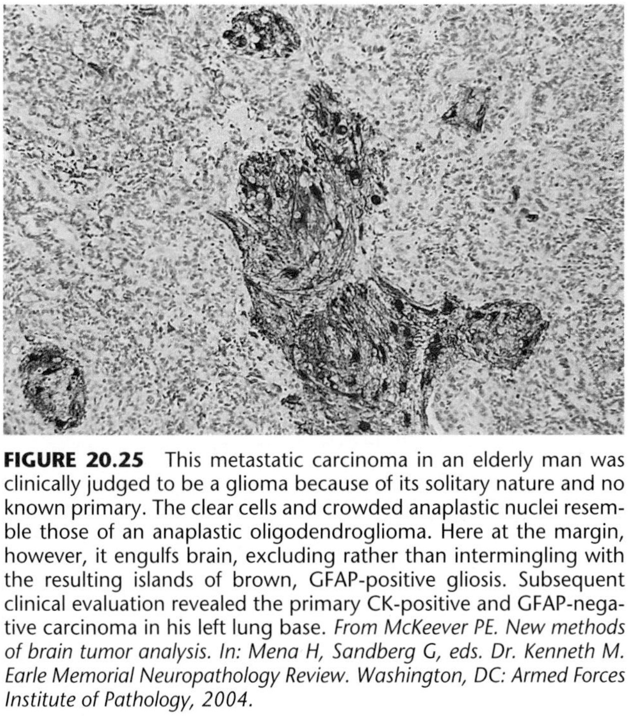

FIGURE 20.25 This metastatic carcinoma in an elderly man was clinically judged to be a glioma because of its solitary nature and no known primary. The clear cells and crowded anaplastic nuclei resemble those of an anaplastic oligodendroglioma. Here at the margin, however, it engulfs brain, excluding rather than intermingling with the resulting islands of brown, GFAP-positive gliosis. Subsequent clinical evaluation revealed the primary CK-positive and GFAP-negative carcinoma in his left lung base. *From McKeever PE. New methods of brain tumor analysis. In: Mena H, Sandberg G, eds. Dr. Kenneth M. Earle Memorial Neuropathology Review. Washington, DC: Armed Forces Institute of Pathology, 2004.*

Anaplastic Oligodendroglioma (Malignant Oligodendroglioma; WHO Grade III)

The features of anaplastic transformation in oligodendroglioma are similar to those in anaplastic ependymoma (Fig. 20.27). However, limited amounts of vascular proliferation are frequently present in oligodendroglioma, and in isolation, they cannot be considered evidence of malignant transformation (see Table 20.6). Vascular proliferation is highlighted by vimentin and CD31 stains.

Anaplastic and low-grade oligodendrogliomas may express neuronal markers and vimentin (Fig. 20.28).

KEY DIAGNOSTIC POINTS

Oligodendrogliomas

- Prepare to use molecular markers to test for 1p and 19q deletions that signal better prognosis and PCV sensitivity.
- Criteria for anaplastic oligodendroglioma are different than for anaplastic astrocytoma. An occasional mitosis and limited vascular proliferation may be found in a grade II oligodendroglioma.
- A few otherwise typical and diffusely invasive oligodendrogliomas may show some cells with positive neuronal markers, particularly synaptophysin.

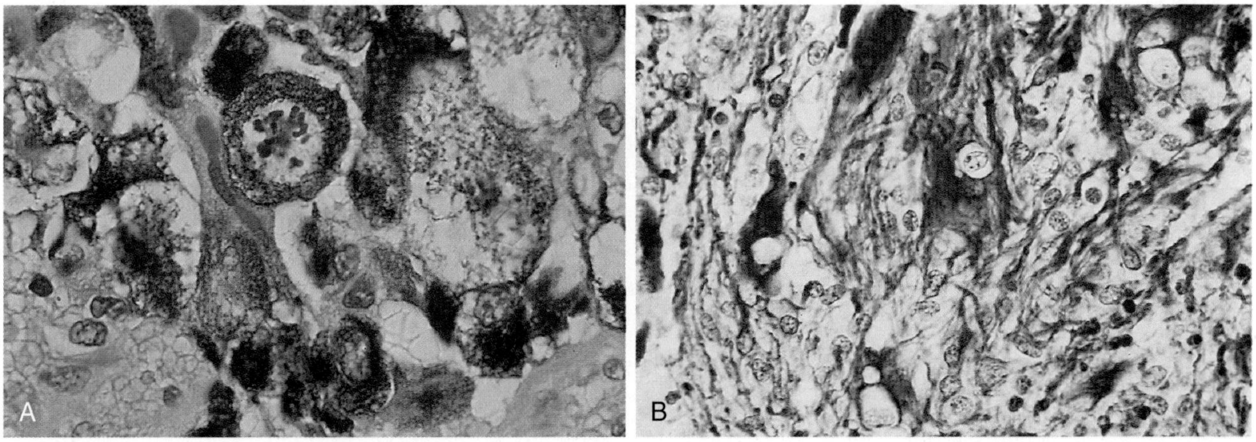

FIGURE 20.26 Glioblastoma versus trapped gliosis. The importance of examining the perikaryon (cytoplasm around the nucleus) for the marker is shown in these two different tumors stained for GFAP. **(A)** GFAP surrounds and touches neoplastic nuclei and a mitosis in the glioblastoma. **(B)** GFAP intimately contacts only reactive astrocytic nuclei in this gliosis trapped by metastatic carcinoma. The carcinoma was CK-positive *(not shown)*. (See Figure 20.24.) *From McKeever PE. New methods of brain tumor analysis. In: Mena H, Sandberg G, eds. Dr. Kenneth M. Earle Memorial Neuropathology Review. Washington, DC: Armed Forces Institute of Pathology, 2004.*

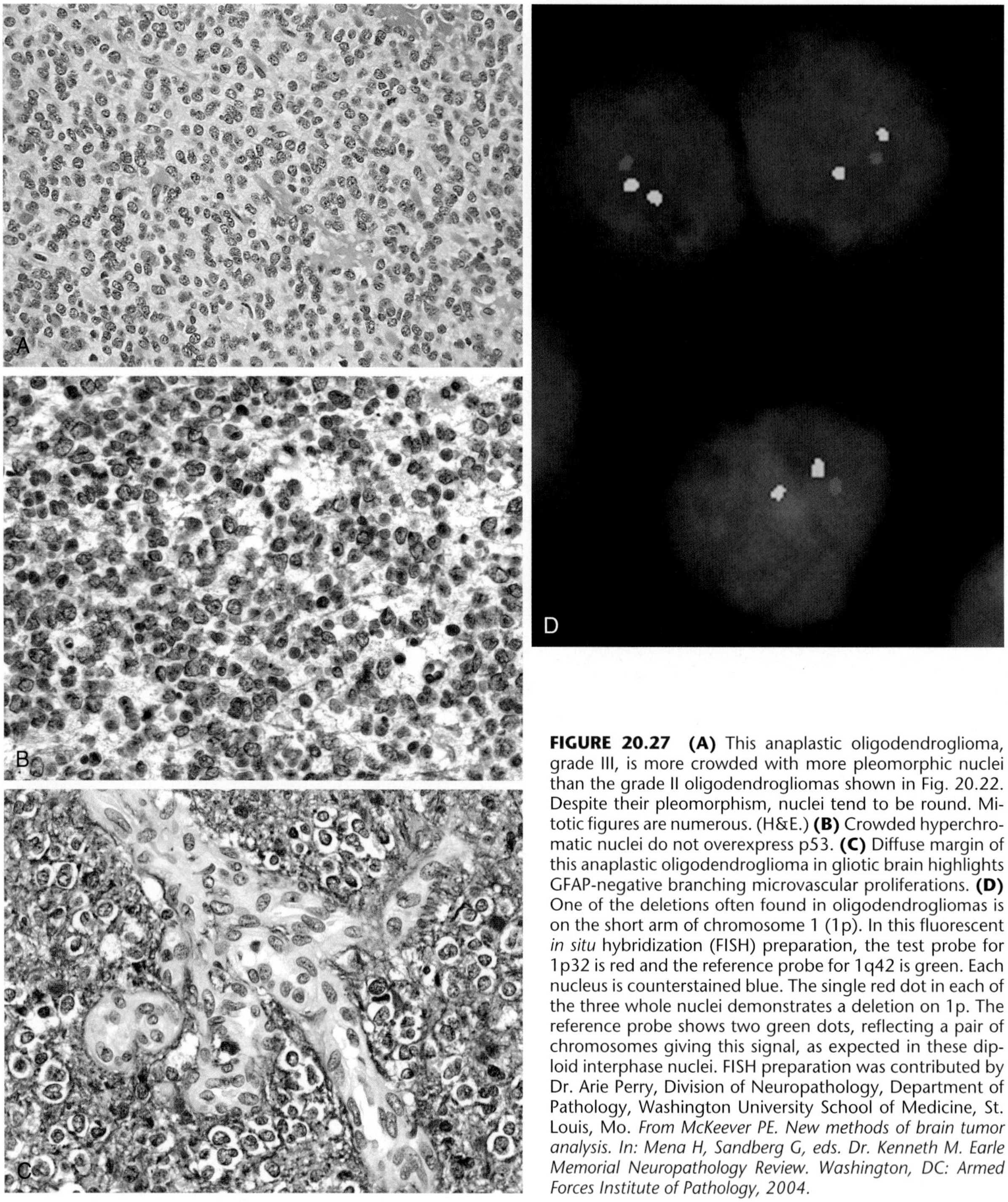

FIGURE 20.27 **(A)** This anaplastic oligodendroglioma, grade III, is more crowded with more pleomorphic nuclei than the grade II oligodendrogliomas shown in Fig. 20.22. Despite their pleomorphism, nuclei tend to be round. Mitotic figures are numerous. (H&E.) **(B)** Crowded hyperchromatic nuclei do not overexpress p53. **(C)** Diffuse margin of this anaplastic oligodendroglioma in gliotic brain highlights GFAP-negative branching microvascular proliferations. **(D)** One of the deletions often found in oligodendrogliomas is on the short arm of chromosome 1 (1p). In this fluorescent *in situ* hybridization (FISH) preparation, the test probe for 1p32 is red and the reference probe for 1q42 is green. Each nucleus is counterstained blue. The single red dot in each of the three whole nuclei demonstrates a deletion on 1p. The reference probe shows two green dots, reflecting a pair of chromosomes giving this signal, as expected in these diploid interphase nuclei. FISH preparation was contributed by Dr. Arie Perry, Division of Neuropathology, Department of Pathology, Washington University School of Medicine, St. Louis, Mo. *From McKeever PE. New methods of brain tumor analysis. In: Mena H, Sandberg G, eds. Dr. Kenneth M. Earle Memorial Neuropathology Review. Washington, DC: Armed Forces Institute of Pathology, 2004.*

Synaptophysin-positive cells are scattered sparsely when present.

Theranostic Applications

MIB1 is useful in predicting good outcome among patients with oligodendrogliomas. An MIB1 LI less than or equal to 5% has been found to correlate with better survival.[106] Vimentin expression and molecular alterations in CDKN2A, PTEN, and EGFR genes correlate with poor prognosis.[70,105]

Beyond Immunohistochemistry: Anatomic Molecular Diagnostic Applications

Molecular characterization of tumors with oligodendroglioma components is being used as a guide to therapy. Chromosomal deletions in 1p and 19q are associated with favorable prognosis and good response to combined PCV chemotherapy—procarbazine, chloroethylcyclohexylnitrosourea (CCNU), and vincristine—for patients with oligodendroglioma and particularly its anaplastic counterpart.[103,104,107] Neurooncologists here

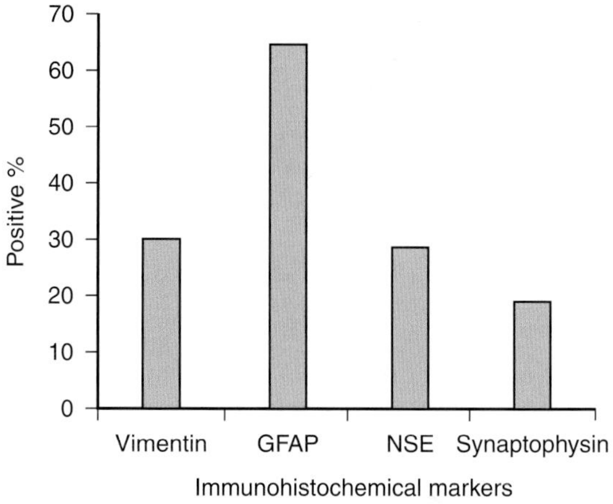

FIGURE 20.28 Immunohistochemical staining responses among more than 80 cases of oligodendrogliomas (grades II and III). GFAP, glial fibrillary acidic protein; NSE, neuron-specific enolase. Bars represent percentages of cases positive for these four markers. *Data from Dehghani F, Schachenmayr W, Laun A, et al. Prognostic implication of histopathological, immunohistochemical and clinical features of oligodendrogliomas: A study of 89 cases. Acta Neuropathol. 1998;95:493-504.*

have dropped vincristine from PCV, preferring PC chemotherapy, and many centers have done the same. Temozolomide is now the first-line chemotherapy for most grade II to IV gliomas.[108] This has occurred without a study proving that temozolomide is superior to PCV or PC, although it is likely that it is at least equal.

Molecular characterization of chromosomal deletions in 1p and 19q is used by some neuropathologists in diagnosis. There has been a new immunohistochemical marker of oligodendroglioma every year or two, and none have lasted. Arguably the best positive marker seems to be deletions on the short arm of chromosome 1 (1p) and the long arm of chromosome 19 (19q).[109,110] Should the absence of at least one sensitive and specific IHC marker for oligodendroglioma cells continue, the combined 1p/19q chromosomal marker will eventually be incorporated into diagnostic criteria for oligodendrogliomas. Chromosomal deletions in 1p and 19q can be detected either by PCR, by ISH enhanced by immunostaining, or by FISH (see Fig. 20.27D).

Anaplastic Oligoastrocytoma (Malignant Mixed Oligodendroglioma-Astrocytoma; WHO Grade III)

Oligoastrocytomas can be anaplastic. Histologic features of cytologic anaplasia, high cell density, conspicuous mitoses, and microvascular proliferation distinguish these anaplastic oligoastrocytomas from grade II oligoastrocytomas. A frequent feature of anaplastic oligoastrocytoma is a prominence of fibrillar, GFAP-positive malignant astrocytes. These may overgrow the oligodendroglial component and may ultimately result in a glioblastoma.

Beyond Immunohistochemistry: Anatomic Molecular Diagnostic Applications

The utility of chemotherapy when deletions are present in 1p and 19q is thought to be higher than when deletions are not present. It is not clear whether oligodendroglioma without deletions is any different from mixed oligoastrocytoma in this regard. Studies of the potential utility of chemotherapy in anaplastic oligoastrocytomas and its relation to 1p/19q status are available.[107,108]

GLIOBLASTOMA MULTIFORME (GLIOBLASTOMA; WHO GRADE IV)

In large part resulting from revelations of its frequent expression of GFAP-positive fibrillar cellular processes, glioblastoma is now considered the most malignant of astrocytomas rather than an embryonal neuroglial malignancy. It often contains focal astrocytoma, less often oligodendroglioma, and rarely ependymoma. The diagnostic criteria for glioblastoma were relaxed in the 1990s. Formerly, the cytologic criteria of anaplastic astrocytoma (mitotic activity, hypercellularity, pleomorphism, nuclear hyperchromasia) plus both vascular proliferation and spontaneous necrosis were required (see Fig. 20.9B). Now, either vascular proliferation *or* spontaneous coagulation necrosis is a sufficient addition to anaplasia for the diagnosis of glioblastoma (see Anaplastic Astrocytoma section for comparison).

If necrosis is absent, *vascular proliferation* (increased density of cells in vascular walls) should be unequivocal; it can be highlighted with vascular endothelial growth factor (VEGF),[111] vimentin, collagen type IV, or fibronectin stain. Other malignant features of glioblastomas are bizarre nuclei, multinucleated cells, and extreme pleomorphism (see Figs. 20.9B, 20.26A, and 20.29). Unfortunately, the heterogeneity of glioblastomas for these histologic features compromises diagnoses obtained on small specimens, such as those obtained with stereotactic needle biopsy, and jeopardizes accurate grading (see Fig. 20.9).[112]

Most confusion arises in distinguishing glioblastoma from malignant meningioma and from carcinoma. Unlike carcinoma and meningioma, glioblastomas contain fibrillar neoplastic cells that express GFAP in their cellular processes (see Figs. 20.1, 20.9B, 20.25, 20.26, and 20.29 and Tables 20.6 to 20.8). The cytologic features of the GFAP-positive cells should be checked for anaplasia to confirm glioblastoma, because either carcinoma or malignant melanoma may trap islands of CNS parenchyma and stimulate gliosis (see Figs. 20.25 and 20.26). Sarcoma is easily confused with glioblastoma on H&E staining, but GFAP reveals the glioblastoma (Fig. 20.29). Although the rapid growth of a glioblastoma may produce a pseudocapsule, neoplastic glia are evident beyond this margin within brain tissue (Fig. 20.30).

Gliosarcoma (WHO Grade IV)

A gliosarcoma is a mixture of glioblastoma and sarcoma (Fig. 20.31). Regions of collagen-positive and GFAP-negative sarcoma cells bridge the glioblastoma in a marbled configuration (see Table 20.5). Differences in collagen messenger RNA and cellular DNA content indicate the extent of variation between these regions.[113,114] Despite the fact that gliosarcomas often seem more circumscribed than the glioblastoma, gliosarcoma can metastasize.[75] Tumor progression from gliosarcoma to pure sarcoma lacking GFAP-positive cells can occur.[115] The glial and mesenchymal elements have similar genetic alterations.[116,117]

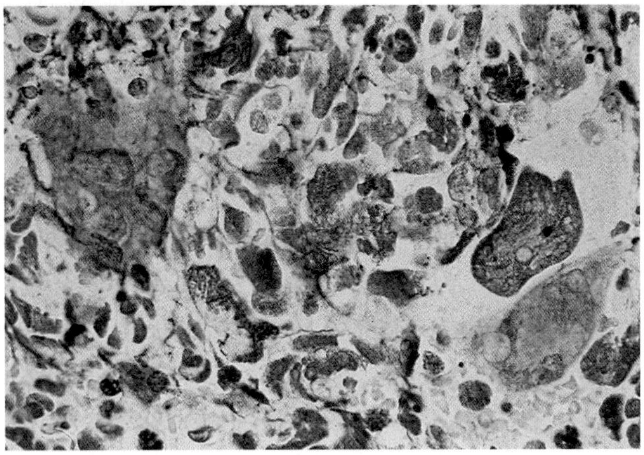

FIGURE 20.29 Extreme pleomorphism of cells and nuclei in a glioblastoma includes a huge brown, GFAP-positive cell with multiple nuclei. Giant cell glioblastomas were called *monstrocellular sarcomas* prior to recognition of their GFAP reactivity. *From McKeever PE. New methods of brain tumor analysis. In: Mena H, Sandberg G, eds. Dr. Kenneth M. Earle Memorial Neuropathology Review. Washington, DC: Armed Forces Institute of Pathology, 2004.*

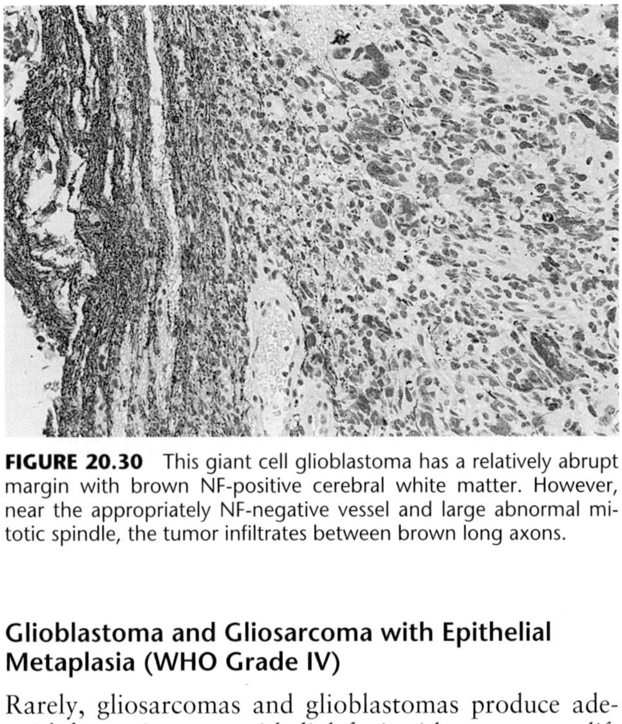

FIGURE 20.30 This giant cell glioblastoma has a relatively abrupt margin with brown NF-positive cerebral white matter. However, near the appropriately NF-negative vessel and large abnormal mitotic spindle, the tumor infiltrates between brown long axons.

Glioblastoma and Gliosarcoma with Epithelial Metaplasia (WHO Grade IV)

Rarely, gliosarcomas and glioblastomas produce adenoid formations or epithelial foci with squamous differentiation and keratin pearls.[3,13] These regions stain immunohistochemically for CK and EMA (see Table 20.7 and Fig. 20.31D). To avoid confusion of this tumor with carcinoma, it is necessary to obtain adequate sampling and to be aware that these regions are focal and that other regions will show the familiar fibrillar, GFAP-positive neoplastic cells of a glioblastoma. It is important to remember that carcinoma cells are GFAP negative.

Glioblastomas manifest other peculiar features. Rare glioblastomas occur with granular cell tumors. Some epithelioid glioblastomas contain diffuse cytoplasmic lipids.[13]

KEY DIAGNOSTIC POINTS

Glioblastomas

- All have some cells that meet cytologic criteria of astrocytoma (long cellular processes, GFAP, elongated nuclei). They often will have additional cells that resemble other types of gliomas.
- All meet cytologic criteria of anaplasia (mitotic activity, hypercellularity, pleomorphism, nuclear hyperchromasia).
- In addition to the above, a glioblastoma must also have either (or both) necrosis or microvascular proliferation.

Theranostic Applications

Two structurally similar varieties of glioblastomas are called primary and secondary glioblastomas. Primary glioblastomas are those that arise *de novo* in older patients. Older patients have higher MIB1 proliferation indices and shorter survival than their younger counterparts.[62] Primary glioblastomas are often associated with CDKN2A deletions, PTEN alterations, and epidermal growth factor receptor (EGFR) gene amplification plus EGFR overexpression.

Secondary glioblastomas are those that arise by progression from lower-grade gliomas. Secondary glioblastomas are associated with *TP53* gene mutations and/or with p53 protein overexpression.[2,13] *TP53* gene mutations and p53 overexpression often, but not always, coincide. EGFR and p53 overexpression can be defined immunohistochemically (Fig. 20.32).

Beyond Immunohistochemistry: Anatomic Molecular Diagnostic Applications

Loss of genetic material in chromosome 10 is the most frequent genetic abnormality in glioblastomas, occurring in about 66% of them. Loss of genetic material in the short arm of chromosome 10 (10p) is nearly always associated with primary glioblastomas.[2] Loss in the long arm (10q) is found in both primary and secondary glioblastomas. These losses can be observed with comparative genomic hybridization,[118] FISH,[119] ISH enhanced with immunostaining,[116] or PCR assay. Amplifications of chromosome 7 DNA are also demonstrated by modifications of these techniques.[120]

Molecular oncology studies show variable responses of glioblastomas to chemotherapy. Some of this is due to O^6 methylguanine DNA methyltransferase (MGMT). MGMT is a DNA repair enzyme. It removes methyl groups from O^6 methylguanine, an abnormal guanine that is harmful to DNA. This is a praiseworthy enzymatic pursuit when protecting normal cells. Unfortunately, MGMT also removes methyl groups from O^6 methylguanine produced in glioblastoma cells by alkylating chemotherapy agents like temozolomide given to kill the tumor. And so, MGMT hinders these important drugs. In an odd twist of fate, however, the MGMT gene promoter is methylated in nearly half of glioblastoma tumors, stopping their production of MGMT and rendering these tumors sensitive to alkylating agents.

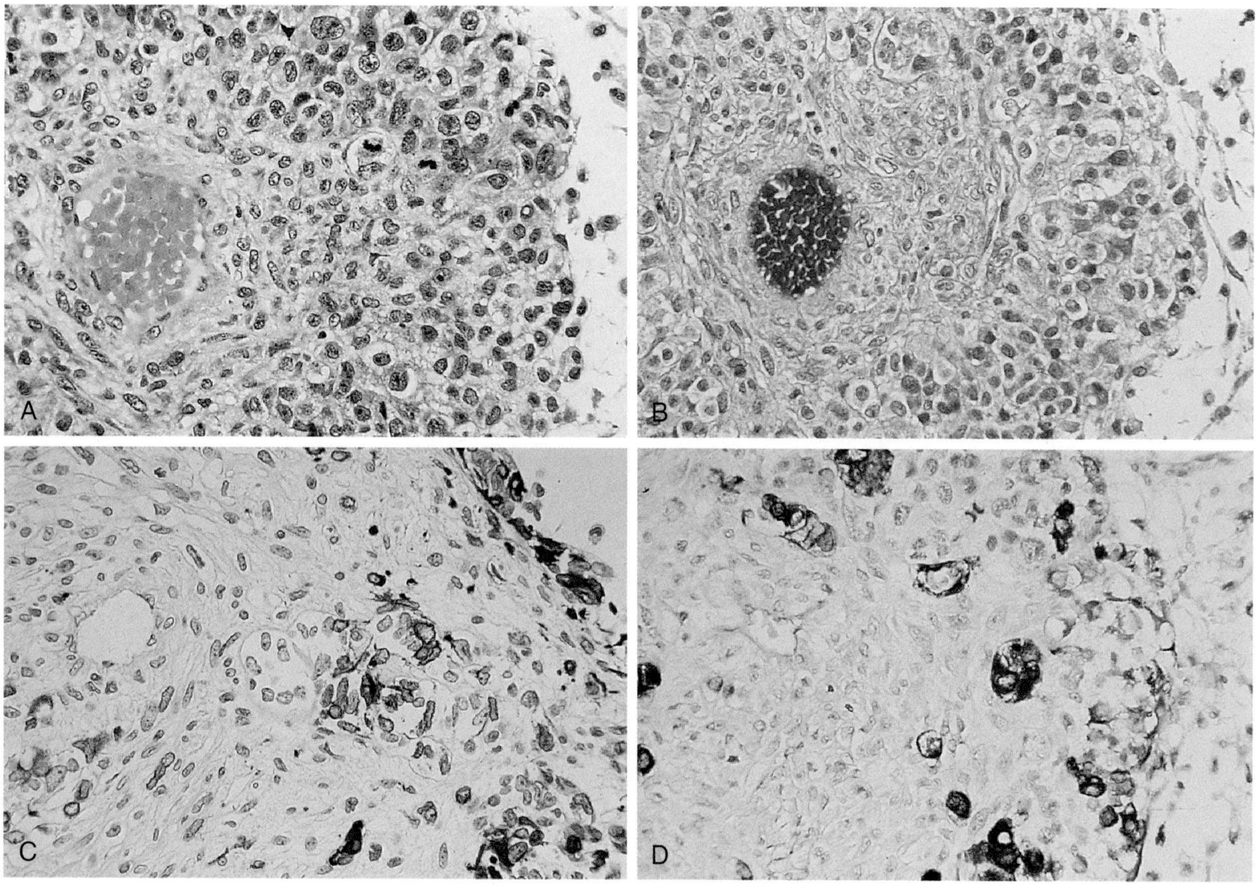

FIGURE 20.31 This gliosarcoma, shown in **(A)** with H&E staining, had regions and bands of collagen-positive, GFAP-negative sarcoma cells and other regions of GFAP-positive, collagen-negative malignant astrocytes. **(B)** Shown under high magnification here, sarcoma cells produce cyan collagen as they wander away from a vessel into tumor parenchyma. (Masson's trichrome stain.) **(C)** A nearby section shows most collagen-associated cells to be GFAP negative, whereas malignant astrocytes further from the vessel are GFAP positive. **(D)** Epithelial metaplasia of brown CAM5.2-positive cells was present in small foci in other regions of this gliosarcoma. *From McKeever PE. New methods of brain tumor analysis. In: Mena H, Sandberg G, eds. Dr. Kenneth M. Earle Memorial Neuropathology Review. Washington, DC: Armed Forces Institute of Pathology, 2004.*

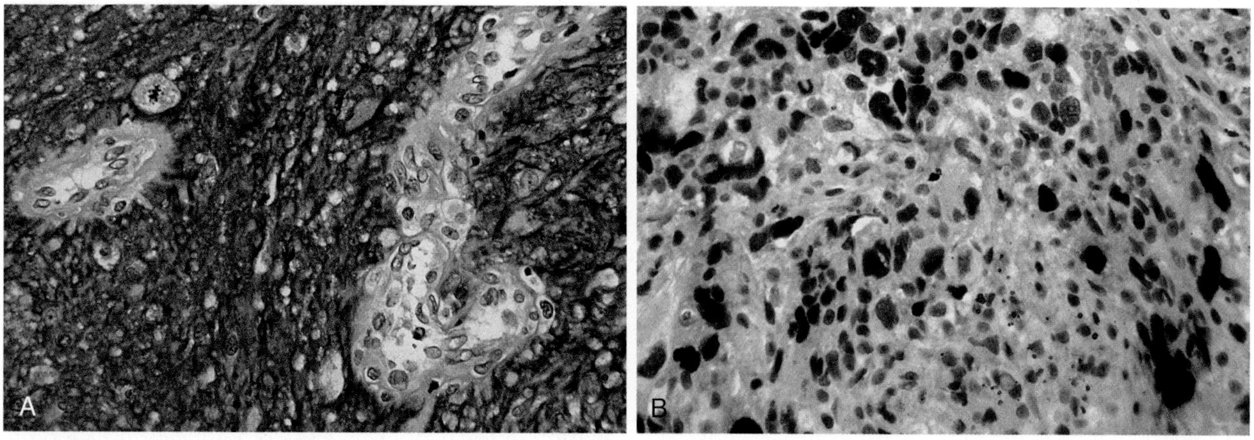

FIGURE 20.32 Molecular marker expression of glioblastomas. This glioblastoma arose *de novo* in a 70-year-old woman with a 2-week history of headaches. It overexpresses epidermal growth factor receptors (EGFR) **(A)** but does not overexpress p53 *(not shown)*. This different glioblastoma progressed from a grade II astrocytoma in a 52-year-old man. It overexpresses p53 **(B)**, but not EGFR *(not shown)*.

Methylation of the MGMT gene promoter can be detected by PCR.[121] If a reliable assay of MGMT gene methylation becomes readily available, it may predict which patients have glioblastomas that are sensitive to temozolomide.

Neuronal Tumors

Neuronal tumors contain an abnormal proliferation of neurons. They range from the most benign gangliocytoma to the anaplastic ganglioglioma and primitive

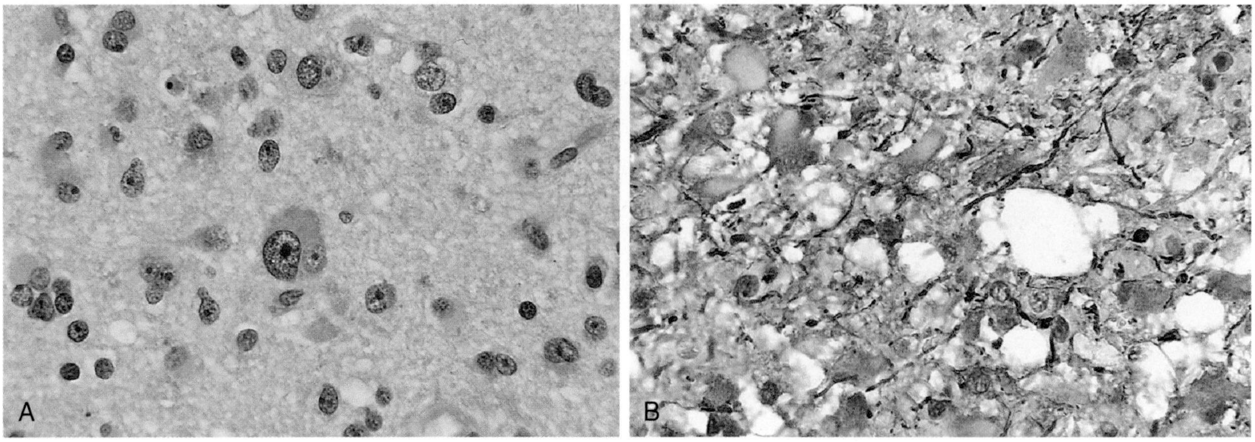

FIGURE 20.33 Ganglioglioma from the parietal lobe of a middle-aged man with progressive unilateral loss of coordination exhibits binucleated ganglion cells with large nucleoli and Nissl substance on H&E **(A)** and NF staining **(B)**. This specimen was prepared with immunoperoxidase anti-NF protein with hematoxylin.

neuroectodermal tumor (PNET; formerly called *ganglioneuroblastoma* and *CNS neuroblastoma*) (see Tables 20.5, 20.7, and 20.8). Most low-grade ganglion cell neoplasms have a better prognosis than gliomas found in the same location, and their proper identification is important.

The identification and evaluation of ganglion cell neoplasms has four important stages:

1. Recognition of neurons (Fig. 20.33)
2. Confirmation that neurons are neoplastic
3. Determination of whether or not glia are present
4. Evaluation of any glia for neoplasia

Many neoplastic cells, particularly cells of glioblastomas, melanomas, and astrocytomas, resemble neurons because of their large size or prominent nucleoli.[122,123] These cells lack NF and synaptophysin markers of neurons (see Fig. 20.30 and 20.41D). The most important step in using NF or synaptophysin to identify a neuron is to trace the marker back to the cell body (perikaryon). Synaptophysin is present in the neuropil, making evaluation of cellular surface staining difficult. Commercial anti-NF and anti-synaptophysin immunoperoxidase markers of neurons must be chosen carefully, and their use must be controlled by staining of normal brain specimens in the same batch of slides and preferably in the same slide as the unknown tumor (see Box 20.2).

While neuron-specific enolase (NSE) has been described as a marker of neuronal tumors in reviews and texts, this author finds that it has better uses than this. The shortcoming for neuronal tumors is its propensity to also stain glial tumors, which commonly need to be distinguished from neuronal tumors.[2,3] Experimental IHC stains such as Neu-N identify neurons by showing their on-target nuclear features rather than their cytoplasmic or confusing surface features.[124,125] In cases refractory to immunohistochemical stains, electron microscopy positively identifies Nissl substance, neurofilaments, neurosecretory granules, and synapses in neoplastic cells.

A common error in determining whether identified neurons are neoplastic is to interpret a field of normal neurons infiltrated by glioma cells as a ganglioglioma. As previously described, the synaptophysin or NF should be traced back to a cell body, and hematoxylin-stained nuclear features should be used to determine whether the cell is neoplastic according to standard criteria. Evidence of neuronal neoplasia includes hypercellularity and disarray of neurons, binucleated neurons, nuclear atypia, and pleomorphism in cells that respond positively to staining for synaptophysin or NF (see Fig. 20.33B). Degenerative changes in such neoplastic neurons may occur.[122] Ganglion cell tumors may show heavy bands of collagen and fibronectin-positive fibrous tissue, or they may show perivascular round cells, but neither of these is invariably present.

GANGLIOCYTOMA (WHO GRADE I), GANGLIOGLIOMA (WHO GRADE I OR II), AND ANAPLASTIC GANGLIOGLIOMA (WHO GRADE III)

Gangliocytoma, ganglioglioma, and anaplastic ganglioglioma may arise anywhere but are most common in the cerebrum, particularly the temporal lobe.

Once a ganglion cell neoplasm has been identified, the glial element must be evaluated (see Table 20.5). A section lightly stained for GFAP with immunoperoxidase (either with less than half the usual time in DAB substrate for manual staining, or with use of a lower primary antibody titer in an automatic stainer) and fully counterstained with hematoxylin facilitates this determination by providing a better view of glial nuclei. If the light brown cells appear reactive, cluster near the margin of the neoplasm, and do not meet the criteria for neoplasia (described in the Astrocytoma section earlier in this chapter), the tumor is a central neurocytoma or gangliocytoma.

Gangliocytomas tend to be benign. They often contain immunocytochemical positivity for at least one neurotransmitter peptide or amine, including somatostatin, corticotropin-releasing hormone, beta-endorphin, galanin, vasoactive intestinal peptide, calcitonin, serotonin, catecholamines, and met-enkephalin.[126]

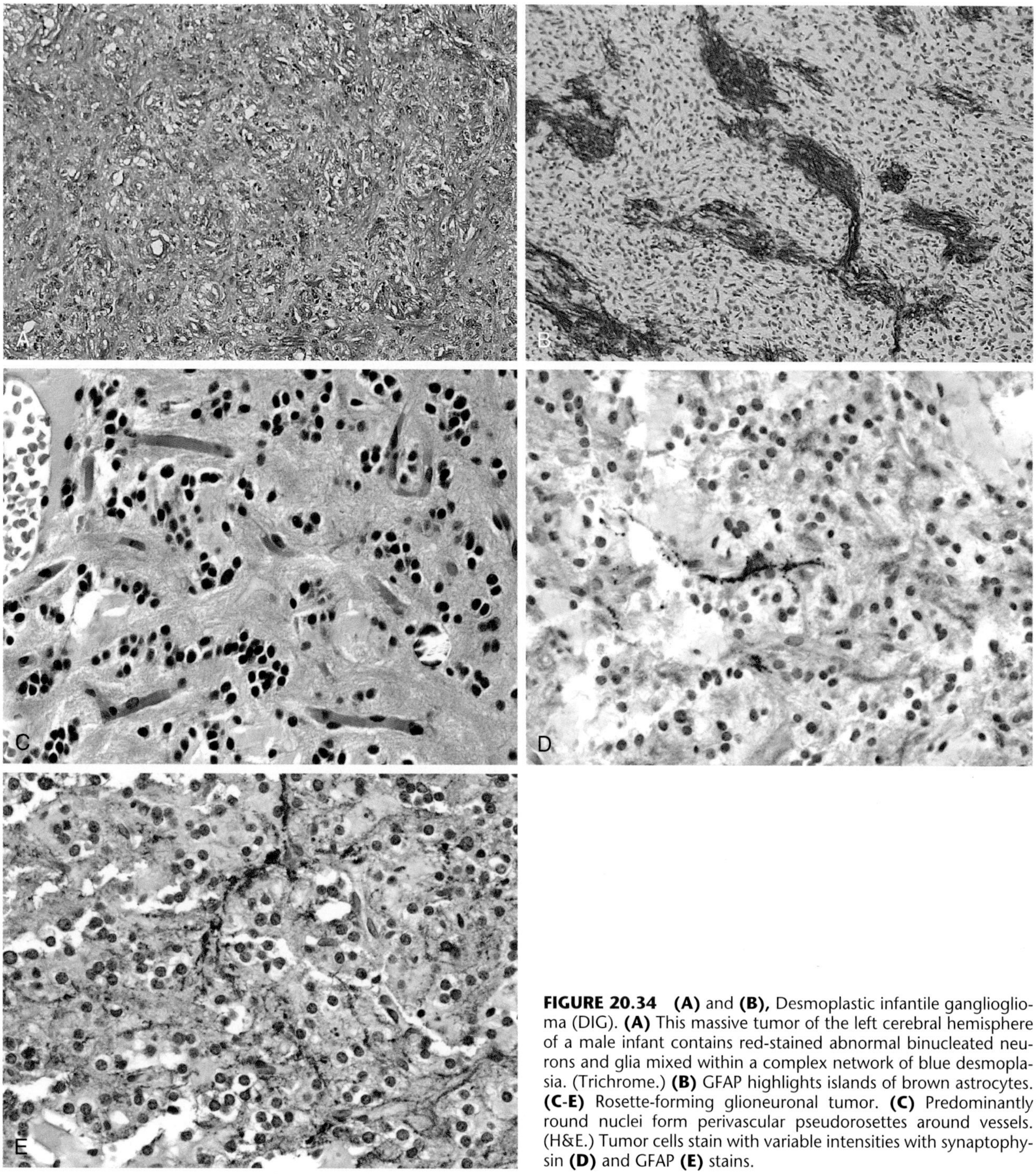

FIGURE 20.34 **(A)** and **(B),** Desmoplastic infantile ganglioglioma (DIG). **(A)** This massive tumor of the left cerebral hemisphere of a male infant contains red-stained abnormal binucleated neurons and glia mixed within a complex network of blue desmoplasia. (Trichrome.) **(B)** GFAP highlights islands of brown astrocytes. **(C-E)** Rosette-forming glioneuronal tumor. **(C)** Predominantly round nuclei form perivascular pseudorosettes around vessels. (H&E.) Tumor cells stain with variable intensities with synaptophysin **(D)** and GFAP **(E)** stains.

If the GFAP-positive cells are neoplastic but not anaplastic, the neoplasm is a ganglioglioma (Fig. 20.34B). If these glial elements are anaplastic (see the sections on Astrocytomas and Glioblastoma earlier in this chapter), the neoplasm is an anaplastic ganglioglioma. The proliferative capacity of the GFAP-positive glial component of ganglion cell tumors is critical to their histologic grade and can be assessed immunohistochemically with MIB1 or PCNA. Usually, the astrocytic component has immunoreactivity for such proliferation markers, and it is routinely low.[13]

DYSPLASTIC GANGLIOCYTOMA OF THE CEREBELLUM (WHO GRADE I)

An unusual variant of a gangliocytoma, dysplastic gangliocytoma of the cerebellum (DGC) is also known as Lhermitte-Duclos disease.[88] Hyperplastic and disordered

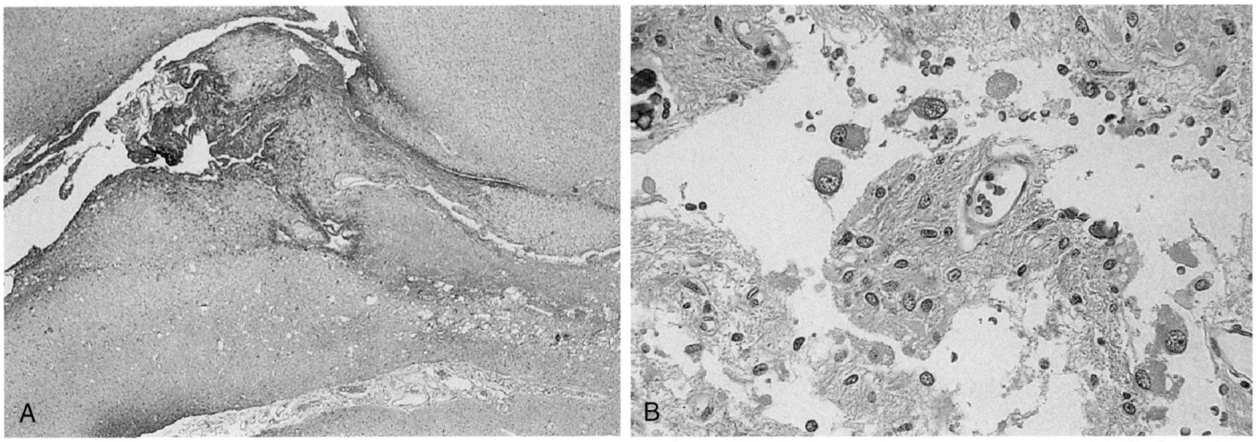

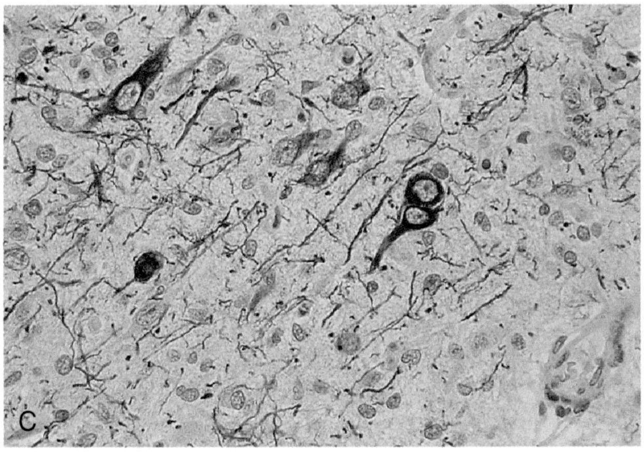

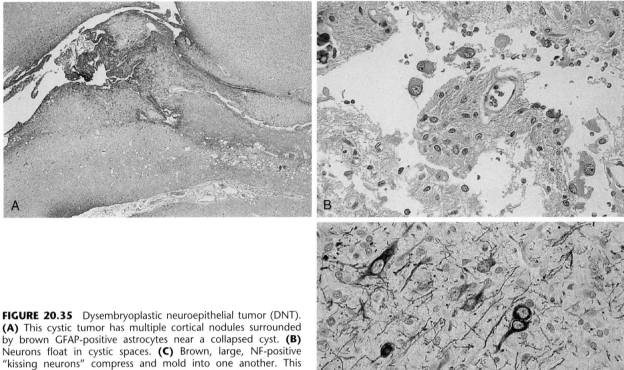

FIGURE 20.35 Dysembryoplastic neuroepithelial tumor (DNT). **(A)** This cystic tumor has multiple cortical nodules surrounded by brown GFAP-positive astrocytes near a collapsed cyst. **(B)** Neurons float in cystic spaces. **(C)** Brown, large, NF-positive "kissing neurons" compress and mold into one another. This specimen is from a 40-year-old man who had long-standing, medically refractory epilepsy and a right frontal multinodular cortical tumor. *From McKeever PE. New methods of brain tumor analysis. In: Mena H, Sandberg G, eds. Dr. Kenneth M. Earle Memorial Neuropathology Review. Washington, DC: Armed Forces Institute of Pathology, 2004.*

synaptophysin-positive granular cell neurons enlarge part of the cerebellum into bizarre "megafolia." This rare tumor looks dysplastic but has recurred after surgery. The growth potential of individual tumors can be monitored by staining for MIB1. Some DGCs are familial, and others are associated with Cowden syndrome or multiple hamartoma-neoplasia syndrome.[127]

DYSEMBRYOPLASTIC NEUROEPITHELIAL TUMOR (WHO GRADE I)

Dysembryoplastic neuroepithelial tumor (DNT) may be the hamartomatous counterpart of a ganglioglioma. It is multinodular within the cerebral cortex, most often in the temporal lobe cortex. Some DNTs are cystic (Fig. 20.35A). Some are incidental findings, but many others are associated with long-standing partial complex seizure disorders in children and young adults.[128]

These tumors have prominent cells that resemble oligodendroglia and NF-positive neurons (or synaptophysin-positive neurons, or both) that often appear to float within Alcian blue-positive acid mucopolysaccharide. These are called *floating neurons* (see Fig. 20.35B). Other large neurons lack their normal spacing (see Fig. 20.35C). GFAP-positive astrocytes are variably present within the tumor and often surround it. This tumor's low MIB1 LI, mature histotopographic appearance, and association with cortical dysplasia suggest a maldevelopmental origin.[13]

Oligodendrogliomas can produce mucopolysaccharide and can even float an occasional normal neuron. Lack of mass effect, discrete cortical location, low MIB1 LI, and lack of brain infiltration typify DNTs and distinguish them from oligodendrogliomas.[2] Evaluating the tumor margin with serial sections analyzed immunohistochemically for NF, MIB1, and synaptophysin shows these features.[59] Neuronal nuclear antigen, if present, may also identify a DNT.[129]

GLIONEURONAL TUMORS

These tumors feature separate GFAP-positive and synaptophysin-positive elements. Currently, glioneuronal tumors include a diverse group of tumors with patterned and almost histiotypic features that include elements of glia and neurons (see Fig. 20.34C-E). The cerebral papillary glioneuronal tumor (PGT) shows layers of glia with compact nuclei next to layers of oligodendroglia-like cells and neurons. Some layers cover vessels, and some look papillary.[130,131] In the posterior fossa, the rosette-forming glioneuronal tumor resembles a PGT with the addition of perivascular pseudorosettes (see Fig. 20.34C) or neurocytic rosettes with fibrillar cores and a more astrocytic glial component.[132] The neurocytic rosettes have fibrillar cores, as do Homer Wright rosettes. Most glioneuronal tumors are grade I, except for the glioneuronal tumor with neuropil-like islands reported to occur within grade II and III diffuse astrocytomas.[2]

Glioneuronal tumors are a heterogeneous group of tumors in need of further definition. When their definition is complete, the glioneuronal tumors may encompass other focally synaptophysin-positive tumors also interpreted as odd variants of gliomas, such as oligodendrogliomas and ependymomas with neuronal differentiation.[104,133,134]

DESMOPLASTIC INFANTILE GANGLIOGLIOMA (WHO GRADE I)

Desmoplastic infantile gangliogliomas (DIGs) often attain considerable size and resemble very fibrous gangliogliomas (see Fig. 20.34A). These neoplasms are found in patients younger than 3 years of age, are frequently cystic, and often involve the meninges.[3] Their substantial differentiation produces a mixture of GFAP-positive glial cells (see Fig. 20.34B), NF-positive and synaptophysin-positive neurons, and vimentin-positive fibrovascular cells. DIGs have a low MIB1 and do not overexpress p53.[135]

CENTRAL NEUROCYTOMA (WHO GRADE II)

Recognized recently, central neurocytoma (CN) has stimulated much interest because of its structural beauty, hidden identity, generally benign prognosis, and fluctuating interpretations (see Fig. 20.23A).[3,136] Its previous WHO grade was grade I, more representative of the benign appearance and low proliferation of nearly all CN. It is the most common neoplasm involving the septum pellucidum in young adults. Although it often has slightly more fibrillarity, CN resembles oligodendroglioma (see Tables 20.5 and 20.6 and Box 20.1). Careful application of immunohistochemical markers facilitates proper identification of the tumor, which for years had been mistaken for a glioma (see Fig. 20.23). CNs express much synaptophysin (see Fig. 20.23B).[58] They are usually GFAP negative but many contain reactive astrocytes. CNs do not amplify EGFR.[137] If the synaptophysin stain is equivocal, electron microscopy is recommended to distinguish central neurocytoma from oligodendroglioma and ependymoma.

Although radiotherapy has been used to treat CN, a good prognosis usually follows total surgical excision.[136] CN rarely show anaplastic features.

CEREBELLAR LIPONEUROCYTOMA

Except for lipids in some of its cells, the rare *cerebellar liponeurocytoma* resembles a CN.[2] Microtubules, 100- to 200-nm dense-core vesicles, and clear vesicles identify its true neuronal lineage.

GANGLIONEUROBLASTOMA AND NEUROBLASTOMA

See the Primitive Neuroectodermal Tumor section later in the chapter.

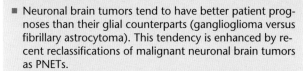

KEY DIAGNOSTIC POINTS

Neuronal Tumors

- Neuronal brain tumors tend to have better patient prognoses than their glial counterparts (ganglioglioma versus fibrillary astrocytoma). This tendency is enhanced by recent reclassifications of malignant neuronal brain tumors as PNETs.
- Key markers of neuronal tumors are synaptophysin and neurofilaments. High-quality hematoxylin counterstain is needed to reveal neoplastic nuclei in positive cells.
- Many neuronal markers including NSE are not reliably specific for neuronal tumors. Test new markers on gliomas before using them to identify neuronal tumors.
- Low-grade neuronal neoplasms resemble hamartomas and dysplasias. Use MIB1 and interval growth on serial radiographs to distinguish the true neoplasms.

Choroid Plexus Epithelial Tumors

Most choroid plexus neoplasms appear in childhood. They can occur in any portion of choroid plexus (see Table 20.6) but are more common in the lateral ventricles of children and the fourth ventricle of adults.[3]

CHOROID PLEXUS PAPILLOMA (WHO GRADE I)

In contrast to papillary ependymoma, the choroid plexus papilloma contains a layer of columnar to cuboidal epithelial cells over a basement membrane and fibrovascular stroma. The type IV collagen and laminin in this stroma contrast with ependymomas, which have solid parenchyma without collagen or laminin (see Tables 20.5 and 20.6; see the Ependymomas section earlier in this chapter). Focal GFAP reactivity in certain choroid plexus papillomas suggests focal ependymal differentiation. This overlap in immunostaining responses includes other markers, although choroid plexus papillomas express substantially more CAM5.2 cytokeratin than ependymomas.[13] The CAM5.2 response is often particularly robust (Fig. 20.36A). Transthyretin is a potential marker of this papilloma (see Fig. 20.36B), but its spectrum of reactivity is broad.[138]

Newer potential markers of choroid plexus papillomas include insulin-like growth factor II (IGF-II) and synaptophysin. IGF-II is found in papillomas but not in normal choroid plexus.[139] Synaptophysin is present in some normal choroid plexus, choroid plexus papilloma, and choroid plexus carcinoma but not in metastatic papillary carcinoma.[140] Both markers may assist in the differential diagnoses of some tumors, but I find them most useful combined with traditional markers. CD44 is preferentially expressed on atypical papilloma and choroid plexus carcinoma and may be a marker of aggressive choroid plexus tumors. Aggressive tumors have higher mean MIB1 LIs of 6%.[141] These various results should be verified with larger series of cases.

Meningiomas and carcinoma enter the differential diagnosis. An epithelial lining of CAM5.2 cytokeratin-positive cells in the choroid plexus papilloma, lack of

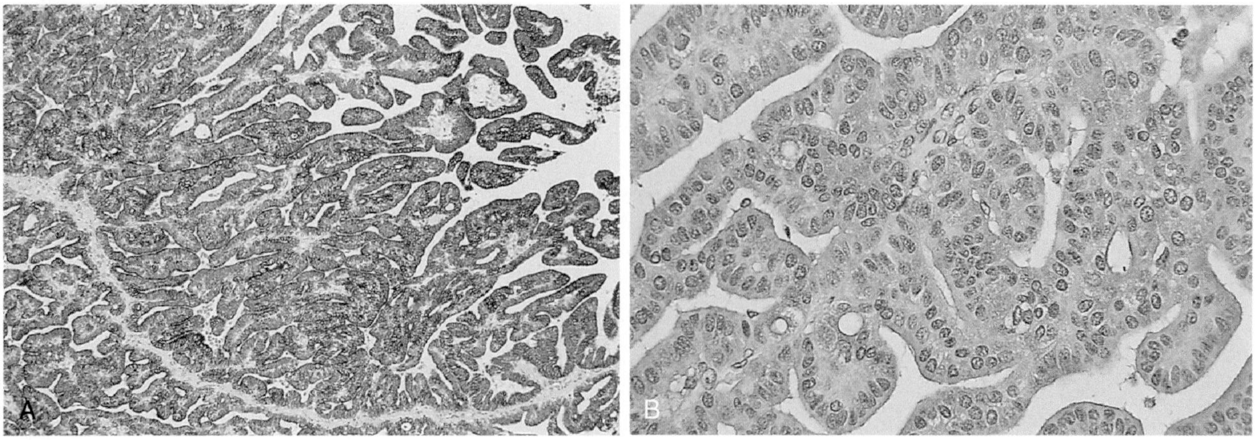

FIGURE 20.36 Choroid plexus papilloma. This choroid plexus papilloma from the lateral ventricle of a child is composed of well-differentiated columnar epithelium resting upon a fibrovascular stroma. It expresses CAM5.2 low molecular weight cytokeratin **(A)** and transthyretin **(B)**. The fibrovascular stroma is easily identified from its negativity for cytokeratin. (Immunoperoxidase anti-CAM5.2 and anti-prealbumin.) *From McKeever PE, Blaivas M. The brain, spinal cord, and meninges. In: Sternberg SS, Diagnostic Surgical Pathology. 2nd ed. New York, NY: Raven Press; 1994:409-492.*

whorls, and lack of syncytial foci distinguish it from papillary meningioma. Secretory meningioma has a focal CK response, but not in an epithelial lining with a fibrovascular core. The choroid plexus papilloma lacks the necrosis and anaplasia seen in metastatic papillary carcinoma.

CHOROID PLEXUS CARCINOMA (WHO GRADE III OR IV)

The choroid plexus carcinoma (anaplastic choroid plexus papilloma) is a rare neoplasm that is most difficult to distinguish from metastatic carcinoma (see Table 20.6). Each of these tumors produces CK, and each may produce transthyretin. A transitional zone between papilloma and carcinoma of the choroid plexus confirms choroid plexus carcinoma. Primary carcinoma of the choroid plexus so closely resembles metastatic carcinoma that the latter must be carefully excluded before the diagnosis of primary choroid plexus carcinoma can be made. Occult pulmonary or gastrointestinal primary tumors are common sources. The paucity of these primary systemic carcinomas in children facilitates diagnosis of choroid plexus carcinoma in a patient in this age group. Some choroid plexus carcinomas express CD44 cell adhesion molecule not seen in the most benign papillomas. The mean MIB1 LI of choroid plexus carcinomas is 14%, which is higher than that of papillomas, but the LI varies between laboratories.[141]

KEY DIAGNOSTIC POINTS

Choroid Plexus Tumors

- A variety of IHC markers are available for choroid plexus (CP) tumors, none of which are ideal. Individual markers lack either sensitivity or specificity, but used as a panel they confirm difficult cases.
- Location and structural features are sufficient to confirm CP papillomas in many cases.
- CP carcinomas are difficult to distinguish from metastatic carcinomas.

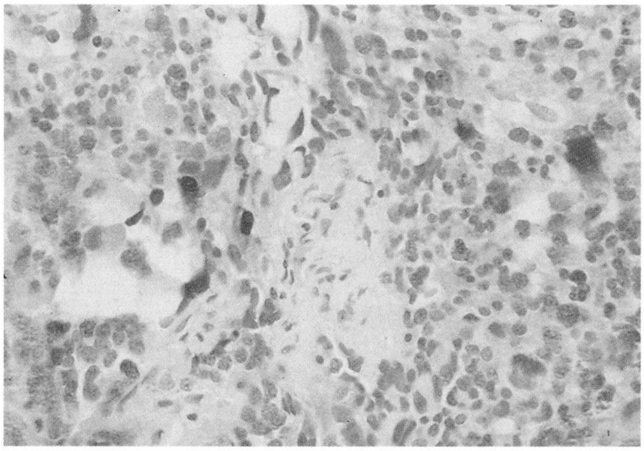

FIGURE 20.37 Pineocytoma. Neoplastic cells with round nuclei include some that express retinal-S antigen. *Courtesy of Dr. Hernando Mena, Armed Forces Institute of Pathology, Washington, DC.*

Beyond Immunohistochemistry: Anatomic Molecular Diagnostic Applications

Earlier in this chapter we discussed LFS, a germline mutation of the *p53* gene on the short arm of chromosome 17. The percentage of choroid plexus tumors associated with LFS is higher than the percentage of astrocytomas associated with LFS.[98-100,142] Consider the possibility of LFS in a patient with a CP tumor, particularly with a CP carcinoma.[99]

Pineal Cell Tumors

Tumors described in this section arise from pineal cells or their precursors. Because tumors that arise from pineal cells are neurons, synaptophysin immunoreactivity is common. Some tumors also react for retinal-S antigen (Fig. 20.37).[143] Many other tumors, including gliomas,

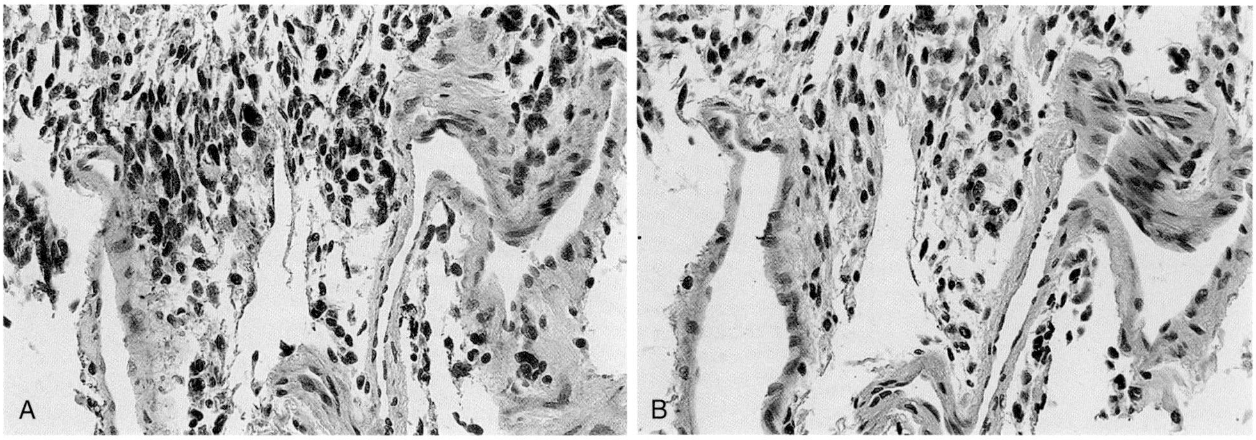

FIGURE 20.38 Crowded malignant cells with pleomorphic and hyperchromatic nuclei in this pineal tumor express synaptophysin **(A)** but not GFAP **(B)** in serial sections of this pineoblastoma.

meningiomas, and germ cell tumors, occur in the pineal region. They are described in their respective sections in this chapter.

PINEOCYTOMA (WHO GRADE I)

Pineocytoma simulates the normal pineal gland (see Table 20.5). Synaptophysin-positive cells with round nuclei are divided by fibrovascular stroma into lobules. Other cells surround fibrillary centers.[88] The cells are fibrillar and often radiate toward the vessels.[143] Immunohistochemical stains for neurofilaments may reveal expansions at the tips of these processes resembling clubs, and electron microscopy shows their similarity to neurons.[3] These neural features distinguish pineocytoma from gliomas. The major source of confusion with this histologic picture is with normal pineal gland. An MIB1 LI higher than normal pineal gland, a specimen larger than the 0.5-cm diameter of the normal pineal gland, or invasion beyond the pineal gland confirms the diagnosis of pineocytoma.

PINEAL CELL TUMOR OF INTERMEDIATE DIFFERENTIATION (LIKELY GRADE II OR III)

Primary pineal cell tumors are less differentiated than pineocytomas and more differentiated than pineoblastomas. They show mitotic activity and moderate crowding of their synaptophysin-positive cells. They may contain regions that resemble pineocytoma near regions like pineoblastoma. Their proliferation is regionally variable, with hot spots of proliferation higher than that of pineocytoma.

PAPILLARY TUMOR OF THE PINEAL REGION (LIKELY GRADE II OR III)

The papillary tumor of the pineal region (PTPR) is a rare tumor found at all ages. It has a prealbumin- and CAM5.2–positive cuboidal epithelium wrapped around vessels and closely resembles a choroid plexus tumor. Some PTPRs may be distinguished by their robust MAP-2 immunoreactivity, lack of membranous Kir7.1, and lack of cytoplasmic stanniocalcin-1 staining.[144] Papillary tumors of the pineal region have an uncertain prognosis and a high risk of local recurrence. They have been treated with surgery and radiotherapy. Their only known prognostic factors are more than 4 mitoses per 10 high-power fields and the extent of surgical resection.[2,145]

PINEOBLASTOMA (GRADE IV)

Pineoblastoma resembles medulloblastoma (Fig. 20.38; see Fig. 20.21) except for its origin in the pineal gland (see Table 20.8). Fibrillary rosettes may be evident and are more common than Flexner-Wintersteiner rosettes. Synaptophysin is most useful in identifying neuronal differentiation in these tumors (see Fig. 20.38A) because NF immunoreactivity is often negative (Box 20.3). Some tumors express retinal-S antigen.[143] It would be interesting to know whether this sight-specific marker is more common in pineoblastomas than in other medulloblastomas.

Embryonal Tumors (All WHO Grade IV)

MEDULLOBLASTOMA

The medulloblastoma is a primitive neuroectodermal tumor that arises in the cerebellum or in the roof of the fourth ventricle (see Box 20.3, Fig. 20.21, and Table 20.8). It is most common in children but also occurs among young adults[146] and rarely in patients older than 35 years.[74] Because medulloblastomas commonly spread along CSF pathways, treatment should be directed at the entire neuraxis. About 5% of medulloblastomas metastasize to a systemic location, particularly to bone marrow, where synaptophysin staining aids their recognition.[13]

Nuclear crowding and high nuclear to cytoplasmic ratio impart a distinctly *blue* macroscopic appearance

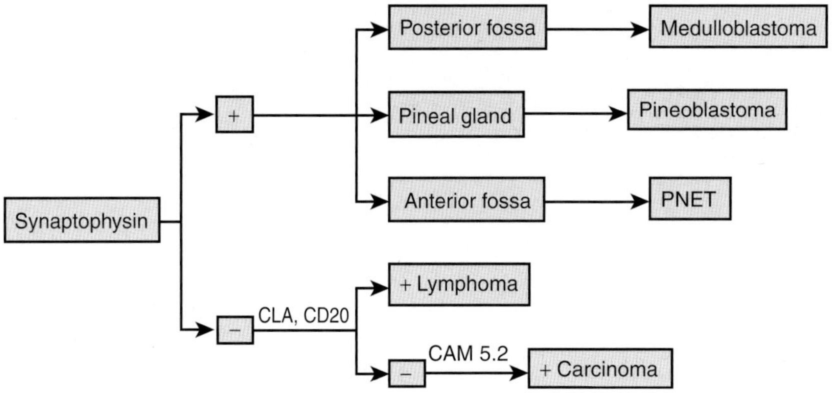

BOX 20.3 Immunohistochemical diagnosis of tumor crowded with malignant nuclei and little cytoplasm.

to the medulloblastoma on H&E staining. These malignant cells have higher nuclear:cytoplasmic ratios than malignant gliomas, and they rarely amplify EGFR.[147,148]

Rosettes that have cores filled with fibrils (Homer Wright rosettes) in the CNS are characteristic of medulloblastomas (see Fig. 20.21A); however, in many biopsy samples of medulloblastoma, rosettes are only vague to nonexistent. In the absence of desmoplasia or large malignant cells, this type is called *classic medulloblastoma*.

Virtually all medulloblastomas express synaptophysin, its most reliable marker of neuronal differentiation, which is not seen in lymphoma and is uncommon in carcinoma (see Fig. 20.21B).[3] Synaptophysin can be focal or diffuse. Special care is needed to trace it back to malignant cells, particularly in gray matter where synaptophysin abounds. One must look for regions of solid tumor and regions where tumor involves white matter. Compare regions of high versus low tumor cell density, and see whether synaptophysin increases with tumor cell density. Inspect individual tumor cells with high magnification and a good nuclear counterstain to determine whether malignant cells have synaptophysin. Cytoplasmic synaptophysin is often present and easier to evaluate than surface staining.

Protein gene product 9.5 (PGP 9.5) is described in texts as another marker of neuronal differentiation of these tumors. S-100 protein may be found in medulloblastomas. In this author's experience, finding PGP 9.5, NSE, and S-100 protein must be carefully interpreted because of its presence in other neoplasms in the differential diagnosis, including most gliomas and some carcinomas.[3] These markers seem to work better for peripheral neuroblastomas than for medulloblastomas. Staining for synaptophysin and the presence of fibrillar cellular processes works best (see Fig. 20.21B). Difficult cases can be examined for their ultrastructure.

This collection of small malignant cells must be distinguished from small cell undifferentiated carcinoma and lymphoma (see Table 20.8). The examiner should look for cellular processes. To indicate medulloblastoma, the fibrillar cellular processes must come directly from the neoplastic cells. Synaptophysin, S-100 protein, and, less often, NF protein stains highlight these processes.

An uncommon variant of medulloblastoma, large cell medulloblastoma, has large cells with prominent nucleoli, nuclear molding, and high rates of mitosis and apoptosis. This variant is aggressive and gives patients a poor prognosis.[2]

Although confirmation by larger studies would be appropriate, evidence suggests that GFAP reactivity in medulloblastoma is associated with longer survival than nonreactivity.[149]

Desmoplastic Medulloblastoma

Regions of medulloblastomas may contain proliferating cells that can be demonstrated by reticulin staining (Fig. 20.39; see Table 20.7). Pale reticulin-free islands of cells with perinuclear halos are often neuroblastic and react positively to staining for synaptophysin (see Fig. 20.39B*)*.[150] Desmoplastic medulloblastoma has been recently redefined to include only nodular medulloblastomas with neuronal and sometimes glial differentiation in the nodules only, and nodules surrounded by highly cellular "desmoplasia" composed of very proliferative cells making reticulin.[2] With standard treatments now employed, this group of tumors has a better prognosis than classic medulloblastoma.

Medullomyoblastoma

Medullomyoblastomas occur in the midline posterior fossa of children and contain smooth or striated muscle fibers.[74] They are mixtures of stainable muscle cells and small neuroectodermal cells resembling medulloblastoma, in contrast to pure primary intracranial rhabdomyosarcomas, which do not contain cells derived from neuroectoderm.[76] Synaptophysin and retinal-S antigen markers facilitate detection of these neuroectodermal cells. Immunoperoxidase stains for desmin and muscle-specific actin markers confirm muscular differentiation (see Table 20.8). Mesodermal elements other than muscle are occasionally found in medulloblastomas and medullomyoblastomas.[13] The medullomyoblastoma has lately been considered a subtype of medulloblastoma.[2]

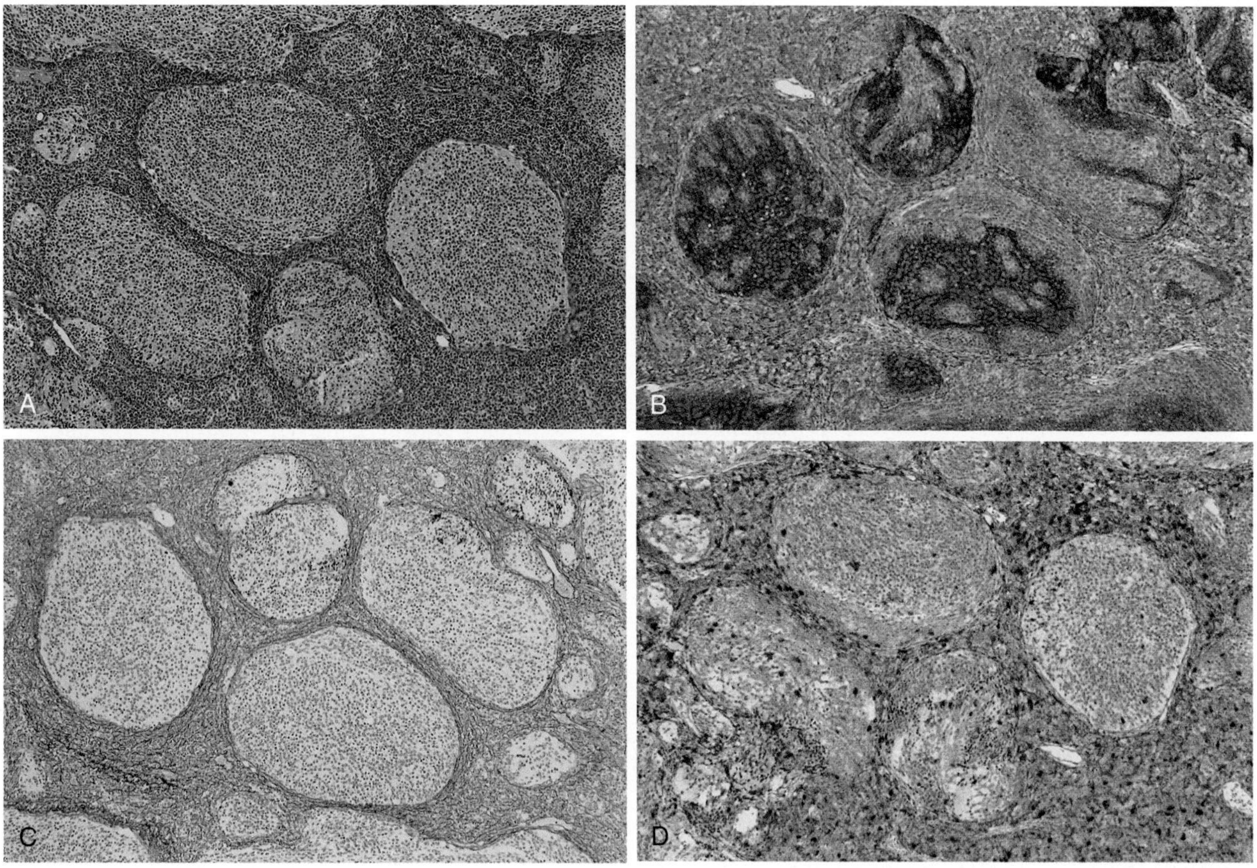

FIGURE 20.39 This desmoplastic medulloblastoma shows pale islands on H&E **(A)** that contain synaptophysin-positive cells **(B)**. Adjacent sections of the same region of tumor show that densely crowded cells form reticulin-positive bands **(C)** around the pale islands and that these bands contain most of the MIB1-positive cells **(D)**.

PRIMITIVE NEUROECTODERMAL TUMOR

The features and differential diagnosis of central nervous primitive neuroectodermal tumor (cPNET) can be found in the Medulloblastoma section earlier in this chapter. Although cerebral PNET, cerebellar medulloblastoma, and pineoblastoma are all primitive neuroectodermal tumors by histology alone, the recent tendency has been to recognize the cerebral tumor as a PNET, the posterior fossa tumor as a medulloblastoma, and the pineal tumor as a pineoblastoma (see Box 20.3). It is this author's opinion that these tumors are all different and that their differences will eventually be revealed with better markers. The cerebral ganglioneuroblastoma and neuroblastoma are called PNET with advanced neuronal differentiation.[2]

Markers of neuronal differentiation such as synaptophysin usually show PNETs with neuronal differentiation (see Box 20.3). Expression of a variety of other ectodermal and neuroectodermal antigens and association with neural tube defects reflect the embryonal nature of these neoplasms.[151]

Peripheral PNETs are intensely immunoreactive with MIC2 (Fig. 20.40) and NSE. Sites of occurrence of pPNET include neural crest derivatives, gonads, chest wall, bone including vertebral column, cranial vault, and cauda equina.[152] Peripheral PNETs are highly aggressive. They recur locally and metastasize to specific organs.[13]

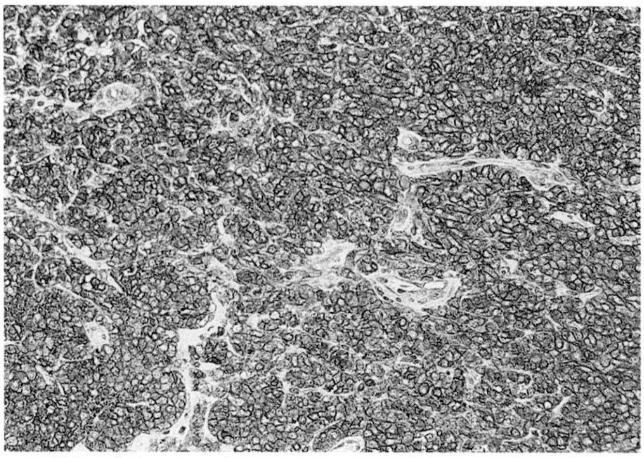

FIGURE 20.40 This peripheral primitive neuroectodermal tumor (pPNET) is diffusely and intensely positive for MIC2.

Beyond Immunohistochemistry: Anatomic Molecular Diagnostic Applications

The medulloblastoma is a CNS primitive neuroectodermal tumor (cPNET) in the cerebellum. The most frequent genetic abnormality associated with medulloblastoma is loss of chromosome arm 17p. This is often seen as an isochromosome 17q (one chromosome composed of two long arms of chromosome 17), which can be detected by ISH enhanced by immunostaining.[147] In a study of 8 cerebral cPNETs and 35 medulloblastomas, no cerebral cPNETs showed this abnormality, whereas 13 medulloblastomas showed it.[153] Cerebral cPNETs are uncommon and numbers are small, but this suggests that cerebral cPNETs are different from medulloblastomas.

In contrast to the cPNET, the peripheral PNET (pPNET) is defined by its t(11;22q24;q12) chromosomal translocation. This 11;22 translocation can be seen with FISH. PCR is an elegant assay for precise definition of the specific chimeric gene of EWS-FLI1.[152]

Earlier in this chapter, I introduced Li-Fraumeni syndrome (LFS), a germline mutation of the *p53* gene on the short arm of chromosome 17. Medulloblastoma and PNET account for about 10% of all brain tumors associated with a germline mutation of the *p53* gene.[2,95]

ATYPICAL TERATOID/RHABDOID TUMOR

Atypical teratoid/rhabdoid tumor (AT/RT) has been defined relatively recently (see Table 20.8). Infants and young children suffer from this highly malignant tumor.[154] Its high frequency of patients younger than 3 years of age may account for 10% of CNS tumors in infants being AT/RT.[155] It occurs throughout the CNS, especially in the posterior fossa. It metastasizes early through the CSF. Malignant cells have a pinker cytoplasm and are more epithelial than those in medulloblastoma. The plethora of immunohistochemical markers that these express contributes significantly to the definition of this tumor (Fig. 20.41). Atypical teratoid-rhabdoid tumor contains multiple intermediate filament (IF) types: nearly always vimentin and EMA, and often focal SMA, GFAP, CK, or other IF types. Synaptophysin and chromogranin may be present. Atypical teratoid-rhabdoid tumors have abnormalities of chromosome 22, particularly involving loss or mutation at the INI1 locus at 22q11.2. The INI1 nuclear protein is lost in most AT/RTs; thus, a loss of INI1 immunostaining can help to distinguish AT/RTs from PNETs and medulloblastoma that retain INI1 expression.[156]

RARE EMBRYONAL TUMORS

The medulloepithelioma looks like carcinoma but occurs in childhood, an unlikely age for carcinoma. The pseudostratified columnar epithelium of medulloepithelioma is crowded with cells that resemble those lining the embryonic neural tube. It rests on a type IV collagen basement membrane and fibrous stroma. The basal layer of the epithelium expresses nestin, vimentin, and microtubule-associated protein type 5 immunoreactivity. Focal differentiation and expression of either GFAP, S-100 protein, NSE (Fig. 20.42), NF protein, CK, or EMA immunoreactivity frequently occur.[157]

The ependymoblastoma usually occurs in the cerebrum of a child (see Table 20.8).[158] It resembles a PNET decorated with well-formed rosettes lined by mitotically active epithelioid cells. Unlike in medulloepithelioma, the rosettes in ependymoblastoma merge into densely cellular malignant cells without a collagenous stroma. Ependymoblastomas contain vimentin. Their GFAP-negative rosettes stain differently from GFAP-positive rosettes in ependymomas.[2,3,76] Ependymoblastoma is more cellular than anaplastic ependymoma and has less vascular proliferation.

KEY DIAGNOSTIC POINTS

Embryonal Tumors

- These multipotential tumors may express almost any neuroectodermal marker, but particularly synaptophysin. Some show additional markers, particularly vimentin.
- Many are seen in childhood.
- There is high cellular density.
- High proliferation is reflected in high MIB1 LI, often above 20%, and frequent mitotic activity.
- Despite their categorical grade of IV, specific diagnosis is important because some entities are very sensitive to radiotherapy or chemotherapy.

Meningeal and Related Tumors

MENINGIOMAS

Meningeal location is a major discriminator of meningioma from other primary intracranial neoplasms (Table 20.9; see Tables 20.5 to 20.7). Meningiomas are attached to dura or falx, which facilitates their recognition. Meningiomas arise less commonly from the choroid plexus and rarely within the CNS parenchyma.[159]

The classic genetic abnormality in meningioma is partial or complete loss of chromosome 22.[1,5] This loss can be detected by chromosomal ISH visualized by immunostaining.

Certain features provide evidence of meningioma. A syncytial appearance is a distinctive feature of meningothelial meningiomas and a focal feature of other subtypes of meningioma (see Fig. 20.40; see Table 20.9). The structural bases of this syncytial appearance are numerous tightly interdigitating cellular processes held together by desmosomes rather than a true syncytium. Meningothelial whorls and psammoma bodies typify meningiomas. The presence of these features on H&E–stained slides diminishes the need for immunohistochemical analysis.[88] Psammoma bodies are concentrically laminated calcifications.

Meningiomas contain EMA,[3] although it is often expressed focally and can be missed in small specimens. EMA positivity plus lack of GFAP distinguishes meningiomas from gliomas (Fig. 20.43; see Fig. 20.1B).[160] A positive EMA is the most decisive IHC marker of meningioma. Expression of progesterone receptors by meningiomas is variable. The intensity of vimentin expression by meningiomas has stimulated its use in these tumors. Vimentin markers should be used only in combination with other markers because many other tumors express

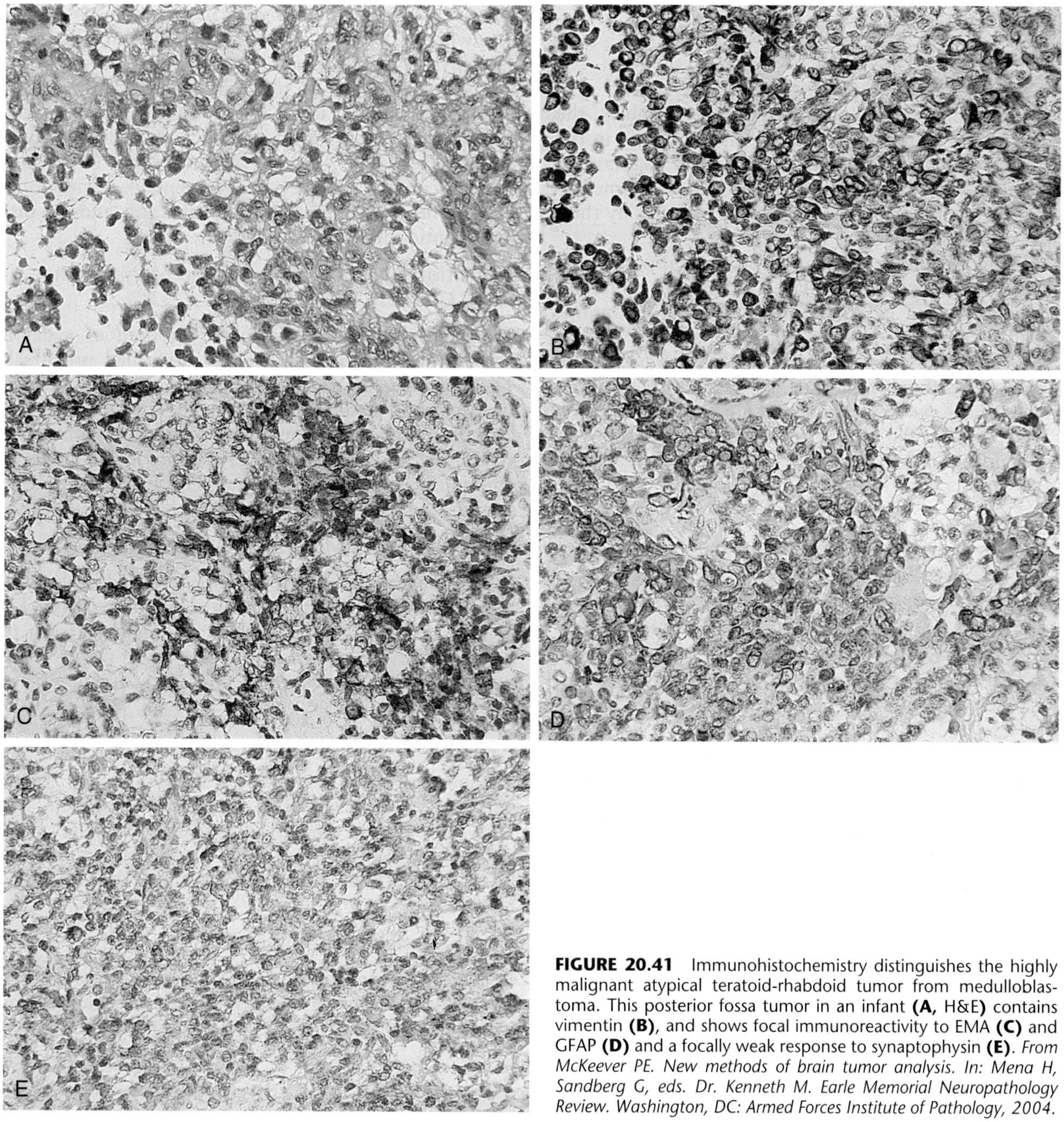

FIGURE 20.41 Immunohistochemistry distinguishes the highly malignant atypical teratoid-rhabdoid tumor from medulloblastoma. This posterior fossa tumor in an infant **(A,** H&E**)** contains vimentin **(B)**, and shows focal immunoreactivity to EMA **(C)** and GFAP **(D)** and a focally weak response to synaptophysin **(E)**. *From McKeever PE. New methods of brain tumor analysis. In: Mena H, Sandberg G, eds. Dr. Kenneth M. Earle Memorial Neuropathology Review. Washington, DC: Armed Forces Institute of Pathology, 2004.*

vimentin. Meningiomas are variable and focal in these three markers, but they often have more reticulin, fibronectin, and collagen in their parenchyma than low-grade gliomas.

Fibrous Meningioma (Fibroblastic Meningioma; WHO Grade I)

Fibrous meningiomas are firm tumors composed of spindle cells (see Table 20.5). They resemble schwannomas, solitary fibrous tumors, fibrillary astrocytomas, and pilocytic astrocytomas.[1,161] Fibrous meningiomas contain parenchymal collagen, often in large, pink bundles on H&E staining that distinguish them from astrocytomas.[3]

The similarity of fibrous meningiomas to schwannomas poses a particular diagnostic problem with tumors in the cerebellopontine angle and around spinal nerve roots. Structures that identify meningiomas in this context include whorls, psammoma bodies, and very thick bundles of collagen. Fibrous meningiomas express EMA, which schwannomas lack. The former usually show more vimentin and less S-100 protein than schwannomas.[3]

Fibrous meningiomas can be distinguished from solitary fibrous tumors (SFTs) by their immunohistochemical profiles.[161,162] Fibrous meningiomas express more EMA, S-100 protein, and glycogen and less CD34 than SFTs (Figs. 20.44 and 20.45).[162]

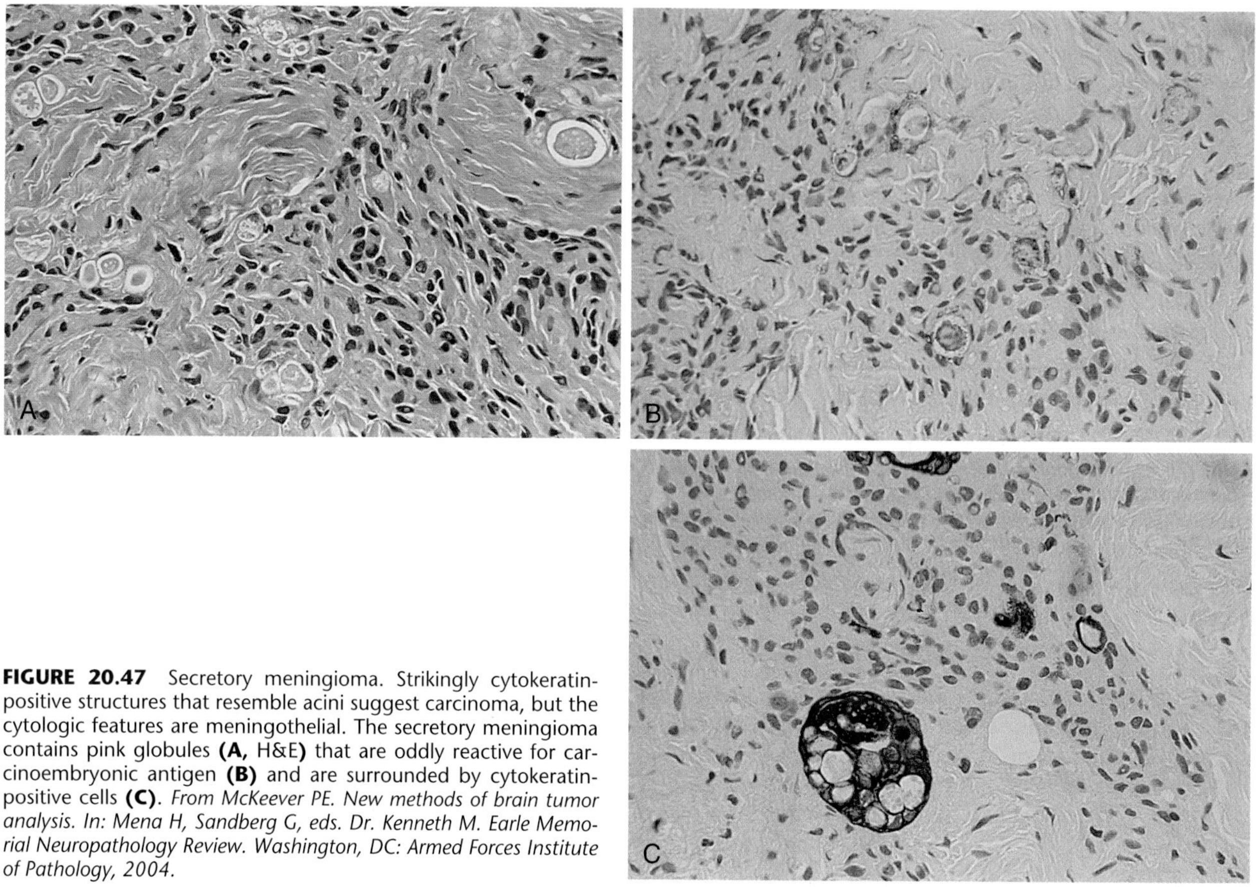

FIGURE 20.47 Secretory meningioma. Strikingly cytokeratin-positive structures that resemble acini suggest carcinoma, but the cytologic features are meningothelial. The secretory meningioma contains pink globules **(A,** H&E**)** that are oddly reactive for carcinoembryonic antigen **(B)** and are surrounded by cytokeratin-positive cells **(C)**. *From McKeever PE. New methods of brain tumor analysis. In: Mena H, Sandberg G, eds. Dr. Kenneth M. Earle Memorial Neuropathology Review. Washington, DC: Armed Forces Institute of Pathology, 2004.*

Clear Cell Meningioma (WHO Grade II as an Intracranial Tumor)

One of the many reasons to subclassify meningiomas is to identify more aggressive variants. The subtype clear cell meningioma is exemplary (Fig. 20.48). Although they look benign, many clear cell meningiomas are biologically aggressive.[2] Their clear cells resemble those in oligodendroglioma and clear cell ependymoma (see Box 20.1).[91] A mixture of clear cells and meningothelial features is a key to its diagnosis.[3] Cytoplasmic glycogen helps to confirm the diagnosis (see Fig. 20.48B and C).[91] Diffusely positive vimentin and focally positive EMA can aid in the identification of its meningothelial origin (see Fig. 20.48F and Table 20.9). This variant is particularly common in the lumbar and cerebellopontine angle regions.[170]

Atypical Meningioma (WHO Grade II)

Specific criteria for the distinction among benign meningioma, atypical meningioma, and anaplastic meningioma have been adopted by the WHO (Table 20.10).[2] Atypical meningioma is a meningioma with 4 to 19 mitotic figures in 10 high-power fields. Alternatively, this diagnosis can be made if three or more of the following histologic features are noted: increased cellularity; small cells with a high nuclear-to-cytoplasmic ratio; large prominent nucleoli; patternless, sheetlike growth; and foci of spontaneous or geographic necrosis. Atypical meningioma is a neoplasm that is likely to be more aggressive than grade 1 meningiomas and to recur locally.

This tumor is recognized as a distinct diagnostic entity with histopathologic features between those of benign and malignant meningiomas. Atypical meningiomas usually retain vimentin and at least slight, focal EMA immunoreactivity. EMA may show in more differentiated foci that often look meningotheliomatous.

Atypical meningiomas tend to be aggressive and to recur locally. Chromosomal abnormalities in addition to standard loss of 22 and increased MIB1 LI may forecast greater aggressiveness.[2,171]

Rhabdoid Meningioma (WHO Grade III)

A highly aggressive tumor, rhabdoid meningioma contains barely cohesive cells that are filled with abundant whorls of filaments that show immunocytochemical reactivity for vimentin.[6,172] These filaments push the meningothelial nuclei to the side of the cell.

Entirely rhabdoid tumors are difficult to distinguish from gemistocytic gliomas. In such cases, vimentin predominance, EMA reactivity, and lack of GFAP reveal their true identity.

Papillary Meningioma (WHO Grade III)

Papillary configurations in meningiomas are associated with high rates of local recurrence and metastases. The papillae have a CD31-positive vascular core.

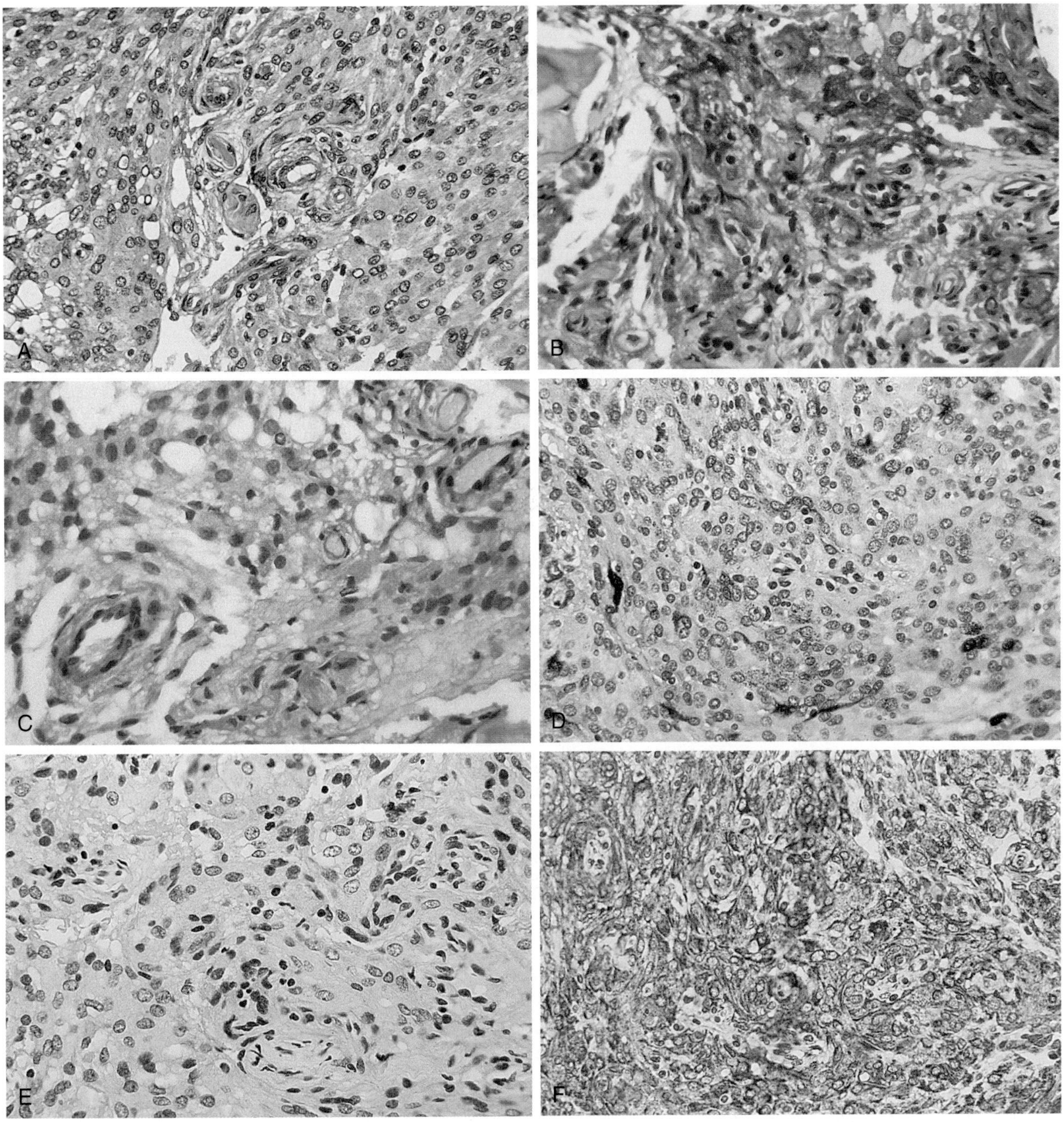

FIGURE 20.48 Clear cell meningioma. This tumor has recurred several times. The clear cell meningioma **(A,** H&E**)** contains red PAS-positive glycogen **(B)** eliminated by enzymes that digest glycogen **(C)**. This one contained scattered S-100 protein–positive cells **(D)** and no CK-positive cells **(E)**. The clear cell meningioma tends to be aggressive and difficult to manage surgically. Like most meningiomas, it is abundantly vimentin-positive **(F)**. *From McKeever PE. New methods of brain tumor analysis. In: Mena H, Sandberg G, eds. Dr. Kenneth M. Earle Memorial Neuropathology Review. Washington, DC: Armed Forces Institute of Pathology, 2004.*

Meningioma cells produce rosettes around these vessels, and, in addition to expected vimentin and S-100 protein, they may express CK.[173]

The recognition of a papillary meningioma in other than the dural locations characteristic of meningioma is difficult. Papillary meningiomas resemble papillary ependymomas, choroid plexus papillomas, and carcinomas.[163] One should look for a high ratio of vimentin to CK and absence of GFAP to identify the meningioma.

Anaplastic Meningioma (Malignant Meningioma) (WHO Grade III)

Anaplastic meningiomas are meningiomas with 20 or more mitoses per 10 high-power fields or regions with malignant cytologic features.[2,3,174] Nuclear staining for *p53* tumor suppressor gene product is evident in 10% of malignant meningiomas. The mean MIB1 LI among 20 tumors in one series was 11.7%, with a wide range between 1% and 24% in individual tumors (MIB PI).[175]

TABLE 20.10 WHO Criteria for Grading of Meningiomas*

Meningioma (Grade I)	Atypical Meningioma (Grade II)	Anaplastic Meningioma (Grade III)
<4 mitotic figures per 10 hpf (0.16 mm²)	Increased mitotic activity: 4-19 per 10 hpf (0.16 mm²)	Increased mitotic activity: >19 per 10 hpf (0.16 mm²)
Fails to meet diagnostic criteria to right	OR >2: Increased cellularity Small cells with high nuclear-to-cytoplasmic ratio Prominent nucleoli Sheetlike and/or patternless growth pattern Foci of spontaneous or geographic necrosis meningiomas	OR: Malignant and/or anaplastic cytologic appearance (e.g., resembling sarcoma, carcinoma, melanoma)
Fits into a well-differentiated subtype (text)	(WHO grade II is assigned to clear cell and chordoid meningiomas)	(WHO grade III is assigned to rhabdoid and papillary meningiomas)

*Brain invasion is not a criterion for increased grade.
hpf, high-power field; *OR*, either mitotic or cytologic criteria needed for diagnosis.
Modified from McKeever PE, Boyer PJ. The brain, spinal cord, and meninges. In: Mills SE, Carter D, Greenson, JK, et al., eds. Sternberg's Diagnostic Surgical Pathology, 4th ed. New York, NY: Lippincott Williams & Wilkins; 2004:399-506.

KEY DIAGNOSTIC POINTS

Meningiomas

- Most are benign, grade I. Location affects their chance for total removal and thus affects individual patient prognosis.
- Grade II and III aggressive meningiomas occur as both specific subtypes (e.g., chordoid, rhabdoid) and as the standard subtypes of meningioma with specific ominous features such as mitotic indices of atypical and malignant meningiomas.
- EMA is the most specific positive marker of meningiomas.
- Virtually all meningiomas express vimentin, but so do many other tumors.

Theranostic Applications

For decades surgeons knew that meningiomas in some women grew during pregnancy. Now we know why: Many meningiomas have progesterone receptors (PR).[176] There are also reasons to assess the PR of meningiomas for patient management, particularly meningiomas that have not been totally removed surgically. PR status may affect decisions about pregnancy (see Fig. 20.46)[1] or taking progesterone supplements. In the future, PR-positive meningiomas may respond to a therapy that blocks the hormone in question.[177] It is worth exploring to determine which higher-grade meningiomas may have decreased or absent PR receptors.[2]

Beyond Immunohistochemistry: Anatomic Molecular Diagnostic Applications

The neurofibromatosis 2 (*NF2*) tumor-suppressor gene is located on the long arm of chromosome 22 at 22q12. It encodes for the Merlin (Schwannomin) protein, which is responsible for the inherited disease neurofibromatosis 2. *NF2* gene mutations predominantly occur in transitional and fibroblastic meningiomas, whereas the meningothelial and secretory meningioma variants are less affected.[178,179] *In situ* hybridization is an efficient and reliable method for routinely assessing *NF2* gene deletion in formalin-fixed, paraffin-embedded tissues.[180] An immunohistochemical assay for Merlin is also available.[178]

HEMANGIOPERICYTOMA (WHO GRADE II OR III)

Hemangiopericytoma is a highly cellular and mitotically active neoplasm that is rich in pericellular reticulin and stainable with anti-type IV collagen. Eighty percent of these tumors recur, and 23% metastasize.[13,181]

Hemangiopericytomas (HPC) are distinguished from benign meningiomas by their hypercellularity, higher mitotic index, and microscopic tendency to bulge into vascular lumens without bursting through the endothelium (see Table 20.8). Although there are exceptions, these tumors tend to lack markers other than the relatively ubiquitous factor XIIIa, mesenchymal markers, and Leu7.[167,182]

The spectrum of immunohistochemical markers for hemangiopericytoma overlaps with that for fibrous meningioma, but lack of EMA has become symbolic of the former (Fig. 20.49).[161] The hemangiopericytoma is distinguished from malignant glioma and metastatic carcinoma by foci of extensive reticulin around individual neoplastic cells. Hemangiopericytoma also lacks the GFAP found in glioma, and its nuclei are less pleomorphic and less spindled than those of fibrosarcoma.

SOLITARY FIBROUS TUMOR

The solitary fibrous tumor (SFT) is a soft tissue tumor (see Chapter 4). It resembles fibrous meningioma but has a different immunohistochemical profile (see Figs. 20.44 and 20.45).[3,161,183] Its parenchymal cells express abundant CD34 and collagen. They lack EMA. IHC is critical in distinguishing SFT from meningioma. SFT and HPC have been said to be the same tumor, a matter that deserves further consideration. SFT is more common in pleura than dura. Malignant transformation of the solitary fibrous tumor may be associated with trisomy 8.[184]

Chordoma and Sarcomas

CHORDOMA

Approximately 40% of chordomas arise in the clivus; 10% arise along cervical, 2% along thoracic, and 2% along lumbar vertebrae; and more than 45% arise in the sacral portions of the spinal canal.[3]

Physaliphorous cells of chordomas contain large characteristic intracytoplasmic vacuoles (Fig. 20.50; see Table 20.6). Because the cells frequently grow in cords, these vacuoles occasionally line up like beads on a string, distinguishing chordoma from chondroid neoplasms, which have individual cells embedded in cartilage.[185] Chordomas contain CK (see Fig. 20.50A), EMA, 5′-nucleotidase, and desmosomes, whereas chondrosarcomas lack these features.[185] Presence of CK is the standard discriminator of chordoma from CK-negative chondrosarcoma.[3]

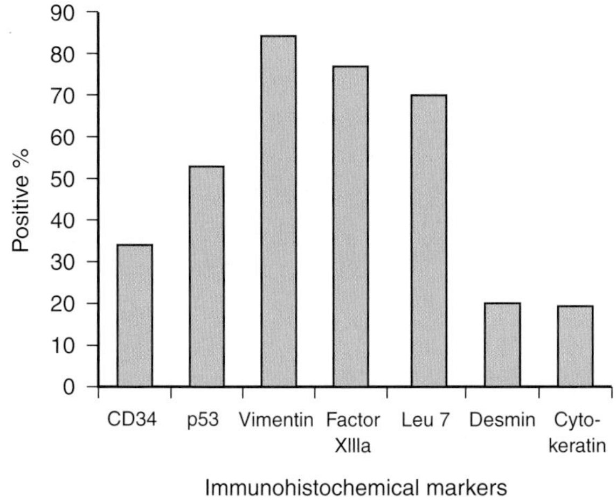

FIGURE 20.49 Immunochemical staining results of 27 meningeal hemangiopericytomas. *Percentages positive are as reported in Perry A, Scheithauer BW, Nascimento AG. The immunophenotypic spectrum of meningeal hemangiopericytoma: A comparison with fibrous meningioma and solitary fibrous tumor of meninges. Am J Surg Pathol. 1997;21:1354-1360.*

Chordoma cells are exuberantly bifilamentous (see Fig. 20.50), containing vimentin and CK in the same cell. The vacuoles of physaliphorous cells contain mucin and glycogen. Their structure is distinct from that of watery perinuclear oligodendroglial halos and the multiplicity of smaller lipid vacuoles of hemangioblastomas (see Figs. 20.22, 20.50, and 20.56B).

Malignant histologic transformation of chordoma is uncommon. Nevertheless, relentless local invasion of clinically sensitive regions results in a poor long-term prognosis.

Chondroid chordomas contain regions of classic chordoma that are positive for EMA, CK, and S-100 as well as chondroid regions that are S-100-positive and lack EMA and CK.[185] The existence of chondroid chordoma has been challenged by some pathologists, who prefer to interpret such tumors as either chordomas or low-grade chondrosarcomas.

SARCOMAS

Sarcomas are rare among brain tumors.[77] Reported incidences of primary intracranial sarcomas vary from 0.08% to 4.3%, and the former percentage is more contemporary.[186] GFAP immunohistochemical analysis has demonstrated that tumors formerly considered sarcomas are actually primary brain tumors, particularly glioblastomas, medulloblastomas, and primary lymphomas.[58]

Causes of some sarcomas are known. Intracranial radiation is a surprisingly common cause of sarcoma.[187 188] Intracranial Kaposi's sarcoma is rare, and most cases are associated with immunodeficiency.[189]

The mesenchymal chondrosarcoma is rare. It originates in the intracranial and spinal meninges and cauda equina in childhood and young adulthood.[190] The

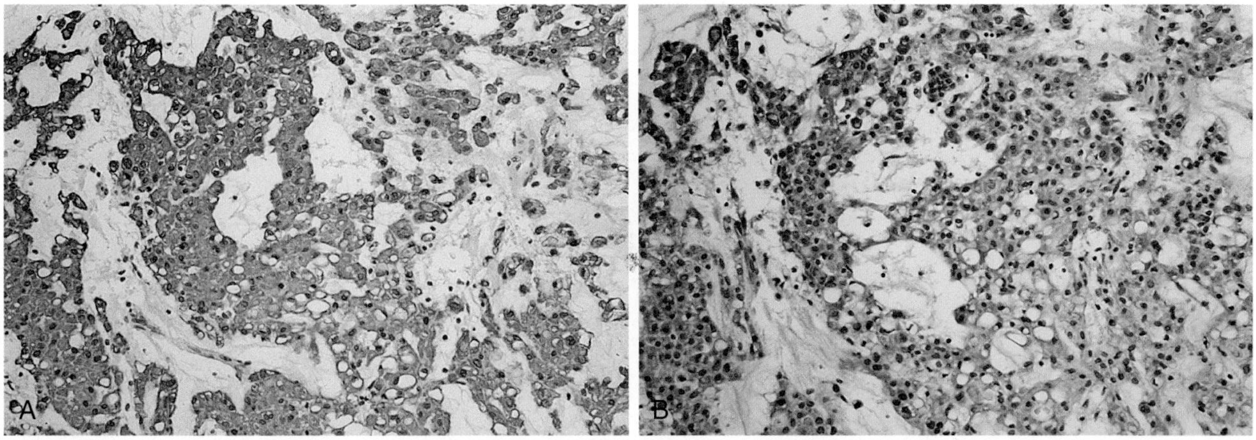

FIGURE 20.50 Chordoma. **(A)** Cords of physaliphorous cells are positive for CK, a most important immunohistochemical feature in distinguishing chordoma from CK-negative chondrosarcoma. **(B)** The tumor also was positive for vimentin. This specimen demonstrates the propensity of chordomas to express more than one intermediate filament.

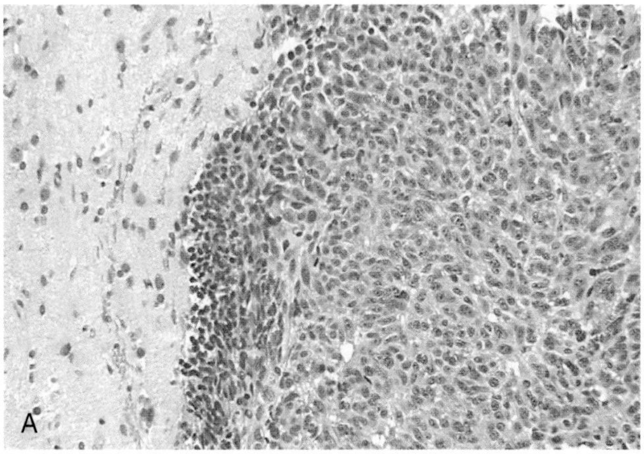

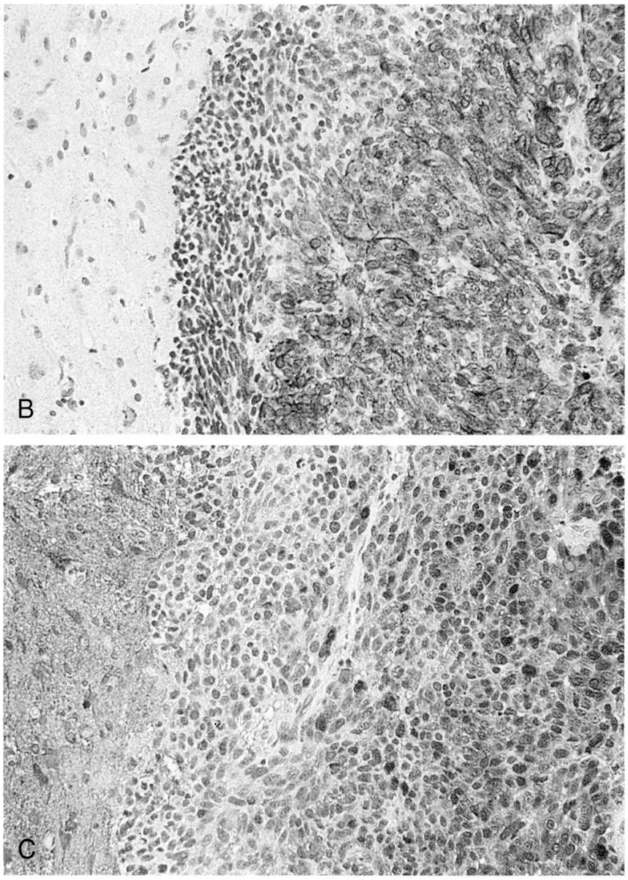

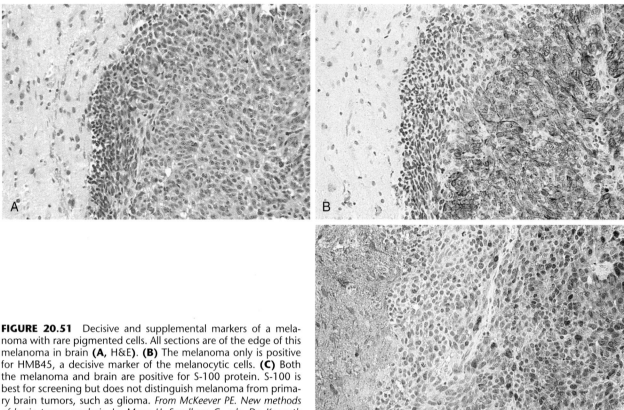

FIGURE 20.51 Decisive and supplemental markers of a melanoma with rare pigmented cells. All sections are of the edge of this melanoma in brain **(A,** H&E**)**. **(B)** The melanoma only is positive for HMB45, a decisive marker of the melanocytic cells. **(C)** Both the melanoma and brain are positive for S-100 protein. S-100 is best for screening but does not distinguish melanoma from primary brain tumors, such as glioma. *From McKeever PE. New methods of brain tumor analysis. In: Mena H, Sandberg G, eds. Dr. Kenneth M. Earle Memorial Neuropathology Review. Washington, DC: Armed Forces Institute of Pathology, 2004.*

mesenchymal chondrosarcoma resembles the hemangiopericytoma except for islands of S-100 protein–positive cartilage.

Poorly differentiated chondrosarcomas are rare and usually involve the meninges. A key feature is evidence of cartilage production, which is often sparse. Presence of S-100 protein as evidence of chondroid differentiation must be interpreted cautiously in meningeal and CNS neoplasms, because most gliomas, chordoma, melanoma, nerve sheath tumors, and an occasional meningioma contain this protein (Fig. 20.51C; see Figs. 20.24 and 20.48D).[3,160]

Primary cerebral rhabdomyosarcomas are rare.[191] Synaptophysin-negative staining differentiates them from synaptophysin-positive medullomyoblastomas.

Lack of GFAP-positive neoplastic glia distinguishes fibrosarcoma from glioblastoma invading the meninges and from gliosarcoma.[3] For specific features that differentiate individual sarcomas, see Chapter 4.

Nerve Sheath Tumors

Benign nerve sheath tumors (WHO grade I) can be subclassified as either schwannoma or neurofibroma, as described in the discussions of these tumors (see Table 20.5). Malignant nerve sheath tumors (WHO grade III or IV) are much more difficult to subclassify when they lose the characteristics of their benign counterparts. Leu7 and S-100 protein markers differentiate nerve sheath tumors from other tumors known to lack these markers.[13,192]

SCHWANNOMA (NEURILEMOMA, NEURINOMA) (WHO GRADE I)

The presence of a noninvasive tumor next to a peripheral nerve suggests the diagnosis of schwannoma. Verocay bodies are more distinctive of schwannomas than the Antoni A and Antoni B patterns but are not seen in all schwannomas.

Bilateral eighth nerve schwannomas indicate neurofibromatosis of NF-2 type. Unusual locations and associations with meningeal proliferation are also seen with NF-2.[193] Both NF-2 and schwannomas are associated with abnormalities in chromosome 22.[1,5]

The histologic appearance of schwannoma is similar to that of fibrous meningioma, tanycytic ependymoma, subependymoma, and astrocytoma. Schwannoma is distinguished from these tumors by its very robust and abundant parenchymal reticulin, which is positive for type IV collagen (see Fig. 20.24A). Schwannomas have continuous basement membranes all along the exterior surfaces of their cells (see Table 20.5). Focal reactivity of some schwannomas with anti-GFAP requires care in the use of these antisera to distinguish the tumors from astrocytomas.[3] However, a negative GFAP response supports the diagnosis of schwannoma.

When they lack the characteristic features of meningioma, like meningeal whorls and psammoma bodies, fibrous meningiomas are more difficult than gliomas to distinguish from schwannomas. Antoni A and Antoni B growth patterns in schwannomas resemble those seen in

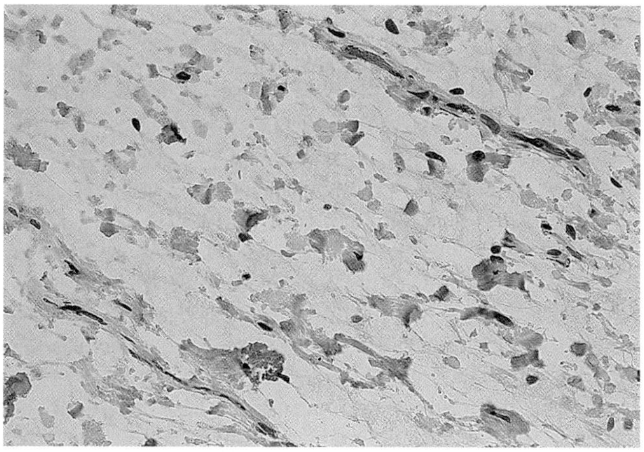

FIGURE 20.52 Neurofibroma. Occasional long brown axons within the tumor are dispersed among proliferating cells. (Anti-NF stain with hematoxylin counterstain.) *Courtesy of Drs. Andrew Flint and Victor Elner, University of Michigan, Ann Arbor, Mich.*

fibrous meningiomas. Schwannomas contain Leu7 and S-100 protein[13] and lack EMA. Reactivity of meningiomas for EMA is therefore a useful discriminator. Both tumors contain S-100 protein, but S-100 is more ubiquitous and abundant in schwannomas (see Fig. 20.24B).[3] There is evidence that sole expression of the beta subunit of S-100 may distinguish eighth nerve schwannomas from some meningiomas.[194] If present, GFAP-positive foci can distinguish a schwannoma from a meningioma. Meningioma cells are GFAP negative.

Beyond Immunohistochemistry: Anatomic Molecular Diagnostic Applications

The *NF2* gene is a tumor suppressor on chromosome 22. Loss of expression of the NF2 protein product, Merlin (Schwannomin), is associated with both sporadic and NF2-related schwannomas.[195] Merlin is a cytoskeleton-associated tumor suppressor protein regulated by phosphorylation at serine 518 (S518). Unphosphorylated Merlin restricts cell proliferation by inhibiting Rac and p21-activated kinase (Pak).[196] In Merlin-deficient schwannoma cells, Rac causes nonfunctional intercellular adhesion in aggregation assays that could cause increased proliferation rates owing to loss of contact inhibition.[197]

NEUROFIBROMA (WHO GRADE I)

The key to recognition of neurofibromas is their involvement within peripheral nerve rather than next to it (see Table 20.5). Neurofibroma differs from schwannoma in having stainable NF-positive axons running through the tumor itself rather than confined to the periphery.[3] This is because the neurofibroma is a swelling of the nerve itself, with a mixture of Schwann cells, fibroblasts, collagen, and mucoid material enclosed in a weakly EMA-positive perineurium. In contrast, schwannomas grow next to and compress the nerve, so that neurofilaments are not evident within the central tumor nidus. The larger the neurofibroma, the more the axons are "diluted" with neoplastic cells. Fortunately, today's anti-NF antibodies can detect individual axons in a "haystack" of tumor tissue (Fig. 20.52).

Neurofibroma may occur as a sporadic tumor or as part of the dominantly inherited tumor syndrome called von Recklinghausen disease or neurofibromatosis-1 (NF-1).[1] Plexiform neurofibromas are multiple swollen fascicles that are associated with NF-1. Other nervous system signs of NF-1 are more than one neurofibroma, optic nerve glioma (more appropriately called *optic nerve pilocytic astrocytoma*), and malignant peripheral nerve sheath tumor with glandular or rhabdomyoblastic regions.[2]

Beyond Immunohistochemistry: Anatomic Molecular Diagnostic Applications

NF1 is caused by constitutional mutations in the *NF1* gene, located in chromosome band 17q11. The *NF1* gene codes for a protein called *neurofibromin*, a GTPase activating protein (GAP) and tumor suppressor protein.[198] Although *NF1* gene involvement in the development of neurofibroma in von Recklinghausen patients has been characterized, it has been harder to prove the significance of inactivation of this gene in sporadic neurofibromas. However, there are well-studied sporadic neurofibromas that have inactivation of both *NF1* gene alleles.[199]

MALIGNANT PERIPHERAL NERVE SHEATH TUMOR

See Chapter 4, Immunohistology of Soft Tissue and Osseous Neoplasms.

Neuroendocrine tumors

See Chapter 10, Immunohistology of Endocrine Tumors.

Germ Cell Tumors

Within the cranial vault, 95% of primary germ cell tumors are found along the midline in the pineal and suprasellar regions, especially the former. About 10% involve both regions, and 25% arise in the suprasellar cistern. The mixed germ cell tumor and lymphoma (gerlymphoma) has only been seen in the sella turcica.[200] Germ cell tumors rarely involve spinal cord or peripheral nerve.[3]

Germinomas are the most common intracranial germ cell neoplasm. There are few differences between intracranial and gonadal germinomas.[201] For details about germ cell tumors, see Chapter 16, Immunohistology of the Prostate, Bladder, Testis, and Kidney, and Chapter 18, Immunohistology of the Female Genital Tract.

Hematopoietic and Lymphoid Neoplasms

LYMPHOMA (WHO GRADE III OR IV)

Primary CNS lymphomas grow within the CNS parenchyma (see Table 20.8). They have a diffuse invasive margin. These lymphomas are nearly always of B-cell origin (Fig. 20.53; see Box 20.3).[1,202-204] Some of these B-cell lymphomas afflict immunosuppressed patients, patients with AIDS, and those with other immunocompromised conditions.[205-207] With few exceptions, AIDS-related lymphomas have poor outcomes.[206,208] Primary CNS lymphomas of T-cell origin are rare.[209]

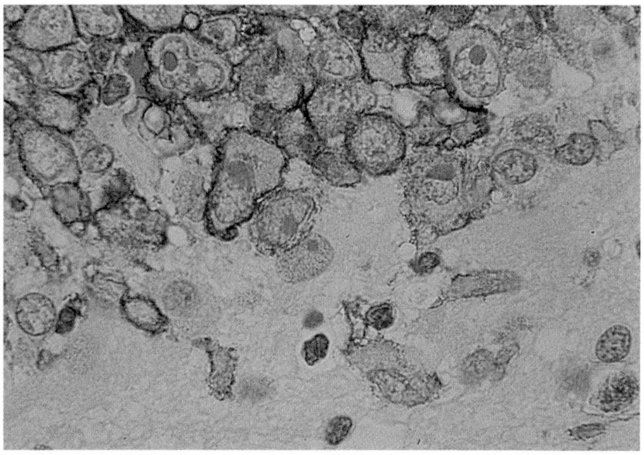

FIGURE 20.53 Primary brain lymphoma. Hematoxylin nuclear counterstain reveals malignant lymphocytes with clumped chromatin and huge nucleoli. The immunohistochemical stain is L26, a B-lymphocyte marker. Malignant lymphocytes were negative for T-cell and macrophage markers (*not shown*). *From McKeever PE. New methods of brain tumor analysis. In: Mena H, Sandberg G, eds. Dr. Kenneth M. Earle Memorial Neuropathology Review. Washington, DC: Armed Forces Institute of Pathology, 2004.*

In paraffin sections, CD20 and CD79a B-cell, and CD3 epsilon and CD45RO T-cell markers should be used along with LCA.[13] Because primary CNS lymphoma invades CNS parenchyma, responses to CNS markers such as GFAP must be interpreted with extreme caution. The nuclear counterstain identifies the non-neoplastic nuclei of gliosis in GFAP-positive cells intermixed among lymphoma cells. Monoclonal staining for B-cell (or, rarely, T-cell) markers helps distinguish lymphoma from CNS inflammation, which is polyclonal (see Fig. 20.3B and C), and from nonlymphoid neoplasms. However, many lymphomas contain polyclonal reactive lymphoid elements, which may be recognized from their smaller size and benign nuclei.[3]

The aforementioned markers are sufficient for most primary CNS lymphomas (see Box 20.1). For details about subclassifying these and other lymphomas, see Chapter 5, Immunohistology of Hodgkin Lymphoma, and Chapter 6, Immunohistology of Non-Hodgkin Lymphoma.

In patients with peripheral lymphoma, secondary involvement of the CNS can occur, with a frequency that has been estimated at 5% to 29% of patients.[3] Secondary involvement may occur anywhere, but it often involves the meninges.

POST-TRANSPLANTATION LYMPHOPROLIFERATIVE DISORDERS Following organ transplantation and associated immunosuppression, a range of post-transplantation lymphoproliferative disorders can develop. Histologic,

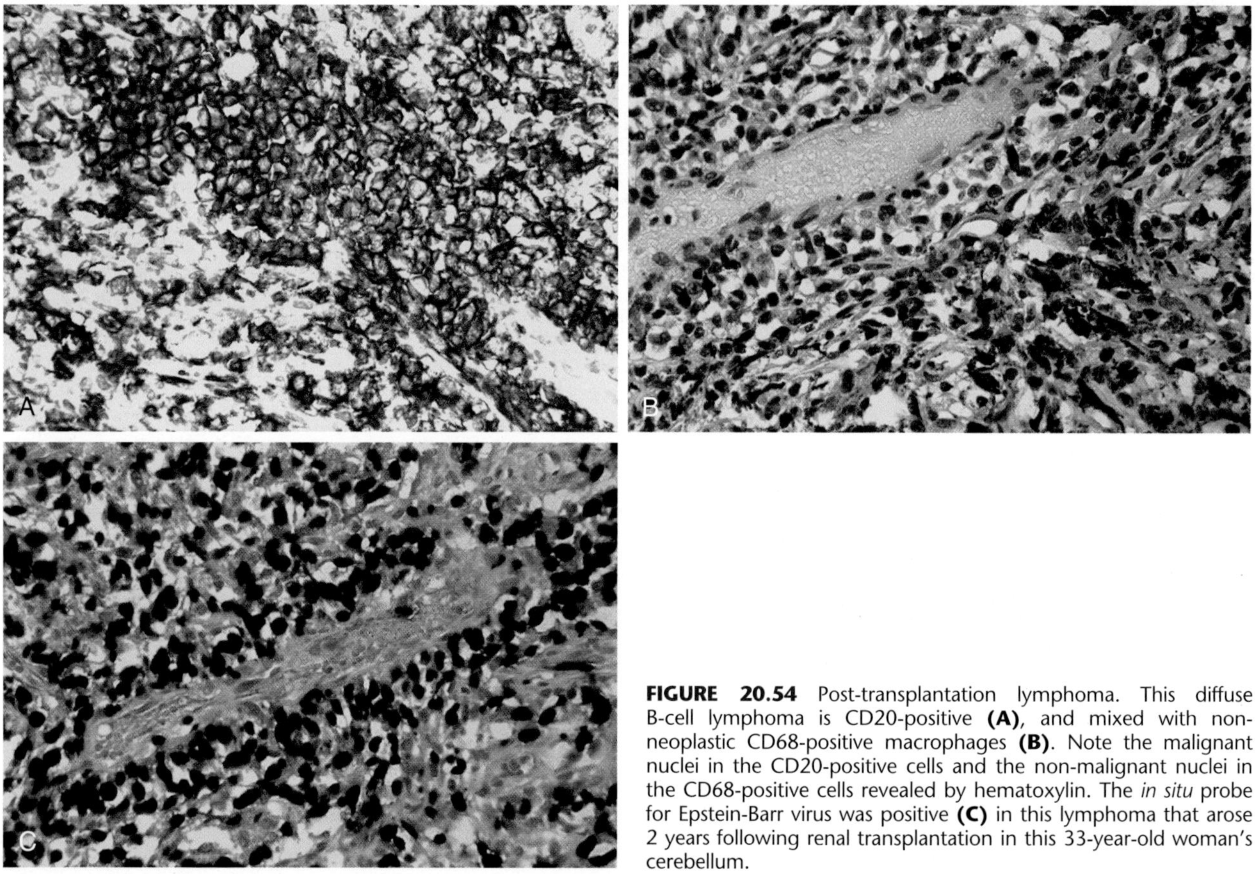

FIGURE 20.54 Post-transplantation lymphoma. This diffuse B-cell lymphoma is CD20-positive **(A)**, and mixed with non-neoplastic CD68-positive macrophages **(B)**. Note the malignant nuclei in the CD20-positive cells and the non-malignant nuclei in the CD68-positive cells revealed by hematoxylin. The *in situ* probe for Epstein-Barr virus was positive **(C)** in this lymphoma that arose 2 years following renal transplantation in this 33-year-old woman's cerebellum.

immunohistochemical, and gene rearrangement studies can distinguish among lymphoid or plasmacytic hyperplasia (polyclonal with no Ig gene rearrangement); atypical hyperplasia or B-cell hyperplasia and lymphoma (monoclonal with Ig rearrangement); and diffuse large B-cell immunoblastic lymphoma (monoclonal) (Fig. 20.54). Epstein-Barr virus can be identified in most cases of post-transplantation lymphoma.[203]

LYMPHOMATOID GRANULOMATOSIS This is a lymphoproliferative disease that resembles vasculitis and neoplasm. Lymphomatoid granulomatosis is an EBV-related process, so that the identification of EBV by *in situ* hybridization or immunoperoxidase aids the diagnosis. Lymphomatoid granulomatosis can progress to lymphoma. There have been claims that all lymphomatoid granulomatosis is lymphoma. CNS involvement is usually seen in conjunction with pulmonary disease.[3]

INTRAVASCULAR LYMPHOMA The CNS is one of the sites of predilection for intravascular lymphoma, a large B-cell lymphoma. The neoplastic cells fill the blood vessel lumina. The clinical presentation mimics vasculitis. Neoplastic cells are positive for CD20.

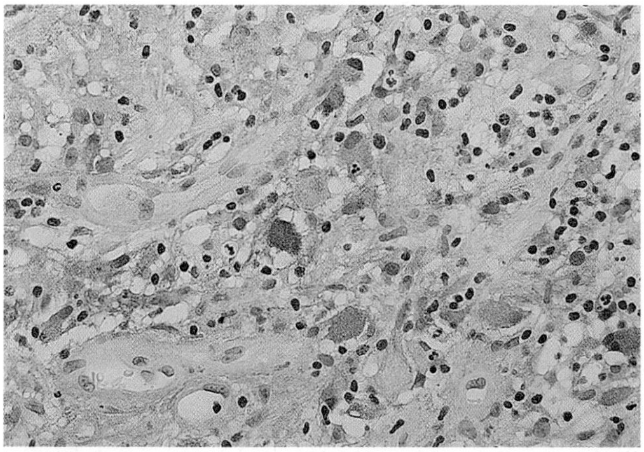

FIGURE 20.55 Histiocytosis. This specimen, from a mass within the brain parenchyma, contains S-100–positive cells. The immunohistochemical stain highlights intracellular leukocytes seen in Rosai-Dorfman disease.

LEUKEMIA

The diagnosis of leukemia within the craniospinal vault is usually established by cytologic examination of CSF.[210] Terminal intraparenchymal CNS hemorrhages reflect blast crises leading to leukocyte counts greater than $300{,}000/mm^3$. This results in intravascular leukostasis. Cerebral vasculitis is rarely associated with leukemia. Focal masses of leukemic cells (chloromas) in the meninges may be heralded by peripheral eosinophilia.[13]

HISTIOCYTOSIS

Histiocytosis occurs predominantly in children and young adults (see Table 20.5).[3] The CNS is often involved secondary to bony involvement or to systemic involvement, often by Langerhans histiocytosis. Non-Langerhans types of histiocytosis also occur (Fig. 20.55).[211,212] Although any region of brain or meninges may be affected, the parasellar region is particularly susceptible.[213] A typical lesion is firm because of the collagen fibers mixed with histiocytes and inflammatory cells. New lesions are less fibrotic than old. Langerhans cells are S-100 protein–positive. The literature suggests that CD1a has good sensitivity in this disease. However, its sensitivity is not quite 100%; therefore a panel of markers is recommended (Table 20.11). Lack of structural GFAP in cellular fibrils distinguishes histiocytes from astrocytes and from ependymal and subependymal cells. Electron microscopy identifies the Birbeck granules of Langerhans cell histiocytosis.[8,10,13]

Histiocytoses less common than Langerhans histiocytoses can be differentiated by their IHC and morphology. Erdheim-Chester disease of the CNS has characteristic Touton giant cells that are CD68 positive and CD1a negative.[203] Rosai-Dorfman disease, or sinus histiocytosis with massive lymphadenopathy, can be seen with or without systemic disease. It is characterized by emperipolesis, which is the engulfment by macrophages of intact leukocytes. The macrophages are CD68 positive, S-100 protein positive, and CD1a negative (see Table 20.11).

TABLE 20.11 Histiocytoses Affecting the Central Nervous System Compared with Macrophages

Disease	Characteristic Histology	CD68 (KP1)	S-100	CD1a	Birbeck Granules (EM)
Macrophage	Foamy epithelioid, multinucleated giant cells	+	–	–	–
Erdheim-Chester	Touton giant cells	+	S[a]	–	–
Rosai-Dorfman	Emperipolesis	+	+	–	–
Langerhans histiocytosis	Reniform nuclei, eosinophilic cytoplasm	+	+	+	+

Key to staining results: +, almost always strong, diffuse positivity; S, sometimes; many positive.
[a]S-100 has been positive in some, but not all, cases of Erdheim-Chester disease.
EM, electron microscopy.
Modified from McKeever PE, Boyer PJ. The brain, spinal cord, and meninges. In: Mills SE, Carter D, Greenson, JK, et al., eds. Sternberg's Diagnostic Surgical Pathology, 4th ed. New York, NY: Lippincott Williams & Wilkins; 2004:399-506.

Miscellaneous Intracranial or Spinal Masses

HEMANGIOBLASTOMA (CAPILLARY HEMANGIOBLASTOMA) (WHO GRADE I)

The capillary hemangioblastoma resembles an endocrine neoplasm (Fig. 20.56). It has close juxtaposition of capillary and stromal cells (see Table 20.7) and occasionally shows secretory granules or expresses erythropoietin.[214] Its pink, vacuolated stromal cells often contain NSE, which is present in neuroendocrine cells.[215] No gland of origin has been found.

Because the hemangioblastoma is nonfibrillar, it should not resemble an astrocytoma. However, the resemblance may occur for two reasons: sampling and artifact. Cerebellar hemangioblastomas are often cystic, with the actual neoplasm embedded somewhere in the wall of the cyst as a mural nodule. Biopsy specimens of the cyst wall may show conspicuously GFAP-positive gliosis (see the Gliosis versus Glioma section later in this chapter).

Sampling a hemangioblastoma can reveal GFAP-positive cells.[216] Some of these cells are reactive astrocytes (common near the periphery of the tumor). However, others are stromal cells (common in the cellular and angioglioma variants of hemangioblastoma), which either take up GFAP from adjacent reactive astrocytes or express their own GFAP.[217] To minimize confusion, the central portion of the solid tumor should be sampled.

Epithelioid hemangioblastoma can resemble paraganglioma[218] or renal cell carcinoma. Hemangioblastomas have more capillaries and much less chromogranin A than paragangliomas.[219] Compared with renal cell carcinoma, hemangioblastoma has more uniform distribution of nuclear chromatin, absence of necrosis, small nucleoli, and intimate arrangement of capillaries and stromal cells (see Fig. 20.56A). This arrangement is accentuated by staining with CD31, CD34, anti–factor VIII, or anti–gamma enolase (NSE).[215] In contrast to renal cell carcinoma, hemangioblastomas tend to stain for NSE, and they do not stain for EMA or CK (see Fig. 20.56B and C).

Beyond Immunohistochemistry: Anatomic Molecular Diagnostic Applications

Many hemangioblastomas are associated with von Hippel-Lindau (VHL) disease. VHL disease should be considered in patients with more than one tumor or a hemangioblastoma in an unusual location.[216] Two hemangioblastomas, one hemangioblastoma and a family history of VHL disease, or one hemangioblastoma and another tumor seen in VHL make the clinical diagnosis of VHL disease. Tumors other than hemangioblastoma seen in VHL are endolymphatic sac tumors, broad ligament or epididymal cystadenoma, pancreatic cysts

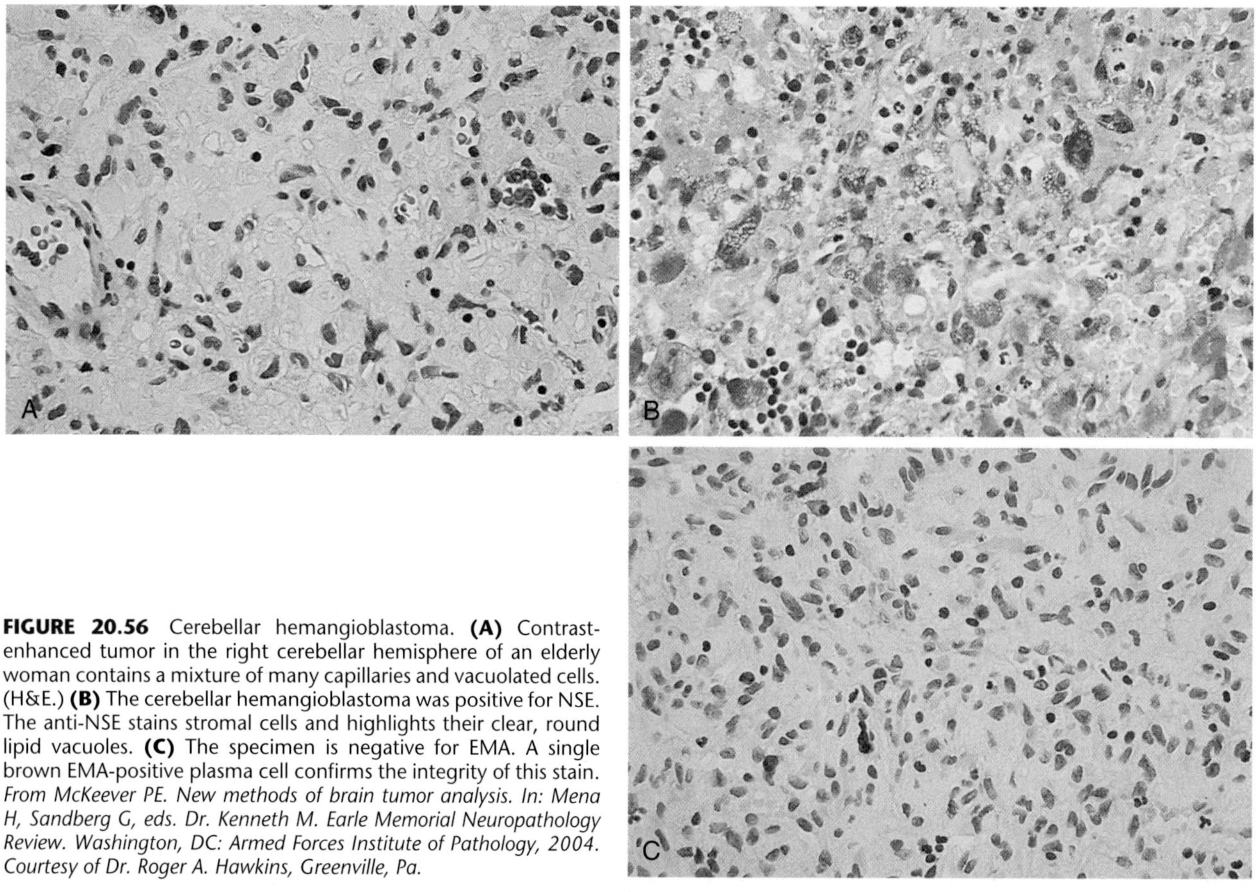

FIGURE 20.56 Cerebellar hemangioblastoma. **(A)** Contrast-enhanced tumor in the right cerebellar hemisphere of an elderly woman contains a mixture of many capillaries and vacuolated cells. (H&E.) **(B)** The cerebellar hemangioblastoma was positive for NSE. The anti-NSE stains stromal cells and highlights their clear, round lipid vacuoles. **(C)** The specimen is negative for EMA. A single brown EMA-positive plasma cell confirms the integrity of this stain. *From McKeever PE. New methods of brain tumor analysis. In: Mena H, Sandberg G, eds. Dr. Kenneth M. Earle Memorial Neuropathology Review. Washington, DC: Armed Forces Institute of Pathology, 2004. Courtesy of Dr. Roger A. Hawkins, Greenville, Pa.*

or tumors, pheochromocytoma, and renal cysts or carcinoma. Renal cell carcinoma is a frequent cause of death in VHL patients.

The VHL gene is on the short arm of chromosome three (3p25-26). An inherited somatic mutation in this tumor suppressor gene creates the chance for a single mutation in the other allele to produce a tumor, following Knudson's hypothesis. To some extent, VHL mutations at certain sites correlate with the propensity of a family to have VHL type 1 (without pheochromocytoma), type 2A (with pheochromocytoma and renal cell carcinoma), type 2B (with pheochromocytoma but without renal cell carcinoma), or type 2C (with only pheochromocytoma).[220] Some sporadic hemangioblastomas are associated with VHL gene abnormalities.[221]

Antibodies to the VHL gene product have been produced. These may aid the diagnosis of clear cell carcinomas and metastatic renal cell carcinoma.[222]

CRANIOPHARYNGIOMA (WHO GRADE I)

This tumor is found within or above the sella turcica. The epithelial appearance of craniopharyngioma is distinctive. A properly sampled craniopharyngioma, including a sample of the solid mass associated with cystic craniopharyngiomas, is difficult to confuse with other brain tumors because of its characteristic epithelium, which may be adamantinomatous, keratinizing, or both (see Tables 20.6 and 20.13).[3] Three of four craniopharyngiomas calcify, a feature helping to distinguish them from metastatic carcinoma, which rarely calcifies in brain and is rarely as differentiated as craniopharyngioma.

Poor sampling of cystic craniopharyngioma may yield a few epithelial cells of unknown origin. In such cases, lack of cytokeratins 8 and 20 favor craniopharyngioma over epithelial cysts common in the same location.[223] Craniopharyngiomas express more high molecular weight keratin than most carcinomas metastatic to brain (Fig. 20.57).

Confusion can arise from sampling of only the intensely GFAP-positive gliotic margin of a craniopharyngioma, which may closely resemble a pilocytic astrocytoma. The highly reactive and fibrillar gliosis surrounding a craniopharyngioma may be distinguished from that of pilocytic astrocytoma on the basis of the even spacing between GFAP-positive cells, the lower cellularity, and the lack of microcysts in the former (see the Gliosis section earlier in this chapter). If a craniopharyngioma nearby is suspected, keratin immunohistochemical analysis may reveal epithelial cells in the gliosis.[224]

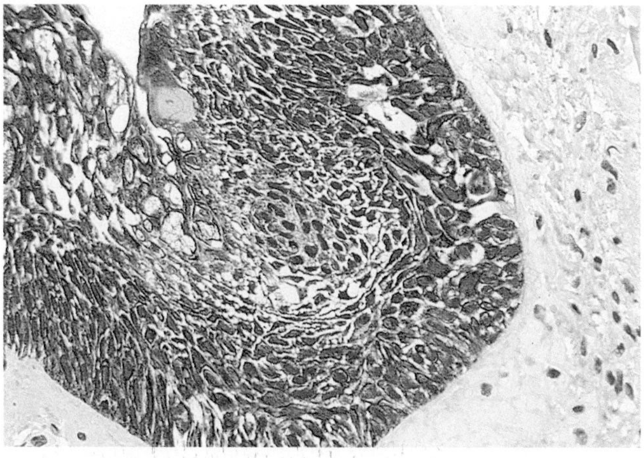

FIGURE 20.57 Most craniopharyngiomas are obvious from their structural features, as was this adamantinomatous craniopharyngioma. Nonetheless, its immunoreactivity for high molecular weight keratin 903 distinguishes it even further and emphasizes the cytoplasm of shrunken epithelial cells (stellate reticulum).

Metastatic Tumors (All Tumors WHO Grade IV)

CARCINOMA

Important characteristics of carcinoma as it relates to the CNS and meninges are its distinctively epithelial structure (Fig. 20.58A; see Table 20.6) and the overwhelming predominance of metastatic over primary carcinomas. Metastatic carcinomas are described in detail in Chapter 8, Immunohistology of Metastatic Carcinomas of Unknown Primary. Rare primary brain carcinomas occur in the choroid plexus, from germ cell tumors of the pineal and suprasellar regions, and from cysts.[3,225] This section emphasizes how to distinguish between carcinomas (see Fig. 20.58B to D) and various primary intracranial tumors (see Box 20.2).

Metastatic carcinoma uncommonly produces neoplastic meningitis. Although its clinical features resemble those of inflammatory meningitis, cytologic examination of the CSF distinguishes the two.[210,225-227]

Many carcinomas metastatic to the CNS and meninges are adenocarcinomas that form acini and produce mucin. Others are small cell or undifferentiated carcinoma. The histologic hallmarks of carcinoma metastatic to the CNS are an epithelial appearance and a *distinct tumor margin* with CNS parenchyma. *Distinct epithelial borders* and lack of fibrillar cytoplasmic processes contrast with the pattern of glioblastoma. Within CNS parenchyma, few neoplasms other than glioblastoma or anaplastic glioma show the intensity of nuclear pleomorphism, profuse mitotic abnormalities, or spontaneous tumor necrosis present in metastatic carcinomas. Carcinomas metastatic to the CNS stain abundantly for CAM5.2 cytokeratin (see Fig. 20.58C), less commonly for 34βE12 keratin, and often for EMA. These features and the lack of GFAP (see Fig. 20.54B) together distinguish carcinomas from gliomas.[3] In distinguishing carcinomas from gliomas, one should avoid the use of AE1/AE3 anti-CK, which cross-reacts with GFAP (see Fig. 20.15). Another common mistake is to interpret gliosis trapped by advancing carcinoma as a GFAP-positive neoplasm (see Figs. 20.25 and 20.26B).

Meningiomas usually contain focal EMA, but so do many carcinomas. Meningiomas rarely contain CAM5.2 CK, except for secretory meningiomas in proximity to their secretory globules. These tumors can often be distinguished from carcinoma on the basis of their focal CK staining (see Fig. 20.47C). Most meningiomas have more diffuse and more intense vimentin staining than carcinomas, and their CK to vimentin ratio is zero or

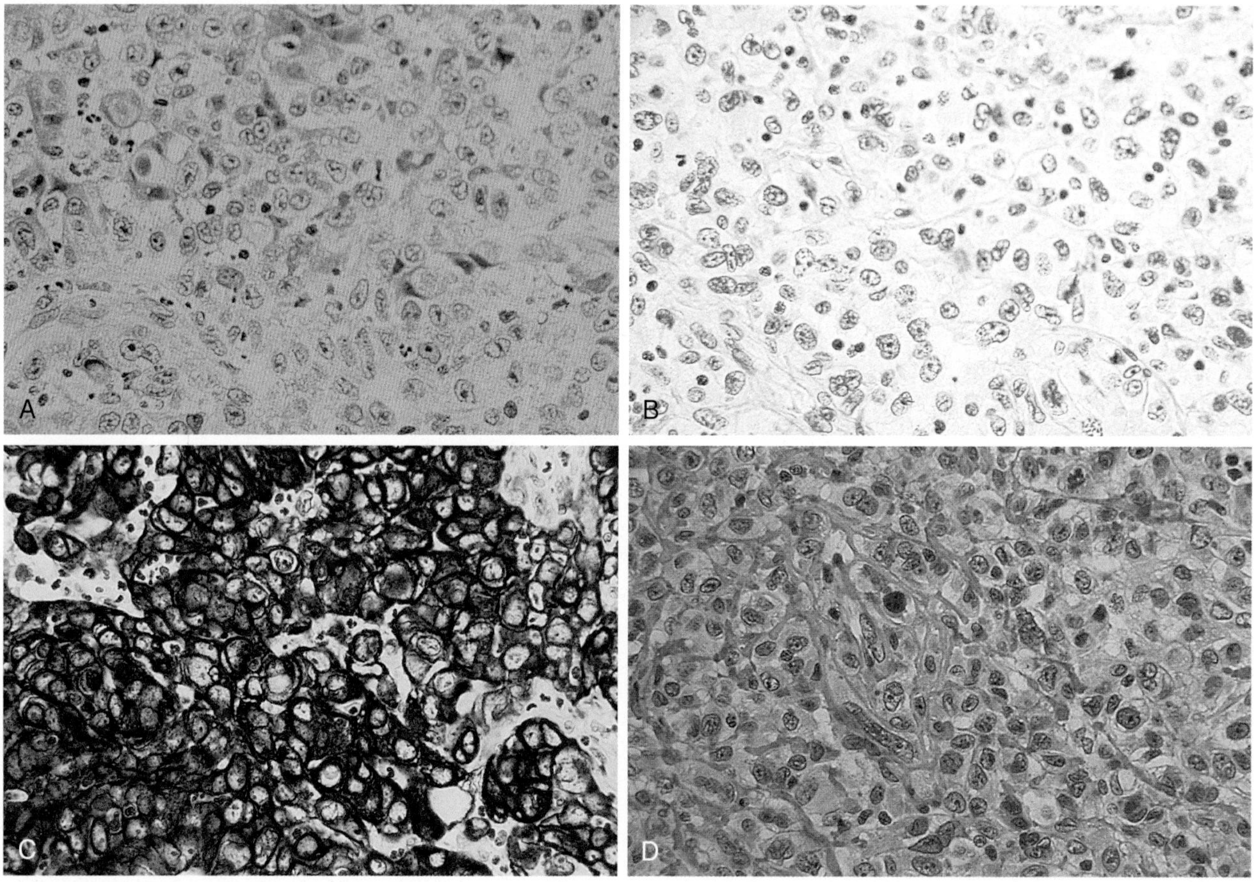

FIGURE 20.58 **(A)** Epithelioid cells in this tumor from the parietal lobe of an elderly woman show distinct borders between cells. (H&E.) These particular epithelioid cells are pleomorphic and contain malignant nuclear features. The algorithm in Box 20.2 offers a way to dissect the differential diagnosis of a brain tumor composed of epithelioid cells. Nearby sections of the tumor shown in **A** are negative for GFAP **(B)**, highly positive for CAM5.2 cytokeratin **(C)**, and negative for S-100 protein **(D)**. It was also positive for EMA and negative for chromogranin A (*not shown*). The diagnostic path in Box 20.2 leads to carcinoma. *From McKeever PE. New methods of brain tumor analysis. In: Mena H, Sandberg G, eds. Dr. Kenneth M. Earle Memorial Neuropathology Review. Washington, DC: Armed Forces Institute of Pathology, 2004.*

at least lower than that of carcinomas. Importantly, all but the most malignant meningiomas lack the abundant and often abnormal mitotic spindles found in metastatic carcinomas.

Renal cell carcinoma metastasis to brain must be distinguished from hemangioblastoma and oligodendroglioma. These neoplasms contain clear cytoplasm and distinct cell borders (see Box 20.1).[91] Presence of EMA and CK distinguishes renal cell carcinoma from cerebellar hemangioblastoma and oligodendroglioma (see the sections on Hemangioblastoma and Oligodendrogliomas earlier in this chapter).[3]

Small cell carcinoma can be very difficult to distinguish from lymphoma and medulloblastoma or PNET (see Box 20.3). EMA or CK is expressed abundantly by small cell carcinoma, infrequently and focally by medulloblastoma, and not by brain lymphoma. Although either small cell carcinoma or medulloblastoma may express synaptophysin, S-100 protein, or NSE, stains for these substances are valuable discriminators for the trained eye; they accentuate the fibrillarity of medulloblastoma, in contrast to the epithelioid cells of small cell carcinoma.

As more precise IHC markers of carcinomas originating in different organs become available, the estimation of the primary origin of a carcinoma in brain has become realistic.[228,229] Thyroid transcription factor-1 (TTF-1) is positive in some lung and many thyroid carcinomas and negative in most other carcinomas.[230] A panel of immunostains for brain should include CAM5.2, CK7, CK20, CEA, and TTF-1. In the right clinical setting, include HER2/neu, ER, and PR, or prostate-specific antigen. The interpretation must be made in accord with the histologic features. Most breast and lung carcinomas in brain are undifferentiated or adenocarcinomas, which are positive for CAM5.2 and CK7, and negative for CK20. Breast cancers are often HER2/neu- or ER-positive. Some lung adenocarcinomas are TTF-1 positive, and such positivity markedly reduces the likelihood of a nonpulmonary primary. A negative TTF-1 is less useful. Colon carcinoma is typically CK20 and CEA positive, and CK7 and TTF-1 negative. The diagnosis of gastric and pancreaticobiliary carcinoma is more challenging, as these show variable CK7 and CK20 expression but are often CEA positive.

Virtually all prostate carcinomas are positive for CAM5.2 and prostate-specific antigen. Prostate carcinomas frequent vertebrae more than CNS. Most renal cell carcinomas (RCCs) are positive for CAM5.2 and negative for CK20; a few are positive for CK7. TTF-1

TABLE 20.12 Differential Diagnosis of a Cyst with Wall of Fibrillar Cells

	Differential Features		
Diagnosis	**Structures**	**Antibody***	**Locations[a]**
Cavitary gliosis	Wall of gliosis	GFAP in glial filaments (+); S-100 (+)	Cerebrum; CNS
Abscess	Wall of granulation tissue; fibrosis (Table 20.5); inflammation and gliosis; purulent contents	Collagen (+); reticulin (+); L26 (S); A6 (S); LCA; k and λ Ig; α-ACT; KP1 (S); microorganisms	Basal frontal and temporal lobes; CNS
Cystic astrocytoma	Wall of pilocytic astrocytoma	GFAP (+); S-100 (+)	Cerebellum; CNS
Hemangioblastoma	Wall of gliosis; mural nodule of hemangioblastoma (Table 20.7)	Factor VIII (S); CD31(S); NSE (S); Wall: GFAP (+)	Cerebellum; CNS
Glial cyst, simple cyst, pineal cyst, wall of syrinx	Wall of gliosis; Rosenthal fibers	GFAP in glial filaments (+); S-100 (+); alpha B-crystalline	Pineal, cerebellum, spinal cord; brainstem
Meningeal cyst	Wall of dura, arachnoid; syncytial cells	Collagen (S); EMA (S)	Spinal epidural surface

*Key to staining results: +, almost always strong, diffuse positivity; *S*, sometimes positive; *R*, rare cells may be positive.
[a]Most common or most specific location is listed first.
α-ACT, alpha-antichymotrypsin; CNS, central nervous system; EMA, epithelial membrane antigen; GFAP, glial fibrillary acidic protein; Ig, immunoglobulin; LCA, leukocyte common antigen; NSE, neuron-specific enolase.
Modified from McKeever PE, Blaivas M. The brain, spinal cord, and meninges. In: Sternberg SS, ed. Diagnostic Surgical Pathology. 2nd ed. New York, NY: Raven Press; 1994:409-492.

is negative. Its large, clear cells and tendency to hemorrhage aid in the identification of RCC.

MELANOCYTIC NEOPLASMS

Metastatic melanoma is the most common melanocytic tumor encountered in the nervous system (see Fig. 20.51). Its histologic features are variable (see Tables 20.5 to 20.7). Melanomas are described in Chapter 6. Melanomas are often strongly positive for S-100 protein (see Fig. 20.51C), a marker of low specificity in brain because it is also seen in many CNS tumors.[231] HMB45 and tyrosinase are the markers recommended as most likely to discriminate melanoma from other brain tumors (see Fig. 20.51B).

Rare meningiomas, schwannomas, ependymomas, neuroblastomas, and PNETs contain melanin.[74] They can be identified from their individually described features.

Primary melanomas confined to the craniospinal vault are rare. Most arise from meningeal melanocytes. They are often found in the meninges, where they may infiltrate the CNS via the perivascular space. Primary melanocytomas are less malignant.[3] They occur in Meckel's cave and elsewhere.

CYSTS

Cysts differ from tumors in their lack of a solid nodule of tissue. This simple fact is critical to distinguishing glial cysts from gliomas and epithelial cysts from cystic craniopharyngiomas. Cysts specific to nervous tissue are emphasized here.[3] Others are described in their primary chapters.

Glial Cyst, Simple Cyst, Pineal Cyst, and Wall of Syrinx

The common denominator of four cysts of various locations and obscure etiologies—glial cyst, simple cyst, pineal cyst, and wall of syrinx—is that the wall is lined only by gliosis (Table 20.12). Histologic characteristics of these cysts are those of gliosis: Highly GFAP-positive stellate cells are uniformly spaced, with vast tangles of GFAP-positive astrocytic processes between them.[232] It is sometimes only with the passage of time that such cysts are proven not to be associated with low-grade astrocytomas.[3]

Neuroepithelial Cyst and Ependymal Cyst

Both the neuroepithelial cyst and ependymal cyst have an epithelioid surface that is positive for S-100 protein and GFAP, resting on a fibrillary glial base that is also positive for these two antibodies.[233] These cysts often occur near a ventricle (Table 20.13). They rarely cause aseptic meningitis.[13]

Colloid Cyst

Location is a key feature of colloid cyst, more precisely called *colloid cyst of the third ventricle* (see Table 20.13). Its location in the third ventricle, usually near the choroid plexus and foramen of Monro, helps distinguish the colloid cyst from other cysts that superficially resemble it but that occur in different locations. This cyst's simple columnar and cuboidal epithelium, which

TABLE 20.13 Differential Diagnosis of a Cyst with Wall Lined by Epithelium

	Differential Features		
Diagnosis	**Structures**	**Antibody***	**Locations[a]**
Cystic craniopharyngioma	Wall of adamantinomatous or incompletely keratinized squamous epithelium; cyst contains "motor oil"	Cytokeratin (+)	Suprasellar; sella
Ependymal cyst	Columnar epithelium usually ciliated	GFAP (+)	Spinal cord; brain
Colloid cyst	Fibrous wall lined by inner ciliated and/or nonciliated simple columnar epithelium; cyst contains colloid and cell ghosts	Cytokeratin (+); EMA	Third ventricle
Dermoid cyst	Epidermoid cyst features plus adnexa of skin; cyst contains sebum, squames, and hair	Keratin (+)	Midline cerebellum; fourth ventricle; skull; spinal dura; cauda equina
Epidermoid cyst	Fibrous wall lined by inner keratinizing stratified squamous epithelium; cyst contains waxy squames	Keratin (+)	CP angle; temporal lobe; spinal dura; pineal; sella; brainstem; CNS
Enterogenous cyst	Lining as above; cyst contains mucin; rests on collagen	Cytokeratin (+); EMA	Spinal cord

*Key to staining results: +, almost always strong, diffuse positivity.
[a]Most common or most specific location is listed first.
CNS, central nervous system; CP, cerebellopontine; EMA, epithelial membrane antigen; GFAP, glial fibrillary acidic protein.
Modified from McKeever PE, Blaivas M. The brain, spinal cord, and meninges. In: Sternberg SS, ed. Diagnostic Surgical Pathology. 2nd ed. New York, NY: Raven Press; 1994:409-492.

may be flattened to squamous epithelium, often contains a mixture of ciliated and nonciliated cells.[234] Motile and sensory cilia suggest olfactory and respiratory epithelium.[235] These cells are positive for CK and EMA. The cyst contents are predominantly carboxymucins, rendering them positive for PAS and Alcian blue.[236]

Dermoid Cyst

Dermoid cysts are frequently midline cysts, possibly arising from embryonic inclusions of skin at the time of closure of the neural groove (see Table 20.13). They occur between the cerebellar hemispheres, in the fourth ventricle, in the lumbosacral region of the cord, and in the skull. These cysts may involve CNS, meninges, or both.[74,76] Ruptured dermoid cysts can cause sterile meningitis and inflammation resembling an abscess. Identification of squamous epithelial cells with CK or cholesterol clefts within the inflammation are clues to its true cause.

Epidermoid Cyst

Epidermoid cysts are more common in lateral than midline sites, but they have been found in many different locations (see Table 20.13). Common locations are the cerebellopontine angle, around the pons, near the sella, within the temporal lobe, in the diploë, and in the spinal canal.[74] Carcinoma rarely arises within an epidermoid cyst.[225]

Enterogenous Cyst

Enterogenous cysts occur throughout the craniospinal vault. Such a cyst is lined by columnar epithelium, which secretes mucus (see Table 20.13). The epithelium resembles intestinal epithelium or, more rarely, bronchial epithelium. It is immunoreactive for keratin and EMA. Some reactivity for CEA and S-100 protein has been noted.[237]

Meningeal Cyst

A cyst that is located in the posterior or lateral epidural space in the spinal canal and that is lined only by fibrous tissue resembling dura and lacking arachnoid membrane is a meningeal cyst or diverticulum (see Table 20.12). A subdural or subarachnoid cyst that has a thinner wall than the epidural cyst and that protrudes toward brain or spinal cord is an arachnoid cyst. Reactivity for vimentin, progesterone receptors, and EMA is common. This immunoreactivity resembles that of arachnoid granulations and meningiomas.[238] Other cysts have variable thickness and are more difficult to categorize.

DEMENTIAS

Dementia, a progressive and persistent alteration and decline of the normal cognitive state, has numerous causes. These include degenerative, infectious, inflammatory, demyelinating, cerebrovascular, neoplastic, and toxic-metabolic diseases. This section deals principally with the most common degenerative diseases (see the sections on Infectious Diseases, Spongiform Encephalopathies, and Cerebrovascular Diseases earlier in this chapter and the CNS Demyelination section later in the chapter). Rare diseases are covered in a recent text.[12]

Specimens intended to determine the etiology of dementia may be submitted along with note of the clinical suspicion of Alzheimer disease or CJD. Any biopsy specimen being evaluated for the etiology of dementia, however, should be processed as if it were CJD until proven otherwise.[8] The processing is as follows: The specimen is split, and a third is sent for Western blot.[9] The rest is fixed in 10% formalin. Then a third of the specimen, which must include a portion of cerebral cortex, is treated with either neat formic acid or 10% formalin plus 20% bleach for primary processing, and the major portion is held in 10% formalin without formic acid or bleach. One should avoid placing any portion of the fresh specimen in bleach without formalin, which would dissolve the tissue. A small portion of cortex is held in glutaraldehyde, in case electron microscopy is needed later. The neat formic acid or formalin-bleach solution inactivates the infective agent and provides tissue preservation adequate to screen for CJD with H&E and GFAP. GFAP is a very stable antigen that resists oxidation. One should look for vacuoles in neurons and gray matter on H&E–stained specimens and for substantial stellate gliosis on GFAP-stained specimens. If these features are not present, the remaining portions of the specimen fixed optimally without bleach can then be processed and stained as needed to investigate other diagnostic possibilities (see Table 20.3).

Neurons are lost in all dementias. Neuronal loss is more difficult to assess than other findings in most biopsy specimens. The assessment requires quantitation more suited to morphometry than to the interpretative eye, and there is anatomic variation in neuronal density. Neuronal loss causes gliosis, which is easier to appreciate than loss of neurons after staining.

Control tissue, consisting of age- and location-matched cerebral cortex obtained from autopsy specimens, provides a valuable baseline for assessing various abnormalities peculiar to dementias. This control is particularly important for assessing cytoplasmic vacuoles, minimal gliosis, and numbers of neurons.

Alzheimer Disease

Minimal criteria necessary to diagnose Alzheimer disease (AD) have been established.[239-241] These criteria refer to counts of argyrophilic plaques and neurofibrillary tangles (NFT) in microscopic fields under a 10× or 20× objective. Chief among the microscopic criteria for Alzheimer disease is the number of argyrophilic plaques (see Table 20.3). Our approach is to count the number of plaques in our case and compare it with the number illustrated in a credible series.[240] The diagnosis of AD requires clinical input, and it should not be attempted on biopsy material without the clinical certainty of dementia.

Neither argyrophilic plaques nor NFT are adequately demonstrated for enumeration by H&E stains. Bielschowsky's silver stain is recommended for staining both argyrophilic plaques and neurofibrillary tangles (Fig. 20.59).[69] Thioflavin S, excited by blue light suitable for fluorescein fluorescence, also reveals these structures.[122] Neurofibrillary tangles are located in neurons and are composed of bihelical filaments.[7,122] These filaments are now being detected immunohistochemically by staining of their protein constituents, tau and ubiquitin (Table 20.14).[3,242] Neurofibrillary tangles are also intensely stained by Alz-50, a monoclonal antibody raised against

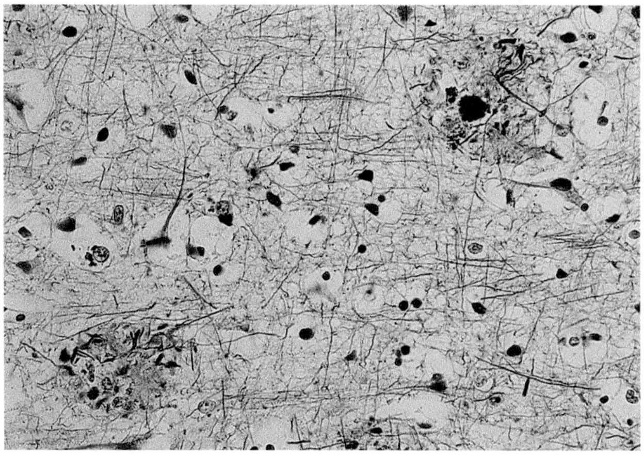

FIGURE 20.59 Alzheimer disease. Two plaques at opposite corners of this specimen contain dark, twisted neurites. Although argyrophilic plaques key to the diagnosis stain with ubiquitin and other immunohistochemical stains, the Bielschowsky silver stain is still the gold standard for this disease. The patient, a middle-aged woman, had displayed progressive dementia for at least 3 years and satisfied the CERAD criteria[240] for diagnosis of Alzheimer disease.

a brain with AD.[243] Antisera to amyloid detect amyloid plaques seen in silver stains as well as congophilic angiopathy when present.[244]

Multi-infarct Vascular Dementia

Cerebral ischemic injury is a common cause of dementia in older adults.[13,245] Combination cases of vascular dementia and Alzheimer disease are also quite frequent. Vascular causes of dementia include subcortical vascular dementia, multi-infarct dementia, ischemic dementia, cerebral autosomal dominant arteriopathy with subcortical infarcts and leukoencephalopathy (CADASIL), and leuko-araiosis (see the Cerebrovascular Diseases section earlier in this chapter).[3]

Lewy Body Diseases

Diffuse cortical Lewy body disease (DCLBD) is a very common disease associated with dementia.[246] Consensus criteria have been developed and validated for the clinical and autopsy diagnosis of DCLBD, and a staging system has been proposed.[247] The hallmark lesion, the Lewy body, is accompanied by neuronal loss and gliosis. In comparison to the Lewy bodies of the brainstem in Parkinson disease, cortical Lewy bodies are difficult to recognize in H&E–stained sections. IHC for ubiquitin or for alpha-synuclein should be done, and the presence of round brown Lewy bodies in cortical neurons should be sought (see Table 20.14). The cingulate gyrus is a good place to find them.[247]

Frontotemporal and Other Dementias

If IHC does not reveal histologic features of AD and DCLBD, the pathologist should consider the frontotemporal dementia group of diseases. Subclassification

TABLE 20.14 Inclusions in Immunophenotypes of Neurodegenerative Diseases

Inclusion	Ubiquitin (HAR)[a]	Tau (HAR)[a]	α-Synuclein (Formic Acid)[a]	β-Amyloid (Formic Acid)[a]
AD tangles	+	+	–	–
AD neuritic plaque	+ Neurites	+ Neurites	S Plaque	+ Plaque
Lewy bodies	+	–	+	–
Pick bodies	+	+	–[b]	–
Frontotemporal dementia or motor neuron disease	+	–	–	–
Multiple system atrophy	+ GCIs	S GCIs	+ GCIs	–

Key to staining results: +, almost always strong, diffuse positivity; *S*, sometimes positive.
[a]Preferred antigen retrieval technique.
[b]Labeling of Pick bodies and neurites has reported with proteinase K antigen retrieval.
AD, Alzheimer disease; GCIs, glial cytoplasmic inclusions; HAR, heat antigen retrieval, microwave in citrate buffer.
Modified from McKeever PE, Boyer PJ. The brain, spinal cord, and meninges. In: Mills SE, Carter D, Greenson, JK, et al., eds. Sternberg's Diagnostic Surgical Pathology, 4th ed. New York, NY: Lippincott Williams & Wilkins; 2004:399-506.

includes Pick disease, corticobasal degeneration, progressive supranuclear palsy, frontotemporal dementia with parkinsonism linked to chromosome 17, and frontotemporal lobar degeneration with or without motor neuron disease.[248]

Most forms of frontotemporal dementia manifest vacuolation of the superficial cortical layers, ballooned neurons, and gliosis. Specific inclusions include silver stain–positive and tau-positive Pick bodies in Pick disease and ubiquitin-positive cytoplasmic inclusions that are tau and α-synuclein negative in frontotemporal lobar degeneration (see Table 20.14).

Additional causes of dementia are Lafora disease, neuronal ceroid lipofuscinosis, adrenoleukodystrophy, and others. Key histologic features of these diseases are outside the scope of this chapter and are covered in other references.[3,12,15]

DEMYELINATION

Unless progressive multifocal leukoencephalopathy (PML) is found in a biopsy specimen, demyelinating diseases are usually investigated clinically and at autopsy (see Table 20.3). Other viral disorders known to cause demyelination are HIV, cytomegalovirus, Epstein-Barr, and varicella-zoster. If the lesion was induced by a virus, amphophilic inclusions may be found, particularly at the periphery of the lesion. Immunohistochemical analysis, ISH, and PCR assay are available for detecting many of these viruses.[40,41,249,250] These are discussed in the Organisms section earlier in this chapter.

Primary and Secondary Demyelination

Primary demyelination affects only the myelin. Primary demyelinating lesions are characterized histologically by destruction of myelin and by abundant foamy KP1-positive macrophages containing myelin debris and lipid droplets. Within the lesion, NF-positive axons are spared (Fig. 20.60). In longitudinal sections of white matter, parallel NF-positive axons are straight and long.

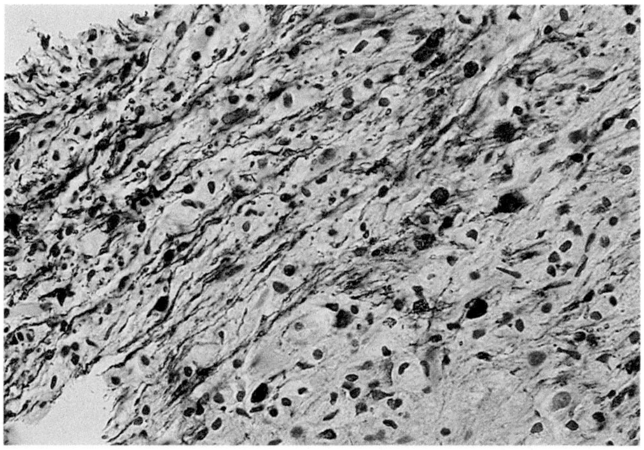

FIGURE 20.60 Primary demyelination with preservation of brown NF-positive axons. Some axons are swollen and are called *spheroids*. Lipid-laden macrophages and gliosis are not stained brown in this section of this brain biopsy specimen, but their pale gray features are still evident.

Secondary demyelination is the loss of myelin secondary to loss of axons. Axonal trophic factors sustain myelin. When the axon is severed or not sustained by its neuron of origin, the axon and then its myelin degenerates. This can happen secondary to infarcts, trauma, toxic, metabolic, or degenerative nervous system diseases. In contrast to primary demyelination, straight and long NF-positive axons are not seen in secondary demyelination. Acutely, the axons crumble into short pieces, and in a few days they are eaten by macrophages and disappear. NF stains thus distinguish secondary from primary demyelination.

CNS Demyelination

In the CNS, the major demyelinating disorder is multiple sclerosis (MS). MS should be differentiated from other disorders in which the histologic appearance of the lesions and the relapsing and remitting clinical course are similar.[7] Acute MS lesions, in addition to plentiful foamy macrophages with increased proteases, have perivascular LCA-positive lymphocytes, EMA-positive and

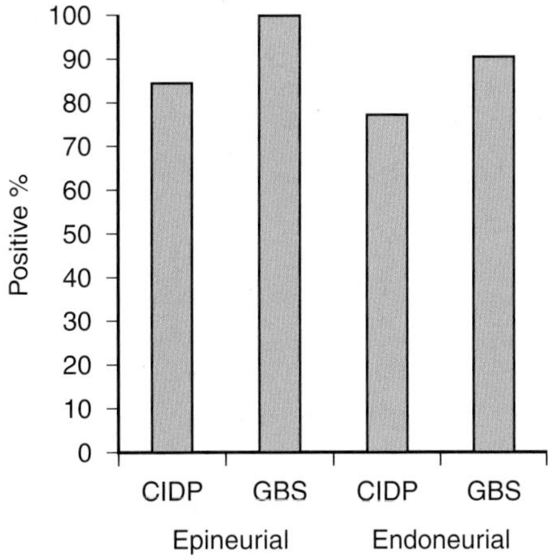

FIGURE 20.61 Locations of T lymphocytes among sural nerve biopsy specimens from 13 cases of chronic inflammatory demyelinating polyneuropathy (CIDP) and 22 cases of Guillain-Barré syndrome (GBS). *Percentages positive are as reported in Schmidt B, Toyka KV, Keifer R, et al. Inflammatory infiltrates in sural nerve biopsies in Guillain-Barré syndrome and chronic inflammatory demyelinating neuropathy. Muscle Nerve. 1996;19:474-487.*

immunoglobulin-positive plasma cells, variable GFAP-positive gliosis, and less endothelial CD34 immunostaining. The macrophages stain positively for class II major histocompatibility complex antigens (HLA-DR [Ia]). They contain myelin debris related to phagocytosis. Oligodendroglia are usually seen only at the periphery of the lesions. Acute plaques can show blood-brain barrier leakage from vessel wall damage with intramural complement on smooth muscle cells and infiltration by HLA-DR–positive macrophages.[13]

Macrophages can accumulate in an active region of white matter demyelination to the extent that they mimic oligodendroglioma and hemangioblastoma (see Box 20.1).[91,251,252] KP1 is used to confirm the presence of macrophages. Oligodendrogliomas have fewer cytoplasmic vacuoles, more central nuclei, and Leu7 and S-100 protein immunoreactivity, features that distinguish them from lipid-laden macrophages. Hemangioblastomas have more factor VIII and CD31-reactive capillaries and less Leu7 (CD57) than oligodendrogliomas. Lipid-laden macrophages in a region of demyelination can be distinguished from neoplasia on the basis of the histochemical or electron microscopic demonstration of small, round globules of phagocytosed myelin.[69]

PNS Demyelination

In peripheral nerve, KP1 (CD68)-positive macrophages engulf myelin and cluster around endoneurial vessels.[253] T lymphocytes that are immunoreactive with CD3, CD4, and CD8 are abundant in the endoneurium, and B lymphocytes are virtually absent in chronic inflammatory demyelinating polyneuropathy (CIDP).[254] T lymphocytes are prominent in both CIDP and Guillain-Barré syndrome (Fig. 20.61).[253] Primary and secondary PNS demyelinations are best distinguished by non-immunohistochemical methods that include teased fiber preparations and electron microscopy.

EPILEPSY

Complex partial seizure disorder (previously called *temporal lobe epilepsy*) may involve the temporal, frontal, parietal, or occipital lobe.[255-259] About 80% of complex partial seizures originate in the temporal lobe; thus, the most common surgical procedure for intractable epilepsy is temporal lobectomy.[255] Staining for neurons and for GFAP, with the use of age-matched temporal-lobe autopsy control tissue, is recommended for detection and neuroanatomic localization of the most common abnormalities, neuronal loss and resulting GFAP-positive gliosis (Figs. 20.62 to 20.64; see Table 20.3).[3] A remarkably effective new stain for highlighting layers of neurons is neuN. It highlights pyramidal neurons in the hippocampus, making it easy to find regions of neuronal loss (see Fig. 20.63).

Neuronal loss triggers gliosis. Both are common in the hippocampus, which is vulnerable to hypoxia (see Fig. 20.62). The large pyramidal neurons are very sensitive.[256] Among these, neurons in Sommer's sector of cornu Ammonis region 1 (CA1) are most sensitive, whereas neurons in CA2 are least sensitive. Neuronal markers, particularly synaptophysin, often are depleted in mirror-image staining to the (increased) GFAP. Surgical fragmentation of some specimens confounds identification of these regions (see Fig. 20.62), but CA4 is obviously enclosed by the series of crowded, small, synaptophysin-positive round neurons of the dentate fascia. Other regions may be evident by their relationship to CA4, the opening of the dentate fascia, and the widening layers of neurons at the subiculum (see Fig. 20.62). Neurofilament and synaptophysin stains aid recognition of neuroanatomic regions in these fragments.

Loss of pyramidal and granular cell neurons in the hippocampus (see Fig. 20.63), large numbers of corpora amylacea (see Fig. 20.64), deposits of hemosiderin pigment in perivascular macrophages, inflammation, focal meningeal fibrosis, calcification, and ferrugination of large pyramidal neurons can be seen in the hippocampus.[3] Cytoarchitectural studies of gray and white matter in resected temporal neocortex may reveal features of neuronal dysgenesis, such as neuronal ectopia, neuronal clustering, and subpial gliosis.[13,257,258]

Deep or surface electrodes are occasionally placed within the region of the future surgical resection in order to monitor and evaluate the seizure activity. The surgeon should inform the pathologist if such electrodes have been used. The electrodes leave a trail of encephalomalacia with chronic inflammation of A6-positive and L26-positive T and B lymphocytes, KP1-positive macrophages, and hemorrhage in the surgical specimen.[258] Surface electrodes cause focal meningitis.

A variety of clinically unsuspected pathologic entities are found in individual specimens. Stereotactic resection of cerebral lesions in partial epilepsy may yield vascular malformations and glial neoplasms. Primary intracerebral tumors manifesting as medically refractory epilepsy are usually low-grade gliomas, mixed tumors with glial or neuronal components or both, hamartomas, or dysembryoplastic neuroepithelial tumors (see Figs. 20.12A, 20.22A, and 20.33).[259,260]

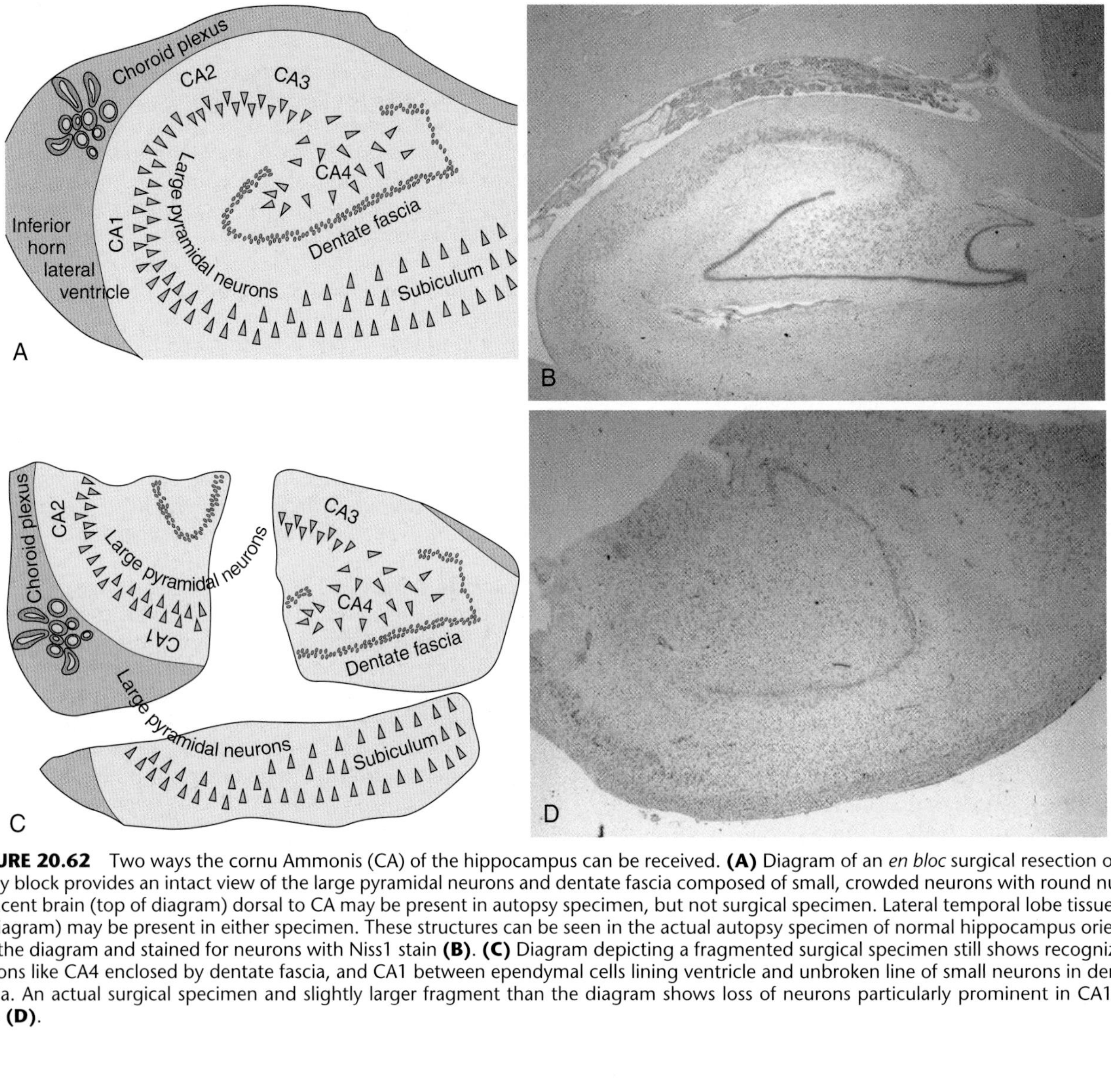

FIGURE 20.62 Two ways the cornu Ammonis (CA) of the hippocampus can be received. **(A)** Diagram of an *en bloc* surgical resection or autopsy block provides an intact view of the large pyramidal neurons and dentate fascia composed of small, crowded neurons with round nuclei. Adjacent brain (top of diagram) dorsal to CA may be present in autopsy specimen, but not surgical specimen. Lateral temporal lobe tissue (left of diagram) may be present in either specimen. These structures can be seen in the actual autopsy specimen of normal hippocampus oriented like the diagram and stained for neurons with Niss1 stain **(B)**. **(C)** Diagram depicting a fragmented surgical specimen still shows recognizable regions like CA4 enclosed by dentate fascia, and CA1 between ependymal cells lining ventricle and unbroken line of small neurons in dentate fascia. An actual surgical specimen and slightly larger fragment than the diagram shows loss of neurons particularly prominent in CA1 and CA4 **(D)**.

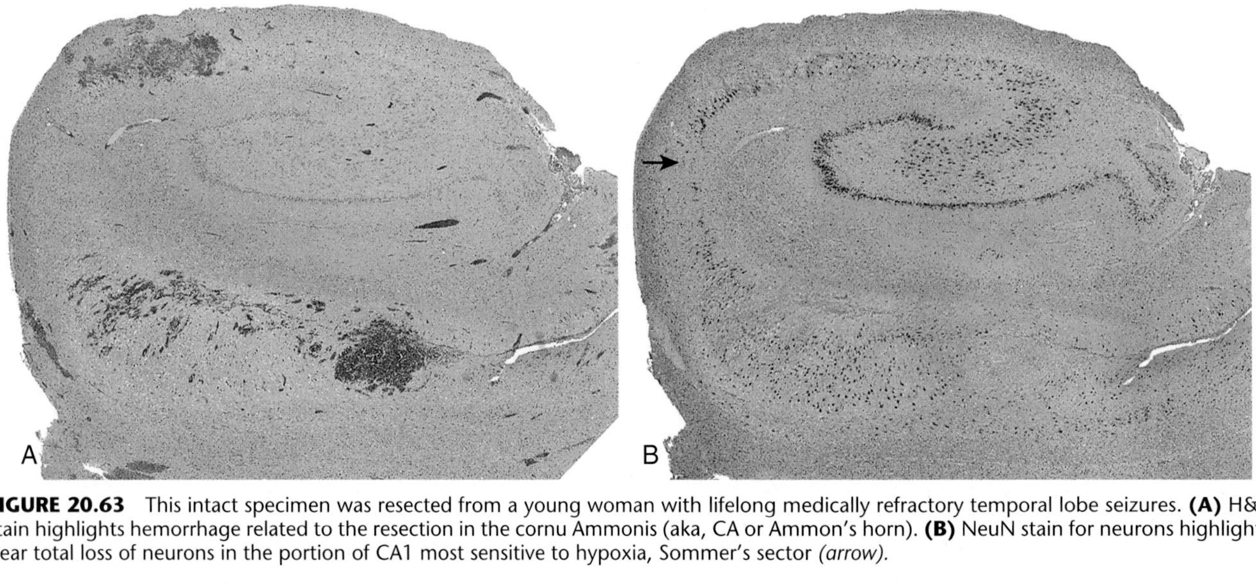

FIGURE 20.63 This intact specimen was resected from a young woman with lifelong medically refractory temporal lobe seizures. **(A)** H&E stain highlights hemorrhage related to the resection in the cornu Ammonis (aka, CA or Ammon's horn). **(B)** NeuN stain for neurons highlights near total loss of neurons in the portion of CA1 most sensitive to hypoxia, Sommer's sector *(arrow)*.

Cortical Malformations

Malformations of the cerebral architecture are seen by the autopsy pathologist, pediatric pathologist, and surgical pathologist. Neuronal markers such as Neu-N, synaptophysin, and NF supplement H&E, S-100, and GFAP in finding these abnormal regions of cortex. They also classify the abnormal cells.[3]

Microdysgenesis is a term for lesions noted only microscopically: (1) focal S-100 protein–positive oligodendroglial clusters, which are often interspersed with (NF-positive) ganglion cells in gray or white matter; (2) oligodendroglial hyperplasia too small and well-differentiated to be oligodendroglioma; and (3) increased numbers of normally scarce neurons in the white matter.

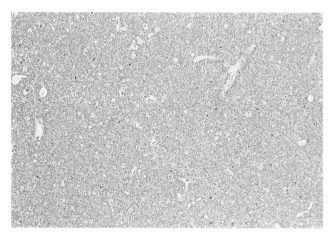

FIGURE 20.64 Pyramidal cell layer of cornu Ammonis region 1 of hippocampus in a patient with decades of partial complex seizures. Two large, clear, GFAP-negative neurons can be seen near a vessel at left side of the field. Other neurons have died. Although there are numerous brown GFAP-positive fibrils of gliosis, the astrocytes are quiescent and have little brown cytoplasm around their nuclei. Round, fuzzy, light purple bodies the size of nuclei are called *corpora amylacea* and are common in such specimens. This neuronal loss and gliosis happened many years ago.

Cortical dysplasia consists of disrupted cortical architecture and abnormally enlarged cells, some with IHC staining of neurons, some with GFAP-positive astrocytes, and some individual cells that stain for both glial and neuronal markers.[75] Cortical tubers, seen with tuberous sclerosis, are cortical dysplasias. Other dysplastic abnormalities are described in the Neuronal Tumors section earlier in this chapter.

PITFALLS IN DIAGNOSIS

Is It Really Negative?

The simple question whether a specimen is really "negative" for the marker in question must be asked to avoid misinterpretation. Whenever possible, one should include a positive control for the marker, as described earlier, within the *same block* as the lesion to be identified (Fig. 20.65). A positive control from a different block does not work as well. If this control tissue does not stain, then the lesion cannot be evaluated with the immunohistochemical stain.

Are the Cells of Interest Positive?

A good nuclear counterstain is essential to correct interpretation of immunohistochemical stain responses. The counterstain distinguishes reactive, neoplastic, and necrotic cells as well as neuroanatomic relationships. Necrotic cells have nuclear pyknosis, karyorrhexis, and karyolysis. Necrotic regions generate false-positive response to immunohistochemical staining. Both features need to be recognized to avoid misinterpretation.

Reactive astrocytosis is associated with many brain tumors. Nuclear features of GFAP-positive cells must be examined to distinguish reactive from neoplastic

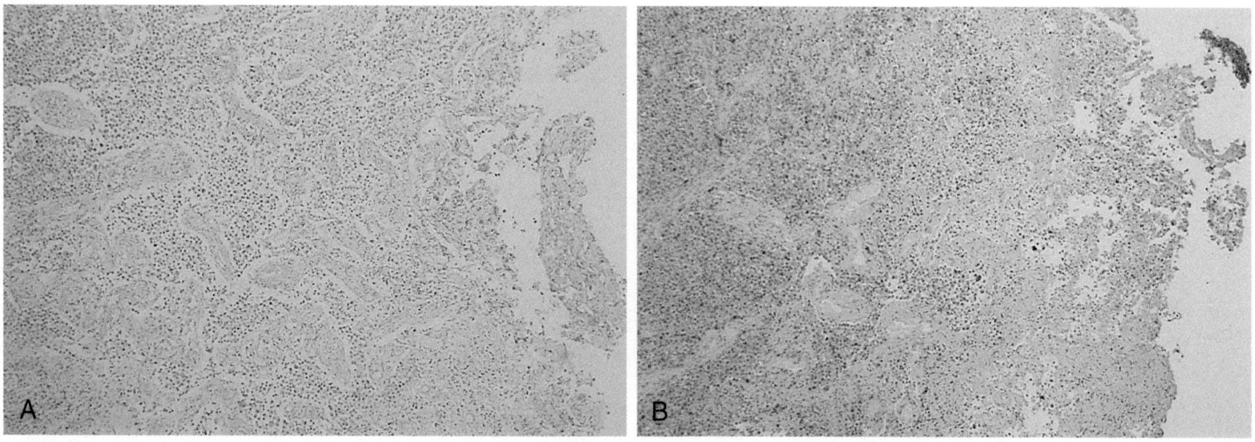

FIGURE 20.65 Importance of internal tissue control for immunohistochemistry. Tiny tissue fragment at the edge of two sections of this tumor specimen and corners of the two illustrations is brain. Brain tissue, which always makes S-100 protein, is the internal positive control. Two procedures were used to test for S-100 protein. **(A)** One procedure for S-100 protein does not stain the tumor, but neither does it stain the brain. **(B)** The second procedure stains the brain fragment dark brown and also stains the tumor. Only the second procedure is a reliable stain for S-100, and it reveals the tumor to be S-100–positive. Subsequent HMB45 staining suggested metastatic melanoma, and ultimately, the cutaneous primary tumor was found. *From McKeever PE. New methods of brain tumor analysis. In: Mena H, Sandberg G, eds. Dr. Kenneth M. Earle Memorial Neuropathology Review. Washington, DC: Armed Forces Institute of Pathology, 2004.*

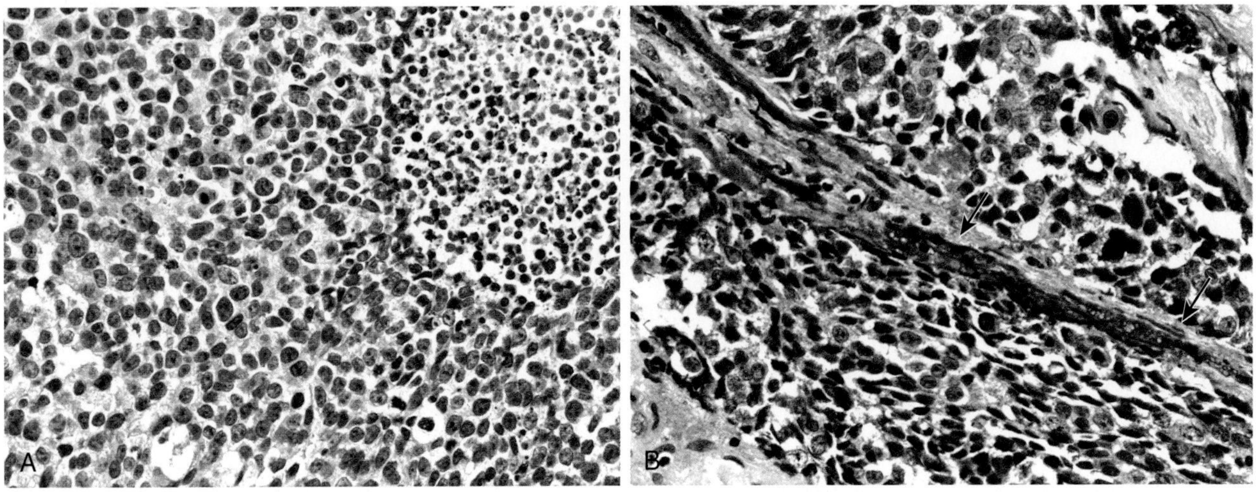

FIGURE 20.66 Sometimes we may wish we had not tried a stain. Both S-100 protein stains are on the same tumor. Neither the primary nor any region of the spinal metastasis of this lung carcinoma stained with S-100 protein **(A)**, except regions near robustly S-100–positive spinal nerve roots **(B)**. This suggests the possibility that this small, acidic molecule may have leaked from damaged nerve *(arrows)* to adjacent carcinoma. This odd pattern of localization suggests restraint in interpretation of the original S-100 protein status of the lung carcinoma.

TABLE 20.15 Types of Swollen GFAP-Positive Cells

Lesion	Interrelationship of GFAP+ Cells	Intracellular Distribution of GFAP	Nuclear Features	Other Tissue Elements
Reactive gliosis	Spaced apart	Low N:C ratios Very fibrillar Longest cell process	Smooth, oval, fine chromatin	NF+ axons are normally spaced
Gemistocytic astrocytoma	Collide, clump	Some long processes	Pleomorphic, elongated, hyperchromatic	NF+ axons are spread apart
Oligodendroglioma with microgemistocytes	Collide, clump	Shortest processes Mixed with negative oligodendroglia	Smooth, round, hyperchromatic	NF+ axons are spread apart

astrocytes (see Fig. 20.26). The immunoreactivity in closest proximity to the definitive nuclei should be checked for correct identification of these cells. This rule has general application to other markers (see Figs. 20.16B and 20.53).

Neoplastic cells have atypical or pleomorphic nuclei. Their chromatin patterns are often distinctive (see Fig. 20.11B). Glioma nuclei are crowded. WHO grade III and higher gliomas and other malignancies show mitoses (see Figs. 20.15A, 20.15C, and 20.26A).

It is important to know the characteristics of the antigen being localized. Structural proteins like all intermediate filament components, histones, and many membrane components tend to remain exactly where they belong in their original cellular compartment (e.g., cytoplasm, nucleus, membrane) after excision, application of saline and formalin, dehydration, and embedding. Small or water-soluble molecules including proteins and peptides may move around during a pathologic process such as invasion or inflammation, or later during specimen handling and processing. S-100 protein is a small and acidic molecule that sometimes moves around (Fig. 20.66). The localization of such molecules requires careful interpretation.

Gliosis versus Glioma

Demyelination may be confused with neoplastic disease because it produces abundant gliosis.[252] Large cells with short chromosomes spread apart in their cytoplasm mimic mitotic activity in a glioma.[251] If numerous lipid-laden KP1-positive macrophages are encountered within parenchyma and around vessels, demyelinating disease should be considered. Appropriate stains for myelin, NF stain for axons (see Box 20.2), and features described in this section should be considered in the interpretation (see Figs. 20.3A, 20.11A and B, and 20.60).

Distinguishing gliosis from glioma can be most difficult (see Fig. 20.9A).[3] Diffuse gliomas infiltrate brain tissue and stimulate their own gliosis, compounding the problem. Swollen GFAP-positive cells can occur in gliosis or gliomas (Table 20.15). Features that distinguish glioma cells from gliosis and normal parenchyma include individual cell variation in GFAP staining, nuclear hyperchromasia (see Fig. 20.11B), nuclear cluster formation, nuclear molding (see Fig. 20.13), mitoses, and calcifications. Mitoses suggest not only that the tumor is a glioma but also that it has a high grade of malignancy. Abnormal variations in size and shape of glial nuclei are common in margins of gliomas.

In astrocytomas, ependymomas, and astrocytic gliomas, GFAP stain is ideal for highlighting glioma cells. GFAP stain delineates the cytoplasm in both gliosis and glioma, facilitating interpretation of these cells. High nuclear to low brown cytoplasmic ratios typify gliomas. Mitotic spindles with chromosomes near each other and surrounded by little cytoplasm (see Fig. 20.26A) are exceptionally rare in gliosis (see Fig. 20.26B). Reactive astrocytes have much lower nuclear to cytoplasmic ratios, abundant dark brown stellate processes, and spaces between them so that they resemble trees in an apple orchard (see Fig. 20.2). There is a possibility that immunohistochemical markers of proliferation, such as MIB1, will help distinguish neoplastic glia from gliosis at these margins.

Gliomas expand, but gliosis contracts. This important feature is difficult to confirm without serial radiographs and *in situ* observation of the confluence of the actual mass and its margin to exclude the possibility of gliosis around another tumor.

Granular *calcifications* scattered among hypercellular glia distinguish glioma from gliosis and normal white matter. Caution is required not to overinterpret calcifications associated with neurons and neuropil within 0.5 cm of a large mass. Although microcysts, calcifications, and mitoses are important diagnostic features of gliomas, they are not seen in every case and are uncommon within the margins of gliomas invading CNS parenchyma.

Another important feature distinguishing the margin of a glioma from gliosis is *cellular density* (see Table 20.2). Some gliomas exhibit *uneven distribution* of cellular density (see Fig. 20.10). Others obscure the junction between gray matter and white matter. Still others spawn secondary structures of Scherer, and the most distinctive are subpial and perineuronal gliomatosis; these secondary structures are collections of neoplastic glia beneath the pia or around neurons.[3] GFAP stain highlights secondary structures from astrocytomas. Secondary structures of oligodendrogliomas show much less synaptophysin than the neuropil of gray matter and are highlighted as lightly staining clusters of cells around neurons or vessels.[59]

Glioma nuclei frequently touch and even indent one another (see Fig. 20.13 and Table 20.15), even among scattered clusters of cells in the diffuse margins of gliomas. Gliosis, however, consists of evenly spaced astrocytes with high GFAP immunoreactivity (see Fig. 20.2). This even spacing is best seen with anti-GFAP staining at low magnification. The low nuclear to cytoplasmic ratio of gliosis is seen at high magnification. Because the nuclei of gliomas are more pleomorphic than normal or gliotic CNS parenchyma, nuclear pleomorphism and hyperchromasia (seen best with a good nuclear counterstain like hematoxylin) help identify a glioma (see Figs. 20.8, 20.9, 20.11, 20.13, and 20.15).[5,88]

Infiltrating versus Non-infiltrating Cells

Non-infiltrating gliomas are often surgically resectable, a characteristic that places a premium on distinguishing them from infiltrating gliomas. This distinction can be difficult in fragmented or incomplete specimens.

After the possibility of neoplastic neurons has been ruled out (see the Neuronal Tumors section earlier in this chapter), neuroanatomic brain tissue constituents are useful markers for distinguishing non-infiltrating from infiltrating gliomas. Axons run close together in parallel in white matter tracts and also are identifiable in gray matter. Noninfiltrating gliomas leave these axons unmolested (see Fig. 20.10B), whereas infiltrating gliomas spread them apart (see Fig. 20.10A) and cause some to swell. Synaptophysin carpets the neuropil of gray matter with tiny brown dots. Synaptophysin-negative glioma cells either stop abruptly or invade this fine carpet.[59]

In specimens that lack discernible brain tissue, information is still available after the tumor has been stained. If axons of non-neoplastic origin are found in the glioma, it is infiltrative (see Fig. 20.13). This feature distinguishes infiltrating gliomas from non-infiltrating gliomas, which have more discrete margins with brain tissue.

Abscess versus Neoplasm

Entities that produce collagen within the CNS may be confused with the wall of an abscess (see Fig. 20.4 and Tables 20.5, 20.7, 20.10, and 20.11). If abscess is suspected during the biopsy procedure, sterile tissue should be sent to microbiology for culture. A negative culture is better than a missed opportunity to find something treatable. Failing culture, stains for microorganisms may help.

Sarcomatous and desmoplastic neoplasms and various cysts with collagenous walls may simulate abscesses (see Figs. 20.31B, 20.34A, and 20.39). These tumors may be distinguished by the lack of an inflammatory component and the presence of a neoplastic component. More problematic are cysts that have ruptured and exuded material foreign to the CNS, such as colloid or squamous epithelial cells. If this material is not detectable on H&E staining within the inflammatory reaction, immunohistochemical stains for cyst wall material, such as CK stains for epithelial cells, assist the interpretation.[224] These other lesions are sterile *in situ* and do not stain for microorganisms as an abscess would (see Box 20.2).

Dysplasia versus Neoplasm

The distinction between cortical dysplasia and gangliocytic neoplasms can be difficult. Presented here are some guidelines for using IHC to distinguish dysplasia from neoplasm. Dysplasias consist of abnormal architecture, such as too many or too few layers of neurons, ectopic neurons, or abnormally large or too small neurons or glia. They may be large, but they do not grow.

Neuronal neoplasms typically manifest more than just architectural abnormalities. Their cytologic abnormalities include binucleation, large and bizarre nuclei, and hyperchromatism. These become evident with neurofilament or synaptophysin stain and a good hematoxylin counterstain. They are easiest to recognize when the suspected lesion is compared to a normal sample of the same region of brain from another case or autopsy material.

Neoplasms have cellular proliferation. The MIB1 stain measures their proliferation potential, many of which show no mitoses. On this author's stains, dysplasia generally falls below a 3% maximal MIB1 LI and neoplasia falls above 3%. Sampling and laboratory techniques can affect this cutoff.

ACKNOWLEDGMENTS

The following colleagues provided particularly valuable assistance. Drs. Philip Boyer, Mila Blaivas, Jeanne Bell, Larry Junck, and Ricardo Lloyd provided key citations. I thank Ms. Elizabeth Wawrzaszek, Ms. Dianna Banka, and Ms. Peggy Otto for their skill and patience in preparing this chapter. Mr. Mark Deming and Ms. Elizabeth Horn Walker carefully prepared the illustrations. Immunohistologists and histopathologists in the University of Michigan Medical Center Pathology Laboratories prepared the fine microscopic slides.

The work described in this chapter is supported in part by NIH CA68545 and CA47558 grants awarded by the U.S. Public Health Service.

REFERENCES

1. McKeever PE. New methods of brain tumor analysis. In: Rushing EJ, Sandberg GD, eds. *Dr. Kenneth M. Earle Memorial Neuropathology Review*. Washington, D.C.: Armed Forces Institute of Pathology; 2008.
2. Louis DN, Ohgaki H, Wiestler OD, et al, eds. *World Health Organization Classification of Tumors: Pathology and Genetics of Tumors of the Nervous System*. Lyon: IARC Press; 2007.
3. McKeever PE, Boyer P. The brain, spinal cord, and meninges. In: Mills SE, Carter D, Greenson JK, et al, eds. *Sternberg's Diagnostic Surgical Pathology*. 4th ed. Philadelphia: Lippincott Williams & Wilkins; 2004:400-503.
4. Firlik KS, Martinez AJ, Lunsford LD. Use of cytological preparations for the intraoperative diagnosis of stereotactically obtained brain biopsies: A 19-year experience and survey of neuropathologists. *J Neurosurg*. 1999;91:454-458.
5. McKeever PE. Laboratory methods in brain tumor diagnosis. In: Nelson JS, Mena H, Parisi J, et al, eds. *Principles and Practice of Neuropathology*. 2nd ed. New York: Oxford University Press; 2003:272-297.
6. Kepes JJ, Moral LA, Wilkinson SB, et al. Rhabdoid transformation of tumor cells in meningiomas: A histologic indication of increased proliferative activity: Report of four cases. *Am J Surg Pathol*. 1998;22:231-238.
7. Graham DI, Lanto PL, eds. *Greenfield's neuropathology*. 7th ed. New York: Edward Arnold; 2002.
8. Garcia JH, Budka H, McKeever PE, et al, eds. *Neuropathology: The diagnostic approach*. Philadelphia: Mosby; 1997.
9. Castellani RJ, Parchi P, Madoff L, et al. Biopsy diagnosis of Creutzfeldt-Jakob disease by Western blot: A case report. *Hum Pathol*. 1997;28:623-641.
10. Mrak RE. The big eye in the 21st century: The role of electron microscopy in modern diagnostic neuropathology. *J Neuropathol Exp Neurol*. 2002;61:1027-1039.
11. Dickson DW, Bergeron C, Chin SS, et al. Office of Rare Diseases neuropathologic criteria for corticobasal degeneration. *J Neuropathol Exp Neurol*. 2002;61:935-946.
12. Dickson DW, ed. Neurodegeneration: *The molecular pathology of dementia and movement disorders*. Basel: ISN Neuropath Press; 2003.
13. McKeever PE. Immunohistology of the nervous system. In: Dabbs D, ed. *Diagnostic Immunohistochemistry*. 2nd ed. Philadelphia: Churchill Livingstone; 2006:746-816.
14. Sundgren PC, Fan X, Weybright P, et al. Differentiation of recurrent brain tumor versus radiation injury using diffusion tensor imaging in patients with new contrast-enhancing lesions. *Magn Reson Imaging*. 2006;24:1131-1142.
15. Ellison D, Love S, Chimelli L, et al. *Neuropathology*. Amsterdam: Elsevier; 2003.
16. McKeever PE, Balentine JD. Macrophage migration through the brain parenchyma to the perivascular space following particle ingestion. *Am J Pathol*. 1978;93:153-164.
17. Danton GH, Dietrich WD. Inflammatory mechanisms after ischemia and stroke. *J Neuropathol Exp Neurol*. 2003;62:127-136.
18. McKeever PE, Fligiel SEG, Varani J, et al. Products of cells cultured from gliomas. IV: Extracellular matrix proteins of gliomas. *Int J Cancer*. 1986;37:867-874.
19. Thomson Jr RB, Bertram H. Laboratory diagnosis of central nervous system infections. *Infec Dis Clin North Am*. 2001;15:1047-1071.
20. Park do Y, Kim JY, Chi KU, et al. Comparison of polymerase chain reaction with histopathologic features for diagnosis of tuberculosis in formalin-fixed, paraffin-embedded histologic specimens. *Arch Pathol Lab Med*. 2003;127:326-330.
21. Kaufman L, Standard PG, Jalbert M, et al. Immunohistologic identification of Aspergillus spp. and other hyaline fungi by using polyclonal fluorescent antibodies. *J Clin Microbiol*. 1997;35:2206-2209.
22. Guarner J, Greer PW, Bartlett J, et al. Congenital syphilis in a newborn: An immunopathologic study. *Mod Pathol*. 1999;12:82-87.
23. Shankar SK, Ravi V, Suryanarayana V, et al. Immunoreactive antigenic sites of Cysticercus cellulosae relevant to human neurocysticercosis—Immunocytochemical localization using human CSF as source of antibody. *Clin Neuropathol*. 1995;14:33-36.
24. Diogo CM, Mendonca MC, Savino W, et al. Immunoreactivity of a cytokeratin-related polypeptide from adult Schistosoma mansoni. *Int J Parasitol*. 1994;24:727-732.
25. Schwartz MA, Selhorts JB, Ochs AL, et al. Oculomasticatory myorrhythmia: A unique movement disorder occurring in Whipple's disease. *Ann Neurol*. 1986;20:677-683.
26. Cadavid D, Barbour AG. Neuroborreliosis during relapsing fever: Review of the clinical manifestations, pathology, and treatment of infections in humans and experimental animals. *Clin Infect Dis*. 1998;26:151-164.
27. Cassady KA, Whitley RJ. Pathogenesis and pathophysiology of viral infections of the central nervous system. In: Scheld WM, Whitley RJ, Durack DT, eds. *Infections of the Central Nervous System*. 2nd ed. Philadelphia: Lippincott-Raven; 1997:7-22.
28. Fleming KA. Analysis of viral pathogenesis by in situ hybridization. *J Pathol*. 1992;166:95-96.
29. Mrak RE, Young L. Rabies encephalitis in humans: Pathology, pathogenesis and pathophysiology. *J Neuropathol Exp Neurol*. 1994;53:1-10.
30. McQuaid S, Cosby SL, Koffi K, et al. Distribution of measles virus in the central nervous system of HIV-seropositive children. *Acta Neuropathol*. 1998;96:637-642.
31. Gray F, Chretien F, Vallat-Decouvelaere AV, et al. The changing pattern of HIV neuropathology in the HAART era. *J Neuropathol Exp Neurol*. 2003;62:429-444.
32. Nath A, Sinai AP. Cerebral toxoplasmosis. *Curr Treat Options Neurol*. 2003;5:3-12.
33. Zimmer C, Daeschlein G, Patt S, et al. Strategy for diagnosis of Toxoplasma gondii in stereotactic brain biopsies. *Stereotact Funct Neurosurg*. 1991;56:66-75.
34. Rhodes RH. Histopathology of the central nervous system in the acquired immunodeficiency syndrome. *Hum Pathol*. 1987;18:636-643.
35. Persons DL, Moore JA, Fishback JL. Comparison of polymerase chain reaction, DNA hybridization, and histology with viral culture to detect cytomegalovirus in immunosuppressed patients. *Mod Pathol*. 1991;4:149-152.
36. Vazeux R, Cumont M, Girard PM, et al. Severe encephalitis resulting from coinfections with HIV and JC virus. *Neurology*. 1990;40:944-948.

37. Daley CL, Small PM, Schecter GF, et al. An outbreak of the tuberculosis with accelerated progression among persons infected with the human immunodeficiency virus. *N Engl J Med.* 1992;4:231-235.
38. Feraru ER, Aronow HA, Lipton RB. Neurosyphilis in AIDS patients: Initial CSF VDRL may be negative. *Neurology.* 1990;40:541-543.
39. Martinez AJ, Visvesvara GS. Free-living, amphizoic and opportunistic amebas. *Brain Pathol.* 1997;7:583-598.
40. Prayson RA, Estes ML. Stereotactic brain biopsy for diagnosis of progressive multifocal leukoencephalopathy. *South Med J.* 1993;86:1381-1394.
41. Hulette CM, Downey BT, Burger PC. Progressive multifocal leukoencephalopathy: Diagnosis by in situ hybridization with a biotinylated JC virus DNA probe using an automated histomatic code-on slide stainer. *Am J Surg Pathol.* 1991;15:791-797.
42. Hulette CM, Earl NL, Crain BJ. Evaluation of cerebral biopsies for the diagnosis of dementia. *Arch Neurol.* 1992;49:28-31.
43. Capellari S, Vital C, Parchi P, et al. Familial prion disease with a novel 144-bp insertion in the prion protein gene in a Basque family. *Neurology.* 1997;49:133-141.
44. Bruce ME, Will RG, Ironside JW, et al. Transmissions to mice indicate that "new variant" CJD is caused by the BSE agent. *Nature.* 1997;389:498-501.
45. Kovacs GG, Head MW, Hegy I, et al. Immunohistochemistry for the prion protein: Comparison of different monoclonal antibodies in human prior disease subtypes. *Brain Pathol.* 2002;12: 1-11.
46. Ironside JW, Sutherland K, Bell JE, et al. A new variant of Creutzfeldt-Jakob disease: Neuropathological and clinical features. *Cold Spring Harb Symp Quant Biol.* 1996;50:523-527.
47. Vinters HV, Secor DL, Pardridge WM, et al. Immunohistochemical study of cerebral amyloid angiopathy. III: Widespread Alzheimer A4 peptide in cerebral microvessel walls colocalizes with gamma trace in patients with leukoencephalopathy. *Ann Neurol.* 1990;28:34-42.
48. Chen ST, Chen SD, Hsu CY, et al. Progression of hypertensive intracerebral hemorrhage. *Neurology.* 1989;39:1509-1514.
49. Kittner SJ, Sharkness CM, Sloan MA, et al. Infarcts with a cardiac source of embolism in the NINDS stroke data bank: Neurologic examination. *Neurology.* 1992;42:299-302.
50. Miettinen M, Lindenmayer AE, Chaubal A. Endothelial cell markers CD31, CD34, and BNH9 antibody to H- and Y-antigens—evaluation of their specificity and sensitivity in the diagnosis of vascular tumors and comparison with von Willebrand factor. *Mod Pathol.* 1994;7:82-90.
51. Takahashi A, Ushiki T, Abe K, et al. Cytoarchitecture of periendothelial cells in human cerebral venous vessels as compared with the scalp vein: A scanning electron microscopic study. *Arch Histol Cytol.* 1994;57:331-339.
52. Lanthier S, Lottie A, Michaud J, et al. Isolated angiitis of the CNS in children. *Neurology.* 2001;56:837-842.
53. Jennekens FG, Kater L. The central nervous system in systemic lupus erythematosus. Parts 1 and 2. *Rheumatology.* 2002;41:605-630.
54. McKelvie PA, Collins S, Thyagarajan D, et al. Meningoencephalomyelitis with vasculitis due to varicella zoster virus: A case report and review of the literature. *Pathology.* 2002;34:88-93.
55. Markus HS, Martin RJ, Simpson MA, et al. Diagnostic strategies in CADASIL. *Neurology.* 2002;59:1134-1138.
56. Fleetwood IG, Steinberg GK. Arteriovenous malformations. *Lancet.* 2002;359:863-873.
57. Hoya K, Asai A, Sasaki T. Expression of myosin heavy chain isoforms by smooth muscle cells in cerebral arteriovenous malformations. *Acta Neuropathol.* 2003;105:455-461.
58. McKeever PE. Insights about brain tumors gained through immunohistochemistry and in situ hybridization of nuclear and phenotypic markers. *J Histochem Cytochem.* 1998;46:585-594.
59. McKeever PE. Neurofilament (NF) and synaptophysin stains reveal diagnostic and prognostic patterns of interaction between normal and neoplastic tissues. Presented at the annual meeting of the Histochemical Society; Bethesda, MD: March 24, 2000.
60. Shi S-R, Cote RJ, Taylor CR. Antigen retrieval immunohistochemistry: Past, present, and future. *J Histochem Cytochem.* 1997;45:327-343.
61. McKeever PE, Ross DA, Strawderman MS, et al. A comparison of the predictive power for survival in gliomas provided by MIB-1, bromodeoxyuridine and proliferating cell nuclear antigen with histopathologic and clinical parameters. *J Neuropathol Exp Neurol.* 1997;7:798-805.
62. McKeever PE, Junck L, Strawderman MS, et al. Proliferation index is related to patient age in glioblastoma. *Neurology.* 2001;56:1216-1108.
63. McKeever PE, Strawderman MS, Yamini B, et al. MIB-1 proliferation index predicts survival among patients with grade II astrocytoma. *J Neuropathol Exp Neurol.* 1998;57:931-936.
64. Hsu DW, Louis DN, Efird JT, et al. Use of MIB-1 (Ki-67) immunoreactivity in differentiating grade II and grade III gliomas. *J Neuropathol Exp Neurol.* 1997;56:857-865.
65. Aboussekhra A, Wood RD. Detection of nucleotide excision repair incisions in human fibroblasts by immunostaining for PCNA. *Exp Cell Res.* 1995;221:326-332.
66. Schiffer D, Cavalla P, Migheli A, et al. Apoptosis and cell proliferation in human neuroepithelial tumors. *Neurosci Lett.* 1995;195:81-84.
67. Taniguchi K, Wakabayashi T, Yoshida T, et al. Immunohistochemical staining of DNA topoisomerase II alpha in human gliomas. *J Neurosurg.* 1999;91:477-482.
68. Chronwall BM, McKeever PE, Kornblith PL. Glial and nonglial neoplasms evaluated on frozen section by double immunofluorescence for fibronectin and glial fibrillary acidic protein. *Acta Neuropathol.* 1983;59:283-287.
69. McKeever PE, Balentine JD. Histochemistry of the nervous system. In: Spicer SS, ed. *Histochemistry in Pathologic Diagnosis.* New York: Marcel-Dekker; 1987:871-957.
70. Reifenberger G, Louis DN. Oligodendroglioma: Toward molecular definitions in diagnostic neuro-oncology. *J Neuropathol Exp Neurol.* 2003;62:111-126.
71. Rodas RA, Fenstermaker RA, McKeever PE, et al. Correlation of intraluminal thrombosis in brain tumor vessels with postoperative thrombotic complications. *J Neurosurg.* 1998;89:200-205.
72. Cheng Y, Pang JC, Ng HK, et al. Pilocytic astrocytomas do not show most of the genetic changes commonly seen in diffuse astrocytomas. *Histopathology.* 2000;37:437-444.
73. Korshunov A, Golanov A, Timirgaz V. Immunohistochemical markers for intracranial ependymoma recurrence. An analysis of 88 cases. *J Neurol Sci.* 2000;177:72-82.
74. Rubinstein LJ. *Tumors of the central nervous system.* Washington, D.C.: Armed Forces Institute of Pathology; 1972.
75. Burger PC, Scheithauer BW, Vogel FS. *Surgical Pathology of the Nervous System and Its Coverings.* 4th ed. New York: Churchill Livingstone; 2002.
76. Burger PC, Scheithauer BW. *AFIP Atlas of Tumor Pathology: Tumors of the Central Nervous System.* 4th Series. Washington, D.C. American Registry of Pathology & Armed Forces Institute of Pathology; 2007.
77. McKeever PE, Blaivas M, Gebarski SS. Sellar tumors other than adenomas. In: Thapar K, Kovacs K, Scheithauer BW, et al, eds. *Diagnosis and Management of Pituitary Tumors.* Totowa, NJ: Humana Press; 2001:387-447.
78. Hayostek C, Shaw EG, Scheithauer BW, et al. Astrocytomas of the cerebellum: A comparative clinicopathologic study of pilocytic and diffuse astrocytomas. *Cancer.* 1993;72:856-869.
79. Forsyth PA, Shaw EG, Scheithauer BW, et al. 51 cases of supratentorial pilocytic astrocytomas: A clinicopathologic, prognostic, and flow cytometric study. *Cancer.* 1993;72:1335-1342.
80. Coakley KJ, Huston J, Scheithauer BW, et al. Pilocytic astrocytomas: Well-demarcated magnetic resonance appearance despite frequent infiltration histologically. *Mayo Clin Proc.* 1995;70:747-751.
81. Clark GB, Henry JM, McKeever PE. Cerebral pilocytic astrocytoma. *Cancer.* 1985;56:1128-1133.
82. Hitotsumatsu T, Iwaki T, Fukui M, et al. Distinctive immunohistochemical profiles of small heat shock proteins (heat shock protein 27 and alpha B-crystallin) in human brain tumors. *Cancer.* 1996;77:352-361.
83. Camby I, Lefranc F, Titeca G, et al. Differential expression of S100 calcium-binding proteins characterizes distinct clinical entities in both WHO grade II and III astrocytic tumours. *Neuropathol Applied Neurobiol.* 2000;26:76-90.

84. Biegel JA. Genetics of pediatric central nervous system tumors. *J Pediatr Hematol Oncol.* 1997;19:492-501.
85. Rao RD, James CD. Altered molecular pathways in gliomas: An overview of clinically relevant issues. *Semin Oncol.* 2004;31:595-604.
86. Bigner SH, Schrock E. Molecular cytogenetics of brain tumors. *J Neuropathol Exp Neurol.* 1997;56:1173-1181.
87. Ho DM, Wong TT, Hsu CY, et al. MIB-1 labeling index in nonpilocytic astrocytoma of childhood: A study of 101 cases. *Cancer.* 1998;82:2459-2466.
88. McKeever PE, Blaivas M, Nelson JS. Diagnosis of nervous system tumors by light microscopic methods. In: Garcia JH, Budka H, McKeever PE, et al, eds. *Neuropathology: The Diagnostic Approach.* Philadelphia: CV Mosby; 1997:193-218.
89. Kimura N, Watanabe M, Date F, et al. HMB-45 and tuberin in hamartomas associated with tuberous sclerosis. *Mod Pathol.* 1997;10:952-959.
90. Levy RA, Allen R, McKeever P. Pleomorphic xanthoastrocytoma presenting with massive intracranial hemorrhage. *AJNR.* 1996;17:154-156.
91. Gokden M, Roth KA, Carroll SL, et al. Clear cell neoplasms and pseudoneoplastic lesions of the central nervous system. *Semin Diagn Pathol.* 1997;14:253-269.
92. Powell SZ, Yachnis AT, Rorke LB, et al. Divergent differentiation in pleomorphic xanthoastrocytoma: Evidence for a neuronal element and possible relationship to ganglion cell tumors. *Am J Surg Pathol.* 1996;20:80-85.
93. Kaulich K, Blaschke B, Numann A, et al. Genetic alterations commonly found in diffusely infiltrating cerebral gliomas are rare or absent in pleomorphic xanthoastrocytomas. *J Neuropathol Exp Neurol.* 2002;61:1092-1099.
94. Martinez-Diaz H, Kleinschmidt-DeMasters BK, Powell SZ, et al. Giant cell glioblastoma and pleomorphic xanthoastrocytoma show different immunohistochemical profiles for neuronal antigens and p53 but share reactivity for class III beta-tubulin. *Arch Pathol Lab Med.* 2003;127:1187-1191.
95. Zhu Y, Guignard F, Zhao D, et al. Early inactivation of p53 tumor suppressor gene cooperating with NF1 loss induces malignant astrocytoma. *Cancer Cell.* 2005;8:119-130.
96. Idbaih A, Boisselier B, Sanson M, et al. Tumor genomic profiling and TP53 germline mutation analysis of first-degree relative familial gliomas. *Cancer Genet Cytogenet.* 2007;176:121-126.
97. Li YJ, Sanson M, Hoang-Xuan K, et al. Incidence of germline p53 mutations in patients with gliomas. *Int J Cancer.* 1995;64:383-387.
98. Broniscer A, Ke W, Fuller CE, et al. Second neoplasms in pediatric patients with primary central nervous system tumors. *Cancer.* 2004;100:2246-2252.
99. Krutilkova V, Trkova M, Fleitz J, et al. Identification of five new families strengthens the link between childhood choroid plexus carcinoma and germline TP53 mutations. *Eur J Cancer.* 2005;41:1597-1603.
100. Rutherford J, Chu CE, Duddy PM, et al. Investigations on a clinically and functionally unusual and novel germline p53 mutation. *Br J Cancer.* 2002;86:1592-1596.
101. Tokunaga A, Onda M, Matsukura N, et al. Li-Fraumeni syndrome. *Nippon Rinsho.* 1995;53:2797-2802.
102. Figarella-Branger D, Gambarelli D, Dollo C, et al. Infratentorial ependymomas of childhood: Correlation between histologic features, immunohistological phenotype, silver nucleolar organizer region staining values and post-operative survival in 16 cases. *Acta Neuropathol.* 1991;82:208-216.
103. Mason WP, Krol GS, DeAngelis LM. Low-grade oligodendroglioma responds to chemotherapy. *Neurology.* 1996;46:203-207.
104. Yong WH, Chou D, Ueki K, et al. Chromosome 19q deletions in human gliomas overlap telomeric to D19S219 and may target a 425 kb region centromeric to D19S112. *J Neuropathol Exp Neurol.* 1995;54:622-626.
105. Dehghani F, Schachenmayr W, Laun A, et al. Prognostic implication of histopathological, immunohistochemical and clinical features of oligodendrogliomas: A study of 89 cases. *Acta Neuropathol.* 1998;95:493-504.
106. Coons SW, Johnson PC, Pearl DK. The prognostic significance of Ki-67 labeling indices for oligodendrogliomas. *Neurosurgery.* 1997;41:878-884.
107. Cairncross G, Berkey B, Shaw E, et al. Phase III trial of chemotherapy plus radiotherapy compared with radiotherapy alone for pure and mixed anaplastic oligodendroglioma: Intergroup RTOG 9402. *J Clin Oncol.* 2006;24:2707-2714.
108. Vogelbaum MA, Berkey B, Peereboom D, et al. RTOG 0131: Phase II trial of pre-irradiation and concurrent temozolomide in patients with newly diagnosed anaplastic oligodendrogliomas and mixed anaplastic oligodendrogliomas: Relationship between 1p/19q status and progression-free survival. *J Clin Oncol.* 2006;24:1517.
109. Perry A, Fuller CE, Banerjee R, et al. Ancillary FISH analysis for 1p and 19q status: Preliminary observations in 287 gliomas and oligodendroglioma mimics. *Front Biosci.* 2003;8:a1-a9.
110. Fuller CE, Schmidt RE, Roth KA, et al. Clinical utility of fluorescence in situ hybridization (FISH) in morphologically ambiguous gliomas with hybrid oligodendroglial/astrocytic features. *J Neuropathol Exp Neurol.* 2003;62:1118-1128.
111. Takekawa Y, Sawada T. Vascular endothelial growth factor and neovascularization in astrocytic tumors. *Pathol Int.* 1998;48:109-114.
112. Paulus W, Peiffer J. Intratumoral histologic heterogeneity of gliomas: A quantitative study. *Cancer.* 1989;64:442-447.
113. Davenport RD, McKeever PE. Ploidy of endothelium in high grade astrocytomas. *Anal Quant Cytol Histol.* 1987;9:25-29.
114. McKeever PE, Zhang K, Nelson JS, et al. Type IV collagen messenger RNA localizes within cells of abnormal vascular proliferations of glioblastoma and sarcomatous regions of gliosarcoma. *J Histochem Cytochem.* 1993;41:1124.
115. McKeever PE, Davenport RD, Shakui P. Patterns of antigenic expression in cultured glioma cells. *Crit Rev Neurobiol.* 1991;6:119-147.
116. Horiguchi H, Hirose T, Kannuki S, et al. Gliosarcoma: An immunohistochemical, ultrastructural and fluorescence in situ hybridization study. *Pathol Int.* 1998;48:595-602.
117. Boerman RH, Anderl K, Herath J, et al. The glial and mesenchymal elements of gliosarcomas share similar genetic alterations. *J Neuropathol Exp Neurol.* 1996;55:973-981.
118. Schröck E, Thiel G, Lozanova T, et al. Comparative hybridization of human malignant gliomas reveals multiple amplification sites and nonrandom chromosomal gains and losses. *Am J Pathol.* 1994;144:1203-1218.
119. McKeever PE, Dennis TR, Burgess AC, et al. Chromosomal breakpoint at 17q11.2 and insertion of DNA from three different chromosomes in a glioblastoma with exceptional glial fibrillary acidic protein expression. *Cancer Genet Cytogenet.* 1996;87:41-47.
120. Liu L, Ichimura K, Pettersson EH, et al. Chromosome 7 rearrangements in glioblastomas: Loci adjacent to EGFR are independently amplified. *J Neuropathol Exp Neurol.* 1998;57:1138-1145.
121. Hegi ME, Diserens AC, Gorlia T, et al. MGMT gene silencing and benefit from temozolomide in glioblastoma. *N Engl J Med.* 2005;352:997-1003.
122. Oberc-Greenwood MA, McKeever PE, Kornblith PL, et al. A human ganglioglioma containing paired helical filaments. *Hum Pathol.* 1984;15:834-838.
123. Wirnsberg GH, Becker H, Ziervogel K, et al. Diagnostic immunohistochemistry of neuroblastic tumors. *Am J Surg Pathol.* 1992;15:49-57.
124. Laeng RH, Scheithauer BW, Altermatt HJ. Anti-neuronal nuclear autoantibodies, types 1 and 2: Their utility in the study of tumors of the nervous system. *Acta Neuropathol.* 1998;96:329-339.
125. Goldbart A, Cheng ZJ, Brittian KR, et al. Intermittent hypoxia induces time-dependent changes in the protein kinase B signaling pathway in the hippocampal CA1 region of the rat. *Neurobiology of Disease.* 2003;14:440-446.
126. Felix I, Bilbao JM, Asa SL, et al. Cerebral and cerebellar gangliocytomas: A morphological study of nine cases. *Acta Neuropathol.* 1994;88:246-251.
127. Lindboe CF, Helseth E, Myhr G. Lhermitte-Duclos disease and giant meningioma as manifestations of Cowden's disease. *Clin Neuropathol.* 1995;14:327-330.
128. Daumas-Duport C, Varlet P, Bacha S, et al. Dysembryoplastic neuroepithelial tumors: Nonspecific histological forms—a study of 40 cases. *J Neurooncol.* 1999;41:267-280.

129. Wolf HK, Buslei R, Blumcke I, et al. Neural antigens in oligodendrogliomas and dysembryoplastic neuroepithelial tumors. *Acta Neuropathol.* 1997;94:436-443.
130. Guo SP, Zhang F, Li QL, et al. Papillary glioneuronal tumor—Contribution to a new tumor entity and literature review. *Clin Neuropathol.* 2008;27:72-77.
131. Gelpi E, Preusser M, Czech T, et al. Papillary glioneuronal tumor. *Neuropathology.* 2007;27:468-473.
132. Pimentel J, Resende M, Vaz A, et al. Rosette-forming glioneuronal tumor: Pathology case report. *Neurosurgery.* 2008;62:E1162-E1163.
133. Rodriguez FJ, Scheithauer BW, Robbins PD, et al. Ependymomas with neuronal differentiation: A morphologic and immunohistochemical spectrum. *Acta Neuropathol.* 2007;113:313-324.
134. Perry A, Scheithauer BW, Macaulay RJ, et al. Oligodendrogliomas with neurocytic differentiation. A report of 4 cases with diagnostic and histogenetic implications. *J Neuropathol Expl Neurol.* 2002;61:947-955.
135. Rout P, Santosh V, Mahadevan A, et al. Desmoplastic infantile ganglioglioma—Clinicopathological and immunohistochemical study of four cases. *Childs Nervous System.* 2002;18:463-467.
136. Figarella-Branger D, Pellissier JF, Daumas-Duport C, et al. Central neurocytomas: Critical evaluation of a small-cell neuronal tumor. *Am J Surg Pathol.* 1992;16:97-109.
137. Tong CY, Ng HK, Pang JC, et al. Central neurocytomas are genetically distinct from oligodendrogliomas and neuroblastomas. *Histopathology.* 2000;37:160-165.
138. Albrecht S, Rouah E, Becker LE, et al. Transthyretin immunoreactivity in choroid plexus neoplasms and brain metastases. *Mod Pathol.* 1991;4:610-614.
139. Kubo S, Ogino S, Fukushima T, et al. Immunocytochemical detection of insulin-like growth factor II (IGF-II) in choroid plexus papilloma: A possible marker for differential diagnosis. *Clin Neuropathol.* 1999;18:74-79.
140. Kepes JJ, Collins J. Choroid plexus epithelium (normal and neoplastic) expresses synaptophysin: A potentially useful aid in differentiating carcinoma of the choroid plexus from metastatic papillary carcinomas. *J Neuropathol Exp Neurol.* 1999;58:398-401.
141. Varga Z, Vajtai I. Prognostic markers in the histopathological diagnosis of tumors of the choroid plexus. *Orv Hetil.* 1998;139:761-765.
142. Kamaly-Asl ID, Shams N, Taylor MD. Genetics of choroid plexus tumors. *Neurosurg Focus.* 2006;20(1):E10.
143. Mena H, Rushing EJ, Ribas JL, et al. Tumors of pineal parenchymal cells: A correlation of histological features, including nucleolar organizer regions, with survival in 35 cases. *Hum Pathol.* 1995;26:20-30.
144. Hasselblatt M, Blumcke I, Jeibmann A, et al. Immunohistochemical profile and chromosomal imbalances in papillary tumours of the pineal region. *Neuropathol Appl Neurobiol.* 2006;32:278-283.
145. Buffenoir K, Rigoard P, Wager M, et al. Papillary tumor of the pineal region in a child: case report and review of the literature. *Childs Nervous System.* 2008;24:379-384.
146. Roberts RO, Lynch CF, Jones MP, et al. Medulloblastoma: A population-based study of 532 cases. *J Neuropathol Exp Neurol.* 1991;50:134-144.
147. Gilhuis HJ, Anderl KL, Boerman RH, et al. Comparative genomic hybridization of medulloblastomas and clinical relevance: Eleven new cases and a review of the literature. *Clinical Neurol Neurosurg.* 2000;102:203-209.
148. Tong CY, Hui AB, Yin XL, et al. Detection of oncogene amplifications in medulloblastomas by comparative genomic hybridization and array-based comparative genomic hybridization. *J Neurosurg Spine.* 2004;100:187-193.
149. Goldberg-Stern H, Gadoth N, Stern S, et al. The prognostic significance of glial fibrillary acidic protein staining in medulloblastoma. *Cancer.* 1991;68:568-573.
150. Katsetos CD, Herman MM, Frankfurter A, et al. Cerebellar desmoplastic medulloblastomas: A further immunohistochemical characterization of the reticulin-free pale islands. *Arch Pathol Lab Med.* 1989;113:1019-1029.
151. Freyer DR, Hutchinson RJ, McKeever PE. Primary primitive neuroectodermal tumor of the spinal cord associated with neural tube defect. *Pediatr Neurosci.* 1989;15:181-187.
152. Mobley BC, Roulston D, Shah GV, et al. Peripheral PNET/Ewing sarcoma in the craniospinal vault: Case report and review. *Hum Pathol.* 2005;37:845-853.
153. Burnett ME, White EC, Sih S. Chromosome arm 17p deletion analysis reveals molecular genetic heterogeneity in supratentorial and infratentorial primitive neuroectodermal tumors of the central nervous system. *Cancer Genet Cytogenet.* 1997;97:25-31.
154. Rorke LB, Packer R, Biegel J. Central nervous system atypical teratoid/rhabdoid tumors of infancy and childhood. *J Neurooncol.* 1995;24:21-28.
155. Biegel JA. Molecular genetics of atypical teratoid/rhabdoid tumor. *Neurosurg Focus.* 2006;20:E11.
156. Nishihira Y, Tan CF, Hirato J, et al. A case of congenital supratentorial tumor: Atypical teratoid/rhabdoid tumor or primitive neuroectodermal tumor? *Neuropathol.* 2007;27:551-555.
157. Khoddami M, Becker LE. Immunohistochemistry of medulloepithelioma and neural tube. *Pediatr Pathol Lab Med.* 1997;17:913-925.
158. Mork SJ, Rubinstein LJ. Ependymoblastoma: A reappraisal of a rare embryonal tumor. *Cancer.* 1985;55:1536-1542.
159. Salvati M, Artico M, Lunardi P, et al. Intramedullary meningioma: Case report and review of the literature. *Surg Neurol.* 1992;37:42-45.
160. Meis JM, Ordonez NG, Bruner JM. Meningiomas: An immunohistochemical study of 50 cases. *Arch Pathol Lab Med.* 1986;110:934-937.
161. Perry A, Scheithauer BW, Nascimento AG. The immunophenotypic spectrum of meningeal hemangiopericytoma: A comparison with fibrous meningioma and solitary fibrous tumor of meninges. *Am J Surg Pathol.* 1997;21:1354-1360.
162. Carneiro SS, Scheithauer BW, Nascimento AG, et al. Solitary fibrous tumor of the meninges: A lesion distinct from fibrous meningioma: A clinicopathologic and immunohistochemical study. *Am J Clin Pathol.* 1996;106:217-224.
163. Kepes JJ. *Meningiomas: biology, pathology, and differential diagnosis.* Chicago: Year Book Medical; 1982.
164. Lattes R, Bigotti G. Lipoblastic meningioma: "Vacuolated meningioma." *Hum Pathol.* 1991;22:164-171.
165. Ito H, Kawano N, Yada K, et al. Meningiomas differentiating to arachnoid trabecular cells: A proposal for histological subtype "arachnoid trabecular cell meningioma." *Acta Neuropathol.* 1991;82:327-330.
166. Kulah A, Ilcayto R, Fiskeci C. Cystic meningiomas. *Acta Neurochir (Wien).* 1991;111:108-113.
167. Winek RR, Scheithauer BW, Wick MR. Meningioma, meningeal hemangiopericytoma (angioblastic meningioma), peripheral hemangiopericytoma, and acoustic schwannoma: A comparative immunohistochemical study. *Am J Surg Pathol.* 1989;13:251-261.
168. Kobata H, Kondo A, Iwasaki K, et al. Chordoid meningioma in a child. *J Neurosurg.* 1998;88:319-323.
169. Probst-Cousin S, Villagran-Lillo R, Lahl R, et al. Secretory meningioma: Clinical, histologic, and immunohistochemical findings in 31 cases. *Cancer.* 1997;79:2003-2015.
170. Alameda F, Lloreta J, Ferrer MD, et al. Clear cell meningioma of the lumbo-sacral spine with chordoid features. *Ultrastruct Pathol.* 1999;23:51-58.
171. Cerdá-Nicolás M, López-Ginés C, Peydró-Olaya A, et al. Histologic and cytogenetic patterns in benign, atypical, and malignant meningiomas: Does correlation with recurrence exist? *Int J Surg Pathol.* 1995;2:301-310.
172. Perry A, Scheithauer BW, Stafford SL, et al. "Rhabdoid" meningioma: An aggressive variant. *Am J Surg Pathol.* 1998;22:1482-1490.
173. Kobayashi S, Haba R, Hirakawa E, et al. Cytology and immunohistochemistry of anaplastic meningiomas in squash preparations: A report of two cases. *Acta Cytol.* 1995;39:118-124.
174. Perry A, Scheithauer BW, Stafford SL, et al. "Malignancy" in meningiomas: A clinicopathologic study of 116 patients, with grading implications. *Cancer.* 1999;85:2046-2056.
175. Prayson RA. Malignant meningioma: A clinicopathologic study of 23 patients including MIB-1 and p53 immunohistochemistry. *Am J Clin Pathol.* 1996;105:719-726.

176. Hatiboglu MA, Cosar M, Iplikcioglu AC, et al. Sex steroid and epidermal growth factor profile of giant meningiomas associated with pregnancy. *Surg Neurol.* 2008;69:356-362.
177. Wolfsberger S, Doostkam S, Boecher-Schwarz HG, et al. Progesterone-receptor index in meningiomas: Correlation with clinicopathological parameters and review of the literature. *Neurosurg Rev.* 2004;27:238-245.
178. Buccoliero AM, Gheri CF, Castiglione F, et al. Merlin expression in secretory meningiomas: Evidence of an NF2-independent pathogenesis? Immunohistochemical study. *Appl Immunohistochem Mol Morphol.* 2007;15:353-357.
179. Hanemann CO. Magic but treatable? Tumours due to loss of merlin. *Brain.* 2008;131:606-615.
180. Begnami MD, Rushing EJ, Santi M, et al. Evaluation of NF2 gene deletion in pediatric meningiomas using chromogenic in situ hybridization. *Int J Surg Pathol.* 2007;15:110-115.
181. Fletcher CD, Unni KK, Mertens F, eds. *World Health Organization Classification of Tumors: Pathology and Genetics of Tumors of Soft Tissue and Bone.* Lyon: IARC Press; 2002.
182. Probst-Cousin S, Rickert CH, Gullotta F. Factor XIIIa-immunoreactivity in tumors of the central nervous system. *Clin Neuropathol.* 1998;17:79-84.
183. Tihan T, Viglione M, Rosenblum MK, et al. Solitary fibrous tumors in the central nervous system: A clinicopathologic review of 18 cases and comparison to meningeal hemangiopericytomas. *Arch Pathol Lab Med.* 2003;127:432-439.
184. Miettinen MM, el-Rifai W, Sarlomo-Rikala M, et al. Tumor size-related DNA copy number changes occur in solitary fibrous tumors but not in hemangiopericytomas. *Mod Pathol.* 1997;10:1194-1200.
185. Persson S, Kindblom LG, Angervall L. Classical and chondroid chordoma: A light-microscopic, histochemical, ultrastructural and immunohistochemical analysis of the various cell types. *Pathol Res Pract.* 1991;187:828-838.
186. Paulus W, Slowik F, Jellinger K. Primary intracranial sarcomas: Histopathological features of 19 cases. *Histopathology.* 1991;18:395-402.
187. Powell HC, Marshall LF, Igneizi RJ. Post-irradiation pituitary sarcoma. *Acta Neuropathol.* 1977;39:165-167.
188. McKeever PE, Blaivas M, Sima AAF. Neoplasms of the sellar region. In: Lloyd RV, ed. *Surgical Pathology of the Pituitary Gland.* Philadelphia: Saunders; 193:141-210.
189. Ariza A, Kim JH. Kaposi's sarcoma of the dura mater. *Hum Pathol.* 1988;19:1461-1463.
190. Rushing EJ, Mena H, Smirniotopoulos JG. Mesenchymal chondrosarcoma of the cauda equina. *Clin Neuropathol.* 1995;14:150-153.
191. Matsukado Y, Yokota A, Marubayashi T. Rhabdomyosarcoma of the brain. *J Neurosurg.* 1975;43:215-221.
192. Scheithauer BW, Woodruff JM, Erlandson RA. *Tumors of the Peripheral Nervous System.* Washington, DC: American Registry of Pathology; 1999.
193. Geddes JF, Sutcliffe JC, King TT. Mixed cranial nerve tumors in neurofibromatosis type 2. *Clin Neuropathol.* 1995;14:310-313.
194. Hayashi K, Hoshida Y, Horie Y, et al. Immunohistochemical study on the distribution of alpha and beta subunits of S-100 protein in brain tumors. *Acta Neuropathol.* 1991;81:657-663.
195. Warren C, James LA, Ramsden R, et al. Identification of recurrent regions of chromosome loss and gain in vestibular schwannomas using comparative genomic hybridisation. *J Med Genet.* 2003;40:802-806.
196. Thaxton C, Lopera J, Bott M, et al. Neuregulin and laminin stimulate phosphorylation of the NF2 tumor suppressor in Schwann cells by distinct protein kinase A and p21-activated kinase-dependent pathways. *Oncogene.* 2008;27:2705-2715.
197. Flaiz C, Utermark T, Parkinson DB, et al. Impaired intercellular adhesion and immature adherens junctions in merlin-deficient human primary schwannoma cells. *GLIA.* 2008;56:506-515.
198. von Deimling A, Krone W, Menon AG. Neurofibromatosis type 1: Pathology, clinical features and molecular genetics. *Brain Pathol.* 1995;5:153-162.
199. Storlazzi CT, Von Steyern FV, Domanski HA, et al. Biallelic somatic inactivation of the NF1 gene through chromosomal translocations in a sporadic neurofibroma. *Int J Cancer.* 2005;117:1055-1057.
200. Valdez R, McKeever P, Finn WG, et al. Composite germ cell tumor and B-cell non-Hodgkin's lymphoma arising in the sella turcica. *Hum Pathol.* 2002;33:1044-1047.
201. Nakagawa Y, Perentes E, Ross GW, et al. Immunohistochemical differences between intracranial germinomas and their gonadal equivalents: An immunoperoxidase study of germ cell tumours with epithelial membrane antigen, cytokeratin, and vimentin. *J Pathol.* 1988;156:67-72.
202. Garvin AJ, Spicer SS, McKeever PE. The cytochemical demonstration of intracellular immunoglobulin: In neoplasms of lymphoreticular tissue. *Am J Pathol.* 1976;82:457-478.
203. Jaffee ES, Harris NL, Stein H, et al, eds. *World Health Organization Classification Of Tumors: Pathology and Genetics of Tumors of Haematopoietic and Lymphoid Tissues.* Lyon: IARC Press; 2001.
204. Lai R, Rosenblum MK, DeAngelis LM. Primary CNS lymphoma: A whole-brain disease? *Neurology.* 2002;59:1557-1562.
205. Davenport RD, O'Donnell LJ, Schnitzer B, et al. Non-Hodgkin's lymphoma of the brain following Hodgkin's disease: An immunohistochemical study. *Cancer.* 1991;67:440-443.
206. Morgello S. Pathogenesis and classification of primary central nervous system lymphoma: An update. *Brain Pathol.* 1995;5:383-393.
207. Carbone A. AIDS-related non-Hodgkin's lymphomas: From pathology and molecular pathogenesis to treatment. *Hum Pathol.* 2002;33:392-404.
208. Kadan-Lottick NS, Skluzacek MC, Gurney JG. Decreasing incidence rates of primary central nervous system lymphoma. *Cancer.* 2002;95:193-202.
209. Ferracini R, Bergmann M, Pileri S, et al. Primary T-cell lymphoma of the central nervous system. *Clin Neuropathol.* 1995;14:125-129.
210. An-Foraker SH. Cytodiagnosis of malignant lesions in cerebrospinal fluid. Review and cytohistologic correlation. *Acta Cytol.* 1985;29:286-290.
211. Deodhare SS, Ang LC, Bilbao JM. Isolated intracranial involvement in Rosai-Dorfman disease: A report of two cases and review of the literature. *Arch Pathol Lab Med.* 1998;122:161-165.
212. Adle-Biassette H, Chetritt J, Bergemer-Fouquet AM, et al. Pathology of the central nervous system in Chester-Erdheim disease: Report of three cases. *J Neuropathol Exp Neurol.* 1997;56:1207-1216.
213. McKeever P, Lloyd RV. Tumors of the pituitary region. In: Garcia JH, Budka H, McKeever PE, eds. *Neuropathology: The Diagnostic Approach.* Philadelphia: CV Mosby; 1997:219-262.
214. Tachibana O, Yamashima T, Yamashita J. Immunohistochemical study of erythropoietin in cerebellar hemangioblastomas associated with secondary polycythemia. *Neurosurgery.* 1991;28:24-26.
215. Feldenzer JA, McKeever PE. Selective localization of gamma-enolase in stromal cells of cerebellar hemangioblastomas. *Acta Neuropathol.* 1987;72:281-285.
216. Rubio A, Meyers SP, Powers JM, et al. Hemangioblastoma of the optic nerve. *Hum Pathol.* 1994;25:1249-1251.
217. McComb RD, Eastman PJ, Hahn FJ, et al. Cerebellar hemangioblastoma with prominent stromal astrocytosis: Diagnostic and histogenetic considerations. *Clin Neuropathol.* 1987;6:149-154.
218. Silverstein AM, Quint DJ, McKeever PE. Intraductal paraganglioma of the thoracic spine. *Am J Neuroradiol.* 1990;11:614-616.
219. Lloyd RV. Immunohistochemical localization of chromogranin in polypeptide hormone producing cells and tumors. In: Lechago J, Kameya T, eds. *Endocrine Pathology Update.* Philadelphia: Field and Wood; 1990.
220. Abbott MA, Nathanson KL, Nightingale S, et al. The von Hippel-Lindau (VHL) germline mutation V84L manifests as early-onset bilateral pheochromocytoma. *Am J Med Genet A.* 2006;140:685-690.
221. Vortmeyer AO, Huang SC, Koch CA, et al. Somatic von Hippel-Lindau gene mutations detected in sporadic endolymphatic sac tumors. *Cancer Res.* 2000;60:5963-5965.

222. Lin F, Shi J, Liu H, et al. Immunohistochemical detection of the von Hippel-Lindau gene product (pVHL) in human tissues and tumors: A useful marker for metastatic renal cell carcinoma and clear cell carcinoma of the ovary and uterus. *Am J Clin Pathol.* 2008;129:592-605.
223. Xin W, Rubin MA, McKeever PE. Differential expression of cytokeratins 8 and 20 distinguishes craniopharyngioma from Rathke cleft cyst. *Arch Pathol Lab Med.* 2002;126:1174-1178.
224. McKeever PE, Spicer SS. Pituitary histochemistry. In: Spicer SS, ed. *Histochemistry in Pathologic Diagnosis.* New York: Marcel-Dekker; 1987:603-645.
225. Wong SW, Ducker TB, Powers JM. Fulminating parapontine epidermoid carcinoma in a four-year-old boy. *Cancer.* 1976;37:1525-1531.
226. Weller M, Stevens A, Sommer N, et al. Tumor cell dissemination triggers an intrathecal immune response in neoplastic meningitis. *Cancer.* 1992;69:1475-1480.
227. Bigner SH, Johnston WW. The cytopathology of cerebrospinal fluid. II: Metastatic cancer, meningeal carcinomatosis and primary central nervous system neoplasms. *Acta Cytol.* 1981;25:461-479.
228. DeYoung BR, Wick MR. Immunohistologic evaluation of metastatic carcinomas of unknown origin: An algorithmic approach. *Semin Diagn Pathol.* 2000;17:184-193.
229. Chu P, Wu E, Weiss LM. Cytokeratin 7 and cytokeratin 20 expression in epithelial neoplasms: A survey of 435 cases. *Med Pathol.* 2000;13:962-972.
230. Srodon M, Westra WH. Immunohistochemical staining for thyroid transcription factor-1: A helpful aid in discerning primary site of tumor origin in patients with brain metastases. *Hum Pathol.* 2002;33:642-645.
231. Cochran AJ, Wen DR. S-100 protein as a marker for melanocytic and other tumors. *Pathology.* 1985;17:340-345.
232. Rushing EJ, Mena J, Ribas JL. Primary pineal parenchymal lesions: A review of 53 cases. *J Neuropathol Exp Neurol.* 1991;50:364.
233. Coca S, Martinez A, Vaquero J, et al. Immunohistochemical study of intracranial cysts. *Histol Histopathol.* 1993;8:651-654.
234. Ho KL, Garcia JH. Colloid cysts of the third ventricle: Ultrastructural features are compatible with endodermal derivation. *Acta Neuropathol.* 1992;83:605-612.
235. McKeever PE, Brissie NT. Scanning electron microscopy of neoplasms removed at surgery: surface topography and comparison of meningioma, colloid cyst, ependymoma, pituitary adenoma, schwannoma and astrocytoma. *J Neuropathol Exp Neurol.* 1977;36:875-896.
236. McKeever PE, Hall BJ, Spicer SS. The origin of colloid cysts of the third ventricle. *J Neuropathol Exp Neurol.* 1978;37:658.
237. Bejjani GK, Wright DC, Schessel D, et al. Endodermal cysts of the posterior fossa: Report of three cases and review of the literature. *J Neurosurg.* 1998;89:326-335.
238. Go KG, Blankenstein MA, Vroom TM, et al. Progesterone receptors in arachnoid cysts: An immunocytochemical study in 2 cases. *Acta Neurochirurg.* 1997;139:349-354.
239. Mirra SS, Heyman A, McKeel D, et al. The Consortium to Establish a Registry for Alzheimer's Disease (CERAD). Part II: Standardization of the neuropathologic assessment of Alzheimer's disease. *Neurology.* 1991;41:479-486.
240. Mirra SS, Hart MN, Terry RD. Making the diagnosis of Alzheimer's disease. A primer for practicing pathologists. *Arch Patho Lab Med.* 1993;117:132-144.
241. National Institute on Aging. Reagan Institute Working Group on diagnostic criteria of the neuropathological assessment of Alzheimer's disease: Consensus recommendations for the postmortem diagnosis of Alzheimer's disease. *Neurobiol Aging.* 1997;18:S1-S2.
242. Feany MB, Dickson DW. Neurodegenerative disorders with extensive tau pathology: A comparative study and review. *Ann Neurol.* 1996;40:139-148.
243. Dwork AJ, Liu D, Kaufman MA, et al. Archival, formalin-fixed tissue: Its use in the study of Alzheimer's type changes. *Clin Neuropathol.* 1998;17:45-49.
244. Lue LF, Brachova L, Civin WH, et al. Inflammation, A beta deposition, and neurofibrillary tangle formation as correlates of Alzheimer's disease neurodegeneration. *J Neuropathol Exp Neurol.* 1996;55:1083-1088.
245. Jellinger KA. Vascular-ischemic dementia: An update. *J Neurol Transm Suppl.* 2002;62:1-23.
246. McKeith IG, Ballard CG, Perry RH, et al. Prospective validation of consensus criteria for the diagnosis of dementia with Lewy bodies. *Neurology.* 2000;54:1050-1058.
247. Braak H, Del Tredici K, Rub U, et al. Staging of brain pathology related to sporadic Parkinson's disease. *Neurobiol Aging.* 2003;24:197-211.
248. McKahann GM, Albert MS, Grossman M, et al. Clinical and pathological diagnosis of frontotemporal dementia: report of the Work Group on Frontotemporal Dementia and Pick's Disease. *Arch Neurol.* 2001;58:1803-1809.
249. Wanschitz J, Hainfellner JA, Simonitsch I, et al. Non-HTLV-I associated pleomorphic T-cell lymphoma of the brain mimicking post-vaccinal acute inflammatory demyelination. *Neuropathol Appl Neurobiol.* 1997;23:43-49.
250. Tachikawa N, Goto M, Hoshino Y, et al. Detection of Toxoplasma gondii, Epstein-Barr virus, and JC virus DNAs in the cerebrospinal fluid in acquired immunodeficiency syndrome patients with focal central nervous system complications. *Intern Med.* 1999;38:556-562.
251. Zagzag D, Miller DC, Kleinman GM, et al. Demyelinating disease versus tumor in surgical neuropathology: Clues to a correct pathologic diagnosis. *Am J Surg Pathol.* 1993;17:537-545.
252. Reith KG, Di Chiro G, Cromwell LD, et al. Primary demyelinating disease simulating glioma of the corpus callosum. *J Neurosurg.* 1981;55:620-624.
253. Schmidt B, Toyka KV, Kiefer R, et al. Inflammatory infiltrates in sural nerve biopsies in Guillain-Barré syndrome and chronic inflammatory demyelinating neuropathy. *Muscle Nerve.* 1996; 19:474-487.
254. Matsumuro K, Izumo S, Umehara F, et al. Chronic inflammatory demyelinating polyneuropathy: Histological and immunopathological studies on biopsied sural nerves. *J Neurol Sci.* 1994;127:170-178.
255. Babb TL, Brown WJ. Pathological findings in epilepsy. In: Engel J, ed. *Surgical Treatment of the Epilepsies.* New York: Raven Press; 1987:511-540.
256. Bruton CJ. The Neuropathology of temporal lobe epilepsy. In: Russel G, Marley E, Williams P, eds. *Maudsley Monographs.* No. 31. London: Oxford Press; 1988:1-94.
257. Prayson RA, Frater JL. Rasmussen encephalitis: A clinicopathologic and immunohistochemical study of seven patients. *Am J Clin Pathol.* 2002;117:776-782.
258. Frater JL, Prayson RA, Morris III HH, et al. Surgical pathologic findings of extratemporal-based intractable epilepsy: A study of 133 consecutive reactions. *Arch Pathol Lab Med.* 2000;124:545-549.
259. Volk EE, Prayson RA. Hamartomas in the setting of chronic epilepsy: A clinicopathologic study of 13 cases. *Hum Pathol.* 1997;28:227-232.
260. Smith DF, Hutton JL, Sandemann D, et al. The prognosis of primary intracerebral tumours presenting with epilepsy: The outcome of medical and surgical management. *J Neurol Neurosurg Psychiatry.* 1991;54:915-920.

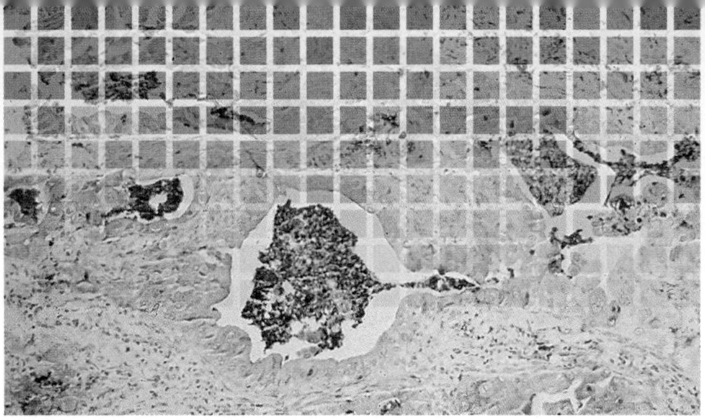

21

Immunocytology

Mamatha Chivukula • David J. Dabbs

- Introduction 890
- Immunocytology Techniques 890
- Specific Organ Cytology 897
- Carcinoma of Unknown Primary 907
- Beyond Immunocytochemistry 910
- Theranostic Applications: ICC for Targeted Therapies 911
- Conclusion 912

INTRODUCTION

The application of immunohistochemistry (IHC) in diagnostic cytopathology in the workup of difficult cases has paralleled the progress seen in surgical pathology and continues to grow. IHC has added a new dimension for cytologic diagnosis. With the use of automation, there has been a great deal of quality improvement in recent years. IHC continues to play an important role in diagnostic cytopathology, and it is evolving as an important adjuvant tool in targeted therapies.

IMMUNOCYTOLOGY TECHNIQUES

Specimen Collection

Cytomorphology forms the basis for determining the most appropriate ancillary technique to use to arrive at a precise diagnosis. The most important tasks for the cytopathologist are to ensure that conventional Romanowsky or Papanicolaou stains have been examined, that a differential diagnosis is generated, and that the appropriate question to be answered by IHC is generated. An array of specimens that can be used for IHC includes exfoliative cell preparations, effusions, direct imprints, fine-needle aspirates, and thin-layer collection samples. These specimens can be processed with air drying or immediate fixation in alcohol, or they can be processed as cytocentrifuge or cell block preparations.

Fixation

Some of the important prerequisites for adequate IHC studies[1] are a well-spread film of cells on a glass slide,[2] adequate fixation,[3] removal of blood and proteinaceous material, and a sensitive, reproducible method of immunocytochemistry (ICC).[4] Wet fixation in alcohol (WFA) must be performed without delay because partial air drying may result in false-positive results. Air-dried smears (ADS) are often more cellular than alcohol-fixed slides because some material often floats off the slide when it is alcohol fixed. Using air-dried slides minimizes cell loss and results in a more even film of cells. Such slides must be fixed immediately before performing IHC, and the types of preferred fixatives vary among cytopathologists. Cold acetone and 95% alcohol[5] are common fixatives, and B5 may be used for lymphoid markers and neuroendocrine antibodies.[6]

Leong and colleagues advocated post-fixation of air-dried smears after testing different fixatives. Though physiologic saline and 96% alcohol with rehydration in normal saline for 30 minutes are the best fixatives, the cytomorphology is crisper and less background staining is seen with the latter.[7,8] A recent study by Fulciniti and associates has shown that formalin post-fixed air-dried smears are reliable and better than the standard wet-fixed smears.[9] The study proposed that the slow dehydration and short rehydration might contribute to a superior interpretation of the results. Our experience showed similar results with preparations that were relatively free of background blood and mucus.[10] The antibodies used with post-fixation are listed in Table 21.1.

An important point to keep in mind is that certain antibodies such as S-100 protein, Hep Par 1, and gross cystic disease fluid protein-15 (GCDFP-15) are leached from alcohol fixatives and often render false-negative results.

Immunohistochemistry: Standardization Issues

The history of standardization attempts is long and is well discussed by Clive Taylor, beginning with his transactions on the Biological Stain Commission and

TABLE 21.1 Antibodies Used with Post-Fixation Technique

Antibody Type	Clone/Code	Producer	Dilution	Antigen Retrieval
Epithelial Markers				
CK7	NCL-CK7 OVTL	Novocastra, Newcastle Upon Tyne, U.K.	1:80	MW
CK20	NCL-CK20 543	Novocastra	1:100	MW
AE1-AE3	NCL-AE1-AE3	Novocastra	1:100	MW
EMA	NCL-EMA	Novocastra	1:400	None
Mesenchymal Markers				
Vimentin	NCL-VIM V9	Novocastra	1:100	MW
SM actin	NCL-SMA	Novocastra	1:80	None
Desmin	NCL-DES-DER II	Novocastra	1:100	Trypsin
Neurofilaments	NCL-NF68-DA2	Novocastra	1:200	MW
Prognostic Markers				
ER	1D5	Dako	1:35	MW pH 9
PR	SP1	Ventana	1:50	MW
HER2	4B5	Ventana	1:80	MW pH 9
Ki-67	NCL-Ki-67-MM1	Novocastra	1:200	MW
Cyclin D 1	P2D11F11	Novocastra	1:50	MW
E-cadherin	NCH-38	Dako	1:100	HCB
EGFR	E30	Dako	1:50	Proteinase K
CD Markers				
CD3	PS1	Novocastra	1:200	MW
CD4	4B2	Novocastra	1:30	MW
CD5	4C7	Novocastra	1:50	MW
CD8	CD5/54/F6	Dako	1:50	MW pH 9
CD10	SS2/36	Dako	1:40	None
CD15	C3D-1	Dako	1:50	MW pH 9
CD20	NCL-CD20-L26	Novocastra	1:50	MW
CD30	Ber-H2	Dako	1:40	MW pH 9
CD45	X16-99	Novocastra	1:20	MW
CD56	CD564	Novocastra	1:100	MW
CD246	ALK1	Dako	1:50	MW pH 9
Myeloperoxidase	Polyclonal	Dako	1:500	MW
Neuroendocrine Markers				
S-100	Polyclonal	Dako	1:400	MW
NSE	BBS/NC/VI-H14	Dako	1:250	MW
HMB45	HMB45	Novocastra	1:60	Trypsin
Calcitonin	M3509	Dako	1:80	None
mCEA	M7072	Dako	1:50	MW

HCB, hot citrate buffer bath treatment; MW, microwave open treatment.

continuing into detailed discussions about the "total test concept" of the IHC tests.[11,12] Currently, most IHC practices in surgical pathology are of diagnostic nature, an exercise that identifies cell lines as epithelial, germ cell, melanoma, hematopoietic, or sarcoma. Rapidly emerging IHC applications are theranostic as well as genomic, and both applications affect the proper treatment of patients.

The Biologic Stain Commission was one of the original agencies to oversee the special stains used in the anatomic pathology laboratory. The agencies that followed include the Clinical Laboratory Standards Institute (CLSI, previously NCCLS), the Food and Drug Administration (FDA), and commissions set up by professional organizations including the College of American Pathologists (CAP). The emphasis of all these organizations has been on consistent, high-quality assay components for IHC. We recognize the fruit of the labor as the "package inserts" that accompany various IHC reagents.

A recent study by members of the Ad-Hoc Committee on Immunohistochemistry Standardization recommends formalin fixative as the standard for immunohistochemical testing, along with a minimum of 8 hours fixative time for prognostic/predictive markers, including estrogen receptor (ER), progesterone receptor (PR), and HER2/neu.[11] These guidelines have been incorporated by the CAP-ASCO committee for breast cancer hormone receptor testing (publication in press). These recommendations follow the simple fact that all clinical validated studies for ER/PR/HER2/neu antibodies have been performed on formalin-fixed paraffin-embedded tissue (FFPE). Alcohol fixatives result in spurious results for ER/PR/HER2/neu and should not be used for those important prognostic and predictive markers. Although alcohol fixatives can be used for other antibodies, it is imperative for the laboratory director to validate protocols to formalin-based results and use appropriate alcohol-based controls if alcohol fixation of cytologic specimens is used. FFPE cell blocks are the preferred samples for IHC. In our laboratory, we have successfully extended our standardization protocols for surgical specimens to cytology specimens.

Rehydration and Storage

Air-dried slides and partially fixed air-dried slides can be rehydrated in normal saline to optimize immunoreactivity as well as cytomorphology.[13–15] Chan and Kung found that the optimal time for rehydration is less than 1 minute, provided that the air-drying time did not exceed 30 minutes.[15] This procedure may be used when cytomorphology is critically important, since air-dried slides can sit for up to 1 week at room temperature and still be used for IHC provided they are fixed immediately before use as already described.[7] Slides for IHC, whether air-dried or fixed, can be stored at −70°C for at least 1 month and still maintain immunoreactivity.[8]

Antigen Retrieval

One of the important methods through which standardization of IHC can be achieved is antigen retrieval. An ideal antigen-retrieval technique is considered to maintain formalin as a standard fixative for both morphology and IHC.[16] High-temperature heating is the most crucial step in this methodology to retrieve the antigens masked by formalin fixation. However, simple methods such as immersing in water or NaOH-methanol solution will yield dramatic retrieval results.[17] Although use of metal ions using zinc and lead[18] in the antigen retrieval solutions has shown improved results in many studies, their environmental toxicity has given way to alternatives such as citrate, Tris, urea, and EDTA. Antigen retrieval has been widely used for detection of ER, PR, MIB1, p53, BCL-2, retinoblastoma gene (pRB), and some cluster designation (CD) markers. Though the literature on the subject of use of antigen retrieval on cytology specimens is still evolving, some important studies have successfully shown that antigen retrieval can be applied to these specimens for a wide range of antibodies.[18] Results are satisfactory and are comparable to their tissue specimen counterparts. Sherman and colleagues have shown a method of "cell transfer" that can facilitate immunostaining on small samples.[19] In a study that compared the effects of heat (using a pressure cooker) on air-dried versus alcohol-fixed smears for cytokeratin (AE1/3, 5D3), cytokeratin 7, cytokeratin 20, neurofibrillary protein (NFP), synaptophysin, ER (clone ID5), PR (clone 1294), and vimentin, it was found that ADS results improved with antigen retrieval. Miller and associates found that fine-needle aspiration biopsy (FNAB) material studied through tissue transfer to adhesive slides, followed by antigen retrieval using the same conditions as for routine paraffin sections, substantially improved ease of interpretation, especially in the air-dried smears.[20]

Fixation for Hormone Receptors

Estrogen receptors (ER) and progesterone receptors (PR) and overexpression of HER2/neu are important prognostic and predictive markers of breast carcinoma. The 1999 CAP consensus statement included the topic of routine performance of hormone receptor analysis and HER2/neu testing, which are usually performed on core needle biopsies or surgical resection specimens.[21] A critically important statement from the NIH consensus conference of December 2000 states, "any nuclear expression of hormone receptors should be regarded as a positive result and render a patient eligible for hormonal therapy."[22] This has enormous implications for treatment purposes. It was not until recently that the need for standardization for pre-analytic variables, particularly tissue fixation, was a critical component of the total test result. Underfixation of tissue cannot be repaired and is the least desirable result of handling tissues in the anatomic pathology laboratory. No amount of antigen retrieval can resurrect a tissue that is under-fixed. Antigens will be lost and false negatives will abound in such situations, regardless of the quality of instrumentation. Over-fixation, on the other hand, can be repaired through a combination of antigen retrieval, antibody titer, and detection systems.[23,24]

The optimal result is to have a standard fixation time, ideally unique for every antigen that one is attempting to detect. For example, as per the CAP-ASCO guidelines, the recommended minimum fixation in 10% neutral buffered formalin for HER2/neu IHC is 6 hours, and for hormone receptors it is 8 hours.

Routinely processed cytologic specimens fixed in formalin (e.g., fine-needle aspiration [FNA]) smears, touch imprints of core needle biopsies, effusions) can also be used to assess the receptor status and HER2 protein by immunohistochemistry.[25]

Estrogen receptor staining on FNA smears using different methods has shown that de-staining the slides with alcohol prior to immunocytostaining significantly reduces the number of cells with positive nuclear staining.[26] Many studies concluded that alcohol may not be an optimal fixative for preserving the ER epitopes, as discussed earlier in this chapter.[26] The available anti-ER antibodies (ID5, 6F11) perform best with formalin fixation (10%) for hormone receptors.[7] Breast prognostic markers MIB1 and c-erbB-2 work well in formalin fixation. It is noted that the immunohistochemical results of ER are highly dependent on fixation time. The minimum fixation time for optimal tissue immunohistochemical results of ER is 8 hours.[27] PreservCyt (Cytyc Corporation, Marlborough, Mass) is a preservative used with the Thin-prep processor (Cytyc Corporation) that stabilizes ER/PR receptors for up to 56 days of storage.[28] The obvious convenience is the ability to collect specimens from clinicians at remote sites. However, primary formalin fixation is essential for ER/PR and HER2/neu because clinical outcome studies are based on results in which tissues were fixed in formalin. Formalin-fixed cell blocks are the venue of choice for ER/PR and HER2/neu owing to better specimen standardization.

Thin-Layer Technique

One can achieve excellent immunostaining results with IHC using the proprietary solutions Cytolyt and PreservCyt, with or without processing on the ThinPrep processor.[29-32] In our experience, lower antibody concentrations can be used, the background is cleaner, immunostaining is crisp,[32] and immunoreactivity is stable even with long-term storage in PreservCyt.[28] It is crucial to assure that the immunostaining pattern is validated to the standard formalin protocol to assure optimum results, and appropriate PreservCyt fixed controls can be used.

Cell Blocks

Cell blocks are all-purpose cellular material that can be used for special stains as well as IHC. The cell blocks can withstand the processing protocols, similar to their paraffin-embedded surgical-tissue-specimen counterparts. In addition to the obvious advantage in studying the tissue architecture, additional tissue sections can be cut for IHC (Fig. 21.1). Ten percent neutral buffered formalin is used for fixation of tissue fragments. Interpretation of the results and storage of the specimen are easier, with unlimited antigen preservation. For these reasons, cell blocks are the superior method for IHC for cytologic specimens. Suspensions or bloody specimens may be fixed in formol-saline to lyse red cells, or the specimen may be collected in RPMI salt solution, treated with a commercial thrombin-plasma agent to organize a clot, and then fixed in 10% formalin and processed like a surgical specimen. The main disadvantage of this method is availability of enough material.

A fully automated rapid cell block (RCB) system introduced recently by Cytyc (Cellient; Hologic Inc., Bedford, Mass) increases overall cellularity in the resulting sections with decreased time and the necessity for fewer reagents to make a cell block.[33] A proprietary tissue cassette and filter assembly designed to capture tissue fragments also permits them to be positioned in a plane for microtomy (Fig. 21.2). Small aliquots of xylene, alcohol, and paraffin are rapidly drawn through the sample to produce a broad, uniform layer of cells embedded in paraffin. The RCB produces a cell block in 15 minutes from residual Thin-prep vials or other specimens and can be used for a variety of gynecological and respiratory tissues, FNA biopsies, body fluids, and other materials. If formalin is not used as the primary fixative, the alternate fixative has to be validated against the formalin-fixed specimen and controls must be used that have been fixed in the alternate material.

The use of cytoscrape cell blocks (SCB) is another valuable technique to prepare cell blocks, especially from stained FNA smears. This technique is useful when cell groups are obscured by clotted blood or when overlapping cell clusters interfere with the cytologic details and make interpretation difficult. The method involves previously stained smears containing thick material that are de-coverslipped in xylene. The slides are passed through two changes of absolute alcohol and water. Papanicolaou-stained smears are de-stained by 1% acid alcohol, whereas Romanowsky-stained smears are de-stained by 2% glacial acetic acid. Then the smears are thoroughly rinsed in running tap water for 2 hours. Slides are carefully scraped with a scalpel blade. The scraped material is meticulously transferred with a forceps in 3% molten agar to form a small button. After the agar solidifies, it is wrapped in Whatman filter paper No. 1 and put in a tissue cassette. The scraped material is refixed in a histologic fixative such as Bouin's fluid or formal saline for 5 to 6 hours and routinely processed to make a paraffin wax block. Sections of 5 μm are cut and stained with hematoxylin and eosin. A recent study that compared SCB with conventional cell blocks found that cytomorphologic details are equally superior in both types of specimen samples. An added advantage with this method is that additional panels of immunostains can be performed on SCB, particularly for cases in which repeat FNA is not feasible.[34,35]

Controls

Positive and negative controls must be performed with each test sample. Tissue controls are typically used in most laboratories for convenience, but the ideal control should be a comparably fixed cytology sample. If tissue controls are used, one must exercise caution in interpretation, because a different set of artifacts is present in tissue compared with cytology samples. Cytologic controls can be obtained on a daily basis from the surgical pathology bench with the use of aspirates or direct imprints. These preparations should be fixed in the same way as the test sample. It is more practical to use cells on the cytology slide as a positive-negative internal control, depending on the antibody and cells that are present.

Specimens of Limited Quality

Immunohistochemistry can be hampered by limited quantity of specimen. There is very limited information in the cytology literature to address this issue. In

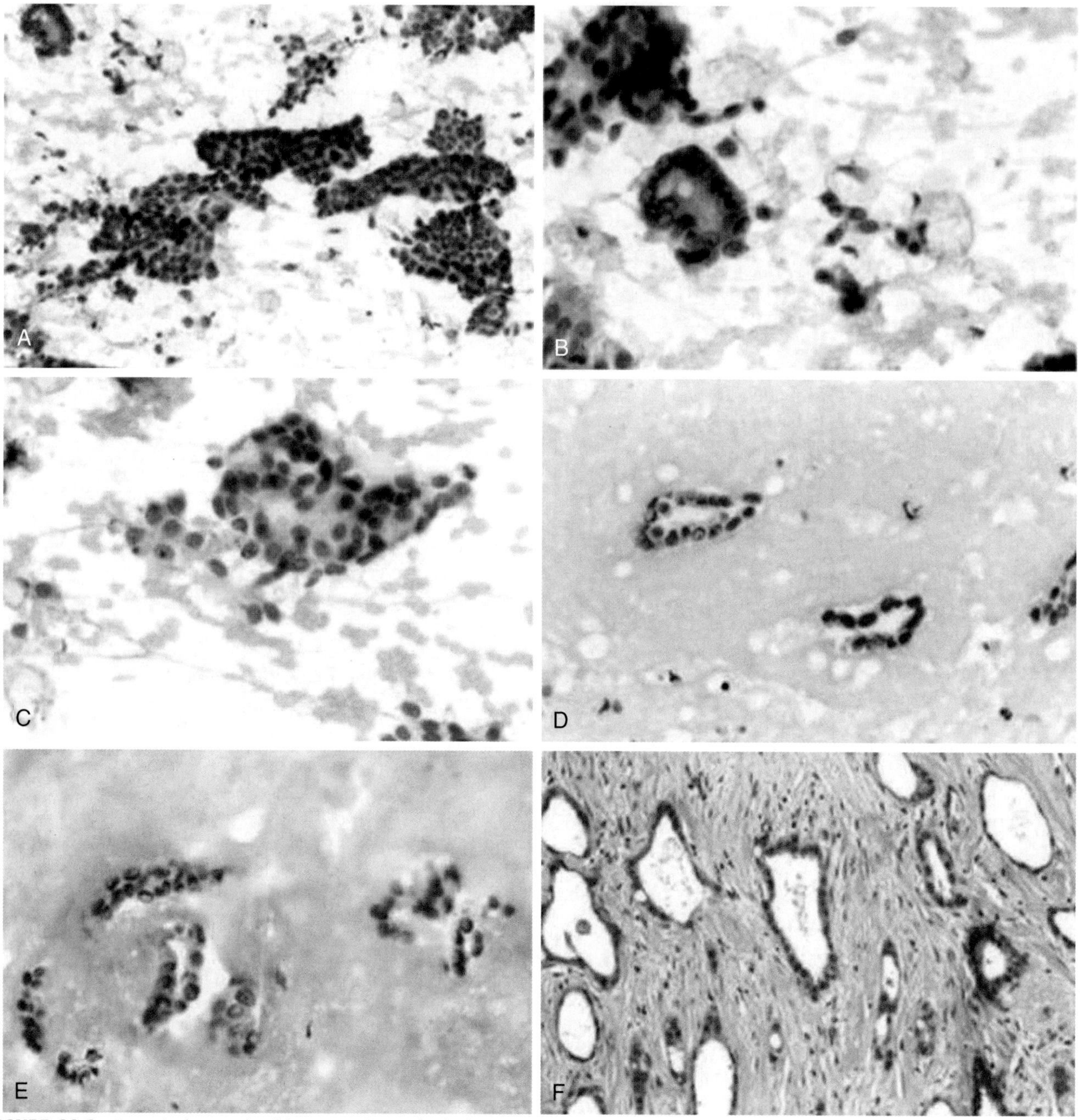

FIGURE 21.1 Papanicolaou-stained breast aspirate of tubular carcinoma illustrating whole tubules en face **(A)**, tubular lumens **(B)**, and comma-shaped glands **(C)**. Cell block of tubular carcinoma **(D)** shows angular glands that are negative for smooth muscle myosin heavy chain **(E)**, confirming the diagnostic impression. **(F)** Tissue from resection of tubular carcinoma.

one study, Dabbs and colleagues described a double-labeling method to address the problem of limited material when more than one antibody is required to make a diagnosis. Immunostaining was performed on these slides with and without a preceding de-colorization step. The results with both types of stains, with or without prior de-colorization, were similar. Immunostaining worked well. Background staining was more of a problem on the air-dried unfixed cases.[10] Thus, recently stained or archived cytology slides can be used for ICC studies, which include commonly used antibodies such as CAM5.2, AE1/AE3, K903, carcinoembryonic antigen (CEA), desmin, HHF-35 (muscle-specific actin), vimentin, CD20, and CD45RO.[10] Given the current recommendation for primary formalin fixative, tissue methodology is still preferred. Cytologic material can also be used in a variation of the dual immunolabeling technique.[36] With this method, cytology slides that were subjected to an immunoperoxidase test and produced a negative result can be subjected to another immunoperoxidase test using a different antibody (Fig. 21.3).[10] It is imperative to use positive and negative controls with both test runs. For example, a poorly differentiated tumor that is tested with leukocyte common antigen and found to be negative may be found to be positive with keratin,

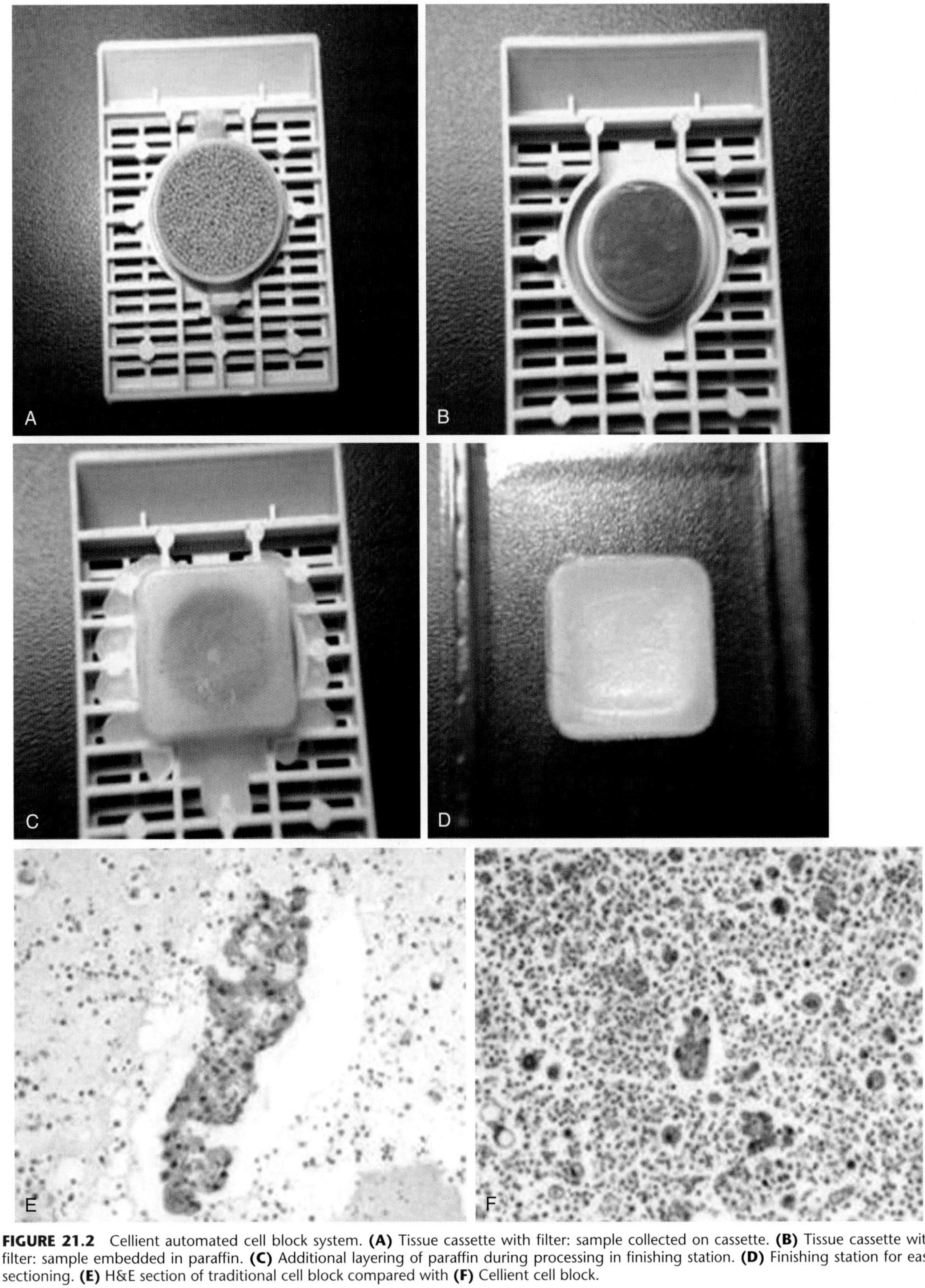

FIGURE 21.2 Cellient automated cell block system. **(A)** Tissue cassette with filter: sample collected on cassette. **(B)** Tissue cassette with filter: sample embedded in paraffin. **(C)** Additional layering of paraffin during processing in finishing station. **(D)** Finishing station for easy sectioning. **(E)** H&E section of traditional cell block compared with **(F)** Cellient cell block.

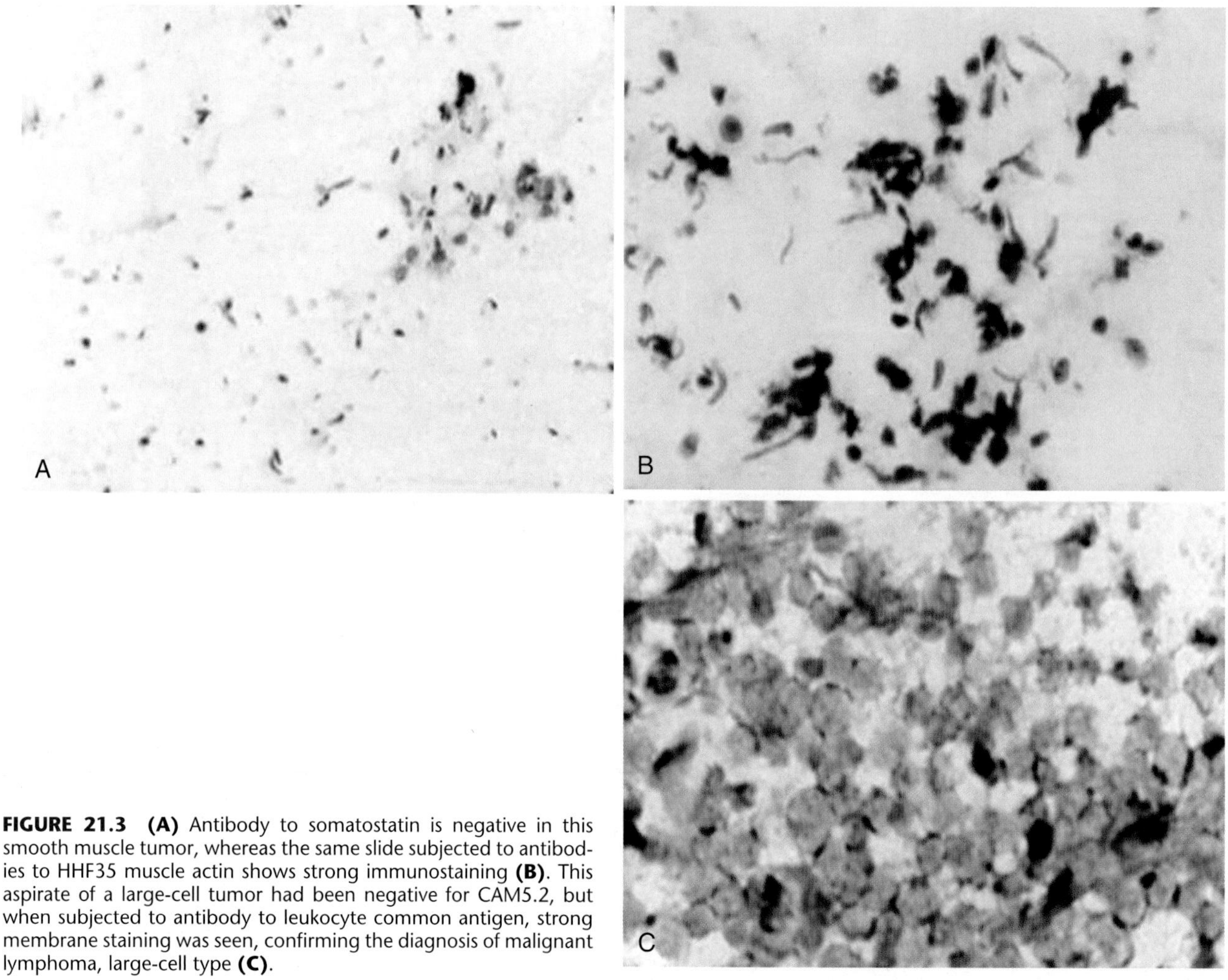

FIGURE 21.3 **(A)** Antibody to somatostatin is negative in this smooth muscle tumor, whereas the same slide subjected to antibodies to HHF35 muscle actin shows strong immunostaining **(B)**. This aspirate of a large-cell tumor had been negative for CAM5.2, but when subjected to antibody to leukocyte common antigen, strong membrane staining was seen, confirming the diagnosis of malignant lymphoma, large-cell type **(C)**.

confirming the carcinomatous nature of the specimen. Antibodies that have been used with this method include CAM5.2, AE1/AE3, K903, GCDFP15, vimentin, CD20, CD45RO, muscle-specific actin (HHF35), desmin, CEA, and S-100.[36] Sherman and associates described the cell transfer technique for use with limited cytologic samples.[19] In this technique, cells are lifted off a slide by re-dissolving them in a new mounting medium. The medium can be removed from the slide, cut into pieces, and re-applied to slides for individual antibody studies (Fig. 21.4). The results of immunostains are generally good, although Hunt and colleagues have described some decreased staining with this method.[37]

Interpretation and Limitations of Immunocytochemistry

As in surgical pathology, the morphologic study of the specimen in concert with the clinicopathologic correlations is of paramount importance in arriving at an accurate diagnosis. No amount of immunostaining will result in a precise diagnosis without a thorough patient workup or tissue examination. A patient workup is only considered complete when immunostaining findings are combined with clinical and other ancillary data.

A plethora of antibodies are available for use in cytology, and none of them is specific for its intended target. Antibodies may be polyclonal or monoclonal, may vary in sensitivity and specificity, or may be dependent on certain types of fixative for proper immunoreactivity. In addition, the differentiation of many tumors exhibits a wide spectrum. For these reasons, it is important to use known positive and negative controls with a panel of multiple antibodies that are known to be positive and negative in the cytologic study. A negative result by itself is of lesser value than a positive result, unless the cytology specimen itself contains known positive and negative control cells.

The pattern of immunostaining will depend on the presence of neoplastic cells, the location (e.g., cell membrane, cytoplasm, or nucleus), proper fixation, background staining, and antibody concentration. Immunostaining for any antigen is rarely uniform in nature. Heterogeneity of immunostaining is the rule rather than the exception, and it is proper to state the pattern, cell localization, and distribution of positive

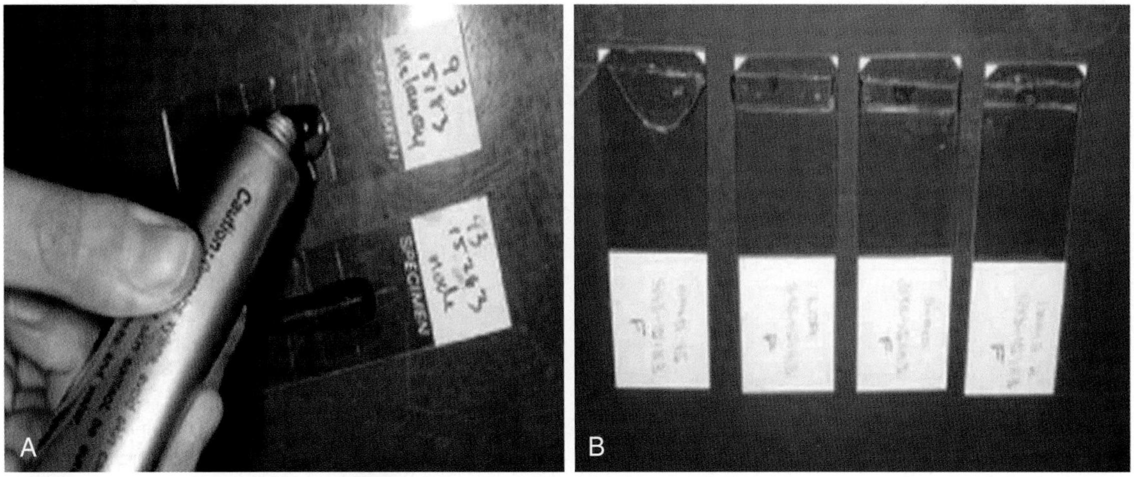

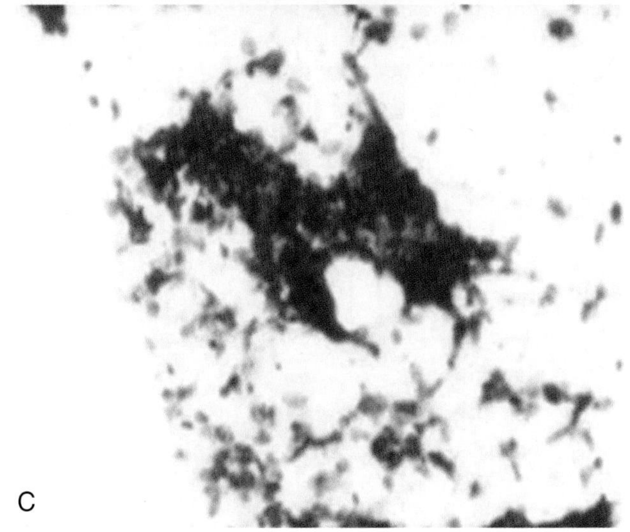

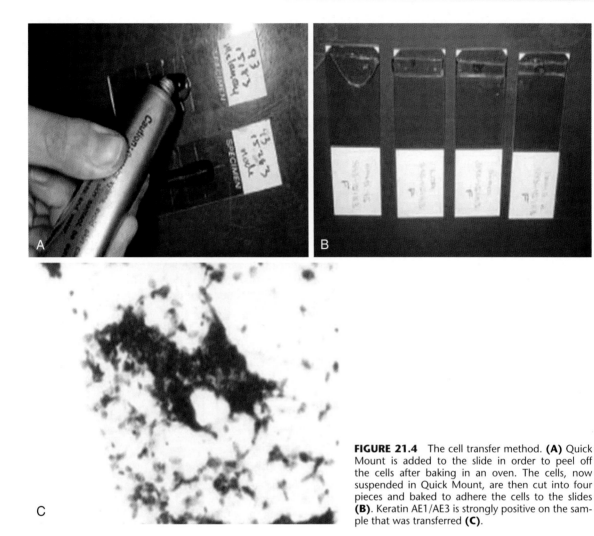

FIGURE 21.4 The cell transfer method. **(A)** Quick Mount is added to the slide in order to peel off the cells after baking in an oven. The cells, now suspended in Quick Mount, are then cut into four pieces and baked to adhere the cells to the slides **(B)**. Keratin AE1/AE3 is strongly positive on the sample that was transferred **(C)**.

and negative immunostaining relative to normal cells that may be present in the sample.

False-positive immunostaining results can be a result of a multitude of factors. First and foremost, the cytopathologist must not mistake normal cellular elements for neoplastic cells, especially in samples in which neoplastic cells are few. The same caution applies to reactive cells in the sample. Air drying of the slide during any step in the immunoperoxidase procedure results in nonspecific antibody binding that can be misinterpreted as positive findings. Necrotic, poorly preserved, and crushed cells must be avoided because nonspecific binding may yield a false-positive result. Care must be taken not to overinterpret the cellular background that is generally seen with polyclonal antibodies. This nonspecific binding to stromal elements can be avoided by carefully assessing the patterns of staining of normal, neoplastic, and stromal elements. Antibodies may cross-react with non–target cell components, or the antibody used may not be as specific as advertised. Only experience and comfort with the antibody in use will satisfy the observer's interpretation in these situations. Improper fixation and incomplete blocking of endogenous peroxidase or biotin activity are well-known sources of false-positive results. Proper blocking with commercial blocking products should eliminate this problem.

False-negative interpretations are also potentially multifactorial in nature. Improper fixation resulting in denaturation or masking of antigen may completely escape the observer. One can eliminate this problem only by ascertaining the working dilution of each antibody and ensuring quality fixation. Antibody concentration is a critical determinant, as concentrations that are too low or too high can cause false-negative and false-positive results, respectively. Insufficient antigen retrieval or even de-colorization of specimens can cause false-negative results. The type of fixation is critical for antibody performance. The best example of false-negative results is for the antibodies to S-100 protein and GCDFP15 for specimens fixed primarily in alcohol fixatives.

SPECIFIC ORGAN CYTOLOGY

Effusion Cytology

Effusion cytology is one of the most challenging areas of cytopathology, wherein IHC serves as a valuable adjunct tool in definitive interpretation. There is a need for ancillary application of IHC, as the sensitivity for diagnosis of the presence of malignant cells has been reported to be as low as 40%.[38]

The native cells (mesothelial cells) of the fluids exhibit a spectrum of cytomorphologic features that sometimes precludes identification of the second population (unknown group) of cells. The most common major practical area where IHC plays an important role is elucidation of reactive mesothelial cells versus adenocarcinoma versus mesothelioma. Several studies have highlighted and proposed panels of antibodies to resolve this issue. These studies indicate that combined use of light microscopic features of cells in effusions, together with IHC based on a *panel* of antibodies comprising both mesothelial and adenocarcinoma markers, can significantly improve diagnostic accuracy.[38-40]

IHC can be performed on various cytology specimens: direct smears—FA or acetone; ADS (fixed with alcohol or post-fixed in formol alcohol); and liquid-based cytology smears (e.g., Thin-prep and Surepath cytospin smears). Storage of effusions at 4°C gives a satisfactory immunohistochemical outcome when a delay in processing of the samples is anticipated.[41] We suggest performing IHC on 10% phosphate-buffered formalin cell-block material because the immunoreactivity pattern of a variety of immunomarkers is changed by different fixation methods. Therefore a standardized method comparable to paraffin-embedded sections can be applied to cytology specimens to achieve optimal results.

MESOTHELIAL MARKERS

Based on several studies in the literature, we will discuss some important markers that can be used in routine practice for positive identification.

Calretinin

The 29-kDa calcium-binding protein is a member of elongation factor (EF) proteins. Calretinin is thought to play a role in the cell cycle. Gotzos[41a] and colleagues were first to report its expression by epithelioid mesotheliomas and epithelioid components of mixed mesotheliomas, and negative results in adenocarcinoma. These results were later confirmed by Doglioni and coworkers, who used calretinin immunostaining in all 44 mesotheliomas, but only rare focal decoration of a variety of adenocarcinomas, and focal staining of 23% of lung adenocarcinomas.[42] The sensitivity of calretinin to distinguish reactive mesothelial cells from adenocarcinoma cells is 100%, and the specificity is up to 80%. Interpretation of this marker is less complex and shows a strong nuclear and cytoplasmic staining pattern. About 10% to 30% of the adenocarcinoma shows immunoreactivity for calretinin.[42] However, the staining pattern observed in the adenocarcinoma cells is focal, less intense, and sometimes a cytoplasmic blush. The intensity and proportion of cells staining for calretinin are much higher in reactive mesothelial cells as compared to malignant mesotheliomas (92% versus 88%).[43,44]

Ordoñez demonstrated a difference in sensitivities of the human recombinant antibodies from Zymed and a guinea pig calretinin from Chemicon.[45] The Zymed antibody sensitivity was 100% compared with a Chemicon sensitivity of 74%. Focal, weak staining of adenocarcinoma was seen in 4% and 9%, respectively. Nagel and colleagues had a similar experience with the study of cytospins. They found that the sensitivity for mesothelial cells was 93%, with 5% of tumor cells immunostaining.[46] In a recent study by Yaziji and associates, calretinin was one of three antibodies (along with BG8 and MOC31) identified in the evaluation of a 12-antibody panel, which was cited to be the most efficient panel for distinguishing epithelioid mesothelioma from adenocarcinoma.[47]

HBME1

The mesothelial cell clone HBME1 is an antibody against cultured mesothelial cells and recognizes an antigen on the microvillus surface. HBME1 has been used as a part of the panel of ICC to distinguish adenocarcinoma from mesothelial cells. Interpretation of this stain is complex compared to calretinin. The staining pattern of mesothelial cells showed a thick bushy membrane pattern and a thin membrane or cytoplasmic staining of adenocarcinoma. There was a gradient in the staining pattern observed in malignant mesothelioma versus adenocarcinoma. The specificity of HBME1 as a mesothelial marker approaches 80%.[44] Although calretinin is superior, HBME1 stains with a stronger intensity in the majority of mesothelial cells.

Cytokeratin 5/6

The 1989 immunohistochemical study by Moll and colleagues[48] confirmed the biochemical study of Blobel and colleagues,[49] in which keratin 5 was found to be a constituent of mesothelioma but not lung adenocarcinoma. Clover and associates found rare, weak staining for CK5/6 in 4 of 27 lung adenocarcinomas with the D5/16B4 antibody clone,[50] whereas Ordoñez found focal staining in up to 7% of non-pulmonary adenocarcinomas and diffuse cytoplasmic staining in all mesotheliomas and squamous cell carcinomas.[51] The sensitivity and specificity of this stain in distinguishing malignant mesothelioma from adenocarcinoma in pleural effusions is 90% to 100%.[51] However, this marker is of no value in differentiating malignant mesothelioma from metastatic pulmonary squamous cell carcinoma. It is important to keep in mind that certain breast carcinomas, particularly the recently described basal phenotype, express CK5/6 as well. Given these data, CK5/6 is only useful for identifying epithelioid malignant mesothelioma and reactive mesothelial cells from adenocarcinoma. A history of the primary carcinoma is also supportive in interpretation of this stain.

Wilms' Tumor Gene 1

Wilms' tumor gene (WT1) is a tumor suppressor gene present on chromosome 11. It was first reported as a candidate for main gene in the development of Wilms' tumor. The immunohistochemical expression of WT1 was demonstrated in a variety of neoplasms. A majority of epithelioid mesotheliomas and a small percentage of sarcomatoid mesotheliomas express WT1. Strong immunoreactivity for WT1 is demonstrated in desmoplastic, small round-cell tumors (DSRT).[52] WT1 represents an

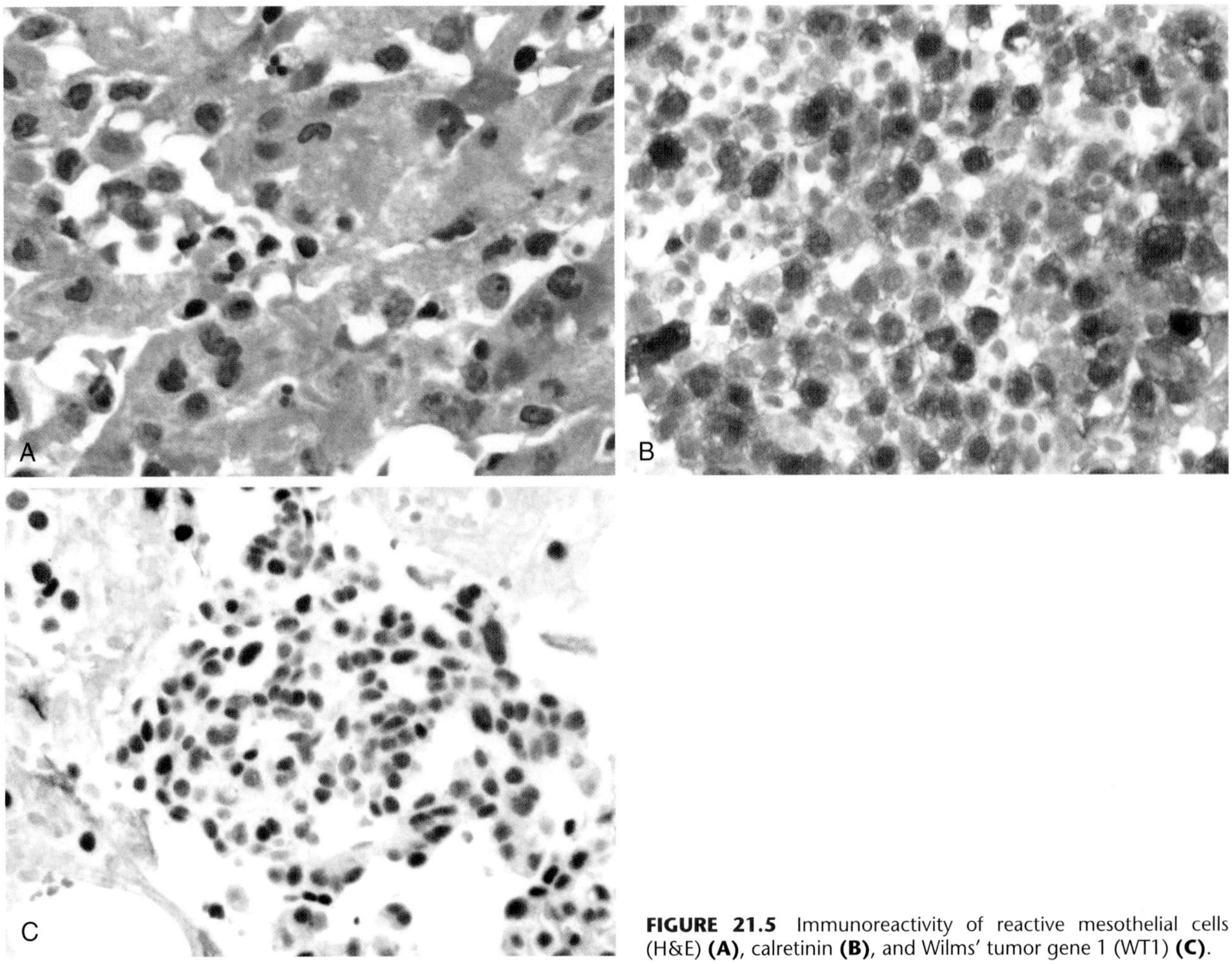

FIGURE 21.5 Immunoreactivity of reactive mesothelial cells (H&E) **(A)**, calretinin **(B)**, and Wilms' tumor gene 1 (WT1) **(C)**.

effective marker for mesotheliomas as well as reactive mesothelial cells in cell block preparations and can aid in the distinction of Wilms' tumor from pulmonary adenocarcinoma. However, in recent years, WT1 has emerged as a highly sensitive and specific marker for carcinomas of müllerian origin. Therefore, one should exercise caution when the metastatic carcinoma is ovarian serous type because a strong nuclear positivity is also seen in reactive and neoplastic mesothelial cells (Fig. 21.5).

D2-40

D2-40 was initially reported to be a marker for lymphatic endothelium but was found to be expressed by benign as well as neoplastic mesothelial cells. D2-40, like WT1, is a sensitive marker. In recent studies, D2-40 was found to be a highly sensitive and specific marker (up to 100%) for malignant mesothelioma (MM). Therefore it is recommended that it be used in a panel to distinguish MM from pulmonary carcinomas in effusion cytology specimens.[53] A recent study that examined the usefulness of old and new markers in evaluating cells in fluid cytologic studies found D2-40 and MOC31 to be very sensitive as well as specific markers for mesothelial and epithelial cell populations. The same study showed that D2-40 was also more sensitive for mesothelial cells than other markers (WT1 or calretinin).[54]

GLUT1

GLUT1, a member of the family of glucose transporter isoforms (GLUT), facilitates the entry of glucose into cells and is expressed in a variety of malignancies. Immunohistochemically, GLUT1 expression demonstrated by membrane staining (sometimes with cytoplasmic staining) is a sensitive and specific immunohistochemical marker that enables the differential diagnosis of reactive mesothelial cells from malignant mesothelioma. It cannot, however, discriminate between malignant mesothelioma and lung carcinoma.[55,56]

XIAP

X-linked inhibitor of apoptosis (XIAP) is a monoclonal antibody shown to be a useful marker for distinguishing malignant from benign groups of cells. XIAP is also demonstrated in a variety of adenocarcinomas (up to 54%). However, weak and focal staining is seen in mesothelial cells (up to 11%).[57]

NON-MESOTHELIAL (ADENOCARCINOMA) MARKERS

The highest sensitivity for adenocarcinomas can be achieved with the staining combination of negative mesothelial markers and positive adenocarcinoma markers (BG-8, MOC31, Ber-EP4, CEA, or B72.3).

MOC31

MOC31 is a monoclonal antibody that has recently become commercially available. MOC31 recognizes an epithelial-associated transmembrane glycoprotein of 40 kD. Squamous cell carcinomas, adenocarcinomas, and small cell carcinomas show a membrane staining pattern. The utility of this marker in distinguishing adenocarcinoma from mesothelial cells has been reported by few studies.[58-60] The sensitivity and specificity of this marker in these studies has been between 78% and 100%. MOC31 expression in malignant mesotheliomas reported in the literature is contradicting, ranging from 0% to 88%; however, the number of cases in these studies was small. In a recent study by Yaziji and associates, MOC31 was identified as a highly specific non-mesothelial marker in addition to BG8 for distinguishing epithelioid mesothelioma from adenocarcinoma.[47] The expression in reactive mesothelial cells is less than 2%, as reported by various studies. MOC31 represents an effective marker for metastatic carcinoma in cell block preparations and also aids in distinguishing between benign and malignant mesothelial cells in these tumors.

BG8

The role of ABH blood antigens in tumor metastasis and in solid tumors has been addressed, with the Lewis-Y antigen precursor postulated as playing a role in tumor spread. BG8, an antibody against Lewis antigen, has been shown in tissue specimens as well as cell block specimens to have a sensitivity and specificity of 86% and 90%, respectively,[44] in differentiating adenocarcinoma from epithelioid mesothelioma. A recent study by Yaziji and colleagues evaluated 12 antibodies for distinguishing epithelioid mesothelioma from adenocarcinoma, and they identified BG8 and MOC31 as highly specific and thus optimal markers for positively identifying adenocarcinoma.[47] BG8 shows a membrane and cytoplasmic staining pattern of adenocarcinoma cells; however, use caution with this stain, as a small percentage of isolated mesothelial cells can show a non-specific positive reaction.[43]

Ber-EP4

Ber-EP4 is a monoclonal antibody that reacts with two glycoproteins on the surface as well as in the cytoplasm of epithelial cells and does not react with mesothelial cells to a significant degree.[65] The role of Ber-EP4 in epithelial malignancies is reported in several studies in the literature, with a sensitivity of more than 90% and a specificity of 90%.[61-67] Ber-EP4 has the advantage of high sensitivity and ease of interpretation because of the high percentage of tumor cells stained, characteristic membranous pattern, and lack of cross-reaction with background inflammatory cells. Exercise caution with this stain because isolated mesothelial cells can show some non-specific focal staining (Fig. 21.6).

Monoclonal CEA

CEA is a 180-kD glycoprotein that is 50% carbohydrate. There are many antibodies available to a variety of epitopes. It is a highly sensitive marker for adenocarcinomas and therefore is used widely in effusion cytology because of its ability to distinguish adenocarcinoma from reactive as well as malignant mesothelial cells. A substantial number of adenocarcinomas stain strongly for CEA. (CEA antibody in effusion cytology has a low sensitivity [55%] and a high specificity [>90%].)[61] Tumor cells that are CEA positive support the diagnosis of adenocarcinoma.[63] A negative result does not exclude adenocarcinoma, because various percentages of carcinomas were negative for CEA in different series of breast carcinomas (e.g., as low as 37% and as high as 70%).[63] Generally, mesothelial cells do not stain, but weak peripheral CEA staining of some reactive mesothelial cells has been reported. Despite weak reactivity expressed by some reactive mesothelial cells and occasional rare cases of benign effusions with strong reactivity,[63] it seems that CEA may be a useful marker for identification of adenocarcinoma cells in effusions. The sensitivity can be increased with the use of other non-mesothelial markers.

TAG-72.3

The mAb B72.3, which is directed against a tumor-associated antigen (TAG-72), is associated with 95% overall recognition for adenocarcinomas on paraffin-embedded effusions, particularly those with origin in the lung,[61] whereas reactive mesothelial cells are negative. Although no reactivity was demonstrated in any cell type in a series of 821 benign effusions,[68] two false-positive cases were noted in a series of 18 benign effusions.[68] Though studies have shown that B72.3 can positively identify adenocarcinoma cells with a sensitivity and specificity of 77% and 98%, respectively, a combination of B72.3 and Ber-EP4 has shown an increased sensitivity and specificity, up to 98%.

CD15 (Leu M1)

CD15 or Lewis X antigen can be identified with the LeuM1 antibody. Monoclonal Abs to Leu-M1 (CD15 granulocyte antigen) and BMA/070 (CD16 natural killer antigen) did not react with mesothelial cells, although they stained carcinoma cells.[61] LeuM1 has a low sensitivity of 29% in identifying adenocarcinoma cells as reported in the literature. False-positive staining of

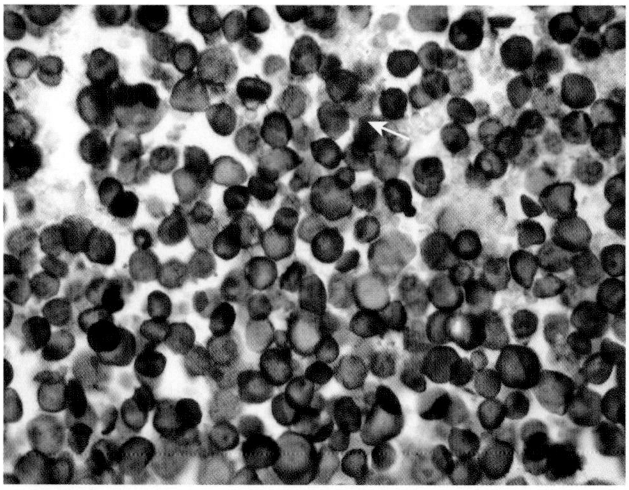

FIGURE 21.6 Strong membrane staining of Ber-EP4 in adenocarcinoma.

LeuM1 with malignant mesothelioma has been reported as result of high hyaluronic acid content.[61] CD15 did not gain popularity as a non-mesothelial marker owing to its low sensitivity as well as its low complementary value with other markers.

SITE-SPECIFIC MARKERS

Thyroid Transcription Factor-1

Thyroid transcription factor-1 (TTF-1) is a homeodomain-containing transcription factor selectively expressed in pulmonary adenocarcinomas, thyroid tumors, and small cell carcinomas (pulmonary and extrapulmonary) with relatively high sensitivity and specificity. TTF-1 is a highly sensitive and specific immunomarker for distinguishing metastatic pulmonary from extrapulmonary adenocarcinoma in effusion cytology specimens, with a sensitivity of 88.2% and specificity of 100%.[68] Anti–TTF-1 can be used as a reliable component of an antibody panel to support the diagnosis of adenocarcinoma of pulmonary origin in patients presenting with metastatic adenocarcinoma in serous fluid(s) with an unknown primary site.[68] In cytologic preparations, TTF-1 is a highly selective marker for pulmonary adenocarcinoma and also can have a role in the distinction between pulmonary adenocarcinoma and mesothelioma.[69,70] It is important to keep in mind that TTF-1 is expressed in a subset of neuroendocrine carcinomas (ovary, breast), in carcinoid tumors of lung origin, and in most thyroid neoplasms (Fig. 21.7).[69]

Estrogen Receptor

Estrogen receptor antibodies have been suggested as a tool to identify metastatic breast carcinoma in effusions from patients without solid tissue metastases. Although reactive mesothelial cells are ER negative, ER is not a sensitive or specific marker by itself. Gynecological carcinomas (vulva, vagina, cervix, endometrium, ovary, and fallopian tube) are often positive for ER in a patchy fashion. A positive ER result can be useful in indicating a breast or gynecological origin, but one must exercise caution when the differential diagnosis includes pulmonary adenocarcinoma, a subset of these tumors may be associated with significant nuclear expression with both 6F11 and 1D5 ER clones (Fig. 21.8).[71,72]

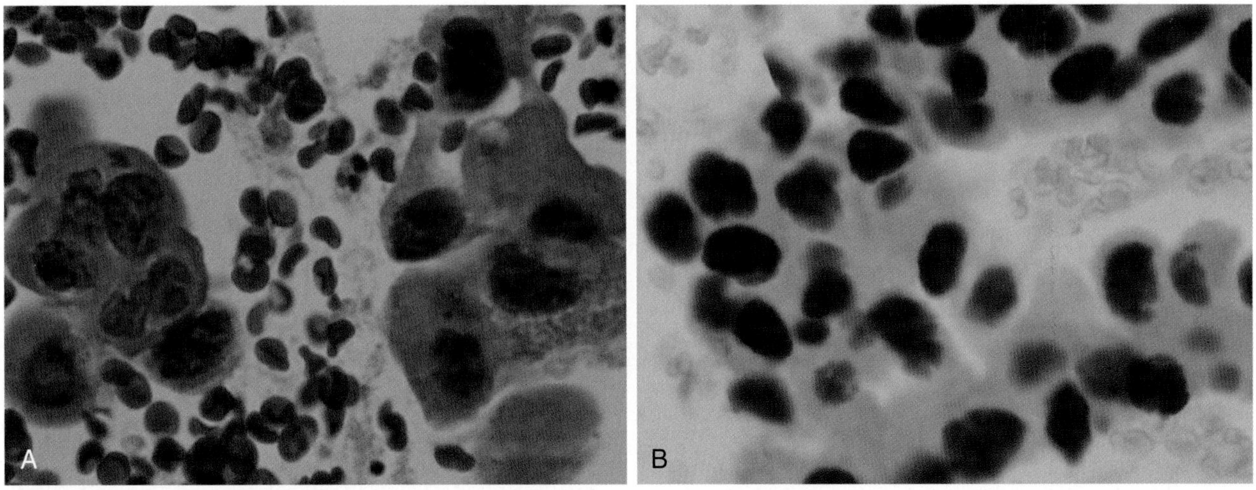

FIGURE 21.7 Metastatic pulmonary adenocarcinoma in pleural effusion: **(A)** cell block demonstrates malignant groups with marked nuclear pleomorphism x40; **(B)** TTF-1 shows a diffuse strong nuclear staining, confirming the lung origin of the adenocarcinoma.

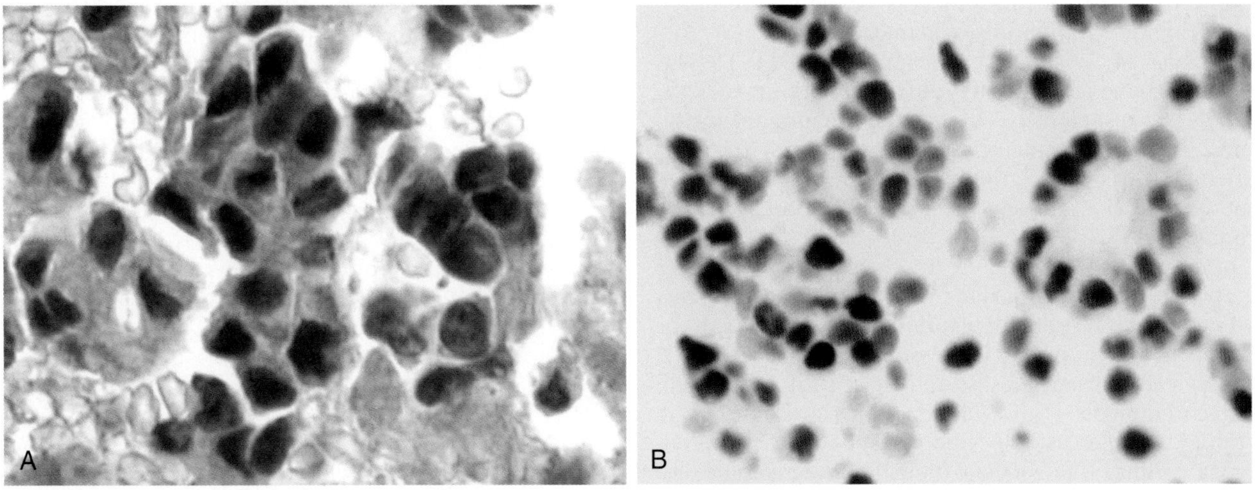

FIGURE 21.8 Cell block of ductal carcinoma demonstrates strong ER staining. **(A)** Cell block demonstrating ductal carcinoma; **(B)** ductal carcinoma showing strong ER expression.

CDX2

CDX2 is a homeobox domain–containing transcription factor that is important in the development and differentiation of the intestine and is expressed in colorectal carcinoma. Results also suggest that strong nuclear staining of CDX2 is a specific and sensitive marker to detect gastrointestinal and pancreatic malignancies in ascites cytologic samples and to differentiate them from reactive mesothelial cells. CDX2 is also seen in mucinous tumors with gastrointestinal differentiation that originate in the lung or ovary.[73-76] A recent study reported a high frequency of CDX2 expression in midgut and foregut carcinoid tumors, making it a marker of neuroendocrine tumors of midgut origin.[77]

Breast Cytology

Therapies for breast carcinoma are changing rapidly in concert with our increasing understanding of the molecular evolution of the disease. Although the diagnosis of breast carcinoma by light microscopy is a relatively straightforward task for the surgical pathologist, therapeutic needs are resulting in increasing demands on the pathologist to correctly diagnose the specific types of breast carcinomas so that appropriate ancillary prognostic and predictive tests will be performed for appropriate therapy. The broad categories of ductal and lobular carcinomas of the breast represent the majority of breast carcinomas, but there are striking differences in morphology, molecular alterations, and treatment strategies for each category. The diagnostic discrimination of ductal from lobular neoplasms is important in many circumstances for therapeutic reasons. Indeed, the diagnosis of breast carcinoma in metastatic sites remains a significant challenge.

GROSS CYSTIC FLUID PROTEIN 15 (GCDFP-15)/(BRST-2)

Gross cystic fluid protein 15 (GCDFP-15) was first described by Haagensen and Pearlman in breast cyst fluid and in the plasma of invasive mammary carcinoma. In an immunohistochemical analysis of 690 neoplasms by Wick and colleagues, GCDFP-15 was shown to have a sensitivity and specificity up to 74% and 95%, respectively, in primary mammary carcinoma.[78,79] The specificity in the metastatic setting was very high (up to 95%); therefore the authors concluded that GCDFP-15 is a specific marker for breast carcinoma.

In another study, GCDFP-15 was found be positive in up to 57% of primary as well as metastatic breast carcinomas.[80] A note of caution: GCDFP-15 can be positive in carcinomas of other organs, such as prostate, salivary, and sweat glands, and in central (bronchial) lung carcinomas.[81] GCDFP-15 is now recognized in cytology samples as a specific marker for breast carcinomas (primary and metastatic); thus, one should use good judgment in situations in which a carcinoma of breast origin is suspected.

MAMMAGLOBIN

Mammaglobin is a gene sequence fragment that was initially isolated by Watson and Fleming. The authors demonstrated expression in 50% of primary breast carcinomas and 62% of metastatic breast carcinomas. On tissue sections, mammaglobin is expressed in 56% of primary breast carcinomas. It is also demonstrated in other tumors such as endometrial adenocarcinomas, salivary gland carcinomas, and endocervical carcinomas *in situ*.[82] Although mammaglobin is studied to a greater extent in tissue sections, there is meager literature on its use in cytologic specimens. A study that examined the potential use of this marker in pleural effusions found that 55% of metastatic breast carcinomas expressed mammaglobin.[83]

Note: The utility of GCDFP-15 and mammaglobin in cytologic specimens is emerging. It is important to note that both mammaglobin and GCDFP-15 have similar sensitivities and specificities. Therefore, in clinical practice, apart from a good clinical history, use of both markers is recommended in order to increase the sensitivity and specificity of the panel to make an accurate diagnosis.

E-CADHERIN AND P120 CATENIN

The E-cadherin complex is composed of the transmembrane E-cadherin protein and the alpha, beta, gamma, and p120 catenins that anchor the E-cadherin protein to the cytoplasmic actin filaments. The catenins are normally located at the junction of the cytoplasm and internal aspect of the cell membrane, where they link with the actin cytoskeleton. They show a variety of cellular molecular abnormalities that may result in the absence of E-cadherin, which is not detectable immunohistochemically and is characteristic of lobular neoplasms. We and others have recently studied the catenin molecular components of the E-cadherin–catenin complex and have discovered a characteristic cytoplasmic redistribution of the catenins in lobular neoplasia.[84,85] In addition to the loss of immunodetectable E-cadherin in lobular neoplasia, a characteristic abnormality in lobular neoplasia is the diffuse upregulation of p120 catenin throughout the cytoplasm, which yields a diffuse cytoplasmic p120 immunostaining pattern. In contrast, ductal neoplasia retains the membrane immunostaining pattern of p120, reflecting the normal construction of the E-cadherin complex, although ductal carcinomas may show reduced membrane immunostaining of E-cadherin complex components. Diffuse signet ring carcinomas of stomach and rectum may also show p120 cytoplasmic immunostaining because they also lack E-cadherin (Figs. 21.9 to 21.11).[85]

Gynecological Cytology

Gynecological cytology is a major area in which application of IHC is growing rapidly. Papanicolaou tests form the bulk of the specimens used primarily for cervical cancer screening. Although colposcopic biopsy is the gold standard for abnormal squamous cells seen on screening, the diagnostic accuracy of detection of human papillomavirus (HPV) infection has been increasing with successful adjuvant methods such as p16^{INK4a} and HPV-DNA testing on cytologic specimens.

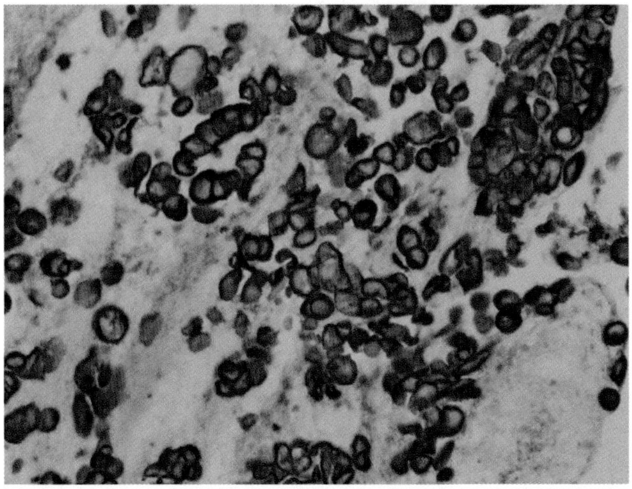

FIGURE 21.9 Infiltrating ductal carcinoma demonstrating strong membranous E-cadherin staining.

MARKERS OF DYSPLASIA

p16^{INK4a}

MOLECULAR PATHOGENESIS OF HUMAN PAPILLOMA VIRUS INFECTION HPV is the major etiologic agent for cervical cancer. Nearly all cervical cancers are high-risk HPV-positive. Women with high-risk HPV-positive infection have an increased risk of developing cervical cancer over time. Viral oncogenes encoding E6 and E7 oncoproteins have the most important role in immortalization and malignant transformation of cervical epithelial cells. E6 oncoprotein binding to p53 leads to subsequent p53 degradation; binding to pro-apoptotic protein BAK leads to resistance to apoptosis, increase in chromosomal instability, and activation of telomerase.

E7 oncoprotein binds to pRb (retinoblastoma protein), which leads to inactivation of G1-S transition control of cell cycle and activation of transcription factor E2F, driving proliferation, inducing centriole amplification, and inducing aneuploidy. p16^{INK4a} over-expression can be used as a biomarker for pre-cancerous and cancerous cervical lesions.

UTILITY OF P16 AS AN ADJUNCT MARKER IN ABNORMAL PAP TESTS Overexpression of p16^{INK4a} has been strongly linked to high-risk HPV infection and is expressed in

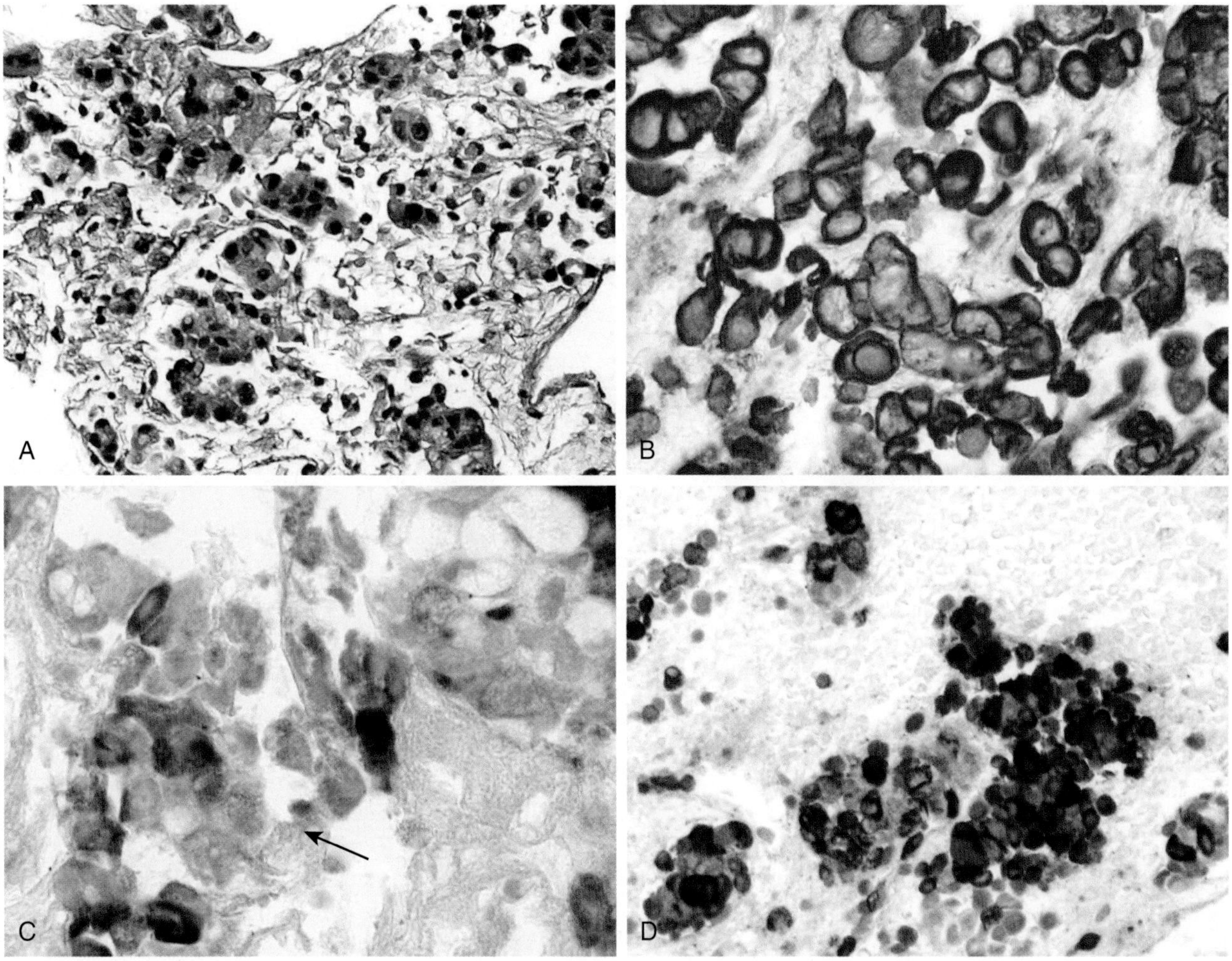

FIGURE 21.10 **(A)** Cell block of metastatic breast carcinoma to bone; tumor cells show positivity for **(B)** cytokeratin 7, **(C)** gross cystic fluid protein 15 (GCDFP-15), and **(D)** mammaglobin.

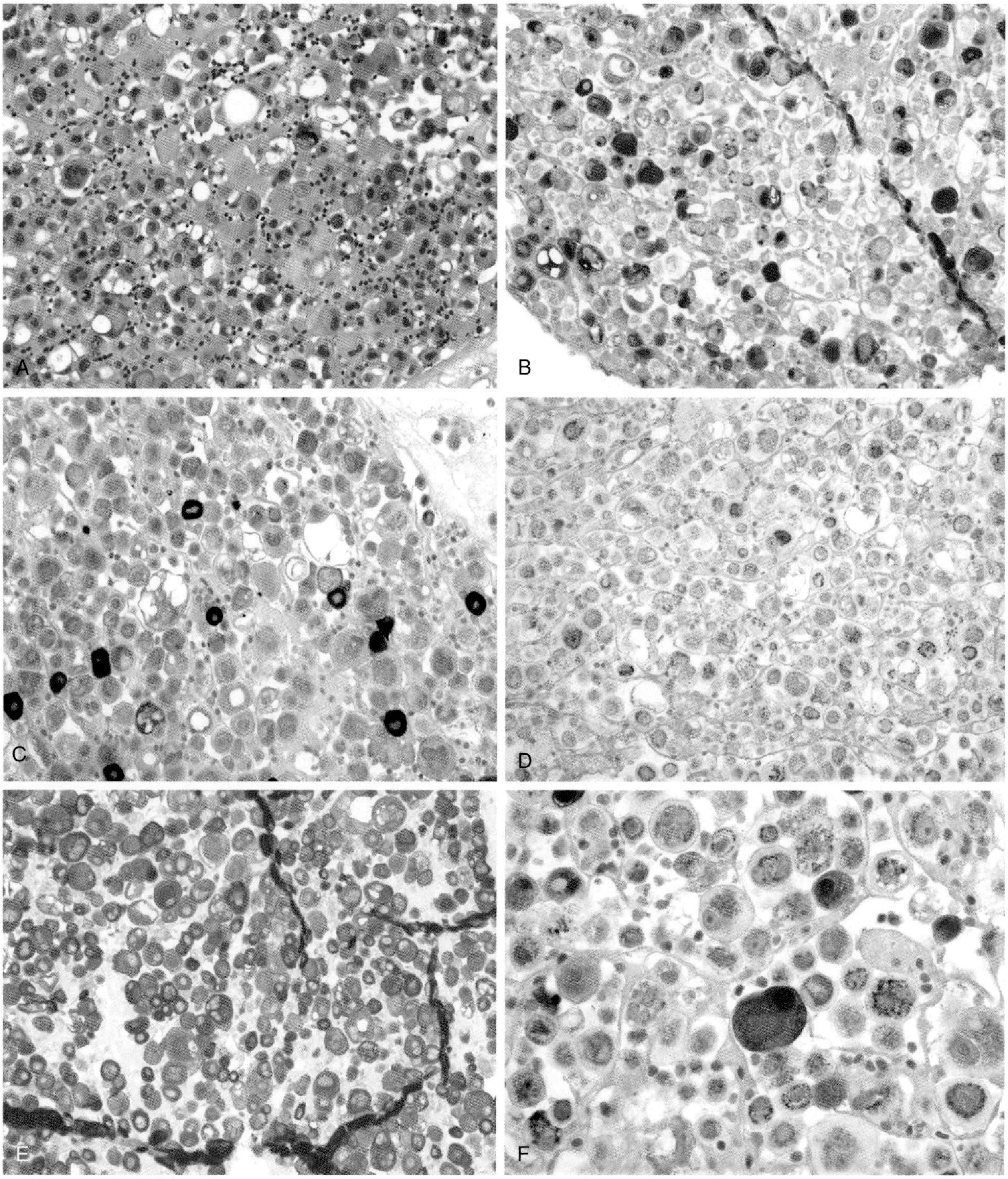

FIGURE 21.11 Pleomorphic lobular carcinoma in pleural effusion: **(A)** cell block preparation. **(B)** Gross cystic disease fluid protein 15 (GCDFP-15). **(C)** Mammaglobin confirms mammary origin. **(D)** Negative E-cadherin. **(E)** p120 cytoplasmic expression confirms lobular origin of tumor cells. **(F)** Non-specific staining in tumor cells and occasional mesothelial show calretinin staining.

dysplastic squamous cells. Over 80 scientific publications demonstrate virtually 100% sensitivity for cervical intraepithelial neoplasia 3 (CIN3) combined with very high specificity for non-malignant disease using CINtec p16 assay, with significant improvements in inter-observer reproducibility and diagnostic accuracy. $p16^{INK4a}$ also consistently discriminates *in situ* and invasive cervical adenocarcinomas from benign endocervical cells. Sensitivity and specificity of $p16^{INK4a}$ expression in adenocarcinoma *in situ* and invasive adenocarcinoma is 94.5% and 100%, respectively.[86-89]

$p16^{INK4a}$ has been successfully demonstrated on Thin-prep and Surepath slides as well as cell blocks.[89-91] Studies show that $p16^{INK4a}$ expression in simultaneously

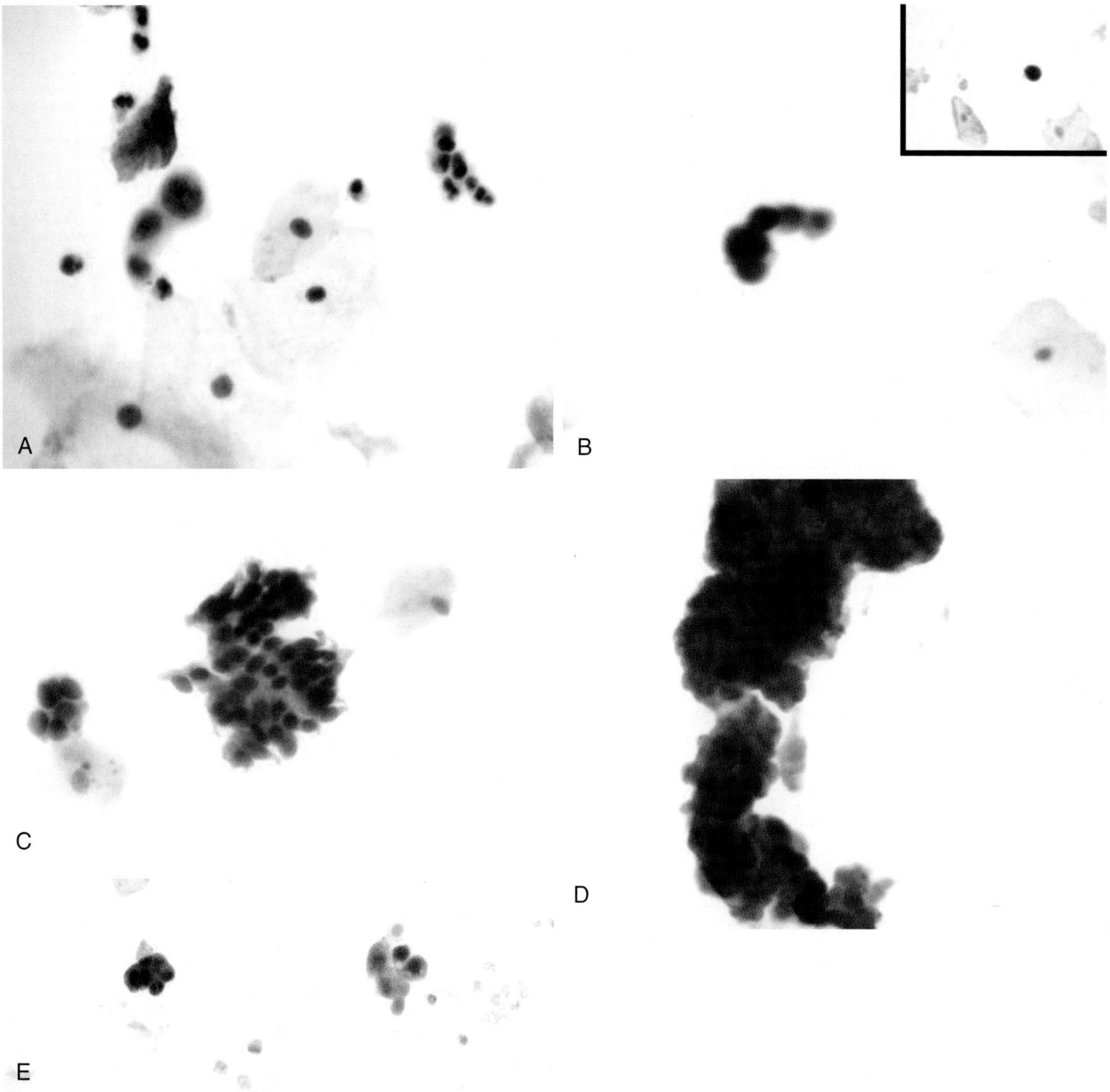

FIGURE 21.12 (A-D) A strong nuclear and cytoplasmic staining of p16 in smears prepared from residual material in the vial from Pap tests. **(E)** Non-specific staining in metaplastic cells.

sampled tissue sections and liquid-based Pap tests carry similar sensitivity and specificity.[92]

Using p16^{INK4a} immunostaining, the sensitivity and specificity of detecting a low-grade squamous intraepithelial lesion (LSIL) is 74%, and for a high-grade squamous intraepithelial lesion (HSIL), it is 97%. A score of more than 10 cells showing predominantly nuclear as well as cytoplasmic staining is considered positive. One study addressed the identification of HSIL in patients with minor cytologic abnormalities (atypical squamous cells of undetermined significance [ASCUS] and/or LSIL group) using nuclear score. It was found that the overall sensitivity and specificity of p16^{INK4a}-positive cells with a nuclear score of greater than 2 for identification of HSIL in ASCUS and LSIL Pap tests combined was 96% and 83%, respectively. These data suggest that the use of p16^{INK4a} as a biomarker combined with nuclear scoring of positive cells in cervical cytology to triage ASCUS and/or LSIL cases allows identification of HSIL with good sensitivity and specificity.[93-96] A caveat with p16^{INK4a} is that some non-specific staining may occur in the metaplastic cells and may also cross-react with *Trichomonas vaginalis* and other organisms as well as endometrial cell nuclei in liquid-based cytology (LBC) specimens. Therefore, it is critical to compare immunostaining with cytomorphology.[97] Figure 21.12 illustrates p16 immunostaining in abnormal Pap tests.

ProEx C

The ProEx C immunocytochemical assay (ProEx C; TriPath Oncology, Burlington, NC) utilizes a cocktail of monoclonal antibodies directed against proteins

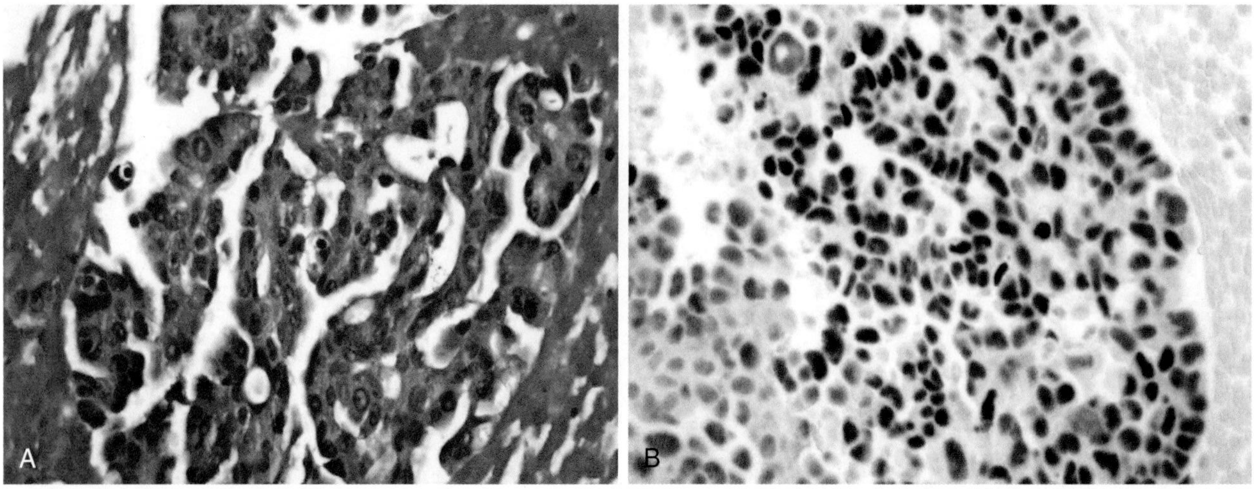

FIGURE 21.13 Utility of Wilms' tumor gene 1 (WT1) as a marker for serous carcinoma in malignant effusions. **(A)** H&E. **(B)** WT1.

associated with aberrant S-phase cell-cycle induction (topoisomerase IIA, mini chromosome maintenance protein 2). Very few studies have addressed the role of ProEx C in liquid-based cytology. One of the few studies showed a 100% positivity for HSIL with ProEx C. It is also interesting to note that 25% of LSILs were positive for ProEx C. This study suggested that the assay should be integrated into a clinical cytology laboratory to increase the positive predictive value of LBC for biopsy-proven HSIL.[98] Although ProEx C is emerging as a promising marker for HSIL, its role in undetermined categories needs to be evaluated further.

MIB1 (Ki-67)

Few studies have compared the expression of p16^{INK4a} and Ki-67 in cervical intraepithelial lesions. One study showed positive scores for Ki-67 and p16^{INK4a} of 68.4% and 100%, respectively, in LSIL, and 94.7% and 100%, respectively, in HSIL. Positive predictive values of these three biomarkers for HPV were 82.4% and 91.4%, respectively. The studies concluded that MIB1 (Ki-67) and p16^{INK4a} are complementary surrogate biomarkers for HPV-related pre-invasive squamous cervical disease.[99]

Utility of Cell Blocks Complementary to Pap Tests

The use of cell blocks in cervicovaginal cytology is rudimentary and underdeveloped. However, some usefulness of cell blocks on residual samples of Pap tests has been reported.[100-102] The diagnostic sensitivity and specificity of cell blocks from the residual samples is shown to be 86% to 100%.[101] Another important use of cell blocks is performing immunohistochemical stains when the Pap test interpretation is equivocal. Very few papers have demonstrated the performance of immunohistochemical stains on cell blocks. A study that looked at the utility of p16 on cell blocks obtained from the residual samples found that the sensitivity of this immunostain was up to 85% in Pap tests with a diagnosis of ASC-H; another similar study with the use of p16 and MIB1 (Ki-67) found the concordance of Pap test and cell block interpretation to be up to 85%.[100-102]

It is important to recognize the growing importance of cell block preparation(s) in cervicovaginal cytology. The use of immunohistochemistry on cell blocks by Kristen and colleagues demonstrated the use of molecular markers along with immunostains. The cell blocks can be useful in certain situations, such as identifying HSIL and differentiating between atrophy and metaplasia. The limitations that are foreseen for use of cell blocks may be insufficient material and added cost of immunostains.

Ovarian Cytology

WILMS' TUMOR GENE PRODUCT

Wilms' tumor gene product (WT1) has been established as a good marker for mesothelial cells. Studies have also demonstrated that WT1 is a highly sensitive and specific marker of serous carcinomas of ovarian surface epithelial origin (both ovarian and extra-ovarian).[103-105] Mucinous and micropapillary breast carcinomas may express WT1 and thus confound the distinction between breast carcinoma and metastatic ovarian serous carcinoma (Fig. 21.13).[106]

THYROID TRANSCRIPTION FACTOR-1

A recent study investigated thyroid transcription factor-1 (TTF-1) expression in 168 cases of primary ovarian epithelial neoplasms and showed TTF-1 positivity in approximately 1.2% of cases. One of these, a mixed serous and endometrioid carcinoma and pure high-grade serous carcinoma, showed strong nuclear staining. Although TTF-1 is still regarded as a sensitive and specific marker for non–small cell carcinoma of primary pulmonary origin, TTF-1 immunoreactivity can occur, albeit rarely, in carcinoma of primary ovarian origin.[107]

SOX9

SOX9 is a transcription factor involved in Sertoli cell differentiation in the testis and is variably expressed in a variety of ovarian tumors (44% of Sertoli cell tumors,

55% of endometrioid borderline tumors, 65% of well-differentiated endometrioid carcinomas, 39% of sertoliform endometrioid carcinomas, and 10% of carcinoid tumors). It therefore is not helpful in the distinction between these epithelial and sex cord–stromal tumors. The role of SOX9 in the pathogenesis of ovarian Sertoli cell tumor requires further study.[108]

HEPATOCYTE NUCLEAR FACTOR-1β

Hepatocyte nuclear factor-1β (HNF-1β) is a transcription factor that directly binds to DNA and is shown to be unregulated in ovarian clear cell carcinomas for unknown reasons. Mesothelial cells and non–clear cell adenocarcinomas are shown to be negative. A distinct nuclear staining is shown in clear cell carcinomas and is considered to be a positive result. HNF-1β is useful in peritoneal fluid cytology to distinguish clear cell carcinomas from other adenocarcinomas. Future studies are needed to evaluate the sensitivity and specificity of this marker in other cytology samples.[109]

CARCINOMA OF UNKNOWN PRIMARY

Carcinoma of unknown primary (CUP) accounts for 3% to 5% of all solid malignancies. The scenarios of CUP presentation are as follows:

1. Metastatic CUP primarily to the liver or to multiple sites
2. Metastatic CUP to lymph nodes
3. Metastatic CUP of peritoneal cavity, including peritoneal papillary serous carcinomatosis in females and peritoneal non-papillary carcinomatosis in males or females
4. Metastatic CUP to the lungs with parenchymal metastases or isolated malignant pleural effusion
5. Metastatic CUP to the bones
6. Metastatic CUP to the brain
7. Metastatic neuroendocrine carcinomas
8. Metastatic melanoma of an unknown primary.

Therapeutic strategies are sparse, and patients presenting with CUP carry a poor prognosis with short survival rates of 1 to 2 years. Identification of the organ of origin of the metastatic tumor may be of some therapeutic significance. Additional clinical history including sex, age, radiologic impression, and pattern of tumor dissemination is a helpful step in evaluation. Body effusions (pleural, peritoneal, and pericardial) are a common presentation of metastasis from an unknown primary. Serous effusions are therefore commonly encountered specimens in cytology for determination of CUP.

It is possible to recognize four different tumor types cytologically in effusions: adenocarcinoma (60%), squamous cell carcinoma (5%), non–small cell carcinoma (30%), and small cell carcinoma (1%).[110] Cytomorphology plays an important role in gearing the ancillary studies (e.g., ICC) for proper interpretation.

Adenocarcinoma is the most common tumor involving the serous membranes.[104] The most common sites of adenocarcinoma presenting as CUP are lung and pancreas (40%), followed by liver, colorectal area, gastric system, and renal tract. The characteristic coexpression patterns of cytokeratin 7 and 20, which have been shown to be of great utility in surgical pathology, have been used in cytology specimens as a first panel of immunostains in identifying the origin of malignant effusions.[40] The majority of lung, breast, gastric, and ovarian adenocarcinomas show a CK7-positive/CK20-negative immunophenotype. TTF-1, a monoclonal antibody, has emerged as a highly sensitive and specific marker in differentiating pulmonary adenocarcinomas from non-pulmonary adenocarcinomas in effusion cytology specimens.[111,112] Strong nuclear staining of TTF-1 in lung adenocarcinomas has a sensitivity of 88% and a specificity of 100%.[111] TTF-1 in conjunction with p63 can be utilized to distinguish pulmonary small cell carcinomas from poorly differentiated squamous cell carcinomas. Ninety-two percent of small cell carcinomas expressed TTF-1, and none expressed p63.[112] The CK7-negative/CK20-positive immunoprofile is highly specific for colorectal origin of adenocarcinoma, though a significant number of gastric and pancreatic adenocarcinomas exhibit this immunoprofile as well.[113,114]

CDX2 is a recent marker that encodes a transcription factor involved in differentiation of colonic epithelium. The sensitivity of expression of CDX2 in colorectal adenocarcinoma is 97%.[74] A weak positivity of CDX2 also is seen in gastric, biliopancreatic, and mucinous ovarian adenocarcinomas. An immunopanel comprising CK7, CK20, TTF-1, and CDX2 is a reasonable panel for CUP in serous effusions. When poorly differentiated, squamous cell carcinoma is difficult to differentiate from poorly differentiated adenocarcinoma. Cytokeratin 5/6, a mesothelial marker, and p63 immunostains are strongly expressed by squamous cell carcinomas and can be added to the panel.[111] Other probable sites of origin such as head and neck, anorectal, and genitourinary sites should be considered.

In males, prostate carcinoma can present rarely as CUP in pleural effusions. Prostate-specific antigen (PSA) can be useful in this situation and can be added to the panel.[115] In females with peritoneal carcinomatosis of unknown origin, the most common site of origin is the müllerian tract, followed by gastrointestinal tract, breast, and lymphoma. Accurate diagnostic markers are needed to accurately determine the likely sites of origin. CA125 is a marker of ovarian carcinoma but can be expressed in a small percentage of gastric and peritoneal carcinomas.[116,117] WT1 can be added to the panel if ovary or breast is considered in the differential diagnosis. It is important to remember that WT1 stains the background mesothelial cells as well.

Non-epithelial Malignancies Presenting as Tumors of Unknown Origin

The common non-epithelial neoplasms that cause malignant effusions include malignant melanomas, lymphomas, sarcomas, germ cell tumors, and some pediatric malignant tumors. The determination of origin of non-epithelial malignancies on purely cytomorphologic

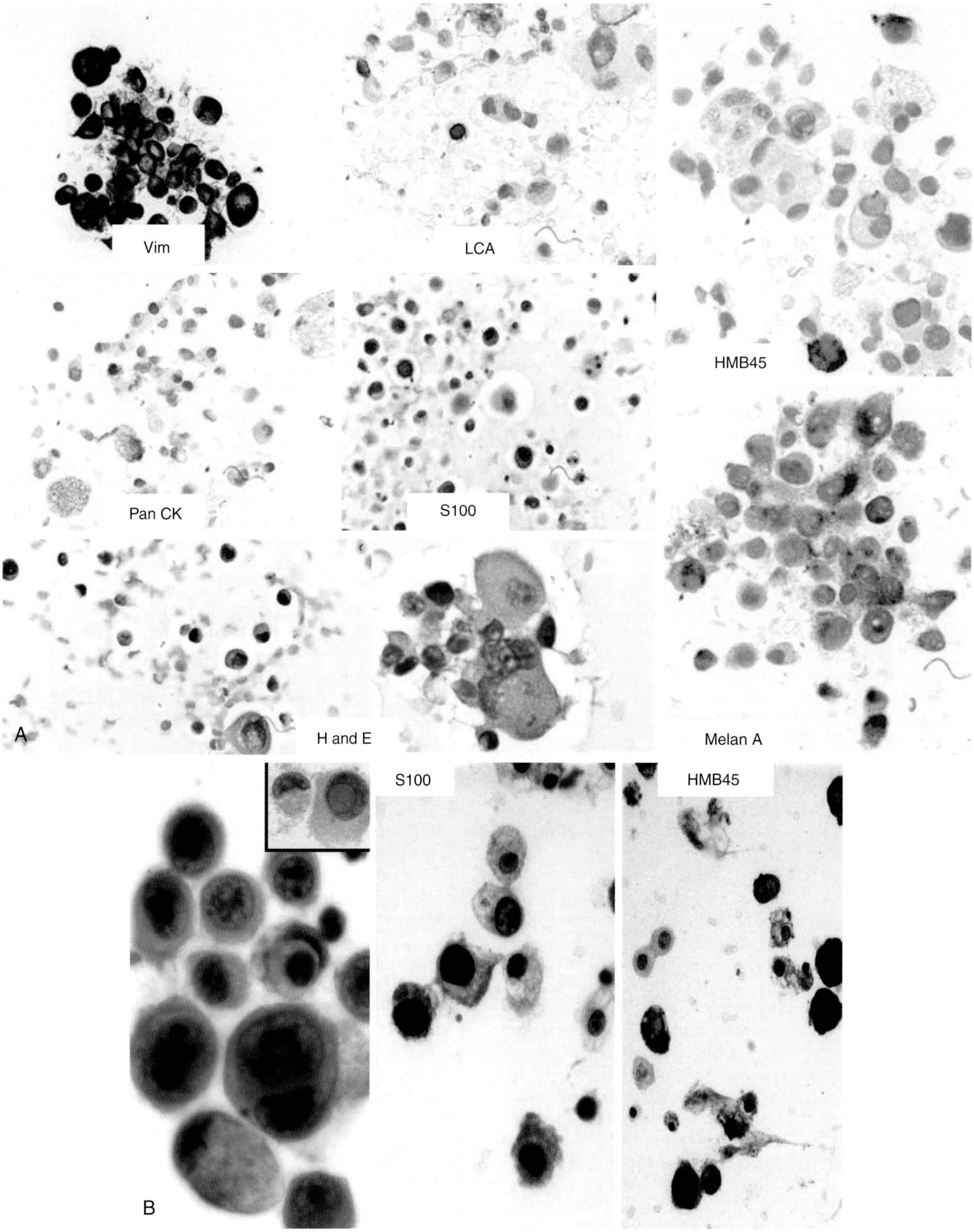

FIGURE 21.14 Metastatic malignant melanoma. **(A)** FNA cytology of an axillary mass. **(B)** Pleural effusion.

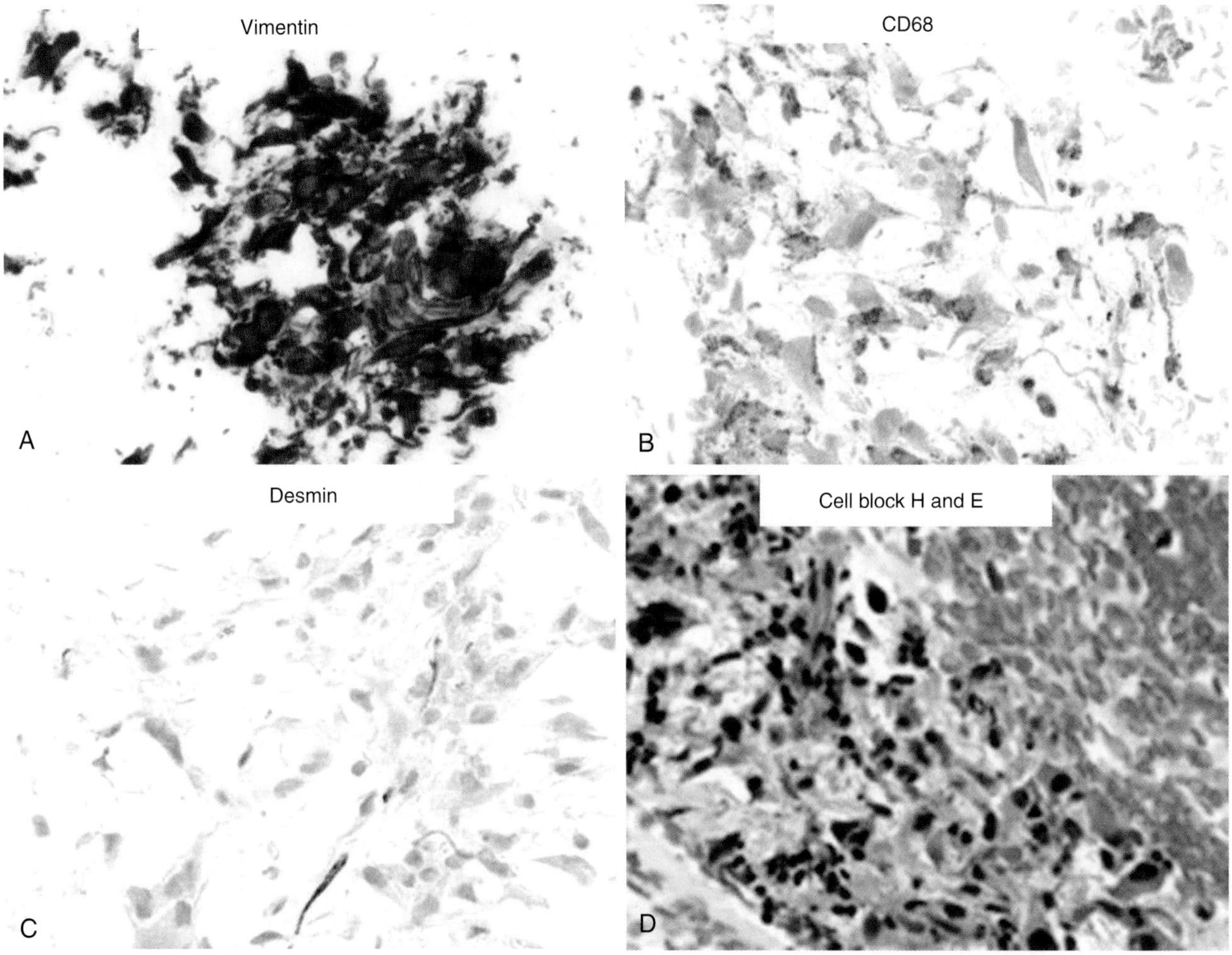

FIGURE 21.15 Malignant fibrous histiocytoma. **(A)** Vimentin, **(B)** CD68, **(C)** desmin, **(D)** cell block.

grounds is difficult. These tumors often exhibit a variety of morphologic features that can differ from those of the original tumor, may overlap with various epithelial tumors, and may preclude the correct diagnosis. IHC plays an important role in identification of these tumors.

MALIGNANT MELANOMA

The incidence of malignant melanoma has increased in recent years. However, effusions due to melanoma are relatively rare and compose only 2% to 3% of malignant effusions.

ICC has proved most practical in the identification of melanoma. The tumor cells are immunoreactive for HMB45 (anti-melanoma), S-100 protein, and other melanoma markers. Vimentin, while positive in melanomas, is also positive in mesotheliomas, sarcomas, and some carcinomas. Malignant melanoma cells are immunoreactive for HMB45 and Melan-A in 60% to 80% of melanomas. Cytokeratin immunoreactivity has been reported in malignant melanoma in 1% to 27% of cases, but immunostaining in these cells is usually weak and focal (Fig. 21.14).[118]

Sarcomas account for only 3% to 6% of malignant effusions. They usually occur in the setting of a known primary tumor, and they rarely present as a tumor of unknown origin. Synovial sarcoma, epithelioid sarcoma, vascular tumors, leiomyosarcoma, endometrial stromal sarcoma, and gastrointestinal stromal tumor (GIST) are some of the sarcomas that can present as tumors of unknown origin (Fig. 21.15).

Malignant effusions caused by non-epithelial neoplasms are more frequently encountered in children than in adults. The most common causes of malignant effusions in children are lymphoma and leukemia, followed by non-epithelial neoplasms including Wilms' tumor, neuroblastoma, Ewing's sarcoma, and embryonal rhabdomyosarcoma.

Germ cell neoplasms are common in pediatric patients as well as young adults. Seminomas are occasionally found in malignant effusions in pleura, peritoneum, and hydrocele sac.[119] Dysgerminoma is the female counterpart of the seminoma and rarely presents in effusions. These tumors can occur as pure tumors or as mixed tumors with other germ cell tumors, and they have potential to metastasize. Cell blocks have been proven to be a useful tool in the immunohistochemical studies performed to diagnose and differentiate components of mixed germ cell tumors.

KI-67

Ki-67 (MIB1) is a monoclonal antigen that interacts with human nuclear antigen Ki-67, which is present in proliferating cells. Studies have shown a good correlation of Ki-67 immunostaining with DNA flow cytometry in tumors. Expression of Ki-67 was shown in 26% of malignant effusions compared with 9% of benign effusions. Ki-67 can be used in difficult effusions to establish the presence of the second population of malignant cells, which needs further workup.[120]

C-MET

C-Met protein is a transmembrane tyrosine kinase that binds the hepatic growth factor (HGF) and plays an important role in the ability to metastasize. C-Met is demonstrated in carcinomas, mesotheliomas, and sarcomas and is also shown to have prognostic significance. Although C-Met is not expressed by benign mesothelial cells, a study performed on cell blocks of malignant and benign effusions shows that it is expressed by reactive mesothelial cells (up to 67%, compared to 100% by malignant cells). Owing to the low specificity, this marker is not of great use in cytologic interpretation.[121]

DPC4

DPC4 (MADH4, SMAD4) is a tumor-suppressor gene on chromosome 18q that has been shown to mediate the downstream effects of TGF-β superfamily signaling, resulting in growth inhibition.[122,123] DPC4 is genetically inactivated in approximately 55% of pancreatic adenocarcinomas.[124,125] Inactivation of the *DPC4* tumor-suppressor gene is relatively specific for pancreatic adenocarcinoma, although it has been shown to be expressed in a small percentage of primary carcinomas of the breast, ovary, colon, and biliary tract.[126-130] DPC4 labeling was observed in 17 of 39 conventional infiltrating pancreatic ductal carcinomas (44%).[126] The utility of DPC4 in immunocytochemistry still needs to be evaluated.

PAX5

PAX5 is a B cell–specific transcription factor. Its expression is detectable as early as the pro–B cell stage and subsequently in all further stages of B cell development until the plasma cell stage, where it is down-regulated. PAX5 is essential for B-lineage commitment in the fetal liver, whereas in adult bone marrow it is required for progression of B cell development beyond the early pro-B (pre-BI) cell stage. Even though there is an excellent correlation between CD20 and PAX5 expression, anti-PAX5 exceeds the specificity and sensitivity of anti-CD20 because of its earlier expression in B-cell differentiation and its ability to detect all committed B cells, including classic Hodgkin lymphoma.[131]

Identification of CUP and tumors of unknown origin is challenging in diagnostic cytopathology. To aid in the diagnostic workup, it is crucial to utilize the clinical history, the cytomorphology of cell groups, and appropriate antibody panels.

The utility of ICC in some of the CUP scenarios is illustrated in Figures 21.16 to 21.18.

BEYOND IMMUNOCYTOCHEMISTRY

IN SITU HYBRIDIZATION ASSAYS FOR DETECTION OF HIGH-RISK HPV

HPV DNA testing can be used in a variety of clinical scenarios. Reflex HPV DNA for ASC-US testing uses either residual liquid-based cytologic specimens or additional samples collected during the initial screening. The only FDA-approved commercially available method for detection of HPV DNA is the Hybrid Capture assay version HC2 (Digene, Gaithersburg, Md), which can detect 13 high-risk types of HPV. Three non–FDA-approved chromogenic ISH assays use signal-amplified colorimetric *in situ* hybridization (CSAC-ISH): the INFORM HPVII and HPVIII (Ventana, Tucson, Ariz) and the GenPoint Kit (Dako, Carpinteria, Calif). CSAC-ISH shows good correlation with PCR analysis, but ISH lacks the sensitivity of PCR and hybrid capture.[132-134]

UroVysion Multiprobe FISH in Urine Cytology

Urine cytology is used in combination with cystoscopy for the diagnosis of primary urothelial carcinomas and to monitor patients for early detection of recurrence. Because a broad overlap of reactive urothelial changes exists with these low-grade neoplasms, the sensitivity of urine cytology for low-grade urothelial neoplasms is 10% to 25%.[135,136] These cases are interpreted as "uncertain." Several studies have been reported to improve the sensitivity in detection of neoplastic cells in urine cytology. However, high false-positive rates and lack of reproducibility are drawbacks of these studies.[137-139]

The FISH technique allows visualization of specific DNA sequences and quantitation of chromosomes and genes, including tumor-specific deletions, amplifications, and aneusomies.[140-143] The UroVysion FISH assay (Abbott Molecular, Des Plaines, Ill) is available for routine urine cytology. The assay is composed of four single-stranded fluorescently labeled nuclei acid probes, including three chromosome enumeration probes (CEPs) for chromosomes 3,7, and 17 and for single locus-specific identifier (LSI) probe 9p21, which are seen frequently in bladder carcinomas. The probes are designated with specific fluorescent dye colors: red (CEP3), green (CEP 7), aqua (CEP 17), and gold (LSI 9p21).[141-144]

The specimen collection, preparation, and interpretation data are available from the package insert of the UroVysion FISH assay.[144]

In many studies, the reported sensitivity and specificity using the UroVysion FISH assay in detection of urothelial neoplasms is more than 90% and is shown to be a better predictor of risk of recurrence irrespective of cystoscopy or cytology. We have successfully adopted the UroVysion test in our laboratory. Figure 21.19 illustrates some examples of positive urine cytology samples.

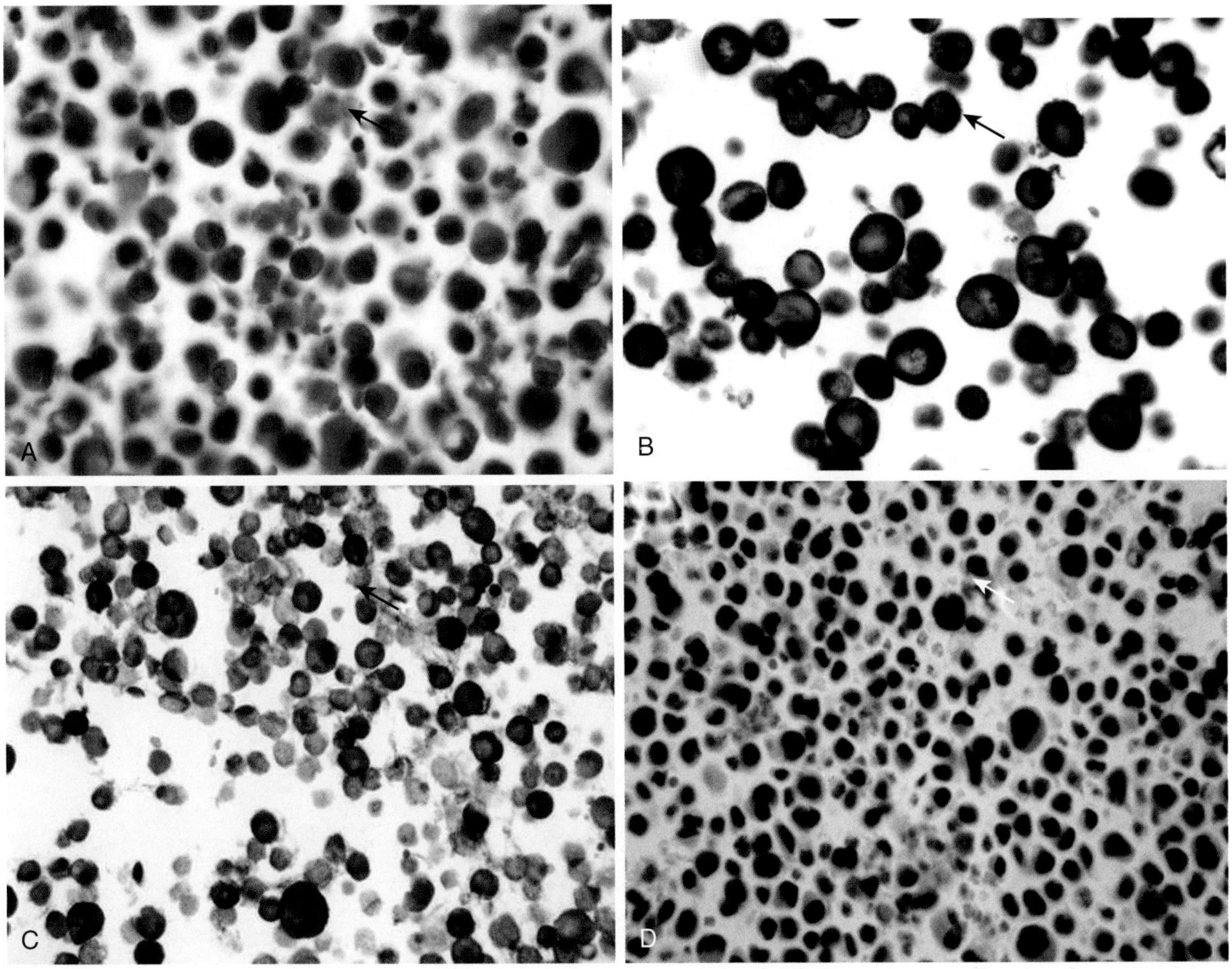

FIGURE 21.16 Carcinoma of unknown primary: **(A)** cell block preparation of ascitic fluid, **(B)** strong CA125 staining, **(C)** calretinin positive in mesothelial cells and negative in tumor cells. **(D)** Wilms' tumor gene 1 (WT1) strongly stains tumor cells, confirming müllerian origin of cells.

TEST FAILURE AND PITFALLS IN INTERPRETATION

Severe inflammation, excess amount of bacteria, crystalluria, hematuria, poor preservation of cells, and poor cellularity (<50 cells) are some of the causes of test failure. Prior radiation therapy in patients with a history of prostate cancer, endometrial cancer, or local/systemic chemotherapy can cause persistent chromosomal aberrations that can lead to erroneous false-positive test results. One should exercise caution to obtain a proper history. Seminal vesicle cells can look highly atypical or aneuploid, which can also lead to similar false-positive results. Presence of the characteristic golden yellow pigment in the cytoplasm serves as a clue for identifying these cells.

THERANOSTIC APPLICATIONS: ICC FOR TARGETED THERAPIES

ICC is becoming an important adjuvant for targeted therapies. These include rituximab for CD20-positive lymphomas, erbitux for epidermal growth factor receptor (EGFR)–positive head and neck and colon cancers, Herceptin for HER2-positive breast cancers, and Gleevac for GISTs.

CD117

c-*kit* (CD117) gene mutations are characteristically seen in GISTs and are shown as increased protein expression on surgical specimens demonstrated by IHC. c-*kit* protein expression can be examined in cytology specimens, but it is critical to use 10% formalin as a primary fixative. Few studies have successfully performed the ICC on cell block material of aspiration specimens (air-dried as well as Romanowsky-stained slides). c-*kit* mutational analysis is also shown in the same study on the cell block material (Fig. 21.20).[145]

HER2/neu

Approximately 15% to 20% of invasive breast carcinomas express HER2/neu and are associated with poor prognosis. Trastuzumab, a humanized monoclonal

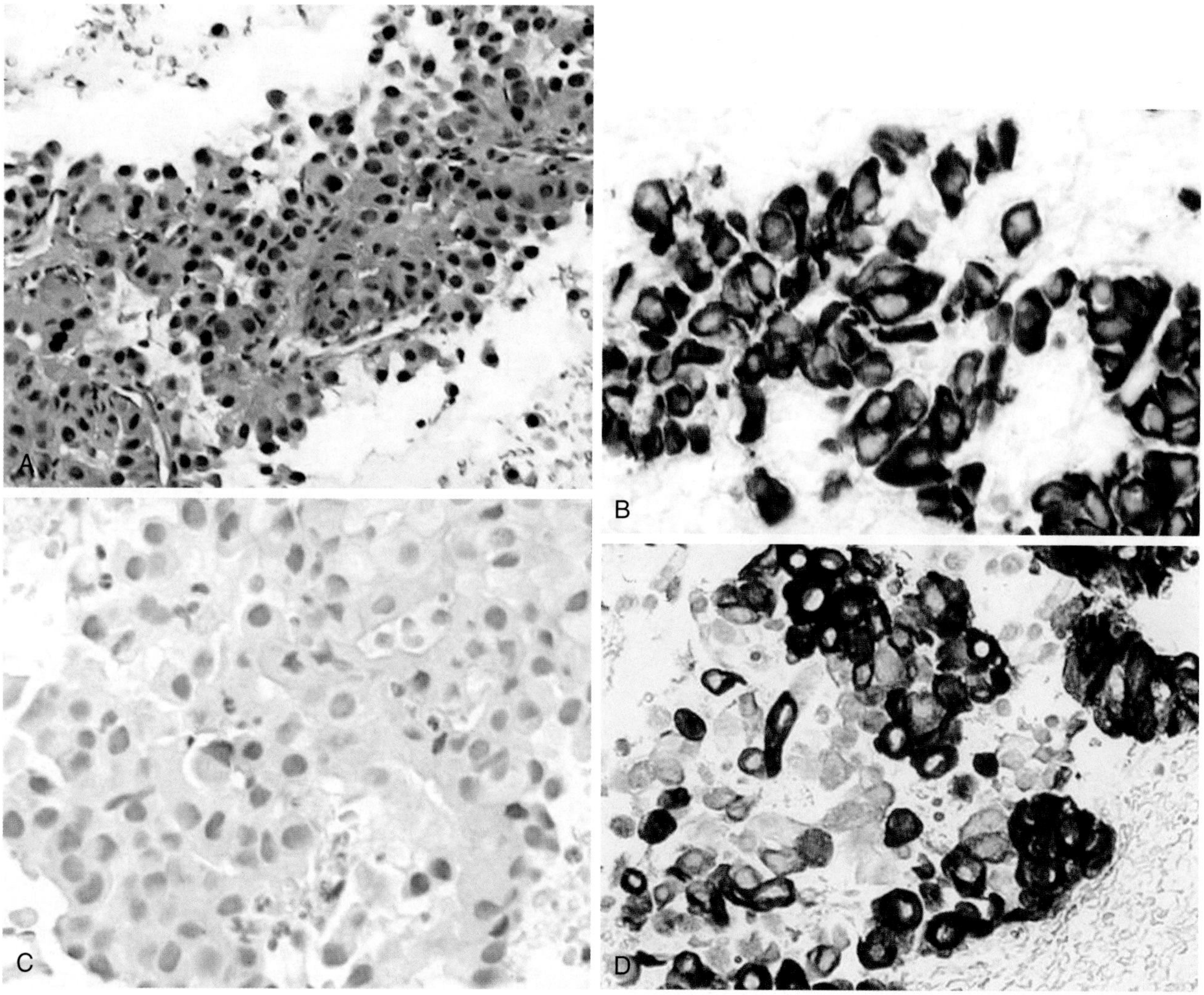

FIGURE 21.17 Carcinoma of unknown primary pancreatic origin **(A)**. FNA cytology of the liver mass **(B)**. Cytokeratin 7 strongly stains tumor cells **(C)**. DPC4 is negative in the tumor cells, indicating the loss of the gene in a subset of pancreatic tumors. **(D)** Cytokeratin 17 is strongly expressed in the tumor cells, confirming pancreatic origin of cells.

antibody directed against the extracellular domain of HER2 protein, has been shown to significantly increase complete pathologic response after adjuvant chemotherapy. Therefore, it is important for the laboratory to assess HER2 status on both histologic and cytologic specimens for management of these patients. HER2/neu protein expression by ICC can be performed on cell blocks, but primary formalin fixation is mandatory (Fig. 21.21).

Chromogenic *in situ* hybridization (CISH) is a recent methodology wherein the HER2/neu gene copies are detected by a silver reaction and visualized by light microscopy. A study that evaluated CISH on ThinPrep-processed fine-needle aspirate specimens found a good concordance between CISH performed on LBC specimens as compared to paraffin-embedded tissue specimens.[146,147]

Epidermal Growth Factor Receptor

EGFR is a cellular transmembrane receptor with tyrosine kinase enzymatic activity, which plays a key role in human cancer. EGFR-dependent signaling is involved in cancer cell proliferation, apoptosis, angiogenesis, invasion, and metastasis. Targeting the EGFR is a valuable molecular approach in cancer therapy. Formalin fixation, ideally in the form of a cell block, is the preferred specimen.

CONCLUSION

In the fast-growing era of technology, diagnostic cytopathology has managed to adopt and incorporate modern ancillary techniques such as ICC to aid in diagnosis. The role of ICC continues to grow not only in arriving at diagnosis but also for targeted therapies. However, the major challenge that remains to be addressed is standardization of immunoreactions within and across laboratories. New guidelines that address fixatives, fixation times, antigen retrieval, and immunodetection methods are being developed. These guidelines will help standardize immunohistochemistry for surgery and cytopathology, with the overall goal of improving quality for every laboratory.

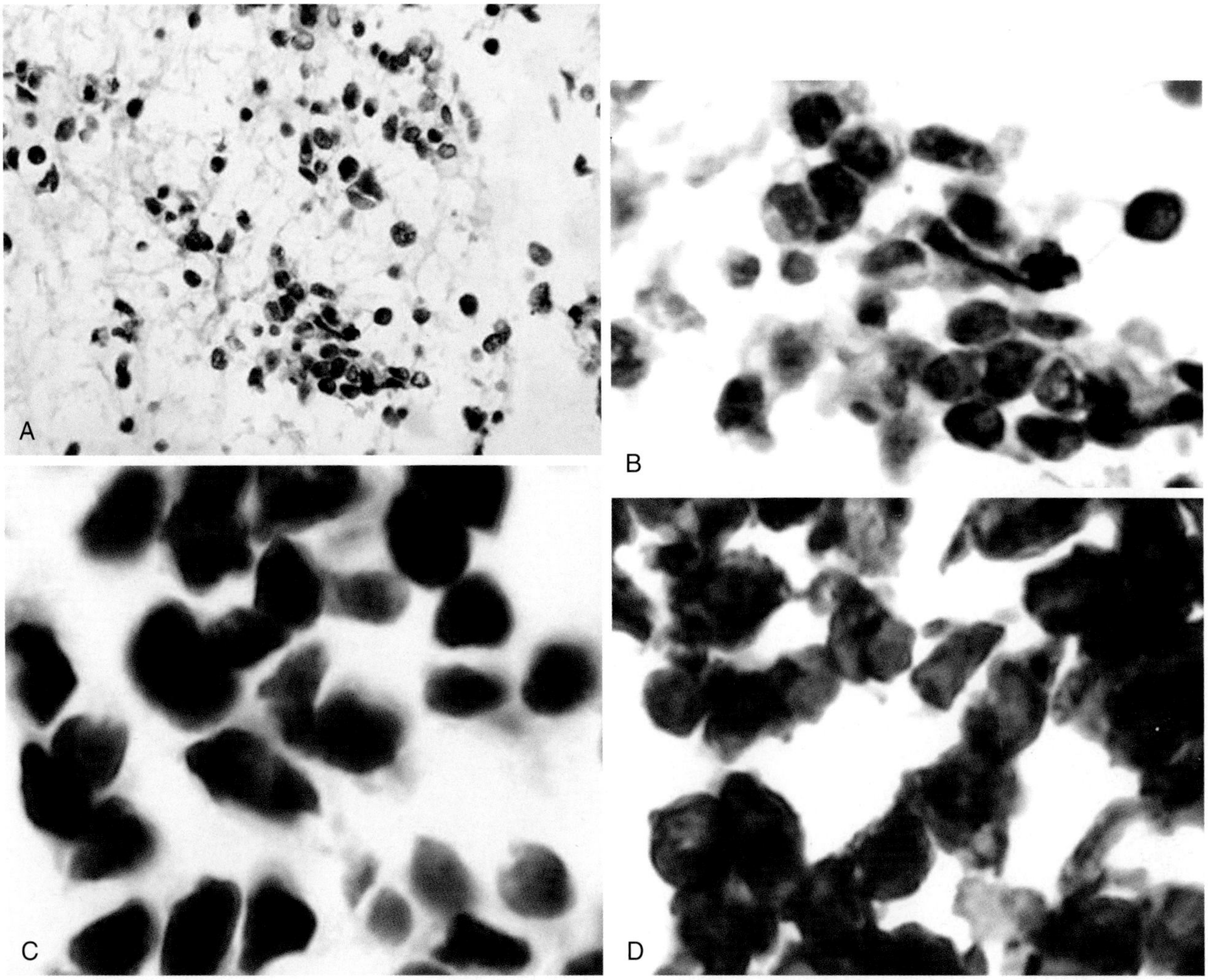

FIGURE 21.18 Carcinoma of unknown primary **(A, B)**. Tumor cells in the pericardial fluid **(C)**. TTF-1 demonstrates a strong nuclear staining **(D)**. Chromogranin is expressed strongly in tumor cells, confirming pulmonary origin, in particular a small cell type.

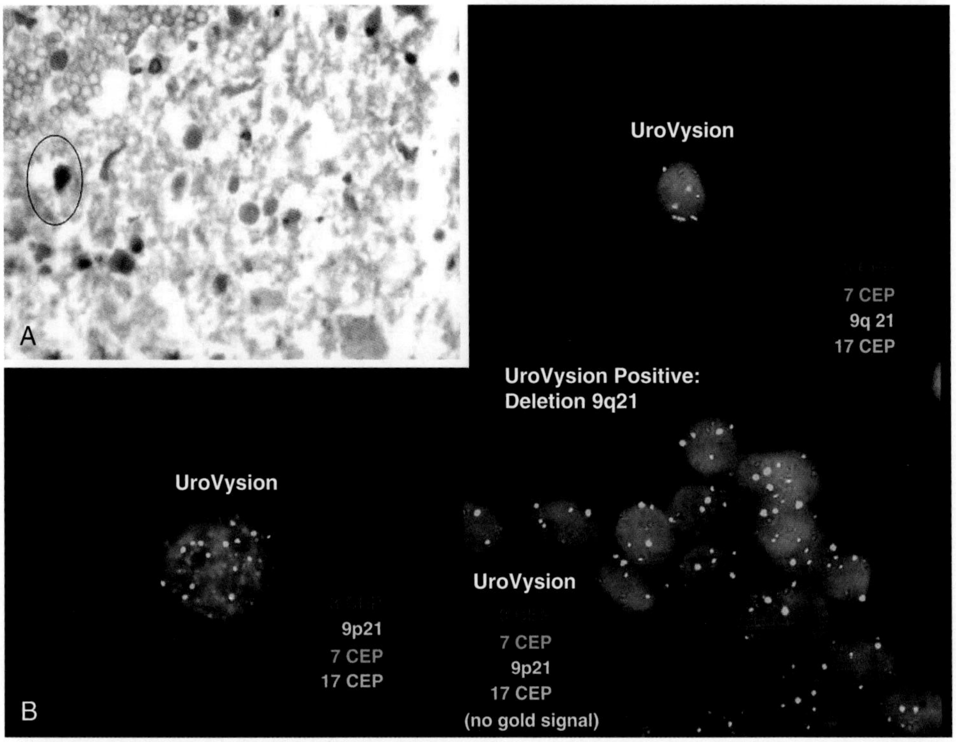

FIGURE 21.19 Urine cytology. **(A)** High-grade TCC cells scattered as single cells in the background of necrotic debris. **(B)** Fluorescently labeled probes including three chromosome enumeration probes (CEPs) for chromosomes 3, 7, and 17 and a single locus-specific identifier (LSI) probe 9p21, which is frequently seen in bladder carcinomas. *Demonstrated by UroVysion.*

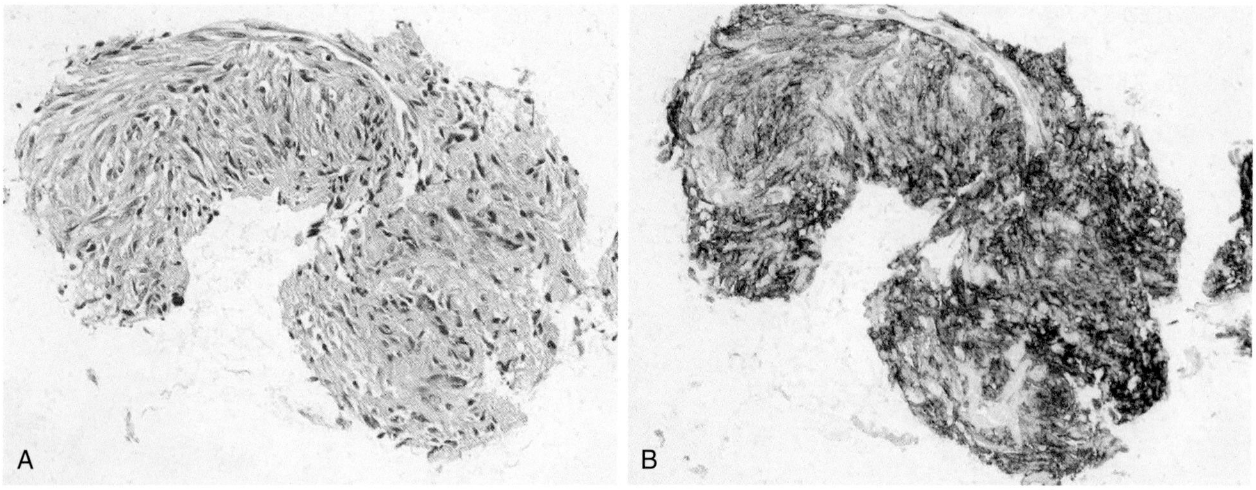

FIGURE 21.20 Fine-needle aspiration biopsy of a gastric wall mass. **(A)** Cell block shows moderately cellular uniform spindle cells with no atypia. **(B)** CD117 is strongly positive in tumor cells and confirms a GIST.

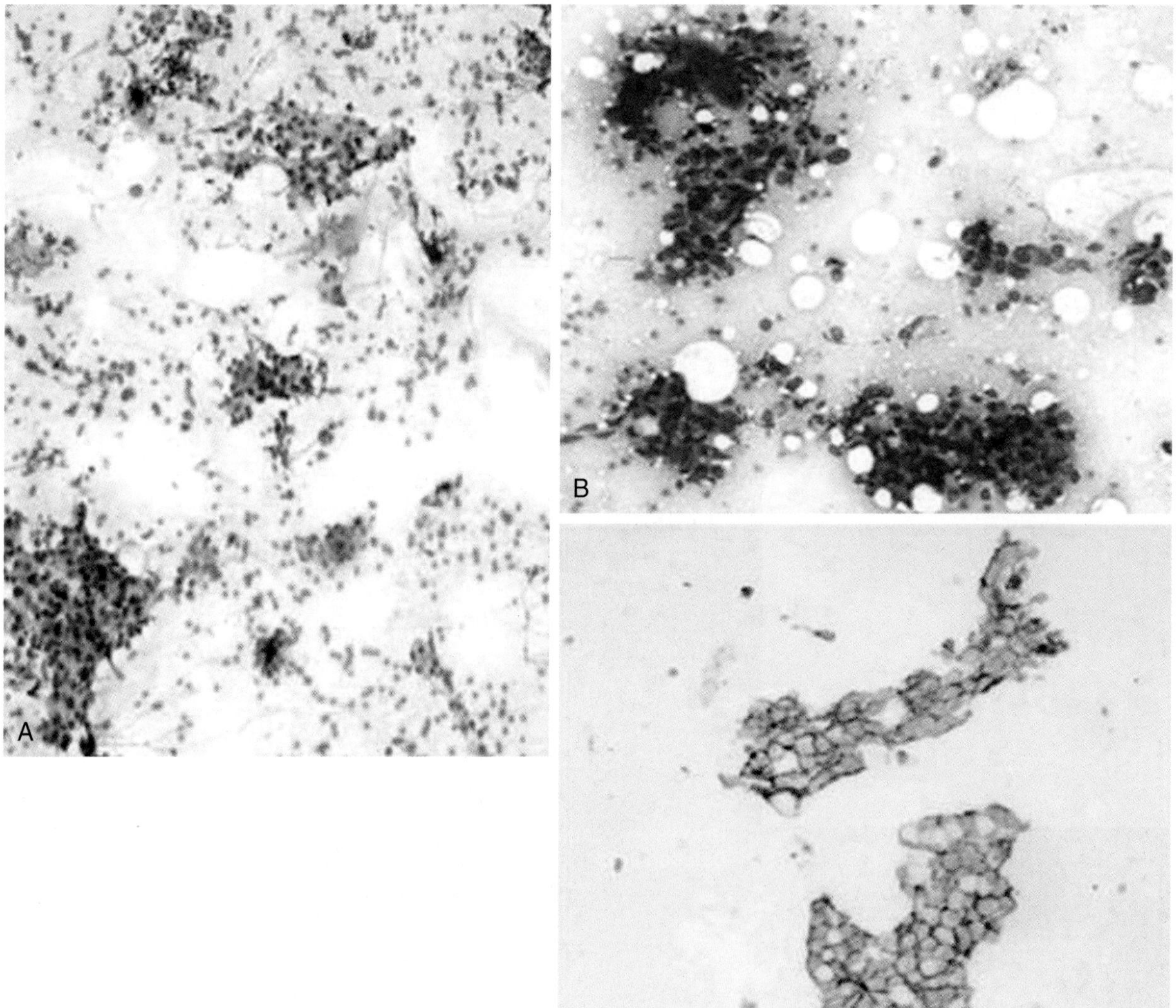

FIGURE 21.21 Fine-needle aspiration biopsy of a breast mass. **(A)** Papanicolaou stain. **(B)** Diff-Quik smears of cytomorphologically invasive ductal carcinoma. **(C)** HER2/neu: moderate complete strong membranous staining (score 2+) (HP). At follow-up, fluorescence *in situ* hybridization showed amplification. Such cytology specimens must be formalin fixed.

ACKNOWLEDGMENTS

The authors would like to thank Jing Yu, MD; Sara Monaco, MD; Walid Khalbuss, MD; and Vinod Shidham, MD, MRCPath for contributing some of the valuable pictures for the chapter.

REFERENCES

1. Chess Q, Hajdu S. The role of immunoperoxidase staining in diagnostic cytology. *Acta Cytol.* 1986;30:1-7.
2. Flens MJ, Valk PVD, Tadema TM, et al. The contribution of immunocytochemistry in diagnostic cytology, comparison and evaluation with immunohistology. *Cancer.* 1990;65:2704-2711.
3. Johnston WW, Szpak CA, Thor A, et al. Techniques in immunocytochemistry, application to diagnostic pathology. *Arch Pathol Lab Med.* 1989;113:641-644.
4. Lai C-R, Pan C-C, Tsay S-H. Contribution of immunocytochemistry in routine diagnostic cytology. *Diagn Cytopathol.* 1996;14:221-225.
5. Schofield J, Krausz T. Metastatic disease and lymphomas. In: Gray W, ed. *Serous Cavities.* London: Churchill-Livingstone; 1995.
6. Nance K, Silverman JF. Immunocytochemical panel for the identification of malignant cells in serous effusions. *Am J Clin Pathol.* 1993;95:867-874.
7. Leong A-Y, Suthipintawong C, Vinyuvat S. Immunostaining of cytologic preparations: A review of technical problems. *Appl Immunohistochem.* 1999;7:214-220.
8. Suthipintawong C, Leong A-Y, Vinyuvat S. Immunostaining of cell preparations: A comparative evaluation of common fixatives and protocols. *Diagn Cytopathol.* 1996;15:167-174.
9. Fulciniti F, Frangella C, Staiano M, et al. Air-dried smears for optimal diagnostic immunocytochemistry. *Acta Cytol.* 2008;52:178-186.
10. Abendroth CS, Dabbs DJ. Immunocytochemical staining of unstained versus previously stained cytologic preparations. *Acta Cytol.* 1995;39:379-386.
11. Goldstein NS, Hewitt SM, Taylor CR, et al. Members of Ad-Hoc Committee on Immunohistochemistry Standardization. Recommendations for improved standardization of immunohistochemistry. *Appl Immunohistochem Mol Morphol.* 2007;15:124-133.
12. Shi SR, Liu C, Taylor CR. Standardization of immunohistochemistry for formalin-fixed, paraffin-embedded tissue sections based on the antigen-retrieval technique: From experiments to hypothesis. *J Histochem Cytochem.* 2007;55:105-109.
13. Randall B, van Amerongen L. Commercial laboratory practice evaluation of air-dried/rehydrated cervico-vaginal smears vs traditionally-fixed smears. *Diagn Cytopathol.* 1997;16:174-176.
14. Ng WF, Choi FB, Cheung LLH, et al. Rehydration of air-dried smears with normal saline: Application in fluid cytology. *Acta Cytol.* 1994;38:56-64.
15. Chan JKC, Kung ITM. Rehydration of air-dried smears with normal saline: Application in fine-needle aspiration cytologic examination. *Am J Clin Pathol.* 1988;89:30-34.
16. Shi SR, Cote RJ, Taylor CR. Antigen retrieval immunohistochemistry: Past, present, and future. *J Histochem Cytochem.* 1997;45:327-343. Review.
17. Shi SR, Key ME, Kalra KL. Antigen retrieval in formalin-fixed, paraffin-embedded tissues: An enhancement method for immunohistochemical staining based on microwave oven heating of tissue sections. *J Histochem Cytochem.* 1991;39:741-748.
18. Boon ME, Kok LP. Breakthrough in pathology due to antigen retrieval. *Mal J Med Lab Sci.* 1995;12:1-9.
19. Sherman ME, Jimenez-Joseph D, Gangi MD, et al. Immunostaining of small cytologic specimens. Facilitation with cell transfer. *Acta Cytol.* 1994;38:18-22.
20. Miller RT, Swanson PE, Wick MR. Fixation and epitope retrieval in diagnostic immunohistochemistry: A concise review with practical considerations. *Appl Immunohistochem Mol Morphol.* 2000;8:228-235.
21. Fitzgibbons PL, Murphy DA, Dorfman DM, et al. Immunohistochemistry Committee, College of American Pathologists Inter laboratory comparison of immunohistochemical testing for HER2: Results of the 2004 and 2005 College of American Pathologists HER2 Immunohistochemistry Tissue Microarray Survey. *Arch Pathol Lab Med.* 2006;130:1440-1445.
22. National Institutes of Health Consensus Development Conference statement. Adjuvant therapy for breast cancer, November 1-3, 2000. *J Natl Cancer Inst Monogr.* 2001:5-15.
23. Chivukula M, Bhargava R, Dabbs DJ. Diagnostic, theranostic and genomic immunohistochemistry standardization issues. *Adv Anat Pathology,* 2008, In Press.
24. Bhargava R, Chivukula M, Beriwal S, et al. Estrogen and progesterone receptors in breast carcinoma: Quantitation is therapeutically important. *Adv Anat Pathol.* 2008;15(5):304-305.
25. McKee GT, Tambouret RH, Finkelstein D. A reliable method of demonstrating HER 2/neu, estrogen receptors, and progesterone receptors on routinely processed cytologic material. *Appl Immunohistochem Mol Morphol.* 2001;9:352-357.
26. Gong Y, Symmans WF, Krishnamurthy S, et al. Optimal fixation conditions for immunocytochemical analysis of estrogen receptor in cytologic specimens of breast carcinoma. *Cancer.* 2004;102:34-40.
27. Goldstein NS, Ferkowicz M, Odish E, et al. Minimum formalin fixation time for consistent estrogen receptor immunohistochemical staining of invasive breast carcinoma. *Am J Clin Pathol.* 2003;120:86-92.
28. Tabbara SO, Sidaway M, Frost AR, et al. The stability of estrogen and progesterone receptor expression on breast carcinoma cells stored as PreservCyt suspensions and as ThinPrep slides. *Cancer Cytopathol.* 1998;84:355-360.
29. Dabbs DJ, Abendroth CS, Grenko RT, et al. Immunocytochemistry on the ThinPrep processor. *Diagn Cytopathol.* 1997;17:388-392.
30. Guiter GE, Gatscha RM, Zakowski MF. ThinPrep vs conventional aspirations of sarcomas: A morphological and immunocytochemical study. *Diagn Cytopathol.* 1999;21:351-354.
31. Leung SW, Bedard YC. Immunocytochemical staining on ThinPrep processed smears. *Mod Pathol.* 1996;9:304-306.
32. Kaplan MA, Segura AM, Wang HH, et al. Evaluation of Cytolyt and PreservCyt as preservatives for immunocytochemistry for cytokeratin in fine needle aspiration. *Appl Immunohistochem.* 1998;6:23-29.
33. Soule N, Mui K, O'Brien M, et al. A rapid automated system for creating paraffin-embedded cell blocks. Abstract 193. *Cancer Cytopathol.* 2006;108(Suppl 5):444-445.
34. Kulkarni MB, Prabhudesai NM, Desai SB, et al. Scrape cell-block technique for fine needle aspiration cytology smears. *Cytopathology.* 2000;11:179-184.
35. Gangane N, Mukerji MS, Anshu Sharma SM. Utility of microwave processed cell blocks as a complement to cervico-vaginal smears. *Diagn Cytopathol.* 2007;35:338-41.
36. Dabbs DJ, Wang X. Immunocytochemistry on cytologic specimens of limited quantity. *Diagn Cytopathol.* 1998;18:166-169.
37. Hunt JL, van de Rijn M, Gupta PK. Immunohistochemical analysis of gel-transferred cells in cytologic preparations following smear division. *Diagn Cytopathol.* 1998;18:377-380.
38. Edwards C, Oates J. OV 632 and MOC-31 in the diagnosis of mesothelioma and adenocarcinoma: An assessment of their use in formalin-fixed and paraffin wax embedded material. *J Clin Pathol.* 1995;48:626-630.
39. To A, Dearnaley DP, Omerod MG, et al. Epithelial membrane antigen: Its use in the cytodiagnosis of malignancy. *Am J Clin Pathol.* 1982;78:214-219.
40. Sack MJ, Roberts SA. Cytokeratins 20 and 7 in the differential diagnosis of metastatic carcinomas in cytologic specimens. *Cytopathology.* 1997;16:132-136.
41. Manosca F, Schinstine M, Fetsch PA, et al. Diagnostic effects of prolonged storage on fresh effusion samples. *Diagn Cytopathol.* 2007;35:6-11.
41a. Gotzos V, Vogt P, Celio MR. The calcium binding protein calretinin is a selective marker for malignant pleural mesothelioma of the epithelial type. *Pathol Res Pract.* 1996;192:137-147.
42. Doglioni C, Dei Tos AP, Laurino L, et al. A novel immunocytochemical marker for mesothelioma. *Am J Surg Pathol.* 1996;20:1037-1046.

43. Politi E, Kandaraki C, Apostolopoulou C, et al. Immunocytochemical panel for distinguishing between carcinoma and reactive mesothelial cells in body cavity fluids. *Diagn Cytopathol.* 2005;32:151-155.
44. Fetsch PA, Simsir A, Abati A. Comparison of antibodies to HBME-1 and calretinin for the detection of mesothelial cells in effusion cytology. *Diagn Cytopathol.* 2001;25:158-161.
45. Ordoñez NG. Value of calretinin immunostaining in differentiating epithelial mesothelioma from lung adenocarcinoma. *Mod Pathol.* 1998;11:929-933.
46. Nagel H, Hemmerlein B, Ruschenberg I, et al. The value of anti-calretinin antibody in the differential diagnosis of normal and reactive mesothelia versus metastatic tumors in effusion cytology. *Pathol Res Pract.* 1998;194:759-764.
47. Yaziji H, Battifora H, Barry TS, et al. Evaluation of 12 antibodies for distinguishing epithelioid mesothelioma from adenocarcinoma: Identification of a three-antibody immunohistochemical panel with maximal sensitivity and specificity. *Mod Pathol.* 2006;19:514-523.
48. Moll R, Dhouailly D, Sun T-T. Expression of keratin 5 as a distinctive feature of epithelial and biphasic mesotheliomas. An immunohistochemical study using monoclonal antibody. *Virchows Arch B Cell Pathol.* 1989;58:129-145.
49. Blobel GA, Moll R, Franke RR, et al. The intermediate cytoskeleton of malignant mesotheliomas and its diagnostic significance. *Am J Pathol.* 1985;121:235-247.
50. Clover J, Oates J, Edwards C. Anti-cytokeratin 5/6: A positive marker for mesothelioma. *Histopathology.* 1997;31:140-143.
51. Ordoñez NG. Value of cytokeratin 5/6 immunostaining in distinguishing epithelial mesothelioma of the pleura from lung adenocarcinoma. *Am J Surg Pathol.* 1998;22:1215-1221.
52. Granja NM, Begnami MD, Bortolan J, et al. Desmoplastic small round cell tumour: Cytological and immunocytochemical features. *Cytojournal.* 2005;2:6.
53. Saad RS, Lindner JL, Lin X, et al. The diagnostic utility of D2-40 for malignant mesothelioma versus pulmonary carcinoma with pleural involvement. *Diagn Cytopathol.* 2006;34:801-806.
54. Bassarova AV, Nesland JM, Davidson B. D2-40 is not a specific marker for cells of mesothelial origin in serous effusions. *Am J Surg Pathol.* 2006;30:878-882.
55. Afify A, Zhou H, Howell L, et al. Diagnostic utility of GLUT-1 expression in the cytologic evaluation of serous fluids. *Acta Cytol.* 2005;49:621-626.
56. Kato Y, Tsuta K, Seki K, et al. Immunohistochemical detection of GLUT-1 can discriminate between reactive mesothelium and malignant mesothelioma. *Mod Pathol.* 2007;20:215-220.
57. Lyons-Boudreaux V, Mody DR, Zhai J, et al. Cytologic malignancy versus benignancy: How useful are the "newer" markers in body fluid cytology? *Arch Pathol Lab Med.* 2008;132:23-28.
58. Morgan RL, De Young BR, McGaughy VR, Niemann TH. MOC-31 aids in the differentiation between adenocarcinoma and reactive mesothelial cells. *Cancer.* 1999;87:390-394.
59. Ordoñez NG. Value of the MOC-31 monoclonal antibody in differentiating epithelial pleural mesothelioma from lung adenocarcinoma. *Hum Pathol.* 1998;29:166-169.
60. Gonzalez-Lois C, Ballestin C, Sotelo MT, et al. Combined use of novel epithelial (MOC-31) and mesothelial (HBME-1) immunohistochemical markers for optimal first line diagnostic distinction between mesothelioma and metastatic carcinoma in pleura. *Histopathology.* 2001;38:528-534.
61. Bailey ME, Brown RW, Mody DR, et al. Ber-EP4 for differentiating adenocarcinoma from reactive and neoplastic mesothelial cells in serous effusions. Comparison with carcinoembryonic antigen, B72.3 and Leu-M1. *Acta Cytol.* 1996;40:1212-1216.
62. Delahaye M, van der Ham F, van der Kwast TH. Complementary value of five carcinoma markers for the diagnosis of malignant mesothelioma, adenocarcinoma metastasis, and reactive mesothelium in serous effusions. *Diagn Cytopathol.* 1997 Aug;17:115-120.
63. Gaffey MJ, Mills SE, Swanson PE, et al. Immunoreactivity for Ber-EP4 in adenocarcinomas, adenomatoid tumors and malignant mesotheliomas. *Am J Surg Pathol.* 1992;16:3-9.
64. Bollinger DJ, Wick MR, Dehner LP, et al. Peritoneal malignant mesothelioma versus serous papillary adenocarcinoma: A histochemical and immunohistochemical comparison. *Am J Surg Pathol.* 1989;13:659-670.
65. Latza U, Niedobitek G, Schwarting R, et al. Ber-EP4: New monoclonal antibody which distinguishes epithelia from mesothelia. *J Clin Pathol.* 1990;43:213-219.
66. Singh HK, Silverman JF, Berns L, et al. Significance of epithelial membrane antigen in the work-up of problematic serous effusions. *Diagn Cytopathol.* 1995;13:3-7.
67. Dejmek A, Hjerpe A. Immunohistochemical reactivity in mesothelioma and adenocarcinoma: A stepwise logistic regression analysis. *APMIS.* 1994;102:255-264.
68. Shield PW, Callan JJ, Devine PL. Markers for metastatic adenocarcinoma in serous effusion specimens. *Diagn Cytopathol.* 1995;11:1-9.
69. Afify AM, al-Khafaji BM. Diagnostic utility of thyroid transcription factor-1 expression in adenocarcinomas presenting in serous fluids. *Acta Cytol.* 2002;46:675-678.
70. Hecht JL, Pinkus JL, Weinstein LJ, et al. The value of thyroid transcription factor-1 in cytologic preparations as a marker for metastatic adenocarcinoma of lung origin. *Am J Clin Pathol.* 2001;116:483-488.
71. Recine MA, Deavers MT, Middleton LP, et al. Serous carcinoma of the ovary and peritoneum with metastases to the breast and axillary lymph nodes: A potential pitfall. *Am J Surg Pathol.* 2004;28:1646-1651.
72. Dabbs DJ, Landreneau RJ, Liu Y, et al. Detection of estrogen receptor by immunohistochemistry in pulmonary adenocarcinoma. *Ann Thorac Surg.* 2002;73:403-405; discussion 406.
73. Kobayashi M, Ueyama Y, Nakanishi H, et al. Immunocytochemical detection using CDX2: An aid for discerning tumor involvement in ascites cytology. *Cancer.* 2006;108:114-118.
74. Kaimaktchiev V, Terracciano L, Tornillo L, et al. The homeobox intestinal differentiation factor CDX2 is selectively expressed in gastrointestinal adenocarcinomas. *Mod Pathol.* 2004;17:1392-1399.
75. Levine PH, Joutovsky A, Cangiarella J, et al. CDX-2 expression in pulmonary fine-needle aspiration specimens: A useful adjunct for the diagnosis of metastatic colorectal adenocarcinoma. *Diagn Cytopathol.* 2006;34:191-195.
76. Saad RS, Essig DL, Silverman JF, et al. Diagnostic utility of CDX2 expression in separating metastatic gastrointestinal adenocarcinoma from other metastatic adenocarcinoma in fine-needle aspiration cytology using cell blocks. *Cancer.* 2004;102:168-173.
77. Jaffee IM, Rahmani M, Singhal MG, et al. Expression of the intestinal transcription factor CDX2 in carcinoid tumors is a marker of midgut origin. *Arch Pathol Lab Med.* 2006;130:1522-1526.
78. Wick MR, Lillemoe TJ, Copland GT, et al. Gross cystic disease fluid protein-15 as a marker for breast cancer: Immunohistochemical analysis of 690 human neoplasms and comparison with alpha-lactalbumin. *Hum Pathol.* 1989;20:281-287.
79. Lee BH, Hecht JL, Pinkus JL, et al. WT1, estrogen receptor, and progesterone receptor as markers for breast or ovarian primary sites in metastatic adenocarcinoma to body fluids. *Am J Clin Pathol.* 2002;117:745-750.
80. Fiel MI, Cernaianu G, Burstein DE, et al. Value of GCDFP-15 (BRST-2) as a specific immunocytochemical marker for breast carcinoma in cytologic specimens. *Acta Cytol.* 1996;40:637-641.
81. Striebel JM, Dacic S, Yousem SA. Gross cystic disease fluid protein-(GCDFP-15): Expression in primary lung adenocarcinoma. *Am J Surg Pathol.* 2008;32:426-432.
82. Bhargava R, Beriwal S, Dabbs DJ. Mammaglobin vs GCDFP-15: An immunohistologic validation survey for sensitivity and specificity. *Am J Clin Pathol.* 2007;127:103-113.
83. Ciampa A, Fanger G, Khan A, et al. Mammaglobin and CRxA-01 in pleural effusion cytology: Potential utility of distinguishing metastatic breast carcinomas from other cytokeratin 7-positive/cytokeratin 20-negative carcinomas. *Cancer.* 2004;102:368-372.
84. Dabbs D, Bhargava R, Chivukula M. The utility of p120 catenin in the diagnosis of lobular Carcinoma of the breast. *Am J Surg Pathol.* 2007;31:427-437.
85. Kalogeraki A, Garbagnati F, Santinami M, et al. E-cadherin expression on fine needle aspiration biopsies of breast invasive ductal carcinomas and its relationship to clinicopathologic factors. *Acta Cytol.* 2003;47:363-367.
86. Agoff SN, Lin P, Morihara J, et al. p16(INK4a) expression correlates with degree of cervical neoplasia: A comparison with Ki-67 expression and detection of high-risk HPV types. *Mod Pathol.* 2003;16:665-673.

87. Hariri J, Øster A. The negative predictive value of p16INK4a to assess the outcome of cervical intraepithelial neoplasia 1 in the uterine cervix. *Int J Gynecol Pathol.* 2007;26:223-228.
88. Schorge JO, Lea JS, Elias KJ, et al. P16 as a molecular biomarker of cervical adenocarcinoma. *Am J Obstet Gynecol.* 2004;190:668-673.
89. Bibbo M, Klump WJ, DeCecco J, et al. Procedure for immunocytochemical detection of P16INK4A antigen in thin-layer, liquid-based specimens. *Acta Cytol.* 2002;46:25-29.
90. Saqi A, Pasha TL, McGrath CM, et al. Overexpression of p16INK4A in liquid-based specimens (SurePath) as marker of cervical dysplasia and neoplasia. *Diagn Cytopathol.* 2002;27:365-370.
91. Bibbo M, DeCecco J, Kovatich AJ. P16INK4A as an adjunct test in liquid-based cytology. *Anal Quant Cytol Histol.* 2003;25:8-11.
92. Yoshida T, Fukuda T, Sano T, et al. Usefulness of liquid-based cytology specimens for the immunocytochemical study of p16 expression and human papillomavirus testing: A comparative study using simultaneously sampled histology materials. *Cancer.* 2004;102:100-108.
93. Pientong C, Ekalaksananan T, Kongyingyoes B, et al. Immunocytochemical staining of p16INK4a protein from conventional Pap test and its association with human papillomavirus infection. *Diagn Cytopathol.* 2004;31:235-242.
94. Wentzensen N, Bergeron C, Cas F, et al. Triage of women with ASCUS and LSIL cytology: Use of qualitative assessment of p16INK4a positive cells to identify patients with high-grade cervical intraepithelial neoplasia. *Cancer.* 2007;111:58-66.
95. Trunk MJ, Dallenbach-Hellweg G, Ridder R, et al. Morphologic characteristics of p16INK4a-positive cells in cervical cytology samples. *Acta Cytol.* 2004;48:771-782.
96. Wentzensen N, Bergeron C, Cas F, et al. Evaluation of a nuclear score for p16INK4a-stained cervical squamous cells in liquid-based cytology samples. *Cancer.* 2005;105:461-467.
97. Pantanowitz L, Florence RR, Goulart RA, et al. Trichomonas vaginalis P16 immunoreactivity in cervicovaginal Pap tests: A diagnostic pitfall. *Diagn Cytopathol.* 2005;33:210-213.
98. Kelly D, Kincaid E, Fansler Z, et al. Detection of cervical high-grade squamous intraepithelial lesions from cytologic samples using a novel immunocytochemical assay (ProEx C). *Cancer.* 2006;108:494-500.
99. Keating JT, Cviko A, Riethdorf S, et al. Ki-67, cyclin E, and p16INK4 are complimentary surrogate biomarkers for human papilloma virus-related cervical neoplasia. *Am J Surg Pathol.* 2001;25:884-891.
100. Negri G, Moretto G, Menia E, et al. Immunocytochemistry of p16INK4a in liquid-based cervicovaginal specimens with modified Papanicolaou counterstaining. *Clin Pathol.* 2006;59:827-830.
101. Gupta S, Halder K, Khan VA, et al. Cell block as an adjunct to conventional Papanicolaou smear for diagnosis of cervical cancer in resource-limited settings. *Cytopathology.* 2007;18:309-315.
102. Liu H, Shi J, Wilkerson M, et al. Immunohistochemical detection of p16INK4a in liquid-based cytology specimens on cell block sections. *Cancer.* 2007;111:74-82.
103. Hylander B, Repasky E, Shrikant P, et al. Expression of Wilms tumor gene (WT1) in epithelial ovarian cancer. *Gynecol Oncol.* 2006;101:12-17.
104. Hwang H, Quenneville L, Yaziji H, et al. Wilms tumor gene product: Sensitive and contextually specific marker of serous carcinomas of ovarian surface epithelial origin. *Appl Immunohistochem Mol Morphol.* 2004;12:122-126.
105. Chivukula M, Kapali M. Expression of Wilms tumor gene (WT-1) in primary peritoneal papillary serous carcinomas. *Mod Pathol.* 2005; Abstract no. 150. Poster: 94th Annual Meeting of United States and Canadian Academy of Pathology, 2005, San Antonio, TX, USA.
106. Karabakhtsian R, Bhargava R. WT-1 expression in primary invasive breast carcinoma: Occasional expression in micropapillary and mucinous subtypes. *Mod Pathol.* 2007;20 (Suppl 2); 38A (abstract 151).
107. Graham AD, Williams AR, Salter DM. TTF-1 expression in primary ovarian epithelial neoplasia. *Histopathology.* 2006;48:764-765.
108. Zhao C, Bratthauer GL, Barner R, et al. Immunohistochemical analysis of sox9 in ovarian Sertoli cell tumors and other tumors in the differential diagnosis. *Int J Gynecol Pathol.* 2007;26:1-9.
109. Kato N, Toukairin M, Asanuma I, et al. Immunocytochemistry for hepatocyte nuclear factor-1beta (HNF-1beta): A marker for ovarian clear cell carcinoma. *Diagn Cytopathol.* 2007;35:193-197.
110. Pomjanski N, Grote HJ, Doganay P, et al. Immunocytochemical identification of carcinomas of unknown primary in serous effusions. *Diagn Cytopathol.* 2005;33:309-315.
111. Jang MJ, Lee DG, Chung MJ. Utility of thyroid transcription factor-1 and cytokeratin 7 and 20 immunostaining in the identification of origin in malignant effusions. *Anal Quant Cytol Histol.* 2001;23:400-404.
112. Wu M, Szporn AH, Zhang D, et al. Cytology applications of p63 and TTF-1 immunostaining in differential diagnosis of lung cancers. *Diagn Cytopathol.* 2005;33:223-227.
113. Ascoli V, Taccogna S, Scalzo CC, et al. Utility of cytokeratin 20 in identifying the origin of metastatic carcinomas in effusions. *Diagn Cytopathol.* 1995;12:303-308.
114. Pereira TC, Saad RS, Liu Y, et al. The diagnosis of malignancy in effusion cytology: A pattern recognition approach. *Adv Anat Pathol.* 2006;13:174-184.
115. Broghamer Jr WL, Richardson ME, Faurest S, et al. Prostatic acid phosphatase immunoperoxidase staining of cytologically positive effusions associated with adenocarcinomas of the prostate and neoplasms of undetermined origin. *Acta Cytol.* 1985;29:274-278.
116. Pinto MM, Bernstein LH, Rudolph RA, et al. Diagnostic efficiency of carcinoembryonic antigen and CA125 in the cytological evaluation of effusions. *Arch Pathol Lab Med.* 1992;116:626-631.
117. Masood S. Use of monoclonal antibody for assessment of estrogen and progesterone receptors in malignant effusions. *Diagn Cytopathol.* 1992;8:161-166.
118. Beaty MW, Fetsch P, Wilder AM, et al. Effusion cytology of malignant melanoma. A morphologic and immunocytochemical analysis including application of the MART-1 antibody. *Cancer.* 1997;81:57-63.
119. Ikeda K, Tate G, Suzuki T, et al. Cytomorphologic features of immature ovarian teratoma in peritoneal effusion: A case report. *Diagn Cytopathol.* 2005;33:39-42.
120. Saleh H, Bober P. Value of Ki67 immunostain in identification of malignancy in serous effusions. *Diagn Cytopathol.* 1999;20:24-28.
121. Zimmerman RL, Fogt F. Evaluation of the c-Met immunostain to detect malignant cells in body cavity effusions. *Oncol Rep.* 2001;8:1347-1350.
122. Dai JL, Turnacioglu KK, Schutte M, et al. Dpc4 transcriptional activation and dysfunction in cancer cells. *Cancer Res.* 1998;58:4592-4597.
123. de Winter JP, Roelen BA, ten Dijke P, et al. DPC4 (SMAD4) mediates transforming growth factor-beta1 (TGF-beta1) induced growth inhibition and transcriptional response in breast tumour cells. *Oncogene.* 1997;14:1891-1899.
124. Moskaluk CA, Hruban RH, Schutte M, et al. Genomic sequencing of DPC4 in the analysis of familial pancreatic carcinoma. *Diagn Mol Pathol.* 1997;6:85-90.
125. Hahn SA, Schutte M, Hoque AT, et al. DPC4, a candidate tumor suppressor gene at human chromosome 18q21.1. *Science.* 1996;271:350-353.
126. Schutte M, Hruban RH, Hedrick L, et al. DPC4 gene in various tumor types. *Cancer Res.* 1996;56:2527-2530.
127. Hoque AT, Hahn SA, Schutte M, et al. DPC4 gene mutation in colitis associated neoplasia. *Gut.* 1997;40:120-122.
128. Hahn SA, Bartsch D, Schroers A, et al. Mutations of the DPC4/Smad4 gene in biliary tract carcinoma. *Cancer Res.* 1998;58:1124-1126.
129. Takagi Y, Kohmura H, Futamura M, et al. Somatic alterations of the DPC4 gene in human colorectal cancers in vivo. *Gastroenterology.* 1996;111:1369-1372.
130. Wilentz RE, Su GH, Dai JL, et al. Immunohistochemical labeling for dpc4 mirrors genetic status in pancreatic adenocarcinomas: A new marker of DPC4 inactivation. *Am J Pathol.* 2000;156:37-43.

131. Torlakovic E, Torlakovic G, Nguyen PL, et al. The value of anti-pax-5 immunostaining in routinely fixed and paraffin-embedded sections: A novel pan pre-B and B-cell marker. *Am J Surg Pathol.* 2002;26:1343-1350.
132. Kong CS, Balzer BL, Troxell ML, et al. p16INK4A immunohistochemistry is superior to HPV in situ hybridization for the detection of high-risk HPV in atypical squamous metaplasia. *Am J Surg Pathol.* 2007;31:33-43.
133. Birner P, Bachtiary B, Dreier B, et al. Signal-amplified colorimetric in situ hybridization for assessment of human papillomavirus infection in cervical lesions. *Mod Pathol.* 2001;14:702-709.
134. Guo M, Hu L, Baliga M, et al. The predictive value of p16(INK4a) and hybrid capture 2 human papillomavirus testing for high-grade cervical intraepithelial neoplasia. *Am J Clin Pathol.* 2004;122:894-901.
135. Koss LG, Deitch D, Ramanathan R, et al. Diagnostic value of cytology of voided urine. *Acta Cytol.* 1985;29:810-816.
136. Bastacky S, Ibrahim S, Wilczynski SP, et al. The accuracy of urinary cytology in daily practice. *Cancer.* 1999;87:118-128.
137. Ross JS, Cohen MB. Ancillary methods for the detection of recurrent urothelial neoplasia. *Cancer.* 2000;90:75-86.
138. Konety BR, Getzenberg RH. Urine based markers of urological malignancy. *J Urol.* 2001;165:600-611.
139. Saad A, Hanbury DC, McNicholas TA, et al. The early detection and diagnosis of bladder cancer: A critical review of the options. *Eur Urol.* 2001;39:619-633.
140. van der Poel HG, Debruyne FM. Can biological markers replace cystoscopy? An update. *Curr Opin Urol.* 2001;11:503-509.
141. Jiang F, Katz RL. Use of interphase fluorescence in situ hybridization as a powerful diagnostic tool in cytology. *Diagn Mol Pathol.* 2002;11:47-57.
142. Halling KC, King W, Sokolova IA, et al. A comparison of cytology and fluorescence in situ hybridization for the detection of urothelial carcinoma. *J Urol.* 2000;164:1768-1775.
143. Placer J, Espinet B, Salido M, et al. Clinical utility of a multiprobe FISH assay in voided urine specimens for the detection of bladder cancer and its recurrences, compared with urinary cytology. *Eur Urol.* 2002;42:547-552.
144. Bubendorf L, Grilli B. UroVysion multiprobe FISH in urinary cytology. *Methods Mol Med.* 2004;97:117-131.
145. Willmore-Payne C, Layfield LJ, Holden JA. c-KIT mutation analysis for diagnosis of gastrointestinal stromal tumors in fine needle aspiration specimens. *Cancer.* 2005;105:165-170.
146. Vocaturo A, Novelli F, Benevolo M, et al. Chromogenic in situ hybridization to detect HER 2/neu gene amplification in histological and ThinPrep-processed breast cancer fine-needle aspirates: A sensitive and practical method in the trastuzumab era. *Oncologist.* 2006;11:878-886.
147. Bozzetti C, Nizzoli R, Guazzi A, et al. HER 2/neu amplification detected by fluorescence in situ hybridization in fine needle aspirates from primary breast cancer. *Ann Oncol.* 2002;13:1398-1403.

INDEX

A

AAM. *See* Aggressive angiomyxoma (AAM)
ABC. *See* Avidin-biotin conjugate (ABC)
Ablative therapy, for renal tumors, 593
Absence, of staining, 28–29
Acanthamoeba, 69
ACC. *See* Acinar cell carcinoma (ACC); Adenoid cystic carcinoma (ACC)
Acid-fast bacilli (AFB) staining, 66
Acidic keratins, 210
Acidophils, 295
Acinar cell carcinoma (ACC), 553–554
Acinar markers, in pancreatic tumors, 542–543
Acquired immunodeficiency syndrome (AIDS), nervous system lesions in, 828–829
Acromegaly, 322
ACT. *See* Alpha-1 antichymotrypsin (ACT)
Actin(s)
 desmin and, 86
 in gastrointestinal stromal tumor, 525
 in gynecologic pathology, 692t
 in mediastinal tumors, 342t, 345f
 in mesothelioma, 423t
 as myogenic marker, 91
 in rhabdomyosarcoma, 669f
 in skin tumors, 480f
Actinic keratosis, 199
Activator protein-2G, in testicular tumors, 644
AD. *See* Alzheimer disease (AD)
Adamantinoma, 123
Adamantinomatous craniopharyngioma, 873f
Ad4BP, in adrenocortical tumors, 314
Adenocarcinoma
 ampullary, 563–564
 anal gland, 518
 bladder, 375t
 bronchioalveolar, 376t
 clear-cell, 516
 colorectal, 376t, 514–516, 517f, 528, 529, 530, 611
 ductal, 544–547
 endocervical, 375t, 696, 700f, 701f
 endometrial, 221t, 375t, 376t
 endometrioid, 704–705
 esophageal, 502
 gastric, 375t, 505–509, 529
 intestinal-type, 269, 563
 invasive, 560–561
 invasive endocervical, 696
 markers, 899
 minimal deviation endocervical, 697–698
 müllerian endometrioid, 517
 pancreatic, 375t
 pancreatic ductal, 544f
Adenocarcinoma *(Continued)*
 peritoneal, 376t
 polymorphous low-grade, 274t, 275–276
 prostate, 375t, 517, 609f
 prostatic metastatic, 283
 signet ring cell, 516
 small intestinal, 511, 512f
 thyroid, 376t
 tubulodesmoplastic pseudo-mesotheliomatous, 441–442
 urinary bladder, 625
Adenohypophysis, 295–297
Adenoid basal carcinoma, 698
Adenoid cystic carcinoma (ACC), 274t, 276, 504, 698
Adenomatoid tumor of fallopian tube, 744
Adenomatoid tumors, 448
Adenosis
 of prostate, 600
 sclerosing, of prostate, 601, 603f
Adenosquamous carcinoma, 548, 561
Adenoviruses, 61–62
Adrenal cortex tumors, 314–316
Adrenal cortical carcinoma, 315f
Adrenal medulla tumors, 317–319
Adrenal neuroblastoma, 318–319
Adrenocortical carcinoma, 375t
Adrenocortical tumors, 236
ADS. *See* Air-dried smears (ADS)
Adult T-cell lymphoma, 179
AE1-3, in epithelial myoepithelial carcinoma, 277f
AE13, in pilar tumors, 470
AEC. *See* Amino-ethyl carbazole (AEC)
Afibrinogenemia, 567
AFP. *See* Alpha-fetoprotein (AFP)
AFX. *See* Atypical fibroxanthoma (AFX)
Aggressive angiomyxoma (AAM), 102
Aggressive meningiomas, 863–866
Aggressive NK-cell leukemia, 179
AIDS. *See* Acquired immunodeficiency syndrome (AIDS)
Air-dried smears (ADS), 890
Albumin, in hepatocellular carcinoma, 570
ALCL. *See* Anaplastic large cell lymphoma (ALCL)
Alfred score, 802f
ALK. *See* Anaplastic lymphoma kinase (ALK)
ALK, in non-Hodgkin lymphoma, 163
Alkaline phosphatase, 4, 5, 23t
Alkaline phosphatase-antialkaline phosphatase (APAAP), 8–9
Allele-specific hybridization, 49
Allele-specific PCR, 49
Alpha$_1$-antichymotrypsin (ACT), 594
Alpha$_1$-antitrypsin deficiency, 567
Alpha B-crystallin, 837, 838f
Alpha-fetoprotein (AFP)
 in cancer of unknown primary site, 237
 in gynecologic pathology, 691t
 in hepatocellular carcinoma, 570
 in mediastinal tumors, 342t
 in ovarian tumors, 723
 in testicular tumors, 644
Alpha-isoform actin, in mediastinal tumors, 342t
Alpha$_2$ macroglobulin, 594
Alpha-methylacyl-CoA racemase (AMACR)
 in cancer of unknown primary site, 234
 in lung tumors, 411–412
 in prostate tumors, 595, 597f
Alpha$_1$ protein inhibitor, 594
Alveolar rhabdomyosarcoma, 104f, 668
Alveolar soft part sarcoma (ASPS), 96, 112f, 115, 213t
Alzheimer disease (AD), 824t, 877, 878t
AMACR. *See* Alpha-methylacyl-CoA racemase (AMACR)
AMF. *See* Angiomyofibroblastoma (AMF)
Amino-ethyl carbazole (AEC), 11, 23
AML. *See* Angiomyolipoma (AML)
Amplification, 9
 chromosomal, 44
 detection phase, 31–34, 35t
 methods, 30–35
 polylabeling, 35t
 polymeric, 35t
 post-detection, 34
 pre-detection, 30–31, 35t
 stepwise, 35t
Ampullary adenocarcinomas, 563–564
Ampullary endocrine neoplasms, 564–565
Anal gland adenocarcinoma, 518
Anal Paget disease, 519
Anal squamous cell carcinoma, 517–518
Anaplastic astrocytoma, 834t, 840
Anaplastic ependymoma, 845
Anaplastic ganglioglioma, 852–854
Anaplastic large cell lymphoma (ALCL), 146, 181
Anaplastic lymphoma, 404t
Anaplastic lymphoma kinase (ALK), 96, 621
Anaplastic meningioma, 862t, 865
Anaplastic oligoastrocytoma, 836t, 849
Anaplastic oligodendroglioma, 835t, 847, 848f
Anaplastic thyroid carcinoma, 302f, 303t
Anaplastic Wilms' tumor, 682f
Androgen receptor protein (ARP)
 in head and neck neoplasms, 257t
 in sebaceous tumors, 468–469
Angioimmunoblastic T-cell lymphoma, 180

Page numbers followed by f indicate figures; t, tables.

Angiomatous meningioma, 862
Angiomyofibroblastoma (AMF), 99–100
Angiomyolipoma (AML), 639–640
Angiosarcoma, 108f, 386–387
Anthrax, 71
Anti-adenocarcinoma antibodies, 721–722
Anti-alpha isoform actin, 87t, 91
Antiandrogen therapy, 602–604
Antibody(ies). *See also* Reagents
  anti-adenocarcinoma, 721–722
  antigens and, 3
  biology of, 83–96
  to caldesmon, 92
  in cholangiocarcinoma, 574t
  in colorectal adenocarcinoma, 515t
  commonly available, 60t
  to desmin, 86
  in direct conjugate-labeled antibody method, 5–6
  in endocrine tumors, 291–295
  to epithelial membrane antigen, 90
  evaluation of, 3
  in gastric adenocarcinoma, 507t
  in gastrointestinal tumors, 500–501
  in gynecologic pathology, 691t
  in head and neck neoplasms, 256, 257t
  in Hodgkin lymphoma, 144–146
  incubation of, 22–23
  keratin, 216t
  lack of specific, 206
  in lung neoplasms, 370–374, 370t
  in malignant melanoma, 189–196
  in mediastinal tumors, 340, 342t–343t
  melanocyte-specific, 193–196
  in mesotheliomas, 416–417, 423t–425t
  in neuroendocrine lung neoplasms, 378–384, 382t
  in non-Hodgkin lymphoma, 157–168
  in pancreatic tumors, 541–544
  in pediatric neoplasms, 662–663
  polyclonal, 3
  in post-fixation technique, 891t
  in prostate tumors, 593–596
  in renal tumors, 632–635
  as specific staining reagents, 2–4
  in testicular tumors, 643–645
  titration of, 11–13, 14t
  troubleshooting variables in, 28t
  tyrosine-related, 195
  units of, 3
  in urinary bladder tumors, 619–621
  validation of, 16–17
Anti-CD31, 88t. *See also* CD31
Anti-CD68, 88t. *See also* CD68
Antidesmin, 87t. *See also* Desmin
Anti-EBV therapy, 151
Anti-epithelial membrane antigen, 87t. *See also* Epithelial membrane antigen (EMA)
Anti-factor VII-related antigen, 88t. *See also* Factor VIII-related antigen
Antigen biology, 83–96
Antigenic determinant, 3
Antigen retrieval (AR), 19–21, 892
  automation in, 27
  in bacterial infection, 59–60
  chromogens and, 23–24
  counterstaining and, 24
  heating conditions, 19–20
  incubation in, 22–23
  microwave heating method for, 22–24
  mounting and, 24
  pH and, 20, 21f
  substrate and, 23–24
  washing in, 22
Antigens, 3
  in endocrine tumors, 291–295
  in gastrointestinal tumors, 500–501
  in head and neck neoplasms, 256
  in Hodgkin lymphoma, 137–144
  keratin, 216t
  in lung neoplasms, 370–374
  in malignant melanoma, 189–196
  in mediastinal tumors, 340
  in non-Hodgkin lymphoma, 157–168
  in pancreatic tumors, 541–544
  in pediatric neoplasms, 662–663
  in prostate tumors, 593–596
  in renal tumors, 632–635
  in testicular tumors, 643–645
  in urinary bladder tumors, 619–621
Antilaminin, 87t
Anti-large cell lymphoma, in mediastinal tumors, 342t
Antimelanoma, in mediastinal tumors, 342t
Anti-muscle-specific actin, 87t, 91. *See also* Muscle-specific actin (MSA)
Antimyogenin, 87t. *See also* Myogenin (MYG)
Antimyoglobin, 87t. *See also* Myoglobin
Antiosteocalcin, 88t. *See also* Osteocalcin (OCN)
Antiosteonectin, 88t. *See also* Osteonectin (ONN)
Antisynaptophysin, 88t. *See also* Synaptophysin
Anti-*Ulex europaeus* I, 88t. *See also Ulex europaeus* I (UEAI)
Antivimentin, 87t. *See also* Vimentin
Anus, 517–519
APAAP. *See* Alkaline phosphatase-antialkaline phosphatase (APAAP)
Appendix, 511–512, 513f, 521–522
AR. *See* Antigen retrieval (AR)
Arbovirus infections, 827–828
ARP. *See* Androgen receptor protein (ARP)
Artifactual staining, 30, 31f
Aspergillosis, invasive, 68
Aspergillus fumigatus, 827
ASPS. *See* Alveolar soft part sarcoma (ASPS)
Astroblastoma, 834t, 840–841
Astrocytomas, 833–841, 834t
Atrophic gastritis, autoimmune type, 505, 506f
Atypical fibroxanthoma (AFX), 480–483
Atypical meningioma, 864
Atypical teratoid-rhabdoid tumor, 837t, 860
Autocrine growth factors, 677
Autoimmune gastritis, 519
Automated sequence analyzer, 49
Automation, 26–27
Avidin-biotin conjugate (ABC), 1, 7, 12f

B

B72.3, in mesothelioma, 430
Bacillus anthracis, 71
Background staining, 4–5, 29–30
Bacterial infections, 64–67
Balamuthia mandrillaris, 69
BALT. *See* Bronchial-associated lymphoid tissue (BALT)
Barrett esophagus (BE), 501–502, 529, 530
Bartonella infections, 65–66
Basal cell carcinoma (BCC), 464–466
Basal cells, 84t
"Basal-like" carcinoma, 781, 782f
Basaloid carcinoma, 397
Basaloid squamous cell carcinoma (BSCC), 258–260, 346, 504
Base pairs, 42
Basic helix-loop helix (BHLH) motif, 92
Basic-neutral keratins, 210
Basophils, 295
BCC. *See* Basal cell carcinoma (BCC)
B-cell chronic lymphocytic leukemia, 169–170
B-cell lymphoma, deep lymphoid infiltrates simulating, 476–477
B-cell lymphoma-1 proteins (BCL-1), in non-Hodgkin lymphoma, 163
B-cell lymphoma-2 proteins (BCL-2), 96
  in follicular lymphoma, 174
  in head and neck neoplasms, 257t
  in mesothelioma, 425t
  in non-Hodgkin lymphoma, 163–164
  in skin lesions, 477
  in thyroid tumors, 308
B-cell lymphoma-6 proteins (BCL-6), 138, 145t, 164
B-cell neoplasms, 169–178
  mature, 169–178
  precursor, 169
B-cell prolymphocytic leukemia, 171
B cells, in non-Hodgkin lymphoma, 157–161
B-cell specific activator protein (BSAP), 142
B-cell transcription factors, 160
BCH. *See* Benign cephalic histiocytosis (BCH)
BCL-2. *See* B-cell lymphoma-2 proteins (BCL-2)
BCL-6, 138, 145t, 164
Benign cephalic histiocytosis (BCH), 478
Benign mimics of prostate adenocarcinoma, 599–602
Benign peripheral nerve sheath tumors, 344
Benign soft-tissue tumors, 97–100
Ber-EP4, 900
  in basal cell carcinoma, 466
  in cancer of unknown primary site, 225
  in mesothelioma, 430
Beta-catenin, 97
  in desmoid tumors, 443
  in gastrointestinal tumors, 500
  in goblet cell carcinoids, 522
  in head and neck neoplasms, 257t
  in pancreatic tumors, 544
  in pleural tumors, 443
  in solid-pseudopapillary neoplasms, 556
  in uterine tumors, 702
BG8, 900
  in cancer of unknown primary site, 225
  in mesothelioma, 431
BHLH. *See* Basic helix-loop helix (BHLH) motif
Bile duct adenoma, 573
Bile duct hamartoma, 573
Bile duct lesions, 573–575
Bile ducts, 565
Biliary cystadenocarcinoma, 575
Biliary cystadenoma, 575
Biologic Stain Commission (BSC), 17
Biology, molecular, 42
Biopsy
  of breast tumors, 796
  of nervous system lesions, 824t
  of renal tumors, 593
  transurethral resection, 619
Biotin, endogenous, 31f
Biotin-avidin detection, 7
Biotin-streptavidin (B-SA), 1, 7–8
Biphasic mesothelioma, 426t
BK virus, 63, 74f
Bladder adenocarcinoma, 375t
Bladder small-cell carcinoma, 376t
Blastomyces dermatitidis, 68

Blocking
of background staining, 4–5
of enzyme activity, 4–5
of non-specific binding, 22
of peroxidase, 4–5
troubleshooting variables in, 28t
BOB.1
in Hodgkin lymphoma, 142
in non-Hodgkin lymphoma, 161
Borderline soft-tissue tumors, 100–102
Borrelia burgdorferi, 827
Botryoid rhabdomyosarcoma, 667–668
BRAF, in thyroid tumors, 309
Brain, metastases to, 207
Brain lymphoma, 869–870
Breast carcinoma, 375t
lymphatic space invasion in, D2-40 detection of, 787
Breast cytology, 902
Breast lymph node assay, 790
Breast tumors
in "basal-like" carcinoma, 781, 782f
biopsy of, 796
cell adhesion in, 773–777
chromogenic *in situ* hybridization in, 799
in ductal carcinoma *in situ*, 764–766
ductal *vs.* lobular carcinoma in, 773–777
E-cadherin in, 774–777, 902
endocrine, 328–329
epidermal growth factor receptor in, 808
ERBB2, 803–804
fibroepithelial, 791–796
fluorescence *in situ* hybridization in, 798–799
FOXA1 in, 809
genomic applications in, 802–806
gross cystic disease fluid protein-15 in, 791
Her2/neu in, 797–799
hormone receptors in, 800–802
in invasive micropapillary carcinoma, 780–785
Ki-67 in, 808
lobular carcinoma variants in, 777–780
luminal A, 803–804
luminal B, 803–804
lymphatic invasion in, 787–790
mammaglobin in, 791, 792f, 902
mesenchymal, 783–784
in metaplastic carcinoma, 781–783
metastasis of, 790–791
molecular classification of, 802–806
myoepithelial cells in, 763–771
in myofibroblastoma, 784
in Paget disease, 785–786
papillary, 770–771
periductal stromal, 796
phyllodes, 792–794
p53 in, 807
p63 in, 764–765
in pleomorphic lobular carcinoma, 777–780
proliferative ductal epithelial, 771–773
in pseudo-Paget disease, 786
recurrence score model for, 806
sentinel lymph node examination in, 787–790
seventy gene profile for, 805
smooth muscle myosin heavy chain in, 763–765
spindle-cell, 783–784
stromal invasion in, 763–771
theranostic applications in, 796–802
in tubulolobular carcinoma, 778–780
two gene ratio model for, 806–807
type identification, 773–785
wound-response model in, 805
Brenner tumors, 729–730
Broad ligament of ovary tumors, 743–744
Bronchial-associated lymphoid tissue (BALT), 387–388
Bronchioalveolar adenocarcinoma, 376t
Bronchioalveolar cell carcinoma, 401f
"Brown revolution," 1
B-SA. *See* Biotin-streptavidin (B-SA)
BSAP. *See* B-cell specific activator protein (BSAP)
BSC. *See* Biologic Stain Commission (BSC)
BSCC. *See* Basaloid squamous cell carcinoma (BSCC)
Burkitt lymphoma, 177–178

C

CA72.4, in sudoriferous tumors, 467
CA125
in gynecologic pathology, 691t
in ovarian tumors, 722, 725f
CA-125, in mesothelioma, 433
Cadherins, 91
in mesothelioma, 423t, 424t, 429, 431
in pancreatic tumors, 543–544
in renal tumors, 633–634
in thyroid tumors, 304
CAIX. *See* Carbonic anhydrase IX (CAIX)
Calbindin, in gastrointestinal endocrine tumors, 320–321
Calcifying fibrous pseudotumor of pleura, 442
Calcitonin
in gastrointestinal endocrine tumors, 320t
in thyroid tumors, 306
Calcitonin gene-related peptide (CGRP), 306
Calcium-binding proteins, in malignant melanoma, 192–193
Caldesmon, 92, 429
in gynecologic pathology, 691t
in uterine tumors, 702–704
Calponin
in head and neck neoplasms, 257t
in spindle-cell sarcomas, 109
Calretinin, 898
in adrenal cortex tumors, 315–316
in cancer of unknown primary site, 227–228
in granulosa cell ovarian tumors, 732
in gynecologic pathology, 691t
in head and neck neoplasms, 257t
in lung neoplasms, 372t
in malignant melanoma, 193
in mesothelioma, 423t, 427
in ovarian fibroma, 732
in ovarian tumors, 722
in pleural tumors, 416f
in Sertoli-Leydig ovarian tumors, 734
in Sertoli ovarian tumors, 734–735
CAM5.2
in gastrointestinal endocrine tumors, 319
in head and neck neoplasms, 257t, 261f
in malignant rhabdoid tumor, 678f
in pancreatic tumors, 541
Campanacci disease, 123
Cancer of unknown primary site (CUPS). *See also* Metastatic disease
alpha-fetoprotein in, 237
alpha-methylacyl-CoA racemase in, 234
BER-EP4 in, 225
BG8 in, 225
biopsy in, 208–209
bone in, 207
brain in, 207
Cancer of unknown primary site (CUPS) *(Continued)*
carcinoembryonic antigen in, 222–223
carcinomas in, 206, 907–910
CD5 in, 237
CD10 in, 235–236
CDX2 in, 231–232, 233f
cell-specific products in, 225–237
chromogranins in, 226
CK1 in, 216t
CK5 in, 216t, 218–219
CK6 in, 218–219
CK7 in, 212–214, 217t
CK8 in, 216t
CK10 in, 216t
CK11 in, 216t
CK13 in, 216t
CK14 in, 216t
CK16 in, 216t
CK18 in, 216t
CK19 in, 212, 216t
CK20 in, 214–217, 216t, 217t, 218t
clinical aspects of, 206–208
C-met in, 910
combined antibody approach in, 237
cytokeratins in, 210–221
diagnostic approach in, 208–209
DPC4 in, 232
economic considerations in, 206–208
epithelial keratins in, 211–217
epithelial line in, 210
epithelial membrane antigen in, 223–225
estrogen receptor/progesterone receptor in, 229–230
germ-cell tumor markers in, 236–237
gross cystic disease fluid protein in, 228–229
hepatocyte paraffin 1 in, 232
inhibin in, 236
Ki-67 in, 910
leu 7 in, 226
liver in, 207
lungs in, 207
lymphoid line in, 209
melan A in, 236
melanocytic line in, 209
melanoma in, 909–910
mesenchymal line in, 210
MOC-31 in, 225
molecular assays in, 243t
multigene expression assays in, 243t
neuroendocrine antibodies in, 226–227
neuron-specific enolase in, 226
Paget disease and, 241–242
pankeratin in, 216t
PAX2 in, 236
PAX5 in, 910
peptide hormones in, 226
peritoneal carcinomatosis and, 241
poorly differentiated, algorithm in, 239f–240f
presentation in, 207
prostatic acid phosphatase in, 233–234
PSA in, 233–234
PSMA in, 234
renal cell carcinoma antigen in, 235
sarcomas presenting as, 213t
screening IHC in, 209–210
special clinical presentations in, 237–242
stepwise approach in, 209–237
supplemental epithelial markers in, 222–225
synaptophysin in, 226
thrombomodulin in, 234–235
thyroglobulin in, 227

Cancer of unknown primary site (CUPS) *(Continued)*
thyroid transcription factor-1 in, 227, 228f
uroplakin III in, 234–235
villin in, 230–231, 233f
vimentin-coexpressing carcinomas in, 221, 222f
Wilms' tumor protein 1 in, 227–228
Candida albicans, 67
Candida infection, 67
"Candle guttering," 840
Capillary hemangioblastoma, 872
Carbonic anhydrase IX (CAIX), in renal tumors, 634–635
Carcinoembryonic antigen (CEA)
in ampullary adenocarcinoma, 563
in cancer of unknown primary site, 222–223
in ductal adenocarcinoma, 545
in endometrioid adenocarcinoma, 704
in gastrointestinal endocrine tumors, 320
in goblet cell carcinoids, 522
in gynecologic pathology, 691t
in head and neck neoplasms, 257t
in hepatocellular carcinoma, 569
in lung neoplasms, 371t, 383f
in malignant melanoma, 191
in mediastinal tumors, 342t
in meningiomas, 863f
in mesothelioma, 424t, 429–430
in pulmonary endocrine tumors, 324
in squamoid corpuscles, 554–555
in squamous cell carcinoma, 465
in thyroid tumors, 304, 308
Carcinoid tumor, mediastinal, 354
Carcinoma
acinar cell, 553–554
adenoid basal, 698
adenoid cystic, 274t, 276, 504, 698
adenosquamous, 548, 561
adrenocortical, 315f, 375t
anal squamous cell, 517–518
anaplastic thyroid, 302f, 303t
basal cell, 464–466
"basal-like," 781, 782f
basaloid, 397
basaloid squamous cell, 258–260, 346, 504
bladder small-cell, 376t
breast, 375t
bronchioalveolar cell, 401f
cervical small-cell, 376t, 703f
choroid plexus, 835t, 856
chromophobe renal cell, 638
clear-cell, 277–278, 706–707
clear-cell hepatocellular, 572
clear-cell ovarian, 728–729
clear-cell renal cell, 636–637
collecting duct, 638, 640f
colloid, 548, 561
desmoplastic, 836t
ductal *in situ*, 764–766
eccrine, 467
embryonal, 738
encapsulated papillary, 771, 772f
endometrial, 704–710
endometrial intraepithelial, 707f
endometrial serous, 705–706
epithelial-myoepithelial, 276–277
Epstein-Barr virus-associated gastric, 529–530
esophageal, 504
esophageal small-cell, 376t
esophageal squamous cell, 502–503

Carcinoma *(Continued)*
fibrolamellar hepatocellular, 572
follicular, 303t, 310
gastrointestinal small-cell, 376t
giant-cell, of lung, 404t
grade III neuroendocrine, small-cell type, 345–346
hepatocellular, 375t, 569–573
hepatoid, 561
high-grade neuroendocrine, 523
histiocytoid breast, 780
intraductal tubular, 552
invasive micropapillary, 780–785
invasive papillary, 563–564
large-cell neuroendocrine
of lung, 404t
of prostate, 606–607
lobular
ductal *vs.,* 773–777
pleomorphic, 777–780
variants, 777–780
lymphoepithelial, 270–271, 270f
lymphoepithelioma-like, 359, 402–403, 404t, 509, 510f
mediastinal small-cell neuroendocrine, 345–346
medullary
hepatocellular, 572
pancreatic, 548
thyroid, 306, 310
medullary thyroid, 306, 310
Merkel cell, 327–328, 375t
metaplastic, 781–783
mixed acinar-endocrine, 557
mucinous tubular and spindle-cell, 638–639
mucoepidermoid, 275
nasopharyngeal, 270–271
neuroendocrine, 266–267, 699, 708–709
neuroendocrine, small-cell, 265t, 266–267, 272–273
neuroendocrine small-cell, 265t, 266–267, 272–273
ovarian mucinous, 375t
ovarian serous, 375t
papillary renal cell, 637–638
papillary squamous cell, 260
papillary thyroid, 299f, 301f, 303t, 305f, 309
parathyroid, 313f, 353
pleomorphic, 384–385
pleomorphic lobular, 777–780
poorly differentiated neuroendocrine, 523, 559
poorly differentiated thyroid, 303t, 310
primary cutaneous neuroendocrine, 471–472
primary thymic, 350–353
prostate, 376t, 874–875
prostatic duct, 605
prostatic intraepithelial, 598f
pseudomesotheliomatous, of lung, 441–442
renal cell, 221t, 449. *See also* Renal tumors
salivary duct, 278–279
salivary gland, 221t, 273–280
sarcomatoid, 384, 426t, 509
sarcomatoid renal cell, 449
sarcomatoid thymic, 359–360
signet ring cell, 376t
sinonasal undifferentiated, 264, 264t, 265t
small-cell, 837t, 874
small-cell neuroendocrine, 265t, 266–267, 272–273, 345–346

Carcinoma *(Continued)*
spindle-cell, 221t, 260–261, 562
spindle-cell hepatocellular, 572
squamous cell, 257–258, 464–466
sweat gland, 466–468
thymic, 350–353
thyroid follicular, 221t
tubulolobular, 778–780
undifferentiated, 270–271, 303t, 310
undifferentiated ductal, 547
undifferentiated nasopharyngeal, 265t
urinary bladder, small-cell, 625–626
urothelial, 517, 607–611, 621–625. *See also* Urinary bladder tumors
uterine endometrioid, 708f
uterine serous, 708f
vaginal, 376t
verrucous, 260
Carcinoma of unknown primary (CUP), 907–910. *See also* Cancer of unknown primary site (CUPS)
Carcinomatous tumors, 375t
Carcinosarcoma, 711–713
CARD. *See* Catalyzed reporter deposition (CARD)
Cassette, tissue, 893, 895f
Catalyzed reporter deposition (CARD), 11
Cathepsin B
in mediastinal tumors, 343t
in skin tumors, 481
Cat-scratch disease, 66
CCC. *See* Clear-cell chondrosarcoma (CCC)
C cells, thyroid tumors and, 305–309
CCR4, 151
CCS. *See* Clear-cell sarcoma (CCS)
CD2
in Hodgkin lymphoma, 139
in nonhematopoietic neoplasms, 405t
in non-Hodgkin lymphoma, 161
CD3, 145t
in Hodgkin lymphoma, 139
in mediastinal tumors, 342t
in mesothelioma, 425t
in nonhematopoietic neoplasms, 405t
in non-Hodgkin lymphoma, 162
in pancreatic medullary carcinoma, 548
CD4
in Hodgkin lymphoma, 139
in nonhematopoietic neoplasms, 405t
in non-Hodgkin lymphoma, 162
in parathyroid tumors, 311
CD5
in esophageal squamous cell carcinoma, 503
in gastrointestinal stromal tumor, 237
in Hodgkin lymphoma, 139
in mediastinal tumors, 342t, 352, 353f
in nonhematopoietic neoplasms, 405t
in non-Hodgkin lymphoma, 162
CD7
in nonhematopoietic neoplasms, 405t
in non-Hodgkin lymphoma, 162
CD8
in Hodgkin lymphoma, 139
in nonhematopoietic neoplasms, 405t
in non-Hodgkin lymphoma, 162
CD10, 100–101
in cancer of unknown primary site, 235–236
in endometrial carcinoma, 709
in gynecologic pathology, 691t
in hepatocellular carcinoma, 570
in müllerian adenocarcinoma, 713f
in non-Hodgkin lymphoma, 164

CD10 *(Continued)*
in renal tumors, 633
in skin tumors, 475f
in uterine tumors, 704
CD14, in non-Hodgkin lymphoma, 165
CD15, 900–901
in gastrointestinal endocrine tumors, 320
in Hodgkin lymphoma, 137, 144, 145t
in lung neoplasms, 371t
in mediastinal tumors, 342t, 358f
in mesothelioma, 424t
in thyroid tumors, 304
CD19
in non-Hodgkin lymphoma, 157, 165
CD20, 145t, 150
in Hodgkin lymphoma, 137
in mediastinal tumors, 342t, 358f
in mesothelioma, 425t
in non-Hodgkin lymphoma, 157–158
CD21
in mediastinal tumors, 343t
in non-Hodgkin lymphoma, 158
CD22, in non-Hodgkin lymphoma, 158
CD23
in mediastinal tumors, 343t
in non-Hodgkin lymphoma, 158
CD25, in non-Hodgkin lymphoma, 158, 165
CD30, 144–145, 145t, 148–149
in embryonal carcinoma, 738f
in gynecologic pathology, 691t
in Hodgkin lymphoma, 137
in mediastinal tumors, 342t
in mesothelioma, 425t
in non-Hodgkin lymphoma, 165
in skin tumors, 474f
CD31, 94
in head and neck neoplasms, 257t
in lung tumors, 386f
in mediastinal tumors, 342t
in mesothelioma, 425t
in serous cystadenoma, 553f
in skin tumors, 487f
CD33, in non-Hodgkin lymphoma, 165
CD34, 93
in epithelial sarcomas, 112
in gastrointestinal stromal tumor, 525
in head and neck neoplasms, 257t
in hepatocellular carcinoma, 570
in mediastinal tumors, 342t, 344f, 363f
in meningiomas, 863f
in mesothelioma, 425t
in skin tumors, 481, 482f
in solitary fibrous tumor, 614f
in stromal tumors of uncertain malignant potential, 612
CD35, in mediastinal tumors, 343t
CD40, 138, 141f, 145t, 150–151
CD43
in mediastinal tumors, 342t
in non-Hodgkin lymphoma, 165–166
CD44
in choroid plexus tumors, 855, 856
in prostate endocrine tumors, 327
in skin tumors, 490
in Wilms' tumor, 681
CD45, 107, 145, 145t
in Hodgkin lymphoma, 137
in mediastinal tumors, 342t, 349, 358f
in mesothelioma, 424t
in neuroblastoma, 666
in non-Hodgkin lymphoma, 166
in ovarian tumors, 723
CD52, in non-Hodgkin lymphoma, 166
CD56, 92–93
in adrenal medulla tumors, 317
in bile duct tumors, 573
in endocrine tumors, 293–294
in gynecologic pathology, 691t
in mediastinal tumors, 345
in nonhematopoietic neoplasms, 405t
in non-Hodgkin lymphoma, 167
in ovarian fibroma, 732
CD57, 92–93
in endocrine tumors, 293
in Hodgkin lymphoma, 138, 145t
in mediastinal tumors, 342t, 345
in non-Hodgkin lymphoma, 167
in pancreatic tumors, 543
in pulmonary endocrine tumors, 324
CD61, in non-Hodgkin lymphoma, 167
CD68
in mediastinal tumors, 343t
in non-Hodgkin lymphoma, 167
in skin tumors, 486f
CD74, 143, 145t, 342t
CD79, in non-Hodgkin lymphoma, 158–159
CD99, 96, 109, 110
in adrenal neuroblastoma, 318
in desmoplastic small round cell tumor, 675f
in Ewing's sarcoma/primitive neuroectodermal tumor, 672f, 673
in gastrointestinal stromal tumor, 525
in granulosa cell ovarian tumors, 732, 733f
in gynecologic pathology, 691t
in head and neck neoplasms, 257t
in malignant rhabdoid tumor, 678f
in mediastinal tumors, 349f
in neuroblastoma, 666
in non-Hodgkin lymphoma, 167
in pediatric neoplasms, 663
in skin tumors, 473f, 482
CD117. *See also* C-kit
in dysgerminoma, 736
in gastrointestinal stromal tumor, 523–525
in gynecologic pathology, 691t
in lung tumors, 413
in mediastinal tumors, 343t, 352
in neuroendocrine lung neoplasms, 382t
in ovarian tumors, 722–723
targeted therapy and, 911, 914f
in testicular tumors, 643–644
CD138, 138
in nonhematopoietic neoplasms, 405t
in non-Hodgkin lymphoma, 159
CD163, in non-Hodgkin lymphoma, 167
CD1A, in non-Hodgkin lymphoma, 164
CD79a, 142
CDC. *See* Collecting duct carcinoma (CDC)
CD11C, in non-Hodgkin lymphoma, 164–165
CDK4. *See* Cyclin-dependent kinase-4 (CDK4)
CDKN2/p16. *See* Cyclin-dependent kinase-4 inhibitor (CDKN2/p16)
CDNA. *See* Complementary DNA (cDNA)
CD45RO, 145t, 342t
CD44v6, in thyroid tumors, 304–305
CDX2, 902
in ampullary adenocarcinoma, 563
in cancer of unknown primary site, 231–232, 233f
in colorectal adenocarcinoma, 514
in endocervical adenocarcinoma, 701f
in endometrioid ovarian tumors, 726
CDX2 *(Continued)*
in gastric adenocarcinoma, 507–508
in gastric neuroendocrine tumors, 520
in gastrointestinal tumors, 500
in gynecologic pathology, 691t
in head and neck neoplasms, 257t
in lung neoplasms, 371t, 372t
in mesothelioma, 425t
in neuroendocrine carcinomas, 406
in ovarian tumors, 725
CEA. *See* Carcinoembryonic antigen (CEA)
Celiac disease, 511, 528
Cell blocks, 893, 895f, 906
Cell cycle markers, endocrine tumors and, 294–295
Cell-membrane proteins, in melanoma, 190–192
Cellular neurothekeoma, 486f
Central nervous primitive neuroectodermal tumor (cPNET), 859–860
Central neurocytoma (CN), 834t, 845f, 846, 855
Cerebellar hemangioblastoma, 872f
Cerebellar liponeurocytoma, 855
Cerebral papillary glioneuronal tumor, 854
Cerebritis, 822t, 826
Cerebrovascular disease, 830–831
Cervical endocrine tumors, 326
Cervical small-cell carcinoma, 376t, 703f
Cervical squamous intraepithelial lesions, 694–696
Cervical tumors, 694–699
Cetuximab, 530
CGH. *See* Comparative genomic hybridization (CGH)
CGRP. *See* Calcitonin gene-related peptide (CGRP)
"Charge-shape" profile, 3
Checkerboard titration, 14t
Chloroethylcyclohexylnitrosourea. *See* Procarbazine, chloroethylcyclohexylnitrosourea, and vincristine (PCV) chemotherapy
4-Chloro-1-naphthol, 5
Cholangiocarcinoma, 375t, 573–575
Cholangitis
immunoglobulin G4-related, 567
primary sclerosing, 566–567
Chondroblastoma, 121–122
Chondroid tumors, 119–122
Chordoid meningioma, 863
Chordoid sarcoma, 122
Chordoma, 119–120, 214t, 835t, 867–868
Choriocarcinoma, 717, 738–739
Choriocarcinomatous differentiation, 509
Choroid plexus carcinoma, 835t, 856
Choroid plexus epithelial tumors, 855–856
Choroid plexus papilloma, 835t, 855–856
Chromogen
freckles, 31f
overview of, 23–24
in tyramine signal amplification, 11
Chromogenic *in situ* hybridization (CISH), 410, 799, 800t
Chromogranins
in cancer of unknown primary site, 226
in cervical endocrine tumors, 326
in cervical small-cell carcinoma, 703f
endocrine tumors and, 292–293
in extra-adrenal neuroblastoma, 319f
in gastrointestinal tumors, 500–501
in gynecologic pathology, 691t
in head and neck neoplasms, 257t, 259t
in mediastinal tumors, 342t, 356f
in mesothelioma, 425t

Chromogranins *(Continued)*
in neuroendocrine lung neoplasms, 378, 382t, 383f
in ovarian tumors, 730
in pancreatic endocrine tumors, 321
in pancreatic tumors, 543
in pulmonary endocrine tumors, 324
Chromophobe renal cell carcinoma (ChromRCC), 638
Chromophobes, 295
Chromosomal deletion, 44, 52–53
Chromosomal rearrangement, 44, 51–52
Chromosomes, 42
ChromRCC. *See* Chromophobe renal cell carcinoma (ChromRCC)
Chronic lymphocytic leukemia, 169–170, 389, 390t
Chymotrypsin, in acinar cell carcinoma, 553
Cirrhosis, 566–567
CISH. *See* Chromogenic *in situ* hybridization (CISH)
CITED1, in thyroid tumors, 303
CJD. *See* Creutzfeldt-Jakob disease (CJD)
CK1
in gastrointestinal stromal tumor, 216t
in urinary bladder tumors, 621
CK4
in head and neck neoplasms, 257t
CK5, 898
in cancer of unknown primary site, 216t, 218–219
in head and neck neoplasms, 257t
in lung neoplasms, 370–371, 370t, 398
in mesotheliomas, 423t
in prostate tumors, 595
in urinary bladder tumors, 621
CK6, 898
in cancer of unknown primary site, 218–219
in head and neck neoplasms, 257t
in lung neoplasms, 370t, 398
in mesotheliomas, 423t
in prostate tumors, 595
CK7
in cancer of unknown primary site, 212–214, 217t
in clear-cell ovarian carcinoma, 728
in colorectal adenocarcinoma, 514
in ductal adenocarcinoma, 544
in endometrioid ovarian tumors, 726
in epithelial neoplasms, 373t
in extrahepatic biliary tract tumors, 560
in gastric adenocarcinoma, 506, 508f
in gastrointestinal tumors, 500
in goblet cell carcinoids, 522
in gynecologic pathology, 691t
in head and neck neoplasms, 257t
in lung neoplasms, 370, 370t, 381t, 402
in mesotheliomas, 423t
in ovarian tumors, 721, 724, 725
in pancreatic tumors, 541
in sarcomatoid mesotheliomas, 436
in transitional cell ovarian tumors, 729
in urinary bladder tumors, 619–620
in urothelial carcinoma, 608
CK8
in cancer of unknown primary site, 216t
in ductal adenocarcinoma, 544
in head and neck neoplasms, 257t
in pancreatic tumors, 541
CK10
in cancer of unknown primary site, 216t
in head and neck neoplasms, 257t
in urinary bladder tumors, 621
CK11, in gastrointestinal stromal tumor, 216t
CK13
in cancer of unknown primary site, 216t
in head and neck neoplasms, 257t
CK14
in cancer of unknown primary site, 216t
in head and neck neoplasms, 257t
in urinary bladder tumors, 621
CK16, in gastrointestinal stromal tumor, 216t
CK18
in gastrointestinal stromal tumor, 216t
in pancreatic tumors, 541
CK19
in cancer of unknown primary site, 212, 216t
in esophageal squamous cell carcinoma, 503, 504f
in pancreatic endocrine tumors, 323, 558f
in thyroid tumors, 301
CK20
in cancer of unknown primary site, 214–217, 216t, 217t
in colorectal adenocarcinoma, 514
in ductal adenocarcinoma, 544
in epithelial carcinomas, 374t
in extrahepatic biliary tract tumors, 560
in gastric adenocarcinoma, 507, 508f
in gastrointestinal endocrine tumors, 319
in gastrointestinal tumors, 500
in goblet cell carcinoids, 522
in gynecologic pathology, 691t
in lung neoplasms, 370t, 371–372, 381t
in mediastinal tumors, 342t
in mesotheliomas, 423t
in neuroendocrine tumors, 520
in ovarian tumors, 721, 725
in pancreatic tumors, 541
in skin endocrine tumors, 327
in transitional cell ovarian tumors, 729
tumors with expression of, 218t
in urinary bladder tumors, 619–620
in urothelial carcinoma, 608
CK903, in prostate tumors, 597f
C-kit. *See also* CD117
in gastrointestinal tumors, 501
in lung tumors, 414–415
in uterine sarcoma, 719
"Classic" trichoepithelioma (CTE), 469–470
Clear-cell adenocarcinoma, 516
Clear-cell carcinoma, 277–278, 706–707
Clear-cell chondrosarcoma (CCC), 122
Clear-cell ependymoma, 844, 845f
Clear-cell hepatocellular carcinoma, 572
Clear-cell meningioma, 864, 865f
Clear-cell neoplasms, 393
Clear-cell ovarian carcinoma, 728–729
Clear-cell renal cell carcinoma, 636–637
Clear-cell sarcoma (CCS), 112f, 113–114, 113f, 213t
CLIP-170/restin, 142
Clusters of differentiation. *See entries at* CD
C-met, 910
CMV. *See* Cytomegalovirus (CMV)
CN. *See* Central neurocytoma (CN)
Coagulant fixatives, 19
Collagenous fibroma, 98
Collagen type IV, 93
Collapsin response mediator proteins (CRMPs)
endocrine tumors and, 325–326
lung tumors and, 415
Collecting duct carcinoma (CDC), 638, 640f
Collection, of specimens, 890
Colloid carcinoma, 548, 561
Colloid cyst, 875–876
Colonic polyps, 513–514
Colorectal adenocarcinoma, 376t, 514–516, 517f, 528, 529, 530, 611
Colorectal neuroendocrine tumors, 522–523
Common acute lymphocyte leukemia antigen (CALLA), 164, 633. *See also* CD10
Comparative genomic hybridization (CGH), 50
Complementary DNA (cDNA), 46
Complete hydatidiform mole, 716–717
Congenital self-healing reticulohistiocytosis (CSHR), 478
Contamination, 13
Controls, 16t, 17, 820, 881f, 893
Control slides, 17–18
Cornea, 84t
Cornu Ammonis (CA), 879, 880f, 881f. *See also entries at* CA
Cortical dysplasia, 881
Cortical malformations, 881
Corticobasal degeneration, 878
Corticotroph cell adenoma, 296t
Counterstaining, 24
COX-1, in thyroid tumors, 304
COX-2
in gastrointestinal tumors, 501
in thyroid tumors, 304
Coxiella burnetii, 67
Coxsackie virus, 827–828
cPNET. *See* Central nervous primitive neuroectodermal tumor (cPNET)
Craniopharyngioma, 836t, 873
Creutzfeldt-Jakob disease (CJD), 824t, 829f, 830
Crimean-Congo hemorrhagic fever, 73f
CRMPs. *See* Collapsin response mediator proteins (CRMPs)
Cross-linking fixatives, 19
Cryptococcus neoformans, 67, 827
Cryptomorphology, 890
CSHR. *See* Congenital self-healing reticulohistiocytosis (CSHR)
CTCL. *See* Cutaneous T-cell lymphomas (CTCL)
CTE. *See* "Classic" trichoepithelioma (CTE)
CTNNB1 mutations, in thyroid tumors, 310
Cultures, 58
CUPS. *See* Cancer of unknown primary site (CUPS)
Curves, standard, 34–35
Cushing's syndrome, 322
Cutaneous angiosarcoma, 487f
Cutaneous large cell lymphoproliferations, 477
Cutaneous lymphohematopoietic disorders, 472–479
Cutaneous nerve sheath tumors, 483–485
Cutaneous pseudopseudolymphomas, 478–479
Cutaneous T-cell lymphomas (CTCL), 475
Cyclin D1
in desmoid tumors, 443
in non-Hodgkin lymphoma, 163
in parathyroid tumors, 311–312
in pleural tumors, 443
Cyclin-dependent kinase-4 (CDK4), 96
Cyclin-dependent kinase-4 inhibitor (CDKN2/p16), 832
Cystic craniopharyngioma, 876t

Cystic seminoma, cystic thymoma *vs.*, 341
Cystic thymoma, cystic seminoma *vs.*, 341
Cysts, central nervous system, 875–876
Cytogenic abnormalities, in non-Hodgkin lymphoma, 170
Cytokeratins, 84–86. *See also specific cytokeratins at* CK
Cytokines, in Hodgkin lymphoma, 143–144
Cytology, specific organ, 897–907
Cytomegalovirus (CMV), 60–61, 829
Cytomegalovirus (CMV) lymphadenitis, 149
Cytotoxic markers, in Hodgkin lymphoma, 139

D

D2-40
  in gynecologic pathology, 691t
  in lung neoplasms, 372t
  in mesothelioma, 425t
  in testicular tumors, 644
D11, in adrenocortical tumors, 314
DA. *See* Ductal adenocarcinoma (DA)
DAB. *See* Diaminobenzidine (DAB) chromogen
DBA 44, in non-Hodgkin lymphoma, 159
DCC. *See* Dextran-coated charcoal (DCC) method
DCIS. *See* Ductal carcinoma *in situ* (DCIS)
DCLBD. *See* Diffuse cortical Lewy body disease (DCLBD)
DdNTPs. *See* Dideoxynucleoside triphosphates (ddNTPs)
Deep lymphoid infiltrates simulating lymphomas, 476–477
DEH. *See* Ductal epithelial hyperplasia (DEH)
Dehydration, inadequate, 27
Deleted in pancreatic carcinoma, Locus-4 (DPC4)
  in cancer of unknown primary site, 910
  in ductal adenocarcinoma, 546
  in gastrointestinal stromal tumor, 232
Deletion, chromosomal, 44, 52–53
Dementias, 876–878
Demyelination, 824t, 878–879
Dendritic cell tumors, 362–364
Dendritic markers, 141–142
Densely granulated growth hormone cell adenoma, 296t
Densely granulated prolactin cell adenoma, 296t
Deoxynucleotidyl transferase, in mediastinal tumors, 350f
Deoxyribonucleic acid (DNA), 42–43
Dermatofibrosarcoma protuberans (DFSP), 93, 480–483
Dermoid cyst, 876
Desmin, 85, 86–87
  in desmoplastic small round cell tumor, 675f, 676f
  in gastrointestinal stromal tumor, 525
  in gynecologic pathology, 691t
  in head and neck neoplasms, 257t
  in malignant melanoma, 189
  in malignant rhabdoid tumor, 678f
  in mediastinal tumors, 342t, 350f, 362f
  in mesothelioma, 423t
  in rhabdomyosarcoma, 669f
  in skin tumors, 480, 483f
  in uterine tumors, 702–704
  in Wilms' tumor, 681f
Desmoglein, 91, 414
Desmoid-type fibromatosis, 525, 526f, 528
Desmoplakin, 91
Desmoplastic amelanotic melanoma, 190f
Desmoplastic carcinoma, 836t
Desmoplastic fibroblastoma, 98
Desmoplastic infantile ganglioglioma (DIG), 853f, 855
Desmoplastic medulloblastoma, 836t, 858, 859f
Desmoplastic small round cell tumor (DSRCT), 106, 107f, 213t, 396, 664t, 674–677
Desmoplastic trichoepithelioma (DTE), 470
Detection phase amplification, 31–34, 35t
Detection system(s)
  alkaline phosphatase-antialkaline phosphatase, 8–9
  avidin-biotin conjugate, 7, 12f
  biotin-avidin, 7
  biotin-streptavidin, 7–8
  direct conjugate-labeled antibody, 5–6, 14t
  EnVision, 10
  enzyme bridge, 6
  enzyme-labeled antigen, 11, 13f
  indirect, 6
  need for, 5
  peroxidase antiperoxidase, 6–7
  polymer-based labeling, 9–11
  PowerVision, 10
  protein A, 11, 12f
  sandwich, 6
  titration of, 11–13
  troubleshooting variables in, 28t
  tyramine signal amplification, 11, 12f
  unlabeled antibody, 6–7
Dextran-coated charcoal (DCC) method, 800
DFSP. *See* Dermatofibrosarcoma protuberans (DFSP)
DGC. *See* Dysplastic gangliocytoma of cerebellum (DGC)
Diaminobenzidine (DAB) chromogen, 10, 23, 24
Dideoxynucleoside triphosphates (ddNTPs), 49
Diffuse astrocytoma, 839
Diffuse cortical Lewy body disease (DCLBD), 877
Diffuse fibrillary astrocytomas, 832f
Diffuse large B-cell lymphoma, 174–177
DIG. *See* Desmoplastic infantile ganglioglioma (DIG)
Digestion, enzyme, 2
Direct conjugate-labeled antibody detection, 5–6, 14t
DNA. *See* Deoxyribonucleic acid (DNA)
DNA-based tissue identity testing, 54–55
DNA microarrays, 50
DNA sequencing analysis, 49, 51
DNTs. *See* Dysembryoplastic neuroepithelial tumors (DNTs)
Dot-blot analysis, 49
Double immunoenzymatic techniques, 24–25
Double stains, 8–9, 36
DPC4. *See* Deleted in pancreatic carcinoma, Locus-4 (DPC4)
DSRCT. *See* Desmoplastic small round cell tumor (DSRCT)
DTE. *See* Desmoplastic trichoepithelioma (DTE)
Ductal adenocarcinoma (DA), 544–547
Ductal carcinoma *in situ* (DCIS), 764–766
Ductal epithelial hyperplasia (DEH), 772, 773f
Duodenal gangliocytic paraganglioma, 565
Duodenal neuroendocrine tumors, 521
Dysembryoplastic neuroepithelial tumors (DNTs), 846, 854
Dysgerminoma, 736, 737t
Dysplasia markers, 903–906
Dysplastic gangliocytoma of cerebellum (DGC), 853–854
Dystrophin, 105

E

Eastern equine encephalitis virus, 64
EBV-LMP1. *See* Epstein-Barr virus latent membrane protein 1 (EBV-LMP1)
ECAD gene, 774–775
E-cadherin, 91, 902
  in breast tumors, 774–777
  in goblet cell carcinoids, 522
  in mesothelioma, 423t, 424t, 429, 431
  in pancreatic endocrine neoplasms, 558
  in pancreatic tumors, 543–544
  p120 and, 775–777, 902
  in solid-pseudopapillary neoplasms, 556
  in thyroid tumors, 304
Eccrine carcinoma, 467
Echovirus, 827–828
Economic considerations, in gastrointestinal stromal tumor, 206–208
Ectopic meningioma, 281–282
Effusion cytology, 897–898
Effusion lymphoma, 176
EGBs. *See* Eosinophilic granular bodies (EGBs)
EGFR. *See* Epidermal growth factor receptor (EGFR)
EHBT. *See* Extrahepatic biliary tract (EHBT) tumors
EHE. *See* Epithelioid hemangioendothelioma (EHE)
Ehrlichia chaffeensis, 74f
Ehrlichioses, 70
EIC. *See* Endometrial intraepithelial carcinoma (EIC)
EIDs. *See* Emerging infectious diseases (EIDs)
ELST. *See* Endolymphatic sac tumor (ELST)
EMA. *See* Epithelial membrane antigen (EMA)
Embryonal carcinoma, 738
Embryonal rhabdomyosarcoma (E-RMS), 102–105, 562–563, 667–668, 669f
Embryonal sarcoma of liver, 576
Embryonal tumors, 857–860
EMC. *See* Epithelial-myoepithelial carcinoma (EMC)
Emerging infectious diseases (EIDs), 69–70
Encapsulated papillary carcinoma, 771, 772f
Encephalitis, 822t, 827
Encephalopathy, 827
Endocervical adenocarcinoma, 375t, 700f, 701f
Endocervical adenocarcinoma *in situ*, 696
Endocrine markers
  in acinar cell carcinoma, 554
  in pancreatic tumors, 543
Endocrine tumor(s)
  adenohypophysis as, 295–297
  adrenal cortex tumors as, 314–316
  algorithm of, 308f
  antibodies in, 291–295
  antigens in, 291–295
  BRAF in, 309
  breast, 328–329
  C cells and, 305–309

Endocrine tumor(s) *(Continued)*
CD57 and, 293
CD56 in, 293–294
cell cycle markers and, 294–295
cervical, 326
chromogranins and, 292–293
CRMPs in, 325–326
CTNNB1 mutations in, 310
enzymes and, 291–292
galectin-3 in, 302–303
gastrointestinal, 319–321
genetic alterations in, 309t
granule proteins and, 292–293
HBME-1 in, 302, 304
histaminase and, 292
hormones and, 291
intermediate filaments in, 294, 300–301
neuron-specific enolase and, 292
overview of, 291
pancreatic, 321–323
parathyroid tumors as, 310–316
PAX-8 in, 300, 302f, 310
pineal gland tumors as, 297–298
pitfalls of IHC in, 295
prostate, 326–327
pulmonary, 323–326
secretogranins and, 292–293
of skin, 327–328
somatostatin receptors in, 294
specific sites for, 295–329
synaptophysin and, 293
of thymus, 329
thyroglobulin in, 298, 307–308
thyroid transcription factor-1 in, 300
thyroid tumors as, 298–310
transcription factors in, 294
Endogenous biotin, 31f
Endolymphatic sac tumor (ELST), 281
Endometrial adenocarcinoma, 221t, 375t, 376t
Endometrial carcinoma, 704–710
Endometrial intraepithelial carcinoma (EIC), 707f
Endometrial metastases, 707–709
Endometrial serous carcinoma, 705–706
Endometrial stromal nodule, 711
Endometrial stromal sarcoma, 214t, 711, 712f
Endometrioid adenocarcinoma, 704–705
Endometrioid ovarian tumors, 726–728
Endothelial markers, 93–95
End-product amplification, 9
Enhanced polymer one-step staining (EPOS), 9–10
Enterogenous cyst, 876
Enteropathy-type T-cell lymphoma, 179
Enteroviruses, 64, 827–828
Enterovirus 71 (EV71) encephalomyelitis, 69–70
EnVision, 10
Enzymatic markers, in pancreatic tumors, 542–543
Enzyme blocking, 4–5
Enzyme bridge technique, 6
Enzyme digestion, 2
Enzyme-labeled antigen method, 11, 13f
Enzymes, endocrine tumors and, 291–292
Eosinophilic granular bodies (EGBs), 837–839
EpCAM, in renal tumors, 633
EPD. *See* Extramammary Paget disease (EPD)
Ependymal cyst, 875, 876t
Ependymoblastoma, 837t, 860
Ependymoma, 834t, 835t, 842–845
Epidermal growth factor receptor (EGFR)
in anaplastic ependymoma, 845
in breast tumors, 808
in glioblastoma, 850
in head and neck neoplasms, 261–262
mutation detection methods for, 410t
in phyllodes tumors, 794
targeted therapy and, 912
theranostic applications of, 409–410
Epidermal tumors, 464–466
Epidermis, 84t
Epidermoid cyst, 876
Epilepsy, 879–881
Epithelia, 84t
Epithelial antigen
in lung neoplasms, 371t
in mediastinal tumors, 342t
Epithelial membrane antigen (EMA), 90–91, 110
in adrenal cortex tumors, 316
in atypical meningioma, 864
in basal cell carcinoma, 466f
in basaloid squamous cell carcinoma, 259
in benign soft-tissue tumor, 98
in cancer of unknown primary site, 223–225
in carcinomas, 224t
in desmoplastic small round cell tumor, 675f, 676f
in endometrioid ovarian tumors, 726
in granulosa cell ovarian tumors, 732
in gynecologic pathology, 691t
in head and neck neoplasms, 257t
in hepatocellular carcinoma, 570
in Hodgkin lymphoma, 138–139, 145t
in invasive micropapillary carcinoma, 780–785
in lung neoplasms, 370t
in malignant melanoma, 191
in malignant rhabdoid tumor, 678f, 679f
in mastoid meningioma, 282f
in mediastinal tumors, 342t
in meningiomas, 860, 863f
in mesothelioma, 423t, 428
in nonepithelial tissues, 224t
in ovarian tumors, 730
in sebaceous tumors, 468
in Sertoli-Leydig ovarian tumors, 734
in Sertoli ovarian tumors, 734–735
in skin tumors, 486f
in squamous cell carcinoma, 464–465
in uterine tumors, 699–700
Epithelial mesothelioma, pleural metastases *vs.*, 238
Epithelial-myoepithelial carcinoma (EMC), 276–277
Epithelial-myoepithelial neoplasm of lung, 396
Epithelial-related markers, 90–91
Epithelioid angiomyolipomas, 119
Epithelioid angiosarcoma, 85, 111–112, 113f
Epithelioid ependymomas, 843
Epithelioid hemangioendothelioma (EHE), 101–102, 223
Epithelioid hemangioendothelioma mimicking mesothelioma, 442
Epithelioid leiomyosarcoma, 112f, 115
Epithelioid malignant peripheral nerve sheath tumors, 114
Epithelioid mesothelioma of mediastinum, 357
Epithelioid monophasic synovial sarcoma, 111
Epithelioid sarcoma (EPS), 111–115, 213t, 488–489
Epithelioid sarcoma-like hemangioendothelioma (ESLH), 102, 487, 488f
Epithelioid trophoblastic tumor (ETT), 717
Epitope, 3
EPOS. *See* Enhanced polymer one-step staining (EPOS)
EPS. *See* Epithelioid sarcoma (EPS)
Epstein-Barr virus, 62f, 109
in head and neck neoplasms, 141f, 261
Hodgkin lymphoma in, 139–141
Epstein-Barr virus-associated gastric carcinoma, 529–530
Epstein-Barr virus latent membrane protein 1 (EBV-LMP1)
in Hodgkin lymphoma, 137
in non-Hodgkin lymphoma, 167
ERBB2 breast tumors, 803–804
ERCC1. *See* Excision repair cross-complementation group 1 (ERCC1)
Erdheim-Chester disease, 392
ERK. *See* Extracellular signal-regulated kinase (ERK)
E-RMS. *See* Embryonal rhabdomyosarcoma (E-RMS)
ER/PR. *See* Estrogen receptor/progesterone receptor (ER/PR)
ERT (extrarenal rhabdoid tumor), 118
ESLH. *See* Epithelioid sarcoma-like hemangioendothelioma (ESLH)
Esophageal adenocarcinoma, 502
Esophageal carcinoma, 504
Esophageal melanoma, 527f
Esophageal neuroendocrine tumors, 519
Esophageal small-cell carcinoma, 376t
Esophageal squamous cell carcinoma, 502–503
ES/PNET. *See* Ewing's sarcoma/primitive neuroectodermal tumor (ES/PNET)
Estrogen receptor/progesterone receptor (ER/PR), 901
in breast tumors, 796, 800–802
in cancer of unknown primary site, 229–230
in endometrial carcinoma, 719
fixation techniques for, 892–893
in gastric adenocarcinoma, 508–509
in lung neoplasms, 372t
in mesothelioma, 424t
in phyllodes tumor, 792
in skin tumors, 489
in uterine tumors, 701–702
ETT. *See* Epithelioid trophoblastic tumor (ETT)
EV71. *See* Enterovirus 71 (EV71) encephalomyelitis
Ewing's sarcoma/primitive neuroectodermal tumor (ES/PNET), 85, 94, 103f, 105–106. *See also* Primitive neuroectodermal tumor (PNET)
in bone, 671–672
in head and neck, 268
pediatric, 664t, 671–674
reagents and, 88t
EWS gene translocation, 673
EWS-WT1 gene fusion, 676
Exaggerated placental site, 717
Excision repair cross-complementation group 1 (ERCC1), 409
Extended incubation, 23
Extra-adrenal paraganglia tumors, 317–319

Extracellular signal-regulated kinase (ERK), 412
Extrahepatic biliary tract (EHBT) dysplasia, 560
Extrahepatic biliary tract (EHBT) tumors, 559–563
Extramammary Paget disease (EPD), 467
Extranodal marginal zone B-cell lymphoma of mucosa-associated lymphoid tissue type, 172–173
Extranodal NK/T-cell lymphoma, nasal type, 179
Extrarenal rhabdoid tumor (ERT), 118
Extraskeletal myxoid chondrosarcoma, 122, 214t
Extratesticular primary germ-cell tumors, 646–647

F

Factor VIII-related antigen, 93, 425t, 571
Factor XIIIa (FXIIIa), 100, 571
Fallopian tube tumors, 743–744
FALs. *See* Fractional allelic losses (FALs)
False positives, 897
Fascin, 145t
  in Hodgkin lymphoma, 141–142
  in pulmonary tumors, 369, 371t
Fat, in mesotheliomas, 436, 438f
"Faux tissue," 35
Female adnexal tumor of wolffian origin, 744
Female genital tract tumors
  adenoid basal carcinoma in, 698
  adenoid cystic carcinoma in, 698
  cervical, 694–699
  endocervical adenocarcinoma in, 696
  gynecological cytology and, 902–907
  in mesothelioma, 742–746
  neuroendocrine carcinomas in, 699
  ovarian
    alpha-fetoprotein in, 723
    anti-adenocarcinoma antibodies in, 721–722
    Brenner, 729–730
    CA125 in, 722
    calretinin in, 722
    CD45 in, 723
    CD117 in, 722–723
    CDX2 in, 725
    CK7 in, 721, 724, 725, 730
    CK20 in, 721, 725
    CK125 in, 725f
    clear-cell, 728–729
    cytokeratins in, 721
    desmoplastic small round cell, 731f
    in dysgerminoma, 736
    endometrioid, 726–728
    epithelial, 724–730
    epithelial membrane antigen in, 730
    fibroma, 732
    germ-cell, 736–742
    granulosa cell, 732–733
    in hepatocyte nuclear factor-1 beta, 728
    human chorionic gonadotropin in, 723
    inhibin in, 722
    Leydig cell, 735
    metastatic, 740–742
    mucinous, 725–726
    neuroendocrine differentiation in, 723–724
    neuron-specific enolase in, 731f
    Oct-4 in, 723
    placental alkaline phosphatase in, 722
    serous, 724
Female genital tract tumors *(Continued)*
    Sertoli, 734–735
    Sertoli-Leydig, 734
    sex cord, 730–735
    S-100 protein in, 723
    steroid, 735
    synaptophysin in, 730
    thecoma, 732
    transitional cell, 729–730
    Wilms' tumor-1 in, 722, 724
    yolk sac, 737, 738f
  ovarian cytology in, 906–907
  p16 in, 690
  uterine
    beta-catenin in, 702
    caldesmon in, 702–704
    carcinosarcoma in, 711–713
    CD10 in, 704
    CDX2 in, 701f
    clear-cell carcinoma in, 706–707
    cytokeratins in, 699–700
    desmin in, 702–704
    endometrial carcinoma in, 704–710
    endometrial serous carcinoma in, 705–706
    endometrial stromal, 711, 712f, 713f
    epithelial membrane antigen in, 699–700
    gastrointestinal stromal, 715
    genomic applications in, 717–718
    gestational trophoblastic, 715–716
    inflammatory myofibroblastic, 715
    leiomyoma in, 710–711
    leiomyosarcoma in, 710–711
    lymphovascular invasion in, 709
    mesenchymal, 710–715
    mismatch repair proteins in, 717–718, 720
    mixed epithelial carcinomas in, 709
    müllerian adenosarcoma in, 713
    myometrial invasion in, 709
    neuroendocrine carcinomas in, 708–709
    perivascular epithelioid cell, 715
    p53 in, 701–702
    PTEN in, 702, 704–705
    resembling ovarian sex cord tumor, 715
    theranostic applications in, 719
    undifferentiated carcinomas in, 709
    undifferentiated sarcoma in, 713–715
    vimentin in, 700
    Wilms' tumor-1 in, 704
  vagina in, 690–694
  vulva in, 690–694
  vulvar granular, 693
  vulvar intraepithelial, 694
  vulvar Paget disease in, 690–693
  vulvar papillary squamous, 693–694
  vulvovaginal mesenchymal, 693
Fetal heavy-chain myosin, 668
FFPE. *See* Formalin-fixed paraggin embedded (FFPE) tissues
Fibrillar mass, differential diagnosis of, 834t–835t
Fibrinogen storage disease, 567–568
Fibroadenoma, phyllodes tumor *vs.*, 794–795
Fibroblastic lesions, in gastrointestinal tract, 526–527
Fibroblastic meningioma, 834t, 861, 863f
Fibroblastic skin tumors, 479–480
Fibroepithelial breast tumors, 791–796
Fibrogenic mediastinum proliferations, 344–345
Fibrohistiocytic markers, 95
Fibrohistiocytic neoplasms, 480–483
Fibrolamellar hepatocellular carcinoma, 572
Fibromatoses, 97–98, 107
Fibronectin, in ductal adenocarcinoma, 545–546
Fibrosarcoma, 107–108, 835t
Fibrosing pleuritis, 440t
Fibrosis, 826, 834t
Fibrous histiocytoma, predominantly epithelial spindle-cell thymoma *vs.*, 343–344
Fibrous meningioma, 861, 863f
Filaggrin, 465
Filamentous proteins. *See* Intermediate filament proteins (IFPs)
FISH. *See* Fluorescence *in situ* hybridization (FISH)
Fixation techniques, 18–21, 890, 892–893
Fixatives
  alternate, 2
  coagulant, 19
  cross-linking, 19
  mercury-based, 670
  troubleshooting variables in, 28t
FLI-1. *See* Friend leukemia integration-1 (FLI-1)
Florid ductal hyperplasia, 772, 773f
Fluorescence *in situ* hybridization (FISH), 45, 49–50, 53f
  chromogenic *in situ* hybridization *vs.*, 800t
  HER2, 798–799
  in lung tumors, 410
  multiprobe, in urine cytology, 910–911, 913f
  in urinary bladder tumors, 629–630
Fluorescence resonance energy transfer (FRET), 47
Focal nodular hyperplasia (FNH), 567
Follicular adenoma, 303t, 310
Follicular carcinoma, 303t, 310
Follicular cell neoplasms, 298–302
Follicular lymphoma, 174, 390, 390t
Folliculostellate cells, 295
Formalin-fixed paraggin embedded (FFPE) tissues, 1
FOXA1, in breast cancer, 809
Fractional allelic losses (FALs), 794
Francisella tularensis, 71–72
Freckles, chromogen, 31f
FRET. *See* Fluorescence resonance energy transfer (FRET)
Friend leukemia integration-1 (FLI-1), 94
  in Ewing's sarcoma/primitive neuroectodermal tumor, 672f, 673, 673f
  in granular cell tumor, 99
  in head and neck neoplasms, 257t
  in pediatric neoplasms, 663
Frontotemporal dementia, 877–878
Fundic gland polyps, 505
Fungal infections, 67–68
FXIIIa. *See* Factor XIIIa (FXIIIa)

G

GADD45a, in lung tumors, 412–413
Galectin-3, in thyroid tumors, 302–303
Galectin-4, in lung tumors, 412
Gallbladder tumors, 559–563
Gangliocytic paragangliomas, 521
Gangliogliocytoma, 852–854
Ganglioglioma, 852–854
Ganglioma, 852f
Ganglion cell tumors, 834t, 836t

Ganglioneuroblastoma, 665
Ganglioneuromas, 344, 665
Gastric adenocarcinoma, 375t, 505–509, 529
Gastric adenocarcinoma with neuroendocrine differentiation, 509
Gastric cardia, 501–502
Gastric/foveolar papillae, 550
Gastric neuroendocrine tumors, 519–520
Gastric-type mucins, 542
Gastrin
 in gastric neuroendocrine tumors, 520
 in gastrointestinal endocrine tumors, 320t
 in pancreatic endocrine tumors, 322, 322f
Gastritis
 atrophic, autoimmune type, 505, 506f
 autoimmune, 519
Gastritis, lymphocytic, 505
Gastrointestinal endocrine tumors (GI-ETs), 319–321
Gastrointestinal small-cell carcinoma, 376t
Gastrointestinal stromal tumor (GIST), 214t, 523–525, 528, 613, 715
Gastrointestinal tumors
 antibodies in, 500–501
 antigens in, 500–501
 in anus, 517–519
 in appendix, 511–512
 in Barrett esophagus, 501–502
 beta-catenin in, 500
 CD117 in, 523–525
 CDX20 in, 500
 chromogranin A in, 500–501
 CK7 in, 500
 CK20 in, 500
 diagnostic panels in, 510–511, 516–517
 in esophageal adenocarcinoma, 502
 in esophageal carcinoma, 504
 genomic applications in, 528
 mesenchymal, 523–528
 neural, 526
 neuroendocrine, 519–523
 presenting as polypoid lesions, 526–528
 in small intestine, 511
 in stomach, 505–511
 theranostic applications in, 528–529
GATA binding protein, in breast cancer, 3, 809
GCA. *See* Giant-cell astrocytoma (GCA)
GCDFP. *See* Gross cystic disease fluid protein (GCDFP)
GCT. *See* Granular cell tumor (GCT)
GCTs. *See* Germ-cell tumors (GCTs)
Gemistocytic astrocytoma, 834t, 839–840, 846, 882t
GeneSearch Breast Lymph Node Assay, 790
Genetic polymorphism, 44
Genomic applications
 in ampullary adenocarcinoma, 564
 in breast tumors, 802–806
 in ductal adenocarcinoma, 546
 in Ewing's sarcoma/primitive neuroectodermal tumor, 674
 in extrahepatic biliary tract tumors, 561
 in gastrointestinal tumors, 528
 in hepatocellular carcinoma, 571–572
 in malignant rhabdoid tumor, 680
 in neuroblastoma, 666
 in ovarian tumors, 745
 in renal tumors, 640–641
 in rhabdomyosarcoma, 671
 in solid-pseudopapillary neoplasm, 555–556
 in urinary bladder tumors, 627–629
 in uterine tumors, 717–718
Germ-cell tumor markers, in gastrointestinal stromal tumor, 236–237
Germ-cell tumors (GCTs)
 classic seminoma *vs.* nonseminomatous, 646
 extratesticular, 646–647
 mediastinal, 353–354
 metastatic, 646–647
 nervous system, 869
 ovarian, 736–742
 testicular, 642–643
Germinomas, 869
Gestational trophoblastic disease, 715–716, 720–721
GFAP. *See* Glial fibrillary acidic protein (GFAP)
Giant-cell astrocytoma (GCA), 834t, 840, 841f
Giant-cell carcinoma, of lung, 404t
Giant-cell glioblastoma, 850f
Giant-cell tumors, 122–123
GI-ETs. *See* Gastrointestinal endocrine tumors (GI-ETs)
GIST. *See* Gastrointestinal stromal tumor (GIST)
Gitter cells, 835t
Glandular psammomatous carcinoid, 564
Glial cysts, 875
Glial fibrillary acidic protein (GFAP), 83, 85, 90
 in anaplastic astrocytoma, 840
 in anaplastic ependymoma, 845
 in ependymomas, 842, 843f
 in ganglioglioma, 853
 in gemistocytic astrocytoma, 839, 840f
 in glioblastoma, 850f
 in gliomas, 832–833
 in gliosarcoma, 850, 851f
 in gliosis, 824–825
 in head and neck neoplasms, 257t
 in infratentorial ependymomas, 844
 in malignant melanoma, 189
 in microgemistocytes, 846
 in myxopapillary ependymoma, 844
 in oligodendrogliomas, 845f, 846, 847, 848f, 849f
 in pilocytic astrocytomas, 839
 in Rosenthal fibers, 837, 838f
 in tancytic ependymomas, 844
Glioblastoma, 836t, 847f
Glioblastoma multiforme, 834t, 849–851
Glioblastoma with epithelial metaplasia, 850
Gliomas
 astrocytomas in, 833–841
 definition of, 832
 differential diagnosis of anaplastic cells in, 837t
 differential diagnosis of epithelioid mass in, 835t–836t
 differential diagnosis of fibrillar mass in, 834t–835t
 eosinophilic granular bodies in, 837–839
 ependymomas in, 842–845
 glial fibrillary acidic protein in, 832–833
 glioblastoma multiforme in, 849–851
 gliosis *vs.*, 882–883
 oligodendroglioma in, 846–849
 Rosenthal fibers in, 833–837, 838f
 S-100 protein in, 839
 treatment of, 832
 tumor margin in, 832–833
Glioneuronal tumors, 854–855
Gliosarcoma, 834t, 849, 851f
Gliosarcoma with epithelial metaplasia, 836t, 850
Gliosis, 822t, 824–825, 833f, 838f, 847f, 882–883
Glomangiopericytoma, 269
Glucagon, in gastrointestinal endocrine tumors, 320t
Glucose oxidase, 5, 23t
Glucose transporter isoform (GLUT), in mesothelioma, 439–440
Glucose uptake and transporter-1 (GLUT-1), 899
 in mesothelioma, 439–440
 in serous cystadenoma, 552–553
Glutathione-transferase alpha, 635
Glypican-3
 in gynecologic pathology, 691t
 in hepatocellular carcinoma, 570
 in lung tumors, 414
GMS. *See* Gomori's methenamine silver (GMS)
Goblet cell carcinoids, appendiceal, 521–522
Gomori's methenamine silver (GMS), 67
Gonadoblastoma, 740
Gonadotroph cell adenoma, 296t
GP100, in malignant melanoma, 193–195
Grade III neuroendocrine carcinoma, small-cell type, 345–346
Granular cell angiosarcoma, 117–118
Granular cell tumor (GCT), 98–99
 in extrahepatic biliary tract, 562
 gastrointestinal, 525
 of head and neck, 271
 of lung, 396
 of skin, 484
 vulvar, 693f
Granule proteins, endocrine tumors and, 292–293
Granuloma, 834t
Granulomatosis, lymphomatoid, 871
Granulomatous lymphadenitis, 150
Granulosa cell ovarian tumors, 732–733
Granzyme B
 in Hodgkin lymphoma, 139
 in non-Hodgkin lymphoma, 167
Gross cystic disease fluid protein (GCDFP), 902
 alcohol leaching of, 890
 in breast tumors, 791
 in cancer of unknown primary site, 228–229
 in lung neoplasms, 372t
 in mesothelioma, 424t
Guillain-Barré syndrome, 879
Gynecological cytology, 902–907

H

Hairy cell leukemia, 171–172
Hantavirus pulmonary syndrome, 69
HBC. *See* Histiocytoid breast carcinoma (HBC)
HBME-1, 898
 in chondroid tumors, 120
 in mesothelioma, 428
 in thyroid tumors, 302, 304
HBV. *See* Hepatitis B virus (HBV)
HCC. *See* Hepatocellular carcinoma (HCC)
HCG. *See* Human chorionic gonadotropin (hCG)
HCV. *See* Hepatitis C virus (HCV)
Head and neck neoplasms
 adenoid cystic carcinoma in, 274t, 276
 antibodies in, 256, 257t
 antigens in, 256
 basaloid squamous cell carcinoma in, 258–260

Head and neck neoplasms *(Continued)*
clear-cell carcinoma in, 277–278
ear in, 280–282
ectopic meningioma in, 281–282
endolymphatic sac tumor in, 281
epidermal growth factor receptor in, 261–262
epithelial-myoepithelial carcinoma in, 276–277
glomangiopericytoma in, 269
intestinal-type adenocarcinoma in, 269
invasive-ectopic pituitary adenoma, 267
low-grade cribriform cystadenocarcinoma in, 279–280
malignant melanoma in, 264–266
metastatic, 283–284
middle ear adenoma in, 280–281
mucoepidermoid carcinoma in, 275
myoepithelioma in, 273–274
nasal cavity in, 262–270
nasopharyngeal angiofibroma in, 271
nasopharyngeal carcinoma in, 270–271
neuroendocrine carcinoma in, 266–267
neuroendocrine carcinoma spectrum in, 272–273
olfactory neuroblastoma in, 263, 264t
overview of, 256
papillary squamous cell carcinoma in, 260
paragangliomas in, 282–283
paranasal sinuses in, 262–270
p53 in, 262
pleomorphic adenoma in, 273
polymorphous low-grade adenocarcinoma in, 274t, 275–276
respiratory epithelial adenomatoid hamartoma in, 262–263
respiratory papillomatosis in, 272
salivary duct carcinoma in, 278–279
salivary glands in, 273–280
sinonasal undifferentiated carcinoma in, 264t, 265t
small-cell neuroendocrine carcinoma in, 265t, 266–267, 272–273
spindle-cell carcinoma in, 260–261
squamoproliferative lesions in, 256–262
squamous cell carcinoma in, 257–258
temporal bone in, 280–282
theranostic applications in, 261–262, 269–270, 280
undifferentiated nasopharyngeal carcinoma, 265t
verrucous carcinoma in, 260
vocal cord nodule in, 272
Heating, microwave, 19–20
Heating conditions, in antigen retrieval, 19–20
Heliobacter pylori, 64–65, 505
Hemangioblastoma, 836t, 872
Hemangioendothelioma, 385–386, 487
Hemangioma, 99
Hemangiopericytoma (HPC), 100, 837t, 862t, 866, 867f
Hematolymphoid malignancies, 107
Hematopoietic determinants, 96
Hematopoietic mediastinal tumors, 356–357
Hepatic adenoma, 568
Hepatic angiomyolipoma, 576
Hepatic epithelioid hemangioendothelioma, 575–576
Hepatic hemangioma, 575–576
Hepatic parenchyma, 565
Hepatitis B virus (HBV), 59, 566
Hepatitis C virus (HCV), 64, 566
Hepatoblastoma, 568–569
Hepatocellular carcinoma (HCC), 375t, 569–573
Hepatocellular neoplasms, 568–573
Hepatocyte nuclear factor-1 beta (HNF-1 beta), 728, 907
Hepatocyte paraffin, 1
in cancer of unknown primary site, 232
in lung neoplasms, 372t
Hepatocytes, 565
Hepatoid carcinoma, 561
Hepatoid differentiation, 509
Hepatosplenic T-cell lymphoma, 179
Hep Par-1
alcohol leaching of, 890
in hepatocellular carcinoma, 569, 570f
Hereditary nonpolyposis colorectal cancer (HNPCC), 548, 706, 745
HER2/neu
in breast tumors, 797–799
in endometrial carcinoma, 719
in head and neck neoplasms, 257t
in lung neoplasms, 402
in pleomorphic lobular carcinoma, 778
targeted therapy and, 911–912, 914f
Herpes simplex encephalitis, 824t, 827
Herpesviruses, 59–61
Heterozygosity, loss of, 44, 52–53
HHV-8, 60
HIF-1. *See* Hypoxia-induced factor-1 (HIF-1)
High-grade neuroendocrine carcinoma, 523
High mobility group A2 (HMGA2) protein, 117
Hirschsprung disease, 512–513
HISL-19, in adrenal neuroblastoma, 318
Histaminase, endocrine tumors and, 292
Histidine decarboxylase, in neuroendocrine lung neoplasms, 378
Histiocytoid breast carcinoma (HBC), 780
Histiocytosis, 835t, 871
Histiocytosis X, 477–478
Histoids, 35
Histoplasma capsulatum, 67
HIV. *See* Human immunodeficiency virus (HIV)
HKN5, in pilar tumors, 470–471
HL. *See* Hodgkin lymphoma (HL)
HL-PTLD. *See* Hodgkin-like post-transplant lymphoproliferative disorder (HL-PTLD)
HMB45
in gynecologic pathology, 691t
in head and neck neoplasms, 257t
in malignant melanoma, 194
in mucosal melanoma, 266f
HMFGPs. *See* Human milk fat globule proteins (HMFGPs)
HMGA2 protein. *See* High mobility group A2 (HMGA2) protein
HNPCC. *See* Hereditary nonpolyposis colorectal cancer (HNPCC)
Hodgkin-like post-transplant lymphoproliferative disorder (HL-PTLD), 146–147, 149f
Hodgkin lymphoma (HL)
antibodies in, 144–146
antigen biology in, 137–144
B-cell specific activator protein and, 142
CD74 and, 143
cytokines in, 143–144
cytotoxic markers in, 139
differential diagnosis of, 148t
Hodgkin lymphoma (HL) *(Continued)*
epithelial membrane antigen, 138–139, 145t
Epstein-Barr virus and, 139–141, 141f
fascin and, 141–142
germinal center markers in, 138
J-chain and, 143
JunB and, 142, 143f, 145t
mixed-cellularity, 359
Oct-2, 142
overview of, 137
post-germinal center markers in, 138
syncytial mediastinal, 355–356
T-cell markers in, 139
types of, 137
Hodgkin/Reed-Sternberg cells (H/RSCs), 137, 140f, 141f
Homer Wright rosettes, 844f, 854, 858
Hormone receptor fixation, 892–893
Hormones
endocrine tumors and, 291
peptide, in cancer of unknown primary site, 226
thymic, 340
Horseradish peroxidase (HRP), 1, 9
HPC. *See* Hemangiopericytoma (HPC)
HPL. *See* Human placental lactogen (HPL)
HPs. *See* Hyperplastic polyps (HPs)
HPT-JT. *See* Hyperparathyroidism-jaw tumor (HPT-JT)
HPV. *See* Human papillomavirus (HPV)
HRP. *See* Horseradish peroxidase (HRP)
HRPT2, in parathyroid tumors, 313
H/RSCs. *See* Hodgkin/Reed-Sternberg cells (H/RSCs)
Human chorionic gonadotropin (hCG)
in choriocarcinoma, 738–739
in gynecologic pathology, 691t
in ovarian tumors, 723
in testicular tumors, 644
Human epithelial antigen
in lung neoplasms, 371t
in mesothelioma, 424t
Human epithelial-related antigen, in mesothelioma, 424t
Human herpes virus 8 (HHV-8), 60
Human immunodeficiency virus (HIV)
nervous system lesions and, 828–829
smooth muscle tumors and, 109
Human milk fat globule proteins (HMFGPs)
in lung neoplasms, 370t
in mesothelioma, 423t, 428
overview of, 90
Human papillomavirus (HPV), 74f, 903
in cervical endocrine tumors, 326
in head and neck BSCC, 259
in head and neck neoplasms, 261
in head and neck SCC, 258
hybridization assays for, 910
p16 and, 690
in respiratory papillomatosis, 272
Human placental lactogen (HPL)
in gynecologic pathology, 691t
in testicular tumors, 644
Hyalinizing trabecular tumor, 299f
Hyaluronan detection, in mesotheliomas, 433
Hybroma technique, 1
Hydatidiform mole, complete, 716–717
Hydrogen peroxide, 5
Hyperparathyroidism-jaw tumor (HPT-JT), 312
Hyperplastic polyps (HPs), 513
Hypofibrinogenemia, 567
Hypoxia-induced factor-1 (HIF-1), 411

I

IBD. *See* Inflammatory bowel disease (IBD)
Identity testing, 54–55
IELs. *See* Intraepithelial lymphocytes (IELs)
IFPs. *See* Intermediate filament proteins (IFPs)
IGCNU. *See* Intratubular germ-cell neoplasia, unclassified (IGCNU)
IGF-II. *See* Insulin-like growth factor-II (IGF-II)
IgG4. *See* Immunoglobulin G4 (IgG4)
IGH V mutational status, 170
IHC. *See* Immunohistochemistry (IHC)
Ileal neuroendocrine tumors, 521
Image analysis systems, 25
Immunocytochemistry. *See* Immunohistochemistry (IHC)
Immunoglobulin G4 (IgG4)-related cholangitis, 567
Immunogold labeling, 5, 23t
Immunohistochemistry (IHC)
  basic principles of, 2
  control in, 16t, 17–18, 820, 881f, 893
  conventional staining *vs.,* 58, 59t
  definition of, 1
  history of, 1
  limitations of, 896–897
  use of, 1
IMTs. *See* Inflammatory myofibroblastic tumors (IMTs)
Inappropriate staining, 27–28
Incubation
  of antibodies, 22–23
  of reagents, 23
Indirect detection, 6
Infections
  bacterial, 64–67
  emerging, 69–70
  fungal, 67–68
  protozoal, 68–69
  terrorism and, 70–72
  viral, 59–64
Infectious mononucleosis, 149
Infinite standard reference controls, 16
Inflammatory bowel disease (IBD), 514
Inflammatory fibroid polyp, 526–527
Inflammatory myofibroblastic tumors (IMTs)
  of bladder, 626–627, 628f
  mediastinal, 345
  uterine, 715
Inflammatory pseudotumor, of lung, 396
Influenza A, 73f
Infratentorial ependymomas, 844
Inhibin
  in adrenocortical tumors, 236, 314
  in granulosa cell ovarian tumors, 733f
  in gynecologic pathology, 691t
  in lung neoplasms, 372t, 402
  in ovarian fibroma, 732
  in ovarian tumors, 722
  in Sertoli-Leydig ovarian tumors, 734
  in Sertoli ovarian tumors, 734–735
  in testicular tumors, 644–645
In situ hybridization (ISH), 72–74
Insulin, in pancreatic endocrine tumors, 321
Insulin-like growth factor-II (IGF-II)
  in choroid plexus papilloma, 855
  in soft-tissue tumors, 100, 105
Integrins, 106
Interferon regulatory factor 4 (IRF4), 160–161
Interfollicular lymphadenitis, 149–150
Interleukin-2 receptor, 151
Intermediate filament proteins (IFPs)
  in endocrine tumors, 294
  in malignant melanoma, 189–190
  overview of, 83–90
  in thyroid tumors, 300–301
Internal controls, 18
Internal reference standards, 18
Interphase FISH, 170
Interpretation, 896–897
Intestinal carcinoid tumor, 376t
Intestinal-type adenocarcinoma (ITAC), 269, 561, 563
Intestinal-type endocervical adenocarcinoma, 697
Intraductal oncocytic papillary neoplasms (IOPNs), 551
Intraductal papillary mucinous neoplasms (IPMNs), 550–551
Intraductal papilloma, 772f
Intraductal tubular carcinoma, 552
Intraepithelial lymphocytes (IELs), 511
Intrapulmonary thymoma, primary, 397–415
Intratubular germ-cell neoplasia, unclassified (IGCNU), 645
Intravascular large B-cell lymphoma, 176
Intravascular lymphoma, 390t, 391, 871
Invasive adenocarcinoma, 560–561
Invasive aspergillosis, 68
Invasive-ectopic pituitary adenoma, 267
Invasive endocervical adenocarcinoma, 696
Invasive micropapillary carcinoma, 780–785
Invasive papillary carcinoma, 563–564
Involucrin, 465
IOPNs (intraductal oncocytic papillary neoplasms), 551
IPMNs (intraductal papillary mucinous neoplasms), 550–551
IRF4. *See* Interferon regulatory factor 4 (IRF4)
ISH. *See In situ* hybridization (ISH)
Islets of Langerhans, 321
ITAC. *See* Intestinal-type adenocarcinoma (ITAC)

J

JAZF1-JJAZ1 translocation, 720
J-chain, 143
JC virus, 63, 64f
JunB, 142, 143f, 145t

K

Kaposiform hemangioendothelioma (KHE), 102
Kaposi's sarcoma, 60, 108f, 111, 385, 386f
Karyometry, in prostate tumors, 617
KD. *See* Kikuchi disease (KD)
Keratin filaments, 210
Keratins, 84–86. *See also specific cytokeratins*
  in adrenal cortex tumors, 315f
  in cancer of unknown primary site, 210–221
  in epithelioid sarcoma, 488
  in head and neck neoplasms, 257t, 259t
  in malignant melanoma, 190f, 191f
  in mediastinal tumors, 342t
  in mesotheliomas, 417–422, 426t
  in sinonasal tumors, 264t
  in thyroid tumors, 300t
KHE. *See* Kaposiform hemangioendothelioma (KHE)
KHN6/7, in pilar tumors, 470–471
Ki-67, 906
  in ampullary endocrine neoplasms, 564
  in breast tumors, 808
  in cancer of unknown primary site, 910
  in endometrial intraepithelial carcinoma, 707f
  in head and neck neoplasms, 259t
  in mediastinal tumors, 343t
  in neuroendocrine carcinomas, 406
  in neuroendocrine lung neoplasms, 382t
  in non-Hodgkin lymphoma, 167–168
  in pancreatic endocrine neoplasms, 557–558
  in phyllodes tumor, 792, 793f
  in prostate tumors, 615–616
Kidney tumors
  ablative therapy for, 593
  in angiomyolipoma, 639–640
  antibodies in, 632–635
  antigens in, 632–635
  biopsy of, 593
  cadherins in, 633–634
  carbonic anhydrase IX in, 634–635
  CD10 in, 633
  in chromophobe renal cell carcinoma, 638
  clear-cell, 636–637
  in collecting duct carcinoma, 638, 640f
  EpCAM in, 633
  genomic applications in, 640–641
  glutathione-transferase alpha in, 635
  in metanephric adenoma, 636
  metastatic, 640
  morbidity in, 631, 632t
  mortality in, 631, 632t
  in mucinous tubular and spindle-cell carcinoma, 638–639
  in papillary renal cell carcinoma, 637–638
  PAX2 in, 633
  PAX8 in, 633, 634f
  prognostic parameters in, 643t
  theranostic applications in, 640–641
  in von Hippel-Lindau disease, 641
Kikuchi disease (KD), 477
KIT mutation status, 530
KRAS gene, 50–51
KRAS mutations
  in ductal adenocarcinoma, 546
  in gastrointestinal tumors, 530
  in intraductal papillary mucinous neoplasms, 550–551
  in mucinous cystic neoplasm, 551
  in serous cystadenoma, 553

L

Labeling index (LI), 831
LAHH. *See* Luminal A-HER2 hybrid (LAHH) breast tumors
Laminin, 93
LANA-1. *See* Latent associated nuclear antigen-1 (LANA-1)
Langerhans cell histiocytosis (LCH), 168, 477–478
Large-cell epithelioid amelanotic malignant melanoma, 190f
Large-cell lymphoproliferations, 477
Large-cell neuroendocrine carcinoma
  of lung, 404t
  of prostate, 606–607
Large-cell non-Hodgkin lymphoma (LCNHL), 355
Large-cell undifferentiated carcinoma of lung, 404t
Large polygonal-cell neoplasms of mediastinum, 350–358

Latent associated nuclear antigen-1 (LANA-1), 60
LBA. *See* Ligand binding assay (LBA)
LBHH. *See* Luminal B-HER2 hybrid (LBHH) breast tumors
LCH. *See* Langerhans cell histiocytosis (LCH)
LCNHL. *See* Large-cell non-Hodgkin lymphoma (LCNHL)
Leiomyomas, 86, 98, 710–711
Leiomyosarcoma (LMS), 84, 86, 108–109, 108f, 362, 710–711
Leishmaniasis, 68–69
LELC. *See* Lymphoepithelioma-like carcinoma (LELC)
Lennert lymphoma, 146
Leptomeningitis, 826
Leptospirosis, 66–67
Leu7
  in gastrointestinal stromal tumor, 226
  in neuroendocrine lung neoplasms, 382t
  in oligodendroglioma, 846
Leukemia
  adult T-cell, 179
  aggressive NK-cell, 179
  B-cell prolymphocytic, 171
  Burkitt, 177–178
  chronic lymphocytic, 169–170, 389
  hairy cell, 171–172
  in nervous system, 871
  in skin, 472–475
  T-cell large granular lymphocytic, 179
  T-cell prolymphocytic, 179
Leu M1. *See* CD15
Lewis X antigen. *See* CD15
Lewis Y antigen, in mesothelioma, 424t
Lewy body diseases, 877
Leydig cell tumor, 647, 735
LFS. *See* Li-Fraumeni syndrome (LFS)
Lhermitte-Duclos disease, 853–854
LHRH. *See* Luteinizing hormone-releasing hormone (LHRH) agonist
LI. *See* Labeling index (LI)
Li-Fraumeni syndrome (LFS), 842, 856
Ligand binding assay (LBA), 800
Light-chain immunoglobulins, 96
  in non-Hodgkin lymphoma, 159
Light chain messenger RNA, in non-Hodgkin lymphoma, 160
Limitations, 896–897
LIP. *See* Lymphocytic interstitial pneumonia-pneumonitis (LIP)
Liponeurocytoma, cerebellar, 855
Liposarcoma variants, 119
Listeria monocytogenes, 827
Liver. *See also entries at* Hepatic
  bile duct lesions in, 573–575
  bile ducts in, 565
  cirrhosis of, 566–567
  diseases of, 565–576
  embryonal sarcoma of, 576
  interstitium of, 566
  metabolic disorders in, 567–568
  metastases to, 207
  neoplastic disease in, 568–576
  neuroendocrine neoplasms in, 575
  normal parenchyma in, 565
  transplantation, 568
  vasculature of, 565
  viral infections of, 566
LMS. *See* Leiomyosarcoma (LMS)
Lobular carcinoma
  ductal *vs.*, 773–777
  pleomorphic, 777–780
  variants, 777–780
Loss of heterozygosity (LOH), 44, 52–53
Low-grade astrocytoma, 839
Low-grade cribriform cystadenocarcinoma, 279–280
Low-grade ependymoma, 843–844
Luminal A-HER2 hybrid (LAHH) breast tumors, 803–804
Luminal A (LUMA) breast tumors, 803–804
Luminal B-HER2 hybrid (LBHH) breast tumors, 803–804
Luminal B (LUMB) breast tumors, 803–804
Lung
  adenocarcinoma, 375t
  desmoplastic small round cell tumor of, 396
  epithelial-myoepithelial neoplasm of, 396
  Erdheim-Chester disease in, 392
  follicular lymphoma in, 390, 390t
  granular cell tumor of, 396
  Hodgkin disease of, 390–391, 390t
  inflammatory pseudotumor of, 396
  Langerhans cell histiocytosis in, 392–393
  lymphomas of, 388–389
  lymphomatoid granulomatosis in, 390t, 391
  lymphoproliferative disorders of, 387–393
  mantle cell lymphoma in, 389–390
  metastases to, 207
  metastasis of cancers in, 283
  placental transmogrification of, 397
  primary effusion lymphoma in, 390t, 392
  pseudomesotheliomatous carcinomas of, 441–442
  pyothorax-associated lymphoma in, 392
  rhabdoid tumor of, 395–396
  salivary gland neoplasm of, 396
  sclerosing hemangioma of, 376t, 394–395
Lung tumors. *See also* Mesothelioma
  antibodies in, 370–374
  antibodies in neuroendocrine, 378–384, 382t
  antigens in, 370–374
  calretinin in, 372t
  carcinoembryonic antigen in, 371t, 383f
  CD15 in, 371
  CD117 in, 413
  CDX2 in, 371t, 372t
  chromogranins in, 378, 382t, 383f
  CK5 in, 370–371, 370t, 398
  CK6 in, 370t, 398
  CK7 in, 370, 370t, 373t, 381t, 402
  CK20 in, 370t, 371–372, 374t, 381t
  C-kit in, 414–415
  collapsin response mediator protein in, 415
  desmoglein 3 in, 414
  D2-40 in, 372t
  epithelial membrane antigen in, 370t
  estrogen receptor/progesterone receptor in, 372t
  fascin in, 369, 371t
  GADD45 in, 412–413
  galectin-4 in, 412
  glypican-3 in, 414
  hepatocyte paraffin in, 372t
  Her2/neu in, 402
  human milk fat globule protein-2 in, 370t
  inhibin in, 372t, 402
  keratin in, 370t, 379t–380t
  mammaglobin in, 372t
  melan-A in, 372t
  mesothelin in, 372t
  minichromosome maintenance protein 2 in, 412
Lung tumors *(Continued)*
  misdiagnosis of, 406
  napsin-A in, 373–374
  neuroendocrine, 323–326, 374–384
  neuroendocrine differentiation in, 407–408
  neuroendocrine markers in, 403–404
  p63 in, 371t, 377t
  primary, 369–396
  prostate acid phosphatase in, 372t
  prostate specific antigen in, 372t
  rare, 384–387
  renal cell carcinoma marker in, 372t
  RON in, 413
  S-100 protein in, 371t, 400, 401f
  surfactant apoprotein A in, 371t, 379t–380t
  thyroglobulin in, 372t
  thyroid transcription factor in, 371t, 372t, 379t–380t, 381t, 383f, 398, 412
  tumor-associated glycoprotein in, 371t
  uroplakin III in, 372t
  vimentin in, 385f
Luteinizing hormone-releasing hormone (LHRH) agonist, 602
Lyme disease, 67, 827
Lymphadenitis
  cytomegalovirus, 149
  granulomatous, 150
  interfollicular, 149–150
Lymphangioleiomyomatosis, 393–394
Lymphocyte-predominant thymoma
  lymphoid hyperplasia *vs.*, 343
  lymphoma *vs.*, 343
Lymphocytic gastritis, 505
Lymphocytic interstitial pneumonia-pneumonitis (LIP), 387
Lymphocytic leukemia, chronic, 169–170
Lymphoepithelial carcinoma, 270–271, 270f
Lymphoepithelioid cell variant of peripheral T-cell lymphoma, 146
Lymphoepithelioma-like carcinoma (LELC), 359, 402–403, 404t, 509, 510f
Lymphohistiocytoid mesothelioma, 446–448
Lymphoid hyperplasia, lymphocyte-predominant hyperplasia *vs.*, 343
Lymphoma, 103f. *See also* Hodgkin lymphoma (HL); Non-Hodgkin lymphoma
  adult T-cell, 179
  anaplastic, 404t
  anaplastic large cell, 146, 181
  Burkitt, 177–178
  as differential diagnosis for anaplastic mass, 837t
  diffuse large B-cell, 174–177
  enteropathy-type T-cell, 179
  extranodal NK/T-cell, nasal type, 179
  follicular, 174, 390, 390t
  hepatosplenic T-cell, 179
  intravascular, 390t, 391, 871
  intravascular large B-cell, 176
  Lennert, 146
  of lung, 388–389
  lymphocyte-predominant thymoma *vs.*, 343
  lymphoepithelioid cell variant of peripheral T-cell, 146
  lymphoplasmacytic, 171
  mantle cell, 174–175, 389–390, 390t
  marginal zone B-cell, MALT type, 389
  mediastinal large B-cell, 174–175
  nervous system, 869–870

Lymphoma *(Continued)*
nodal marginal B-cell, 173–174
peripheral T-cell, unspecified, 180–181
pleural, 444
primary cutaneous large B-cell, 177
primary effusion, 176, 390t, 392
primary mediastinal B-cell, 146
pyothorax-associated, 390t, 392
in skin, 472–475
small-cell lymphocytic, 389
splenic marginal zone B-cell, 171
subcutaneous panniculitis-like T-cell, 179–180
T-cell/histiocyte-rich B-cell, 177
T-cell-rich B-cell, 146
Lymphomatoid granulomatosis, 178, 390t, 391, 871
Lymphomatoid papulosis (LYP), 478–479
Lymphoplasmacytic lymphoma, 171
Lymphoproliferative disorders of lung, 387–393
Lymphovascular invasion (LVI), 709
Lynch syndrome, 745
LYP. *See* Lymphomatoid papulosis (LYP)
Lysozyme, in mediastinal tumors, 342t

M

Macrophages, 822t, 825–826
Magnetic resonance imaging (MRI), of nervous system lesions, 821
MAGs. *See* Myelin-associated glycoproteins (MAGs)
Malignancy grading, of nervous system tumors, 831–832
Malignant ependymoma, 835t
Malignant epithelioid mesothelioma of mediastinum, 357
Malignant fibrous histiocytoma (MFH), 115, 480–483
Malignant mediastinal germ-cell tumors, 353–354
Malignant melanoma (MM)
antibodies in, 189–196
antigens in, 189–196
in brain, 868f
calcium-binding proteins, 192–193
calretinin, 193
in cancer of unknown primary site, 909–910
carcinoembryonic antigen in, 191
cell-membrane proteins in, 190–192
cutaneous granular cell tumor *vs.*, 199
desmoplastic amelanotic, 190f
differential diagnosis of, 197–200
as differential diagnosis of fibrillar mass, 835t
epithelial determinants in, 191
in gastrointestinal tract, 526
GP100 in, 193–195
hematopoietic markers in, 191–192
HMB-45 in, 194
keratin in, 190f, 191f
large-cell epithelioid amelanotic, 190f
melanocytic nevus variants *vs.*, 197
metastatic *vs.* malignant glioma, 198–199
microphthalmia transcription factor protein in, 195
NB84 in, 192
neuroendocrine markers in, 196
overview of, 189
pigmented actinic keratosis *vs.*, 199
placental-like alkaline phosphatase in, 191
PMel 17 in, 193–195
PNL2 in, 195–196
Malignant melanoma (MM) *(Continued)*
putatively prognostic markers for, 196–200
rhabdoid, 197
sarcomatoid, 197
sarcomatoid amelanotic, 190f
sentinel lymph node biopsies for metastatic, 196
of sinonasal tract, 264–266
small-cell amelanotic, 190f
soft-tissue sarcomas *vs.*, 199
tumor-associated glycoprotein-72 in, 191
tyrosinase-related antibodies in, 195
vimentin in, 190f
vulvar, 691
Malignant meningiomas, 863–866
Malignant mixed müllerian tumor (MMMT), 700
Malignant mixed oligodendroglioma-astrocytoma, 849
Malignant oligodendroglioma, 847, 848f
Malignant paragangliomas, 282–283
Malignant peripheral nerve sheath tumor (MPNST), 84–85, 107, 108f, 109–110, 114, 214t
Malignant rhabdoid tumor (MRT), 664t, 677–680
Malignant small-cell mediastinal neoplasms, 345–350
Mallory's bodies, 566
MALT. *See* Mucosa-associated lymphoid tissue (MALT) lymphoma
Mammaglobin, 902
in breast carcinoma, 791, 792f
in lung neoplasms, 372t
Mammalian achaete-scute complex-like protein (MASH)
in pancreatic endocrine tumors, 323
in skin endocrine tumors, 328
in small-cell lung cancer *vs.* Merkel cell carcinoma, 408–409
Mammaprint, 805
Mammary Paget disease, 785–786
Mammosomatotroph cell adenoma, 296t
Mantle cell lymphoma, 174–175, 389–390, 390t
Marginal zone B-cell lymphoma of MALT type, 389, 390t
Margins
in ependymomas, 842
in epithelioid ependymomas, 843
in gliomas, 832–833
MART. *See* Melan-A tyrosinase (MART)
MASH. *See* Mammalian achaete-scute complex-like protein (MASH)
Mature B-cell neoplasms, 169–178
Mature T-cell neoplasms, 178–181
MCM2. *See* Minichromosome maintenance protein 2 (MCM2)
MCNs. *See* Mucinous cystic neoplasms (MCNs)
MCS. *See* Mesenchymal chondrosarcoma (MCS)
MDR1. *See* Multidrug resistance protein (MDR1)
ME1, in mesothelioma, 427–428
MEA. *See* Middle ear adenoma (MEA)
MEC. *See* Mucoepidermoid carcinoma (MEC)
MECs. *See* Myoepithelial cells (MECs)
Mediastinal large B-cell lymphoma, 174–175
Mediastinal leiomyosarcoma, 362
Mediastinal malignant mesothelioma, sarcomatoid, 361
Mediastinal small-cell neuroendocrine carcinoma, 345–346
Mediastinal solitary fibrous tumor, 362
Mediastinal tumor(s)
algorithmic immunohistochemistry in, 340–341
antibodies in, 340, 342t–343t
antigens in, 340
basaloid squamous cell, 346
carcinoid, 354
cystic thymoma *vs.* cystic seminoma in, 341
dendritic cell, 362–364
differential diagnosis of thymoma variants in, 341–344
germ-cell, 353–354
hematopoietic, 356–357
large-cell non-Hodgkin, 355
large polygonal-cell, 350–358
malignant epithelioid mesothelioma, 357
metastatic, 357–358
mixed small and large cell, 358–359
neuroblastoma, 346
paragangliomas as, 354–355
parathyroid carcinoma as, 353
primitive neuroectodermal, 346
prognostic markers in, 364
rhabdomyosarcoma, 346–348
small-cell, malignant, 345–350
small-cell lymphoma, 348–350
spindle-cell, 359–362
syncytial, Hodgkin, 355–356
types of, 238–242
Mediastinum, 340
Medullary carcinoma
hepatocellular, 572
pancreatic, 548
Medullary thyroid carcinoma, 306, 310
Medulloblastoma, 837t, 844f, 857–858
Medulloepithelioma, 835t, 860, 862f
Medullomyoblastoma, 858
Melan A
in adrenocortical tumors, 236, 314
in lung neoplasms, 372t
Melan-A tyrosinase (MART)
in bone tumors, 96
in malignant melanoma, 194
in mediastinal tumors, 342t
Melanocyte-specific monoclonal antibodies, 193–196
Melanocytic nevus, 197
Melanoma. *See* Malignant melanoma (MM)
Melanoma antigen, in mesothelioma, 425t
Melanophages, pigmented, 31f
MELF. *See* Microcystic, elongated, and fragmented (MELF) pattern
Membrane-bound B-cell antigen, in mediastinal tumors, 342t
MEN1. *See* Multiple endocrine neoplasia, type 1 (MEN1)
MEN2. *See* Multiple endocrine neoplasia, type 2 (MEN2)
Meningeal cyst, 876
Meningeal tumors, 860–867
Meningiomas, 860–866
as differential diagnosis for epithelial mass, 835t
fibroblastic, 834t
keratin expression in, 220
transitional, 836t
Meningitis, 826
Meningotheliomatous meningioma, 862, 863f
Mercury-based fixatives, 670
Merkel cell carcinoma, 327–328, 375t

Mesenchymal breast tumors, 783–784
Mesenchymal chondrosarcoma (MCS), 103f, 106, 867–868
Mesenchymal cytokeratin subclasses, 85t
Mesenchymal lesions of gastrointestinal tract, 523–528
Mesenchymal skin tumors, 479–489
Mesonephric remnants, 694
Mesonephroma, 728
Mesothelial hyperplasia, mesothelioma *vs.*, 438, 439t
Mesothelial markers, 898–899
Mesothelin
  in ductal adenocarcinoma, 546
  in lung neoplasms, 372t
  in mesothelioma, 425t, 429
Mesothelioma
  antibodies int, 423t–425t
  antigen, 423t
  cadherins in, 429
  calretinin in, 427
  carcinoembryonic antigen in, 429–430
  cytokeratin profiles in, 426t
  diagnosis of, considerations in, 434–440
    pitfalls in, 444–450
  fat in, 436, 438f
  fibrosing pleuritis *vs.*, 440t
  HBME-1 in, 428
  heterologous elements in, 436
  hyaluronan detection in, 433
  immunostains in, 435t
  LeuM1 in, 430
  lymphohistiocytoid, 446–448
  mesothelial hyperplasia *vs.*, 438, 439t
  negative markers for, 429–433
  pleomorphic, 438
  pleural metastases *vs.*, 238
  positive markers for, 415–429
  pulmonary adenocarcinoma *vs.*, 445t
  sarcomatoid, 435–436
  thrombomodulin in, 428–429
  variabilities in, 444–450
  variants, 418–422
  vascular neoplasm *vs.*, 448, 451f
  vimentin in, 427
  X-link inhibitor of apoptosis protein in, 439
Mesothelioma-like tumors of pleura, 441
Messenger RNA (mRNA), 43
Metabolic disorders, in liver, 567–568
Metanephric adenoma, 636
Metaplastic carcinoma, 781–783
Metastatic disease. *See also* Cancer of unknown primary site (CUPS)
  adrenal, 316
  to bladder, 622–624
  to bone, 207
  to brain, 207
  from breast, 790–791
  endometrial, 707–709
  in germ cells, 646–647
  to head and neck, 283–284
  to kidney, 640
  to liver, 207
  from lungs, 283
  to lungs, 207
  mediastinal, 357–358
  in melanoma, 196, 198–199
  to nervous system, 873–875
  to ovaries, 740–742
  in pleura, 238
  renal cell, 283
  from renal cell carcinoma, 449
  in sentinel lymph node, 788
Methanol-hydrogen peroxide combination, 5
Methylguanine DNA methyltransferase (MGMT), 850–851
MF. *See* Mycosis fungoides (MF)
MFH. *See* Malignant fibrous histiocytoma (MFH)
MGMT. *See* Methylguanine DNA methyltransferase (MGMT)
MIC2 protein, 96
Microarrays, 50
Microcystic, elongated, and fragmented (MELF) pattern, 710
Microdysgenesis, 881
Microgemistocytes, 846, 882t
Microphthalmia transcription factor protein (MTFP), in malignant melanoma, 195
MicroRNA (miRNA), 244
Microsatellite instability (MSI)
  in colorectal adenocarcinoma, 515
  detection, 53–54
  in ductal adenocarcinoma, 546
  in ovarian tumors, 746
Microsatellites, 42
Microwave heating, 19–20
Middle ear adenoma (MEA), 280–281
Minichromosome maintenance protein 2 (MCM2), 412
Minimal deviation endocervical adenocarcinoma, 697–698
Minute pulmonary meningothelial nodules (MPMN), 397
Mismatch repair (MMR) proteins, 717–718, 720
Mixed acinar-endocrine carcinoma, 557
Mixed-cellularity Hodgkin disease, 359
Mixed oligodendroglioma-astrocytoma, 846–847
Mixed small-cell and large-cell malignancies, 358–359
MLPS. *See* Myxoid liposarcoma (MLPS)
MMMT. *See* Malignant mixed müllerian tumor (MMMT)
MMR. *See* Mismatch repair (MMR) proteins
MOC-31, 900
  in cancer of unknown primary site, 225
  in gastrointestinal tumors, 501
  in hepatocellular carcinoma, 570
  in mesothelioma, 430–431
Mole, complete hydatidiform, 716–717
Molecular assays, gastrointestinal stromal tumor and, 243t
Molecular biology, 42
Molecular diagnostic applications, 72–74
Molecular testing
  specimen requirements in, 44–45
  techniques for, 45–50
Monoclonal antibody therapy, 150
Monocytoid cell aggregates, 168
Mononucleosis, infectious, 149
Monophasic spindle-cell synovial sarcoma, 110–111
Monophasic synovial sarcoma (MSS), 107, 110
Monosynovial sarcoma, 108f
Mounting slides, 24
MPMN. *See* Minute pulmonary meningothelial nodules (MPMN)
MPNST. *See* Malignant peripheral nerve sheath tumor (MPNST)
MPO. *See* Myeloperoxidase (MPO)
MRI. *See* Magnetic resonance imaging (MRI)
MRNA. *See* Messenger RNA (mRNA)
MRT. *See* Malignant rhabdoid tumor (MRT)
MS. *See* Multiple sclerosis (MS)
MSA. *See* Muscle-specific actin (MSA)
MSI. *See* Microsatellite instability (MSI)
MSS. *See* Monophasic synovial sarcoma (MSS)
MTAs. *See* Multi-tissue arrays (MTAs)
MTFP. *See* Microphthalmia transcription factor protein (MTFP)
MTSC. *See* Mucinous tubular and spindle-cell carcinoma (MTSC)
MUC. *See* Mucin-related antigens (MUCs)
Mucinous appendiceal neoplasms, 511–512, 513f
Mucinous cystadenoma, 560
Mucinous cystic neoplasm (MCNs), 551
Mucinous tubular and spindle-cell carcinoma (MTSC), 638–639
Mucin-related antigens (MUCs)
  in ampullary adenocarcinomas, 563
  in ductal adenocarcinoma, 544–545
  in gastric adenocarcinoma, 508
  in gastrointestinal tumors, 501
  in intraductal oncocytic papillary neoplasm, 551
  in intraductal papillary mucinous neoplasm, 550
  in intraductal tubular carcinoma, 552
  in pancreatic intraepithelial neoplasia, 549
  in pancreatic tumors, 541–542
  in thyroid tumors, 304
Mucins, in pancreatic tumors, 542
Mucoepidermoid carcinoma (MEC), 275
Mucosa-associated lymphoid tissue (MALT), 387
Mucosa-associated lymphoid tissue (MALT) lymphoma, 172–173
Müllerian adenosarcoma, 713, 714f
Müllerian endometrioid adenocarcinoma, 517
Multidrug resistance protein (MDR1), in adrenal cortex tumors, 316
Multigene expression assays, in gastrointestinal stromal tumor, 243t
Multi-infarct vascular dementia, 877
Multiple endocrine neoplasia, type 1 (MEN1), 519, 557, 558
Multiple endocrine neoplasia, type 2 (MEN2), 306
Multiple myeloma oncogene 1 (MUM1), 160–161
Multiple sclerosis (MS), 878–879
Multiple system atrophy, 878t
Multipotential-subserosal cells, 415–416
Multi-tissue arrays (MTAs), 17–18
Multi-tissue control slides, 17–18
MUM1. *See* Multiple myeloma oncogene 1 (MUM1)
Muscle-specific actin (MSA)
  in gastrointestinal stromal tumor, 525
  in malignant rhabdoid tumor, 678f, 679f
  in mediastinal tumors, 342t, 345f
  in mesothelioma, 423t
  in rhabdomyosarcoma, 669f
  in uterine tumors, 702–704
Mutations
  overview of, 44
  small-scale, detection of, 50–51
MXPE. *See* Myxopapillary ependymoma (MXPE)
MYCN amplification, in neuroblastoma, 667
Mycobacterium tuberculosis infection, 66
Mycosis fungoides (MF), 180, 475

Myelin-associated glycoproteins (MAGs), 92
Myelitis, 826
Myeloid/histiocyte antigen, in mediastinal tumors, 343t
Myeloperoxidase (MPO)
  in mediastinal tumors, 343t
  in non-Hodgkin lymphoma, 168
  in skin tumors, 474f
MYG. *See* Myogenin (MYG)
Myo-D1, 91–92, 104, 342t, 670f
Myoepithelial cells (MECs), breast tumors and, 763–771
Myoepithelioma, 121, 273–274
Myofibroblastic mediastinal proliferations, 344–345
Myofibroblastic skin tumors, 479–480
Myofibroblastoma of breast, 784
Myogenic regulatory patterns, 663
Myogenin (MYG), 91–92, 104, 342t, 668–669, 670, 670f
Myoglobin, 91, 668
Myomelanocytoma, 118f, 119
Myometrial invasion, 709
Myosin
  desmin and, 86
  in gynecologic pathology, 692t
  II, 91
  in rhabdomyosarcoma, 668
Myxoid liposarcoma (MLPS), 119
Myxopapillary ependymoma (MXPE), 835t, 843f, 844–845, 845f

N

NA. *See* Nephrogenic adenoma (NA)
Naegleria fowleri, 69
NAF. *See* Nasopharyngeal angiofibroma (NAF)
Napsin-A, in lung tumors, 373–374
Nasal cavity neoplasms, 262–270
Nasopharyngeal angiofibroma (NAF), 271
Nasopharyngeal carcinoma (NPC), 270–271
National Cancer Institute (NCI), 15
NB84
  in adrenal neuroblastoma, 318
  in malignant melanoma, 192
NBC. *See* Nuclear beta-catenin (NBC)
NBF. *See* Neutral buffer formalin (NBF)
NCI. *See* National Cancer Institute (NCI)
Negative controls, 16t, 17
Neoplasms
  cytokeratins in, 85t
  keratins and, 84–86
Nephroblastoma. *See* Wilms' tumor
Nephrogenic adenoma (NA), 626
Nerve sheath tumors, 868–869
Nervous system cysts, 875–876
Nervous system lesions
  in AIDS, 828–829
  biopsies of, 824t
  in cerebrovascular disease, 830–831
  clear-cell, differential diagnosis of, 823b
  clinical perspective of, 821–824
  differential diagnosis of, infiltrating parenchyma, 822t
  fibrosis in, 826
  gliosis in, 824–825, 833f
  in infectious disease, 826–828
  macrophages in, 825–826
  non-neoplastic, 824–831
  perivascular inflammation in, 825–826
  radiography of, 821–824
  in small vessel disease, 830–831
  in spongiform encephalopathies, 829–830
  in vascular malformation, 831
Nervous system tumors
  abscess *vs.,* 883
  chordomas in, 867–868
  choroid plexus epithelial, 855–856
  dysplasia *vs.,* 883–884
  embryonal, 857–860
  germ-cell, 869
  gliomas in, 832–851
    astrocytomas in, 833–841
    definition of, 832
    differential diagnosis of anaplastic cells in, 837t
    differential diagnosis of epithelioid mass in, 835t–836t
    differential diagnosis of fibrillar mass in, 834t–835t
    eosinophilic granular bodies in, 837–839
    ependymomas in, 842–845
    glial fibrillary acidic protein in, 832–833
    glioblastoma multiforme in, 849–851
    oligodendroglioma in, 846–849
    Rosenthal fibers in, 833–837, 838f
    S-100 protein in, 839
    treatment of, 832
    tumor margin in, 832–833
  grading of, 831–832
  histiocytosis in, 870–871
  leukemia in, 871
  lymphoma in, 869–870
  meningeal, 860–867
  metastatic, 873–875
  nerve sheath, 868–869
  neuronal, 851–855
  PCNA in, 831
  pineal cell, 856–857
  sarcomas in, 867–868
NESP-55, in gastrointestinal tumors, 501
Nestin, 105
Neural cell adhesion molecule, 92–93, 293–294
Neural lesions, 526
Neurilemmoma, 868–869
Neurinoma, 868–869
Neuroblastoma, 837t
  adrenal, 318–319
  of mediastinum, 346
  olfactory, 263
  pediatric, 663–667
Neurocysticercosis, 827
Neurocytoma, central, 834t, 845f, 846, 855
Neuroendocrine adenomas, 280–281
Neuroendocrine carcinoma, 266–267, 699, 708–709
Neuroendocrine carcinoma spectrum, 272–273
Neuroendocrine markers
  in cancer of unknown primary site, 226–227
  in malignant melanoma, 196
Neuroendocrine prostatic neoplasms, 605–607
Neuroendocrine small-cell carcinoma, 265t, 266–267, 272–273
Neuroendocrine tumors of gastrointestinal tract, 519–523
Neuroepithelial bodies, 323
Neuroepithelial cyst, 875
Neurofibrillary tangles (NFTs), 877
Neurofibromas, 98, 483–485, 835t, 869
Neurofibromatosis type 1 (NF1), 319
Neurofilament proteins (NFPs), 83, 85, 89–90
Neuronal tumors, 851–855
Neuron-specific enolase (NSE)
  in adrenal neuroblastoma, 318
  in bone tumors, 96
  in cancer of unknown primary site, 226
  in desmoplastic small round cell tumor, 675f
  in Ewing's sarcoma/primitive neuroectodermal tumor, 672f, 673f
  in gastrointestinal endocrine tumors, 319
  in malignant rhabdoid tumor, 678f
  in mediastinal tumors, 342t
  in mesothelioma, 425t
  in neuroendocrine lung neoplasms, 378, 382t
  in neuronal tumors, 852
  in oligodendrogliomas, 849f
  in ovarian tumors, 731f
  overview of, 292
  in pancreatic tumors, 543
Neurothekeomas (NTKs), 484–485, 486f
Neutral buffer formalin (NBF), 19
NFPs. *See* Neurofilament proteins (NFPs)
Nipah virus, 70
NLPHL. *See* Nodular lymphocyte predominance Hodgkin lymphoma (NLPHL)
Nodal marginal zone B-cell lymphoma, 173–174
Nodular fasciitis, 107
Nodular ganglioneuroblastoma, 665
Nodular hyperplasia, 303t
Nodular lymphocyte predominance Hodgkin lymphoma (NLPHL), 137, 139f. *See also* Hodgkin lymphoma (HL)
Nodular lymphoid infiltrates of uncertain nature, 388
Non-Hodgkin lymphoma, 146–147
  ALK in, 163
  antibodies in, 157–168
  antigens in, 157–168
  B cells in, 157–161
  B-cell transcription factors in, 160
  BCL-1 in, 163
  BCL-2 in, 163–164
  BCL-6 in, 164
  CD1A in, 164
  CD11C in, 164–165
  CD2 in, 161
  CD3 in, 162
  CD4 in, 162
  CD5 in, 162
  CD7 in, 162
  CD8 in, 162
  CD10 in, 164
  CD14 in, 165
  CD19 in, 165
  CD21 in, 158
  CD22 in, 158
  CD23 in, 158
  CD25 in, 158, 165
  CD30 in, 165
  CD33 in, 165
  CD43 in, 165–166
  CD45 in, 166
  CD52 in, 166
  CD56 in, 167
  CD61 in, 167
  CD68 in, 167
  CD79 in, 158–159
  CD99 in, 167
  CD138 in, 159
  CD163 in, 167
  classification of, 156, 169
  cyclin D1 in, 163

Non-Hodgkin lymphoma *(Continued)*
cytogenic abnormalities in, 170
DBA 44 in, 159
diagnosis of, 156
interferon regulatory factor 4 in, 160–161
Ki-67 and, 167–168
MUM1 in, 160–161
myeloperoxidase in, 168
other malignancies and, 168–169
overview of, 156–157
PAX5 in, 161
pulmonary, 389
T-bet in, 162–163
T cells in, 161–163
T-cell transcription factors in, 162–163
terminal deoxynucleotidyl transferase in, 168
Nonlymphoid tumors, 148–149
Non-mesothelial markers, 899–901
Nonseminomatous germ-cell tumors, 646
Non-specific background staining, 4–5, 29–30
Non-specific binding, blocking of, 22
NPC. *See* Nasopharyngeal carcinoma (NPC)
NSE. *See* Neuron-specific enolase (NSE)
NTKs. *See* Neurothekeomas (NTKs)
Nuclear beta-catenin (NBC), 97
Null cell adenoma, 296t
Numerical chromosome change, 44

O

OBF.1, 142
OCN. *See* Osteocalcin (OCN)
Oct-2
in Hodgkin lymphoma, 142
in non-Hodgkin lymphoma, 161
Oct-3/4, in mediastinal tumors, 343t
Oct-4
in dysgerminoma, 736
in gynecologic pathology, 692t
in ovarian tumors, 723
in testicular tumors, 643
OFMT. *See* Ossifying fibromyxoid tumor (OFMT) of soft parts
Olfactory neuroblastoma (ONB), 263, 264t
Oligoastrocytoma, 836t, 846–847, 849
Oligodendroglioma, 835t, 845f, 846–849, 882t
ONB. *See* Olfactory neuroblastoma (ONB)
Oncocytoma, 296t
renal, 635–636
Oncogenes
in ductal adenocarcinoma, 546
in prostate tumors, 616–617
and skin tumors, 490
thyroid tumors and, 301–302
Oncoproteins, in pancreatic tumors, 541–542
Onco*type* DX, 806
ONN. *See* Osteonectin (ONN)
Organ cytology, specific, 897–907
OS. *See* Osteosarcoma (OS)
Ossifying fibromyxoid tumor (OFMT) of soft parts, 101
Osteoblastic differentiation markers, 95–96
Osteocalcin (OCN), 95, 122
Osteoclast-like giant cells, in undifferentiated carcinoma, 547, 548f
Osteofibrous dysplasia, 123
Osteonectin (ONN), 95–96, 122
Osteosarcoma (OS), 122, 664t, 682–683
Ovarian cytology, 906–907
Ovarian mucinous carcinoma, 375t
Ovarian serous carcinoma, 375t
Ovarian tumors
alpha-fetoprotein in, 723
anti-adenocarcinoma antibodies in, 721–722
Brenner, 729–730
CA125 in, 722
calretinin in, 722
CD45 in, 723
CD117 in, 722–723
CDX2 in, 725
CK7 in, 721, 724, 725, 730
CK20 in, 721, 725
CK125 in, 725f
clear-cell, 728–729
cytokeratins in, 721
desmoplastic small round cell, 731f
in dysgerminoma, 736
endometrioid, 726–728
epithelial, 724–730
epithelial membrane antigen in, 730
fibroma, 732
germ-cell, 736–742
granulosa cell, 732–733
in hepatocyte nuclear factor-1 beta, 728
human chorionic gonadotropin in, 723
inhibin in, 722
Leydig cell, 735
metastatic, 740–742
mucinous, 725–726
neuroendocrine differentiation in, 723–724
neuron-specific enolase in, 731f
Oct-4 in, 723
placental alkaline phosphatase in, 722
serous, 724
Sertoli, 734–735
Sertoli-Leydig, 734
sex cord, 730–735
Sox9 in, 906–907
S-100 protein in, 723
steroid, 735
synaptophysin in, 730
thecoma, 732
transitional cell, 729–730
Wilms' tumor-1 in, 722, 724
yolk sac, 737, 738f
Overnight incubation, 23

P

p16, 903–905. *See also* Human papillomavirus (HPV)
in cervical small-cell carcinoma, 703f
in female genital tract tumors, 690
in gynecologic pathology, 692t
in urinary bladder tumors, 621
in uterine sarcoma, 719
p53
in anaplastic ependymomas, 845
in breast tumors, 807
in endometrial intraepithelial carcinoma, 707f, 719
in extrahepatic biliary tract tumors, 560
in gastrointestinal tumors, 501
in gynecologic pathology, 692t
in head and neck neoplasms, 262
in mediastinal tumors, 343t, 352
in meningiomas, 863f
in mesotheliomas, 433
in ovarian tumors, 730
in pancreatic intraepithelial neoplasia, 549
in parathyroid tumors, 312
in urinary bladder tumors, 621
in uterine tumors, 701–702
in Wilms' tumor, 682f
p57, in gynecologic pathology, 692t
p63
in breast tumors, 764–765
in ductal adenocarcinoma, 545f
in epithelial myoepithelial carcinoma, 277f
in gastrointestinal tumors, 501
in head and neck neoplasms, 259t, 261f
in lung neoplasms, 371t, 377t
in mesothelioma, 425t
in prostate tumors, 596, 599f
in squamous cell carcinoma, 465f
in urinary bladder tumors, 620
in urothelial carcinoma, 608
PA. *See* Pleomorphic adenoma (PA)
Paget disease
anal, 519
of breast, 785–786
in cancer of unknown primary site, 241–242
extramammary, 467
vulvar, 690–693
PAH. *See* Postatrophic hyperplasia (PAH)
PAI. *See* Plasminogen activator inhibitor (PAI)
PAL. *See* Pyothorax-associated lymphoma (PAL)
Pancreatic adenocarcinoma, 375t
Pancreatic ductal adenocarcinoma, 544f
Pancreatic endocrine neoplasms (PENs), 321–323, 557–559
Pancreatic gastrinoma, 322f
Pancreatic intraepithelial neoplasia (PanIN), 549–550
Pancreatic polypeptide, in gastrointestinal endocrine tumors, 320t
Pancreatic tumors
acinar cell, 553–554
acinar markers in, 542–543
adhesion molecules in, 543–544
antibodies in, 541–544
antigens in, 541–544
beta-catenin in, 544
chromogranins in, 543
colloid, 548
ductal adenocarcinoma in, 544–547
E-cadherin in, 543–544
endocrine, 557–559
endocrine markers in, 543
enzymatic markers in, 542–543
exocrine, 544–556
glandular and ductal markers in, 541–542
intraductal oncocytic papillary, 551
intraductal papillary mucinous, 550–551
medullary, 548
mucinous cystic, 551
neuron-specific enolase in, 543
overview of, 541
poorly differentiated neuroendocrine, 559
solid-pseudopapillary, 555–556
synaptophysin in, 543
trypsin in, 542
Pancreatobiliary papillae, 550
Pancreatoblastoma, 554–555
PanIN. *See* Pancreatic intraepithelial neoplasia (PanIN)
Pankeratin, in gastrointestinal stromal tumor, 216t
PAP. *See* Peroxidase-antiperoxidase (PAP)
Papillary ependymomas, 844
Papillary glioneuronal tumor (PGT), 854
Papillary lesions, breast, 770–771
Papillary meningioma, 864–865
Papillary renal cell carcinoma (PRCC), 637–638

Papillary squamous cell carcinoma (PSCC), 260
Papillary thyroid carcinoma, 299f, 301f, 303t, 305f, 309
Papillary tumor of pineal region (PTPR), 857
Parachordoma, 121
Paracrine growth factors, 677
Parafibromin, in parathyroid tumors, 313
Paragangliomas
  differential diagnosis of, 272t
  duodenal gangliolytic, 565
  malignant, 282–283
  mediastinal, 354–355
Paranasal sinus neoplasms, 262–270
Parathyroid adenoma, 313f
Parathyroid carcinoma, 313f, 353
Parathyroid hormone (PTH)
  in mediastinal tumors, 354
  parathyroid tumors and, 311
Parathyroid tumors, 310–316
Parvovirus B19, 62, 73f
PAS. *See* Periodic acid-Schiff (PAS)
PAS-positive microphages, 65
PAX2
  in gastrointestinal stromal tumor, 236
  in renal tumors, 633
PAX5
  in cancer of unknown primary site, 910
  in non-Hodgkin lymphoma, 161
PAX8
  in renal tumors, 633, 634f
  in thyroid tumors, 300, 302f, 310
PBC. *See* Primary biliary cirrhosis (PBC)
P120 catenin, 775–777, 902
PCNA
  in mediastinal tumors, 343t
  in nervous system tumor grading, 831
PCNC. *See* Primary cutaneous neuroendocrine carcinoma (PCNC)
PCR. *See* Polymerase chain reaction (PCR)
PCV. *See* Procarbazine, chloroethylcyclohexylnitrosourea, and vincristine (PCV) chemotherapy
PDSS. *See* Poorly differentiated small-cell synovial sarcoma (PDSS)
PEComas, 393
Pediatric neoplasms
  antibodies in, 662–663
  antigens in, 662–663
  desmoplastic small round cell, 674–677
  Friend leukemia integration-1 in, 663
  malignant rhabdoid, 677–680
  myogenic regulatory patterns and, 663
  neuroblastic, 663–667
  osteosarcoma in, 682–683
  overview of, 662
  in Wilms' tumor, 680–682
  Wilms' tumor 1 in, 663
Penicillium marneffei, 68
PENs. *See* Pancreatic endocrine neoplasms (PENs)
Peptide hormones, in gastrointestinal stromal tumor, 226
Peptidylglycine alpha-amidating enzyme, in gastrointestinal endocrine tumors, 320
Perforin
  in Hodgkin lymphoma, 139
  in non-Hodgkin lymphoma, 167
Periductal stromal tumor, 796
Perikaryon, 847f
Perineuromas, 484, 526
Perineuronal oligodendroglia, non-neoplastic, 838f
Periodic acid-Schiff (PAS), 67
Peripheral nerve sheath tumors (PNSTs), 98, 484
Peripheral nervous system demyelination, 879
Peripheral T-cell lymphoma, unspecified, 180–181
Peritoneal adenocarcinoma, 376t
Peritoneal carcinomatosis, 241
Perivascular epithelioid cell tumor, 118f, 119, 715
Perivascular inflammation, 825–826
Perivascular rosettes, 842
Peroxidase
  background staining and, 29
  blocking of, 4–5
  chromogens, 23t
  hydrogen peroxide and, 5
Peroxidase-antiperoxidase (PAP), 1, 6–7
PET. *See* Predominantly epithelial thymoma (PET)
P30/32 glycoprotein, 96
PGP9.5. *See* Protein gene product 9.5 (PGP9.5)
PGT. *See* Papillary glioneuronal tumor (PGT)
PH, antigen retrieval and, 20, 21f
Phenylhydrazine, 5
Pheochromocytomas, 317
Phosphotungstic acid hematoxylin (PTAH), 839
Phyllodes tumor, 792–795
Pick disease, 878
Pigmented melanophages, 31f
Pilar tumors, 469–471
Pilocytic astrocytoma, 833–839, 834t
PIN. *See* Prostatic intraepithelial carcinoma (PIN)
Pineal cell tumors, 856–857
Pineal cyst, 875
Pineal gland tumors, 297–298
Pineal parenchymal tumors of intermediate differentiation (PPT-ID), 298
Pineoblastomas, 297–298, 837t, 857
Pineocytomas, 297–298, 834t, 857
Pituitary adenomas, 296t, 297f, 846
Placental alkaline phosphatase (PLAP)
  in mediastinal tumors, 342t, 355f
  in ovarian tumors, 722
  in testicular tumors, 644, 645f
Placental-like alkaline phosphatase (PLAP)
  in gynecologic pathology, 692t
  in malignant melanoma, 191
  in testicular tumors, 644
Placental site nodule, 717
Placental site trophoblastic tumor (PSTT), 717
Placental transmogrification of lung, 397
Plague, 72
PLAP. *See* Placental alkaline phosphatase (PLAP); Placental-like alkaline phosphatase (PLAP)
Plasma cell myeloma, 172
Plasmacytoma, 172, 220
Plasminogen activator inhibitor (PAI), 808
Pleomorphic adenoma (PA), 273, 274t
Pleomorphic carcinoma, 384–385
Pleomorphic dedifferentiated liposarcoma, 116–117
Pleomorphic leiomyosarcoma, 115–116
Pleomorphic liposarcoma, 116–117
Pleomorphic lobular carcinoma, 777–780
Pleomorphic malignant peripheral nerve sheath tumor, 116, 117
Pleomorphic mesothelioma, 438
Pleomorphic rhabdomyosarcoma, 116, 117f
Pleomorphic tumors of soft tissue, 115–117
Pleomorphic xanthoastrocytoma (PXA), 834t, 841, 842f
Pleural calcifying fibrous pseudotumor, 442
Pleural lymphomas, 444
Pleural metastases, epithelial mesothelioma *vs.,* 238
Pleural neoplasms, 415–417. *See also* Mesothelioma
Pleural primary desmoid tumors, 442–444
Pleural solitary fibrous tumor, 440–441
Pleural thymomas, primary, 444
Pleuritis, fibrosing, 440t
Pleuropulmonary blastoma, 444
PLGA. *See* Polymorphous low-grade adenocarcinoma (PLGA)
PMBCL. *See* Primary mediastinal B-cell lymphoma (PMBCL)
PMel, in malignant melanoma, 17, 193–195
PML. *See* Progressive multifocal leukoencephalopathy (PML)
PNET. *See* Ewing's sarcoma/primitive neuroectodermal tumor (ES/PNET); Primitive neuroectodermal tumor (PNET)
Pneumocystis carinii, 67
Pneumocystis jirovecii, 68
PNL2, in malignant melanoma, 195–196
PNSTs. *See* Peripheral nerve sheath tumors (PNSTs)
Podoplanin (PPN), 94
  in endometrial carcinoma, 709
  in epithelial sarcomas, 112
  in mediastinal tumors, 343t, 355f
  in testicular tumors, 644
Point mutations, 50–51
Polar spongioblastoma, 834t
"Polyclonal antibody," 3
Polylabeling amplification, 35t
Polymerase chain reaction (PCR), 9, 45–47, 50–51
Polymer-based labeling, 9–11
Polymeric amplification, 35t
Polymorphism, 44
Polymorphism analysis
  restriction fragment length, 47–48
  single-strand conformation, 48
Polymorphous low-grade adenocarcinoma (PLGA), 274t, 275–276
Polyomaviruses, 63, 64f, 74f
Polyphenotypic small round-cell tumors, 106–107
Poorly differentiated neuroendocrine carcinoma, 523, 559
Poorly differentiated small-cell synovial sarcoma (PDSS), 107
Poorly differentiated thyroid carcinoma, 303t, 310
Popcorn cells, 137, 140f
Positive controls, 16t, 17
Positives, false, 897
Postatrophic hyperplasia (PAH), 599–600, 602f
Post-detection amplification, 34
Post-fixation technique, 890, 891t
Post-transplantation lymphoproliferative disorders, 870
PowerVision system, 10
PPN. *See* Podoplanin (PPN)
PPT-ID. *See* Pineal parenchymal tumors of intermediate differentiation (PPT-ID)
PRCC. *See* Papillary renal cell carcinoma (PRCC)
Precursor B-cell neoplasms, 169
Precursor T-cell neoplasms, 178

Pre-detection amplification, 30–31, 35t
Predominantly epithelial thymoma (PET), fibrous histiocytoma *vs.*, 343–344
Preincubation, 4
Preparation
sample, 13–15
tissue, 18–19
Primary biliary cirrhosis (PBC), 566–567
Primary cutaneous CD30 positive T-cell lymphoproliferative disorders, 180
Primary cutaneous large B-cell lymphoma, 177
Primary cutaneous neuroendocrine carcinoma (PCNC), 471–472
Primary demyelination, 878
Primary desmoid tumors of pleura, 442–444
Primary effusion lymphoma, 176, 390t, 392
Primary intrapulmonary thymoma, 397–415
Primary mediastinal B-cell lymphoma (PMBCL), 146, 149f
Primary pleural thymomas, 444
Primary pulmonary Hodgkin disease, 390–391, 390t
Primary sarcoma, 385
Primary sclerosing cholangitis (PSC), 566–567
Primary thymic carcinoma, 350–353
Primitive neuroectodermal tumor (PNET). *See also* Ewing's sarcoma/primitive neuroectodermal tumor (ES/PNET)
central nervous, 859–860
mediastinal, 346
Procarbazine, chloroethylcyclohexylnitrosourea, and vincristine (PCV) chemotherapy, 832, 846, 848–849
ProEx C, 905–906
Progesterone receptor proteins (PRPs). *See also* Estrogen receptor/progesterone receptor (ER/PR)
in mucinous cystic neoplasm, 551, 552f
in skin tumors, 489
Progressive multifocal leukoencephalopathy (PML), 824t, 829
Progressive supranuclear palsy, 878
Prolactin, sparsely granulated, 296t
Proliferative ductal epithelial lesions, 771–773
Prostate adenocarcinoma, 375t, 517, 609f
Prostate carcinoma, 376t, 874–875
Prostate endocrine tumors, 326–327
Prostate-specific acid phosphatase (PSAP)
in neuroendocrine prostatic neoplasms, 605
in prostate tumors, 595
in urothelial carcinoma, 608
Prostate-specific antigen (PSA)
in cancer of unknown primary site, 233–234
in lung neoplasms, 372t
in mesothelioma, 424t
in neuroendocrine prostatic neoplasms, 605
in prostate tumors, 594
in urothelial carcinoma, 608
Prostate-specific membrane antigen (PSMA)
in gastrointestinal stromal tumor, 234
in neuroendocrine prostatic neoplasms, 605
in prostate tumors, 594–595
Prostate tumors
alpha-methylacyl-CoA racemase in, 595, 597f
angiogenesis in, 616
antiandrogen therapy for, 602–604
Prostate tumors *(Continued)*
antibodies in, 593–596
antigens in, 593–596
in colorectal adenocarcinoma, 611
early detection markers in, 618–619
in gastrointestinal stromal tumors, 613
genomic approaches in, 617–618
karyometry in, 617
mesenchymal, 612–613
morphometry in, 617
neuroendocrine, 605–607
neuroendocrine differentiation in, 617
oncogenes in, 616–617
post-therapy changes in, 602–605
prognostic factors in, 615–618
proliferation index in, 615–616
prostate-specific acid phosphatase in, 595
prostate-specific antigen in, 594
prostate-specific membrane antigen in, 594–595
prostatic acid phosphatase in, 595
radiation therapy for, 604–605
recurrent chromosomal rearrangements in, 614
in smooth muscle, 613
solitary fibrous, 613, 614f
stromal, of uncertain malignant potential, 612
theranostic applications in, 613–619
therapy targets in, 618–619
tumor suppressor genes in, 616–617
urothelial carcinoma in, 607–611
Prostatic acid phosphatase (PSAP)
in cancer of unknown primary site, 233–234
in gastrointestinal endocrine tumors, 320
in lung neoplasms, 372t
in mesothelioma, 424t
in prostate tumors, 595
in stromal carcinoids, 739
Prostatic adenocarcinoma, metastatic, 283
Prostatic adenosis, 600
Prostatic atrophy, 599–600, 601f
Prostatic duct carcinoma, 605
Prostatic hyperplasia, postatrophic, 599–600, 602f
Prostatic intraepithelial carcinoma (PIN), 598f
Prostatic sclerosing adenosis, 601, 603f
Prostatic xanthoma, 602, 603f
Prostein (P501S)
in neuroendocrine prostatic neoplasms, 605, 606
in prostate tumors, 595
in urothelial carcinoma, 608
Protein(s)
cell-membrane, 190–192
intermediate filament, 83–90
mismatch repair, 717–718
in molecular biology, 44
neurofilament, 83, 89–90
Protein A, 11, 12f, 13f
Protein gene product 9.5 (PGP9.5), 96
in embryonal tumors, 858
in endocrine tumors, 292
Protein YY, 739
Protocol validation, 15–18
Protozoal infections, 68–69
PRPs. *See* Progesterone receptor proteins (PRPs)
P501S. *See* Prostein (P501S)
PSA. *See* Prostate-specific antigen (PSA)
Psammomatous meningioma, 862
PSAP. *See* Prostate-specific acid phosphatase (PSAP)
PSC. *See* Primary sclerosing cholangitis (PSC)
PSCC. *See* Papillary squamous cell carcinoma (PSCC)
Pseudomesotheliomatous carcinoma of lung, 441–442
Pseudomesotheliomatous epithelioid hemangioendothelioma, 442
Pseudomyxoma peritonei, 726
Pseudoneoplastic look-alikes, 149–150
Pseudoneoplastic lymphoid skin lesions, 475–476
Pseudo-Paget disease, in breast, 786
Pseudopseudolymphomas, cutaneous, 478–479
PSMA. *See* Prostate-specific membrane antigen (PSMA)
PSTT. *See* Placental site trophoblastic tumor (PSTT)
PTAH. *See* Phosphotungstic acid hematoxylin (PTAH)
PTEN, in uterine tumors, 702, 704–705
PTH. *See* Parathyroid hormone (PTH)
PTPR. *See* Papillary tumor of pineal region (PTPR)
Pulmonary blastoma, 385
Pulmonary endocrine tumors, 323–326
Pulmonary Langerhans cell histiocytosis, 392–393
Pulmonary meningothelial nodules, 397
Pulmonary non-Hodgkin lymphoma, 389
PXA. *See* Pleomorphic xanthoastrocytoma (PXA)
Pyloric gland-type adenomas, 559
Pyothorax-associated lymphoma (PAL), 390t, 392
Pyrophosphate, 49
Pyrosequencing, 49

Q

Q fever, 67
QIRS. *See* Quantifiable Internal Reference Standards (QIRS)
QPCR. *See* Quantitative PCR
Quality, of specimens, 893–896
Quality control, 13–18
Quantifiable Internal Reference Standards (QIRS), 18
Quantitative PCR, 47

R

Rabies, 64, 828
Radial scar, 766, 768f
Radiation therapy, for prostatic adenocarcinoma, 604–605
Rapamycin, 641
RAS mutations, in thyroid tumors, 310
RB. *See* Retinoblastoma (RB) protein
RCC. *See* Renal cell carcinoma (RCC)
Reactive gliosis, 882t
Reagents. *See also* Antibody(ies)
antibodies as, 2–4
fresh, 13
incubation of, 23
in soft-tissue tumor studies, 87t–88t
validation of, 15–18
REAH. *See* Respiratory epithelial adenomatoid hamartoma (REAH)
REAL. *See* Revised European American Lymphoma (REAL) classification
Real-time PCR, 47, 50–51
Rectal neuroendocrine tumors, 522–523
Rectum, in Hirschsprung disease, 512–513

Recurrence score model, for breast tumors, 806
Reference standards, 16, 34–35
Refractory celiac disease, 528
Rehydration, 892
Renal angiomyolipoma, 642f, 643t
Renal cell carcinoma antigen
  in cancer of unknown primary site, 235
  in lung neoplasms, 372t
  in parathyroid tumors, 311
Renal cell carcinoma metastasis, 283, 874
Renal cell carcinoma (RCC), 221t, 449. *See also* Renal tumors
Renal oncocytoma, 635–636
Renal tumors
  ablative therapy for, 593
  in angiomyolipoma, 639–640
  antibodies in, 632–635
  antigens in, 632–635
  biopsy of, 593
  cadherins in, 633–634
  carbonic anhydrase IX in, 634–635
  CD10 in, 633
  in chromophobe renal cell carcinoma, 638
  clear-cell, 636–637
  in collecting duct carcinoma, 638, 640f
  EpCAM in, 633
  genomic applications in, 640–641
  glutathione-transferase alpha in, 635
  in metanephric adenoma, 636
  metastatic, 640
  morbidity in, 631, 632t
  mortality in, 631, 632t
  in mucinous tubular and spindle-cell carcinoma, 638–639
  in papillary renal cell carcinoma, 637–638
  PAX2 in, 633
  PAX8 in, 633, 634f
  prognostic parameters in, 643t
  theranostic applications in, 640–641
  in von Hippel-Lindau disease, 641
Respiratory epithelial adenomatoid hamartoma (REAH), 262–263
Respiratory papillomatosis, 272
Restin, 142
Restriction fragment length polymorphism (RFLP) analysis, 47–48
Restriction sites, 47–48
Retinoblastoma (RB) protein
  in parathyroid tumors, 312
  in urinary bladder tumors, 621
Reverse transcriptase, 46
Reverse transcriptase polymerase chain reaction (RT-PCR), 46–47, 790
Revised European American Lymphoma (REAL) classification, 156
RFLP. *See* Restriction fragment length polymorphism (RFLP) analysis
RFs. *See* Rosenthal fibers (RFs)
Rhabdoid meningioma, 864
Rhabdoid tumor, of lung, 395–396
Rhabdomyomas, 86, 99
Rhabdomyosarcomas (RMS), 86, 102–103, 108f
  cancer of unknown primary site and, 213t
  desmoplastic small round cell tumor *vs.*, 676–677
  in head and neck, 267
  mediastinal, 346–348
  pediatric, 664t, 667–671
Ribonucleic acid (RNA), 43–44, 45
Ribosomal RNA (rRNA), 43
Richter's transformation, 147
Rituxan, 157
Rituximab, 150
RMS. *See* Rhabdomyosarcomas (RMS)
Rocky Mountain spotted fever (RMSF), 65
RON, in lung tumors, 413
Rosenthal fibers (RFs), 833–837, 838f
Rosettes, 842, 844f, 854, 858
Rotavirus, 64
Rotterdam assay, 805–806
RRNA. *See* Ribosomal RNA (rRNA)
RT-PCR. *See* Reverse transcriptase polymerase chain reaction (RT-PCR)

S

Salivary duct carcinoma (SDC), 278–279
Salivary gland carcinoma, 221t, 273–280
Salivary gland neoplasm of lung, 396
Sample preparation, 13–15
Sandwich detection, 6
Sarcoma
  alveolar soft part, 96, 112f, 115, 213t
  chordoid, 122
  clear-cell, 112f, 113–114, 113f, 213t
  embryonal, of liver, 576
  endometrial stromal, 214t, 711, 712f
  epithelioid, 111–115, 213t, 488–489
  epithelioid monophasic synovial, 111
  Ewing's, 85, 94, 103f, 105–106
    in bone, 671–672
    in head and neck, 268
    pediatric, 664t, 671–674
    reagents and, 88t
  Kaposi's, 60, 108f, 111, 385, 386f
  monophasic spindle-cell synovial, 110–111
  monophasic synovial, 107, 110
  monosynovial, 108f
  poorly differentiated small-cell synovial, 107
  primary, 385
  small-cell synovial, 103f
  spindle-cell, 107–115
  synovial, 213t, 376t, 444, 677
Sarcomatoid amelanotic melanoma, 190f
Sarcomatoid carcinoma, 384, 426t, 509
Sarcomatoid mediastinal malignant mesothelioma, 361
Sarcomatoid mesothelioma, 426t, 435–436
Sarcomatoid renal cell carcinoma, 449
Sarcomatoid thymic carcinoma (STC), 359–360
Sarcomatoid thymic yolk sac tumor, 362
Sarcomeric control proteins, 91
SARS. *See* Severe acute respiratory distress syndrome (SARS)
SARS-associated coronavirus, 70, 71f
SCA. *See* Serous cystadenoma (SCA)
SCC. *See* Squamous cell carcinoma (SCC)
Schistosomiasis, 827
Schwannian differentiation markers, 92–93
Schwannomas, 98, 525, 835t, 868–869
Sclerosing adenosis of breast, 767f, 769f
Sclerosing adenosis of prostate, 601, 603f
Sclerosing cholangitis, 566–567
Sclerosing epithelioid fibrosarcoma (SEF), 112f, 114–115
Sclerosing hemangioma of lung, 376t, 394–395
SCNEC. *See* Small-cell neuroendocrine carcinoma (SCNEC)
SCTAT. *See* Sex cord tumor with annular tubules (SCTAT)
SDC. *See* Salivary duct carcinoma (SDC)
Sebaceous tumors, 468–469
Secondary demyelination, 878
Secondary tumors of testis, 648
Secretogranins, endocrine tumors and, 292–293
Secretory meningioma, 864f
SEF. *See* Sclerosing epithelioid fibrosarcoma (SEF)
SEGA. *See* Subependymal giant-cell astrocytoma (SEGA)
Sentinel lymph node (SLN), 787–788
Sentinel lymph node biopsy (SLNB), 196, 787–790
Sentinel lymph node metastasis (SLNM), 788
Serologic assays, 58
Serotonin
  in adrenal medulla tumors, 317
  in gastrointestinal endocrine tumors, 320t
  in pancreatic endocrine neoplasms, 557
Serous cystadenoma (SCA), 552–553
Sertoli cell tumors, 647, 734–735, 906–907
Sertoli-Leydig cell ovarian tumors, 734
Sessile serrated adenoma (SSA), 513
Seventy gene profile, for breast tumors, 805
Seventy-six gene profile, for breast tumors, 805–806
Severe acute respiratory distress syndrome (SARS), 70, 73f
Sex chromosomes, 42
Sex cord stromal tumors, 730–735
Sex cord tumors, 647–648
Sex cord tumor with annular tubules (SCTAT), 735
Sézary syndrome, 180
SFT. *See* Solitary fibrous tumor (SFT)
Signet ring cell adenocarcinoma, 516
Signet ring cell carcinoma, 376t
Signet ring gastrointestinal stromal tumor, 525
Silent adenoma, 296t
Silent corticotroph cell adenoma, 296t
Simple epithelial keratins, 211–217
Single nucleotide polymorphism (SNP), 44, 48
Single-strand conformation polymorphism (SSCP) analysis, 48, 51
Sinonasal-type hemangiopericytoma, 269
Sinonasal undifferentiated carcinoma (SNUC), 264, 264t, 265t
Site-specific markers, 901–902
Skeletin. *See* Desmin
Skin lesions, special pseudoneoplastic lymphoid, 475–476
Skin leukemia, 472–475
Skin lymphoma, 472–475
Skin tumors
  carcinoembryonic antigen in, 465
  CD10 in, 475f
  CD30 in, 474f
  CD99 in, 473f
  endocrine, 327–328, 471–472
  epidermal, 464–466
  epithelial, 464–472
  epithelial membrane antigen in, 464–465
  estrogen and progesterone receptor proteins in, 489
  fibroblastic, 479–480
  granular cell, 484
  mesenchymal, 479–489
  myeloperoxidase in, 474f
  myofibroblastic, 479–480
  nerve sheath, 483–485
  oncogenes in, 490
  pilar, 469–471
  sebaceous, 468–469

Skin tumors *(Continued)*
smooth muscle differentiation in, 483
special topics in, 489–490
sudoriferous, 466–468
vascular, 485–486
Slides, mounting, 24
SLN. *See* Sentinel lymph node (SLN)
SLNB. *See* Sentinel lymph node biopsy (SLNB)
SLNM. *See* Sentinel lymph node metastasis (SLNM)
Small bowel neuroendocrine tumors, 520–521
Small-cell amelanotic melanoma, 190f
Small-cell carcinoma, 837t, 874
Small-cell lymphocytic lymphoma, 389, 390t
Small-cell malignant lymphomas of mediastinum, 348–350
Small-cell neuroendocrine carcinoma (SCNEC), 265t, 266–267, 272–273, 345–346
Small-cell osteosarcoma, 103f
Small-cell rhabdomyosarcoma, 105f
Small-cell synovial sarcoma, 103f
Small intestinal adenocarcinomas, 511, 512f
Small lymphocytic leukemia, 169–170
Small round cell mesenchymal tumors, 489
Small round cell neoplasms, 102, 103f
Small-scale mutation detection, 50–51
Small vessel disease, 824t, 830–831
SMMHC. *See* Smooth muscle myosin heavy chain (SMMHC)
Smooth muscle actin, in gynecologic pathology, 692t
Smooth muscle myosin, in gynecologic pathology, 692t
Smooth muscle myosin heavy chain (SMMHC), 763–765
Smooth muscle neoplasms, of gastrointestinal tract, 525–526
Snap-frozen tissue, 44
SNP. *See* Single nucleotide polymorphism (SNP)
SNUC. *See* Sinonasal undifferentiated carcinoma (SNUC)
Sodium azide, 5
Soft-tissue tumors
benign, 97–100
borderline, 100–102
chondroid, 119–121
giant cell, 122–123
malignant, 102–117
pleomorphic, 115–117
Solid-pseudopapillary neoplasm (SPN), 555–556
Solitary fibrous tumor (SFT), 93, 100–101, 362, 525, 613, 866–867
Solitary fibrous tumor-hemangiopericytoma, 343–344
Solitary fibrous tumor of pleura, 440–441
Somatic chromosomes, 42
Somatostatin
in gastrointestinal endocrine tumors, 320t
in pancreatic endocrine tumors, 321–322
in thyroid tumors, 307
Somatostatinomas, 321–322
Somatostatin receptors, in endocrine tumors, 294
S-100 protein, 92, 109
in adrenal cortex tumors, 316
alcohol leaching of, 890
in ampullary endocrine neoplasms, 564
in ductal adenocarcinoma, 546
in gastrointestinal stromal tumor, 525
S-100 protein *(Continued)*
in gynecologic pathology, 692t
in head and neck neoplasms, 259t
in lung neoplasms, 371t, 400, 401f
in malignant melanoma, 192–193
in mammary Paget disease, 786
in mediastinal tumors, 342t, 356f
in meningiomas, 863f
in mesothelioma, 425t
in ovarian tumors, 723
in pilocytic astrocytomas, 839
in skin tumors, 484
in soft-tissue tumors, 101
in thyroid tumors, 305
Sox9, 906–907
SP-A. *See* Surfactant apoprotein A (SP-A)
Sparsely granulated growth hormone cell adenomas, 296t
Sparsely granulated prolactinoma, 296t, 297f
SPCC. *See* Spindle-cell carcinoma (SPCC)
Specific organ cytology, 897–907
Specimen collection, 890
Specimen quality, 893–896
Specimen requirements, 44–45
Spermatocytic seminoma, 647
Spindle-cell angiosarcoma, 111
Spindle-cell breast neoplasms, 783–784
Spindle-cell carcinoid tumor of thymus, 360–361
Spindle-cell carcinoma (SPCC), 221t, 260–261, 261f, 562
Spindle-cell cholangiocarcinoma, 574
Spindle-cell differentiation, 509
Spindle-cell hepatocellular carcinoma, 572
Spindle-cell lipoma, 93, 98
Spindle-cell mediastinal tumors, 359–362
Spindle-cell rhabdomyosarcoma, 667
Spindle-cell sarcomas, 107–115
Splenic marginal zone B-cell lymphoma, 171
SPN. *See* Solid-pseudopapillary neoplasm (SPN)
Spongiform encephalopathies, 829–830
Spongioblastoma, polar, 834t
Sporothrix schenckii, 68
Squamoid corpuscles, 554–555
Squamoproliferative lesions, 256–262
Squamous cell carcinoma (SCC), 257–258, 464–466
Squamous epithelia, 84t
SSA. *See* Sessile serrated adenoma (SSA)
SSCP. *See* Single-strand conformation polymorphism (SSCP) analysis
Staining
absence of, 28–29
acid-fast bacilli, 66
antibodies as specific reagents, 2–4
artifactual, 30, 31f
automation in, 26–27
background, 29–30
blocking non-specific background, 4–5
double, 8–9, 36
enhanced polymer one-step, 9–10
inappropriate, 27–28
internal control, 18
two-step, 10
validation of, 15–18
weak, 17, 28t, 29
Standard curves, 34–35
Standardization, 13–18, 890–892
STC. *See* Sarcomatoid thymic carcinoma (STC)
Steatohepatitis, 566
Stepwise amplification, 35t
Steroid cell tumor, 735
Storage, 892
Streptavidin, 7–8
Stromal tumors of uncertain malignant potential (STUMPs), 612
Struma ovarii, 739
STUMPs. *See* Stromal tumors of uncertain malignant potential (STUMPs)
Subcutaneous panniculitis-like T-cell lymphoma, 179–180
Subependymal giant-cell astrocytoma (SEGA), 840
Subependymoma, 834t, 844
Substance P, in gastrointestinal endocrine tumors, 320t
Substrate, chromogen and, 23–24
Sudoriferous tumors, 466–468
Sugar tumor, 393
Suprasellar oligodendrogliomas, 846
Surfactant apoprotein A (SP-A)
in lung neoplasmst, 371t, 379t–380t
in mesothelioma, 425t
Surfactant protein A, in thyroid tumors, 300
Sweat gland carcinoma, 466–468
Synaptic vesicle proteins, 293
Synaptophysin, 96
in adrenal cortex tumors, 315f
in cancer of unknown primary site, 226
in cervical small-cell carcinoma, 703f
endocrine tumors and, 293, 298f
in Ewing's sarcoma/primitive neuroectodermal tumor, 672f
in gastrointestinal stromal tumor, 525
in gastrointestinal tumors, 501
in gynecologic pathology, 692t
in malignant rhabdoid tumor, 678f, 679f
in mediastinal tumors, 342t, 349f
in medulloblastoma, 844f
in mesothelioma, 425t
in neuroendocrine lung neoplasms, 378, 382t
in oligodendroglioma, 846, 849f
in ovarian tumors, 730
in pancreatic endocrine tumors, 321
in pancreatic tumors, 543
in pheochromocytomas, 317
in pineal cell tumors, 857f
in primary thymic carcinoma, 354
in pulmonary endocrine tumors, 324
Syncytial mass differential diagnosis, 862t
Syncytial mediastinal Hodgkin disease, 355–356
Syncytial meningioma, 862, 863f
Synovial sarcoma, 213t, 376t, 444, 677
Syphilis, 66, 827
SYT/SSX fusion, 51–52

T

TAG. *See* Tumor-associated glycoprotein (TAG)
Tancytic ependymoma, 834t, 844
Targeted therapies, 911–912
T-bet, in non-Hodgkin lymphoma, 162–163
T-cell/histiocyte-rich B-cell lymphoma, 177
T-cell large granular lymphocytic leukemia, 179
T-cell markers, in Hodgkin lymphoma, 139
T-cell neoplasms, 178–181
T-cell prolymphocytic leukemia, 179
T-cell-rich B-cell lymphoma, 146
T cells, in non-Hodgkin lymphoma, 161–163
T-cell transcription factors, in non-Hodgkin lymphoma, 162–163
TdT. *See* Terminal deoxynucleotidyl transferase (TdT)

Temporal lobe epilepsy, 879–881
Temsirolimus, 641
Tendon sheath fibroma, 98
Teratoid-rhabdoid tumor, atypical, 837t, 860
Terminal deoxynucleotidyl transferase (TdT), 168
Terrorism, 70–72
Test battery, 20, 21t
Testicular tumors
  activator protein-2G in, 644
  alpha-fetoprotein in, 644
  antigens in, 643–645
  CD117 in, 643–644
  diagnosis of, 645–648
  germ-cell, 642–643
  human chorionic gonadotropin in, 644
  human placental lactogen in, 644
  inhibin A in, 644–645
  intratubular germ-cell, 645
  Leydig cell, 647
  Oct-4 in, 643
  placental alkaline phosphatase in, 644, 645f
  placental-like alkaline phosphatase in, 644
  podoplanin in, 644
  secondary, 648
  Sertoli cell, 647
  sex cord, 647–648
TGB. *See* Thyroglobulin (TGB)
Theranostic applications
  in adrenal cortex tumors, 316
  in astrocytomas, 842
  in breast tumors, 796–802
  in cervical tumors, 699
  in diffuse large B-cell lymphoma, 174
  in endometrial carcinoma, 719
  in Ewing's sarcoma/primitive neuroectodermal tumor, 674
  in gastrointestinal tumors, 528–529
  in glioblastomas, 850
  in head and neck neoplasms, 261–262, 269–270, 280
  in Hodgkin lymphoma, 150–151
  in meningiomas, 866
  in neuroblastoma, 666–667
  in non-Hodgkin lymphoma, 170
  in oligodendroglioma, 848
  in ovarian tumors, 745
  in prostate tumors, 613–619
  in pulmonary endocrine tumors, 324–326
  in renal tumors, 640–641
  in rhabdomyosarcoma, 671
  in skin endocrine tumors, 328
  in thyroid tumors, 310
  in urinary bladder tumors, 627–629
  in uterine sarcoma, 719
  in Wilms' tumor, 681–682
Thin-layer technique, 893
Thrombomodulin (TMN)
  in cancer of unknown primary site, 234–235
  in Ewing's sarcoma/primitive neuroectodermal tumor, 94
  in mesothelioma, 423t, 428–429
  in urinary bladder tumors, 620
Thymic carcinoma, 350–353
Thymic hormones, 340
Thymic yolk sac tumor, sarcomatoid, 362
Thymoma, primary intrapulmonary, 397–415
Thymus
  endocrine gland tumors of, 329
  spindle-cell carcinoid tumors of, 360–361
Thyroglobulin (TGB)
  in cancer of unknown primary site, 227
  in lung neoplasms, 372t
  in mesothelioma, 424t
  in thyroid tumors, 298, 307–308
Thyroid adenocarcinoma, 376t
Thyroid follicular carcinoma, 221t
Thyroid transcription factor-1 (TTF-1), 901
  in cancer of unknown primary site, 227, 228f
  in esophageal squamous cell carcinoma, 503
  in hepatocellular carcinoma, 570
  in lung neoplasms, 371, 372t, 379t–380t, 381t, 383f, 398, 412
  in mesothelioma, 424t
  in neuroendocrine prostatic neoplasms, 606
  in ovarian cytology, 906
  in prostate endocrine tumors, 327
  in pulmonary endocrine tumors, 323–324
  in struma ovarii, 739
  in thyroid tumors, 300
  in tumors, 376t
Thyroid transcription factor-2 (TTF-2), in thyroid tumors, 300
Thyroid tumors, 298–310
Thyrotroph cell adenoma, 296t
TIA-1, 139
Tissue, troubleshooting variables in, 28t
Tissue cassette, 893, 895f
Tissue fixation techniques, 18–21
Tissue identity testing, 54–55
Tissue preparation, 18–19
Titin, 91
Titration, 11–13, 14t
TLE. *See* Transducin-like enhancer (TLE)
TMN. *See* Thrombomodulin (TMN)
Tonofibrils, 83
Tonofilaments, 83
"Total test," 14t, 15
Toxoplasmosis, 68, 824t
TP53 mutations, 547
Transcription factors, in endocrine tumors, 294
Transducin-like enhancer (TLE), 96
Transfer RNA, 43
Transitional cell ovarian tumors, 729–730
Transitional meningioma, 836t, 862
Transplant patients
  CMV in, 60–61
  liver, 568
  lymphoproliferative disorders in, 870
Transurethral resection biopsy (TURB), 619
Transurethral resection of prostate (TURP), 600
Trapped gliosis, 847f. *See also* Gliosis
Trichoepithelioma
  classic, 469–470
  desmoplastic, 470
TRNA. *See* Transfer RNA
Tropheryma whippelii, 827
Tropomyosin, 91
Troponin, 91
Troubleshooting, 27–30
Trypsin
  in acinar cell carcinoma, 553, 554f
  in pancreatic tumors, 542
TS. *See* Tuberous sclerosis (TS)
TSA. *See* Tyramine signal amplification (TSA)
TSC. *See* Tuberous sclerosis complex (TSC)
TSGs. *See* Tumor suppressor genes (TSGs)
TTF-1. *See* Thyroid transcription factor-1 (TTF-1)
TTF-2. *See* Thyroid transcription factor-2 (TTF-2)
Tuberculosis, 66, 827
Tuberin, 840
Tuberous sclerosis (TS), 840
Tuberous sclerosis complex (TSC), 639
Tubulodesmoplastic pseudomesotheliomatous adenocarcinoma, 441–442
Tubulolobular carcinoma, 778–780
Tularemia, 71–72
Tumor-associated glycoprotein (TAG), 191
  in lung neoplasms, 371t
  in mesothelioma, 424t
Tumor suppressor genes (TSGs)
  in ductal adenocarcinoma, 546
  in prostate tumors, 616–617
  in thyroid tumors, 301–302
TURB. *See* Transurethral resection biopsy (TURB)
TURP. *See* Transurethral resection of prostate (TURP)
Two gene ratio model, for breast tumors, 806–807
Two-step staining, 10
Tyramine signal amplification (TSA), 9, 11, 12f
Tyrosinase
  in mediastinal tumors, 342t
  in mucosal melanoma, 266f
Tyrosinase-related antibodies, in malignant melanoma, 195

U

UEAI. *See Ulex europaeus* I (UEAI)
UEC. *See* Uterine endometrioid carcinoma (UEC)
Ulex europaeus I (UEAI), 88t, 94, 113f
Undifferentiated carcinoma, 270–271, 303t, 310
Undifferentiated ductal carcinoma, 547
Undifferentiated nasopharyngeal carcinoma (UNPC), 265t
Unlabeled antibody detection, 6–7
UNPC. *See* Undifferentiated nasopharyngeal carcinoma (UNPC)
UPA. *See* Urokinase plasminogen activator (uPA)
Urinary bladder adenocarcinoma, 625
Urinary bladder small-cell carcinoma, 625–626
Urinary bladder tumors
  anaplastic lymphoma kinase in, 621
  antibodies in, 619–621
  antigens in, 619–621
  benign mimics in, 626–627
  biopsy of, 619
  CK7 in, 619–620
  CK20 in, 619–620
  deaths from, 619
  fluorescence *in situ* hybridization in, 629–630
  genomic applications in, 627–629
  inflammatory myofibroblastic, 626–627, 628f
  p16 in, 621
  p53 in, 621
  p63 in, 620
  predictive markers in, 630–631
  retinoblastoma protein in, 621
  theranostic applications in, 627–629
  thrombomodulin in, 620
  uroplakin III in, 620
Urine cytology, 910–911, 913f
Urokinase plasminogen activator (uPA), 808

Uroplakin III
in cancer of unknown primary site, 234–235
in lung neoplasms, 372t
in urinary bladder tumors, 620
Urothelial carcinoma, 517, 607–611, 621–625. *See also* Urinary bladder tumors
UroVysion, 910–911, 913f
USC. *See* Uterine serous carcinoma (USC)
Uterine endometrioid carcinoma (UEC), 708f
Uterine serous carcinoma (USC), 708f
Uterine tumors
beta-catenin in, 702
caldesmon in, 702–704
carcinosarcoma in, 711–713
CD10 in, 704
clear-cell carcinoma in, 706–707
cytokeratins in, 699–700
desmin in, 702–704
endometrial carcinoma in, 704–710
endometrial serous carcinoma in, 705–706
endometrial stromal, 711, 712f, 713f
epithelial membrane antigen in, 699–700
gastrointestinal stromal, 715
genomic applications in, 717–718
gestational trophoblastic, 715–716
inflammatory myofibroblastic, 715
leiomyoma in, 710–711
leiomyosarcoma in, 710–711
lymphovascular invasion in, 709
mesenchymal, 710–715
mismatch repair proteins in, 717–718, 720
mixed epithelial carcinomas in, 709
müllerian adenosarcoma in, 713
myometrial invasion in, 709
neuroendocrine carcinomas in, 708–709
perivascular epithelioid cell, 715
p53 in, 701–702
PTEN in, 702, 704–705
resembling ovarian sex cord tumor, 715
theranostic applications in, 719
undifferentiated carcinomas in, 709
undifferentiated sarcoma in, 713–715
vimentin in, 700
Wilms' tumor-1 in, 704

V

Vagina, 690–694
Vaginal carcinoma, 376t
Validation, 15–18
Varicella-zoster (VZV), 59–60
Vascular dementia, 877
Vascular endothelial growth factor receptor-3 (VEGFR3), 95
Vascular malformation, 831
Vascular neoplasms, of skin, 485–486
VC. *See* Verrucous carcinoma (VC)
VEGFR3. *See* Vascular endothelial growth factor receptor-3 (VEGFR3)
Verrucous carcinoma (VC), 260
VHL. *See* Von Hippel-Lindau disease (VHL)
VHL gene, in serous cystadenoma, 553
Villin
in cancer of unknown primary site, 230–231, 233f
in colorectal adenocarcinoma, 514
in gastric adenocarcinoma, 507–508
in gastrointestinal tumors, 501
Villous/intestinal papillae, 550
Vimentin, 85, 87–90, 113f
in anaplastic ependymoma, 845
coexpression in cancer of unknown primary site, 221, 222f
in desmoplastic small round cell tumor, 675
in Ewing's sarcoma/primitive neuroectodermal tumor, 672f
in gynecologic pathology, 692t
in lung neoplasms, 385f
in malignant melanoma, 189, 190f
in malignant rhabdoid tumor, 678f
in mediastinal tumors, 342t
in meningiomas, 860–861, 863f
in mesotheliomas, 423t, 427
in oligodendrogliomas, 849f
in skin tumors, 480f
in squamous cell carcinoma, 465f
in thyroid tumors, 308–309
in uterine tumors, 700
Vincristine. *See* Procarbazine, chloroethylcyclohexylnitrosourea, and vincristine (PCV) chemotherapy
Viral hemorrhagic fevers, 62–63
Viral infections, 59–64
Vocal cord nodule, 272
Von Hippel-Lindau disease (VHL), 319, 641, 872–873
Von Willebrand factor, 93
Von Willebrand syndrome, 93
Vulva, 690–694
Vulvar granular cell tumor, 693, 693f
Vulvar intraepithelial neoplasia (VIN), 691, 694
Vulvar melanoma, 691
Vulvar Paget disease, 690–693, 692f
Vulvar papillary squamous lesions, 693–694
Vulvovaginal mesenchymal lesions, 693
VZV. *See* Varicella-zoster (VZV)

W

Wall of syrinx, 875
Washing, in antigen retrieval, 22
Watery diarrhea, hypokalemia, and achlorhydria (WDHA), 322
Weak staining, 17, 28t, 29
Weibel-Palade bodies (WPBs), 93
West Nile virus (WNV) encephalitis, 69
Wet fixation in alcohol (WFA), 890
Whipple's disease, 65, 827
Wilms' tumor, 664t, 680–682
Wilms' tumor-1 (WT1), 95, 112, 898–899
in cancer of unknown primary site, 227–228
in desmoplastic small round cell tumor, 675f, 676f
in gynecologic pathology, 692t
in lung neoplasms, 372t
in mesothelioma, 425t, 429
in ovarian tumors, 722, 724
in pediatric neoplasms, 663
in uterine tumors, 704
in Wilms' tumor, 681f
WNV. *See* West Nile virus (WNV) encephalitis
Wound-response model, in breast tumors, 805
WPBs. *See* Weibel-Palade bodies (WPBs)
WT1. *See* Wilms' tumor-1 (WT1)

X

Xanthogranuloma, 835t
Xanthoma, prostatic, 602, 603f
X-link inhibitor of apoptosis protein (XIAP)
in mesothelioma, 439
overview of, 899

Y

Yersinia pestis, 72
Yolk sac differentiation, 509
Yolk sac tumor
ovarian, 737, 738f
sarcomatoid thymic, 362

Z

Zollinger-Ellison syndrome, 519, 521